BRIEF CONTENTS

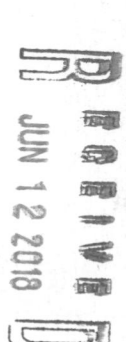

NEWARK CAMPUS LIBRARY - COTC

i

NEWARK CAMPUS LIBRARY - COTE

NINTH EDITION

Essentials *for* Nursing Practice

Patricia A. Potter, RN, MSN, PhD, FAAN
Formerly, Director of Research
Patient Care Services
Barnes-Jewish Hospital
St. Louis, Missouri

Anne Griffin Perry, RN, MSN, EdD, FAAN
Professor Emerita
School of Nursing
Southern Illinois University—Edwardsville
Edwardsville, Illinois

Patricia A. Stockert, RN, BSN, MS, PhD
President, College of Nursing
Saint Francis Medical Center College of Nursing
Peoria, Illinois

Amy M. Hall, RN, BSN, MS, PhD, CNE
Dean, School of Nursing
Franciscan Missionaries of Our Lady University
Baton Rouge, Louisiana

ELSEVIER

ELSEVIER

3251 Riverport Lane
St. Louis, Missouri 63043

ESSENTIALS FOR NURSING PRACTICE, NINTH EDITION   ISBN 978-0-323-48184-7

Copyright © 2019, Elsevier Inc. All Rights Reserved.

No part of this publication may be reproduced or transmitted in any form or by any means, electronic or mechanical, including photocopying, recording, or any information storage and retrieval system, without permission in writing from the publisher. Details on how to seek permission, further information about the Publisher's permissions policies and our arrangements with organizations such as the Copyright Clearance Center and the Copyright Licensing Agency, can be found at our website: www.elsevier.com/permissions.

This book and the individual contributions contained in it are protected under copyright by the Publisher (other than as may be noted herein).

Notice

Practitioners and researchers must always rely on their own experience and knowledge in evaluating and using any information, methods, compounds or experiments described herein. Because of rapid advances in the medical sciences, in particular, independent verification of diagnoses and drug dosages should be made. To the fullest extent of the law, no responsibility is assumed by Elsevier, authors, editors or contributors for any injury and/or damage to persons or property as a matter of products liability, negligence or otherwise, or from any use or operation of any methods, products, instructions, or ideas contained in the material herein.

Previous editions copyrighted 2015, 2011, 2007, 2003, 1999, 1995, 1991, 1987.

Herdman, T.H. & Kamitsuru, S. (Eds.) Nursing Diagnoses—Definitions and Classification 2012-2014 Copyright © 2014, 1994-2014 NANDA International. Used by arrangement with John Wiley & Sons, Inc. In order to make safe and effective judgments using NANDA-I nursing diagnoses, it is essential that nurses refer to the definitions and defining characteristics of the diagnoses listed in the work.

International Standard Book Number: 978-0-323-48184-7

Director: Tamara Myers
Content Development Manager: Lisa P. Newton
Senior Content Development Specialist: Tina Kaemmerer
Publishing Services Manager: Jeff Patterson
Senior Project Manager: Jodi M. Willard
Design Direction: Paula Catalano

Printed in Canada

Last digit is the print number: 9   8   7   6   5   4   3   2   1

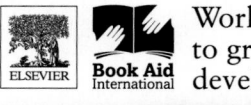

Working together to grow libraries in developing countries

www.elsevier.com • www.bookaid.org

CONTRIBUTORS

Carolyn Wright Boon, MSN, BSN
Assistant Professor
Saint Francis Medical Center College of
    Nursing
Peoria, Illinois

Linda Cason, DNP, MSN, BSN
Clinical Nurse Specialist
Deaconess Hospital, Inc.
Evansville, Indiana

Lori Catalano, JD, MSN, RN, CCNS, PCCN
Assistant Professor of Clinical Nursing
College of Nursing
University of Cincinnati
Cincinnati, Ohio

Edith Claros, PhD, MSN, RN, APHN-BC
PMHNP Track Coordinator and Associate
    Professor
School of Nursing
MCPHS University
Worcester, Massachusetts

Janice C. Colwell, RN, MS, CWOCN, FAAN
Advanced Practice Nurse
Surgery
University of Chicago Medicine
Chicago, Illinois

Margaret Ecker, RN, MS
Nurse Consultant
Los Angeles, California;
Director of Nursing Quality, retired
Kaiser Permanente Los Angeles
Los Angeles, California

Jane Fellows, MSN, CWOCN
Wound/Ostomy CNS
Advanced Clinical Practice
Duke University Health System
Durham, North Carolina

Linda Felver, PhD, RN
Associate Professor
School of Nursing
Oregon Health & Science University
Portland, Oregon

Susan Fetzer, BA, BSN, MSN, MBA, PhD, CNL
Professor
College of Health and Human Services
University of New Hampshire
Durham, New Hampshire;
Director of Research
Patient Care Services
Southern New Hampshire Medical Center
Nashua, New Hampshire

Victoria N. Folse, PhD, APN, PMHCNS-BC, LCPC
Director and Professor; Caroline F. Rupert
    Endowed Chair of Nursing
School of Nursing
Illinois Wesleyan University
Bloomington, Illinois

Lorri A. Graham, DNP, RN
Associate Professor
Saint Francis Medical Center College of
    Nursing
Peoria, Illinois

Susan Hendricks, EdD, MSN, RN, CNE
Associate Dean for Undergraduate Programs
School of Nursing
Indiana University
Indianapolis, Indiana

Cassandra Horack, MS, PSL, BSN
Vice President Quality and Safety
OSF HealthCare Saint Francis Medical
    Center
Peoria, Illinois

Noël Marie Kerr, PhD
Assistant Professor
School of Nursing
Illinois Wesleyan University
Bloomington, Illinois

Jerrilee Lamar, PhD, RN, CNE
Associate Professor of Nursing
Dunigan Department of Nursing and
    Health Sciences
University of Evansville
Evansville, Indiana

Nancy Laplante, PhD, RN, AHN-BC
Associate Professor
School of Nursing
Widener University
Chester, Pennsylvania

Angela McConachie, FNP, DNP
Assistant Professor
Faculty
Goldfarb School of Nursing at Barnes-
    Jewish College
St. Louis, Missouri

Judith A. McCutchan, ASN, BSN, MSN, PhD
Adjunct Faculty
Nursing
University of Evansville
Evansville, Indiana

Staci McIntosh, MS, RD
Assistant Professor (Lecturer)
Department of Nutrition and Integrative
    Physiology
University of Utah
Salt Lake City, Utah

Emily McKenna, APN, CNS
INI Neurology
OSF HealthCare Saint Francis Medical
    Center
Peoria, Illinois

Jill Parsons, PhD, RN
Associate Professor
Nursing
MacMurray College
Jacksonville, Illinois

Theresa Pietsch, PhD, RN, CRRN, CNE
Associate Professor
Division of Nursing & Health Sciences
Neumann University
Aston, Pennsylvania

Sandra L. Richmond, DNP, MS, RN, CSN
Dean, School of Nursing and Health
    Sciences
Pennsylvania College of Technology
Williamsport, Pennsylvania

Anita Shoup, DNP, RN, CNS-SP, CNOR
Assistant Professor; Coordinator,
    Simulation/Experiential Learning
Nursing
Heritage University
Toppenish, Washington

REVIEWERS

Michelle Aebersold, PhD, RN, CHSE, FAAN
Clinical Associate Professor and Director of
    Simulation
University of Michigan School of Nursing
Ann Arbor, Michigan

Lezley Anderson, MA, MSN, RN
Assistant Professor
Saint Francis Medical Center College of
    Nursing
Peoria, Illinois

**Colleen Andreoni, DNP, MSN, ANP-BC,
FNP-BC**
Advanced Practice Nurse
Board Certified Nurse Practitioner
Northwestern Medicine Regional Medical
    Group
Chicago, Illinois

Suzanne L. Bailey, PMHCNS-BC, CNE
Associate Professor of Nursing
University of Evansville
Evansville, Indiana

Leigh Ann Bonney, PhD, RN, CCRN
Associate Professor
Saint Francis Medical Center College of
    Nursing
Peoria, Illinois

Denise Branchizio, DNP, MSN, RN
Assistant Professor of Nursing
New Jersey City University
Jersey City, New Jersey

Anna M. Bruch, RN, MSN
Nursing Professor
Illinois Valley Community College
Oglesby, Illinois

Sheryl Buckner, PhD, RN, ANEF
Assistant Professor/Lab Director
University of Oklahoma Earl and Frances
    Ziegler College of Nursing
Oklahoma City, Oklahoma

Pat Callard, DNP, RN, CNL
Associate Professor of Nursing
College of Graduate Nursing
Western University of Health Sciences
Pomona, California

Kim Clevenger, EdD, MSN, RN, BC
Associate Professor of Nursing
Morehead State University
Morehead, Kentucky

Tracy Colburn, RN, MSN, C-EFM
Associate Professor of Nursing
Lewis and Clark Community College
Godfrey, Illinois

Barbara A. Coles, PhD, RN-BC, LHRM
Adjunct Professor
American Public University System
Charles Town, West Virginia

Janice C. Colwell, RN, MS, CWOCN, FAAN
Advanced Practice Nurse
Surgery
University of Chicago Medicine
Chicago, Illinois

Pamela Cook, PhD(c), MSN, RN, CNS
Assistant Professor
Bloomsburg University
Bloomsburg, Pennsylvania

Eileen Costantinou, MSN, RN-BC
Practice Specialist, Senior Coordinator
Barnes-Jewish Hospital
St. Louis, Missouri

Graciela Lopez Cox, MSN, RN
Assistant Professor
Samuel Merritt University
Sacramento, California

**Pamela A. Dettenmeier, PhD(c), DNP,
ANP-BC**
Associate Professor of Medicine
Director CPAP Adherence Clinic
Adult Nurse Practitioner
Division of Pulmonary, Critical Care &
    Sleep Medicine
Saint Louis University
St. Louis, Missouri

Holly Johanna Diesel, PhD, RN
Associate Professor and Academic Chair of
    the Accelerated and RN to BSN Program
Goldfarb School of Nursing at Barnes-
    Jewish College
St. Louis, Missouri

Christine R. Durbin, PhD, JD, RN
Associate Professor and Chair, Primary Care
    & Health Systems Department
Southern Illinois University School of
    Nursing
Edwardsville, Illinois

Amber Essman, DNP, MSN, FNP-BC, CNE
ARNP
Confluence Health;
Visiting Professor
Chamberlain College of Nursing
Moses Lake, Washington

Kelly L. Fisher, PhD, RN, FNAP
Dean, School of Nursing
Endicott College
Beverly, Massachusetts

**Linda R. Garner, PhD, RN, APHN-BC,
CHES**
Associate Professor
Southeast Missouri State University
Cape Girardeau, Missouri

Linda Hansen-Kyle, PhD, RN, CCM
Chair (Retired) Second Degree Program
Azusa Pacific University
Azusa, California;
University of San Diego
San Diego, California;
University of Phoenix
Tempe, Arizona

Nicole M. Heimgartner, MSN, RN, COI
Vice President
Connect: RN2ED
Dayton, Ohio

Kathleen C. Jones, MSN, RN, CNS
Associate Professor of Nursing
Walters State Community College
Morristown, Tennessee

Shari Kist, PhD, RN, CNE
Associate Professor
Goldfarb School of Nursing at Barnes-
    Jewish College
St. Louis, Missouri

**Kimberly Leppert, MSN, RN, ACNS-BC,
CNOR, ONC**
Surgery Clinical Supervisor
Swedish Health Services-Ballard
Seattle, Washington

Kathryn A. Lever, RN, MSN, WHNP-BC
Associate Professor of Nursing
Dunigan Family School of Nursing and
    Health Sciences
University of Evansville
Evansville, Indiana

Mary M. Lopez, PhD, RN
Associate Dean, Research
Western University of Health Sciences
Pomona, California

Angela McConachie, DNP, FNP
Assistant Professor
Goldfarb School of Nursing at Barnes-
    Jewish Hospital
St. Louis, Missouri

Janis Longfield McMillan, RN, MSN, CNE
Associate Clinical Professor
Northern Arizona University
Flagstaff, Arizona

Pamela Molnar, RN, CEN
Decatur Morgan Hospital
Decatur, Alabama

Katrin Moskowitz, DNP, FNP
Doctor of Nursing Practice
Meriden, Connecticut

Katie Murphy, RN, MSN, PHN
Virtual Nurse Educator
Quintiles/Abbvie
Chicago, Illinois

Wendy R. Ostendorf, RN, MS, EdD, CNE
Professor of Nursing
Neumann University
Aston, Pennsylvania

Veronica (Ronnie) Peterson, BA, BSN, MS
Manager of Clinical Support
UW-Medical Foundation
Madison, Wisconsin

Victoria Plagenz, PhD, MS, BSN
Assistant Professor
University of Great Falls
Great Falls, Montana

Melissa Anne Radecki, MSN, NEd, RN, PCCN
Nursing Instructor
Florida Southern College
Lakeland, Florida

Cherie R. Rebar, PhD, MBA, RN, COI
Affiliate Faculty
Indiana Wesleyan University
Marion, Indiana;
Consultant
Xavier University School of Nursing
Cincinnati, Ohio

Anita K. Reed, MSN, RN
Chair, Community Health Practice
St. Elizabeth School of Nursing
Saint Joseph's College
Lafayette, Indiana

Jill R. Reed, PhD, APRN-NP
Assistant Professor
University of Nebraska Medical Center,
    College of Nursing
Kearney, Nebraska

Rhonda J. Reed, MSN, RN, CRRN
Learning Resource Center Director—
    Technology Coordinator
Indiana State University
Terre Haute, Indiana

Maura C. Schlairet, EdD, MA, MSN, RN, CNL
Professor of Nursing, Bioethicist
College of Nursing and Health Sciences
Valdosta State University
Valdosta, Georgia

Susan Parnell Scholtz, RN, PhD
Associate Professor of Nursing
Moravian College
Bethlehem, Pennsylvania

Elizabeth Sibson-Tuan, MS, RN
Bay Area Preceptor Coordinator
Samuel Merritt University
Oakland, California

Crystal Slaughter, DNP, APN, ACNS-BC
Associate Professor
Saint Francis Medical Center College of
    Nursing
Peoria, Illinois

Emily G. Smith, DNP, RN, CRRN, CNE, FNAP
Assistant Professor
Endicott College
Beverly, Massachusetts

Mindy Stayner, PhD, MSN, RN
Professor
Northwest State Community College
Chamberlain College of Nursing
Capella University
Archbold, Ohio

Laura M. Streeter, BSN, RN, SCRN, GCPH
Stroke Program Nurse
University of Missouri Health System
Columbia, Missouri

Linda Turchin, RN, MSN, CNE
Associate Professor of Nursing
Fairmont State University
Fairmont, West Virginia

Claudia C. Turner, MSN, RN
Professor of Nursing
Temple College
Temple, Texas

Heidi Tymkew, PT, DPT, MHS, CCS
Clinical Specialist
Barnes-Jewish Hospital
St. Louis, Missouri

Kim Webb, MN, RN
Adjunct Nursing Instructor
Pioneer Technology Center
Ponca City, Oklahoma

Anne M. Welsh, MSN-Ed, RN
Assistant Professor
Lewis and Clark Community College
Godfrey, Illinois

Estella J. Wetzel, MSN, APRN, FNP-C
Family Nurse Practitioner
AANP, OAAPN
Dayton, Ohio

Laura M. Willis, DNP, APRN, FNP-C
Co-President, Connect: RN2ED
Beavercreek, Ohio;
Family Nurse Practitioner
Urbana, Ohio

Paige Wimberley, PhD, APRN, CNS, CNE
Associate Professor of Nursing
Arkansas State University
Jonesboro, Arkansas

Valerie Yancey, PhD, RN
Associate Professor
Southern Illinois University Edwardsville
Edwardsville, Illinois

Jean Yockey, PhD, FNP-BC, CNE
Assistant Professor
University of South Dakota
Vermillion, South Dakota

CONTRIBUTORS TO PREVIOUS EDITIONS

Jeanette Spain Adams, RN, PhD, CRNI, APRN

Michelle Aebersold, PhD, RN

Elizabeth A. Ayello, RN, BSN, MS, PhD, CS, CETN

Marjorie Baier, RN, PhD

Sylvia Baird, RN, BSN, MM

Brenda A. Battle, MBA, BSN, RN

Lois Bentler-Lampe, RN, MS

Peggy Breckenridge, MSN, FNP

Judith C. Brostron, RN, BA, JD, LLM

Victoria M. Brown, RN, BSN, MSN, PhD, HNC

Jeri Burger, RN, PhD

Gale Carli, MSN, MSHed, BSN, RN

Rhonda Comrie, PhD, RN

Kelly Jo Cone, RN, BSN, MS, PhD

Roslyn Corcoran, RN, BSN

Eileen Costantinou, RN, MSN, BC

Ruth Curchoe, RN, MSN, CIC

Rick Daniels, RN, BSN, MSN, PhD

Carolyn Ruppel D'Avis, RN, BSN, MSN

Christine Durbin, RN, JD, PhD

Sharon J. Edwards, RN, BSN, MSN, PhD

Martha Keene Elkin, RN, MSN, IBCLC

Linda Fasciani, RN, BSN, MSN

Susan J. Fetzer, RN, BA, BSN, MSN, MBA, PhD

Leah Frederick, MS, RN, CIC

Cynthia S. Goodwin, RN, BSN, MSN

Lois C. Hamel, BS, MS

Janis Waite Hayden, RN, EdD

Maureen Huhmann, MS, RD

Tara Hulsey, RN, PhD, CNE, FAAN

Judith Ann Kilpatrick, RN, MSN, DNSc

Carl A. Kirton, RN-C, BSN, MA, ACRN, ANP

Lori Klingman, RN, MSN

Kristine L'Ecuyer, RN, MSN, CCNS

Kathryn A. Lever, RNC, MSN, WHNP-BC

Ruth Ludwick, RN, BSN, MSN, PhD, RN-C

Suzanne Lugerner, RN, MS, LN, CNSC, CNS

Mary Kay Knight Macheca, RN, BSN, MSN(R), CS, CDE

Deborah L. Marshall, RN, MSN

Carol McGinnis, DNP, RN, CNS, CNSC

Rita G. Mertig, RNC, MS, CNS

Mary Dee Miller, RN, BSN, MS, CIC

Elaine Neel, BSN, MSN

Geralyn A. Ochs, RN, ADN, BSN, MSN

Marsha Evans Orr, RN, MS, CS, CNSN

Wendy R. Ostendorf, MS, EdD

Dula F. Pacquiao, EdD, RN, CTN

Nancy Panthofer, RN, BSN, MSN

Elizabeth S. Pratt, RN, MSN, ACNS-BC

Julia Balzer Riley, RN, MN, AHN-C, CET®

Kristine A. Rose, RN, MSN

Janice J. Rumfelt, BSN, MSN, EdD, RNC

Marilyn Schallom, MSN, CCRN, CCNS

Matthew R. Sorenson, RN, PhD

Sharon Souter, RN, BSN, MSN

Elizabeth Speakman, RN, EdD

Rachel E. Spector, BS, MS, PhD, CTN, FAAN

Susan Speraw, RN, PHD, CNP

Donna L. Thompson, MSN, CRNP, FNP-BC, CCCN

Jelena Todic, MSW, LCSW

Riva Touger-Decker, PhD, RD, FADA

Ann Tritak, RN, EdD

Ellen Wathen, PhD, RN, BC

Pamela Becker Weilitz, DNP, APRN, ANP-BC

Joan Domigan Wentz, MSN, RN

Paige Wimberley, PhD, APN, CNS, CNE

Terry L. Wood, PhD, RN, CNE

Rita Wunderlich, PhD, RN, CNE

Valerie Yancey, RN, PhD

Barbara Yoost, RN, BSN, MSN, CNS

I wish to dedicate this edition of Essentials to the many friends who make up my family. Each one contributes in so many ways to support and value the work I am able to do. Special thanks to Ruth, a wonderful listener and advocate; Jim, a valued friend and kind man; Bess, always adding humor and love to my life; and Anne, a consummate writing colleague and lifelong mentor.
Patricia A. Potter

To all nursing faculty and professional nurses who work each day to advance clinical nursing. Your commitment to nursing education and nursing practice inspires us all to be the guardians of the discipline.

I also want to thank my husband Bob for his loving support.
Anne Griffin Perry

I was blessed to have an incredible nursing role model in my life—my mother, Evelyn M. Clark, RN. Your dedication and service to nursing inspired me to pursue my career as a professional nurse. Your unwavering support of my endeavors provided a foundation for me to continue to grow in my nursing role. Your encouragement and pride in my accomplishments was tremendous. Thank you for starting me on my path to a long and satisfying career in nursing and nursing education. I love you and miss you!
Patricia A. Stockert

To my family, especially Greg, Jacob, Isaac, and Mom and Dad. Thank you for your love, support, and patience, without which I would not be able to chase my dreams. Thank you also to the nursing faculty at Franciscan Missionaries of Our Lady University. Your never-ending compassion and commitment to nursing education inspires me every day. And finally, to my Varsity Sports running friends, who keep me grounded and who have helped me integrate into my new community. Despite all those really hot and long runs, y'all haven't killed me yet!
Amy M. Hall

The nursing profession is always responding to dynamic change and continual challenges. Today's nurses must be prepared to adapt to the continual changes occurring in health care. They play a vital role in the delivery of multidisciplinary health care services. The practice arena is changing—moving more to the community setting. The focus of care is also changing, with more emphasis being placed on health promotion and restorative care. Even the patients are changing—more cultural diversity exists, and the percentage of older adult patients continues to increase. Patients are far more involved in and informed about health care.

Despite—or perhaps because of—these changes, it is essential that the basics of nursing remain the foundation of practice. Nurses must be knowledgeable and professional. They must be both technically proficient and personally caring. And they must be able to synthesize a broad array of knowledge and experience when providing care for their patients.

We continue to cover all of the fundamental nursing concepts, skills, and techniques that students must master before moving on to other areas of study. In addition, we address changes in practice that affect how and where nurses use the skills and knowledge they acquire.

FEATURES

We have designed this text to welcome the new student to nursing, communicate our own love for the profession, and promote learning and understanding. We know that today's students are busy and, too often, are overwhelmed by all that they must learn and do. They want their texts to focus on the most current, factual, and essential content and skills. We want to ensure that these students are ready to continue with their education and will ultimately be prepared for all of the challenges of practice. To this end, we have included the following key features:

- Students will appreciate the **clear, engaging writing style.** The narrative actually addresses the reader, making this textbook more of an active instructional tool than a passive reference. Students will find that even complex technical and theoretical concepts are presented in a language that is easy to understand.
- The **attractive, functional design** will appeal to today's visual learner. The clear, readable type and bold headings make the content easy to read and follow. Each special element is consistently color keyed so students can readily identify important information.
- Hundreds of **large, clear, full-color photographs and drawings** reinforce and clarify key concepts and techniques.
- The **five-step nursing process** serves as the organizing framework for all clinical chapters. This logical, consistent framework for narrative discussions is further enhanced by special boxes that highlight assessment, care plans, and evaluation of outcome achievement.
- **Ongoing case studies** in each chapter introduce "real-world" patients, families, and nurses. The chapter follows

the case study through the steps of the nursing process, helping students see how to apply the process, as well as critical thinking, to the care of patients. Cases take place in both acute and community settings and include patients and nurses from a variety of cultural backgrounds.

- **Nursing Care Plans** guide students on how to conduct an assessment and analyze the defining characteristics that indicate nursing diagnoses. The plans include NIC and NOC classifications to familiarize students with this important nomenclature. The evaluation sections of the plans show students how to evaluate and then determine the outcomes of care.
- **Concept Maps** included in clinical chapters show you the associations among multiple nursing diagnoses for a patient with a selected medical diagnosis, as well as their relationship to nursing interventions.
- The implementation narrative consistently addresses health promotion, acute care, and restorative and continuing care to reflect a focus on **community-based nursing** and **health promotion.**
- Information related to the **Quality and Safety Education for Nurses (QSEN)** initiative is highlighted with activities integrated into each chapter. These activities incorporate one of the six key competencies and relate back to the progressive chapter case study scenarios.
- **More than 35 nursing skills** are presented in a clear, two-column format with steps and rationales. Skills include delegation guidelines and clinical decision points that alert students to steps that require special assessment or specific technique for safe and effective administration.
- **Procedural guidelines** provide streamlined step-by-step instructions for performing very basic skills.
- Care of the **older adult** and **patient teaching** are stressed throughout the narrative and are also highlighted in special boxes.
- **Learning aids** to help students identify, review, and apply important content in each chapter include Objectives, Key Terms, Key Points, and Review Questions.
- **Printed lists** on the inside back cover provide information on locating specific assets in the book, including Skills, Procedural Guidelines, Nursing Care Plans, and Patient Teaching boxes.

New to This Edition

- A **new chapter on "Complementary, Alternative, and Integrative Therapies"** addresses content that is now included on the NCLEX® examination.
- A **new Reflective Learning** section in each chapter helps students better understand and reflect on their clinical and simulation experiences as they move through their first nursing course.
- **Evidence-Based Practice** boxes have been updated with new PICO questions. These boxes provide a summary of nursing research evidence related to that specific topic and then explain its implications for nursing practice. These

boxes have been updated to reflect current research topics and trends.

LEARNING SUPPLEMENTS FOR STUDENTS

- The **Evolve Student Resources** are available online at http://evolve.elsevier.com/Potter/essentials and include the following valuable learning aids organized by chapter:
  - Review Questions with Answers and Rationales
  - Answers to QSEN Activity Scenarios
  - Case Studies with Questions
  - Printable Key Points
  - Video Clips
  - Interactive Skills Performance Checklists
  - Fluids and Electrolytes Tutorial
  - Audio Glossary
  - Concept Map Creator
  - Conceptual Care Map
  - Calculation Tutorial
  - Answers to Student Study Guide
  - Content Updates
- A thorough **Study Guide** by Patricia A. Castaldi provides students with a wide variety of exercises and activities to enhance learning and comprehension. This study guide features case studies with related questions; chapter review sections with matching, fill-in-the-blank, and multiple-choice questions; study group questions; and instructions for creating and using study charts.
- **Virtual Clinical Excursions** is an exciting workbook and CD-ROM experience that brings learning to life in a virtual hospital setting. The workbook guides students as they care for patients, providing ongoing challenges and learning opportunities. Each lesson in *Virtual Clinical Excursions* complements the textbook content and provides an environment for students to practice what they are learning. This CD/workbook is available separately or packaged at a special price with the textbook.

TEACHING SUPPLEMENTS FOR INSTRUCTORS

- The **Evolve Instructor Resources** (available online at http://evolve.elsevier.com/Potter/essentials) are a comprehensive collection of the most important tools instructors need, including the following:
  - **TEACH for Nurses** ties together every chapter resource you need for the most effective class presentations, with sections dedicated to objectives, teaching strategies, nursing curriculum standards (including QSEN/NLN Competencies, BSN Essentials, and Nursing Concepts), instructor chapter resources, student chapter resources, and an in-class case study discussion. Teaching Strategies include relationships between the textbook content and discussion items. Examples of student activities, online activities, and large group activities are provided for more "hands-on" learning.
  - The **Test Bank** contains a revised set of more than 950 questions with answers coded for NCLEX® Client Needs category, nursing process, and cognitive level. The Exam-View software allows instructors to create new tests; edit, add, and delete test questions; sort questions by NCLEX® category, cognitive level, nursing process step, and question type; and administer and grade online tests.
  - **PowerPoint Presentations** include over 1400 slides for use in lectures. Art is included within the slides, and progressive case studies include discussion questions and answers.
  - The **Image Collection** contains hundreds of illustrations from the text for use in lectures.
- **Simulation Learning System** is an online toolkit that helps instructors and facilitators effectively incorporate medium- to high-fidelity simulation into their nursing curriculum. Detailed patient scenarios promote and enhance the clinical decision-making skills of students at all levels. The system provides detailed instructions for preparation and implementation of the simulation experience, debriefing questions that encourage critical thinking, and learning resources to reinforce student comprehension. Each scenario in *Simulation Learning System* complements the textbook content and helps bridge the gap between lectures and clinicals. This system provides the perfect environment for students to practice what they are learning in the text for a true-to-life, hands-on learning experience.

MULTIMEDIA SUPPLEMENTS FOR INSTRUCTORS AND STUDENTS

- **Nursing Skills Online 4.0** contains 19 modules rich with animations, videos, interactive activities, and exercises to help students prepare for their clinical lab experience. The instructionally designed lessons focus on topics that are difficult to master and pose a high risk to the patient if done incorrectly. Lesson quizzes allow students to check their learning curve and review as needed, and the module exams feed out to an instructor grade book. Modules cover Airway Management, Blood Therapy, Bowel Elimination/Ostomy, Cardiac Care, Closed Chest Drainage Systems, Enteral Nutrition, Infection Control, Maintenance of IV Fluid Therapy, IV Fluid Therapy, Administration of Parenteral Medications: Injections and IV Medications, Non-parenteral Medication Administration, Safe Medication Preparation, Safety, Specimen Collection, Urinary Catheterization, Caring for Central Vascular Access Devices (CVAD), Vital Signs, and Wound Care. Available alone or packaged with the text.
- **Mosby's Nursing Video Skills: Basic, Intermediate, Advanced, 4th edition,** provides 126 skills with overview information covering skill purpose, safety, and delegation guides; equipment lists; preparation procedures; procedure videos with printable step-by-step guidelines; appropriate follow-up care; documentation guidelines; and interactive review questions. Available online, as a student DVD set, or as a networkable DVD set for the institution.

ACKNOWLEDGMENTS

The ninth edition of *Essentials for Nursing Practice* is the result of a continued collaboration among all authors, contributors, and editorial team members. Having professional colleagues to work with, trust, and challenge one another is a gift—one that ensures a timely and accurate text.

This textbook cannot be created without the support, guidance, and creative direction from our editorial team, designer, and production staff. Likewise, no book is successful without the hard work and dedication of its marketing team. We are also very fortunate regarding the manner in which staff from the electronic media division of Elsevier has produced products that complement the text and ensure its success. We wish to make special mention of some important individuals.

Tamara Myers, Director, is a dedicated professional who continually challenges the author team to create a state-of-the-art revision. Her enthusiasm and knowledge creates an environment for the writing, editorial, and production teams to develop a relevant and creative textbook that reflects contemporary nursing practice.

Tina Kaemmerer, Senior Content Development Specialist, is a dedicated professional whose organizational skills ensure that this project remains on target. She effectively collaborates with all members of the writing team in tracking manuscript through the publication process, in problem solving, and in being an invaluable resource for authors, contributors, and the production team.

Paula Catalano, our Book Designer, has developed a visually distinctive textbook design. Her expertise created a text that is visually appealing yet easy for our readers to use. Paula is also credited for her creativity and vision for the design of the cover art and her direction in implementing the overall design of the text.

Many thanks and gratitude go to members of the Production Team. Jodi Willard, Senior Project Manager, is a tireless and dedicated professional. As an accomplished project manager, she keeps us on deadline while ensuring consistency in formatting, presentation, and style. Her sense of humor and ability to always remain calm under pressure are invaluable attributes. She is one of a kind. Jeff Patterson, Publishing Services Manager, has contributed support throughout the editing and final pages.

A tip of the hat must always go to the sales and marketing team, headed by Julie Burchett and Megan Atencio, who provided us direction early in the planning stage of *Essentials for Nursing Practice*. Their knowledge of market trends and needs helps us to make revisions of high quality.

Many thanks to our contributors, clinicians, and educators, who share their experiences and knowledge about nursing practice in helping to create informative, accurate, and current information. Their knowledge of their own clinical specialties ensures we have a state-of-the-art textbook. We are fortunate to be associated with excellent nurse authors who are able to convey standards of nursing excellence through the printed word.

A heartfelt thanks to our many reviewers for their expertise, candor, knowledge of the literature, and astute comments that assist us in developing a text with high standards that reflect professional nursing practice today.

After many years of collaboration, we find ourselves very fortunate and humble. *Essentials for Nursing Practice* and the other textbooks we have been able to develop have made important contributions to nursing practice. It remains a work of love.

Patricia A. Potter
Anne Griffin Perry
Patricia A. Stockert
Amy M. Hall

CONTENTS

Professional Nursing

evolve MEDIA RESOURCES

http://evolve.elsevier.com/Potter/essentials

- Audio Glossary
- QSEN Activity and Review Questions Answers

OBJECTIVES

- Discuss the characteristics of professionalism in nursing.
- Discuss the importance of education in professional nursing practice.
- Describe the purpose of professional standards of nursing practice.
- Describe the roles and career opportunities for nurses.
- Discuss the influence of social, political, and economic changes on nursing practices.

KEY TERMS

advanced practice registered nurse (APRN), p. 9
American Nurses Association (ANA), p. 2
caregiver, p. 8
certified nurse-midwife (CNM), p. 9
certified registered nurse anesthetist (CRNA), p. 9
clinical nurse specialist (CNS), p. 9
code of ethics, p. 6

continuing education, p. 6
genomics, p. 11
in-service education, p. 6
International Council of Nurses (ICN), p. 10
licensed practical nurse (LPN), p. 5
licensed vocational nurse (LVN), p. 5
National League for Nursing (NLN), p. 10
nurse administrator, p. 10

nurse educator, p. 9
nurse practitioner (NP), p. 9
nurse researcher, p. 10
nursing, p. 2
patient advocate, p. 8
professional organization, p. 10
Quality and Safety Education for Nurses (QSEN), p. 10
registered nurse (RN), p. 5

Nursing is an art and a science. As a professional nurse, you learn to deliver care artfully with compassion, caring, and respect for each patient's dignity and personhood. As a science, nursing practice is based on a body of knowledge that is continually changing with new discoveries and innovations. When you integrate the science and art of nursing into your practice, the quality of care you provide to your patients is at a level of excellence that benefits patients and their families. Your patients' health care needs are multidimensional. Thus, your care reflects patients' needs as well as the needs and values of society and professional standards of care. In addition, your care should integrate evidence-based practices to provide the highest level of care.

The patient is the center of your practice. The patient includes the individual, family, and/or community. Patients have a wide variety of health care needs, experiences, vulnerabilities, and expectations; this is what makes nursing both challenging and rewarding. Making a difference in your patients' lives is fulfilling. For example, you help a dying patient find relief from pain, help a young mother learn parenting skills, or find ways for older adults to remain independent in their homes. Nursing offers personal and professional rewards every day.

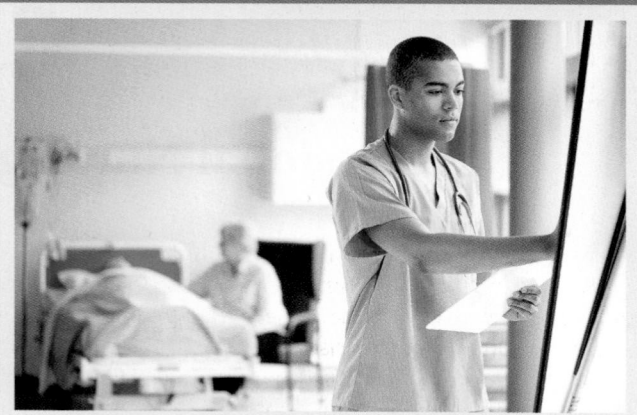

CASE STUDY *Lucas*

Copyright © sturti/Getty Images.

Lucas is a nursing student assigned to provide care for a 52-year-old patient, Mr. Thompson, at the residential hospice home. Mr. Thompson came to the hospice home with metastatic pancreatic cancer. Lucas focused his nursing care plan on comfort care for Mr. Thompson. Mrs. Thompson told Lucas that she was worried that her husband would be experiencing pain. This morning Lucas is participating in the interdisciplinary team meeting to discuss Mr. Thompson's care management.

As a nurse, you can choose a variety of career paths including clinical practice, education, research, management, administration, and entrepreneurship. As a student, it is important for you to understand the scope of nursing practice and how nursing influences the lives of your patients. You are required to provide nursing care according to standards of practice and follow a code of ethics (ANA, 2015a; Fowler, 2015b). Professional practice includes knowledge from social and behavioral sciences, biological and physiological sciences, and nursing theories. In addition, nursing practice incorporates ethical and social values, professional autonomy, and a sense of commitment and community. The **American Nurses Association (ANA)** defines **nursing** as *the protection, promotion, and optimization of health and abilities; prevention of illness and injury; facilitation of healing; alleviation of suffering through the diagnosis and treatment of human response; and advocacy in the care of individuals, families, groups, communities, and populations* (ANA, 2015a). The International Council of Nurses (ICN) (2016) has another definition: *Nursing encompasses autonomous and collaborative care of individuals of all ages, families, groups and communities, sick or well and in all settings. Nursing includes the promotion of health; prevention of illness; and the care of ill, disabled, and dying people. Advocacy, promotion of a safe environment, research, participation in shaping health policy and in patient and health systems management, and education are also key nursing roles.* Both definitions support the importance that nursing holds in providing safe, patient-centered health care to the global community.

Expert clinical nursing practice is a commitment to the application of knowledge, ethics, standards of practice, and clinical experience. Your ability to interpret clinical situations and make complex decisions is the foundation for your nursing care and the basis for the advancement of nursing practice and the development of nursing science (Benner, 1984; Benner et al., 1997; Benner et al., 2010). Clinical expertise takes time and commitment. Critical thinking skills are essential to nursing (see Chapter 8). When providing nursing care, you need to make clinical judgments and decisions about your patients' health care needs based on knowledge, experience, and standards of care. Critical thinking and reflection help you gain and interpret scientific knowledge, integrate knowledge from clinical experiences, and become a lifelong learner (Benner et al., 2010). This includes integrating knowledge from basic science and nursing knowledge bases, applying knowledge from past and present experiences, applying critical thinking attitudes to a clinical situation, and implementing intellectual and professional standards (see Chapter 8). When you provide well-thought-out care with compassion and caring, you provide each of your patients the best of the science and art of nursing care (see Chapter 7).

HISTORY OF NURSING

Since the beginning of the profession, nurses have studied and tested new and better ways to help patients. Patients are most vulnerable when they are injured, sick, or dying. Today nurses are active in determining the best practices for patient care related to problems such as skin care management, pain control, nutritional management, and care of older adults. Nurse researchers are leaders in expanding knowledge in nursing and other health care disciplines. Their work provides evidence for practice to ensure that we have the best available evidence to support our practices (see Chapter 7).

Nurses are also active in social policy and political arenas. With their professional organizations, they lobby for health care legislation. For example, nurses have lobbied for laws promoting smoke-free environments and stronger anti-tobacco laws, setting up anti-gang coalitions, establishing safer environments for walking and physical fitness in their communities, and advocating for breastfeeding (Mason et al., 2016).

Knowledge of the history of the nursing profession increases your ability to understand the social and intellectual origins of the discipline. Although it is not practical to describe all the historical aspects of professional nursing, some of the more significant milestones are described in the following paragraphs.

Florence Nightingale

In *Notes on Nursing: What It Is and What It Is Not,* Florence Nightingale established the first nursing philosophy based on health maintenance and restoration (Nightingale, 1860). She saw the role of nursing as having "charge of somebody's health" based on the knowledge of "how to put the body in such a state to be free of disease or to recover from disease" (Nightingale, 1860). She developed the first organized training program for nurses in 1860, the Nightingale Training

School for Nurses at St. Thomas' Hospital in London. Nightingale volunteered during the Crimean War in 1853 and traveled the battlefield hospitals at night carrying her lamp; thus she was known as the "lady with the lamp." As a result of Nightingale's organization and improvement of the sanitation facilities at the battlefield hospitals, the mortality rate at the Barracks Hospital in Scutari, Turkey, was reduced from 42.7% to 2.2% in 6 months (Donahue, 2011). Perhaps one of Nightingale's greatest contributions was the maintenance of statistics to show the efficacy of her strategies.

The Civil War to the Beginning of the Twentieth Century

The Civil War (1860–1865) stimulated the growth of nursing in the United States. Clara Barton, founder of the American Red Cross, cared for soldiers on the battlefields, cleansing their wounds, meeting their basic needs, and comforting them in death. Dorothea Lynde Dix, Mary Ann Ball (Mother Bickerdyke), and Harriet Tubman also influenced nursing during the Civil War (Donahue, 2011). Dix and Bickerdyke organized hospitals and ambulances, appointed nurses, cared for the wounded soldiers, and managed supplies. Tubman was active in the Underground Railroad movement and helped lead more than 300 slaves to freedom (Donahue, 2011).

The first professionally educated African-American nurse was Mary Mahoney. She was concerned with relationships between cultures and races. As a nursing leader, she brought forth an awareness of cultural diversity and respect for the individual, regardless of background, race, color, or religion.

Isabel Hampton Robb helped found the Nurses' Associated Alumnae of the United States and Canada in 1896. This organization became the ANA in 1911. She authored many nursing textbooks and was one of the original founders of the *American Journal of Nursing* (Donahue, 2011).

Nursing in hospitals expanded in the late nineteenth century. However, nursing in the community did not increase significantly until 1893, when Lillian Wald and Mary Brewster opened the Henry Street Settlement, which focused on the health needs of poor people who lived in tenements in New York City (Donahue, 2011).

Twentieth Century

In the early twentieth century, nursing evolved toward developing a scientific, research-based defined body of nursing knowledge and practice. Nurses began to assume expanded and advanced practice roles to meet society's needs. Mary Adelaide Nutting, the first professor of nursing at Columbia University Teachers College, was instrumental in the affiliation of nursing education with universities (Donahue, 2011). In addition, the Goldmark Report concluded that nursing education needed increased financial support.

As nursing education developed, nursing practice also expanded, and the Army and Navy Nurse Corps were established. By the 1920s nursing specialization started to develop. The last half of the century saw specialty-nursing organizations such as the American Association of Critical Care Nurses, Association of Operating Room Nurses (AORN), Infusion Nurses Society (INS), and Emergency Nurses Association (ENA) created. In 1990 the ANA established the Center for Ethics and Human Rights (see Chapter 6). The Center provides a forum to address the complex ethical and human rights issues confronting nurses and designs programs to increase ethical competence in nurses (Fowler, 2015b).

Twenty-First Century

Today the nursing profession faces multiple challenges. Nurses and nurse educators are revising nursing practice and school curricula to meet the ever-changing needs of society including bioterrorism, emerging infections, and disaster management. Advances in technology and informatics (see Chapter 10), the aging population, the high-acuity level of care of hospitalized patients, and early discharge from health care institutions require nurses in all settings to have a strong and current knowledge base. In addition, nursing and the Robert Wood Johnson Foundation are taking a leadership role in developing standards and policies for end-of-life care through the *Last Acts Campaign* (see Chapter 27). The End-of-Life Nursing Education Consortium (ELNEC) offered collaboratively by the American Association of Colleges of Nursing (AACN) and the City of Hope Medical Center has brought end-of-life care and practices into nursing curricula and professional continuing education programs for practicing nurses (AACN, 2016).

INFLUENCES ON NURSING

Multiple external forces affect nursing today including health care reform and costs, demographic changes of the population, increasing numbers of medically underserved individuals, need for emergency preparedness, workplace issues, and the nursing shortage.

Health Care Reform and Costs

Health care reform affects how health care is paid for and delivered. In the future there will be greater emphasis on health promotion, disease prevention, and illness management. More services will be provided in community-based care settings. As a result, more nurses will be needed to practice in community care centers, patients' homes, schools, and senior centers. This will require expert nurses to assess for resources, service gaps, and how patients adapt to return to their communities. Nursing needs to respond by assessing for resources, changing nursing education, helping patients adapt to new health care delivery methods, and providing care to safely return patients to their homes.

Skyrocketing health care costs present challenges to the profession, consumer, and health care delivery system. As a nurse you are responsible for providing the patient with the best-quality care in an efficient and economically sound manner including following established protocols, exercising timely well-planned patient discharge from a care setting, and judiciously using supplies and equipment. The challenge is to use health care and patient resources wisely. Chapter 3 summarizes reasons for the rise in health care costs and its implications for nursing.

Demographic Changes

The U.S. Census Bureau (2015) predicts that between 2014 and 2060, there will be a steady rise in the population, although this increase will slow in future decades as fertility rates decline over these years. This change requires expanded health care resources. Add to the population change a steady increase in the percentage of the population of people 65 years of age and older. By 2030 it is estimated that one in five persons will be 65 years of age or older (U.S. Census Bureau, 2015). It is also predicted that by 2044 more than half of the U.S. population will be part of a minority group (U.S. Census Bureau, 2015). To effectively meet all the health care needs of the expanding minority and aging populations, changes in how care is provided are needed, especially in the area of public health. The population is shifting from rural areas to urban centers, and more people are living with chronic and long-term illness (RWJF, 2014). Outpatient settings are expanding, and more people want to receive outpatient and community-based care and remain in their homes or community (see Chapters 3 and 4).

Medically Underserved Population

Unemployment, underemployment and low-paying jobs, mental illness, poor health care access in rural areas, homelessness, and health care costs all contribute to increases in the medically underserved population. Caring for this population is a global issue; the social, political, and economic factors of a country affect both access to care and resources to provide and pay for these services. In the United States, some of the medically underserved population are individuals who are poor and on Medicaid. Others are part of the working poor (e.g., they cannot afford their own insurance, but they make too much money to qualify for Medicaid and as a result do not receive any health care). Patients who are medically underserved and who have low health literacy are less likely to participate in decision making regarding their care often because they do not understand the medical information provided (Seo et al., 2016). Today nurses and schools of nursing are developing partnerships to improve health outcomes in underserved communities. Nurses work in these community-based settings providing health promotion and disease prevention.

Need for Emergency Preparedness

The world is a changing place; the threats of terrorism are continuous. Many health care agencies, schools, and communities have educational programs to prepare for nuclear, chemical, or biological attacks and other types of disasters. Nurses play an active role in emergency preparedness ranging from participation in vaccine research, to decontamination in times of biological attack, to triage for mass casualty, to participation in crisis response units. Nurses provide emergency preparedness education and prepare for disasters at the local, state, and federal levels (Zerwekh and Garneau, 2015).

Workplace Issues

Nurses are faced with multiple issues and hazards in the workplace. For example, they are at risk for ergonomic hazards that result in musculoskeletal injuries such as back injury and repetitive motion disorders (ANA, 2016). When looking for a new position, evaluate the workforce protection and safety plan that the hospital or health care organization has in place (Zerwekh and Garneau, 2015).

Another issue facing nurses is workplace violence. Workplace violence takes the form of bullying and acts of verbal or nonverbal aggression or harassment from co-workers and sometimes patients and families. Nurses who experience workplace violence often develop anger, fear, anxiety, post-traumatic stress disorder symptoms, guilt, or shame (Huber, 2014). Respect for the dignity and rights of all co-workers is an ethical responsibility for all nurses (NCSBN, 2016). The ANA calls for "zero tolerance" to violence of any kind within the workplace. The ANA recommends evidence-based interventions to prevent violence and to promote the health and safety of nurses (ANA, 2015c). Know the policies of your institution on prevention or response to workplace violence.

Nursing Shortage

There is an ongoing nursing shortage in the United States, which results from insufficient qualified registered nurses (RNs) to fill vacant positions, the aging population of nurses, and a growing need for health care services (AACN, 2014). An increased number of nurses are retiring; 55% of nurses are aged 50 or older (AACN, 2014; NCSBN, 2016). This shortage affects all nursing care settings, including hospitals, long-term care facilities, administration, and nursing education (AACN, 2014); it also represents challenges and opportunities for the profession. Many dollars are invested in strategies aimed at increasing student enrollment in nursing programs and recruiting a well-educated, critically thinking, motivated, and dedicated nursing workforce (Benner et al., 2010; AACN, 2014). At the same time hospitals, the largest employer of nurses, seek ways to improve nurse retention. There is a direct link between RN staffing and nursing care with positive patient outcomes including reduced complication rates and a more rapid return of the patient to an optimal functional status (Box 1.1) (Choi and Staggs, 2014; Giuliano et al., 2016).

With fewer nurses in the workplace, it is important for you to learn to use your patient contact time efficiently and professionally. Time management, therapeutic communication, patient education, and compassionate implementation of psychomotor skills are just a few of the essential skills you need. Most important, ensure your patients leave the health care setting with a positive image of nursing and a feeling that they received quality care. Your patient should never feel rushed or that he or she was unimportant. If a certain aspect of patient care requires 15 minutes of contact, it takes the same amount of time to deliver the care in an organized manner as it would in a rushed, harried manner.

BOX 1.1 EVIDENCE-BASED PRACTICE

PICO Question: Are patient outcomes improved in hospitals with adequate nursing staffing versus hospitals with lower nursing staffing?

SUMMARY OF EVIDENCE

There is a growing body of research that shows that nurse staffing does impact patient outcomes, patient survival, and the occurrence of adverse events. A secondary data analysis from 661 hospitals showed that there was a significantly lower 30-day readmission rate for patients with heart failure in hospitals that had high nurse staffing, thus reducing health care costs (Giuliano et al., 2016). Higher nurse staffing was also found to significantly increase the survival of patients in an intensive care unit (West et al., 2014). Patients experiencing an in-hospital cardiac arrest were more likely to survive when there was a decreased patient-to-nurse ratio (McHugh et al., 2016). Cho et al. (2016) found that larger numbers of patients assigned to a nurse increased the occurrence of medication errors, pressure injury formation, and falls with injuries. Studies demonstrating the positive impact that nurse-to-patient ratios have on outcomes provide nursing administrators with evidence to support hiring of qualified professional nurses.

APPLICATION TO NURSING PRACTICE

- Consider the nurse-to-patient ratio when looking at a hospital or unit for employment.
- Adequate nursing levels help to improve the nursing work environment (Cho et al., 2016).
- Improved working conditions increase the likelihood of patient survival in emergency events (McHugh et al., 2016).
- Continuing research needs to be conducted to study the economic impact of nurse staffing and improved patient outcomes (Giuliano et al., 2016).

PROFESSIONALISM

Nursing is a profession. A person who acts professionally is conscientious in actions, knowledgeable in the subject, and responsible to self and others. This means that as a nurse you administer patient-centered care in a safe, conscientious, and knowledgeable manner. Professions possess the following characteristics:

- An extended education of members and a basic liberal education foundation
- A theoretical body of knowledge leading to defined skills, abilities, and norms
- Provision of a specific service
- Autonomy in decision making and practice
- A code of ethics for practice

Nursing shares each of these characteristics, offering an opportunity for the growth and enrichment of all its members.

Licensed Practical Nurse/Licensed Vocational Nurse Education

A licensed practical nurse (LPN) or licensed vocational nurse (LVN) is educated in basic nursing techniques and direct patient care. The LPN/LVN is a nurse who completes a practical nursing program and passes a licensure examination (NCLEX-PN®). The LPN/LVN practices under the supervision of an RN or other licensed person. The responsibilities and scope of practice are set by each state board of nursing. An LPN/LVN, or in Canada an RN assistant (RNA), generally receives 1 year of education and clinical preparation in a community college or other agency. Some RN programs allow an LPN to enter the program at an advanced level.

Registered Nurse Education

As a profession nursing requires that its members possess a significant amount of education. There are various educational routes for becoming a registered nurse (RN). Currently in the United States an individual becomes an RN by earning an associate degree, diploma, or baccalaureate degree program in nursing and by passing the NCLEX-RN® examination. The baccalaureate degree is required as the entry to practice standard for RNs in all provinces of Canada except Quebec (Canadian Nurses Association [CAN], 2016a). Nursing education provides the solid foundation for practice, and it responds to changes in health care created by scientific and technological advances.

Advanced Education

Some roles for RNs require advanced graduate degrees. A graduate degree provides the advanced clinician with strong skills in nursing science and theory, with an emphasis on the basic sciences and research-based clinical practice related to a specialty. A master's degree in nursing (e.g., Master of Arts in Nursing [MA], Master of Nursing [MN], or Master of Science in Nursing [MSN]) is for RNs seeking roles such as nurse educator, nurse administrator, clinical nurse leader, nursing informatics specialist, or advanced practice registered nurse (APRN). Some programs require the RN to have a Bachelor of Science in Nursing (BSN) degree before entry; other programs offer entrance to associate degree–prepared nurses who take bachelor's level courses as they progress through the curriculum toward the master's degree.

Some roles within nursing require doctoral degrees. There are two doctorate degree in nursing options for nurses. The Doctor of Philosophy (PhD) has a focus on research, and the Doctor of Nursing Practice (DNP) has a focus on advanced clinical practice. The health care industry needs nurses prepared at the doctorate level with advanced academic and clinical preparation to educate nursing students and participate as members of the interdisciplinary health care team to provide evidence-based, competent, safe patient care (IOM, 2010). Nurses with doctorates advance the profession by promoting evidence-based practice, developing practice guidelines, conducting and disseminating research, developing and testing theory, educating future nurses, and influencing public policy and health care planning.

Continuing and In-Service Education

Continuing education programs are one way to promote and maintain current nursing skills, gain new knowledge about the latest research and practice developments, gain certification credits to specialize in a specific practice area, meet requirements for continuing licensure as a nurse, and obtain new skills and techniques reflecting the changes in the health care delivery system. **Continuing education** involves formal, organized educational programs offered by universities, hospitals, state nurses associations, professional nursing organizations, and educational and health care institutions. Examples include a program on caring for older adults with dementia offered by a university or a program on safe medication practices offered by a hospital. Often these programs provide attendees with some type of continuing education credit.

In-service education programs contain instruction or training provided by a health care agency or institution designed to increase the knowledge, skills, and competencies of nurses and other health care professionals employed by the institution. Often in-service programs focus on new technologies or fulfill required competencies of the organization. For example, a hospital offers an in-service program on safe principles for administering chemotherapy or a program on cultural sensitivity.

Theory

Professional nursing practice and knowledge have developed in part through nursing theories (global views that help to describe, predict, or prescribe activities for the practice of nursing). Theoretical models provide frameworks for how nurses practice. Some nursing school curricula integrate a theoretical model. Some nursing organizations adopt a nursing theory as the foundation for their standards of nursing care. Examples of theories used in education and practice are Orem's self-care deficit theory, Benner's primacy of caring, and Watson's Theory of Human Caring. The ongoing development of nursing theory or nursing science involves generating knowledge to advance and support nursing practice and health care (Alligood, 2014).

Service

Nursing is a service profession and a vital and indispensable part of the health care delivery system. Nurses in practice maintain a consumer-based and service-based focus. Patients are more knowledgeable about their health care problems, options, and rights. As a nurse you work with patients and families individualizing care while incorporating their preferences and expectations. Show respect by providing care on time, displaying a caring attitude, and considering patients' cultural and social differences. Collaborate with necessary health care providers to ensure continuation of care from one setting to the next.

Autonomy and Accountability

Autonomy is essential to professional nursing and involves the initiation of independent nursing interventions without medical orders. Autonomy means that a person is reasonably independent and self-governing in decision making and practice. You reach autonomy through experience, advanced

education, and the support of an organization that values the independent role of the nurse. With increased autonomy comes greater responsibility and accountability for the performance of nursing care activities. Accountability means that you are professionally and legally responsible for the type and quality of nursing care provided. To be autonomous and accountable carries the responsibility to keep current and competent in nursing and scientific knowledge and skills.

Code of Ethics

Nursing's **code of ethics** defines the principles that nurses use to provide patient-centered care (see Chapter 6). In addition, nurses incorporate their own values and ethics into practice. The ANA's *Code of Ethics for Nurses: With Interpretive Statements* (2015b) provides a guide for carrying out nursing responsibilities to ensure high-quality nursing care and provide for the ethical obligations of the profession.

Developing Professionalism in Your Career

It is important that you work to develop professionalism early in your nursing career. Professionalism in appearance and behaviors is critical to earning recognition and respect as a nurse (Splendore et al., 2016). The use of social media is prevalent with both nursing students and professional nurses (Mamocha et al., 2015). You need to be very aware of your use of social media and practice e-professionalism (Westrick, 2016). Social media has positive uses for providing patient education, providing communication, and fostering professional connections (NCSBN, 2011). However, inappropriate use of social media violates legal, ethical, and professional standards. Research has shown that there are an increasing number of incidents of nursing students and practicing nurses posting unprofessional content, such as patients' personal health information (PHI), on social media sites (Westrick, 2016). Cyberbullying was also found to have occurred against both peers and faculty (Mamocha et al., 2015). As a nurse you must be aware of social media ethical and professional standards that you need to follow. Be aware of both personal and professional information that you share on social media sites. You will violate state and federal laws if you share patient health information on social media sites (NCSBN, 2011). Check your agency or school policy on use of social media to ensure that you are acting professionally when using social media (Brown, 2016). To protect yourself and your patients, follow the guidelines on use of social media established by the ANA and National Council of State Boards of Nursing (ANA, 2011; NCSBN, 2011; Westrick, 2016).

It is important that you display professionalism when applying for nursing positions. Professional communication dictates that you send a cover letter when submitting your resume, a thank-you letter for the interview opportunity, and a resignation letter if you are leaving your position (Yoder-Wise, 2014). The professional letter and resume that you submit is often the first impression you make on the individual who is hiring nurses. Make sure that your letters are professional in appearance, using appropriate paper and good grammar with no misspellings. Your resume should be typed, printed on high-quality paper, accurate, error-free, and grammatically correct (Yoder-Wise, 2014).

For your interview, dress in professional clothing. Do not wear scrubs. Be prepared for the interview and be prepared to answer questions that are related to "how you handled a challenging situation" or discussing your strengths and opportunities for improvement. Other questions may focus on how your education has prepared you for the position for which you are interviewing. Turn off and put away all your electronic devices so that you are not distracted by them during the interview. Avoid eating, drinking, and chewing gum during the interview.

The first impression that you make on patients is often related to your appearance. Your uniform is a form of non-verbal communication with patients (Splendore et al., 2016). Your uniform should be clean, be odor-free, and fit appropriately conveying a professional appearance. Make sure that you follow your agency dress code so that you are professional in your appearance when providing care to patients. Nursing uniforms have a positive impact on the patient experience (Splendore et al., 2016).

NURSING PRACTICE

You will have an opportunity to practice in a variety of settings, in many roles within those settings, and with caregivers in other related health professions. State and provincial Nurse Practice Acts (NPAs) establish specific legal regulations for practice. The ANA is concerned with nursing practice, public recognition of the significance of nursing practice to health care, and implications for nursing practice regarding trends in health care. The ANA definition of nursing illustrates the consistent need for nurses to promote the well-being of their patients individually or in groups and communities (Fowler, 2015a). State and provincial NPAs establish specific legal regulations for nursing practice. Professional organizations such as the ANA establish professional standards for practice.

Nurse Practice Acts

In the United States each State Board of Nursing oversees its NPA. The NPA regulates the scope of nursing practice for the state and protects public health, safety, and welfare. This includes protecting the public from unqualified and unsafe nurses. Although each state has its own NPA that defines the scope of nursing practice, most NPAs are similar. The definition of nursing practice published by the ANA is representative of the scope of nursing practice as defined in most states. During the last decade, many states have revised their NPAs to reflect the growing autonomy of nursing, minimum education requirements, certification requirements, and the expanded roles and scope of practice of APRNs.

Licensure and Certification

Licensure. In the United States RN candidates must pass the NCLEX-RN® examination administered by the individual State Boards of Nursing to obtain a nursing license. Regardless of educational preparation, the examination for RN licensure is exactly the same in every state in the United States to provide a standardized minimum knowledge base for nurses. As of January 2015, new graduates of Canada's 10 provinces/territories must also pass the NCLEX-RN® to become an RN (CNA, 2016b). Whether nurses are able to practice in a state or province other than their own depends on the agreement between the states or provinces involved.

Certification. Beyond the NCLEX-RN®, some nurses work toward certification in a specific area of nursing practice. Minimum practice requirements are set based on the certification. National nursing organizations such as the American Nurses Credentialing Center (ANCC) have many types of certification to enhance your career such as certification in medical-surgical or geriatric nursing. After passing the initial examination, you maintain your certification by ongoing continuing education and clinical or administrative practice.

STANDARDS OF NURSING PRACTICE

Nursing is a helping, independent profession that provides services that contribute to the health of people. Three essential components of professional nursing are care, cure, and coordination. The *care* aspect is more than "to take care of"; it is also "caring about." Caring is relational and requires you as a nurse to understand a patient's needs so that you can individualize nursing therapies (see Chapter 20). When you promote health and healing, you are practicing the *cure* aspect of professional nursing. To cure is to help patients understand their health problems, manage their symptoms and cope. The cure aspect involves the administration of treatments and the use of clinical nursing judgment in determining, on the basis of patient outcomes, whether the plan of care is effective. *Coordination* of care involves organizing and timing medical and other professional and technical services to meet the holistic needs of a patient. Often a patient requires many services simultaneously for care to be effective. A professional nurse also supervises, teaches, and directs all individuals involved in nursing care.

As an independent profession, nursing sets its own standards for practice. These standards define competent nursing care and how nurses exercise the care, cure, and coordination aspects of nursing. Clinical, academic, and administrative nurse experts develop standards of nursing practice. As an example, the ANA has published *Nursing: Scope and Standards of Practice* (2015a). Within this document are Standards of Professional Performance and Standards of Practice for professional nurses (see http://www.nursingworld.org/scopeandstandardsofpractice).

In the practice setting it is important to have objective guidelines for providing and evaluating nursing care. Standards of nursing care are developed and established on the basis of strong scientific research and the work of clinical nurse experts. A standard of care describes the common level of professional nursing care to achieve quality nursing practice. An organization sometimes adopts a general set of standards for nursing care such as organizational protocols, policies, or procedures. For example, an organization has a written nasogastric tube protocol based on research findings. This protocol spells out the expected nursing care for patients with nasogastric tubes in that organization. Individual nursing units or work groups also establish standards of care to address the unique needs of patients in their care. For example, an oncology nursing unit develops standards of care for pain management and palliative care for patients with cancer. More important, standards of care establish the guidelines for nursing excellence within an organization.

RESPONSIBILITIES AND ROLES OF THE NURSE

As a nurse you are responsible for obtaining and maintaining specific knowledge and skills for a variety of professional roles and responsibilities. Nurses provide care and comfort for patients in all health care settings. Their concern for meeting patients' needs remains the same whether care focuses on health promotion and illness prevention, disease and symptom management, family support, or end-of-life care.

Caregiver

As **caregiver** you help patients maintain and regain health, manage disease and symptoms, and attain a maximal level function and independence through the healing process. You provide evidence-based nursing care to promote healing through both physical and interpersonal skills. Healing involves more than achieving improved physical well-being. You need to meet all health care needs of a patient by providing measures that restore the patient's emotional, spiritual, and social well-being. As a caregiver you help the patient and family set goals and assist them with meeting these goals with minimal financial cost, time, and energy.

Most nurses provide direct patient care in an acute care setting, whereas some pursue a specific area of specialty practice such as pediatrics, critical care, or emergency care. Many specialty care areas require some experience as a medical-surgical nurse and certification in advanced cardiac life support and critical care, emergency nursing, or trauma nursing.

As health care returns to the home care setting, there are increased opportunities for you to provide direct care in a patient's home or community. Use the nursing process and critical thinking skills to provide care that is restorative, curative, and evidence-based. Educate your patients and families to promote health maintenance and self-care. In collaboration with other health care team members, focus your care on returning patients to their home at an optimal functional status.

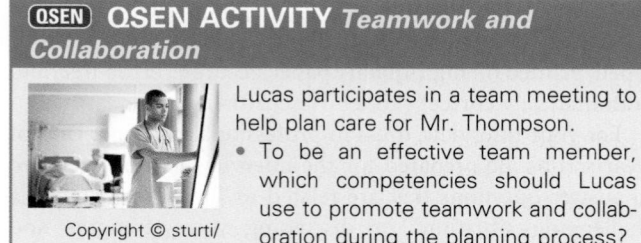

QSEN QSEN ACTIVITY *Teamwork and Collaboration*

Lucas participates in a team meeting to help plan care for Mr. Thompson.
- To be an effective team member, which competencies should Lucas use to promote teamwork and collaboration during the planning process?

Copyright © sturti/ Getty Images.

evolve   Answers to QSEN Activities can be found on the Evolve website.

Advocate

As a **patient advocate** you protect your patient's human and legal rights and provide assistance in asserting these rights if the need arises. As an advocate you act on behalf of your patient, securing and standing up for your patient's health care rights (Kowalski, 2016). For example, you provide information to help a patient decide whether or not to accept a treatment, or you find an interpreter to help family caregivers communicate their concerns. You sometimes need to defend patients' rights in a general way by speaking out against policies or actions that put patients in danger or conflict with their rights.

Educator

As an educator you explain concepts and facts about health, describe the reason for routine care activities, demonstrate procedures such as self-care activities, reinforce learning or patient behavior, and evaluate patients' progress in learning. Sometimes patient teaching is unplanned and informal (see Chapter 12). For example, during a casual conversation you respond to questions about the reason for an intravenous infusion, a health issue such as smoking cessation, or necessary lifestyle changes. Other teaching activities are planned and more formal such as when you teach your patient to self-administer insulin injections. Always use teaching methods that match your patient's capabilities and needs, and incorporate other resources such as family members or caregivers in teaching plans (see Chapter 25).

Communicator

Your effectiveness as a communicator is central to the nurse-patient relationship. It allows you to know your patients, including their strengths and weaknesses and their needs; and when possible, to know the family's concerns and needs. Communication is essential for all nursing roles and activities. You routinely communicate with patients and families, other nurses and health care professionals, resource persons, and the community. Without clear communication it is impossible to give comfort and emotional support, give care effectively, make decisions with patients and families, protect patients from threats to well-being, coordinate and manage patient care, assist patients in rehabilitation, or provide patient education. The quality of communication is a critical factor in meeting the needs of individuals, families, and communities (see Chapter 11).

Leader

Leaders are found in all areas of nursing and at all levels, functioning in both formal and informal settings. As a leader, you will work with others to create a vision and then make decisions and take action to achieve this vision. You will assess the situation, identify strategies using the best evidence, and guide others toward the vision (Yoder-Wise, 2014). Your behaviors and attitudes will impact those that you lead. As a leader, you must inspire others. A good leader should have the skills of self-awareness, self-management, social awareness, and relationship management (Huber, 2014). Effective leadership requires you to grow through ongoing personal development and good communication skills. One strategy to develop your leadership skills is to select a mentor who models effective leadership. Your mentor can be your role model, coach, and teacher (Yoder-Wise, 2014).

Manager

Today's health care environment is fast paced and complex. Nurse managers need to establish an environment for collaborative patient-centered care to provide safe, quality care with positive patient outcomes. A manager coordinates the activities of members of the nursing staff in delivering nursing care and has personnel, policy, and budgetary responsibility for a specific nursing unit or agency. The manager uses appropriate leadership styles to create a nursing environment for the patients and staff that reflects the mission and values of the health care organization (see Chapter 13).

Career Development

Innovations in health care, expanding health care systems and practice settings, and the increasing needs of patients have created new nursing roles. Today most nurses practice in hospital settings, community-based care, ambulatory care, and nursing homes or extended care settings.

Nursing allows you to commit to lifelong learning and career development to provide patients the state-of-the-art care they need. Career roles are specific employment positions or paths. Because of increasing educational opportunities for nurses, the growth of nursing as a profession, and a greater concern for job enrichment, the nursing profession offers expanded roles and different kinds of career opportunities. Your career path is limitless. You will probably switch career roles more than once. Take advantage of the different clinical practice and professional opportunities. These career opportunities include APRNs, nurse educators, nurse administrators, and nurse researchers.

Advanced Practice Registered Nurse. The advanced practice registered nurse (APRN) is the most independently functioning nurse. An APRN has a master's degree or Doctor of Nursing Practice (DNP) degree in nursing; advanced education in pathophysiology, pharmacology, and physical assessment; and certification and expertise in a specialized area of practice (AACN, 2006, 2011). In 2008, the APRN Consensus Work Group and the National Council of State Boards of Nursing APRN Advisory Committee developed the Consensus Model for APRN Regulation: Licensure, Accreditation, Certification and Education. The Consensus model identified that the title of APRN is for nurses with advanced graduate–level knowledge prepared in one of four roles: clinical nurse specialist (CNS), nurse practitioner (NP), certified nurse-midwife (CNM), and certified registered nurse anesthetist (CRNA). The educational preparation for the four roles is in at least one of the following six populations: adult-gerontology, pediatrics, neonatology, women's health/gender related, family/individual across life span, and psychiatric mental health. APRNs function within their area of practice to plan or improve the quality of nursing care for patients and their families.

Clinical Nurse Specialist. The clinical nurse specialist (CNS) is an APRN who is an expert clinician in a specialized area of practice. The specialty may be identified by a population (e.g., geriatrics), setting (e.g., critical care), disease specialty (e.g., diabetes), type of care (e.g., rehabilitation), or type of problem (e.g., pain) (NACNS, 2016). The CNS practices in all health care settings.

Nurse Practitioner. The nurse practitioner (NP) is an APRN who provides health care to a group of patients, usually in an outpatient, ambulatory care, or community-based setting. The major NP categories are acute care, adult, family, pediatric, women's, psychiatric mental health, and geriatric. The NP provides comprehensive care, directly managing the medical care of patients who are healthy or have chronic conditions, and establishes a collaborative provider-patient relationship, working with a specific group of patients or with patients of all ages and health care needs.

Certified Nurse-Midwife. The certified nurse-midwife (CNM) is an APRN who is educated in midwifery and is certified by the American College of Nurse-Midwives. The practice of nurse-midwifery involves providing independent care for women during normal pregnancy, labor, and delivery and care for the newborn. It includes providing some gynecological services such as routine Papanicolaou (Pap) tests, family planning, and treatment for minor vaginal infections.

Certified Registered Nurse Anesthetist. A certified registered nurse anesthetist (CRNA) is an APRN with advanced education earned in a nurse anesthesia accredited program. Nurse anesthetists provide surgical anesthesia under the guidance and supervision of an anesthesiologist, who is a physician with advanced knowledge of surgical anesthesia.

Nurse Educator. A nurse educator works primarily in schools or programs of nursing, staff development departments of health care agencies, and patient education departments. They usually have a specific clinical, administrative, or research specialty and advanced clinical and educational experience. A faculty member in a school of nursing is responsible for teaching current nursing practice, trends, theory, and necessary skills in laboratories and clinical settings to educate students to become professional nurses.

Nurse educators in educational programs of nursing usually have graduate degrees in nursing and additional education such as a doctorate or an advanced degree in nursing, education, or administration such as a Master of Business Administration (MBA).

Nurse educators in staff development departments of health care institutions provide educational programs for nurses within their institutions. These programs include orientation of new personnel, critical care nursing courses, assisting with clinical skill competency, safety training, instruction about new equipment or procedures, and participation in developing nursing policies and procedures.

The primary focus of the nurse educator in a patient education department of an agency is to teach patients and their families how to self-manage their illness or disability. These nurse educators are usually specialized and certified such as a Certified Diabetes Educator (CDE) or an ostomy care nurse and see only a specific population of patients.

Nurse Administrator. A nurse administrator manages patient care and the delivery of specific nursing services within a health care agency. Nursing administration often begins with positions such as the assistant nurse manager. Experience and additional education sometimes lead to a middle-management position such as nurse manager of a specific patient care area or house supervisor or an upper-management position such as assistant or associate director or director of nursing services.

Nurse manager positions usually require at least a baccalaureate degree in nursing, and director and nurse executive positions generally require a master's degree. Chief nurse executives and vice president positions in large health care organizations often require preparation at the doctoral level. Nurse administrators frequently have advanced degrees such as Master of Nursing Administration, MBA, Master of Hospital Administration (MHA), Master of Public Health (MPH), or Master of Health Service Administration.

In today's health care organizations directors may have responsibility for more than nursing units or manage a particular service or product line such as medicine or cardiology. Management of a service line often includes directing supportive functions and the health care personnel within areas such as medicine clinics, diagnostic departments, or outpatient care settings.

Vice presidents of nursing or chief nurse executives often have responsibilities for all clinical functions within a hospital. This may include all ancillary personnel who provide and support patient care services. The nurse administrator needs to be skilled in business and management and understand all aspects of nursing and patient care. Functions of administrators include budgeting, staffing, strategic planning of programs and services, employee evaluation, and employee development.

Nurse Researcher. The nurse researcher investigates problems to improve nursing care and further define and expand the scope of nursing practice (see Chapter 7). The nurse researcher often works in an academic setting, hospital, or independent professional or community service agency. The preferred educational requirement is a doctoral degree, with at least a master's degree in nursing.

PROFESSIONAL NURSING ORGANIZATIONS

A professional organization deals with issues of concern to individuals practicing in the profession. In North America two major professional nursing organizations are the National League for Nursing (NLN) and the ANA. The NLN advances excellence in nursing education to prepare nurses to meet the needs of a diverse population in a changing health care environment.

The purposes of the ANA are to improve standards of health and the availability of health care, foster high standards for nursing, and promote the professional development and general and economic welfare of nurses. The ANA is part of the International Council of Nurses (ICN). The objectives of the ICN parallel those of the ANA: promoting national associations of nurses, improving standards of nursing practice, seeking a higher status for nurses, and providing an international power base for nurses. The ANA is active in political, professional, and financial issues affecting health care and the nursing profession. It is a strong lobbyist in professional practice issues.

Nursing students may take part in organizations such as the National Student Nurses' Association (NSNA) in the United States and the Canadian Student Nurses' Association (CSNA) in Canada. These organizations consider issues of importance to nursing students such as career development and preparation for licensing. The NSNA often cooperates in activities and programs with the professional organizations.

Some professional organizations focus on specific areas such as critical care, nursing administration, nursing research, or nurse-midwifery. These organizations seek to improve the standards of practice, expand nursing roles, and foster the welfare of nurses within the specialty areas. In addition, professional organizations present educational programs and publish journals.

TRENDS IN NURSING

Nursing is a dynamic profession that grows and evolves as society and lifestyles change, as health care priorities and technologies change, and as nurses themselves change. The current philosophies and definitions of nursing have a holistic focus, which addresses the needs of the whole person in all dimensions, in health and illness, and in interaction with the family and community. Additionally, there is a definitive focus on patient safety in all care settings.

Quality and Safety Education for Nurses

The Robert Wood Johnson Foundation sponsored the Quality and Safety Education for Nurses (QSEN) initiative to respond to reports about safety and quality patient care by the Institute of Medicine (IOM) (QSEN Institute, 2014a).

TABLE 1.1	QUALITY AND SAFETY EDUCATION FOR NURSES
COMPETENCY	**DEFINITION WITH EXAMPLES**
Patient-centered care	Recognize the patient or designee as the source of control and full partner in providing compassionate and coordinated care based on respect for patient's preferences, values, and needs. *Examples: Involve family and friends in care. Elicit patient's values and preferences. Provide care with respect for diversity of the human experience.*
Teamwork and collaboration	Function effectively within nursing and interprofessional teams, fostering open communication, mutual respect, and shared decision making to achieve quality patient care. *Examples: Recognize the contributions of other health team members and patient's family members. Discuss effective strategies for communicating and resolving conflict. Participate in designing methods to support effective teamwork.*
Evidence-based practice	Integrate best current evidence with clinical expertise and patient and/or family preferences and values for delivery of optimal health care. *Examples: Demonstrate knowledge of basic scientific methods. Appreciate strengths and weaknesses of scientific bases for practice. Appreciate the importance of regularly reading relevant journals.*
Quality improvement	Use data to monitor the outcomes of care processes, and use improvement methods to design and test changes to continuously improve the quality and safety of health care systems. *Examples: Use tools such as flow charts and diagrams to make process of care explicit. Appreciate how unwanted variation in outcomes affects care. Identify gaps between local and best practices.*
Safety	Minimize risk of harm to patients and providers through both system effectiveness and individual performance. *Examples: Examine human factors, basic safety design principles, and commonly used unsafe practices. Value own role in preventing errors.*
Informatics	Use information and technology to communicate, manage knowledge, mitigate error, and support decision making. *Examples: Navigate an electronic health record. Protect confidentiality of protected health information in electronic health records.*

Adapted from QSEN Institute: Pre-licensure KSAs, 2014, http://qsen.org/competencies/pre-licensure-ksas/.

QSEN addresses the challenge to prepare nurses with the competencies needed to continuously improve the quality of care in their work environments (Table 1.1). The QSEN initiative encompasses the competencies of patient-centered care, teamwork and collaboration, evidence-based practice, quality improvement, safety, and informatics (QSEN Institute, 2014a). For each competency there are targeted knowledge, skills, and attitudes (KSAs). Different KSAs apply for nursing students in prelicensure as well as graduate nursing programs (QSEN Institute, 2014b; Sherwood and Zomorodi, 2014).

As you gain experience in clinical practice, you encounter situations in which your education helps you to make a difference in improving patient care. Whether that difference in care is to provide evidence for implementing care at the bedside, identify a safety issue, or study patient data to identify trends in outcomes, each of these situations requires competence in patient-centered care, safety, or informatics.

Emerging Technologies

As a nurse you will be affected by emerging technologies found in today's health care environment. These technologies have the potential to change nursing practice. New technologies provide more accurate, noninvasive assessment tools; help you to implement evidence-based practices; collect and trend patient outcome data; and use clinical decision support systems. The electronic health record (EHR) is an efficient method to document and manage patient health care information (see Chapter 10). Computerized physician/provider order entry (CPOE) is a critical patient safety initiative (Houston, 2014). Additionally, the availability and use of telehealth and telemedicine functions to provide health care are increasing (NCSBN, 2016). Genomic information combined with technology can improve health outcomes, quality, and safety and reduce health care costs (McCormick and Calzone, 2016). Technological innovations help family caregivers monitor and manage home environments of older adults, enable older adults to stay in their homes but stay connected to their support systems, and help with decision support and care coordination (Andruszkiewicz and Fike, 2015–2016). Younger nurses entering the workforce today have a high aptitude for technology. When surveyed, these nurses indicated that they would like to receive their health care through mobile devices and telehealth (NCSBN, 2016).

Genomics

Genetics is the study of inheritance, or the way traits are passed down from one generation to another. Genes carry the instructions for making proteins, which direct the activities of cells and functions of the body that influence traits such as hair and eye color. **Genomics** is the study of all the genes in a person and interactions of these genes with one another and with that person's environment (McCormick and Calzone, 2016). Using genomic information allows health care providers to determine how genomic changes contribute to patient conditions and influence treatment decisions such as assessment and symptom management and titration of medications based on a patient's response (McCormick and Calzone, 2016). For example, when a family member has colon cancer before the age of 50, it is likely that other family members are at risk for developing this cancer. Knowing this information is important for family members who may need a colonoscopy before age 50 and repeat colonoscopies more often than patients who are not at risk. In this case nurses play an essential role in identifying a patient's risk factors through assessment and counseling patients about what this genomic finding means to them personally and to their family. Nurses need to increase their knowledge of genomics in order to provide effective, individualized genetic and genomic information and resources to their patients (Sharoff, 2016).

Public Perception of Nursing

Nursing is a crucial health care profession. As frontline health care providers, nurses practice in all health care settings and constitute the largest number of health care professionals. They provide skilled, specialized, knowledgeable care; improve the health status of the public; and ensure safe, effective quality care (ANA, 2015b). The Gallup survey continues to find that survey participants ranked nurses highest among professionals for honesty and ethics (Advisory Board, 2015).

Consumers of health care are more informed than ever, and with the Internet consumers have access to more health care and treatment information. This information affects the perception the public has of nursing. For example, the media frequently highlights incidents of preventable medical errors such as medication and surgical errors. Publications such as *To Err Is Human* (IOM, 2000) describe strategies for government, health care providers, industry, and consumers to reduce preventable medical errors. When you care for patients, realize how your approach to care influences public opinion. Always act in a competent professional manner.

Effect of Nursing on Politics and Health Policy

Involvement of nurses in politics is receiving greater emphasis in nursing curricula, professional organizations, and health care settings. Professional nursing organizations at both the national and the state level employ lobbyists to urge U.S. Congress and state legislatures to improve the quality of health care (Mason et al., 2016).

You can influence policy decisions at all governmental levels. One way to get involved is by participating in local and national efforts (Mason et al., 2016). This involvement is critical in exerting nurses' influence early in the political process. The future is bright when nurses become serious students of social needs, activists in influencing policy to meet those needs, and generous contributors of time and money to nursing organizations and candidates who support efforts to improve access to and quality of health care (Mason et al., 2016).

KEY POINTS

- A profession possesses the characteristics of extended education, theory, service, autonomy, and a code of ethics.
- The essential components of professional nursing are care, cure, and coordination.
- During your education begin to develop professionalism through an ongoing understanding of what denotes appropriate appearance and behaviors, ethical practices (including those associated with social media), and standards of practice.
- Nursing standards of care offer evidence-based guidelines for nurses to provide and evaluate care.
- State or provincial boards of nursing regulate the scope of nursing practice and protect the public health, safety, and welfare with its established Nurse Practice Act.
- Nursing responds to the health care needs of society, which are influenced by economic, social, and cultural variables of a specific era.
- Changes in society such as increased technology, new demographic patterns, consumerism, health promotion, and the women's and human rights movements lead to changes in nursing.
- Nursing definitions reflect the practice of nursing by identifying the domain of nursing practice and guiding research, practice, and education.

REFLECTIVE LEARNING

- Reviewing the history of nursing, discuss a key influence or event that you feel impacted the advancement of the nursing profession.
- Consider your clinical day and discuss the nursing roles you functioned in today. Was there anything that you would do differently or improve?
- Thinking back on your clinical day, which QSEN competency knowledge, skills, or attitudes did you use while providing care today?

REVIEW QUESTIONS

1. You are preparing a presentation for your nursing course on the topic of professional standards of care. Which statements best describe professional standards of care? (Select all that apply.)
   1. Describe a competent level of behavior in the professional role
   2. Protect the patient's confidentiality
   3. Are based on scientific research
   4. Provide the foundation for decision making for nurses
   5. Define the principles of right and wrong to provide patient care

2. The nurse is providing a patient and caregiver information about the low-sodium diet ordered by the health care provider. The nurse uses teach-back to determine the patient's understanding of the diet. Which professional nursing role is demonstrated by the nurse?
   1. Manager
   2. Educator
   3. Researcher
   4. Caregiver
3. The nurse participates in a team care conference for a patient. The nurse listens to the registered dietitian and physical and occupational therapists detail the plan for the patient. The nurse then describes the patient's concerns about walking to the group. This is an example of which QSEN competency?
   1. Patient-centered care
   2. Safety
   3. Teamwork and collaboration
   4. Evidence-based practice

4. The nurse is preparing a presentation on the nursing profession and factors that are creating impact. Which are key factors impacting professional nursing today that should be included in the presentation? (Select all that apply.)
   1. Increasing prevalence of workplace violence
   2. Increased need for knowledge on emergency preparedness
   3. The rising rate of the medically underserved population
   4. Shift of the population from urban settings to rural areas
   5. Increased number of nurses reaching retirement age
5. A nurse has responsibility for the nursing budget, develops strategic programs, and oversees staffing for all clinical departments in a hospital. The nurse is practicing in which nursing role?
   1. Nurse manager
   2. Nurse administrator
   3. Nurse educator
   4. Nurse researcher

evolve

Additional Review Questions, as well as rationales for all Review Questions, can be found on the Evolve website.

1. 1, 3, 4; 2. 2; 3. 3; 4. 1, 2, 3, 5; 5. 2.

REFERENCES

Advisory Board: *Why nurses again top Gallup's list of "most trusted" professionals*, 2015. The Advisory Board Company, https://www.advisory.com/daily-briefing/2015/01/05/why-nurses-again-top-gallups-list-of-most-trusted-professionals.

Alligood MR: *Nursing theory: utilization and application*, ed 5, St Louis, 2014, Elsevier.

American Association of Colleges of Nursing (AACN): *The essentials of doctoral education for advanced nursing practice*, Washington, DC, 2006, The Association.

American Association of Colleges of Nursing (AACN): *The essentials of master's education for advanced practice nursing*, Washington, DC, 2011, The Association.

American Association of Colleges of Nursing (AACN): *AACN nursing shortage fact sheet*, 2014. http://www.aacn.nche.edu/media-relations/NrsgShortageFS.pdf.

American Association of Colleges of Nursing (AACN): *ELNEC fact sheet*, 2016. http://www.aacn.nche.edu/elnec/about/fact-sheet.

American Nurses Association (ANA): *Social networking principles toolkit*, 2011. http://nursingworld.org/FunctionalMenuCategories/AboutANA/Social-Media/Social-Networking-Principles-Toolkit.

American Nurses Association (ANA): *Nursing: scope and standards of practice*, ed 3, Silver Spring, MD, 2015a, The Association.

American Nurses Association (ANA): *Code of ethics for nurses with interpretive statements*, Silver Spring, MD, 2015b, The Association.

American Nurses Association (ANA): *Incivility, bullying, and workplace violence. ANA Position Statement*, 2015c. http://www.nursingworld.org.

American Nurses Association (ANA): *Handle with care fact sheet*, 2016. http://www.nursingworld.org/MainMenuCategories/ANAMarketplace/Factsheets-and-Toolkits/FactSheet.html.

Andruszkiewicz G, Fike K: Emerging technology trends and products: how tech innovations are easing the burden of family caregiving, *Generations* 39(4):64, 2015–2016.

APRN Consensus Work Group, the National Council of State Boards of Nursing APRN Advisory Committee: *Consensus Model for APRN Regulation: Licensure, Accreditation, Certification and Education*, 2008. http://www.nursecredentialing.org/Certification/APRNCorner/APRN-FAQ.

Benner P: *From novice to expert: excellence and power in clinical nursing practice*, Menlo Park, CA, 1984, Addison-Wesley.

Benner P, Tanner CA, et al: The social fabric or nursing knowledge, *Am J Nurs* 97(7):16, 1997.

Benner P, et al: *Educating nurses: a call for radical transformation*, Stanford, CA, 2010, Carnegie Foundation for the Advancement of Teaching.

Brown DW: Social media policies for employers and employees: regulatory and statutory considerations, *J Nurs Reg* 6(4):45, 2016.

Canadian Nurses Association (CNA): *Becoming an RN*, 2016a. https://

www.cna-aiic.ca/en/becoming-an-rn/education.

Canadian Nurses Association (CNA): *RN exam*, 2016b. https://www.cna-aiic.ca/en/becoming-an-rn/rn-exam.

Cho E, et al: The relationships of nurse staffing level and work environment with patient adverse events, *J Nurs Scholarsh* 48(1):74, 2016.

Choi J, Staggs VS: Comparability of nurse staffing measures in examining the relationship between RN staffing and unit-acquired pressure ulcers: a unit-level descriptive, correlational study, *Int J Nurs Stud* 51:1354, 2014.

Donahue MP: *Nursing: the finest art—an illustrated history*, ed 3, St Louis, 2011, Mosby.

Fowler DM: *Guide to nursing's social policy statement: understanding the profession from social contract to social covenant*, Silver Spring, MD, 2015a, American Nurses Publishing.

Fowler DM: *Guide to the Code of Ethics for nurses with interpretive statements: development, interpretation and application*, Silver Spring, MD, 2015b, The Association.

Giuliano KK, et al: The relationship between nurse staffing and 30-day readmission for adults with heart failure, *J Nurs Admin* 46(1):25, 2016.

Houston C: Technology in the health care workplace: benefits, limitations, and challenges. In Houston CJ, editor: *Professional issues in nursing: challenges and opportunities*, ed 3, Philadelphia, 2014, Lippincott Williams & Wilkins.

Huber DL: *Leadership & nursing care management*, ed 5, St Louis, 2014, Elsevier.

Institute of Medicine (IOM): *To err is human*, Washington, DC, 2000, The Institute.

Institute of Medicine (IOM): *The future of nursing: leading change, advancing health*, Washington, DC, 2010, National Academies Press.

International Council of Nurses (ICN): *ICN definition of nursing*, 2016. http://www.icn.ch/who-we-are/icn-definition-of-nursing/.

Kowalski K: Professional behavior in nursing, *J Contin Educ Nurs* 47(4):158, 2016.

Mamocha S, et al: Unprofessional content posted online among nursing students, *Nurse Educ* 40(3):119, 2015.

Mason DJ, et al: *Policy & politics in nursing and health care*, ed 7, St Louis, 2016, Elsevier.

McCormick KA, Calzone KA: The impact of genomics on health outcomes, quality, and safety, *Nurs Manage* 47(4):23, 2016.

McHugh MD, et al: Better nurse staffing and nurse work environments associated with increased survival of in-hospital cardiac arrest patients, *Med Care* 54(1):74, 2016.

National Association of Clinical Nurse Specialists (NACNS): *CNS FAQs*, 2016, http://nacns.org/html/cns-faqs.php.

National Council of State Boards of Nursing (NCSBN): *A nurse's guide to the use of social media*, Chicago, IL, 2011, NCSBN.

National Council of State Boards of Nursing (NCSBN): A changing environment: 2016 NCSBN environmental scan, *J Nurs Reg* 6(4):4, 2016.

Nightingale F: *Notes on nursing: what it is and what it is not*, London, 1860, Harrison & Sons.

QSEN Institute: *The evolution of the Quality and Safety Education for Nurses (QSEN) initiative*, 2014a. http://qsen.org/about-qsen/project-overview/.

QSEN Institute: *Pre-licensure KSAs*, 2014b. http://qsen.org/competencies/pre-licensure-ksas/.

Robert Wood Johnson Foundation (RWJF): *More newly licensed nurse practitioners choosing to work in primary care, Federal study finds*. RWJF, Human Capital Blog, June 10, 2014. http://www.rwjf.org/en/blogs/human-capital-blog/2014/06/more_newly_licensed.html.

Seo J, et al: Effect of health literacy on decision-making preferences among medically underserved patients, *Med Decis Making* 36:550, 2016.

Sharoff L: Holistic nursing in the genetic/genomic era, *J Holist Nurs* 34(2):146, 2016.

Sherwood G, Zomorodi M: A new mindset for quality and safety: the QSEN competencies redefine nurses' roles in practice, *J Nurs Adm* 44(10):510, 2014.

Splendore R, et al: Dress for respect: a shared governance approach, *Nurs Manage* 47(4):51, 2016.

U.S. Census Bureau: *Projections of the size and composition of the U.S. population: 2014 to 2060*, 2015. http://www.census.gov/content/dam/Census/library/publications/2015/demo/p25-1143.pdf.

West E, et al: Nurse staffing, medical staffing and mortality in intensive care: an observational study, *Int J Nurs Stud* 51:781, 2014.

Westrick SJ: Nursing students' use of electronic and social media: law, ethics, and e-professionalism, *Nurs Educ Perspect* 37(1):16, 2016.

Yoder-Wise PS: *Leading and managing in nursing*, ed 5 Revised Reprint, St Louis, 2014, Elsevier.

Zerwekh J, Garneau AZ: *Nursing today: transition and trends*, ed 8, St Louis, 2015, Saunders.

Health and Wellness

evolve MEDIA RESOURCES

http://evolve.elsevier.com/Potter/essentials

- Audio Glossary
- QSEN Activity and Review Questions Answers

OBJECTIVES

- Discuss the health belief, health promotion, basic human needs, and holistic health models of health and illness and their relationship to patients' attitudes toward health and health practices.
- Describe the variables influencing health beliefs, health practices, and illness behaviors.
- Describe health promotion and illness prevention activities.
- Compare and contrast the three levels of prevention.

- Explain how different types of risk factors affect a person's health.
- Describe a nurse's role in helping patients modify their health risks and change their health behaviors.
- Describe variables that influence illness behavior.
- Explain how illness affects a patient and family.
- Discuss the nurse's role in caring for people, communities, and populations in various states of health and illness.

KEY TERMS

acute illness, p. 24
chronic illness, p. 24
health, p. 15
health belief model, p. 16
health beliefs, p. 16
health education, p. 20

health promotion, p. 17
health promotion model, p. 16
holistic health, p. 19
illness, p. 24
illness behavior, p. 24
illness prevention, p. 20

Maslow's hierarchy of needs, p. 17
primary prevention, p. 20
risk factor, p. 21
secondary prevention, p. 21
tertiary prevention, p. 21

Nurses play a key role in helping individuals, families, communities, and populations become or remain healthy. Nurses are considered to be health experts because they are caregivers, advocates, and educators. Health information is readily available through electronic and print media. However, people often have difficulty determining which information is accurate and helpful. Because health information is so readily available now and because of your expertise in health, your patients, family, and friends will frequently ask you questions about how to use this information to become healthier. If you can help a person remain well, you can reduce how frequently that person accesses health care, which reduces health care costs. Thus it is very

important for nurses to help patients make changes to improve their health and wellness.

DEFINITION OF HEALTH

The World Health Organization (WHO) defines health as a "state of complete physical, mental and social well-being and not merely the absence of disease or infirmity" (1947, 2017). Every person has a different definition of health (Pender, et al., 2011). A person who is free from disease is not necessarily healthy (Pender, 1996). **Health** is a state of being influenced by a person's values, personality, and lifestyle. For many people, health is defined by the circumstances surrounding

CASE STUDY *Charlie*

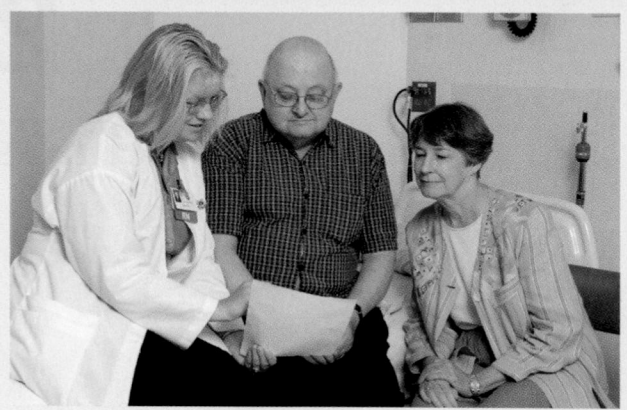

Charlie is a 56-year-old retired Navy officer who was recently diagnosed with hyperlipidemia (high cholesterol) and hypertension. Knowing that he has a family history of cardiac disease, Charlie has always tried to eat the right foods and exercise, but since retiring he has had difficulty consistently making healthy food choices and exercising regularly. Charlie's doctor told him he needs to lose 30 lb. Charlie has difficulty exercising daily. His wife still works full time, and they often eat out during the week because of her busy schedule.

   Charlie comes to the clinic today for a routine visit after starting on medication to reduce his cholesterol. Liz, the cardiac nurse educator, is working with Charlie. Charlie's total cholesterol level has decreased since starting his medication, but his triglycerides are still high. His blood pressure is also still running on the high side of normal. Liz plans to help Charlie increase his exercise and improve his eating habits to help him develop a healthier lifestyle and reduce his risk for cardiovascular disease. She plans to assess his understanding of his cardiac risk factors and lifestyle choices and evaluate his readiness to make behavior changes to help him better manage his health.

their life rather than their physical condition (Pender et al., 2011). Nurses individualize nursing care by considering the whole person and the environment to help patients reach their health goals. Individual perceptions of health are affected by a person's health beliefs and change as a person ages. For example, the definition of health for older people is often affected by the ability to function independently, the presence of or management of symptoms, acceptance of current health status, being connected to others, and having energy (Song and Kong, 2015).

MODELS OF HEALTH AND ILLNESS

Models help you understand complex ideas such as health and illness. Thus you use models to understand the relationships between health and illness and your patients' attitudes toward health and health practices. Health beliefs influence health practices. Health beliefs are a person's ideas, opinions, and attitudes about health and illness. They are sometimes based on facts or misinformation, common sense or myths,

good or bad experiences, or reality or false expectations. Health beliefs influence health behavior and positively or negatively affect a patient's level of health. Nurses use a variety of health models to understand patients' beliefs, attitudes, and values about health and illness to provide effective health care. They also allow you to understand and predict patients' health behavior.

Health Belief Model

The health belief model (Fig. 2.1) addresses the relationship between a person's beliefs and behaviors (Rosenstoch, 1974; Becker and Maiman, 1975). It helps you understand and predict how patients will behave in relation to their health and how successful they will be in following suggested therapy or illness management plans. Positive health behaviors are activities related to maintaining, attaining, or regaining health and preventing illness. Common positive health behaviors include getting immunizations, using prescribed and over-the-counter medications properly, maintaining proper sleep patterns, exercising regularly, and eating healthy foods. Implementing positive health behaviors depends on an individual's awareness of how to live a healthy life and the ability and willingness to carry out these behaviors. Negative health behaviors include activities that are harmful such as smoking, abusing drugs or alcohol, adopting a sedentary lifestyle, and refusing to take necessary medications.

   The first component of the health belief model involves an individual's perception of susceptibility to an illness. The second component is a patient's perception of the seriousness of that illness. Demographic and sociopsychological variables, perceived threats of an illness, and cues to action (e.g., mass media campaigns and advice from family, friends, and medical professionals) influence and modify this perception. The third component, the likelihood that a patient will take preventive action, results from a patient's perception of the benefits of and barriers to taking action. Preventive actions include lifestyle changes, increased participation in recommended medical therapies, and a search for medical advice or treatment. *For example, to apply the health belief model when caring for a patient like Charlie who has a risk for coronary artery disease (CAD), Charlie first needs to recognize that family history increases the chances of developing CAD. He needs to believe that CAD is serious to change existing behaviors and implement healthy changes such as following a low-fat diet and increasing exercise to reduce the risk for CAD.*

   The health belief model helps you understand patients' perceptions, beliefs, and behavior and plan care that will most effectively help patients maintain or restore health and prevent illness. Understand that each patient's view of health and wellness and individual belief systems influence the ability to make lasting changes in health status. Do not make judgments when you encounter views and beliefs that differ from your own.

Health Promotion Model

The health promotion model (Fig. 2.2) (Pender, 1982, 1996; Pender et al., 2011) defines health as a positive, dynamic state,

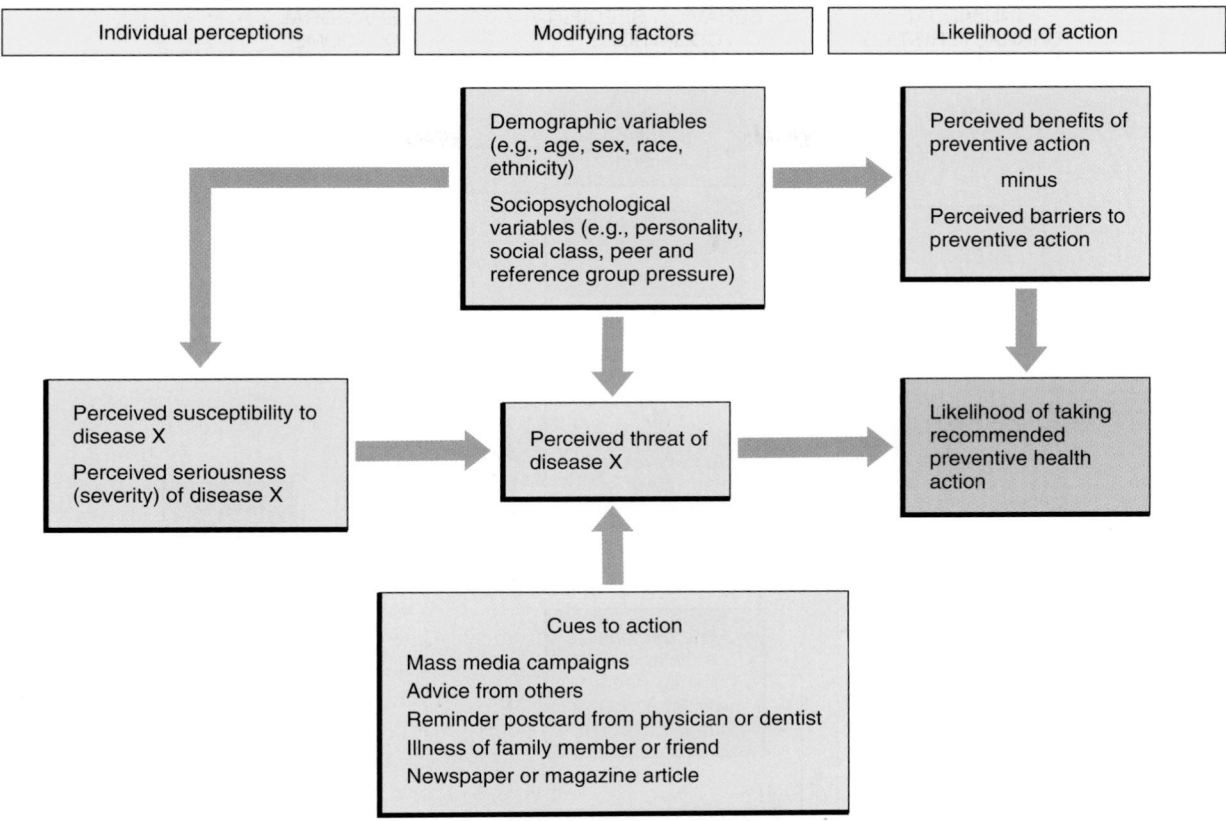

Individual perceptions	Modifying factors	Likelihood of action

FIG 2.1 Health belief model. (Data from Becker MH, Maiman LA: Sociobehavioral determinants of compliance with health and medical care recommendations, *Med Care* 13[1]:10, 1975.)

not merely the absence of disease. The model is a framework that integrates the perspectives of nursing with behavioral science and factors that influence health behaviors. You use it with individuals, not communities.

Health promotion is behavior motivated by the desire to increase well-being and actualize human health potential, whereas health protection is behavior motivated by a desire to avoid illness, detect it early, or maintain function within the constraints of an illness (Pender et al., 2011). This model describes the multidimensional nature of people as they interact within their environment to pursue health (Pender et al., 2011). The model focuses on three areas:

1. Individual characteristics and experiences
2. Behavior-specific cognitions and affect
3. Behavioral outcomes

It also organizes cues into a pattern to explain the likelihood of a patient developing health promotion behaviors (Pender et al., 2011). You can use this model to help your patients carry out healthy behaviors in their daily lives.

Basic Human Needs Model

Maslow's hierarchy of needs (Maslow, 1954) helps you understand an individual's motivation to achieve optimal health. This model explains the basic needs of patients and families, their behaviors, and their readiness to take part in health activities. Maslow's original model describes human needs using a hierarchical pyramid divided into five levels

(Fig. 2.3). According to Maslow, individuals have to meet lower level needs before they are able to satisfy higher level needs. As people meet the needs of one level, they move up to the next level. Unmet needs motivate human behavior.

A person needs to meet basic *physiological* needs such as oxygen, water, food, sleep, and shelter before progressing to higher level needs. When basic needs are not met, an affected person feels sick or irritated or experiences pain or discomfort. These feelings motivate an individual to satisfy the need (Maslow, 1970, 1987). The second level on the hierarchy of needs consists of *safety and security needs,* which include establishing stability and consistency. These psychological needs include the security of a home and a family. For example, a woman in an abusive relationship is unable to move to the next level of love and belongingness because she is constantly concerned for her safety. The third level on the hierarchy, *love and belongingness,* is a desire to belong to groups. It consists of the need to feel love by others and to be accepted. The fourth level deals with the need for *self-esteem.* Self-esteem results from mastery of a task and includes the recognition gained from others. The highest level of needs on the hierarchy is *self-actualization,* which is the desire to become everything that one is capable of becoming. Individuals at this level are concerned with maximizing their potential.

Maslow (1970) expanded his model to include cognitive, aesthetic, and transcendence needs to incorporate needs

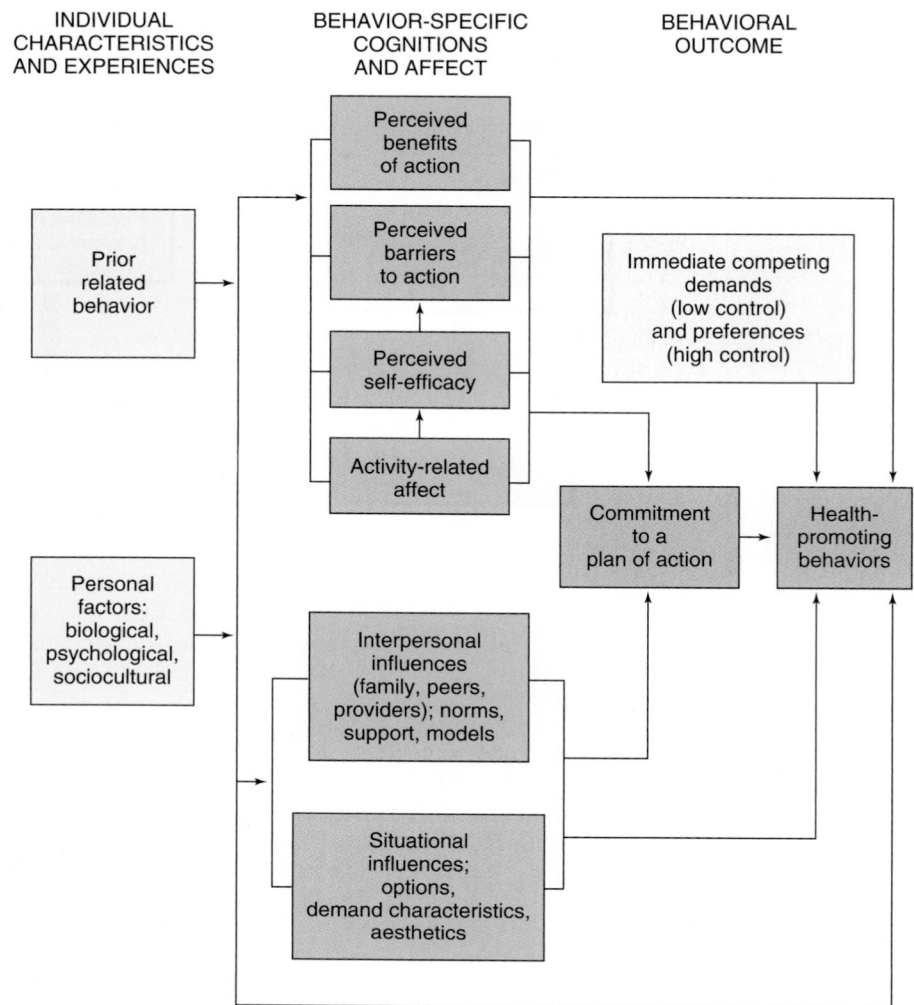

FIG 2.2 Health promotion model. (From Pender NJ, Murdaugh CL, Parsons MA: *Health promotion in nursing practice*, ed 5, Upper Saddle River, NJ, 2006, Prentice Hall.)

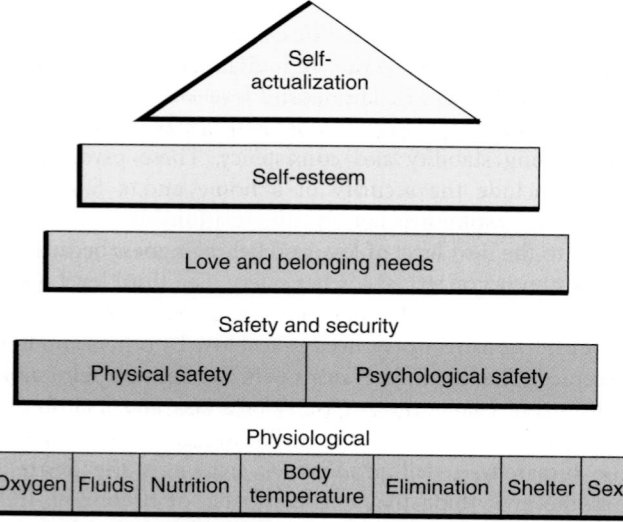

FIG 2.3 Maslow's hierarchy of needs. (From Maslow AH, Frager RD, Fadiman J: *Motivation and personality*, ed 3. Copyright ©1987. Reprinted by permission of Pearson Education, Inc., New York, New York.)

that could not be explained by his original model. In the expanded model, cognitive and aesthetic needs come between esteem and self-actualization needs (McLeod, 2016). According to Maslow (1970), cognitive needs are hard-wired in all of us and include the needs for knowledge, understanding, meaning, and predictability. Aesthetic needs are universal and include the appreciation and search for beauty and balance. Cognitive and aesthetic needs help explain why patients respond better when they understand their health problems (Lorig et al., 2016) and when they are in attractive surroundings with peaceful colors (Slatyer et al., 2015). Transcendence needs refer to the need to help others achieve self-actualization and are the highest needs (McLeod, 2016).

You can use Maslow's hierarchy as a framework when addressing patient needs and prioritizing patient care. Unless a patient's basic needs are met, higher levels in the pyramid are not relevant. Patients approach life differently (Bracken et al., 2015). *For example, Charlie in the case study can afford to purchase food, he has a safe home environment, and he has a good relationship with his wife, but he is having trouble changing his eating habits to reduce his cholesterol. While interviewing Charlie, Liz determines that Charlie has low self-esteem. Liz implements interventions to enhance Charlie's self-esteem to help him realize he needs to change his eating behaviors.*

The requirements to satisfy the needs of each level of the hierarchy vary from person to person. Therefore you need to thoroughly assess the individual needs of each patient. For example, in caring for patients with psychological issues such as depression or risk for suicide, safety and security needs are a priority. As a nurse, you need to provide all patients with physical and psychological safety (Bracken et al., 2015).

Holistic Health Model

A person's health is affected by the relationship between the body, mind, and spirit. Thus nurses and all members of the health care team need to take a holistic view of health by considering the dynamic interaction between the emotional, spiritual, social, cultural, and physical aspects of an individual's wellness (Chapa et al., 2014). **Holistic health** views a person as a biopsychosocial and spiritual being (Edelman et al., 2014). The intent of the holistic health model is to empower patients to engage in their own recovery and assume some responsibility for health maintenance (Edelman et al., 2014).

The holistic health model includes a variety of techniques recognizing that personal health choices powerfully affect an individual's health. Some of the most widely used holistic interventions include aromatherapy, biofeedback, breathing exercises, and guided imagery (see Chapter 19). Most holistic therapies are easy to learn and apply to almost any setting and all stages of health and illness. For example, you use reminiscence to help relieve anxiety in an older patient dealing with memory loss or meditation with a patient dealing with the difficult side effects of chemotherapy. You help patients recognize the many options available and help them make choices to enhance health.

HEALTHY PEOPLE DOCUMENTS

For the past 30 years, *Healthy People* has established evidenced-based objectives to (1) achieve high-quality, longer lives free of disease, disability, injury, and premature death; (2) eliminate health disparities; (3) create social and physical environments that promote health for all people; and (4) promote quality of life, healthy development, and healthy behaviors across the life span (Healthy People 2020, 2017). The objectives are updated every 10 years to meet a wide range of health needs, encourage collaboration in communities, help individuals make informed health decisions, and measure the impact of prevention activities.

Healthy People 2020 includes 26 leading health indicators divided among 12 topic areas to provide a way to assess the health of people in the United States in key areas; encourage collaboration across diverse groups; and motivate action for individuals, communities, and the nation (Healthy People 2020, 2017). The goal is to achieve or make improvements for each objective by 2020.

VARIABLES INFLUENCING HEALTH BELIEFS AND HEALTH PRACTICES

Peoples' beliefs about their own health, their health practices, and the manner in which they care for themselves ultimately influence their health status. Health beliefs are a person's ideas and attitudes about health (Tovar and Clark, 2015). These beliefs often directly influence health practices whether there is evidence to support them or not. Health practices are activities that individuals perform to care for themselves (Schofield et al., 2016). They include activities of daily living such as bathing and brushing teeth and formal activities such as taking medications and visiting the health care provider for routine checkups. Today health care focuses on the role of patients and their responsibility for self-care. The ability to care for oneself is as important for healthy living as managing a complex medical regimen for a chronic illness. Many variables influence patients' health beliefs, health practices, and self-care. Internal and external variables influence how a person thinks, acts, and will deal with an illness. Consider the effect of these internal and external variables and incorporate appropriate interventions based on a person's unique characteristics when you deliver nursing care.

Internal Variables

Developmental Stage. Our concept of illness depends on our developmental stage (see Chapter 23). Knowledge of the stages of growth and development help you predict your patient's response to an actual illness or the threat of future illness. Your educational interventions need to be age appropriate as well as developmentally appropriate to be effective. For example, you use different techniques to teach healthy diet choices to a child versus an adult. You also use different techniques for people whose developmental age differs from their chronological age.

Intellectual Background. A person's beliefs about health are shaped in part by knowledge (or misinformation) about body functions and illnesses, educational background, and past experiences. Cognitive abilities shape the *way* a person thinks, including the ability to understand factors involved in illness and apply knowledge of health and illness to personal health practices.

Emotional Factors. A person's degree of anxiety or stress influences health beliefs and practices. How people handle stress throughout each phase of life influences their personal reaction to illness. A person who generally is very calm may have little emotional response during illness, whereas a person normally unable to cope with stress may overreact to illness or deny the presence of symptoms and does not take therapeutic action (see Chapter 26).

Spiritual Factors. Spirituality is a cultural factor reflected in how a person lives his or her life including the values and beliefs exercised, the relationships established with family and friends, and the ability to find hope and meaning in life. Spiritual health often provides motivation to engage in health-promoting activities and enhances mental and physical health during times of illness (Conway-Phillips and Janusek, 2014; Jim et al., 2015; Salsman et al., 2015). You need to understand patients' spiritual beliefs to incorporate them effectively in nursing care (see Chapter 22).

External Variables

Culture broadly reflects the whole of human behavior, including ideas, beliefs, and values about health and illness; ways of relating to one another; language and manners of speaking; and work and lifestyle practices (Ball et al., 2015). A variety of cultural factors influence a patient's health beliefs and practices.

Family Role and Practices. The roles and organization of a family defines the relationship of insiders and outsiders and includes concepts related to family goals and priorities and how each member defines health and illness and values preventive health practices (Chapter 21). There is usually a person in the family responsible for health-related decisions For example, parental health beliefs, attitudes, perceptions, and misperceptions have a direct effect on a family's health practices. The family's socioeconomic status, family structure, and parental practices also affect a family's health (Adamo and Brett, 2014). A person raised in a family that believes in the importance of preventive care such as dental checkups twice a year is more likely to continue those health practices as an adult, whereas parents who have misconceptions and unhealthy perceptions about diet quality often contribute to eating habits that lead to obesity (Adamo and Brett, 2014).

Socioeconomic Factors. Socioeconomic factors are social determinants of health that increase the risk for illness and influence how a person defines and reacts to illness (see Chapter 21). Socioeconomic variables also determine how and where patients access medical care and receive treatment, how they pay for their health care, and the potential reimbursement to the health care agency or patient (Lessard et al., 2016). Poor access to health care is one social determinant of health that contributes to health disparities. Economic variables affect a patient's level of health by increasing the risk for disease and influencing how or at what point the patient enters the health care system. In addition, economic status affects a person's participation in treatment to maintain or improve health (Hefei et al., 2015). A person who has high utility bills, a large family, and a low income may give a higher priority to food and shelter than to prescribed drugs or treatment or foods for special diets.

HEALTH PROMOTION, WELLNESS, AND ILLNESS PREVENTION

Health promotion is a key component of public health and uses a variety of strategies, such as health education, legislation, and policy, to help individuals, groups, and communities increase control over and improve their health. It also focuses on improving quality of life, reducing premature death, and reducing costs of medical treatment through its focus on prevention.

Health promotion policies or legislation affect all people in a community, state, or country even if the people affected by the policies or laws are not aware of them. For example, bars in a county are required by law to ban smoking to reduce exposure to secondhand smoke. Other health promotion strategies require individuals, groups, or communities to engage in and adopt specific health behaviors. For example, smoking cessation programs require patients to be actively involved in improving their present and future levels of wellness while decreasing their risk for disease.

Health promotion, health education, and illness prevention help patients maintain and improve their health, decrease the incidence of illness, and minimize the effects of illness or disability. Health promotion activities such as routine exercise and good nutrition help patients maintain or enhance their present levels of health and reduce their risks for developing certain diseases. Health education teaches people how to care for themselves in a healthy way and includes topics such as physical awareness, stress management, and self-responsibility (Box 2.1). Illness prevention protects patients from actual or potential threats to health, such as obtaining immunizations. Health promotion, health education, and illness prevention are closely related and sometimes overlap. All are focused on the future; the differences between them involve motivations and goals. Health promotion activities motivate people to reach more stable levels of health. Health education helps patients achieve new understanding and control of their lives. Illness prevention activities help people avoid declines in health or functional level.

Illnesses, particularly chronic illnesses, increase the cost of health care. Improving self-management and providing preventive services reduce health care needs and costs. Therefore you need to educate your patients about improving their ability to improve and manage their health. You do this by helping them recognize the effects their choices have on their health. *In the case study, Liz determines Charlie needs more health education. Liz teaches him the importance of diet and exercise to manage his cholesterol and prevent long-term complications. She works with Charlie and his wife to develop heart-healthy food choices.*

Three Levels of Prevention

There are three levels of prevention in public health and health promotion. As a nurse, you will provide care in all three levels.

Primary prevention is true prevention. Its goal is to reduce the incidence of disease (Edelman et al., 2014; Stanhope and Lancaster, 2016). Many primary prevention activities (e.g., federally funded immunization programs, water treatment) are supported by the government. You provide primary prevention when you provide interventions such as health education to reduce the risk of developing

BOX 2.1 PATIENT TEACHING

Reducing Cardiac Risk

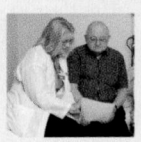 Because she knows that couples with a positive relationship often experience better health, Liz decides to focus her teaching on reducing the risk of developing cardiac disease with Charlie and his wife.

OUTCOME

- By the end of the visit, Charlie will develop a plan to reduce his cardiac risk factors that is supported by his wife.

TEACHING STRATEGIES

- Make sure that Charlie and his wife understand his risk for cardiac disease.
- Ensure that Charlie understands how risk-reduction strategies such as exercise can improve his health (Resnick et al., 2014).
- Provide education to Charlie and his wife about risk factor reduction such as a low-fat diet, regular aerobic exercise, and taking medications as prescribed (Sher et al., 2014).
- Allow time for Charlie and his wife to discuss any challenges they experience with communication or their relationship (Sher et al., 2014).
- Work with the couple to help Charlie set achievable and realistic goals for change (Sher et al., 2014).
- Help Charlie and his wife develop problem-solving skills together. Give them problems to solve, such as medication adjustment when Charlie becomes ill or adaptation of diet when a favorite food is not available.
- Identify community resources available to Charlie (e.g., walking track, fitness facilities).

EVALUATION

- Use the principles of teach-back to evaluate the couple's learning.
  - "Tell me what changes in your diet the two of you can use to help reduce Charlie's risk for heart disease."
  - "Describe how Charlie can increase his activity level."
  - "Tell me how you will work together to make behavioral and relationship changes to help Charlie improve his health."

type 2 diabetes. Other examples of primary prevention include ensuring communities have safe water sources, implementing bloodborne pathogen regulations, and inspecting restaurants to ensure safe food handling (Stanhope and Lancaster, 2016). *For Charlie, primary prevention means reducing his cholesterol through diet and exercise to prevent the development of cardiac disease.*

Secondary prevention focuses on preventing the spread of disease, illness, or infection once it occurs (Edelman et al., 2014; Stanhope and Lancaster, 2016). Nurses who practice secondary prevention identify and treat people who have new cases of a disease or identify people who have been exposed to a disease but do not have the disease yet. Examples of secondary prevention activities include health screenings and contacting health care employees after exposure to a patient

with an unknown diagnosis of tuberculosis. Screening activities may lead to primary prevention interventions such as providing health teaching. *Secondary prevention for Charlie involves having him come to the clinic every year to have his fasting blood sugar and lipid blood levels drawn.*

Tertiary prevention focuses on reducing complications of long-term disease and disabilities through treatment and rehabilitation (Edelman et al., 2014; Stanhope and Lancaster, 2016). It involves preventing further disability or reduced functioning. Tertiary prevention helps patients achieve as high a level of functioning as possible, despite limitations caused by illness or impairment. For example, you provide tertiary prevention when you help patients who have had a stroke adapt to their impaired mobility so that they can walk and prepare meals again.

Risk Factors

A risk factor is any attribute, quality, trait, or environmental condition that increases vulnerability of an individual, community, or population to an illness or accident. Risk factors do not cause diseases or accidents, but they increase the chance that an individual, community, or population will experience a particular disease or accident. You assess for risk factors to identify a patient's health status. A person's knowledge of risk factors sometimes influences health beliefs and practices. People can modify some risk factors such as dietary choices, whereas other risk factors such as genetics or age are nonmodifiable.

Nonmodifiable Risk Factors. Nonmodifiable risk factors such as age, gender, genetics, and family history cannot be changed. Use your knowledge of nonmodifiable risk factors to provide secondary prevention. Age increases susceptibility to certain illnesses and accidents. For example, children are at risk for accidental deaths due to drowning. The risk for heart disease, diabetes, and many cancers increases with age for both genders. Box 2.2 discusses ways to support health promotion in older adults.

A person's gender sometimes is a risk factor for disease or accidents. For example, the risk for asthma is higher in boys than girls. However, by the age of 20, the number of men and women who have asthma is about equal, and by age 40, more women have asthma. Men have a higher risk for cardiovascular disease (CVD) than premenopausal women. However, after menopause, the risk for CVD is similar between men and women.

An individual's family history and genetics are also risk factors for some illnesses. Breast, ovarian, and colon cancer appear to have a genetic link. A person with a family history of diabetes or CVD has a higher risk of developing these diseases. Sometimes it is difficult to determine if the family link to illness is related to genetics, lifestyle choices, or environmental exposure, or a combination of these factors. For example, you are caring for a female patient with obesity who develops high blood pressure. Her parents have high blood pressure, and her husband smokes. It is challenging for you to determine which risk factor—lifestyle, genetics, or

BOX 2.2　CARE OF THE OLDER ADULT

Importance of Health Promotion

- Because individuals are living longer, health promotion activities are important to help maintain function and independence and improve quality of life.
- Partner with appropriate community partners (e.g., churches, agencies that address health inequities) and ensure people providing the education represent the characteristics and/or ethnicity of the participants (Boutaugh et al., 2015).
- Focus on self-care abilities and practices that foster health while aging and living with a chronic illness (Boutaugh et al., 2015).
- Emphasize the need to engage in physical and social activity (Resnick et al., 2014).
- Monitor older adults, especially those 75 years of age and older, for high blood pressure, obesity, and diabetes (Resnick et al., 2014).
- Promote self-care activities that maintain and improve functional status including management of chronic illnesses (Boutaugh et al., 2015).
- Ensure health promotion interventions are individualized (Resnick et al., 2014). For example, use the stages of behavior change model (see Table 2.1) to identify older adults who are open to participating in health promotion activities.

BOX 2.3　EVIDENCE-BASED PRACTICE

PICO Question: Are individualized developmentally appropriate health promotion interventions effective in increasing patients' activity levels?

SUMMARY OF EVIDENCE

Being physically active is important in preventing many health issues such as obesity, cardiovascular disease, cancer, and type 2 diabetes. Many people of all ages do not participate in regular physical activity. Nurses are in key positions to provide health education to patients, families, and communities to promote physical activity. Walking is an activity that people of all ages can usually do and is effective in helping people lose weight or maintain a healthy weight (Adams et al., 2015; Yan et al., 2015). Current evidence shows that effective health promotion interventions are individualized and take a patient's age and developmental level into consideration. Interventions that are effective with younger people are not typically effective with older adults. When high school–age and college-age patients receive positive, individualized text messages regularly that encourage exercise such as walking and address barriers, goal-setting, motivation, and connection with others, the messages are frequently effective in helping patients increase the number of steps they take every day and engage in regular physical activity (Yan et al., 2015; Thompson et al., 2016). Community-based groups that encourage walking and exercise are often effective in helping middle-aged and elderly patients increase their physical activity (Resnick et al., 2014; Adams et al., 2015). Health promotion interventions that emphasize connections with others are effective in patients of all ages (Resnick et al., 2014; Thompson et al., 2016).

APPLICATION TO NURSING PRACTICE

- Ensure the health education you provide to your patients is connected to their developmental needs (Yan et al., 2015).
- Include connections with significant others when designing health promotion strategies for patients of all ages (Resnick et al., 2014).
- Encourage patients to set realistic, measurable goals, and encourage them to use pedometers if possible to count their steps daily (Adams et al., 2015).

environmental toxins—caused her condition, or if all factors were involved.

Modifiable Risk Factors. Some risk factors such as lifestyle practices and health-related behaviors can be modified. Although some practices can positively affect health, practices with potential negative effects are risk factors. Examples of modifiable risk factors include overeating or poor nutrition, insufficient rest and sleep, and poor personal hygiene. Other habits that put a person at risk for illness include tobacco use, alcohol or drug abuse, and activities involving a threat of injury such as drinking alcohol or texting while driving. Some habits are risk factors for specific diseases. For example, excessive sunbathing increases the risk for skin cancer, and being overweight increases the risk for CVD. Examples of modifiable behavioral risk factors that are leading causes of mortality in the United States include tobacco use, obesity, lack of physical activity, poor control of blood pressure, high cholesterol, and not being immunized for influenza (Johnson et al., 2014). Modifiable risk factors especially for people who are 10 to 24 years of age include behaviors that lead to unintentional injuries (e.g., texting while driving, bullying); use of tobacco, alcohol, and other drugs; sexual behaviors leading to unintended pregnancy and sexually transmitted infections; unhealthy diet choices; and physical inactivity (Kann et al., 2016). Current evidence emphasizes the need for preventive care and shows the effect that lifestyle choices have on our health care system, our economy, and our communities.

Lifestyle behavior choices affect people throughout their life. For example, a teenager whose nutritional choices lead to obesity will most likely experience the effects of obesity later in life. Patients of all ages are vulnerable to the influences of unhealthy lifestyle patterns. You can influence the choices your patients make to prevent or change unhealthy behaviors and promote healthy lifestyle patterns. Therefore you need to understand the relationship between growth and development, lifestyle behaviors, and your patients' health status. Use developmentally appropriate evidence-based interventions when teaching about wellness-promoting lifestyle behaviors (Box 2.3).

Environment. The environment is affected by physical, chemical, biological, social, and psychosocial factors. Our environment includes the physical space in which we live; the air, water, soil, and food that is all around us; and the biological, chemical, and radiological exposures we experience. All of these can increase the likelihood that certain illnesses will occur. Some home environments increase the risk that a person will contract and spread infections, whereas some cancers are more likely to develop when people live near toxic waste disposal sites. Environmental exposure rarely occurs one time, in one location, and from one source because we are constantly interacting with our environment (Stanhope and Lancaster, 2016).

Risk Factor Identification. You identify modifiable and nonmodifiable risk factors to help patients understand what they need to modify or eliminate to promote wellness and prevent illness. Health risk appraisals assess individuals, families, or communities for the presence of factors that increase specific health threats. You will often find risk factors through patient interviews and reading medical records. You need to link the risk factors you identify with educational programs and other community resources to help people make lifestyle changes to reduce their risks. *In the case study, Liz determines Charlie has several nonmodifiable risk factors for CVD: advanced age, gender, and family history (World Health Federation, 2016). She implements health teaching to help Charlie understand how these factors affect his health.*

Changing Health Behaviors. Once you identify a patient's risk factors, you implement appropriate and relevant health education and counseling to help a person change a risky health behavior or implement a new behavior to modify the risk for a disease or injury. It is essential to engage and collaborate with patients when determining which changes they perceive they need to make or are willing to make. Patients typically will not change a behavior unless they see a need and are motivated and supported to change. This will also often require family caregiver support.

Aim your attempts to help a patient stop a health-damaging behavior (e.g., tobacco use or alcohol misuse) or adopt a healthy behavior (e.g., make healthy food choices or exercise) (Pender et al., 2011). Changing health behavior, especially long-term lifestyle habits, is difficult. Adopting healthy behaviors to reduce risk factors requires patients to change. As a nurse, you are challenged to motivate and facilitate health behavior change in working with individuals, families, and communities (Edelman et al., 2014). Use evidence-based guidelines such as the clinical guidelines and recommendations published by the Agency for Healthcare Research and Quality (AHRQ) (2014), when helping your patients make health behavior changes.

You will better help your patients make difficult behavioral changes if you apply knowledge about the process of change. Current evidence supports that many people go through a series of five stages of behavior change (Table 2.1), ranging from precontemplation, when a person has no intention to change, to the maintenance stage, when a person maintains a changed behavior (Prochaska, et al., 2014; pro-change, 2016). Change typically is not a linear process; most people relapse and recycle through the stages of change frequently

TABLE 2.1	STAGES OF BEHAVIOR CHANGE
STAGE	**DEFINITION**
Precontemplation	Does not intend to make changes within the next 6 months. Patient is unaware of the problem or underestimates it. "There is nothing that I really need to change."
Contemplation	Considering a change within the next 6 months. Patient says that he or she is seriously considering a change. "I have a problem, and I really think I need to work on it."
Preparation	Has tried to make changes, but without success. Patient intends to take action in the next month. "I started to exercise regularly, but it didn't last long. I'll probably try again in a few weeks."
Action	Actively engaged in strategies to change behavior. This stage sometimes lasts up to 6 months. It requires commitment of time and energy. "I am really working hard to stop smoking."
Maintenance	Sustained change over time. This stage begins 6 months after action has started and continues indefinitely. It is important to avoid relapse. "I need to avoid people who smoke so I'm not tempted to start smoking again."

(pro-change, 2016). When relapse occurs, a person returns to the contemplation or precontemplation stage before attempting change again. Although patients will often feel like relapse is a failure, you need to help them view it as a learning process. Patients can apply what they learned in their next attempt to change. Health promotion interventions have a greater effect if you time them appropriately to match a patient's specific stage of change (Box 2.4). For example, teaching a patient who is in the contemplation stage and does not routinely eat fruits and vegetables to immediately begin eating five fruits and vegetables a day is not effective. It is better to encourage this patient to think about the costs and benefits of eating five fruits and vegetables a day to help the patient move into the preparation stage.

Health care professionals design interventions and wellness strategies for people in all stages of behavior change. For example, current evidence shows that initiating tobacco cessation in hospital settings is very successful (Prochaska et al., 2014). However, if there are no resources or programs available or patients are not aware of available programs, they miss

BOX 2.4   APPLICATION OF THE STAGES OF THE BEHAVIOR CHANGE MODEL

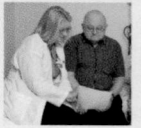

Instead of telling Charlie how much he needs to exercise, Liz applies the stages of behavior change with Charlie to help him become more active. She begins by asking Charlie how he feels about exercise and what his plans are. Charlie states, "I know that exercise is good for me, and I probably should start working on it." Liz determines Charlie is in the contemplation stage based on his response. She plans her teaching to help Charlie see the benefits of exercise, create a plan to fit exercise into his schedule, and find out what kind of activity he prefers. She asks him to bring a list of pros and cons about starting an exercise routine and plans to try some exercises with him at their next appointment. With this process she anticipates Charlie will move into the preparation stage of behavior change within the next month.

the opportunity to make a behavior change to improve their health. Patients maintain changes over time when you help them integrate the changes into their daily routine. True change comes from a patient's desire to change. Maintenance of healthy lifestyles prevents hospitalizations and potentially lowers the cost of health care. Your advice and support may help patients adapt to a healthier lifestyle.

ILLNESS

Illness is not the same as disease. Disease is a pathophysiological process, whereas illness is a state in which a person's physical, emotional, intellectual, social, developmental, or spiritual functioning is diminished or impaired compared with previous experience. A person can feel ill in the presence or absence of disease. For example, cancer is a disease. Some patients with cancer feel ill, whereas others continue to function as usual. Some patients with breast cancer feel well physically but experience spiritual distress. Many patients find health within illness. Sometimes illness motivates an individual to adopt positive health behaviors. Although you need to be familiar with different types of diseases and their treatments, be concerned more with illness, which includes the effects of disease and treatments on a person's functioning and well-being in all dimensions.

Acute and Chronic Illness

Acute and chronic illnesses affect many dimensions of functioning. An acute illness is usually short-term. The symptoms appear abruptly, are intense, and often subside after a relatively short period. A chronic illness usually lasts longer than 6 months. Patients fluctuate between maximal functioning and serious health relapses that are sometimes life threatening.

Because of advances in public health, medicine, and biomedical technology, acute and infectious diseases are no longer major causes of death, disease, and disability in the United States. Chronic illnesses (e.g., diabetes, heart disease, stroke, cancer, arthritis, obesity) are the most common, costly, and preventable of all health problems in the United States (CDC, 2016). You need to learn how to help patients prevent and manage their chronic illness or disabilities to enhance wellness and improve patients' quality of life (tertiary prevention).

Self-Management

Programs that teach chronic disease management must use a holistic approach and include family caregivers when appropriate. The Chronic Disease Self-Management Program (CDSMP) is one of the most widely used evidence-based programs for people with a variety of chronic illnesses (Lorig et al., 2014). CDSMP is community-based and includes self-management education workshops led by people with the chronic illness. It upholds that people with different chronic illnesses have similar self-management needs and problems, that people can learn how to become responsible for the daily management of their diseases, and that people who are confident and knowledgeable about their disease management will have positive health outcomes (Lorig et al., 2014). Taking responsibility for living well with illness strengthens patients. Therefore encourage patients to ask questions about their health care and make informed decisions. The process of learning self-management skills is crucial when learning to live with a chronic illness. The management of chronic illnesses promotes health within illness and addresses human comfort and quality of life (Lorig et al., 2016; Williams et al., 2016). You are able to reduce the impact of chronic illness on an individual and society by providing quality, comprehensive, patient-centered care (Risendal et al., 2014).

Variables Influencing Illness Behavior

People have different attitudes and reactions to illness. Medical sociologists call this reaction illness behavior. People who are ill generally adopt illness behaviors (cognitive, affective, and behavioral reactions) that are influenced by sociocultural and social psychological factors. Illness behaviors affect how people monitor their bodies, define and interpret their symptoms, take remedial actions, and use the health care system. Although people react to an illness in a variety of ways, patients often use illness behavior displayed in sickness to manage difficulties in life (Mechanic, 1995). People who have more positive coping skills, greater social support, and a good perceived health status tend to report less illness behaviors (Thomas and Borrayo, 2014). Internal and external variables affect illness behavior. The influences of these variables affect how likely a patient is to seek health care and participate in therapy, which ultimately affects health outcomes.

Internal Variables. Internal variables are patients' perceptions of symptoms and the nature of illnesses. If patients believe that the symptoms of their illnesses disrupt their normal routine, they are more likely to seek health care assistance than if they do not perceive the symptoms as disruptive.

If they believe that the symptoms are serious or perhaps life threatening, they are also more likely to seek assistance. A person awakened by crushing chest pains in the middle of the night generally views this symptom as potentially serious and life threatening and will probably be motivated to seek assistance. However, some patients fear serious illness and react by denying it and not seeking medical assistance.

External Variables. External variables influencing a patient's illness behavior include the visibility of symptoms, social group, cultural variables, accessibility of the health care system, and social support. The visibility of the symptoms of an illness affects body image and illness behavior. A patient with a visible symptom or a recognizable symptom such as crushing chest pain, intense headache, or a high fever is more likely to seek assistance than a patient who has symptoms that are less visible or recognizable such as the nonspecific symptoms associated with ovarian cancer (e.g., fatigue, bloating, trouble eating, and feeling full quickly) (Mechanic, 1995).

Patients' social groups help them accept or deny the threat of illness. Families, friends, and co-workers all influence patients' illness behavior. Patients often react positively to social support while practicing positive health behaviors. How patients perceive health and the effects of disease and its interpretation vary according to a patient's culture and family.

Economic variables are social determinants of health that influence the way a patient reacts to illness. Financial difficulty will often lead a patient to delay treatment. This is especially common in patients who are uninsured or underinsured. The health care system is a socioeconomic system that patients enter, interact within, and exit. For many patients, entry into the system is complex or confusing, and some patients seek nonemergency medical care in an emergency department because they do not have access through insurance or do not know how to obtain health services otherwise. The physical proximity of patients to a health care agency often influences how soon they enter the system after deciding to seek care.

IMPACT OF ILLNESS ON PATIENT AND FAMILY

An illness of a family member affects the function of an entire family unit. A patient and family commonly experience behavioral and emotional changes and changes in body image, self-concept, family roles, and family dynamics.

Behavioral and Emotional Changes

Individual behavioral and emotional reactions depend on the nature of an illness, a patient's attitude toward the illness, the reaction of others to the illness, and the variables of illness behavior. Short-term, non–life-threatening illnesses evoke few behavioral changes in the functioning of a patient or family. For example, a parent who has a severe cold lacks the energy and patience to spend time in family activities and prefers not to interact with the family. This is a behavioral change, but it is subtle and does not last long. Some even consider such a change a normal response to illness.

Severe illness, particularly one that is life threatening, leads to more extensive emotional and behavioral changes such as anxiety, shock, denial, anger, and withdrawal. These are common responses to the stress of illness. You develop interventions to help patients and families cope with and adapt to this stress because the stressors usually cannot be changed.

Impact on Body Image

Body image is the subjective concept of physical appearance. Our perception of body image changes as we grow and develop (see Chapter 24). Some illnesses result in changes in physical appearance. Patients and families react differently to these changes. Their reactions depend on the type of changes (e.g., the loss of a limb or an organ), the adaptive capacity of a family, the rate at which changes take place, and the support services available.

When a profound change in body image occurs, such as after a mastectomy or leg amputation, a patient generally adjusts by experiencing phases of the grief process (see Chapter 27). Initially the change or impending change shocks the patient. As the patient and family recognize the reality of the change, they become anxious and sometimes withdraw. As they acknowledge the change, they gradually move toward accepting their loss. During rehabilitation, the patient is ready to learn how to adapt to the change in body image.

Impact on Self-Concept

Self-concept is your mental self-image of all aspects of your personality. It depends in part on body image and roles but also includes other aspects of psychology and spirituality. Self-concept is important in relationships with other family members. A patient whose self-concept changes because of illness is sometimes no longer able to meet family expectations, leading to tension or conflict. As a result, family members change their interactions with the patient. While providing care, you observe changes in a patient's self-concept (or in the self-concepts of family members) and develop a care plan to help a patient adjust to the changes resulting from the illness (see Chapter 24).

Impact on Family Roles and Family Dynamics

People have many roles in life such as wage earner, decision maker, professional, and parent. When an illness occurs, the roles of the patient and family change (see Chapter 25). Patients and their families generally adjust more easily to subtle, short-term changes caused by minor acute illness, such as when a child gets strep throat. However, long-term changes caused by sudden acute and severe health problems (e.g., stroke or head injury from a motor vehicle accident) or the diagnosis of a chronic illness (e.g., type 1 diabetes or cancer) require an adjustment process similar to the grief process (see Chapter 27). A patient and family often need specific counseling and guidance to help them cope with the role changes.

Family dynamics is the process by which the family functions, makes decisions, gives support to individual members, and copes with everyday changes and challenges. Because of the effects of illness, family dynamics often change. Another family member sometimes needs to assume a patient's usual roles and responsibilities. This often creates tension or anxiety in the family. Include the whole family as appropriate while helping patients attain their maximal level of functioning and well-being (see Chapter 25).

THE NURSE'S ROLE IN HEALTH AND ILLNESS

Patients receive care related to their health and illness needs in all health care settings. Although nurses are often the key members of the health care team to provide information to patients about health, wellness, and illness, patients' needs are very complex. Thus as a nurse, you need to collaborate with other members of the health care team to successfully improve the health of individuals, families, and communities. Value, respect, and trust the other members of the health care team as you work together to develop an appropriate plan of care. Ensure that a patient's interests are at the center of the plan. Understand how each team member can contribute to a patient's health or illness care and determine how you can best work together to help your patient. Effective teams communicate with and listen to each other clearly and frequently (Interprofessional Education Collaborative Expert Panel, 2011; AHRQ, 2016).

QSEN **QSEN ACTIVITY** *Teamwork and Collaboration*

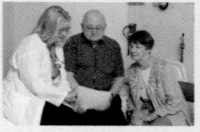 Charlie has been attending cardiac education classes at the clinic for several weeks now. He finds the classes helpful, but he does not understand why so many different people are part of the education team. He has been seeing a nurse, a registered dietitian, a psychologist, and a relaxation therapist. He thinks that it might be easier to just have one person do it all.
- How would you explain to Charlie the role of each health care professional on his patient care team?

evolve Answers to QSEN Activities can be found on the Evolve website.

You will use your knowledge of various models of health and illness and apply concepts of growth and development to provide individualized effective care that promotes optimal patient outcomes and helps patients achieve the highest level of health possible. Your role in promoting health will vary based on your patient's needs. Regardless of your practice setting (e.g., hospital, long-term care, school, health department), you will synthesize what you know to make evidence-based and effective clinical decisions that affect your patient's care. Whether you are caring for a patient who is healthy or ill, it is important to assess and take your patient's

expectations into consideration while developing a plan of care. Understanding your patient's definition of health builds a trusting and therapeutic relationship, enhancing your ability to help your patients make positive lifestyle choices or behavioral changes. Ensure that health teaching meets your patient's needs, and provide patient education at a literacy level that your patient can understand (see Chapter 12). You will use the nursing process to develop and implement appropriate nursing care directed at helping your patients achieve or maintain health or adapt to illness (see Chapter 9). Evaluate the effectiveness of your care, taking into consideration whether or not your care met your patient's expectations. Modify health teaching and health promotion interventions as needed to best meet your patient's needs.

KEY POINTS

- Health and wellness are not merely the absence of disease and illness. A person's state of health, wellness, or illness depends on his or her values, attitudes, personality, and lifestyle.
- Unmet needs motivate human beings. Basic human needs must be met before an individual is able to focus on higher level needs.
- The health promotion model focuses on behaviors motivated by the desire to increase well-being and actualize human potential.
- Holistic health models of nursing promote optimal health by incorporating active participation of patients in improving their health state. Holistic nursing interventions complement standard medical therapy.
- Consider internal and external variables that influence patients' health beliefs and practices when planning nursing care.
- Health promotion activities maintain or enhance health. Wellness education teaches patients how to care for themselves. Illness prevention activities protect against health threats and thus maintain an optimal level of health.
- Nursing incorporates health promotion, wellness, and illness prevention activities rather than simply treating illness.
- The three levels of prevention are primary (prevention of disease or illness), secondary (minimize spread of disease of illness), and tertiary (long-term management of conditions).
- Risk factors threaten health, influence health practices, and are important considerations in illness prevention activities. Some risk factors are modifiable, whereas others are nonmodifiable.
- Improvement in health often requires a change in health behaviors.
- Illness behavior influences how patients respond to illness. Patients who cope better tend to respond better to illnesses.
- Illness has many effects on the patient and family, including changes in behavior and emotions, family roles and dynamics, body image, and self-concept.

REFLECTIVE LEARNING

- Understanding a person's risk factors helps you determine important information to teach to help that person prevent potential illnesses. Reflect on a patient you recently cared for or think about someone in your family. What actual or potential health problems does this person have? What risk factors contributed to these problems? Can they be modified or not? What health behaviors can this person implement to limit any risk factors?

- Interview a patient or someone you know who is the process of changing a health behavior. Ask what behavior this person is thinking about (e.g., smoking cessation, starting an exercise program, losing weight). Find out if the person has begun to make changes yet. Identify which stage of behavior change this person is in based on the information you gain from the interview (see Table 2.1).

- Reflect on your own health. How do you define health? Do you consider yourself healthy or not? Explain your answer. What health behaviors would you like to change or implement right now? For example, do you exercise regularly, do you typically make healthy food choices, and are you getting an appropriate amount of sleep right now? Develop a plan to make a behavior change geared toward improving your health status. What are the benefits and possible barriers you will face when you make this change?

REVIEW QUESTIONS

1. Some nursing students are giving flu vaccines to older adults at a retirement village. What level of prevention are the students providing?
   1. Primary prevention
   2. Secondary prevention
   3. Tertiary prevention
   4. Rehabilitation
2. An interprofessional health care team is developing a health education program for a middle school. Which health topics are consistent with the goals of *Healthy People 2020*? (Select all that apply.)
   1. Determining the best treatment for strep throat
   2. Explaining why it is important to get immunizations as scheduled
   3. Teaching about healthy snacks
   4. Describing why genetically modified foods are controversial
   5. Teaching different ways to fit exercise into the daily routine
   6. Explaining the problems related to lead exposure in the environment

3. When creating a plan of care for a patient with a new below-the-knee amputation, the nurse will consider which factors? (Select all that apply.)
   1. The patient and family may grieve the loss of the leg.
   2. The patient may have difficulty coping with the change in the appearance of his body.
   3. The patient may experience a change in self-concept that will lead to conflict within the family.
   4. The patient and family will adjust very quickly and will experience no changes in family dynamics.
   5. The loss of the leg will affect only the patient, as the patient is most affected by the change in health status.
4. Which priority nursing intervention is most important to help a patient meet the goal of smoking cessation?
   1. Determine if the patient wants to stop smoking.
   2. Provide information on the health risks caused by smoking.
   3. Include a psychologist to help with implementing this major lifestyle change.
   4. Suggest the patient use nicotine-replacement therapy to help with nicotine cravings.
5. The nurse is assessing a patient who has decided to begin running and exercising regularly. Which patient statement reflects the action phase?
   1. "I really need to start working out and running to improve my health."
   2. "I went to a gym to talk with a personal trainer and have developed a fitness plan I think will work for me."
   3. "I have been getting up early at least 3 days a week for the past month to exercise for at least 30 minutes every day."
   4. "Now that I have been exercising regularly for the past 7 months, I can tell I have a lot more energy and I have lost weight."

evolve

Additional Review Questions, as well as rationales for all Review Questions, can be found on the Evolve website.

1. 1; 2, 3, 5, 6; 3. 1, 2, 3; 4. 1; 5. 3.

REFERENCES

Adamo K, Brett K: Parental perceptions and childhood dietary quality, *Matern Child Health J* 18(4):978, 2014.

Adams T, et al: A community-based walking program to promote physical activity among African American women, *Nurs Womens Health* 19(1):26, 2015.

Agency for Healthcare Research and Quality (AHRQ): *Clinical guidelines and recommendations*, 2014, http://www.ahrq.gov/professionals/clinicians-providers/guidelines-recommendations/index.html.

Agency for Healthcare Research and Quality (AHRQ): *TeamSTEPPS® 2.0*, 2016, http://www.ahrq.gov/teamstepps/instructor/index.html.

Ball JW, et al: *Seidel's guide to physical examination*, ed 6, St Louis, 2015, Elsevier.

Becker MH, Maiman LA: Sociobehavioral determinants of compliance with health and medical care recommendations, *Med Care* 13(1):10, 1975.

Boutaugh ML, et al: Closing the disparity gap: the work of the Administration on Aging, *Generations* 38(4):107, 2015.

Bracken N, et al: Facilitators of HIV medical care engagement among former prisoners, *AIDS Educ Prev* 27(6):566, 2015.

Centers for Disease Control and Prevention (CDC): *Chronic disease overview*, 2016, https://www.cdc.gov/chronicdisease/overview/.

Chapa DW, et al: Pathophysiological relationships between heart failure and depression and anxiety, *Crit Care Nurse* 34(2):14, 2014.

Conway-Phillips R, Janusek L: Influence of sense of coherence, spirituality, social support and health perception on breast cancer screening motivation and behaviors in African American women, *ABNF J* 25(3):72, 2014.

Edelman CL, et al: *Health promotion throughout the life span*, ed 8, St Louis, 2014, Mosby.

Healthy People 2020, 2017, https://www.healthypeople.gov/2020/About-Healthy-People.

Hefei W, et al: Effect of Medicaid expansions on health insurance coverage and access to care among low-income adults with behavioral health conditions, *Health Serv Res* 50(6):1787, 2015.

Interprofessional Education Collaborative Expert Panel: *Core competencies for interprofessional collaborative practice: report of an expert panel*, 2011, http://www.aacn.nche.edu/education-resources/ipecreport.pdf.

Jim HSL, et al: Religion, spirituality, and physical health in cancer patients: a meta-analysis, *Cancer* 121(21):3760, 2015.

Johnson NB, et al: *CDC national health report: leading causes of morbidity and mortality and associated behavioral risk and protective factors—United States, 2005-2013*, 2014, http://www.cdc.gov/mmwr/preview/mmwrhtml/su6304a2.htm.

Kann L, et al: Youth risk behavior surveillance—United States 2015, *MMWR Surveill* 65(SS-6):1, 2016. http://www.cdc.gov/mmwr/volumes/65/ss/ss6506a1.htm.

Lessard LN, et al: Pollution, poverty, and potentially preventable childhood morbidity in central California, *J Pediatr* 168:198, 2016.

Lorig K, et al: Effectiveness of the chronic disease self-management program for persons with a serious mental illness: a translation study, *Community Ment Health J* 50(1):96, 2014.

Lorig K, et al: Benefits of diabetes self-management for health plan members: a 6-month translation study, *J Med Internet Res* 18(6):e164, 2016.

Maslow AH: *Motivation and personality*, New York, 1954, Harper & Row.

Maslow AH: *Motivation and personality*, ed 2, New York, 1970, Harper & Row.

Maslow AH: *Motivation and personality*, ed 3, Upper Saddle River, NJ, 1987, Prentice Hall.

McLeod S: *Maslow's hierarchy of needs*, 2016, http://www.simplypsychology.org/maslow.html.

Mechanic D: Sociological dimensions of illness behavior, *Soc Sci Med* 41(9):1207, 1995.

Pender NJ: *Health promotion and nursing practice*, Norwalk, CT, 1982, Appleton-Century-Crofts.

Pender NJ: *Health promotion in nursing practice*, ed 3, Stamford, CT, 1996, Appleton & Lange.

Pender NJ, et al: *Health promotion in nursing practice*, ed 6, Upper Saddle River, NJ, 2011, Prentice Hall.

pro-change: *The transtheoretical model*, 2016, http://www.prochange.com/transtheoretical-model-of-behavior-change.

Prochaska JJ, et al: Efficacy of initiating tobacco dependence treatment in inpatient psychiatry: a randomized controlled trial, *Am J Public Health* 104(8):1557, 2014.

Resnick B, et al: The impact of PRAISEDD on adherence and initiation of heart health behaviors in senior housing, *Public Health Nurs* 31(4):309, 2014.

Risendal B, et al: Adaptation of the chronic disease self-management program for cancer survivors: feasibility, acceptability, and lessons for implementation, *J Cancer Educ* 29(4):762, 2014.

Rosenstoch I: Historical origin of the health belief model, *Health Educ Monogr* 2:334, 1974.

Salsman JM, et al: A meta-analytic approach to examining the correlation between religion/spirituality and mental health in cancer, *Cancer* 121(21):3769, 2015.

Schofield R, et al: Comparing personal health practices: individuals with mental illness and the general Canadian population, *Can Nurse* 112(5):23, 2016.

Sher T, et al: The partners for life program: a couples approach to cardiac risk reduction, *Fam Process* 53(1):131, 2014.

Slatyer S, et al: Finding privacy from a public death: a qualitative exploration of how a dedicated space for end-of-life care in an acute hospital impacts on dying patients and their families, *J Clin Nurs* 24(15/16):2164, 2015.

Song M, Kong E: Older adults' definitions of health: a metasynthesis, *Int J Nurs Stud* 52(6):1097, 2015.

Stanhope M, Lancaster J: *Public health nursing: population-centered health care in the community*, ed 9, St Louis, 2016, Elsevier.

Thomas JJ, Borrayo EA: The combined influence of psychosocial factors on illness behavior among women, *Women Health* 54(6):530, 2014.

Thompson D, et al: Texting to increase adolescent physical activity: feasibility assessment, *Am J Health Behav* 40(4):472, 2016.

Tovar E, Clark MC: Knowledge and health beliefs related to heart disease risk among adults with type 2 diabetes, *J Am Assoc Nurse Pract* 27(6):321, 2015.

Williams EM, et al: Intervention to improve quality of life for African-American lupus patients (IQAN): study protocol for a randomized controlled trial of a unique a la carte intervention approach to self-management of lupus in African Americans, *BMC Health Serv Res* 16:1, 2016.

World Health Federation: *Cardiovascular disease risk factors*, 2016, http://www.world-heart-federation.org/cardiovascular-health/cardiovascular-disease-risk-factors/.

World Health Organization (WHO) Interim Commission: *Chronicle of WHO*, Geneva, 1947, The Organization.

World Health Organization (WHO): *Constitution of WHO principles*, 2017, http://www.who.int/about/mission/en/.

Yan AF, et al: mHealth text messaging for physical activity promotion in college students: a formative participatory approach, *Am J Health Behav* 39(3):395, 2015.

The Health Care Delivery System

evolve MEDIA RESOURCES

http://evolve.elsevier.com/Potter/essentials

- Audio Glossary

- QSEN Activity and Review Questions Answers and Rationales

OBJECTIVES

- Describe the six levels of health care.
- Discuss the factors that affect a person's access to health care.
- Explain the concept of "pay for value" used to reward hospitals financially.
- Explain the relationship between levels of health care and levels of prevention.
- Discuss the features of an integrated health care system.
- Discuss the types of settings in which professionals provide various levels of health care.

- Discuss the role of nurses in various health care settings.
- Describe the elements of discharge planning.
- Explain approaches nurses can use to improve patient satisfaction.
- Discuss the nursing implications regarding issues facing the health care system.
- Describe the effects of health disparities on the health of a community.

KEY TERMS

acute care, p. 30
adult day care centers, p. 39
assisted living, p. 38
diagnosis-related group (DRG), p. 40
discharge planning, p. 34
health care disparities, p. 44
home care, p. 36
hospice, p. 39

Medicaid, p. 37
Medicare, p. 37
Minimum Data Set (MDS), p. 38
patient-centered care, p. 42
Patient Protection and Affordable Care Act, p. 29
primary care, p. 31
prospective payment system (PPS), p. 40

rehabilitation, p. 37
respite care, p. 39
restorative care, p. 36
secondary health care, p. 33
skilled nursing facility, p. 38
tertiary health care, p. 33

The health care delivery system has changed significantly in the last 3 decades. Efforts have been made to reduce the costs of health care while improving access to the health care system and ensuring high-quality outcomes. Until recently, however, the costs of health care skyrocketed each year. Millions of Americans had limited access to health care, there were limited incentives for people to engage in healthy behaviors, and participants had no accepted method for measuring and evaluating health care outcomes.

Initiatives in the current Patient Protection and Affordable Care Act and the work of agencies such as the National Quality Forum (NQF), the Centers for Medicare and Medicaid Services (CMS), and The Joint Commission (TJC) are significantly improving the U.S. health care system (CMS,

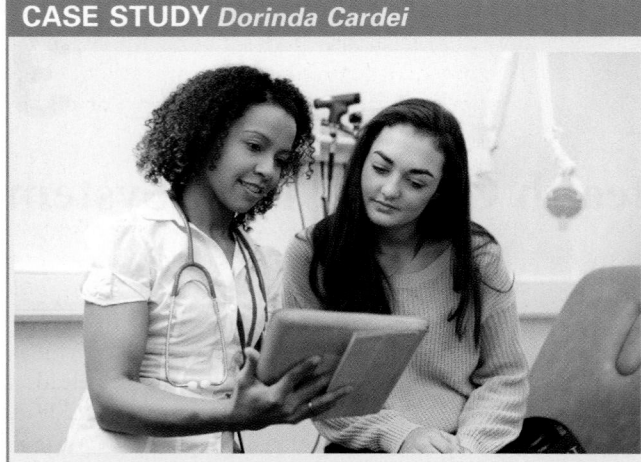

Copyright © bowdenimages/iStock/Thinkstock.

CASE STUDY *Dorinda Cardei*

Dorina Cardei is a 17-year-old girl who was born in the United States and whose parents are from Romania. She is a junior at a local high school. She has two brothers and lives at home with her parents. Her mother, Sylvana, is a part-time cashier at a local grocery store. Her father, Alex, works as a maintenance man at a local hospital. Both of her parents have chronic health problems. Sylvana has hypertension and is overweight, and Alex has had several injuries to his knees, causing osteoarthritis. Dorina reports that her family is very close and that her parents work together to meet all the needs of their children.

Dorina has had asthma since she was 5 years old. She sometimes has difficulty controlling the disease because of the cost of her medications. Her parents recently were able to obtain insurance through the federal exchange marketplace. Now Dorina can get the medications she needs. She visits the clinic today and is learning when and how to use an inhaler. She reports having some recent difficulty breathing, especially during gym class.

Corrine is a nurse who recently began working at the outpatient clinic as an advanced practice nurse. Corrine last worked at a pediatrician's office. Dorina's difficulty in managing her asthma is significant for Corrine because Corrine's daughter also has asthma. In addition, Corrine cared for children with asthma and helped patients access the health care system during her work in the pediatrician's office.

2015a). For example, national health expenditures from 2011 to 2013 grew at the slowest rate since record keeping began. As of 2014, costs continued to decrease even though millions gained insurance coverage (CMS, 2015a). Other important improvements are as follows (CMS, 2015a):
- Health outcomes are improving (for example, patient harm has dropped 17% since 2011).
- Hospital readmissions for select medical conditions fell by 8% during 2012–2013.
- Health care providers are much more engaged in developing innovative care models.

You should know these facts so that you can answer the questions patients or their families ask about health care costs and how they might affect the care they or their family members receive.

As you begin your career in nursing, you will soon realize that the U.S. health care system is very complex and constantly changing. You will better succeed in your career if you understand the functioning of the health care system and the role nurses play. Nursing is a caring discipline. The profession's values are rooted in helping people to regain, maintain, or improve their health; prevent illness; and find comfort and dignity at the time of death. Today, the health care system overall is trying to move in the same direction.

As a result of health care transformations, the practice of nursing is changing. The American Nurses Association (ANA) takes this position: "Registered nurses are educated and practice within a holistic framework that views the individual, family, and community as an interconnected system that can keep us well and help us heal. Registered nurses are fundamental to the critical shift needed in health services delivery, with the goal of transforming the current 'sick care' system into a true 'health care' system" (ANA, 2014).

TRADITIONAL LEVELS OF HEALTH CARE

The U.S. health care system delivers six levels of care: preventive, primary, secondary, tertiary, restorative, and continuing care. Levels of care describe the scope of services and settings delivered by health care providers to patients in all stages of health and illness. You need to understand how the health care industry organizes and delivers these levels of care. Box 3.1 highlights the types of services available to patients and families at each level of care.

Each level of care has different requirements and opportunities for a nurse. For example, in your role within a primary care setting, you will be involved in patient assessment. You will identify changes in chronic conditions or the development of new acute conditions. You will teach new mothers how to care for their babies or young adults how to use an inhaler. In a continuing care setting, you will apply gerontology nursing principles to help patients adapt to permanent health changes so that they can remain active and engaged.

Levels of care are not the same as levels of prevention (see Chapter 2). Levels of prevention describe the focus of health-related activities in a care setting. These include health promotion and disease prevention (primary prevention), curing of disease (secondary prevention), and reducing complications (tertiary prevention).

At every level of care, nurses and other health care providers offer a variety of prevention services. For example, a nurse working in a specialized **acute care** (secondary/tertiary) hospital setting monitors the recovery of a patient following open heart surgery while also providing health promotion information to the family caregiver concerning diet and exercise. Health care reform has led to changes unique to each level of care. For example, the health care industry now places greater emphasis on wellness. Thus the industry directs more resources toward primary and preventive care. Wellness care focuses on the health of populations

BOX 3.1   EXAMPLES OF HEALTH CARE SERVICES

PREVENTIVE CARE

- Adult screenings for blood pressure, cholesterol, tobacco use, and cancer
- Pediatric screenings for hearing, vision, autism, and developmental disorders
- Human immunodeficiency virus (HIV) screening for adults at higher risk
- Wellness visits
- Immunizations
- Diet counseling
- Mental health counseling and crisis prevention
- Community legislation (seat belts, air bags, bike helmets)

PRIMARY CARE (HEALTH PROMOTION)

- Diagnosis and treatment of common illnesses
- Ongoing management of chronic health problems
- Prenatal care
- Well-baby care
- Family planning
- Patient-centered medical home

SECONDARY (ACUTE CARE)

- Urgent or emergency care
- Acute medical-surgical care: ambulatory, hospital
- Radiological procedures

TERTIARY CARE

- Highly specialized: intensive care, inpatient psychiatric facilities
- Specialty care (such as neurology, cardiology, rheumatology, dermatology, oncology)

RESTORATIVE CARE

- Rehabilitation programs (such as cardiovascular, pulmonary, orthopedic)
- Sports medicine
- Spinal cord injury programs
- Home care

CONTINUING CARE

- Long-term care: assisted living, nursing centers
- Psychiatric and older-adult day care

and communities rather than simply curing an individual's disease. In wellness care, nurses help lead communities and health care systems in coordinating resources to better serve their populations. Finding strategies to better address patient needs at all levels of care is critical to improving the health care system.

Integrated Health Care Delivery

Some individual health care systems provide services at all levels of health care. However, the health care system has largely been very reactive, focusing primarily on acute care. Integrated health care systems are shifting to more holistic paradigms for optimizing population health (Strandberg-Larsen and Krasnik, 2009). At the core of this shift is provision of a coordinated continuum of services that support patients with chronic conditions and improve the health status of specific populations.

There is no single model for an integrated health care system. In a systematic review of existing systems, two types of integrated health care systems were found: (1) an organizational structure that follows economic imperatives such as combining financing with all providers, from hospitals, clinics, and physicians to home care and long-term care facilities; and (2) a structure that supports an organized care delivery approach (coordinating care activities and services into seamless functioning) (Strandberg-Larsen and Krasnik, 2009).

The patient-centered medical home model is an example of an integrated health care system. Instead of focusing on symptom- and illness-based episodic care, this model provides comprehensive, coordinated primary care for patients of all ages (American Academy of Family Physicians, 2017). The patient-centered medical home model strengthens the physician-patient relationship with coordinated, individualized care. In this approach, just as a quarterback leads a football team, a patient's primary health care provider leads the health care team, enlisting the skills and knowledge of health care professionals from various services. These professionals often include nurses, medical assistants, nutritionists, social workers, pharmacists, and other caregivers. Members of a patient-centered medical home care team are linked by information technology, electronic health records (EHRs), and system-best practices to ensure that patients receive care when and where they need it and how they want it. Patient centeredness is a unifying principle. It describes an ongoing, active partnership between a personal primary care physician or nurse practitioner who leads a team of professionals dedicated to providing proactive, preventive, and long-term care management through all stages of a patient's life (American Academy of Family Physicians, 2017).

Preventive and Primary Health Care Services

Whether you work in a traditional health care system or one that has an integrated delivery of care approach, you need to understand your role and how it complements the delivery of a specific level of care. Health promotion is the level of prevention delivered in preventive and primary care settings such as schools, physicians' offices, outpatient clinics, occupational health settings, and nursing centers (Table 3.1).

Health promotion is a key to quality health care. Effective health promotion programs help patients develop healthier lifestyles. The Centers for Disease Control and Prevention (CDC, 2015a) notes that employees who adopt healthy behaviors through health promotion programs not only reduce their risk for developing disabling or life-threatening diseases and their associated costs but also improve their everyday quality of life including their physical, mental, and emotional health.

The focus of health promotion is to keep people healthy through personal hygiene, good nutrition, clean living environments, regular exercise, rest, and the adoption of positive health attitudes. Health promotion programs reduce the costs of health care by reducing the incidence of disease and minimizing complications, thereby reducing the need to use expensive health care resources. In contrast, preventive care is more disease oriented and focuses on reducing and controlling risk factors for disease through activities such as immunization and diet counseling.

TABLE 3.1   HEALTH PROMOTION IN PREVENTIVE AND PRIMARY CARE SETTINGS

TYPE OF SERVICE	PURPOSE	AVAILABLE PROGRAMS/SERVICES
School health	Comprehensive programs integrate health promotion principles into a school curriculum. Services emphasize program management, interdisciplinary collaboration, and community health principles. Research shows a link between the health outcomes of young people and their academic success (CDC, 2015b).	Health education Physical education and physical activity Nutrition environment and services Health services Physical environment Social and emotional climate Counseling, psychological, and social services Employee wellness Family engagement Community involvement
Occupational health	The workplace is an important setting for delivering comprehensive health protection, health promotion, and disease/accident prevention programs. Americans working full time spend an average of more than one-third of their day, 5 days per week at the workplace (CDC, 2015a). The goal is to increase worker productivity, reduce absenteeism, reduce health risks, and reduce use of expensive medical care.	Environmental surveillance Create company policies that promote healthy behaviors such as a tobacco-free campus policy Work environment: offer healthy foods through vending machines or cafeterias Physical assessment and health screening Health education classes Communicable disease control Counseling
Physicians' offices	Physicians' offices provide primary health care and diagnose and treat acute and chronic illnesses. Practitioners are beginning to focus more on health promotion practices. Advanced nurse practitioners often partner with a physician in managing a patient population.	Routine physical examination Health screening Diagnostics Disease management
Nurse-managed clinics	Nurse-managed clinics or centers deliver nursing services with a focus on health promotion and health education, chronic disease assessment and management, and support for self-care and caregivers. Clinics often are associated with a school, college, department of nursing, federally qualified health center, or independent nonprofit health care agency (AACN, 2014).	Day care Clinical education site for other health care providers in school Physical examinations, cardiovascular checks Prevention services: diabetes and osteoporosis screenings, smoking cessation programs, and immunizations. Health risk appraisal Wellness counseling Employment readiness Acute and long-term care management
Block and parish nursing	Nurses deliver health care services to patients (e.g., older adults or those unable to leave their home) within their own religious communities. Nurses provide services that are unavailable in traditional health care systems.	Running errands/transportation Respite care Counseling Spiritual health: balancing body and mind health to achieve overall wellness
Community centers	Centers provide comprehensive and cost-effective primary care and supportive services that promote access to health care. Services are often provided to a specific patient population (such as well-baby care, mental health care, diabetes care) within underserved communities. Centers are sometimes affiliated with a hospital, medical school, church, or other community organization. Care offered by community centers is culturally appropriate and delivered in languages that many people in the community speak (Center for American Progress, 2010).	Physical assessment and health screening Nutrition education Translation services Dental care Mental health services Care coordination and case management Specialty care (such as orthopedic, cardiac, or podiatric care Disease management Health education

At the primary care level, health care providers deliver interventions that improve health outcomes for an entire population. The primary level of health care includes:

- Medical health care services
- Health education
- Nutritional counseling
- Maternal/child health care
- Family planning
- Control of diseases

Community-based primary health care programs consider societal and environmental factors when addressing the health needs of communities (see Chapter 4). *In the case study, Dorina Cardei visits the same primary care clinic as her mother. Dorina is seeing a health care provider to learn to use an inhaler, and Mrs. Sylvana Cardei is visiting the dietitian. Corrine knows that diet is an important factor in controlling Mrs. Cardei's blood pressure and keeping her healthy. Corrine tells the dietitian what she has learned about the family's eating habits and preferences.*

Secondary and Tertiary Care

The traditional reason people use health care services such as a hospital is to diagnose and treat illness. When the nature or severity of a condition makes primary care insufficient, secondary and tertiary care often becomes necessary. The difference between secondary and tertiary care arises from the complexity of a patient's medical needs. Secondary health care is provided by a specialist or agency on referral by a primary health care provider. It requires more specialized knowledge, skill, or equipment than the primary care physician or nurse practitioner can provide.

Tertiary health care is specialized consultative care, usually provided on referral from secondary medical personnel. However, changes in medical cost reimbursement, improved technology, and less invasive treatments have often made secondary and tertiary care available at the primary care level. For example, more surgeons are performing simple surgeries in outpatient surgical centers or office suites. However, if a patient develops a problem that the surgeon or primary health care provider is unable to treat and/or intensive nursing care is needed, the patient needs a medical specialist, often resulting in hospitalization. Secondary and tertiary care, also called *acute care,* typically are expensive, especially if a patient has waited to seek care until after symptoms have developed.

Hospitals. During 2014, more than 34 million patients were admitted to American Hospital Association–registered hospitals. An additional 33 million patients were admitted to community hospitals (AHA, 2017). Even allowing for the fact that some patients are admitted multiple times during a year, a large percentage of the U.S. population receives health care in a hospital each year. Hospitalized patients are acutely ill and need comprehensive, specialized secondary and tertiary health care.

Hospitals vary in the services they offer. Small rural hospitals offer general inpatient services but have limited emergency and diagnostic services. In comparison, large urban medical centers offer comprehensive, state-of-the-art diagnostic services, trauma and emergency care, surgical intervention, intensive care units (ICUs), inpatient services, and rehabilitation facilities. Larger hospitals hire professional staff from a variety of specialties such as nursing, social service, respiratory therapy, physical and occupational therapy, and speech therapy. Most patients who require these services are having acute episodes of illness. As a nurse, you must be able to think critically and identify patients' changing problems quickly and accurately. This is challenging when you are assigned multiple patients at one time, depending on your unit. You need to be able to deliver an array of nursing interventions effectively. You also must be able to plan and coordinate care with other health care providers quickly and competently.

Many hospitals use evidence-based practice guidelines and clinical protocols (see Chapter 7). You must keep current on evidence-based practices to improve patient outcomes. You will constantly evaluate whether care is effective and how to improve it. *In the case study, Dorina develops a severe asthma attack at home. Her mother learned from the clinic staff to call 911. Dorina is taken to the emergency department at a community hospital. The emergency health care providers stabilize her. The nurse in the emergency department wants to provide primary care while Dorina is in the emergency department. She talks with Dorina and her family to learn what triggers her asthma attacks and how Dorina might learn to reduce those triggers.*

According to the American Hospital Association (2016-2017), delivering the right care, at the right time, and in the right setting is the core mission of hospitals across the United States. To fulfill this mission, hospitals focus much time on supporting quality and safety initiatives. An example of a quality initiative is patient satisfaction. Patient satisfaction is challenging to achieve in a stressful setting such as an inpatient nursing unit. Patients expect you to treat them courteously and respectfully and involve them in decisions affecting their care. More hospitals are adopting models of patient-centered care, which involves providing care that is respectful of and responsive to individual patient preferences, needs, and values and ensuring that patient values guide all clinical decisions (IOM, 2001). A patient-centered care model requires nurses to be more engaged with patients and to incorporate patients and families early into the decision-making process. As a nurse, you play a key role in bringing respect and dignity to your relationship with each patient. You must learn your patients' needs and expectations early to form effective partnerships. This ultimately improves the nursing care you deliver, which results in patient satisfaction.

Health care payers such as CMS and private insurers expect patients who are hospitalized to be treated and discharged within a projected time. Hospitals are reimbursed based on the quality and timeliness of care. If you work in a hospital, you must use resources efficiently to limit costs and help your patients recover and return home. For example, you collaborate with members of the interprofessional health care team such as case managers, physical therapists, physicians, and social workers to plan a quick yet realistic transition to home or to another health care agency.

Discharge Planning. Discharge planning is a coordinated, interdisciplinary process that develops a plan for continuing care after a patient leaves a health care agency. Studies have shown that patients tend to be discharged "quicker and sicker" from hospitals. This sometimes results in adverse events during the immediate postdischarge period (Mabire et al., 2013). Such problems include medication prescribing errors, poor communication between hospital and primary care providers, and lack of coordination with community health care services. The focus of discharge planning is to ensure that a patient transitions to the setting in which his or her health care needs can be appropriately met.

According to the Department of Health and Human Services and Centers for Medicare and Medicaid Services (DHHS CMS) (2014), patients within acute care hospitals have an average length of stay (LOS) of only 2 to 3 days. Thus *discharge planning with coordination of services must begin the moment a patient is admitted to a hospital.* As a nurse, you will play a large role in discharge planning by knowing a patient's plan of care (developed by the interdisciplinary team) as soon as possible, informing the patient and family caregivers of that plan, encouraging their participation, acting on the plan, and evaluating progress. Discharge planning involves the following elements (DHHS CMS, 2014):

- Determining the appropriate posthospital destination for a patient. A case manager or social worker usually selects this setting based on a patient's health care needs, self-care capacity, insurance, and place of residence.
- Identifying a patient's needs for a smooth and safe transition from the acute care hospital/post–acute care facility to his or her discharge destination. Nurses, therapists (physical, occupational, speech), health care providers, and dietitians usually identify these needs.
- Beginning the process of meeting a patient's needs while the patient is still hospitalized with approaches such as early mobility protocols, health education, and new medication regimens.

With a well-developed discharge plan, a patient continues progressing toward the goals of his or her plan of care after discharge without experiencing unavoidable complications or unrelated illnesses or injuries (DHHS CMS, 2014). As a nurse, participate in discharge planning by anticipating and identifying each patient's continuing needs before the actual time of discharge and by coordinating efforts to achieve an appropriate discharge plan.

The DHHS CMS does not require discharge planning for outpatients, including patients who go to an emergency department and are not admitted as hospital inpatients. At the same time, hospitals help some outpatients, such as patients in the emergency department or same-day surgery, by providing some discharge planning services (DHHS CMS,

---

BOX 3.2 DISCHARGE PLANNING MODELS

CARE TRANSITIONS PROGRAM (COLEMAN ET AL., 2006)
Emphasizes the role of a transition coach in managing/facilitating the discharge of a patient to home or to a rehabilitation center. Model is based on four pillars: (1) medication self-management, (2) patient-centered record, (3) follow-up, and (4) indicators of worsening medical condition. Each pillar has different interventions depending on the stage of the hospitalization.

TRANSITIONAL CARE MODEL (NAYLOR ET AL., 2009)
Emphasizes comprehensive discharge planning and follow-up for chronically ill, high-risk, older patients. Model contains six key components: (1) in-hospital assessment and development of the discharge care plan by a transitional care nurse/advanced practice nurse/gerontological nurse; (2) discharge preparation by a multidisciplinary care team; (3) patient participation (communication between nursing staff and the patient) in the process, decision making, discharge planning, and discharge education; (4) continuity of care and communication between health care providers; (5) predischarge assessment; and (6) postdischarge follow-up.

HIGH INTENSITY CARE MODEL (GRACE TEAM CARE, INDIANA UNIVERSITY)
The team is headed by both a nurse practitioner and a social worker. This team works together to support the primary care physician and, following best practice protocols, fully address a patient's health conditions. The focus is to help patients manage their health conditions, coordinate their health care, and achieve optimal health (Michigan Care Management Resource Center, 2017). This achieves patients' goals from the convenience and security of their own home (Counsell, 2015).

2014). Box 3.2 describes models of discharge planning that focus on a patient and his or her family caregiver.

Some patients are more in need of discharge planning because of their health-related risks. For example, some patients have poor health literacy, limited financial resources, or limited family support; others have long-term disabilities or chronic illnesses; and older adults sometimes have cognitive and/or hearing impairments affecting their ability to understand discharge instructions. There are also barriers to effective discharge planning including ineffective communication (e.g., from health care provider to provider or from health care provider to patient), lack of role clarity among health care team members (e.g., responsibility and follow-up), and lack of resources (e.g., rehabilitation and nursing home beds) (Okoniewska et al., 2015). You reduce barriers to discharge planning by clearly communicating about the plan of care with patients, families, and members of the health care team. Change-of-shift hand-offs and hourly bedside rounds are ways to keep all health care providers and patients informed (see Chapter 11). Communicate clearly both verbally and in the entries you make in the EHR (see Chapter 10). Clarify any role confusion (e.g., between the case manager and yourself) to be sure elements of the plan are completed.

Discharge instructions prepare the patient for transition from a hospital to the next level of care, such as home, rehabilitation, or long-term care. Nurses offer useful and relevant information that prepares patients and their family caregivers for postdischarge care. To develop discharge instructions, you need to understand the proper timing for discharge, engage the patient and family caregiver in the process, and know the health care team's plan of care. Patients have difficulty learning when they are experiencing pain, nausea, confusion, or other disabling symptoms. Family caregivers are excellent resources when a patient desires their help. Always involve patients and family caregivers in decisions about a patient's discharge destination (Mabire et al., 2013). Provide discharge instruction as early as possible so that you and other health care team members can reinforce the information several times to improve learning. For example, when a patient receives care that follows a standard protocol, you can easily anticipate the treatment and the patient's estimated discharge date. When a patient has multiple complications, the plan of care and estimated discharge date might not be clear. Begin explaining discharge instruction as soon as you know the plan of care. The following are required discharge instruction topics (TJC, 2017): Discharge medications, follow-up care if needed, a list of all medications changed and/or discontinued, dietary needs, and follow-up tests or procedures.

In the case study, Dorina was not admitted to the hospital. However, discharge planning was needed. In the discharge plan, the nurse enters a plan of care focusing on information she gave to Dorina and family members about asthma triggers. The EHR in this health care system is linked to Corrine's medical clinic. This sharing of information supports continuity of care by relaying essential information to Corrine and other health care providers so they can reinforce patient education and reduce Dorina's readmissions to the emergency department.

Some patients take passive roles when they receive instructions. They might be satisfied when a nurse, physician, or therapist rushes through an explanation and finishes by simply inquiring, "Any questions?" This often leads the patient to automatically answer "no." Health care providers may not have invited this patient to actively participate in the health care plan. A patient-centered approach does more. The health care provider *invites* the patient to participate: "I want to make sure that I've helped you understand everything you need to know about your illness. Patients usually have questions because their situations are complicated. Could you tell me what you understand, and then I can help clarify …?"

The teach-back approach (see Chapter 12) is an excellent way to ensure that a patient understands instructions. Comprehensive discharge instruction ensures that patients know what to do when they get home, how to perform care activities, and what to do when problems develop.

Discharge planning often leads to referrals to other health care providers, especially when specific therapies are planned, such as physical therapy. Some tips for making a successful referral follow:

- Engage the patient and family caregiver in the referral process, including selecting the care provider. Explain the reason for the referral, the service to be provided, and how the service will be provided.
- Make the referral as soon as possible.
- Give the care provider receiving the referral as much information as possible about the patient. This prevents unnecessary duplication of assessment (e.g., current vital signs or pain status) and omission of important information.
- The care provider such as a physical therapist, social worker, dietitian, or radiologist makes recommendations for the patient's care. Understand these recommendations and incorporate them into the treatment plan as soon as possible.

Intensive Care. An ICU or critical care unit is a hospital unit in which patients who are critically ill and unstable are closely monitored and intensively treated. A patient who is critically ill can experience changes by the minute, so health care providers must have specialized knowledge and skill. ICUs have advanced technology such as computerized cardiac monitors and high-tech ventilators. Although regular nursing units have many of these devices, patients within ICUs are monitored and maintained on multiple devices at the same time. Nursing and medical staff members within an ICU are proficient in critical care principles and techniques. The ICU is the most expensive site for delivery of medical care. This site is costly because each nurse is usually assigned no more than one or two patients and because patients usually require many treatments and procedures.

Mental Health Facilities. According to the National Alliance on Mental Illness (NAMI) (2017), about 1 in 5 adults in the United States—43.8 million, or 18.5%—experiences mental illness in a given year. Perhaps more concerning is the report that only 41% of adults in the United States with a mental health condition received mental health services in the past year (NAMI, 2017). Patients who have emotional and behavioral problems such as depression, mood disorders, violent behavior, and eating disorders require special counseling and treatment in psychiatric facilities. However, during the period from 2009 to 2011, massive cuts to non-Medicaid state mental health spending totaled more than $1.8 billion (Honberg, 2011). As a result, states have cut vital mental health services for tens of thousands of youth and adults living with the most serious mental illnesses. These services include community- and hospital-based psychiatric care, housing, and access to medications (Honberg, 2011). Individuals with serious mental illness are more likely to have a chronic disease and as a result die on average 25 years earlier than others, largely as a result of treatable medical conditions (NAMI, 2017).

Psychiatric agencies are located in a variety of settings, including hospitals, independent outpatient clinics, and private mental health hospitals. They offer inpatient and outpatient services, depending on the severity of a patient's problem. Patients enter mental health facilities voluntarily or involuntarily. Patients who are hospitalized usually have short stays intended to stabilize them before transfer to outpatient treatment centers. Patients with mental illness receive a comprehensive multidisciplinary treatment plan that engages patients and their families. Medical, nursing, social work, and activity therapy providers collaborate to develop a plan of care that enables a patient to become more functional within his or her community. At discharge from inpatient facilities, patients usually receive referrals for follow-up care at clinics or with counselors.

Rural Hospitals. Lack of access to health care in rural areas is a serious problem. Approximately 10% of physicians practice in rural areas in the United States, whereas nearly one-fourth of the population lives in these areas (NRHA, 2017). Americans living in rural areas face a unique combination of factors that create health care disparities not found in urban areas. These factors include economic factors (e.g., Americans in rural areas are more likely to live below the poverty level), cultural and social differences, lower levels of education, lack of attention to the problems by legislators, and isolation of living in remote rural areas (NRHA, 2017).

Many rural hospitals have failed economically and closed. To address this problem, the Balanced Budget Act of 1997 changed the designation of some rural hospitals to Critical Access Hospital (CAH) when certain criteria were met (DHHS CMS, 2014). A CAH is in a rural area (35 miles from another hospital) and provides 24-hour emergency care. It has no more than 25 inpatient beds and provides temporary care for 96 hours or less to patients needing stabilization before transfer to a larger hospital. Physicians, advanced practice nurses, or physician assistants staff a CAH. The CAH provides inpatient care to acutely ill or injured patients before they are transferred to better-equipped agencies. Basic radiological and laboratory services are also available. To improve care for patients residing in rural areas, rural hospitals are expected to (HealthIT.gov, 2015):

- Improve access to services including urgent care services and meet unmet health needs in isolated rural communities
- Engage rural communities in developing rural health care systems
- Develop collaborative delivery systems in rural communities as the hubs of rural health care
- Create protocols for coordinating care transition by aligning urban health care systems
- Be the subject matter experts and coordinators for the health care environment of providers, patients, and staff

Health care reform has enabled urban health care systems to branch out and establish affiliations or mergers with rural hospitals. The rural hospitals provide a referral base to the larger tertiary care medical centers. Nurses who work in rural hospitals or clinics often function independently without a physician. These nurses must be competent in physical assessment, clinical decision making, and emergency care. Advanced practice nurses such as nurse practitioners and clinical nurse specialists use medical protocols and establish collaborative agreements with staff physicians.

Restorative Care

Patients recovering from acute illnesses or who have chronic illnesses or disabilities require services designed to restore their health. Continuing care is needed until they return to their previous level of function or reach a new level of function allowed by their illness or disability. Restorative care helps a patient regain maximal functional status, improving quality of life and promoting independence and self-care. The current emphasis on early hospital discharge means that most patients require some level of restorative care. For example, some surgical patients require ongoing wound care and activity and exercise management until they have recovered enough to resume normal activities of daily independent living.

Restorative care settings have increased their intensity of care because patients are leaving hospitals earlier. Patients in a home or rehabilitation setting often still receive intravenous fluids (see Chapter 18), aggressive pain control (see Chapter 34), and enteral nutrition (see Chapter 35). The restorative health care team is interprofessional and includes the patient and family caregiver. In restorative care settings, nurses recognize that success depends on effective and early partnering with patients and their families. Patients and families need to clearly understand the goals for physical recovery, the rationale for any recommended physical restrictions, and the purpose and potential risks associated with therapies. The more you engage patients and families in restorative care, the more likely they are to follow treatment plans and achieve optimal function.

Home Care. Home care provides medically related professional and paraprofessional services and equipment to patients and families in their homes. This care consists of part-time, medically necessary skilled care (e.g., nursing, physical therapy, occupational therapy, and speech-language therapy) that is ordered by a physician (CMS, 2016). Home health care is the fastest growing health care service in the United States because of the greater emphasis placed on keeping patients in their homes (ANA, 2014). Services include health maintenance, education, illness prevention, diagnosis and treatment of disease, palliation, and rehabilitation.

A typical home health nurse has a baccalaureate degree and provides holistic care to patients across the life span, from prenatal care to care after death and from intermittent care to 24-hour care (ANA, 2014). In addition to performing the nursing process in making relevant clinical decisions, the home health nurse often helps patients manage their health-related resources and financial costs.

Home health nurses must have expertise in assessment. Nurses who work in Medicare-certified home care agencies use this expertise to conduct patient-specific comprehensive assessments at a patient's start of care, at 60-day follow-up examinations, at discharge, and before and after an inpatient agency stay (Research Data Assistance Center [ResDac], 2012). This comprehensive assessment, Home Health Outcome and Assessment Information Set (OASIS), consists of a group of standardized core items included in a comprehensive assessment for an adult receiving home care. OASIS forms the basis for measuring patient outcomes for the purposes of outcome-based quality. Data items within OASIS include sociodemographic, environmental, support system, health status, functional status, and health service utilization characteristics of a patient (ResDac, 2012). The OASIS assessment tool gathers the data items needed to measure both outcomes and patient risk factors in the home setting.

Home health care focuses on the goal of helping patients and their family caregivers achieve independence. Home care addresses recovery from and stabilization of illness in the home. In addition, home care identifies problems related to lifestyle, safety, environment, family dynamics, and health care practices in the home. Home care agencies employ skilled and intermittent professional services, such as wound care, administering parenteral and enteral nutrition, administering medications and blood therapy, and home care aide services. These services usually are delivered once or twice a day up to 7 days a week.

Approved home care agencies usually receive reimbursement for services from government programs such as Medicare and Medicaid, private insurance, and private payers. The U.S. government strictly regulates reimbursement for home care services. An agency cannot simply charge whatever it wants for its services and expect to receive that amount. Government programs set the amount of reimbursement for most professional services.

Home care nurses have their own patient caseloads and deliver highly individualized nursing care. They help patients adapt to many permanent or temporary physical limitations to help patients assume a daily home routine that is as normal as possible. Home care requires a strong knowledge base in many areas such as family dynamics (see Chapter 25), cultural competency (see Chapter 21), spiritual values (see Chapter 22), and communication principles (see Chapter 11).

Rehabilitation. The World Health Organization (WHO) defines rehabilitation as the process aimed at enabling people with disabilities to reach and maintain their optimal physical, sensory, intellectual, psychological, and social functional levels. Rehabilitation provides people with disabilities the tools they need to attain independence and self-determination (WHO, 2017).

Patients need rehabilitation after a physical or mental illness, injury, or chemical addiction. Rehabilitation was once offered mostly to patients with illnesses or injury to the nervous or musculoskeletal system, but the health care system has expanded its scope of services. Today specialized rehabilitation services such as cardiovascular and pulmonary rehabilitation programs help patients and families adjust to changes in lifestyle and learn to function within the limits of their disease. Drug rehabilitation centers help patients recover from drug dependence and return to the community as healthy citizens.

Rehabilitation first focuses on preventing complications related to an illness or injury such as promoting early mobility after surgery. As a patient's condition stabilizes, rehabilitation focuses on returning the patient to the maximum possible function and independence (e.g., by determining the need for assist devices such as walkers or canes). Rehabilitation settings include rehabilitation institutions, outpatient settings, and the home. Patients who need long-term rehabilitation, such as patients who have had strokes or spinal cord injuries, have severe disabilities that damage their ability to carry out the activities of daily living.

Outpatients receive treatment at appointments during the week but remain at home the rest of the time. Specific rehabilitation services are provided in the home to help the patient reach the greatest possible function and independence.

Continuing Care

The term *continuing care* describes a variety of health, personal, and social services provided over a long period to people who are disabled, who never were functionally independent, or who have a terminal disease. The need for continuing health care services in the United States is growing. People are living longer. Thus many people with long-term health care needs do not have any family caregivers. A decline in the birth rate, the aging of family caregivers, and the increasing rates of divorce and remarriage complicate this problem.

Continuing care is provided in many settings, including institutions such as nursing centers, group homes, and retirement communities; community-based centers such as adult day care and senior centers; or the home (e.g., home care, home-delivered meals, and hospice. Elder care services provide an alternative for a patient who does not need continuous nursing care but needs some assistance to stay independent. These services offer companionship, assistance with activities of daily living, and food preparation.

Nursing Centers. The language of long-term care is confusing and constantly changing. *Nursing home* was the dominant term for long-term care settings (Meiner, 2015). With the Omnibus Budget Reconciliation Act of 1987, *nursing facility* became the term for nursing homes and other agencies that provide long-term care. Now *nursing center* is the most appropriate term. A nursing center typically provides 24-hour intermediate and custodial care for residents of any age with chronic or debilitating illnesses. Services provided by Medicaid-certified nursing centers include the following (Medicaid.gov, n.d.):

- Skilled nursing
- Rehabilitation
- Long-term care

These three services provide 24-hour licensed nursing, rehabilitation, medically related social services, pharmaceutical services, dietary services individualized to the needs of each resident, a professionally directed program of activities to meet the interests and needs for the well-being of each resident, emergency dental services, room and bed maintenance services, and routine personal hygiene items and services. A skilled nursing facility must care for its residents in a manner and an environment that promotes maintenance or enhancement of the quality of life of each resident (Legal Information Institute, 2010).

Most people living in nursing centers are older adults. A nursing center may be a resident's temporary or permanent home with surroundings made as homelike as possible. Residents receive a planned, systematic, and interdisciplinary approach to care to help them reach and maintain their highest level of function. Nursing centers must comply with the Omnibus Budget Reconciliation Act of 1987 and its minimum requirements to receive payment from Medicare and Medicaid. Government regulations require that staff members in nursing centers comprehensively assess each resident and make care planning decisions within a prescribed period. Care focuses on a resident's functional ability (such as the ability to perform activities of daily living and instrumental activities of daily living) and long-term physical and psychosocial well-being.

A nursing center must have a Resident Assessment Instrument (RAI) completed for each resident. The RAI helps the nursing center staff gather definitive information on a resident's strengths and needs, which they must address in an individualized care plan (CMS, 2015b). The RAI has three components: Minimum Data Set (MDS) Version 3.0, Care Area Assessment (CAA) process, and RAI Utilization Guidelines (Box 3.3). The components of the RAI provide information about a resident's functional status, strengths, weaknesses, and preferences and offer guidance on further assessment when problems are identified (CMS, 2015b). MDS Version 3.0 gives an initial overview of a resident's health care needs and identifies a resident's potential problems, strengths, and preferences. CAAs are triggered by individual MDS item responses that reveal the need for additional assessment. These item responses identify problems, known as "triggered care areas," which form a critical link between the MDS and decisions about care planning. CAAs help facilities identify and use tools that are grounded in current clinical standards of practice such as evidence-based or expert-endorsed research, clinical practice guidelines, and resources.

Information gathered from the RAI provides a national database for nursing centers that enables policy makers to better understand the health care needs of patients requiring long-term care. MDS and CAAs help nurses select interventions that best meet the health care needs of this growing population.

Assisted Living. Assisted living is one of the fastest growing industries in the United States. Assisted living offers an attractive long-term care setting with a homier environment and greater resident autonomy than nursing facilities. Patients require some assistance with activities of daily

---

BOX 3.3   COMPONENTS OF THE RESIDENT ASSESSMENT INSTRUMENT (RAI)

MINIMUM DATA SET (MDS)

A core set of screening, clinical, and functional status elements including common definitions and coding categories, which forms the foundation of a comprehensive assessment for all residents of Medicare or Medicaid certified nursing centers. Elements include:

- Resident's background
- Cognitive, communication/hearing, and vision patterns
- Physical functioning and structural problems
- Mood, behavior, and activity pursuit patterns
- Psychosocial well-being
- Bowel and bladder continence
- Disease diagnoses and other health conditions
- Mood and behavior patterns
- Activity pursuit patterns
- Oral/nutritional and dental status
- Skin condition
- Medication use
- Treatments and procedures

CARE AREA ASSESSMENT (CAA) PROCESS

This process helps the assessor systematically interpret the information recorded on the MDS. Once a care area is triggered, nursing center providers use current, evidence-based clinical resources to conduct an assessment of the potential problem and determine whether or not to care plan for it. The CAA process helps the clinician focus on key issues.

- **Care Area Triggers (CATs)** are specific resident responses for one or a combination of MDS elements. The triggers identify residents who have or are at risk for developing specific functional problems and require further assessment.
- **Care Area Assessment** is the further investigation of triggered areas to determine if the care area triggers require interventions and care planning.
- **CAA Summary** provides a location for documentation of the care areas triggered from the MDS and the decisions made during the CAA process regarding whether or not to proceed to care planning.

UTILIZATION GUIDELINES

The Utilization Guidelines provide instructions for when and how to use the RAI.

Adapted from Centers for Medicare and Medicaid Services (CMS): *Long-term care facility resident assessment instrument 3.0 user's manual version 1.13,* 2015, https://www.cms.gov/Medicare/Quality-Initiatives-Patient-Assessment-Instruments/NursingHomeQualityInits/Downloads/MDS-30-RAI-Manual-V113.pdf.

---

living but remain relatively independent within a partially protective setting. A group of residents live together; each resident has his or her own room with personal possessions, and the residents share dining and social areas.

Facilities range from hotel-like buildings with hundreds of units to modest group homes that house a handful of older adults. Assisted living provides independence, security, and

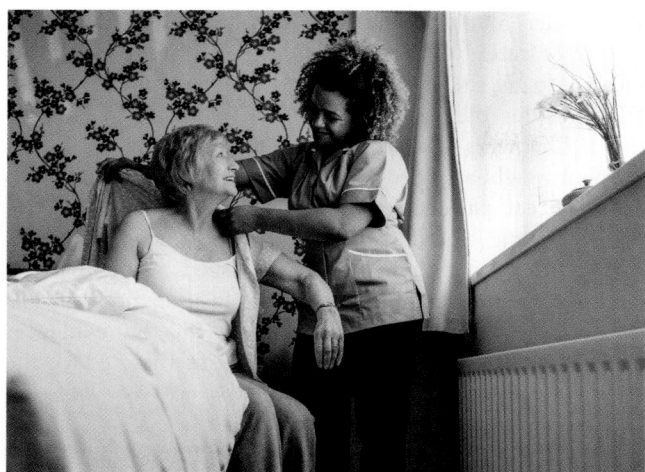

FIG 3.1 Delivering nursing services in assisted-living facilities promotes physical and psychosocial health. (Copyright © DGLimages/iStock/Thinkstock.)

privacy all in one setting (Fig. 3.1). Services include medication management, exercise, educational activities, social activities, laundry and housekeeping services, assistance with meals and personal care, and 24-hour oversight. Some facilities assist with medication administration. An assisted-living center does not directly provide nursing care, but a home care nurse can visit a resident.

Respite Care. Caring for family members within the home creates great physical and emotional burdens for family caregivers. This is especially true when the family member who needs assistance is physically or cognitively limited. The family caregiver is usually an adult who not only has the responsibility for providing care to a loved one, such as a spouse, parent, or sibling, but also often maintains a full-time job, raises a family, and manages the routines of daily living.

Respite care is a service that offers short-term relief by providing family caregivers a temporary rest from caregiving (Alzheimer's Association, 2017). As a nurse who works in a home health setting, you can recommend respite services to the family caregivers of your patient. Respite care is provided in many ways, such as at home by a friend, family member, volunteer, or paid service; or in a community-based setting such as adult day care or a residential facility (Alzheimer's Association, 2017). Residential respite care facilities provide 24-hour care, allowing family caregivers to take an extended break for a few days or to take a vacation. Research shows that family caregivers are more likely to use respite care when they trust the respite care service providers and perceive their family member will experience improved well-being because of the social interaction and meaningful activity provided by the service (Stirling et al., 2014).

Adult Day Care Centers. Adult day care centers offer a variety of health and social services to specific patient populations who live alone or with family in the community. Services are offered during the day and enable family members to maintain their lifestyles and employment while still providing home care for their relatives (Meiner, 2015). Some day care centers exist independently, whereas others operate within a hospital or nursing center.

Frequently patients who use these centers do not require hospitalization but need continuous health care services while family caregivers are at work. These patients include:

- Older adults who need daily physical rehabilitation
- Individuals with emotional illnesses who need daily counseling
- Individuals with chemical dependence problems who are involved in rehabilitation programs

The centers usually operate 5 days a week during typical business hours and charge by the day. Adult day care centers allow patients to retain independence by living at home and potentially reduce health care costs by avoiding or delaying admission to a nursing center. Additional services offered in day care settings include transportation to and from the center, assistance with personal care, nursing, and therapeutic services (e.g., counseling and physical therapy, meals, and recreational activities) (Meiner, 2015).

Nurses who work in day care centers provide continuity between care delivered in the home and care delivered in the center. To provide adequate support to patients, these nurses know a community's needs and resources. The patients often spend only a few hours a week in the day care setting.

Hospice. A hospice is a system of family-centered care that enables patients with terminal illnesses to live with comfort, independence, and dignity while helping to manage the stress caused by the illness. Hospice care is provided in a setting that best meets the needs of each patient and family including a patient's home, nursing center, assisted-living center, freestanding hospice, and hospital. The focus of hospice care is palliative care, not curative treatment (see Chapter 27). A hospice benefits patients in the terminal phase of any disease such as cardiomyopathy, multiple sclerosis, acquired immunodeficiency syndrome (AIDS), and cancer.

A patient receiving hospice care is in the terminal phase of illness; the patient, family, and physician agree that no further treatment will reverse the disease process. Staff members collaborate to provide care that ensures death with dignity. Hospice care is usually not provided 24 hours a day, 7 days a week. Instead, hospice provides intermittent nursing visits to assess, monitor, and treat symptoms as well as teach family caregivers the skills they need to care for the patient. Team members are available around-the-clock to answer questions or visit anytime the need for support arises. Services continue without interruption if a patient's care setting changes. While every effort is made to provide hospice care at home, sometimes patients require more specialized care and need to be admitted to an inpatient hospice that provides 24-hour care.

The patient and family must accept that the hospice will not use emergency measures such as cardiopulmonary resuscitation to prolong life. The focus is on symptom management and ensuring the patient's comfort. The hospice multidisciplinary team works together continuously with the patient's primary health care provider to develop and maintain a patient-directed, individualized plan of care. Chapter 27 provides more detail on hospice care.

HEALTH CARE COSTS AND QUALITY

It is currently impossible to separate two initiatives facing health care institutions: managing costs and achieving high-quality patient care. Health care payers such as Medicare, Medicaid, and private insurers have tried to manage costs for many years using different payment models (Table 3.2). The Social Security Act establishes a system of payment for the operating costs of acute care hospital inpatient stays under Medicare Part A (Hospital Insurance) based on preset rates (CMS, 2017c). This payment system is referred to as the inpatient prospective payment system (PPS). Under the inpatient PPS, each case is categorized into a diagnosis-related group (DRG). Each DRG has a payment weight assigned to it based on the average resources used to treat patients covered by Medicare in that DRG (CMS, 2017c). Regardless of the amount a hospital spends to care for a patient, the DRG-established payment is the amount the hospital receives. The DRG payment groups are still used, but many payers now demand that evidence-based standards of care be followed to further reduce the cost of health care.

TABLE 3.2   COMMON HEALTH CARE PAYMENT MODELS IN THE UNITED STATES

Among current health care payment models, quality is a key component. Most health care cost reimbursement arrangements tie the final payment to achievement of key quality metrics.

Fee-for-Service	• This is the most traditional health care payment model. • Patients or payers are required to reimburse the health care provider for each service performed. • There is no incentive to implement preventive care strategies, prevent hospitalization, or take any other cost-saving measures.
Pay-for-Coordination	• The insurer coordinates care between the primary care provider and specialists. • Coordinating care helps patients and their families manage a unified plan of care and can thus reduce redundancy in expensive tests and procedures.
Pay for Performance (P4P)	• Health care providers are compensated only if they meet certain metrics for quality and efficiency. • Physician reimbursement is tied to quality benchmark measures (e.g., unplanned hospital admissions, preventive care and screening).
Bundled Payment or Episode-of-Care Payment	• The insurer determines expected services for bundles of care or episodes. • Health care providers are reimbursed for specific care bundles or episodes of care rather than for individual services. • Efficiency and quality of care are encouraged because only a set amount of money will pay for the entire episode of care
Upside Shared Savings Programs (CMS or Commercial)	• The insurer determines the expected cost of care for patients. • Health care providers are given incentives for treating specific patient populations. • A percentage of any net savings from a patient's care is given to the provider. • This model is most common with MSSP Accountable Care Organizations, but all MSSP participants must move to a downside model after 3 years.
Downside Shared Savings Programs (CMS or Commercial)	• Similar to the Upside Shared Savings Programs (see above), except the health care provider shares in any costs **or** savings related to patient care. If patient care is more expensive than anticipated, the provider is penalized, but if patient care is less expensive than expected, the provider gets a larger share of the savings. • Because providers are taking on greater risk with this model, their potential earnings are potentially higher than in an upside-only program.
Partial or Full Capitation	• Patients are assigned a per-member per-month (PMPM) payment based on their age, race, sex, lifestyle, medical history, and benefit design. • Payment rates are tied to expected usage regardless of whether the patient visits their health care provider more often or less often. • A provider is given a certain amount of money for each person covered under the system, whether or not the people who are covered access or use care. • As with bundled payment models, health care providers have an incentive to help patients avoid expensive procedures and tests to maximize their compensation. • Only certain types or categories of services are paid on a capitation basis.

CMS, Centers for Medicare and Medicaid Services; *MSSP,* Medicare Shared Savings Program.
Adapted from McKesson Corporation: *What payment models exist?* 2017, http://www.mckesson.com/population-health-management/resources/what-payment-models-exist/.

The U.S. Congress created the CMS Innovation Center to test "innovative payment and service delivery models to reduce program expenditures ... while preserving or enhancing the quality of care" for people who receive Medicare, Medicaid, or Children's Health Insurance Program (CHIP) benefits (CMS, 2017a). The Innovation Center supports the following priorities: testing new payment and service delivery models, evaluating results and advancing best practices, and engaging a broad range of stakeholders to develop additional models for testing. One example of an initiative supported by the Innovation Center is the creation of Medicare Accountable Care Organizations (ACOs). ACOs are groups of physicians, hospitals, and other health care providers who come together voluntarily to give coordinated high-quality care to their Medicare fee-for-service (FFS) beneficiaries and reduce unnecessary costs (CMS, 2017d). As of 2015, 424 ACOs participate in the CMS Shared Savings Program (CMS, 2015a).

The current Affordable Care Act ties payment to organizations offering Medicare Advantage plans to the quality ratings of the coverage they offer. If hospitals perform poorly in quality scores, they receive lower payments for services. Quality outcome measures include patient satisfaction, more effective management of care by reducing complications and readmissions, and improving care coordination. Examples of reforms that incent or "pay for value" and that are designed to build a health care system to better serve the U.S. population include (CMS, 2015a):

- *Hospital Value-Based Purchasing:* This program links a portion of a hospital's Medicare payments (1.5% of base operating DRG payment) for inpatient acute care to the hospital's performance in important quality measures. The Hospital Consumer Assessment of Healthcare Providers and Systems (HCAHPS) is the standardized survey instrument and data collection methodology CMS requires for measuring patients' perceptions of hospital care. HCAHPS is a patient satisfaction measure that sets a national standard for collecting or publicly reporting patients' perceptions. HCAHPS data enable users to make valid comparisons across all hospitals (HCAHPS, n.d.).
- *Hospital Readmissions Reduction Program:* This CMS program reduces Medicare payments to hospitals with excess patient readmissions within 30 days of hospital discharge. It is designed to encourage patient safety and care quality. The Hospital Readmissions Reduction Program increased the maximum reduction in payments in 2015 to 3% of base DRG amounts. The conditions that are regulated under this program include heart attack, heart failure, pneumonia, chronic obstructive pulmonary disease, and knee and hip replacements (National Quality Forum, 2017a). Nurses are a vital part of interdisciplinary teams. These team members collaborate to design treatment and discharge instruction protocols to reduce unnecessary patient readmissions.
- *Bundled Payments for Care Improvements:* Certain health care organizations are testing whether bundling payments for episodes of care (e.g., inpatient stays in an acute care hospital) can better coordinate care for Medicare patients

and reduce Medicare costs. This initiative focuses on improving care of people who have specific conditions. Bundling payments for services that patients receive across a single episode of care such as heart bypass surgery is one way to encourage physicians and hospitals to better coordinate care during hospitalization and after discharge (CMS, 2015a). Bundling links payments for the multiple services patients receive during an episode of care (e.g., medical, radiological, and therapeutic). Health care institutions enter into payment arrangements that include financial and performance accountability for an episode of care (CMS, 2017b).

Patient Satisfaction

Patient satisfaction is the responsibility of all health care providers. This is more important than ever because patient satisfaction measures are linked to hospital reimbursement. Patient perceptions of the quality of their health care are incorporated into quality assessment. As a result, health care organizations have made patient-centered care a major component of their health care missions (Al-Abri and Al-Balushi, 2014). Hospitals now report patient satisfaction scores for patient care units monthly. All health care staff members help identify satisfaction trends and determine ways to improve quality of care. Hospitals and other health care agencies use a variety of instruments to measure patient satisfaction, such as (Al-Abri and Al-Balushi, 2014):

- Instruments provided by private vendors. These usually are not published, and their reliability and validity are unclear.
- Public and standardized instruments such as patient satisfaction questionnaires: PSQ-18 and consumer assessment health plans (e.g., HCAHPS). Such instruments have the advantage of good reliability and validity; however, they have a limited scope of survey questions.
- Internally developed instruments. These are derived mainly from questions extracted from other instruments.

HCAHPS, developed by CMS and the Agency for Healthcare Research and Quality (AHRQ), is a patient satisfaction tool used by many hospitals to collect and publicly report data for comparison purposes (HCAHPS, n.d.). The HCAHPS survey has 32 questions that ask patients to respond about communication with physicians, communication with nurses, responsiveness of hospital staff, pain management, communication about medicines, discharge information, cleanliness of the hospital environment, quietness of the hospital environment, transition of care, and willingness to recommend the hospital (HCAHPS, n.d.). The survey also includes four screening questions and seven demographic items, which are used for adjusting the mix of patients across hospitals and for analytical purposes.

Recently, the factors that affect patient satisfaction, including relational communication techniques, hourly rounding (Box 3.4), and bedside shift report, have been the focus of many research studies (Radtke, 2013). Common factors that

BOX 3.4 EVIDENCE-BASED PRACTICE

PICOT Question: In acute care hospitals, does the use of hourly rounding by registered nurses influence patient satisfaction?

SUMMARY OF EVIDENCE

Patient satisfaction is a key measurement that affects both hospital quality ratings and reimbursement. Nurses spend a great deal of time with patients and thus have a large influence on patients' perceptions of their experiences and level of satisfaction. A systematic review of studies examining the effects of hourly rounding shows that evidence supporting the use of hourly rounding in inpatient care is of low to moderate strength because the studies were not conducted in a consistent manner (Mitchell et al., 2014). However, evidence from this study suggests that purposeful, hourly rounding improves patients' perceptions of nursing staff responsiveness in units where this may have been a problem. Hourly rounding can reduce patient falls and use of nurse call system and improves patient satisfaction scores. Hourly nurse rounding is possibly also a cost-effective intervention because it reduces injuries related to patient falls and pressure injuries, both of which often extend hospital length of stays (Brosey and March, 2014).

APPLICATION TO NURSING PRACTICE

- Proactive and regular checks of hospitalized patients during hourly rounds may reduce patient anxiety and minimize uncertainty that a nurse will be available to assist with basic needs.
- The use of a script or structure of tasks to be performed during rounding may be beneficial. Those tasks correspond to the "four P's": bathroom ("potty"), positioning, pain control, and proximity of personal items (Meade et al., 2006).
- The approach to rounding may differ by patient care setting (such as hourly rounding, rounding every 30 minutes [emergency department], or involvement of RN or nursing assistive personnel).

positively affected patient satisfaction in these studies included interpersonal skills, especially the courtesy and respect of health care providers, as well as the communication skills of explanation and clear information. These factors were more influential than other technical skills such as clinical competency and hospital equipment (Al-Abri and Al-Balushi, 2014).

Patient satisfaction is an issue in all health care settings. When the Cardei family returns to the health clinic, Corrine asks if they are satisfied with the information given to Dorina about asthma triggers. Corrine previously learned that Mr. and Mrs. Cardei sometimes struggle to understand health care terms. Corrine learns that Dorina has some questions about the triggers because she feels that she had insufficient time in the emergency department to learn the information. Corrine reviews the asthma triggers with all members of the family.

ISSUES IN HEALTH CARE DELIVERY FOR NURSING

Your familiarity with the issues facing health care will help you understand the expectations, programs, and policies used in the institution where you begin your nursing career. For example, controlling health care costs has been a major issue for the last 2 decades and has affected the way nursing care is provided and the staffing models used in hospitals. These issues will not only affect the choices you make in your career but will also affect the quality of care provided to all patients.

Nursing Shortage

The American Association of Colleges of Nursing (AACN) warns of a shortage of registered nurses (RNs) that is expected to intensify as baby boomers age and the need for health care grows (AACN, 2017). The problem is complicated by the fact that nursing schools across the United States are struggling to expand their capacity to meet the rising demand for RNs. In addition, aging nurses are retiring from the workforce. The AACN noted important shortage indicators:

- The Bureau of Labor Statistics (BLS) Employment Projections for 2012–2022 shows RNs among the top occupations in terms of job growth through 2022 (BLS, 2013). The RN workforce is expected to grow 9% (increase of 526,800) by 2022. The BLS also predicts the need for 525,000 replacement nurses in the workforce, bringing the total number of RN job openings to 1.05 million by 2022.
- The Institute of Medicine (IOM) report entitled *The Future of Nursing: Leading Change, Advancing Health* (2010) called for an 80% increase in the number of baccalaureate-prepared nurses in the workforce and doubling the population of nurses with doctoral degrees. The current nursing workforce falls far short of these recommendations, with only 55% of RNs prepared at the baccalaureate or graduate degree level.
- With the passage of the Patient Protection and Affordable Care Act in 2010, more than 32 million Americans are gaining access to health care services, including services provided by RNs and advanced practice registered nurses (APRNs) (AACN, 2017).

The nursing shortage opens great opportunities for every nurse. If you pursue further education and watch trends in health care, you will be able to find employment in any professional position you choose.

Patient-Centered Care

In a landmark report, *Crossing the Quality Chasm,* the IOM defines patient-centered care as "care that is respectful of and responsive to individual patient preferences, needs, and values and (ensures) that patient values guide all clinical decisions" (IOM, 2001). Hospitals across the United States have been implementing patient-centered care strategies, specifically delivery of care models (see Chapter 13).

Patient-centered care is much more than simply "individualizing" patient care. A critical component of patient-centered care is the nurse, patient, and family care-giver partnering to identify the patient's health care needs within the context of the patient's lifestyle. Patient-centered care also requires the entire health care team to collaborate so that the patient and family caregiver are engaged in the care process and associated decisions. This is a major shift in how care is delivered, empowering the patient and family caregiver to participate in the plan of care. Following are the eight principles of patient-centered care (National Council of State Boards of Nursing, n.d., Picker Institute, 2013), based on input from patients, families, and health care experts:

1. **Respect for patients' values, preferences, and expressed needs.** Engage patients in decision making, recognizing that they are individuals with their own unique values and preferences. Treat patients with dignity, respect, and sensitivity to their cultural values and autonomy.

2. **Coordination and integration of care.** Coordinate care to reduce patients' feelings of vulnerability:
   - Coordinate clinical care
   - Coordinate ancillary and support services
   - Coordinate frontline patient care

3. **Information and education.** Improve communication with patients and families:
   - Provide information on clinical status, progress, and prognosis
   - Provide information on processes of care
   - Provide information to facilitate autonomy, self-care, and health promotion

4. **Physical comfort.** Provide physical comfort throughout the care experience including pain management, assistance with activities and daily living needs, and providing comforting hospital surroundings and environment.

5. **Emotional support and alleviation of fear and anxiety.** Professional caregivers need to pay attention to patients' fear and anxiety:
   - Anxiety over physical status, treatment, and prognosis
   - Anxiety over the effect of the illness on themselves and family
   - Anxiety over the financial impact of illness

6. **Involvement of family and friends.** Support family and friends in taking a role in a patient's experience. Family dimensions of patient-centered care include:
   - Providing accommodations for family and friends
   - Involving family and close friends in decision making
   - Supporting family members as caregivers
   - Recognizing the needs of family and friends

7. **Continuity and transition.** Offer support and resources so that patients can care for themselves after discharge or receive the assistance they need:
   - Provide understandable, detailed information about topics such as medications, physical limitations, and dietary needs
   - Coordinate and plan treatment and services to continue after discharge
   - Provide information about access to clinical, social, physical, and financial support continually

8. **Access to care.** Patients need to know they can access care when it is needed, especially ambulatory care:
   - Access to hospitals, clinics, and physician offices
   - Availability of transportation
   - Ease in scheduling appointments
   - Availability of appointments when needed
   - Accessibility of specialists or specialty services when a referral is made
   - Clear instructions provided on when and how to get referrals

---

QSEN ACTIVITY *Patient-Centered Care*

Alex Cardei falls while working on a ladder at work in the hospital. He fractured his right leg and is admitted through the emergency department for surgery.
- Based on what you know about the Cardei family, identify three ways to promote patient-centered care while he is hospitalized.

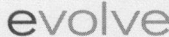 Answers to QSEN Activities can be found on the Evolve website.

Magnet Recognition Program

The American Nurses Credentialing Center (ANCC, 2017) established the Magnet Recognition® Program to honor health care organizations that achieve excellence in nursing practice. Health care organizations that apply for Magnet® status must demonstrate quality patient care, nursing excellence, and innovation in professional practice. The professional work environment must allow nurses to practice with a sense of empowerment and autonomy to deliver quality nursing care. The Magnet® Model is an empirical model consisting of Model Components—Transformational Leadership, Structural Empowerment, Exemplary Professional Practice, New Knowledge, Innovation and Improvements, and Empirical Outcomes—embedded within the context of ever-present Global Issues in Nursing and Health Care. The Magnet® Model serves as a framework for the Magnet Recognition Program's® emphasis on the impact of organizational structure and process to achieve superior performance as evidenced by outcomes (Table 3.3).

Institutions must present strong evidence that they have achieved these model components in order to achieve Magnet® status. Magnet® status requires nurses to use evidence-based practice and engage in research activities. Hospitals that have achieved Magnet® status foster positive work environments and nurse satisfaction, which can improve nurse retention (Renter and Allen, 2014).

Technology in Health Care

Technological advances continually affect health care organizations and change the ways nurses deliver evidence-based care to patients (Simpson, 2012). Emerging technologies that will change nursing practice include genetics and genomics, less invasive and more accurate tools for diagnosis and

TABLE 3.3 MAGNET® MODEL

FORCES OF MAGNETISM	EMPIRICAL DOMAINS OF EVIDENCE	MAGNET® MODEL COMPONENTS
1. Quality of Nursing Leadership 3. Management Style	Leadership	Transformational Leadership
2. Organizational Structure 4. Personnel Policies and Programs 10. Community and the Healthcare Organization 12. Image of Nursing 14. Professional Development	Resource Utilization and Development	Structural Empowerment
5. Professional Models of Care 8. Consultation and Resources 9. Autonomy 11. Nurses as Teachers 13. Interdisciplinary (Interprofessional) Relationships 6. Quality of Care: Ethics, Patient Safety, and Quality Infrastructure 7. Quality Improvement	Professional Practice Model Safe and Ethical Practice Autonomous Practice Quality Processes	Exemplary Professional Practice (EP)
6. Quality of Care: Research- and Evidence-Based Practice 7. Quality Improvement	Research	New Knowledge, Innovations, and Improvements (NK)
6. Quality of Care	Outcomes	Empirical Quality Outcomes

From American Nurses Credentialing Center: *Magnet Model,* 2017, http://www.nursecredentialing.org/Magnet/ProgramOverview/New-Magnet-Model.

treatment, three-dimensional printing, robotics, biometrics, EHRs (see Chapter 10), and computerized physician/provider order entry and clinical decision support (Huston, 2013). Technology makes your work easier in many ways, but it does not replace your judgment. For example, when you manage an IV infusion smart pump, you monitor the device to ensure that it infuses on schedule and without complications despite its numerous automatic settings. An infusion device infuses at a constant rate, but you must confirm the rate is calculated correctly. An infusion device sets off an alarm if the infusion slows, making it important for you to respond to the alarm and fix the problem. Technology does not replace a nurse's astute, critical eye and clinical judgment.

Robotics is a form of emerging technology that will greatly affect how nursing is practiced in the future. Experts estimate that robotic use will grow because of workforce shortages, a growing elderly population, and a call for higher quality care not subject to human limitations (Huston, 2013). Robotic applications include food service, medication distribution, infection control, surgery, and diagnosing patients (Maleski, 2014). Another area with great potential for impacting nursing is the use of robots as direct care providers (Huston, 2013). Maleski (2014) reports that there are daily care robots designed to support older patients and people with disabilities in activities such as preparing and serving meals and daily care tasks. In addition, exoskeleton-powered robots can help patients with paraplegia stand with the goal of reducing morbidity and augmenting physical therapy. The implications for nursing are significant. Nursing must be on the front line in deciding how robotics are used to advocate for patients and families as well as ensure professional standards of care are delivered.

Telemedicine is a technology that relies on interactive video and uses medical information gathered and reviewed at one site (such as a hospital, home, clinic, or urgent care center) and transmits treatment recommendations to another site to improve a patient's clinical health status (American Telemedicine Association, 2016). A variety of applications and services use two-way video, smartphones, wireless tools, and other forms of telecommunications technology. However, varying state policies on telemedicine use and reimbursement pose an obstacle to wider adoption of this emerging practice (Urbina, 2013). Research shows that specific telemedicine applications (such as the Hospital at Home model and management of chronic illness) save patients, providers, and payers money compared with traditional approaches (American Telemedicine Association, 2015).

Health Care Disparities

The National Quality Forum (2017b) reports that health care disparities are linked to inadequate resources, poor patient-provider communication, a lack of culturally competent care (see Chapter 21), and inadequate access to patient language services, among other factors. The health care system and the many professionals who serve patients must address these factors and reduce their effect so that all patients receive equal treatment. One strategy is to establish and support policies that positively influence social and economic conditions and

BOX 3.5   SOCIAL DETERMINANTS OF HEALTH

- Availability of resources to meet daily needs (such as safe housing, local food markets, pharmacy)
- Access to educational, economic, and job opportunities
- Access to health care services
- Quality of education and job training
- Availability of community-based resources in support of community living and opportunities for recreational and leisure activities
- Transportation options
- Public safety
- Social support
- Social norms and attitudes (such as discrimination, racism, distrust of health care providers)
- Exposure to crime, violence, and social disorder
- Socioeconomic conditions (such as concentrated poverty and stressful conditions that accompany it)
- Residential segregation
- Language/literacy
- Access to mass media and emerging technologies
- Culture

Adapted from *Healthy People 2020: Social determinants of health,* 2017. https://www.healthypeople.gov/2020/topics-objectives/topic/social-determinants-of-health.

support changes in individual behavior, such as pursuing healthy diets and adhering to medication regimens.

Healthy People 2020 recognizes that health starts in our homes, schools, workplaces, and communities. One of the *Healthy People 2020* goals for the decade is to "Create social and physical environments that promote good health for all" (*Healthy People 2020,* 2017). Nurses practice in a wide variety of settings that require an awareness of the social determinants of health and that contribute to health disparities (Box 3.5) (see Chapter 21). Nursing plays a key role in promoting access to health care and offering appropriate teaching resources to patients and families.

KEY POINTS

- Levels of health care describe the scope of services and settings in which health care is delivered to patients in all stages of health and illness.
- The primary level of health care includes medical health care services, health education, nutritional care, maternal/child health care, family planning, and control of diseases.
- Nurses and other health care providers offer preventive services at every level of health care.
- Hospitals deliver health care to patients who are acutely ill and need comprehensive specialized secondary and tertiary health care.
- Access of rural Americans to health care is affected by economic factors (rural Americans are more likely to live below the poverty level), cultural and social differences, educational shortcomings, lack of recognition of the problem by legislators, and the isolation of living in remote rural areas.

- The holistic model of care is used within integrated health care systems and delivers a coordinated continuum of services that supports patients with chronic conditions and improves the health of specific populations.
- Expertise in assessment is a critical competency of home health nurses.
- The Patient Protection and Affordable Care Act pays hospitals for value by tying payment from Medicare Advantage plans to the quality ratings of the coverage they offer.
- Hospital value-based purchasing is an example of pay for value and is promoted by the Centers for Medicare and Medicaid Services.
- Preventive services are health-related activities delivered in a care setting and include health promotion and disease prevention (primary prevention), curing disease (secondary prevention), and reducing complications (tertiary prevention).
- Barriers to effective discharge planning include ineffective communication, lack of role clarity among health care team members, and lack of resources.
- In restorative care settings, nurses know that success depends on their effective and early partnering with patients and their families.
- As a nurse, you can promote patient satisfaction through interpersonal skills including courtesy, respect, and good communication skills.
- The nursing shortage opens vast opportunities to nurses. If you pursue further education and follow trends in health care, many professional options will be available to you.

REFLECTIVE LEARNING

- Consider a patient you cared for recently while in a clinical area. Identify three social determinants of health that might affect that patient's access to health care.
- Spend some time in the clinical area shadowing a registered nurse. Describe three approaches that the nurse uses to deliver patient-centered care.
- Interview a patient during your clinical day and determine whether he or she is satisfied with the level of care received. Avoid using yes/no questions to elicit their perceptions.

REVIEW QUESTIONS

1. Which of the following describe characteristics of an integrated health care system? (Select all that apply.)
   1. The focus is holistic.
   2. Participating hospitals follow the same model of health care delivery.
   3. The system coordinates a continuum of services.
   4. The focus of health care providers is finding a cure for patients.
   5. Members of the health care team link electronically to use the electronic medical record to share the patient's health care record.

2. A school nurse has been following a 9-year-old student who has behavioral problems in class. The student acts out and does not follow teacher instructions. The nurse plans to meet with the student's family and learn more about social determinants of health that might be affecting them. Which of the following factors are appropriate for this type of assessment? (Select all that apply.)
   1. The student's seating placement in the classroom
   2. The level of support parents offer when the student completes homework
   3. The level of violence in the family's neighborhood
   4. The age at which the child first began having behavioral problems
   5. The cultural values about education held by the family
3. A hospital that supports models of care that encourage professional engagement, commitment to professional development, and engagement of professional staff members in community health activities meets which component of the Magnet model?
   1. Exemplary professional practice
   2. Transformational leadership
   3. Structural empowerment
   4. Empirical outcomes

4. Which of the following are common barriers to effective discharge planning? (Select all that apply.)
   1. Ineffective communication among providers
   2. Lack of role clarity among health care team members
   3. Sufficient number of hospital beds to manage patient volume
   4. Patient's long-term disabilities
   5. Patient's cultural background
5. A nurse newly hired at a community hospital learns about hourly rounding during orientation. Which of the following are known evidence-based outcomes from hourly rounding? (Select all that apply.)
   1. Reduction in nurse staffing requirements.
   2. Improved patient perceptions of nursing staff responsiveness
   3. Reduction in patient falls
   4. Increased costs
   5. Reduction in patient use of nurse call system

evolve

Additional Review Questions, as well as rationales for all Review Questions, can be found on the Evolve website.

1, 3, 5; 2, 3, 5; 3, 4, 1, 2; 5, 2, 3, 5.

REFERENCES

Al-Abri R, Al-Balushi A: Patient satisfaction survey as a tool towards quality improvement, *Oman Med J* 29(1):3–7, 2014.

Alzheimer's Association: *Alzheimer's and dementia caregiver center: respite care*, 2017. https://www.alz.org/care/alzheimers-dementia-caregiver-respite.asp.

American Academy of Family Physicians: *Patient-centered medical home*, 2017. http://www.aafp.org/about/policies/all/medical-home.html.

American Association of Colleges of Nursing (AACN): *Nursing shortage*, 2017. http://www.aacn.nche.edu/media-relations/fact-sheets/nursing-shortage.

American Association of Colleges of Nursing (AACN): *Policy brief: nurse-managed health clinics: increasing access to primary care and educating the healthcare workforce*, 2014. http://www.aacn.nche.edu/government-affairs/FY13NMHCs.pdf.

American Hospital Association: *Fast facts on US hospitals*, 2017. http://www.aha.org/research/rc/stat-studies/fast-facts.shtml.

American Hospital Association: *Quality and patient safety*, 2016-2017. http://www.aha.org/advocacy-issues/quality/index.shtml.

American Nurses Association (ANA): *Health care transformation: the Affordable Care*

Act and more, 2014. http://nursingworld.org/MainMenuCategories/Policy-Advocacy/HealthSystemReform/HealthCareReformResources/More-on-Health-Care-Reform/AffordableCareAct.pdf.

American Nurses Credentialing Center (ANCC): *Magnet Model*, 2017. http://www.nursecredentialing.org/Magnet/ProgramOverview/New-Magnet-Model.

American Telemedicine Association: *About telemedicine*, 2016. https://www.americantelemed.org/about/telehealth-faqs.

American Telemedicine Association: *Research outcomes: telemedicine's impact on healthcare cost and quality*, 2015. https://pdfs.semanticscholar.org/c16e/8540a99c5ed82373adc7374541ade81f092c.pdf.

Brosey L, March KS: Effectiveness of structured hourly nurse rounding on patient satisfaction and clinical outcomes, *J Nurs Care Qual* 30(2): 2014. https://www.researchgate.net/publication/265863446_Effectiveness_of_Structured_Hourly_Nurse_Rounding_on_Patient_Satisfaction_and_Clinical_Outcomes.

Bureau of Labor Statistics (BLS): *Economic news release*, 2013. http://www.bls.gov/news.release/ecopro.t08.htm.

Center for American Progress: *The importance of community health centers: engines of economic activity and job creation*, 2010. https://www.americanprogress.org/issues/healthcare/report/2010/08/09/8195/the-importance-of-community-health-centers/.

Centers for Disease Control and Prevention (CDC): *Workplace health promotion: health outcome measures*, 2015a. http://www.cdc.gov/workplacehealthpromotion/model/evaluation/outcomes.html.

Centers for Disease Control and Prevention (CDC): *Whole school, whole community, whole child (WSCC): a collaborative approach to learning and health*, 2015b. http://www.cdc.gov/healthyschools/wscc/index.htm.

Centers for Medicare and Medicaid Services (CMS): *Better care, smarter spending, healthier people: improving our health care delivery system*, 2015a. https://www.cms.gov/Newsroom/MediaReleaseDatabase/Fact-sheets/2015-Fact-sheets-items/2015-01-26.html.

Centers for Medicare and Medicaid Services (CMS): *Long-term care facility resident assessment instrument 3.0 user's manual version 1.13*, 2015b. https://www.cms.gov/Medicare/Quality-Initiatives-Patient-Assessment

-Instruments/NursingHomeQualityInits/
Downloads/MDS-30-RAI-Manual
-V113.pdf.

Centers for Medicare and Medicaid Services
(CMS): *Home health quality initiative*,
2016. https://www.cms.gov/Medicare/
Quality-Initiatives-Patient-Assessment
-Instruments/HomeHealthQualityInits/
index.html?redirect=/HomeHealth
QualityInits/.

Centers for Medicare and Medicaid Services
(CMS): *About the CMS innovation center*,
2017a. https://innovation.cms.gov/about/
index.html.

Centers for Medicare and Medicaid Services
(CMS): *Bundled payments for care
improvements: general information*,
2017b. https://innovation.cms.gov/
initiatives/bundled-payments/.

Centers for Medicare and Medicaid Services
(CMS): *Acute inpatient PPS*, 2017c.
https://www.cms.gov/Medicare/
Medicare-Fee-for-Service-Payment/
AcuteInpatientPPS/index.html?redirect=/
acuteinpatientpps/.

Centers for Medicare and Medicaid Services
(CMS): *Shared savings programs*, 2017d.
https://www.cms.gov/Medicare/
Medicare-Fee-For-Service-Payment/
sharedsavingsprogram/index.html.

Coleman EA, et al: The care transitions
intervention: results of a randomized
controlled trial, *Arch Intern Med*
166:1822–1828, 2006.

Counsell S: *10 key components of a
post-discharge care model*, June 2015.
http://www.beckershospitalreview.com/
quality/10-key-components-of-
a-post-discharge-care-model.html.

Department of Health and Human Services
Centers for Medicare and Medicaid
Services (DHHS CMS): *Discharge
planning*, 2014. https://www.cms.gov/
Outreach-and-Education/Medicare
-Learning-Network-MLN/MLNProducts/
Downloads/Discharge-Planning-Booklet
-ICN908184.pdf.

HealthIT.gov: *Benefits for critical access
hospitals and other small rural hospitals*,
2015. https://www.healthit.gov/
providers-professionals/benefits-critical
-access-hospitals-and-other-small
-rural-hospitals.

*Healthy People 2020: Social determinants of
health*, 2017. https://www.healthypeople
.gov/2020/topics-objectives/topic/social
-determinants-of-health.

Honberg R: *State mental health cuts: a
national crisis, National Alliance on
Mental Illness*, 2011. https://
www.nami.org/getattachment/

About-NAMI/Publications/Reports/
NAMIStateBudgetCrisis2011.pdf.

Hospital Consumer Assessment of
Healthcare Providers and Systems
(HCAHPS): *CAHPS Hospital Survey*,
n.d.. http://www.hcahpsonline.org.

Huston C: The impact of emerging
technology on nursing care: "warp speed
ahead," *Online J Issues Nurs* 18(2):2013.

Institute of Medicine (IOM): *Crossing the
quality chasm: a new health system for the
21st century*, Washington, DC, 2001,
National Academies Press.

Institute of Medicine (IOM): *The future of
nursing: leading change, advancing health*,
Washington, DC, 2010, National
Academies Press.

Legal Information Institute: 42 U.S. Code §
1395i-3. *Requirements for, and assuring
quality of care in, skilled nursing facilities*,
2010. https://www.law.cornell.edu/
uscode/text/42/1395i-3.

Mabire C, et al: Effectiveness of nursing
discharge planning interventions on
health-related outcomes in elderly
inpatients discharged home: a systematic
review protocol, *JBI Database System Rev
Implement Rep* 11(8):2013.

Maleski DA: *Health care robotics: automated
devices to handle tough hospital tasks*,
Health Facilities Management, 2014.
http://www.hfmmagazine.com/articles/
1328-health-care-robotics.

Meade CM, et al: Effects of nursing rounds:
on patients' call light use, satisfaction,
and safety, *Am J Nurs* 106(9):58–70, 2006.

Medicaid.gov: *Nursing facilities (NF)*, n.d..
https://www.medicaid.gov/medicaid
-chip-program-information/by-topics/
delivery-systems/institutional-care/
nursing-facilities-nf.html.

Meiner SE: *Gerontologic nursing*, ed 5,
St Louis, 2015, Mosby.

Michigan Care Management Resource
Center: *High intensity care model*, 2017.
http://micmrc.org/programs/high
-intensity-care-model.

Mitchell MD, et al: Hourly rounding to
improve nursing responsiveness: a
systematic review, *J Nurs Adm* 44:
462–472, 2014.

National Alliance on Mental Illness (NAMI):
Mental health by the numbers, 2017.
http://www.nami.org/Learn-More/
Mental-Health-By-the-Numbers.

National Council of State Boards of Nursing:
Transition to practice, n.d., https://www
.ncsbn.org/transition-to-practice.htm.

National Quality Forum: *National efforts to
reduce readmissions are helping more
patients heal at home*, 2017a. http://

www.qualityforum.org/Readmissions_-_
Home_vs_Hospitals.aspx.

National Quality Forum: *Disparities*, 2017b.
http://www.qualityforum.org/Topics/
Disparities.aspx.

National Rural Health Association (NRHA):
About rural health care, 2017. http://
www.ruralhealthweb.org/go/left/
about-rural-health/what-s-different
-about-rural-health-care.

Naylor MD, et al: Translating research into
practice: transitional care for older adults,
J Eval Clin Pract 15(6):1164–1170, 2009.

Okoniewska B, et al: Barriers to discharge in
an acute care medical teaching unit: a
qualitative analysis of health providers'
perceptions, *J Multidiscip Healthc*
8:83–89, 2015.

Picker Institute: *Principles of patient-centered
care*, 2013. http://pickerinstitute.org/
about/picker-principles/.

Radtke K: Improving patient satisfaction
with nursing communication using
bedside shift report, *Clin Nurse Spec*
27(1):19–25, 2013.

Renter M, Allen A: How Magnet®
designation affects nurse retention: an
evidence-based research project,
Am Nurse Today 9(3):2014. https://
americannursetoday.com/how-magnet
-designation-affects-nurse-retention-an
-evidence-based-research-project/.

Research Data Assistance Center (ResDac):
*The Home Health Outcome and
Assessment Information Set (OASIS)*,
2012. https://www.resdac.org/resconnect/
articles/129.

Simpson RL: Technology enables
value-based nursing care, *Nurs Adm Q*
36(1):85, 2012.

Stirling C, et al: Why carers use adult day
respite: a mixed method case study, *BMC
Health Serv Res* 14:245, 2014.

Strandberg-Larsen M, Krasnik A:
Measurement of integrated healthcare
delivery: a systematic review of methods
and future research directions, *Int J
Integr Care* 9:e01, Published online
February 4, 2009.

The Joint Commission (TJC): *2017
comprehensive accreditation manual for
hospitals*, Oakbrook Terrace, IL, 2017,
The Commission.

Urbina Z: *Healthcare IT Connect, top 12
health information technology issues*,
2013. http://www.healthcareitconnect
.com/list-top-12-health-information
-technology-issues/.

World Health Organization (WHO): *Health
topics: rehabilitation*, 2017. http://www
.who.int/topics/rehabilitation/en/.

4

Community-Based Nursing Practice

evolve MEDIA RESOURCES

http://evolve.elsevier.com/Potter/essentials
- Audio Glossary

- QSEN Activity and Review Questions Answers and Rationales

OBJECTIVES

- Explain the relationship between public and community health nursing.
- Differentiate community health nursing from community-based nursing.
- Describe the role of the community health nurse.
- Discuss the role of the nurse in community-based practice.

- Explain the characteristics of patients from vulnerable populations that influence a nurse's approach to care.
- Describe competencies important for success in community-based nursing practice.
- Describe elements of a community assessment.

KEY TERMS

community-based nursing, p. 51
community health nursing, p. 50

incidence rates, p. 50
population, p. 50

public health nursing, p. 50
vulnerable populations, p. 51

CASE STUDY *Homeless in the Community*

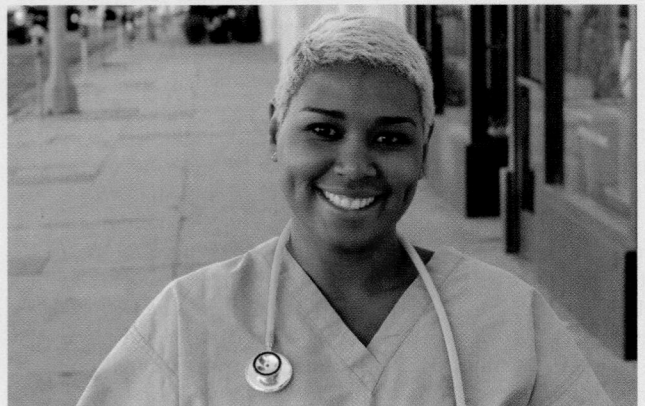

Copyright © ajr_images/iStock/Thinkstock.

Shanise Prezi is a registered nurse and works at a community health center located within an impoverished area of a culturally diverse medium-size city. The center is dedicated

to improving the health and well-being of underserved, low-income residents in the community by providing and coordinating accessible and comprehensive quality health care. There are many health needs affecting the community, which is composed of people who are Hispanic, Arabic, Albanian, African American, and Portuguese. The health problems and needs of the community include tobacco use, substance abuse, mental health, and homelessness. Many of the patients who visit the center are homeless or at risk for becoming homeless. There is a lack of preventive health care practices due to language barriers, lack of insurance, economic factors, and poor health literacy. Shanise reflects daily about her work and experiences at the center. She realizes there is a need to reach out to stakeholders to further assess the needs of her community. Shanise discusses her concerns with the public health nurse, several church and city leaders, business leaders, and community groups. Together they identify access to health care and homelessness as primary concerns.

Community-based care is a model of care that emphasizes the provision of integrated, coordinated, and continuous health care services in a community with a focus on the care of illnesses. Care of patients in acute care settings is short-term. Therefore health care delivery services in the community are essential and provide access where people and their families live, work, socialize, and learn. Community-based health care takes place in health clinics, provider offices, home health, or school-based clinics (Stanhope and Lancaster, 2016). Community-based health care is a collaborative, evidence-based model designed to meet the health needs of every member of the community.

The terms *community health nursing* and *public health nursing* are used interchangeably to encompass a population focus with special attention to advocacy, community organizing, health education, political reform, and policy development (ANA, 2013). It is not setting specific. Whether community based or public health focused, health promotion and disease prevention at each level (primary, secondary and tertiary) are at the heart of professional nursing practice (see Chapter 2).

Throughout the history of nursing, many nurses have established and met the public health needs of communities, their patients, and their families. Within community health settings, nurses are leaders in assessing, planning, implementing, and evaluating the types of public and community health services their communities need. Community health nursing and community-based nursing are part of the health care delivery system (see Chapter 3) necessary to improve and maintain the health of the general public.

A healthy community includes elements that maintain a high quality of life and productivity. Safety and access to health care services enable people to function productively in their community (USDHHS, 2017). As community health care partnerships evolve, nurses are in strategic positions to play an important role in health care delivery and improve the health of communities.

ACHIEVING HEALTHY POPULATIONS AND COMMUNITIES

The U.S. Department of Health and Human Services Public Health Service designed the *Healthy People Initiative* to improve the overall health status of people living in the United States and establishes ongoing health care goals (Fig. 4.1; also see Chapter 2). The overall goals of *Healthy People 2020* are to increase the life expectancy and quality of life and eliminate health disparities through an improved delivery of health care services (USDHHS, 2017).

Improved delivery of health care occurs through the assessment of the health care needs of individuals, families, and members of the community; development and implementation of public health policies; and improved access to care. Assessment includes systematic data collection about the population, monitoring the health status of the population, and accessing information about the community

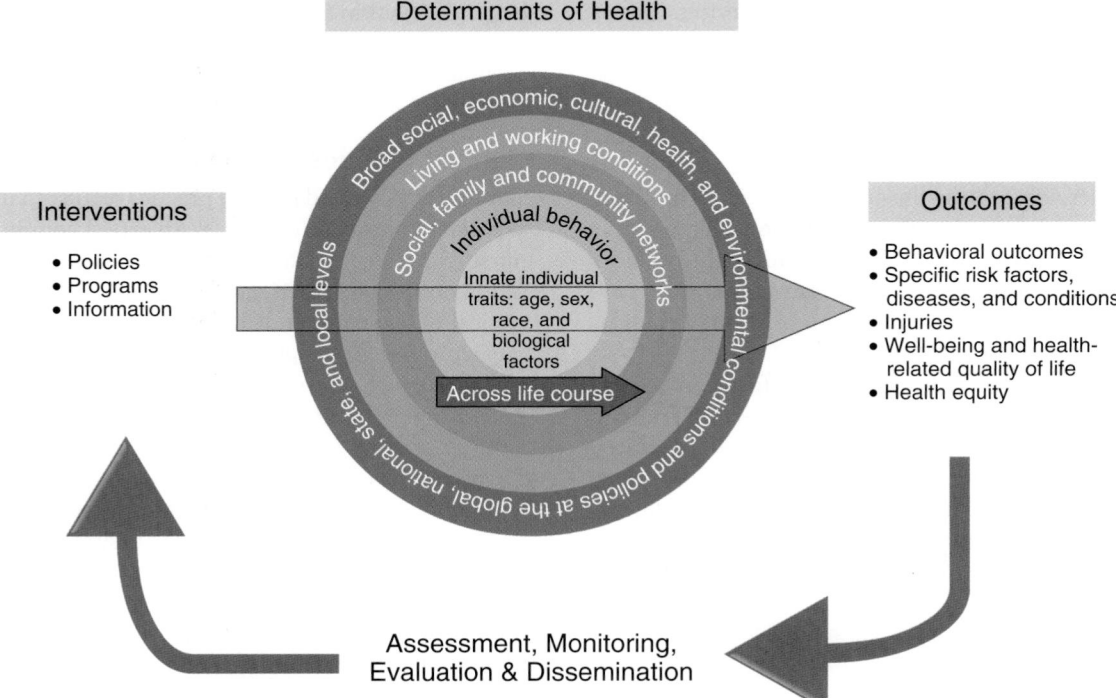

FIG 4.1 Action model for achieving *Healthy People 2020* Goals. (From U.S. Department of Health and Human Services, Public Health Service: *Phase 1 Report: recommendations for the framework and format of Healthy People 2020*. http://www.healthypeople.gov/HP2020/advisory/Phase1/summary.htm.)

(Stanhope and Lancaster, 2016). Results of data analysis lead to development of community health promotion programs such as exercise programs for school-aged children to reduce the risks for childhood obesity, nutrition education for expectant mothers, and smoking cessation programs for adolescents. In addition, assessment helps to gather information on incidence rates such as identifying and reporting new infections, determining adolescent pregnancy rates, and reporting the number of motor vehicle collisions by teenage drivers.

Community health professionals (e.g., public health nurses) are involved in developing and implementing public policy to improve the health of the community. Research-based findings help to design and implement health-related policies for the community. For example, a group of public health nurses find data identifying an increased incidence in motor vehicle collision fatalities when the driver is between 16 and 18 years old and driving after midnight. They use these data to work with local legislators to develop driving restrictions for new teenage drivers to reduce motor vehicle fatalities.

Improved access to care ensures that essential community-wide health services are available and accessible to the total community (Stanhope and Lancaster, 2016). Examples include coordination of prenatal health care and well-baby immunization programs for people who are uninsured. Population-based public health programs center on interventions aimed at disease prevention, health protection, and health promotion. These strategies provide the foundation for health care services at all levels (see Chapter 3).

Chapter 3 described six levels of health services. Except for secondary acute care and tertiary care, community-based services can be offered within existing health care services. For example, a rural community has a hospital that meets the acute care needs of its patients. While completing a community assessment, a community health nurse notices that there are few services to meet the needs of expectant mothers, reduce teenage smoking, or provide nutritional support for older adults. The nurse uses these data to begin building community-based primary care and preventive care programs that provide these services to improve the health of specific populations in the community.

The principles of public health practice focus on achieving a healthy environment in which all individuals, families, and their communities can live (Stanhope and Lancaster, 2016). Nursing plays a role in providing all levels of the health services. By using public health principles, you are able to better understand the environment in which patients live and the types of interventions necessary to help keep them healthy.

PUBLIC HEALTH NURSING

A public health nursing focus requires understanding the needs of a population, or a collection of individuals who have one or more personal or environmental characteristics in common (Stanhope and Lancaster, 2016). Examples of populations include high-risk infants, homeless people, and a cultural group such as Native Americans.

As a public health nurse, you need to understand factors that influence health promotion and health maintenance of populations, trends and patterns influencing the incidence of disease within these populations, environmental factors, such as pollution, that contribute to health and illness, and the political processes used to affect public policy. For example, you use data regarding car accidents involving adolescents' use of cell phones or texting while driving to lobby for support of a policy ban on texting while driving.

COMMUNITY HEALTH NURSING

Community health nursing is nursing care provided in the community with the primary focus on the health care of populations (e.g., high-risk infants, homeless people) in the community. The goal is to preserve, protect, promote, or maintain health to create and maintain healthy conditions in which all people live (Stanhope and Lancaster, 2016). The emphasis is on improving the quality of health and life within that community. Additionally, community health nurses provide direct care services to subpopulations within that community. These subpopulations are often a clinical focus in which a nurse has gained expertise. A community health nurse who works as a case manager follows older adults recovering from stroke and sees the need for community rehabilitation services; or a nurse administers immunoglobulin (IG) to a susceptible group of people in the community with the objective of managing and preventing the spread of hepatitis A within the community. By focusing on subpopulations, a community health nurse cares for the community as a whole and considers the individual or family to be only one member of a group at risk (Stanhope and Lancaster, 2016).

Nursing Practice in Community Health

Community-focused nursing practice requires a unique set of skills and knowledge (Box 4.1). An expert community health nurse comes to understand the needs of a population or community through experiences with individual families and clinical understanding of health and illness and by creating opportunities for people to live healthier physically, mentally, and socially. The nurse uses critical thinking to apply knowledge of public health principles, community health nursing, family dynamics (see Chapter 25), and communication (see Chapter 11) to identify the best approaches to collaborating with individuals and families within the population.

Successful community health nursing practice involves building relationships with members of a community and responding to changes within a community. When a community health nurse notices an increase in the number of grandparents assuming child care responsibilities, the nurse works collaboratively with local schools to establish a program to assist and support grandparents in the caregiving role. Community health nurses also work in partnership with community members and health care providers to explore resources and establish goals. They promote and maintain

BOX 4.1 SYNTHESIS IN PRACTICE

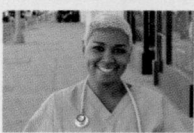

Copyright ©
ajr_images/iStock/
Thinkstock.

Shanise observes that the patients who are homeless and come to the free clinic tend to walk to the clinic and carry their belongings with them. When the patients come to the clinic, Shanise uses assessment skills to obtain as much information from the patients at the time of the visit. She asks her patients about medical conditions or medications taken. Many patients have a history of mental illnesses and substance abuse, and they do not usually carry wallets with them, as the wallets are easily stolen in the shelters or on the streets. They do not have cell phones and cannot obtain medicines because pharmacies normally require an address and a phone number.

Shanise practices the ethical principle of beneficence and believes it is very important to take a caring, nonjudgmental, and holistic approach in the care of her patients. She recognizes there is much stigma around mental illnesses and homelessness and works collaboratively with staff and health providers at the clinic to deliver compassionate and coordinated care based on respect. Shanise understands that these patients are not likely to follow up for preventive care. She explores strategies to strengthen the clinic services and sustain the program over time.

a community's health by planning, evaluating, negotiating, and supporting programs focusing on prevention of illness, injury, and disability (Stanhope and Lancaster, 2016).

Community health nurses often work with complex systems (e.g., welfare system) and encourage them to be more responsive to the needs of a population. Developing your skills of patient advocacy, communicating people's concerns, and designing new systems in cooperation with existing systems will help you make nursing practice in the community effective.

COMMUNITY-BASED NURSING

You provide community-based nursing in community settings such as the home, a health center, or clinics where the focus is on the nursing care of ill individuals or families. You work in home health to care for patients recovering from acute illnesses or who are disabled or chronically ill (see Chapter 3). In these settings, you provide care that focuses on the safety needs of individuals and families and enhance their ability for self-care and independent decision making (Stanhope and Lancaster, 2016). Use critical thinking when caring for an individual patient and family—assessing health status, selecting nursing interventions, and evaluating outcomes of care. When providing direct care services where patients live, work, and play, it is important to be knowledgeable about the diverse needs of the individual and family and appreciate differences in style and ethnic and cultural practices. For example, you work in a home health care setting

with a patient who is newly diagnosed with diabetes to create a comprehensive plan for the patient's health. As the nurse-patient relationship evolves, you begin to understand the patient's habits or lifestyle patterns and learn how these change when the patient is with friends and co-workers. Knowing the community and available resources (e.g., medical supply shops for glucose monitoring and local diabetes association support groups) helps you provide comprehensive support for the patient's needs. Ultimately, as a community-based nurse, you help patients and their families assume responsibility for their health care decisions.

Vulnerable Populations

In the community setting, nurses care for patients from diverse cultures and backgrounds and with various health conditions. However, changes in the health care delivery system have made high-risk groups the community health nurse's principal patients. For example, visiting low-risk mothers and babies is unlikely. Instead you are more likely to make home visits to adolescent mothers or mothers with substance-use disorders.

Vulnerable populations are groups of patients who are more likely to develop health problems as a result of excess risks, limited access to health care services, and dependency on others for care. Vulnerable populations include individuals living in poverty, older adults, homeless people, people in abusive relationships, people with substance-abuse problems and/or mental illnesses, and new immigrants. Often vulnerable individuals belong to more than one group, with cumulative effects on their health. Some individuals who are homeless also have chronic physical conditions, mental illnesses, and substance-use disorders. These individuals typically have poorer outcomes than patients who are not homeless and have readily available access to resources and health care services.

The special needs of vulnerable populations create challenges when caring for patients with increasingly complex acute and chronic health conditions. You need to determine community needs and appropriate interventions that will be successful in improving a community's level of health. Communication skills and caring practices are critical in identifying and understanding patients' perceptions of their problems and planning successful health care strategies. Box 4.2 summarizes guidelines to follow when assessing members of vulnerable population groups.

Immigrant Populations. The immigrant population in the United States, based on census bureau data for 2014 and 2015, is 42.4 million people; this is the largest number in American history (Ziegler and Camarota, 2016). This growth creates potential for multiple health issues and health care needs, posing significant legal and health policy issues. For some immigrants, access to health care is limited because of legal status; language barriers; and lack of benefits, resources, and transportation. In addition, some immigrant populations have specific health care risks such as hepatitis B, tuberculosis, or dental problems. Immigrant populations often

BOX 4.2   GUIDELINES FOR ASSESSING MEMBERS OF VULNERABLE POPULATION GROUPS

SETTING THE STAGE

- Create a comfortable, nonthreatening environment.
- Obtain information about the culture to gain an understanding of practices, beliefs, and values that affect health care.
- Understand the meaning of the patient's language and nonverbal behavior to complete a culturally competent assessment (see Chapter 21).
- Be sensitive to the fact that patients often have priorities other than their health care such as financial, legal, or social issues. Help them with these concerns before beginning a health assessment. If the patient needs financial assistance, consult a social worker. If there are legal issues, provide the patient with a resource. Do not attempt to provide financial or legal advice yourself.

NURSING HISTORY OF AN INDIVIDUAL OR FAMILY

- Because you often have only one opportunity to conduct a nursing history, obtain an organized history of all the essential information needed to help the individual or family during that visit.
- Collect data on a comprehensive form that focuses on the specific needs of the vulnerable population. However, be flexible so as not to overlook important health information. For example, when with an adolescent mother, obtain a nutritional history on both the mother and the baby. Be aware of the developmental needs of the adolescent mother, and listen to her social needs as well.
- Identify both developmental and health care needs. Remember, the goal is to collect enough information to provide family-centered care.
- Identify any risks to the patient's immune system. This is especially important for vulnerable patients who are homeless and sleep in shelters.

PHYSICAL EXAMINATION AND HOME ASSESSMENT

- Complete as thorough a physical and/or home assessment as possible. However, collect only data that will be important when providing care to the patient and family.
- Be alert for signs of physical or substance abuse (e.g., inappropriately clothed to hide bruising, underweight, runny nose).
- When assessing a patient's home, observe: Is there adequate water and plumbing? What is the status of the utilities? Are foods and perishables stored properly? Are there signs of insects or vermin? Is the paint peeling? Are the windows and doors adequate? Are there water stains on the ceiling? Is there evidence of a leaky roof? What is the temperature? Is it comfortable? Observe the outside environment: Are there vacant houses and/or lots nearby? Is there a busy intersection? What is the crime level?

Modified from Stanhope M, Lancaster J: *Public health nursing: population-centered health care in the community,* ed 9, St Louis, 2016, Elsevier.

practice nontraditional healing practices. It is important that you understand how these practices interfere with or complement traditional therapies. It is crucial for you to work collaboratively with a patient's health care provider to listen to the patient, explain perceptions, and acknowledge differences (see Chapter 21). You and the health care provider need to collaborate with the patient to develop a treatment plan that is sensitive to the physical, psychological, and safety needs of the patient, family, or community.

Poor and Homeless People.   People who live in poverty are more likely to live in poor living environments, work at high-risk jobs, have lack of access to adequate nutritious foods, and have multiple stressors in their lives such as poor or unreliable transportation (Box 4.3). Homeless patients have even fewer resources than poor patients. They are usually jobless, do not have shelter, and must cope with finding food and a place to sleep at night. Chronic health problems worsen because they do not get nutritious meals and do not have a place to store medications, if they can afford them. In addition, they lack a healthy balance of rest and activity because of walking throughout the day to meet basic needs. For many individuals, the quickest access to health care is the emergency department to receive treatment for worsening conditions. In the community setting, it is important to help these patients identify available resources, determine their eligibility for assistance, and implement interventions to improve their health status.

QSEN QSEN ACTIVITY *Patient-Centered Care*

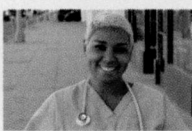

Copyright © ajr_images/iStock/ Thinkstock.

Shanise leads a group that is establishing a community-organized free health care clinic run by volunteers and donations. Nursing and medical students with faculty from area schools participate. The free clinic provides a nutritious snack, bottled water, foot care, immunizations, and needed checkups to patients during their visit. Many of the patients visiting the clinic are homeless and at risk of foot ulcers, foot infections, and injury because of poor hygiene, long periods of standing or walking, and ill-fitting shoes. Shanise provides guidance to the nursing students in all aspects of patient care. Together, they bring the patients into the examination rooms, take their vital signs, examine their feet, and wash their feet with soap and water and dry them well. They offer them new socks and boots, which are donated by local businesses. They encourage the patients to seek shelter during extreme weather. Additionally, they provide simple, language-appropriate health education materials and information on local state-assisted housing resources and make referrals as necessary.

- How can Shanise make sure that the nursing students involve their patients in their recommendations and make sure they are appropriate to their environment?

evolve   Answers to QSEN Activities can be found on the Evolve website.

BOX 4.3 EVIDENCE-BASED PRACTICE

PICO Question: Do community health centers that provide community-centered care produce better patient outcomes compared with centers that do not provide community-centered care?

SUMMARY OF EVIDENCE

The poor and homeless populations of all ages continue to increase (National Center for Health Statistics, 2016) leading to an increase in their health care needs. Federally funded community health centers (CHCs) provide comprehensive primary care health services to "safety net" patients (i.e., patients who are medically underserved and who experience substantial barriers to accessing health care) (Laws et al., 2014). More than 7000 CHCs in the United States and U.S. territories serve approximately 22 million people (Laws et al., 2014). An analysis of CHC program patients show that 6 in 10 patients are female, approximately 33% are children, and working-age adults make up the largest share of the CHC patient population (Shin et al., 2015). More than half (57%) of CHC patients who report their race and ethnicity are people of color (Shin et al., 2015).

The quality of care in CHCs is very good. Recent studies show that racial and ethnic disparities in the rates of low-birth-weight infants are small in magnitude in CHCs and are narrower compared to disparities in the total population (Lebrun et al., 2013). CHCs are also associated with reduced disparities in health care based on race and ethnicity and insured status and also with reduced disparities in health (O'Malley et al., 2005; Shi et al., 2013). In addition, CHCs have been associated with reductions in older adult mortality rates, and the increased use of primary care and access to lower-cost medications provided by CHCs were likely important mechanisms for success (Bailey and Goodman-Bacon, 2015).

Effective community health centers provide a health safety net for the poor and homeless populations (White and Newman, 2015). Many centers provide primary and urgent care services. Within these centers there are resources to determine the health care needs of the community, identify health education needs, and provide child care and parenting classes. Highly successful centers assess for and respect the needs of the target community; provide safe, effective primary and urgent care services; and assist patients to safe shelters or into transitional housing arrangements (White and Newman, 2015).

APPLICATION TO NURSING PRACTICE

- Promptly identify and assess people who are newly homeless and provide them with timely health and social interventions to enhance the chances for improved health status (White and Newman, 2015).
- Obtain an ongoing, comprehensive listing of homeless shelters and transitional housing that is age and gender appropriate and know which resources to use to help a newly homeless person obtain placement in an appropriate residence.
- Ensure patients have transportation and resources to access the lower-cost medications made available, and provide literacy-appropriate education regarding medication use.

People With Mental Illness. It is important to explore health and socioeconomic problems when caring for patients with mental illnesses such as depression, bipolar disorder, and personality disorders (e.g., borderline, obsessive-compulsive, antisocial). It is common for people in poverty to suffer depression (Kurtzelben, 2012). When a patient has a pervasive mental illness, such as having severe impairment in development or communication, the illness affects many aspects of the patient's life and requires medication therapy, counseling, housing, and vocational assistance. Many patients with pervasive mental illnesses are homeless or have poor housing. Others lack the ability to maintain employment or care for themselves on a daily basis. In addition, they are at greater risk for abuse and assault.

Patients who are mentally ill are no longer routinely hospitalized in long-term psychiatric institutions. Instead the goal is to offer resources within their community. Although comprehensive service networks are in every community, many patients with mental illnesses still go untreated or they are provided with fewer and more fragmented services, with little skill in surviving and functioning within the community. Collaboration with multiple community resources is a key to helping people with pervasive mental illnesses receive adequate health care (Stanhope and Lancaster, 2016).

Older Adults. Because people are living longer, and because of the impact of the number of baby boomers, there has been an increase in the older adult population. Thus more patients have chronic diseases such as hypertension, cancer, and dementia. There is a greater demand for health care services provided in community settings (Table 4.1). Successful disease management and symptom control of chronic conditions help patients maintain or increase their quality of life. For the older adult population, it is important to view health promotion and disease management within a broad context. In the United States, more than 25% of patients living with HIV are older than age 50 and remain sexually active (CDC, 2017). Understand what health means to older adults and the steps they can take to promote healthy lifestyles and maintain their own health (see Chapter 23).

COMPETENCY IN COMMUNITY-BASED NURSING

You need a variety of skills and talents to be successful in community-based practice. In addition to helping patients with their health care needs and developing relationships within the community, you need skills in promoting health, preventing disease, and caring for the health of the community. Use critical thinking and the nursing process (see

TABLE 4.1 MAJOR HEALTH PROBLEMS IN OLDER ADULTS AND COMMUNITY HEALTH NURSING ROLES AND INTERVENTIONS

PROBLEM	COMMUNITY HEALTH NURSING ROLES AND INTERVENTIONS
Hypertension	Monitor blood pressure and weight; educate about nutrition and antihypertensive drugs; teach stress management techniques; promote a good balance between rest and activity; establish blood pressure screening programs; assess current lifestyle and promote lifestyle changes; promote dietary modifications by using techniques such as a diet diary
Cancer	Obtain health history; promote monthly breast self-examinations and annual Pap tests and mammograms for older women; promote regular physical examinations; encourage smokers to stop smoking; correct misconceptions about processes of aging; provide emotional support and quality of care during diagnostic and treatment procedures
Arthritis	Educate about management of activities, correct body mechanics, availability of mechanical appliances, and adequate rest; promote stress management; counsel and assist the family to improve communication, role negotiation, and use of community resources; help persons avoid the false hope and expense of arthritis fraud
Visual impairment (e.g., loss of visual acuity, eyelid disorders, opacity of the lens)	Provide support in a well-lighted, glare-free environment; use printed aids with large, well-spaced letters; help clean eyeglasses; help make arrangements for vision examinations and obtain necessary prostheses; teach to be cautious of false advertisements
Hearing impairment (e.g., presbycusis)	Speak with clarity at a moderate volume and pace, and face individual when performing health teaching; help make arrangements for hearing examination and obtain necessary prostheses; teach to be cautious of false advertisements
Depression	Use motivational approaches to encourage adherence to treatment with medication and therapy. Also encourage participation in physical activity to meet CDC recommendations for exercise. Discuss opportunities for older adults to increase their social interactions.
Alzheimer's disease	Maintain high-level functioning, protection, and safety; encourage human dignity; demonstrate to the primary family caregiver techniques to dress, feed, and toilet adult; provide frequent encouragement and emotional support to caregiver; act as an advocate for older adult when dealing with respite care and support groups; protect older adult's rights; provide support to maintain family caregivers' physical and mental health; maintain family stability; recommend financial services if needed
Dental problems	Perform oral assessment and refer to dentist as necessary; emphasize regular brushing and flossing, proper nutrition, and dental examinations; encourage older adults with dentures to wear and take care of them; calm fears about dentist; help provide access to financial services (if necessary) and dental care facilities
Substance and alcohol abuse	Get drug use history; educate adult about safe storage, risks for medication, drug-drug, drug-alcohol, and drug-food interactions; give general information about drug (e.g., drug name, purpose, side effects, dosage); instruct adult about presorting techniques (using small containers with one dose of drug that are labeled with specific times to take drug). Counsel about substance abuse; promote stress management to avoid need for drugs or alcohol, and arrange for and monitor detoxification if appropriate
Sexually transmitted infections	Perform a full sexual risk assessment and bring awareness regarding risk factors and susceptibility to HIV/AIDS; educate about safe sexual practices such as abstinence and use of condoms and refer as necessary for HIV testing

AIDS, Acquired immunodeficiency syndrome; *HIV,* human immunodeficiency virus.

Data from Stanhope M, Lancaster J: *Public health nursing: population centered health care in the community,* ed 9, St Louis, 2016, Elsevier; Mauk KL: *Gerontological nursing: competencies for care,* ed 4, Boston, 2014, Jones & Bartlett.

Chapters 8 and 9) to provide individualized nursing care for patients and their families.

Caregiver

Caregiving is the most important role. You develop appropriate, individualized nursing care within the context of a patient's and family caregiver's community to achieve long-term successful health outcomes. Work with the patient and family caregiver to develop a caring partnership to recognize actual and potential health care needs and identify community resources. As a caregiver, you build a healthier community that is safe and helps the population achieve and maintain an improved quality of life and optimal health status.

Case Manager

Being a case manager means you make an appropriate plan of care based on your assessment of patients and families and coordinate needed resources and services for a patient's well-being across a continuum of care (see Chapter 3). Generally a community-based case manager assumes responsibility for the case management of multiple patients. This usually involves patients who need coordination of different health care services (e.g., patients with mental illnesses and patients with complex medical conditions). The greatest challenge is coordinating the activities of many different providers and payers in different settings throughout a patient's continuum of care. An effective case manager anticipates obstacles and opportunities that exist within a community that will influence the ability to find solutions for the patient's and family's needs. Case management with individual patients and families reveals the overall picture of health services and the health status of a community.

Educator

Community-based nurses teach their patients individually or in groups. With the goal of helping patients assume responsibility for their own health care, the role of educator is important in a community-based setting. Patients and families need to gain knowledge and skills to care for themselves (see Chapter 12). When practicing in a community, you assess a patient's learning needs and readiness to learn, adapt teaching skills to instruct within the home setting, and make the learning process meaningful. Evaluate learning by reviewing a patient's level of knowledge and ability to teach back and perform specific skills, following up with phone calls and referring the patient to community support and self-help groups. Evaluation of patient learning occurs over time and requires patience and commitment.

Epidemiologist

Community health nurses use basic principles of epidemiology such as tracking health problems; collecting and analyzing data to identify disease trends, outbreaks of illnesses, and disease incidence rates; and planning strategies to prevent or contain disease outbreaks. Consider the following scenario. Several people in a community are newly diagnosed with hepatitis A. A community health nurse conducts interviews with the people who became ill and identifies an infected food handler at the restaurant where the food was consumed. In collaboration with the health department, the restaurant closes while the kitchen is thoroughly sanitized. The nurse educates all employees about sanitation practices and coordinates postexposure immunization clinics. In addition, the nurse provides education about illness prevention to the community.

COMMUNITY ASSESSMENT

When practicing in a community setting, it is important to learn how to assess the community. Community assessment requires you to systematically collect data about a population to monitor the health status of the population and make information available about the health of the community (Stanhope and Lancaster, 2016). The community is the environment in which people live and work. Without an adequate understanding of that environment, any effort to promote community health and institute necessary change is unlikely to be successful. The community has three components or parts: structure or locale, the people or population, and social systems. A complete assessment involves a careful look at each component to begin to identify needs for health policy, health program development, and service provision (Box 4.4).

Include a patient's living environment and neighborhood during your assessment. When assessing the structure or locale, conduct a windshield survey by traveling around a neighborhood or community. Observe its design, location of services, and locations where residents meet. A public library or local health department is a great source for accessing statistics to assess the demographics of the community. Once you have a thorough understanding of the community structure or locale, perform individual patient assessments against that background. Assess a patient's home for safety. Does the home have secure locks on doors? Are windows secure and

---

BOX 4.4 COMMUNITY ASSESSMENT

STRUCTURE
- Name of community or neighborhood
- Geographic boundaries
- Emergency services
- Water and sanitation
- Housing
- Economic status (e.g., average household income, number of residents on public assistance)
- Availability of public transportation system

POPULATION
- Age distribution
- Gender distribution
- Growth trends
- Density
- Educational level
- Predominant ethnic groups
- Predominant religious groups

SOCIAL SYSTEM
- Educational system
- Government
- Communication system
- Welfare system
- Volunteer programs
- Health system

intact? Is lighting along walkways and entryways working? Be aware of the level of community violence and the resources that are available to the patient when help is necessary.

Finally, investigate the social systems within a community. To get information about existing social systems such as schools or health care facilities, visit various sites and learn about their services. Which types of health promotion resources such as smoking cessation or weight management programs are available? Are any day care or adult day care resources available? Which types of health and wellness activities are available in the schools? Which types of safety programs are sponsored by the police department? Knowing the social systems within a community increases your ability to help the community or individuals within that community improve their level of health. In addition, identifying the lack of these programs provides necessary data when advocating for resources for new social programs.

CHANGING PATIENTS' HEALTH

In community-based practice you care for patients from diverse backgrounds and in diverse settings. It is relatively easy over time to become familiar with the resources that are available within a particular community setting and identify the unique needs of individual patients. However, the challenge becomes promoting and protecting a patient's health within the context of the community. Can a patient with lung disease have the quality of life necessary when the patient's community has a serious environmental pollution problem? Likewise it is important to bring together the resources necessary to improve the continuity of care that patients receive (Box 4.5). Be a leader in reducing the duplication of

---

BOX 4.5   EVALUATION

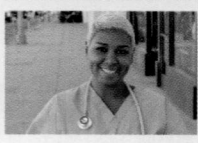

Copyright © ajr_images/iStock/ Thinkstock.

Since the start of the free clinic a year ago, the number of clinical and nonclinical volunteers has increased to include other health disciplines. The state grant allowed the free clinic services to expand providing vaccinations, disease screening and prevention, translators, health education and promotion, and assistance with screening to help qualify applicants for Medicaid and other state-run programs. The free clinic is affiliated with the medical center, which provides diagnostic testing related to sexual health, prenatal care, diabetes, and colon cancer. The church provides space for volunteer-run English as a second language classes and parenting classes for young parents. Shanise reflects on the hard work she, stakeholders, and all the volunteers have done. She realizes that she has established trusting nurse-patient relationships with many of them. Many patients are keeping appointments, and several are returning to follow up. She believes in the importance of including the community and its leaders in all aspects of program building from the assessment of needs through program development and evaluation.

---

health care services and locating the best services for a patient's needs.

A starting point for effective community-based nursing is establishing strong caring relationships with patients and their families (see Chapter 20). Understanding the day-to-day activities of family life helps you adapt nursing interventions. Consider the time of day a patient goes to work, the availability of the spouse and patient's parents to provide child care, and the family values that shape views about health. Once you gain a picture of a patient's life, you can develop patient-centered interventions to promote health and prevent disease.

KEY POINTS

- The principles of public health nursing practice focus on helping individuals and communities achieve a healthy living environment.
- Community-based health care focuses on the provision of comprehensive, culturally competent, quality primary care to underserved and vulnerable populations.
- Essential public health functions include assessment, policy development, and access to resources.
- When population-based health care services are effective, there is a greater likelihood that health education and promotion will contribute efficiently to health improvement at the individual and family levels.
- A community health nurse considers the individual or family to be only one member of a group while providing care to the community as a whole.
- A successful community health nursing practice involves building relationships with the community and being responsive to changes within the community.
- Vulnerable populations have needs that challenge nurses who care for their complex acute and chronic conditions.
- Chronic health problems are common and worsen among homeless people because they have few resources.
- Essential competencies for a community-based nurse include caregiving, case management, patient education, and basic understanding of epidemiology.
- Assessment of a community includes three elements: structure or locale, people, and social systems.

REFLECTIVE LEARNING

Think of a new skill that you learned while in clinical or a skill that you put into practice with a patient, family, or a group of people in the community.
- What were your feelings about the experience?
- What did you learn from the experience?
- What would you do differently in the future?

REVIEW QUESTIONS

1. While assessing an immigrant community, the nurse identifies that the children are undervaccinated. The nurse notes that there is a health clinic within a 3-mile radius. The nurse meets with the community leaders and explains the need for immunizations and educates them about the location of the clinic and the process for accessing health care resources. Together they develop a plan for improving the rate of vaccinations. Which of the following practices is the nurse providing? (Select all that apply.)
   1. Educating about community resources
   2. Teaching about illness prevention
   3. Promoting autonomy and independence
   4. Improving the health care of the children in the community
   5. Managing chronic illness in the community
2. An 82-year-old patient who experienced a stroke and will be using a wheelchair is being discharged home from the hospital. The family wants to care for the patient at home but does not have the resources for 24-hour care. Which action by the community-based nurse who is a case manager is most appropriate?
   1. Telling the family that a long-term care facility would be the best choice for a patient in a wheelchair
   2. Making multiple referrals to a variety of community-based services
   3. Organizing a community fundraising event to pay for needed services
   4. Contacting local nurses in the community to provide assistance to the family
3. A community health nursing instructor and a group of students are organizing a health fair for the homeless population in a large urban setting. Funding is very limited and will not cover costs for space or transportation. Assuming that space is available at no cost at the following sites, where should the students suggest that the health fair be located?
   1. At the city's homeless shelter
   2. At the inner-city church
   3. At the largest inner-city police station
   4. At the local community college

4. Which actions display effective nursing practice in the community? (Select all that apply.)
   1. Educating families of young children about the effects of lead paint in the home
   2. Conducting a blood pressure clinic at a senior health care center
   3. Prescribing treatments for patients when physicians are unable
   4. Forming partnerships with families in the community to share common goals
   5. Assessing a patient who reports cough and fever for 2 days
5. Following a community assessment, a nurse identifies an area near an industrial park with increased respiratory illnesses. The community asks the nurse to come and speak about environmental trends associated with respiratory disease and how the community can reduce its risks. This is an example of which competencies? (Select all that apply.)
   1. Caregiver
   2. Case manager
   3. Epidemiologist
   4. Educator
   5. Environmentalist

evolve

Additional Review Questions, as well as rationales for all Review Questions, can be found on the Evolve website.

1. 1, 2, 4; 2. 2; 3. 1; 4. 1, 2, 4; 5. 3, 4.

REFERENCES

American Nurses Association (ANA): *Public health nursing scope and standards of practice*, ed 2, Washington, DC, 2013, The Association.

Bailey M, Goodman-Bacon A: The war on poverty's experiment in public medicine: community health centers and the mortality of older Americans, *Am Econ Rev* 105(3):1067, 2015.

Centers for Disease Control and Prevention (CDC): *HIV among people 50 and over*, 2017, http://www.cdc.gov/hiv/group/age/olderamericans/index.html.

Kurtzelben D: *Americans in poverty at greater risk for chronic health problems*, 2012, https://www.usnews.com/news/articles/2012/10/30/americans-in-poverty-at-greater-risk-for-chronic-health-problems.

Laws R, et al: The Community Health Applied Research Network (CHARN) data warehouse: a resource for patient-centered Outcomes Research and Quality Improvement in Underserved, safety net populations, *EGEMS* 2(3):1097, 2014.

Lebrun L, et al: Racial/ethnic differences in clinical quality performance among health centers, *J Ambul Care Manage* 36(1):24, 2013.

National Center for Health Statistics: *Health, United States, 2015, with special feature on racial and ethnic health disparities*, 2016, http://www.cdc.gov/nchs/data/hus/hus15.pdf.

O'Malley A, et al: Health center trends, 1994-2001: what do they portend for the federal growth initiative, *Health Aff* 24(2):465, 2005.

Shi L, et al: Reducing disparities in access to primary care and patient satisfaction with care: the role of health centers, *J Health Care Poor Underserv* 24(1):56, 2013.

Shin P, et al: *Community health centers: a 2013 profile and prospects as ACA implementation proceeds.* March 17, 2015, Kaiser Family Foundation. http://www.kff.org/report-section/community-health-centers-a-2013-profile-and-prospects-as-aca-implementation-proceeds-executive-summary/.

Stanhope M, Lancaster J: *Public health nursing: population-centered health care in the community*, ed 9, St Louis, 2016, Elsevier.

U.S. Department of Health and Human Services (USDHHS): *Healthy People 2020*, 2017, http://healthypeople.gov/2020/about/default.aspx.

White BM, Newman SD: Access to primary care services among the homeless: a synthesis of the literature using the equity of access to medical care framework, *J Prim Care Community Health* 6(2):77–87, 2015.

Ziegler K, Camarota S: *Center for Immigration Studies: immigrants in the United States*, 2016. http://cis.org/Immigrants-in-the-United-States?gclid=CLTficXD0dQCFROXfgodCwUMSA.

Legal Principles in Nursing

evolve MEDIA RESOURCES

http://evolve.elsevier.com/Potter/essentials

- Audio Glossary

- QSEN Activity and Review Questions Answers and Rationales

OBJECTIVES

- Describe the legal responsibilities and role of nurses regarding federal and state laws that affect health care.
- Explain the legal concepts of standard of care and informed consent.
- Describe the purpose of standards of care for nurses.

- Explain the concept of negligence, and identify the elements of professional negligence.
- Define the legal relationships of nurse-patient, nurse–health care provider, nurse-nurse, and nurse-employer.
- Identify nursing interventions to improve patient safety.

KEY TERMS

administrative law, p. 60
assault, p. 61
battery, p. 61
common law, p. 60
criminal law, p. 61
defendant, p. 62
due process, p. 61
felony, p. 61
Good Samaritan laws, p. 64
health care proxy, p. 67

informed consent, p. 65
intentional torts, p. 61
living wills, p. 67
malpractice, p. 62
misdemeanor, p. 61
negligence, p. 61
never events, p. 64
Nurse Practice Act, p. 59
occurrence report/incident
    report, p. 64

plaintiff, p. 62
power of attorney for health
    care, p. 67
rapid improvement event (RIE), p. 64
regulatory agencies, p. 59
risk management, p. 64
standards of care, p. 62
statutory law, p. 60
surrogate, p. 67
torts, p. 61

Look at any news website or publication and you will see examples of health care providers who are involved in malpractice court cases. In general, providing safe, competent nursing care to your patients protects you from legal action. How do you achieve this? By making sure that you are always practicing nursing care according to standards of practice. This includes using clinical reasoning skills and understanding the legal boundaries within which you practice.

Nurses frequently practice under several sources and jurisdictions of law simultaneously. In addition to understanding the federal laws that apply to health care in general, you need to understand how different regulatory agencies and your state's Nurse Practice Act affect how you practice. Understanding the legal limits of nursing and the standards of care that affect nursing practice allows you to know your responsibilities as a patient advocate to protect patients from harm. This chapter provides general information that is applicable to a wide variety of health care settings. If you have specific questions or are involved in a lawsuit related to your practice, consult with your own attorney or with the attorney for your employing institution.

CASE STUDY *Lynette Donovan*

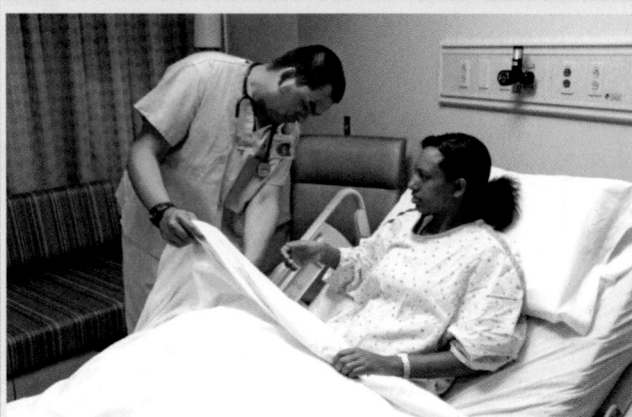

Lynette Donovan, a 15-year-old girl, was a passenger in a motor vehicle collision and is admitted to the hospital with a fractured right femur. Lynette tells the nurses on the trauma unit that her right leg felt numb, was swollen, and looked blue within an hour of when the emergency department health care provider applied a cast to that leg. The nurses assessed Lynette's right leg and determined that these symptoms indicated impaired circulation in the extremity with the cast. The nurses were unable to reach the emergency department health care provider or the physician on call despite several phone calls. They did not call other providers or notify the nursing supervisor of the patient's situation (*Darling v. Charleston Community Memorial Hospital,* 1965).

David is a 23-year-old nursing student newly assigned to the nursing unit and to care for Lynette. During his initial assessment, he notes that the patient's right leg is swollen, slightly discolored, and slightly malodorous. Lynette seems very anxious and upset. She asks David, "Why won't anyone fix my leg?"

LEGAL LIMITS OF NURSING

Sources of Law

Three types of law govern nursing practice: common law, statutory law, and administrative law. **Common law** is based on judicial decisions, or case law precedent, and includes both federal and state court decisions (Garner, 2014). A well-known example of a judicial decision that guides health care practice is *Roe v. Wade* (1973), in which the U.S. Supreme Court identified time periods when elective termination of a pregnancy is legal. One of the most important state court decisions impacting health care was *Schloendorff v. Society of New York Hospital* (1914), which established principles of informed consent for health care.

Statutory law consists of statutes that have been enacted by legislative bodies at the federal and the state levels (Garner, 2014). A commonly known federal statute is the Health Insurance Portability and Accountability Act (HIPAA) of 1996. HIPAA established standards to keep medical records and other personal health information confidential. The most recent federal law significantly affecting health care is the Patient Protection and Affordable Care Act (ACA) (2010).

BOX 5.1 FEDERAL STATUTES IN NURSING PRACTICE

Americans With Disabilities Act (ADA) (1995): Civil rights law that protects disabled individuals regarding access to public services, health care, and employment. It was extended to include individuals with HIV infection.

Patient Protection and Affordable Care Act (ACA) (2010): Law intended to increase the affordability and quality of health insurance for Americans without it, decrease the number of uninsured Americans, and reduce the costs of health care. It created exchanges in the states that allow patients to purchase health insurance.

Emergency Medical Treatment and Active Labor Act (EMTALA) (1986): "Antidumping" law that requires screening of patients in an emergency department and appropriate stabilization before transfer of the patient to another health care agency.

Health Insurance Portability and Accountability Act (HIPAA) (1996): Law that protects a patient from losing health insurance because of preexisting illnesses when changing jobs. It also sets rules regarding release of a patient's protected health information and carries both civil and criminal penalties for violations.

Patient Self-Determination Act (PSDA) (1991): Law that requires health care agencies to provide information to all patients regarding advance directives and to document advance directives in the medical record.

Federal Nursing Home Reform Act (1987): Law that gives nursing home residents the right to be free of unnecessary and inappropriate restraints.

National Organ Transplant Act (1984): Law that prohibits purchase or sale of organs. It also provides immunity from civil and criminal actions against the hospital and health care providers and immunity from liability for the donor's estate.

Mental Health Parity Act (1996): Law that prohibits health plans from placing lifetime or annual limits on mental health benefits.

HIV, Human immunodeficiency virus.

The ACA reformed health care in a variety of ways including requiring that all Americans obtain health insurance, expanding Medicaid eligibility, and creating state health insurance exchanges. This and other federal statutes affecting health care practice are outlined in Box 5.1.

Nurse Practice Acts regulate the practice of nursing and are examples of state laws that impact health care. Although Nurse Practice Acts vary from state to state, they all authorize a State Board of Nursing, set standards for nursing education programs, set standards and the scope of nursing practice, define titles and licenses including requirements for licensure, and set grounds for disciplinary action against nurses including defining violations and remedies (National Council of State Boards of Nursing [NCSBN], 2016).

Administrative law consists of rules and regulations developed and enforced by state regulatory agencies including the State Boards of Nursing. State Boards of Nursing are authorized by state Nurse Practice Acts to set rules, regulations, and guidelines that specifically define the standard of care in nursing practice. Much of a state's Nurse Practice Act is further defined and described in its administrative code. For example, Illinois statutory law defines professional nursing (Professional Nursing, 2015), but the state sets out specific rules for nurses to follow in its administrative code including standards of professional conduct (Standards of Professional Conduct, 2015). In addition to State Boards of Nursing, the administrative code contains rules and regulations from Boards of Pharmacy, Medicine, and other health care professions.

To practice nursing, you must be licensed by the State Board of Nursing of the state in which you wish to practice. Nurse licensure is attained by meeting the educational requirements set by your State Board of Nursing and having a passing score on the National Council Licensure Examination (NCLEX®). Once obtained, a nursing license must be renewed, usually every 2 years. Many states require obtaining continuing education units for license renewal, and some prescribe what should be included as part of the continuing education to be completed. For example, Ohio requires nurses to complete 24 hours of continuing education every 2 years including at least 1 hour of education related to the Ohio Nurse Practice Act.

Your nursing license in one state does not allow you to practice outside of that state unless it is part of the Nursing Licensure Compact (NLC). Many states belong to the NLC; you are free to practice in any of these states as long as you conform to that state's Nurse Practice Act. You can find more information on the National Council of State Boards of Nursing (NCSBN) website (www.ncsbn.org).

A State Board of Nursing has the power to suspend or revoke a nurse's license if the nurse's conduct violates provisions of the licensing statute. Criminal law violations, even if unrelated to nursing, may jeopardize your licensure status. For example, a nurse who is convicted of driving under the influence of alcohol must report this to the State Board of Nursing, and the Board can then determine if this affects the nurse's ability to practice. The Board can look at any conduct of the nurse including previous academic conduct to determine whether that nurse may be licensed. Because a nursing license is a property right under the law, the State Board of Nursing must fulfill the constitutional duty of **due process** in any disciplinary proceeding. Due process requires a State Board of Nursing to notify the nurse of the listed charges or violations and conduct a hearing at which the nurse may hear the evidence of the charges and offer a defense with or without the assistance of legal counsel (Garner, 2014). In license hearings a panel of members of a State Board of Nursing conducts the hearing instead of a judge. Depending on your state administrative rules, you may file an appeal of the State Board of Nursing judgment in a state administrative court. In any licensing proceeding nurses should exercise the right to legal counsel to ensure full protection of their rights.

Criminal Law

Criminal law refers to federal or state statutory laws that define as a crime certain actions that inflict or threaten substantial harm to individuals or the public interest without justification (Garner, 2014). Criminal laws are separated into misdemeanors or felonies. A **misdemeanor** is a crime that, although injurious, does not inflict serious harm. For example, parking your car in a designated no parking zone is a misdemeanor violation of a traffic law. Nontraffic misdemeanors include such crimes as petty theft (e.g., shoplifting), which is typically theft of less than about $500. A conviction or guilty plea to a misdemeanor usually results in a penalty of a monetary fine, forfeiture of license or, rarely, brief imprisonment. A **felony** is a serious offense that results in significant harm to another person or society in general. Felony crimes carry penalties of monetary restitution, imprisonment for greater than 1 year, or death (Pozgar, 2016). Examples of Nurse Practice Act violations that may carry criminal penalties include practicing nursing without a license and misuse of controlled substances.

Torts

Torts are civil wrongful acts or omissions against a person or a person's property that are compensated by awarding monetary damages to the individual whose rights were violated (Pozgar, 2016). Torts are characterized as either intentional or unintentional. Nursing practice is implicated by some intentional and unintentional torts.

Intentional torts are deliberate acts of wrongful conduct (Pozgar, 2016). An example of an intentional tort in health care is assault and battery. Even though assault and battery can be criminal statutory violations, they are also tort injuries and can occur in health care. The definitions of assault and battery are the same in both criminal and tort law. **Assault** is an intentional threat toward another person that places the person in reasonable fear of harmful, imminent, or unwelcome contact (Pozgar, 2016). No actual contact is required for an assault to occur. An example of an assault in nursing practice is to threaten to restrain a patient for an x-ray procedure when the patient has refused consent. **Battery** is intentional offensive touching without consent or lawful justification (Pozgar, 2016). The touching may be harmful to the patient by causing an injury, or it may be merely offensive to the patient's dignity. Battery generally always includes an assault. An example of a battery in health care is when a patient has consented to a right knee surgery and the surgeon performs surgery on the patient's left knee. An example of an assault and battery is to threaten to restrain a competent patient for an unconsented x-ray procedure and then to restrain him or her.

False imprisonment is an intentional tort that may occur when the nurse restrains a patient, either chemically or physically, without following hospital policy or procedure. Always follow agency policies (e.g., the need for a physician's order) and manufacturer's recommendations for proper use of the restraint. Agencies must provide training on the proper use and application of restraints used by the agency. Liability for improper or unlawful restraint lies both with the nurse and the health care agency.

Negligence is an unintentional tort. **Negligence** is conduct that falls below the generally accepted standard of care that a reasonably prudent person would provide under similar circumstances (Garner, 2014). An example of negligence is a driver's failure to stop at a clearly identified stop sign. Malpractice is an example of negligence, sometimes referred to as professional negligence. The law defines nursing **malpractice** as the failure to use the same care that a reasonably prudent nurse would use under the same or similar circumstances (Garner, 2014). To establish the elements of malpractice, the patient and/or family, or **plaintiff**, must prove the following: (1) there was a provider-patient relationship between the nurse, or **defendant**, and the patient; (2) the nurse breached the duty owed to the patient under that relationship; (3) the patient's injury was due to the nurse's breach of duty; and (4) the patient has accrued damages (physical or monetary) because of the injury. Negligent acts may result in lawsuits against hospitals and nurses (Box 5.2). The negligent act may be as simple as failing to check a patient's armband and then administering medication to the wrong patient. Failure to monitor a patient's condition appropriately and communicate changes in the patient's condition to the health care provider that result in injury to the patient are examples of negligent acts that may result in malpractice. One recent case involved nurses who failed to notify an obstetrician that an infant was in distress during labor. A cesarean section was performed, but the delay caused a lack of oxygen flow to the infant that resulted in cerebral palsy (*Ciechoski v. Phoenixville Hospital Co.*, 2014). The best way to avoid being liable for malpractice is to give nursing care that meets the accepted standard of care. In a malpractice lawsuit the judge and jury use nursing standards of care to measure nursing conduct and determine whether the nurse acted as a reasonably prudent nurse would act under the same or similar circumstances. Box 5.3 describes the steps of a typical malpractice lawsuit.

BOX 5.2   COMMON SOURCES OF NEGLIGENCE

Be aware of the common negligent acts that have resulted in lawsuits against hospitals and nurses:

1. Medication errors that result in injury to patients, including medicating the wrong patient
2. IV therapy errors resulting in infiltration or phlebitis
3. Burns to patients caused by equipment, bathing, or spills of hot liquids and foods
4. Falls resulting in injury to patients
5. Failure to use aseptic technique when required
6. Errors in sponge, instrument, or needle counts in surgical cases, meaning that an item was left in a patient
7. Failure to give a report or giving an incomplete report to oncoming shift personnel
8. Failure to adequately monitor a patient's condition
9. Failure to notify a health care provider of a significant change in a patient's status
10. Failure to clarify an ambiguous order
11. Failure to question or clarify an inaccurate or incorrect order

---

STANDARDS OF CARE

Standards of care (see Chapter 1) are legal guidelines for minimally safe and adequate nursing practice (Neil, 2015; Pozgar, 2016). They are defined by the following: (1) State Nurse Practice Acts, (2) state and federal hospital licensing laws and accreditation rules, (3) professional and specialty organizations (American Nurses Association [ANA], 2015), and (4) formal policies and procedures of health care agencies. Formal policies and procedures of a health care agency are specific guidelines and directions for nursing care and are usually found on an agency's intranet portal or in a policy and procedure manual. The procedure for following the "chain of command" to notify a health care provider of a serious change in patient status is frequently a part of the nursing unit policy and procedure manual. *In the case study, the nurses caring for Lynette could have consulted agency policy and procedure to determine whom to contact if they were unable to reach her health care provider in a timely manner.* Standards of care change regularly to reflect current scientific or technological advances (Neil, 2015).

It is important that you know the nursing scope of practice and the policies and procedures of your employing health care agency because these are the standards of care to which your actions will be compared if you are in a malpractice trial. If you become a specialized nurse such as a nurse anesthetist, intensive care nurse, certified nurse midwife, or operating room nurse, you are held to the standard of care and skill exercised by professionals in the specialty area. Nursing experts (nurses with extensive experience in the area or issue in question) testify to the appropriate standard of care as indicated by the policy and procedure manual, your professional organization, or the State Nurse Practice Act and compare your conduct to these standards. Many states have developed "apology statutes" that encourage a health care provider to disclose errors or unanticipated outcomes to a patient and/or family without admitting liability. These statutes are designed to improve communication and decrease litigation (Westrick and Jacob, 2016). It is always important to be up to date about agency policies and procedures; state and federal laws; current legal issues; standards of care from professional associations; and any new rules, regulations, or case law that affect your nursing practice.

Malpractice Insurance

Malpractice insurance provides you with an attorney, the payment of attorney's fees, and the payment of any judgment or settlement if a patient sues you for malpractice. If you work for a health care agency, the insurance of that agency covers you during your employment if you are practicing within your scope of practice and follow the agency policies and procedures. If your agency determines that you were not following policy and procedures, the agency malpractice insurance will not cover you. Additionally if you plan on practicing nursing outside of your employing agency, you need to purchase additional malpractice insurance. For example, if a family friend asks you to provide nursing care in his or

BOX 5.3 ANATOMY OF A LAWSUIT

Petition—elements of the claim: The plaintiff outlines what the defendant nurse did wrong and how, as a result of that alleged negligence, the plaintiff was injured. *In the case study, the petition would state that the nurses failed to provide adequate care to the patient by failing to treat the changing condition (change in circulation to leg) appropriately.*

Answer: The nurse admits or denies each allegation in the petition. Anything that is not admitted must be proved. *In the case study, the nurses admit or deny that they were able to provide further appropriate care to the patient to meet the standard of care during her change in condition.*

Discovery: The process of uncovering all the facts of the case involves using interrogatories, requests for production of the medical records in question, and depositions. The patient and all health care staff listed in the lawsuit or called as witnesses are asked questions by counsel for the plaintiff and the defense. They answer under oath, and their testimony is recorded and kept for reference in the trial.

- *Interrogatories:* Written questions requiring answers under oath usually concern witnesses, insurance experts, and which health care providers the plaintiff saw before and after the event.
- *Requests for production:* Each party asks for full disclosure of all documents including medical records that may pertain to the lawsuit. The defendant obtains all the plaintiff's relevant medical records for treatment before and after the incident. Everything documented by the nurses and the health care provider in the medical record is open to examination by both the plaintiff and the defendants. Remember that occurrence reports are not part of the medical record.
- *Witnesses' depositions:* Questions are posed to witnesses under oath to obtain all relevant, nonprivileged information about the case.
- *Parties' depositions:* The plaintiff and defendants (health care provider, nurse, and hospital personnel) are almost always deposed.

- *Other witnesses' depositions:* Factual witnesses, both neutral and biased, are deposed to obtain information and their version of the case. Witnesses may include family members on the plaintiff's side and other medical personnel (e.g., nurses) on the defendant's side.
- *Treating health care providers' depositions:* Before subsequent treating, health care providers' depositions may be taken to establish issues such as those concerning preexisting conditions, causation, the nature and extent of injuries, and permanency.

Expert witnesses: The plaintiff selects experts to establish the essential legal elements of the case against the defendant. The defendant selects experts to establish the appropriateness of the nursing care. Nursing experts are asked to testify to the reasonableness or inappropriate actions of the health care staff once the patient's condition began to change. The expert is asked to compare the actions of the nursing staff to the standard of care, which is what the reasonably prudent nurse in the same situation would have done.

Trial: The trial usually occurs at least 1 to 3 years after the filing of the petition. Approximately 5% of cases are actually tried before a judge; most are dismissed or settled. Settlement means that compensation has been paid for the case to be dismissed.

PROOF OF NEGLIGENCE
- The nurse owed a duty to the patient. This is satisfied if there was a health care provider–patient relationship.
- The nurse did not carry out the duty or breached it (failed to use the degree of skill and learning ordinarily used under the same or similar circumstances by members of the profession).
- The patient sustained an injury, either physical or financial.
- The patient's injury was caused by the nurse's failure to carry out that duty.
- The patient's injury resulted in compensable damages that can be quantified such as medical bills, lost wages, pain, and suffering.

QSEN ACTIVITY *Safety*

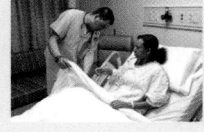

David has completed his clinical experience for the day. As the circulation to Lynette's right leg continued to worsen, an amputation of her leg became necessary. David observed the surgery and now returns to post-conference. The nursing instructor asks David to describe his experience. When he finishes relating the facts of the case, the instructor asks the group to describe which actions should have been taken by the nursing staff to have a better patient outcome.

- If you were a nursing student in this post-conference, identify the actions that you think the nurses should have taken and place them in their order of priority.

evolve Answers to QSEN Activities can be found on the Evolve website.

her home, the hospital malpractice insurance does not cover you if the family friend files suit against you. If you work for an agency that employs nurses who contract with health care agencies, you may not be covered by malpractice insurance.

Malpractice insurance carriers are required by federal law to report all malpractice insurance verdicts and settlements made to the National Practitioner Data Bank (NPDB). Because this data bank includes information on advanced practice nurses, it indirectly affects the practice of nursing. Costs of malpractice claims against RNs decreased in the 5-year period ending in 2015, with claims now averaging $201,000 total paid per claim rather than the $250,000 average for the 5-year period ending in 2010 (Nurses Service Organization, 2015).

Documentation

It is necessary to apply legal principles when documenting patient assessments, planning, interventions, and evaluations to avoid liability. Frequently a nurse's notes are the first thing that an attorney reviews when a lawsuit is filed. As a nurse, you need to document as fully as possible because your documentation of your nursing care is your only record of what was done for a patient and serves as proof that you acted reasonably and safely (see Table 10.1). Chapter 10 outlines the principles to follow to make your documentation thorough, accurate, clear, and timely. Trials over health care disputes that involve using the medical record as a source of information generally occur 2 to 3 years after the event. Most individuals have difficulty remembering events over a period of time. Therefore your nursing notes, documented at the time of the event, are viewed as better evidence of the facts of the event than anyone's memory. Nurses' notes composed without regard to detail or hospital standards of documentation do not reflect well on your credibility or appearance of accountability to a judge or jury (Catalano, 2014).

When there is a deviation from the standard of care such as when a patient or visitor falls or an error is made, you document the event or incident in the form of an occurrence report/incident report. You complete an occurrence report when anything unusual happens that could potentially cause harm to a patient, visitor, or employee. Most health care agencies provide specific forms for this purpose (see Chapter 10). Objectively record the details of the event and any other information required by the form. Occurrence reports are not kept in patients' medical records, although they may be admissible evidence in lawsuits in some jurisdictions (*In re Intracare Hospital*, 2007; *Tibbs v. Bunnell*, 2014). Other jurisdictions such as Ohio and Michigan have enacted laws that specifically protect these reports from being evidence in lawsuits, even if their completion was documented in the medical record. *As a general rule, however, do not document in the nurses' notes that an occurrence report was completed.* Follow the policy of your agency to determine what to do with the occurrence report after it is completed. Also be sure to report the occurrence to the appropriate person (e.g., the charge nurse, your manager).

Risk Management and Quality Improvement

The underlying rationale for quality improvement and risk-management programs is the development of an organizational system of ensuring appropriate, quality health care. Risk management involves several components, including identifying possible risks, analyzing them, acting to reduce them, and evaluating the measures taken to reduce them (Barger, 2014). The Joint Commission requires the use of quality improvement and risk-management procedures (The Joint Commission [TJC], 2016). Both quality improvement and risk management require thorough documentation.

Risk managers review occurrence reports to determine areas of patient risk. For example, if a certain kind of problem has occurred repeatedly, such as patients falling when being transferred to stretchers, educational methods could be developed to help prevent the problem in the future.

Patient safety and improved care are the ultimate goals of risk management and quality assurance. Patient safety

issues are the focus of attention by accrediting agencies such as The Joint Commission (2016) and public interest groups such as the National Academy, Health and Medicine Division, formerly known as the Institute of Medicine. Never events are preventable errors, which may include falls, catheter-associated urinary tract infections, and health care–associated pressure injuries (Agency for Healthcare Research and Quality [AHRQ], 2016a). The federal government and health care insurance companies have not reimbursed health care agencies for these preventable medical errors since 2007. Never events are rare, but a large number of them are fatal to patients (AHRQ, 2016a) and thus are carefully monitored, with evidence-based strategies implemented for prevention. Becoming involved in developing and monitoring the policies and procedures of the agency in which you work helps to develop a system and a culture of patient safety.

One way that a culture of patient safety is maintained is through rapid improvement events. A rapid improvement event (RIE) or rapid improvement assessment is a method used by businesses including health care agencies to change a process quickly to solve a problem or improve efficiency. People involved in the process come together to determine solutions for improvement, and one idea is quickly implemented and evaluated to determine if it was effective. If it was not effective, another solution is implemented. RIEs have been used in health care to decrease emergency department wait times, decrease inpatient fall rates, improve communication with patients and families, and facilitate discharge processes (Martin et al., 2009; Wolf et al., 2013).

GOOD SAMARITAN LAWS

Good Samaritan laws exist in almost every state to encourage nurses and other health care providers to help in emergency situations (Morris, 2014). These laws limit liability and offer legal immunity if a nurse helps at the scene of an accident. For example, if you stop at the scene of an automobile accident and give appropriate emergency care such as applying pressure to a bleeding extremity and stopping a hemorrhage, you are acting within accepted standards, even though proper equipment was not available. If the patient subsequently develops complications as a result of your actions, you are immune from liability as long as you acted without gross negligence and within your scope of practice. The statutes also provide that a nurse can assist a minor in an emergency at the scene of an accident or a competitive sports event before obtaining the parent's consent. Good Samaritan laws provide immunity to a nurse who does what is reasonable to save a person's life; however, if you perform a procedure for which you have no training, you are liable for any injury resulting from that act. Therefore provide only care that is consistent with your level of expertise. In addition, once you have committed to providing emergency care to a patient, you are responsible for following through (i.e., to safely transfer the care of the patient to individuals who can provide needed care such as emergency medical technicians [EMTs] or emergency department staff).

CONSENT

A patient's signed consent form is necessary for admission to a health care agency, invasive procedures including surgery, and participation in research studies. A patient signs a general consent form for treatment when he or she is admitted to the hospital or other health care agency. A patient or the patient's representative must sign separate special consent forms before anyone performs specialized procedures. **Informed consent** is a patient's agreement to allow a procedure such as surgery based on a full disclosure of the risks, benefits, alternatives, and consequences of refusal (Beauchamp and Childress, 2012). Informed consent requires that you ensure that a patient has all relevant information required to decide about undergoing treatment, that the patient is capable of understanding the relevant information, and that the patient gives consent.

Written informed consent is needed when a patient is going to have an invasive medical procedure such as surgery. The health care provider who is performing the surgery or medical procedure is legally responsible for providing information about the procedure and obtaining a patient's informed consent (Rock and Hoebeke, 2014). A nurse assumes the responsibility of witnessing a patient's signature on a consent form. When you provide consent forms for patients to sign, ask them if they understand the procedures for which they are giving consent. If patients deny any understanding or if you suspect that they do not understand, notify the health care provider and your nursing supervisor immediately.

Documentation of written informed consent includes the following:

- The patient's signature
- The witnesses' signatures
- The date and time of signing
- Verification that the patient voluntarily signed the consent
- Verification that the patient discussed the risks, benefits, alternatives, and the right to refuse the procedure with the health care provider
- Verification that the patient understands the procedure and has had all questions answered satisfactorily

Follow general guidelines when the health care provider obtains legal consent to medical treatments (Box 5.4). Take special consideration for a patient who is deaf or illiterate or speaks a foreign language because the duty of informed consent remains the same (Pozgar, 2016). In each instance, be sure that the patient understands the document being signed. There may be cases in which you need a professional interpreter.

It is also important to be sensitive to the cultural issues of consent and understand the way in which patients and their families communicate to make important decisions. The cultural beliefs and values of your patients are sometimes very different from your own or the culture in which you are comfortable. Show respect by not imposing your cultural values on your patients or their families. For example,

---

BOX 5.4 STATUTORY GUIDELINES FOR LEGAL CONSENT FOR MEDICAL TREATMENT

Individuals who may consent to medical treatment are governed by state law but generally include the following:

I. Adults
   A. Any competent individual 18 years of age or older for himself or herself
   B. Any parent for his or her unemancipated minor
   C. Any guardian for his or her ward
   D. Any adult for the treatment of his or her minor brother or sister (if an emergency and parents are not present)
   E. Any grandparent for a minor grandchild (if an emergency and parents are not present)
II. Minors (younger than 18 years of age)
   A. Ordinarily minors may not consent to medical treatment without a parent. However, emancipated minors may consent to medical treatment without a parent. Emancipated minors include the following:
      1. Minors who are designated emancipated by a court order
      2. Minors who are married, divorced, or widowed
      3. Minors who are in active military service
   B. Unemancipated minors may consent to medical treatment if they have specific medical conditions, as follows:
      1. Pregnancy and pregnancy-related conditions (Various states differ in characterizing a pregnant minor as either emancipated or unemancipated. Know the rules of your state in this matter.)
      2. A minor parent for his or her custodial child
      3. STI information and treatment
      4. Substance abuse treatment
      5. Outpatient and/or temporary sheltered mental health treatment

STI, Sexually transmitted infection.

---

traditional Islamic and Jewish cultures have strict guidelines concerning consent for postmortem examinations and handling of the dead. In general, decision making by a member of a traditional Asian or Hispanic culture is done by the family together and not by the individual seeking treatment. However, remember that each patient is a unique individual; therefore it is necessary to assess the patient's preferences for how to handle consent. When your patient refuses a treatment, it is necessary to make him or her aware of the consequences of his or her refusal.

When a competent patient refuses care or treatment, it is important to recognize that this act is legitimately his or her right. Inform the health care provider of the patient's refusal to receive care and document the situation in the medical record.

If you or a health care provider performs a procedure on a patient without informed consent, the person who performed the procedure can be liable for battery. You do not need to have written informed consent when performing most nursing care. However, it is important that you explain to a patient what you are going to do and ensure that the patient accepts the care you are going to provide. For example, you tell a patient you are going to take the patient's blood pressure and the patient puts his or her arm out. This is called implied consent.

Parents are normally the legal guardians of pediatric patients; therefore they sign consent forms for treatment. If the parents are divorced, the parent with legal custody gives consent. When a parent refuses medically necessary treatment for a child, health care providers sometimes petition the court to intervene on the child's behalf. Using the standard known as "the best interests of the child," courts may overrule parental decisions (Carbone, 2014). Although there is no standard definition of the best interests of the child, courts generally consider the child's ultimate safety and well-being as the most important factors. Children, most often adolescents younger than age 16 years, may be characterized as emancipated or unemancipated minors. This characterization refers to their legal standing as competent adults. Even though an emancipated minor has not achieved the legal age of consent, he or she may give consent for procedures and treatment (Pozgar, 2016). Emancipation is certified by a legal document. Some states may characterize some adolescents as emancipated when certain conditions such as pregnancy exist. In this case the adolescent mother is considered competent to consent to treatment for herself and her child. When there is a question about an adolescent's capacity to consent to a procedure, contact the nursing supervisor for guidance.

If a patient is unconscious, you need to obtain consent from a person legally authorized to give consent on his or her behalf. In an emergency, however, health care providers may provide care to patients without consent if it is presumed that a reasonable person would have agreed to the same or similar treatment (Rock and Hoebeke, 2014). A patient who is legally incompetent needs to have the consent of a legal guardian, which is determined through a legal proceeding. If a mentally ill person refuses treatment, involuntary admission (determined by a judge at a legal proceeding) is limited to situations in which a patient is determined to be dangerous to self or others (Pozgar, 2016). A patient's consent for voluntary psychiatric unit admission is also required. These patients retain the right to refuse treatment until a court has determined that they are incompetent to decide for themselves.

Restraints

A physical restraint is any manual method, physical or mechanical device, or material or equipment that immobilizes or reduces the ability of a patient to move freely (Springer, 2015). The use of restraints has been associated with serious complications and even death. It is imperative for you to know when and how to use and safely apply restraints. The Resident's Rights section of the Omnibus Budget Reconciliation Act (Resident's Rights, 1988) regulates the use of physical or chemical restraints in long-term care nursing agencies. The Joint Commission (2016) sets guidelines for the use of restraints in hospitals. These regulations set the standard that all patients have the right to be free from seclusion and physical or chemical restraints except to ensure the patient's safety in emergency situations. They further describe the procedures to follow to restrain any patient including who orders restraints, when to enter the order, and how often to renew the order. The standards specifically prohibit restraining patients for staff convenience, punishment, or retaliation (Springer, 2015). The regulations also describe documentation of restraint use and follow-up assessments. The documentation needs to describe all of the less restrictive interventions attempted before using a physical or chemical restraint (see Chapter 30). Liability for improper or unlawful restraint lies with the nurse and the health care agency.

Death and Dying

There are legal responsibilities for nurses to assume when caring for patients during the process of death and dying. Carefully document all events that occur, including patient status, any interventions or supportive care measures delivered, and the patient's response while caring for a dying patient. There are two standards for the determination of death: cardiopulmonary death and brain death (Uniform Determination of Death Act, 1980). The cardiopulmonary standard requires failure of a patient's circulatory and respiratory functions. The brain death standard requires irreversible failure of all functions of the entire brain including the brainstem. The reason for the development of the two definitions is to set the legal standard for determining death in all situations. The definitions are helpful to health care providers when there is a question of whether to continue life support or when the discussion of organ donation is appropriate.

You are legally obligated to treat your deceased patient's remains with dignity and care (see Chapter 27). Spiritual and cultural beliefs also need to be considered when handling patient's remains (see Chapters 21 and 22). Wrongful handling causes emotional harm to survivors and can be the basis of a civil lawsuit. In one litigated case survivors sued when a mislabeling of bodies led to an Orthodox Jewish person being prepared for a Roman Catholic funeral and a Roman Catholic person being prepared for an Orthodox Jewish burial (*In re Schiller*, 1977).

Advance Directives

You may encounter legal issues associated with caring for patients who are terminally ill, severely debilitated, or in a persistent vegetative state (permanently comatose). One of these legal issues involves the right to refuse medical treatment and the withholding of food and nutrition. The doctrine of informed consent is the basis of the right to refuse treatment. The Supreme Court has held that a competent person has the right to refuse medical treatment, including lifesaving food and nutrition (*Cruzan v. Director Missouri Department of Health,* 1990).

Advance directives include living wills and durable powers of attorney for health care. **Living wills** are documents that provide instructions about a patient's wishes in certain situations, including withholding or withdrawing life-sustaining procedures in patients who are terminally ill. If a patient has executed a durable **power of attorney for health care**, the document designates an individual, also known as a **health care proxy** or a **surrogate**, who can give consent for health care treatment when the patient is no longer able. State law may designate a surrogate decision maker such as a spouse, who acts as a substitute when no documented preference exists. Each state providing for living wills or advance directives has its own requirements for executing them. In general you need two witnesses who are not relatives or health care providers when a patient signs the document. Only a competent patient can revoke advance directives. Health care providers who ignore valid living wills, advance directives, or the directions of a health care power of attorney may be subject to civil liability. The Patient Self-Determination Act (1991) requires health care institutions to inquire about the presence of advance directives, give patients information on advance directives, and document whether a patient states that he or she has an advance directive.

If a health care provider has documented in the progress notes that a patient is deteriorating and the health care provider and the patient have made the decision not to administer cardiopulmonary resuscitation, the health care provider should enter a "do not resuscitate" (DNR) order. Health care providers need to regularly review DNR orders in case a patient's condition warrants a change. Be familiar with the policies of your institution and procedures concerning DNR orders, as there may be specific regulations about nurses entering telephone orders for DNR status.

Organ and Tissue Donation

A signed consent is necessary before donating a patient's body, tissues, or organs for medical use (Uniform Anatomical Gift Act, 2006). In some states a person signs the back of his or her driver's license in the presence of witnesses, indicating consent to having his or her body donated. Consent is valid as long as the license is valid. Generally a hospital is not liable for honoring a patient's consent for organ donation despite the family's objection. However, in practice, health care institutions typically honor a family's wishes even if they conflict with the patient's organ donation consent. At the time of death, a health care provider (sometimes the nurse) will ask a patient's family if they would like the patient to be considered for organ donation. If they agree, each agency will then have procedures for the nurse to follow. Be familiar with your own agency's procedures that describe how you proceed after a patient's death.

Autopsies

An autopsy requires consent by a patient before his or her death or by a close family member at the time of the patient's death (Autopsy Consent, 1998). The priority for giving consent for autopsies is (1) the patient, in writing before death; (2) durable power of attorney for health care (if named); (3) surviving spouse; and (4) surviving child, parent, brother, or sister in the order named. State statutes specify that you need to notify the coroner when there are reasonable grounds to believe that a patient died as a result of violence, homicide, suicide, accident, or death occurring in any unusual or suspicious manner. You also notify the coroner or medical examiner if a patient's death is unforeseen and sudden and a health care provider has not seen the patient in a certain amount of time (determined by state law). In these "coroner's cases," an autopsy is typically performed.

Confidentiality and Privacy

HIPAA (1996) sets standards regarding the electronic exchange of private and sensitive health information. Known as the Privacy Rules (Carter, 2017), these standards create patient rights to consent to use and disclose protected health information, inspect and copy one's medical record, and amend mistaken or incomplete information. In addition, the standards require all hospitals and health agencies to have specific policies and procedures in place to ensure compliance with the standards. The policies and procedures need to provide reasonable safeguards to protect written and verbal communications about patients. Although HIPAA does not require such things as soundproof rooms in hospitals, it does mean that nurses and health care providers need to avoid discussing patients in public hallways and provide reasonable levels of privacy when communicating with and about patients in any matter. HIPAA violations have civil and criminal sanctions. Patient confidentiality is a right of all patients, and it is a privilege when a patient entrusts you with his or her personal health information. Dealing with deliberate violations of a patient's confidential personal health information by other staff members is a difficult situation. The best actions to take are to advise the staff members to stop, inform the nursing supervisor, and complete an occurrence report.

Issues of disclosure, privacy, and confidentiality are important concerns when working with patients or peers infected with bloodborne illnesses such as human immunodeficiency virus (HIV) infection or acquired immunodeficiency syndrome (AIDS), hepatitis, and sexually transmitted illnesses. You care for these patients in every segment of your nursing practice. Use Standard Precautions as a standard of care when caring for all patients (see Chapter 14). The Americans With Disabilities Act (ADA) (1995) applies to people with AIDS. This federal law protects the rights of people who are disabled and those who have HIV. Health care workers and other employees who refuse to work with people who have HIV leave companies open to indirect charges of discrimination if the employer does not monitor the work environment. The ADA regulations protect patient privacy by giving individuals the opportunity to decide whether to disclose their disability. As a health care worker, it is not a requirement for you to be tested for HIV or other infectious diseases such as hepatitis B as a condition of employment. While a few cases have held that the health care provider is obligated to disclose the fact that he or she is infected with such infectious diseases (see *Estate of Behringer v. Med. Ctr. at Princeton*, 1991), a publication from the Centers for Disease Control and Prevention (CDC) stated that such disclosures are no longer required or even recommended (CDC, 2012).

Confidentiality and Social Media

Confidential patient information should be shared only with other health care providers within the confines of the provider-patient relationship. The act of keeping a patient's information confidential and safe forms the basis of the trust relationship between a patient and nurse. A patient also has an expectation to be treated with dignity and respect, which forms the basis of the patient's right to privacy. Whenever a nurse breaks a patient's trust by disclosing confidential information or violating a patient's right to privacy, the nurse-patient relationship is unalterably changed. This change affects not only that patient and that nurse but also the profession of nursing (ANA, 2011). It is important for any professional to collaborate and share professional development education and exchange ideas regarding the practice issues facing today's nursing professionals. However, when a professional nurse fails to demonstrate respect for the boundaries that must exist between a patient and a professional nurse or between professionals, the nursing profession loses credibility with the public it serves (NCSBN, 2011).

Posting on social media sites, even when patients or colleagues are not specifically described, breaches a patient's trust and may be a form of lateral violence with respect to co-workers (ANA, 2011). Inappropriate use of a patient's confidential information or image may be reported to the State Board of Nursing, and the nurse could face disciplinary charges (NCSBN, 2011). The ANA has developed a Social Media Policy (ANA, 2011), which recommends that, **when using social media sites, a nurse should never name or describe a patient, never post an image of a patient, and never disparage a fellow employee or employer.** In addition, the professional nurse has an obligation to report breaches of privacy and confidentiality. A nurse should become knowledgeable about his or her employer's policies on the use of social media as well as any rules or guidelines provided by the State Board of Nursing. The NCSBN also publishes guidelines on the use of social media by nurses (NCSBN, 2014). As a student nurse, be aware of potential employers' use of social media. Many hospitals are now using social media as they hire new graduates. Even if there is not a breach of confidentiality, if the student has posted "unwisely," the employer may choose to use that information as a representation of the student's professional behavior.

OTHER LEGAL ISSUES IN NURSING PRACTICE

Nurses face issues that can become liability concerns. Thus you need to anticipate these issues so that you are better prepared to deal with any problems that arise.

Health Care Provider Orders

A health care provider is responsible for directing the medical treatment of a patient. You are responsible for carrying out that medical treatment unless the order is in error, violates hospital policy, or is harmful to the patient. Therefore assess all provider orders; if you determine that they are erroneous or harmful, obtain further clarification from the health care provider (Fig. 5.1). For example, if an order indicates that a medication should be given but you note in the admission assessment that the patient reports taking the medication in the past and developing a rash, you have a responsibility to seek clarification from the health care provider. If the health care provider confirms the order but you still believe that it is inappropriate, inform the nurse manager or the nursing supervisor. *Do not carry out an order* if there is a risk that harm will come to your patient. Your supervisor will help resolve the questionable order. If you knowingly carry out the questionable order without obtaining any supporting consultation from your supervisor or administrative staff, you are legally responsible for the harm suffered by your patient. It is always important to put the patient's interests first while still attempting to maintain a collegial approach in providing ordered health care treatments. Notifying the appropriate health care provider through the chain of command is a long-standing and accepted practice when resolving an issue related to a questionable order (Pozgar, 2016).

Before the advent of electronic medical records (EMR), errors could occur because of incorrect transcription of written orders from a health care provider. Now most orders

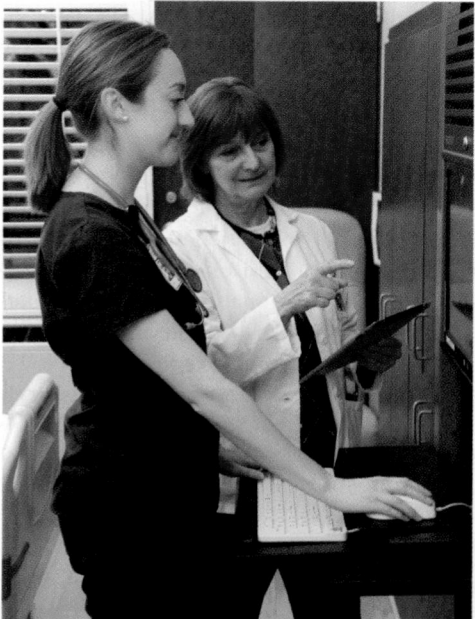

FIG 5.1 If an order creates questions, the nurse clarifies it with the physician or health care provider.

are entered electronically. Verbal or telephone orders are not recommended because they leave possibilities for error. If a verbal or telephone order is necessary in an emergency, make sure the order is repeated to the health care provider and make sure that the health care provider writes down the order and signs it as soon as possible, usually within 24 hours (TJC, 2016) (see Chapter 10).

Nursing Students

Nursing students are responsible for any of their actions that cause harm to patients (*Dimora v. Cleveland Clinics Foundation*, 1996). When a patient is injured as a direct result of your actions, you, your instructor, the staff nurses working with you, and the hospital or health care agency all may share the liability for the incorrect action. Faculty members are responsible for instructing and observing their students, but in some situations staff nurses also share these responsibilities. As a nursing student, no one should assign you to perform tasks for which you are unprepared. Your instructors should carefully supervise you as you learn new procedures. Every nursing school should provide clear definitions of student responsibility. During the clinical rotation, generally the school liability insurance covers you; however, always check with your school regarding the specific coverage.

If you work as an employee of a health care agency while you are in nursing school, perform only those tasks that appear in your job description. For example, even if you have learned how to administer intramuscular medications as a nursing student, do not perform this task as a nurse's aide. Even the act of delivering a patient his or her oral medication is outside the scope of your practice as a nurse's aide or nursing assistant.

Patient Abandonment and Assignment Issues

You will encounter inadequate staffing during times of nursing shortages and staff downsizing when agencies seek to achieve cost containment. The Joint Commission (2016) and laws of many states require institutions to have guidelines for the number of staff needed to care for patients. In California, state law provides for the exact number of nurses required in different levels of care such as intensive care units and general medical units (Staff to Patient Ratios, 1999). Liability issues exist if a health care agency does not have enough RNs to provide competent and safe care and if a patient is injured as a result of negligent care by any personnel. If you are assigned to care for more patients than is reasonable for safe care, notify your nursing supervisor. If you are required to accept the assignment, document this information in writing and provide the document to nursing administrators. Although documentation does not relieve you of responsibility if patients suffer harm because of inattention, it shows that you attempted to act appropriately. Whenever you document information about short staffing, keep a copy of the document. Do not walk out when staffing is inadequate because this act could be regarded as patient abandonment. It is important to know the policies of your institution and procedures for handling inadequate staffing before such a situation arises. RNs are always responsible for making nursing care judgments based on the nursing process. Even when an RN delegates care to unlicensed assistive personnel or licensed practical nurses, the nurse maintains responsibility for patient outcomes. The nurse transfers responsibility only when there has been a hand-off to another nurse (Box 5.5).

Nurses practicing in acute care and long-term care agencies may be required to "float" from the area in which they normally practice to other nursing units. If you float, inform your supervisor if you lack experience in caring for the types of patients on the new nursing unit. Request an orientation to the unit and assistance from a nurse experienced in the area if possible. When you float you are held to the same standard of care as nurses who regularly work on that unit. A supervisor is liable if a staff nurse is assigned to a patient for whom he or she cannot safely care. In one case the court noted that if employers float nurses out of their usual work area of practice, the employers need to provide training and education to prepare the nurses to work in the other areas (*Winkelman v. Beloit Memorial Hospital*, 1992).

Controlled Substances

The Comprehensive Drug Abuse Prevention and Control Act (1970) was initiated to control and regulate hospital drug distribution systems of narcotics, antidepressants, hypnotics, sedatives, stimulants, and hallucinogens. You administer controlled substances only under the direction of a licensed health care provider, including advanced practice nurses in many states.

Controlled substances are securely locked away, and only authorized personnel (nursing and pharmacy staff) have access to them. Because they are generally under electronic lock (with fingerprint or password access only), dispensing, wasting, and storage of controlled substances are closely monitored. Be sure to follow your agency's rules for wasting surplus medication. There are criminal penalties for the misuse of controlled substances. There have been cases in which providers have illegally prescribed and dispensed controlled substances. If you are employed by such a provider and fail to report these activities, you are legally accountable for aiding and abetting the provider.

Reporting Obligations

It is mandatory for all health care providers to report incidents such as child, spousal, or elder abuse; rape; gunshot wounds; attempted suicide; and certain communicable diseases. To encourage reports of suspected cases, states provide legal immunity for the reporter if the person makes the report in good faith. Health care professionals who do not report suspected child abuse or neglect are liable for civil or criminal legal action. You are also required to report unsafe or impaired professionals. Required reporting information varies among states; become familiar with the appropriate statutes in your state and the policies and procedures of your employing health care agency.

BOX 5.5 EVIDENCE-BASED PRACTICE

PICO Question: Does bedside hand-off report compared with traditional end-of-shift report positively impact patient outcomes including patient safety?

SUMMARY OF EVIDENCE

Inadequate communication is the root cause of most health care errors, especially when health care team members share information during change-of-shift reports, transfer reports, and cross-coverage reports. Risk management and quality improvement teams are always looking for ways to improve patient safety and reduce health care errors. One area of communication breakdown found by these teams was during patient hand-offs—reports that occur when patient care is transferred from one provider to another to transfer the responsibility for the patient to the oncoming person. Bedside hand-off reports aim to improve patient safety by increasing the clarity of communication and having the patient confirm the plan of care.

Interviews were conducted with 13 baccalaureate-prepared nurses from a 31-bed pediatric unit to explore how nurses communicate safety issues and improve patient safety during hand-off reports (Groves et al., 2016). The nurses had between 0.75 and 5 years of experience and worked both day shift and night shift. Results showed that a bedside hand-off report was perceived to improve patient safety in three ways: early assessment of the patient, direct visualization of the patient, and a single-patient focus. However, research on the use of hand-off reports has included few clinical trials and thus has not defined best practices across multiple settings. A systematic review conducted in 2010 has identified effective practices in various settings (Riesenberg et al., 2010). Ultimately both actual and potential errors were caught earlier, and improvements were seen in patient safety.

APPLICATION TO NURSING PRACTICE

- Conduct a hand-off by limiting interruptions and distractions.
- Verify that the person receiving the report understands and accepts the transfer of responsibility.
- Delay such a transfer if there are concerns about patient status or stability.
- Use specialized hand-off tools that use a standardized format, such as SBAR (Situation-Background-Assessment-Recommendation), to reduce the likelihood of missing information.
- Report information in the same order every time and use a verification process (such as reading back) to ensure that the information is both received and understood.
- Include patient and family in plans and goals.
- Encourage participants in hand-offs to engage in discussion about the patient (AHRQ, 2016b).

KEY POINTS

- RNs are licensed by the state in which they practice.
- Under the law, you are required to follow standards of care, which originate in Nurse Practice Acts, the guidelines of professional organizations, and documented policies and procedures of employing institutions.
- You are responsible for performing procedures correctly and exercising professional judgment when you carry out physician or health care provider orders.
- All patients are entitled to confidential health care and freedom from unauthorized release of information.
- The civil law system is concerned with the protection of a person's private rights, and the criminal law system deals with the rights of individuals and society as defined by legislative statutes.
- You are liable for malpractice if the following are established: (1) you (defendant) owe a duty to the patient (plaintiff) because of a provider-patient relationship, (2) you did not carry out or you breached that duty, (3) the patient was injured, and (4) your failure to carry out that duty caused the patient's injury.
- Informed consent must meet the following criteria: (1) the person giving consent is competent and of legal age; (2) the consent is given voluntarily; (3) the person giving consent thoroughly understands the procedure, its risks and benefits, and alternative procedures; and (4) the person giving consent has a right to have all questions answered satisfactorily.

- You are obligated to follow a health care provider's order unless you believe that it is in error, violates hospital policy, or is possibly harmful to a patient, in which case you make a formal report explaining the refusal.
- You file an occurrence report in any unusual situation that will potentially cause harm to a patient; such reports are also for quality improvement and risk management.
- Legal issues involving death include documenting all events surrounding the death, treating a deceased person with dignity, and obtaining timely consent for an autopsy from the decedent or close family member.
- Depending on state laws, nurses are required to report possible criminal activities such as child abuse and certain communicable diseases.

REFLECTIVE LEARNING

- At clinical, you hear the nurses talking about their patients in the nurses' station all day, and sometimes visitors and other staff are within hearing range. What implications does this have? What would you say or do about it?
- What would you do if someone called you and asked you about your patient's treatment plan or how the patient was doing?
- Think about a situation where your patient was scheduled for surgery. What would you do if he told you he had more questions about a procedure and was not sure if he needed it, even though he had already signed the consent form?

REVIEW QUESTIONS

1. Your patient has a discharge order. You check his blood pressure before he gets dressed and find that his blood pressure has decreased significantly from that morning. You call the provider and leave a message about the blood pressure, but no one returns your call. What should you do next?
   1. Recheck the patient's blood pressure and complete the discharge process if his blood pressure has returned to normal.
   2. Complete the discharge process because the provider would have returned your call if the discharge was cancelled.
   3. Notify the nursing supervisor of the need for the patient's discharge to be delayed until the provider returns the call.
   4. Complete the discharge process, but tell the patient to check his blood pressure in the morning and notify the provider of the results.
2. A patient has just returned from surgery and has an order for insulin, but the patient does not have diabetes. When you ask the nurse, the nurse tells you that the surgeon who ordered it must have felt that the patient needed the medication and to give the insulin. What should you do in this situation?
   1. Give the insulin, but document that the patient's nurse was consulted.
   2. Give the insulin, but only if the patient agrees to it.
   3. Hold the insulin until the patient is able to eat.
   4. Hold the insulin until someone clarifies the order with the surgeon.
3. You are a new graduate nurse working on a medical/surgical unit. One morning, you are floated to the labor and delivery unit for the day because it is very short-staffed. You tell your charge nurse that you are uncomfortable working on a unit so different from your own. The charge nurse tells you that the labor and delivery charge nurse will make sure you have easy patients and will help you with anything you need. What should you do?
   1. Refuse to accept the assignment and go home for the day.
   2. Obtain hand-off report on the new patients and determine whether you can safely care for them.
   3. Notify the charge nurse on the labor and delivery unit of your concerns so that all the nurses can help you.
   4. Call the nursing supervisor about your concerns and take the assignment only if your concerns are documented in writing.
4. You are a new graduate nurse talking to a nursing student about the standards of care on the cardiac unit. The student nurse asks you if the standards of care are set by the State Board of Nursing. Your answer to the student nurse is that the standards of care incorporate which of the following? (Select all that apply.)
   1. State Nurse Practice Acts
   2. Health care provider orders
   3. Recommendations from professional nursing organizations
   4. Policies and procedures of the health care agency
   5. Evidence-based practice recommendations
5. You are working on an adolescent unit and know that some minors can legally give consent for their health care. Which of the following minors could give consent for a procedure? (Select all that apply.)
   1. A 17-year-old who is in the armed forces
   2. A 16-year-old whose grandmother has custody of him
   3. A 15-year-old with a chronic medical condition
   4. A 17-year-old who is married
   5. A 14-year-old seeking treatment for a sexually transmitted infection

evolve

Additional Review Questions, as well as rationales for all Review Questions, can be found on the Evolve website.

1, 3; 2, 4; 3, 4; 4, 1, 3, 4, 5; 5, 1, 4, 5.

REFERENCES

Agency for Healthcare Research and Quality (AHRQ): *Patient safety primer: never events*, 2016a. https://psnet.ahrq.gov/primers/primer/3/never-events.

Agency for Healthcare Research and Quality (AHRQ): *Handoffs and sign outs*, 2016b. https://psnet.ahrq.gov/primers/primer/9/handoffs-and-signouts.

American Nurses Association (ANA): *Principles for social networking and the nurse*, Silver Spring, MD, 2011, The Association.

American Nurses Association (ANA): *Scope and standards of practice*, ed 3, Silver Spring, MD, 2015, The Association.

Barger DM: Risk management revisited, *Nurs Manage* 45(5):26, 2014.

Beauchamp TL, Childress JF: *Principles of biomedical ethics*, ed 7, Oxford, UK, 2012, Oxford University Press.

Carbone J: Legal applications of the "best interest of the child" standard: judicial rationalization or a measure of institutional competence, *Pediatrics* 134(S2):S111, 2014.

Carter PI: *HIPAA compliance handbook, 2017 edition*, New York, NY, 2017, Wolters Kluwer.

Catalano LA: What you need to know about electronic documentation, *Am Nurse Today* 9(11):24, 2014.

Centers for Disease Control and Prevention: Updated CDC recommendations for the management of hepatitis B virus–infected health-care providers and students, *MMWR Morb Mortal Wkly Rep* 61(RR-3):1, 2012.

Garner B: *Black's law dictionary*, ed 10, St Paul, MN, 2014, Thompson West Publishing.

Groves PS, et al: Handing off safety at the bedside, *Clin Nurs Res* 25(5):473, 2016.

Martin SC, et al: Rapid improvement event: an alternative approach to improving care delivery and the patient experience, *J Nurs Care Qual* 24(1):17, 2009.

Morris E: Liability under "good Samaritan" laws, *AAOS Now* 2014.

National Council of State Boards of Nursing (NCSBN): *White paper: a nurse's guide to the use of social media*, 2011. https://www.ncsbn.org/Social_Media.pdf.

National Council of State Boards of Nursing (NCSBN): *Social media guidelines for nurses*, 2014. https://www.ncsbn.org/347.htm.

National Council of State Boards of Nursing (NCSBN): *Nurse Practice Act, rules and regulations*, 2016. https://www.ncsbn.org/nurse-practice-act.htm.

Neil H: Legally: what is quality care? Understanding nursing standards, *Medsurg Nurs* 24(S1):S14, 2015.

Nurses Service Organization: *Nurse professionals' liability exposures: 2015 claim report update*, 2015.

Pozgar GD: *Legal and ethical issues for health professionals*, ed 4, Burlington, MA, 2016, Jones & Bartlett.

Riesenberg LA: Nursing Handoffs: a systematic review of the literature, *AJN* 110(4):24–34, 2010.

Rock MJ, Hoebeke R: Informed consent: whose duty to inform?, *Medsurg Nurs* 23(3):189, 2014.

Springer G: When and how to use restraints, *Am Nurse Today* 10(1):2015.

The Joint Commission (TJC): *Facts about The Joint Commission*, 2016. https://www.jointcommission.org/facts_about_the_joint_commission/.

Westrick SJ, Jacob N: Disclosure of errors and apology: law and ethics, *J Nurse Pract* 12(2):120, 2016.

Wolf L, et al: Fall prevention for inpatient oncology using lean and rapid improvement event techniques, *HERD* 7(1):85, 2013.

Statutes

Americans With Disabilities Act (ADA), 42 USC §121.010-12213 (1995).

Autopsy Consent, Mo Rev Stat, §194.115 (1998).

Comprehensive Drug Abuse Prevention and Control Act, Pub L No. 91-513, 84 Stat §1236 (1970).

Emergency Medical Treatment and Active Labor Act (EMTALA) (1986).

Federal Nursing Home Reform Act (1987).

Health Insurance Portability and Accountability Act of 1996 (HIPAA), Pub L No. 104 (1996).

Mental Health Parity Act (1996).

National Organ Transplant Act, Pub L No. 98-507 (1984).

Patient Protection and Affordable Care Act (ACA), Pub L No. 111-148 (2010).

Patient Self-Determination Act, 42 CFR 417 (1991).

Professional Nursing, 225 Ill Comp Stat 65/50 (2015).

Resident's Rights, Medicaid Statute, 42 USCA §1396R (1988).

Staff to Patient Ratios, Calif Assembly Bill 394 (1999).

Standards of Professional Conduct, Ill Admin Code Tit 68, Pt 1300.350 (2015).

Uniform Anatomical Gift Act (2006).

Uniform Determination of Death Act (1980).

Cases

Ciechoski v. Phoenixville Hospital Co., 1931 EDA (Chester County Circuit Ct 2014) (verdict upheld 2015).

Cruzan v. Director Missouri Department of Health, 497 US 261 (1990).

Darling v. Charleston Community Memorial Hospital, 33 Ill 2d 326, 331, 211 NE2d 253 (1965).

Dimora v. Cleveland Clinics Foundation, 114 Ohio App 3d 711 (1996).

Estate of Behringer v. Med. Ctr. at Princeton, 592 A.2d 1251 (NJ Super Ct Law Div 1991).

In re Intracare Hospital, 2007 WL 2682268 (Tex App, September 13, 2007).

In re Schiller, 148 NJ Super 168 (1977).

Roe v. Wade, 410 US 113 (1973).

Schloendorff v. Society of New York Hospital, 105 NE 92 (NY 1914).

Tibbs v. Burnell, 448 SW 3d (Ky 2014).

Winkelman v. Beloit Memorial Hospital, 484 NW2d 211 (Wisc 1992).

evolve MEDIA RESOURCES

http://evolve.elsevier.com/Potter/essentials

- Audio Glossary

- QSEN Activity and Review Questions Answers and Rationales

OBJECTIVES

- Discuss the foundations of ethics and ethical practice in nursing.
- Discuss the principles of health care ethics.

- Describe patient advocacy and the nurse's role.
- Describe the process for recognizing and resolving an ethical dilemma.

KEY TERMS

advocacy, p. 76
autonomy, p. 74
beneficence, p. 75
bioethics, p. 74
deontology, p. 77
ethical dilemma, p. 77

ethics, p. 73
ethics of care, p. 78
feminist ethics, p. 77
fidelity, p. 75
justice, p. 75
morals, p. 73

multidisciplinary ethics
   committee, p. 78
nonmaleficence, p. 75
utilitarianism, p. 77
value, p. 74

ETHICS

Ethics refers to standards of conduct, particularly right and wrong behavior (*American Heritage Dictionary of English Language*, 2016). A fundamental concern of ethics is the effect of our actions on others. The study of ethics includes the study of personal behavior and issues of character such as kindness, tolerance, and generosity. In health care, professional groups establish standards of ethical behavior that guide individual providers about right and wrong actions. Because of these standards, the public comes to trust that providers have the best interests of patients in mind. These standards also provide guidance for the navigation of difficult situations that can arise in the presence of suffering, health care decisions near the end of life, disagreements about what constitutes right and wrong behaviors, and issues of social justice.

Nursing knowledge about patients uniquely positions nurses to contribute to ethical discussions and debates. Your clinical practice is strengthened by your ongoing knowledge about professional standards of practice and the ethical principles that guide the navigation of difficult situations. Nursing excellence comprises elements greater than the sum of your clinical skills. In this chapter, you will learn about common ethical terms and the philosophical foundations that shape and nurture professional nursing practice.

Basic Definitions

Ethical issues differ from legal issues. Legal issues are resolved by reference to laws that are usually concrete and publicly determined. Breaking a law results in a public consequence such as a ticket for speeding or jail time for stealing. However, ethics has a broader base of interest than the law, referring more to issues of behavior and character. The terms *ethics* and *morals* sometimes are used interchangeably. **Morals** usually refer to judgment about behavior, based on specific beliefs, and ethics refers to the study of the ideals of right and wrong

CASE STUDY

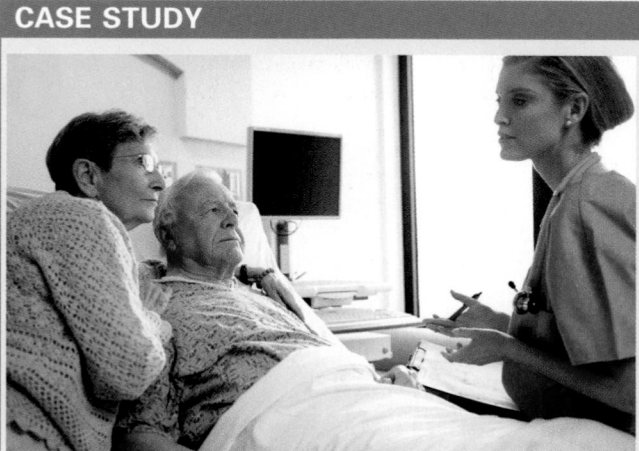

Copyright © monkeybusinessimages/iStock/Thinkstock.

Albert Timmons, a 92-year-old man, is admitted to a medical-surgical unit for management of pneumonia. He is in hospice and has advanced dementia. His family is supportive and present. The primary goal of the admission is comfort. Medications on admission include morphine for pain, risperidone to reduce hallucinations, and lorazepam for agitation as needed. Mr. Timmons has been on these medications for about 1 year.

The admitting nurse is not familiar with risperidone. On review, she learns that use of it in older-adult patients is not officially approved (National Institutes of Health [NIH], 2015). Its primary use is for patients with schizophrenia or bipolar disorder. Side effects of long-term use in older-adult patients include increased risk of stroke and death. Furthermore, discontinuing risperidone requires a slow taper over several days or weeks because without a taper, the patient can experience increased disorientation and hallucinations. The nurse discusses her findings with the admitting physician. The physician challenges the nurse's proposal to discontinue the medication, citing his past experiences with patients on risperidone and the fact that the patient is in hospice care. He eventually agrees to stop the medication but without tapering it first. What are the nurse's ethical obligations at this point?

TABLE 6.1	PRINCIPLES OF HEALTH CARE ETHICS
PRINCIPLE	**DEFINITION**
Autonomy	Independence; self-determination; self-reliance
Justice	Fairness or equity
Fidelity	Faithfulness; striving to keep promises
Beneficence	Actively seeking benefits; promotion of good
Nonmaleficence	Actively seeking to do no harm

The study of **bioethics** represents a branch of ethics within the field of health care. The study of bioethics has grown over the last 50 years, beginning with the emergence of technologies related to organ transplant. When researchers perfected kidney transplant procedures in the early 1970s, only a limited number of kidneys were available for transplant compared with the number of patients in need. This lack of resources became an immediate ethical concern. The health care community in the United States began to grapple with this issue by means of ethical discussion in local and national groups.

Changing medical technologies continue to require societies to face difficult ethical questions. Why should we do genetic testing for diseases we cannot cure? How shall we define quality of life? Who should decide? In the study of bioethics, health care professionals agree to negotiate these difficult and important questions by referring to a common set of ethical principles.

Ethical Principles

Health care providers agree to common ethical principles that guide professional practice and decision making (see Table 6.1). **Autonomy** refers to a person's independence. As a principle in bioethics, providers agree to respect an individual's right to determine a course of action. The respect pertains to patients as well as to providers. For example, before surgery a patient is required to sign a consent form. The purpose of the consent is to verify in writing that the health care team respects the patient's independence by obtaining the patient's permission to proceed. Respect for autonomy becomes complicated when the patient is a child or when the patient is cognitively impaired by disease, age, or trauma. Although the health care team turns to the individual who is identified as legally responsible for the patient, the ethical goal remains: determine the best interests of the patient, from the patient's point of view, out of a respect for autonomy.

Respect for autonomy also refers to providers and provider relationships with institutions. What happens when a provider is asked to perform duties that conflict with religious or personal beliefs? Institutions provide policies to accommodate respect for providers by reassigning or modifying duties when religious beliefs conflict with duties. The reassignment is conducted, however, only in a way that protects the patient from abandonment and only when patient

behavior. *In the case study the nurse can use ethical standards of practice such as fidelity, beneficence, and nonmaleficence (Table 6.1) to guide her decisions about how to proceed with the issues that she faces with Mr. Timmons and his physician.*

Values play an important role in understanding ethics. A **value** is a personal belief about the worth a person holds for an idea, a custom, or an object. The values that the person holds reflect cultural and social influences. For example, a person who makes a living in a rural place may value the environment differently than someone who visits rural areas for recreation. Ethical codes grow from shared values, negotiated and discussed over time through religious groups, ethnic groups, or work groups. As you enter the nursing profession, you undergo a similar process of learning shared values. Clarity about your values and your own point of view will guide you in making effective ethical decisions.

care is not compromised. Concern for patient well-being remains the primary concern.

What happens when a provider is concerned that an institution's practices are unsafe? Institutional whistle blower protections prohibit retaliation against an employee who makes a legitimate report about clinical safety issues. These protections represent expressions of respect for provider autonomy.

Justice refers to the principle of fairness. In health care the term reflects a commitment to fair treatment and fair distribution of health care resources. How to ensure a fair distribution, however, is not always clear. Access to care is uneven in the United States. Poverty and race remain strong predictors of access, quality, and treatment efficacy. For example, according to an analysis of U.S. cities, a person's zip code has a greater impact on health outcomes than a person's genetic code (Box 6.1). The principle of justice is at the heart of the national discussion in the United States about health care reform and access to care.

Fidelity refers to the agreement to keep promises and is based on the virtue of caring. For example, if you assess a patient for pain and then offer a plan to manage the pain, the principle of fidelity encourages you to do your best to provide follow-up that includes continuous reevaluation of pain levels. In this way you keep your promise to improve patient comfort. *In the case study, the nurse makes an unspoken but important promise to advocate for Mr. Timmons' well-being, which is why she questioned the ongoing use of risperidone for the patient.*

The principle of **beneficence** refers to taking positive action to help others. It encourages you to do good for a patient. The agreement to act with beneficence requires that the best interest of a patient remains more important than self-interest and that you act thoughtfully to understand patient needs and work actively to help meet those needs.

Nonmaleficence refers to the fundamental agreement to do no harm. It is closely related to the principle of beneficence. The health care provider tries to balance the risks and benefits of care, while striving at the same time to do the least harm possible. The principle of nonmaleficence promotes a continuing effort to consider the potential for harm and to minimize harm, even when it may be necessary to promote health. In the case study, the agreement to do no harm is at stake: when do the benefits of the medication become risks that will cause more harm than benefit? The answer may not always be clear, but the commitment to negotiate questions of benefit and harm remains constant.

Codes of Ethics

The American Nurses Association (ANA) *Code of Ethics for Nurses* (2015) lays out principles and obligations that shape professional nursing practice including responsibility, accountability, respect for confidentiality, competency, judgment, and advocacy. The ANA Ethics Council comprises national leaders in nursing ethics who craft the code in collaboration with international health communities including the United Nations, World Medical Association, and Inter-

---

BOX 6.1 EVIDENCE-BASED PRACTICE

PICOT Question: How does race contribute to health outcomes for persons of color in the United States?

In health care, we commit to the principle of justice (i.e., to find a way to ensure fair distribution of services and equal access to quality outcomes). The commitment is clearly articulated in the American Nurses Association (ANA) *Code of Ethics for Nurses* (2015). The fact that health care outcomes remain uneven in the United States presents us with an ethical challenge. Although solutions may be complex, we remain professionally committed as members of the health care team to seeking a solution.

SUMMARY OF EVIDENCE

In an editorial titled "Being Black Is Bad for Your Health," researchers describe current analysis of what they refer to as a "daunting health equity challenge" for the United States. Analysis of demographics in Miami and Philadelphia and other metropolitan areas shows that a person's zip code has a greater impact on good health than a person's genetic code (Center on Society and Health, 2016). Black children have at least a 500% higher death rate from asthma compared with white children (Akinbami et al., 2014; Lavizzo-Mourey and Williams, 2016). According to data collected by the Centers for Disease Control and Prevention and the Agency for Healthcare Research and Quality, African Americans are 20% less likely to receive treatment for depression than white people, 30% more likely than white people to die of heart disease or stroke, and 40% more likely than white people to die of breast cancer (Families USA, 2014). Providers need to recognize the link between racism and poor health and work together to close the gap so that everyone has the best opportunity to achieve good health (Lavizzo-Mourey and Williams, 2016).

APPLICATION TO NURSING PRACTICE

- Consider how issues of race impact all your patients (Lavizzo-Mourey and Williams, 2016).
- Consider how your nursing practice may be affected by racial prejudice (Families USA, 2014).
- Apply your commitment to patient advocacy by participating in public policy discussions and actions in your community (ANA, 2015).
- Make a commitment to learn more about health disparities, and support innovative efforts to resolve them.

---

national Council of Nurses (ICN) (2012). (See Box 6.2 for the ICN Code of Ethics.)

Responsibility refers to reliability and dependability in the performance of duties. As the case study illustrates, when administering a medication, a nurse is responsible for conducting an accurate assessment of a patient's need for the medication, acquiring the patient's consent for receiving the medication, giving the medication safely, and evaluating the patient's response to it. By agreeing to act responsibly over time, you gain trust from patients, colleagues, and society.

Accountability refers to the ability to answer for your actions. You are accountable to yourself, first and foremost, for your own actions and behaviors. As a professional nurse,

---

BOX 6.2   THE ICN CODE OF ETHICS FOR NURSES

PREAMBLE

Nurses have four fundamental responsibilities: to promote health, prevent illness, restore health, and alleviate suffering. The need for nursing is universal. Inherent in nursing is respect for human rights, including cultural rights and the right to life and choice, to dignity, and to be treated with respect. Nursing care is respectful of and unrestricted by considerations of age, colour, creed, culture, disability or illness, gender, sexual orientation, nationality, politics, race, or social status. Nurses render health services to the individual, the family, and the community and coordinate their services with those of related groups.

ELEMENTS OF THE CODE

1. Nurses and People

The nurse's primary professional responsibility is to people requiring nursing care. In providing care the nurse promotes an environment in which the human rights, values, customs, and spiritual beliefs of the individual, family, and community are respected. The nurse ensures that the individual receives sufficient information on which to base consent for care and related treatment. The nurse holds in confidence personal information and uses judgment in sharing this information. The nurse shares with society the responsibility for initiating and supporting action to meet the health and social needs of the public, in particular those of vulnerable populations. The nurse advocates for equity and social justice in resource allocation, access to health care, and other social and economic services. The nurse demonstrates professional values such as respectfulness, responsiveness, compassion, trustworthiness, and integrity.

2. Nurses and Practice

The nurse carries personal responsibility and accountability for nursing practice and for maintaining competence by continual

learning. The nurse maintains a standard of personal health such that the ability to provide care is not compromised. The nurse uses judgment regarding individual competence when accepting and delegating responsibility. The nurse at all times maintains standards of personal conduct that reflect well on the profession and enhance public confidence. In providing care the nurse ensures that use of technology and scientific advances is compatible with the safety, dignity, and rights of people. The nurse strives to foster and maintain a practice culture promoting ethical behaviour and open dialogue.

3. Nurses and the Profession

The nurse assumes the major role in determining and implementing acceptable standards of clinical nursing practice, management, research, and education. The nurse is active in developing a core of research-based professional knowledge. The nurse is active in developing and sustaining a core of professional values. The nurse, acting through the professional organization, participates in creating and maintaining safe, equitable social and economic working conditions in nursing. The nurse practices to sustain and protect the natural environment and is aware of its consequences on health. The nurse contributes to an ethical organizational environment and challenges unethical practices and settings.

4. Nurses and Co-workers

The nurse sustains a collaborative and respectful relationship with co-workers in nursing and other fields. The nurse takes appropriate action to safeguard individuals, families, and communities when their health is endangered by a co-worker or any other person. The nurse takes appropriate action to support and guide co-workers to advance ethical conduct.

ICN, International Council of Nurses.
From International Council of Nurses: *The ICN code of ethics for nurses,* 2012, http://www.icn.ch/images/stories/documents/about/icncode_english.

---

you are then first and foremost accountable to the patients you serve. You are also accountable to your workplace and to the larger community. You exercise accountability by taking ownership of your actions, making a reasoned judgment about what is right, and then acting accordingly. *In the case study, the nurse demonstrates accountability to Mr. Timmons by questioning the physician's order when she determines that a medication order could harm Mr. Timmons.* Finding the balance between competing obligations is not always easy or clear, but the commitment to understand how and why you are accountable remains constant.

A responsible nurse is competent in knowledge and skills. Your competence ensures the provision of safe nursing care. The agreement to practice with competence is described in the ANA *Code of Ethics for Nurses* (2015). State regulations for nursing practice commonly include regulations about competence. As a responsible nurse, for example, you will ensure that your knowledge about the risks and benefits of medications is current before you administer them. Because you are competent, the patient can trust that the medications you offer are safe. In the case study, the nurse does not simply follow a physician's order; she demonstrates competence by

taking time to look up a new medication before administering it. Beyond your clinical competence, the *Code of Ethics for Nurses* lays out a justification for workplace competencies that include collaboration, participatory development of workplace policies and procedures, and advocacy in the public arena.

Judgment refers to the ability to form an opinion and to draw sound conclusions based on your study of the situation. To practice critical thinking, you learn to practice good judgment in nursing school (see Chapter 8). You continue to improve your judgment skills throughout your career.

Advocacy involves speaking up for patients. The ANA *Code of Ethics for Nurses* (2015) explains that a nurse "promotes, advocates for, and protects the rights, health, and safety of the patient." Your advocacy is inspired by your relationship with patients. You come to know your patients while performing nursing care that brings you into intimate contact with them such as performing special procedures, teaching new skills, and preparing for discharge. You gain specific information about patients that is unique to nursing and part of the larger picture of the whole patient. As such, the nursing contribution is essential to the success of the overall plan of care. In the case study, the nurse's willingness to challenge an order represents a fundamental act of patient advocacy.

Advocacy can also take the form of engagement with public policy. Your work with individual patients exposes you to elements that shape health care outcomes in the larger world. As a result, you become a respected public voice on public policy. Local Nurse Practice Acts, health care reform policy, mental health issues, and public health issues are just a few examples of how a nurse's voice makes a difference. For example, the study of health care disparities in the United States (see Box 6.1) sheds light on demographic elements that impact health outcomes. Those elements may seem to be beyond your control at first. However, your willingness to learn more and to become engaged with solutions represents a powerful kind of patient advocacy. Provision 9 of the ANA *Code of Ethics for Nurses* (2015) specifically calls for your engagement with issues of social justice as an expression of your professional nursing role: "The profession of nursing, collectively through its professional organizations, must articulate nursing values, maintain the integrity of the profession, and integrate principles of social justice into nursing and health policy."

Developing a Personal Point of View

Your point of view is shaped by your personal values. Values vary among people and change over time. Understanding your own values while at the same time acknowledging the values of others can help to resolve conflict during decision making.

An ethical dilemma exists when the right thing to do is not clear, when members of the health care team cannot agree on the right thing to do, or when the health care team and the patient and/or family disagree on a course of action. Whether the dilemma involves disagreement or lack of clarity about the right action, resolution involves negotiating differing points of view. You will become a stronger negotiator by making sure you can articulate your own point of view from the start. You can then turn to the patient to determine the patient's point of view. A clear understanding of a patient's point of view helps you advocate for the patient even if the patient's opinions differ from yours. When you understand your own opinions and beliefs as well as the opinions and beliefs of your patient, you are able to join your colleagues in collaborative discussion.

When the situation concerns issues such as health, personal habits, and quality of life, all participants in a discussion benefit from clarity about personal values and a willingness to look beyond personal preferences for shared values. Your respect for the point of view of others, especially when it differs from your own, is essential in the successful navigation of ethical deliberation.

ETHICAL THEORY

Traditional theories of ethics provide a foundation for navigating ethical problems in health care (Beauchamp and Childress, 2012). This section contains descriptions of common ethical philosophies that overlap in some areas and compete in others. In your everyday work as a nurse, you may encounter discussions that refer to one or another of these philosophies. Your personal values, personal experiences, and relationships with others influence which of these or which combination of them helps you to navigate ethical issues in your daily life.

Deontology

This system of ethics is perhaps most familiar to health care practitioners. Deontology defines actions as right or wrong based on principles such as truth and justice (Beauchamp and Childress, 2012). With deontology, you focus less on consequences, ethically speaking, and more on reason and "right-making characteristics" such as respect for autonomy, truthfulness, and justice (see Table 6.1) (Beauchamp and Childress, 2012). If an act is just, respects autonomy, and provides good, the act is ethical. Deontology depends on a mutual understanding of justice, autonomy, and goodness.

Utilitarianism

You use a utilitarian ethic when determining the value of something based primarily on its usefulness. This philosophy is also known as consequentialism because of its emphasis on outcomes. The greatest good for the greatest number of people is the guiding principle for action in this system. As with deontology, utilitarianism relies on the application of the principles of "good" and "greatest." Difficulties arise when people have conflicting definitions of "greatest good." Utilitarianism guides us to measure the effect, or consequences, that an act will have. By comparison, deontology focuses less on consequences and looks to the presence of right-making characteristics (Beauchamp and Childress, 2012).

Virtue Ethics

A focus on the character of an individual is at the heart of virtue ethics. A virtue is a character trait that is socially valued (Beauchamp and Childress, 2012). Virtue ethics values the motivation of the individual over simple obedience to principles such as beneficence or respect for autonomy. Virtue ethics need not compete with theories such as utilitarianism or deontology, but it does guide us to examine motives even as we try to establish principles of right action and to nurture the presence of virtuous characteristics such as sympathy and kindness (Beauchamp and Childress, 2012). *In the case study, the nurse demonstrates a virtue of sympathy for Mr. Timmons' well-being when she decides to challenge the physician's order for the sake of Mr. Timmons' well-being. That virtue probably motivates her actions to question the physician order as much as her respect for the principle of beneficence.*

Feminist Ethics

Feminist ethics proposes that we routinely ask how ethical decisions will affect women as a way to repair a history of inequality (Lindeman, 2005). Writers with a feminist perspective tend to concentrate more on practical solutions than on theory. For example, when deciding whether to perform a possibly futile procedure on a dying patient, feminist ethics might guide us to look at a patient's relationships with family and friends to determine the ethically right thing to do. How would a patient's ability to engage in relationships be affected? If the patient is a parent, how would the patient's relationship to the children be affected by the intervention? These questions might surface less often if the discussion is framed solely by conventional ethical principles.

Critics of feminist ethics worry about the lack of appeal to ethical principles. Without guidance from principles such as autonomy and beneficence, they argue, solutions to ethical questions could become situational and too dependent on perceptions that can be temporal and fleeting.

Ethics of Care

Nel Noddings, an early proponent of the ethics of care, used the term *one-caring* to identify the individual who provides care and *cared-for* to refer to the patient. In adopting this language, Noddings hoped to emphasize the role of feelings. Ethics of care strives to address issues beyond individual relationships by raising ethical concerns about the structures within which individual caring occurs such as hospitals or universities (Noddings, 2013). Its principles apply to all members of a health care community and not just to nurses. Ethics of care suggests that health care workers resolve ethical dilemmas by paying attention to relationships and stories of the participants and by promoting a fundamental act of caring.

Casuistry

Casuistry, or case-based reasoning, turns away from conventional principles of ethics to determine best actions and focuses instead on an "intimate understanding of particular situations" (Beauchamp and Childress, 2012). This approach to ethical discourse depends on finding consensus more than an appeal to philosophical principle. Building consensus is an act of discovery, where collective wisdom guides a group to the best possible decision. As a strategy for solving dilemmas, consensus building promotes respect and agreement rather than a particular philosophy or moral system itself.

HOW TO PROCESS AN ETHICAL DILEMMA

Ethical dilemmas can be deeply distressing for patients, families, and providers. A guide for processing ethical dilemmas, based on ethical principles and shaped by the ANA *Code of Ethics for Nurses* (2015), serves to promote successful resolution.

Most health care institutions establish a multidisciplinary ethics committee to process ethical dilemmas with representatives from nursing, medicine, professional disciplines, and the community at large. Besides individual case consultation, the mission of an ethics committee usually includes education and policy recommendation. Any involved person, including nurses, patients, and families of patients, can request consultation with an ethics committee.

Ethical issues can be processed in settings other than a committee. Other venues include family conferences, staff meetings, and one-on-one meetings with patients and

---

BOX 6.3 HOW TO PROCESS AN ETHICAL DILEMMA

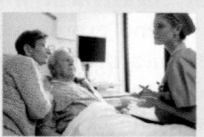
Copyright © monkey businessimages/ iStock/Thinkstock.

STEP 1. IS THIS AN ETHICAL DILEMMA?
When the question remains perplexing even after careful review of pertinent information, an ethical dilemma may exist.

STEP 2. GATHER ALL INFORMATION RELEVANT TO THE CASE.
Gathering facts is critical to an effective process. An overlooked fact sometimes provides quick resolution or affects the options available. Patient, family, institutional, and social perspectives are important sources of relevant information.

STEP 3. EXAMINE AND DETERMINE YOUR VALUES AND OPINIONS ABOUT THE ISSUES.
This step ensures that you distinguish between your personal values and those of the other participants and allows you to become a more open listener.

STEP 4. STATE THE PROBLEM CLEARLY.
A clear statement of the dilemma is not always easy but facilitates next steps.

STEP 5. CONSIDER POSSIBLE COURSES OF ACTION.
To respect all sides of an issue, list potential actions, especially when the list will reflect opinions that conflict.

STEP 6. NEGOTIATE THE OUTCOME.
Sometimes a course of action that seemed unlikely at the beginning of the process takes on new possibility during discussion. Negotiation requires a confidence in your own point of view and a deep respect for the opinions of others.

STEP 7. EVALUATE THE ACTION.
Did the interventions provide for compromise that is acceptable to all? An ethical dilemma is often complicated emotionally as well as clinically. It is important to review outcomes to ensure that the process has worked.

---

co-workers. Whatever the venue, nurses provide a valuable and unique perspective.

Resolving an ethical dilemma is similar to the nursing process because it benefits from systematic thinking (Box 6.3). In the case study, the nurse faces a difficult situation where the physician's order seems contrary to safe practice, but the nurse is uncertain about challenging the order. A standard process for resolving an ethical dilemma can help create a satisfying plan of action.

Step 1: Is This an Ethical Dilemma?
The first step guides you to determine if the problem is actually an ethical one. Start by distinguishing ethical problems from issues about procedure, legality, or medical diagnosis, as these other categories are more easily solved by reference to policy or law.

In the case study, the nurse faces a difficult decision. If she follows the order as it is written, she may cause harm to Mr.

Timmons. Legal and procedural issues are at stake, but the nurse's main concern is ethical. She agrees with the physician's order to discontinue risperidone, but without a proper tapering, discontinuing the medication will likely harm Mr. Timmons. She knows she can challenge the order, but the physician has already listened to her recommendation to taper the medication and was reluctant to stop it in the first place. Why should she continue to challenge the order, and how can she best justify her challenge?

Step 2: Gather All Relevant Information

Accurate and complete information is essential for the ethical process to go forward. Sometimes gathering information resolves the situation without further deliberation.

In the case study, the nurse looked up information about the medication as a first step. It might also be helpful to learn more from the family about why Mr. Timmons was put on it in the first place. Because Mr. Timmons has advanced dementia, the nurse needs to know who is making medical decisions for the patient. She could discuss the situation with her colleagues and her supervisor to find out what other providers have experienced with discontinuing this medication. She might also try to learn more about how this physician has managed the medication in the past.

Step 3: Examine and Determine Your Values and Opinions About the Issues

The distinction between personal opinion and the opinions of others can be helpful in reaching resolution. People reach different conclusions about the same situation with no malice intended toward other people. Remembering this helps you to be an effective participant.

The nurse might reflect on her values about end-of-life care. If Mr. Timmons is on hospice care and actively dying, will withdrawal side effects really impact his clinical course? What if she finds that the description of withdrawal in the literature is different from the experience of others on her unit? Has the family been involved with the decision about the medication? How does the surrogate decision maker feel about the issue? Does the nurse manager of the unit have an opinion on the matter? What is the physician's experience about the off-label use of this medication in older-adult patients? By taking time to explore and learn more about values and opinions, the perception of conflict with the physician's order may become easier to manage or understand.

Step 4: State the Problem Clearly

After reviewing relevant information, develop a statement of the problem. Discussions will remain more focused and constructive when all parties agree on a statement of the problem.

What is the best course of action for Mr. Timmons in regard to comfort and dignity? How important is the recommendation to taper risperidone over time?

Step 5: Consider Possible Courses of Action

In trying to resolve a dilemma, it can help to list the possible actions, even if you are not sure which is right.

The nurse could speak with her colleagues and her supervisor and other physicians to find out more about the practice and past experiences of others. The nurse could converse with the physician and state her reasons again for challenging the order.

The best outcome at this point would be to reach an agreement on action with the physician. If the nurse and the physician cannot agree, the nurse could voice her concerns to her manager and consider other steps for reaching resolution.

Step 6: Negotiate the Outcome

In the case study, the only wrong answer would be to comply with an order without regard to the consequences for Mr. Timmons. The nurse is ethically and professionally obligated to act in the patient's best interest.

Step 7: Evaluate the Action

Once a resolution for an ethical dilemma is determined, action can move forward. Taking time to evaluate the outcome will ensure that the act was effective and right, and if not, further discussion can help to promote further resolution.

In the case study, in seeing the situation through to a positive outcome for Mr. Timmons, the nurse will sustain her ethical commitment to "protect the health, safety, and rights of the patient" (ANA, 2015).

QSEN QSEN ACTIVITY *Teamwork and Collaboration*

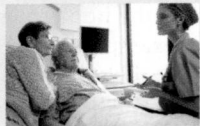

Copyright © monkey businessimages/ iStock/Thinkstock.

In the case study, the nurse faces a difficult decision: to comply with an order that she considers might be harmful to Mr. Timmons or challenge the ordering physician to rewrite the order. The QSEN competency that often comes into play when ethical issues are at stake is teamwork and collaboration. Collaboration, however, implies more than simply remaining courteous and supportive. It can sometimes mean taking a deep breath, getting the facts and opinions lined up, and challenging a colleague.

- How would you deal with the situation that the nurse faces in the case study?
- What would you do to prepare for your action?
- What ethical principles would inspire your action?

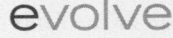 evolve Answers to QSEN Activities can be found on the Evolve website.

ETHICAL ISSUES IN NURSING

This section describes ethical issues common in health care today.

Care at the End of Life

Working with patients who are near the end of life can be an inspiring experience. Nurses and others say they feel "that it is a privilege to spend time with the dying, to be allowed into a person's life and a family's life when they are at their rawest and most vulnerable, and when they most need help" (MacFarquhar, 2016). It can also involve difficult ethical challenges. Questions often come up about the appropriateness of interventions that prolong life but increase suffering. For example, a patient with terminal cancer may become too weak to swallow safely and the possibility of a gastrostomy tube comes up as a way to provide nourishment and avoid risk for aspiration pneumonia. However, the safe delivery of nourishment to prevent pneumonia could, at the same time, prolong the pain and suffering from the cancer. Gathering all information relevant to the case is the usual first step for resolving ethical questions. What is the patient's perception of the prognosis? What are the religious or spiritual concerns of the patient and the patient's family and circle of friends? What are the surgical risks and benefits from placement of the gastrostomy tube? What is the medical risk for aspiration pneumonia? Is the patient competent to make the decision? If not, who is?

Your role as a patient's nurse is invaluable. You will provide a unique point of view about the patient's status and the family's ability to cope. Whether the resolution flows from a family conference or in a formal ethics consultation, your contributions to the discussion will reflect your professional role as a nurse and your ethical commitment to respect the patient's journey.

Disability and Difference

Until recently, discussions about disability focused on a medical model where the goal was to define the impairment and devise a medical intervention. For example, when a person develops a neurological disorder that makes ambulation difficult or impossible, the goal in the medical model would be to craft interventions that attempt to fix or minimize the neurological deficit. A newer proposal suggests that we define disability as a "poor fit between the individual and the social, material, and technological environment" (Kukla, n.d.). Between the two models of disability, medical and social, we can see that disability could be managed by changing the body and/or the environment. In the example of a person with neurological disease, the focus could extend beyond medical or surgical interventions and include ensuring public policy that optimizes life with the disease by ensuring access to public places, workplace tolerance, and access to care. Changes in public policy reflect these changes in approach. For example, since implementation of the Americans with Disabilities Act (ADA) in 1990, public places such as restaurants and buses are now accessible to people who use wheelchairs (U.S. Department of Justice [USDOJ], n.d.). Most school districts no longer separate children who are physically or mentally challenged but rather integrate them into mainstream classrooms. Antidiscrimination laws enhance the economic security of people with physical, mental, or emotional challenges. These changes result in the greater integration of persons with disabilities into general society. The models themselves challenge our notion of "disabled" in the first place.

Philosophically, the conversation has shifted from one about a focus on what is wrong with an individual to a conversation about how best to nurture capabilities of all humans, regardless of their circumstances. This capabilities approach, as it is called, "begins with a commitment to the equal dignity of all people, whatever their class, religion, caste, race, or gender, and it is committed to the attainment, for all, of lives that are worthy of that equal dignity"

(Nussbaum, 2011). As a nurse, your professional commitment to advocacy is outlined in the ANA *Code of Ethics for Nurses*, especially Provision 1: "The nurse practices with compassion and respect for the inherent dignity, worth, and unique attributes of every person" (ANA, 2015). Your ethical obligation to respect patient autonomy also guides you to treat patients with this kind of equal dignity.

Social Media

Online apps such as Facebook, Twitter, Snapchat, and Instagram offer great networking tools for nurses, but the benefits come with risks. On one hand, social media provides opportunities to enhance conversation between nurses who work together but whose off-work paths rarely cross. Social media can help foster a sense of team that can be a real asset for the workplace. For patients, online communication with providers offers powerful support, especially for patients who live long distances from providers or whose ability to travel is compromised.

On the other hand, the risk of exposure of private information is tremendous and often not well understood. Professional boundaries can be violated when nurses share feelings, opinions, or images about a workplace in online public venues. For example, online groups may be a place where colleagues post news about work-related classes, parties, and important social milestones such as marriages or births. However, even when they are designed to be private, access by others can occur inadvertently. When private postings become public, they can cross an ethical line when details include personal feelings about co-workers or other workplace troubles. That kind of public news can undermine workplace cohesion. Also, it can upset patients and their families and jeopardize their trust in your ability to care for them.

Even a well-intentioned effort to support a family by agreeing to become a Facebook friend can backfire. Other families may see evidence of your friendship and worry why you are not friends with them too. Posting selfies of you with a patient can be a source of pride and accomplishment for you but distressing for a family who strives for privacy. Your commitment to respect patient autonomy and your professional obligation for accountability and responsibility are at stake with social media, and extreme caution is advised.

The ANA crafted a position statement regarding social networking (ANA, 2011). In addition, the National Council for State Boards of Nursing (NCSBN) developed a white paper and video lessons outlining suggested safe practices (2014). Most workplace policies now address issues of social media and provide guidelines that will help to protect you and your patients.

CONCLUSION

As a nurse, you bring a unique voice to quality patient care and to the health of the community at large. The privilege to serve as an advocate for patients flows from your study of the ethical foundations of your profession. Your willingness to embrace ethical practice will nurture your development as an informed, collaborative, and generous professional nurse.

KEY POINTS

- Principles of ethics include autonomy, justice, fidelity, beneficence, and nonmaleficence.
- The ANA *Code of Ethics for Nurses* guides nursing practice and nursing behaviors.
- Professional nursing promotes accountability, responsibility, and advocacy.
- An ethical nurse maintains competence in practice and assumes responsibility for nursing judgments.
- The primary goal of advocacy is to support patient well-being at the bedside, within organizations, and in the larger world of public policy and politics.
- Professional nurses commit to provide high-quality health care to patients, the community, and society.
- Ethical issues often arise from differences in values, changing professional roles, and technological advances that challenge commonly held notions of health and well-being.
- A standard process for managing ethical dilemmas helps to resolve difficult situations in a collaborative way that nurtures workplace relationships.
- A nurse's point of view provides a unique and valuable voice in the management of ethical issues.

REFLECTIVE LEARNING

- Thinking back on a recent clinical experience, describe specific actions in your practice that reflected a respect for patient autonomy.
- Consider the clinical history of a patient you cared for recently. Describe how you think the concept of justice is reflected in the patient's access to care. How will the patient's access to care before and after admission impact the patient's quality of life?
- Describe an action that you took or witnessed during a clinical experience that illustrates the concept of advocacy. What was easy about the action? What was challenging?

REVIEW QUESTIONS

1. The ANA *Code of Ethics for Nurses* articulates that the nurse "promotes, advocates for, and strives to protect the health, safety, and rights of the patient." This promise to protect includes a promise to protect patient privacy. On the basis of this principle, if you participate in a public online social network such as Facebook, could you post images of a patient's x-ray film if you obscured or deleted all patient identifiers? Indicate the right answer with the best rationale.
   1. Yes. Patient privacy would not be violated because patient identifiers were removed.
   2. Yes. Respect for autonomy implies that you have the autonomy to decide what constitutes privacy.
   3. No. A viewer might identify the patient based on other comments that you make online about the patient's condition and your place of work.
   4. No. The principle of justice requires you to allocate resources fairly.

2. You decide to write an editorial to your local newspaper expressing your opinion about disparities in access to health care in your community. Which provisions from the ANA *Code of Ethics for Nurses* could you use to strengthen your editorial? (Select all that apply.)
   1. Provision 2: The nurse's primary commitment is to the patient, whether an individual, family, group, community, or population.
   2. Provision 6: The nurse, through individual and collective effort, establishes, maintains, and improves the ethical environment of the work setting and conditions of employment that are conducive to safe, quality health care.
   3. Provision 8: The nurse collaborates with other health professionals and the public to protect human rights, promote health diplomacy, and reduce health disparities.
   4. Provision 9: The profession of nursing, collectively through its professional organizations, must articulate nursing values, maintain the integrity of the profession, and integrate principles of social justice into nursing and health policy.
   5. The ANA *Code of Ethics for Nurses* applies to nursing practice, and it is therefore inappropriate to refer to specific provisions when discussing public policy.

3. A nurse is caring for a 36-year-old patient with a brain tumor who is dying. The patient has undergone surgery and chemotherapy, but nothing has worked so far to stop the growth of the tumor. The physician offered the patient one further treatment plan that could prolong life for a few weeks, but the treatment has painful side effects. The patient tells his nurse that he is at peace with the prognosis and wants to stop all further treatment. The nurse is troubled by the patient's response. She feels confident that the side effects could be managed, and, for her, refusing treatment violates a belief in the sanctity of life. Which of the following accurately describes ethical principles at stake in this situation? (Select all that apply.)
   1. Even though the patient does not want it, making sure that the patient gets all possible treatments including experimental treatments will show a commitment to justice for this patient.
   2. Respect for the patient's autonomy is a fundamental ethical commitment and needs to be taken into consideration when making clinical decisions with a patient.
   3. The principle of beneficence implies that the providers need to ensure the patient receives the treatment because it could possibly work to the patient's benefit.
   4. The nurse will remain committed to advocacy for this patient, speaking for the patient's point of view even though it conflicts with her own beliefs. Her commitment reflects a professional commitment to fidelity.
   5. The nurse's concern about managing difficult side effects represents the practice of nonmaleficence, the commitment to do no harm.

4. Which of the following actions illustrate accountability? (Select all that apply.)
    1. A patient undergoes a surgical procedure that is new to the agency. The nurse asks the manager to provide an in-service about the procedure.
    2. A health care provider writes orders for pain-management medication even though the patient has been free of pain for 3 days. Out of respect for the health care provider's authority, a nurse administers the medications.
    3. During annual budget preparation at an agency, a nurse advocates for annual pay increases for the staff.
    4. A patient reports she does not have health insurance and will not be able to pay for her discharge medications. A nurse requests that a social worker meet with this patient to find a way to maximize available health care benefits.
    5. The policy on a patient care unit requires repositioning of patients every 2 hours. During busy shifts, the nursing staff is unable to keep up with the practice requirement. Whenever this happens, a nurse notifies the manager and discusses possible remedies.

5. A nurse is caring for a 32-year-old patient with Down syndrome, a genetic disorder that includes impaired cognition. The patient's parents are deceased. He lives in a group home and works part time as a bagger at a grocery store. What actions does the nurse take during discharge planning to show respect for the patient's inherent dignity and worth? (Select all that apply.)
    1. Make sure written materials are written at an appropriate reading level
    2. Contact the group home to ensure that a caregiver is involved with discharge plans
    3. Allow the patient extra time for return demonstrations of your teaching plan
    4. Assume he is unable to understand instruction and focus on needs other than education
    5. Let his supervisor at the grocery story know about the patient's discharge medications

evolve

Additional Review Questions, as well as rationales for all Review Questions, can be found on the Evolve website.

1, 3; 2, 1, 3, 4; 3, 2, 4, 5; 4, 1, 5; 5, 1, 2, 3.

REFERENCES

Akinbami LJ, et al: Trends in racial disparities for asthma outcomes among children 0 to 17 years, 2001-2010, *J Allergy Clin Immunol* 134(3):547, 2014.

American Heritage Dictionary of English Language, ed 5, Boston, 2016, Houghton-Mifflin.

American Nurses Association (ANA): *Fact sheet: navigating the world of social media*, Silver Spring, MD, 2011, The Association, http://www.nursingworld.org/FunctionalMenuCategories/AboutANA/Social-Media/Social-Networking-Principles-Toolkit/Fact-Sheet-Navigating-the-World-of-Social-Media.pdf.

American Nurses Association (ANA): *Code of ethics for nurses with interpretative statements*, Washington, DC, 2015, The Association, http://nursingworld.org/DocumentVault/Ethics-1/Code-of-Ethics-for-Nurses.html.

Beauchamp T, Childress J: *Principles of biomedical ethics*, ed 7, New York, 2012, Oxford University Press.

Center on Society and Health: *Mapping life expectancy*, Virginia Commonwealth University, 2016, http://www.societyhealth.vcu.edu/work/the-projects/mapping-life-expectancy.html.

Families USA: *African American health disparities compared to Non-Hispanic Whites*, 2014, http://familiesusa.org/sites/default/files/product_documents/HSI-Health-disparities_african-americans-infographic_062414_final.png.

International Council of Nurses: *The ICN code of ethics for nurses*, revised 2012, http://www.icn.ch/images/stories/documents/about/icncode_english.pdf.

Kukla R: *PHLX101-02 Introduction to bioethics: two models of disability*, Kennedy Institute of Ethics, Georgetown University, n.d., https://bioethicsarchive.georgetown.edu/phlx101-02/course.html#units/disability/two-models-of-disability.

Lavizzo-Mourey R, Williams D: Being black is bad for your health, *US News and World Report*, April 14, 2016, http://www.usnews.com/opinion/blogs/policy-dose/articles/2016-04-14/theres-a-huge-health-equity-gap-between-whites-and-minorities.

Lindeman H: *An invitation to feminist ethics*, New York, 2005, McGraw-Hill Humanities.

MacFarquhar L: A tender hand in the presence of death, *The New Yorker*, July 11 and 18, 2016, http://www.newyorker.com/magazine/2016/07/11/the-work-of-a-hospice-nurse.

National Council for State Boards of Nursing (NCSBN): *Social media guidelines for nurses*, 2014, https://www.ncsbn.org/347.htm.

National Institutes of Health (NIH): *MedlinePlus: Risperidone*, 2015, https://medlineplus.gov/druginfo/meds/a694015.html.

Noddings N: *Caring: a relational approach to ethics and moral education*, Berkeley, CA, 2013, University of California Press.

Nussbaum M: What makes a good life, *The Nation*, May 2, 2011.

U.S. Department of Justice (USDOJ): *Information and technical assistance on the Americans with Disabilities Act*, n.d., https://www.ada.gov/2010_regs.htm.

Evidence-Based Practice

evolve EVOLVE MEDIA RESOURCES

http://evolve.elsevier.com/Potter/essentials

- Audio Glossary
- QSEN Activity and Review Questions Answers and Rationales

OBJECTIVES

- Discuss the relationship between evidence-based practice and the improvement of the safety and quality of nursing practice.
- Discuss the QSEN competencies for evidence-based practice.
- Describe the steps of evidence-based practice.
- Develop a PICO or PICOT question.
- Discuss the levels of evidence in the literature.
- Explain how critiquing the scientific literature leads to best evidence for practice changes.
- Discuss ways to apply evidence in nursing practice.
- Discuss ways to measure outcomes for an evidence-based practice change.
- Identify ways to sustain knowledge in evidence-based practice.
- Explain the relationship among nursing research, evidence-based practice, and quality improvement.

KEY TERMS

active errors, p. 95
bias, p. 88
clinical guidelines, p. 87
evidence-based practice (EBP), p. 84
hypotheses, p. 90

latent errors, p. 95
nursing-sensitive outcome, p. 92
peer-reviewed, p. 86
performance improvement (PI), p. 95
PICO (or PICOT), p. 86

quality improvement (QI), p. 95
reliable, p. 84
sentinel event, p. 95
valid, p. 89
variables, p. 90

Many nurses practice nursing according to what they learn in nursing school, their experiences in practice, and the policies and procedures of their institutions. This level of practice alone is not acceptable. Nursing practice is in an "age of accountability," in which nursing care impacts the quality, safety, and cost of health care (White and Spruce, 2015; Jun et al., 2016). People today are often more informed about their own health and the incidence of medical errors within health care institutions. Health care organizations are required to show their commitment to each health care stakeholder (e.g., patients, insurance companies, government agencies) to reducing health care error and improving safety by putting into place evidence-based safe practices (National Quality Forum [NQF], 2017). Nurses and other health care providers can no longer accept and practice the status quo. Greater attention must be given to why certain health care approaches are used, which ones work, and which ones do not. Research priorities identified by nurse administrators include the economic value of nursing, the design of nursing practice and care delivery models, patient safety and outcomes, and creating a healthy practice environment (Scott et al., 2016). Evidence-based practice (EBP) guides nurses and other health care providers in making effective, timely, and appropriate clinical decisions.

CASE STUDY *Cathy and Tom*

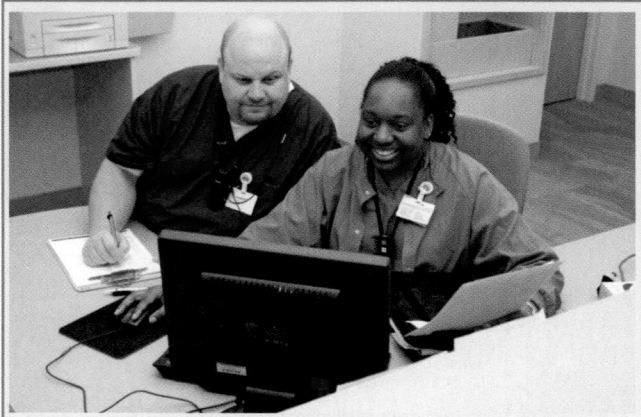

Cathy and Tom are two nurses who work in the medical intermediate care unit. They are members of the unit practice committee (UPC), which consists of a group of staff nurses, pharmacist, respiratory therapist, infection control practitioner, and physician. A UPC provides an ongoing forum for all clinicians in the department to discuss practice issues and explore ways to make improvements. The committee meets monthly to discuss practice issues on the unit and received a copy of the monthly report on the quality indicators for their unit. Cathy notes that the incidence of central line–catheter-associated bloodstream infections (CLABSIs) has steadily increased during the last 3 months. Patients with central venous catheters (CVCs) used to deliver fluids and medications over extended periods of time (see Chapter 18) are becoming infected, but why? Tom questions if the problem is related to the type of dressing placed over catheters or the way that sites are cleansed before insertion. The measurement of CLABSIs is considered a "Never Event," meaning that the hospital will not be reimbursed for the care of patients who have this hospital-acquired complication (Centers for Medicare and Medicaid Services, 2015). Thus it is important for the UPC to find ways to prevent CLABSIs from occurring.

The UPC decides to explore these questions as part of its evidence-based practice process. The first step is to develop a clinical question to efficiently search the scientific literature. Tom volunteers to do the search with the aid of the hospital librarian. The aim is to determine what evidence is available so that the committee can make an informed decision about standards needed to reduce CLABSIs in patients.

A CASE FOR EVIDENCE-BASED PRACTICE

Evidence-based practice (EBP) is a problem-solving approach to clinical practice that combines the conscientious use of best evidence in combination with a clinician's expertise, patient preferences and values, and available health care resources in making decisions about patient care (Melnyk and Fineout-Overholt, 2015). Put in simpler terms, EBP addresses a clinical problem by seeking the very best scientific and clinical evidence available for treating or managing the problem and implementing changes in practice. Some examples of using research-based findings include using a sliding board to transfer a patient from bed to stretcher instead of lifting and using the research-based Braden scale (see Chapter 38) to routinely assess a patient's risk for skin breakdown. Research shows that EBP enhances the patient experience, decreases cost, and improves patient outcomes (Crabtree et al., 2016; Godlock et al., 2016; McNeil, 2016). Use of EBP competencies by nurses and advanced practice nurses further improves the quality and consistency of health care (Melnyk et al., 2014).

Nurses regularly face important clinical decisions when caring for patients (e.g., "Why do I use this approach in providing patient care? Is a change needed? Is there a way to improve patient outcomes?"). Implementing health care processes or practices that are known to work (evidence based) in a reliable way is a feature of "quality care" and effective timely and appropriate clinical decisions (Peterson et al., 2014). Implementing new knowledge into practice requires a systematic approach that applies evidence to improve clinical and administrative practice. The National Academy, Health and Medicine Division, formerly known as the Institute of Medicine, released in its report, *The Future of Nursing*, recommendations that EBP is a nursing practice competency (IOM, 2010). EBP is also one of the Quality and Safety Education for Nurses (QSEN) competencies, with the overall goal for the QSEN initiative being to meet the challenge of preparing future nurses to have the knowledge, skills, and attitudes (KSAs) necessary to continuously improve the quality and safety of the health care systems within which they work (QSEN, 2014). The knowledge, skills, and attitudes embedded in the QSEN EBP competency are (QSEN, 2014):

- Knowledge
  - Demonstrating knowledge of basic scientific methods and processes
  - Describing EBP to include components of research evidence, clinical expertise, and patient and family values
  - Describing reliable sources for locating evidence reports and clinical practice guidelines
- Skills
  - Base individualized care plan on patient values, clinical expertise, and evidence
  - Read original research and evidence reports related to area of practice
  - Locate evidence reports related to clinical practice topics and guidelines
- Attitudes
  - Value the need for ethical conduct of research and quality improvement (QI)
  - Value the concept of EBP as integral to determining best clinical practices.

As a nursing student, you diligently read your textbooks and the assigned scientific articles. A good textbook incorporates current evidence into the practice guidelines and procedures it describes. Although a textbook relies on the scientific literature, sometimes information on a topic is outdated by the time a book is published. Therefore it is important to also seek out scientific articles that are available on almost any topic involving nursing practice. However, not all articles present topics that are "research based." This means that some nursing practices are not based on findings from well-designed research studies because the findings are inconclusive or researchers have not yet studied the practices. Your challenge is to obtain the very best, most current information at the right time, when you need it for patient care. To assist with finding the best evidence, health care organizations are implementing virtual libraries, which consist of a room with computers and Internet to research the latest evidence.

The best scientific evidence comes from well-designed, systematically conducted research studies found in scientific, peer-reviewed journals. Researchers are usually able to conclude whether a new treatment or approach truly makes a difference at the completion of a research study. However, much of that evidence never reaches the bedside. There are still nurses in practice settings, in contrast to educational settings, who may not have easy access to databases for scientific literature. Instead, they often care for patients on the basis of tradition or convenience (Hanrahan et al., 2015). However, during the last 10 years more health care settings have adopted EBP as an expectation in policy and procedure updating and in developing new clinical protocols. Hospitals that achieve Magnet designation are required to adopt EBP and research to fulfill the requirements of "New Knowledge Innovations and Improvements" standards (ANCC, 2008).

There are other sources of information to use in EPB that involve non–research-based evidence such as the following:
- Performance improvement (PI) and risk-management data
- International, national, and local standards of care
- Infection control data
- Benchmarking
- Retrospective or concurrent chart reviews
- Clinicians' expertise

It is important to always seek out research evidence rather than to depend solely on non–research-based evidence. When you face a clinical problem, ask yourself where the best evidence is to help you find the best solution in caring for patients.

Even when you use the best evidence available, application and outcomes differ based on your patients' values, state of health, preferences, concerns, and expectations. The correct application of EBP involves ethical and accountable professional nursing practice. To be successful in sustaining EBP, health care institutions need to have a strategic implementation plan (Hanrahan et al., 2015). Use critical thinking skills to determine which evidence is appropriate and related to your patients' clinical situations. For example, a single research article involving older adults shows that the use of therapeutic touch is effective in reducing patients' perceptions of abdominal pain. However, if your patients have cultural beliefs that discourage use of touch, you probably need to search for a different evidence-based therapy that your patients will accept. Using your clinical expertise and considering patients' values and preferences ensure that you appropriately apply the evidence available.

EVIDENCE-BASED PRACTICE STEPS

EBP is a systematic approach to rational decision making that aligns nursing practices with the best available scientific knowledge. A step-by-step approach ensures that you obtain the strongest available evidence to apply in patient care. Melnyk and Fineout-Overholt (2015) recommend the following seven-step process for EBP:

0. Cultivate a spirit of inquiry.
1. Ask a clinical question in PICO(T) format.
2. Search for the most relevant and best evidence.
3. Critically appraise the evidence you gather.
4. Integrate the best evidence with your clinical expertise and patient preferences and values in making a practice decision or change.
5. Evaluate the outcomes of practice decision or change based on evidence.
6. Communicate the outcomes of the EBP decision or change.

Fleiszer et al. (2016) offer a critical additional step of sustaining knowledge use and practice changes. This means continuing practices or procedures within an organization that successfully lead to the routine use of evidence in practice.

Cultivate a Spirit of Inquiry

Changes in health care are often made slowly because multiple barriers often prevent implementation of EBP. When your care is not evidence based, your patients will sometimes experience poor outcomes. Questioning and analyzing current clinical practices and believing in the value of EBP leads to the consistent use of EBP in nursing practice. For an institution to be successful at implementing and sustaining EBP changes, there must be a culture that promotes and supports a spirit of inquiry (Melnyk and Fineout-Overholt, 2015). Health care institutions, such as Magnet hospitals, that have cultures and environments that promote and support EBP demonstrate the following: a culture where nurses are encouraged to question practice, EBP mentors to mentor other nurses in the process, an infrastructure that supports inquiry and provides tools to support EBP, nursing leaders that value EBP, and recognition programs for nurses for their work in EBP (Melnyk and Fineout-Overholt, 2015).

Ask the Clinical Question in PICOT Format

Always think about your practice when caring for patients. Question what does not make sense to you and what you think needs clarification. Think about a problem or area of interest that recurs, is time-consuming, or is not logical. These thoughts are part of an ongoing spirit of inquiry into best practice. The University of Iowa Model for EBP suggests using problem-focused and knowledge-focused triggers to think critically about clinical and operational nursing-unit issues (Titler et al., 2001; Dontje, 2007). A problem-focused trigger is one you face while caring for patients or a trend you see on a nursing unit. *For example, Cathy and Tom identified from the quality indicator report that the trend in CLABSIs increased over each of the last 3 months. Data gathered from a* health care setting allow you to examine clinical trends and form questions. Most hospitals keep monthly records on key quality or performance indicators such as medication errors or infection rates. All Magnet hospitals maintain the National Database of Nursing Quality Improvement (NDNQI). The database has information on falls, pressure injury incidence, and nurse satisfaction. Quality-management and risk-management data do not give you evidence for finding a solution to a problem. Rather the data inform you about the nature or severity of problems, which then allows you to form practice questions. Other examples of problem-focused triggers include a patient injury following a fall or a postoperative patient who develops a stage 3 pressure injury.

A knowledge-focused trigger is a question that arises because of new information available on a topic. Examples are "What is the current evidence for the best way to educate patients with low health literacy?" and "Which approaches are effective in reducing delirium in patients in a critical care unit?" Important sources of new scientific information include the standards and practice guidelines available from national agencies or organizations such as the Agency for Healthcare Research and Quality (AHRQ), the American Pain Society (APS), and the American Association of Critical Care Nurses (AACN). Other sources of knowledge-focused triggers include recent research publications and nurse experts within an organization.

When you ask a clinical question, you want to make it concise so that it leads you to a reasonable number of scientific articles to review. You do not have time to read 100 articles to find the handful that are most helpful. You also do not want to make a practice change based on only one article. You want to be able to read the best four to six articles that specifically address your practice question. That is why it is best to use a PICO (or PICOT) format to state questions (Melnyk and Fineout-Overholt, 2015) (Box 7.1). Using a structured format for clinical questions helps you identify the key words that guide a successful literature search. *For example, Cathy and Tom first went to the literature with a general background question: "Which factors cause CLABSI in CVCs?" They were quickly frustrated when they found numerous articles about different factors that influence CLABSIs in CVCs. They decided to write two focused PICO questions: (1) "Does the use of 2% chlorhexidine (I) compared with alcohol (C) for cleansing central catheter insertion sites in hospitalized patients (P) reduce the incidence of CLABSI (O) within 6 months (T)?" (2) "Does the use of sterile barrier techniques during catheter insertion (I) compared with sterile gloving only (C) reduce the incidence of CLABSI (O) in postoperative surgical patients (P)?"* A well-designed PICO(T) question does not have to include all elements of the P, I, C, O, and T sequence; but the aim is to ask a question that contains as many of the PICO(T) elements as possible. For example, including a time element is not necessary when the intervention or phenomenon you are interested in is not time dependent. Asking a PICO(T) question allows you to focus on the time frame for reaching outcomes from the interventions that pertain to your question.

BOX 7.1   DEVELOPING A PICO OR PICOT QUESTION

P = Patient population or area of interest
  Identify your patients (family, clinical staff) by age, gender, ethnicity, disease, and experience or health problem.
I = Intervention of interest
  Which intervention do you want to use in practice (e.g., a treatment, diagnostic test, educational approach)?
C = Comparison of interest
  What is the usual standard of care or current intervention that you now use in practice?
O = Outcome
  What result do you wish to achieve or observe as a result of an intervention (e.g., change in patient/family caregiver behavior, physical finding, patient perception)?
T = Time
  How much time does it take to demonstrate an outcome (e.g., the time it takes for the intervention to achieve an outcome or how long participants are observed)?

The questions you ask in a PICO(T) format identify knowledge gaps within a clinical situation. When you create well–thought out questions, you discover evidence that is missing to guide clinical practice. Remember, do not be satisfied with clinical routines. Always question and use critical thinking to consider better ways to provide patient care.

Less precise questions (e.g., "What is the best way to reduce CLABSI?" "What is the best way to measure blood pressure?") are background questions that lead to many irrelevant articles and other sources of information, making it difficult to find the best evidence. However, it is sometimes necessary to begin with a background question if you do not yet have the knowledge to form a more specific PICO(T) question. The PICO(T) format allows you to ask questions that are intervention focused. Some questions that arise in nursing practice do not always contain all the PICO(T) elements. An example is a "meaning-focused" question such as "How do women with breast cancer (P) rate their quality of life (O)?" This question contains only a P and an O. These types of questions are frequently raised in daily nursing practice.

Search for the Best Evidence

Once you have a clear and concise PICO(T) question, you are ready to search for evidence. Thousands of resources are available to aid in your search, including government and professional websites, agency procedure manuals, PI data, existing clinical practice guidelines, and computerized bibliographical databases. Do not hesitate to ask for help to find appropriate evidence. Your faculty is always a key resource. When you are assigned to a health care setting, consider using experts such as advanced practice nurses, staff educators, risk managers, and infection control nurses.

When you go to the scientific literature for evidence, always seek the assistance of a medical librarian. A medical librarian knows the databases that are available to you (Box 7.2). The databases are repositories of published scientific studies, including peer-reviewed research. A *peer-reviewed*

BOX 7.2 SEARCHABLE SCIENTIFIC LITERATURE DATABASES AND SOURCES

CINAHL	Cumulative Index of Nursing and Allied Health Literature; includes studies in nursing, allied health, and biomedicine http://www.cinahl.com/
MEDLINE	Studies in medicine, nursing, dentistry, psychiatry, veterinary medicine, and allied health http://www.ncbi.nim.nih.gov
PsycINFO	Studies in psychology and related health care disciplines http://www.apa.org/psycinfo/
Cochrane Database of Systematic Reviews	Full text of regularly updated systematic reviews prepared by the Cochrane Collaboration; includes completed reviews and protocols http://www.cochrane.org/reviews
National Guidelines Clearinghouse	Repository for structured abstracts (summaries) about clinical guidelines and their development; also includes condensed version of guidelines for viewing http://www.guideline.gov/
PubMed	Health science library at the National Library of Medicine offers free access to journal articles http://www.nlm.nih.gov
Worldviews on Evidence-Based Nursing	Electronic journal containing articles that provide a synthesis of research and an annotated bibliography for selected references http://onlinelibrary.wiley.com/journal/10.1111/(ISSN)1741-6787

article is one submitted for publication and reviewed by a panel of experts familiar with the topic or subject matter of the article. The librarian helps translate your PICO(T) question into the language or key words that yield the best evidence. When conducting a search, you enter and manipulate different key words until you get the combination that gives you the articles you want to read about your question. *For example, Cathy and Tom's first PICO question includes the key words "catheter-associated bloodstream infection," "surgical patients," "chlorhexidine," and "alcohol."* When you enter a word to search into a database, be prepared for some confusion with the evidence you obtain. The vocabulary in published articles is often vague. The word you select sometimes has one meaning to one author and a very different meaning to another. A medical librarian can help you learn how to choose alternative words (e.g., "surgery" versus "surgical patients") or terms that identify your PICO(T) question and thus ensure that you obtain evidence about your specific question.

MEDLINE and the Cumulative Index of Nursing and Allied Health Literature (CINAHL) are among the best-known comprehensive databases and represent the scientific knowledge base of health care (Melnyk and Fineout-Overholt, 2015). Some databases are available through vendors at a cost, whereas others are free of charge. As a student, you have access to the databases purchased by your school. Vendors such as OVID usually offer several different databases. Databases are also available free on the Internet. The *Cochrane Database of Systematic Reviews* is a valuable resource of high-quality evidence. It includes the full text of regularly updated systematic reviews and protocols for reviews currently underway. Collaborative review groups prepare and maintain the reviews. The AHRQ supports the National Guidelines Clearinghouse (NGC) database. It contains clinical guidelines (i.e., systematically developed statements about a plan of care for a specific set of clinical circumstances involving a specific patient population). Examples of clinical guidelines on NGC include nursing care of dyspnea and treatment of adults with low back pain. The NGC is invaluable when you want to develop a plan of care for a patient (see Chapter 9).

The pyramid in Fig. 7.1 represents one example of the hierarchy of available evidence. The level of rigor or the amount of confidence you have in the findings of a study decreases as you move down the pyramid (Ingham-Broomfield, 2016). At this point in your nursing career, you cannot be an expert on all aspects of the types of research studies conducted. But you can learn enough about the types of studies to help you know which ones have the best scientific evidence. Understanding the hierarchy of evidence helps you decide if evidence from a source is relevant, valid, and appropriate for use in practice. At the top of the pyramid are systematic reviews or meta-analyses, which are state-of-the-science summaries from an individual researcher or panel of experts. These research summaries are the perfect answers to PICO(T) questions because the researchers have rigorously summarized all current evidence on the question.

A good systematic review reports the findings from a literature search on a topic and tells you what evidence exists about your question. In a systematic review the researcher summarizes all studies conducted on a particular topic and reports if the current evidence supports a change in practice or if further study is needed. In the Cochrane Library all entries include information on meta-analyses or systematic reviews. A meta-analysis uses statistics to show the effect of an intervention on an outcome. A systematic review uses no statistics to draw conclusions.

A randomized controlled trial (RCT) is the highest level of experimental research. In an RCT a researcher tests an intervention (e.g., method for intravenous [IV] site care or patient education) against the usual standard of care. Researchers assign subjects in an experiment to either a control or a treatment group randomly. In other words, all subjects have an equal chance to be in either group. The treatment group receives the experimental intervention, and the control group receives the usual standard of care. The researchers measure both groups for the same outcomes and

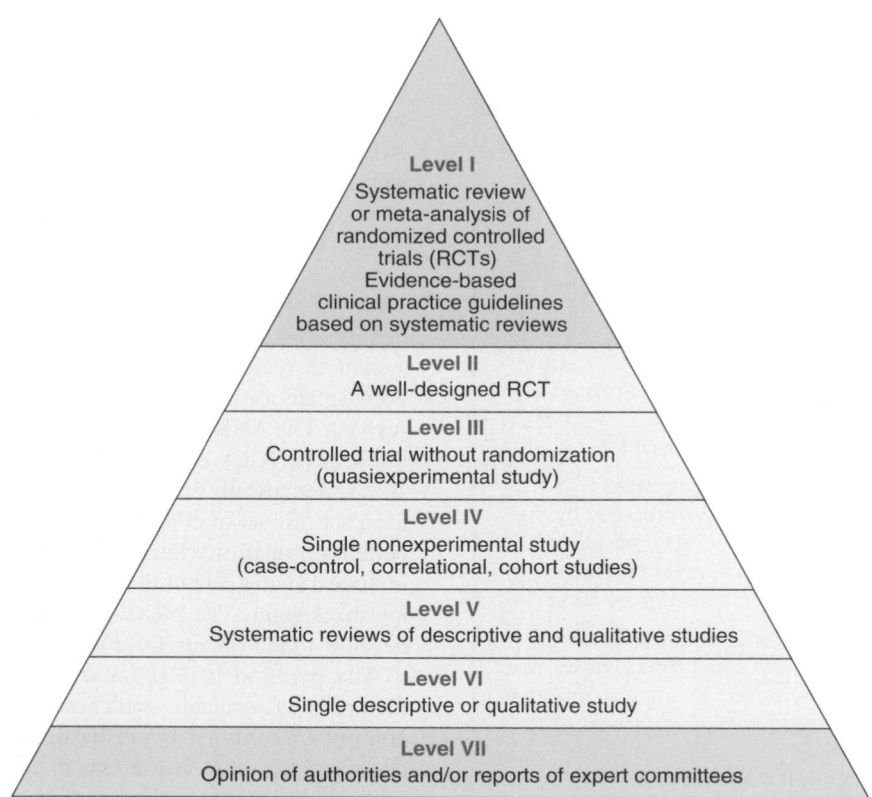

Level I
Systematic review
or meta-analysis of
randomized controlled
trials (RCTs)
Evidence-based
clinical practice guidelines
based on systematic reviews

Level II
A well-designed RCT

Level III
Controlled trial without randomization
(quasiexperimental study)

Level IV
Single nonexperimental study
(case-control, correlational, cohort studies)

Level V
Systematic reviews of descriptive and qualitative studies

Level VI
Single descriptive or qualitative study

Level VII
Opinion of authorities and/or reports of expert committees

FIG 7.1 Levels of evidence. (From LoBiondo-Wood G, Haber J: *Nursing research,* ed 9, St Louis, 2018, Elsevier.)

then perform statistical tests to see if the experimental intervention made a significant difference. When an RCT is completed, the researcher knows if the intervention leads to better outcomes than the standard of care.

A single RCT is not as conclusive as a review of several RCTs on the same question. However, a single RCT that tests the intervention included in your question yields very useful evidence. If an RCT is not available on your question, use results from other research studies such as descriptive or qualitative studies to answer your PICO(T) question (Box 7.3). The use of clinical experts may be at the bottom of the evidence pyramid, but do not consider clinical experts to be poor sources of evidence. Expert clinicians use evidence frequently as they build their own practice, and they are rich sources of information for clinical problems.

Health care agencies gather data about clinical practice trends such as NDNQI indicators. Typically, quality-management and risk-management data do not give you evidence for finding a solution to a problem, but the trending of the data (such as number of falls or type of medication errors over a period of 6 months) informs you about the nature or severity of problems occurring within the health care setting. Access to quality data helps you refine or redirect your PICO(T) question.

Critically Appraise the Evidence

With the help of the hospital librarian, Tom searched three databases: PubMed, CINAHL, and Cochrane Database of Systematic Reviews. He found a systematic review summary on

central line dressings from the Cochrane Database and an article from the highly regarded New England Journal of Medicine reporting a cohort study showing a reduction in CLABSIs after use of a bundling of several interventions (including use of chlorhexidine and barrier precautions). Cathy helped by searching the Centers for Disease Control and Prevention (CDC) website for clinical guidelines on central line catheters. Once they obtained the full text of all articles (not just the abstracts), Cathy and Tom distributed them to members of the UPC for critical review and evaluation.

Critically reviewing and analyzing the available evidence requires a systematic approach. You need to review each source of evidence (article, clinical guideline, expert summary) to determine its value, feasibility, and utility of evidence for making a practice change. This requires you to review each source of evidence carefully to determine its scientific worth, determine the strength of any study methods (when appropriate), identify the level of evidence from each source, summarize your findings, and determine if the evidence is conclusive regarding your practice question. *The surgical intensive care unit (ICU) UPC committee reviews the articles and clinical guidelines on CLABSIs and decides if there is convincing evidence for the use of chlorhexidine instead of alcohol in cleansing catheter sites. The team also determines if the use of barrier precautions during catheter insertion makes a difference in infection rates.*

To begin it is important to understand basic research terminology such as sample, bias, dependent variable, and independent variable (Grove et al., 2015). In addition, know how

BOX 7.3 TYPES OF RESEARCH STUDIES IN NURSING

- *Randomized controlled trial*—Participants in a study are randomly assigned to one of two groups and tested for the same outcome to determine if there is a difference in the effect of a treatment or intervention compared with a standard of care. It is the classic experiment and most rigorous level of research.
- *Quasi-experimental study*—Type of study that aims to determine whether a program or intervention has the intended effect on its participants. A true experiment includes (1) *pretest-posttest design*, (2) a *treatment group* and a *control group*, and (3) *random assignment* of study participants; however, quasi-experimental studies lack one or more of these design elements.
- *Descriptive*—A researcher uses statistical measures to analyze data (e.g., survey responses, physical measures) to describe phenomena affecting patients or health care professionals.
- *Case control study*—Study that compares patients who have a disease or outcome of interest with patients who do not have the disease or outcome. The researcher looks back (retrospectively) to compare how frequently the exposure to a risk factor is present in each group to determine the relationship between the risk factor and disease.
- *Cohort study*—Study that follows over time one or more populations (called *cohorts*) to determine which patient characteristics (risk factors) are associated with a disease or outcome.
- *Qualitative*—Analysis of interviews, observations, or surveys to measure people's perceptions, feelings, or views of phenomena about which little is known.

BOX 7.4 RATING EVIDENCE

Evidence-based practice is ranked by the way the evidence was collected by the researcher or clinician. The following is an example of a rating system from strongest to weakest evidence (LoBiondo-Wood and Haber, 2014):

Level 1: Systematic reviews or meta-analyses of randomized and nonrandomized clinical trials; evidence-based clinical practice guidelines based on systematic reviews

Level 2: Well-designed single randomized and nonrandomized clinical trials

Level 3: Controlled trials without randomization (quasi-experimental studies)

Level 4: Single nonexperimental studies such as correlational, cohort, or case control studies

Level 5: Systematic review of descriptive and qualitative studies

Level 6: Single descriptive or qualitative studies

Level 7: Opinions from authorities and/or reports from expert committees

to rank the different types of study designs (Box 7.4) to understand how **valid** the findings of a study or information are in making conclusions about your PICO(T) question. The University of Colorado (2014) has a useful *Research and Evidence Based Practice Manual*, ed 3, with a glossary of research terms and other useful information.

As a student new to nursing, it takes time to acquire the skills to critique research evidence. When you read an article from a scientific journal, do not let the statistics or technical wording cause you to put the article down and walk away. To determine its worth to practice, consider:

- What is the level of evidence?
- How well was a study (if research article) conducted?
- How useful are the findings to practice?

When rating the evidence from a study, you determine the type of study based on an evidence hierarchy similar to the one shown in Fig. 7.1. Then you use a numbering system (see Box 7.4) for rating. For example, evidence from a systematic review is rated 1, evidence from a randomized trial is rated 2, and published clinical articles are rated lower, 6 (LoBiondo-Wood, 2017). Combining all articles gives you a sense of the highest level of evidence you have.

Read each article carefully to decide how well the study was conducted. When reading through a scientific study, summarize key elements. Many EBP committees use critical appraisal guides or useful checklists for evaluating studies (Spruce et al., 2016). A guide lists questions about essential elements of research (e.g., purpose, sample size, setting, method of study). It is important to know the elements of scientific articles to decide the value and relevance to your PICO(T) question. Evidence-based articles (research and clinical) include the following elements:

- *Abstract:* An abstract is a brief summary of the article that quickly tells you if the article is research or clinically based. An abstract summarizes the purpose of the study or clinical review, the type of study, major themes or findings, and the implications for nursing practice.
- *Introduction:* The introduction of a scientific article describes its purpose and the importance of the topic for the audience who reads it. There is usually brief supporting evidence as to why the topic is important from the author's point of view.

Together the abstract and introduction tell you if you want to continue to read the entire article. You know if the topic of the article is similar to your PICO(T) question or related closely enough to provide you useful information. Continue to read the next elements of the article.

- *Literature review or background:* A good author offers a detailed background of previous studies and the level of evidence or clinical information that exists about the topic of the article. The literature review explains what led the author to conduct a study or report on the clinical topic. This section of an article is very valuable. Perhaps the article itself does not address your specific PICO(T) question the way you want, but it can lead you to other more useful articles. Once you read the literature review, you should have a good idea of how past research led to the researcher's question. *For example, one article Tom found described a study designed to test the effects of aseptic practices on CLABSI. This study reviewed literature that describes the nature of CLABSI and the patients most at risk, the type of factors shown previously in the literature to contribute to CLABSI, and previous interventions used to prevent CLABSI.*

- *Manuscript narrative:* The "middle section" or narrative of a manuscript differs according to the type of evidence-based article it is (Melnyk and Fineout-Overholt, 2015). A clinical article describes a clinical topic, which often includes a description of a patient population, the nature of a certain disease or health problem, how patients are affected, and the appropriate nursing therapies. An author sometimes writes a clinical article to explain how to use a therapy or new technology. A research article contains several subsections within the narrative, including:
  - *Purpose statement:* This statement explains the focus or intent of a study. It identifies which concepts are researched including research questions (what the researcher intends to learn from the study) or **hypotheses** (predictions made about the relationship among study **variables**) (e.g., characteristics or traits that vary among subjects). An example of a research question is: "Does the use of chlorhexidine 2% compared with povidone-iodine reduce CLABSI in patients with CVCs?" With this question the author is studying the variables (independent) of chlorhexidine and povidone-iodine solutions as they affect the outcome (dependent variable) of CLABSI. In contrast, a hypothesis might state: Chlorhexidine 2% for site care reduces the incidence of CLABSI in patients with CVCs.
  - *Methods or design:* This section explains how researchers organize and conduct studies to answer research questions or test hypotheses. This is where you learn which type of study it is (e.g., RCT, case control, qualitative study). You also learn how many subjects (sample) or people are in a study. Generally, the more subjects included in a study, the stronger the findings because a larger sample makes it easier to detect an effect from an intervention. However, sample sizes are usually small in qualitative studies. In health care studies subjects often include patients, family members, or health care staff. The methods section also tells you the setting where a study was conducted, which may affect your interest in the findings. Remember, language in the methods section is sometimes confusing. Use a faculty member as a resource to help interpret this section.
  - *Analysis:* This section explains how the data collected in a study are analyzed. If quantitative data such as physical measurements and scores on surveys are collected, statistical results from the study are explained. Statistics can be confusing. Focus on learning if the researcher found differences between groups or if an association was found between different variables. For example, if a researcher tests a new fall-prevention strategy, did the strategy reduce falls more than the standard approach to care? The researcher reports a *p* value. The *p* value (usually set at 0.05) is a probability level that tells you whether the difference between two groups was likely related to the intervention or if it was simply a difference by chance. When the statistic shows that the value was less than the *p* value ($p<0.05$), the result was likely the result of the intervention (less than

5% probability caused by chance). If a study involved collection of qualitative information such as audio-taped interviews or open-ended surveys, the analysis describes the major themes from the data. This section helps to determine if a study was conducted in a way that allows you to trust the results and use them to inform practice (Grove et al., 2015).

- *Results or conclusions:* Clinical and research articles have a summary section. In a clinical article the author explains the clinical implications for the topic presented. In a research article the author describes the findings from the study and explains whether a hypothesis is supported or how a research question is answered. Were the results clinically relevant (pertinent or connected to the clinical situation being studied)? A good author also discusses any limitations to a study in the results section. Study limitations are valuable in helping you decide if you want to apply the evidence with your patients.
- *Clinical implications:* A research article includes a section that explains if the findings from the study have clinical implications. The researcher explains how to apply findings in a practice setting for the type of subjects studied.

After you have critically reviewed each article for your PICO(T) question, combine the findings from all the articles to determine the state of the evidence. If you used a critical appraisal guide for each article, summarize information in all the forms into a final evaluation table. As you complete the evaluation table, use critical thinking to consider the scientific rigor or strength of the combined evidence and how well it answers your area of interest. Consider the evidence in light of your patient's concerns, values, preferences, and available health care resources. Your review of articles offers a snapshot conclusion of the combined evidence on your PICO(T) question. As a new nurse, you learn to judge whether to use the evidence for a specific patient or group of patients who usually have complex health care situations (Melnyk and Fineout-Overholt, 2015). Ethically it is important to consider evidence that benefits patients and does no harm.

After appraising all articles, the surgical ICU UPC focuses on the systematic review, cohort study, and CDC clinical guidelines as offering the most information about the use of chlorhexidine and other interventions for preventing CLABSI. The committee collaborates by discussing their conclusions, reviews the results of the final evaluation table, and applies their clinical expertise. They consider the types of patients they see in the ICU and determine if the evidence is strong enough for use in practice. The systematic review article (evidence level 1) did not address chlorhexidine use but concluded that there is no definitive advantage of transparent IV dressings over gauze for preventing CLABSI. Although level 7 evidence, the clinical guidelines from the CDC contained recommendations categorized on the basis of strength of existing scientific data and applicability. The CDC guidelines reported that research has shown no difference between transparent and gauze dressings in causing bloodstream infection and highly recommends use of chlorhexidine for IV site care and the use of sterile barriers during catheter insertion. The cohort study (evidence level 4) showed a significant reduction in CLABSI in ICUs that used a bundle of interventions, including rigorous hand hygiene, chlorhexidine site care, and sterile barriers. The data from all studies apply to adult patients who are critically ill. The committee recommended adopting practice changes to include chlorhexidine site care, sterile barrier precautions for catheter insertion, and reinforcement of strict hand hygiene during all forms of central line site care.

Integrate the Best Evidence

Once you decide that the evidence is strong and applicable to your patients and clinical situation, incorporate it into practice. The easiest step is to take the evidence you find and apply it in your plan of care for a patient (see Chapter 9). Use the source of evidence as the scientific rationale for the intervention you plan to try. For instance, you are assigned to work in a long-term care nursing center, and you care for a patient with dementia who wanders. Your review of the literature offers strong evidence on techniques that can successfully reduce wandering. You decide to use several techniques from the articles you reviewed during your next clinical assignment to see if it reduces wandering in your assigned patient.

When you work as a part of a hospital committee or task force, sometimes EBP change occurs on a larger scale. One strategy to engage nurses in the EBP process is the formation of a Nursing Clinical Effectiveness Committee (McKeever et al., 2016). Once you identify evidence to make a practice change, an organized collaborative effort is needed to bring appropriate administrators and staff all on board. A Nursing Clinical Effectiveness Committee can help overcome barriers to implementation of EBP (McKeever et al., 2016). Engagement brings all stakeholders (individuals who have an interest or concern in the practice change) together to explain why the evidence-based interventions are important. For example, administrators want to know if the practice change improves patient outcomes and lowers costs. Staff nurses want to know if the practice change improves patient outcomes and how it will affect the way they provide care. Health care providers also want to know how the practice change affects the way they provide care. To integrate evidence into practice, education of all those involved in the practice change must occur. This requires approaches such as teaching seminars, informational newsletters, and ongoing discussions during staff and UPC meetings.

The actual execution of a practice change requires planning, especially if it occurs on a large scale, involving more than one nursing unit or work area. The staff who are implementing a practice change must work closely with the individuals who will be adopting the new practice to anticipate what is needed to make a change successful (e.g., new documentation forms, a change in the way information is communicated between disciplines). It is always best to trial a new practice change by conducting a 3-month pilot before implementation on a large scale. The results of the pilot tell you if the practice change can be implemented easily and if it results in desired outcomes. Staff buy in is important to the success

of the pilot project and sustaining the change. Nurses are more likely to use an EPB if they perceive the practice to be useful and relevant (Jun et al., 2016).

A common approach used for integrating evidence into practice is to incorporate new evidence into policies and procedures (P&P). Many organizations have adopted an EBP approach when reviewing all P&P. A key feature of a practice environment that supports the use of best evidence is requiring clinical practice policies and procedures to be evidence based (Hanrahan et al., 2015; Jun et al., 2016). Many organizations involve staff nurses and research-prepared advanced practice nurses to review scientific articles relevant to P&P and make appropriate revisions. P&P are important tools for supporting hospital-based nurses in using evidence in their everyday practice and promoting positive patient outcomes.

After reviewing the evidence on CLABSI, the surgical ICU UPC committee decides to revise the P&P for central catheter insertion and maintenance. Cathy and Tom recommend that the committee be responsible for conducting in-service sessions to educate all staff about the new P&P. A brief explanation about the change is also placed in the unit's monthly newsletter. The bundle of interventions (hand hygiene, chlorhexidine use, and full barrier precautions) is implemented after the staff have the opportunity to ask questions about the new P&P in staff meetings. The ICU implements the new P&P with the UPC committee monitoring the monthly reports on CLABSI to determine if infection rates change. In addition, the UPC does spot audits of staff practices to be sure that the new interventions are being followed consistently to ensure that the change in practice is sustained.

You can use evidence in a variety of other ways through teaching tools, clinical practice guidelines, and new assessment or documentation tools. Depending on the amount of change needed to apply evidence in practice, it becomes necessary to involve a few key staff from a given nursing unit. It is important to consider the setting in which you want to apply the evidence. Is there support from all staff? Does the practice change fit within the scope of practice in the clinical setting? Are there resources (time, equipment, staff) available to make a change? As a nursing student integrating evidence, your focus begins with searching for and applying best evidence to improve the care that you directly provide your patients. Using an EBP approach improves your skills and knowledge as a nurse and your patients' outcomes.

Evaluate the Outcomes of the Practice Decision or Change

When you plan to integrate evidence into practice, it is essential to decide how you will evaluate the outcomes. Remember the "O" in your PICO(T) question. It represents the outcomes you choose to measure as you integrate the evidence. These outcomes tell you how well the evidence-based intervention works. Sometimes your evaluation is as simple as determining if the expected outcome you set for a specific patient is met (see Chapter 9) after using a new evidence-based technique in care. For example, when using a new approach to preoperative teaching, does a patient learn what to expect after surgery?

When an EBP change occurs on a larger scale, an evaluation of outcomes is more formal. For example, *evidence of factors that reduce the incidence of CLABSI leads the surgical ICU to adopt the new P&P for central line catheter care. To evaluate the procedure, the members of the EBP committee track the outcome of incidence of CLABSI over a course of time before and then after the practice change (e.g., 3 to 6 months). A preintervention and postintervention measure is needed to determine change. In this case the CLABSI measure is collected monthly by the hospital. In addition, the staff collects data to describe both the patients who develop CLABSI and the patients who do not.* This comparative information is valuable in determining the effects of the procedure and whether modifications are necessary. Often outcome measures are not routinely collected by an institution, requiring staff to identify the outcomes and the methods for measurement and then collect the outcome data required.

The evaluation of an EBP change determines if a practice change is desirable, if you need to modify your intervention, or if you need to discontinue a practice change. Unforeseen variables sometimes lead to results that you do not anticipate. *For example, the changes made in the protocol developed by Cathy and Tom might lead to an increase in CLABSIs. If this is not determined during evaluation, the practice will continue, and patients will suffer.* Never implement a practice change without evaluating its effects. Often an EBP change is stopped when the outcome measurements show poor outcomes.

Outcomes Measurement

An outcome is an observable effect of an intervention (see Chapter 9). Outcome measures determine if a patient progresses or if a practice change was beneficial or effective. In the example of the surgical ICU, the outcome measure is the monthly incidence of CLABSI before and after the practice change. This measure informs the ICU EBP committee if the new catheter-care procedure effectively reduces CLABSI.

Nurses work with many members of the health care team. As a result, it is often difficult to associate an outcome with an intervention by a specific health care discipline. However, a nursing-sensitive outcome focuses on how patients and their health care problems are affected by nursing interventions (Heslap and Lu, 2014; Press Ganey 2017). These outcomes look at the effects of interventions within the scope of nursing practice. Examples of nursing-sensitive outcomes include:

- Symptoms (e.g., pain, fatigue, nausea).
- Functional status (e.g., activity tolerance, ability to perform activities of daily living).
- Safety (e.g., incidence of falls, infections, pressure injuries).
- Psychological distress (e.g., anxiety, depression).

Patient education is a very common nursing intervention. Measuring educational outcomes occurs at several levels: reaction, learning, and behavior. When a nurse teaches a class to a group of patients or even one on one, a reaction outcome is one that evaluates how the learner feels about an educational activity. Did the patient enjoy the teaching experience?

TABLE 7.1 **OUTCOME MEASUREMENT**	
OUTCOME	**MEASUREMENT APPROACH**
Patient loses 10 lb in 2 months.	Weight
Patient describes side effects of antihypertensive medication.	Patient interview
Patient is satisfied with nursing care.	Patient satisfaction survey
Patient expresses less fatigue after a 4-week exercise program.	Self-report fatigue scale
Incidence of methicillin-resistant *Staphylococcus aureus* decreases among surgical patients.	Medical record laboratory reports

Did class members perceive that the nurse was competent in teaching? A learning outcome measures a patient's KSAs developed as a result of education. An example is a return demonstration. Perhaps the most important type of outcome resulting from patient education is a behavioral outcome, which evaluates the extent to which learners change their behavior due to education. For example, does a patient begin to follow the right meal plan at home or adhere to a medication schedule following patient education?

When identifying an outcome to evaluate a practice change, consider the type of measurement to use. Will you observe a patient behavior (e.g., taking a medication or performing an exercise or skill) or collect a physiological measure (e.g., weight or blood pressure)? Will measurement require you to conduct an interview, audit an existing medical record, or check results in a laboratory report? If you do not choose the correct measurement approach, you will not be certain if an outcome was met (Table 7.1). For example, if your practice change is a new relaxation technique for reducing patients' pain, your outcome of reduced pain is measured by using a pain-rating scale. If a practice change is a new type of breathing mask to reduce pressure injuries on the face, the outcome of pressure injury incidence is measured using observation.

An outcome measure must be appropriate for patients or families. When you implement an EBP change, will you observe patients, or will you ask the patients to complete a survey or questionnaire? Consider if an outcome measure is too difficult for a patient to complete because of factors such as pain, fatigue, or level of consciousness.

You will be more successful in implementing EBP when outcome measurement plans are acceptable and important to the clinicians involved. This means including colleagues in any EBP project from the beginning when you select outcome measures. It is also important to be consistent and accurate when collecting outcome measures. Any clinicians who are involved in outcome measurement need proper training in data measurement and collection. For example, if outcome measurement involves a new device such as a pulse oximeter, each data collector must demonstrate competency in the use of the oximeter. Individuals who collect outcome data must collect it in the same way. For example, if you decide to use a new patient satisfaction survey, EBP team members need to administer the tool and use the same set of guidelines for administering it to patients. Competence and consistency in measurement help ensure quality outcome data. Outcome measurement contributes to the body of evidence and strengthens the process of EBP.

Process Measurement

When you implement a practice change, you sometimes want to monitor if the process or protocol was implemented as planned. This requires a process measurement. *For example, when the surgical ICU implements the use of chlorhexidine for central line catheter care, a process outcome is tracking documentation to see if chlorhexidine was used for site care.* Process indicators (e.g., chart audit data or observations of staff using a protocol) simply tell you if an intervention was completed, but the information is useful in deciding if your approach to a practice change is working.

Communicate the Outcomes of the Evidence-Based Practice Decision

After collecting outcome measures to evaluate an EBP change, it is necessary to communicate results. If you implement an evidence-based intervention at an individual patient level, you let the patient know the results of your therapy. Is the patient's wound showing signs of healing? Has the patient correctly learned how to self-administer an injection? When your practice change occurs on a larger unit level, the first group to whom you communicate results is the clinical staff of a patient care unit. The EBP team should share results in a larger staff meeting or perhaps in a unit-based newsletter. Clinicians enjoy and appreciate seeing the results of a practice change. In addition, the practice change more likely is sustainable (i.e., remaining in place) when the staff see the benefits from a change.

It is important for a health care agency to benefit as much as possible from EBP. A nursing unit or clinical area that makes an EBP change needs to communicate the results to the entire agency. Communication sometimes occurs during grand rounds or agency level committees. Communicating with nurses and other clinicians from different units increases the likelihood they will decide to make the same type of practice change. As a professional nurse, it is critical for you to contribute to the growing knowledge of nursing practice. When you are involved in an EBP change, consider how you can communicate your results to the profession at large. Becoming involved in professional societies or organizations allows you to present EBP changes in scientific abstracts or poster or podium presentations.

Sustain Knowledge Use

Sustaining an EBP practice change is a challenge. Health care institutions are bombarded by change from government and accrediting agencies, internal administrative initiatives, and the ongoing demands of delivering safe and effective patient care. When a new practice change is introduced, it is important that it is incorporated into the culture and practice

---

BOX 7.5   EVIDENCE-BASED PRACTICE

PICO Question: Does the use of targeted strategies improve nurses' implementation and sustained use of EBP?

SUMMARY OF EVIDENCE

Nurses' implementation and sustained use of EBP continues to be a challenge. Critical to this is that leaders in the institution must actively engage in and role model EBP behaviors and provide mentorship to other nurses (Warren et al., 2016b). Specific strategies effectively increase and sustain EBP use. For example, EBP practices are more likely to be sustained by nurses when units have nursing leaders who align vision, use integrated strategies, and conduct EBP activities (Fleiszer et al., 2016). Forming health care agency or unit committees such as Nursing Clinical Effectiveness or EBP committees within Shared Governance Councils was found to be effective in engaging nurses at the unit level in EBP (Gallagher-Ford, 2014; McKeever et al., 2016). Ongoing strategic communication from nursing leaders related to research and EBP increased nurses' interest and willingness to adopt innovative practices (Mortenius et al., 2016). Nurses must be engaged in EBP to continue to impact and improve health care costs and patient outcomes.

APPLICATION TO NURSING PRACTICE

- Be familiar with a nursing leader's vision as it relates to strategies and activities for EBP in the agency (Fleiszer et al., 2016).
- Form an EBP team with other nurses to help create a culture of inquiry in your agency (Kitson and Harvey, 2016).
- Watch for strategic communication from leadership about research and EBP improvements within your agency (Mortenius et al., 2016).
- As a student, partner with a nurse on the unit to search the literature to answer a practice improvement question and share your findings with the other nurses (Raines, 2016).

---

environment of an organization. It is important for health care institutions to use targeted strategies to sustain use of EBP decisions and changes (Box 7.5). *Once the surgical ICU adopts the new P&P for central line catheter care, they do not stop there. The committee posts the monthly CLABSI outcome measure on the conference room bulletin board for all staff to see. Members of the UPC conduct occasional audits to be sure that the processes of using chlorhexidine and sterile barriers are being followed by staff members. When the CLABSI measure trends back up, the UPC committee discusses the results and reviews the causes for each patient situation.* Translating new knowledge into practice requires transformational nursing leadership (see Chapter 13) that provides the resources to develop EBP education for nurses to increase EBP knowledge, a toolkit to standardize nursing practices, participation on interdisciplinary EBP teams, and role modeling of EBP behaviors (Warren et al., 2016a, 2016b).

NURSING RESEARCH

After completing a thorough appraisal of the scientific literature, you sometimes find a gap in knowledge. If there is insufficient evidence to answer your PICO(T) question and make a practice change, the best way to answer your question is through the research process. At this time in your career you are not conducting research, but it is important for you to understand the process. Research is a systematic process that asks and answers questions to generate new knowledge. This knowledge provides a scientific basis for nursing practice and validates the effectiveness of interventions.

In the past much of the information used in nursing practice was borrowed from other disciplines such as biology, physiology, and psychology. Often this information was applied to nursing without testing or comparing ways of caring for patients. For example, nurses use several methods to help patients sleep. Interventions such as giving a patient a backrub, making sure that the bed is clean and comfortable, and preparing the environment by dimming the lights are frequently used and in general are logical, commonsense approaches. However, when you consider these measures in greater depth, questions arise about their applications. For example, are they the best methods to promote sleep? Do different patients in different situations require other interventions to promote sleep?

Research is an orderly series of steps that allow a researcher to move from asking a research question to finding the answer. It is more rigorous than EBP because a researcher must review all previous research related to his or her area of interest and select a relevant research question that can be studied. The aim of a study is to build on existing knowledge. A formal proposal is written to address the purpose of a study, the subjects, and the setting that are involved; how the subjects will be enrolled into the study; the actual methods for conducting the study; and the plan for analysis of study data.

All researchers must protect the rights of human subjects and obtain informed consent from the participants (Stausmire, 2014). An individual participant must know the purpose of any research, what it involves (time and activity), and all risks and benefits and be assured that participation is voluntary. Research studies must be approved by an institutional review board (IRB), also called a *human subjects committee*.

An actual research project takes time. The researcher and research team members follow an orderly and systematic process for enrolling subjects, obtaining their informed consent, administering any initial testing measures (e.g., physical measurements, observations, surveys, focus group discussions), applying any intervention (when appropriate to a study), collecting any final data, and analyzing the study results. Table 7.2 outlines briefly the elements of a research study that involves a pretest and posttest design. As in the case of EBP, a person conducting research disseminates or communicates the results of a research study by presenting at scientific conferences (poster or podium presentations) or publishing study results.

Once completed, the research process contributes new knowledge to the practice of nursing. A researcher attempts to design a study so the knowledge gained can later be applied repeatedly to other similar groups of patients. Nursing research creates the evidence for EBP. The highest level of evidence comes from well-designed experimental research studies (see Box 7.4). Nursing research improves nursing practice and raises the standards for the profession. Promoting EBP and research increases your scientific knowledge base for practice. The recipients of these improvements to practice are your patients, their families, and the communities in which they live.

TABLE 7.2   EXAMPLE OF A RESEARCH STUDY (PRETEST AND POSTTEST DESIGN)

Research Question: Does the use of a new bed sensor system reduce the number of falls and fall-related injuries in older adults living in a nursing home?

TYPE OF STUDY	QUASI-EXPERIMENTAL STUDY WITH PRETEST AND POSTTEST DESIGN
Study design	This study involved testing a new bed sensor system designed to alert staff when patients try to exit their bed. A group of 40 patients in a nursing home agreed to participate in the study. The outcome measures for the study were the number of falls and fall-related injuries.
Study procedure	Patients volunteered to participate and signed informed consents. A brief survey was collected to record patients' ages, medical conditions, medications, and use of ambulatory devices. Patients' medical records provided pretest outcome data (i.e., the number of falls and fall-related injuries that the patients had experienced over the 3 months before the study). All patients were placed on beds with the new alarm system. Nursing home staff were trained on use of the sensors. The researchers collected data on any falls and fall-related injuries for 3 months (the length of the study).
Data analysis	The researchers ran statistical tests to learn if patients fell less often or had fewer injuries after the sensor system was implemented. The researchers also analyzed if patients who did fall had different characteristics (e.g., age, disease, medications) compared with patients who did not fall.
Results	There were fewer patient falls during the 3 months after implementing the new sensor system compared with the 3 months before implementation. The difference was statistically significant. Although the number of fall-related injuries also declined, this finding was not statistically significant. Adults with ambulatory deficits (unstable gait, balance) fell more often.
Implications	Sensor systems may help reduce patient falls. More research is needed involving clinical trials with control and treatment groups.

QUALITY IMPROVEMENT AND PERFORMANCE IMPROVEMENT

Near the bottom of the evidence pyramid (see Fig. 7.1) is quality or performance data. Every health care organization gathers data on health outcome measures to determine their quality of care. Examples of quality data include fall rates, number of medication errors, incidence of pressure injuries, and infection rates. Quality data trends often trigger EBP projects and research.

Quality improvement (QI) and performance improvement (PI) are formal approaches to analyze health care–related processes. The two terms frequently are used interchangeably. An organization monitors specific quality outcomes and, when findings suggest potential problems, it institutes formal QI/PI initiatives. Also, in many cases trends from QI data reveal problems that lead to EBP projects. QI/PI projects usually occur more quickly than an EBP or research project. An organization analyzes and evaluates current performance data to solve system problems (e.g., supply delivery, appointment scheduling), people problems (e.g., staffing ratios, communication protocols), or clinical problems (e.g., surgical incision infection rates, patient injuries from falls). When interprofessional teams participate in PI activities, they may or may not use research findings to develop strategies; however, an evidenced-based approach is advised when dealing with clinical problems.

Health care organizations routinely promote efforts for improving patient care processes and outcomes, particularly with respect to reducing medical errors and enhancing patient safety. QI and PI are the continuous and ongoing efforts to achieve measurable improvements in the efficiency, effectiveness, performance, accountability, outcomes, and other indicators of quality services or processes.

Quality Improvement/Performance Improvement Programs

QI is a competency within the QSEN model. It begins with the use of data to monitor the outcomes of care processes (e.g., medication administration or surgical wound care). When problems are revealed, improvement methods are designed and tested to continuously improve the quality and safety of health care within a health care agency (QSEN, 2014). A well-organized QI/PI program focuses on processes or systems that significantly contribute to outcomes of a specific organization (Stausmire, 2014). Included in any QI/PI program is a plan on how to sustain measurable improvements over time (Stausmire, 2014). Facilities need an organization-wide, systematic approach to ensure that everyone supports a continuous QI/PI philosophy. This begins with an organizational culture in which all staff members understand their responsibility toward maintaining and improving quality. Typically, in health care many people are involved in single processes of care. For example, medication delivery involves the health care provider who prescribes medications, the secretary who communicates new orders being written, the pharmacist who prepares the dosage, the transporter who delivers medications,

and the nurse who prepares and administers the drugs. When an organization identifies a need to improve the medication administration process, all professions involved in medication administration need to be engaged in the QI/PI process. Because most health care processes are interprofessional, all members of the health care team must collaborate in QI/PI activities. As a member of the nursing team, you participate in recognizing trends in practice, identifying when recurrent problems develop, and initiating opportunities to improve the quality of care.

The QI/PI process begins at the staff level, where all disciplines become involved in identifying quality problems. This requires staff members to know the outcomes measured by the organization and the practice standards or guidelines that define quality. Unit QI/PI committees review quality data and the activities or services considered to be most important in providing quality care to patients. One way to identify the greatest opportunity for improving quality is to consider activities that are high volume (greater than 50% of the activity of a unit); high risk (potential for trauma or death); and problem areas for patients, staff, or the institution. For example, on an orthopedic nursing unit hip surgery volume is high, adults older than 80 years of age have more postoperative complications, and family members are dissatisfied with patients' pain control. Any one of these factors could become the focus of a QI/PI project.

Another example is The Joint Commission's annual patient safety goals (TJC, 2018), which provide an excellent focus for QI/PI initiatives (see Chapter 30). Sometimes a problem is presented to a committee in the form of a sentinel event, an unexpected occurrence involving death or serious physical or psychological injury of a patient. After a sentinel event, the unit conducts a root cause analysis (RCA). The goal of the RCA is to review all information and identify how the event occurred through identification of active errors (i.e., the acts that personnel perform) and why it occurred through identification and analysis of latent errors (i.e., the organization or steps of the process). Once a committee defines the problem, it applies a formal model for exploring and resolving quality concerns. There are several models for QI and PI (Table 7.3). Health care organizations today are changing current organizational culture toward the concept of a "just culture." An organization with a "just culture" values the reporting of errors and focuses on the processes that lead to the error. A "just culture" also values nurses' critical thinking and problem-solving skills and the nurses' work on improving patient care processes (Kennedy, 2016).

QI combined with EBP is the foundation for excellent patient care and outcomes. Once a QI committee makes an EBP change, it is important to communicate results to staff from all appropriate departments. Practice changes will likely not last when QI committees fail to report findings and the results of interventions. Regular discussions of QI activities through staff meetings, newsletters, and memos are good communication strategies. Often a QI study reveals information that prompts organization-wide change. An organization must be responsible for responding to the problem with the appropriate resources. Revision of P&Ps,

TABLE 7.3 EXAMPLES OF PERFORMANCE IMPROVEMENT MODELS

PERFORMANCE IMPROVEMENT MODEL	SUMMARY DESCRIPTION
1. Balanced scorecard	A multidimensional framework for managing strategy by linking objectives, initiatives, targets, and performance measures across key organization perspectives.
2. Root cause analysis (RCA)	A structured method used to analyze serious adverse events. A central tenet of RCA is to identify underlying problems that increase the likelihood of errors, while avoiding the trap of focusing on mistakes by individuals.
3. Six Sigma	A disciplined methodology for process improvement that deploys a wide set of tools based on rigorous data analysis to identify sources of variation in performance and ways of reducing them.
4. *Plan-Do-Study-Act* (PDSA)	An experiential learning method that involves analyzing a quality problem and testing a change by developing a plan to test the change (*Plan*), carrying out the test (*Do*), observing and learning from the consequences (*Study*), and determining which modifications should be made to the test (*Act*).

QSEN QSEN ACTIVITY *Evidence-Based Practice*

The Nursing Practice Council notes that the incidence of falls with injuries has increased on all units in the agency over the last year. When checking its Fall Prevention Protocol, the Council notes it was last reviewed 4 years ago. The Council knows that falls with injuries is a nursing-sensitive outcome (NDNQI) and established a goal to reduce the incidence of falls in the upcoming year.

• How should the Nursing Practice Council proceed?

evolve   Answers to QSEN Activities can be found on the Evolve website.

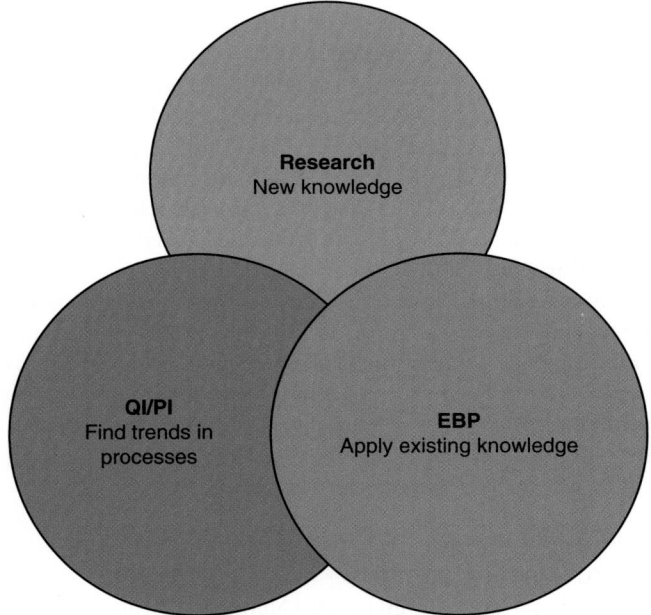

FIG 7.2 The relationship between research, evidence-based practice *(EBP),* and performance improvement *(PI).* QI, Quality improvement.

modification of standards of care, and new support services are examples of ways an organization responds.

RELATIONSHIP BETWEEN EVIDENCE-BASED PRACTICE, RESEARCH, AND QUALITY IMPROVEMENT

EBP, research, and QI are closely interrelated (Fig. 7.2). All three processes require you to use the best evidence to provide the highest quality of patient care. As a nurse, you are professionally accountable to know the differences and which process to select when facing clinical problems or when you desire to improve patient care. Although you will use all three practices in your nursing career, it is important to know how the processes are similar and how they differ (Table 7.4). Checklists are available that you can use to decide if your intended project is a QI project or research (Stausmire, 2014). When implementing an EBP project, it is important to first review evidence from appropriate research and QI data. This information helps you better understand the extent of a problem in practice and your organization. QI data inform you about how processes work within an organization and offer information about how to make EBP changes. EBP and QI sometimes provide opportunities for research. To increase the likelihood of success of EBP on your clinical unit, use combined QI and research methodologies (Granger and Shah, 2015).

Here is an example of how the three processes interrelate to improve nursing practice: *A nursing unit is experiencing a decrease in patient satisfaction with pain management over the last several months. QI data identify factors associated with pain management (e.g., the types of pain medications typically ordered, patient reports of pain relief after administration of pain medications). A thorough analysis of QI data leads a unit-based quality council team of nurses to conduct a literature review and implement the best evidence available to improve their pain-management protocol for the type of patients on the unit. The staff implement the revised protocol and evaluate its results. Despite the implementation of the revised pain-management protocol, patient satisfaction data continue to be lower than desired. Thus staff decide to conduct a research study to further investigate this clinical problem and improve patient care.*

TABLE 7.4   SIMILARITIES AND DIFFERENCES AMONG EVIDENCE-BASED PRACTICE, RESEARCH, AND QUALITY IMPROVEMENT

	EVIDENCE-BASED PRACTICE	RESEARCH	QUALITY IMPROVEMENT
Purpose	Use of information from research, professional experts, personal experience, and patient preferences to determine safe and effective nursing care with the goal of improving patient care and outcomes	Systematic inquiry answers questions, solves problems, and contributes to the generalizable knowledge base of nursing; it may or may not improve patient care	Improves local work processes to improve patient outcomes and efficiency of health systems; results usually not generalizable
Focus	Implementation of evidence already known into practice	Evidence is generated to find answers for questions about nursing practice	Measures effects of practice and/or practice change on specific patient population
Data sources	Multiple research studies, expert opinion, personal experience, patients	Subjects or participants have predefined characteristics that include or exclude them from the study; researcher collects and analyzes data from subjects	Data from patient records or patients who are in a specific area such as on a patient care unit or admitted to a particular hospital
Who conducts the activity?	Practicing nurses and possibly other members of the health care team	Researchers who may or may not be employed by the health care agency and usually are not a part of the clinical health care team	Employees of a health care agency such as nurses, physicians, and pharmacists
Is activity part of regular clinical practice?	Yes	No	Yes
Is IRB approval needed?	Sometimes	Yes	Sometimes
Funding sources	Internal, from health care agency	Funding is usually external such as a grant	Internal, from health care agency

IRB, Institutional review board.

KEY POINTS

- EBP guides nurses and other health care providers in making effective, timely, and appropriate clinical decisions.
- The best scientific evidence comes from well-designed, systematically conducted research studies.
- Application and outcomes of EBP differ based on patients' values, state of health, preferences, concerns, and expectations.
- The steps of EBP include the following: Cultivate a spirit of inquiry, ask a clinical question in PICOT format, search for the most relevant and best evidence, critically appraise the evidence, integrate the best evidence, evaluate the outcomes of the practice change, communicate results of the change, and sustain knowledge use.
- Using problem-focused and knowledge-focused triggers to think critically about clinical and operational nursing unit issues helps you define a PICO(T) question.
- Using the PICO(T) format for clinical questions helps you identify key words for a successful literature search.
- Understanding the hierarchy of evidence helps you decide if evidence from a source is relevant, valid, and appropriate for use in practice.
- Critically appraising or analyzing the available evidence requires a systematic approach with each source of evidence to determine its value, feasibility, and usefulness of evidence for making a practice change.
- The use of outcome measurement to evaluate an EBP change determines if a practice change is desirable, if you need to modify your intervention, or if you need to discontinue a practice change.
- After appraising the evidence for a PICO(T) question, if the question is unanswered and there is a gap in knowledge, the research process is the next option.
- The aim of a research study is to build on existing knowledge using either quantitative or qualitative methods.
- QI involves the review of quality data and identifying activities for improving the quality of a health care organization.
- Although EBP, research, and QI are closely related, they are separate processes.

REFLECTIVE LEARNING

- While on the clinical unit, talk to a staff nurse about the QI activities on the nursing unit. Report on the focus of the unit's QI activities to improve patient outcomes.
- Think about the nursing care that you provided to your patients on the clinical unit today. What questions came to your mind about the practices that you were doing? Formulate one of the questions in PICO(T) format.

- After asking the PICO(T) question, search the literature and find two or three research studies on the topic. What is the current state of the evidence related to your question?

REVIEW QUESTIONS

1. Place the steps of the EBP process in the appropriate order.
   1. Critically appraise the evidence you gather.
   2. Ask the clinical question in PICOT format.
   3. Evaluate the outcomes of the practice decision or change.
   4. Search for the most relevant and best evidence.
   5. Cultivate a spirit of inquiry.
   6. Integrate the evidence.
   7. Communicate the outcomes of the EBP change.
   8. Sustain the EBP change.
2. A patient in the intensive care unit experiences a sentinel event related to central line catheter care that resulted in serious injury. What quality improvement technique should the unit engage in to identify errors that led to the sentinel event?
   1. Six sigma
   2. Root cause analysis
   3. PDSA
   4. Balanced scorecard
3. Which of the following are outcomes measurements? (Select all that apply.)
   1. A nurse teaches a patient how to administer an injection and then observes the patient do a return demonstration.
   2. A nurse implements a new pain-management protocol and checks patients' charts to confirm if interventions are being provided.
   3. A nursing unit adopts a set of strategies for reducing pressure injuries, and the UPC members use direct observation of the skin to measure incidence of pressure injuries.
   4. A nursing unit implements a new fall prevention protocol and checks the monthly performance data for incidence of falls on the unit.
   5. A nursing unit implements a patient rounding program, and the charge nurse watches the unlicensed personnel to see if hourly rounding is being done on patients.

4. The nurses on a medicine unit have seen an increase in the number of pressure injuries developing in their patients. The nurses decide to initiate a quality improvement project using the PDSA model. Which of the following is an example of "Plan" from that model?
   1. Orienting patients to the unit's practice of hourly rounding on patients
   2. Reviewing the incidence of pressure injuries in patients cared for using the protocol
   3. Based on findings from patients who developed ulcers, implementing an evidence-based skin care protocol on all units
   4. Meeting with all disciplines to develop a multidisciplinary approach for reducing pressure injuries
5. A nurse is using the QSEN competency of EBP when working with the unit council to initiate a change related to pain management. Which behaviors demonstrate the nurse practicing behaviors associated with EBP? (Select all that apply.)
   1. Initiates plan for self-development as a team member
   2. Reads original research related to pain management
   3. Demonstrates effective use of strategies to reduce risk of harm to self or others
   4. Values EBP as critical to the develop of pain management guidelines for the unit
   5. Describes to the unit council reliable sources for locating clinical guidelines
   6. Applies technology and information management tools to support safe processes of care

evolve

Additional Review Questions, as well as rationales for all Review Questions, can be found on the Evolve website.

1. 5, 2, 4, 1, 6, 3, 8, 7; 2. 2; 3. 1, 3, 4, 4; 4. 5; 2, 4, 5.

REFERENCES

American Nurses Credentialing Center (ANCC): *A new model for ANCCs Magnet Recognition program*, 2008, http://www.nursecredentialing .org/documents/magnet/newmodel brochure.aspx.

Centers for Medicare and Medicaid Services (CMS): *Hospital acquired conditions*, 2015, https://www.cms.gov/Medicare/ Medicare-Fee-for-Service-Payment/ HospitalAcqCond/Hospital-Acquired _Conditions.html.

Crabtree E, et al: Improving patient care through nursing engagement in evidence-based practice, *Worldviews Evid Based Nurs* 13(2): 172, 2016.

Dontje KJ: Evidence-based practice: understanding the process, *Topics in Advanced Practice Nursing eJournal* 7(4), 2007. http://www.medscape.com/ viewarticle/567786.

Fleiszer AR, et al: Nursing unit leaders' influence on the long-term sustainability of evidence-based practice improvements, *J Nurs Manag* 24:309, 2016.

Gallagher-Ford L: Leveraging shared governance councils to advance evidence-based practice: the EBP council journey, *Worldviews Evid Based Nurs* 12(1):61, 2014.

Godlock G, et al: Implementation of an evidence-based patient safety team to prevent falls in inpatient medical units, *Medsurg Nurs* 25(1):17, 2016.

Granger BB, Shah BR: Blending quality improvement and research methods for implementation science, part I: design and data collection, *AACN Adv Crit Care* 26(3):268, 2015.

Grove SK, et al: *Understanding nursing research: building an evidence-based practice*, ed 6, St Louis, 2015, Elsevier.

Hanrahan K, et al: Sacred cow gone to pasture: a systematic evaluation and integration of evidence-based practice, *Worldviews Evid Based Nurs* 12(1):3, 2015.

Heslap L, Lu S: Nursing-sensitive indicators: a concept analysis, *J Adv Nurse* 70(11): 2469, 2014.

Ingham-Broomfield R: A nurses' guide to the hierarchy of research designs and evidence, *Aust J Adv Nurs* 33(3):38, 2016.

Institute of Medicine (IOM): *The future of nursing: leading change, advancing health*, Washington, DC, 2010, Institute of Medicine.

Jun J, et al: Barriers and facilitators of nurses' use of clinical practice guidelines: an integrative review, *Int J Nurs Stud* 60:54, 2016.

Kennedy B: Team concepts: towards a just culture, *Nurs Manage* 47(6):13, 2016.

Kitson AL, Harvey G: Methods to succeed in effective knowledge translation in clinical practice, *J Nurs Scholarsh* 48(3):294, 2016.

LoBiondo-Wood G: *Nursing research*, ed 9, St Louis, 2017, Elsevier.

McKeever S, et al: Engaging a nursing workforce in evidence-based practice: introduction of a nursing clinical effectiveness committee, *Worldviews Evid Based Nurs* 13(1):85, 2016.

McNeil A: Using evidence to structure discharge planning, *Nurs Manage* 47(5):22, 2016.

Melnyk BM, et al: The establishment of evidence-based practice competencies for practicing registered nurses and advanced practice nurses in real-world clinical settings: proficiencies to improve healthcare quality, reliability, patient outcomes, and costs, *Worldviews Evid Based Nurs* 11(1):5, 2014.

Melnyk BM, Fineout-Overholt E: *Evidence-based practice in nursing and healthcare: a guide to best practice*, ed 3, Philadelphia, 2015, Lippincott Williams & Wilkins.

Mortenius H, et al: Strategic communication intervention to stimulate interest in research and evidence-based practice: a 12-year follow-up study with registered nurses, *Worldviews Evid Based Nurs* 13(1):42, 2016.

National Quality Forum (NQF): *NQF's strategic direction 2016-2019: lead, prioritize, and collaborate for better health care measurement*, 2017, http://www .qualityforum.org/NQF_Strategic _Direction_2016-2019.aspx.

Peterson MH, et al: Choosing the best evidence to guide clinical practice: application of AACN levels of evidence, *Crit Care Nurse* 34(2):58, 2014.

Press Ganey: *Nursing Quality (NDNQI)*, 2017, http://www.pressganey.com/ solutions/clinical-quality/nursing-quality.

Quality and Safety Education for Nurses (QSEN) Institute: *Pre-licensure KSAs*, 2014, http://qsen.org/competencies/ pre-licensure-ksas/.

Raines DA: A collaborative strategy to bring evidence into practice, *Worldviews Evid Based Nurs* 13(3):253, 2016.

Scott ES, et al: Nursing administration research priorities, *J Nurs Adm* 46(5): 238, 2016.

Spruce L, et al: AORN's revised model for evidence appraisal and rating, *AORN J* 103:60, 2016.

Stausmire JM: Quality improvement or research—deciding which road to take, *Crit Care Nurse* 34(6):58, 2014.

The Joint Commission (TJC): *2018 National Patient Safety Goals*, 2018, https:// www.jointcommission.org/standards _information/npsgs.aspx.

Titler MG, et al: The Iowa model of evidence-based practice to promote quality care, *Crit Care Nurs Clin North Am* 13(4):497, 2001.

University of Colorado: *Research and Evidence Based Practice Manual*, ed 3, 2014, http://evidencebasednurse .weebly.com/uploads/4/2/0/8/42081989/ prof-ebp-2014-practice-outcomes -manual.pdf.

Warren JI, et al: The strengths and challenges of implementing EBP in healthcare systems, *Worldviews Evid Based Nurs* 13(1):15, 2016a.

Warren JI, et al: Three-year pre-post analysis of EBP integration in a Magnet-designated community hospital, *Worldviews Evid Based Nurs* 13(1):50, 2016b.

White S, Spruce L: Perioperative nursing leaders implement clinical practice guidelines using the Iowa Model of Evidence-Based Practice 1.3, *AORN J* 102:51, 2015.

CHAPTER

8

Critical Thinking

evolve MEDIA RESOURCES

http://evolve.elsevier.com/Potter/essentials

- Audio Glossary

- QSEN Activity and Review Questions Answers and Rationales

OBJECTIVES

- Describe the characteristics of a critical thinker.
- Discuss the importance of clinical judgment in a nurse's ability to make clinical decisions.
- Describe how reflection improves clinical decision making.
- Describe the components of a critical thinking model for clinical decision making.

- Discuss critical thinking skills used in nursing practice.
- Discuss the critical thinking attitudes used in clinical decision making.
- Explain how experience and professional standards influence a nurse's critical thinking.
- Discuss the relationship of the nursing process to critical thinking.

KEY TERMS

clinical decision making, p. 107
clinical inferences, p. 107
clinical judgment, p. 101
critical thinking, p. 101

decision making, p. 105
diagnostic reasoning, p. 105
nursing process, p. 108
problem solving, p. 105

reflection, p. 102
scientific method, p. 105
workarounds, p. 111

Every day you think critically without realizing it. If your computer flashes an error warning, you think about the actions you took before the error, consider possible causes of the problem, and correct a key stroke error or reboot the computer. If you decide to walk your dogs, go to the door, and notice that it is raining, you change into your raincoat. These examples show how you use basic critical thinking skills every day.

As a professional nurse, you care for patients with unique, complicated health care problems that can change within minutes. Thus critical thinking is embedded in your everyday routine, as it involves knowing as much as possible about each patient and sorting out the information into patterns to clarify problems, recognize changes, and make appropriate decisions under pressure (Rueskin, 2015). Critical thinking is an essential process for safe, efficient, and skillful nursing intervention (Papathanasiou, 2014). Sound critical thinking enables you to face each new experience and problem involving a patient's care with open-mindedness, confidence, and continual inquiry. This skill enables you to avoid common mistakes and proceed in the most logical manner.

As Jessica arrives at Mr. Myers' bedside, she performs an assessment to collect information relevant to his condition: vital signs, his self-report of pain and ability to turn (log roll), the condition of his surgical dressing, the status of the IV and urinary catheter, and his ability to move his extremities. She also asks Mr. Myers whether he has any questions and whether he understands the elements of postoperative monitoring. Jessica analyzes the information she gathers, reviews the progress note

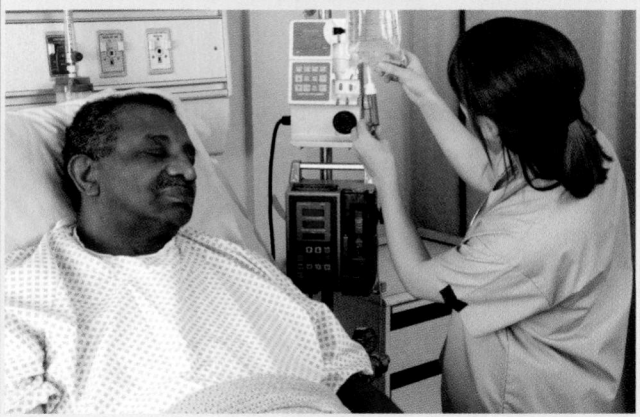

CASE STUDY *William Myers*

Copyright © monkeybusinessimages/iStock/Thinkstock.

William Myers is a 60-year-old man who had surgery to correct a spinal deformity. He just arrived on the neurosurgery patient care unit from the recovery room. He has an IV infusion of D_5NS running at 80 mL/hr. An indwelling urinary catheter is in place and draining clear amber-colored urine. The nurse, Jessica, is a recently graduated nurse who has worked on the unit for about 6 months. She enters the room to introduce herself and begin an assessment of Mr. Myers' condition. The patient's medical record shows he received oxycodone 10 mg for pain while in the recovery room. Jessica considers what to include in an assessment of her patient's condition.

reported by nurses from the recovery room, and determines the nursing care priorities for Mr. Myers.

Critical thinking is not a simple, step-by-step, linear process. It is a thinking process that you will develop as you gain clinical nursing experience.

CLINICAL JUDGMENT IN NURSING PRACTICE

Why is the nursing role so important to health care? Nurses make the decisions and judgments that help ensure that patients receive the most appropriate, timely, and effective interventions to maintain or restore their health. A **clinical judgment** is a conclusion about a patient's needs, concerns, or health problems and/or the decisions to take or avoid action, use or modify standard approaches, or improvise new approaches based on the patient's response (Tanner, 2006). Clinical decision making separates professional nurses from nursing assistive personnel (NAP). For example, an RN observes for changes in patients' conditions, recognizes changes and potential problems as they arise, and takes quick action when a patient's clinical condition worsens. Nurses direct technical personnel to perform basic aspects of care based on patient need; technical personnel do not have the knowledge or critical thinking skills to analyze when or why patients' clinical needs change. Good clinical decision making requires you to investigate and analyze all aspects of a clinical

situation or problem and then apply scientific and nursing knowledge to choose the best course of action.

In 2006, Dr. Christine Tanner described a research-based model of clinical judgment in nursing. It included the following conclusions:

- Clinical judgments are influenced more by the nurse's experience and knowledge than by the objective data about the situation at hand. This means experience is crucial.
- Sound clinical judgment partly relies on knowing the patient and his or her typical pattern of responses as well as an engagement with the patient and his or her concerns.
- Clinical judgments are influenced by the context of clinical situations and the culture of patient care units.
- Nurses use a variety of reasoning patterns alone or in combination, including reflection.

Critical thinking and good clinical judgment enable you to creatively seek knowledge, act quickly when conditions change, and make quality decisions to protect your patient's well-being. This process requires you to be flexible and able to recognize important aspects of an undefined clinical situation, interpret their meanings, and respond appropriately (Tanner, 2006).

Critical Thinking Defined

As Jessica assesses Mr. Myers, she learns that his vital signs are stable and that his self-report of pain is at a level 6. He tells Jessica that he had back pain for more than 3 years before finding a surgeon who would correct his deformity. Jessica knows that the manipulation of tissue during spinal surgery can cause considerable discomfort. Mr. Myers is reluctant to turn in bed. Jessica knows that the standard of care for patients who have had spinal surgery is to begin a mobility protocol within the first 12 hours after surgery. However, after questioning Mr. Myers, Jessica learns that his doctor has not told him about the protocol. As she considers the difficulty Mr. Myers might experience in tolerating increased activity, she reviews the medical orders for postoperative analgesics. She decides on the best time to give Mr. Myers an analgesic so that she can begin to get him out of bed and start the mobility protocol. In this example, Jessica observes the patient's clinical situation. She asks questions and reflects on her previous experiences caring for patients who had spinal surgery. She considers what she learned from managing their postoperative pain and preventing complications related to immobility. Jessica makes a clinical decision by applying critical thinking.

A critical thinker identifies the important data in each clinical situation, imagines and explores alternatives, considers ethical principles and care standards, and makes informed decisions about patient care. **Critical thinking** is a continuous process characterized by open-mindedness, continual inquiry, and perseverance combined with a willingness to look at each unique patient situation and identify the assumptions that are true and relevant. Critical thinking includes recognizing an issue (e.g., patient problem), analyzing information related to the issue (e.g., clinical and historical data about the patient), evaluating information (including assumptions and evidence), and drawing conclusions. An effective nurse engages in critical thinking by fully assessing a patient's health condition (see Chapter 9), meaning that a nurse learns as much as possible about the patient from many sources to form a clear holistic view of a patient's problems and the approaches for resolving them. Critical thinking allows you to focus on the important issues at hand in any clinical situation and make decisions that produce desired outcomes (Raterink, 2011).

You begin to learn critical thinking early in your practice. For example, Jessica first learned about the importance of early mobility after surgery when she read the nursing and scientific literature on the concepts of mobility and deconditioning. While caring for previous patients, she learned that pain reduces mobility. Critical thinking is a way of thinking about a situation by asking:

- "Why does the patient have this condition"?
- "Are the signs and symptoms demonstrated by the patient what I would expect for the condition or situation?"
- "What do I really know about this patient's situation?"
- "What options do I have?"
- "What factors can contribute to comfort?"

Evidence-based knowledge (knowledge based on research or clinical expertise) makes nurses better informed critical thinkers (see Chapter 7). Thinking critically and learning about the concepts of deconditioning, mobility, and comfort prepare Jessica to better anticipate Mr. Myers' needs, identify problems more quickly, and provide appropriate care.

Critical thinking requires cognitive skills, the habit of asking questions, the dedication to stay well informed, honesty in facing personal biases, the willingness to reconsider conclusions, and the ability to think clearly about issues (Facione, 1990). Table 8.1 summarizes core critical thinking skills that, when applied to nursing, show the complex nature of clinical decision making.

Learning to think critically helps you care for patients by acting as their advocate and making informed choices about their care. Facione and Facione (1996) identified concepts for critical thinking (Table 8.2). These concepts are still current and essential to the use of critical thinking skills. Critical thinking is more than just problem solving. It is an attempt to continually improve your effectiveness in facing patient care problems.

Reflection

As you care for patients, you will often review your practice experience to describe, analyze, and evaluate it (Barksby et al., 2015). You might ask yourself:

- How did I act?
- Why did I take such an action?
- What could I have done differently?
- What should I do in a similar situation in the future?

This is **reflection,** a part of critical thinking that involves purposefully reviewing a situation to discover its purpose or meaning. As a nurse you will reflect on the purpose and meaning of each patient's situation as well as the purpose and meaning of your actions in that situation.

BOX 8.1   MODEL FOR REFLECTION

REFLECT: This model can be used individually or as a process shared with others.

R	**Recall** the events:	Review the facts about a situation, and describe what happened.
E	**Examine** your responses:	Think about or discuss your thoughts and actions at the time of the situation.
F	Acknowledge **Feelings:**	Identify any feelings you had during the situation.
L	**Learn** from the experience:	Review and highlight what you learned from the situation, for example, your patient's responses and your actions.
E	**Explore** options:	Think about or discuss your options for similar situations in the future.
C	**Create** a plan of action:	Create a plan for action in future similar situations.
T	Set a **Timescale:**	Set a time by which your plan of action will be completed.

Adapted from Barksby J, et al: A new model of reflection for clinical practice, *Nurs Times* 111(34/35):21-23, 2015.

Reflection means recalling patient care situations to explore the factors that influenced your actions in handling each situation. Reflection is like replaying a video. It is not intuitive. It means visualizing a past situation and taking time to honestly review everything you remember about the situation. This reflection allows you to gain new knowledge and raise questions about your practice, which can lead to a search for better evidence for practice (Barksby et al., 2015). Research shows that reflective reasoning improves the accuracy of making diagnostic conclusions (Mamede et al., 2012). This means that gathering information about a patient, reflecting on the meaning of your findings, and exploring the possible meaning of those findings improves your ability to identify a patient's problems (see Chapter 9). Reflection helps you to focus on learning and self-awareness and to avoid simply retelling an event (Barksby et al., 2015). Box 8.1 lists steps of a model for using reflection in your practice.

Knowing the Patient

Clinical learning is a lifelong process. Learning to know patients results from working with many patients over time, hearing accounts of their experiences with illness, observing them, and coming to understand how they typically respond (Tanner, 2006). *For example, even though Jessica worked as a nurse for only 6 months, she is developing a level of knowing having worked with patients on the neurosurgical unit. She is becoming familiar with the clinical signs that indicate a worsening condition in patients who have had brain or spinal surgery. She has observed the behavioral and physiological changes that occur in these patients and thus is beginning to*

TABLE 8.1 CORE CRITICAL THINKING SKILLS
(Peter A. Facione – Modified From the 1990 APA Delphi Report)

Interpretation	Interpretation is the process of discovering, determining, or assigning meaning. Interpretation skills can be applied to anything (e.g., written messages, charts, diagrams, maps, graphs, memes, and verbal and nonverbal exchanges). People apply their interpretive skills to behaviors, events, and social interactions when deciding what they think something means in a given context.
Analysis	Analytical skills are used to identify assumptions, reasons, themes, and the evidence used in making arguments or offering explanations. Analytical skills enable us to consider all the key elements in any given situation and to determine how those elements relate to one another. People with strong analytical skills notice important patterns and details. People use analysis to gather the most relevant information from spoken language, documents, signs, charts, graphs, and diagrams.
Inference	Inference skills enable us to draw conclusions from reasons, evidence, observations, experiences, or our values and beliefs. Using Inference, we can predict the most likely consequences of the options we may be considering. Inference enables us to see the logical consequences of the assumptions we may be making. Sound inferences rely on accurate information. People with strong inference skills draw logical or highly reliable conclusions using all forms of analogical, probabilistic, empirical, and mathematical reasoning.
Evaluation	Evaluative skills are used to assess the credibility of the claims people make or post, and to assess the quality of the reasoning people display when they make arguments or give explanations. We can also apply our evaluation skills to assess the quality of many other elements that are important for good thinking, such as analyses, interpretations, explanations, inferences, options, opinions, beliefs, hypotheses, proposals, and decisions. People with strong evaluation skills can judge the quality of arguments and the credibility of speakers and writers.
Explanation	Explanation is the process of justifying what we have decided to do or what we have decided to believe. People with strong explanation skills provide the evidence, methods, and considerations they actually relied on when making their judgment. Explanations can include our assumptions, reasons, values, and beliefs. Strong explanations enable others to understand and to evaluate our decisions.
Self-Regulation	Self-Regulation in the context of critical thinking relates to monitoring and, if necessary, correcting any mistakes that may have occurred in the process of interpreting, analyzing, inferring, evaluating, or explaining. Self-regulation occurs throughout the critical thinking process; it is not confined to the ending point only. As soon as an individual or a thinking team identifies an error as a result of the process of self-monitoring, that error can be corrected so that the overall process of critical thinking can again begin to move forward toward its culmination, which is the considered judgment about what to believe or what to do in any given context. Self-regulation can focus any of the elements in that process, including how the problem was framed, what was accepted as evidence, what methods were employed, what the guiding theoretical considerations were, and what level of closure was deemed appropriate for regarding the problem as having been solved or the decision as having been made. Self-regulation is the skill which separates critical thinking from un-critical thinking.

Copyright © 2017 Facione, PA, Gittens, C., and Measured Reasons, LLC, Hermosa Beach, CA. All rights reserved.

recognize changes in each new patient. In addition, she is learning that each patient is unique and has values, beliefs, and cultural factors that affect the response to illness. Knowing each patient as an individual with a unique pattern of responses enables you to individualize your responses and interventions (Tanner, 2006).

Knowing your patients occurs by engaging with them, acting responsibly, and providing excellent care. Show concern for patients and their families' well-being so that you can learn who they are, how illness has affected their lives, and how that knowledge should affect your approach to care. Make the patient and family partners in care. To make good clinical decisions, you must understand not only the pathophysiological and diagnostic aspects of a patient's clinical presentation and disease but also the effect of the illness on the patient and family and their physical, social, and emotional strengths and coping resources. Always approach

your clinical work informed, and do not consider it simply a task-based, detached exercise. Reflect on your practice and knowledge to learn to think like a nurse.

LEVELS OF CRITICAL THINKING IN NURSING

Your ability to think critically grows as you gain knowledge and experience in nursing practice. Kataoka-Yahiro and Saylor (1994) developed a critical thinking model (Fig. 8.1) that includes three levels of critical thinking in nursing: basic, complex, and commitment.

Basic Critical Thinking

Beginning nursing students are very task oriented, focusing on performing skills and organizing nursing care activities correctly. At the basic level of critical thinking, a student trusts that experts have the right answers for every problem.

TABLE 8.2	CONCEPTS FOR A CRITICAL THINKER
CONCEPT	**COMPONENT**
Truth seeking	Seek the true meaning of a situation. Be courageous, honest, and objective about asking questions. *Case study: Jessica asks Mr. Myers more questions about how he usually deals with pain and the meaning pain has in this particular situation.*
Open-mindedness	Be tolerant of different views and be sure that you clearly know your patients' views. Be aware of your own biases and respect the right of others to have different opinions. *Case study: Jessica asks Mr. Myers to tell her the approaches he would like to use to become mobile after surgery. Mr. Myers tells Jessica that he fears walking too soon and hurting his back.*
Analyticity	Be alert to potentially problematic situations; anticipate possible results or consequences (e.g., how should a patient respond to a certain treatment?); value reason; use evidence-based knowledge. *Case study: Jessica points out to Mr. Myers that he has had back pain for some time and explains that evidence shows that persistent low back pain leads to exercise intolerance and further loss of functional capacity (Atalay et al., 2012). His ability to regain mobility quickly will reduce the risk of further decline.*
Systematicity	Be organized and focused and work hard in answering your questions. Organize inquiry based on priorities of care. *Case study: Jessica focuses on pain assessment and gives Mr. Myers additional analgesia after consulting with Mr. Myers and his surgeon to identify the best medication considering Mr. Myers' previous pain history.*
Self-confidence	Trust your own reasoning processes. *Case study: Jessica believes that by managing Mr. Myers' pain well, she will build trust with him as she prepares him for the mobility protocol and use of relaxation techniques.*
Inquisitiveness	Be eager to acquire knowledge and explanations even when applications of the knowledge are not immediately obvious. Value learning for learning's sake. *Case study: Jessica decides to take some time and talk with Mr. Myers' wife about her husband's experience with pain and his coping strategies.*
Maturity	Multiple solutions are acceptable. Reflect on your own judgments; develop cognitive maturity. *Case study: Jessica consults with a physical therapist who also is willing to talk with Mr. Myers about the importance of early mobility. Jessica and the physical therapist will form a plan for physical therapy and nursing staff to implement an ambulation schedule during Mr. Myers' waking hours.*

Copyright © monkeybusinessimages/ iStock/Thinkstock.

Modified from Facione N, Facione P: Externalizing the critical thinking in knowledge development and clinical judgment, *Nurs Outlook* 44:129, 1996.

Thinking is concrete and based on a set of rules or principles. For example, a student might rely on a hospital procedure manual or a clinical simulation guideline for inserting a nasogastric tube. The student follows the steps of the procedure without learning how to adjust his or her approach when a problem arises or a patient has a unique need (e.g., a patient has a deviated nasal septum or has difficulty swallowing). The student does not have enough experience to anticipate how to individualize or adapt the procedure when various problems arise. At this level, answers to complex problems are perceived as either right or wrong (e.g., the nasogastric tube will not advance because it is coiled in the throat), and a single solution usually resolves each problem (e.g., removing the tube and starting over). Such basic critical thinking is an early step in the development of reasoning (Kataoka-Yahiro and Saylor, 1994). A basic critical thinker learns to accept the diverse opinions and values of experts (e.g., instructors and staff nurse role models). However, inexperience, weak competencies, and inflexible attitudes can slow a nurse's ability to move to the next level of critical thinking.

Complex Critical Thinking

As a complex critical thinker, you begin to rely less on experts in daily care. You learn to analyze data and examine choices more independently. Your thinking abilities and initiative to look beyond expert opinion begin to increase. As your critical thinking skills grow, you learn that you must consider alternative and perhaps even conflicting solutions. *In the case study, Jessica learns from Mrs. Myers that Mr. Myers dislikes taking pain medication and that he experienced great distress at home before taking an analgesic. Bringing an analgesic to the bedside and urging Mr. Myers to take it might not be an effective approach. Jessica begins to consider possible nonpharmacological approaches to combine with an analgesic that will help Mr. Myers (see Chapter 34). Knowing his attitude about pain also might change Jessica's method of explaining the importance of pain control.*

In complex critical thinking, you learn to synthesize knowledge. This means that you combine your experience and knowledge of patients to develop a new thought or idea. When you consider therapies for patients, you realize that each option has benefits and risks that factor into your choice. Your thinking becomes more creative and innovative. At this level, you are more willing to consider deviations from standard protocols or procedures and to provide more individualized care.

Commitment

The third level of critical thinking is commitment (Kataoka-Yahiro and Saylor, 1994). In commitment, you anticipate the need to make choices without assistance from others. You

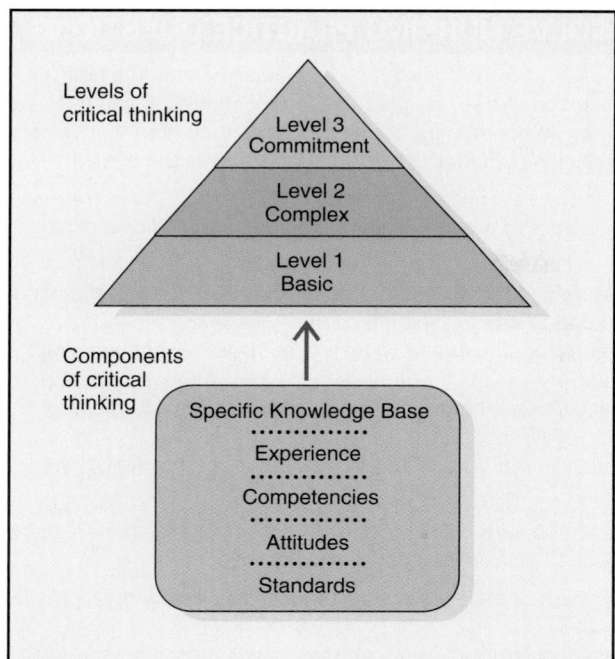

FIG 8.1 Critical thinking model for nursing judgment. (Redrawn from Kataoka-Yahiro M, Saylor C: A critical thinking model for nursing judgment, *J Nurs Educ* 33[8]:351, 1994. Modified from Glaser E: *An experiment in the development of critical thinking,* New York, 1941, Bureau of Publications, Teachers College, Columbia University; Miller J, Malcolm N: Critical thinking in the nursing curriculum, *Nurs Health Care* 11:67, 1990; Paul R: *The art of redesigning instruction.* In Willsen J, Blinker AJA, editors: *Critical thinking: how to prepare students for a rapidly changing world,* Santa Rosa, CA, 1993, Foundation for Critical Thinking.)

accept accountability for the decisions you make. As a nurse, you do more than just consider the complex alternatives that might resolve a problem. At the commitment level, you choose an action or belief based on the alternatives available and stand by your choice. Sometimes the choice is to avoid or delay acting.

Jessica decides that relaxation might be a valuable exercise for Mr. Myers to learn because it will allow him to have some control over his pain. Because of what she has learned about Mr. Myers, Jessica conducts a discussion with him and his wife, explaining the importance of pain control and having him agree to trying relaxation after a dose of analgesic. Jessica knows relaxation exercises are difficult to perform if pain has not been managed.

CRITICAL THINKING COMPETENCIES

Kataoka-Yahiro and Saylor (1994) describe critical thinking competencies as the cognitive processes a nurse uses to make judgments about the clinical care of patients. The three competencies are general critical thinking, specific critical thinking in clinical situations, and specific critical thinking in nursing.

General critical thinking processes are not unique to the nursing profession. They include the scientific method,

problem solving, and decision making. Specific critical thinking competencies in clinical health care situations include clinical inference, diagnostic reasoning, and clinical decision making. The specific critical thinking competency in nursing is the nursing process (see Chapter 9), which involves each of the three specific critical thinking competencies.

General Critical Thinking Competencies

Scientific Method. The scientific method is a way to solve problems through reasoning. It is a systematic, ordered approach to gathering data and solving problems. Professionals use it in nursing, medicine, and a variety of other health care disciplines. This approach looks for the truth or verifies that a set of facts agrees with reality. Nurse researchers use the scientific method when testing research questions in nursing practice situations. The scientific method has five steps:

1. Identifying the problem
2. Collecting data
3. Forming a question or hypothesis
4. Testing the question or hypothesis
5. Evaluating results of the test or study

The scientific method is one formal way to approach a problem, plan a solution, test the solution, and come to a conclusion. Table 8.3 gives an example of a nursing practice issue solved by application of the scientific method in a research study.

Problem Solving. You face problems every day. When a problem arises, you obtain information, combine it with what you already know, and develop a solution. Patients routinely present problems in practice. A traditional approach for solving problems is to clarify the problem, identify possible causes, assess and identify alternatives, choose one, implement it, and evaluate whether the problem was solved.

Jessica wants to help Mrs. Myers know what to expect and prepare for when Mr. Myers returns home. Even though he is expected to become actively mobile while in the hospital, he likely will still have some mobility limitations when he returns home. Jessica learns that the family lives in a two-story home with bedrooms upstairs. Mr. Myers will likely be unable to climb stairs initially. Jessica could give Mrs. Myers a pamphlet on postoperative restrictions, discuss with the family how to arrange a temporary sleeping place for Mr. Myers, or consult with the physician and physical therapist about referring the family to rehabilitation. After discussing the problem with the family, Jessica decides to discuss the alternative of rearranging the home setting and having Mrs. Myers attend the hospital mobility assistance class offered by the physical therapists.

A systematic approach to problem solving makes it more likely that you will find an appropriate solution. Effective problem solving includes evaluating a solution over time to be sure that it continues to be effective. If a problem recurs, you try various options. Solving a problem in one situation adds to your clinical experience and enables you to apply the knowledge in future patient situations.

TABLE 8.3   USING THE SCIENTIFIC METHOD TO SOLVE NURSING PRACTICE QUESTIONS

Clinical Problem: The incidence of a health care–associated infection, *Clostridium difficile* infection, has increased on a hospital general medicine patient care unit. The nursing staff on the unit practice committee, an infection control specialist, and a clinical nurse specialist in medicine have met to discuss factors that may be contributing to the problem. They note that visitors are inconsistent in the use of antiseptic hand rubs. A staff member questions whether the use of hand rubs is the best approach for this type of infection.

Identify the problem.	• The incidence of *C. difficile* has increased among patients on a general medicine patient care unit.
Collect data.	• Staff members review the literature about the nature of *C. difficile* infection and the hand antiseptic techniques recommended to prevent the infection. • Staff members search the literature for studies that investigated hand-hygiene practices of visitors of hospitalized patients. • Staff members review performance improvement reports to monitor the occurrence of *C. difficile* on the unit. • The infection control specialist is asked to discuss the trends within the hospital in the incidence of *C. difficile*.
Form a research question to study the problem.	• Does visitor use of antiseptic hand rub with chlorhexidine versus handwashing with soap and water reduce the incidence of *C. difficile* infection in medical patients?
Answer the question.	• The nurse specialist and a small team of staff members create a 4-month study approved by the hospital research board. • Patients' visitors are asked to use a chlorhexidine rub on their hands before entering and leaving patient rooms. • Visitors switch to handwashing with soap and water for the next 2 months. • The infection control specialist tracks the incidence of *C. difficile* infection over the 4 months.
Evaluate the results of the study. Does the study answer the research question?	• Compare the incidence of *C. difficile* infection for the 2-month period when each hand-hygiene method was used. • Results showed a decline in number of *C. difficile* infections when visitors used chlorhexidine.

Decision Making. When you face a problem and choose a course of action from several options, you are making a decision. Decision making focuses on resolving a problem. Following a set of criteria helps you make a thorough and thoughtful decision. The criteria may be personal, may be based on an organizational policy, or, in the case of nursing, may be based on a professional standard.

For example, a person practices decision making when he or she chooses a health care provider. To make a decision, the individual must recognize and define the problem (the need for a health care provider) and assess all options (e.g., consider recommended health care providers or choose one whose office is close to home). The person weighs the options against a set of personal criteria (experience, friendliness, reputation, location), tests possible options (talks directly with health care providers), and makes a decision. This process leads to informed conclusions that are supported by evidence and reason. Decision making goes hand in hand with problem solving.

Specific Critical Thinking Competencies

Diagnostic Reasoning and Inference. Diagnostic reasoning depends on your state of readiness to apply critical thinking (Levett-Jones et al., 2010). You must be committed to doing diagnostic reasoning well. It is influenced by your attitudes, philosophical perspective, and preconceptions about nursing. For example, if you do not value a holistic approach to nursing, you will likely not complete thorough assessments of your patients. Preconceptions and inaccurate assumptions such as "most people who are poor have an alcohol use disorder" or "people who are obese are not motivated to improve their health" will negatively affect your reasoning. You must reflect on and question your assumptions and prejudices when you engage in diagnostic reasoning to become a competent thinker and to ultimately improve patient outcomes. Diagnostic reasoning involves a combination of gathering and analyzing information (Delany and Golding, 2014).

As you collect information about a patient in a clinical situation, diagnostic reasoning begins. It is the analytical process for determining a patient's health problems. You must accurately recognize a patient's health problems before you choose solutions and implement actions. *When Jessica first gathers information about Mr. Myers, she learns a great deal: he is having pain and difficulty turning. According to his wife, he is generally resistant to taking analgesics. Jessica also knows Mr. Myers is on a mobility protocol, but he is uninformed about it. Jessica's responsibility as a nurse is to analyze this information and diagnose the patient's health problems accurately, identify the priorities, and then take action.*

Diagnostic reasoning requires you to assign meaning to the behaviors and physical signs and symptoms a patient presents. This begins when you interact with a patient, make physical or behavioral observations, and review medical history information. An expert nurse sees the context of a patient situation (e.g., a patient who has a long history of back pain is now recovering from surgery, is uniformed about postoperative care, and will require routine analgesics for reliable pain management). The nurse observes patterns and themes (e.g., symptoms that include wincing and moaning and the inability of the patient to describe what early mobility requires him to do). Once diagnostic reasoning is complete and problems are identified, the nurse makes clinical decisions quickly (e.g., control pain first so the patient can later attend and learn about the mobility protocol and be able to get out of bed). The information a nurse collects and analyzes leads to a diagnosis of a patient's condition and the appropriate interventions.

Nurses do not make medical diagnoses; they make nursing diagnoses (see Chapter 9). They do, however, assess and monitor patients closely and compare patients' signs and symptoms with signs and symptoms that are common to a medical diagnosis. This type of diagnostic reasoning helps health care providers pinpoint a problem and select proper therapies more quickly.

As a part of diagnostic reasoning, you make **clinical inferences**. You learn to draw conclusions from related pieces of patient data and previous experience with similar evidence. An inference is a conclusion the nurse draws from data before making a nursing diagnosis. *For example, Jessica notices Mr. Myers' wincing, his difficulty in turning, and his self-report pain score; she reflects on previous patients who return from back surgery showing a clear pattern of acute pain. Jessica uses her experience and patient data that she has gathered to logically identify a problem.*

As a student, you confirm your judgments with more experienced nurses or your instructor. Your judgment can be wrong at times, but consulting with nurse experts gives you feedback to support future clinical judgments. Often you cannot make a precise diagnosis during your first meeting with a patient. You may sense that the patient has a problem, but you lack sufficient data to make a specific diagnosis. Some patients' physical conditions limit their ability to tell you about their symptoms. Some patients choose not to share sensitive and important information during your initial assessment. Patients' behaviors and physical responses often become observable after your initial assessment. When you are uncertain of a diagnosis, continue collecting data from all possible sources. You must critically analyze changing clinical situations on a continuous basis until you can determine a patient's unique situation. Diagnostic reasoning takes practice and must become part of your routine thinking in nursing practice.

Clinical Decision Making. Clinical decision making or reasoning is a problem-solving activity that involves diagnostic reasoning as well as deciding on the appropriate therapeutic actions specific to a patient's situation and wishes (Delany and Golding, 2014). When you face a clinical problem such as a patient who has an area of redness over the heel, you form a diagnostic conclusion that identifies the problem (impaired skin integrity and possible early formation of a pressure injury); then you choose the best nursing interventions (skin care, turning, and reducing heel pressure). Nurses make clinical decisions to improve a patient's health or maintain wellness. This means minimizing the severity of the problem or resolving the problem completely. **Clinical decision making** requires problem solving and reasoning so you can choose the options that produce the best patient outcomes based on a patient's condition and priority of the problem.

Part of developing expertise in clinical decision making comes from knowing your patients. Expert nurses develop a level of knowing that enable them to recognize patterns of patient symptoms and responses. You begin to acquire this expertise by learning to assess patients thoroughly and by actively engaging with them. You investigate and reflect on all your clinical observations and then apply nursing and scientific knowledge to choose a course of action. For example, an expert nurse who has worked on a general surgery unit for many years knows that when a patient's blood pressure falls, it becomes necessary to further assess the patient. The nurse checks the patient's pulse and level of consciousness and quickly reviews recent laboratory tests to detect any internal hemorrhage (which could result in a fall in blood pressure, rapid pulse, a change in consciousness, or a decrease in blood count). An expert nurse can do this more quickly than a new nurse because the expert nurse has developed pattern recognition.

The expert nurse has a combination of experience, time spent in a specific clinical area, and the quality of relationships formed with patients that enables him or her to know clinical situations and quickly anticipate and select the proper course of action (Tanner, 2006). Spending more time with each patient to thoroughly observe and measure normal and abnormal findings is a way to know your patient better. In addition, consistently monitoring patients as problems develop helps you see how clinical changes evolve over time.

Select nursing interventions based on clinical knowledge and specific information that you collect from your patients, including:

- Initial assessment data about a patient's status and situation, including data collected by actively listening to a patient discuss his or her health care needs
- Knowledge of a patient's clinical variables (e.g., age, severity of the problem, preexisting disease conditions) and how the variables are linked
- Knowledge of a patient's current health risks (e.g., smoking, alcohol use, lack of immunization) related to the problem
- A judgment about the likely course and outcomes of the diagnosed problem

- Additional relevant data about a patient's needs with respect to the activities of daily living, functional capacity, and social resources
- Knowledge about the nursing intervention options available and the way in which specific interventions may affect a patient's situation

Always keep the patient your center of attention as you make clinical decisions. Making an accurate clinical decision allows you to set care priorities. Because patients bring different variables to a situation, an activity or treatment is often a higher priority in one situation than in another. *For example, Jessica knows that Mr. Myers ultimately will need to become engaged and active in the mobility protocol. To achieve this goal, she has two immediate priorities: manage Mr. Myers' pain and provide information and support to gain his involvement. These priorities must be met before she can effectively implement the mobility protocol.*

Do not assume that a particular condition is a priority. For example, you expect that a patient immediately out of surgery will experience pain, and pain treatment is often a priority of nursing care. However, if the patient is experiencing anxiety with heightened pain perception, the nurse must focus on relieving anxiety before pain-relief measures can be effective.

Clinical decision making is challenging because nurses care for multiple patients in a fast-paced and unpredictable environment. When you work in a busy setting, use criteria such as the clinical condition of a patient, Maslow's hierarchy of needs (see Chapter 2), risks involved in treatment delays, and patients' expectations of care to decide which patients have higher priorities. Applying critical thinking to clinical decision making enables you to attend to a high-priority patient and perhaps delegate less essential tasks to an NAP. Skillful, prioritized clinical decision making allows you to manage the various problems associated with groups of patients.

The Nursing Process as a Competency

Nurses apply the nursing process as a competency when delivering patient care (Kataoka-Yahiro and Saylor, 1994). The American Nurses Association (ANA) (2010) standards set forth the framework for critical thinking in the application of the five-step nursing process (Fig. 8.2): assessment, diagnosis, planning, implementation, and evaluation (see Chapter 9). The purpose of the nursing process is to diagnose and treat human responses (e.g., patient symptoms, need for knowledge, or emotional stress) to actual or potential health problems (ANA, 2010). Using this process enables nurses to help patients meet agreed-on outcomes for better health. The nursing process requires a nurse to use the general and specific critical thinking competencies described earlier in this chapter to focus on a specific patient's unique needs. The format of the nursing process is unique to the discipline of nursing and sets a common language for nurses to "think through" patients' clinical problems (Kataoka-Yahiro and Saylor, 1994). Table 8.4 provides a summary of the nursing process, and Chapter 9 contains a detailed description of the nursing process.

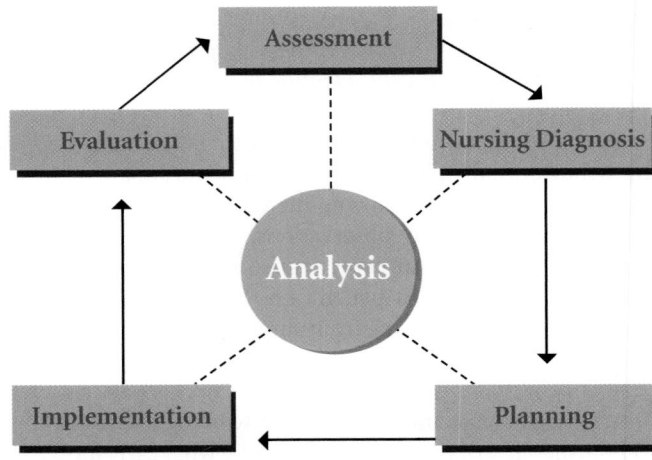

FIG 8.2 Five-step nursing process model.

CRITICAL THINKING MODEL

Because critical thinking is complex, a model helps explain the steps in making clinical decisions and judgments about your patients. Kataoka-Yahiro and Saylor (1994) developed a model of critical thinking for nursing judgment based in part on previous works by Paul (1993), Glaser (1941), and Miller and Malcolm (1990) (see Fig. 8.1). The model defines the outcome of critical thinking: nursing judgment that is relevant to nursing problems in a variety of health care settings. The model includes five elements of critical thinking in nursing judgment: competence (e.g., problem-solving and clinical decision-making ability), knowledge, experience, attitudes, and standards (intellectual and professional). The five model elements combine to guide nurses in making clinical decisions leading to safe, effective nursing care (Box 8.2).

Competence

The first element of critical thinking is competence. Nurses perform competent critical thinking as they apply the nursing process. Throughout this text, the model shows you how to apply critical thinking as part of the nursing process.

Specific Knowledge Base

A second element of the critical thinking model is a nurse's knowledge base. A nurse's knowledge base varies according to his or her educational experience (e.g., type of basic nursing education, continuing education courses, and additional college education and degrees). In addition, a nurse builds knowledge by reading nursing literature (especially research-based literature) to maintain current knowledge of nursing science. Knowledge prepares a nurse to better anticipate and identify patient problems by understanding their origin and nature.

Your exposure to knowledge comes from your educational experiences and your collaboration and work at the side of knowledgeable colleagues. Your knowledge base includes information and theory from the basic sciences, humanities, behavioral sciences, science from other health care disciplines,

TABLE 8.4 SUMMARY OF THE NURSING PROCESS

COMPONENT	PURPOSE	STEPS
Assessment	To gather, verify, and communicate data about a patient so a database can be established	Collect nursing health history. Perform physical examination. Collect laboratory data. Validate or confirm that data are correct. Cluster data by common themes or problem areas. Document data.
Nursing diagnosis	To identify a patient's health care needs in the form of nursing diagnoses	Analyze and interpret data. Identify patient problems. Form nursing diagnoses. Document nursing diagnoses.
Planning	To work with a patient, his or her family, and health care team members, to set priorities of care, identify patient-centered goals and expected outcomes, and prescribe an individualized approach to care	Identify and mutually set goals with the patient. Establish expected outcomes. Select nursing interventions. Document a nursing plan of care. Collaborate with other health care providers.
Implementation	To carry out nursing interventions specified by the plan of care	Perform nursing interventions. Reassess patient. Review and modify existing care plan.
Evaluation	To determine extent to which interventions helped achieve goals of care	Compare patient response with expected outcomes. Analyze reasons for results and conclusions. Modify care plan.

BOX 8.2 COMPONENTS OF CRITICAL THINKING IN NURSING

I. Specific knowledge base in nursing
II. Experience in nursing
III. Critical thinking competencies
  A. General critical thinking competencies
  B. Specific critical thinking competencies in clinical situations
  C. Specific critical thinking competency in nursing—the nursing process
IV. Attitudes for critical thinking
  A. Confidence
  B. Independence
  C. Fairness
  D. Responsibility
  E. Risk taking
  F. Discipline
  G. Perseverance
  H. Creativity
  I. Curiosity
  J. Integrity
  K. Humility
V. Standards for critical thinking
  A. Intellectual standards
    1. Clear: Plain and understandable (e.g., clear communication)
    2. Precise: Exact and specific (e.g., focusing on a problem and possible solution)

    3. Specific: To mention, describe, or define in detail
    4. Accurate: True and free from error; getting to the facts (objective and subjective)
    5. Relevant: Essential and crucial to a situation (e.g., a patient's situation)
    6. Plausible: Reasonable or probable
    7. Consistent: Expressing consistent beliefs or values
    8. Logical: Engaging in correct reasoning by moving from what one believes in a given instance to the conclusions that follow
    9. Deep: Containing complexities and multiple relationships
    10. Broad: Covering multiple viewpoints
    11. Complete: Thorough thinking and evaluation
    12. Significant: Focusing on what is important and not trivial
    13. Adequate (for purpose): Satisfactory in quality or amount
    14. Fair: Open-minded and impartial
  B. Professional standards
    1. Ethical criteria for nursing judgment
    2. Criteria for evaluation
    3. Professional responsibility

Modified from Kataoka-Yahiro M, Saylor C: A critical thinking model for nursing judgment, *J Nurs Educ* 33(8):351, 1994. Data from Paul R: The art of redesigning instruction. In Willsen J, Blinker AJA, editors: *Critical thinking: how to prepare students for a rapidly changing world,* Santa Rosa, CA, 1993, Foundation for Critical Thinking.

and nursing science. This broad knowledge base gives you a holistic view of patients and their health care needs. Your depth of knowledge affects your ability to think critically about nursing problems. This is one reason why thoroughly knowing your patients is a vital part of critical thinking. *In the case study, Jessica is a new nurse who continues to enjoy learning. She asks her manager if she can join the patient care unit's evidence-based practice committee. She decides to take an online class in nursing informatics. These experiences help her better understand the scientific articles she reads. Although she is new to nursing, Jessica's preparation and knowledge help her make the clinical decisions needed to care for Mr. Myers and other patients.*

Experience

Nursing is a practice discipline. You develop the knowledge of nursing through practice—the hands-on care of patients. Experience is the body of knowledge you gain from talking and listening to patients and families, observing their courses of illness, providing interventions, and seeing the effects. You learn from these experiences by reflecting actively on your experiences alone and with faculty and fellow students. You need clinical learning to become competent at clinical decision making.

Clinical experience is the application of nursing knowledge. Textbook approaches and simulation exercises lay an important foundation for practice, but you must adapt your practice to each setting, the unique qualities of each patient, and the experiences you gain from caring for previous patients. Benner (1984) noted that an expert nurse understands the context of a clinical situation, recognizes signs suggesting patterns, and interprets them as relevant or irrelevant. This level of competency comes with experience and a commitment to learning. Perhaps the best lesson you can learn is to value all patient experiences. Each clinical experience becomes a stepping stone to building knowledge and stimulating innovative thinking.

QSEN **QSEN ACTIVITY** *Patient-Centered Care*

- How might experience affect a nurse's development of communication skills with patients and their families?
- Describe three ways to build your communication skills in clinical situations.

evolve Answers to QSEN Activities can be found on the Evolve website.

Attitudes for Critical Thinking

The fourth element of the critical thinking model is attitudes (see Box 8.2). There are 11 attitudes that define a critical thinker and his or her success in approaching a problem (Paul, 1993; Papathanasiou et al., 2014). To become a critical thinker, you must be motivated to develop the attitudes and dispositions of a fair-minded thinker. For example, when a patient complains of anxiety before a diagnostic procedure, a curious nurse seeks information and an explanation by asking several questions to learn what the patient does not know and the nature of the patient's concerns (Kaddoura, 2013). The nurse shows discipline in forming questions and performing a thorough assessment to learn the source of the patient's anxiety.

Assessing the reliability of information is also an important stage of critical thinking. In this step, the nurse confirms the accuracy of the information collected by checking other evidence and informants (e.g., when a patient self-reports having fallen at home, the nurse confirms the patient's story about the incident with the family caregiver and learns what factors were associated with the fall and how the patient responded).

Critical thinking attitudes give you methods for approaching a problem or making a decision. Table 8.5 summarizes the ways nurses use critical thinking attitudes in practice situations. A summary of each critical thinking attitude follows.

Confidence. To be confident is to feel secure in your ability to accomplish a task or goal such as performing a nursing procedure or making a diagnostic decision. Confidence grows with experience as you recognize your strengths and limits. You gradually shift your focus from your own needs (e.g., remembering the steps for performing a procedure such as inserting an IV safely) to the patient's needs (e.g., adapting the approach to IV insertion to accommodate the excess swelling in the patient's arm).

When you are not confident in performing a nursing skill, you become anxious. This anxiety prevents you from attending to a patient, and this anxiety can be perceived by your patient. Always be aware of the extent and limits of your knowledge. If you have a question about a procedure, discuss it with your nursing instructor or preceptor first before performing the procedure on a patient. Patient safety is always the top priority. When an experienced nurse shows willingness to disagree with an action or expresses a doubt about an action he or she is considering, the nurse acts as a role model to colleagues and inspires them to develop their own confidence (Papathanasiou et al., 2014).

Thinking Independently. As you gain knowledge, you learn to consider a wide range of ideas and concepts before forming an opinion or making a judgment. You also are no longer limited by what you learned in school, and you become open minded in considering interventions (Papathanasiou et al., 2014). Independent thinking does not mean that you ignore other people's ideas. Instead you consider all sides of a situation. By the same token, a critical thinker does not accept another person's ideas without question. When thinking independently, you challenge the ways others think and look for rational and logical answers to problems. An independent thinker applies evidence-based practices (see Chapter 7) when facing clinical decisions. You must be willing to seek answers to difficult questions as well as obvious ones.

TABLE 8.5   CRITICAL THINKING ATTITUDES AND APPLICATIONS IN NURSING PRACTICE

CRITICAL THINKING ATTITUDE	APPLICATION IN PRACTICE
Confidence	Learn how to introduce yourself to a patient. For example: "Mrs. Tyms, I'm Chuck Lord, your nurse for this shift. I'll be responsible for your nursing care and will work with your doctor to make sure that you're comfortable." Speak with conviction when you begin a treatment or procedure. Do not let a patient think that you are not sure how to perform care safely. Always be prepared (e.g., organize equipment and provide comfort measures) before beginning a nursing activity.
Thinking independently	Read the nursing literature, especially when there are different opinions on a subject. Ask colleagues and expert staff nurses to share their ideas about nursing interventions.
Fairness	Listen to both sides in any discussion. If a patient or family member complains about a colleague, listen to the story and then speak with the colleague. Weigh all the facts.
Responsibility and accountability	Ask for help if you are not sure about how to perform a task. Report any problems immediately. Follow standards of practice in the care you give.
Risk taking	If your knowledge leads you to question a health care provider's order, speak up. Offer alternative approaches to nursing care when colleagues are having little success with patients.
Discipline	Be thorough in everything you do. Use established criteria for activities such as assessment and evaluation. Take time to be thorough.
Perseverance	Be wary of an easy answer. If colleagues give you information about a patient but some information is missing, clarify the facts or talk to the patient directly. If the same problems recur on a nursing division, bring colleagues together, look for a pattern, and find a solution.
Creativity	Seek different approaches when interventions are not working. For example, a patient may need a different positioning technique or a different instructional approach.
Curiosity	Always ask "why." A clinical sign or symptom can indicate a variety of problems. Learn more about the patient to help you make the right clinical judgments.
Integrity	Recognize when your opinions conflict with those of your patient. Review your position and work with the patient to reach agreement on how best to reach a positive outcome.
Humility	Recognize times when you need more information to make a decision. When you are new to a clinical division and unfamiliar with the patients, ask for an orientation to the area. Ask nurses regularly assigned to the area for assistance. Read professional journals regularly to keep updated on approaches to care.

Fairness. A critical thinker deals with situations fairly. This means that bias or prejudice does not enter into a decision. For example, regardless of what you think about illicit drug use, you do not allow your attitudes to affect the way you deliver care to patients who abuse drugs. Fairness requires that you look at each situation objectively and consider all viewpoints to understand the situation completely before making a decision. Use your imagination to help you develop an attitude of fairness. For example, imagining being in your patient's situation helps you see it through his or her eyes and appreciate its complexity.

Responsibility and Accountability. When caring for patients, you are responsible for correctly performing nursing care activities consistent with standards of practice. Standards of practice are the minimum acceptable level of performance needed to ensure high-quality care. For example, you do not take shortcuts or workarounds when you administer medications to a patient (e.g., failing to identify a patient or preparing medication doses for multiple patients at the same time). You are responsible for following the "six rights" of medication administration (see Chapter 17).

A professional nurse is responsible for performing nursing interventions competently. When you are competent, you make better clinical decisions about your patients. As a nurse, you are answerable, or accountable, for your decisions and the outcomes of your actions. This means that you must recognize ineffective nursing care and know the limits and scope of your practice.

Risk Taking. People often associate risk taking with danger. Using your cell phone while driving on a highway is a risk that might result in injury to you and drivers around you. However, risk taking is not always negative. Risk taking is desirable, particularly when the result can be a positive outcome. A critical thinker will take certain risks in attempting to solve problems. The willingness to take risks comes from experience with similar problems. In nursing, risk taking often produces innovations in patient care. In the past, nurses have taken risks by trying new approaches to skin care, wound care, and pain management. Some of these attempts produced interventions that are more effective than traditional approaches. When taking a risk, you must consider all options, be knowledgeable of the new intervention, identify any potential danger to a patient, and then act in a well-reasoned, logical, and thoughtful manner. In the end the evaluation of patient outcomes is critical.

Discipline. A disciplined thinker misses few details and follows a systematic approach in collecting information, making decisions, and taking action. *For example, Jessica asks Mr. Myers to rate his incisional pain on a scale of 0 to 10. Instead of asking only that question, Jessica conducts a systematic pain assessment and asks, "What makes the pain worse? Where does it hurt the most? Has anything helped to relieve the pain?"* Being disciplined and thorough in gathering information helps you identify problems more accurately and select the most appropriate nursing interventions. Disciplined thinking does not lessen your creativity but rather ensures that your decision making is systematic, accurate, and comprehensive.

Perseverance. A critical thinker is determined to find effective solutions to patient care problems. Perseverance is especially important when problems remain unresolved or when they recur. You must learn as much as possible about a particular problem and try various approaches to care. Perseverance also means that you continually look for additional resources until you find a successful approach. A critical thinker who perseveres is not satisfied with minimal effort but constantly tries to achieve high-quality patient care.

Creativity. Creativity arises from original thinking. This means you find solutions outside of the standard routines of care while still following standards of practice. Creativity helps you think of new options and approaches. A patient's clinical problems, living environment, and social support systems are just a few factors that can make the simplest nursing procedure more complicated. However, they also can be assets. *Jessica talks with Mr. and Mrs. Myers to learn whether Mr. Myers would be comfortable with his wife coaching him through relaxation exercises. The exercises are a way to help Mr. Myers relax more fully and enhance the effects of his pain medications. A coach reinforces the value of the exercise and is able to spend time so the patient does not rush the exercise. The two agree and allow Jessica to instruct them in relaxation exercise options.* Creativity means tailoring unique approaches to a patient's specific needs.

Curiosity. A critical thinker's favorite question is "Why?" As you care for a patient, you learn a lot of information. As you analyze this patient information, data patterns begin to emerge. Patterns may be unclear, new to you, or very unusual. Curiosity motivates you to question further, investigate the clinical situation in all possible directions, and obtain all the information needed to make a decision. For example, even if a patient who has had a recent myocardial infarction complains about chest pain, it is essential to be curious and consider other possible sources for the pain such as a pulled or strained muscle.

Integrity. Critical thinkers quickly and thoroughly question and test their own knowledge and beliefs against the knowledge and beliefs of others (Papathanasiou et al., 2014).

This shows a willingness to admit and understand inconsistencies between one's own beliefs and the beliefs of other colleagues. Your integrity as a nurse builds trust in you from your co-workers. Nurses face many dilemmas in everyday clinical practice (e.g., organizing care for multiple patients, choosing the correct size of a urinary catheter for a patient, being unable to respond to a patient's nurse call system while changing a different patient's wound dressing). Everyone occasionally makes a mistake or omits care activities. A person of integrity is honest and willing to admit to any mistakes or inconsistencies in his or her performance, behavior, and beliefs. A professional always tries to follow the highest standards of nursing practice.

Humility. Always know and admit the limits in your knowledge and skill. Critical thinkers admit their knowledge gaps and try to find the knowledge they need to make proper decisions. A nurse is often an expert in one area of clinical practice (e.g., general surgery) but a novice in another area (e.g., orthopedics). You put a patient's safety and welfare at risk if you cannot admit your inability to solve a practice problem. You must rethink a situation, seek additional knowledge (e.g., literature, clinical experts), and use the information to form an opinion and draw a conclusion.

Standards for Critical Thinking

The fifth element of the critical thinking model includes intellectual and professional standards (Kataoka-Yahiro and Saylor, 1994).

Intellectual Standards. Paul (1993) identified 14 intellectual standards (see Box 8.2) universal to critical thinking. An intellectual standard is a guideline or principle for rational thought. You apply these standards when you use the nursing process competency. When you consider a patient problem, you apply intellectual standards such as precision, accuracy, and consistency to ensure that all clinical decisions are sound. A thorough use of intellectual standards in clinical practice ensures that you avoid performing critical thinking haphazardly. When you reflect on your thinking, you can begin to recognize when you are unclear, imprecise, or inaccurate.

*Jessica administers a pain medication, and 45 minutes later Mr. Myers has his first ambulation session. After returning to bed, Mr. Myers reports fatigue and says to Jessica, "Will I ever get back to walking without feeling so worn out?" Jessica is a new nurse but knows not to make any unrealistic promises to the patient. She also knows that the surgery performed on Mr. Myers is usually highly successful. She is **precise** in her response: "Fatigue is normal after the first time you walk, but the mobility protocol will help you gain strength and endurance." Jessica raises a **relevant** question: "What bothers you the most about feeling fatigued right now?" Mr. Myers expresses concern that he might be unable to manage self-care at home. Jessica responds in a **significant** manner: "Remember we talked with the therapist about how to rearrange your home to make it easier to be mobile? Your wife is going to the mobility assistance class this afternoon."*

Professional Standards. Professional standards for critical thinking include ethical criteria for nursing judgments (e.g., advocacy, patient autonomy, and beneficence), evidence-based criteria used for assessment and evaluation (Box 8.3), and criteria for professional responsibility (Paul, 1993). Applying professional standards requires you to use critical thinking for the good of individuals or groups (Kataoka-Yahiro and Saylor, 1994). Standards of practice improve patient outcomes and thus maintain a high level of care.

Excellent nursing practice is a reflection of ethical standards (see Chapter 6). Patient care requires more than just the application of scientific knowledge and performing skills. Being able to focus on a patient's values and beliefs helps you make clinical decisions that are just, faithful to a patient's choices, and beneficial to a patient's well-being. Critical thinkers maintain a sense of self-awareness through conscious awareness of their beliefs, values, and feelings and the multiple perspectives that patients, family members, and professional peers bring to clinical situations.

Critical thinking also requires the use of evidence-based criteria for making clinical judgments. These criteria are often based on scientific research findings—practices that clinical experts developed or that institutions developed through performance improvement initiatives. For example, Dr. Barbara Braden applied evidence from her research to develop the Braden Scale, which is used in many practice settings to predict pressure injury risk (see Chapter 38). Other examples are the clinical practice guidelines from the Agency for Healthcare Research and Quality (AHRQ) and the performance measures from the National Quality Forum (NQF) (e.g., asthma assessment and urinary incontinence management in older adults). The NQF performance measures are used to assess the performance of a health care institution against recognized standards. An NQF-endorsed performance measure reflects rigorous scientific and evidence-based review, input from patients and their families, and the perspectives of people throughout the health care industry (NQF, 2016).

The standards of professional responsibility that a nurse tries to achieve are the standards cited in Nurse Practice Acts, institutional practice guidelines, and standards of practice of professional organizations (e.g., the ANA Scope and Standards of Practice [http://www.nursingworld.org/scopeandstandardsofpractice]). These standards raise the bar for the responsibilities and accountabilities that nurses assume in guaranteeing quality health care to the public.

Developing Critical Thinking Skills

Although you will need time to develop critical thinking skills in nursing, start now by actively engaging patients who are in your care. Apply the principles of the critical thinking model that have been presented in this chapter. Many factors in health care settings can pose barriers to critical thinking (Box 8.4). Rising patient acuity, decreasing length of stay, and conflicts in professional relationships are just some of the factors that can challenge even experienced nurses who are adept at critical thinking. Berkow et al. (2011) argue that critical thinking is essential to nursing practice in that nurses must learn to readily see a holistic picture of their patients' conditions to recognize emerging clinical patterns.

One practice that can help you become a critical thinker is reflective journaling. Reflective journaling involves keeping a written record of your clinical experiences in your own words in a personal journal. Returning to the journal after each clinical experience gives you the chance to record the perceptions you had during patient care and develop the ability to apply theory to practice. Using a journal also improves your observational and descriptive skills. Writing skills improve as you learn to clearly describe concepts applied in practice (e.g., suffering, resilience, or hope). A journal helps you increase your experiential learning during clinical experiences (Silvia et al., 2013). Ask and answer these questions in your daily journal entry:

- What did I learn from the experience?
- Did I respond appropriately in this situation? If not, how should I have responded?
- Were there consequences to my actions? What were they, and whom did they affect?
- Why did I react as I did? What was I thinking at that moment?
- How might I react differently in the future?
- Was I working from just instinct or from evidence-based practices?

BOX 8.3 EXAMPLES OF OUTCOMES AND CORRESPONDING EVALUATION CRITERIA

OUTCOME: PAIN RELIEF
Evaluation Criteria
Character of pain, including the following: onset (When did it start?), duration (How long does it last during an episode? How long has the pain been bothering the patient?), location (Which area of body is involved?), severity (How intense is the pain based on objective measurement using a visual analog scale?), type or description of pain (Is it aching, burning, cramping?), precipitating factors (What causes the pain to begin?), relieving factors (What helps to reduce or eliminate the pain?), other related symptoms (Does the patient experience nausea, dizziness, blurred vision?).

OUTCOME: IMPROVED PHYSICAL FUNCTION
Evaluation Criteria
Ability to perform activities of daily living (e.g., bathing, grooming, toileting) *or instrumental activities of daily living* (e.g., writing checks, buying groceries, cleaning home).

OUTCOME: PATIENT LEARNING
Evaluation Criteria
Patient recall of information (Can patient describe how to perform a skill or describe when to notify a health care provider about health changes?), *patient's ability to perform learned skill correctly* (Can patient demonstrate the skill learned?), *patient's success in adapting knowledge or skill in the home* (While the nurse visits the home, does the patient apply knowledge correctly?).

BOX 8.4   **EVIDENCE-BASED PRACTICE**

PICO Question: What are the effects on critical thinking and decision making among acute care nurses who work in stressful work environments versus nonstressful environments?

SUMMARY OF EVIDENCE
Regions of the brain including cortex, amygdala, and brainstem interact in both mental and physiological states (Critchley et al., 2013). Thus cognitive and emotional processes are affected by autonomic nervous system responses during stress. Stress is common among health care workers, resulting from workload demands, ineffective working relationships among nurses and with physicians, gaps in leadership support, and professional conflict (Hayward et al., 2016). Nurses must understand the relationship between the stress of caregiving and the cognitive and decision-making processes and empathy important to nursing practice (Critchley et al., 2013). Stress affects the accuracy of problem solving as well as the ability to speak fluently and clearly, to remember, and to manage emotions. Negative mood and stress affect what and how nurses communicate to one another (Pfaff, 2012). Stress increases the risk that inaccurate information will be conveyed. A high stress level can ultimately cause nurses to resign (Hayward et al., 2016).

APPLICATION TO NURSING PRACTICE
- Promote collaborative practice; engage with peers in discussions about ways to enhance working relationships (Hayward et al., 2016).
- Learn to recognize when you are feeling stressed; be mindful of your body reactions (e.g., tense muscles, impatience, fatigue) (Critchley et al., 2013).
- Take a time out. Do a quick relaxation exercise or find a place where colleagues are not bombarding you with questions.
- Participate in opportunities to make decisions about practice activities and issues.
- Attend a stress management class at work.

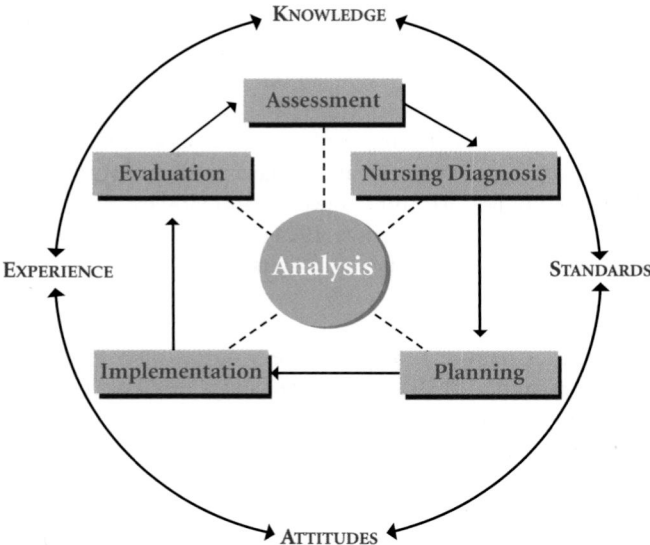

FIG 8.3 Synthesis of critical thinking with the nursing process competency.

interventions, evaluation measures) and represent relationships in a visual format. Current evidence shows the value of concept maps in improving the critical thinking of nursing students (Moattari et al., 2014). You can use a concept map to organize or link information about a patient in a unique and meaningful way. You will see examples of these maps throughout this text. Chapter 9 offers examples of concept maps with details about their development.

CRITICAL THINKING SYNTHESIS

Critical thinking is a reasoning process in which you reflect on and analyze your own thoughts, actions, and knowledge and use this information to make decisions about patient care. To be a good critical thinker, you must know patients and have the dedication and desire to grow intellectually. As a beginning nurse, you must learn the steps of the nursing process and combine them with the elements of critical thinking (Fig. 8.3). These two processes go hand in hand in making clinical decisions. This text provides a model for using critical thinking in nursing practice and emphasizes the components of critical thinking to help you better understand their relationship to the nursing process.

KEY POINTS

- Good clinical decision making requires you to investigate and reflect on all aspects of a problem and then to apply scientific and nursing knowledge to choose the best course of action.
- Critical thinking requires recognizing that a patient has a problem, analyzing information related to the problem (e.g., clinical and historical data about a patient), evaluating information (including assumptions and evidence), and drawing conclusions.

When you begin caring for a patient with multiple health problems, you may initially have difficulty sorting out the multiple problems and how they are interrelated. With knowledge and practice, you learn to assess for problems and develop a nursing diagnosis for each one. However, you will need complex critical thinking skills to see how the problems are related and to develop a holistic view of the patient.

Concept maps help you do this. A concept map is a visual representation of meaningful relationships between concepts (e.g., patient problems or nursing diagnoses and interventions), which then form propositions. Concept maps are visual road maps that highlight the meanings of these relationships (Hunter Revell, 2012). The maps encourage students to comprehensively observe their patients and organize and process the complex information (Moattari et al., 2014). The maps come in many different designs, but the primary purpose of a concept map is to gather relevant data about a patient (e.g., assessment data, nursing diagnoses, health needs, nursing

- When you care for patients on a given day, reflection means reviewing your practice experience so that you can describe, analyze, and evaluate it.
- You learn to know patients by engaging them, caring for them over time, hearing accounts of their experiences with illness, observing them, and coming to understand how they typically respond to treatments.
- The critical thinking model includes three levels of critical thinking in nursing that you develop with time and experience: basic, complex, and commitment.
- The scientific method is a systematic and ordered approach that uses reasoning to solve problems.
- You must use the intellectual standards of clinical practice to ensure that you do not perform critical thinking haphazardly.
- To become a critical thinker, you must be motivated to develop critical thinking and clinical judgment skills, as well as the 11 attitudes of the critical thinking model.
- In complex critical thinking, you learn to analyze and examine alternatives independently and take initiative to solve problems.
- The specific critical thinking competency in nursing is the nursing process, which involves clinical inference, diagnostic reasoning, and clinical decision making.
- Professional standards for critical thinking in nursing include ethical criteria for nursing judgments, evidence-based criteria used for assessment and evaluation, and criteria for professional responsibility.

▮ REFLECTIVE LEARNING

Apply the following questions to your own clinical and school experiences.

- Consider a conversation you have had with the family of one of your patients. Apply the REFLECT model to analyze the experience.
- Select three of the critical thinking attitudes in the critical thinking model and apply them in the assessment of your next patient. Discuss your results with a faculty member or fellow student.
- Keep a journal of your clinical experiences for a week. Record notes on examples where you used interpretation, inference, and evaluation.

▮ REVIEW QUESTIONS

1. A nurse asks a student nurse to irrigate a patient's feeding tube. The student has not performed the procedure other than in simulation laboratory. The student approaches her clinical instructor and asks a clarifying question about the amount of saline to use in the procedure. This is an example of which critical thinking attitude?
   1. Risk taking
   2. Confidence
   3. Consistency
   4. Curiosity

2. A nurse enters a heated discussion with a colleague over a work schedule change. The nurse has a patient who asked for a pain medication 20 minutes earlier. Another patient calls the nurse to request assistance. The nurse feels tension in her neck and around her eyes, and she takes a 10-second time out. This shows the nurse is aware of which of the following? (Select all that apply.)
   1. Stress affects accuracy of problem solving.
   2. During stressful events, it is easier to communicate concise information.
   3. The level of stress can affect the nurse's ability to speak clearly.
   4. Stress improves recall of information.
   5. Managing emotions is difficult during stress.

3. You can use the REFLECT model to improve learning after providing patient care. Place the steps of this model in the correct order.
   1. Think about your thoughts and actions at the time of the situation.
   2. Review the knowledge you gained from the experience.
   3. Review the facts of the situation.
   4. Set a schedule for completing your plan of action.
   5. Consider options for handling a similar situation in the future.
   6. Recall any feelings you had at the time of the situation.
   7. Create a plan for future situations.

4. One element of clinical decision making is knowing the patient. Which of the following activities affect a nurse's ability to know patients better? (Select all that apply.)
   1. Caring for similar groups of patients over time
   2. Reading the evidence-based practices appropriate to patients
   3. Learning how patients typically respond to a particular clinical situation
   4. Observing patients
   5. Engaging with patients experiencing illness

5. While preparing medications for a patient, the nurse compares the name of the medication on the label with the name of the medication on the physician's order. At the bedside, the nurse checks the patient's name against the order as well. The nurse is following which critical thinking attitude?
   1. Responsible
   2. Complete
   3. Accurate
   4. Broad

evolve

Additional Review Questions, as well as rationales for all Review Questions, can be found on the Evolve website.

1. 2; 1, 3, 5; 3. 3, 1, 6, 2, 5, 7, 4; 4. 1, 3, 4, 5; 5. 1.

REFERENCES

American Nurses Association (ANA): *Nursing's social policy statement: the essence of the profession*, Washington, DC, 2010, The Association.

Atalay A, et al: Deconditioning in chronic low back pain: might there be a relationship between fitness and magnetic resonance imaging findings?, *Rheumatol Int* 32(1):21–25, 2012.

Barksby J, et al: A new model of reflection for clinical practice, *Nurs Times* 111(34/35):21–23, 2015.

Benner P: *From novice to expert*, Menlo Park, CA, 1984, Addison Wesley.

Berkow S, et al: Assessing individual frontline nurse critical thinking, *J Nurs Admin* 41(4):168, 2011.

Critchley HD, et al: Interaction between cognition, emotion, and the autonomic nervous system, *Handb Clin Neurol* 117:597, 2013.

Delany C, Golding C: Teaching clinical reasoning by making thinking visible: an action research project with allied health clinical educators, *BMC Med Educ* 14:20, 2014. http://bmcmededuc.biomedcentral.com/articles/10.1186/1472-6920-14-20.

Facione N, Facione P: Externalizing the critical thinking in knowledge development and clinical judgment, *Nurs Outlook* 44:129, 1996.

Facione P: *Critical thinking: a statement of expert consensus for purposes of educational assessment and instruction. The Delphi report: research findings and recommendations prepared for the American Philosophical Association*, Washington, DC, 1990, ERIC. ERIC Doc No. ED 315-423.

Glaser E: *An experiment in the development of critical thinking*, New York, 1941, Bureau of Publications, Teachers College, Columbia University.

Hayward D, et al: A qualitative study of experienced nurses' voluntary turnover: learning from their perspectives, *J Clin Nurs* 25(9-10):1336–1345, 2016.

Hunter Revell SM: Concept maps and nursing theory: a pedagogical approach, *Nurse Educ* 37(3):131, 2012.

Kaddoura M: New graduate nurses' perceived definition of critical thinking during their first nursing experience, *Educ Res Q* 36(3):3, 2013.

Kataoka-Yahiro M, Saylor C: A critical thinking model for nursing judgment, *J Nurs Educ* 33(8):351, 1994.

Levett-Jones T, et al: Learning to think like a nurse, *HNE Handover for Nurses and Midwives* 3(1):15–20, 2010.

Mamede S, et al: Reflection as a strategy to foster medical students' acquisition of diagnostic competence, *Med Educ* 46(5):464–472, 2012.

Miller M, Malcolm N: Critical thinking in the nursing curriculum, *Nurs Health Care* 11:67, 1990.

Moattari M, et al: Clinical concept mapping: does it improve discipline-based critical thinking of nursing students?, *Iran J Nurs Midwifery Res* 19(1):70–76, 2014.

National Quality Forum (NQF): *Measuring performance*, 2016. http://www.qualityforum.org/Measuring_Performance/Measuring_Performance.aspx.

Papathanasiou IV, et al: Critical thinking: the development of an essential skill for nursing students, *Acta Inform Med* 22(4):283–286, 2014.

Paul R: The art of redesigning instruction. In Willsen J, Blinker AJA, editors: *Critical thinking: how to prepare students for a rapidly changing world*, Santa Rosa, CA, 1993, Foundation for Critical Thinking.

Pfaff M: Negative affect reduces team awareness: the effects of mood and stress on computer-mediated team communication, *Hum Factors* 54(4):5601, 2012.

Raterink G: Critical thinking: reported enhancers and barriers by nurses in long-term care: implications for staff development, *J Nurs Staff Dev* 27(3):136, 2011.

Rueskin M: *The importance of critical thinking skills in nursing*, 2015. http://www.rasmussen.edu/degrees/nursing/blog/understanding-why-nurses-need-critical-thinking-skills/.

Silvia B, et al: The reflective journal: a tool for enhancing experience based learning in nursing students in clinical practice, *J Nurs Educ Pract* 3(3):2013. http://www.sciedu.ca/journal/index.php/jnep/article/viewFile/1388/1067.

Tanner CA: Thinking like a nurse: a research-based model of clinical judgment in nursing, *J Nurs Educ* 45(6):204–211, 2006.

evolve MEDIA RESOURCES

http://evolve.elsevier.com/Potter/essentials
- Audio Glossary

- QSEN Activity and Review Questions Answers and Rationales

OBJECTIVES

- Describe each step of the nursing process.
- Explain the relationship between critical thinking and each step of the nursing process.
- Describe how developing relationships with patients improves the assessment process.
- Discuss approaches to data collection in nursing assessment.
- Differentiate between subjective and objective data.
- Describe the types of conclusions resulting from data analysis.
- Discuss how a nursing diagnosis guides nursing practice.
- Explain how a nurse uses defining characteristics and etiological factors to individualize a nursing diagnosis.

- Describe differences among health-promotion, problem-focused, and risk nursing diagnoses.
- Describe the criteria used in setting priorities.
- Discuss the differences between a goal and an expected outcome.
- Identify examples of nursing-sensitive outcomes.
- Develop a plan of care based on a nursing assessment.
- Discuss the process of selecting nursing interventions.
- Explain the relationship among goals of care, expected outcomes, and evaluative measures when evaluating and revising nursing care.

KEY TERMS

CASE STUDY *Mrs. Tillman*

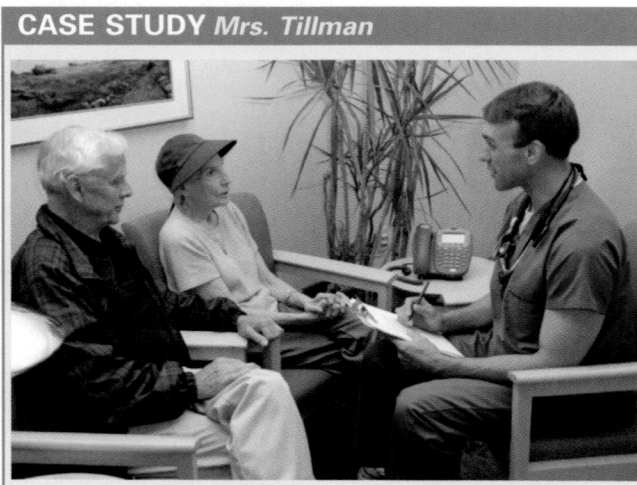

Rich is a nursing student who is assigned to care for Mrs. Jane Tillman, a 72-year-old woman with metastatic breast cancer. She recently retired after working for 40 years as a school teacher. She was treated with chemotherapy and radiation for her cancer. Recent magnetic resonance imaging (MRI) revealed that the cancer spread to her lungs. Rich sees Mrs. Tillman and her husband Greg during the patient's visit to the outpatient cancer care clinic. He observes the patient sighing deeply and looking down as she talks with her husband. Rich knows from reading the medical record that the couple was recently told about the prognosis of Mrs. Tillman's cancer. He also reviewed information about chemotherapy and radiation therapy to learn about the various complications and health problems these therapies can cause. He prepares to use the nursing process to determine Mrs. Tillman's current health status and plan nursing therapies. His first step will be a thorough assessment, which includes an interview with the patient and her husband and a health examination of the patient.

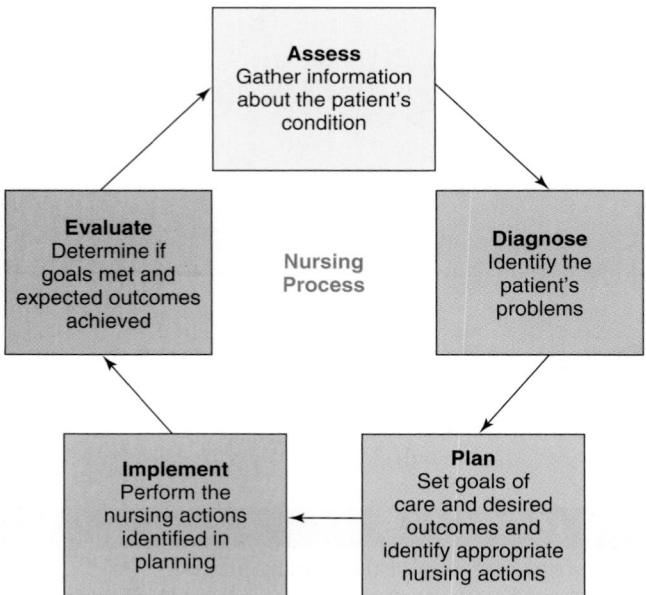

FIG 9.1 Five-step nursing process.

coordinated care based on respect of a patient's preferences, values, and needs" (QSEN Institute, 2014).

The nursing process is a standard of practice that, when followed correctly, protects nurses against legal problems related to nursing care. It allows you to provide timely, appropriate, and individualized care to your patients.

The five steps of the nursing process are assessment, nursing diagnosis, planning, implementation, and evaluation (Fig. 9.1). Initially you learn how to apply the process step-by-step. However, as you gain more clinical experience and care for more than one patient, you learn to move back and forth among the steps of the process. In so doing, you use critical thinking to make judgments about your patients' clinical situations, preferences, and needs. As a result, you individualize your approaches to care (Burman et al., 2013).

The nursing process is a form of scientific reasoning. Using the nursing process helps you to systematically organize and conduct your practice. You learn to make inferences from a patient's response to a health problem or generalize about a patient's functional state of health. Through the assessment process a pattern of a patient's health problems begins to form, and you gather more data to identify a patient's specific problems. Clearly defining your patient's problems provides a basis for planning and implementing relevant nursing interventions and evaluating the outcomes of care. Each time you meet a patient, you apply the nursing process, just as Rich will do throughout this chapter.

INTRODUCTION

The nursing process is a critical thinking process that professional nurses use to apply the best available evidence to caregiving and the promotion of human functions and responses to health and illness (American Nurses Association [ANA], 2010). It is the fundamental blueprint for patient care. Patient-centered care improves patient assessment, patient education, patient adherence to interventions, patient outcomes, and patient satisfaction (Bertakis and Azari, 2011; Burman et al., 2013). The Quality and Safety Education for Nurses (QSEN) Institute defines patient-centered care as the process of "recognizing a patient or designee as the source of control and full partner in providing compassionate and

ASSESSMENT

Assessment is the thorough systematic collection of patient data. The data reveal a patient's past and current health status, functional status, and past and present coping patterns (Carpenito-Moyet, 2017). Assessment requires you to apply critical thinking to have a clear picture of a patient's condition. Nursing assessment has two steps:

1. Collection and verification of data from a primary source (the patient) and secondary sources (e.g., family caregiver, friends, health professionals, medical record)
2. Interpretation and validation of data to ensure a complete database.

When you assess your patient, you collect and organize patient information into a detailed **database.** This database includes information about a patient's perceived needs, health problems, and responses to these problems. In addition, the data reveal related health issues, health practices, goals, values, and expectations about the health care delivery system.

To establish this database, you first apply knowledge that helps identify what to assess. For example, your knowledge of the physical, biological, and social sciences prepares you to ask relevant questions about a patient's health status and response to illness. You use this knowledge to collect relevant physical assessment data related to a patient's clinical condition.

Critical thinking attitudes and intellectual standards allow you to ask pertinent questions, clarify data, and gather further data for validation (see Chapter 8). Then you see the data patterns that reflect problems. Your experience allows you to recognize and anticipate what to assess. This experience leads you to ask the right questions. The answers to those questions will give you the most relevant and useful information.

An assessment database includes a patient's comprehensive **health history.** This history includes information about the patient's physical and developmental status, emotional health, social practices and resources, goals, values, lifestyle, and expectations about the health care system. The database also includes physical examination findings and a summary of results from laboratory and diagnostic testing. The knowledge you gather about a patient's medical diagnosis and treatment from the literature and medical record is also part of the database that leads you to fully understand your patient's condition and health care needs.

Critical thinking is a vital part of the assessment. As you gather data about a patient you synthesize relevant knowledge, recall prior clinical experiences, apply critical thinking standards and attitudes, and use professional standards of practice to direct your assessment in a meaningful and purposeful way (see Chapter 8).

Rich introduces himself to Mrs. and Mr. Tillman and explains his role in the clinic. "I am a nursing student assigned to you today. I want to take some time to talk with you and ask you a few questions to see how you're doing. Then I need to examine you by taking your blood pressure, listening to your lungs, and performing some other measures to get a good idea of your condition. I will share what I find with your doctor.

Then I want to work with you to put a plan together for your care. Is that okay with you?" Mrs. Tillman responds hesitantly, "Well, I guess so. I'm just not sure what to expect." Rich responds, "Well, let's start there. Tell me what you've been told by your doctor." Mrs. Tillman answers, "My breast cancer has spread; it's in my lungs." Rich notes, "I noticed you were sighing a minute ago. You look a bit down." Mrs. Tillman responds, "I'm so tired. I've gone through two different courses of chemotherapy and then radiation, and the cancer came back. Lately I just haven't had the energy to do what I like to do around the house. My husband and I are worn out." Mr. Tillman responds, "Yes, cancer is just exhausting." Rich replies, "It sounds as though this has been difficult for both of you. Mrs. Tillman, you say you're tired. Tell me how you spend a typical day. I want to learn about the symptoms you're having from your cancer and treatment."

As he listens, Rich reflects and considers the physical examination techniques that he will use later to explore each symptom. He wants to be sure that he collects all relevant assessment data without causing Mrs. Tillman unnecessary fatigue.

Rich has set the stage for an initial nursing assessment. He knows that a terminal disease can cause considerable grief and many physical changes. He wants to explore Mrs. Tillman's symptom experience and learn her feelings about her cancer so that he clarifies her emotional reaction to her cancer and prognosis. He applies critical thinking by asking relevant questions. The answers to those questions will help reveal a clear picture of how cancer affects Mrs. Tillman and her husband on a daily basis. His knowledge base also guides his assessment of Mrs. Tillman's symptoms because cancer and its treatment cause a variety of physical and psychological changes. Good communication skills and critical thinking prepare Rich to gather information for a complete, accurate, and relevant database (Palos, 2014).

Clinical experience contributes to assessment skills. For example, if you cared for a patient with heart disease in the past, you know the type of factors that precipitate or signal chest pain. As a result, you thoroughly assess the patient for conditions that typically precede a patient's chest pain. Your previous experience with abnormal assessment findings and your personal observation of assessments performed by skilled nurses increase your proficiency in assessing these conditions. You also learn to apply standards of practice and accepted standards of "normal" physical assessment data when assessing a patient. These standards help you collect the right kind of information and provide you with a standard against which to compare your findings. The use of attributes such as curiosity, perseverance, and risk taking ensures that your database is thorough and complete.

Data Collection

When you assess a patient, think critically about what to assess (i.e., the information you need to know to provide individualized, safe, effective care). Determine which questions or measurements are appropriate based on your clinical knowledge and experience. Once you start, select additional questions and measurements based on your patient's responses. When you meet a new patient, make a quick observational overview

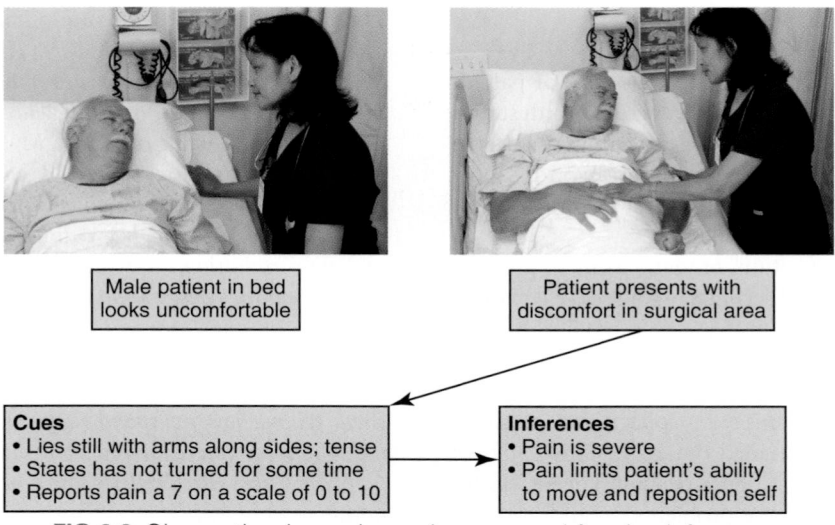

Male patient in bed looks uncomfortable

Patient presents with discomfort in surgical area

Cues
• Lies still with arms along sides; tense
• States has not turned for some time
• Reports pain a 7 on a scale of 0 to 10

Inferences
• Pain is severe
• Pain limits patient's ability to move and reposition self

FIG 9.2 Observational overview using cues and forming inferences.

TABLE 9.1	FOCUSED PATIENT ASSESSMENT		
FACTORS TO ASSESS	**QUESTIONS**	**PHYSICAL ASSESSMENT**	
Ability to perform routine tasks	Tell me how your fatigue affects your daily activities.	Observe how quickly patient responds to questions.	
	Describe what you did in a typical day before you had cancer. How has this changed?	Observe posture and body movements.	
Extent to which lack of energy affects her physically	Tell me how feeling tired affects your interest in social activities.	Observe facial and other nonverbal expressions.	
	Do you have more energy after you sleep or rest?		

or screening. For example, a community health nurse assesses a patient's neighborhood and community, a surgical nurse focuses on a patient's pain control and surgical wound healing, and a home care nurse focuses on a patient's environment, health care resources, and ways to cope with illness.

You learn to differentiate important data from the total data collected. A **cue** is information that you obtain through use of your senses. An **inference** is your judgment or interpretation of these cues (Fig. 9.2). For example, the cue of Mrs. Tillman expressing a sense of feeling tired and not having energy for daily routines leads Rich to infer a problem with activity. Anything a patient says and any behaviors you observe are important cues. You can miss cues when you conduct your initial overview. Thus you always need to be observant and interpret cues from the patient to guide your eventual assessment.

After the observational overview, you begin to focus on assessment cues and patterns of information that suggest problem areas. However, it is essential to conduct a comprehensive assessment when you can. An assessment moves from the general to the specific.

A comprehensive assessment can follow several approaches. One approach uses a structured database format, based on an agency's electronic health record (EHR). A second approach

to assessment is the problem-focused approach. For example, you might focus on a patient's report of feeling tired. Then you ask the patient follow-up questions to clarify and expand. For example, Rich asks Mrs. Tillman whether her lack of energy affects her ability to perform routine tasks and the extent to which it affects her physically (Table 9.1). Once he completes his initial assessment, he thoroughly analyzes the extent and nature of Mrs. Tillman's sense of feeling tired. This enables him to identify her health problem correctly so that he can develop a comprehensive treatment plan.

Whichever approach you use for assessment, you begin to cluster cues, make inferences, and identify emerging patterns and potential problems. To do this well, you must always try to stay a step ahead of the assessment. For example, if you suspect that a patient has a particular health problem (e.g., fatigue), you pose questions that deal with responses typically seen with fatigue.

Remember your inferences must always have supporting cues. Inferences lead you to more questions. When you ask a question or make an observation of a patient, the information branches to an additional series of questions or observations (Fig. 9.3). Failing to anticipate assessment questions results in an incomplete assessment, or you might fail to recognize cues and dismiss relevant problems. Knowing how

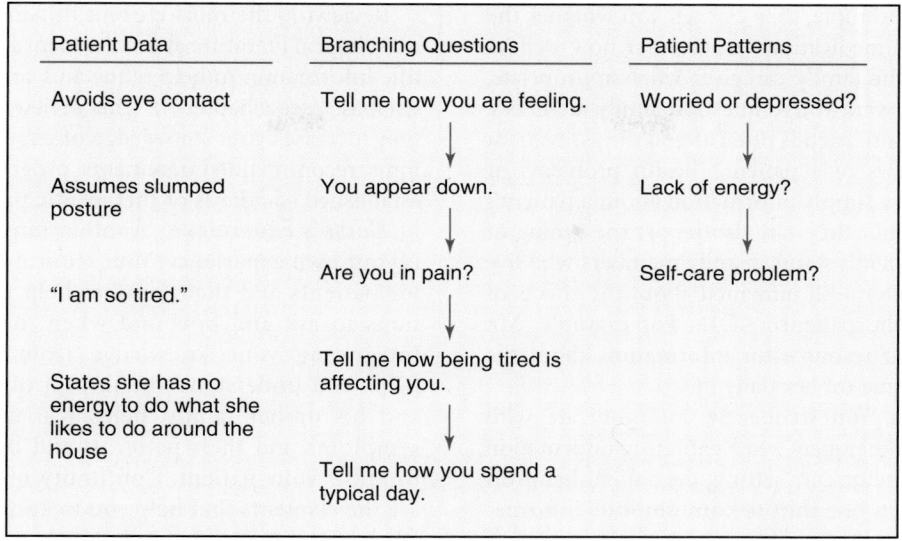

Patient Data	Branching Questions	Patient Patterns
Avoids eye contact	Tell me how you are feeling.	Worried or depressed?
Assumes slumped posture	You appear down.	Lack of energy?
"I am so tired."	Are you in pain?	Self-care problem?
States she has no energy to do what she likes to do around the house	Tell me how being tired is affecting you.	
	Tell me how you spend a typical day.	

FIG 9.3 Example of branching logic for selecting assessment questions.

to probe and frame questions is a skill that grows with experience. You learn which questions are relevant to a specific sign, symptom, or situation while at the same time making sure the assessment is complete.

Types of Data. There are two primary sources of data, subjective and objective. **Subjective data** are patients' verbal descriptions of their health problems, such as feelings of fear, anxiety, fatigue, physical discomfort, or mental stress. Patients are the only source of subjective data. For example, Mrs. Tillman's comments about being worn out and dealing with a difficult experience are subjective findings. Only patients provide subjective data.

Objective data are observations or measurements of a patient's health status. Inspection of the condition of a wound or observation of a patient's posture and gait are examples of objective data. Base your measurements of objective data on an accepted standard, such as the Fahrenheit or Celsius measure on a thermometer, centimeters on a measuring tape, or known characteristics of behaviors. For example, after listening to Mrs. Tillman describe her fatigue and its effects, Rich assesses her ability to walk a short distance to gather more data about how fatigue impacts her physical activity, such as change in heart rate or distance walked.

Sources of Data. You obtain data from a variety of sources. When you collect data, you apply critical thinking intellectual standards (e.g., clear, precise, and consistent) to correctly interpret your findings. Each data source provides information about the patient's level of wellness, risk factors, health practices and goals, and patterns of health and illness.

Patient. A patient is usually your best source of information. A patient who is conscious, alert, and able to answer questions appropriately provides the most accurate information about health care needs, lifestyle patterns, present and past illnesses, perception of symptoms, and changes in activities of daily living (ADLs).

Always consider the setting for your assessment. A patient experiencing acute pain in an emergency department will not offer the same depth of information as one who comes to an outpatient clinic for a routine checkup. When you communicate with your patient, always be attentive and show a caring presence with patients (see Chapter 20). Patients are more likely to fully reveal the nature of their health care problems when you show interest and focus solely on the patient and his or her concerns (Palos, 2014).

Know your patient's health literacy level. Health literacy includes specific cognitive and social skills that help determine the motivation and ability of individuals to gain access, understand, and use information in ways to promote and maintain good health (see Chapter 12). A patient with limited health literacy has difficulty obtaining, processing, and understanding basic health information (Agency for Healthcare Research and Quality [AHRQ], 2016). Because of limited health literacy your patient may not fully understand some of your assessment questions, especially if your questions are clinical and use a lot of medical terminology. If English is not the patient's first language or the patient cannot speak English, he or she will be unable to understand you or your questions. As a result, the risk of obtaining incomplete, inaccurate assessment data increases.

Family and Significant Others. Family members and significant others are the primary sources of information for infants, children, critically ill adults, patients with decreased mental capacity, and patients who are unconscious or have reduced cognitive function. In cases of severe illness or emergencies, families are often the only available sources of information for nurses and other health care providers. The family caregiver and significant others are also good secondary sources of information for patients who are able to communicate. These additional sources confirm information that the patient provides. For example, they can tell you whether the patient regularly takes medications at home or how well he or she eats). Include the family caregiver when appropriate. The patient might not want you to question family members. However, spouses or close friends often attend the assessment and provide their views of a patient's health problems or needs. Not only do they supply information about a patient's current health status, but they can also report the timing of any changes in the patient's status. Family members who live with the patient are often well informed about the effects of health problems on the patient's ADLs. For example, Mr. Tillman is an excellent resource for information about the effect of his wife's fatigue on her daily life.

Health Care Team. You frequently communicate with other health care team members when gathering information about patients. In the acute care setting, the patient hand-off is the way for nurses on one shift to communicate information to nurses or other health care providers on oncoming shifts (see Chapter 10). The hand-off is an interactive process of passing patient-specific information from one caregiver to another for the purpose of ensuring patient-centered care and safety (Chaboyer et al., 2010; Boykins, 2014). Communicating effectively during the hand-off provides an opportunity for you to collect initial information about patients assigned to your care including their health care needs and concerns and to clarify any medications or care procedures (Jahne, 2015). When nurses and other health care providers consult with one another about a patient's condition, all of them typically contribute information about the patient. This information includes the patient's adjustment to the health care environment, the patient's reactions to treatment, the results of diagnostic procedures or therapies, and the patient's responses to visitors. Every member of the health care team is a source of information about the patient.

Medical Records. The medical record is a source of a patient's medical history, laboratory and diagnostic test results, and current physical findings and a health care provider's treatment plan. The records contain baseline and ongoing information about a patient's response to illness and progress to date. The Health Insurance Portability and Accountability Act (HIPAA) of 1996, which became effective in 2003, has a privacy rule to set standards for the protection of health information (U.S. Department of Health and Human Services [USDHHS], 2017). Information in a patient's record is confidential. Each health care agency has policies governing how health care providers can share information. A nurse can review a patient's medical record for assessment data but needs to know the agency policies governing how to share the information with other staff.

Other Records and the Scientific Literature. Educational, military, and employment records often contain pertinent health care information (e.g., immunizations or prior illnesses). If a patient received treatment at a community clinic or another hospital, the nurse must obtain written permission from the patient or guardian before seeing the records. HIPAA regulations dictate specifically how to obtain an information release (USDHHS, 2017). Consult agency policies.

Reviewing the most current nursing, medical, and pharmacological literature about a patient's illness provides scientific information to help refine and complete the assessment database (see Chapter 7). This review of scientific information increases your knowledge of expected signs and symptoms, recommended treatments, prognosis of the illness, and established standards of therapeutic practice.

Nurse's Experience. Another important source of data is your own experience. Your clinical experiences in caring for patients and their families help you choose the questions to ask and how and when to ask these questions. Integrating your knowledge from clinical experiences helps you understand the impact of disease on a patient and his or her family, helps you understand signs and symptoms and their patterns, and builds on your ability to know your patient. Continuity of care and experience are the elements that help you to know your patient better. When patient care is fragmented, your knowledge of the patient declines, and patient-centered care is compromised (Zolnierek, 2014).

Methods of Data Collection. As a nurse, you use the patient interview as the tool to assess a patient's health history. Once you have collected data, you proceed to a physical examination.

Patient-Centered Interview. The first step in establishing a patient-centered database is to collect subjective information by interviewing a patient. An interview is an organized conversation with a patient (see Chapter 11). The interview focuses on a patient's health history and obtaining information about the current illness (Ball et al., 2015). During the initial interview you have the opportunity to:

1. Introduce yourself to the patient, explain your role, and explain the roles of others who will provide care.
2. Establish a caring patient-centered relationship.
3. Explain how you will conduct the interview (for example, first you will ask about the patient's current concerns and then collecting other information).
4. Gain insight about the patient's concerns and worries.
5. Determine the patient's goals and expectations of the health care delivery system.
6. Obtain cues to identify topics requiring further investigation and data collection.

Later interviews allow you to further assess a patient's situation and focus on specific problem areas. The interview also helps patients explain their own interpretations and understandings of their conditions. Therefore you and the patient are partners during the interview; you do not control it.

Always prepare for the interview. Collect all available information about the patient and create a comfortable environment for the interview. For example, review the information you learn during the hand-off report, and plan to interview the patient during rounds and before you begin to deliver patient care. In a hospital, you often need to relieve a patient's symptoms before the patient can talk comfortably with you. In a patient's home, choose a location that is as quiet and private as possible.

The interview consists of three phases: orientation, working, and termination.

Orientation Phase Including Setting an Agenda. During the orientation phase you establish trust and confidence with a patient. Begin by introducing yourself and your position and explaining the purpose of the interview and why you are collecting data. Assure the patient that all the information and protected health information will remain confidential and be used only by health care professionals who provide the patient's care (see Chapter 10). HIPAA regulations require patients to sign an authorization before you collect personal health data (USDHHS, 2017). The patient usually signs this form in the admitting or screening areas before you meet the patient.

One important goal of the initial interview is to explain to the patient the reason you want to understand the patient's needs. *In their initial discussion Rich explains to Mrs. Tillman that he wants to develop a plan of care, and to do this, he wants to understand more about the effects of her cancer during a typical day. Rich also tells Mrs. Tillman that he wants to learn more about her symptoms.*

Another goal of the interview is to begin developing a relationship that enables the patient to become an active partner in care decisions. As the orientation phase proceeds, the patient usually becomes more comfortable in speaking with you.

You first gather demographic data (such as date of birth, gender, address, and family members' names and addresses) as specified by the institution. Because this information is the least personal topic, it helps initiate the therapeutic relationship and eases the transition into the working phase of the interview.

Working Phase—Collecting Assessment or Nursing Health History. Start an assessment or nursing health history with open-ended questions rather than yes/no questions. Open-ended questions encourage patients to tell their story in detail. During the working phase you gather information about the patient's health status. Stay focused, orderly, and unhurried. Obtain the patient's health history using a variety of communication techniques to promote a clear interaction (see Chapter 11) and construct a thorough database (Box 9.1). Techniques you can use include active listening, paraphrasing, and summarizing.

Rich begins the working phase of his interview by focusing on Mrs. Tillman's report of "feeling worn out." He addresses her concerns, immediately makes her a partner in the interview, and then focuses on details that will reveal the effect her cancer is having on her life.

> *Rich:* "You say you're worn out. Can you tell me how you spend a typical day?"
>
> *Mrs. Tillman:* "When I first wake up, I actually feel pretty good. I'm able to get through breakfast and most of my bath before I start to feel tired."
>
> *Rich:* "Uh-huh, go on." (Active listening and probing)
>
> *Mrs. Tillman:* "I used to do my errands midmorning, but I seem to lose energy and feel worn out before I can run my errands. My husband decided to retire this year. He helps me a lot."

> **BOX 9.1   BASIC COMPONENTS FOR A NURSING HEALTH HISTORY**
>
> - *Biographical information:* Age, address, occupation and working status, marital status, family members, source of health care, and insurance.
> - *Reasons for seeking health care:* Goals of care, expectation of the services and care delivered, and expectations of the health care team and system.
> - *Present illness or health concern:* Onset, symptoms, nature of symptoms (e.g., sudden or gradual), duration, precipitating factors, relief measures, and weight loss or gain.
> - *Health history:* Prior illnesses throughout development, injuries, and hospitalizations; surgeries; blood transfusions; allergies; immunizations; habits (e.g., smoking, caffeine intake, alcohol intake, and alcohol or drug abuse); prescribed and self-prescribed medications; over-the-counter medications; work habits; relaxation activities; and sleep, exercise, and eating or nutritional patterns.
> - *Family history:* Health status of immediate family and living relatives; cause of death of relatives; and risk factor analyses for cancer, heart disease, diabetes mellitus, kidney disease, hypertension, and mental disorders.
> - *Environmental history:* Hazards, pollutants, and physical safety.
> - *Psychosocial and cultural history:* Primary language, cultural group, community resources, mood, attention span, and developmental stage.
> - *Review of systems:* Head-to-toe review of all major body systems and patient's knowledge of and compliance with health care (e.g., frequency of breast or testicular self-examination or last visual acuity examination). (Another option for an approach is to use *functional health patterns* as the method for organizing assessment data.)

> *Rich:* "You say you lose energy and feel worn out. Tell me how you feel." (Paraphrase and open-ended question)
>
> *Mrs. Tillman:* "I just feel this sensation that I can't do any more. I'm too weak to move. I often need a nap midmorning. Isn't that ridiculous? The cancer has just weakened me so much."
>
> *Rich:* "How you feel is not ridiculous, Mrs. Tillman. Please tell me how you feel after you nap." (Open-ended question)

Rich explores how Mrs. Tillman's cancer physically affects her. He also gathers information from Mr. Tillman. All this information guides him in identifying Mrs. Tillman's health problems and choosing appropriate nursing therapies.

The first interview with a patient is often the longest. Ongoing interviews occur each time you interact with your patient. They do not need to be as extensive. The ongoing interviews are just as important, however, because they update the patient's status and focus on changes in previously identified problems and new problems.

Termination Phase—Ending the Interview. As in the other phases of the interview, the termination phase requires skill on the part of the interviewer. Give your patient a clue that the interview is coming to an end. For example, you might say, "There are just two more questions" or "We'll be finished in 5 to 6 minutes." This helps a patient maintain direct attention without being distracted by wondering when the interview will end. This approach also gives the patient a chance to ask questions. When ending the interview, summarize the important points and ask your patient if the summary is accurate. End the interview in a friendly manner, telling the patient when you will return to provide care. *For example, Rich states, "Thanks, Mrs. Tillman. You've given me a clear picture of your health and how you've been affected. It's important for you to understand how we expect the cancer will affect you and how we can help you manage your symptoms. Is that OK? I hope to develop a plan of care that will manage your difficulty breathing and your fatigue. Do you have any questions?"*

Interview Techniques. The way you conduct an interview is just as important as the questions you ask. To ensure a successful interview, select a comfortable environment, provide for the patient's comfort, and use effective communication techniques (see Chapter 11). During the interview direct the flow of conversation so that you obtain accurate and complete information and the patient can contribute freely. Ideally you want patients to tell their stories about their health problems so that you can obtain as many details as possible.

Some interviews are focused, whereas others are comprehensive. Listen to the patient and consider the information shared. This helps you direct a patient to give more detail or to discuss a topic that probably reveals a possible problem. Because a patient's report includes subjective information, validate data from the interview later with objective data. *For example, Mrs. Tillman reports that she often feels too weak to move. Rich later measures her muscle strength and tolerance to walking.*

Remember that patients also obtain information during interviews. You may be the first health care provider the patient has encountered. If you establish a positive nurse-patient relationship, the patient will feel comfortable asking you questions about planned treatments, diagnostic procedures, and need for resources. Patients need this information to make decisions about their health care.

A good interview environment is free of distractions, unnecessary noise, and interruptions. A patient is more likely to be candid if an interview is private (i.e., out of earshot of other patients, visitors, and staff). Timing is important in avoiding interruptions. If possible, set aside a 15- to 30-minute period when no other activities are planned. Another option in a busy hospital setting is to set aside two 15-minute periods during your shift. Help the patient feel relaxed and unhurried. Before you begin the interview, be sure that the patient is comfortable. Comfort factors include toileting, providing adequate light and warmth, and positioning. Sit facing the patient to encourage eye contact. During the interview observe your patient for signs of discomfort or fatigue.

When the interview includes a health history, encourage the patient to use his or her own words to describe the health problem and its likely cause. Patients are usually the best source of their health history.

Begin by asking the patient a question to elicit his or her story. For example, say, "Tell me why you came to the hospital today" or "Tell me about the problems you're having." Open-ended questions prompt patients to describe a situation in more than one or two words. This technique leads to a discussion in which patients actively describe their health status. Open-ended questions strengthen the nurse-patient relationship because they show that you want to invest time in hearing the patient's thoughts. Encourage the patient to tell the story all the way through.

Reinforce your interest by using good eye contact, listening skills, and back-channeling. Back-channeling is the practice of giving positive comments such as "all right," "go on," or "uh-huh" to the speaker. These indicate that you have heard what the patient said and are interested in hearing the full story.

After patients tell their story, use a problem-seeking interview technique. This approach takes the information provided in the patient's story and more fully describes and identifies specific problem areas. For example, focus on the symptoms that the patient identifies and ask closed-ended questions that limit his or her answers to one or two words such as "yes" or "no" or a number or frequency of a symptom. For example, ask, "How often do you feel really tired or fatigued?" or "After taking a nap, do you feel more rested?" As closed-ended questions reveal more information, you ask the patient to discuss historical information in more detail.

A good interviewer leaves with a complete story that contains enough information to understand the patient's perceptions of his or her health status and the information needed to help identify nursing diagnoses and/or collaborative health problems. Always clarify or validate any information that is unclear.

Observation. Observation is a powerful assessment tool. During an interview and physical examination closely observe a patient's verbal and nonverbal behaviors. This information is important and adds depth to the objective database. Determine whether data obtained by observation match the patient's words. For example, if a patient expresses no concern about an upcoming diagnostic test but appears anxious and irritable, verbal and nonverbal data conflict. Your observations lead you to persist in gathering the information needed to resolve conflicting data and form accurate conclusions about the patient's condition.

Observation also provides information about a patient's level of function—the physical, developmental, psychological, and social aspects of everyday life. Observing the patient's level of function is different from the observation you perform during the interview. At this point you observe the patient's ability to perform tasks such as self-feeding, hygiene, or making a decision.

Physical Examination. A physical examination allows the nurse to examine the patient's body to determine his or her state of health. It involves use of the techniques of inspection, palpation, percussion, auscultation, and smell.

A complete examination includes a patient's height, weight, vital signs (see Chapter 15), general appearance and behavior, and a head-to-toe examination of all body systems (see Chapter 16).

Diagnostic and Laboratory Data. Diagnostic and laboratory test results identify or confirm conditions suspected or identified during the nursing health history and physical examination. For example, during the health history the patient reports having had a bad cold for 6 days and currently has a productive cough with dark yellow sputum and mild shortness of breath.

During a physical examination you notice an elevated temperature, increased respirations, and decreased breath sounds in the right lower lobe. You review the results of a complete blood count (CBC) and note that the white blood cell count is elevated, indicating an infection. In addition, the radiologist's report of a chest x-ray examination shows the presence of a right lower lobe infiltrate. Such findings in combination suggest that the patient has the medical diagnosis of pneumonia and the associated nursing diagnosis of *Impaired Gas Exchange.* When a patient collects and monitors laboratory data at home such as with routine blood glucose monitoring for diabetes, ask the patient about the routine results to determine the patient's response to illness and the effects of treatment measures. Compare laboratory data with the established norms for a particular test, age-group, and gender.

Cultural Considerations in Assessment

Good assessment techniques are important to patient-centered care, especially when you are caring for patients from cultural backgrounds different from your own (Box 9.2). Make a conscious effort to understand your patient's culture, including values, beliefs, lifestyle practices, language, and ways of relating to friends and family. This information will assist you in providing quality care. You must act within different value systems and with respect and understanding for the patient without imposing your own attitudes and beliefs (see Chapter 21). Culture affects the way individuals express their feelings, both verbally and nonverbally. When you learn the ways people of different cultures communicate, you will likely perform a better assessment and gather better information from these patients (Darnell and Hickson, 2015). You show respect for your patient when you apply sensitive communication techniques. Speaking at eye level, maintaining a proper distance, and listening carefully all demonstrate respect for your patient.

Interpreting and Validating Assessment Data

Assessment requires you to use critical thinking to continuously interpret information and make accurate judgments. You want to identify any abnormal findings, recognize that further observations are needed to clarify information, and begin to identify the patient's problems. Once you have collected your data, validate the data you obtained. This helps you to more accurately analyze and interpret a patient's clinical picture. **Validation** of assessment data is the comparison

---

⊕ BOX 9.2 PATIENT-CENTERED CARE

The nursing process is a good method for implementing patient-centered care. To be effective, it is important during the assessment phase to ask a patient and family members useful questions that explore the patient's illness or health care problem in the context of the patient's culture (Ball et al., 2015). Involvement of families encourages sharing of information and planning of care to improve the well-being of the patient (Flagg, 2015).

IMPLICATIONS FOR PRACTICE
- When talking about a patient's illness try to understand it "through the patient's eyes":
  - What do you think is wrong with you?
  - What do you call your problem?
  - What worries you most about your illness?
  - What types of treatments or health practices do you use?
- When talking about treatments:
  - What should we do to eliminate your problem?
  - Which types of treatments do you use?
  - What benefit do you expect from the treatment?
- When there is a cross-cultural difference between you and your patient, ask yourself these questions (Suhonen et al., 2011; Darnell and Hickson, 2015):
  - What is unique to the patient's culture and its impact on the treatment plan?
  - Are there risk factors for cultural misunderstanding? When there is a risk, try to reduce or correct it.
  - Are there resources within the agency and community to help you to provide culturally competent care to the patient and family?

---

of data with another source to confirm data accuracy. *For example, Rich observes Mrs. Tillman crying and logically infers that the crying is related to her cancer diagnosis. Making such an initial inference is not wrong, but problems can result if you do not validate the inference with the patient. Rich should ask, "I notice that you've been crying. Can you tell me about it?" By doing so, Rich discovers the real reason for Mrs. Tillman's crying.*

You must also ask your patient to validate the information you gathered during the interview and health history. For example, when a patient describes joint pain, ask the patient to rate the pain on a scale of 0 to 10, ask what precipitates the pain, and ask what measures the patient uses to reduce the pain.

Validate findings from physical examination and observation of patient behavior by comparing data in the medical record and consulting with other health team members or family caregivers. Validation often leads you to gather more assessment data and occasionally to reassess previously covered areas to clarify vague or ambiguous data. The nurse continually analyzes and thinks about the patient's database to fully understand the patient's problems, measure their extent, and discover possible relationships between them.

Rich gathers initial data about Mrs. Tillman's physical health after focusing on her fatigue and its effects on her ability to perform daily activities. He applies critical thinking in his assessment by considering the typical effects of cancer. He also considers the effects of chemotherapy and other therapies Mrs. Tillman has received.

The patient has reported taking frequent naps and feeling a lack of energy for performing routine chores or engaging in any social activities. Rich also learns a great deal about Mrs. Tillman's feelings about having advanced-stage cancer.

Rich uses intellectual standards, including precision (specific feelings about prognosis), consistency, accuracy (using a self-report scale to measure the patient's perceptions of her quality of life), and completeness (probing to learn how her feelings affect her relationship with her husband).

Rich learns that Mrs. Tillman worries about her husband. She tells Rich, "He means so much to me. The doctor has told me what to expect. I know this is going to be very hard for him." Rich could make several inferences from this comment, but he applies the critical thinking attitude of discipline and validates his inferences, "You sound worried about your husband. Please describe what's bothering you." Mrs. Tillman confirms Rich's assessment: "I'm worried about Greg because he tries so hard to help me. I'm worried that he'll get worn out too."

Data Documentation and Communication

Communicating your assessment findings, either verbally or through documentation, is the last step of a complete assessment. Timely, thorough, and accurate communication of facts is vital to ensuring continuity and quality patient care. If you fail to report or record an assessment finding or problem interpretation, it is lost and unavailable to anyone else caring for the patient (see Chapter 10). If you do not report specific information, you leave another health care team member uninformed and often with only general impressions. Observing, reporting, and recording of a patient's status are legal and professional responsibilities. The Nurse Practice Acts in all states and the American Nurses Association (ANA) policy statement (2010) require accurate data collection and recording as independent functions essential to the role of a professional nurse.

NURSING DIAGNOSIS

After you review and validate the data collected in a patient assessment, the next step of the nursing process is to form diagnostic conclusions that identify a patient's problems and the level of care required. When a nurse forms an accurate diagnostic conclusion, nursing therapies will be appropriate and effective. A diagnostic conclusion takes one of two forms: a nursing diagnosis or a collaborative problem.

A nursing diagnosis is a clinical judgment concerning a human response to health conditions and/or life processes or vulnerability for that response by an individual, family, or community that a nurse is licensed and competent to treat (Herdman and Kamitsuru, 2014b). A nursing diagnosis provides the basis for the selection of nursing interventions to achieve outcomes for which the nurse is accountable (Herdman and Kamitsuru, 2014b).

Never confuse a medical diagnosis with a nursing diagnosis. A medical diagnosis is the identification of a disease condition based on an evaluation of physical signs, symptoms, history, and diagnostic tests and procedures. A medical diagnosis stays constant as long as the disease condition remains. Health care providers are licensed to treat diseases or pathological processes described in medical diagnostic statements. An advanced practice nurse can also treat medical diagnoses but does not perform surgery.

In contrast, a patient's responses to cancer such as symptoms of pain and nausea and insufficient knowledge about treatment are nursing diagnoses that nurses manage. What makes a nursing diagnostic process unique is having patients involved in the process when possible.

A collaborative problem is an actual or potential physiological complication that nurses monitor to detect the onset of changes in a patient's status (Carpenito-Moyet, 2017). When collaborative problems develop, nurses intervene in cooperation with social workers, dietitians, or personnel from other health care disciplines.

The Canadian Interprofessional Health Collaborative (2010) defines interprofessional collaboration as a partnership between a team of health care providers (such as nurses, health care providers, therapists, and dietitians) and a patient in a participatory collaborative and coordinated approach for shared decision making about the patient's health care issues. Nurses manage collaborative problems such as hemorrhage or infection using both physician-prescribed and nursing-prescribed interventions. For example, a patient who has a surgical wound is at risk for developing an infection. Thus a physician or advanced practice nurse prescribes antibiotics. The nurse monitors the patient for signs of infection, provides meticulous wound care, and administers the prescribed antibiotics.

Nurses use scientific and nursing knowledge and their experience to analyze and interpret assessment data to identify the patient's unique nursing diagnoses and collaborative problems.

Critical Thinking and the Nursing Diagnostic Process

The nursing diagnostic process requires you to use critical thinking. This involves logically analyzing and interpreting assessment data about a patient to form a clinical judgment, in this case a nursing diagnosis. The nursing diagnostic process flows from the assessment process and includes data clustering, interpreting and analyzing, identifying patient needs, and formulating the nursing diagnosis or collaborative problem (Fig. 9.4).

When you analyze assessment data accurately, you identify patients' problems and make clinical decisions about their care. You begin analysis and interpretation of assessment data by organizing all your data into meaningful and usable data clusters. A data cluster is a set of signs or symptoms gathered during assessment that you group together in a logical way. During clustering, a cue or an individual sign, symptom, or finding stands out more than others. Clustering also requires

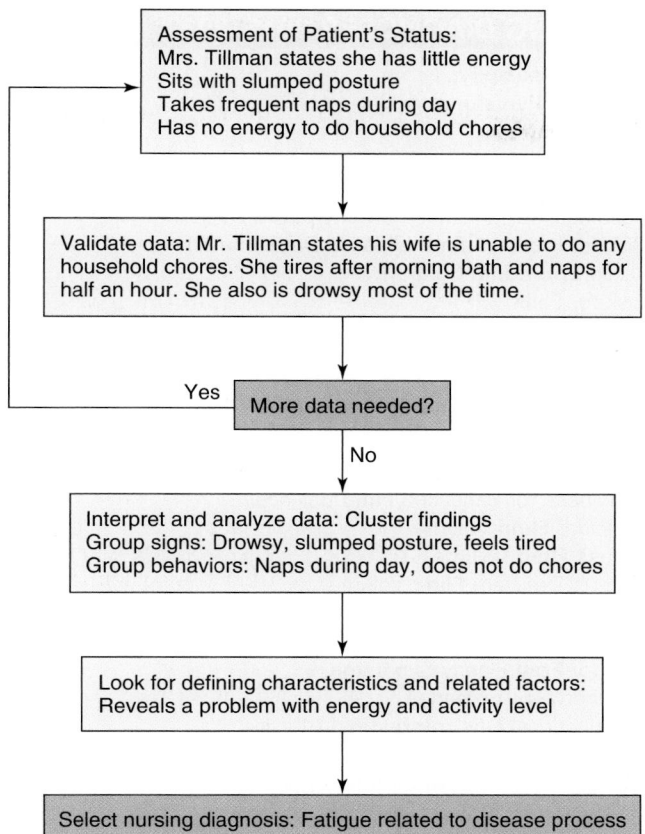

Assessment of Patient's Status:
Mrs. Tillman states she has little energy
Sits with slumped posture
Takes frequent naps during day
Has no energy to do household chores

Validate data: Mr. Tillman states his wife is unable to do any household chores. She tires after morning bath and naps for half an hour. She also is drowsy most of the time.

Yes

More data needed?

No

Interpret and analyze data: Cluster findings
Group signs: Drowsy, slumped posture, feels tired
Group behaviors: Naps during day, does not do chores

Look for defining characteristics and related factors: Reveals a problem with energy and activity level

Select nursing diagnosis: Fatigue related to disease process

FIG 9.4 Nursing diagnostic process for Mrs. Tillman.

your knowledge of the signs and symptoms and how they support the nursing diagnoses (Herdman and Kamitsuru, 2014a). For example, Mrs. Tillman talks about feeling fatigued and "worn out," taking frequent naps, and being unable to perform usual activities such as preparing meals. These cues show a pattern.

Data analysis and interpretation involve recognizing patterns or trends in the clustered data, comparing them with standards, and coming to a reasoned conclusion about the patient's response to a health problem. Rich compares Mrs. Tillman's signs and symptoms with normal standards for a woman her age. The typical woman might feel rested, sleeping through the night, and being able to perform daily routines. Mrs. Tillman's clinical picture suggests that her cancer is producing a pattern of fatigue that affects her activity level.

You use reasoning and judgment to identify the assessment data that explains a patient's health status. Patients often present multiple cues, suggesting more than one type of health problem or need. You may need to gather additional data to clarify your interpretation. *For example, Mrs. Tillman tells Rich that she has many unanswered questions, even though her doctor has talked about the way her cancer will progress. She says, "I wish I could just not wake up one morning." Rich infers that Mrs. Tillman dreads the ways cancer will affect her. He seeks further information: "Let's talk about what your doctor said about the cancer." "He says that further chemotherapy*

likely will not be effective. I can expect to have trouble breathing and possibly pain, but he said he will be sure to give me what I need," Mrs. Tillman says.

Rich clarifies, "You sound a bit uncertain. Are you concerned that you'll suffer?"

Mrs. Tillman begins to cry. "Yes, oh yes, that is my greatest fear. I really don't know what to expect." Rich further clarifies, "Has anyone talked to you about palliative care?" Mrs. Tillman responds, "No. What does that mean?"

In seeking data patterns, Rich decides that Mrs. Tillman is having difficulty accepting her impending death and has insufficient understanding of her health care options. These problems intensify her pattern of fatigue.

Formulating the Nursing Diagnosis

After a nurse identifies the patterns of data that reveal a patient's health problems, the nurse must identify these problems in a way that will be clear to all health care providers. NANDA International (NANDA-I) has developed a model for organizing nursing diagnoses for documentation, auditing, and communication purposes. Researchers continually develop new diagnoses and add them to the NANDA-I listing (Box 9.3). The use of standard formal nursing diagnoses serves the following purposes (Gallagher-Lepak, 2014):

- Provides a precise definition that gives all members of the health care team a common language for understanding patient needs
- Allows nurses to communicate what they do among themselves, with other health care professionals, and with the public
- Distinguishes the nurse's role from that of physicians and other health care providers
- Helps nurses focus on the scope of nursing practice
- Fosters the development of knowledge and nursing science

When you finished assessing your patient, review all assessment data and compare the clusters and patterns of data with the clinical criteria that supports a nursing diagnosis. Defining characteristics are observable cues and inferences that cluster as manifestations of a problem-focused or health promotion diagnosis or syndrome. These are the clinical criteria or assessment findings that support an actual nursing diagnosis (Gallagher-Lepak, 2014). NANDA-I–approved nursing diagnoses have identified sets of defining characteristics that support identification of each nursing diagnosis (Herdman and Kamitsuru, 2014b). As you gain clinical experience you become familiar with the defining characteristics for the more common nursing diagnoses in your practice. This helps you identify nursing diagnoses. Box 9.4 shows an example of an approved nursing diagnosis and its associated defining characteristics and related factors. As you analyze clusters of data you begin to consider possible nursing diagnoses that may apply to your patient. *For example, Rich reviews findings pertaining to Mrs. Tillman, who reported feeling fatigue. The defining characteristics of tiredness and fatigue apply to the nursing diagnoses of Fatigue and Activity Intolerance. However, Rich's assessment probed further and revealed Mrs. Tillman's*

BOX 9.3 NANDA-INTERNATIONAL–APPROVED NURSING DIAGNOSES 2015–2017

Activity Intolerance
Risk for **Activity** Intolerance
Ineffective **Activity** Planning
Risk for Ineffective **Activity** Planning
Decreased Intracranial **Adaptive Capacity**
Ineffective **Airway** Clearance
Risk for **Allergy** Response
Anxiety
Risk for **Aspiration**
Risk for Impaired **Attachment**
Autonomic Dysreflexia
Risk for **Autonomic** Dysreflexia
Disorganized Infant **Behavior**
Readiness for Enhanced Organized Infant **Behavior**
Risk for Disorganized Infant **Behavior**
Risk for **Bleeding**
Risk for Unstable **Blood** Glucose Level
Disturbed **Body** Image
Risk for Imbalanced **Body** Temperature
Readiness for Enhanced **Breastfeeding**
Ineffective **Breastfeeding**
Interrupted **Breastfeeding**
Insufficient **Breast** Milk
Ineffective **Breathing** Pattern
Decreased **Cardiac** Output
Risk for Decreased **Cardiac** Output
Risk for Impaired **Cardiovascular** Function
Caregiver Role Strain
Risk for **Caregiver** Role Strain
Ineffective **Childbearing** Process
Readiness for Enhanced **Childbearing** Process
Risk for Ineffective **Childbearing** Process
Impaired **Comfort**
Readiness for Enhanced **Comfort**
Readiness for Enhanced **Communication**
Acute **Confusion**
Chronic **Confusion**
Risk for Acute **Confusion**
Constipation
Perceived **Constipation**
Risk for **Constipation**
Chronic Functional **Constipation**
Risk for Chronic Functional **Constipation**
Contamination
Risk for **Contamination**
Compromised Family **Coping**
Defensive **Coping**
Disabled Family **Coping**
Ineffective **Coping**
Ineffective Community **Coping**
Readiness for Enhanced **Coping**
Readiness for Enhanced Community **Coping**
Readiness for Enhanced Family **Coping**
Death Anxiety
Readiness for Enhanced **Decision Making**
Decisional Conflict
Ineffective **Denial**
Impaired **Dentition**
Risk for Delayed **Development**
Diarrhea

Risk for **Disuse** Syndrome
Deficient **Diversional** Activity
Risk for **Dry** Eye
Risk for **Electrolyte** Imbalance
Impaired **Emancipated** Decision-Making
Readiness for Enhanced **Emancipated** Decision Making
Risk for Impaired **Emancipated** Decision Making
Labile **Emotional** Control
Risk for **Falls**
Dysfunctional **Family** Processes
Interrupted **Family** Processes
Readiness for Enhanced **Family** Processes
Fatigue
Fear
Ineffective Infant **Feeding** Pattern
Readiness for Enhanced **Fluid** Balance
Deficient **Fluid** Volume
Excess **Fluid** Volume
Risk for Deficient **Fluid** Volume
Risk for Imbalanced **Fluid** Volume
Frail Elderly Syndrome
Risk for **Frail** Elderly Syndrome
Impaired **Gas** Exchange
Dysfunctional **Gastrointestinal** Motility
Risk for Dysfunctional **Gastrointestinal** Motility
Risk for Ineffective **Gastrointestinal** Perfusion
Grieving
Complicated **Grieving**
Risk for Complicated **Grieving**
Risk for Disproportionate **Growth**
Deficient Community **Health**
Risk-Prone **Health** Behavior
Ineffective **Health** Maintenance
Ineffective **Health** Management
Readiness for Enhanced **Health** Management
Ineffective Family **Health** Management
Impaired **Home** Maintenance
Readiness for Enhanced **Hope**
Hopelessness
Risk for Compromised **Human** Dignity
Hyperthermia
Hypothermia
Risk for **Hypothermia**
Risk for Perioperative **Hypothermia**
Ineffective **Impulse** Control
Functional Urinary **Incontinence**
Overflow Urinary **Incontinence**
Reflex Urinary **Incontinence**
Stress Urinary **Incontinence**
Urge Urinary **Incontinence**
Risk for Urge Urinary **Incontinence**
Bowel **Incontinence**
Risk for Sudden **Infant** Death Syndrome
Risk for **Infection**
Risk for **Injury**
Risk for Corneal **Injury**
Risk for Perioperative-Positioning **Injury**
Risk for Thermal **Injury**
Risk for Urinary Tract **Injury**
Insomnia

BOX 9.3 NANDA-INTERNATIONAL–APPROVED NURSING DIAGNOSES 2015–2017—cont'd

Neonatal **Jaundice**
Risk for Neonatal **Jaundice**
Deficient **Knowledge**
Readiness for Enhanced **Knowledge**
Latex Allergy Response
Risk for **Latex** Allergy Response
Sedentary **Lifestyle**
Risk for Impaired **Liver** Function
Risk for **Loneliness**
Risk for Disturbed **Maternal/Fetal Dyad**
Impaired **Memory**
Impaired Bed **Mobility**
Impaired Physical **Mobility**
Impaired Wheelchair **Mobility**
Impaired **Mood** Regulation
Moral Distress
Nausea
Unilateral **Neglect**
Noncompliance
Imbalanced **Nutrition:** Less than Body Requirements
Readiness for Enhanced **Nutrition**
Obesity
Impaired **Oral** Mucous Membrane
Risk for Impaired **Oral** Mucous Membrane
Overweight
Risk for **Overweight**
Acute **Pain**
Chronic **Pain**
Labor **Pain**
Chronic **Pain** Syndrome
Impaired **Parenting**
Readiness for Enhanced **Parenting**
Risk for Impaired **Parenting**
Risk for **Peripheral** Neurovascular Dysfunction
Disturbed **Personal** Identity
Risk for Disturbed **Personal** Identity
Risk for **Poisoning**
Post-Trauma Syndrome
Risk for **Post-Trauma** Syndrome
Readiness for Enhanced **Power**
Powerlessness
Risk for **Powerlessness**
Risk for **Pressure** Injury
Ineffective **Protection**
Rape-Trauma Syndrome
Risk for **Reaction** to Iodinated Contrast Media
Ineffective **Relationship**
Risk for Ineffective **Relationship**
Readiness for Enhanced **Relationship**
Impaired **Religiosity**
Readiness for Enhanced **Religiosity**
Risk for Impaired **Religiosity**
Relocation Stress Syndrome
Risk for **Relocation** Stress Syndrome
Risk for Ineffective **Renal** Perfusion
Impaired **Resilience**
Readiness for Enhanced **Resilience**
Risk for Impaired **Resilience**

Parental **Role** Conflict
Ineffective **Role** Performance
Readiness for Enhanced **Self-Care**
Bathing **Self-Care** Deficit
Dressing **Self-Care** Deficit
Feeding **Self-Care** Deficit
Toileting **Self-Care** Deficit
Readiness for Enhanced **Self-Concept**
Chronic Low **Self-Esteem**
Risk for Chronic Low **Self-Esteem**
Situational Low **Self-Esteem**
Risk for Situational Low **Self-Esteem**
Self-Mutilation
Risk for **Self-Mutilation**
Self-Neglect
Sexual Dysfunction
Ineffective **Sexuality** Pattern
Risk for **Shock**
Impaired **Sitting**
Impaired **Skin** Integrity
Risk for Impaired **Skin** Integrity
Sleep Deprivation
Readiness for Enhanced **Sleep**
Disturbed **Sleep** Pattern
Impaired **Social** Interaction
Social Isolation
Chronic **Sorrow**
Spiritual Distress
Risk for **Spiritual** Distress
Readiness for Enhanced **Spiritual** Well-Being
Impaired **Standing**
Stress Overload
Risk for **Suffocation**
Risk for **Suicide**
Delayed **Surgical** Recovery
Risk for Delayed **Surgical** Recovery
Impaired **Swallowing**
Ineffective **Thermoregulation**
Impaired **Tissue** Integrity
Risk for Impaired **Tissue** Integrity
Ineffective Peripheral **Tissue** Perfusion
Risk for Ineffective Peripheral **Tissue** Perfusion
Risk for Decreased Cardiac **Tissue** Perfusion
Risk for Ineffective Cerebral **Tissue** Perfusion
Impaired **Transfer** Ability
Risk for **Trauma**
Risk for Vascular **Trauma**
Impaired **Urinary** Elimination
Readiness for Enhanced **Urinary** Elimination
Urinary Retention
Risk for Self-Directed **Violence**
Risk for Other-Directed **Violence**
Impaired Spontaneous **Ventilation**
Dysfunctional **Ventilatory** Weaning Response
Impaired **Verbal** Communication
Impaired **Walking**
Wandering

From Herdman TH, Kamitsuru S, editiors: *Nursing diagnoses—definitions and classification 2015–2017.* Copyright © 2014, 1994–2014 NANDA International. Used by arrangement with John Wiley & Sons, Inc. In order to make safe and effective judgments using NANDA-I nursing diagnoses, it is essential that nurses refer to the definitions and defining characteristics of the diagnoses listed in this work.

| BOX 9.4 | **EXAMPLE OF A NANDA INTERNATIONAL–APPROVED NURSING DIAGNOSIS WITH DEFINING CHARACTERISTICS AND RELATED FACTORS** |

Diagnosis: Fatigue

DEFINING CHARACTERISTICS	RELATED FACTORS (EXAMPLES)
Impaired ability to maintain usual physical activity	Psychological: Anxiety, stress, depression
Impaired ability to maintain usual routines	Physiological: Physical deconditioning, malnutrition
Insufficient energy	Environmental: Humidity, lights, noise
Lethargy	Situational: Negative life events, occupation
Increase in rest requirements	

Used with permission from Herdman TH, Kamitsuru S, editors: *NANDA International nursing diagnoses: definitions & classification 2015-2017*, Oxford, 2014, Wiley Blackwell.

inability to maintain usual levels of activity or routines, pointing him toward the nursing diagnosis of Fatigue. The absence of certain defining characteristics suggests that you must reject a nursing diagnosis under consideration. Carefully review all defining characteristics that support or eliminate a nursing diagnosis.

While focusing on patterns of defining characteristics, you also compare a patient's pattern of data with data that are consistent with normal, healthful patterns. Use accepted norms as the basis for comparison and judgment. These norms include laboratory and diagnostic test values, professional standards, and normal anatomical or physiological limits. When you compare patterns, determine whether the patient's grouped signs and symptoms are normal for the patient and within the range of healthful responses.

As you isolate the defining characteristics that are not within healthy norms, you identify a patient need or problem. *For example, Rich assessed Mrs. Tillman's verbal report of feeling tired and lacking energy. These symptoms are not necessarily common for a 72-year-old woman and indicate a basic problem involving the patient's ability to participate in normal activity.*

Rich also learned that Mrs. Tillman sometimes has difficulty completing routine chores and requires frequent naps during the day. Rich recognized that Mrs. Tillman had a problem, but he reviewed the NANDA-I classifications to define her problem more specifically. He looked first at the domain of activity/rest. NANDA-I has a variety of nursing diagnoses that can apply to activity/rest (e.g., Activity Intolerance, Risk for Activity Intolerance, Fatigue, *and* Impaired Walking).

After carefully reviewing Mrs. Tillman's presenting symptoms, Rich selected Fatigue. *The key to Rich's diagnosis was his*

assessment showing that the patient's lack of energy affected her daily activities.

It is critical to identify the correct diagnostic label for a patient's need. A nurse usually moves from general to specific. It helps to think of the problem identification phase as the identification of a general health care problem and the formulation of the nursing diagnosis as the identification of a specific health problem. When you begin to identify a problem, review the NANDA-I domains to help you focus on nursing diagnoses pertinent to a particular domain.

Types of Nursing Diagnoses. NANDA-I identifies three types of nursing diagnoses: problem-focused diagnoses, risk diagnoses, and health promotion diagnoses. A problem-focused diagnosis is a clinical judgment concerning an undesirable human response to a health condition and/or life process that exists in an individual, family, group, or community (Gallagher-Lepak, 2014). Selecting a problem-focused diagnosis means that there are sufficient assessment data to support the nursing diagnosis. In Mrs. Tillman's case, *Fatigue* and *Death Anxiety* are problem-focused nursing diagnoses.

A risk nursing diagnosis is a clinical judgment concerning the vulnerability of an individual, family, group, or community for developing an undesirable human response to health conditions and/or life processes (Gallagher-Lepak, 2014). These diagnoses do not have related factors or defining characteristics because they have not yet occurred. Instead a risk diagnosis has risk factors. Risk factors are the environmental, physiological, psychosocial, genetic, and chemical elements that place a person at risk for a health problem. *Risk for Falls* is an example of a risk diagnosis.

A health promotion nursing diagnosis is a clinical judgment concerning motivation and desire to increase well-being and actualize human health potential. These responses are expressed by a readiness to enhance specific health behaviors and can be used in any health state. Health promotion responses may apply to an individual, family, group, or community (Gallagher-Lepak, 2014). This readiness is supported by defining characteristics (Herdman and Kamitsuru, 2014a). *Readiness for Enhanced Comfort* is an example of a health promotion diagnosis.

Components of a Nursing Diagnosis. The identification of a nursing diagnosis flows from the assessment and diagnostic processes. Throughout this text nursing diagnoses are worded in a two-part format: the diagnostic label followed by a statement of a related factor (Table 9.2). This two-part format provides a diagnosis that is relevant for a specific patient.

Diagnostic Label. The diagnostic label is the name of the nursing diagnosis as approved by NANDA-I, and it describes the essence of a patient's response to a health condition in as few words as possible (see Box 9.3). Each NANDA-I–approved diagnosis also has a definition. The definition describes the characteristics of the particular human response. Use these definitions to help you identify a patient's correct diagnoses.

TABLE 9.2	NANDA INTERNATIONAL NURSING DIAGNOSIS FORMAT	
DIAGNOSTIC LABEL	**RELATED FACTORS (EXAMPLES LISTED)**
Fatigue	• Psychological: Anxiety, depression, stressors • Physiological: Malnutrition, physical deconditioning • Environmental: Humidity, lights, ambient noise • Situational: Negative life events, occupational demands
Death Anxiety	• Perceived imminence of death • Anticipation of pain • Anticipation of suffering • Discussions on topic of death • Uncertainty of prognosis

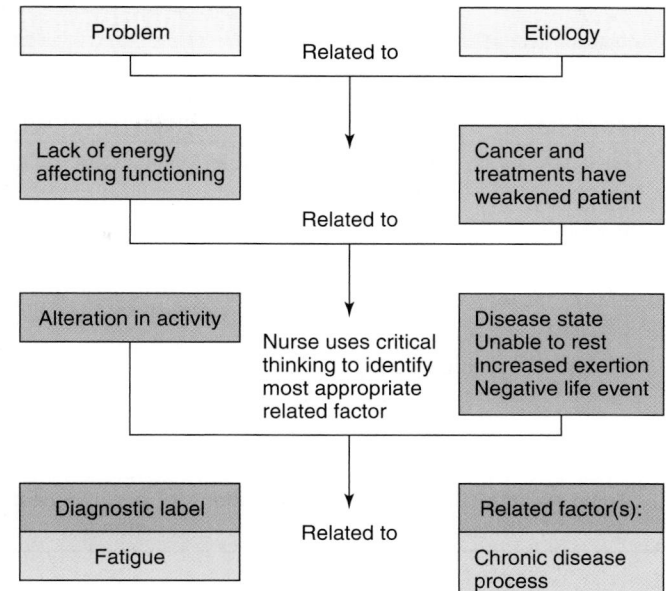

FIG 9.5 Relation between diagnostic label and etiology (related factor). (Redrawn from Hickey P: *Nursing process handbook,* St Louis, 1990, Mosby.)

The definitions are especially helpful when selecting between two diagnoses with similar defining characteristics. The diagnostic labels include descriptors that further support the nursing diagnosis. For example, the diagnosis *Impaired Physical Mobility* includes the descriptor *impaired*. The term *impaired* describes the nature of or change in mobility that best describes the patient's response. Examples of other descriptors are *compromised, decreased, delayed,* or *ineffective*.

Related Factor. The **related factor** is an integral component of all problem-focused nursing diagnoses. The related factor is associated with a patient's actual or potential response to the health problem and can change by using specific nursing interventions (Herdman and Kamitsuru, 2014b). The related factor comes from the patient's assessment data. Thus the assessment data must be accurate. A related factor provides context for the defining characteristics (see Box 9.4). It is a condition associated with or contributing to the diagnosis. For example, a nursing diagnostic statement applicable to Mrs. Tillman includes the diagnostic label (e.g., *Fatigue*) and the related factor (e.g., *chronic disease process*).

Related factors include four categories: pathophysiological (biological or psychological), treatment-related, situational (environmental or personal), and maturational (Carpenito-Moyet, 2017). The "related to" phrase does not always imply a cause-and-effect relationship. It indicates that the etiology contributes to or is associated with the problem (Fig. 9.5). The "related to" phrase requires you to use critical thinking skills to individualize the nursing diagnosis and select appropriate nursing interventions.

Related factors are not listed for risk diagnoses (such as *Risk for Infection, Risk for Falls,* and *Risk for Injury*). The diagnosis is supported by various risk factors. For example, Mrs. Tillman has sleeplessness, metastatic disease, and lack of strength. These risk factors all contribute to her increased vulnerability for a *Risk for Falls* nursing diagnosis.

The **etiology** is always within the domain of nursing practice and a condition that responds to nursing interventions. Nurses sometimes record medical diagnoses as the etiologies of nursing diagnoses. This is incorrect. Nursing interventions cannot change a medical diagnosis. For example, in Mrs. Tillman's case nursing interventions cannot change cancer. Thus the diagnosis of *Fatigue related to cancer* is incorrect. Instead, you direct nursing interventions toward behavior or conditions that you can treat or manage. For example, the nursing diagnosis *Fatigue related to chronic disease process* is correct. Rich, Mrs. Tillman's nurse, can develop interventions that are known to help manage fatigue related to the chronic and progressive nature of cancer.

Table 9.3 demonstrates the association between a nurse's assessment of a patient, the clustering of defining characteristics, and the formulation of two different nursing diagnoses. The diagnostic process results in the formation of a total diagnostic statement that enables a nurse to develop an appropriate, patient-centered plan of care. The defining characteristics and relevant etiologies are from NANDA-I (Herdman and Kamitsuru, 2014b).

Definition. NANDA-I approves a definition for each diagnosis following clinical use and testing. The definition describes the characteristics of the human response identified. For example, the definition of the diagnostic label *Fatigue* is an "overwhelming sustained sense of exhaustion and decreased capacity for physical and mental work at usual level" (Herdman and Kamitsuru, 2014b). Always refer to a definition to help you further identify a patient's diagnosis.

PES Format. Some health care agencies prefer a three-part nursing diagnostic label. In this case the diagnostic label consists of the NANDA-I label, the related factor, and

TABLE 9.3 FORMULATION OF NURSING DIAGNOSES

ASSESSMENT ACTIVITIES	DEFINING CHARACTERISTICS (CLUSTERING CUES)	NURSING DIAGNOSIS	ETIOLOGIES ("RELATED TO")
Ask patient to describe usual daily physical activities.	Impaired ability to maintain usual level of physical activity	Fatigue	Chronic disease process
Observe patient during care activities.	Lethargy Drowsiness		
Question patient about frequency of rest periods.	Increase in rest requirements		
Ask patient to talk about any concerns or worries related to diagnosis of cancer.	Fear of suffering related to dying	Death Anxiety	Anticipation of suffering
Have patient describe her emotions.	Reports deep sadness		
Ask patient to discuss how she thinks her illness will affect her relationship with her husband.	Reports worry about impact of her own death on significant others		

the defining characteristics (Ackley and Ladwig, 2016). A problem-focused nursing diagnosis, including a diagnostic label and the related factor exhibited by defining characteristics, is best practice (Herdman and Kamitsuru, 2014b). This approach makes a diagnosis even more specific to the patient. The acronym *PES* stands for *problem, etiology,* and *symptoms*. Following is an example using the nursing diagnosis in Mrs. Tillman's care plan:

P (Problem) NANDA-I label: *Death Anxiety*
E (Etiology or related factors): Anticipation of suffering
S (Symptoms or defining characteristics): Increased expression of worries, difficulty breathing (examples)
PES diagnostic statement: *Death Anxiety* related to anticipation of suffering, evidenced by increased expression of worries, difficulty breathing.

Cultural Relevance of Nursing Diagnoses. When you select nursing diagnoses, always consider your patient's culture, which in its broadest sense reflects the whole of human behavior, including ideas, beliefs, values, ways of relating to one another, language and manners of speaking, and work and lifestyle practices (Ball et al., 2015; Flagg, 2015) (see Chapter 21). Consideration of the patient's culture is more than just knowing the cultural differences; it is assessing how those cultural differences affect patient-centered care (Ball et al., 2015; Flagg, 2015). Lai et al. (2013) noted that certain NANDA-I nursing diagnoses were difficult for nurses to apply considering the cultural beliefs of a Chinese health care setting, which emphasizes holistic harmony and balance. The patient's culture influences health care preferences and a patient's desire to resolve health care problems (Burman et al., 2013; Nielsen et al., 2015).

A patient's culture influences the type of health care problems that he or she experiences as well as the importance of those problems (Nielsen et al., 2015). When you make a nursing diagnosis, consider the effect of culture on the related factor in the diagnostic statement. For example, *Impaired*

Verbal Communication related to cultural differences reflects a diagnostic conclusion that considers a patient's unique cultural needs. *Deficient Knowledge* is a common nursing diagnosis and may be related to a patient's culture. When a nurse is aware of the effects of culture on a patient's health care practices, the nurse can improve the cultural effectiveness of the nursing diagnoses by asking some of the following questions:

- How has this health problem affected you and your family?
- What worries you most about this problem?
- What do you believe will help or fix the problem?
- What health care practices do you use to keep yourself and family well?

Using a patient-centered approach when asking these questions helps you see the patient's problems through his or her eyes (Cope, 2015). This leads you to culturally relevant nursing diagnoses and interventions (Lai et al., 2013; Nielsen et al., 2015).

Concept Mapping Nursing Diagnoses. Your patients usually will have multiple nursing diagnoses. When you care for multiple patients prioritizing and focusing on all patients' multiple diagnoses becomes challenging. Developing a concept map helps you critically think about your patients' nursing diagnoses, their relationship to one another, and their effect on the nursing care plan (Pilcher, 2011; Lhussier et al., 2015). Concept mapping helps you logically organize and link data about a patient's multiple diagnoses. The concept map graphically represents the connections between concepts (such as a nursing diagnosis) that relate to a central subject (such as a patient's health problems). As you apply each step of the nursing process your concept map includes more detail about planned interventions (see Planning section).

Fig. 9.6 shows the first part of a concept map for Mrs. Tillman. It includes the patient's assessment findings and four nursing diagnoses. As Rich forms the concept map, he begins to see relationships among the nursing diagnoses. For

CONCEPT MAP

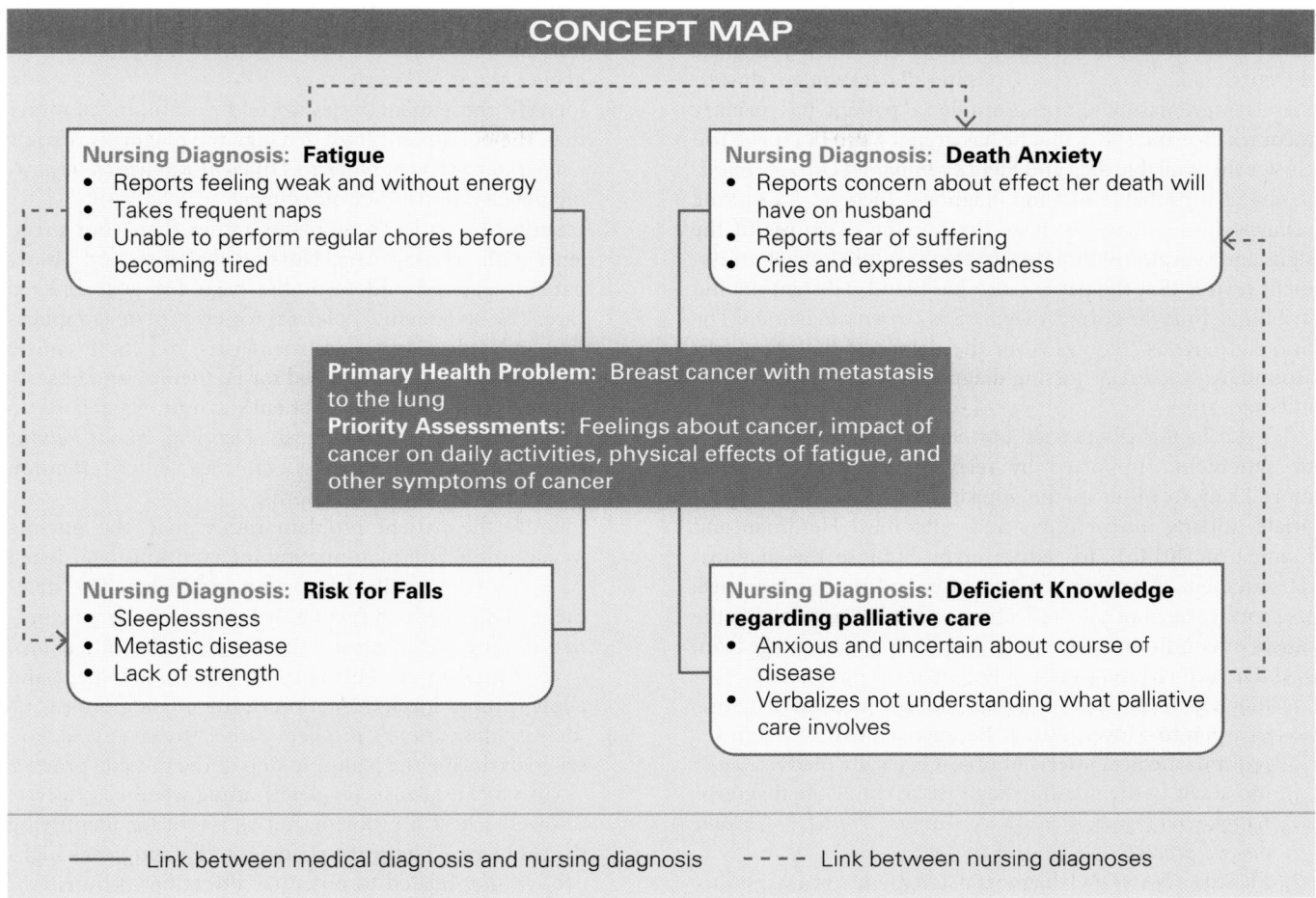

Nursing Diagnosis: Fatigue
- Reports feeling weak and without energy
- Takes frequent naps
- Unable to perform regular chores before becoming tired

Nursing Diagnosis: Death Anxiety
- Reports concern about effect her death will have on husband
- Reports fear of suffering
- Cries and expresses sadness

Primary Health Problem: Breast cancer with metastasis to the lung
Priority Assessments: Feelings about cancer, impact of cancer on daily activities, physical effects of fatigue, and other symptoms of cancer

Nursing Diagnosis: Risk for Falls
- Sleeplessness
- Metastic disease
- Lack of strength

Nursing Diagnosis: Deficient Knowledge regarding palliative care
- Anxious and uncertain about course of disease
- Verbalizes not understanding what palliative care involves

——— Link between medical diagnosis and nursing diagnosis   - - - - Link between nursing diagnoses

FIG 9.6 Concept map with nursing diagnoses.

example, Mrs. Tillman's *Death Anxiety* makes it more difficult for her to sleep, and this results in *Fatigue*. Fatigue in turn is a risk factor that increases the *Risk for Falls*. Finally, the diagnoses of *Deficient Knowledge* and *Death Anxiety* also are related. Having a poor understanding of her conditions heightens Mrs. Tillman's anxiety. Being anxious can make it hard for her to sleep. This concept map will show you how the diagnoses relate to one another.

Sources of Diagnostic Errors. Errors can occur in the diagnostic process during data collection, data interpretation, clustering, and statement of the nursing diagnosis. Apply methodical critical thinking to make an accurate nursing diagnosis.

Errors in Data Collection. To avoid errors in data collection, be knowledgeable of, and skillful in, all assessment techniques. Ensure that data are complete and accurate, and collect data in an organized way. The following practice tips are essential in avoiding data collection errors:

- Review your level of comfort and competence with interview and physical assessment skills before you begin the data collection step.
- Approach assessment in steps. Focus on completing the patient history and interview before starting the examination. Consider focusing on a single body system to learn how to perform an examination. Then move to a more complex head-to-toe examination.
- Review your assessments in clinical or classroom settings to gain feedback and learn to revise an assessment or gather more information.
- Organize the examination. Prepare the patient and environment for the examination (see Chapter 16).

Errors in Interpretation and Analysis of Data. After you complete the data collection step, review your database to determine whether it is accurate and complete. Review your data to validate that measurable, objective physical findings support the subjective data. For example, when a patient reports "difficulty breathing," you auscultate lung sounds and assess respiratory rate and rhythm.

When data are not validated, the result is a mismatch between clinical cues and the nursing diagnosis. Consider any conflicting cues and determine whether you have sufficient cues to form a diagnosis.

Consider the patient's cultural background or developmental stage when you interpret the meaning of cues. For example, male and female patients might express pain very differently. Misinterpreting the patient's expression of pain could easily lead to an inaccurate diagnosis.

Errors in Data Clustering. Errors result when you cluster data prematurely, incorrectly, or not at all. When you make the nursing diagnosis before grouping all data you are clustering data prematurely. For example, a patient has urinary incontinence and states that he has urgency and nocturia. You cluster the available data and identify *Impaired Urinary Elimination* as a probable nursing diagnosis. Incorrect clustering occurs when you try to make the nursing diagnosis fit the signs and symptoms obtained. In this example further assessment reveals that the patient also has bladder distention and dribbling; thus the correct diagnosis is *Urinary Retention.* The nursing diagnosis comes from the data, not the other way around. An incorrect nursing diagnosis affects the quality of nursing care.

Errors in the Diagnostic Statement. A correct diagnostic statement, supported by relevant assessment data, is more likely to result in the appropriate selection of appropriate nursing interventions and outcomes (Herdman and Kamitsuru, 2014b). To reduce errors, phrase the diagnostic statement in appropriate, concise, and precise language. Use correct terminology reflecting a patient's response to the illness or condition. Use standardized nursing language from NANDA-I to ensure accuracy. Follow these guidelines:

1. Identify the patient's response, not the medical diagnosis (Carpenito-Moyet, 2017). Because a medical diagnosis requires medical interventions, it is legally inadvisable to include it in the nursing diagnosis. Change the diagnosis *Fatigue related to cancer* to *Fatigue related to chronic disease process.*

2. Identify a NANDA-I diagnostic statement, not a symptom. Identify nursing diagnoses from a cluster of defining characteristics that apply to a patient. A single symptom is insufficient for identifying a problem. For example, shortness of breath alone does not identify a diagnosis. In contrast, shortness of breath, pain on inspiration, and productive cough in a postoperative patient form the cluster for *Ineffective Breathing Pattern related to increased airway secretions.*

3. Identify a treatable related factor or risk factor, rather than a clinical sign or chronic problem that is not treatable through nursing intervention. Identifying a related factor allows you to select nursing interventions for resolving the etiology of the problem or minimizing the patient's risk. A diagnostic test or chronic dysfunction is not an etiology that a nursing intervention can treat. A patient with cancer often develops anemia, reflected in low red blood cell counts. The diagnosis *Fatigue related to low red blood cell counts* is an incorrect diagnostic statement. *Fatigue related to chronic disease process* is appropriate because it allows you to focus interventions on the physical responses common in chronic progressive disease.

4. Identify the problem caused by the treatment or diagnostic study rather than the treatment or study itself. Patients can respond to diagnostic tests and medical treatments in many ways. These responses are the area of nursing concern. The patient who has severe chest pain and is scheduled for a cardiac catheterization may have a nursing diagnosis of *Anxiety related to lack of knowledge about cardiac catheterization.*

5. Identify the patient response to the equipment rather than the equipment itself. Change the diagnosis *Anxiety related to cardiac monitor* to *Deficient Knowledge regarding the need for cardiac monitoring.*

6. Identify the patient's problems rather than your problems with nursing care. Nursing diagnoses are always patient-centered and form the basis for goal-directed care. The statement, "potential for electrolyte complications related to severe gastroenteritis" directs the nurse to focus on the patient's need for IV therapy and observing and controlling the patient's symptoms related to gastroenteritis. The diagnosis *Deficient Fluid Volume related to severe vomiting and diarrhea* centers attention on patient signs and symptoms.

7. Identify the patient problem rather than the nursing intervention. You plan nursing interventions later when you plan care to alleviate patient problems. The statement, "Offer bedpan frequently because of altered elimination patterns" changes to the diagnosis *Diarrhea related to food intolerance.* This corrects the misstatement and allows proper implementation of the nursing process.

8. Identify the patient's problem rather than the goal. You set goals during the planning step of the nursing process. Goals serve as a basis for determining whether you have resolved a health problem, not as a tool for identifying the problem. Change the statement, "Patient needs high-protein diet related to potential alteration in nutrition" to *Imbalanced Nutrition: Less Than Body Requirements related to inadequate protein intake.* This diagnosis identifies the correct etiology and enables you to then plan a proper treatment.

9. Make professional rather than prejudicial judgments. Base nursing diagnoses on subjective and objective patient data rather than on your personal beliefs and values. Remove your judgment from *Impaired Skin Integrity related to poor hygiene habits* by changing the nursing diagnosis to *Impaired Skin Integrity related to lack of knowledge about perineal care.*

10. Avoid legally inadvisable statements that imply blame, negligence, or malpractice (Carpenito-Moyet, 2017). The diagnosis *Chronic Pain related to insufficient pain medication* implies that the health care provider prescribed inadequate analgesia prescription. The correct way to identify the problem is to write *Chronic Pain related to incorrect adherence of analgesic schedule.*

11. Identify the problem and etiology to avoid a circular statement. Circular statements are vague and give no direction to nursing care. Change the diagnosis *Acute Pain related to alteration in comfort* to the specific patient problem and cause: *Acute Pain related to incisional trauma.*

12. Identify only one patient problem in a diagnostic statement. Problems have different expected outcomes. Including multiple problems in a nursing diagnosis

causes confusion during the planning step. However, it is permissible to include multiple etiologies contributing to one patient problem. For example, you might restate *Pain and Anxiety related to difficulty in ambulating* as two nursing diagnoses. These could be *Impaired Physical Mobility related to pain in right knee* and *Anxiety related to fear of falling.*

Documentation and Informatics

After identifying a patient's nursing diagnoses, enter them on his or her written plan of care or in the EHR of the health care agency. Start-of-the art EHRs contain the following:

- NANDA-I–approved nursing diagnoses, interventions, and outcomes
- Related or risk factors
- Defining characteristics (Herdman and Kamitsuru, 2014b).

With this type of EHR the nurse enters assessment data, and the computer organizes the data into clusters. This feature improves the nurse's ability to select accurate nursing diagnoses. Once the diagnoses are identified, the computer system will direct the nurse to possible outcomes and interventions to select for the patient. This helps to make the patient care plan more theoretically based. When agencies use EHR systems that do not use NANDA-I, entry of nursing diagnoses is more tedious.

List nursing diagnoses chronologically as you identify them. When you initiate a care plan, always list the diagnoses in order from highest priority to lowest. The highest priority diagnosis depends on a patient's condition and the nature of the nursing diagnosis. (For example, an acute physical health problem ranks above a long-term, chronic health problem.)

Add nursing diagnoses to the list and date each nursing diagnosis. When caring for a patient, always review the list of nursing diagnoses and identify the diagnoses with the highest priority, regardless of chronological order.

PLANNING

After you identify a patient's nursing diagnoses and collaborative problems, you begin the planning step of the nursing process. Planning involves setting priorities, identifying patient-centered goals and expected outcomes, and prescribing nursing interventions. The most important principle in planning is the individualization of a plan of care for each patient's unique needs. The nursing diagnoses you select direct your selection of nursing interventions and goals and outcomes you hope to achieve. The individualized nursing diagnoses and problems that you identify direct your selection of individualized nursing interventions and the goals and outcomes you hope to achieve (Flagg, 2015; Nielsen et al., 2015).

Establishing Priorities

A single patient often has multiple diagnoses and collaborative problems. Eventually you will care for multiple patients at one time. You must be able to set priorities for these patients carefully and wisely to ensure timely, safe, and effective care.

Priority setting is the ordering of nursing diagnoses or patient problems considering their urgency and importance to establish an order for nursing actions. In other words, you must provide some types of care before others. By ranking nursing diagnoses in order of importance, you attend to your patient's most important needs and better prioritize your care activities.

A priority list helps you anticipate and sequence nursing interventions when a patient has multiple problems. Together with your patients, you select mutually agreed-on priorities based on the urgency of the problem, the patient's safety and desires, and the nature of the treatment indicated. Establishing priorities is not just a matter of numbering the nursing diagnoses based on severity or physiological importance.

Classify priorities as high, intermediate, or low. Nursing diagnoses that, if left untreated, result in harm to the patient or others have the highest priority. One way to prioritize diagnoses is to consider Maslow's hierarchy of needs. For example, you want to attend to a patient's oxygen, fluid, and nutrition needs before you focus on shelter or sexual needs. However, it is always important to consider each patient's unique case. High priorities are sometimes both psychological and physiological. Avoid classifying only physiological nursing diagnoses as high priority.

Consider Mrs. Tillman's case. The nursing diagnosis of *Death Anxiety* is a high-priority diagnosis because it has the potential to impair Mrs. Tillman's ability to participate in her own care and maintain a healthy relationship with her husband. Intermediate-priority nursing diagnoses involve the nonemergent, non–life-threatening needs of a patient. In Mrs. Tillman's case, *Fatigue* is an intermediate diagnosis. Mrs. Tillman's activity problem is linked to the progressive nature of her cancer. Her fatigue will be an ongoing challenge, but not a life-threatening issue. Energy conservation and management therapies are important but not critical.

Low-priority nursing diagnoses are patient needs that are usually directly related to a specific illness or prognosis but also affect a patient's future well-being. Rich, Mrs. Tillman's nurse, knows that she will have more health care needs as her disease progresses. Her husband, the family caregiver, may assume even more responsibility for in-home care. *Deficient Knowledge regarding palliative care related to inexperience* is a relevant diagnosis but currently of lower priority than the other diagnoses. In future clinic visits Rich will plan a discussion about palliative care with the Tillman family.

Priorities change as the patient's condition changes. Each time you begin a sequence of care such as the beginning of a nursing care shift or during a clinic visit, you must reorder priorities. Continually assess the patient to determine the status of a patient's nursing diagnoses. Following the order of priorities helps to ensure that you meet your patients' needs in a timely and effective way.

Priority setting includes prioritizing specific interventions that you plan to use with the patient. For example, as Rich considers the high-priority diagnosis of *Death Anxiety,* he decides whether to counsel Mrs. Tillman first or conduct a care conference with the patient, her husband, and the clinic nurse practitioner. Rich must prioritize interventions to be most effective in meeting desired goals and outcomes. It is always important to involve the patient in priority setting. In some situations you and the patient assign different priority rankings to nursing diagnoses and collaborative problems. Resolve these differences through open communication. When a patient's physiological and emotional needs are at stake, you must assume primary responsibility for setting priorities.

Ethical care must factor into priority setting. When ethical issues cloud priorities, you must maintain an open dialogue with the patient, family, and other health care providers. For example, when caring for patients with cancer and other disabling illnesses, discuss the situation with the patient and understand his or her expectations. Understand your professional responsibility in providing care, and work with the health care team, patient, and family caregivers when developing a patient-centered care plan.

Critical Thinking in Setting Goals and Expected Outcomes

After you identify a nursing diagnosis for your patient, ask yourself the following questions:

- What is the best approach to address and resolve the problem?
- What does my patient need to achieve? What are the goals and expected outcomes?
- How will I know when my patient has achieved them?

Goals and expected outcomes are specific statements of patient behavior or physiological responses that you select to resolve a nursing diagnosis or collaborative problem. They serve two purposes: to set a clear direction for the selection and use of nursing interventions and to set specific measures for evaluating the effectiveness of the interventions.

Goals of Care. A patient-centered goal is a broad statement that describes a desired change in a patient's condition or behavior. For Mrs. Tillman, who has a diagnosis of *Fatigue related to chronic disease process,* a goal of care would be "Patient will achieve improved energy level within 2 weeks." A goal is realistic and based on patient needs and resources.

A patient goal is a predicted resolution of a problem, evidence of progress toward problem resolution, progress toward improved health status, or continued maintenance of good health or function (Carpenito-Moyet, 2017).

Each goal is time limited so the health care team has a common time frame for problem resolution. The time frame depends on the nature of the problem, etiology, overall condition of the patient, and treatment setting. A *short-term goal* is an objective behavior or response that you expect the patient to achieve in a short time, usually less than a week. In an acute care setting, you may set goals to be achieved within just a few hours. For example, "Patient will maintain a balanced fluid status within the next 12 hours." A *long-term goal* is an objective behavior or response that you expect the patient to achieve over a longer period, usually several days, weeks, or months. Goal setting establishes the framework for the nursing care plan. Table 9.4 shows the progression from nursing diagnoses to goals and expected outcomes, which you individualize to meet patient needs.

Goals are often based on standards of care or clinical guidelines established for minimal safe practice. For example, the Infusion Nurses Society (INS) has standards of care to prevent the IV complication of phlebitis. When a nurse cares for a patient with a peripheral IV catheter, the goal "The IV site will remain free of phlebitis" is established based on sound nursing practice standards.

Role of the Patient in Goal Setting. Always collaborate with your patients when setting goals. Mutual goal setting involves the patient and family caregiver (when appropriate) in prioritizing the goals of care and developing a plan of action to achieve those goals. Unless goals are mutually set and include a clear plan of action, patients or family caregivers will not participate. Patients need to understand and see the value of nursing therapies even though they are often totally dependent on you as the nurse. When developing goals, you act as an advocate or supporter for the patient when developing nursing interventions to promote the patient's return to health or prevent further deterioration when possible.

Expected Outcomes. For Rich to determine if Mrs. Tillman has shown progress and achieved the goal of an

TABLE 9.4	EXAMPLES OF GOAL SETTING WITH EXPECTED OUTCOMES FOR MRS. TILLMAN	
NURSING DIAGNOSES	**GOALS**	**EXPECTED OUTCOMES**
Fatigue related to chronic disease process	Mrs. Tillman will achieve an improved energy level within 2 weeks.	Patient's self-report of fatigue is 3 or less on a scale of 0 to 10 in 2 weeks. Patient is able to increase some daily activities in 1 week.
Death Anxiety related to anticipation of suffering	Mrs. Tillman will express belief that she will gain a stable level of comfort in 3 weeks.	Patient seeks information about palliative care treatment in 1 week. Patient reports acceptable comfort level in 2 weeks. Patient participates in health care decisions in 1 week.

improved energy level within 2 weeks, expected outcomes are necessary. An expected outcome is the measurable change in the patient that must be achieved to reach a goal. Expected outcomes provide a focus or direction for nursing care because they are the desired physical, psychological, behavioral, social, emotional, developmental, or spiritual responses that show resolution of a patient's health problems. Expected outcomes must also be singular.

For example, in Mrs. Tillman's case measurable outcomes for the goal of improved energy level include "Patient's self-report of fatigue is 3 or less on a scale of 0 to 10" and "Patient is able to complete bathing without taking rest periods." These outcomes help Rich determine the success of selected interventions that effectively lessen Mrs. Tillman's fatigue. An outcome includes measurable criteria (e.g., 3 or less on a scale of 0 to 10, completes bathing without taking rest) to evaluate goal achievement (Table 9.5). Achieving outcomes means that a goal has been met.

Typically all health care providers contribute to achievement of patient outcomes. A nursing-sensitive outcome is a measurable patient or family state, behavior, or perception largely influenced by and sensitive to nursing interventions (Moorhead et al., 2013). Examples of nursing-sensitive outcomes include reduction in pain severity, incidence of pressure injuries, and incidence of falls. In comparison, outcomes largely influenced by medical interventions include patient mortality and hospital readmission.

Outcomes are measurable, reliable, valid, suited to the patient, and sensitive to change (Moorhead et al., 2013). Consider the example of Mrs. Tillman's problem of fatigue. One outcome measure is a self-report fatigue scale. The scale provides an objective measure of the patient's level of fatigue. Current evidence shows self-report scales are reliable (consistently measure an outcome) and valid (accurately measure an outcome). A self-report scale is easy for a patient to complete without causing anxiety or physical distress as in the case of an exercise test for fatigue. The patient's perceptions of fatigue change over time and are reflected by differences in the fatigue scale.

You normally develop several expected outcomes for each nursing diagnosis and goal. The reason for multiple outcomes is that sometimes one nursing action is not enough to resolve a patient problem. The listing of step-by-step expected outcomes guides you in planning interventions. Always write expected outcomes sequentially with time frames. Time frames give you progressive steps in which to move a patient toward recovery. They also give an order for when to perform nursing interventions. In addition, time frames set limits for problem resolution.

Nursing Outcomes Classification. Health care agencies are very interested in measuring nursing-sensitive outcomes because of the effect they have on patient outcomes, quality of care, and health care costs. The *Nursing Outcomes Classification (NOC),* published by the Iowa Intervention Project, classifies, identifies, labels, and validates nursing-sensitive outcomes (Moorhead et al., 2013). NOC links evidence-based outcomes to every NANDA-I nursing diagnosis (Moorhead et al., 2013). NOC-suggested outcomes describe the focus of nursing care and provide ways to measure the success of nursing interventions (see Table 9.5). NOC helps you select appropriate nursing interventions to improve the quality of care for individuals, families, and communities in all health care settings (Moorhead et al., 2013). Using a common language allows nurses to plan effective patient care and provides a standardized way to measure the success of nursing interventions. In addition, the use of NOC facilitates the evaluation of the effects of nursing interventions over time and across a variety of health care settings.

Guidelines for Writing Goals and Expected Outcomes. Goals and expected outcomes direct your nursing care. After you set a patient-centered goal for a nursing diagnosis, the expected outcomes set the desired physiological, psychological, behavioral, social, developmental, or spiritual responses that measure the resolution of the patient's health problem.

Use the *SMART* acronym (specific, measureable, attainable, realistic, timed) as an approach for writing goals and expected outcomes.

1. *Specific:* Outcomes and goals reflect a specific patient behavior or response that you expect as a result of nursing interventions. A proper goal statement is, "Patient will ambulate independently in 3 days." A proper outcome statement is "Patient ambulates in the hall 3 times a day by 4/22." A common error is to write an outcome as an intervention, such as, "Ambulate patient in the hall 3 times a day."

TABLE 9.5	EXAMPLES OF NANDA INTERNATIONAL NURSING DIAGNOSES AND SUGGESTED NOC LINKAGES	
NURSING DIAGNOSIS	SUGGESTED NOC OUTCOMES (EXAMPLES)	OUTCOME INDICATORS (EXAMPLES)
Fatigue	Activity tolerance	Walking pace Ease of performing ADLs Pulse rate with activity Ease of breathing with activity
	Energy conservation	Balances activity and rest Uses naps to restore energy Adapts lifestyle to energy level
Deficient Knowledge regarding palliative care	Knowledge of treatment regimen	Rationale for treatment Self-care responsibilities for ongoing treatment Expected effects of treatment

ADLs, Activities of daily living; *NOC, Nursing Outcomes Classification.*

In addition, the outcome must address only one behavior or response. For example, an outcome might read, "Patient's lungs are clear to auscultation, and respiratory rate is 24 breaths/min by 8/22." How would you evaluate the outcome when you determine that the lungs are clear but the respiratory rate is 28 breaths/min? You would be unable to determine whether the expected outcome has been achieved.

By splitting the statement into two parts, "Lungs are clear to auscultation by 8/22" and "Respiratory rate is 24 breaths/min by 8/22," you can determine whether the patient achieves each outcome separately. This focus on a single outcome enables you to determine whether you need to modify the plan of care.

2. *Measurable:* You must be able to measure or observe whether a change takes place in a patient's status. Examples such as, "Body temperature remains 98.6° F" and "Apical pulse remains between 60 and 100 beats/min" allow you to objectively measure changes in a patient's status. Do not use vague qualifiers such as "normal," "acceptable," "stable," or "sufficient" in the expected outcome statement. Vague terms make it difficult to determine a patient's response to care. Terms describing quality, quantity, frequency, length, or weight allow you to accurately evaluate if outcomes are met.

3. *Attainable:* A goal and an outcome are more attainable when mutually set with the patient. This ensures that the patient and nurse agree on the direction and time limits of care. Mutual goal setting increases a patient's motivation and cooperation. As a patient advocate you apply standards of practice, patient safety, and basic human needs when helping patients set goals.

4. *Realistic:* Set goals and expected outcomes that a patient can achieve. Achieving a goal gives a patient a sense of accomplishment. This sense of accomplishment further increases the patient's motivation and cooperation. When you establish realistic goals, consider the resources of the health care agency, family, and patient. For example, do the patient's cultural beliefs affect the goals you set? Does the patient have the necessary resources in the home to successfully meet the goals?

5. *Timed:* A time limit is set for each goal and outcome so the health care team has a common time frame for problem resolution. For example, "Patient will be able to ambulate the hospital corridor in 2 days." Time frames help you and your patient determine if progress is being made at a reasonable rate. If not, revision of the plan of care is necessary.

Critical Thinking in Planning Nursing Care

During planning you make clinical decisions by choosing the nursing interventions most appropriate to your patient's nursing diagnoses and collaborative problems. The actual implementation of these interventions occurs during the implementation phase of the nursing process. Choosing suitable nursing interventions involves critical thinking applied in decision making. To select interventions you need to be competent in three areas: (1) knowing the scientific rationale, or reason, for the interventions; (2) possessing the necessary psychomotor and interpersonal skills to perform the interventions; and (3) being able to function within a particular setting to use the available health care resources effectively (Bulechek et al., 2013).

Types of Interventions. Nursing interventions include three categories: nurse-initiated, health care provider–initiated, and collaborative interventions. Nurse-initiated interventions are independent nursing interventions or actions that nurses initiate. These do not require direction or an order from another health care professional. Nurse-initiated interventions (independent nursing interventions) are autonomous actions based on scientific rationales. Examples include elevating an edematous extremity, offering counseling on coping, and instructing patients about medication side effects. These interventions benefit patients in a predicted way related to nursing diagnoses and patient goals (Bulechek et al., 2013). They require no supervision or direction from others. Every U.S. state has developed a Nurse Practice Act that defines the legal scope of nursing practice (see Chapter 5). According to state Nurse Practice Acts, independent nursing interventions pertain to ADLs, health education and promotion, and counseling.

Health care provider–initiated interventions are dependent nursing interventions or actions that require an order from a health care professional. Such interventions are based on a health care provider's response to treat or manage a medical diagnosis. Advanced practice nurses who have collaborative agreements with physicians or who are licensed independently by state Nurse Practice Acts also write dependent interventions. As a nurse, you intervene by carrying out the independent provider's written and/or verbal orders. Administering a medication, implementing an invasive procedure, and preparing a patient for diagnostic tests are examples of dependent nursing interventions.

Each dependent nursing intervention involves specific nursing responsibilities and technical nursing knowledge. When you perform the intervention you must also know the types of observations and precautions to take for the intervention to be delivered safely and correctly. For example, when administering medications you are responsible for knowing the classification of the drug, its physiological action, normal dosage, and side effects as well as nursing interventions related to its action or side effects (see Chapter 17). When a health care provider orders diagnostic testing, you are responsible for scheduling the test, preparing the patient, and knowing the normal findings and associated nursing implications.

Collaborative interventions, or interdependent nursing interventions, are therapies that require the combined knowledge, skill, and expertise of multiple health care professionals. When you plan care for a patient, you review the necessary interventions and determine whether the collaboration of other health care professionals is necessary. In the case study, Rich decides to have an interdisciplinary conference with the health care team to discuss a palliative care plan for Mrs. Tillman. Interdisciplinary conferences bring together professionals from all disciplines involved in the patient's care so that they can jointly establish and execute the most appropriate plan of care.

Selection of Interventions. Never select interventions for a patient randomly. For example, patients with the diagnosis of *Anxiety* do not always need care in the same way with the same interventions. You treat *Anxiety related to the uncertainty of results from a diagnostic test* differently from *Anxiety related to a threat of loss of a loved one.* When choosing interventions, consider the following six factors: (1) desired patient outcomes, (2) characteristics of the nursing diagnosis, (3) evidence base (research or clinical practice guidelines) for the intervention, (4) feasibility of implementing the intervention, (5) acceptability to the patient, and (6) your own competency (Box 9.5) (Bulechek et al., 2013).

When choosing interventions review resources such as evidence in the literature, standard protocols or guidelines, the Nursing Interventions Classification (NIC), critical pathways, and current textbooks. Collaborating with other health care professionals is also useful, especially when a patient moves from one setting to another, such as hospital to home or hospital to a rehabilitation agency (Lemetti et al., 2015). Review your patient's needs, values, priorities, and previous experiences to select the nursing interventions that have the best potential for achieving the expected outcomes.

Nursing Interventions Classification. Just as with the standardized NOC, the Iowa Intervention Project developed a set of nursing interventions that provides a level of standardization to enhance communication of nursing care across all health care settings and to compare outcomes (Bulechek et al., 2013). The NIC model includes three levels: domains, classes, and interventions for ease of use. The seven domains (level 1) are the highest level of the model, using broad terms (e.g., *physiological, safety*) to organize the more specific classes and interventions (Table 9.6). The second level of the model includes 30 classes, which offer useful clinical categories to refer to when selecting interventions. The third level includes interventions, defined as any treatment based on clinical judgment and knowledge that a nurse performs to enhance patient outcomes (Bulechek et al., 2013). Each intervention has a variety of nursing activities from which to choose (Box 9.6). The NIC interventions link with NANDA-I nursing diagnoses. For example, Mrs. Tillman has the problem of *Fatigue,* which falls under the domain of Physiological: Basic and the class of Activity and Exercise Management. Under the class of Activity and Exercise Management, there are a variety of interventions to choose from (e.g., Energy Management, Exercise Therapy: Ambulation). When you refer to an intervention within NIC such as energy management, there are numerous nursing activities or interventions to choose from (see Mrs. Tillman's Care Plan [see Fig. 9.7]). NIC is a valuable resource for selecting interventions for your unique patients.

Systems for Planning Nursing Care

In every health care setting, the nurse is responsible for developing a plan of nursing care for each patient. The plan of care can take one of several forms (e.g., standardized care plan, computerized plan). EHRs typically include

---

BOX 9.5 SELECTING NURSING INTERVENTIONS

CHARACTERISTICS OF THE NURSING DIAGNOSIS
- Interventions should alter the etiological (related to) factor associated with the diagnostic label.
- When an etiological factor cannot change, direct interventions toward treating the signs and symptoms (e.g., NANDA-I defining characteristics).
- For potential or high-risk diagnoses, direct interventions at altering or eliminating risk factors for the nursing diagnoses.

EXPECTED OUTCOMES
- Specify expected outcomes before choosing interventions.
- Identify for each patient the outcomes that can be reasonably expected and attained as the result of nursing care.
- Use the Nursing Outcomes Classification to specify outcomes.

EVIDENCE BASE
- Know the research base for an intervention.
- Research will indicate the effectiveness of using an intervention with certain types of patients.
- When research is not available, use scientific principles (e.g., safety) or consult experts.

FEASIBILITY OF THE INTERVENTION
- A specific intervention has the potential for interacting with other interventions.
- Consider cost: Is the intervention clinically effective and cost-efficient?
- Consider time: Are time and personnel resources available?

ACCEPTABILITY TO THE PATIENT
- An intervention must be acceptable to the patient and family caregiver and match a patient's goals, beliefs, health care values, and culture.
- Promote informed choice; help a patient know how he or she is expected to participate.

CAPABILITY
- Be prepared to carry out the intervention.
- Be competent in knowing the scientific rationale for the intervention, possessing necessary psychomotor and interpersonal skills, and being able to function in the particular setting.

Modified from Bulechek GM, et al: *Nursing interventions classification (NIC),* ed 6, St Louis, 2013, Mosby.

TABLE 9.6   NURSING INTERVENTIONS CLASSIFICATION (NIC) TAXONOMY

DOMAIN 1	DOMAIN 2	DOMAIN 3
Level 1 Domains		
1. **Physiological: Basic** Care that supports physical functioning	2. **Physiological: Complex** Care that supports homeostatic regulation	3. **Behavioral** Care that supports psychosocial functioning and facilitates lifestyle changes
Level 2 Classes		
A *Activity and Exercise Management:* Interventions to organize or assist with physical activity and energy conservation and expenditure	H *Drug Management:* Interventions to facilitate desired effects of pharmacological agents	O *Behavior Therapy:* Interventions to reinforce or promote desirable behaviors or alter undesirable behaviors
B *Elimination Management:* Interventions to establish and maintain regular bowel and urinary elimination patterns and manage complications caused by altered patterns	I *Neurological Management:* Interventions to optimize neurological functions	P *Cognitive Therapy:* Interventions to reinforce or promote desirable cognitive functioning or alter undesirable cognitive functioning
C *Immobility Management:* Interventions to manage restricted body movement and the sequelae	J *Perioperative Care:* Interventions to provide care before, during, and immediately after surgery	Q *Communication Enhancement:* Interventions to facilitate delivering and receiving verbal and nonverbal messages
D *Nutrition Support:* Interventions to modify or maintain nutritional status	K *Respiratory Management:* Interventions to promote airway patency and gas exchange	R *Coping Assistance:* Interventions to assist another to build on own strengths, adapt to a change in function, or achieve a higher level of function
E *Physical Comfort Promotion:* Interventions to promote comfort using physical techniques	L *Skin/Wound Management:* Interventions to maintain or restore tissue integrity	S *Patient Education:* Interventions to facilitate learning
F *Self-Care Facilitation:* Interventions to provide or assist with routine activities of daily living	M *Thermoregulation:* Interventions to maintain body temperature within a normal range	T *Psychological Comfort Promotion:* Interventions to promote comfort using psychological techniques
G *Electrolyte and Acid-Base Management:* Interventions to regulate electrolyte/acid-base balance and prevent complications	N *Tissue Perfusion Management:* Interventions to optimize circulation of blood and fluids to the tissue	

From Bulechek GM, et al: *Nursing interventions classification (NIC),* ed 6, St Louis, 2013, Mosby.

BOX 9.6   EXAMPLES OF LEVEL 3 INTERVENTIONS AND ACTIVITIES FOR ACTIVITY AND EXERCISE MANAGEMENT

ACTIVITY AND EXERCISE MANAGEMENT
Interventions to organize or assist with physical activity and energy conservation and expenditure

Level 3 Interventions
- Body Mechanics Promotion
  Examples of Nursing Activities for Body Mechanics Promotion: Instruct to use a firm mattress, assist to demonstrate appropriate sleeping positions, assist to avoid sitting in same position for prolonged periods.
- Energy Management
- Exercise Promotion
- Exercise Therapy: Ambulation
- Teaching Prescribed Activity/Exercise

Examples of Linked Nursing Diagnoses
- Activity Intolerance
- Fatigue
- Impaired Physical Mobility

From Bulechek GM, et al: *Nursing interventions classification (NIC),* ed 6, St Louis, 2013, Mosby.

a documentation system for nursing care plans. These programs use standardized nursing language, including NANDA, NOC, and NIC taxonomies. This enables nurses and other health care providers to quickly identify a patient's needs and situation. Although EHR plans often follow a standard format, you customize each plan to the needs of the unique patient. Patients also benefit from standardized language because it promotes continuity of care and standardizes communications.

A **nursing care plan** includes nursing diagnoses, goals and/or expected outcomes, and individualized nursing interventions. This plan promotes continuity of care because it allows all health care providers to identify a patient's needs and interventions and reduces the risk for incomplete, incorrect, or inaccurate care. The plan is a guideline for coordinating nursing care, promoting continuity of care, and listing outcome criteria for the evaluation of care.

Besides addressing a patient's short-term problems, the care plan also addresses the patient's long-term needs. You incorporate the goals of the care plan into discharge planning. All patients benefit from this level of continuity of care, especially those who need long-term rehabilitation in the community and those who require home care. Same-day surgeries and earlier discharges from hospitals also require

DOMAIN 4	DOMAIN 5	DOMAIN 6	DOMAIN 7
4. Safety Care that supports protection against harm	**5. Family** Care that supports the family unit	**6. Health System** Care that supports effective use of the health care delivery system	**7. Community** Care that supports the health of the community
U *Crisis Management:* Interventions to provide immediate short-term help in both psychological and physiological crises V *Risk Management:* Interventions to initiate risk-reduction activities and continue monitoring risks over time	W *Childbearing Care:* Interventions to assist in understanding and coping with the psychological and physiological changes during the childbearing period Z *Childrearing Care:* Interventions to assist in rearing children X *Life Span Care:* Interventions to facilitate family unit functioning and promote the health and welfare of family members throughout the life span	Y *Health System Mediation:* Interventions to facilitate the interface between patient/family and the health care system a *Health System Management:* Interventions to provide and enhance support services for the delivery of care b *Information Management:* Interventions to facilitate communication among health care providers	c *Community Health Promotion:* Interventions that promote the health of the whole community d *Community Risk Management:* Interventions that assist in detecting or preventing health risks to the whole community

you as the nurse to begin planning discharge needs from the moment a patient enters a health care agency. The adaptation of the care plan enhances the continuity of nursing care between nurses working in hospital settings and nurses working in community agencies (Nielsen et al., 2015). Fig. 9.7 provides an example of the care plan format used throughout this text.

Hand-Off Reporting. Part of planning is transferring essential information from one nurse to another. This is often called hand-off reporting, which offers a health care provider accepting the care of a patient the opportunity to ask questions to clarify and confirm important details about the patient's plan of care, patient progress, and continuing needs during the transfer of information. A correctly formulated nursing care plan facilitates a hand-off report as one nurse communicates to another nurse (see Chapter 10). You learn to focus your reports on the nursing care, treatments, and expected outcomes documented in your care plans. During end-of-shift hand-off or when transferring a patient, you can discuss the care plan and the patient's overall progress with the next caregiver. Thus all nurses are able to discuss current and relevant information about the patient's plan of care.

Student Care Plans. Student care plans help you learn the problem-solving technique, the nursing process, skills of written communication, and organizational skills needed for nursing care. Most important, the student care plan enables you to apply knowledge gained from the nursing and medical literature and the classroom to a practice situation.

Students typically write care plans for each nursing diagnosis, using a columnar format with columns for assessment findings, goals, expected outcomes, nursing interventions with supporting rationales, and evaluative outcome criteria. The student care plan is more detailed than a care plan in a hospital or community health care agency because its purpose is to teach the process of planning care. Each nursing school uses a different format for its student care plans.

Concept Mapping. In the Nursing Diagnosis section, you were introduced to a concept map for Mrs. Tillman that displayed relevant assessment data and four interrelated nursing diagnoses. To complete Mrs. Tillman's concept map, you add individualized nursing interventions (Fig. 9.8). As you further develop the concept map, you must think critically, organize information, understand complex relationships among nursing diagnoses and nursing interventions,

CARE PLAN   Death Anxiety

ASSESSMENT

Rich learns in his initial discussions with Mrs. Tillman that she feels a sense of dread and uncertainty about the course of cancer. Mrs. Tillman shares her emotions through crying and sadness in the way she looks down and has difficulty talking about her condition. She admitted to Rich that her greatest fear is not knowing if she might suffer from her disease. Rich knows from his review of pathophysiology the probable course of the patient's disease and the type of palliative care treatments her physician will recommend. He decides to assess further the extent of her death anxiety.

ASSESSMENT ACTIVITIES	FINDINGS*
Ask Mrs. Tillman to discuss her concerns about the effect her illness will have on her husband.	Patient is **concerned about strain on her husband** and that he will begin to have more physical problems.
Have Mrs. Tillman explain what she fears most about having a terminal illness.	Patient states that she **fears loss of her mental thought processes and pain**
Question Mrs. Tillman about her desire to be able to make decisions regarding palliative care.	Patient expresses fear of ***powerlessness*** and having little control over what will happen.

*Defining characteristics/risk factors** are shown in **bold** type.

NURSING DIAGNOSIS: Death Anxiety related to anticipation of suffering

PLANNING

GOAL	EXPECTED OUTCOMES (NOC)†
	Anxiety Level
Mrs. Tillman will state, within 3 weeks, that she believes she will have a comfortable death.	Patient will verbalize feeling less anxious about the course of her disease in 1 week.
	Patient uses relaxation techniques when anxiety heightens by 2 weeks.
	Participation in Health Care Decisions
	Patient is able to specify her priorities in palliative care plan in 2 weeks.
	Patient and husband establish end-of-life care plan in 3 weeks.

†Outcomes classification labels from Moorhead S, et al, editors: *Nursing outcomes classification (NOC)*, ed 5, St Louis, 2013, Mosby.

INTERVENTIONS (NIC)‡	RATIONALE
Anxiety Reduction	
Plan a palliative care conference with patient, husband, and health care team and provide factual information on treatment options and availability of respite care for husband.	Information that helps patients understand their condition, disease course, and the benefits and burdens of treatment options reduces anxiety (Suhonen et al., 2011). Interventions designed to meet individualized needs preserves autonomy and lessens uncertainty (Suhonen et al., 2011).
Instruct patient in guided imagery and passive relaxation exercises.	Patients with advanced disease such as cancer require a moderate expenditure of energy to perform active progressive relaxation exercise. This can increase a person's existing fatigue. Passive relaxation and guided imagery are more appropriate options (Koithan, 2017).
Explore community resources for a short-term education group for Carl that teaches self-care tools to reduce stress.	Education groups help caregivers develop self-care tools to reduce stress, charge negative self-talk, communicate more effectively, and make difficult decisions (Cope, 2015; Flagg, 2015).

FIG 9.7 Nursing care plan.

CARE PLAN   Death Anxiety—cont'd

INTERVENTIONS (NIC)‡	**RATIONALE**
Explain specifically how palliative care measures will reduce symptoms patient is most anxious about.	You can lessen anxiety in terminally ill patients by explaining and managing underlying causes of anxiety (Matzo and Sherman, 2015). For example, improving a patient's breathing and oxygenation helps to decrease anxiety (McClurg, 2017).
Decision-Making Support	
Provide information requested by patient, and help to identify advantages and disadvantages of all alternatives.	Respect for a patient's autonomy involves a commitment to support a patient's ability to make decisions in a well-informed way.
Facilitate a discussion between patient and husband about end-of-life treatment preferences regarding life-extending treatment.	Difficult end-of-life decisions complicate the survivor's grief and create family divisions. When these decisions are handled well and patient's symptoms are controlled, families experience a meaningful conclusion to the loved one's death (McClurg, 2017).

‡Intervention classification labels from Bulechek GM et al, editors: *Nursing interventions classification (NIC)*, ed 6, St Louis, 2013, Mosby.

EVALUATION

NURSING ACTIONS	**PATIENT RESPONSE/FINDING**	**ACHIEVEMENT OF OUTCOME**
Question Mrs. Tillman about level of anxiety she feels.	Patient states she feels less worried about suffering. "I know what I'm facing, and I know what they can give me when I have trouble breathing."	Patient obtaining control over anxiety; accepting course of her disease.
Ask Mr. Tillman if Mrs. Tillman practices guided imagery at home.	Husband reports patient uses guided imagery each afternoon for a period of 20 minutes.	Patient is applying anxiety control technique effectively in the home.
Have Mrs. Tillman discuss her feelings about an end-of-life care plan.	Patient is planning to discuss feelings with husband. Has not finalized plan yet. Wants to know more about respite care for husband.	Further discussion and support necessary to help patient and husband finalize an end-of-life care plan.

FIG 9.7, cont'd

and integrate theoretical knowledge into practice (Daley and Torre, 2010; Lhussier et al., 2015).

Fig. 9.8 is a visual representation of Mrs. Tillman's diagnoses and the nursing interventions for each diagnosis. Using a concept map will help you make better clinical decisions, develop better clinical judgment, and provide better patient-centered care (Gerdeman et al., 2013). It forms a picture of each patient's diagnoses and the interconnections between the assessment data and nursing interventions associated with the patient problems.

Concept mapping also helps you develop reflective thinking skills (Box 9.7). These skills will help you understand that patient care, patient information, nursing diagnoses, interdisciplinary interventions, and patient outcomes all are interrelated and prioritized to produce a plan of care.

As Mrs. Tillman's nurse, Rich's next step is to plan interventions for each of her nursing diagnoses. At the same time,

he must recognize that each intervention can apply to more than one diagnosis (see Fig. 9.8).

Use these tips to help you develop a complete concept map:
1. Begin by reviewing the patient's clinical assessment data. Verify that this information is current.
2. Review all information about the patient's health problems, treatments, and medications in course textbooks, scientific literature, and other related resources.
3. Review any standardized nursing care plans, clinical pathways, protocols, or patient education materials developed for patients on the nursing unit.
4. Prepare the concept map by first developing a skeleton diagram of the patient's health problems. Write the patient's primary health problems and key assessment priorities in the middle of the map. Next add boxes for the patient's nursing care needs like spokes on a wheel.

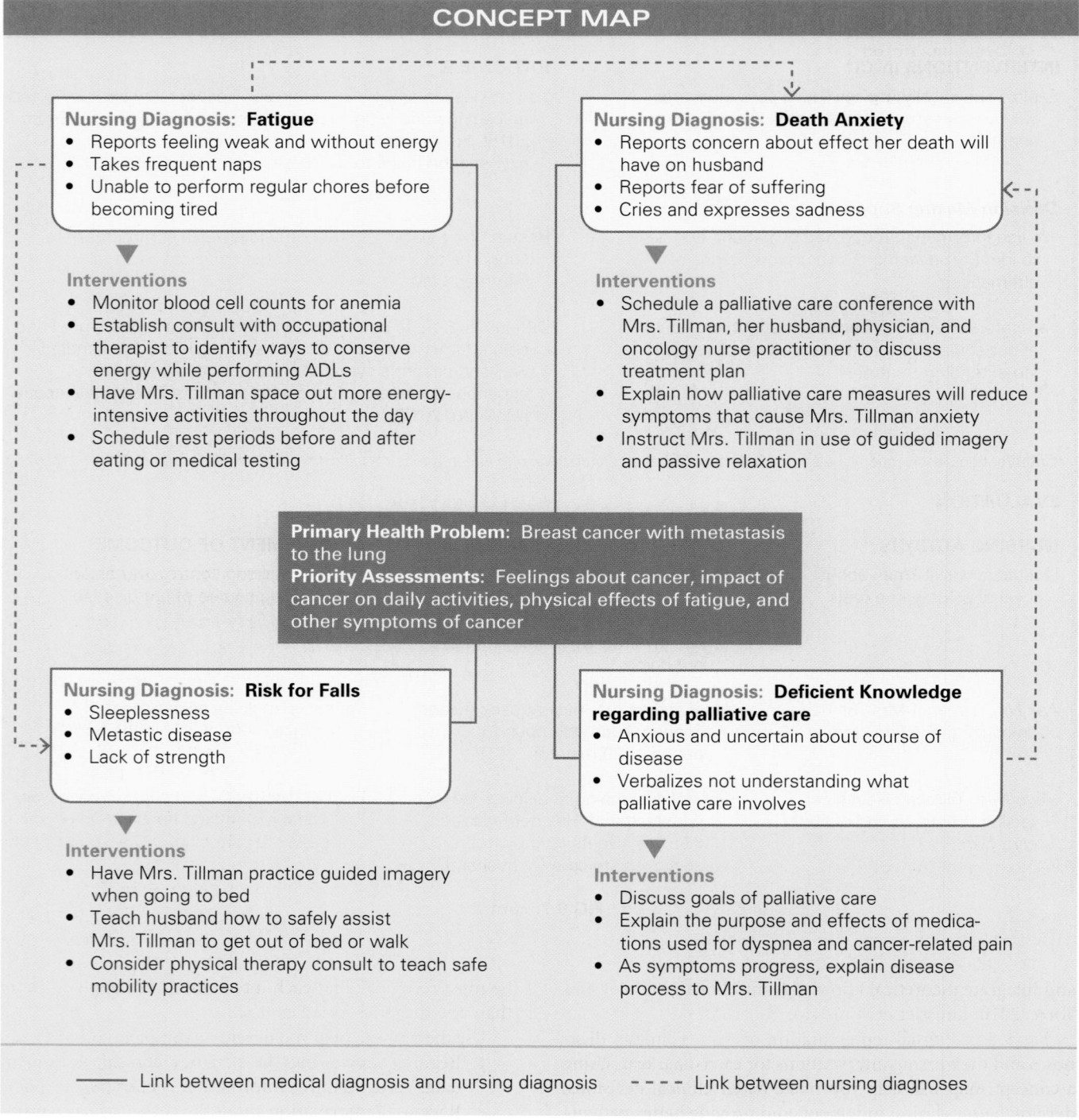

CONCEPT MAP

Nursing Diagnosis: Fatigue
- Reports feeling weak and without energy
- Takes frequent naps
- Unable to perform regular chores before becoming tired

Interventions
- Monitor blood cell counts for anemia
- Establish consult with occupational therapist to identify ways to conserve energy while performing ADLs
- Have Mrs. Tillman space out more energy-intensive activities throughout the day
- Schedule rest periods before and after eating or medical testing

Nursing Diagnosis: Death Anxiety
- Reports concern about effect her death will have on husband
- Reports fear of suffering
- Cries and expresses sadness

Interventions
- Schedule a palliative care conference with Mrs. Tillman, her husband, physician, and oncology nurse practitioner to discuss treatment plan
- Explain how palliative care measures will reduce symptoms that cause Mrs. Tillman anxiety
- Instruct Mrs. Tillman in use of guided imagery and passive relaxation

Primary Health Problem: Breast cancer with metastasis to the lung
Priority Assessments: Feelings about cancer, impact of cancer on daily activities, physical effects of fatigue, and other symptoms of cancer

Nursing Diagnosis: Risk for Falls
- Sleeplessness
- Metastic disease
- Lack of strength

Interventions
- Have Mrs. Tillman practice guided imagery when going to bed
- Teach husband how to safely assist Mrs. Tillman to get out of bed or walk
- Consider physical therapy consult to teach safe mobility practices

Nursing Diagnosis: Deficient Knowledge regarding palliative care
- Anxious and uncertain about course of disease
- Verbalizes not understanding what palliative care involves

Interventions
- Discuss goals of palliative care
- Explain the purpose and effects of medications used for dyspnea and cancer-related pain
- As symptoms progress, explain disease process to Mrs. Tillman

—— Link between medical diagnosis and nursing diagnosis   - - - - Link between nursing diagnoses

FIG 9.8 Concept map with interventions. *ADLs,* Activities of daily living.

5. In each box identify and group clinical assessment data that seem to form patterns. Do not worry if you have difficulty labeling nursing diagnoses at first. It is important to first recognize the major nursing care focus for the patient. Remember that sometimes symptoms apply to more than one nursing diagnosis. Repeat symptoms under different categories when appropriate.

6. Analyze relationships among the nursing diagnoses. Draw lines between nursing diagnoses to show relationships. The links must be accurate, meaningful, and complete. You must be able to explain how the nursing diagnoses are related. For example, Mrs. Tillman's nursing diagnoses of *Death Anxiety* and *Deficient Knowledge* are interrelated. In addition, her *Fatigue* nursing diagnosis influences her *Risk for Falls* nursing diagnosis.

BOX 9.7 EVIDENCE-BASED PRACTICE

PICO Question: Do educational activities using concept mapping compared with standard lecture improve students' critical thinking competencies?

SUMMARY OF EVIDENCE

Concept mapping can be used as an outcome-based strategy to develop and improve critical thinking (Jaafarpour et al., 2016). Concept mapping improves clinical decision making because it requires the student to actively participate in the learning process (Pilcher, 2011; Hsu et al., 2016). The use of concept maps in the clinical setting facilitates the acquisition and use of nursing and scientific knowledge (Gerdeman et al., 2013). In one study, students developed concept maps for patients assigned during their clinical rotations. As the students gained more clinical experience, they were able to draw on the knowledge acquired from previous concept maps to improve critical thinking and plan patient-centered care. The concept maps also helped students to identify multiple concerns affecting patients. The use of concept

maps encourages interprofessional collaboration (Daley and Torre, 2010). Concept maps help students better understand how different health care disciplines interact to provide individualized patient care in a timely and cost-effective manner.

APPLICATION TO NURSING PRACTICE

- An actual or simulated learning concept map improves pre-clinical preparation and increases student self-confidence in both simulated laboratory and clinical settings (Samawi et al., 2014).
- Consistent use of concept maps in clinical practice and discussion with faculty facilitate clinical decision making (Pilcher, 2011; Gerdeman et al., 2013).
- Concept maps encourage understanding of complex relationships between patients' health care problems, outcomes of care, and nursing interventions (Hsu et al., 2016).
- Use of concept maps between multiple health care disciplines fosters a holistic view of patients and better understanding of multiple concerns (Daley and Torre, 2010).

7. List on the map the nursing interventions that you select to attain the outcomes for each nursing diagnosis.
8. While caring for your patient, write down the patient's responses to each nursing activity. Also write your clinical impressions and inferences about the patient's progress toward expected outcomes and the effectiveness of interventions. Use the concept map as a working tool and revise as needed.

Consulting Other Health Care Professionals

Planning requires consultation with other members of the health care team. Consultation can occur at any step in the nursing process, but you consult most often during planning and implementation. During these steps, you are more likely to identify a problem requiring additional knowledge, skills, or community or agency resources.

Consultation is a process in which you seek the expertise of a specialist to help you identify methods of handling problems in patient care or implementation of therapies. For example, you might consult a clinical nurse specialist. Consultation is based on the problem-solving approach, and the consultant is the stimulus for change. An experienced nurse often is a valuable consultant when you face an unfamiliar patient care situation. Through consultation and collaboration, you use the best available resources to individualize nursing actions to produce expected outcomes.

When to Consult. You consult when you identify a problem that you cannot solve using your own knowledge, skills, and resources. Consulting with other care providers increases your knowledge about the patient's problems and helps you learn skills and use additional resources.

A good time to consult with another health care professional is when you cannot identify the patient's precise

problem. An objective consultant enters the situation and more clearly assesses the patient and identifies the problem. Sometimes consultations occur with other health care providers in your clinical area; however, phone consultations are also effective.

How to Consult. Begin with your own understanding of a patient's clinical problems. The following list contains important steps to follow in the consultation process:

- Identify the general problem area.
- Choose an appropriate nurse, social worker, dietitian, or other professional to help you identify the problem.
- Provide the consultant with relevant information and resources about the problem area. Include a relevant summary of the problem, methods used to resolve the problem so far, and outcomes of the methods. Share information from the patient's medical record and conversations with nurses, other members of the health team, and the patient's family caregiver.
- Do not prejudice or influence consultants. Consultants help to identify and resolve a nursing problem. Biasing or prejudicing can block problem resolution. Avoid bias by not overloading consultants with subjective and emotional conclusions about a patient and problem.
- Be available to discuss the consultant's findings and recommendations. When you request a consultation, provide a private, comfortable atmosphere for the consultant and the patient. However, this does not mean that you leave the environment. A common mistake is turning the whole problem over to the consultant. The consultant is not there to take over the problem but to help you resolve it. When possible, request the

consultation for a day when both you and the consultant are working and during a time when there are few distractions.

- Include the consultant's recommendations in the care plan. The success of the advice depends on the implementation of the problem-solving strategies. Follow up with the consultant about the outcomes.

IMPLEMENTATION

Implementation, the fourth step of the nursing process, begins after you develop the care plan. It involves providing care to patients. Implementation is the performance of nursing interventions necessary for achieving the goals and expected outcomes of nursing care. A nursing intervention is any treatment based on clinical judgment and knowledge that a nurse performs to enhance patient outcomes (Bulechek et al., 2013). Ideally the nurse uses evidence-based nursing interventions (see Chapter 7). Interventions include both direct and indirect care measures provided to individuals, families, and the community.

Direct care interventions are treatments performed through interactions with patients. Examples are medication administration, insertion of an IV catheter, and counseling during a time of grief. Indirect care interventions are treatments performed away from but on behalf of the patient or group of patients (Bulechek et al., 2013). Examples are actions aimed at managing the patient's environment (safety and infection control), documentation, and interdisciplinary collaboration.

Both direct and indirect care interventions fall under the categories discussed earlier: independent nursing (nurse-initiated), dependent nursing (health care provider–initiated), and collaborative interventions. For example, the direct care intervention of patient education is an independent nursing intervention. The indirect intervention of consultation is a collaborative intervention.

Standard Nursing Interventions

Health care settings offer opportunities for nurses to create and individualize patient care plans. Although it is critical for each patient to have his or her own unique set of interventions, many health care systems have mechanisms for standardizing the more common types of interventions or approaches to care. Many patients have common health problems. Thus standardized interventions assist nurses to intervene more efficiently. Standard interventions are set at a level of excellence for practice. Nurse-initiated and health care provider–initiated standardized interventions include clinical practice guidelines, protocols, standing orders, and NIC. The ANA defines standards of professional nursing practice, which include standards for the implementation step of the nursing process (ANA, 2010).

Clinical Practice Guidelines and Protocols. A clinical practice guideline or protocol is a systematically developed set of statements. Guidelines are based on an authoritative examination of current scientific evidence. The guideline helps nurses and other health care providers choose appropriate interventions for specific clinical circumstances. Guidelines are key tools for improving the quality of patient care.

The AHRQ National Guideline Clearinghouse (NGC) is a resource for evidence-based clinical practice guidelines (NGC, n.d.). This site is continually updated and provides nurses and other health care providers easy access to current guidelines on many topics such as low back pain, dizziness, or deep vein thrombosis.

Clinicians within a health care agency review the scientific literature and their own standard of practice to create a clinical practice guideline. Some guidelines are already developed by national health groups such as the National Institutes of Health, INS, and NGC. These clinical guidelines are available to any clinician or agency that wishes to adopt evidence-based guidelines in patient care.

Ongoing review of scientific literature and best practices leads to the development of care bundles for a variety of conditions. A care bundle is a group of interventions related to a disease process or condition. These interventions, when executed together, result in better patient outcomes than when implemented individually. The aim for the care bundle is to ensure that patients receive quality care and achieve positive outcomes while preventing the most common complications associated with their diagnoses (Goldstone et al., 2015). Examples of care bundles include, but are not limited to, sepsis management, prevention of central line–associated bloodstream infection (CLABSI), and prevention of ventilator-associated pneumonia (VAP). As you move through clinical practice you will study specific bundles in later chapters of this text.

In acute care settings it is common to find clinical protocols that outline independent nursing interventions for specific conditions. Examples are protocols for admission and discharge, pressure injury care, and fall prevention. Protocols are also used in interdisciplinary settings for diagnostic testing and physical, occupational, and speech therapies.

A standing order is a preprinted document containing orders for conducting routine therapies, monitoring guidelines, or diagnostic procedures for specific patients with identified clinical problems. A standing order directs the specific interventions to be used in specific clinical settings. Licensed, prescribing health care providers in charge of care at the time of implementation approve and sign standing orders. These orders are common in critical care settings and other specialized practice settings in which patients' needs can change rapidly and require immediate attention. For example, a standing order might specify certain medications such as diltiazem or propranolol for an irregular heart rhythm. After assessing a patient and identifying the irregular rhythm, the critical care nurse gives the specified medication without first notifying the health care provider because his or her initial standing order covers the nurse's action. After completing a standing order, the nurse notifies the health care provider. Standing orders are also common in the community health setting, where nurses face situations that do not permit immediate contact with a physician or health care provider. Standing orders give you the legal protection to intervene appropriately in the patient's best interest.

Nursing Intervention Classification Interventions.

The NIC system developed by the University of Iowa differentiates nursing practice from practice of other health care professionals by offering a language that nurses can use to describe sets of actions in delivering nursing care (see Table 9.6). The NIC interventions offer a level of standardization to improve communication of nursing care across settings and compare outcomes.

Critical Thinking in Implementation

Selecting nursing interventions for your patient is part of clinical decision making. Strong clinical reasoning and decision-making skills help you accurately identify appropriate nursing interventions for a patient's specific nursing diagnoses and achieve appropriate patient outcomes. The critical thinking model discussed in Chapter 8 provides a framework for decision making when implementing nursing care. Your knowledge about your patient's health problems leads you to select appropriate therapies. For example, in Mrs. Tillman's case, knowledge of the disease course of metastatic cancer assists Rich in selecting interventions for pain relief, fatigue, and breathing alterations. His knowledge of the NIC classification directs him to select specific care activities for each of Mrs. Tillman's nursing diagnoses.

Apply prior clinical experiences in performing specific interventions. Consider which interventions have worked before and which have not worked in previous clinical situations. Be aware of both professional and agency standards of practice. Standards of practice offer guidelines for selection of interventions, their frequency, and the determination of whether the procedures may be delegated. In Mrs. Tillman's case, the NGC has a guideline for cancer pain management that would be very helpful (NGC, n.d.). As you perform any nursing intervention, apply intellectual standards. For example, when teaching patients a self-care procedure your language should be relevant, clear, and logical to promote patient learning (see Chapter 12). All critical thinking attitudes such as confidence, creativity, and discipline apply to implementation. A beginning student needs supervision from an instructor or experienced nurse to guide the decision-making process for implementation.

Implementation Process

Preparation for implementation ensures efficient, safe, and effective nursing care. Perform these five preparatory activities: reassess the patient, review and revise the existing nursing care plan, organize resources and care delivery, anticipate and prevent complications, and implement nursing interventions.

Reassessing the Patient.

Patient assessment is a continuous process that occurs each time you interact with a patient. When you gather new data and identify a new nursing diagnosis you might need to reestablish priorities and modify the care plan. Creating a concept map helps you understand the relationship between nursing diagnoses and interventions. You also modify a plan when you resolve a patient's health care need. Just before implementing a nursing activity, reassess your patient. This is a partial assessment and sometimes focuses on one dimension such as level of comfort or on one system such as the cardiovascular system. The reassessment helps you decide if the proposed nursing activity is still appropriate for the patient's level of wellness. For example, you plan to assist a patient with ambulation after lunch. However, a reassessment reveals shortness of breath and increased fatigue. The occurrence of these signs and symptoms requires you to help the patient back to bed.

Reviewing and Revising the Care Plan.

Reassessment allows you to validate the patient's nursing diagnoses, review the care plan, and determine whether the nursing interventions are still appropriate. If the patient's status has changed and the nursing diagnosis and related interventions are no longer appropriate, modify the nursing care plan. An out-of-date or incorrect care plan puts the quality of nursing care at risk. Reviewing and modifying the care plan enables you to provide timely nursing interventions to best meet a patient's current needs.

There are four steps to modifying the written care plan:
1. Revise data in the assessment section to reflect a patient's current status. Date any new data to inform other health team members of the time that the change occurred.
2. Revise nursing diagnoses. Delete diagnoses that are no longer relevant and add and date any new diagnoses. Revise related factors and the patient's goals, outcomes, and priorities as needed.
3. Revise specific interventions that correspond to the new nursing diagnoses and goals. This revision should reflect the patient's present status.
4. Choose the method of evaluation for determining whether the patient achieved his or her outcomes.

Rich prepares to have a discussion with Mrs. Tillman and her husband about palliative care. Before he begins, Rich reassesses Mrs. Tillman's level of anxiety to learn more specifically about what is contributing to her worry about suffering. She explains that she has a general sense of dread and does not want to have a lot of pain. Her worries keep her from sleeping at night on a regular basis. Rich probes this further and with additional information identifies the nursing diagnosis of Disturbed Sleep Pattern. He revises his plan to focus instruction on planned comfort measures.

Organizing Resources and Delivering Care.

Organize time, equipment, and personnel to prepare for implementing nursing actions. Organizing equipment and personnel makes timely, efficient, and skilled patient care possible. Preparing for care delivery also includes preparing the environment and patient for nursing interventions.

Time Management. Providing patient-centered care is the focus of your nursing practice. You will practice within work environments that are part of the sociocultural context of a health care organization (see Chapter 13). These are busy environments, and you will assume dual roles: a patient care provider and an organizational employee. In this dual role you need to be aware of efficiency and cost control of the organization. You need to provide timely, safe, competent, and efficient care. This conveys caring and concern to your patient. Poor patient care results when you are hurried, experience interruptions, or are disorganized.

Equipment. Most nursing procedures require some equipment or supplies. Decide which supplies are necessary and determine their availability before you start implementation. Equipment should be in safe working order. Place supplies in a convenient, uncluttered location for easy access during the procedure. Be sure extra supplies are available in case of errors or accidents, but do not take them into a patient's room or open them unless they are needed. Unused equipment left in rooms must be thrown away as a loss to an agency. Wise use of supplies controls health care costs. After a procedure return any unopened supplies.

Personnel. Nursing care delivery models determine how nursing personnel deliver patient care (see Chapter 13). For example, the accountabilities of an RN in a team nursing model differ from the accountabilities of an RN in a primary nursing model. A team nurse is accountable for the specific shift in which he or she works. A primary nurse is accountable for the nursing care that a patient receives during his or her length of stay or course of visits. You are responsible for determining whether to perform an intervention or delegate it to another member of the nursing team. Your ongoing assessment of a patient directs the decision about delegation and not the intervention alone. For example, you know nursing assistive personnel (NAP) can competently ambulate patients. However, you learn that a patient experienced an increased pulse rate after walking during the previous shift; thus you decide to personally assist the patient with ambulation and evaluate his or her cardiac status.

Patient care staff work together as patients' needs demand it. If a patient makes a request such as for use of a bedpan, position the patient on the pan if you have time rather than trying to find NAP. When interventions are complex or physically difficult, you may need assistance from colleagues. For example, you are more effective in performing procedures when NAP help you position a patient and hand you supplies during the procedure.

Environment. A patient care environment needs to be safe and conducive for implementing therapies. Patient safety is your first concern. When the patient has sensory deficits, physical disabilities, or an alteration in level of consciousness, arrange the environment to prevent injury (e.g., provide assistive devices such as walkers or eyeglasses, rearrange furniture and equipment, and make rooms free of clutter). Make sure that lighting is adequate to perform procedures correctly.

Patient. Before you deliver interventions, be sure your patients are as physically and psychologically comfortable as possible. For example, symptoms such as nausea or pain interfere with a patient's full concentration and cooperation. Offer comfort measures before initiating interventions to help the patient participate more fully. If you need a patient to be alert, give a dose of pain medication to relieve discomfort but not impair mental faculties (e.g., ability to follow instruction, reasoning, and communication). If a patient is fatigued, delay ambulation until after he or she has had a chance to rest. Be aware of the patient's level of endurance and plan the amount of activity that the patient can tolerate comfortably. Even if symptoms are not a factor, make the patient physically comfortable during interventions. Start any intervention by controlling environmental factors, positioning, and taking care of other physical needs (e.g., elimination).

Knowing a patient's psychosocial needs enables you to create a supportive emotional climate. Some patients feel reassured by having a significant other present for encouragement and moral support. Other strategies include planning sufficient time or multiple opportunities for patients to work through and vent feelings and anxieties. Adequate preparation allows a patient to obtain maximal benefit from each intervention.

Anticipating and Preventing Complications. Risks to patients come from both illness and treatment. Observe for and recognize these risks, adapt your choice of interventions to each situation, evaluate the relative benefit of the treatment versus the risk, and take risk-prevention measures. Many conditions place patients at risk for complications. For example, a patient who had a stroke has limited mobility and is at risk for developing pressure injury.

Nurses are often the first ones to detect changes in patients' conditions. Your knowledge of pathophysiology and previous patient care experiences help identify or anticipate possible complications. A thorough assessment reveals the level of a patient's current risk. Scientific rationales for the effectiveness of certain interventions (e.g., turning and use of pressure-relief devices) to prevent or minimize complications help you select the most useful preventive measures. Some nursing procedures pose risks for patients. Be aware of potential complications and take precautions. For example, the patient with a urinary catheter is at risk for infection. In this situation implementing catheter-associated urinary tract infection (CAUTI) guidelines for urinary tract infection prevention reduces infection risk (see Chapter 36).

Identifying Areas of Assistance. Certain patient care situations require you to obtain assistance by seeking additional personnel, knowledge, or nursing skills. Before beginning care, review the plan to determine the need for assistance and the type required. Sometimes you need help performing a procedure, providing comfort measures, or preparing a patient for a procedure. For example, when you care for a patient who is overweight and immobilized, you require safe patient handling equipment and additional personnel to safely turn and position the patient. Be sure to determine in advance the number of additional personnel and when you need them. Discuss your need for assistance with potential resources such as other nurses or NAP.

You require additional knowledge and skills in situations in which you are less familiar or experienced. For example, seek additional knowledge when you give a new medication or implement a new procedure. You find such information in a hospital formulary or procedure book. If you are still uncertain about the new medication or procedure, ask other members of the health care team for help.

Because of the continual growth in health care technology, you may lack the skills needed to perform a new procedure. When this occurs, first locate information about the procedure in the literature and in the agency's policies and procedures. The agency's policies and procedures are usually available online or in print. Second, collect all equipment necessary for the procedure. Last, ask another nurse who is experienced in performing the procedure to provide assistance and guidance. The assistance can come from another staff nurse, supervisor, educator, or nurse specialist. Requests for assistance are common, are part of the learning process, and continue during education and into professional development.

Implementation Skills. Nursing practice requires cognitive, interpersonal, and psychomotor (technical) skills. You need each of these skills to implement direct and indirect nursing interventions. You are responsible for knowing when one type of implementation skill is preferred over another and for having the necessary knowledge and skill to perform each.

Cognitive Skills. Cognitive skills involve the application of critical thinking in the nursing process. Always use good judgment and sound clinical decision making when performing any intervention. This ensures that no nursing action is automatic. Always think and anticipate so that you individualize patient care appropriately. Know the rationale for therapeutic interventions and understand normal and abnormal physiological and psychological responses. Know the evidence to ensure that you deliver the most current and relevant nursing interventions.

Interpersonal Skills. Interpersonal skills are essential to effective nursing action. Develop a trusting relationship, express caring, and communicate clearly with the patient and family caregiver (see Chapter 11). Effective communication is critical for keeping patients informed, for teaching, and for supporting patients who have challenging emotional needs. Your interpersonal skills should enable you to perceive a patient's verbal and nonverbal communications accurately. As a member of the health care team, you must communicate patient problems and needs clearly, intelligently, and promptly.

Psychomotor Skills. Psychomotor skills require the integration of cognitive and motor activities. For example, when you take a pulse you must understand anatomy and physiology (cognitive) and assume the proper positioning and use of touch to detect the pulse correctly (motor). With time and practice you learn to perform skills correctly, smoothly, and confidently. This is critical in establishing patient trust. You are responsible for acquiring necessary psychomotor skills. In

the case of a new skill, assess your level of competency and obtain the necessary resources to ensure that the patient receives safe treatment.

Direct Care

Nurses provide a wide variety of direct care measures (i.e., activities that nurses perform with patient interaction). Remain sensitive to a patient's clinical condition, values and beliefs, expectations, and cultural views. All direct care measures require competent, safe practice. Show a caring approach when you provide direct care.

Activities of Daily Living. Activities of daily living (ADLs) are activities usually performed during a normal day and include ambulation, eating, dressing, bathing, and grooming. A patient's need for assistance with ADLs may be temporary or permanent. A patient with impaired mobility because of bilateral arm casts has a temporary need for assistance. After the casts are removed, the patient gradually regains the strength and range of motion needed to perform ADLs. A patient with an irreversible injury to the cervical spinal cord is paralyzed and thus has a permanent need for assistance. It is unrealistic to plan a rehabilitation goal for this patient to be independent with ADLs. Instead, through restorative care the patient learns new ways to perform ADLs to be less dependent on others.

When an assessment reveals that a patient is experiencing fatigue, a limitation in mobility, confusion, or pain, assistance with ADLs is likely needed. This assistance ranges from partial to complete care. Always consider a patient's preferences when assisting with ADLs. Consulting with a physical or occupational therapist may be helpful. Involving the patient in planning the timing and types of interventions can also increase the patient's self-esteem and willingness to become more independent.

Instrumental Activities of Daily Living. Illness or disability sometimes alters a patient's ability to be independent in society. Instrumental activities of daily living (IADLs) include skills such as shopping, preparing meals, handling finances (e.g., writing checks), and taking medications. Nurses in home care and community nursing often help patients find new ways to perform IADLs. Family caregivers and friends can be excellent resources for assisting patients. In acute care you must anticipate the effect of patients' illnesses on their ability to perform IADLs so that you can make appropriate referrals.

Physical Care Techniques. You routinely perform a variety of physical care techniques in patient care. Physical care techniques involve the safe and competent administration of nursing procedures (e.g., inserting a urinary catheter, performing range-of-motion exercises). The specific knowledge and skills needed to perform these procedures are in subsequent clinical chapters of this text. Common methods for administering physical care techniques appropriately include protecting you and the patient from injury, using proper infection control practices, staying organized, and positioning patients correctly. When you apply physical care during a procedure, know the clinical practice guidelines and how to perform the procedure, the standard frequency, and the expected outcomes.

Lifesaving Measures. A lifesaving measure is a physical care technique that you use when a patient's physiological or psychological state is threatened. The purpose of lifesaving measures is to restore physiological and psychological balance. Such measures include administering emergency medications, performing cardiopulmonary resuscitation, and protecting a violent patient. When an inexperienced nurse encounters a situation requiring emergency measures, it is critical to obtain the assistance of an experienced professional.

Counseling. Counseling helps patients use a problem-solving process to recognize and manage stress and facilitate interpersonal relationships. As a nurse, you counsel patients to accept actual or impending changes resulting from stress. Counseling includes emotional, intellectual, spiritual, and psychological support (see Chapters 26 and 27). Examples of counseling strategies are behavior modification, bereavement counseling, biofeedback, and crisis intervention. A patient and family caregiver who need nursing counseling may have normal adjustment difficulties and are upset or frustrated, but they are not necessarily psychologically disabled. A good example is the case of Mr. Tillman, who faces normal grief and the uncertainty of how cancer will affect his wife and his relationship with her.

Nurse counseling encourages patients to examine available alternatives and make useful and appropriate choices. When patients can examine alternatives, they develop a sense of control and can better manage stress. Patients with severe depression, schizophrenia, or other psychiatric diagnoses require specialized therapy provided by mental health care nurses, social workers, psychologists, or psychiatrists.

Teaching. Teaching is an important nursing responsibility. The teaching-learning process is an active interaction between the teacher and learner in which you, the teacher, address specific learning objectives.

The focus of teaching is intellectual growth or the acquisition of new knowledge or psychomotor skills. You teach correct principles, procedures, and techniques of health care to inform patients about their health status and prepare them for self-care (see Chapter 12). When patients are unable to assume self-care, nurses focus teaching efforts on family caregivers. Teaching takes place in all health care settings. As a nurse, you are responsible for assessing the learning needs and readiness of patients and family caregivers, and you are accountable for the quality of education you deliver. Know your patients; be aware of the cultural and social factors that influence their willingness and ability to learn. Know your patient's health literacy level. Can he or she read directions or make calculations that are necessary for self-care skills?

Controlling for Adverse Reactions. An adverse reaction is a harmful or unintended effect of a medication, diagnostic test, or therapeutic intervention. Adverse reactions can follow any nursing intervention. Learn to anticipate them and know which adverse reactions to expect. Nursing actions that control for adverse reactions reduce or counteract the reaction. For example, when applying a moist heat compress, you want to prevent burns to the patient's skin. First assess the area requiring the compress. After applying the compress, check the area every 5 minutes for any adverse reaction such as excessive reddening of the skin from the heat. When administering a medication, understand the known and potential side effects of the drug. After administration of the medication, evaluate the patient's response for adverse effects. Remember that certain drugs are available to counteract side effects. Although adverse reactions are uncommon, they do occur. You must recognize the signs and symptoms of an adverse reaction and intervene promptly.

Preventive Measures. Preventive nursing actions promote health and prevent illness. Prevention includes promoting a patient's health potential, applying prescribed measures (e.g., immunizations), health teaching, and identifying risks for illness and/or trauma. Consider Mrs. Tillman's situation. Rich worries that, with her fatigue and the progressive nature of her cancer, she is likely to become weaker and less mobile and have an increased risk for falling. He recommends preventive measures to make the Tillman's home setting safer. He assesses their home environment and chooses the interventions (e.g., installing grab bars in the bath and rearranging furniture) that will improve Mrs. Tillman's safety and ability to move about in her home. All patients need nursing interventions aimed at promoting health and preventing illness. As changes in the health care system continue, there is and will be greater emphasis on health promotion and illness prevention.

Indirect Care

Indirect care measures are actions that support the effectiveness of direct care measures (Bulechek et al., 2013). Many measures are managerial in nature such as emergency cart maintenance and supply management. Much of a nurse's time is spent in indirect care activities such as consultation and preparing a hand-off report. These activities promote communication of patient information. Accurate communication ensures that direct care activities are planned and coordinated with proper resources. Delegation of care to NAP is another indirect care activity. Proper delegation ensures that the right care providers perform the right tasks so that RNs and NAP work most efficiently for their patients.

Communicating Nursing Interventions. Communicate all patient interventions in an electronic, written, or oral format (see Chapter 10). Electronic health records (EHRs) or written charts have sections for individualized interventions, which are part of a patient's nursing care plan and permanent medical record. All entries usually have a brief description of pertinent patient assessment findings, the specific interventions, and the patient's response. A patient's medical record validates that a procedure or intervention was performed, and provides valuable information to subsequent caregivers. Some institutions have interdisciplinary care plans, which represent the contributions of all disciplines caring for a patient. Enter your nursing interventions into the plan, documenting the treatment and patient's response (see Chapter 10). Effective communication and teamwork among all health care professionals reduce medical errors and prevent adverse events. Miscommunication is often the root cause for most reported or sentinel events that occur in health care organizations. (ECRI, 2017).

Delegating, Supervising, and Evaluating Work of Other Staff Members. The nurse who develops the care plan frequently does not perform all the nursing interventions. Nurses delegate some activities to other members of the health care team (see Chapter 13). Remember that an RN delegates components of care but not the nursing process itself (ANA and National Council of State Boards of Nursing [NCBSN], 2012). You can assign noninvasive and repetitive interventions to certified nurse assistants and other NAP. These activities include skin care, ambulation, grooming, and hygiene measures. Licensed practical nurses (LPNs) perform these measures in addition to medication administration and many invasive tasks. For example, LPNs may perform dressing care and catheterization.

The nursing tasks or activities that members of the nursing team perform under the direction of an RN are identified according to legal parameters defined by each state in its Nurse Practice Act and by the scope of practice and standards established by professional nursing organizations (ANA, 2010). When you delegate aspects of care to another staff member, you are responsible for assigning the task and ensuring that the staff member completes the task according to the standard of care. You are also responsible for delegating direct care interventions to personnel competent to provide the care.

EVALUATION

Evaluation is the crucial step of determining whether a patient's condition or well-being improved after an intervention was delivered (see Fig. 9.7). During evaluation you examine the patient's condition or situation and then decide whether change has occurred.

The evaluation determines if the nursing care was effective. Apply all that you know about a patient and the patient's condition together with experience with previous patients. You conduct this evaluation to determine if expected outcomes are met, not if nursing interventions were completed. *For example, in Rich's plan of care for Mrs. Tillman, he established the outcome of "The patient will verbalize feeling less anxious about the course of her disease within 1 week." Rich implements educational interventions to improve Mrs. Tillman's knowledge and anxiety-reduction exercises.* Evaluation

does involve questioning Mrs. Tillman about her feelings toward her disease. Evaluation *does not* involve observation of her performing anxiety-reduction exercises. Expected outcomes are the standards against which you judge if goals have been met and care is successful.

Critical Thinking and Evaluation

Critical thinking is key to evaluation. Evaluation is an ongoing process that you conduct while caring for a patient. After you complete an intervention, use evaluative measures to gather subjective and objective data from the patient, family, and health care team members. This includes reviewing knowledge about a patient's current condition, treatment, and resources available for recovery. By referring to previous experiences caring for similar patients, you are in a better position to know how to evaluate outcomes of care. Then apply critical thinking attitudes and standards to determine whether outcomes of care are achieved. If outcomes are met, the overall goals for the patient are also met.

The evaluation process includes a before-and-after comparison. Compare patient behavior and responses assessed before delivering nursing interventions with behavior and responses that occur after administering nursing care. *For example, Rich's initial assessment revealed Mrs. Tillman's sense of anxiety about her impending death and uncertainty about her course of illness. On a subsequent clinic visit he considers the following questions: Has the patient's condition improved? Can the patient improve, or are there physical or psychological factors preventing recovery? To what degree does the patient's emotional health influence response to therapies? To evaluate Mrs. Tillman's progress, he asks her how she now feels about the cancer and its anticipated effects. She is able to talk about her cancer without crying. She also tells Rich, "I think I have a better idea of what to expect; but, more important, I know my doctor will do all he can to make me comfortable." The evaluation shows that the patient has a better sense of control over her condition.*

During evaluation you make clinical decisions and continually redirect nursing care. For example, when evaluating a patient for a change in pain severity, you apply knowledge of disease processes, physiological responses to interventions, and the correct procedure for measuring pain severity to interpret whether a change has occurred and if it is desirable. If a patient continues to report pain at a higher level on the pain scale than expected, you consult with the health care provider to increase an analgesic dose or try different noninvasive approaches to help the patient relax and concentrate less on the pain. You continue to evaluate until the patient achieves pain relief.

When expected outcomes are met, you conclude that the nursing interventions effectively met the patient's goals. Negative evaluations or undesired results indicate that the interventions were not effective in meeting the outcomes of care (e.g., resolving the actual problem or avoiding a potential problem). Sometimes new data reveal that a patient's condition altered the patient's ability to meet the expected outcome. As a result, change the care plan and try different therapies or a different approach in administering existing therapies.

This sequence of critically evaluating and revising therapies continues until you and the patient appropriately resolve the problems. Outcomes must be realistic and adjusted based on the patient's prognosis and nursing diagnoses. Evaluation is dynamic and ever changing, depending on a patient's nursing diagnoses and condition. A patient whose health status continuously changes requires more frequent evaluation. In addition, priority diagnoses are usually evaluated first. For example, you evaluate a patient's *Acute Pain* before evaluating the status of *Deficient Knowledge*.

Evaluation Process

The evaluation process includes five elements: (1) comparing achieved effect with goals and outcomes, (2) collecting data to determine if your patient met the criteria or standards, (3) interpreting and summarizing findings, (4) recognizing errors or unmet outcomes, and (5) revising the care plan as needed.

Comparing Achieved Effect With Goals and Outcomes.
Evaluation is most effective when you know what to observe or measure. During evaluation you compare your findings with the goals and expected outcomes set for your patient. Critical thinking directs you to analyze evaluation data. Did the patient reach a level of wellness or recovery that was reflected in the goals of care? Are there factors that prevent achievement of goals? Has the patient's condition changed?

Collecting Data.
Evaluate a patient's response to nursing care using evaluative measures, which are simply assessment skills and techniques (e.g., auscultation of lung sounds, observation of a patient's skill performance, or discussion of the patient's feelings). In fact, evaluative measures are the same as assessment measures, but you perform them after the nursing intervention at the point of care when you prepare to make decisions about a patient's status and progress. The intent of the original assessment is to identify what, if any, problem exists. The purpose of the evaluation is to determine whether the identified problems have remained the same, improved, worsened, or otherwise changed.

In many clinical situations, you need to collect evaluative measures over a period of time to determine if a pattern of improvement or change exists. For example, observing a pressure injury one time will not sufficiently determine if the area of impaired skin integrity is healing. You want to see consistency in change. For example, over a period of 2 days is the pressure injury decreasing in size? Is the amount of drainage declining? Recognizing a pattern of improvement or decline allows you to reason and decide if the patient's problems are resolved.

The primary source of data for evaluation is the patient. However, you also use input from the family and other caregivers. For example, you ask a family caregiver to report on the amount of food a patient eats during a meal or how well

the patient is able to sleep during the night. You sometimes consult with colleagues about how patients responded to therapies (e.g., pain-control measures) during a previous shift. In addition to outcomes, it is important to evaluate if you met a patient's expectations of care. You evaluate patients about their perceptions of care such as, "Did you receive the type of pain relief you expected? Were you able to feel comfortable?" This level of evaluation is important to determine the patient's satisfaction with care and strengthen partnering between you and the patient.

Interpreting and Summarizing Findings.
An expert nurse recognizes relevant evidence, even if it does not match clinical expectations, and makes judgments about the patient's condition. To develop clinical judgment, you learn to match the results of evaluative measures with expected outcomes to determine whether or not a patient's status is improving. When interpreting findings you compare the patient's behavioral responses and the physiological signs and symptoms you expect to see with those you actually see during evaluation. To objectively evaluate the degree of success in achieving outcomes of care, use the following steps:

1. Examine the outcome criteria to identify the exact desired patient behavior or response.
2. Measure the patient's actual behavior or response.
3. Compare the established outcome criteria with the actual behavior or response.
4. Judge the degree of agreement between outcome criteria and the actual behavior or response.
5. If there is no agreement (or only partial agreement) between outcome criteria and patient response, why did they not agree? What barriers prevented achievement of outcomes?

Evaluation is easier to perform after you have cared for a patient over a period of time. You can then make subtle comparisons of patient responses and behaviors. When you have not had the chance to care for a patient over an extended time, you can improve your evaluation by referring to previous experiences and asking colleagues familiar with the patient to confirm evaluation findings.

Remember to evaluate each expected outcome and its place in the sequence of care. If you do not, you will have trouble identifying the unmet outcomes. This prevents you from revising and redirecting the plan of care when necessary.

Recognizing Errors or Unmet Outcomes.
During evaluation recognizing errors or unmet outcomes requires you to have an open mind, to actively pursue truth, to be patient and confident, and to engage in self-reflections (Shu-Yuan et al., 2013). You cannot assume that all your interventions will be successful. Applying your observational skills, critical thinking intellectual standards, and knowledge help you recognize the actual results of nursing interventions. You reflect on your patient care and identify possible reasons for unmet outcomes. Was the intervention specific for the patient's health care need? Did the patient's status change? Did the patient have an adverse reaction? During reflection use problem-solving

techniques to analyze and explain unmet outcomes and to identify new interventions to achieve a desired outcome.

Revising the Care Plan.
The result of the evaluation helps you decide whether to discontinue or revise the plan of care. If your patient meets a goal successfully, discontinue that part of the care plan. Unmet and partially met goals require you to continue intervention. During the evaluation process you often modify or add nursing diagnoses with appropriate goals and expected outcomes and then establish interventions. You must also redefine priorities. This is an important step in critical thinking (i.e., knowing how the patient is progressing and how problems either resolve or worsen).

Discontinuing a Care Plan. After you determine that expected outcomes and goals were met, you confirm this evaluation with the patient whenever possible. If you and the patient agree, you discontinue that part of the care plan. Documentation of a discontinued plan ensures that other nurses will not unnecessarily continue interventions for that portion of the plan of care. Continuity of care assumes that care provided to patients is relevant and timely. You waste time when you do not communicate achieved goals.

Modifying a Care Plan. When goals are not met, you must identify the factors that interfered with achieving them. A change in a patient's condition, needs, or abilities makes modifications to the care plan necessary. For example, *while monitoring Mrs. Tillman's level of fatigue, Rich learns during a follow-up visit that Mrs. Tillman is now having difficulty breathing. Her respiratory rate is elevated and shallower than her last visit. She confirms that she experiences shortness of breath, especially when climbing stairs at home. Her breathing difficulty has also aggravated her sense of fatigue. Mrs. Tillman explains, "I sometimes don't have the energy just to dress and eat." Rich knows that the breathing problem is related to progression of the cancer and thus establishes a new diagnosis,* Impaired Gas Exchange related to damaged alveolar capillary membrane.

A failure to achieve a goal can also result from an error in nursing judgment or a failure to follow each step of the nursing process. Patients often have multiple problems. Always remember the possibility of overlooking or misjudging something. When a goal is not achieved, no matter what the reason, repeat the entire nursing process sequence for that nursing diagnosis to discover changes the plan needs. Reassess the patient, determine accuracy of the nursing diagnosis, establish new goals and expected outcomes, and select new interventions.

When you modify a plan you must completely reassess all patient factors relating to the nursing diagnosis and etiology. Apply critical thinking as you compare new data about the patient's condition with previous data. Knowledge from previous experiences helps you direct the reassessment process. Caring for patients who have had similar health problems gives you a strong background of knowledge to use for anticipating patient needs and knowing what to assess. Reassessment ensures that the database is accurate and relevant (standards for critical thinking). It also reveals any missing link or piece of information that was overlooked and perhaps responsible for preventing goal achievement.

After reassessment determine which nursing diagnoses are accurate for the situation. Ask yourself whether you selected the correct diagnosis and whether the diagnosis and the etiological factors are current. Revise the problem list to reflect the patient's changed status. You may make a new diagnosis. You base nursing care on an accurate list of nursing diagnoses. Accuracy is more important than the number of diagnoses selected. As the patient's condition changes, the diagnoses do as well.

When you modify a care plan, also review the goals and expected outcomes for needed changes. Examine the goals for unchanged nursing diagnoses. Are they still appropriate? A change in one diagnosis may affect others. For example, if Mrs. Tillman now has *Impaired Gas Exchange*, it likely will require Rich to alter goals and outcomes with respect to her diagnosis of *Fatigue*. It is also important to determine that each goal and expected outcome is realistic for the problem, etiology, and time frame. Unrealistic expected outcomes and time frames make goal achievement difficult.

Clearly document goals and expected outcomes for new or revised nursing diagnoses so that all team members are aware of the revised care plan. When the goal is still appropriate but has not yet been met, you may change the evaluation date to allow more time. You may also decide at this time to change interventions. For example, when a patient's wound does not heal with a transparent dressing, you choose a different dressing material such as a colloid dressing. All goals and expected outcomes are patient centered, with realistic expectations for patient achievement.

The evaluation of interventions examines two factors: the appropriateness of the interventions selected and the correct application of the intervention. The appropriateness of an intervention is based on the standard of care for a patient's

---

QSEN QSEN ACTIVITY *Patient-Centered Care*

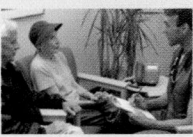

Mrs. Tillman and her husband decide to use a hospice program affiliated with the health care agency. As part of this program, her acute care nurse Rich consults with the hospice nurse assigned to the Tillman family. Mrs. Tillman is dying and is no longer responsive; her husband is at her bedside. Although symptom management and skilled nursing care remain a care priority for Mrs. Tillman, Mr. Tillman's emotional and physical needs are now the top priority of care. Rich and the hospice nurse decide that they must assess Mr. Tillman's emotional status and support and his ability to meet his basic needs.

- Which skills of assessment do they need to use to determine Mr. Tillman's needs?
- How do Rich and the hospice nurse validate Mr. Tillman's needs and individualize a patient-centered plan of care?

evolve   Answers to QSEN Activities can be found on the Evolve website.

health problem. A standard of care is the minimum level of care accepted to ensure high quality of care to patients. Standards of care define the types of therapies typically administered to patients with specific problems or needs. For example, if a patient who is receiving chemotherapy for leukemia has the nursing diagnosis *Nausea related to pharyngeal irritation,* the standard of care established by a nursing department for this problem includes pain-control measures, mouth-care guidelines, and diet therapy. The nurse reviews the standard of care to determine if the right interventions have been chosen or if additional ones are needed.

You may need to increase or decrease the frequency of interventions when you revise a care plan. Use clinical judgment based on previous experience and a patient's actual response to therapy. For example, if a patient continues to have congested lung sounds, you increase the frequency of coughing and deep-breathing exercises to remove secretions.

During evaluation you may find that some planned interventions deliver an inappropriate level of nursing care. If you need to change the level of care, substitute a different action verb, such as *assist* in place of *provide*, or *demonstrate* in place of *describe*. For example, assisting a patient with walking requires a nurse to be at the patient's side during ambulation, whereas providing an assistive device suggests that the patient is more independent. Sometimes the level of care is appropriate, but the interventions are unsuitable because of a change in the expected outcome. In this case discontinue the interventions and plan new ones.

Make any changes in the plan of care based on the nature of the patient's unfavorable response. Consulting with other health care providers often yields suggestions for improving the approach to care delivery. Practicing nurses are usually excellent resources because of their experience. Simply changing the care plan is not enough. Implement the new plan and reevaluate the patient's response to the nursing actions. Remember, *evaluation is continuous.*

▌ KEY POINTS

- The nursing process has five steps: assessment, nursing diagnosis, planning, implementation, and evaluation.
- Using critical thinking skills with each step of the nursing process helps to develop and refine clinical decision making.
- When you first meet a patient, you conduct an initial assessment screening and then focus on cues and patterns of information to complete a more comprehensive assessment.
- Subjective data are obtained from the patient's perception of a sign or symptom (e.g., level of pain or shortness of breath).
- Objective data are obtained for specific validated measures (e.g., body temperature, blood pressure).
- Data analysis involves recognizing patterns or trends, comparing data with standards, and forming a reasoned conclusion about the meaning of the data.

- Data clustering organizes assessment data into meaningful clusters of defining characteristics or sets of signs and symptoms.
- The diagnostic process includes analysis and interpretation of data, identification of patient and family needs, and formulation of nursing diagnoses and collaborative problems.
- Nursing diagnoses provide the basis for selection of nursing interventions to achieve outcomes for which a nurse is accountable.
- The absence of certain defining characteristics following a patient assessment suggests that you reject a nursing diagnosis under consideration.
- Nursing diagnostic errors may lead to inappropriate and/or inadequate nursing care.
- During the planning component, you determine patient goals, establish priorities, develop expected outcomes of nursing care, and write a nursing care plan.
- The NOC has labels for describing the focus of nursing care and includes indicators for use in measuring success with interventions.
- A nurse begins a care plan by first addressing the nursing diagnoses that have the highest priority.
- The care plan is a guideline for patient care so that all members of the health care team can quickly understand the care given.
- A concept map organizes and links data about a patient's multiple diagnoses in a logical way.
- There are three types of nursing interventions: nurse-initiated, physician-initiated, and collaborative.
- The NIC is a comprehensive standardized classification of the interventions that nurses use in the care of patients.
- You evaluate by comparing the patient's response to nursing actions with expected outcomes established during planning.
- When goals of care are not met, you identify factors that interfere with goal achievement, reassess the patient's condition, revise existing or develop new nursing diagnoses, and select appropriate interventions.

▌ REFLECTIVE LEARNING

- Think about a recent clinical experience, list three objective assessment findings and two or three subjective findings. Reflect on these findings and ask yourself if you collected complete and correct data and if you considered your patient's culture when collecting these data. How could you improve your assessment of these findings?
- Given your assessment findings listed in the previous question, identify at least two nursing diagnostic labels. Be sure you include relevant defining characteristics collected during assessment.
- Using the same clinical experience, develop expected outcomes and nursing interventions for the patient and/or family caregiver. Reflect on why you chose these outcomes.

REVIEW QUESTIONS

1. A nurse working on a cardiac unit is assigned an 84-year-old patient who was just admitted with symptoms of lung infection. When the nurse enters the room, the nurse notices that the patient is short of breath. The patient continues to cough and has a respiratory rate of 36 breaths/min. The patient is anxious and states "I am scared." The nurse does an initial preliminary assessment and follows up 30 minutes later. The nurse's knowledge about the patient results in which of the following assessment approaches? (Select all that apply.)
   1. Problem-focused approach
   2. Structured comprehensive approach
   3. Emotion-focused approach
   4. Using multiple visits to gather a complete patient database
   5. Focusing on the functional health pattern of role-relationship

2. A patient has a pressure injury resulting from urinary incontinence and sustained pressure over the coccyx. The nursing plan of care includes a goal of "Pressure injury heals in 3 weeks." Which of the following is an evaluation measure for this goal? (Select all that apply.)
   1. Turn patient every 90 minutes.
   2. Measure the diameter of the pressure injury.
   3. Measure urine output.
   4. Monitor patient's report of discomfort during turning.
   5. Measure depth of pressure injury.

3. A nurse completes a respiratory assessment on a patient who had abdominal surgery 1 day ago. During the assessment, the nurse auscultates crackles in both lower lobes, and the patient coughs, producing light yellow sputum. The patient's body temperature is 37.0° C (98.6° F), pulse is 110 beats/min, respiratory rate is 28 breaths/min, and blood pressure is 118/82 mm Hg. Pulse oximetry was 99% and is now 93%. The nurse identifies a nursing diagnosis of *Impaired Gas Exchange*. Which of following goals is appropriate for this patient?
   1. Patient's pulse oximetry will be greater than 95%.
   2. Instruct patient to deep breathe and cough every 2 hours.
   3. Patient's lungs will be clear to auscultation.
   4. Patient will be able to sleep through the night.

4. During the implementation step of the nursing process, a nurse reviews and revises the nursing care plan. Place the following steps of review and revision in the correct order.
   1. Review the care plan.
   2. Decide whether the nursing interventions remain appropriate.
   3. Reassess the patient.
   4. Compare assessment findings to validate existing nursing diagnosis.

5. Which of the following statements correctly describes the evaluation process? (Select all that apply.)
   1. Evaluation is an ongoing process.
   2. Evaluation usually reveals obvious changes in a patient.
   3. Evaluation involves making clinical decisions.
   4. Evaluation requires the use of assessment skills.
   5. Evaluation is performed only when the patient's condition changes.

evolve

Additional Review Questions, as well as rationales for all Review Questions, can be found on the Evolve website.

1. 1, 4; 2, 2, 5; 3, 3; 4, 3, 4, 1; 2, 5; 1, 3, 4.

REFERENCES

Ackley BJ, Ladwig GB: *Nursing diagnosis handbook*, ed 11, St Louis, 2016, Mosby.

Agency for Healthcare Research and Quality (AHRQ): *Health literacy measurement tools (revised)*, 2016. http://www.ahrq.gov/professionals/quality-patient-safety/quality-resources/tools/literacy/index.html.

American Nurses Association (ANA): *Nursing's social policy statement: the essence of the profession*, ed 3, Washington, DC, 2010, The Association.

American Nurses Association (ANA) and the National Council of State Boards of Nursing (NCBSN): *Joint statement on delegation*, 2012. https://www.ncsbn.org/Delegation_joint_statement_NCSBN-ANA.pdf.

Ball JW, et al: *Seidel's guide to physical examination*, ed 8, St Louis, 2015, Mosby.

Bertakis KD, Azari R: Determinants and outcomes of patient-centered care, *Patient Educ Counsel* 85(10):46, 2011.

Boykins A: Core communication competencies in patient-centered care, *ABNF J* 25(2):40, 2014.

Bulechek GM, et al: *Nursing interventions classification (NIC)*, ed 6, St Louis, 2013, Mosby.

Burman ME, et al: Linking evidence-based nursing practice and patient-centered care through patient preferences, *Nurs Adm Q* 37(3):231, 2013.

Canadian Interprofessional Health Collaborative: *A national interprofessional competency framework*, February 2010. http://www.cihc.ca/files/CIHC_IPCompetencies_Feb1210.pdf.

Carpenito-Moyet LJ: *Nursing diagnosis: application to clinical practice*, ed 15, Philadelphia, 2017, Lippincott Williams & Wilkins.

Chaboyer W, et al: Bedside nursing handover: a case study, *Int J Nurs Pract* 16(1):27, 2010.

Cope DG: Cultural competency in nursing research, *Oncol Nurs Forum* 42(3):305, 2015.

Daley BJ, Torre DM: Concept maps in medical education: an analytical literature review, *Med Educ* 44:440, 2010.

Darnell LK, Hickson SV: Culturally competent patient-centered nursing care, *Nurs Clin North Am* 50(1):99, 2015.

ECRI Institute: *Top 10 patient safety concerns for healthcare organizations*, 2017. https://www.ecri.org/EmailResources/PSRQ/Top10/2017_PSTop10_ExecutiveBrief.pdf.

Flagg AJ: The role of patient-centered care in nursing, *Nurs Clin North Am* 50(1): 75, 2015.

Gallagher-Lepak S: Nursing diagnosis basics. In Herdman TH, Kamitsuru S, editors: *NANDA International nursing diagnoses: definitions & classification 2015-2017*, Oxford, 2014, Wiley Blackwell.

Gerdeman JL, et al: Using concept mapping to build clinical judgement skills, *J Nurs Educ Pract* 13(1):11, 2013.

Goldstone L, et al: Bundle up: introducing care bundles to increase knowledge and confidence of senior nursing students, *Teach Learn Nurs* 10(3):143, 2015.

Herdman TH, Kamitsuru S: From assessment to diagnosis. In Herdman TH, Kamitsuru S, editors: *Nursing diagnoses: definitions & classification 2015-2017*, Oxford, 2014a, Wiley Blackwell.

Herdman TH, Kamitsuru S, editors: *Nursing diagnoses: definitions & classification 2015-2017*, Oxford, 2014b, Wiley Blackwell.

Hsu LL, et al: Randomized comparison between objective-based lectures and outcome-based concept mapping for teaching neurological care to nursing students, *Nurse Educ Today* 37:83, 2016.

Jaafarpour M, et al: Does concept mapping enhance learning outcome of nursing students?, *Nurse Educ Today* 36:129, 2016.

Jahne J: Palliative care: patient-centered assessment and communication to improve quality of life, *N M Nurse* 60(4):4, 2015.

Koithan MS: Complementary and alternative therapies. In Potter PA, et al, editors: *Fundamentals of nursing*, ed 9, St Louis, 2017, Mosby.

Lai W, et al: Does one size fit all? Exploring the cultural applicability of NANDA-I nursing diagnoses to Chinese nursing practice, *J Transcult Nurs* 24(1):43, 2013.

Lemetti T, et al: Collaboration between hospital and primary care nurses: a literature review, *Int Nurs Rev* 62:248, 2015.

Lhussier M, et al: Care planning for long-term conditions a concept mapping, *Health Expect* 18:605, 2015.

Matzo M, Sherman D: *Palliative care nursing: quality care to the end of life*, ed 4, New York, 2015, Springer.

McClurg EL: The experience of loss, death, and grief. In Potter PA, et al, editors: *Fundamentals of nursing*, ed 9, St Louis, 2017, Mosby.

Moorhead S, et al: *Nursing outcomes classification (NOC)*, ed 5, St Louis, 2013, Mosby.

National Guideline Clearinghouse (NGC): *Guidelines, Agency for Healthcare Research and Quality*, n.d. http://www.guideline.gov.

Nielsen LS, et al: Patient-centered care of cultural competence: negotiating palliative care at home for Chinese Canadian immigrants, *Am J Hosp Palliat Care* 32(4):372, 2015.

Palos GR: Care, compassion, and communication in professional nursing: art, science, or both, *Clin J Oncol Nurs* 18(2):247, 2014.

Pilcher J: Teaching and learning with concept maps, *Neonatal Netw* 30(5):336, 2011.

QSEN Institute: *Pre-licensure KSAS*, 2014. http://qsen.org/competencies/pre-licensure-ksas/.

Samawi Z, et al: Using high-fidelity simulation and concept mapping to cultivate self-confidence in nursing students, *Nurs Educ Perspect* 35(6): 408, 2014.

Shu-Yuan C, et al: Identifying critical thinking indications and critical thinker attributes in nursing practice, *J Nurs Res* 21(3):204, 2013.

Suhonen R, et al: Nurses' perceptions of individualised care: an international comparison, *J Adv Nurs* 67(9):1895, 2011.

U.S. Department of Health and Human Services (USDHHS): *Summary of the health information privacy rule*, 2017. http://www.hhs.gov/hipaa/for-professionals/privacy/laws-regulations/index.html.

Zolnierek CD: An integrative review of knowing the patient, *J Nurs Scholarsh* 46(1):3, 2014.

Informatics and Documentation

evolve MEDIA RESOURCES

http://evolve.elsevier.com/Potter/essentials

- Audio Glossary
- QSEN Activity and Review Questions Answers and Rationales

OBJECTIVES

- Identify key reasons for reporting and documenting patient care.
- Describe the concept of informatics and its relationship to the delivery of quality care.
- Compare paper-based and electronic documentation.
- Discuss legal and ethical implications associated with documentation.
- Discuss advantages of computerized documentation.
- Discuss methods for maintaining privacy and confidentiality of protected health information.

- Discuss the relationship between informatics and quality health care.
- Identify key reasons for documenting patient care.
- Describe guidelines for effective documentation in a variety of health care settings.
- Discuss legal guidelines for documentation.
- Compare different methods and forms used for documentation.
- Discuss the purpose for incident (event or occurrence) reports and why the existence of such reports should not be documented in the medical record.

KEY TERMS

CASE STUDY *Mr. Roland*

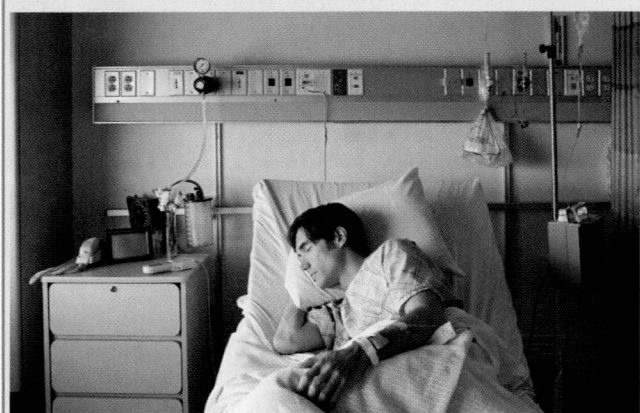

Copyright © XiXinXing/iStock/Thinkstock.

Chris is admitting Mr. Roland to the medical unit. During hand-off report received over the phone, the emergency department (ED) nurse gave the following information to Chris: "Mr. Roland is a 46-year-old construction worker who had a traumatic injury to his left lower leg and has been home on disability for the last month. He is 5' feet, 8 inches tall and weighs 200 lb. He stated he had sharp pain in his left lower leg for the last 2 days when he came to the ED. His left lower leg is swollen with large areas of redness over the anterior and medial areas that are warm and tender to touch. A diagnosis of deep vein thrombosis (DVT) was confirmed with venous ultrasound, and he has orders for treatment with bed rest and initiation of anticoagulation therapy with a continuous heparin infusion.

Chris signs on to the computer and opens Mr. Roland's electronic medical record (EMR) to review the admission orders and enter information about Mr. Roland's medical history when completing admission documentation. Chris documents that Mr. Roland has smoked one pack of cigarettes per day for the last 20 years, that he has a family history of heart disease, and that he takes a beta blocker for high blood pressure.

Reviewing the medical record, Chris notes that the ED nurse documented he inserted a 20-gauge peripheral IV in Mr. Roland's left lower forearm and converted it to a saline lock before transferring Mr. Roland to the medical unit. Chris assesses the peripheral IV site, which is free from redness, swelling, and drainage. The IV site is patent when flushed with 5 mL of sterile normal saline. Implementing the admitting orders, Chris uses the bar code medication administration function in the EMR to document administration of the provider-ordered loading dose of heparin 7300 units IV push and the initiation of a continuous heparin infusion at 3600 units/hr via the existing peripheral IV site. After Chris documents this care in the EMR, he uses the alcohol-based hand cleanser from the wall dispenser (one of the "five moments for hand hygiene") before he leaves Mr. Roland's room (World Health Organization, 2017).

Documentation is a key communication strategy between health care professionals and a vital element of nursing practice (Penoyer et al., 2014). Health care documentation consists of all information entered into a medical record, which may be electronic, paper, or a combination of both formats. The information you enter into the medical record communicates the type and frequency of patient care provided, and provides accountability for the care provided by each member of the health care team. It is necessary to document all the nursing care you provide for each patient including assessment data, interventions, and patient responses in the medical record.

The health care environment creates many challenges for accurately documenting patient care. Quality patient care depends on a nurse's ability to communicate effectively as part of an interprofessional team. You are held accountable for the accuracy of the documentation you enter into the patient's record. Regulations from agencies such as The Joint Commission (TJC) and the Centers for Medicare and Medicaid Services (CMS) require health care institutions to monitor and evaluate the quality and appropriateness of patient care (Center for Clinical Standards and Quality/Survey Certification Group, 2014; TJC, 2017). Audits of information that nurses and other health care providers document in the medical record are one way that monitoring and evaluation of the quality of care are carried out.

On October 1, 2008, the CMS implemented a policy under which hospitals are no longer reimbursed for the treatment of 11 specific hospital-acquired conditions (HAC) or preventable adverse events commonly known as never events (Department of Health and Human Services, 2008). Four of these preventable adverse events are considered "nurse-sensitive": stage III and IV pressure injuries, falls with injury, catheter-associated urinary tract infections (CAUTIs), and central line–catheter-associated bloodstream infections (CLABSI) (Bae and Yoder, 2015). Therefore, it is crucial that your documentation accurately reflects the status of the patient, especially on admission, transfer, or discharge. This chapter will help you understand the current systems and standards for health care documentation and be prepared to document effectively.

HEALTH CARE INFORMATICS

Health care informatics is the "application of computer and information science in all basic and biomedical sciences to facilitate the acquisition, processing, interpretation, optimal use, and communication of health-related data. The focus is the patient and the process of care and the goal is to enhance the quality and efficiency of care provided" (Hebda and Czar, 2013).

Health Care Information System

A health care information system (HIS) is a group of systems used within a health care organization to support and enhance health care. An HIS consists of two major types of information systems: a clinical information system (CIS) and an administrative information system. Together the two systems operate to make the entry and communication of data and information more efficient. Individual health care agencies sometimes use one or several CISs and administrative information systems. Administrative information systems include databases such as payroll, financial, and quality assurance systems.

Clinical Information System

A clinical information system (CIS) includes monitoring systems; order entry systems; and laboratory, radiology, and pharmacy systems. A monitoring system includes devices that automatically monitor and record biometric measurements (e.g., vital signs, oxygen saturation, cardiac index, stroke volume) in acute care, critical care, and specialty care areas. Some of these devices electronically send measurements directly to a nursing documentation system, decreasing nursing workload.

One example of an order-entry system is a computer program that allows nurses to order supplies and services from another department such as sterile supplies from the central supply department. This eliminates the use of written order forms and expedites the delivery of needed supplies to a nursing unit.

Another example is a computerized provider order entry (CPOE) system that allows health care providers to directly enter orders for patient care into a medical record from any computer in the hospital information system. Advanced CPOE systems have built-in reminders and alerts to help a health care provider select the most appropriate medication or diagnostic test. The direct entry of orders by providers eliminates safety issues related to illegible handwriting and transcription errors. In addition, a CPOE system potentially speeds the implementation of ordered diagnostic tests and treatments, which contributes to quality care and better patient outcomes. Use of a CPOE system has been shown to improve productivity and cost-effectiveness in the communication and implementation of health care provider orders. More importantly, most CPOE systems have significant potential to reduce medication errors associated with illegibility and inappropriate drug use and dosing (Hebda and Czar, 2013).

One of the primary goals of the National Academy of Medicine (formerly the Institute of Medicine), is to improve the quality of care and reduce medication errors. Many believe CPOE is the answer. When a provider puts an order entry into the electronic health record (EHR), the order is sent immediately to the appropriate department. The direct order eliminates issues related to illegible handwriting and transcription errors (Mostashari, 2013).

NURSING INFORMATION SYSTEMS

Nurses need to be knowledgeable in the science and application of nursing informatics. Nursing informatics is broadly defined as the "use of information and computer technology to support all aspects of nursing practice, including direct delivery of care, administration, education, and research" (Hebda and Czar, 2013). Nursing informatics is also recognized as a specialty area of nursing practice at the graduate level. Nurses who specialize in informatics have advanced knowledge in information management and demonstrate proficiency with informatics to support all areas of nursing practice including quality improvement, research, project management, and system design (Hebda and Czar, 2013). Through the application of nursing informatics, technology is put to practical use to enhance bedside care and education. The application of nursing informatics results in an efficient and effective nursing information system that facilitates the integration of data, information, and knowledge to support patients, nurses, and other providers in patient care decision making.

Nursing competence in health care informatics is a priority as health care providers and agencies across the United States shift to the use of electronic documentation. You need informatics competencies to deliver safe and efficient care and to facilitate the implementation of evidence-based practice. Professional organizations such as the National Academy of Medicine Division, Robert Wood Johnson Foundation, Quality and Safety Education for Nurses (QSEN) Institute, and National League for Nursing recommend that all nurses acquire a minimal level of awareness and competence in informatics and the use of information technology (Fig. 10.1). QSEN defined the scope of RN competencies for informatics as "the use of information and technology to communicate, manage knowledge, mitigate error, and support decision making" and outlined specific knowledge, skills, and attitudes that prelicensure nursing students need to learn in order to use informatics technology to provide patient care in an effective and safe manner (QSEN Institute, 2014). The American Association of Colleges of Nursing established a framework that outlines curricular goals and informatics competencies for baccalaureate, master's, and doctoral programs of nursing (Hebda and Czar, 2013).

Competence in informatics is not the same as computer competency. To become competent in informatics, you must use evolving methods of discovering, retrieving, and using information in practice (Hebda and Czar, 2013). You must also recognize when information is needed and have the skills to find, evaluate, and use that information effectively. Learn

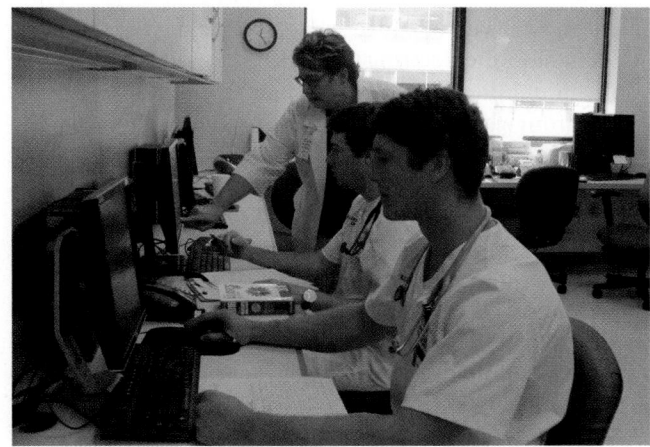

FIG 10.1 Nursing students and nursing faculty at computer screen.

how to use clinical databases within your institution and apply the information so that you can deliver high-quality, appropriate patient care. Patients' records contain multiple types of data, and you need to know how to record, interpret, and report data and use critical thinking to apply your knowledge when providing patient care.

You will collect data including numbers, characters, or facts according to a perceived need for analysis and possible action. You gain knowledge from gathering and using information from several sources. For example, you review several consecutive assessments of a wound documented within the EHR. Reviewing changes in the descriptions of the wound's edges, color of drainage, and measurements over several days allows you to evaluate and identify a pattern that indicates that the wound is not healing. Based on evidence available in the scientific literature, you apply knowledge of wound care principles and intervene to develop new nursing interventions to manage the patient's wound and promote healing.

Clinical Decision Support Systems

A clinical decision support system (CDSS) is a computerized program used within the health care setting to aid and support clinical decision making. The knowledge base within a CDSS contains rules and logic statements that link information required for clinical decisions to generate tailored recommendations for individual patients, which are presented to health care providers as alerts, warnings, or other information for consideration (Lee, 2013). For example, an effective CDSS notifies health care providers of patient allergies before entering a medication order using CPOE to increase patient safety during the medication ordering process.

CDSSs also improve nursing care. When patient assessment data are combined with patient care guidelines, nurses are better able to implement evidence-based nursing care, resulting in improved patient outcomes. When used to support nursing decisions, these programs are called a *nursing CDSS (NCDSS)*. For example, Fig. 10.2 is a model that illustrates how an NCDSS provides nurses with knowledge or specific information at appropriate times to enhance patient care. Using this model, an example of an NCDSS would be a program built within the computer system in which a nurse enters patient data obtained while performing a skin assessment in the clinical setting to review alternatives for pressure injury prevention displayed through the decision support system from which the best evidence-based nursing interventions are selected, thus supporting clinical decision making (Hebda and Czar, 2013). Use of nursing-specific CDSSs has not been implemented as often as CDSSs in other disciplines. However, CDSSs are in development for acute care nursing settings (Ahamed et al., 2016; Rudolph et al., 2016).

Typically, a health care agency uses one or several CISs and administrative information systems. For example, a small community hospital uses a nursing information system; an order entry system; and laboratory, radiology, and pharmacy systems to coordinate its core patient care services. Nurses use a computer to document their care, locate and review laboratory test results, order sterile supplies, and enter health care

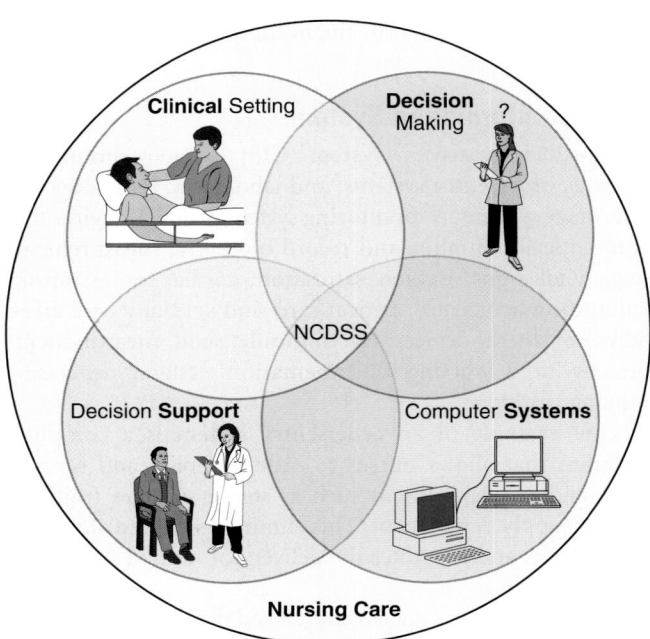

FIG 10.2 Model of a nursing clinical decision support system (NCDSS). (Courtesy Frank Lyerla.)

provider orders for x-ray films and patient medications (Hebda and Czar, 2013).

CONFIDENTIALITY OF MEDICAL RECORD AND PATIENT INFORMATION

Nurses are legally and ethically obligated to keep information about patients confidential. Only members of the health care team who are directly involved in a patient's care have legitimate access to the medical record. You discuss a patient's diagnosis, treatment, assessment, and any personal conversations only with members of the health care team who are specifically involved in the patient's care. Do not share information with other patients or with health care team members who are not caring for the patient. Patients have the right to request copies of their medical records and read the information. Each institution has policies that describe how medical records are shared with patients or other people who request them. In most situations, patients are required to give written permission for release of their medical information.

The Health Insurance Portability and Accountability Act (HIPAA) of 1996 was the first federal legislation to provide protection for patient records; it governs all areas of patient information and management of that information. To eliminate barriers that potentially delay access to care, HIPAA requires providers to notify patients of privacy policies and to obtain written acknowledgment from patients indicating they received this information. Under HIPAA, the Privacy Rule requires that disclosure or requests regarding health information are limited to the specific information required for a particular purpose (Hebda and Czar, 2013). For example, if you need a patient's home telephone number to reschedule

QSEN ACTIVITY *Informatics*

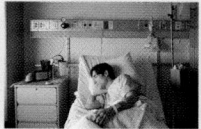

Copyright © XiXinXing/
iStock/Thinkstock.

Mr. Roland has been hospitalized for 3 days and is still receiving a continuous heparin infusion of 1300 units/hr via the peripheral IV located in his left lower forearm. Chris is working from 1500 to 2300 today and learns during the hand-off report that Mr. Roland's most recent partial thromboplastin time (PTT) is 90 seconds, indicating that the current dose of heparin infusing at 1300 units/hr is therapeutic (Pagana et al., 2015). The plan of care is to establish therapeutic anticoagulation levels using warfarin, an oral anticoagulant, so the heparin infusion can be discontinued. Mr. Roland will be discharged with a prescription for warfarin, which he will take for 6 months until his DVT is resolved. He received his first dose of warfarin 10 mg PO yesterday evening.

It is 1800, and Mr. Roland's next dose of warfarin 10 mg PO is due. Chris logs on to the computer located in Mr. Roland's room and opens the medication administration record in his EHR. As Chris scans the package of warfarin using the bar code medication administration function, a warning statement, "Review most recent PT/INR results before administration," pops up on the computer screen. Chris switches screens in the EHR to review Mr. Roland's laboratory results. Chris notes that Mr. Roland's most recent prothrombin time (PT) is 23 seconds, and the international normalized ration (INR) is 2.3, indicating that the dose of warfarin that Mr. Roland received yesterday evening was too high and that he is increased at risk for bleeding (Pagana et al., 2015). The abnormal results are displayed in red font in the EHR, and a notation reading "Critical Value" is displayed next to each of the results displayed in red.

- What is the most appropriate action to take in this situation?

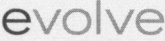 Answers to QSEN Activities can be found on the Evolve website.

an appointment, access to the medical records is limited solely to telephone information. Of equal importance under HIPAA is the Security Rule, which specifies administrative, physical, and technical safeguards for 18 specific elements of **protected health information (PHI)** in electronic form (U.S. Government Publishing Office [GPO], 2017).

Sometimes nurses use health care records for data gathering, research, or continuing education. This is permitted as long as you use a record as specified and permission is granted. When you are a student learning in a clinical setting, maintaining patient **confidentiality** and compliance with HIPAA are required as part of professional practice. You can review patient medical records only for information needed to provide safe and effective patient care. For example, when you are assigned to care for a patient, you need to review the patient's medical record and the **interprofessional plan of care.** You *do not* share this information with classmates (except for clinical conferences) and *do not* access the medical records of other patients on the unit. Access to an **electronic health record (EHR)** is traceable through user log-in

information. It is unethical to view medical records of other patients, and breaches of confidentiality will lead to disciplinary action by employers and potentially dismissal from work or nursing school. To protect patient confidentiality, you must ensure that any electronic or written materials you use in your student clinical practice *do not* include patient identifiers (e.g., name, room number, date of birth, demographic information). *Never* print material from an EHR for personal use; any information printed must be for professional use only and should not include identifiable information.

Security Mechanisms for Privacy and Confidentiality

There are legal implications associated with the use of electronic documentation. It is possible for anyone to access a computer within a health care agency and gain information about almost any patient. Under HIPAA, ensuring appropriate access to and confidentiality of PHI is the responsibility of all persons working in health care. Therefore protection of information and computer systems is one of your top priorities. PHI includes health information that identifies the individual such as demographic data; facts that relate to an individual's past, present, or future physical or mental health condition; provision of care; and payment for the provision of care (Hebda and Czar, 2013; Amer, 2015).

Most computer information system security mechanisms use a combination of logical and physical restrictions to protect information. For example, an automatic sign-off is a safety mechanism that logs a user off a computer system after a specified period of inactivity (Hebda and Czar, 2013). Other security measures include firewalls and the installation of antivirus and spyware-detection software. A **firewall** is a combination of hardware and software that protects private network resources (e.g., the information system of the hospital) from outside hackers, network damage, and theft or misuse of information.

Physical security measures include placing computers or file servers in restricted areas or using privacy filters for computer screens that are visible to visitors or other people without access. This form of security has limited benefit, especially if an organization uses mobile wireless devices such as notebooks, tablets, personal computers (PCs), and smartphones. These devices are easily misplaced or lost, falling into the wrong hands. Some organizations use motion detectors or alarms with these devices to help prevent theft.

Access or log-in codes along with passwords are frequently used for authenticating authorized access to electronic records. A **password** is a collection of alphanumeric characters and symbols that a user types into a computer sign-on screen before accessing a program after the entry and acceptance of an access code or user name. Strong passwords use combinations of letters, numbers, and symbols that are difficult to guess. When using a health care agency computer system, it is essential that you do not share your computer password with anyone under any circumstances. A good system requires frequent changes in personal passwords to prevent unauthorized persons from tampering with records. A password does not appear on the computer screen when it is typed, and it should not be known to anyone but the user and information system administrators (Hebda and Czar, 2013). Most health care personnel are given access only to patients in their work area. Some staff (e.g., administrators or risk managers) have authority to access all patient records. To protect patient privacy, health care agencies track who accesses patient records and when they access them. Failure to comply with HIPAA can result in civil and criminal penalties for health care agencies and providers. Depending on the nature of a violation, civil penalties can result in minimal fines of $100 to $50,000 per violation and maximum fines of $50,000 per violation with an annual maximum of $1.5 million (American Medical Association [AMA], 2017). Thus employers have policies for disciplinary action, including loss of employment, that are implemented when nurses or other health care personnel inappropriately access patient information.

Handling and Disposal of Health Care Information

Maintaining the confidentiality of medical records is a fundamental responsibility of all members of the health care team. It is essential to safeguard any information that is printed from the record or extracted for report purposes. For example, you print a copy of a nursing activities work list to use in planning while providing patient care. You refer to information on the list and write notes to record into the computer and share later during hand-off report. Information on the list is PHI; you do not leave it out for view by unauthorized persons. Destroy (e.g., shred) anything that is printed when the information is no longer needed. Nursing students should not print information from the medical record to take away from the clinical agency to complete written assignments for clinical. Instead, patient information needed for clinical assignments should be transcribed to academic forms or notebooks directly from viewing the medical record on the computer screen or the physical chart. All patient data must be de-identified when transcribed onto forms or used for academic papers for clinical courses in nursing school. Any information that is transcribed and must be removed from the clinical setting and any documents that must be printed out must be kept secure and destroyed through shredding or disposal in a locked receptacle as soon as possible.

Historically, information printed from a patient record and/or faxed to other health care providers has been the primary source for accidental, unauthorized disclosure of PHI. All papers containing PHI (e.g., Social Security number, date of birth or age, patient's name or address) must be destroyed after use or after being faxed. Most agencies have shredders or locked receptacles for shredding and later incineration. Nurses also work in settings where they may be responsible for erasing files from a computer hard drive that contain calendars, schedules for surgery or diagnostic procedures, or other daily records that contain PHI (Hebda and Czar, 2013). You are responsible to know and follow the record disposal policies in the agency where you work.

Health care facilities and departments have policies for the use of fax machines that specify the kinds of information that can be faxed, who can receive faxed information, where information can be sent, and the process used to verify that information was sent to and received by the appropriate person or persons. Information sent by fax should not exceed what was requested or required for immediate clinical needs. Following are some steps to take to enhance fax security (Hebda and Czar, 2013):

- Confirm fax numbers are correct before sending a fax to be sure that you direct information to the proper individual or agency.
- Use a cover sheet for all faxes containing health care information. This eliminates the need for the recipient to read the information to determine to whom a fax needs to be delivered. This is especially important if a fax machine serves a number of different users.
- Authenticate at both ends before transmitting data to verify that source and destination are correct. Use the cover sheet to list intended recipients, the sender, and the phone and fax numbers. Verify the fax number on the transmittal confirmation sheet.
- Use preprogrammed speed-dial keys to eliminate the chance of a dialing error and misdirected information.
- Utilize the encryption feature on the fax machine. Encoding transmissions makes it impossible to read confidential information without the encryption key.
- Place fax machines in a secure area, and limit machine access to designated individuals.
- Log fax transmissions. This feature is often available electronically on the machine.

INTERPROFESSIONAL COMMUNICATION WITHIN THE HEALTH CARE TEAM

The health care record provides the most reliable way for members of the interprofessional health care team to communicate about patient needs and response to care and therapies; clinical decision making; and the content and outcomes of consultations, patient education, and discharge planning. The record is the most current and accurate continuous source of information about a patient's health care status; the plan of care needs to be clear to anyone who accesses the record. Information communicated in the health care record allows health care providers to know a patient thoroughly, facilitating safe, effective, timely, and patient-centered clinical decision making. To enhance communication and promote safe patient care, you document assessment findings and patient information as soon as possible after you provide care (e.g., immediately after providing a nursing intervention or completing a patient assessment).

The quality of patient care depends on your ability to communicate with other members of the health care team (see Chapter 11). Regardless of whether documentation is entered electronically or on paper, each member of the health

BOX 10.1 EVIDENCE-BASED PRACTICE

PICO Question: Does use of structured content and tools within an electronic medical record during bedside patient hand-off improve caregiver communication and reduce patient adverse effects?

SUMMARY OF EVIDENCE

Communication of patient information from one clinician to another during clinical hand-off provides for continuity of care. These moments when responsibility and accountability for a patient are transferred from one clinician to another have significant potential to impact patient safety (Anderson et al., 2015). The Joint Commission estimates that 80% of serious medical errors involve miscommunication between caregivers during change of shift or patient transfers (Joint Commission Center for Transforming Healthcare, 2012). The hand-off (especially face-to-face hand-off) report between nurses at a patient's bedside is one strategy suggested to improve patient safety (Mardis et al., 2016). A recent study by Johnson et al. (2016) demonstrated that use of a structured content tool with the electronic clinical information system during bedside hand-off resulted in a significant increase in the transfer of critical patient information without an increase in time needed for hand-off report.

APPLICATION TO NURSING PRACTICE

- Face-to-face hand-off at the bedside is believed to be an effective method for increasing patient safety during the patient hand-off between nurses and other caregivers (Mardis et al., 2016).
- Multiple mnemonics, such as SBAR (Situation-Background-Assessment-Recommendation) and I PASS the BATON (Introduction, Patient, Assessment, Situation, Safety concerns, Background, Actions, Timing, Ownership, and Next) help nurses provide an organized hand-off report (see Box 11.4) (Mardis et al., 2016).
- Use of electronic tools within the electronic medical record to facilitate completion of bedside report shows promise as one way to increase patient safety by improving the quality of patient hand-off (Johnson et al., 2016).

care team must document patient care in an accurate, timely, concise, and effective manner to develop and maintain an effective, organized, and comprehensive plan of care. When a plan is not communicated to all members of the health care team, care becomes fragmented, tasks are repeated, and delays or omissions in care often occur (Box 10.1).

PURPOSES OF RECORDS

The health care record is a valuable source of data for all members of the health care team. Data entered into the health care record serve many purposes, including communication, legal documentation, reimbursement, education, and research. Health care record data are used for auditing, monitoring, and evaluating care provided (Beach and Oates, 2014; Chand and Sarin, 2014; Griffith, 2015) to support the process needed for quality and performance improvement.

Health care records also serve as sources of research data and as learning resources for nursing and health care education.

Communication

A patient's medical record provides information to all members of the health care team, communicates patient needs and progress toward meeting desired patient outcomes, and maintains continuity of care. The record includes a patient's assessment and responses to interventions and changes made in the plan of care. It is the most current and accurate source of information about a patient's health care status. This information prepares you to know a patient thoroughly so that you can make timely and appropriate care decisions.

Legal Record of Patient Care

Accurate documentation is one of the best defenses for legal claims associated with nursing care. Documentation is an important professional responsibility. To limit liability, your documentation needs to follow organizational standards, which include a clear description of individualized and goal-directed nursing care you provide based on your nursing assessment. You need to document in a timely manner. When documenting, follow agency standards. Documenting all aspects of the nursing process is a critical nursing responsibility that limits nursing liability by providing evidence that you maintained and exceeded practice standards while taking care of patients (Lewis et al., 2017).

Mistakes in documentation that commonly result in malpractice include (1) failing to record pertinent health or drug information, (2) failing to record nursing actions, (3) failing to record medication administration, (4) failing to record drug reactions or changes in patients' conditions, (5) incomplete or illegible records, and (6) failing to document discontinued medications. Table 10.1 provides guidelines for avoiding these mistakes and gives some examples of basic criteria for legally sound documentation in a medical record.

Health Care Reimbursement

Documentation by all members of the health care team is used to determine the severity of illness, the intensity of services received, and the quality of care provided during an episode of care. Insurance companies use this information to determine payment or reimbursement for health care services. **Diagnosis-related groups (DRGs)** are classifications based on a hospitalized patient's primary and secondary medical diagnoses that are used as the basis for establishing Medicare reimbursement for patient care. Hospitals are reimbursed a predetermined dollar amount by Medicare for each DRG. Private insurance carriers and auditors from federal agencies review records to determine the reimbursement that a patient or a health care agency receives (Hall et al., 2015). Accurate documentation of nursing services provided as well as supplies and equipment used in a patient's care clarifies the type of treatment a patient received and supports accurate and timely reimbursement to a health care agency and/or patient.

TABLE 10.1 GUIDELINES FOR LEGALLY SOUND DOCUMENTATION

GUIDELINES FOR ELECTRONIC AND WRITTEN DOCUMENTATION	RATIONALE	CORRECT ACTION
Do not document retaliatory or critical comments about a patient or care provided by another health care professional. Do not enter personal opinions.	Statements can be used as evidence for nonprofessional behavior or poor quality of care.	Enter only objective and factual observations of a patient's behavior or the actions of another health care professional. Quote all patient statements.
Correct all errors promptly.	Errors in recording can lead to errors in treatment or may imply an attempt to mislead or hide evidence.	Avoid rushing to complete documentation; be sure that information is accurate and complete.
Record all facts.	Record must be accurate, factual, and objective.	Be certain that each entry is factual and thorough. A person reading your documentation needs to be able to determine that a patient received adequate care.
Document discussions with providers that you initiate to seek clarification regarding an order that is questioned.	If you carry out an order that is written incorrectly, you are just as liable for prosecution as the health care provider.	Do not record "provider made error." Instead document that "Dr. Smith was called to clarify order for analgesic." Include the date and time of the phone call, with whom you spoke, and the outcome.
Document only for yourself.	You are accountable for information that you enter into a patient's record.	Never enter documentation for someone else (*exception:* caregiver has left unit for the day and calls with information that needs to be documented; include date and time of entry and reference specific date and time to which you are referring and name of source of information in entry; include that information was provided via telephone).
Avoid using generalized, empty phrases such as "status unchanged" or "had good day."	This type of documentation is subjective and does not reflect patient assessment.	Use complete, concise descriptions of assessments and care provided so that documentation is objective and factual.
Begin each entry with date and time and end with your signature and credentials.	This ensures that the correct sequence of events is recorded; signature documents who is accountable for care delivered.	Do not wait until the end of shift to record important changes that occurred several hours earlier; sign each entry according to agency policy (e.g., M. Marcus, RN).
Protect the security of your password for computer documentation.	This maintains security and confidentiality of patient medical records.	Once logged into a computer, do not leave computer screen unattended. Log out when you leave the computer. Make sure that a computer screen is not accessible for public viewing.
Guidelines Specific to Written Documentation		
Do not erase, apply correction fluid, or scratch out errors made while recording.	Charting becomes illegible: it appears as if you were attempting to hide information or deface a written record.	Draw single line through error, write word error above it, and sign your name or initials and date it. Then record note correctly.
Do not leave blank spaces or lines in a written nurses' progress note.	This allows another person to add incorrect information in open space.	Chart consecutively, line by line; if space is left, draw a line horizontally through it and place your signature and credentials at the end.

Quality Improvement

Hospitals are required to establish quality improvement programs to conduct objective, ongoing reviews of patient care and to establish standards for quality care (TJC, 2017). Health care record audits help to determine whether standards of care were met and to identify areas for improvement and staff development. For example, a quality improvement nurse may monitor a unit's records to determine if nurses consistently and accurately documented implementation of fall precautions or evaluation of pain measures. Any deficiencies identified are then shared with all members of the nursing staff so that changes in policy or practice can occur.

Research

Some nurses use data in patient records for statistical analysis (e.g., frequency of clinical disorders, complications, use of specific medical and nursing therapies, clinical outcomes achieved during care for specific illnesses, and patient mortality). After obtaining appropriate agency approvals, a nurse researcher reviews patients' records in a research study to collect information on a particular health problem. Analysis of the data contributes to evidence-based nursing practice and quality health care (Polit and Beck, 2017). For example, if a nurse researcher suspects that early ambulation decreases the complication rate in postoperative patients, the researcher reviews the records of select surgical patients to compare the rates of postoperative complications with early versus late ambulation.

Nursing Education

A patient's record contains a variety of information (e.g., medical and nursing diagnoses, signs and symptoms of disease, successful and unsuccessful treatments, diagnostic findings, and patient behaviors). Reading a patient care record is an effective way to learn the nature of a condition and a patient's response to it. Review of patients with similar medical problems allows you to identify patterns and trends. Such information builds your clinical knowledge. As you identify patterns associated with specific diseases and conditions, you are able to anticipate the type of care your patients require and how patients respond to treatment.

GUIDELINES AND STANDARDS FOR QUALITY NURSING DOCUMENTATION

Whether the transfer of patient information occurs through verbal reports or electronic or written documents, you need to follow basic guidelines and standards for nursing documentation. Every health care organization has standards that govern the type of information nurses document and for which they are held accountable. Agency standards or policies often dictate the frequency of documentation such as how often you record a nursing assessment or a patient's level of pain. You are responsible for knowing the standards of your health care organization to ensure that you provide complete and accurate documentation. Nurses are expected to meet the standard of care for every nursing task they perform. Information in patient health care records can be used as evidence in a court of law to demonstrate whether nursing standards of practice were, or were not, met (Lavin et al., 2015).

In addition, your documentation needs to conform to the standards of the National Committee for Quality Assurance (NCQA) and accrediting bodies such as TJC to maintain institutional accreditation and to minimize liability. Health care organizations usually incorporate accreditation standards into policies and revise documentation systems and forms to suit these standards. Current documentation standards require that all patients admitted to a health care agency be assessed for physical, psychosocial, environmental, self-care, spiritual, cultural, knowledge level, and discharge planning needs. Your documentation needs to demonstrate application of the nursing process, describe clinical decision making, and include evidence of patient and family teaching and discharge planning (TJC, 2017). In addition to HIPAA standards, health care documentation is affected by standards from state and federal regulatory agencies, the Department of Justice, and CMS.

Quality nursing documentation is necessary to enhance efficient, individualized patient care and has five important characteristics: factual, accurate, current, organized, and complete. According to Beach and Oates (2014), it is easier to maintain these characteristics in your documentation if you continually seek to express ideas clearly and succinctly by doing the following:

- Stick to the facts
- Write in short sentences
- Use simple, short words
- Avoid the use of jargon or abbreviations

Factual

A factual record contains descriptive, objective information about what a nurse observes, hears, palpates, and smells. Avoid vague terms such as *appears, seems,* or *apparently.* These words suggest you are stating an opinion; they do not accurately communicate facts and do not inform other caregivers about the details regarding the behaviors exhibited by a patient. Objective data are obtained through direct observation and measurement and include description of a patient's behaviors, for example, *"BP 90/50, heart rate 115 and regular, patient diaphoretic and holding both hands over abdominal dressing."* The only subjective data included in the record are statements made by a patient. When recording subjective data, you document a patient's exact words within quotation marks whenever possible. Include objective data to support subjective data so that your documentation is as descriptive as possible. For example, instead of documenting *"the patient seems anxious,"* provide objective signs of anxiety and document the patient's statement about the feelings experienced: *"the patient's heart rate is 110 beats/min, respiratory rate is slightly labored at 22 breaths/min, and the patient states 'I feel very nervous.'"*

Accurate

Using exact measurements establishes accuracy and helps you determine if a patient's condition has changed in a positive or negative way. For example, a description such as *"Intake, 360 mL of water"* is more accurate than *"Patient drank an adequate amount of fluid."* Documenting that an abdominal incision is *"Approximated, 5 cm in length without redness, drainage, or edema"* is more descriptive than *"large abdominal incision healing well."* Documentation of concise data is clear and easy to understand. Avoid using unnecessary words and irrelevant detail. For example, the fact that the patient is watching television is necessary only when this activity is significant to the patient's status and plan of care.

Use abbreviations carefully to avoid misinterpretation and promote patient safety. TJC (2015) developed a list of "do not use" abbreviations that is used by all health care providers to promote patient safety. In addition, TJC requires that health care institutions develop a list of standard abbreviations, symbols, and acronyms to be used by all members of the health care team when documenting or communicating patient care and treatment. To minimize errors, spell out abbreviations in their entirety when they become confusing.

Correct spelling demonstrates a level of competency and attention to detail. Many terms are easily misinterpreted (e.g., *dysphagia* or *dysphasia*). Some spelling errors result in serious treatment errors (e.g., the names of medications such as lamotrigine and terbinafine or hydromorphone and hydrocodone are similar). Transcribe medication information carefully to ensure a patient receives the correct medication.

All health care record entries should be dated and timed, and the author of each entry must be able to be identified (TJC, 2017). Each entry in a patient's record must end with the caregiver's full name or initials and credentials/title/role such as "Jane Woods, RN." If initials are used in a signature, the full name and credentials/title/role of the individual needs to be documented at least once in the health care record to allow others to readily identify that individual. As a nursing student, enter your full name and nursing student abbreviation, such as "David Jones, NS" or "David Jones, SN." The abbreviation for *nursing student* varies between *NS* for *nursing student* or *SN* for *student nurse*. Include information about your educational institution at the end of your signature when required by agency policy.

Current

Timely entries are essential in a patient's ongoing care, as delays in documentation can lead to unsafe patient care. Many health care agencies keep records or computers near a patient's bedside to facilitate immediate documentation of information. Document the following activities or findings at the time of occurrence:

- Vital signs
- Pain assessment
- Administration of medications and treatments
- Preparation for diagnostic tests or surgery including preoperative checklist

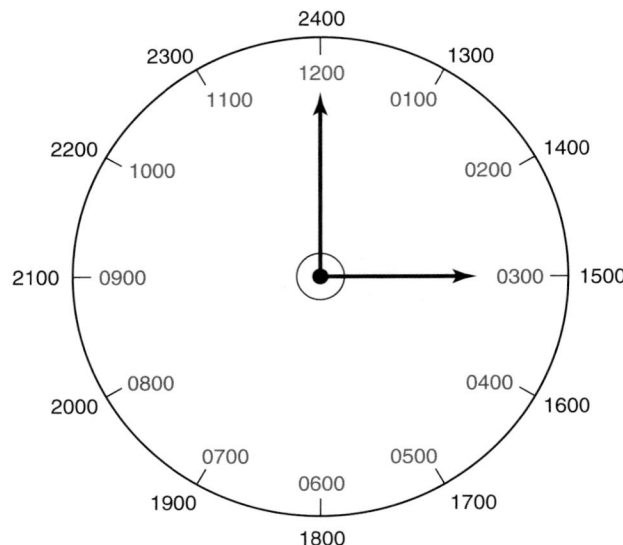

FIG 10.3 Comparison of 24 hours of military time with the hourly positions on the clock face for civilian time.

- Change in patient's status and who was notified (e.g., health care provider, manager, patient's family)
- Admission, transfer, discharge, or death of a patient
- Treatment for sudden change in a patient's status
- Patient's response to treatment or intervention

Most health care agencies use military time, a 24-hour system that avoids misinterpretation of a.m. and p.m. times (Fig. 10.3). Instead of two 12-hour cycles in standard time, the military clock is one 24-hour time cycle. The military clock ends with midnight at 2400 and begins at 1 minute after midnight as 0001. For example, 10:22 a.m. is 1022 military time, and 10:22 p.m. is 2222 military time.

Organized

Information entered in a health care record facilitates communication when it is documented in a logical order. Documentation is also more effective when notes are concise, clear, and to the point. To document notes about complex situations in an organized fashion, first think about the situation, and then make decisions about what information and words you need to include before beginning to enter data in the health care record. Application of your critical thinking skills and the nursing process will help you document clearly and comprehensively in a logical order. For example, an organized entry would describe a patient's pain, your assessment and interventions, and the patient's response to treatment.

Complete

You need to ensure the information within a recorded entry or a report is complete, containing appropriate and essential information. Follow established criteria and standards for thorough communication within the health care record or when reporting certain health problems or nursing activities (Table 10.2). Your written entries in a patient's health care record describe the nursing care you administer and the

TABLE 10.2 CRITERIA FOR DOCUMENTATION AND REPORTING

TOPIC	CRITERIA TO REPORT OR RECORD
Subjective assessment data	Patient's description of episode in quotation marks, for example: *"I feel like an elephant is sitting on my chest, and I can't catch my breath."* Describe in patient's own words onset, location, and description of condition (severity; duration; frequency, precipitating, aggravating, and relieving factors), for example: *"The pain in my left knee started last week after I knelt on the ground. Every time I bend my knee I have a shooting pain on the inside of the knee."*
Objective assessment data (e.g., rash, tenderness, breath sounds) or descriptions of patient behavior (e.g., anxiety, confusion, hostility)	Onset, location, description of condition, for example: 1100: 2-cm raised pale red area noted on back of left hand. Onset, precipitating factors, behaviors exhibited (e.g., pacing in room, avoiding eye contact with nurse), patient statements, for example: repeatedly stating *"I have to go home now."*
Nursing interventions, treatments, and evaluation (e.g., enema, bath, dressing change)	Time administered, equipment used, patient's response (subjective and objective response) compared with previous treatment, for example: denied incisional pain during abdominal dressing change, ambulated 300 feet in hallway without assistance.
Medication administration	At time of administration when using a computerized bar-code medication administration program (or immediately after administration), document time medication given, medication name, dose, route, preliminary assessment (e.g., pain level, vital signs), patient response or effect of medication; for example: 1500: Reports *"throbbing headache all over my head."* Rates pain at 6 (0-to-10 scale). Acetaminophen 650 mg given PO. 1530: Patient reports pain level 2 (0-to-10 scale) and states *"the throbbing has stopped."*
Patient and/or family teaching	Information presented, method of instruction (e.g., discussion, demonstration, videotape, booklet), and patient response, including questions and evidence of understanding such as teach-back, return demonstration, or change in behavior.
Discharge planning	Measurable patient goals or expected outcomes, progress toward goals, need for referrals.

patient's response. An example of a thorough nurse's note for Mr. Roland, the patient described in the case study, follows:

1915: Adhering to bed rest as ordered. Left lower extremity is swollen; calf circumference is 30 inches. Areas of redness that are warm and tender to touch are noted over anterior (3 cm by 4 cm) and medial areas (3 cm by 3 cm) of left leg. Left lower leg elevated on one pillow. Heparin infusing at 3600 units/hr via 20-gauge peripheral IV in left lower forearm. Site without redness, swelling, or drainage. Verbalizes sharp throbbing leg pain rated at 8 on a 0-to-10 scale. Pedal pulses 3+ bilaterally. Capillary refill in toes of both feet is less than 3 seconds. Oxycodone/acetaminophen 2 tablets (PO) given for pain as ordered. Chris Turno, RN.

2000: States "The pain medication really helped." Rates pain in left lower leg at 4 on a 0-to-10 scale. Comfort level goal is 4/10. Chris Turno, RN.

Flow sheets (graphic records) document routine activities such as daily hygiene care, vital signs, and pain assessments. You need to describe these data in greater detail when they are relevant such as when a change in functional ability or status occurs. For example, if your patient's blood pressure, pulse, and respirations are elevated above expected values following a walk down the hall, document additional description about the patient's status and response to the walk in the appropriate place in the health care record (e.g., nurse's notes).

METHODS OF DOCUMENTATION

Regardless of whether documentation is entered electronically or on paper, each health care agency selects a documentation system that reflects the philosophy of nursing at that agency. The same system is used throughout a specific agency and sometimes is used throughout a health care system as well.

The Shift to Electronic Documentation

Historically, health care professionals documented on paper health care records. Paper records are episode oriented, with a separate record for each patient visit to a health care agency. Key information such as patient allergies, current medications, and complications from treatment may be lost from one episode of care (e.g., hospitalization or clinic visit) to the next, jeopardizing a patient's safety (Hebda and Czar 2013).

To facilitate communication among health care providers and improve patient safety, the American Recovery and Reinvestment Act (ARRA) of 2009 set a goal that all health care records would be kept electronically as of 2014 (IRS, 2016). Since 2011, the Health Information Technology for Economic and Clinical Health Act (HITECH), enacted under Title XIII of ARRA, has been a major driver in the adoption and use of EHRs across the United States. HITECH established provisions to promote the meaningful use of health information technology (HIT) to improve the quality and value of health care (HITECH, 2017). Although the goal set by ARRA that all health care records would be kept electronically by 2014 has not yet been fully met, the adoption of EHRs has accelerated rapidly since the passage of HITECH.

As of May 2013, more than 293,000 eligible medical providers and more than 3900 eligible hospitals in the United States received incentive payments from the Medicare and Medicaid EHR Incentive Programs, and more than 220,000 of eligible professionals and more than 3000 of eligible hospitals achieved the requirements for meaningful use of electronic patient data. Those numbers represented nearly 80% of eligible hospitals and more than half of physicians and other eligible professionals (Mostashari, 2013).

Although the terms *EHR* and *EMR* are frequently used interchangeably in practice, there are differences between them. The EMR contains patient data gathered in a health care setting at a specific time and place and is part of the EHR. The EHR is a digital version of patient data found in traditional paper records. The term *EHR* is increasingly used to refer to a longitudinal (lifetime) record of all health care encounters for an individual patient. To meet agreed-on standards, EHRs are expected to have the following attributes or components (Hebda and Czar, 2013):

- Provide a longitudinal or lifetime patient record by linking all patient data from previous health care encounters.
- Contain a problem list that indicates current clinical problems for each health care encounter, the number of occurrences associated with all past and current problems, and the current status of each problem.
- Use of accepted, standardized measures to evaluate and record health status and functional levels.
- Provide a method for documenting the clinical reasoning or rationale for diagnoses and conclusions that allows clinical decision making to be tracked by all providers who access the record.
- Support confidentiality, privacy, and audit trails.
- Provide continuous access to authorized users at any time, and allow multiple health care providers access to customized views of patient data at the same time.
- Support links to local or remote information resources such as databases using the Internet or intranet resources based within an organization.
- Support the use of decision analysis tools.
- Support direct entry of patient data by physicians.
- Include mechanisms for measuring the cost and quality of care.
- Support existing and evolving clinical needs by being flexible and expandable.

A unique feature of an EHR is its ability to integrate all patient information into one record, regardless of the number of times a patient enters a health care system. An EHR also includes results of diagnostic studies that may include diagnostic images (e.g., x-ray or ultrasound images) and decision support software programs. Because an unlimited number of patient records potentially can be stored within an EHR system, health care providers can access clinical data to identify quality issues, link interventions with positive outcomes, and make evidence-based decisions (Weis and Levy, 2014). The key advantages of an EHR for nursing include a means for nurses to compare current clinical data about a patient with data from previous health care encounters, maintain ongoing symptom management, and provide an ongoing record of health education provided to a patient and the patient's response to that information (Ozkaynak et al., 2017).

Problem-Oriented Medical Record

A problem-oriented medical record (POMR) is a system of organizing documentation that places primary focus on patients' individual problems. Data are organized by problem or diagnosis. Ideally each member of the health care team contributes to one interprofessional list of identified patient problems, which coordinates a common plan of care. Some EHR systems are organized using POMR components. The POMR has the following major sections: database, problem list, care plan, and progress notes.

Database. The database section contains all available assessment information pertaining to a patient (e.g., history and physical examination, the nurse's admission history and ongoing assessment, the dietitian's assessment, laboratory reports, and radiological test results). It is the foundation for identifying patient problems and planning care. As new data become available, the database is revised. It accompanies patients through successive hospitalizations or clinic visits.

Problem List. After analyzing data, health care team members identify problems and make a single problem list. The problem list includes a patient's physiological, psychological, social, cultural, spiritual, developmental, and environmental needs. Team members list the problems in chronological order and file the list in a patient's record to organize patient care. Team members add new problems as they arise. When a problem is resolved, the text of that problem is highlighted or lined out, and the date is recorded.

Care Plan. Disciplines involved in a patient's care develop a care plan or plan of care for each problem (see Chapter 9). Nurses document the plan of care in a variety of formats. Regardless of the format used, most plans of care include nursing diagnoses, expected outcomes, and interventions.

Progress Notes. Health care team members monitor and record the progress made toward resolving a patient's problems in progress notes using one of several formats or structured notes.

Narrative Documentation

Narrative documentation is the format traditionally used by nurses and health care providers to record patient assessment, clinical decisions, and care provided. It simply uses a story-like format to document information. In an electronic nursing information system, this is accomplished through use of free text entry or menu selections (Hebda and Czar, 2013). Narrative documentation sometimes is time-consuming and repetitious. It requires the reader to sort through information to locate desired data. However, some nurses believe that in certain situations use of this method provides better detail of individual patient assessment findings and/or complex patient situations (Kerr, 2013). Health care providers review nursing documentation for details about changes in a patient's condition (Penoyer et al., 2014). One of the limitations of electronic documentation is the limited use of narrative documentation. Some areas of the EHR are designed to allow the use of multiple checkboxes or drop-down lists, which some believe may not adequately convey the details of significant events that result in a change in patient condition (Kerr, 2013; Penoyer et al., 2014). EHRs that incorporate options for narrative descriptions in a format that can be easily retrieved and reviewed may augment clinician communication and interprofessional understanding for patient care.

Examples include traditional narrative documentation, subjective-objective-assessment-plan (SOAP) note documentation, problem-intervention-evaluation (PIE) notes, and focus charting using the data-action-response (DAR) format. SOAP, PIE, and focus charting are several other methods of documentation that were implemented when paper medical records were the norm. Box 10.2 provides a short description of each of these methods and an example note using each method based on the case study.

Charting by Exception

The philosophy behind charting by exception (CBE) is that all standards are met unless otherwise documented. The method was introduced in the early 1980s, and although the philosophy behind the method has consistently raised professional concern (Kerr, 2013), many computerized nursing documentation systems currently use a CBE design. Exception-based documentation systems incorporate standards of care and interventions and use clearly defined criteria for nursing assessment and documentation of "normal" findings. These predefined statements used to document nursing assessment of body systems are called "within defined limits" (WDL) or "within normal limits" (WNL) definitions. They consist of written criteria for a "normal" assessment for each body system. Automated documentation within a computerized documentation system allows nurses to select a WDL statement or to choose other statements from a drop-down menu that allow description of any unexpected assessment findings or assessment findings that deviate from the WDL definition (Hebda and Czar, 2013). You write a progress note only when a patient's assessment does not meet the standardized criteria for "normal" in one or more body systems. When changes in a patient's condition develop, the progress note narrative should include a thorough and precise description of the effects of the changes on the patient and the actions taken to address the changes.

Case Management and Critical Pathways

The case management model of delivering care incorporates an interprofessional approach to documenting patient care. Critical pathways (also known as clinical pathways, practice guidelines, or CareMap tools) are interprofessional care plans that identify patient problems, key interventions, and expected outcomes within an established time frame (American Health Consultants, 2015). Critical pathway documents facilitate integration of care because all members of the health care team use the same document to monitor a patient's progress during each shift or, in the case of home care, every visit. Many organizations summarize the standardized plan of care into a critical pathway for a specific disease or condition. Evidence-based critical pathways can improve patient outcomes. For example, use of critical pathways has been shown to improve adherence to evidence-based guidelines for administration of antibiotics for community-acquired pneumonia (Almatar et al., 2016) and to improve clinical outcomes for management of pain in patients with sickle cell disease (Ender et al., 2014).

Critical pathways eliminate nurses' notes, flow sheets, and nursing care plans because the document integrates all relevant information. Unexpected outcomes, unmet goals, and interventions not specified within the critical pathway are called variances. A variance occurs when the activities on the critical pathway are not completed as predicted or a patient does not meet the expected outcomes. Variances sometimes result from a change in a patient's health or because of other health complications not associated with the primary reason for which a patient requires care. Once you identify a variance, you modify the patient's care to meet the needs associated with the variance. A positive variance occurs when a patient makes progress faster than expected (e.g., use of a Foley catheter is discontinued a day earlier than anticipated). An example of a negative variance is when a patient develops pulmonary complications after surgery, requiring oxygen therapy and monitoring with pulse oximetry. All variances to expected outcomes are documented on the critical pathway document (Box 10.3). Documentation allows trends to be identified and analyzed, which can provide data to develop an effective action plan to respond to identified patient problems. Over time health care teams sometimes revise critical pathways if similar variances reoccur.

COMMON RECORD-KEEPING FORMS

Nurses use a variety of electronic or paper documentation forms. The categories or data fields within a form are usually derived from institutional standards of practice or guidelines established by accrediting agencies.

Nursing Admission History

A nurse completes a nursing admission history form when a patient is admitted to a nursing unit. The fields in the form guide you through a comprehensive assessment to identify relevant nursing diagnoses or problems. Completion of this

BOX 10.2   EXAMPLES OF NURSING DOCUMENTATION IN DIFFERENT FORMATS

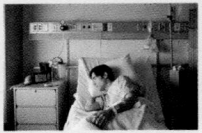

Copyright © XiXinXing/
iStock/Thinkstock.

Case Study Continuation: Chris needs to document the information obtained from Mr. Roland during the admission process. Following are some examples of how to document this information using various methods of documentation that were widely used before implementation of the electronic health record:

NARRATIVE NOTE

- Patient stated "My leg is so swollen. I'm worried about this blood clot." Is asking questions about medications and treatment plan. Discussed importance of bed rest and the reason for treatment with heparin infusion. Explained need for daily blood tests to check anticoagulation levels. Provided brochure on anticoagulation therapy for DVT. Used teach-back method to validate that patient understands plan of care; he is able to describe that the heparin infusion will be stopped when his PT/INR is therapeutic on warfarin and that he can expect to take warfarin for approximately 6 months after discharge until clot in his leg is fully resolved.

SOAP

- The acronym **SOAP** stands for:
  - **S:** Subjective data (patient statements)
  - **O:** Objective data (data that are measured and observed)
  - **A:** Assessment (nursing diagnosis or problem based on the data)
  - **P:** Plan (what the caregiver plans to do)
- Example of SOAP note:
  - **S:** "My leg is so swollen. I'm worried about this blood clot."
  - **O:** Asking questions about medications and treatment plan.
  - **A:** *Knowledge Deficit related to lack of knowledge about how DVT is treated.*
  - **P:** Provide brochure on anticoagulation therapy for DVT. Explain rationale for bed rest and daily blood tests to check anticoagulation levels. Explain that heparin infusion will be stopped when PT/INR is therapeutic on warfarin and that he will need to continue taking warfarin for approximately 6 months after discharge until clot in his leg is fully resolved.

PIE

- A PIE note differs from a SOAP note in that it has a specific nursing focus:

- **P:** Identifies a nursing diagnosis
- **I:** Describes interventions that will be used to address the problem
- **E:** Describes the nursing evaluation
- Example of PIE note:
  - **P:** *Knowledge Deficit related to lack of knowledge about how deep vein thrombosis (DVT) is treated.*
  - **I:** Provide brochure on anticoagulation therapy for DVT. Explain rationale for bed rest and daily blood tests to check anticoagulation levels. Explain that heparin infusion will be stopped when PT/INR reaches therapeutic levels on warfarin and that he will need to continue taking warfarin for approximately 6 months after discharge until DVT is fully resolved.
  - **E:** Stated "My leg is so swollen. I'm worried about this blood clot, but I understand how it is being treated." Able to teach back and verbalized that the heparin infusion will be stopped when PT/INR is therapeutic on warfarin and that he can expect to take warfarin for approximately 6 months after discharge until clot in his leg is fully resolved.

FOCUS CHARTING

- **Focus charting** involves the use of DAR notes:
  - **D:** Data (both subjective and objective)
  - **A:** Action or nursing intervention
  - **R:** Response of the patient (i.e., evaluation of effectiveness).
- DAR notes address patient concerns such as a sign or symptom, condition, nursing diagnosis, behavior, significant event, or change in a patient's condition.
- Example of focus charting note:
  - **D:** Patient stated, "My leg is so swollen. I'm worried about this blood clot. Do you know how they are going to treat it?"
  - **A:** Provided brochure on anticoagulation therapy for DVT. Explained rationale for bed rest and daily blood tests to check anticoagulation levels. Explained that heparin infusion will be stopped when PT/INR is therapeutic on warfarin.
  - **R:** Able to teach back and verbalized that heparin infusion will be stopped when his PT/INR reaches therapeutic levels on warfarin and that he can expect to take warfarin for approximately 6 months after discharge until DVT is fully resolved.

---

form provides baseline data that are used for comparison when a patient's condition changes.

Flow Sheets and Graphic Records

Acute care and critical care units commonly use flow sheets and graphic records to document physiological data and provision of routine care. Within a computerized documentation system, these forms allow you to quickly and easily enter patient assessment data, such as vital signs, admission and/or daily weights, and percentage of meals eaten. They also facilitate documentation of routine care such as hygiene measures,

ambulation, and safety and restraint checks. These documents provide current patient information that is accessible to all members of the health care team so that patient trends can be easily identified. If you document an unusual occurrence or significant change in patient condition on a flow sheet, you should also describe the details of that occurrence or change in a progress note. For example, if a patient's blood pressure becomes dangerously high, you first complete and record a focused assessment on the flow sheet, and then you document the action taken and the patient's response in a progress note.

BOX 10.3 EXAMPLE OF VARIANCE DOCUMENTATION

- A critical pathway for routine postoperative care is being used for a 56-year-old patient who had abdominal surgery yesterday. One of the expected outcomes for postoperative day 1 on the critical pathway document is "Afebrile with lungs clear bilaterally." This patient has an elevated temperature, has decreased breath sounds bilaterally in the bases of both lobes of the lungs, and is slightly confused.
- The following is an example of how this variance is documented on the pathway:
- "Breath sounds diminished bilaterally at the bases. T 100.4, P 92, R 28/min, pulse oximetry 84% on room air. Daughter states patient is "confused" and did not recognize her when she arrived a few minutes ago. Oxygen 2 L nasal cannula started per provider-ordered Respiratory Protocol. Oxygen saturation improved to 92% after 5 minutes. Physician notified of change in status. Daughter remains at bedside."

Patient Care Summary

Many computerized documentation systems generate a **patient care summary** document that you review and sometimes print for each patient at the beginning and/or end of each shift to use as a worksheet for organizing care and in giving hand-off report. The document automatically updates and provides the most current information that was entered into the EHR and usually includes the following information:

- Basic demographic data (e.g., age, religion)
- Health care provider's name
- Primary medical diagnosis
- Medical and surgical history
- Current orders from the health care provider (e.g., dressing changes, ambulation, glucose monitoring)
- Nursing care plan
- Nursing orders (e.g., education needed, symptom relief measures, counseling)
- Scheduled tests and procedures
- Safety precautions used in a patient's care
- Factors that affect patient independence with activities of daily living
- Nearest relative/guardian or person designated as a patient's health care power of attorney to contact in an emergency
- Emergency code status (e.g., indication of do not resuscitate order)
- Allergies

Standardized Care Plans

Many computerized documentation systems include **standardized care plans** that facilitate the creation and documentation of a nursing and/or interprofessional plan of care. Each standardized plan facilitates safe and consistent care for an identified problem by describing or listing institutional standards and evidence-based guidelines that are easily accessed and included in a patient's EHR. After completing a nursing assessment, the nurse identifies and selects the standardized plans that are appropriate for the patient and are to be included in an individualized plan of care within the EHR. Most computer documentation systems allow these care plans to be modified by creating individualized interventions, goals, and outcomes for each patient.

Standardized care plans are useful when conducting quality improvement audits. They also improve continuity of care among professional nurses. When they are used, the nurse remains responsible for providing individualized care to each patient. Standardized care plans cannot replace a nurse's professional judgment and decision making. You update care plans on a regular basis to ensure that the documents are appropriate and evidence-based.

Discharge Summary Forms

Nurses help ensure cost-effective care and appropriate reimbursement by preparing patients for a safe, effective, and timely discharge from a health care institution. Developing a comprehensive plan for a safe discharge relies on interprofessional discharge planning. This process includes identification of key clinical outcomes and appropriate timelines for reaching them, the appropriate level of care for discharge, and all necessary resources.

Ideally discharge planning begins at admission. By identifying discharge needs early, nursing and other health care professionals begin planning for discharge to the appropriate level of care, which sometimes includes support services such as home care and any equipment needs. Involve the patient and family in the discharge planning process so they have the necessary information and resources to return home or move to the next level of care. Discharge documentation includes medications, diet, community resources, follow-up care, and the name of a person to contact for questions or in case of an emergency. All this information is included in a discharge summary document that is printed out and given to the patient on discharge. The information remains in the EHR as a record of the discharge teaching that was provided (Box 10.4).

Acuity Rating Systems

Nurses use **acuity ratings** to determine the hours of care and number of staff required for a given group of patients every shift or every 24 hours. A patient's acuity level, usually determined by assessment data an RN enters into a computer program, is based on the type and number of nursing interventions (e.g., IV therapy, wound care, or ambulation assistance) required by that patient over a 24-hour period. Although acuity ratings are not part of a patient's health care record, nursing documentation within the health care record provides evidence that supports the assessment of an acuity rating for an individual patient.

The acuity level is a classification used to compare one or more patients with another group of patients. An acuity system classifies patients from 1 (independent in all but one or two aspects of care; almost ready for discharge) to 5 (totally

BOX 10.4 DISCHARGE SUMMARY INFORMATION

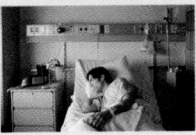

Copyright © XiXinXing/ iStock/Thinkstock.

Mr. Roland is scheduled for discharge this afternoon; his prescription for warfarin was called into his local pharmacy. Chris used the teach-back technique to ensure that Mr. Roland understands why he needs to take his daily dose of warfarin at the same time every evening and why he needs to get his blood drawn every week (so that his warfarin dose can be adjusted as needed). Chris considers some of the following key points when providing discharge information:

- Use clear, concise descriptions in the patient's own language.
- Provide step-by-step instructions for how to perform any procedures the patient or family caregiver will be doing independently (e.g., emptying a urinary catheter drainage bag or self-administration of an injectable medication).
- Identify precautions to follow when performing self-care or administering medications.
- List signs and symptoms of complications that should be reported to a health care provider.
- List names and phone numbers of health care providers and community resources that the patient can contact.
- Identify any unresolved problems, including plans for follow-up and continuous treatment.
- List actual time of discharge, mode of transportation, and who accompanied the patient.

Example of discharge documentation: "Discharge teaching completed. Patient verbalized understanding of the plan of care with warfarin for anticoagulation therapy through use of teach-back technique. Verbalized understanding of need to contact provider for fever higher than 101.5, increased swelling or redness of leg, and if pain in affected leg increases and/or does not subside with use of prescribed pain medication. Instructed to schedule follow-up appointment with health care provider within 1 week. Provider's office phone: 333-333-3333. Discharged to home via wheelchair at 1530, accompanied by wife.

dependent in all aspects of care; requiring intensive care). Using this system, a patient returning from surgery requiring frequent monitoring and extensive care has an acuity level of 3 compared with another patient awaiting discharge after a successful recovery from surgery who has an acuity level of 1. Accurate acuity ratings justify the number and qualifications of staff needed to safely care for patients. The patient-to-staff ratios established for a unit depend on a composite gathering of 24-hour acuity data for all patients receiving care.

DOCUMENTATION IN HOME CARE SETTINGS

Documentation in the home care setting is different from other areas of nursing. The use of laptop and tablet computers makes it possible for home health care records to be available in multiple locations (i.e., the patient's home and the home care agency), improving accessibility to information and facilitating interprofessional collaboration. Medicare has specific guidelines to establish eligibility for home care reimbursement. Information used for reimbursement is gathered from documentation of care provided in the home care setting. Documentation is both the quality control and the justification for reimbursement from Medicare, Medicaid, or private insurance companies. Information in the home care health care record includes patient assessment, referral and intake forms, the interprofessional plan of care, a list of medications, and reports to third-party payers. Nurses must document all their services for payment (e.g., direct skilled care, patient teaching, skilled observation, and evaluation visits) (TJC, 2017).

Nurses use two different data sets to document the clinical assessments and care provided in the home care setting. Assessment using the Outcome and Assessment Information Set (OASIS) is required for all patients age 18 years and older (with the exception of prenatal or postnatal patients) who are receiving skilled care through a home health agency that is reimbursed by Medicare or Medicaid (Shang et al., 2015). OASIS includes a comprehensive admission assessment and calculates clinical, functional, and service scores to provide justification for reimbursement of services (Allender et al., 2014). The Omaha System consists of three components, Problem Classification Scheme, Intervention Scheme, and Problem Rating Scale for Outcomes, and provides a useful model for comprehensive evaluation of nursing care and evaluates the quality of nursing care provided in the home care setting (Allender et al., 2014).

DOCUMENTATION IN LONG-TERM CARE SETTINGS

Long-term health care settings include skilled nursing facilities (SNFs), in which patients receive 24-hour-a-day care including housing, meals, specialized (skilled) nursing care, and treatment services, and long-term care facilities, in which patients with chronic conditions receive 24-hour-a-day care including housing, meals, personal care, and basic nursing care. Requirements for documentation in these facilities are governed by individual state regulations, TJC, and CMS. CMS mandates use of the Resident Assessment Instrument (RAI), which includes the Minimum Data Set (MDS) and the Care Area Assessment (CAA) to document data in long-term care facilities. MDS assessment forms are completed on admission and then periodically within specific guidelines and time frames for all residents in certified nursing homes (Ahn et al., 2015).

MDS data also determine the reimbursement level under the prospective payment system for Medicare Part A residents in an SNF. Communication among nurses; social workers; dietitians; and recreational, speech, physical, and occupational therapists is essential. Documentation in the long-term care setting supports an interprofessional approach to the assessment and planning process for all patients. Compliance with state and federal requirements as well as reimbursement for care provided in a long-term care facility is dependent on accurate completion of the required documentation to justify the care provided (Hebda and Czar, 2013; Voyer et al., 2014).

REPORTING

Reports are oral, written, or audiotaped exchanges of information between members of the health care team. A report reflects a summary of activities or observations seen, performed, or heard by the health care provider. Common reports given by nurses include hand-off reports, change-of-shift reports, and transfer reports.

Hand-Off Report

A hand-off report occurs any time one health care provider transfers care of a patient to another health care provider. The purpose of hand-off reports is to provide better continuity and individualized care for patients (Anderson et al., 2015). A hand-off is the process of transferring responsibility for patient care from one provider to another. For example, if you find that a patient breathes better in a certain position, you relay that information to the next nurse caring for the patient (Mardis et al., 2016).

Standardizing communication during hand-off reports helps ensure patient safety. Face-to-face hand-off communication includes up-to-date information about a patient's condition, required care, treatments, medications, services, and any recent or anticipated changes. In addition, these reports reduce patient care errors (Johnson et al., 2016).

When a hand-off report is given, it is essential for staff to have an opportunity for last-minute updates to clarify information or to receive information on care events or changes in a patient's condition. Properly performed, a hand-off report provides for patient safety and continuity of care.

An effective hand-off report is quick and efficient. A good report provides a baseline for comparisons and indicates the kind of care anticipated for the next nurse who will be caring for the patient. An organized and concise approach helps you set goals and anticipate patient needs and lessens the chance of overlooking important information (Johnson et al., 2016). A sample format frequently includes background information (name, age, and medical diagnosis); primary health problem; unusual occurrences; discharge planning issues; identification of significant changes in measurable terms (e.g., pain scale); observations; findings; times when new, STAT, or prn medications were given; care required such as medications that need to be started, when to assess the effectiveness of STAT or prn medications, or when a dressing needs to be changed next; progress with teaching interventions; and family involvement. It is especially important to report any recent changes or priority situations concerning the patient's condition. Do not include normal findings or routine information retrievable from other sources or derogatory or inappropriate comments about a patient or family.

Change-of-Shift Report

The change-of-shift report is a type of hand-off report that occurs at the end of each shift. This report provides the transfer of relevant information from nurses who have completed a shift of care to nurses about to begin a shift of care. Shift reports occur in a variety of ways.

Sometimes nurses walk with each other from one patient's room to the next. This is called *walking rounds*. Walking reports given in person or during rounds allow you to obtain immediate feedback when questions arise about a patient's care. When you make rounds, the patient and family members can participate in any discussions and care decisions. However, be careful about mentioning information that the patient should not hear (e.g., new laboratory or diagnostic reports not yet explained by the health care provider).

Nurses also give reports orally. Oral reports occur in person with staff members from both shifts participating. Reports can be audiotaped before the end of the shift by the nurse going off duty; the incoming staff listens to the report before assuming patient care. Audiotaped reports often enhance efficiency and minimize social interactions. However, the audiotaped report does not provide the opportunity to raise questions or obtain feedback about the patient's nursing care needs.

Transfer Reports

Patients frequently transfer from one unit to another or to another agency to receive different levels of care. For example, they transfer from intensive care units to general nursing units when the level of care no longer requires intense monitoring. A transfer report is another type of hand-off report that involves the nurse on the sending unit communicating information about a patient to the nurse on the receiving unit. Nurses usually give transfer reports by phone or in person. When giving a transfer report, include the following information:

1. Patient's name, age, date of birth, health care provider(s), and medical diagnosis
2. Summary of medical progress up to the time of transfer
3. Current health status (physical and psychosocial)
4. Allergies
5. Emergency code status
6. Family support
7. Current nursing diagnoses or problems and care plan
8. Any critical assessments or interventions to be completed shortly after transfer (helps receiving nurse establish priorities of care)
9. Up-to-date reconciled medication list (TJC, 2017, 2018)
10. Need for any special equipment such as isolation equipment, suction equipment, or traction

At the completion of the transfer report, the receiving nurse clarifies information by asking questions about the patient's status. Some institutions require a written transfer report sheet that includes information communicated in the transfer report.

Documentation of Telephone Reports, Telephone Orders, and Verbal Orders

Document every phone call you make to a health care provider. Your documentation needs to include when the call was made, the number called, who made the call (if you did not make the call), who was called, to whom information was given, what information was given, and what information was received. For example: *"09/30/2016 (21:30): Called Dr. Bank's office at 123-456-7890. Spoke with L. Matthews, RN, who will inform Dr. Banks that Mr. Andrews' potassium level drawn at 2000 was 5.9 mEq/dL. Informed that Dr. Banks will call back after he is finished seeing his current patient. R. Jenner, RN."*

Telephone Reports. A telephone report needs to include clear, accurate, and concise information. TJC reported that in 2011 verbal and written communication among staff and with patients was listed as one of the 10 most frequently identified root causes of medical errors, also called *sentinel events* (TJC, 2012). To improve communication, some institutions use SBAR (Situation-Background-Assessment-Recommendation), a communication strategy designed to improve patient safety (see Chapter 11). SBAR standardizes telephone communication of significant events or changes in the patient's condition.

Telephone Orders and Verbal Orders. Telephone orders (TOs) occur when a health care provider gives therapeutic orders over the phone to an RN. Verbal orders (VOs) occur when a health care provider gives therapeutic orders to an RN while they are standing in proximity to one another. Use of VOs is discouraged except in urgent or emergent situations. TOs and VOs usually occur at night or during emergencies; they should be used only when absolutely necessary and not for the sake of convenience. In some situations, it is wise to have a second person listen to TOs; some agency policies require it. Check your agency's policy. Box 10.5 provides guidelines that promote accuracy when receiving TOs or VOs.

A nurse receiving a TO or VO enters the complete order into the computer using the CPOE software or writes it out on a physician's order sheet for entry in the computer as soon as possible. After a nurse transcribes an order, the nurse uses the read-back process and documents the process to provide evidence that the information received (e.g., call back instructions and/or therapeutic orders) was verified with the provider. For example: *"09/30/2016 (1015), Change IV fluid to lactated Ringer with potassium 20 mEq/L to run at 125 mL/hr. TO: Dr. Knight/K. Noll, RN, telephone order read back."* The health care provider later verifies the TO or VO legally by co-signing it within a time frame (e.g., 24 hours) as set by agency policy.

Incident or Occurrence Reports

An incident or occurrence is any event that is not consistent with the routine, expected care of a patient or the standard procedures in place on a health care unit or within an agency.

BOX 10.5   GUIDELINES FOR TELEPHONE AND VERBAL ORDERS

- Only authorized staff (who are identified in a written policy by each agency) receive and record telephone and verbal orders.
- Clearly identify the patient's name, room number, and diagnosis.
- Use clarification questions to avoid misunderstandings.
- Write TO (telephone order) or VO (verbal order), date and time received, name of patient, the complete order transcribed exactly as stated, and the name of physician or health care provider and nurse.
- Read back all telephone and verbal orders to physician or health care provider (TJC, 2015).
- Follow agency policies; some institutions require telephone and verbal orders to be reviewed and signed by two nurses.
- The health care provider cosigns each telephone and verbal order within the time frame required by each agency (usually 24 hours).

Examples include patient falls, needlestick injuries, medication administration errors, accidental omission of ordered therapies, a visitor losing consciousness, and any circumstances that lead to injury or pose a risk for patient injury such as a "near miss." A near miss is an incident in which no property was damaged and no patient or personnel were injured, but with a slight shift in time or position, damage or injury could have occurred (Occupational Safety and Health Administration [OSHA], n.d.).

An incident report (occurrence report) is completed whenever an incident occurs. Incident reports are an important part of the quality improvement program of a unit or agency; however, they are not part of the health care record. Incident reports contain confidential information; distribution of the report is limited to the individuals responsible for reviewing the forms. Follow agency policy when completing an incident report, and file the report with your agency's risk-management department. Analysis of incident or occurrence reports helps identify system and/or individual human issues in which educational or in-service programs or changes in policies and procedures are needed to reduce the risk of future occurrences.

When an incident occurs, document an objective description of what happened, what you observed, and the follow-up actions taken including notification of the patient's health care provider in the patient's health care record. Remember to evaluate and document the patient's response to the incident in the health care record as well. Do not label this as an "incident," "near miss," or "sentinel event" in the health care record, and do not make any reference to these types of documents. A notation about an incident, near miss, or sentinel event report in a patient's health care record makes it easier for a lawyer to argue that the reference makes the incident report part of the health care record and therefore admissible for attorney review.

KEY POINTS

- In response to federal regulations, documentation of health care information continues to shift to electronic rather than paper-based documentation systems.
- Computerized health care records improve continuity of care by providing the ability to compare data from various health care encounters.
- Computerized health care information systems provide patient data in an accessible and organized manner.
- The security of health care computer systems and protection of the confidentiality of patients' health information must remain a top priority.
- The health care record is a confidential, legal, and continuing account of a patient's health care status. It is available to all members of the health care team involved in the patient's care to facilitate communication.
- The health care record provides a legal and financial record of care, aids in clinical education and research, and guides professional and organizational performance improvement.
- Nursing informatics facilitates the integration of data, information, knowledge, and wisdom to support patients, nurses, and other providers in decision making in all roles and settings.
- Accurate and timely record keeping requires objective documentation of data with precise measurements, correct spelling, and proper use of abbreviations.
- Effective nursing documentation limits liability through objective description of what happened to a patient and clearly indicates that individualized, goal-directed nursing care was provided based on nursing assessment.
- Nursing documentation supports reimbursement to health care agencies through accurate accounting of the use of services and equipment and medications administered.
- Documentation standards for nurses who work in home health care settings are set by Medicare guidelines that establish reimbursement for home health care.
- Documentation in long-term health care settings is interprofessional and closely linked with financial requirements of outside agencies.
- The major purposes of hand-off reports are patient safety, enhanced communication between health care professionals, and continuity of care.
- When information relevant to care is communicated by telephone, verification of information through use of a read-back process should be documented in the health care record.
- Incident (occurrence/event) reports objectively describe any event not consistent with the routine care of a patient. These reports are confidential and are used for quality improvement within an agency. Information about an incident report should never be documented in a patient's health care record.

REFLECTIVE LEARNING

- Using a recent clinical experience, describe how a clinical decision support system could support evidence-based clinical decision making and nursing actions.
- Reflect on a recent clinical experience and describe how the hand-off report helped or could have helped to provide continuity of care.
- There is an increase of wound infections on a surgical floor. Describe what data you will collect from the agency's nursing information system. Discuss why this information is important to collect.

REVIEW QUESTIONS

1. You work in a health care agency that uses an EHR. Which nursing action is appropriate?
   1. Allow a temporary staff member to use your computer user name and password.
   2. Remain logged in to a computer when you leave to administer a medication.
   3. Allow a health care provider to quickly enter an order using the computer you are currently logged into to document patient care.
   4. Prevent others from seeing a display monitor that contains patient information.
2. A hospital uses military time for documentation. At 10:15 p.m. a nurse administered a dose of morphine 1 mg IV prn to a patient who reports a pain level of 8 on a 0-to-10 scale. How does the nurse document the administration time of the medication?
   1. 1015 hours
   2. 10:15 o'clock
   3. 10:15 p.m.
   4. 2215 hours
3. At the end of a shift, a nurse is giving a hand-off report about a patient named Mrs. Lennon to another nurse. Which pieces of information are appropriate to include in the hand-off report? (Select all that apply.)
   1. "Mrs. Lennon is 45 years old. She was admitted yesterday after an open cholecystectomy."
   2. "Mrs. Lennon has really been difficult today. She has been using her nurse call system constantly, and nothing I've done has pleased her."
   3. "Mrs. Lennon is allergic to strawberries, fentanyl, and sulfa medications."
   4. "Mrs. Lennon has a urethral catheter in place that has drained 450 mL of clear, light yellow urine."
   5. "Mrs. Lennon has received tramadol 100 mg PO every 8 hours for pain and has consistently rated her pain from 5 to 6 on a 1-to-10 scale this shift.
   6. "Mrs. Lennon has a dressing over her right upper quadrant incision that has a moderate amount of old, dark red drainage. I was not able to change the dressing this shift because of inadequate staffing."

4. A patient is being discharged to an acute rehabilitation facility. You need to print some information from the patient's health care record and fax it to that facility. What actions do you take to maintain privacy and confidentiality of the patient's information in providing the health care record information to the acute rehabilitation facility? (Select all that apply.)
   1. Confirm that the fax number you have for the acute rehabilitation facility is correct before sending the fax.
   2. Use a cover sheet that indicates the specific person at the acute rehabilitation facility to whom you are directing the patient information.
   3. Utilize the encryption feature on the fax machine to encode the information making it impossible for staff at the acute rehabilitation facility to read the information you fax unless they have the encryption key.
   4. Rip up the information you printed out to fax and place it in a standard trash can.
   5. Place the information you printed out to fax in the patient's paper-based chart.
   6. Place the information you printed out to fax in a secure canister marked for shredding.

5. A nurse is changing the dressing on the wound of a patient who had abdominal surgery yesterday. Assessment shows new findings that are different than what was documented by the previous nurse. After documenting specifics about the wound, the nurse contacts the surgeon to communicate the changes. What is the most appropriate way to document this conversation?
   1. "Health care provider notified about change in assessment of abdominal incision. A. Carron, RN"
   2. "10-3-16, 18:30: Contacted Dr. Sylvana by phone. Notified about new 2-cm opening at bottom of abdominal incision and large amount of serosanguineous drainage. No orders received. Dr. Sylvana stated she would be in to assess patient within the next hour. A. Carron, RN"
   3. "10-3-16: Notified health care provider by phone that there is a new opening in the patient's incision. A. Carron, RN."
   4. "18:30: Contacted Dr. Sylvana by phone. Notified about changes in abdominal incision. A. Carron, RN."

evolve

Additional Review Questions, as well as rationales for all Review Questions, can be found on the Evolve website.

1, 4; 2, 4; 3, 1, 3, 4, 5, 6; 4, 1, 2, 3, 6; 5, 2.

REFERENCES

Ahamed T, et al: Towards a methodology for nursing-specific clinical decision support systems, *J Decis Syst* 25:23, 2016.

Ahn H, et al: Bodily pain intensity in nursing home residents with pressure ulcers: analysis of National Minimum Data Set 3.0, *Res Nurs Health* 38:207, 2015.

Allender JA, et al: *Community and public health nursing: promoting the public's health*, ed 8, Philadelphia, 2014, Lippincott Williams & Wilkins.

Almatar M, et al: Clinical pathway and monthly feedback improve adherence to antibiotic guideline recommendations for community-acquired pneumonia, *PLoS ONE* 11:e0159467, 2016.

Amer K: Informatics: ethical use of genomic information and electronic medical records, *Online J Issues Nurs* 20:10, 2015.

American Health Consultants: They're back! Clinical pathways are in favor again, *Hosp Case Manag* 23:13, 2015.

American Medical Association (AMA): *HIPAA violations and enforcement*, 2017. https://www.ama-assn.org/practice -management/hipaa-violations -enforcement.

Anderson J, et al: Nursing bedside clinical handover—an integrated review of issues and tools, *J Clin Nurs* 24:662, 2015.

Bae SH, Yoder LH: Implementation of the Centers for Medicare & Medicaid Services nonpayment policy for preventable hospital-acquired conditions in rural and nonrural U.S. hospitals, *J Nurs Care Qual* 30:313, 2015.

Beach J, Oates J: Maintaining best practice in record-keeping and documentation, *Nurs Stand* 28:45, 2014.

Center for Clinical Standards and Quality/ Survey Certification Group: *Requirements for hospital medication administration, particularly intravenous (IV) medications and post-operative care of patients receiving IV opioids*, Baltimore, MD, 2014, Department of Health and Human Services, Centers for Medicare and Medicaid Services.

Chand S, Sarin J: Electronic nursing documentation, *Int J Inf Dis Technol* 4:328, 2014.

Department of Health and Human Services: *State Medicaid Director Letter*, SMDL #08-004, Baltimore, MD, 2008, Center for Medicaid and State Operations.

Ender KL, et al: Use of a clinical pathway to improve the acute management of vaso-occlusive crisis pain in pediatric sickle cell disease, *Pediatr Blood Cancer* 61:693, 2014.

Griffith R: Understanding the code: keeping accurate records, *Br J Community Nurs* 20:511, 2015.

Hall ES, et al: Variation in neonatal inpatient charges at the State and Local level, *Hosp Top* 93:27, 2015.

Hebda T, Czar P: *Handbook of informatics for nurses & healthcare professionals*, Upper Saddle River, NJ, 2013, Pearson Education, Inc.

HITECH: *Answers: Meaningful use*, 2017. http://www.hitechanswers.net/ chr-adoption-2/meaningful-use/.

Internal Revenue Service (IRS): *The American Recovery and Reinvestment Act (ARRA) of 2009: Information center*, 2016. https://www.irs.gov/uac/the -american-recovery-and-reinvestment -act-of-2009-information-center.

Johnson M, et al: Reducing patient clinical management errors using structured content and electronic nursing handover, *J Nurs Care Qual* 31:245, 2016.

Joint Commission Center for Transforming Healthcare: *Hand-off communication*, 2012. https://www.jointcommission.org/ assets/1/6/tst_hoc_persp_08_12.pdf.

Kerr N: Creating a protective picture: a grounded theory of RN decision-making when using a charting-by-exception documentation system, *Medsurg Nurs* 22:110, 2013.

Lavin M, et al: Health information technology, patient safety, and professional nursing care documentation in acute care settings, *Online J Issues Nurs* 20:6, 2015.

Lee S: Features of computerized clinical decision support systems supportive of nursing practice, *Comput Inform Nurs* 31:477, 2013.

Lewis SL, et al: *Medical-surgical nursing: assessment and management of clinical problems*, St Louis, 2017, Elsevier.

Mardis T, et al: Bedside shift-to-shift handoffs: a systematic review of the literature, *J Nurs Care Qual* 31:54, 2016.

Mostashari F: *Statement by Farzad Mostashari, MD, ScM, National Coordinator, Office of the National Coordinator for Health Information Technology, U.S. Department of Health and Human Services (HHS) on Health IT before Committee on Finance, U.S. Senate, Wednesday*, July 17, 2013.

Occupational Safety and Health Administration (OSHA): *Incident investigation*, n.d. https://www.osha .gov/dcsp/products/topics/ incidentinvestigation/index.html.

Ozkaynak M, et al: Use of electronic health records by nurses for symptom management in inpatient settings: a systematic review, *Comput Inform Nurs* 35(9):465, 2017.

Pagana KD, et al: *Mosby's diagnostic and laboratory test reference*, ed 12, St Louis, 2015, Elsevier.

Penoyer DA, et al: Use of electronic health record documentation by healthcare workers in an acute care hospital system, *J Healthc Manag* 59:130, 2014.

Polit DF, Beck CT: *Essentials of nursing research: appraising evidence for nursing practice*, ed 8, Philadelphia, 2017, Lippincott, Williams & Wilkins.

QSEN Institute: *QSEN competencies*, 2014. http://qsen.org/competencies/ pre-licensure-ksas/#informatics.

Rudolph JL, et al: Validation of a delirium risk assessment using electronic medical record information, *J Am Med Dir Assoc* 17:244, 2016.

Shang J, et al: Infection in home health care: results from national Outcome and Assessment Information Set data, *Am J Infect Control* 43:454, 2015.

The Joint Commission (TJC): Sentinel Events statistics for 2011, *Jt Comm Perspect* 32(5):5, 2012.

The Joint Commission (TJC): Patient safety, *Joint Commission Online*, 2015. http:// www.jointcommission.org/assets/1/23/ jconline_April_29_15.pdf.

The Joint Commission (TJC): *2017 Comprehensive accreditation manual for hospitals*, Oakbrook Terrace, IL, 2017, The Commission.

The Joint Commission (TJC): *2018 National Patient Safety Goals*, Oakbrook Terrace, IL, 2018, The Commission. https:// www.jointcommission.org/standards _information/npsgs.aspx.

US Government Publishing Office (GPO): *Electronic Code of Federal Regulations (eCFR)*, 2017. http://www.ecfr.gov/ cgi-bin/text-idx?c=ecfr&tpl=/ecfrbrowse/ Title45/45cfr164_main_02.tpl.

Voyer P, et al: Nursing documentation in long-term care settings: new empirical evidence demands changes be made, *Clin Nurs Res* 23(4):442, 2014.

Weis JM, Levy PC: Copy, paste, and cloned notes in electronic health records, *Chest* 145(3):632, 2014.

World Health Organization: *Clean care is safer care: five moments for hand hygiene*, 2017. http://www.who.int/gpsc/tools/ Five_moments/en/.

evolve MEDIA RESOURCES

http://evolve.elsevier.com/Potter/essentials
- Audio Glossary
- QSEN Activity and Review Questions Answers and Rationales

OBJECTIVES

- Describe the elements of the communication process.
- Describe the levels of communication and their uses in nursing.
- Differentiate aspects of verbal and nonverbal communication.
- Identify features and expected outcomes of the nurse-patient relationship.
- Describe a nurse's focus within each phase of a therapeutic nurse-patient relationship.
- Describe behaviors and techniques that affect communication.
- Describe standardized communication tools used to facilitate safe, complete, and organized communication.
- Discuss the principles of plain language for promoting health literacy.
- Explain the focus of communication within each phase of the nursing process.
- Discuss effective communication for patients of varying developmental levels.
- Explain techniques used to assist patients with special communication needs.

KEY TERMS

active listening, p. 192
AIDET, p. 184
assertive communication, p. 194
channel, p. 179
communication, p. 179
compassion fatigue, p. 187
connotative meaning, p. 180
denotative meaning, p. 180
empathy, p. 192

environment, p. 180
feedback, p. 179
hand-off report, p. 185
interpersonal communication, p. 180
interpersonal variables, p. 179
intrapersonal communication, p. 180
lateral violence, p. 187
message, p. 179
metacommunication, p. 182

nonverbal communication, p. 181
presence, p. 189
public communication, p. 180
receiver, p. 179
sender, p. 179
SBAR, p. 185
therapeutic communication, p. 184
touch, p. 195
verbal communication, p. 180

Communication is essential to achieve positive patient outcomes and is a deliberate nursing intervention for engaging patients and families in their own nursing care. Therapeutic communication conveys caring and facilitates positive change through the nursing process. Effective communication with all members of the health care team supports quality and safety initiatives and enhances patient satisfaction. Effective communication among the health care team strengthens nurses' engagement within their work units and organizations and improves nurse retention (Arnold and Boggs, 2016).

You use nonverbal, verbal, and technological skills to communicate in both personal and professional situations. Even without speaking, you send and receive information

CASE STUDY *Elmer "Bud" Johnson*

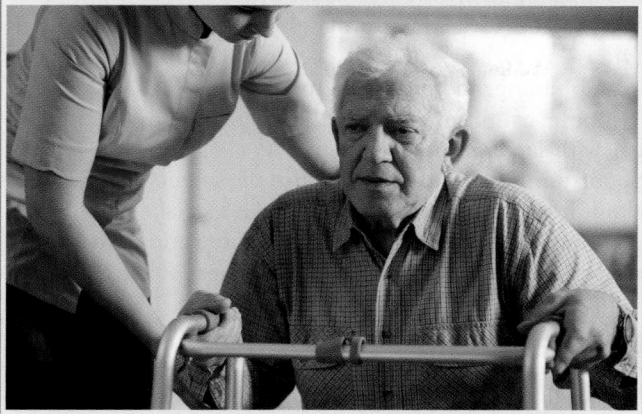

Copyright © KatarzynaBialasiewicz/iStock/Thinkstock.

Elmer "Bud" Johnson is a 72-year-old white man who is recovering from a fall with a femur fracture. He currently is a patient on a rehabilitation unit. Bud has significant peripheral neuropathy that has affected his gait for many years. He is a Vietnam War veteran who also has a history of addiction to narcotics that began during his military service, but he has been free of narcotic use for the past 20 years. After Bud fell, however, he was given narcotics for several days postoperatively. He sees himself as a fighter and is determined to regain full mobility. The goals for his rehabilitation are to restore safe ambulation (with or without an assistive device), restore independence in activities of daily living, and maintain narcotic-free pain control. Bud experienced a bitter divorce and has been living alone for the past 15 years. He has one grown daughter who lives more than 500 miles away. His main activity had been work as an auto mechanic. He retired about 5 years ago. His current support network consists of a few friends who are also veterans and part of a group that participates in events and rallies for veterans.

Marianne is a 45-year-old nurse whose father was also a veteran. Marianne became interested in nursing as a career that would allow her flexibility in work hours and the ability to help people. She enjoys working with older adults and finds satisfaction in seeing patients meet their rehabilitation goals.

continually through posture, gestures, or facial expressions. You communicate in person, in writing, over the telephone or by text, through fax and electronic mail, in the electronic health record (EHR), and with social media such as Facebook and Twitter. Communication in all these modes is a dynamic and often complex process.

THE POWER OF COMMUNICATION

As with any aspect of treatment, communication may result in both harm and good. Your posture, expressions, gestures, and every word you choose and phrase you speak can hurt or heal through the messages they send. Therapeutic communication empowers others and enables people to make health-promoting choices. Failure to communicate effectively leads to serious problems such as health care errors and

increased liability and threatens professional credibility. Inappropriate or missing communication causes delays in health care delivery; contributes to medical errors; and may increase the cost to the patient, the health care agency, and society.

Self-awareness is important for effective communication (Arnold and Boggs, 2016). As you know more about yourself, you are able to relate to others more effectively. Reflection on your interactions increases your understanding of the communication process and improves your ability to communicate with your patients.

In the case study, Marianne reflects on her perception of older adults when she first began to work as a nurse. Initially she had thought that older adults were likely to be confused or dull. She now realizes that each of the patients she cares for has a unique life story; each patient is an individual. Bud, for example, shared some of his experiences in Vietnam with Marianne as well as his struggle with pain and addiction when he returned stateside. These conversations have deepened her awareness of her own father's wartime experience as well as his coping strategies used at home.

BASIC ELEMENTS OF THE COMMUNICATION PROCESS

In your professional nursing role you learn to pay attention to each aspect of the communication process so your interactions are purposeful and effective. The basic elements of the communication process are the following:

- The **sender** is the person who delivers the message. The roles of sender and receiver change back and forth as two persons interact.
- You send a message to the **receiver**. The message prompts a response. The more the sender and receiver have in common and the closer the relationship, the more likely it is that the receiver will accurately perceive the sender's meaning and respond appropriately.
- The **message** is the content of the conversation including verbal and nonverbal information that the sender expresses. The most effective message is clear, organized, and expressed in a manner familiar to both the sender and the receiver.
- The message that the receiver returns to the sender is **feedback**. Feedback indicates whether the receiver understood the meaning of the sender's message. Your positive intent is not enough to ensure accurate reception of a message. Seek verbal and nonverbal feedback from the receiver to be sure that the receiver understands the message.
- The **channel** is the means of conveying and receiving messages through visual, auditory, and tactile senses. For example, your facial expression sends a visual message, and spoken words travel through auditory channels. Usually the more channels the sender uses to convey a message, the more clearly the receiver will understand the message.
- **Interpersonal variables** influence communication, as the sender and receiver continually influence one another. A

nurse's communication with a patient or another professional may be affected by interpersonal factors such as educational level, role in the health care environment, or socioeconomic status; communication of a patient or family member with the nurse will also be affected by interpersonal factors. A patient may respond differently to a nurse who is significantly younger or older. A family member's response to the nurse leader may be different than the person's response to a student nurse.

- The environment is the physical and emotional climate in which an interaction takes place. Each environmental factor can enhance or distract from a satisfying nurse-patient communication. If the environment includes significant background noise or insufficient light, the ability of the patient to attend to the communication is often impaired. Similarly, if other people are present, the communication may be impaired or enhanced. Patients sometimes withhold information or feelings if others in the area are not known or trusted but are set at ease by the presence of a different person. If the patient is not physically or emotionally comfortable in the environment, communication will be less than ideal. For example, if the environment is not at a comfortable temperature, the patient may be ill at ease, impacting the quality of the interaction. The more appropriate the environment, the more successful the communication exchange.

LEVELS OF COMMUNICATION

As a nurse, you communicate at different levels. You communicate with yourself, other individuals, and groups. Each level of communication is important and affects your nursing practice. Even though you have been communicating all your life, effective nursing communication is a complex skill that improves with practice and feedback through reflection and the responses of others.

Intrapersonal communication, also called *self-talk*, is a powerful form of communication that occurs within an individual. Both you and your patients engage in self-talk by forming thoughts internally. These thoughts strongly influence perceptions, feelings, behavior, self-concept, and performance. Self-talk is a mental rehearsal for difficult tasks or situations so that individuals deal with them more effectively. An example is reflection, which you can use to think back on previous patient care situations so that you consider effective and ineffective approaches that you used previously (see Chapter 8). Be aware of the nature and content of your own thinking, and seek to replace negative, self-defeating thoughts with realistic and positive ones. Your intrapersonal "self-talk" affects the way others perceive you in your professional role. Use positive self-talk to boost your confidence as a nurse.

Interpersonal communication is interaction that occurs between two people or within a small group. It refers to nonverbal and verbal behavior within a social context and includes the use of symbols and cues to give and receive meaning. Because the message received is sometimes different from the intended message, validate or mutually negotiate the meaning for all involved. Effective interpersonal communication includes idea and information sharing, problem solving, expressing feelings, making decisions, accomplishing goals, team building, and personal growth.

Public communication is the interaction of one individual with large groups of people. As a nurse, you may have opportunities to speak with groups of patients or consumers about health-related topics. You make special adaptations in eye contact, posture, gestures, voice inflection, and use of media materials to communicate messages effectively.

FORMS OF COMMUNICATION

You send messages in many ways: verbally, nonverbally, concretely, and symbolically. People express themselves through language, movements, gestures, voice inflection, facial expressions, and use of space. Many forms of communication combine to create meaning in a sender's message.

Verbal Communication

Verbal communication involves the spoken or written word. Verbal language conveys specific meaning as you combine words. The following sections discuss the most important aspects of verbal communication.

Vocabulary. Communication is unsuccessful if a receiver cannot translate a sender's words and phrases. You will work with people of various cultures who speak different languages. Even people who speak the same language use subcultural variations of words. For example, *dinner* means a midday meal for some, whereas others use *dinner* to mean the last meal of the day. Because medical terms are often misunderstood, you need to use plain language when communicating with people outside the health care field. This means avoiding jargon, using the active voice (e.g., "When you get up …"), and keeping your sentences and explanations brief (Wittenberg et al., 2015).

For many individuals with limited English proficiency (LEP), the inability to communicate in English is the primary barrier to accessing health information and services. These patients require you to use professional interpreters who are able to speak the person's primary language. Health information for people with LEP needs to be communicated plainly in their primary language, using words and examples that make the information understandable (Nordby, 2016).

Denotative and Connotative Meaning. A word sometimes has several meanings. Individuals who use a common language share the denotative meaning of a word. The word *baseball* has the same meaning for all individuals who speak English, but the word *code* denotes cardiac arrest primarily to health care providers. The connotative meaning is the shade or interpretation of the meaning of a word, which is influenced by the thoughts, feelings, or ideas that people have about the word. Families who are told that a loved one is in serious condition might believe that death is near, but to nurses the term *serious* may simply describe the nature of the illness and not the prognosis.

Pacing. Talking rapidly, using awkward pauses, or speaking extremely slowly and deliberately conveys an unintended message. Consider the following exchange:

> *Patient:* "Do you know if the doctor found anything wrong with me?"
> *Nurse:* "No ... but I'm sure if he did ... he would have come to explain things to you." (Then very rapidly) "Now let's get back to what we were doing."

Long pauses and a rapid shift to another subject may give the impression that you are hiding the truth. Speak slowly, enunciate clearly, and use pauses to stress a particular point or give the listener time to understand.

Intonation and Volume. Tone of voice and volume dramatically affect the meaning of a message, and emotions directly influence tone of voice. A simple question or statement can express enthusiasm, anger, or concern. Be aware of your intonation and volume to avoid sending unintended patronizing or critical messages. If a patient interprets your message as uncaring or condescending, communication is blocked. Pay attention to a patient's intonation and volume for information about his or her emotional state or energy level.

Clarity and Brevity. Effective communication is simple, short, and to the point to minimize confusion. Avoid phrases such as "you know," "right," or "OK?" at the end of every sentence. Give examples to clarify messages for the receiver. Use short sentences and words that express an idea simply and directly.

Timing and Relevance. Timing is critical in communication. Even if a message is clear, poor timing prevents it from being effective. Do not begin routine teaching when a patient is in severe pain, short of breath, or in emotional distress. The best time for interaction is when a patient expresses an interest in communicating because relevant messages are more effective. When a patient is facing emergency surgery, discussing the risks of smoking is less relevant than discussing what the staff will do to prepare the patient for surgery.

Nonverbal Communication

Nonverbal communication includes messages sent through body language without using words. Nonverbal forms of communication include facial expressions; vocal cues; eye contact; and cues such as gestures, posture, touch, odor, physical appearance, dress, silence, and the use of time (Arnold and Boggs, 2016). Nonverbal communication often reveals true feelings because you may be less censored about nonverbal reactions. A patient who says he feels fine but frowns while moving and holds his body rigidly is probably in pain. Nonverbal cues add meaning to verbal communication and help you judge the reliability of verbal messages. Nonverbal behav-

iors vary in different cultures, so gestures or expressions that are acceptable in one culture may have a different meaning and be considered rude in another culture (Arnold and Boggs, 2016). When communicating with a person from an unfamiliar culture, you need to clarify the meaning of gestures or other nonverbal cues.

Because you communicate using nonverbal messages often without awareness, you need to be aware of your own nonverbal behavior. Be sure that your nonverbal and verbal messages match and convey care and concern. If you say that a patient is getting better but demonstrate an expression of doubt, you do not relieve a patient's anxiety.

Personal Appearance. Physical characteristics, manner of dress and grooming, and jewelry are indicators of well-being, personality, social status, occupation, religion, culture, and self-concept. First impressions are largely based on appearance. Your physical appearance influences a patient's perception of you as a professional and the care you will deliver. You wear uniforms, scrubs, laboratory coats, business suits, or street clothes, depending on your role. Although your dress may not reflect your abilities, it takes longer to establish trust if your clothing detracts from a professional image. Tattoos and body piercings are becoming common in society. However, both can affect the perceptions patients have about your professionalism; they are examples of interpersonal variables, and patients will respond to them. In a study of hospitalized patients, patient care providers with visible tattoos and/or body piercings were not perceived as caring, confident, reliable, attentive, cooperative, professional, efficient, or approachable as providers without tattoos and/or body piercings (Westerfield et al., 2012). Female providers with tattoos were perceived as less professional than male providers with similar tattoos. In many health care settings any tattoos must be covered by a uniform.

Posture and Gait. The way people sit, stand, and move is a form of self-expression. Posture and gait reflect emotions, self-concept, and health status. An erect posture and a quick, purposeful gait communicate a sense of well-being and confidence. A slumped posture and slow, shuffling gait may indicate depression or fatigue. Leaning forward conveys attention. Leaning backward in a more relaxed manner shows less interest or indicates caution.

Facial Expression. A sender's facial expressions often become the basis for judgments by the receiver. However, because of the diversity in facial expressions, meanings may be misunderstood. Facial expressions reveal, contradict, or suppress true emotions. People are often unaware of the messages their expressions send. When facial expressions are unclear, seek verbal feedback about the sender's intent. A patient who frowns after receiving information may be confused, angry, disapproving, or simply unable to hear you clearly or concentrating on a reply. In this case say, "I notice you're frowning," and have the patient clarify his or her response.

Patients watch nurses closely. Consider the effect that your facial expression has on a patient who asks, "Am I going to die?" The slightest change in the eyes, lips, or face reveals your true feelings. Practice avoidance of showing overt shock, disgust, dismay, or other distressing reactions in a patient's presence.

Eye Contact. Many individuals, regardless of sociocultural differences, maintain eye contact during conversation. By maintaining eye contact, you communicate respect and a willingness to listen. Lack of eye contact may indicate deference, anxiety, defensiveness, discomfort, or a lack of confidence in communicating. You may find that some individuals respond to eye contact by looking away, looking down, or becoming uncomfortable; this may be a cultural difference or may be related to a personal characteristic. Adjust your eye contact to promote an interaction that is comfortable for the patient. If you are in doubt, you may ask the patient about his or her preferences.

Eye movements communicate feelings and emotions. Wide eyes express frankness, terror, and innocence. Downward glances show avoidance or modesty. Raised upper eyelids reveal displeasure, and a constant stare may be associated with hatred or coldness. Avoid significant nurse-patient conversation that involves you looking down on a person; take time to sit down and make eye contact at the same level with a patient. This conveys equality and caring in your nurse-patient relationship. Equalizing the eye level with an angry person can diffuse a situation.

Gestures. A salute, thumbs up, fist bump, and tapping foot are types of gestures. Hands, shoulders, and feet emphasize, punctuate, and clarify the spoken word. Gestures alone carry specific meanings, or they may create messages with other communication cues. A finger pointed toward a person may communicate several different meanings; however, if for example you frown and have a stern tone of voice, the gesture becomes a sign of accusation or threat.

Territoriality and Space. Territoriality is the need to gain, maintain, and defend one's exclusive right to space. *Territory* can be separated and made visible to others such as by a fence around a yard. *Personal space* is invisible, is individual, and travels with a person. During interpersonal interaction people maintain varying distances between themselves, depending on the nature of the relationship and situation. When personal space is threatened, people respond defensively and communicate less effectively. Examples of nursing actions within the four zones of personal space are listed in Box 11.1 (Kneisl and Trigoboff, 2013).

Because of the nature of caregiving, you must frequently move into a patient's territory and personal space. Convey confidence, gentleness, and respect for privacy, especially when actions require intimate contact. Knock before you enter a room. As you leave, ask if the patient wants the door open or closed. Ask if you can reposition the bed table and clarify which items the patient wants within reach.

BOX 11.1   NURSING ACTIONS WITHIN THE ZONES OF PERSONAL SPACE AND TOUCH

ZONES OF PERSONAL SPACE

Intimate Zone (0 to 18 inches)
- Holding a crying infant
- Performing physical assessment
- Bathing, grooming, dressing, feeding, and toileting a patient
- Changing a patient's dressing

Personal Zone (18 inches to 4 feet)
- Sitting at patient's bedside
- Taking patient's nursing history
- Teaching an individual patient
- Exchanging hand-off communication at change of shift

Social Zone (4 to 12 feet)
- Making rounds with a health care provider
- Sitting at the head of a conference table
- Teaching a class for patients with diabetes
- Conducting a family support group

Public Zone (12 feet and greater)
- Speaking at a community forum
- Testifying at a legislative hearing
- Lecturing to a class of students

ZONES OF TOUCH

Social Zone (Permission Not Needed)
- Hands
- Arms
- Shoulders
- Back

Consent Zone (Permission Needed)
- Mouth
- Wrists
- Feet

Vulnerable Zone (Special Care Needed)
- Face
- Neck
- Front of body

Intimate Zone (Great Sensitivity Needed)
- Genitalia
- Rectum

FACTORS INFLUENCING COMMUNICATION

Contextual factors influence the nature of communication and interpersonal relationships (Box 11.2). Awareness of these factors helps you to make sound decisions during the communication process.

Metacommunication is the exploration of all factors that influence communication. Awareness of influencing factors helps you better understand what is communicated (Arnold and Boggs, 2016). *For example, Bud tells Marianne, "I am getting along OK without pain medicine," but he has tight facial features and is grimacing while speaking.* Your nursing knowledge and experience with assessing patients' pain will make you sensitive to cultural and personal variations that affect communication. When you become aware that a patient's verbal and nonverbal behaviors do not match, this will prompt you to explore the situation further. *For example, Marianne responds to Bud, "It looks like you may be having*

BOX 11.2 FACTORS INFLUENCING COMMUNICATION

PSYCHOPHYSIOLOGICAL CONTEXT—INTERNAL FACTORS INFLUENCING COMMUNICATION
- Physical health (e.g., pain, hunger, weakness, dyspnea)
- Emotional status (e.g., anxiety, anger, depression, fear)
- Growth and development status (e.g., age and developmental stage)
- Unmet needs (e.g., safety/security; love/belonging; grief resolution)
- Attitudes, values, and beliefs (e.g., confidence in health care providers; meaning of illness)
- Perceptions and personality (e.g., optimistic/pessimistic; trusting/nontrusting)
- Self-concept and self-esteem (e.g., positive/negative)

RELATIONAL CONTEXT—NATURE OF RELATIONSHIP BETWEEN PARTICIPANTS
- Social, helping, or working relationship
- Level of trust and self-disclosure between participants
- Degree of sharing among participants
- Shared history of participants
- Balance of power and control

SITUATIONAL CONTEXT—REASON FOR COMMUNICATION
- Information exchange
- Goal achievement
- Problem resolution
- Expression of feelings

ENVIRONMENTAL CONTEXT—PHYSICAL SURROUNDINGS IN WHICH COMMUNICATION OCCURS
- Degree of privacy
- Comfort and safety level
- Noise level
- Presence of distractions

CULTURAL CONTEXT—SOCIOCULTURAL ELEMENTS THAT AFFECT INTERACTION
- Educational level of participants
- Language and self-expression patterns
- Customs and expectations

some pain, by the expression on your face.” Bud then clarifies, *“Yes, I am having some pain, but I can bear it and I don't want to use narcotics for pain control, since it was so hard to shake that habit after Vietnam.”* This analysis of all aspects of communication is metacommunication.

Culture is an important factor influencing communication (see Chapter 21). Culture affects how people communicate, understand, and respond to health information (Mott-Coles, 2014). Your cultural and linguistic competence contribute to a patient's health literacy. Your competence in responding to patients from different cultures will depend on your ability to recognize their cultural beliefs, values, attitudes, traditions, language preferences, and health practices and to apply that

knowledge to produce a positive health outcome when you communicate with them. Try to understand their situation through their eyes. This perspective makes communication more relevant and appropriate to each patient's situation and increases the likelihood of giving patients the information they need for desirable outcomes (Nordby, 2016).

Health Literacy

The health of many of the millions of patients we care for may be at risk because of the challenges in understanding and acting on health information (Literacy Inc., 2017; Weiss, 2015). According to a study conducted in 2015 by the U.S. Department of Education and the National Institute of Literacy, 32 million adults in the United States cannot read above a fifth-grade level, and 19% of high school graduates cannot read (U.S. Department of Education, 2016). The average American reads at the eighth- or ninth-grade level. The language that health care providers choose to use when communicating with patients when speaking and writing significantly impacts whether they understand basic health information and the services needed to make appropriate health decisions. Follow these tips when communicating with patients whom you suspect have health literacy problems:

- Organize what you want to say so that the most important points come first. For example, when teaching about a medication, start with its purpose, the dose a patient is to take, and the time to take the medicine. Follow with information about side effects and what to report to a health care provider.
- Break complex information into understandable chunks. For example, say, “This medicine is for your heart. We want you to take a dose once a day. The best time is in the morning about an hour after you usually have breakfast.”
- Plan multiple short teaching sessions instead of one long session.
- Use simple language, avoiding jargon and defining technical terms (e.g., use the term *tablets* instead of medication).
- Use the teach-back method (see Chapter 12) to gather important information about patient understanding
- Use the active voice. An example of active voice is “One of the nurses will give you a prescription before you go home.” An example of passive voice is “The prescription for your medicines is being prepared by one of the nurses.”

The Nurse-Patient Relationship

In the case study, as Marianne works with Bud, she develops a therapeutic relationship. They work together to manage his pain without the use of narcotics. Marianne recognizes Bud's courage and integrity. Marianne knows that active listening skills are essential to understand Bud's life experience and perceptions, including his personal insights and aspirations for rehabilitation. In the working phase of the therapeutic relationship, Marianne poses open-ended questions that encourage Bud to reflect.

Marianne asks, "What are your needs at this time?" and "Tell me about your hopes for the future." Bud talks about wanting to become strong enough to remain in his second floor apartment. He is concerned that he will have no one to help him as he becomes less able to manage his own affairs, and he does not want to burden his daughter.

You develop helping relationships between you and your patients through caring and skill involving effective communication. Through therapeutic communication, an interactive dynamic process involving verbal and nonverbal exchanges between a nurse and patient, you develop a relationship with a patient to meet health-related goals (Arnold and Boggs, 2016). Box 11.3 summarizes the four phases of the nurse-patient relationship. A therapeutic relationship requires you to help your patients clarify needs and goals, solve problems, and cope with situational or maturational crises. You also help them explore the meaning of their illness experience and sort out responses to stressful situations to increase their coping skills (Arnold and Boggs, 2016). Creating a therapeutic environment depends on your ability to communicate, provide comfort, and help patients meet their needs. Comforting strategies include gentle humor, physical comfort measures, emotionally supportive statements, and therapeutic touch. You provide information, support patients' active decision making, and offer opportunities for patients to engage in social exchange. As a nurse, your time with each patient may be limited. Nonetheless, you can still achieve a therapeutic relationship. Use each interaction as an opportunity to build rapport and convey caring whether you are completing your assessment, providing technical care, or responding to a nurse call system. Aim to listen carefully to what a patient says, and pay attention to the unspoken message. Respond with empathy and attentiveness to the patient's physical and emotional needs.

AIDET. One important tool for initiating and structuring a therapeutic relationship is derived from the work of the Studer Group (n.d.). Used widely and known to health care workers simply as *AIDET,* this acronym provides you with prompts for effective communication during an interaction with patients. It is especially valuable in enabling you to communicate important information in a short period of time. You can use the AIDET tool in any inpatient or outpatient setting. Each letter stands for part of a communication pattern that ensures that patients receive clear communication:

- **Acknowledge:** Recognize and greet the patient and individuals accompanying the patient. Provide a warm greeting with eye contact and open welcoming body language.
- **Introduce yourself:** Provide your name, department, and job role on your initial visit. Reinforce your role on

---

BOX 11.3 NURSING INTERVENTIONS DURING PHASES OF THE THERAPEUTIC RELATIONSHIP

PREINTERACTION PHASE—BEFORE MEETING THE PATIENT
- Review available data including medical and nursing histories.
- Talk to other caregivers who may have information about the patient.
- Anticipate health concerns or issues that may arise.
- Identify a location and setting that fosters comfortable, private interaction.
- Plan enough time for initial interaction.

ORIENTATION PHASE—WHEN YOU AND THE PATIENT MEET AND GET TO KNOW ONE ANOTHER
- Set the tone for the relationship by adopting a warm, empathetic, caring manner.
- Recognize that the initial relationship may be casual, uncertain, and tentative.
- Expect the patient to test your competence and commitment.
- Closely observe and expect to be closely observed by the patient.
- Begin to make inferences and form judgments about the patient's messages and behavior.
- Assess the patient's health status.
- Prioritize patient problems and identify patient goals.
- Clarify the patient's role and your role.

- Form contracts with the patient to specify roles.
- Let the patient know when the relationship will end.

WORKING PHASE—WHEN YOU AND THE PATIENT WORK TOGETHER TO SOLVE PROBLEMS AND ACCOMPLISH GOALS
- Encourage and help the patient express feelings about his or her health.
- Encourage and help the patient with self-exploration.
- Provide information needed to understand and change behavior.
- Encourage and help the patient to set goals.
- Take actions to meet the goals set with the patient.
- Use therapeutic communication skills to facilitate successful interactions.
- Use appropriate self-disclosure and confrontation.

TERMINATION PHASE—DURING THE ENDING OF THE RELATIONSHIP
- Remind the patient that termination is near.
- Evaluate goal achievement with the patient.
- Reminisce about the relationship with the patient.
- Separate from the patient by relinquishing responsibility for his or her care.
- Achieve a smooth transition for the patient to other caregivers as needed.

subsequent visits. During an initial communication, include details about your experience or skills that will assure the patient of your competence. When appropriate, include positive statements about other health care personnel who will also be involved in the patient's care.

- **Duration:** The patient wants to understand how long an appointment, treatment, test, or procedure will take, including likely periods of waiting. Provide the most accurate information you can. Sometimes, the length of the wait or the treatment cannot be estimated. In this case provide a time period within which you will check back in with the patient. When appropriate, explain when the patient should expect to hear about the results or needed follow-up from a test or procedure.
- **Explanation:** Discuss the reason for an appointment, test, intervention, or action with the patient. Clarify what will happen and what the patient should expect. Ask, "What questions do you have? Tell me what you would like to know."
- **Thanks:** Demonstrate sincere appreciation to the patient and others. Convey to the patient that it has been an honor to be entrusted with his or her health care (Lerner, 2015).

Nurse–Health Team Member Relationships

Effective communication with other members of the health care team positively influences teamwork and staff satisfaction and improves quality of patient care and safety. To ensure quality and promote a culture of safety, health care organizations must address behaviors that threaten the performance of the health care team including interpersonal skills and professionalism (Gluyas, 2015; Mascioli, 2016). Breakdown in communication among health care professionals is a key cause of serious injuries and death in health care settings (Lim and Bernstein, 2014). Many of the 2017 National Patient Safety Goals from The Joint Commission (TJC, 2018) such as patient identification, improving staff communication, and reconciling medications are directly or indirectly related to communication.

Reporting. Reports are an exchange of information among health care team members. A report reflects a summary of activities or observations seen, performed, or heard by a health care provider. Key types of reports nurses provide include a telephone report, incident report, and hand-off report (see Chapter 10). A risk for miscommunication exists when patients move from one nursing unit to another or from one provider to another. A hand-off report is the verbal and written exchange of pertinent information during this transition of care (Pettit and Duffy, 2015). Open and accurate communication, particularly during hand-offs, is essential to prevent errors. The purpose of a hand-off report is to provide safe and effective continuity of care. Following a hand-off report, responsibility for patient care is transferred from one person to another.

A change of shift report is one type of hand-off report. Other hand-off reports occur when a patient is being moved from one department or area to another for a period of time. When you perform a hand-off report, you share essential information to provide for patient safety and continuity of care. Use an organized and concise approach to ensure that key information is not omitted and excess detail does not add confusion (Anderson et al., 2015). A standardized approach to a hand-off report may be used as a tool. One standardized hand-off acronym is I PASS THE BATON (Box 11.4).

Similar to a hand-off report, a telephone conversation also benefits from use of common language and format. When you are communicating critical information, one commonly used tool that helps prevent misunderstandings and creates a culture of safety is SBAR (pronounced S-BAR). This tool is used in telephone and verbal reports. SBAR communication has become a best practice for standardizing communication

BOX 11.4	I PASS THE BATON: AN EXAMPLE OF A STANDARDIZED HAND-OFF TOOL	
I	Introduction	Introduce yourself and your role/job (include patient)
P	Patient	Name, identifiers, age, sex, and location
A	Assessment	Present chief complaint, vital signs, symptoms, and diagnosis
S	Situation	Current status/circumstances including code status, level of (un)certainty, recent changes, and response to treatment
S	Safety	Critical laboratory values and/or reports, socioeconomic factors, allergies, and alerts (e.g., falls, isolation)
THE		
B	Background	Comorbidities, previous episodes, current medications, and family history
A	Actions	Explain what actions were taken or are required; provide rationale
T	Timing	Level of urgency and explicit timing and prioritization of actions
O	Ownership	Identify who is responsible (person/team) including patient/family caregivers
N	Next	What will happen next? What are anticipated changes? What is the plan? Are there contingency plans?

(QSEN) QSEN ACTIVITY *Patient-Centered Care*

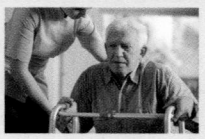

Copyright © KatarzynaBialasiewicz/ iStock/Thinkstock.

The rehabilitation unit staff conduct patient-centered bedside shift reports, according to the evidence-based guidelines created by the Agency for Healthcare Research and Quality (AHRQ) and consistent with QSEN. Providing patient-centered care recognizes the patient as the source of control and as a full partner in providing compassionate and coordinated care (Cronenwett et al., 2007). Marianne and the other nurses on the unit identified several ways to improve communication among the health care team and with patients including moving the location of the change-of-shift report to the bedside and establishing nurse-physician huddles at the bedside (Davis, 2015).

- As the nurse caring for Bud, state the plain language you will use to describe the rationale behind conducting hand-off communication at the bedside.
- How, if at all, do you adapt your communication with your coworkers, as Bud can hear and participate in everything you say?
- Describe one strategy for responding to differences of opinion regarding the goals of Bud's care for the next shift.

evolve Answers to QSEN Activities can be found on the Evolve website.

among health care providers. SBAR stands for *Situation, Background, Assessment,* and *Recommendation* (see Chapter 10). Information about both SBAR and I PASS THE BATON is available from the Agency for Healthcare Research and Quality (AHRQ, n.d.) as a part of TeamSTEPPS.

In the case study, Bud begins to experience warmth, redness, and pain in the right calf area. Marianne assesses Bud and then calls the health care provider. Recognizing the potential complication of a deep vein thrombosis (DVT), she communicates the change in Bud's health status (situation) and his recent fall/ fracture history including his peripheral neuropathy (background). Marianne then reports the results of her assessment: there is redness, swelling, tenderness, and a positive Homans' sign on Bud's right lower extremity (assessment). She then requests action to verify or rule out her suspicious findings that may suggest a DVT is developing (recommendation).

Because of Marianne's assessment and call, an ultrasound ordered by the physician confirms a DVT. The decision is made to transfer Bud to the acute care unit of the hospital for treatment. Marianne calls the acute care unit charge nurse, Tim Brown, to provide a hand-off report. She includes up-to-date information about Mr. Johnson's condition, including care, treatments, medications, and recent symptoms.

Teamwork. Effective communication with the health care provider and other health team members ensures patient safety and promotes optimal patient outcomes (Box 11.5). Nurses and other health care professionals work as a team. Effective communication and teamwork among nurses in a

BOX 11.5 EVIDENCE-BASED PRACTICE

PICO Question: Do hand-off reports compared with traditional end-of-shift reports reduce sentinel events and/ or errors among hospitalized patients?

SUMMARY OF EVIDENCE

Effective communication with a health care provider and other members of the health care team promotes optimal patient outcomes. The Joint Commission (TJC) reported that breakdowns in communication and leadership were among the top three most frequently identified root causes of sentinel events during 2014 (TJC, 2015). Sentinel events are unexpected occurrences that result in patient death or serious injury. Communication when the patient is handed over from one provider to another or from one setting to another is especially a problem. Intimidating and disruptive behaviors affect communication and must not be tolerated in health care settings (Anderson et al., 2015). Keebler et al. (2016) conducted a meta-analysis of research studies on the effects of standardized hand-off procedures on patient, provider, and organizational outcomes with a sample of 36 qualifying studies. The research showed a positive impact on all three types of outcomes.

APPLICATION TO NURSING PRACTICE

- Intimidating and disruptive behaviors affect communication and must not be tolerated in health care settings (Anderson et al., 2015).
- Develop common language for critical information for hand-off communications and communication of changes in a patient's condition.
- Use a communication tool such as SBAR to standardize communication (Institute for Healthcare Improvement [IHI], n.d.).
- Use a standardized format for change of shift report and hand-off communication (Agency for Healthcare Research and Quality [AHRQ], n.d.).
- Use a standardized format such as I PASS THE BATON or SBAR for report when patients are transferred to other units or facilities (IHI, n.d.).
- Provide the opportunity for questions and confirmation of understanding of communication.
- Have face-to-face communication when possible.
- Read back all health care provider prescriptions or orders or other pertinent information.
- Create a culture of teamwork and communication focused on patient safety that eliminates disruptive behavior (Pettit and Duffy, 2015).
- Work in multidisciplinary teams to develop common language.
- Develop skills in assertive communication and conflict management.

work setting is essential. Teamwork also affects nurse recruitment and retention. Social, informational, and therapeutic interactions help team members build morale, accomplish goals, and strengthen working relationships. Collegial relationships among all health care providers are characterized by communication elements of openness, accuracy, timeliness, and understanding to support professional nursing practice (Gluyas, 2015).

Interprofessional collaboration is characterized by effective communication, respect, trust, and availability and is a key factor in reducing error and improving patient outcomes (Pettit and Duffy, 2015). Interdisciplinary care rounds and huddles improve teamwork by bridging the communication gap among care providers, reducing caregiver stress, facilitating the communication of consistent health information to patients and caregivers, and promoting conflict resolution (Davis et al., 2015). Taking the term from sports teams, huddles are short meetings that include key care providers held to quickly discuss and respond to patient care needs or new problems. Nursing personnel may huddle partway through a shift to monitor a situation on the unit and provide additional assistance in areas of need. Sometimes interprofessional colleagues huddle to identify discharge planning strategies.

Effects of Stress. Compassion fatigue is defined as a combination of secondary traumatic stress and burnout experienced by professional and lay caregivers (see Chapter 26) (Houck, 2014; Perry and Edwards, 2015). Secondary traumatic stress is the emotional trauma you experience when witnessing patients' traumatic experiences and stories of pain, fear, and suffering. Being empathic increases your risk for secondary traumatic stress. Burnout occurs when your perceived demands of caregiving outweigh the resources (e.g., staffing, supplies, time) you have available. Nurses working closely with patients experiencing challenging illnesses often experience compassion fatigue. Recognition of this sense of stress is key to overcoming it (Houck, 2014). When you experience ongoing stressful patient relationships, you may disengage as a protective response; symptoms include anger, fatigue, feelings of inadequacy, cynicism, and impaired relationships in the workplace. This disengagement can also occur when perceived stress comes from challenging interprofessional relationships. Health care providers do not always voice concerns about patients and often avoid conflict with other health care workers in clinical settings, negatively impacting patient safety (Lim and Bernstein, 2014).

Lateral violence (also called *horizontal violence*) sometimes occurs in nurse-nurse interactions and includes behaviors such as withholding information, making snide remarks, and demonstrating nonverbal expressions of disapproval such as raising eyebrows or making faces. It can be a result of compassion fatigue or other factors. Nonetheless, these behaviors are uncivil and may undermine the unit culture. New graduates and nurses new to a unit are most at risk to experience lateral or horizontal violence. Challenged with the task of making the transition from student to practitioner, new graduates often lack the confidence and social skills that may ward off interpersonal conflict (Weaver, 2013). The following is an example of lateral violence: You may attempt to explain the scientific reason behind a procedure that you learned at school, but older nurse colleagues may joke about or deride your knowledge. Another example is a nurse may

---

BOX 11.6   SUGGESTED RESPONSES TO UNCIVIL PEER BEHAVIORS

COPING RESPONSES TO LACK OF CIVILITY AND LATERAL VIOLENCE BY PEERS

- Confront an uncivil peer in a quiet and private area, using assertive communication techniques described in this chapter. Do not engage in front of patients or colleagues, as this is not civil.
- **Paraphrasing:** When a colleague says something disparaging to you, you may try paraphrasing the response back in a questioning tone, "You're telling me that my time management skills are inadequate?"
- **Verbalizing the implied message:** When a colleague implies something negative, by a verbal or a nonverbal gesture such as eye rolling or smirking, you may respond by saying, "I see by your remark/facial expression that you have more to say about this. Please tell me what you are thinking."
- **Using humor:** When you may have erred or not responded well and others are either talking behind your back or teasing you, you can use humor that acknowledges the situation and takes the pressure off all parties.
- **Using "CUS" communication:** Use the TeamSTEPPS CUS method (AHRQ, n.d.) to respond to uncivil remarks or behaviors that undermine safety. For example, "I am *Con*cerned that when I indicated that I needed help with this urgent assessment, the only response I got was a comment that it was *my* patient." Then if no response, "I feel *Un*comfortable that there was no backup for a difficult situation." Then, "The well-being of all our patients is of primary concern, and this lack of response caused a *Safety* risk."
- **Creating opportunities for a welcoming culture:** Be a leader in creating a welcoming unit culture by consistent courteous communication, inviting others to engage with you, and by showing warmth and thanks.

---

complain about your lack of skill in front of a patient. All nurses require conflict resolution skills to address problems in the work environment, better manage the stressors that contribute to compassion fatigue, and respond to uncivil behaviors such as lateral violence. See Box 11.6 for suggested strategies. Nurses need to develop resiliency skills in stress and conflict management, including the ability to confront and respond to negative behaviors professionally.

COMMUNICATION WITHIN CARING RELATIONSHIPS

Therapeutic communication strengthens all caring relationships established within the professional role. You create caring and helping relationships with the qualities and behavior explained in this section.

Establishing a Therapeutic Relationship

Professionalism. A patient's acceptance of you as a professional often depends on your professional and caring image. Verbal and nonverbal behaviors influence the helping relationship. Professional appearance, demeanor, and behavior are important in establishing trustworthiness and competence. When you act professionally, you communicate that you have assumed the professional helping role, you are clinically skilled, and your focus is on the patient. Inappropriate appearance and behavior in individuals who hold a professional role harm the image of nursing. Consider the level of trust a patient feels with each nurse in the following examples.

In the acute care unit, Bud meets Annie Robbins, a nurse who walks in late and begins to adjust Bud's intravenous drip without introducing herself or washing her hands. She is smacking gum, wearing a very large necklace and earrings, and has long brightly colored false nails. She turns to Bud to obtain vital signs. Bud is becoming worried that he will not receive proper treatment, based on this employee's demeanor (he cannot see her name tag and is unsure of who she is). He says, "When will I see the doctor?" Annie replies that the doctor is always late, a statement that is not accurate and casts doubt on the quality of the care that Bud will receive.

Tim Brown, the charge nurse, enters Bud's area. He is organized, prepared, clean, and well groomed, with a visible name tag and no distracting scent, jewelry, or mannerisms. Tim enters the room, washes his hands, and introduces himself using the AIDET acronym. Tim then uses effective communication skills to assess the situation, providing information to Bud about what will happen next, explaining that a test will be performed to visualize the area where there may be a blood clot and that the health care provider will then confer with him about appropriate treatment. Bud feels a sense of relief flood over him because of this warm, informative, and professional communication.

Courtesy. Professional courtesy conveys respect for others and oneself. When you use the AIDET approach in your interactions, courtesy is ensured (Lerner, 2015). Remember to acknowledge adults by name to show your respect for the dignity and uniqueness of the other person, including use of a title and the patient's last name. Use of a first name is appropriate for children. Ask adult patients how they would like you to address them and let them know your personal preference as well. Other ways you demonstrate courtesy include saying "please" and "thank you" and apologizing for making an error or causing someone distress. These all are parts of professional communication. When you are discourteous, patients and staff perceive you as rude or insensitive. This sets up barriers between you and your patients and causes friction or tension among team members.

Showing genuine interest in a patient as a person is important in establishing a therapeutic relationship. As you get to know a patient and family, use limited social conversation to make connections. Commenting on a patient's choice of music, television show, reading materials, or personal items in the room can demonstrate interest; however, you must move beyond social conversation to discuss issues or concerns

affecting the patient's health. When establishing rapport, begin by asking an open-ended question about the patient's illness experience.

Avoid Terms of Endearment and Excessive Socializing. Calling a patient "honey," "dear," "Grandpa," or "sweetheart" rather than by a given name is inappropriate. Such casual familiarity from caregivers offends most people. Avoid referring to patients by diagnosis, room number, or another attribute. When you refer to patients by characteristics rather than their names, it is demeaning and depersonalizing and sends the message that you do not care enough about the person to know him or her as an individual. Spending too much time socializing undermines opportunities to establish a professional presence.

Confidentiality. Always safeguard a patient's right to privacy by carefully protecting confidential information. Reassure patients that you will keep information private, and keep that promise. Resist the temptation to share exciting or shocking information. Do not share information with people who are genuinely interested and concerned but have no legal right to the information as in the following example:

> *Patient:* "What's wrong with my roommate? She seems so sick."
> *Nurse:* "I know you're concerned about Mrs. Hoover, but I can't share any personal information about her."

If you need to report health information to others, tell the patient in advance, if possible. Sharing personal information or gossiping about others violates the ethical code and practice standards of nursing. It sends the message that you are not trustworthy and damages interpersonal relationships.

Trust. Trust is an essential building block of a therapeutic relationship. You foster trust when you demonstrate consistency, reliability, honesty, and competence. This means following through and doing what you say you will do. Trusting another person involves risk and vulnerability; however, it also fosters open, therapeutic communication and enhances the expression of feelings, thoughts, and needs. Do not compromise trust by sending the message to patients that you are "too busy." Such a response becomes a protective excuse for not becoming involved with them. It may also be a symptom of compassion fatigue. Being untrustworthy or dishonest seriously damages relationships and violates legal and ethical standards of practice. Do not withhold key information, lie, or distort the truth.

Acceptance and Respect. Conveying acceptance means that you are nonjudgmental and demonstrate unconditional respect. As a nurse, you are expected to provide high-quality care regardless of social or economic status, personal attributes, or the nature of an illness. Acceptance includes giving positive feedback, making sure that verbal and nonverbal cues match, and using touch appropriately. Being empathetic, restating, and avoiding arguments also show acceptance and respect.

Presence. The concept of presence is an interpersonal process that is characterized by sensitivity, holism, intimacy, vulnerability, and adaptation to unique circumstances (Turpin, 2014). Presence involves conveying closeness and a sense of caring. By being present for another person when needed, you offer your presence even when a patient does not express the need verbally. You do this by showing a caring attitude, demonstrating your willingness to listen and talk, or just being physically present (see Chapter 20). Do not avoid a patient whose behavior is troublesome. Such avoidance often increases a patient's negative behavior. Being *task oriented,* or making a technical procedure (e.g., administration of a medicine) your priority, is another way of not being emotionally available. You miss opportunities to assess patients, explore their concerns, calm anxiety, demonstrate empathy, teach, or involve patients in care. Patients perceive you as cold, uncaring, and unapproachable when you are task oriented. As a student, it is difficult to integrate therapeutic communication when you perform technical skills because of the need to focus on the procedure. In time you learn to do both and promote more satisfactory interactions. Consider the quality of care given in each of the following scenarios.

Nurse A silently enters the patient's room: "It's time for your pain shot."

The patient, Mr. Stewart, is mildly startled and grimaces. Nurse A again tells him that she has a pain shot but does not offer further explanation. She quickly reaches for his arm, gives the injection, disposes of her supplies, and leaves the room without asking if the patient has other needs.

Nurse B calls the patient's name as she enters the room: "Mr. Stewart, I have your pain medication. Are you feeling as uncomfortable as you look?"

Patient: "Yes, my back feels like a knife went through it. Will the pain ever go away?"

Nurse B lays syringe down and sits by patient: "It's common to have some pain the first few days after surgery, but I'll work with you to keep you comfortable. This medicine should help. I'll give the shot and then show you how to move in bed so the pain won't get worse. I'll check back with you to confirm that you're more comfortable."

Nurse B assessed the patient's need for a caring presence, set aside her own task, and became available for the patient. Notice that this intervention was brief yet more effective than the intervention of Nurse A. Question the assumption that nurses do not "have time" for caring connections. Caring is essential for effective care.

COMMUNICATION WITHIN THE NURSING PROCESS

In the nursing process, you use communication to gather information for developing nursing diagnoses, planning your care, implementing nursing interventions, and evaluating your care (see Chapter 9). You also use the nursing process when patients experience problems with communication.

BOX 11.7 COMMUNICATION EXAMPLES THROUGHOUT THE NURSING PROCESS

ASSESSMENT
- Verbal interviewing and history taking
- Visual observation of nonverbal behavior
- Visual, auditory, and tactile data gathering during physical examination
- Review of written medical records, diagnostic tests, and literature review

NURSING DIAGNOSIS
- Intrapersonal analysis of assessment findings
- Interpersonal validation of health care needs and priorities with patient and family
- Review of written and electronic documentation of nursing diagnosis

PLANNING
- Interpersonal team and interprofessional health planning sessions
- Interpersonal discussions with patient and family to determine methods of implementation
- Review of written or electronic documentation of expected outcomes and overall plan of care
- Review of written and/or verbal referrals to health care professionals

IMPLEMENTATION
- Verbal discussion with other health professionals
- Verbal, visual, auditory, and tactile health teaching
- Provision of support through therapeutic communication techniques
- Contact with other health resources
- Entering written and/or electronic documentation of patient's progress in medical record

EVALUATION
- Acquisition of verbal and nonverbal feedback
- Written analysis of actual and expected outcomes
- Identification of factors affecting outcomes
- Modification and update of written or electronic care plan
- Verbal and/or written explanation of revisions to patient

Although the nursing process is a reliable framework for delivering comprehensive patient care, it does not work well unless you master the art of therapeutic communication. Successful communication occurs with knowledge from the literature, experiences, and observation of others' communication skills. You also use communication techniques during the problem-solving process with team members to resolve problems or accomplish goals within the clinical setting (Box 11.7).

■■■ ASSESSMENT

Use communication during the assessment phase of the nursing process to gather information about a patient. Your initial assessment will not be accurate and complete if you do not identify and address patient and family communication needs. The time you spend assessing patients is a good time to establish the rapport needed for good communication. You collect data about a patient's medical history and current problem or concern using therapeutic communication techniques. *For example, Tim Brown follows up his initial meeting with Bud by completing a history and physical examination, paying special attention to Bud's calf. Beginning with an open-ended question about Bud's symptoms, Tim explores factors that possibly led to the problem and current symptoms. He completes a focused physical examination, explaining what he is doing to Bud. Tim follows his assessment with a description of what will happen next and seeks to answer any questions or concerns that Bud has.* Systematically collect data and organize the data you collect. Document information you obtain from a patient, family, and significant others.

Physical and Emotional Factors.

Assess physical or psychological factors that influence communication. Many health conditions limit communication, including facial trauma, cancer of the larynx or trachea, aphasia after a stroke, Alzheimer disease, and heavy sedation. Various symptoms make communication difficult such as pain, high anxiety, and breathing difficulties. Certain mental illnesses cause patients to have impaired communication such as pressured speech, constant verbalization of the same words or phrases, or a slow speech pattern. Review a patient's medical record for relevant information. The medical record describes any physical barriers to speech, neurological deficits, and pathophysiological conditions affecting hearing or vision. Also review the medication record. Opiates, antidepressants, antipsychotics, hypnotics, and sedatives cause patients to slur words or use incomplete sentences. Communicate directly with patients and family members to fully assess communication difficulties and build a plan to enhance communication.

Developmental Factors.

Consider a patient's developmental level when assessing communication. An infant's self-expression is limited to crying, body movement, and facial expression. Older children express their needs more directly. Pay attention to your nonverbal behavior when working with children. Sudden movements, threatening gestures, and loud noises can be frightening. Include the parents as sources of information about the child's health.

Older Adult Considerations. Advancing age can influence communication. Problems with hearing, vision, or speech are barriers to communication. Assess the hearing ability and visual acuity of older adults (see Chapter 16). Get an older adult's attention before you begin your assessment questions. Face the patient and stand or sit on the same level so the patient can read your lips. Speak slowly and clearly and use techniques that adapt to patients' sensory losses (see Chapter 39). Give older adults enough time to ask questions. Remember, do not assume that an older adult has communication impairments or limited cognition.

Sociocultural Factors.

When caring for patients from diverse cultural backgrounds, recognize how to adapt your communication approach. Show respect for all people regardless of their age, gender, religion, socioeconomic group, sexual orientation, or ethnicity. Recognize and attend to any personal biases or prejudices that might interfere with patients' care. Take cultural issues into account and work to be culturally sensitive and competent (see Chapter 21). Accept patients' rights to adhere to cultural customs and norms. People of various cultures use different types of verbal and nonverbal cues to convey meaning. Make a conscious effort not to interpret messages through your own cultural perspective; instead consider the context of the other individual's background. Avoid stereotyping people from other cultures or making jokes about them.

Consider the cultural sensitivity that the nurses demonstrate in the case study. *The nurses caring for Bud Johnson benefit from understanding that each person's sociocultural background may be diverse, even if one's language, ethnicity, or appearance does not demonstrate obvious differences. For example, returning from Vietnam with injuries as well as symptoms of posttraumatic stress disorder (PTSD), Bud spent several years experiencing erratic behavior, nightmares and flashbacks, suicidal ideas, and narcotic addiction. In those first years, Bud was unable to hold a job, lost his marriage, and felt a deep sense that his country had betrayed him. Being open to listening to a patient's life experiences and perceptions without jumping to conclusions is key to empathetic understanding within and across cultures and situations.*

Cultural insensitivity in communication takes many forms, including making fun of another's beliefs, practices, ethnicity, language, or dress. Telling jokes that make fun of ethnic groups, stereotyping obese patients, patronizing, and incorrectly interpreting culturally based behavior are examples of being culturally insensitive. Listen to patients' stories. Respect their views, opinions, and attitudes. Do not behave in ways that offend the cultural practices of others.

Language.

Language barriers sometimes exist with foreign-born patients and patients who speak English as a second language. It is essential that you assess a patient's understanding of all communication and obtain a professional interpreter to ensure accurate communication (see Chapter 21). Do not allow family members to interpret important information that you need to obtain from patients or to provide to patients, as misunderstanding can occur, and you will not know how accurately the messages have been delivered or received.

Gender.

Gender influences how we think, act, feel, and communicate. Being unaware of or insensitive to potential gender communication patterns can block the development of a therapeutic nurse-patient relationship. Assess the communication patterns of each individual, and do not make assumptions simply based on gender. There may be differences in male and female communication patterns in health care settings, although gender does not need to be a barrier in developing therapeutic communication with patients (Arnold and Boggs, 2016).

■■■■ NURSING DIAGNOSIS

After collecting assessment data from a patient, cluster pertinent defining characteristics and any risk factors for patterns and problems. Success in accurately identifying a patient's communication problems ensures the formulation of accurate nursing diagnoses. Nursing diagnoses for patients with communication difficulties often include the following:

- *Compromised Family Coping*
- *Ineffective Coping*
- *Readiness for Enhanced Family Coping*
- *Powerlessness*
- *Impaired Social Interaction*

Impaired Verbal Communication is a problem-focused nursing diagnosis that describes a patient who has limited or no ability to communicate verbally. It is defined as difficulty or inability to use or understand language in interpersonal reactions (Herdman and Kamitsuru, 2014). A patient with this diagnosis has related factors such as the inability to articulate words, difficulty forming words, and difficulty understanding. This diagnosis is useful for a wide variety of patients with special problems and needs related to communication. The related factor for a problem-focused diagnosis focuses on the cause of the communication disorder. In the case of impaired verbal communication, a related factor might be physiological, mechanical, anatomical, psychological, cultural, or developmental. Be accurate in choosing a related factor or risk factor for a diagnosis so that the interventions you select will effectively resolve the patient's problem.

■■■■ PLANNING

Once you identify the nature of a patient's communication problem, you must consider several factors to design a plan of care. For example, motivation improves communication. Patients often need encouragement to select and then try different communication strategies. In addition, select interventions and communication techniques appropriate for a patient's age, cultural background, and practices. When considering the best ways to communicate, work collaboratively with a patient to select possible methods. Give patients adequate time to practice new communication approaches. It also helps to plan practice sessions in a quiet, private environment. When possible, involve the family in selecting approaches that foster communication with the patient.

Goals and Outcomes. A plan of care supporting effective communication ultimately helps a patient to communicate his or her needs. Work with the patient to identify expected outcomes. Then ensure that the goals are relevant and realistic, specific, and measurable. After you have implemented your interventions and the patient has participated in care, evaluate outcomes to determine if the patient's goal was achieved. *The goals for Bud's rehabilitation were to restore safe ambulation (with or without an assistive device), restore independence in activities of daily living, and maintain narcotic-free pain control. Examples of associated expected outcomes include:*

- Patient ambulates 30 feet safely without an assistive device within 24 hours.
- Patient dresses himself without assistance by discharge.
- Patient maintains acceptable levels of pain control without reliance on narcotic pain relief by discharge.

Patients who have difficulty sending, receiving, and interpreting messages sometimes have difficulty developing healthy interpersonal relationships. Plan interventions that help patients improve their communication skills. For example, writing down key points or participating in role play helps patients rehearse situations in which they have difficulty communicating.

Setting Priorities. Include your patient in setting goals and expected outcomes. You will not make any progress if you select goals that your patient does not value. The patient should agree with the aims of nursing care. You cannot address all problems at the same time; consider which is most important and take the patient's perspective into account when prioritizing. Always maintain an open line of communication so that a patient can express any immediate needs or problems. Keep the nurse call system in reach for the patient restricted to bed or provide appropriate alternative communication devices such as a message board or Braille computer. If you plan to have a lengthy discussion with a patient, be sure to take care of his or her physical needs first to avoid interruptions. Make a patient comfortable by ensuring that any symptoms are under control.

Collaborative Care. Remember to include family caregivers during the planning and implementation phases of the nursing process. This collaboration supports the family and patient. When you collaborate with patients and family caregivers, they accept and commit to the treatment plan, and thus the patient is more likely to be successful in meeting mutually identified goals. Collaboration also promotes communication among family members to facilitate positive patient-family relationships. Encourage collaboration by asking others for ideas and suggestions about how to reach goals. This gives them the opportunity to express themselves and strengthens problem-solving ability.

In addition, collaborate with other health care providers who have expertise in communication strategies. Speech therapists help patients with aphasia. Professional interpreters are invaluable when a patient speaks a foreign language. Mental health advanced practice nurses help to communicate with angry or highly anxious patients.

■■■■ IMPLEMENTATION

Nurses use communication techniques that are appropriate to meet the individual needs of patients when carrying out plans of care. Before learning how to adapt communication methods to help patients with serious communication impairments, it is necessary to learn therapeutic communication techniques that are the foundation of professional communication. It is also important to understand which communication techniques create barriers to effective interaction. Principles of effective communication are the same whether you are promoting health or providing acute, restorative, or continuing care.

Therapeutic Communication Techniques. Therapeutic communication techniques are specific responses that encourage the expression of feelings and ideas and convey acceptance and respect. These techniques offer a variety of responses for you to appropriately use in different situations. Although some of the techniques may seem artificial or unnatural at first, your skill and comfort increase with practice and experience.

Conveying Empathy. Empathy is the ability to understand and accept another person's perspective (Arnold and Boggs, 2016). You can never totally know another's experiences because you are not in that person's situation, but you can try to understand and acknowledge what the person is experiencing. Empathic statements reflect an understanding of what a patient communicated and inform the patient that you heard both the feeling and the factual content of the communication. This allows a patient to validate or clarify feelings and perceptions.

Empathic responses are neutral and nonjudgmental and foster shared respect. Use them to establish trust in very difficult situations. *In the case study Bud stated that he did not want to come to rely on narcotics, as he had worked very hard to turn his life around after he became addicted to narcotic pain relievers. An empathic response from Tim is, "It sounds like you feel very strongly that regardless of your pain, you do not want to use narcotic pain relievers."*

Active Listening. Active listening means being attentive to what a patient is saying both verbally and nonverbally. Active listening facilitates patient communication. The ancient Greek philosopher Epictetus stated, "We have two ears and one mouth so we may listen more and talk less." That is good advice for nurses. Active listening enhances trust because a nurse communicates acceptance and respect for a patient. Several nonverbal skills facilitate attentive listening. Plan adequate time for in-depth conversation, based on the type of conversation you will have. Sit facing the patient, use an open posture, lean in toward the patient, and make eye contact. Ask an open-ended question, and refrain from talking too much. Focus first on understanding your patient's point of view accurately.

Sharing Observations. Nurses make observations by commenting on a patient's appearance and how he or she sounds or acts. Stating observations often helps a patient communicate without the need for extensive questioning, focusing, or clarification. This technique helps start a conversation with quiet or withdrawn persons. Do not state observations that will embarrass or anger a patient such as telling someone, "You're a mess!" Even if such an observation is made with humor, a patient can misinterpret the intent.

Sharing observations differs from making assumptions, which means drawing unnecessary conclusions about the other person without validating them. Making assumptions puts a patient in the position of having to contradict you. Examples include your interpretation of a patient's fatigue as depression and assuming that untouched food indicates lack of interest in meeting nutritional goals. Making observations is a gentler and safer technique: "I see you didn't eat any breakfast," "You are clenching your jaw," or a positive observation such as, "I see you've been organizing your papers."

Using Silence. It takes time and experience to become comfortable with silence. Most people have a natural tendency to fill empty spaces with words, but sometimes silence is useful when decisions that require much thought need to be made. Practice remaining mindfully present, but stay silent and listen when interacting with a patient. Silence is especially therapeutic during times of sadness or grief.

Providing Information. Providing relevant information helps your patients make informed decisions, experience less anxiety, and feel safe and secure. Speak in simple language and translate medical terms. When offering options, stress that the patient has the right to make decisions. Provide information that enables others to understand what is happening and what to expect. *For example, Tim Brown tells Bud that another ultrasound of his calf is scheduled to evaluate the effectiveness of his treatment. Tim includes how long it will take and how long it will take to get the results of the test.*

Clarifying. Clarifying validates if a person interpreted a message correctly. Any time a message is unclear or ambiguous, try to restate it or ask the other person to restate it, explain further, or give an example of what he or she means. *For example, when Bud asks whether the test for a blood clot will be painful, Tim responds, "The ultrasound test that your doctor has ordered is not painful. It involves moving a wand across parts of your body and uses sound waves to visualize your bloodstream for blockages."*

Focusing. Focusing directs conversation to a specific topic or issue when a discussion becomes unclear. It limits the area to which the sender can respond. Use it when the sender rambles or introduces many unrelated topics in the same conversation. *For example, when Bud begins to ramble about the many painful medical tests and treatments that he had in the past following his injuries in the Vietnam War, Tim uses a focusing response to bring the conversation to the present, "Are you concerned that your current problem may become very complicated and painful?"*

Paraphrasing. Paraphrasing is restating the sender's message in the receiver's own words to make sure that the receiver has received information accurately. Be careful not to change the meaning when you paraphrase. Confirm the meaning with the patient. *For example, Bud states, "I've been walking more, and I don't need as much help as I did before." Tim replies, "You feel you're getting stronger and more independent?"*

Summarizing. Summarizing is a concise review of main ideas from a discussion. It brings a sense of satisfaction and closure to an individual conversation or during the termination phase of a nurse-patient relationship. By reviewing a conversation, you focus on key issues and obtain additional relevant information as needed. *For example, Bud completes his testing and returns to the acute care unit. Tim Brown summarizes what happened in the diagnostic center and the health care provider's brief report to the patient, stating, "Today we assessed your right calf area because you had a deep vein thrombosis, or a clot in your right calf vein. As your health care provider reported, there is swelling in the vein, but no clot formation is evident right now. This tells us your treatment is working. We will remove your IV (intravenous catheter) and send you back to rehabilitation. The doctor is going to order a prescription for medication to help prevent this inflamed area from developing another clot. You will start taking this new medication when you get back to the rehabilitation unit."*

Self-Disclosure. You may use self-disclosure during the working phase of a helping relationship. Self-disclosures are personal statements intentionally revealed to the other person to assist the patient. The purpose is to model and educate, foster a therapeutic alliance, validate reality, and encourage autonomy (Stuart, 2013). Keep self-disclosures brief, relevant, and appropriate, and do not introduce your *current* personal concerns or problems into the conversation, as this may turn the conversation to focus on your problem. Make these statements to benefit the patient, not you, and use them sparingly so that the patient remains the focus of the interaction. *Bud is transferred back to rehabilitation, and Marianne is again assigned to his care. Bud voices reluctance to have help at home, even though he can see that he is not able to do everything he needs to for self-sufficiency. Marianne responds with self-disclosure, "After I had surgery a few years ago it was hard for me to have someone help me with daily tasks I had always done myself. I have always been independent. Is that how it is for you?"*

Instilling Hope. Nurses recognize that hope is essential for healing and learn to communicate a "sense of possibility" to others (see Chapter 22). You give hope by commenting on the positive aspects of the other person's behavior, performance, or response. Sharing a realistic vision of the future and reminding others of their resources and strengths also strengthen hope. You can reassure patients that there are many kinds of hope and that meaning and personal growth can come from illness experiences.

Nontherapeutic Communication Techniques.
Certain communication techniques hinder or damage professional relationships. These specific techniques are nontherapeutic and often cause recipients to use defenses to avoid being hurt or negatively affected. Nontherapeutic techniques discourage further expression of feelings and ideas and often result in negative responses or behaviors in others.

Inattentive Listening. Behaviors and nonverbal expressions such as fidgeting, breaking eye contact, daydreaming during conversation, and pretending to listen convey the message that what the sender has to say is not important. These behaviors discourage conversation and damage trust.

Further examples are looking at your watch, tapping your foot impatiently, and documenting at the computer with your back to the patient.

Overusing Medical Vocabulary. Health care professionals have their own culture and language. Using technical words in discussions with patients can cause confusion and anxiety. Avoid excessive use of such terms or translate them into lay terms (e.g., medicine instead of medication, what you eat or drink instead of intake, get worse or better instead of progressive).

Prying or Asking Personal Questions. Asking irrelevant personal questions simply to satisfy your curiosity is inappropriate and invasive. Limit questions to health-related information.

Giving Approval or Disapproval. Do not impose your own attitudes, values, beliefs, and moral standards on others while in the professional helping role. People have the right to be themselves and make their own decisions. Avoid using terms such as *should, ought, good, bad, right,* or *wrong.* Agreeing, disagreeing, or sharing your opinion sends the subtle message that you are making value judgments about patient decisions. Instead offer options and help the other person anticipate the consequences of decisions. The problem and its solution belong to the patient, not you.

> *Bud:* "I really want to live at home in my apartment, but I am not sure I can manage the stairs, and fully take care of myself."
> *Marianne:* "I don't think it's a good idea for you to live alone. You should consider assisted living."

A better response is, *"It sounds like you want to live independently but recognize some of the barriers that you will need to overcome."* Giving approval or disapproval should be differentiated carefully from providing health care information and education, which are important nursing functions. *For example, as Bud and Marianne discuss living arrangements, it would be appropriate for Marianne to teach Bud about home safety strategies to prevent falls or to share information about community resources that may provide him with assistance.*

Changing the Subject. Changing the subject is a common problem when you are uncomfortable with a topic, but it is insensitive and tends to block further communication.

Automatic Responses. Clichés or stereotypical remarks such as, "You're never given more than you can handle," tend to belittle a patient's feelings and minimize the importance of his or her message. These automatic phrases communicate that you are not taking concerns seriously or responding thoughtfully.

False Reassurance. When a patient is seriously ill or distressed, you may be tempted to offer hope with statements such as, "I'm sure everything will be okay." Although you may be trying to be kind, false reassurance discounts the patient's concerns or situation and tends to block communication.

Asking for Explanations. Sometimes asking "why" implies an accusation and results in resentment, insecurity, and mistrust. Try to phrase questions without using "why." You could say, "Tell me about the problems you're having with your medicines," rather than, "Why aren't you taking the medicines the doctor prescribed?"

Arguing. Challenging or arguing with someone's perception of a situation denies that his or her perceptions are real. It implies that they are lying, misinformed, or uneducated. Instead be open and listen to the other person's views and opinion.

Being Defensive. When patients express criticism, listen to what they have to say. Listening does not imply agreement. To discover reasons for a patient's anger or dissatisfaction, you need to listen with a nonjudgmental approach. By avoiding defensiveness, you are able to defuse anger and uncover deeper concerns. Rather than saying, "None of the nurses would intentionally ignore you," you respond, "You feel the nurses are ignoring you."

Sympathy. Sympathy is the concern, sorrow, or pity that you feel for a patient when you personally identify with his or her needs. In contrast to empathy, which tries to understand a patient's experience, sympathy takes a subjective look at the patient's world. Sharing sympathy with another feels good, creates a bond, and minimizes differences; however, it can prevent effective problem solving and impair good judgment. When you share a patient's needs, you are assuming that his or her feelings are similar to your own, and you are unable to help the patient select realistic solutions for problems.

Decision Making and Communication. As a nurse, you constantly make decisions about what, when, where, why, and how to send messages to others. Deciding which techniques best fit each unique nursing scenario is challenging. Many situations that arise in a complex and demanding practice environment challenge your decision-making skills and call for careful use of therapeutic techniques. Practice helps; therefore take the initiative to discuss and role play these scenarios before facing them in the clinical setting. When you are unsure of how to respond initially, try to focus on actively listening to what the patient is saying, and use fewer verbal responses.

Assertiveness and Autonomy. Assertive communication is based on a philosophy of protecting individual rights and responsibilities. It includes the ability to be self-directive in acting to accomplish goals and advocate for others. An assertive response promotes self-esteem and upholds personal and professional rights. Feelings of security, competence, power, and professionalism characterize assertive responses. Assertive statements convey a message without resorting to sarcasm, whining, anger, blaming, or manipulation. Assertive responses are good tools to deal with criticism, change, negative conditions in personal or professional life, and conflict or stress in relationships. Negative interactions among nurses such as interactions that include horizontal or lateral violence adversely affect communication and collaboration. Aggression between health care workers undermines the culture of safety (Lim and Bernstein, 2014).

Assertive responses often contain "I" messages, such as "I want," "I need," "I think," or "I feel." Simple assertive messages are usually stated in three parts, referencing the nurse, the other individual's behavior, and its effect.

Nurse to nurse: "I notice you have been late to work three times this week. When you're late for work, I have to stay late, and that makes me late picking up my children from the babysitter."

Nurse to supervisor: "I'm confused to hear you say I'm not performing well because I was told by my preceptor that I was meeting expectations. Please give me some examples of what you mean."

Avoiding Passive Responses. Passive responses avoid issues or conflict. Some characteristics of being passive are expressing feelings of sadness, depression, anxiety, and hopelessness.

For example, a nurse responds to an angry, aggressive worker: "My opinion doesn't matter, do whatever you think." A better response is, "Let's take a few minutes to talk about the situation, as this has been difficult. What can we do to make things better?"

Avoiding Aggressive Responses. Aggressive responses provoke confrontation at the other person's expense. Some characteristics of aggression are expressing feelings of anger, frustration, resentment, and stress.

For example, an aggressive response by a nurse to an angry patient is, "You can't talk to me that way." A better response is, "I want to hear your concerns and help you have a positive experience. Can we talk about them now, or should I come back later?"

Humor. Humor is a coping strategy that adds perspective and helps you and a patient adjust to stress. Laughter is a diversion from stress-related tension. It provides a sense of well-being and more of a feeling of control or mastery. Humor provides emotional support to patients and humanizes the illness experience. Laughter provides both a psychological and a physical release for you and the patient; promotes open, relaxed interaction; and reinforces our shared experience. However, humor may not always be therapeutic or suitable to a patient care situation.

You assess whether humor is appropriate by noticing if patients use it in their conversations. Start with small examples to see if this is helpful. To offer positive humor, share humorous incidents or situations or share puns or simple jokes that are not offensive. Positive humor is associated with hope, love, and joy, with the intent to bring people closer. Avoid negative humor, which is inappropriate in a health care setting. Ethnic, religious, sexist, ageist, or put-down humor creates distance. Realize that humor sometimes backfires; not everyone appreciates a humorous approach because of negative moods, stress, or physical discomfort. Your patient may view a humorous remark as one that makes light of a difficult situation and may not find this helpful. If your patient leads with a small humorous remark, such as, "If you raise this bed up any higher I will be standing at the pearly gates of heaven," you may respond with a bit of laughter. It would be very appropriate to respond in a supportive manner. For example, you could respond, "I'm going to bring this bed down to earth now; we plan to work hard to keep you safe and well during your stay here."

Sometimes health care providers use dark, negative humor after difficult or traumatic situations to relieve tension and stress. This response may seem callous or uncaring by individuals not involved in the situation. Avoid using such humor within earshot of patients or their loved ones. Understand that humor is a release, but timing, content, and receptivity are important in the use of therapeutic humor (Arnold and Boggs, 2016).

Responding to Aggressive Behavior. Health care providers must be prepared to respond to patients who become verbally or physically aggressive. Patients who have cognitive impairments such as delirium or dementia are at risk for displaying a violent response. Other risk factors include patients who arrive into a health care system through the emergency department, who are male, who are older than 65 years of age, and whose history includes violence (Williamson et al., 2013). Keep safety in mind when interacting with patients who are likely to be aggressive; your safety as well as the safety of the patient and others in the environment must be ensured. Preventive communication strategies include the following: approach the patient slowly and in full view, maintain a calm demeanor, use very short and simple words, avoid rushing the patient, and seek the patient's affirmation before activities involving close personal space are attempted. When entering a patient's room, place yourself nearer to the door than the patient in case you must exit quickly. Allow the patient to verbally express frustration without becoming defensive. Respond to the patient's concern in a helpful manner. When responding to a patient who is currently physically violent, safety is paramount. Remove others from the immediate area and obtain help. Do not approach such a patient alone or without a plan that provides for the safe deescalation of the patient.

Touch. Touch is one of a nurse's most powerful forms of communication. Nurses are privileged to experience more of this intimate form of personal contact than almost any other professional. Touch conveys affection, emotional support, encouragement, and personal attention (Fig. 11.1). Therapeutic touch such as holding a hand is important for vulnerable patients who are experiencing severe illness with its accompanying physical and emotional losses. Sometimes touch is misinterpreted. Always be sensitive to a patient's response to touch. Following are examples of inappropriate and appropriate use of touch:

In a cancer support group the wife of a patient tearfully describes how overwhelmed she is feeling.

Inappropriate touch: A nurse moves too quickly and tries to hug the wife without permission. The wife backs off and struggles to hold back more tears.

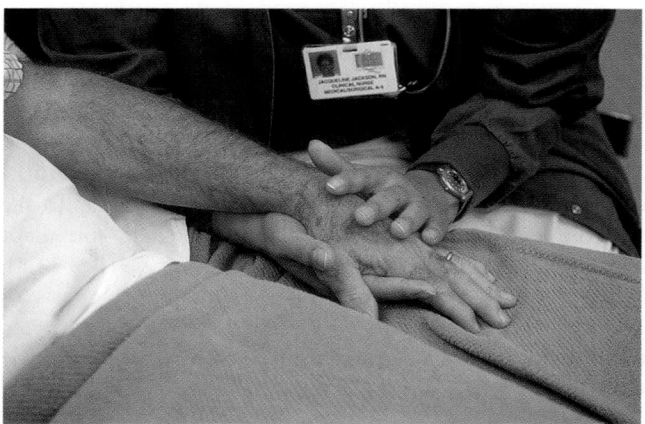

FIG 11.1 A nurse uses touch to communicate.

Appropriate touch: A nurse says, "I see you're distressed (while placing her hand gently on the patient's shoulder)." The nurse attends to both the patient's verbal and nonverbal response to this touch.

Another concern is the confusion about the use of touch with patients from other cultures (see Chapter 21). Look for cues that indicate a patient welcomes touch. We use touch to awaken patients, get their attention, or add emphasis to explanations. Touch sometimes conveys understanding better than words or gestures, but it is important to ask a patient what he or she prefers and what is culturally appropriate or forbidden.

Because much of what you do involves touching patients, learn to use touch wisely. The zones of touch are described in Box 11.1. Touch delivered in the social or consent zone causes less anxiety than touch delivered in the vulnerable or intimate zone. Students initially find giving intimate care stressful, especially with patients of the opposite sex. Shift your focus from personal discomfort and focus on the intent to provide sensitive nursing care. Trust that you will become more comfortable with experience. Remember that a patient who is ill and dependent must permit closer physical contact than is normally tolerated and may be uncomfortable with touch. Remain sensitive to your own responses and to patients' feelings. If a patient refuses to hold your hand while in pain or pulls away from physical contact, this signals that he or she is uncomfortable with being touched. People perceive touch negatively when it is given without consent; used within a hostile or mistrusting relationship; or delivered to a vulnerable, intimate, or painful area of the body. Your touch should never be angry, rough, violent, overly stimulating, threatening, overly tentative, sexual, or unnecessarily painful.

Communicating With Patients With Special Needs. Many health-related and developmental issues contribute to impaired communication. Promoting effective communication in nonvocal patients includes thoroughly assessing communication needs, identifying alternative communication strategies, and creating an individualized plan of care (Rodriguez et al., 2016). This includes a patient who is ventilator dependent and cannot speak or an infant who is limited to crying, body movement, and facial expression. Patients who are deaf or hard of hearing or who have LEP require individualized communication approaches. In addition, patients who are unresponsive or heavily sedated are sometimes unable to send or receive verbal messages.

A patient who cannot communicate effectively has difficulty expressing needs and responding appropriately to the environment. Such patients benefit greatly when you adapt communication techniques to their circumstances (Box 11.8). When caring for a patient with the nursing diagnosis of *Impaired Verbal Communication related to a language barrier,* the priority is to have a professional interpreter available. If this cannot be achieved, provide the patient a list with pictures of simple words in the patient's language. The patient's use of these key images enables him or her to communicate basic needs such as food, water, toileting, rest, and need for pain relief. Collaborate with team members and family members when appropriate to design the best communication strategies.

Effective communication improves the quality of your patient's interpersonal relationships and well-being. If a patient uses ineffective communication techniques that interfere with coping or interpersonal relationships, intervene to help him or her send, receive, and interpret messages more

---

BOX 11.8 COMMUNICATING WITH PATIENTS WHO HAVE SPECIAL NEEDS

PATIENTS WHO ARE HEARING IMPAIRED

- Ensure that patient has access to working hearing aids and glasses.
- Reduce environmental noise and distractions.
- Speak at a normal volume and avoid shouting.
- Rephrase instead of repeat if misunderstood.
- Punctuate speech with facial expression and gestures.
- Provide a sign language interpreter if needed.

PATIENTS WHO ARE VISUALLY IMPAIRED

- Ensure that patient has access to glasses—corrective lenses and/or magnifying lenses.
- Communicate verbally before touching the patient.
- Orient the patient to sounds in the environment.
- Ensure that lighting is adequate for patient to see speaker.
- Identify yourself when entering the room and notify patient when leaving the room.
- Modify written handouts to accommodate degree of visual impairment.
- Offer audiotapes for instructional information.

PATIENTS WHO ARE MUTE, UNABLE TO SPEAK, OR CANNOT SPEAK CLEARLY

- Answer nurse call system in person.
- Listen attentively, be patient, and do not interrupt or finish patient's sentences.
- Ask simple questions that require "yes" or "no" answers.
- Allow time for understanding and responses.
- Use visual cues (e.g., words, pictures, objects) when possible.
- Allow only one person to speak at a time.
- Use normal volume and do not shout or speak too loudly.
- Let patient know if you do not understand.
- Use communication aids as needed:
  - Pad and felt-tipped pen or Magic Slate
  - Flash cards
  - Communication board with words, letters, or pictures denoting basic needs
  - Computer toy ("speak and spell" type) for children
  - Call bells or alarms
  - Sign language
  - Use of eye blinks or movement of fingers for simple responses ("yes" or "no")
- Be attentive and responsive to restless physical movements.

PATIENTS WHO ARE COGNITIVELY IMPAIRED

- Reduce environmental distractions while conversing.
- Prioritize communication over other tasks.
- Get patient's attention before speaking.
- Use simple sentences and avoid long explanations.
- Avoid shifting from subject to subject.
- Ask one question at a time.
- Allow time for patient to respond.
- Include family and friends in conversations when appropriate.

PATIENTS WHO ARE UNRESPONSIVE

- Call patient by name during interactions.
- Communicate both verbally and by touch.
- Speak to patient as though he or she could hear.
- Explain all procedures and sensations.
- Provide orientation to person, place, and time as needed.

PATIENTS WHO DO NOT SPEAK ENGLISH

- Speak to patient in a normal tone of voice (shouting may be interpreted as anger).
- Establish a method for patient to signal desire to communicate (nurse call system or bell).
- Avoid using family members, especially children, as interpreters.
- Provide professional interpreter/translator as needed:
  - Use a person familiar with patient's culture and with health care if possible.
  - Allow plenty of time for interpreter to transmit messages.
  - Communicate directly to patient and family rather than to interpreter.
  - Ask one question at a time.
  - Avoid making comments to interpreter about the patient or family (they may understand some English).
- Develop a communication board, pictures, or cards using words translated into English for patient to make basic requests (e.g., pain medication, water, elimination).
- Have a dictionary (e.g., English/Spanish) available if patient can read.
- Provide written materials in English and in patient's primary language.

effectively. Be a communication role model and teacher to help patients express needs, feelings, and concerns. Help patients develop social interaction skills and communicate thoughts and feelings clearly. This helps them interpret messages sent from others, increasing their autonomy and assertiveness. Methods such as role-playing allow patients to practice situations in which they have difficulty communicating.

Providing Alternative Communication Methods. Patients with physical communication barriers (e.g., patients with a laryngectomy or endotracheal tube) may be unable to speak, or the clarity of speech may be so poor that they need alternative methods of communication (see Box 11.8). To decrease frustration, provide simple communication methods and allow the patient time to respond. The patient must be physically able to use the method you provide (e.g., electronic or physical communication boards or pencil and pad). Patients who are unable to speak are at risk for injury unless they are able to communicate personal needs quickly.

Communicating With Children. Communication with a child requires knowledge of developmental tasks and milestones as well as special considerations to develop a working relationship with the child and family. Confirm that information communicated by the parents is consistent with other reports, including from the child. Offer the child toys or materials so that the parent gives full attention to your information gathering. Give periodic attention to infants and younger children as they play to include them. An older child can be actively involved in communication. Consider the influence of development on language and thought processes.

Children, particularly young children, are especially responsive to nonverbal messages. Sudden movements or gestures can be frightening. Remain calm and gentle and, if possible, let a child make the first move. Use a quiet, friendly, confident tone of voice. A child feels helpless in most situations involving health care personnel, which makes it particularly important to facilitate the presence of parents. When giving explanations or directions, use simple, direct language and be honest. To minimize fear and anxiety, prepare a child by explaining what to expect and seeking input from parents when appropriate. Avoid overly lengthy or involved explanations, and, similar to adults, meet a child at eye level.

Drawing and playing with young children allows them to communicate nonverbally (making the drawing) and verbally (explaining the picture). Use a child's drawing as a basis for beginning a conversation (Fig. 11.2).

Communicating With Older Adults. When you are communicating with older adults, avoid use of language that implies that the older adult is feeble; for example, do not speak in a singsong, high-pitched or overly loud voice, and do not use terms that imply the older adult is cute or childlike. Although some older adults experience some loss of sensory function that interferes with sending or receiving messages clearly, each patient is an individual. Many older adults who have some sensory losses adapt to sensory losses and learn to communicate effectively. Other older adults require moderate adaptation. When obvious deficits exist, maximize existing motor and sensory function to help patients communicate

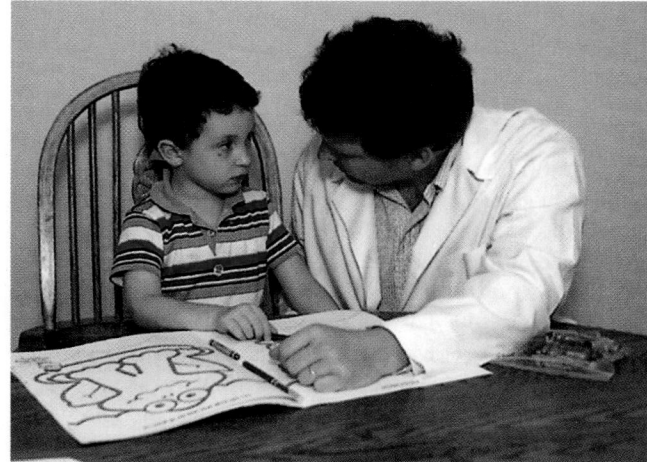

FIG 11.2 Drawing helps children communicate.

BOX 11.9 CARE OF THE OLDER ADULT

Improving Communication

When communicating with older adults, the primary goal is to establish a reliable communication system that all health care team members easily understand. Ideally an interprofessional model delivers effective care for older adults. Communication with older adults requires special attention. Be aware of the physical, psychological, and social changes of aging. Use the following interventions to assist with impaired communication with older adults:

- During conversation maintain a quiet environment that is free from background noise.
- Avoid shifting from subject to subject; allow time for conversation.
- Be an attentive listener. Use explorative questions to facilitate conversation.
- Avoid long sentences to explain the subject. Try to keep it short, simple, and to the point.
- Allow older adults the opportunity to reminisce. Reminiscing has therapeutic properties that increase the sense of well-being.
- If you are experiencing problems understanding a patient, let the patient know, and facilitate methods that help him or her speak more clearly. Consult with a speech therapist if necessary.
- Include a patient's family and friends in conversations, particularly in subjects known to the patient.
- Be aware of cultural differences among patients.

---

more effectively (see Box 11.8). You can make some simple modifications in your approach and the environment to improve communication with older adults (Box 11.9). Identify these challenges and work with patients to enhance effective communication (Hanson, 2014).

■■■■ EVALUATION

You and the patient determine the success of the plan of care together by evaluating patient communication outcomes. Ask yourself if you understood what your patient communicated, if your patient had the opportunity to express feelings and concerns, and if your patient has unresolved needs.

Patient Outcomes. Evaluate whether communication interventions were effective by comparing the expected outcomes you established in the plan of care with your patient's actual outcomes you observe. If your patient meets jointly established outcomes, you have resolved the goals of care and the nursing diagnosis. When outcomes remain unmet, you may revise the existing plan with new goals, outcomes, or interventions. For example, if using a pen and paper is frustrating for a patient who is nonverbal and whose handwriting is shaky, you revise the care plan to include use of a picture board instead. In this case observing the patient's handwriting and asking other caregivers about the patient's success in communicating needs are your evaluation measures. Remember that careful evaluation requires you to make observations similar to those in your original assessment. For example, after initially assessing the extent of a patient's ability to hear the spoken word and providing various interventions to promote hearing, you return to evaluate his or her ability to hear any interaction or instruction. It is also helpful to question the patient about whether needs were adequately met.

You should reflect and evaluate the effectiveness of your own communication by reflecting on the success of your verbal and nonverbal interactions with patients. This is useful in determining how your communication style might improve.

Patient Expectations. Review evaluation findings to decide if the patient's expectations of care were met. This is an important part of the evaluation process. Ask patients and their families for input about goal achievement, factors that affected outcomes, and suggestions for changes in the plan of care. *Marianne consistently asked Bud if his expectations for care were being met: Were the pain management strategies effective? Bud was pleased that his nurses were open to working with him to achieve pain management by using nonpharmacological therapies such as relaxation and massage and by avoiding narcotics.*

Avoiding patient input during evaluation and care plan modification leads to a task-oriented (nurse centric) rather than a patient-centered approach to nursing care. It denies the patient's right to see the total picture of care and be involved in all phases of the nursing process. Thus ensure you value and encourage your patient's participation when evaluating outcomes of care.

KEY POINTS

- Communication is a powerful therapeutic tool and an essential nursing skill used to influence others and achieve positive health outcomes.

- Nurses consider many contexts and factors influencing communication when making decisions about what, when, where, how, why, and with whom to communicate.
- Communication is most effective when the receiver and sender accurately perceive the meaning of one another's messages.
- Effective verbal communication requires appropriate intonation, clear and concise phrasing, proper pacing of statements, and proper timing and relevance of a message.
- Effective nonverbal communication complements and strengthens the message conveyed by verbal communication.
- Strengthen helping relationships by establishing trust, empathy, autonomy, confidentiality, and professional competence.
- Effective communication techniques are facilitative and tend to encourage the other person to openly express ideas, feelings, or concerns.
- Ineffective communication techniques inhibit or block the other person's willingness to openly express ideas, feelings, or concerns.
- Nurses who are experiencing compassion fatigue often have difficulty relating with patients and co-workers.
- A nurse blends social and informational interactions with therapeutic communication techniques so that others explore feelings and manage health issues.
- The language that health care providers choose to use when communicating with patients can significantly impact whether patients understand basic health information.
- When using therapeutic humor, consider timing, receptivity, and content of the humorous intervention.
- When responding to an angry or aggressive patient, remain calm and unhurried, approach the patient slowly and in view, and seek the patient's approval before coming close.
- Older adults with sensory, motor, or cognitive impairments require adaptation of communication techniques to make up for their loss of function and special needs.

REFLECTIVE LEARNING

- Consider your most recent experience providing care to a patient. Describe the way you introduced yourself. Did you follow the AIDET guidelines? Which parts did you complete fully and which were not included? What do you think the effect was on the patient care experience?
- Consider a time when you noticed that a patient was upset. Describe the patient's verbal and nonverbal behavior. What was the problem the patient was concerned about? Evaluate your response to the situation. How did the patient respond?
- Consider a time when you provided or observed a hand-off interaction. Describe the strategy used by the professional who was providing report. Was a structured approach used? From your perspective, what was the quality of the hand-off?

REVIEW QUESTIONS

1. A nurse is caring for a patient who had surgery 2 days ago and has not yet had a bowel movement. Upon assessment, the nurse finds bowel sounds are present in all four quadrants, abdomen is slightly distended, and patient reports feeling uncomfortably full. The patient has been scheduled for discharge tomorrow. The nursing history on admission noted that the patient had a history of constipation and takes stool softeners. The nurse prepares to call the health care provider to request a medication for constipation. Place the following in the correct order for an SBAR communication related to this concern.
   1. Would you prescribe a medication for relief of constipation?
   2. Mr. John Smith had surgery 3 days ago, and he has not yet had a bowel movement. He is slated for discharge tomorrow.
   3. Mr. Smith reports that he has a history of constipation and often takes stool softeners at home.
   4. Mr. Smith has bowel sounds in all four quadrants and has passed flatus today. His abdomen is slightly distended, and he reports feeling uncomfortably full.

2. A family member angrily tells the nurse, "No one told me that my husband was back in his room after surgery. I have been waiting and worrying for 3 hours!" How should the nurse reply?
   1. "Well, the recovery room nurse is supposed to take care of that before sending the patient back to us. I will be sure to let her know about your frustration."
   2. "I am sorry we did not notify you more quickly. It sounds like you have been really worried about your husband."
   3. "At least your husband's surgery went well. That is something positive to think about."
   4. "I would be angry, too, if no one told me that my husband was back in his room after surgery."

3. A patient recovering from a surgery that has a decreased ability to speak has activated her nurse call system. How should the nurse respond?
   1. Use the intercom and ask the patient, "What do you need?"
   2. Respond in person and speak loudly and carefully.
   3. Respond in person and ask simple questions that can be answered with a gesture.
   4. Use the intercom and use simple sentences.

4. A nurse is providing a hand-off report related to a patient leaving the medical-surgical unit for a diagnostic procedure. What should the nurse providing the report include? (Select all that apply.)
   1. Timing and administration of new, STAT, and prn medications
   2. Recent laboratory and test results
   3. Perceptions of the patient's family situation
   4. Discharge planning issues
   5. The patient's need for an interpreter

5. A nurse is being uncivil by speaking poorly about a new nurse in front of a patient. What should the charge nurse who overhears this do?
   1. Promptly counter the negative statement by the uncivil nurse with a positive statement
   2. Immediately correct the uncivil nurse's poor judgment in speaking about the new nurse in front of the patient
   3. Speak privately with the uncivil nurse about not providing evaluative judgments about others, especially in front of patients
   4. Immediately write up the uncivil nurse for inappropriate communication skills

evolve

Additional Review Questions, as well as rationales for all Review Questions, can be found on the Evolve website.

1. 2, 3, 4, 1; 2. 2; 3. 3; 4. 1, 2, 5; 5. 3.

REFERENCES

Agency for Healthcare Research and Quality (AHRQ): *TeamSTEPPS: strategies and tools to enhance performance and patient safety*, n.d. http://www.ahrq.gov/professionals/education/curriculum-tools/teamstepps/index.html.

Anderson J, et al: Nursing bedside clinical handover—an integrated review of issues and tools, *J Clin Nurs* 24(5/6):662, 2015.

Arnold EC, Boggs KU: *Interpersonal relationships: professional communication skills for nurses*, ed 7, St Louis, 2016, Elsevier.

Cronenwett L, et al: Quality and safety education for nurses, *Nurs Outlook* 55(3):122, 2007.

Davis C, et al: Safety alert: protecting yourself and others from violence, *Nursing* 45(1):55, 2015.

Davis M: Bed huddles improve communication and patient safety, *MedSurg Matters* 24(5):2, 2015.

Gluyas H: Effective communication and teamwork promotes patient safety, *Nurs Stand* 29(49):50, 2015.

Hanson RM: Is elderly care affected by nurse attitudes?" A systematic review, *Br J Nurs* 23(4):225, 2014.

Herdman TH, Kamitsuru S, editors: *NANDA International: nursing diagnoses: definitions and classification 2015-2017*, Oxford, 2014, Wiley Blackwell.

Houck D: Helping nurses cope with grief and compassion fatigue: an educational intervention, *Clin J Oncol Nurs* 18:454, 2014.

Institute for Healthcare Improvement (IHI): *SBAR technique for communication: a situational briefing model*, n.d. http://www.ihi.org/knowledge/Pages/Tools/SBARTechniqueforCommunicationASituationalBriefingModel.aspx.

Keebler JR, et al: Meta-analyses of the effects of standardized handoff protocols on patient, provider, and organizational outcomes, *Hum Factors* 58(8):1187, 2016.

Kneisl CR, Trigoboff E: *Contemporary psychiatric-mental health nursing,* ed 3, Boston, 2013, Pearson.

Lerner M: The promise, *Radiol Manage* 37(2):23, 2015. http://www .radiologymanagement-digital.com/ radiologymanagement/03042015?pg=25 #pg25.

Lim F, Bernstein I: Civility and workplace bullying: resonance of Nightingale's persona and current best practices, *Nurs Forum* 49(2):124, 2014.

Literacy Inc: *About us,* 2017. http:// literacyinc.com/about-us/.

Mascioli S: Spotlight on the 2016 National Patient Safety Goals for hospitals, *Nursing* 46(5):52, 2016.

Mott-Coles S: Patients' cultural beliefs in patient-provider communication with African American women and Latinas diagnosed with breast cancer, *Clin J Oncol Nurs* 18(4):443, 2014.

Nordby H: Communication and the interpretive principle of charity in nurse-patient interaction, *Res Theory Nurs Pract* 30(2):176, 2016.

Perry B, Edwards M: A qualitative study of compassion fatigue among family caregivers in long-term care homes, *Perspectives (Montclair)* 38(3):14, 2015.

Pettit AM, Duffy JJ: Patient safety: creating a culture change to support communication and teamwork, *J Legal Nurse Consulting* 26(4):23, 2015.

Rodriguez C, et al: Enhancing the communication of suddenly speechless critical care patients, *Am J Crit Care* 25(3):e40, 2016.

Stuart GW: *Principles and practice of psychiatric nursing,* ed 10, St Louis, 2013, Elsevier.

Studer Group: *AIDET® patient communication,* n.d. https://www .studergroup.com/aidet.

The Joint Commission (TJC): *Joint commission on-line: patient safety,* 2015. http://www.jointcommission.org/ assets/1/23/jconline_April_29_15.pdf.

The Joint Commission (TJC): *2018 National Patient Safety Goals,* Oakbrook Terrace, IL, 2018. The Commission, https:// www.jointcommission.org/standards _information/npsgs.aspx.

Turpin R: State of the science of nursing presence revisited: knowledge for preserving nursing presence capability, *Int J Human Caring* 18(4):14, 2014.

U.S. Department of Education, *National Institute of Literacy: Illiteracy statistics,* 2016. http://www.statisticbrain.com/ number-of-american-adults-who -cant-read/.

Weaver KB: The effects of horizontal violence and bullying on new nurse retention, *J Nurses Prof Dev* 29(3):138, 2013.

Weiss B: Health literacy: what do you need to do?, *Am Fam Physician* 92(2):84, 2015.

Westerfield HV, et al: Patients' perceptions of patient care providers with tattoos and/or body piercings, *J Nurs Adm* 42(3):160, 2012.

Williamson R, et al: Patient factors associated with incidents of aggression in a general inpatient setting, *J Clin Nurs* 23(7/8):1144, 2013.

Wittenberg E, et al: Enhancing communication related to symptom management through plain language, *J Pain Symptom Manage* 50(5):707, 2015.

evolve MEDIA RESOURCES

http://evolve.elsevier.com/Potter/essentials
- Audio Glossary
- QSEN Activity and Review Questions Answers and Rationales

OBJECTIVES

- Identify common topics for a patient's health education needs.
- Describe the concepts of teaching and learning.
- Identify a nurse's role in teaching and learning
- Describe the domains of learning.
- Describe the difference between readiness to learn and ability to learn.
- Apply the nursing process to the process of teaching.
- Describe the characteristics of an environment that promotes learning.
- Identify the principles of effective teaching and learning.

- Describe how to incorporate a patient's culture into the teaching plan of care.
- Discuss ways to adapt teaching approaches for patients with low health literacy.
- Describe ways to incorporate teaching with routine nursing care.
- Identify methods for evaluating learning.
- Describe how to use the teach-back method.
- Describe appropriate documentation of teaching and learning.

KEY TERMS

Being a patient educator is one of the most important professional nursing roles because education is essential to patient safety, health, and well-being. Factors such as shorter hospital stays, the focus on reducing hospital readmissions within 30 days, and the increased demand on nurses' time support the importance of providing timely quality patient education. Nurses need to find the most effective way to educate patients because health care consumers continue to be more assertive in seeking information, understanding their health needs, and finding resources available within the health care system. Patient education is important because the patient must be informed to consent to treatment. In particular, a patient has the right to know and be informed of diagnosis and prognosis of illness, treatment options, how to perform care activities in the home, and risks associated with treatment. A well-designed, comprehensive teaching plan that fits a patient's unique learning needs improves quality of care, reduces health care costs, helps patients make informed decisions about their health care, and allows them to become healthier and more independent.

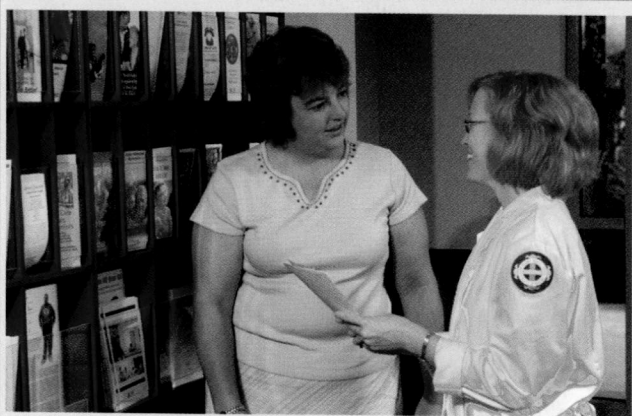

Latinka Drusko is a 55-year-old accountant. She immigrated to the United States from Bosnia in 1991 and has two grown sons who live close to her. Her husband died recently. Latinka is overweight and smokes 1 to 1½ packs of cigarettes a day. She is visiting her advanced practice nurse at a community clinic for her annual physical.

Ashley is a 23-year-old nursing student assigned to care for Latinka. During their first visit, Latinka states, "I'd like to get some information to help me become healthier. I would like to stop smoking and lose weight. Do you think you can help me?" Ashley gives Latinka some written material and sets up a time when they can meet later.

STANDARDS FOR PATIENT EDUCATION

Education has been a part of the nurse's role since the days of Florence Nightingale (Miller and Stoeckel, 2016). Patient education is considered a basic nursing competency by the American Association of Colleges of Nursing (AACN), National League for Nursing (NLN), Quality and Safety Education for Nurses (QSEN) Institute, and National Academy of Medicine (NAM) (formerly the Institute of Medicine [IOM]). The American Hospital Association (AHA) created the Patient's Bill of Rights. One of the rights is the right to information about one's diagnosis, treatment, and prognosis that is understandable, current, and relevant (Miller and Stoeckel, 2016). The American Nurses Association (ANA) (2015) specifically addresses a patient's right to self-determination and the nurse's obligation to assess the patient's understanding in Provision 1.4 of the *Code of Ethics for Nurses*. A nurse's role in patient education is becoming increasingly important because patients receive health care from several providers and specialties (Choi, 2015). Nurses provide information about illnesses and health and facilitate communication between a patient and the health care team to promote continuity of care. As a nurse, you need to ensure that patient and family education takes place, evaluate if learning occurred, and document all steps of the process.

PURPOSES OF PATIENT EDUCATION

Healthy People 2020 identifies patient education as a key intervention to improve health behaviors (U.S. Department of Health and Human Services [USDHHS], 2017a). The goal of patient education is to promote, retain, and restore health (Miller and Stoeckel, 2016). Patient education involves not only prevention but also treatment and management of illness. To prevent illness, patients must have information regarding health promotion activities. Patients need to understand how health promotion activities such as obtaining a flu shot or having a mammogram can help prevent illness. Patients and their family caregivers must learn skills to help manage diseases such as how to take medications to control high blood pressure.

Maintenance and Promotion of Health and Illness Prevention

By providing health education to patients, you promote positive, informed changes in habits and encourage patients to adapt habits that not only prevent disease and disability but also promote optimal health (Miller and Stoeckel, 2016). Nurses are in a unique position to act as educators because they have the most contact with patients. Patient education takes place in many settings in which nurses actively engage patients in learning how to manage their health, such as schools, hospitals, home, and the workplace (Box 12.1). Self-management is associated with improvements of health outcomes, especially for patients with chronic medical conditions such as diabetes or cardiovascular disease (Panagioti et al., 2014). For example, in childbearing classes expectant parents learn about physical and psychological changes in the woman and about fetal development. After learning about normal childbearing, the mother is more likely to engage in physical exercise, and the father is more likely to support the mother during her pregnancy.

Restoration of Health

Patients who are injured or ill need information or skills to improve or restore their level of health (see Box 12.1). Patients who are recovering from illness or adapting to chronic illness are often receptive to health education and usually motivated to learn whatever is necessary to resume their normal life (Miller and Stoeckel, 2016). However, patients who are acutely ill benefit from information that focuses on their immediate problems. As a nurse, you need to identify a patient's current health state and readiness to learn to motivate him or her to learn (Bastable, 2014). Family caregivers and friends frequently contribute to a patient's return to health and need to know as much as the patient. However, do not assume that you should involve them. Assess a patient's relationships and level of involvement with others before including family members or friends in patient education.

Coping With Impaired Functioning

Not all patients fully recover from illness or injury. Patients who need to learn to cope with permanent health changes need new knowledge and skills to continue activities of daily living (see Box 12.1). For example, a patient who loses the ability to move the left arm after a stroke needs to learn how to do activities of daily living with the right hand. You must

BOX 12.1 TOPICS FOR HEALTH EDUCATION

HEALTH MAINTENANCE AND PROMOTION AND ILLNESS PREVENTION

- First aid
- Avoidance of risk factors (e.g., smoking, alcohol)
- Growth and development
- Hygiene
- Immunizations
- Prenatal care and normal childbearing
- Nutrition
- Exercise
- Safety (e.g., in home, car, workplace, hospital)
- Screening (e.g., blood pressure, vision, cholesterol level)
- Lifestyle changes to reduce risk factors (e.g., smoking cessation, substance abuse treatment)

RESTORATION OF HEALTH

- Patient's disease or condition
  - Anatomy and physiology of body system affected
  - Cause of disease
  - Origin of symptoms
  - Expected effects on other body systems
  - Prognosis
  - Limitations on function
  - Rationale for treatment
  - Expected duration of care
- Medications
- Tests and therapies
- Nursing measures
- Surgical intervention
- Hospital or clinic environment
- Hospital or clinic staff
- Long-term care
- How patient can participate in care

COPING WITH IMPAIRED FUNCTION

- Home care
  - Medications
  - Diet
  - Activity
  - Self-help devices
- Rehabilitation of remaining function
  - Physical therapy
  - Occupational therapy
  - Speech therapy
- Prevention of complications
  - Knowledge of risk factors
  - Implications of noncompliance with therapy
  - Environmental alterations

also consider chronic illness when planning patient education. Patients who are chronically ill often experience fluctuations in receptiveness to learning over time that are due to their perception that their illness is controlling them (Bastable, 2014).

In the case of serious illness or injury such as a heart attack or spinal cord injury, a patient's family caregiver often partners with the patient and learns how to help him or her

manage health care needs (Bastable, 2014). Begin teaching as soon as you identify a patient's needs and determine that the family caregiver is willing to help. Provide information to help families cope with and adapt to emotional effects when your patients have long-term functional limitations.

TEACHING AND LEARNING

Teaching occurs when you deliberately communicate information to a learner to enable him or her to meet identified learning needs. In the case of patients, teaching enables patients to acquire the knowledge and skills for improving health behaviors. The objective of patient teaching is to help a learner adopt desired behaviors to achieve healthy outcomes (Bastable, 2014). Nurses often provide education during teachable moments as they administer nursing care. Examples of teachable moments include during medication administration, after medical appointments, before procedures, and during patient transportation.

Compare the steps of the teaching process with steps of the communication process (Table 12.1; see Chapter 11). As a nurse, you are the sender who wants to communicate a message to the receiver, your patient. Many intrapersonal variables influence your style and approach. Attitudes, values, cultural preferences, emotions, and knowledge influence the way you send messages. Evaluating past experiences with teaching helps you choose the best way to present information with each new patient (Bastable, 2014).

The receiver in the teaching-learning process is the learner. Intrapersonal variables affect a patient's readiness and ability to learn. Language, attitudes, literacy level, cultural background, and values influence the ability to understand a message. The ability to learn also depends on emotional and physical health, stage of development, and previous knowledge.

Learning is the purposeful acquisition of new knowledge, attitudes, behaviors, or skills (Bastable, 2014). It is a complex process, especially if a patient is learning new skills, changing existing attitudes, transferring knowledge to new situations, or solving problems. Generally teaching and learning begin when a person identifies a need for knowing or acquiring an ability to do something. Teaching is most effective when it responds to a learner's immediate needs. The teacher identifies these needs by asking questions and determining the learner's interests. After you identify what you need to teach, consider developing specific learning objectives. A learning objective describes what a patient will be able to do after successful instruction. Learning objectives clearly state the purpose of the teaching and the expectations of the teaching sessions. Both the patient and the nurse need to work together to create the learning objectives so that they are relevant and meaningful. The patient should believe that the learning objectives are achievable and realistic.

Role of a Nurse in Teaching and Learning

All nurses act as educators. This responsibility is outlined in the *Code of Ethics for Nurses* (ANA, 2015) and the *Patient Care Partnership* (AHA, 2006). Both documents support patients'

TABLE 12.1 COMPARISON OF COMMUNICATION AND TEACHING PROCESSES

COMMUNICATION	TEACHING
Referent	
Idea that initiates reason for communication	Perceived need to provide a person with information, establishment of relevant learning objectives by teacher
Sender	
Person who conveys message to another	Teacher who performs activities to help a person learn
Intrapersonal Variables (Sender)	
Knowledge, values, emotions, and sociocultural influences that affect sender's thoughts	Teacher's philosophy of education (based on learning theory), knowledge of teaching content, teaching approach, experiences in teaching, emotions and values
Message	
Information expressed or transmitted by sender	Content or information taught
Channels	
Methods used to transmit message (visual, auditory, touch)	Methods used to present content (visual and auditory materials, touch, taste, smell)
Receiver	
Person to whom message is sent	Learner
Intrapersonal Variables (Receiver)	
Knowledge, values, emotions, and sociocultural influences that affect receiver's thoughts	Willingness and ability to learn (physical and emotional health, cultural background, education, experience, developmental level)
Feedback	
Information revealing that true meaning of message was received	Determination of whether learner achieved learning objectives

rights to make informed decisions about their care, which requires accurate, complete, and relevant information. Furthermore, the *Speak Up Initiatives* (The Joint Commission [TJC], 2017) help patients become more involved in their care and more aware of their right to know about the care they will receive in a language they can understand. You enhance patient safety by teaching patients their role in preventing medical errors.

Your responsibility is to provide information that your patients and their families need. To increase the effectiveness of education, you present information by engaging patients enthusiastically, including the use of appropriate humor, problem-solving activities, and role modeling, and by using examples and technology (Bastable, 2014).

To be an effective educator, engage your patients as partners in learning. Do not merely pass on facts. *For example, in the case study when Ashley considers her approaches for teaching Latinka, she individualizes her educational approach based on Latinka's desire and interest in making a behavior change, her existing knowledge about the effects of smoking, and her preferences for ways to learn. By engaging Latinka in the teaching and learning experience, Ashley achieves greater success in making her teaching relevant and meaningful to Latinka.* Carefully determine what your patients need to know and provide education when they are ready to learn. Then evaluate the outcomes of teaching; for example, Can patients plan a medication schedule over 24 hours? Do patients prepare the right foods for their prescribed diet? Do patients know their activity restrictions?

DOMAINS OF LEARNING

Learning occurs in three domains: (1) cognitive (understanding), (2) affective (attitudes), and (3) psychomotor (motor skills).

Cognitive learning includes what a patient needs to know and understand. All intellectual behaviors are in the cognitive domain, including:

- Acquisition of knowledge
- Comprehension (ability to understand)
- Application (using abstract ideas in concrete situations)
- Analysis (relating ideas in an organized way)
- Synthesis (recognizing parts of information as a whole)
- Evaluation (judging the worth of a body of information)

Affective learning includes a patient's feelings, attitudes, opinions, and values. Research shows that you need to include the affective domain in teaching because it includes a patient's personal attitudes, beliefs, behaviors, and emotions (Miller and Stoeckel, 2016). Learning objectives in the affective domain include influencing attitudes and motivating the learner.

Psychomotor learning occurs when patients acquire skills that require the integration of knowledge and physical skills. Examples of psychomotor learning are learning how to administer insulin injections, use inhalers, and swipe a magnet across a vagal nerve stimulator (VNS). As patients begin to complete psychomotor skills with more confidence, they are able to perform the behaviors in more complex or different situations (e.g., using a walker to walk across a street curb). Adaptation occurs when a patient changes a response as a result of unexpected problems. This results in originating behavior, which involves creating new patterns of behavior.

Some learning topics involve all domains, whereas others involve only one. Patients often need to learn in each domain.

For example, patients diagnosed with high blood pressure need to understand how high blood pressure affects the body and what they can do to lower it (cognitive domain). Patients begin to accept the chronic nature of high blood pressure by learning positive ways to cope with their illness (affective domain). Many patients learn to take their blood pressure at home. This requires them to learn how to use a sphygmomanometer for home use (psychomotor domain). When you understand each learning domain, you are better prepared to use appropriate teaching techniques and apply the basic principles of learning.

BASIC LEARNING PRINCIPLES

To teach effectively and efficiently you first need to understand how people learn. Learning depends on the motivation to learn, the ability to learn, learning styles, and the learning environment. The ability to learn depends on a patient's physical and cognitive characteristics, developmental level, physical wellness, and intellectual thought processes. Remember that people have different preferences for learning and that they learn information in different ways and at different speeds.

Motivation to Learn

Motivation is an internal state that helps arouse, direct, and sustain human behavior (Miller and Stoeckel, 2016). A patient's motivation to learn is influenced by the patient's belief of the need to know something. Patients who need knowledge for survival have a stronger motivation to learn than patients who need it for promoting health (Bastable, 2014). Patients who are motivated to learn are often actively involved in decisions about their care and thus are better able to manage their health care. If a person does not want to learn, it is unlikely that learning will occur.

An attentional set is the mental state that allows a learner to focus on and understand the information being taught. Before learning anything, patients must be able to pay attention to or concentrate on the information they will learn. Physical discomfort, anxiety, fatigue, nausea, and environmental distractions make it more difficult for patients to concentrate and thus interfere with learning. You determine a patient's level of comfort by assessing verbal and nonverbal cues and by using objective symptom assessment tools (e.g., pain scale) before beginning a teaching plan. Teach only when your patient can focus on the information.

Anxiety, an uneasiness or uncertainty resulting from anticipating a threat or danger, decreases a patient's ability to attend. Learning requires a change in behavior, often leading to anxiety. A mild level of anxiety motivates learning as abstract thinking and enhances information processing (Bastable, 2014). However, high levels of anxiety disable a person, creating an inability to attend to anything other than relieving the anxiety. If a patient is highly anxious, you can help decrease anxiety before education by using techniques such as guided imagery or using appropriate humor (Bastable, 2014) (see Chapter 11).

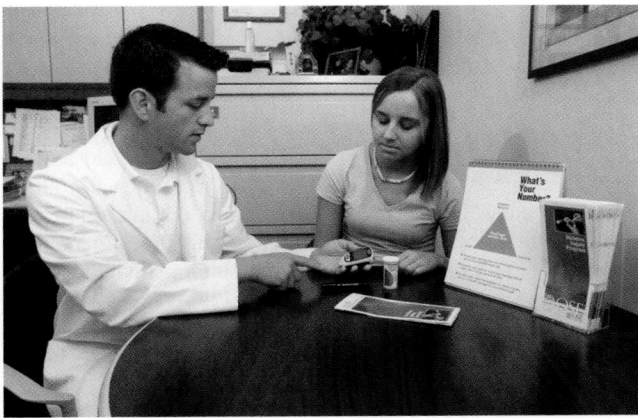

FIG 12.1 Nurse instructing patient with a glucose meter.

Health education often involves changing attitudes and values that are not easy to change simply by teaching facts. You enhance learning by actively involving patients and allowing them to make decisions during an educational session (Edelman and Mandle, 2014). Help patients adapt what they need to learn to their day-to-day lifestyle. For example, to help a patient with diabetes learn to monitor blood glucose levels, have the patient choose a blood glucose meter that is easy to use and affordable, and then observe the patient use it. You also attempt to incorporate the patient's lifestyle into a schedule for blood glucose testing (Fig. 12.1). In addition, knowing your patient's culture (see Chapter 21) and health beliefs (see Chapter 2) helps you develop patient-centered interventions to motivate your patients to learn (Box 12.2). Using a model such as the ACCESS model helps you to focus on cultural factors that influence patient education. The six aspects of the model are:

1. **Assessment** of a patient's lifestyle, health beliefs, cultural traditions, and health practices
2. **Communication** with awareness of the many variations in verbal and nonverbal responses
3. **Cultural negotiation and compromise** that encourages awareness of various characteristics of a patient's culture and one's own biases
4. **Establishment** of respect for a patient's cultural beliefs and values; establishment of a caring rapport as the basis for a therapeutic relationship
5. **Sensitivity** to how patients from diverse backgrounds perceive their care needs and the various patterns of communications (terms, concepts, tone, and style of communication) they use.
6. **Safety** that enables patients to feel culturally secure and avoids disempowerment of their cultural identity; respecting and nurturing the unique cultural identity of the individuals is necessary (Purnell, 2014).

Readiness to Learn

Readiness to learn is based on a patient's willingness and ability to engage in learning (Miller and Stoeckel, 2016). Assess a patient's readiness to learn through discussion with

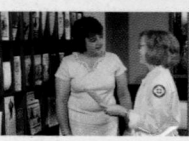

BOX 12.2   PATIENT-CENTERED CARE

Ashley recognizes that she knows very little about Bosnian culture. Therefore before she next meets with Latinka, Ashley takes some time to read about it. She finds that during the 1990s approximately 300,000 people from Bosnia immigrated to the United States because of the Balkan wars. The immigrants were older and experienced significant trauma related to the war. Many women experienced violence personally or witnessed violence toward their family and friends. Thus they have a higher incidence of mental illnesses. People from Bosnia tend to have strong ties with their families and communities. Common values include hospitality, spontaneity, owning a home, and telling stories. Bosnians have unique health concerns. Researchers estimate that Bosnian refugees living in the United States are three times more likely to smoke than U.S.-born residents; they also tend to believe their risk for developing long-term complications from smoking is lower than other populations (Sabic et al., 2014). Folk and family remedies are often passed down from mother to daughter. Common treatments include using herbal teas for colds or the flu. Bosnians who attend religious services tend to have lower levels of anxiety (Hasanovic and Pajevic, 2015). Physical activity often helps reduce the negative effects of stress caused by life events (Heaney et al., 2014). Ashley uses this information about Bosnian culture and the positive effects of physical activity to develop a culturally competent plan that focuses on helping Latinka lose weight and stop smoking.

IMPLICATIONS FOR PRACTICE

- Ashley has a better understanding of Bosnian culture, but she recognizes that not all Bosnian people are the same. Therefore she assesses Latinka's values and her beliefs about the American health care system.
- Ashley asks Latinka about her experiences with the war in Bosnia and is prepared to deal with sensitive issues related to mental health.
- Ashley uses her knowledge about Bosnian refugees and their attitudes about smoking to develop a patient-centered and culturally sensitive plan to help Latinka stop smoking (Sabic et al., 2014).
- Ashley explores healthy coping strategies such as attending religious services and participating in regular exercise to help Latinka better deal with her feelings and fears (Hasanovic and Pajevic, 2015; Heaney et al., 2014).

the patient. Many factors affect readiness to learn. For example, patients cannot learn when they are unwilling or unable to accept the reality of illness. A loss of health is usually very difficult for patients to accept. Grief is a complex process that patients experience during illness (see Chapter 27). People experience the stages of grief at different rates. It is important to properly time patient teaching to ease a grieving patient's adjustment to illness or disability (Table 12.2). Introduce a teaching plan when your patient enters the stage of acceptance, which is most compatible with learning. Continue to teach as long as the patient remains in a stage

conducive to learning. For example, a patient is recently diagnosed with seizures after a motor vehicle accident and you overhear the patient telling his wife that the result of his electroencephalogram (EEG) is wrong. It is inappropriate to initiate teaching with the patient regarding his new prescription for an antiseizure medication. Instead, you need to educate the patient about his testing and results.

A patient's health status also affects the readiness for education. Patients move along a continuum of health. As the patient moves along the continuum, his or her willingness to learn changes as well (Miller and Stoeckel, 2016). A patient who is acutely ill is concerned with survival. Conditions such as delirium, anxiety, fatigue, or pain interfere with thinking. At these times, the family caregiver often becomes the recipient of the education. Simple facts addressing immediate needs are most important. For example, a patient in pain is receptive to education about the use of a patient-controlled analgesia (PCA) pump but not how to use crutches.

Ability to Learn

A patient's developmental level and cognitive and physical capabilities influence the ability to learn. Consider the following important factors while developing a teaching plan.

Developmental Capability

Learning, similar to developmental growth, is an evolving process. Therefore consider your patient's stage of development and intellectual abilities so that your teaching will be successful. Learning occurs more readily when new information complements existing knowledge. Assess a patient's level of knowledge, intellectual skills, and literacy level before beginning a teaching plan. For example, before reviewing a teaching booklet about healthy food choices, determine your patient's understanding of nutrition and his or her reading and comprehension skills.

Age-Group

Age often reflects the developmental capability for learning and learning behaviors that a patient can acquire. Without proper biological, motor, language, and personal-social development, many types of learning cannot take place (see Chapter 23). Adapt your teaching approach based on a patient's developmental level (Box 12.3). When teaching a child, it is very important to match the information you provide with the child's developmental stage. As people mature into adulthood they often become more self-directed and able to identify their own learning needs. Enhance learning by encouraging an adult learner to reflect on personal and life experiences. Consider generational differences as well. For example, many baby boomers prefer visual aids and focusing on one topic at a time, whereas younger patients prefer using technology.

Physical Capability

The ability to learn depends on a person's level of physical development and overall physical health. To learn a psychomotor skill, your patient needs to have the necessary level of strength, coordination, and sensory acuity. For example, it is

TABLE 12.2 RELATIONSHIP BETWEEN PSYCHOSOCIAL ADAPTATION TO ILLNESS AND LEARNING

STAGE	PATIENT'S BEHAVIOR	LEARNING IMPLICATIONS	RATIONALE
Denial or disbelief	Patient avoids discussion of illness ("There's nothing wrong with me") and disregards physical restrictions. Patient suppresses and distorts information that has not been presented clearly.	Provide support, empathy, and careful explanations of all procedures while they are being done. Let patient know that you are available for discussion. Explain situation to family. Teach in present tense (explain current therapy).	Patient is not prepared to deal with problem. Any attempt to convince or tell patient about illness results in further anger or withdrawal. Provide only information patient pursues or absolutely requires.
Anger	Patient blames and complains and often directs anger at nurse.	Do not argue with patient but listen to concerns. Teach in present tense. Reassure family of patient's normality.	Patient needs opportunity to express feelings and anger. Patient is still not prepared to face future.
Bargaining	Patient offers to live better life in exchange for promise of better health. ("If God lets me live, I promise to be more careful.")	Continue to introduce only reality. Teach only in present tense.	Patient is still unwilling to accept limitations.
Resolution	Patient begins to express emotions openly, realizes that illness has created changes, and begins to ask questions.	Encourage expression of feelings. Begin to share information needed for future and set aside formal times for discussion.	Patient begins to perceive need for assistance and is ready to accept responsibility for learning.
Acceptance	Patient recognizes reality of condition, actively pursues information, and strives for independence.	Focus teaching on future skills and knowledge required. Continue to teach about present occurrences. Involve family in teaching information for discharge.	Patient is more easily motivated to learn. Acceptance of illness reflects willingness to deal with its implications.

BOX 12.3 TEACHING METHODS BASED ON PATIENT'S DEVELOPMENTAL CAPACITY

INFANT
- Repetition and continuity are essential; keep routines (e.g., feeding, bathing) consistent.
- Hold infant firmly while smiling and speaking softly to convey sense of trust.
- Have infant touch different textures (e.g., soft fabric, hard plastic).

TODDLER
- Use play to teach a procedure or activity (e.g., handling examination equipment, applying bandage to doll).
- Offer picture books that describe story of children in hospital or clinic.
- Use simple words such as *cut* instead of *laceration* to promote understanding.

PRESCHOOLER
- Use role playing, imitation, and play to make it fun for pre-schoolers to learn.
- Encourage questions and offer simple explanations and demonstrations.
- Encourage children to learn together through pictures and short stories about how to perform hygiene.

SCHOOL-AGED CHILD
- Teach psychomotor skills needed to maintain health. (Complicated skills such as learning to use a syringe take considerable practice.)
- Offer opportunities to discuss health problems and answer questions.

ADOLESCENT
- Help adolescent learn about feelings and need for self-expression.
- Use teaching as collaborative activity.
- Allow adolescents to make decisions about health and health promotion (safety, sex education, substance abuse).
- Use problem solving to help adolescents make choices.

YOUNG OR MIDDLE-AGED ADULT
- Encourage participation in teaching plan by setting mutual goals.
- Encourage independent learning.
- Offer information so that patient understands effects of health problem.

OLDER ADULT
- Teach when patient is alert and rested.
- Involve patient in discussion or activity.
- Focus on wellness and the patient's strength.
- Use approaches that enhance reception of stimuli for patients with sensory alterations (see Chapter 39).
- Keep teaching sessions short.

unrealistic for you to teach your patient to transfer from a bed to a wheelchair if he or she has insufficient upper body strength. To learn psychomotor skills, your patient requires the following characteristics:

- Size (height and weight sufficient for the task to be performed or the equipment to be used [e.g., crutch walking])
- Strength (ability of the patient to follow strenuous exercise program)
- Coordination (ability to maintain balance or having the dexterity needed for complicated motor skills such as using utensils or changing a bandage)
- Sensory acuity (visual, auditory, tactile, gustatory, and olfactory—sensory resources needed to receive and respond to messages taught)

Any condition (e.g., fatigue, breathing difficulty, depression) that drains a person's energy impairs the ability to learn. Medications such as pain medications often influence the ability to learn. Postpone teaching when an illness becomes aggravated by complications such as pain, fever, or respiratory difficulty. While providing care, assess a patient's energy level by noting his or her willingness to communicate, amount of activity initiated, and responsiveness to questions. Stop teaching if a patient tires; resume teaching when the patient feels rested. Offer several short teaching sessions rather than one long session.

Learning Environment

Learning takes place in a variety of environments. Always assess the physical environment and ensure it is as conducive to learning as possible (Miller and Stoeckel, 2016). Choose settings (e.g., small classroom, office) that help patients focus attention on their learning task.

The ideal environment that promotes learning is a room that has good lighting and ventilation, appropriate furniture, and a comfortable temperature (Fig. 12.2). A room that is too cold, hot, stuffy, or crowded makes patients too uncomfortable to pay attention. Comfortable furniture eliminates distractions such as the need to change position or shift body weight. It is also important to choose a quiet setting that offers privacy and few interruptions. If a patient desires,

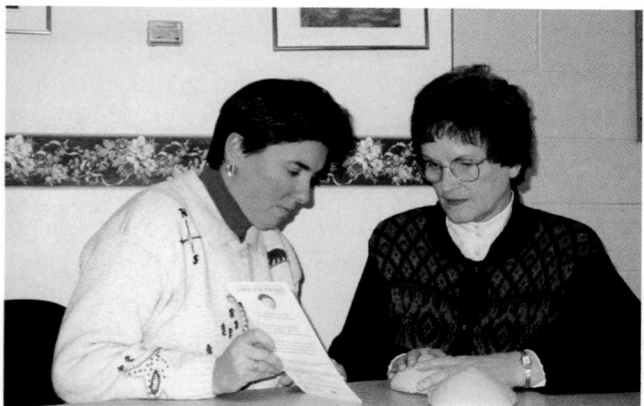

FIG 12.2 Choosing a comfortable, pleasant environment enhances the learning experience. Nurse is explaining breast self-examination procedure to patient.

include family members (especially the primary family caregiver) in discussions. However, remember that some patients are reluctant to engage in discussions about their illness when family members are present. Ask patients for permission to have family caregivers participate.

Teaching a group of patients requires a room that is an appropriate size and allows everyone to be seated comfortably and within hearing distance of the teacher. If the room is too large, participants are often tempted to sit outside the group along the perimeter. Arranging the group to allow participants to observe one another (e.g., in a circle) further enhances learning. More effective communication occurs as learners observe the verbal and nonverbal interactions of others.

INTEGRATING NURSING AND TEACHING PROCESSES

The teaching process parallels the nursing process (see Chapter 9). Both processes use the same steps (Table 12.3). Both processes require critical thinking (Box 12.4). The two processes differ in that the nursing process focuses on providing care, whereas the education process focuses on teaching (Bastable, 2014). Also, the outcomes of the processes are different. The outcomes of the nursing process include physical and psychosocial needs of the patient being met. The outcomes of the teaching process include changes in knowledge and skills. There are many models for patient education that you can use when developing education, including the ASSURE model. The acronym *ASSURE* stands for *a*nalyze the learner, *s*tate the objectives, *s*elect the instructional methods and materials, *u*se the instructional methods and materials, *r*equire learner performance, and *e*valuate the teaching plan (Bastable, 2014).

■ ■ ■ ASSESSMENT

An effective assessment for teaching provides the basis for individualized patient instruction. Apply critical thinking and consider what you know from your general nursing assessment (e.g., patient's condition, medications, physical status) to further explore and assess the patient's learning needs.

Ability to Learn. Begin your approach to teaching with an assessment of a patient's learning needs, readiness to learn, and preferred learning styles (Bastable, 2014). An individualized assessment ensures a more relevant and accurate approach to patient education (Table 12.4).

Patient Expectations. Because you need to focus education on the individual needs of a patient, gather information from the patient, analyze the information, and incorporate the information into a plan for patient education. It is also essential to understand what your patient expects to learn. For example, if your patient is a teenage boy newly diagnosed with type 1 diabetes mellitus, ask what he expects to learn about taking care of himself at home and while at school. Does he expect to self-administer the insulin, or is the

TABLE 12.3 COMPARISON OF NURSING AND TEACHING PROCESSES

BASIC STEPS	NURSING PROCESS	TEACHING PROCESS
Assessment	Collect data about patient's physical, psychological, social, cultural, developmental, and spiritual needs from patient, family, all databases, medical record, nursing history, and literature.	Gather data about patient's learning needs, literacy level, cultural background, motivation, ability to learn, and teaching resources from patient, family, learning environment, and all databases.
Nursing diagnosis	Identify appropriate nursing diagnoses.	Identify patient's learning needs on basis of three domains of learning.
Planning	Develop individualized care plan. Set diagnosis priorities based on patient's immediate needs.	Establish learning objectives stated in behavioral terms. Identify priorities regarding learning needs. Collaborate with patient on teaching plan.
Implementation	Collaborate with patient on care plan. Perform nursing care therapies. Include patient as active participant in care. Involve family caregiver in care as appropriate.	Identify type of teaching method to use. Implement teaching methods. Actively involve patient in learning activities. Include family caregiver participation as appropriate.
Evaluation	Identify success in meeting desired outcomes and goals of nursing care.	Determine outcomes of teaching-learning process. Measure patient's ability to achieve learning objectives. Reteach as needed.

BOX 12.4 SYNTHESIS IN PRACTICE

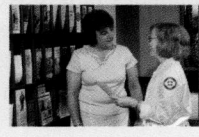

Ashley will be caring for Latinka during the rest of her clinical rotation. As Ashley assesses Latinka's educational needs, she reviews Latinka's health concerns and requests for information. Ashley knows that people learn best when you provide the information they want. She also wants to provide culturally competent patient education. Therefore she knows that assessing Latinka's perceptions of being overweight, being an immigrant in the United States, and how she is affected by the American health care system is a priority before she begins teaching about losing weight and smoking cessation.

Ashley's parents decided to stop smoking and have not smoked for 6 months. Ashley talks with her parents to find out which strategies were most helpful in their effort to quit smoking. She recalls that her mother gained about 10 lbs. She also read a research article that found that several women in the study gained weight after they quit smoking. Because Latinka expressed an interest in losing weight and quitting

smoking, Ashley decides that she needs to help Latinka develop healthy strategies that do not involve food to cope with nicotine withdrawal symptoms.

Ashley knows that she has the ethical responsibility to provide culturally sensitive patient teaching. She needs to accept Latinka and respect her beliefs and attitudes when providing patient teaching. Ashley found patient education handouts about smoking cessation, but the handouts were designed for Caucasian Americans and African Americans, not for Bosnians. Therefore she decides to take the printed information home with her and make revisions so that the information reflects Latinka's cultural preferences. Ashley also makes sure that the information is written in words that are easy to understand. She realizes that if Latinka cannot read English well, she will need the printed information translated into Bosnian. Ashley is excited to learn more about Latinka and who she is as an individual. After establishing a caring relationship with Latinka, Ashley begins to assess Latinka's health needs and learning styles so that she can put together an effective, individualized teaching plan.

expectation that a parent or school nurse will give the injections? Also assess your patient's expectations in all three learning domains. Questions such as "What do you think is important for you to know to take care of yourself?" allow the patient to be an active participant in planning self-care. Learning needs change, depending on your patient's health status. Assessment of learning needs is an ongoing activity. Examples of key areas of assessment are (1) questions raised by a patient or family about health issues; (2) a patient's understanding of current health status, implications of illness, types of therapy, and prognosis; (3) information or skills needed to perform self-care; (4) experiences that influence a patient's need to learn; and (5) information necessary for family caregivers to meet a patient's needs.

Motivation to Learn. Assess a patient's motivation to learn: Is the patient prepared and willing to learn based on the acuity and severity of his or her health risks or problems? Ask questions that relate to a patient's learning behaviors, health beliefs, cultural attitudes about health care providers, knowledge of health problems, and information to be learned. Other factors to assess include a patient's socioeconomic background, perception of the health problem, and perceived ability to perform health behaviors.

Teaching Environment. Ensure the environment is favorable to learning. Assess for distractions, noise, a patient's comfort level (e.g., sitting or lying, the need to use the toilet), and the availability of rooms and equipment. In the home

TABLE 12.4	FOCUSED PATIENT ASSESSMENT	
FACTORS TO ASSESS	**QUESTIONS**	**PHYSICAL ASSESSMENT**
Learning needs	Tell me what you know about your illness and its treatment. What would you like to know that would help you better manage your disease at home?	Observe expression on patient's face (e.g., puzzled, attentive, distracted).
Resources for learning	Who is the primary person who can help you at home? Will you have any trouble getting to the local health department to obtain teaching materials?	Observe for signs of anxiety when discussing home and transportation issues.
Ability to learn	Do you wear glasses or contacts? Do you have trouble seeing words printed in the newspaper? Do you have any difficulties hearing when someone speaks to you?	Observe where patient holds reading material and for squinting of eyes when reading. Observe whether patient turns head when attempting to listen.

setting, you need to assess lighting, space, and the availability of equipment.

Learning Styles. Learning styles are the ways in which learners most efficiently and effectively perceive, process, store, and recall information (Bastable, 2014). You assess learning styles by observation, interviews, and administering learning style assessments. An example of a learning style assessment is the VARK questionnaire (Bastable, 2014). This questionnaire provides patients with information regarding their learning preferences. It consists of 16 questions with four options. A patient can select more than one option for each question. This instrument is available in either an online or printed version. The VARK questionnaire has four learning preferences: visual, aural, read/write, and kinesthetic. The VARK questionnaire is easy for patients to use. It helps create a dialogue between you and your patient regarding the patient's preferred learning style.

There are two subsets of visual learning: linguistic and spatial. Linguistic learners prefer written information (e.g., computer-based instructions, books, articles). Spatial learners prefer visual aids (e.g., pictures, models, demonstrations). Auditory learners favor listening and speaking. They often repeat back the information to themselves or to others. Kinesthetic/tactile learners are physically active and gain skills and knowledge through manipulation. They write, draw pictures, and manipulate models of information.

Resources for Learning. Identify resources for learning, which often include the support of family caregivers or significant others. Determine who the patient's primary caregiver is in the home and whether the patient wishes to include the person in instruction.

The family influences the health and health behavior of the patient. For example, you provide a male patient with information regarding dietary changes required because of a medication such as avoiding foods rich in vitamin K while taking warfarin (Coumadin). If you give the education regarding dietary changes to the patient, it may not be successful if his wife is the primary cook at home. Thus you need to assess the readiness of family caregivers (as there may be more than one) to learn, when appropriate, to help care for a patient. Determine family caregivers' perceptions of a patient's illness and their willingness to help provide care. Determine the resources available in the home (e.g., running water, heating, access to transportation) and the teaching tools needed based on the patient's needs and ability to learn.

Language and Cultural Factors. Assess the language a patient most commonly uses. Sometimes you will need a translator to complete your assessment (see Chapter 21). TJC requires hospitals to provide qualified professional translators, whether the translator is physically present or available via telephone or interpreter care. Do not use family members as translators because they may not be able to translate important terms needed in obtaining informed consent or education, and many concepts are not easily translated.

Taking a patient's culture into account is essential in the educational assessment of a patient. Culture is a reflection of the whole of human behavior, including ideas, beliefs, and values; ways of relating to one another; language and manners of speaking; and work and lifestyle practices (Ball et al., 2015) (see Chapter 21). In terms of illness, patients often feel a loss of control, which often makes them hold on tighter to their cultural and family beliefs. In the United States, the decision maker is the adult patient. However, it is important to recognize that not all cultures have a strong emphasis on patient autonomy, and many cultures consider the family as a collective decision maker. You need to assess a patient's perception of health and illness, the use of traditional remedies and folk practitioners, the patient's perceptions of western medicine, the role of the family and family member relationships, and lastly the perception of emotional support (Bastable, 2014). For example, explore the significance prescribed medications and therapies has for a patient and consider alternative therapies he or she may use.

Health Literacy. Current evidence shows that health literacy is a key component that affects a patient's health care experience (National Institutes of Health [NIH], 2017). Therefore, you need to assess your patients' health literacy before providing instruction. Health literacy is defined by the National Academy of Medicine (NAM, formerly IOM) as an individual's ability to obtain, process, and understand basic health information and services to make appropriate and informed health decisions (Toronto and Weatherford, 2016). Approximately 90 million people in the United States have basic or below basic health literacy skills, which means they have difficulty understanding basic health information and making decisions regarding health care (Miller and Stoeckel, 2016). Individuals with low health literacy are at greater risk for adverse health outcomes and are less likely to adhere to medical recommendations. People with low health literacy come from all age ranges, races, and socioeconomic and educational backgrounds (Miller and Stoeckel, 2016). Low health literacy is not always easy for nurses to recognize. Simply asking patients if they can read often does not work because they do not feel comfortable admitting that they cannot read.

Current evidence supports using evidence-based assessment tools such as the Single-Item Literacy Screener (SILS). This tool asks questions such as "How often do you have to have someone help you read instructions, pamphlets, or other written material from your doctor or pharmacy?" and "How confident do you feel in filling out medical forms by yourself?" (Brice et al., 2014). Another assessment tool, the Newest Vital Sign (NVS) (http://www.pfizer.com/health/literacy/public_policy_researchers/nvs_toolkit), is available in English or Spanish; takes 3 minutes to complete; and screens a patient's general literacy level, numeracy skills, and comprehension of health-related written materials. Other assessment data that indicate low health literacy include a patient's inability to complete forms, read a prescription label, or adhere to a treatment plan or a patient's displaying uncooperative behavior, asking no questions, or asking for help from the family (Driessnack et al., 2014).

Special Needs of Children. Children pass through several developmental stages (see Chapter 23). You need to assess a child's cognitive and psychomotor abilities, physical strength, coordination, and reading level (see Box 12.3). Involve the parents during your assessment to better understand a child's needs, especially when children are very young and unable to care for themselves.

Middle Age Considerations. Middle age is a time in which it becomes important for adults to begin to build positive health habits (e.g., diet, exercise, lifestyle practices) to be better prepared for the older adult stage of life. Middle-aged adults must adapt their physical and psychological changes with their social roles. For example, does their tolerance to exercise enable them to participate in sports activities? Is there a need to select friends who are less involved in risky social behaviors? Assess a patient's understanding of what healthy behaviors involve and whether he or she accepts what changes may be necessary to adopt those behaviors.

Older Adult Considerations. The population of older adults continues to increase, and their care is becoming more complex. Thus use the best evidence when assessing an older adult's learning needs (Box 12.5). Older adults experience numerous physical and psychological changes as they age. Assess each patient for sensory changes that require modification of teaching methods (Miller and Stoeckel, 2016). For example, if you assess decreased visual acuity in your patient, use large-print materials to provide and reinforce patient teaching.

BOX 12.5 EVIDENCE-BASED PRACTICE

PICO Question: In patients with heart failure, does use of the teach-back method during discharge prevent hospital readmission compared with a standard discharge process?

SUMMARY OF EVIDENCE

Heart failure affects approximately 5 million patients in the United States (Dastoom et al., 2016). Care related to patients with heart failure costs 50% to 79% more compared with care given to other patients. It is estimated to cost the United States more than $35 billion per year (Dastoom et al., 2016). As a result of changes in repayment, hospitals are now penalized for readmissions, which is driving hospitals to look for solutions to prevent 30-day readmissions. Current research focuses on interventions to reduce readmission rates for different patient populations, especially patients with heart failure (Vesterlund et al., 2015). Teach-back allows nurses to confirm that learning has occurred. Discharge teaching can positively affect readmission rates (Vesterlund et al., 2015). In one study, the number of patients who were readmitted with heart failure was reduced by 56.2% for patients who received group education with the teach-back method before discharge (Dastoom et al., 2016).

APPLICATION TO NURSING PRACTICE

- Use the teach-back method to assess a patient's ability to manage heart failure and address gaps in knowledge before discharge (Dastoom et al., 2016).
- The amount of time a nurse and other members of the health care team spend providing patient education positively contributes to a patient's ability to answer questions correctly when evaluating the effectiveness of education sessions (Dastoom et al., 2016).
- Involve multiple disciplines in providing discharge information including dietary and therapies (Vesterlund et al., 2015).
- Along with the teach-back technique, implement other interventions during discharge to prevent readmission such as making follow-up phone calls to provide continuity of care and giving informational packets to patients (Vesterlund et al., 2015; Dastoom et al., 2016).

NURSING DIAGNOSIS

After assessing information related to your patient's ability and need to learn, interpret data and cluster defining characteristics to form nursing diagnoses that reflect the patient's specific learning needs. If a patient has several learning needs, the nursing diagnoses guide priority setting.

Several North American Nursing Diagnosis Association International (NANDA-I) nursing diagnoses apply to learning needs. When the diagnosis is *Deficient Knowledge,* the diagnostic statement describes the specific type of learning need and related factor (e.g., *Deficient Knowledge regarding psychomotor learning related to newly ordered injectable medication*). Some diagnoses are very similar to one another. Thus in order to identify the correct problem-focused diagnosis, you must analyze the patient's defining characteristics carefully. For example, when you care for a patient who is not physically active because the patient does not understand the importance of physical activity, the nursing diagnosis is *Sedentary Lifestyle related to deficient knowledge of health benefits of physical exercise.* However, if this same patient is having difficulty completing activities of daily living because of increased weight and the patient needs to know how to adapt activities to meet health needs, the nursing diagnosis is *Activity Intolerance related to generalized weakness,* and your plan of care would include patient education regarding how to improve endurance.

When you manage or eliminate health care problems through education, the related factor of a problem-focused and health promotion diagnostic statement refers to knowledge deficits. Include the specific type of learning need when possible. For example, when an older-adult patient is not taking a medication at the appropriate time because she does not understand how the medication works (*Noncompliance with medication schedule related to deficient knowledge*), focus on explaining the action of the medication and its purpose. Other nursing diagnoses (e.g., *Acute Pain, Fear*) indicate that barriers to learning exist. In these situations, delay teaching until you resolve the priority nursing diagnosis. Other examples of nursing diagnoses that indicate learning needs include the following:

- *Ineffective Denial*
- *Ineffective Health Maintenance*
- *Ineffective Health Management*
- *Risk-Prone Health Behavior*
- *Ineffective Family Health Management*

PLANNING

After determining nursing diagnoses, identify your patient's learning needs and develop a teaching care plan. When helping a patient change a health behavior, remember that knowledge alone does not change behavior. Discuss factors that facilitate and inhibit learning with your patient during planning. For the plan to be effective, collaborate with the patient, family caregiver(s), and other members of the health care team. The plan needs to include topics for instruction, teaching resources (e.g., equipment or booklets), recommendations for involving the family caregiver(s), and teaching objectives.

Goals and Outcomes. It is very important to set clear goals and measurable outcomes so that you can effectively establish and later evaluate and revise a teaching plan as needed. Include the patient if possible when establishing learning goals and outcomes. Expected outcomes guide the choice of teaching strategies and who is involved in the plan. Learning objectives are either short term (relating to immediate learning needs) or long term (relating to permanent adaptation to a health problem). Each objective is a statement of a single behavior that identifies a patient's ability to do something after a learning experience.

In some health care settings you develop written teaching plans. Include topics for instruction and resources, recommendations for involving family, and objectives of the teaching plan in these cases. Some plans are very detailed, whereas others are in an outline format (Box 12.6). Remember that the more specific your plan is, the easier it is to follow.

BOX 12.6   PATIENT TEACHING

Healthy Food Choices

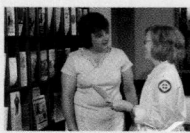 Before planning educational sessions, Ashley assesses what Latinka expects to learn while they are together. Latinka asks Ashley to help her make healthier food choices. Ashley begins by assessing what Latinka normally eats. She completes a diet history. The Bosnian diet is high in animal fats and has a Turkish influence. Meat, bread, vegetables, stews, cheese, legumes, fish, eggs, coffee, sweetened fruit juices, and sweet cakes are common in the Bosnian diet. Using this information, Ashley develops the following teaching plan for Latinka.

OUTCOME

At the end of the teaching session, Latinka will identify three ways to make her diet lower in fat and calories.

TEACHING STRATEGIES

- Review Latinka's favorite recipes and meals and make suggestions for food substitutions that make meals healthier (e.g., eat fruit instead of drinking sweetened fruit juice; use ground turkey, low-fat cheese, and vegetable oil; and decrease number of eggs used in recipes).
- Encourage Latinka to increase the number of legumes and fresh vegetables in her diet, while decreasing the amount of sweet bread she eats.
- Provide Latinka with culturally sensitive teaching handouts on healthy food choices.
- Summarize what was taught.
- Make a follow-up appointment to reinforce teaching.

EVALUATION

- Use the principles of teach-back to evaluate patient/family caregiver learning:
  - "Tell me what food substitutions you used to make your recipes healthier."
  - "What types of foods do you plan to increase and decrease in your diet?"
  - "Tell me three healthy meal options you can make this week."

Setting Priorities. Learning objectives identify the expected outcomes of a planned learning experience, which help establish priorities for learning. Focus on what the patient needs to know, his or her nursing diagnoses, and previous knowledge. As a nurse, you are ultimately responsible for ensuring that all teaching needs have been met. Usually patient safety is a teaching need that is most important. For example, a patient with newly diagnosed hypertension and angina needs to learn about newly prescribed medications, which typically include nitroglycerin for angina and an antihypertensive medication, such as an angiotensin-converting enzyme (ACE) inhibitor. In this situation knowledge regarding the early identification of chest pain and appropriate use of nitroglycerin are the learning priorities.

Timing. When is the right time to teach? When a patient first enters a clinic or hospital? At discharge? At home? Each time point is appropriate because patients have learning needs as long as they stay in the health care system. There are times in which it is not appropriate to provide teaching such as when a patient receives bad results from a diagnostic test. Plan to teach when a patient is most attentive, receptive, and alert. The frequency of sessions depends on each patient's abilities and the complexity of the information that is being taught.

The length of teaching sessions also affects learning. Prolonged sessions cause patients to lose concentration and attentiveness, especially older-adult patients. It is easier to maintain patients' interests when educational sessions are shorter (e.g., lasting 10 to 15 minutes) and more frequent. Nonverbal cues such as poor eye contact or slumped posture indicate that a patient has lost concentration. If you note a loss of concentration, stop the session.

Organizing Teaching Material. Consider the order of information presented. Organize material so that it progresses from simple to complex because a person learns simple facts and concepts before learning how to make associations or complex interpretations of ideas. For example, to teach a woman how to feed her husband who has a gastric tube (see Chapter 35), first teach her how to measure the tube feeding and manipulate the equipment. Once you accomplish this, teach her how to administer the feeding.

Because patients are more likely to remember information taught in the beginning of a teaching session, present essential information first. Informative but less critical content follows the essential information. Use repetition and summarize key points to reinforce learning.

Collaborative Care. Although you are the primary member of the health care team responsible for patient education, your patients' educational needs are often highly complex. Collaboration with other health care professionals is required to successfully meet patient needs. For example, refer a patient with a new diagnosis of chronic renal failure to a dietitian for dietary teaching. Patients in acute care settings often require assistance from discharge planners, case managers, and community agencies to be successfully discharged to home. It is your responsibility to collaborate with and include these interdisciplinary health care team members in the teaching plan. A variety of educational resources is available in the community including diabetes education clinics, prenatal classes, and support groups. Encourage your patients to use these resources and reinforce information provided.

■ ■ ■ IMPLEMENTATION

Implementation of a teaching plan requires you to use critical thinking while you analyze assessment data and nursing diagnoses and apply teaching and learning principles. Remember that each interaction with a patient is an opportunity to teach. You implement teaching strategies that integrate all styles of learning to fully engage the patient and enhance learning. Use evidence-based interventions to create an effective and active learning environment and maximize opportunities for learning. Because learning situations vary, there is no single correct way to teach.

Teaching Approaches. Teaching may be provided in a variety of ways, but it is important to choose a teaching approach that matches your patient's needs and learning style. A patient's learning needs change over time. Modify your teaching approach as you care for a patient over time.

Telling. Use the telling approach when teaching limited information such as when you are preparing a patient for an emergent diagnostic procedure. Outline the task a patient needs to do and give explicit instructions. There is no time for feedback with this method.

Participating. When using the participating approach, you and the patient participate in the learning process together. The patient helps decide content and how best to present it, and you guide and counsel the patient. For example, a parent with a child diagnosed with sickle cell disease works with you to manage the child's pain. You select pain management approaches that will likely be effective at times when the child's pain is the worst. At the end of each teaching session you review the objectives with the parent and child and plan or revise what you will cover the next time you meet.

Entrusting. The entrusting approach gives patients the opportunity to manage their self-care. A patient accepts responsibilities and correctly performs a task while you observe the patient's progress and remain available for assistance. For example, a patient who is receiving continuous intravenous pain medication at home for end-stage cancer requires a higher dose of pain medication. The patient understands the dosage of the medication and how the medication pump works. You help the patient determine an appropriate new pain medication dosage and allow him or her to adjust the settings on the medication pump.

Reinforcing. Reinforcement is using a stimulus that increases the probability of a response. A learner who receives reinforcement before or after a desired learning behavior will likely repeat the behavior. Feedback is a common form of reinforcement. Reinforcers are positive or negative. Positive reinforcement such as a smile or praise and support produces the desired responses. Although negative reinforcement (e.g., frowning) may work, people usually respond better to positive reinforcement.

Three types of reinforcers are social, material, and activity. Use social reinforcers (e.g., smiles, compliments, words of encouragement, or physical contact) to acknowledge a learned behavior. Examples of material reinforcers are food, toys, and music. They work best with young children. Activity reinforcers (e.g., physical therapy) rely on the principle that a person is motivated to engage in an activity if there is an opportunity to participate in more desirable activity on completion of this first activity. Choosing an appropriate reinforcer involves careful thought and attention to individual preferences. Never use reinforcers as threats. Reinforcement is not effective with every patient.

Incorporating Teaching With Nursing Care.

As you gain confidence in your knowledge and clinical skills, you find that you are able to teach more effectively while you provide care to your patients. For example, you educate your patient on the actions of medications while you administer them. When you follow a teaching plan informally, your patient feels less pressure to perform, and learning becomes more of a shared activity. Teaching during routine care is efficient and cost-effective and makes the information more relevant.

Teaching Methods.

Active participation enhances learning. By actively experiencing a learning event, your patient is more likely to retain knowledge. A teaching method is the way you deliver information and is based on a patient's learning needs and preferences (Box 12.7). For example, older adults learn and remember more if the material is relevant to their needs and abilities and is provided at an appropriate pace (Box 12.8) (Miller and Stoeckel, 2016). The instructional method you choose depends on the time available for teaching, the setting, the resources available, and your comfort level with teaching.

One-on-One Discussion. Whenever you teach a patient at the bedside, in a health care provider's office, or in the home, you share information through one-on-one discussion. You provide information informally, allowing the patient to ask questions or share concerns. Use various teaching aids during the discussion, depending on the patient's learning needs.

Group Instruction. Group instruction offers an economical way to teach several patients at one time and allows patients to develop a network of social support (Miller and Stoeckel, 2016). Group instruction often involves both lecture and discussion. Lectures are efficient in helping groups of patients learn about a subject. After hearing information from a lecture, learners need the opportunity to share ideas and seek clarification. Group discussions allow patients and

---

BOX 12.7   TEACHING METHODS BASED ON PATIENT'S LEARNING NEEDS

COGNITIVE

Discussion (One-on-One or Group)
- Involves nurse and patient or nurse with several patients
- Promotes active participation and focuses on topics of interest to patient
- Allows peer support
- Enhances application and analysis of new information

Lecture
- More formal method of instruction because teacher controls it
- Helps learner acquire new knowledge and gain comprehension

Question-and-Answer Session
- Designed specifically to address patient's concerns
- Helps patient apply knowledge

Role-Play, Discovery
- Allows patient to actively apply knowledge in controlled situation
- Promotes synthesis of information and problem solving

Independent Project (Computer-Assisted Instruction), Field Experience
- Allows patient to assume responsibility for completing learning activities at own pace
- Promotes analysis, synthesis, and evaluation of new information and skills

AFFECTIVE

Role Play
- Allows expression of values, feelings, and attitudes

Discussion (Group)
- Allows patient to acquire support from others in group
- Permits patient to learn from others' experiences
- Promotes responding, valuing, and organization

Discussion (One-on-One)
- Allows discussion of personal, sensitive topics of interest or concern

PSYCHOMOTOR

Demonstration
- Provides presentation of procedures or skills by nurse
- Permits patient to incorporate modeling of nurse's behavior
- Allows nurse to control questioning during demonstration

Practice
- Gives patient opportunity to perform skills using equipment
- Provides repetition

Return Demonstration
- Permits patient to perform skills as nurse observes
- Is excellent source of feedback and reinforcement

Independent Project, Game
- Requires teaching method that promotes adaptation and origination of psychomotor learning
- Permits learner to use new skills

BOX 12.8 **CARE OF THE OLDER ADULT**

Effective Teaching Strategies for the Older Adult

- Provide individualized information that is based on what the patient needs to know.
- Present information slowly in frequent sessions.
- Include family caregivers when necessary.
- Repeat information frequently.
- Reinforce teaching with audiovisual material, written exercises, and practice.
- Emphasize the older adult's current concerns and past positive coping strategies (Touhy and Jett, 2016).
- Allow more time for learner to express himself or herself, demonstrate learning, and ask questions (Edelman and Mandle, 2014).
- Establish measurable and realistic short-term goals.
- Establish follow-up sessions.
- Base new information on patient's previous level of learning.

families to learn from one another as they share common experiences.

Preparatory Instruction. Patients frequently face unfamiliar tests or procedures that create anxiety. Providing information about procedures helps them feel less anxious because they understand what to expect during a procedure. When preparatory instructions accurately describe actual experiences, patients usually cope more effectively with the stress from the procedure and therapies. The following are guidelines for giving preparatory explanations:

1. Describe physical sensations during the procedure but do not evaluate them. For example, when drawing a blood specimen, explain that the patient will feel a sticking sensation as the needle punctures the skin.
2. Describe the cause of the sensation, preventing false impressions of the experience. For example, explain that a needle insertion burns because alcohol used to cleanse the skin enters the puncture site.
3. Prepare patients only for aspects of the experience that have commonly been noticed by other patients. For example, explain that it is normal for a tight tourniquet (applied during an intravenous needle insertion) to cause a person's hand to tingle and feel numb.

Demonstrations. Use demonstrations when teaching psychomotor skills. An effective demonstration requires planning. Include the following steps in a demonstration:

1. Assemble and organize equipment.
2. Perform each step in sequence while analyzing the knowledge and skills involved.
3. Determine when to give explanations, considering the patient's learning needs.
4. Judge the proper speed and timing of the demonstration based on the patient's cognitive abilities and anxiety level.

Demonstrate the procedure or skill under the same conditions that the patient will experience at home and in the same order in which the patient will perform it. Encourage the patient to ask questions so that he or she clearly understands each step. To enable the patient to easily observe each step, perform demonstrations slowly and avoid rushing. Give the patient the opportunity to practice the procedure under supervision. At the end of the session have the patient perform a **return demonstration,** allowing the patient to complete the procedure independently to show competence. When appropriate, also have family caregivers perform return demonstrations, especially when they are likely the ones who will provide the skill at home.

Analogies. Learning occurs when a teacher translates complex language or ideas into words or concepts that a patient understands. **Analogies** add to verbal instruction by providing familiar images that make complex information more real and understandable (Miller and Stoeckel, 2016). For example, comparing arterial blood pressure to the flow of water through a hose is an analogy that is useful when explaining hypertension to a patient. When using analogies, know the concept; keep the analogy simple and clear; and be aware of the patient's background, experience, and culture. Analogies work only if the other person understands the comparison.

Role Play. During role play your patients play themselves or someone else in a situation. Patients learn required skills and feel more confident in performing them independently following the role play. For example, you are teaching a family caregiver effective communication strategies to use with an older, confused parent. You pretend to be the parent who is having difficulty getting dressed. The caregiver responds to you in this situation. At the end of the session you help the caregiver evaluate the response and determine if an alternative approach would have been more effective.

Simulation. Simulation is a useful technique for teaching problem solving, application, and independent thinking. During individual or group discussion you present a problem or situation for patients to solve. For example, you ask patients with heart disease to plan a meal low in cholesterol.

Use of Technology. Communication and patient teaching does not happen only in person; it also occurs electronically. Most Americans have access to the Internet, and about 56% of people own a smartphone (Miller and Stoeckel, 2016). As technology continues to improve, more people are online and use online resources to enhance their health. For example, some hospitals use Twitter to improve communication to share news and health information with the community (Gomes and Coustasse, 2015). A trend in the hospital setting is to use technology through TV networks and tablets to provide self-paced and self-directed learning (Sawyer et al., 2016). The patient completes surveys on admission, and then the nurse launches education modules for the patient; the program is evaluated using review questions at the end of each topic segment. Another technology platform called the GetWellNetwork uses the television in a patient's room (Kompany et al., 2016). The GetWellNetwork delivers age-appropriate education, including interactive education for children. Technology is also used in the outpatient setting to provide education. Placing education

QSEN **QSEN ACTIVITY** *Informatics*

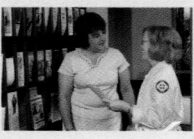

Latinka tells Ashley that she recently purchased a new smartphone and is excited about it. She asks Ashley if there are any apps that she can use to help her stop smoking, eat better, and manage her weight. Ashley knows that these apps help patients change their behaviors and better understand how to make positive changes at the same time.

- Conduct a literature search and find at least one smartphone app that Ashley could suggest that Latinka use to stop smoking, improve her diet, and manage her weight. Why is it important for Ashley to evaluate these apps and help Latinka decide which ones to use?

evolve Answers to QSEN Activities can be found on the Evolve website.

materials in waiting rooms using tablets helps improve patient satisfaction, which increases compliance with treatment plans and future appointments (Stribling and Richardson, 2016).

Maintaining Attention and Participation. All the senses are channels for presenting information. Patients learn best when you use multiple senses while you teach. In addition, your actions can increase learner attention and participation. When conducting a discussion with a patient, change the tone and intensity of your voice, make eye contact, and use gestures that accentuate key points of discussion.

Illiteracy and Other Disabilities. Medical terms are very confusing. Thus you need to provide information in words that your patients are able to understand. People who have problems with illiteracy or other learning disabilities often have difficulty analyzing instructions and synthesizing information. Use a variety of resources (e.g., audiotapes, videos, drawing pictures) with patients who have low health literacy or other difficulties learning (Box 12.9).

Sometimes you provide education to patients who have sensory alterations (see Chapter 39). When caring for patients who are hearing impaired, you may need to include a sign language interpreter to help implement your interventions or use a white board to write messages to each other. Visual impairments also affect the teaching strategy you use. Patients who are blind or have reduced vision often have acute listening skills. To enhance communication and decrease anxiety, tell the patient that you are there, and do not shout during teaching sessions.

Cultural Awareness. Health education materials often fail to address a patient's cultural beliefs, values, language, perceptions, and attitudes. Be aware of a patient's cultural background, beliefs, and ability to understand instructions. In some cases, you need to provide information written in the patient's native language.

BOX 12.9 PATIENT TEACHING STRATEGIES FOR PATIENTS WITH LIMITED HEALTH LITERACY

- Make time for one-on-one educational sessions. Speak clearly and listen carefully.
- Individualize teaching materials (e.g., reading level, use of graphics, photographs) to meet a patient's needs and match his or her reading level; if you do not know a patient's reading level, provide information at a fifth-grade or lower level.
- Keep a lesson simple. In general, introduce no more than four topics (USDHHS, n.d.).
- Provide information in a variety of ways (e.g., written, on a computer, videotape, audiotape).
- Make teaching materials visually appealing. For written materials, use at least 12-point font and avoid using all capital letters, italics, and fancy script (USDHHS, n.d.).
- Use simple words that a patient can understand (e.g., shot instead of injection, walk instead of ambulate, medicine instead of medication). Avoid long or run-on sentences (USDHHS, n.d.).
- Use the active voice when providing instructions (e.g., tell patient to "take medicine before bedtime" instead of "medicine should be taken at bedtime").
- Use examples (e.g., what to do when feeling bad, how to set up a pill counter at home) to keep a patient an active participant in learning.
- Present the most important information first, and summarize it at the end of the session.
- Space out information to decrease intimidation.
- Use pictures or illustrations when possible.
- Encourage patients to ask questions during the teaching session.
- Ask specific questions (e.g., "When will you take this medicine each day?") and ask patient to "teach back" or "show back" what you have taught to evaluate learning. Examples are "We discussed the problems you need to call your doctor about; tell me what those are" and "I explained the type of foods that are high in salt; give me three examples."
- Observe patient's ability to perform any desired behaviors or self-care activities.

Cultural awareness helps you provide culturally sensitive health care and patient education. For example, how you explain guidelines for safe sex varies if a patient is heterosexual versus homosexual. A patient from a lower socioeconomic background will require nutritional education with a different focus on foods than a patient who has unlimited financial resources and is able to purchase any type of food.

Effective educational strategies often require the use of different patterns of communication. When educating patients of different ethnic groups, do the following:

- Become aware of the distinctive aspects of each culture (Mott-Coles, 2014).
- If an interpreter is necessary, determine your patient's beliefs about using an interpreter. First, in some

BOX 12.10   EVALUATION

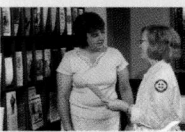

After Ashley and Latinka met for the first time, Latinka decided to quit smoking on her birthday, which was in 1½ weeks. During that time Ashley made an appointment for Latinka to see the advanced practice nurse at the health department so she could get a prescription for nicotine patches. Ashley and Latinka decided to meet 4 weeks after Latinka started her smoking cessation plan.

Today Ashley and Latinka meet to evaluate how the teaching plan is going. Ashley completes a physical assessment and asks Latinka questions about her progress to date. Latinka states that she is less short of breath and has more energy now that she is not smoking. Latinka's sons, who also smoked, decided to quit with their mom as a birthday present. Latinka states, "If one of us feels like smoking, we call one another for help. It's really nice that we can support one another." Ashley reinforces that having a good support system at home will help Latinka continue not to smoke. Latinka also relates that the nicotine patch is working well. She still suffers from nicotine withdrawal symptoms but says, "They aren't that bad if I use my patches."

Because Ashley is also concerned about Latinka's weight-management plan, she asks her about her level of exercise and diet choices since the last time they met. Latinka says that she walks with her sons 2 days a week and with her neighbor another 2 days a week. She has also been experimenting with her recipes. She made her famous *burek,* which is a Bosnian meat pie. She used egg whites instead of egg yolks and ground sirloin instead of ground beef. She added more vegetables to her recipe and decreased the amount of butter she used. Latinka said, "I thought it was good, but I wasn't sure if it matched up to my old recipe. So I served it to my boys, and they didn't even notice the difference."

Ashley reviews healthy coping strategies with Latinka and provides reinforcement for all the positive changes made so far. They decide to meet again in 4 weeks. Ashley asks Latinka if there is anything that Latinka would like to review at their next appointment. Latinka says, "I want to review all the good things that will happen to me now that I'm not smoking. I also want to talk about what I'm going to do with all the money I'm saving now that I don't smoke. I might even bring you a sample from my new stew recipe." Latinka tells Ashley that she is so glad that Ashley is her nurse. Ashley feels a sense of satisfaction. She has helped Latinka make healthy changes, and she looks forward to learning more about Bosnian culture.

DOCUMENTATION NOTE

"Outcomes of education plan assessed. Reports quit smoking about 4 weeks ago on birthday. Sons have quit smoking also, providing support for one another. Has symptoms of nicotine withdrawal, but reports that nicotine replacement patch is helpful in minimizing symptoms. Verbalized increased feelings of energy and less shortness of breath. Walking 4 days a week with sons and neighbor. Is successfully experimenting with healthy substitutions in family recipes. Has asked to review short-term benefits associated with smoking cessation and will review diet information at next visit."

---

cultures, it is inappropriate to discuss private health-related issues with people of the opposite sex or people who are younger. Always use a professional interpreter who understands medical terminology.

- Demonstrate respect for your patient and the family, address them using their appropriate titles, and pronounce their names correctly.
- Use culturally relevant teaching resources and approaches (Mott-Coles, 2014).

■■■ EVALUATION

Patient Outcomes. Patient education is not complete until you evaluate the outcomes of the teaching-learning process. Studies show that patients forget about 40% to 80% and misunderstand about 50% of information taught during office visits (Agency for Healthcare Research and Quality [AHRQ], 2015). Additionally, the IOM Committee of Health Literacy reported that many patients are hesitant to admit they do not understand what was taught to them (Caplin and Saunders, 2015). Thus it is important to determine if your patient achieved learning objectives set during the planning stage (Box 12.10). Regardless of information you provide to patients, use the **teach-back** method (Box 12.11), as it enables you to immediately confirm patient understanding, which improves compliance (Caplin and Saunders, 2015). Many

BOX 12.11   TEACH-BACK METHOD OF EVALUATION

Use the following questions to evaluate patient understanding of education. Ask the questions in an open-ended, respectful manner and modify them as needed (AHRQ, 2015).

- "I want to be sure that I explained this clearly. How should you take this medication?"
- "Let's review the main side effects of (insert name of medication). What two things do you need to watch for?"
- "We've talked a lot today about (insert appropriate topic). I want to be sure that I've explained everything clearly. What changes in (insert appropriate topic/condition/routine/person) will you call the health care provider about?"
- "On days when you and your wife (or husband) go out, what will you do about taking your (insert name of medication)?"
- "After talking today, what will your daily routine look like?"
- "Please use this model to show me how you'll do (procedure)."

health care organizations such as AHQR, National Quality Forum, TJC, and Institute for Healthcare Improvement encourage nurses to use the teach-back method. When using the teach-back method, you ask a patient questions to determine what he or she learned from the education session (AHRQ, 2015). Do not use "yes" or "no" questions; use open-ended questions. For example, an incorrect would be, "Can you tell me how increasing your activity, taking your medications, and decreasing salt in your diet can help control your high blood pressure?" Correct questions would be, "Tell me how increasing your activity, taking your medications, and decreasing salt in your diet can help control your high blood pressure" and "What can you tell me about changes you can make in your diet to help lower your cholesterol?"

Modify the teaching plan if evaluation indicates that a knowledge or skill deficit still exists. Alternative teaching methods often help to clarify information or strengthen skills that the patient was unable to comprehend or perform originally. Evaluation reveals new learning needs or new factors that may interfere with the patient's ability to learn. Similar to the nursing process, the teaching process is continuous and ever changing.

Patient Expectations. After receiving education to manage health promotion activities, disease processes, and physical and functional limitations, patients return to their homes and communities. It is important to have a method to evaluate a patient's expectations regarding patient education. Ask patients if they believe they have learned what is needed to manage their health care in the home. Have patient's describe how they have adapted any instructions you have provided and whether they feel satisfied with the information. If patients' expectations are not met, it is more likely that they will not continue to follow the prescribed treatment plan, will be less independent, and perhaps will ignore signs and/or symptoms indicating a need to make an appointment with their health care provider.

DOCUMENTATION OF PATIENT TEACHING

Because patient teaching often occurs informally (e.g., during medication administration or physical examination), it is difficult to document it consistently. However, because nurses are professionally and legally responsible for providing accurate and timely information to patients, quality documentation is essential. Documentation also helps members of the health care team coordinate patient education. Document the following information about patient education:

1. *Assessment data and related nursing diagnoses:* Provide information and support for goals and outcomes.
2. *Interventions planned and used:* Planned education provides continuity of care. Specifically describe subject matter and what has been presented so that other nurses can follow up and reinforce teaching (e.g., "verbalized side effects of digoxin").
3. *Evaluation of learning:* Document evidence of learning (e.g., a return demonstration of coughing and deep breathing). This informs staff about the patient's progress and determines material that you still need to teach. Always use the teach-back method.
4. *Ability of patient and/or family caregiver to manage care:* Identify needs for outpatient or home care follow-up after discharge. Appropriate referrals meet the patient's needs better.

KEY POINTS

- Health education is aimed at the promotion, restoration, and maintenance of health.
- Teaching is most effective when it is responsive to a learner's needs and requires the learner's active involvement.
- Teaching is a form of interpersonal communication, with teacher and student actively involved in a process that increases the student's knowledge and skills.
- Teaching a patient a specific behavior involves incorporation of behaviors from all three learning domains.
- A person's health beliefs influence the willingness to gain the knowledge and skills necessary to maintain health.
- Patients of different age-groups require different teaching strategies because of developmental capabilities.
- Presentation of teaching content progresses from simple to more complex ideas.
- Assess the reading ability and the ability of the patient to understand health information before providing patient education.
- Patient teaching is culturally sensitive and individualized to meet the needs of each patient.
- A patient is an active participant in a teaching plan, agreeing to the plan, helping to choose instructional methods, and recommending times for instruction.
- A combination of teaching methods improves a learner's attentiveness and involvement.
- Match teaching methodologies to a patient's learning needs.
- Learning objectives describe what a person is to learn in behavioral terms.
- Evaluate a patient's learning by using the teach-back method and observing the performance of expected learning behaviors under desired conditions.

REFLECTIVE LEARNING

- Reflect on a recent experience you had teaching a patient in clinical. What topic did you teach? What teaching method did you use? Evaluate what went well and what could be improved in the future.
- Find a patient education resource online, such as medication information, and evaluate it. Is it written in a way that patients can understand? Is it organized logically? Is the font used easy to read? What would you change to improve it?
- Locate an application on your smartphone or tablet that a patient may download to help promote management of a chronic illness such as hypertension or diabetes. Evaluate the application in terms of usefulness. Is it easy to use? How can a patient use the application to improve his or her health? What do you think are the pitfalls and benefits of encouraging patients to use health technology such as this application?

REVIEW QUESTIONS

1. Which scenario best describes the first step in the teaching process? (Select all that apply.)
   1. A nurse asks a new mother what she understands about her home care of her cesarean-section incision including activity restrictions and incision care.
   2. A nurse gives a patient who had a stroke a magnet that lists the warning signs of a stroke.
   3. A nurse provides education regarding a new blood pressure medication to a patient before discharge.
   4. A nurse gathers information regarding the home and school life of a 10-year-old patient who recently had an appendectomy.
   5. After a patient reads an informational pamphlet, the nurse has the patient explain the correct way to take a newly ordered diabetes medication.

2. A 3-year-old child is diagnosed with type 1 diabetes. The provider starts the patient on injections of insulin at her endocrinology appointment. How does the nurse best explain the injection to the child?
   1. The nurse speaks only to the parents because a 3-year-old child cannot comprehend what is being said regarding medication.
   2. The nurse verbally reviews information with both the patient and the parents.
   3. The nurse uses a doll to show the child how the injection works.
   4. The nurse demonstrates the injection on the child.

3. Which scenario best demonstrates that learning has taken place? (Select all that apply.)
   1. A nurse reviews the warning symptoms of a stroke.
   2. A patient describes how to set up her pill organizer for the week.
   3. A patient attends a spinal cord injury support group.
   4. A nurse gives a patient written information regarding a new medication.
   5. A patient demonstrates how to take his blood pressure at home using his home machine.

4. A nurse is preparing to teach a patient about sleep apnea. Which action is most appropriate for the nurse to perform first?
   1. Show the patient how the CPAP machine works
   2. Assess what the patient already knows about sleep apnea
   3. Evaluate the outcomes of the education session
   4. Set mutual goals for the education session

5. A nurse is teaching an older-adult patient about poststroke seizures. Which teaching technique is most appropriate to use?
   1. A pamphlet with large font in green ink
   2. Speaking in a high-pitched voice
   3. Short sessions during which the nurse provides the most important information at the beginning and end of the education session
   4. An hour-long lecture including symptoms of a seizure, safety during a seizure, types of seizures, and information regarding medications used to treat seizures

evolve

Additional Review Questions, as well as rationales for all Review Questions, can be found on the Evolve website.

1. 1, 4; 2. 3; 3. 3, 5; 4. 2; 5. 3.

REFERENCES

Agency for Healthcare Research and Quality (AHRQ): *Health literacy universal precautions toolkit*, ed 2, 2015. https://www.ahrq.gov/professionals/quality-patient-safety/quality-resources/tools/literacy-toolkit/healthlittoolkit2-tool5.html.

American Hospital Association (AHA): *The patient care partnership*, 2006. http://www.aha.org/content/00-10/pcp_english_030730.pdf.

American Nurses Association (ANA): *Code of ethics for nurses with interpretive statements*, 2015. http://nursingworld.org/DocumentVault/Ethics-1/Code-of-Ethics-for-Nurses.html.

Ball JW, et al: *Seidel's guide to physical examination*, ed 8, St Louis, 2015, Elsevier.

Bandura A: *Self-efficacy: the exercise of control*, New York, 1997, WH Freeman.

Bastable S: *Nurse as educator: principles of teaching and learning for nursing practice*, ed 4, Sudbury, MA, 2014, Jones & Bartlett.

Brice JH, et al: Single-item or two-item literacy screener to predict the S-TOFHLA among adult hemodialysis patients, *Patient Educ Couns* 94(1):71, 2014.

Caplin M, Saunders T: Utilizing Teach-Back to reinforce patient education: a step-by-step approach, *Orthop Nurs* 34(6):365, 2015.

Centers for Disease Control and Prevention (CDC): *Build your quit plan*, 2017a. http://www.cdc.gov/tobacco/campaign/tips/quit-smoking/guide/quit-plan.html.

Centers for Disease Control and Prevention (CDC): *Health care professionals: help your patients quit smoking*, 2017b. https://www.cdc.gov/tobacco/campaign/tips/partners/health/hcp/index.html.

Choi PP: Patient advocacy: the role of the nurse, *Nurs Stand* 29(41):52, 2015.

Dastoom M, et al: The effects of group education with the Teach-Back Method on hospital readmission rates of heart failure patients, *Jundishapur J Chronic Dis Care* 5(1):e30377, 2016.

Driessnack M, et al: Using the "Newest Vital Sign" to assess health literacy in children, *J Pediatr Health Care* 28(2):165, 2014.

Edelman CL, Mandle CL: *Health promotion throughout the life span*, ed 7, St Louis, 2014, Mosby.

Gomes C, Coustasse A: Tweeting and treating: how hospitals use twitter to improve care, *Health Care Manag (Frederick)* 34(3):203, 2015.

Hasanovic M, Pajevic I: Religious moral beliefs inversely related to trauma experiences severity and presented posttraumatic stress disorder among Bosnia and Herzegovina war veterans, *J Relig Health* 54(4):1403, 2015.

Heaney JL, et al: Physical activity, life events stress, cortisol, and DHEA: preliminary findings that physical activity may buffer against the negative effects of stress, *J Aging Phys Act* 22(4):465, 2014.

Kompany L, et al: Children's Specialized Hospital and GetWellNetwork collaborate to improve patient education and outcomes using an innovative approach, *Pediatr Nurs* 42(2):95, 2016.

Miller MA, Stoeckel PR: *Client education: theory and practice*, Sudbury, MA, 2016, Jones & Bartlett.

Mott-Coles S: Patients' cultural beliefs in patient-provider communication with African American women and Latinas diagnosed with breast cancer, *Clin J Oncol Nurs* 18(4):443, 2014.

National Institutes of Health (NIH): *Health literacy*, 2017. https://www.nih.gov/institutes-nih/nih-office-director/office-communications-public-liaison/clear-communication/health-literacy.

Panagioti M, et al: Self-management support interventions to reduce health care utilization without compromising outcomes: a systematic review and meta-analysis, *BMC Health Serv Res* 14(1):356, 2014.

Purnell LD: *Guide to culturally competent health care*, Philadelphia, 2014, FA Davis.

Sabic D, et al: Bosnian refugees: screening and treatment in an immigrant population, *J Am Osteopath Assoc* 114:617, 2014.

Sawyer T, et al: Implementing electronic tablet-based education of acute care patients, *Crit Care Nurse* 36(1):60, 2016.

Schuck K, et al: Predictors of cessation treatment outcome and treatment moderators among smoking parents receiving quitline counselling or self-help material, *Prev Med* 69:126, 2014.

Stribling JC, Richardson JE: Placing wireless tablets in clinical settings for patient education, *J Med Libr Assoc* 104(2):159, 2016.

The Joint Commission (TJC): *Speak up initiatives*, 2017. http://www.jointcommission.org/speakup.aspx.

Toronto CE, Weatherford B: Registered nurses' experiences with individuals with low health literacy: a qualitative descriptive study, *J Nurses Prof Dev* 32(1):8, 2016.

Touhy TA, Jett K: *Ebersole and Hess' toward healthy aging: human needs and nursing response*, ed 9, St Louis, 2016, Mosby.

U.S. Department of Health and Human Services (USDHHS): *Quick guide to health literacy*, n.d. https://health.gov/communication/literacy/quickguide/quickguide.pdf.

U.S. Department of Health and Human Services (USDHHS): *HealthyPeople 2020*, 2017a. http://www.healthypeople.gov/2020/default.aspx.

U.S. Department of Health and Human Services (USDHHS): *Using nicotine replacement therapy*, 2017b. https://smokefree.gov/tools-tips/medications-can-help-you-quit/using-nicotine-replacement-therapy.

Vesterlund M, et al: Tailoring your heart failure project for success in rural areas, *Qual Manag Health Care* 24(2):91, 2015.

Managing Patient Care

evolve MEDIA RESOURCES

http://evolve.elsevier.com/Potter/essentials

- Audio Glossary
- QSEN Activity and Review Questions Answers and Rationales

OBJECTIVES

- Differentiate among the types of nursing care delivery models.
- Describe the elements of decentralized decision making.
- Discuss the ways in which a nurse manager supports staff involvement in a decentralized decision-making model.
- Discuss ways to apply clinical care coordination skills in nursing practice.
- Describe strategies to work effectively as a member of an interprofessional health care team.
- Discuss principles to follow in the appropriate delegation of patient care activities.

KEY TERMS

accountability, p. 225
authority, p. 224
autonomy, p. 224
case management, p. 223
decentralized management, p. 224

delegation, p. 230
patient- and family-centered care, p. 223
primary nursing, p. 223
responsibility, p. 224

team nursing, p. 223
total patient care, p. 223
transformational leadership, p. 222

CASE STUDY *Jennifer*

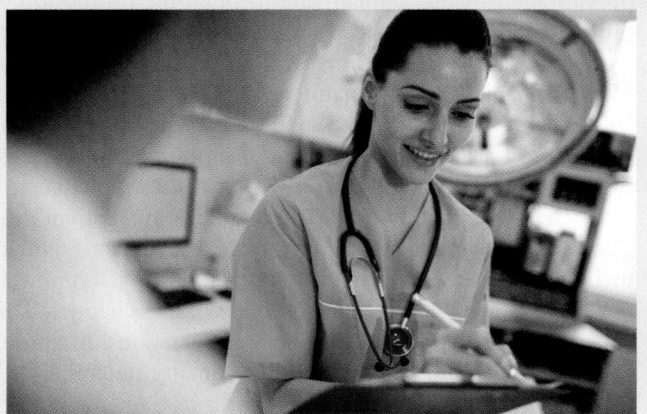

Copyright © wavebreakmedia/iStock/Thinkstock.

Jennifer is a nursing student assigned to care for three patients today. Mrs. Sinclair, her first patient, will have surgery at 1 p.m. to repair her fractured right hip. It is the first time she has had surgery. It is now 11:30 a.m. The operating room (OR) notified Jennifer that OR staff will pick up Mrs. Sinclair in 30 minutes. Jennifer enters Mrs. Sinclair's room to complete the preoperative checklist and make final preparations for surgery. She finds Mrs. Sinclair moving about restlessly in bed and reluctant to talk. At the same time the nurse call system at the bedside comes on, and the unit clerk notifies Jennifer that her second patient, Mr. Timmons, finished his lunch and is ready for his pain medication so he can ambulate down the hall. Mr. Timmons had abdominal surgery 2 days ago for removal of a colon tumor. Her third patient, Mr. Dodson, has a postoperative wound infection. He is due for his next dose of antibiotic medication and needs his dressing changed.

As a nursing student, it is important for you to gain the necessary knowledge, skills, and attitudes that ultimately allow you to practice as an entry-level nurse. The National Council of State Boards of Nursing (NCSBN) (2016a) develops licensure examinations for RNs, licensed practical nurses (LPNs), and licensed vocational nurses (LVNs) to ensure entry-level nurses can safely practice nursing. Despite variation in Nurse Practice Acts and professional nursing standards, you will be expected to have certain knowledge, skills, and attitudes when you enter the nursing profession (Box 13.1). Regardless of where you practice or the type of nursing you practice, you implement professional standards of care, use health care resources appropriately, and collaborate with the health care team. Delivering nursing care within the health care system is challenging because of high patient acuity; the complex nature of health care; and the changes that influence health professionals, patients, and health care organizations (see Chapter 3). As you develop the knowledge, skills, and attitudes to become a nurse, you learn what it takes to effectively manage the care of multiple patients and to take the initiative as a leader among your professional colleagues.

BOX 13.1 EXPECTED ENTRY-LEVEL NURSE KNOWLEDGE, SKILLS, AND ATTITUDES

- Value placing the patient at the center of care.
- Respect patients' rights, beliefs, culture, spirituality, preferences, values, and needs.
- Be a patient advocate.
- Understand the health care system and processes to promote safety, reduce harm, and enhance efficiency and effectiveness.
- Manage care of patients.
- Think critically using the nursing process.
- Use data to monitor outcomes, assess problems, identify and implement solutions, evaluate care, and follow up appropriately.
- Communicate effectively with patients and health care team members, and document events and activities surrounding patient care appropriately in written and/or electronic records.
- Use evidence-based practices when providing patient care.
- Promote change in behavior when needed using appropriate teaching and learning strategies.
- Demonstrate nursing knowledge and display confidence in knowledge base.
- Work effectively in nursing and interprofessional teams, recognizing the contributions of all team members, encouraging open communication, and fostering shared decision making.
- Recognize own limitations and seek help as needed.

Modified from NCSBN: *NCLEX-RN® examination test plan for the National Council Licensure Examination for Registered Nurses,* 2015. https://www.ncsbn.org/RN_Test_Plan_2016_Final.pdf; QSEN Institute: *Pre-licensure KSAS,* 2014. http://qsen.org/competencies/pre-licensure-ksas/.

BUILDING A NURSING TEAM

Nurses want to work in a setting that has positive leaders, provides access to resources that help them accomplish their work, and supports healthy relationships between colleagues (Read and Laschinger, 2015). Your education and commitment to practice within established standards help you work as a member of a cohesive and strong nursing team that values mentoring, integrity, and respect for teamwork. An empowering work environment brings out the best in nurses. It concentrates on effective patient care systems (e.g., patient assessment, referral mechanisms, and collaboration among nurses and health care providers), supports risk taking and innovation, focuses on results and rewards, and offers professional opportunities for growth and advancement. Effective team development requires team building and training, trust, communication, and a workplace that facilitates collaboration (Huber, 2014).

Nurse managers play a critical role in developing successful teams that work together (LeBlanc, 2014). Nurse managers who use transformational leadership focus on creating work environments that allow individuals to work to their highest potential and bring positive change to the work environment through their use of reflection, intellectual stimulation, and using the best evidence to guide their decisions (Roberts-Turner et al., 2014). Transformational leaders hold their staff accountable and influence their staff by acting as a positive role model. The *TEEAMS* approach is one way a nurse manager can implement transformational leadership. In this approach a manager spends *time* with the staff; *empowers* the staff; is *enthusiastic* about enhancing the team; *appreciates* team members for a job well done; *manages* the team, holding members accountable; and *supports* the team in their stressful environment (LeBlanc, 2014). A transformational leadership approach improves nurse job satisfaction; enhances teamwork, collaboration, and communication; and reduces errors thus promoting patient safety (Lievens and Vlerick, 2014; Roberts-Turner et al., 2014; Buck and Doucette, 2015).

Another way leaders create an empowering work environment is through the Magnet Recognition Program. The Magnet Recognition Program recognizes organizations that provide high-quality patient care through the promotion of professional nursing practice and innovations in nursing care (American Nurses Credentialing Center [ANCC], 2017). A Magnet hospital has a dynamic and positive organizational culture. Magnet hospitals have transformational nursing leaders; foster interprofessional collaboration and professional practice; and integrate evidence-based practice and research into policies, procedures, processes, and patient care. The nurses have autonomy over their practice and control their practice environment. A Magnet hospital empowers the nursing team to be innovative and make changes. This culture produces a strong collaborative relationship among team members and improves patient quality outcomes (see Chapter 3).

The Institute of Medicine (IOM) (2004) (now the National Academy of Medicine) challenged health care environments to shift their focus to patient safety. Because nurses are experts in patient assessment and evaluation and spend a great deal of time in direct patient contact, they are key team members to help transform the health care environment. As a part of this transformation, all health care professionals need to be educated to deliver patient-centered care using evidence-based practice, quality improvement approaches, and informatics (IOM, 2001). Nurses need to deliver safe, effective quality patient care through collaboration as a member of an interdisciplinary team (IOM, 2011).

It takes an excellent nurse manager and nursing staff to create and maintain an enriching work culture and environment. Together a manager and the nursing staff share a philosophy of care for their unit. A philosophy of care incorporates the values and concerns of the professional nursing staff and guides the way they view and care for patients. For example, a philosophy addresses the purpose of the nursing unit, how staff will work with patients and families, and the standards of care for the work unit. It is a vision for how to practice nursing. Integral to the philosophy of care is the selection of a nursing care delivery model and management structure that supports professional nursing practice.

NURSING CARE DELIVERY MODELS

A nursing care delivery model allows you to help your patients achieve desirable outcomes and satisfaction with care (Huber, 2014). Since Florence Nightingale, nurses have used a variety of nursing care delivery models to provide care. Nursing care delivery models contain the common components of nurse-patient relationship, clinical decision making, patient assignments and work allocation, interprofessional communication, and management of the environment of care (Huber, 2014). Classic nursing care models sometimes used today include team nursing and primary nursing. Newer models usually used today include patient- and family-centered care, total patient care, and case management.

Team nursing provides care through a group of people led by a nurse. Members of the group collaborate to provide care as planned by the team leader. Communication in this model is hierarchical (e.g., charge nurse to team leader and team leader to team members). Variations of team nursing include modular nursing and pod nursing (Huber, 2014). In this delivery care model nurses and other care providers on the unit are grouped together to provide care in one geographical area or "pod" of the patient care unit. Nurses often work together as partners, fostering teamwork (Friese et al., 2014). This model works well when the team leader has effective leadership skills (Huber, 2014).

In **primary nursing** one RN assumes the responsibility for a caseload of patients. The same nurse provides care for the same patients during their stay in a health care agency or while receiving nursing care, and other nurses cannot change the care plan without discussing it with the primary nurse. In the hospital, this model puts the RN at the bedside and promotes collaboration among health care team members. However, primary nursing is not always cost-effective in acute

care settings; thus it is typically used today in home care or community and public health (Huber, 2014).

Patient- and family-centered care promotes mutual partnerships among the patient, family, and health care team. The patient or family is at the center of the model (QSEN Institute, 2014). Four concepts are included in the patient- and family-centered care model (Institute for Patient- and Family-Centered Care [IPFCC], n.d.): (1) *dignity and respect* to ensure patient and family choices are respected and care is provided based on knowledge, beliefs, values, and cultural preferences of the patient and family; (2) *information sharing,* which ensures health care providers communicate and share information to allow patients and families to effectively participate in their care and have input into decision making; (3) *participation,* which encourages and supports patients and families to participate in their care in making decisions; and (4) *collaboration,* which ensures health care leaders collaborate with patients and families when developing, implementing, and evaluating policies and programs (IPFCC, n.d.). When using this model, nurses include patients and families in hand-off reports and in interprofessional rounds (see Chapter 3) (IPFCC, n.d.; Stelson et al., 2016).

Total patient care was the original care delivery model developed during Florence Nightingale's time. Nurses in this model provide all aspects of care for assigned patients. Because there is one nurse who provides all the care to a small number of patients, patients usually receive comprehensive, consistent, and holistic care. Patient satisfaction is usually high with this model. However, because many RNs are needed to staff a unit that uses this model, it is not usually cost-effective on general patient care units (Huber, 2014). Thus today total patient care is usually used only in critical care areas where nurses deliver total care to one or two patients (Yoder-Wise, 2015).

Case management emerged in the 1980s because health care organizations needed to provide complex cost-effective care. Case management requires collaboration in meeting the health needs of a patient and family. The process includes assessment, planning, facilitation, care coordination, evaluation, and advocacy (Case Management Society of America, 2016). Case managers coordinate and link health care services to patients and their families with the goal of promoting quality cost-effective outcomes (see Chapter 3). Clinicians, either as individuals or as part of a team, oversee the management of patients with specific case types (e.g., patients with complex nursing and medical problems such as diabetes or brain injury) across levels of care, focusing on length of stay and improving clinical outcomes (Lannin et al., 2014). Case managers are usually held accountable for cost management and quality standards. In the hospital, a case manager coordinates a patient's acute care and follows the patient after discharge home. For example, a case manager gathers a patient, family, social services, dietitian, and physical therapist together to plan the discharge of a patient following a stroke. Case managers do not provide direct care. Instead they collaborate with and supervise the care that other staff members deliver. Additionally, they actively coordinate patient discharge planning. Many organizations use critical pathways, which are multidisciplinary treatment plans, in a case-management delivery system to improve patient and institutional outcomes (Yoder-Wise, 2015). Advantages of case management include cost-effectiveness, focus on patients' complex health needs, efficiency in discharge planning, and multidisciplinary collaboration (Yoder-Wise, 2015).

DECISION MAKING

Effective decision making is critical for an effective manager and leader (Huber, 2014). A nursing manager directs and supports staff in applying an organization's nursing philosophy. A nurse executive supports managers by creating a nursing governance structure along with policies and procedures to help achieve organizational goals. It takes a committed nurse executive, an excellent manager, and empowered nursing staff to create an enriching work environment.

Decentralized management allows decisions to be made at the staff level. Shared governance is the typical decentralized structure used within health care organizations today (Huber, 2014). Health care organizations achieve more when they actively involve employees at all levels. Advantages of decentralization include increased morale and improved interpersonal relationships among staff. Staff members feel more important and are willing to become involved in the identity and successes of the health care organization.

Decentralization also promotes creativity in problem solving (Brunges and Foley-Brinza, 2014). As a result, it is critical for nurse managers to create and lead effective nursing units or groups. Nursing managers assume diverse responsibilities (Box 13.2). To make shared governance work, managers move decision making toward the staff level. On a nursing unit, it is important for all staff members (RNs, LPNs, and LVNs), nursing assistive personnel (NAP), and unit secretaries to feel involved, particularly with issues affecting their ability to care for patients and the quality of care provided. Decision making includes responsibility, authority, autonomy, and accountability (Yoder-Wise, 2015).

Responsibility refers to the duties or tasks that you are required or expected to do. As a professional nurse, a position description outlines your responsibilities in patient care and your expected level of participation as a member of a nursing unit. Responsibility reflects ownership and obligation; the individual who oversees the employee gives responsibility, and the employee accepts it. For example, a staff nurse is responsible for assessing all assigned patients, developing a plan of care that addresses each of a patient's nursing diagnoses, and implementing care strategies. The nurse is also responsible for involving a patient and family in care and for making sure that other staff members know what care they are responsible for performing. As the staff delivers the plan of care, the nurse is responsible for evaluating if the plan is successful and what to do when it is not successful. This responsibility becomes a nurse's work ethic in delivering excellent patient care.

BOX 13.2 RESPONSIBILITIES OF THE NURSE MANAGER

- Help staff establish annual goals for the unit and the systems needed to accomplish goals.
- Monitor professional nursing standards of practice on the unit.
- Develop an ongoing staff development plan, including one for new employees.
- Recruit new employees (interview and hire).
- Conduct routine staff evaluations.
- Establish self as a role model for positive customer service (customers include patients, families, and other health care team members).
- Serve as an advocate for the nursing staff to the administration of the organization.
- Submit staffing schedules for the unit.
- Conduct regular patient rounds and help to solve patient or family complaints.
- Establish and implement a quality improvement (QI) plan for the unit.
- Review and recommend new equipment needs for the unit.
- Conduct regular staff meetings.
- Conduct rounds with health care provider.
- Establish and support necessary staff and interdisciplinary committees.

Autonomy is freedom of choice and responsibility for those choices. Autonomy, consistent with the scope of professional nursing practice, maximizes your effectiveness as a nurse (Yoder-Wise, 2015). As a professional nurse, you make independent decisions about patient care, plan patient care within the scope of professional nursing practice, implement nursing interventions, and provide patient and family caregiver education without physician permission (Weiland, 2015). Autonomy also refers to your workplace. As a nurse, you have the ability to make independent decisions about the work of your unit such as scheduling or unit governance. Autonomy is not an absolute but occurs in degrees. For example, you have the autonomy to develop a discharge teaching plan based on specific patient needs for your patients and family caregivers. However, your unit does not use self-scheduling; as a result, you do not have the autonomy to create your own work schedule.

Authority refers to the official power to act. It provides a nurse power to make final decisions and give instructions related to the decisions (Yoder-Wise, 2015). By using authority in bringing a nursing team together, a nurse determines if collaboration was successful, if continuity in teaching occurred, and if a patient and family understood the information. For example, you discover that members of the nursing team did not follow through on a discharge teaching plan for an assigned patient. You have the authority to consult your team members to learn why they did not follow recommendations on the plan of care and to choose appropriate teaching strategies for the patient that all members of the team will follow.

Accountability refers to individuals being responsible for their actions. It involves follow-up and a reflective analysis of decisions and an evaluation of their effectiveness. As a nurse, this means you will take responsibility to provide excellent patient care by following standards of practice and your institution's policies and procedures. You assume responsibility for the outcomes, actions, judgments, and omissions when providing that care (Krautscheid, 2014). You are not accountable for overall outcomes of patient care, but you are accountable for your actions. You will sometimes delegate responsibility, but you remain accountable for your patients' outcomes (Yoder-Wise, 2015).

A successful decentralized nursing unit exercises responsibility, autonomy, authority, and accountability on an ongoing basis. An effective manager sets expectations for the staff to make decisions. Staff members need to feel comfortable in expressing differences of opinion and challenging ways in which the team functions. They do this while recognizing their own responsibility, autonomy, authority, and accountability. Ultimately shared governance allows a nursing unit to achieve its vision of professional nursing care.

Staff Involvement

When transformational leadership and decentralized decision making exist on a nursing unit, all staff members actively participate in unit activities. Because the work environment promotes participation, all staff members benefit from the knowledge and skills of the entire work group. Better patient- and family-centered care results when staff members value the knowledge and contributions of colleagues. A nursing manager supports staff involvement in a variety of ways:

1. *Establishment of nursing practice or problem-solving committees:* Staff committees establish and maintain professional nursing practice on a unit. Practice committees review and revise standards of care, develop policies and procedures, and resolve patient satisfaction issues. These activities ensure the delivery of quality patient- and family-centered care on the unit. A senior staff member usually chairs a committee. Managers are not always members of the committee, but they receive regular reports of committee progress. The nature of work on the nursing unit determines committee membership. Sometimes members of other disciplines (e.g., pharmacy, respiratory therapy, or clinical nutrition) participate on practice committees.

2. *Interprofessional collaboration among nurses and health care providers:* Interprofessional collaboration among nurses and health care providers is critical to the delivery of quality, safe patient care and creation of a positive work culture for practitioners (Glymph et al., 2015; Interprofessional Education Collaborative [IPEC], 2016). Interprofessional collaboration involves bringing representatives of various disciplines together to work with patients and families to deliver quality care (Fig. 13.1) (IPEC, 2016). Interprofessional team members bring different points of view and knowledge when identifying, clarifying, and

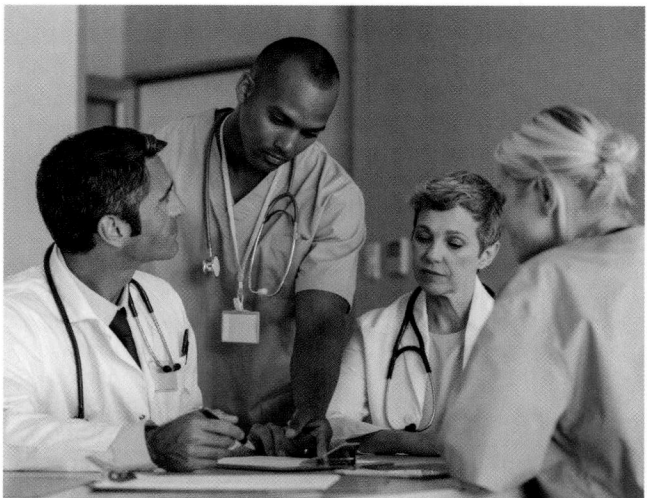

FIG 13.1 Interdisciplinary team collaborating on practice issues. (Copyright © Ridofranz/iStock/Thinkstock.)

solving complex patient problems. A nurse plays a key role within the team, helping coordinate patient care and facilitating communication among the team members (QSEN Institute, 2014). Open communication, cooperation, trust, mutual respect, and understanding of team members' roles and responsibilities are critical for successful interprofessional collaboration (Kear and Ulrich, 2015; IPEC, 2016). Education and team training of health care practitioners builds effective teams and improves interprofessional collaboration. IPEC (2016) identified four competencies needed by health care practitioners to be effective team members in interprofessional collaboration. The development of these competencies comes through interprofessional education (Box 13.3). Competencies needed for effective interprofessional collaboration include:

a. *Values/ethics for interprofessional practice:* Work with individuals of other professions to maintain a climate of mutual respect and shared values.

b. *Roles/responsibilities:* Use the knowledge of one's own role and roles of other professions to appropriately assess and address the health care needs of patients and to promote and advance the health of populations.

c. *Interprofessional communication:* Communicate with patients, families, communities, and professionals in health and other fields in a responsive and responsible manner that supports a team approach to the promotion and maintenance of health and prevention and treatment of disease.

d. *Teams and teamwork:* Apply relationship-building values and the principles of team dynamics to perform effectively in different team roles to plan, deliver, and evaluate patient-/population-centered care and population health programs and policies that are safe, timely, efficient, effective, and equitable.

3. *Interprofessional rounding:* Many health care organizations use interprofessional rounding to improve patient care coordination and communication among the health

BOX 13.3 EVIDENCE-BASED PRACTICE

PICO Question: Do active learning strategies that include interprofessional education improve interprofessional collaboration knowledge, skills, and attitudes in health care professionals compared with traditional learning activities?

SUMMARY OF EVIDENCE

A key component of delivering high-quality, safe patient care is interprofessional collaboration (IPC) (Sweigart et al., 2016). Effective communication is a critical aspect of IPC. Active learning strategies, such as role-playing and simulation, enhance learning because they engage learners in their own learning, simulate real-life situations, and provide a safe learning environment (Rossler and Kimble, 2016). Research shows that interprofessional education simulation activities in both live and virtual simulations are effective in improving the perceived need for collaboration, competency, and autonomy (Fung et al., 2015; Sweigart et al., 2016). For example, nursing students participating in simulation activities with medical students indicated that participating in interprofessional simulation activities improved communication skills by providing opportunities to practice speaking to physicians, patients, and families (Turrentine et al., 2016). Debriefing sessions after simulations offer another strategy to learn IPC (Fung et al., 2015). Students enrolled in a virtual Team-STEPPS course demonstrated slight improvement in teamwork attitudes related to team structure and significant improvements in teamwork attitudes related to leadership, situation monitoring, mutual support, and communication (Sweigart et al., 2016).

APPLICATION TO NURSING PRACTICE

- Participate in active learning experiences that include interdisciplinary health care students and/or professionals and focus on teamwork to enhance your ability to work as a team (Fung et al., 2015; Rossler and Kimble, 2016; Sweigart et al., 2016).
- Understand the roles of other interprofessional team members to improve your effectiveness as a member of the IPC team (Rossler and Kimble, 2016; Turrentine et al., 2016).
- Actively participate in interprofessional learning opportunities to enhance your knowledge, skills, and attitudes related to teamwork and collaboration such as problem solving, conflict resolution, communication, and shared decision making (Sweigart et al., 2016; Turrentine et al., 2016).
- Educators need to continue to develop instruments to measure knowledge, skills, and attitudes surrounding interprofessional education and practice to better understand the effectiveness of these active learning strategies (Reising et al., 2015).

QSEN QSEN ACTIVITY *Teamwork and Collaboration*

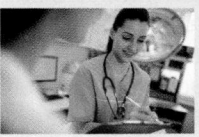

Copyright © wavebreakmedia/ iStock/Thinkstock.

Jennifer participates in the interprofessional rounding session that occurred in Mrs. Sinclair's room on the morning of her discharge. In addition to Jennifer, the team included Mrs. Sinclair, her family, physician, physical therapist, and nurse. During the rounds the team recognized the expertise of the various disciplines, listened to every team member, and treated each member with respect.

- Describe the behaviors displayed by the team that promoted effective teamwork.
- Why was it important for Mrs. Sinclair and her family to be involved in the rounds?

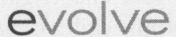 Answers to QSEN Activities can be found in the Evolve Media Resources.

care team. During rounding members of the health care team share important patient information, answer questions asked by other team members, discuss patients' clinical progress, plan for discharge, discuss family caregiver needs, and focus all team members on the same patient and family caregiver goals (Nichols et al., 2015). Interprofessional rounding has also helped decrease medical errors and improve quality of care (Glymph et al., 2015; Wilder et al., 2016). For interprofessional rounding to be successful, health care team members need to be flexible, trust each other, and treat each other with respect.

4. *Staff communication:* In the present health care environment, it is difficult for a manager to send a clear, accurate, and timely message to all members of a nursing staff. Lack of communication about planned changes on a unit often leads to mistrust among staff members. Effective managers do not assume total responsibility for all communication. Instead they use a variety of approaches to ensure quick and accurate communication of information to all staff members. For example, a manager distributes biweekly newsletters of current unit or health care agency activities and posts minutes of staff and practice committee meetings in a convenient location for all staff members to read. Managers hold staff meetings when they need to discuss important issues affecting the unit or the health care agency. When a change within a unit is needed, a manager will often assign each member of a committee or task force working on the change the responsibility to communicate directly to specific staff members. This ensures all staff members understand the need to change and have the opportunity to voice their concerns and offer their ideas.

5. *Staff education:* It is impossible to remain knowledgeable about current medical and nursing practice trends without ongoing education. The nurse manager is responsible to give staff members the necessary opportunities to remain competent in their practice. This involves planning in-service training sessions, sending staff members to professional conferences, and having staff members present case studies or practice issues during staff meetings.

LEADERSHIP SKILLS FOR NURSING STUDENTS

As you begin your clinical assignments, it is important to learn how to care for patients and become a responsible and productive team member. Start by always being responsible and accountable for the care you provide. Become a leader by making good clinical decisions and learning from your mistakes. Seek help, collaborate closely with professional nurses, and strive to improve your performance during each patient interaction. Use the knowledge, skills, and attitudes presented in the following paragraphs to become a competent professional. You need to think critically and solve problems in the clinical setting. Thinking critically allows you to provide higher quality care, meet the individual needs of patients and their family caregivers, consider alternatives to problems, understand the rationale for performing nursing interventions, and evaluate the effectiveness of care. Clinical experiences help you develop and expand your critical thinking skills (Benner et al., 2010, 2011).

Clinical Care Coordination

As you progress through your nursing courses, you will gain the knowledge and skills necessary to deliver patient care competently and in a timely and effective manner. In the beginning you will probably care for only one patient, but eventually you will be able to care for groups of patients. Clinical care coordination allows you to safely and effectively care for multiple patients at one time. To coordinate the care of multiple patients, you need to learn how to make clinical decisions, set priorities, gain organizational skills, use resources, manage time, and evaluate the outcomes of your care. This requires critical reflection, critical reasoning, and clinical judgment (Benner et al., 2010). These are important steps in developing caring relationships with your patients and their family caregivers. Use a critical thinking approach by applying your knowledge and previous experiences into your clinical decision-making process (see Chapter 8).

Clinical Decisions. When you begin caring for a patient, always conduct a focused but complete assessment of your patient's condition and ask what outcomes the patient expects to achieve. This information allows you to know your patient, understand your patient's situation, and recognize your patient's responses during care. Assessment data also help you make accurate clinical decisions about your patient's needs (see Chapter 8). Making clinical decisions requires you to be thorough. Failing to make accurate clinical judgments often results in undesirable patient outcomes (Shelestak et al., 2015).

To become better at making clinical decisions, build relationships with the staff in every clinical experience. Display a positive attitude and seize every learning opportunity. Your attitude is very important in gaining the best learning and clinical experiences (Hooper et al., 2016). Always attend to a patient, listen to what the patient is telling you, look for any cues (obvious or subtle) that point to a pattern of findings, and direct your assessment to explore the pattern further. Accurate clinical decision making keeps you focused on the proper course of action, especially when a patient's condition changes. Never hesitate to ask for help to verify your assessment findings or modify a patient's plan of care when your assessment findings reveal a change in your patient's clinical condition.

Organizational Skills. Implementing a plan of care requires you to be effective and efficient. Effective use of time means doing the right things, whereas efficient use of time means doing things right. Effective use of time helps you prepare and organize your care. Efficient use of time conserves effort and minimizes interruptions. One way to be efficient is by combining various nursing activities (i.e., doing more than one thing at a time). As you address your patient's priorities, certain organizational skills ensure that you become more efficient. This takes practice. For example, during medication administration or while obtaining a specimen, combine therapeutic communication skills, patient teaching, and assessment and evaluation. Try to establish and strengthen relationships with patients and use any patient contact as an opportunity to teach or give important information. Always assess a patient's behaviors and responses to therapies to determine if any new problems are developing and to evaluate responses to interventions.

A nursing procedure is easier to perform if you are well organized. A well-organized nurse prepares by having all necessary equipment and supplies available. Prepare a patient by ensuring a patient is comfortable, positioned correctly for the procedure, and well informed to increase the likelihood that the procedure will go smoothly. Sometimes you need the assistance of colleagues to perform or complete a procedure (e.g., helping to turn a patient for an enema or handing supplies during a dressing change). Have the work area organized and preliminary steps completed before asking colleagues for help. Then clearly communicate to the colleague how to help.

You plan and deliver care based on established priorities. However, events that interfere with your plans sometimes occur. Your priorities at this time conflict with the priorities of other health care personnel. Always keep a patient's needs at the center of care. For example, just as you begin to give a patient a bath, the x-ray film technician enters the room to take a chest x-ray. Once the technician takes the x-ray, the phlebotomist comes to draw a sample of blood. The patient experienced symptoms earlier that required the x-ray and laboratory work. In this case completing the diagnostic tests is more important than the patient's bath. In another example a patient is waiting to visit family, and a routine chest x-ray was ordered. The patient's condition is stable, and the x-ray technician is willing to return later to take the x-ray. In this case, your priority is to complete the patient's bath quickly so the family is able to visit. The x-ray can be done later.

Priority Setting. As you begin to make clinical judgments (including nursing diagnoses), you begin to better understand all your patient's needs. Decide which patient needs or problems to address first while planning care (see Chapter 9). It is important to prioritize in all caregiving situations because it allows you to see relationships between patient problems and avoid delays in action (Hendry and Walker, 2004).

Priority setting is not the ordering of a list of patient care tasks, but rather a way to organize your care. You integrate tasks in your priority setting when you have multiple tasks to perform for either a single patient or a group of patients. According to Maslow's hierarchy of needs, you need to meet a patient's physiological needs such as oxygen, food, water, sleep, and elimination first. After meeting the physiological needs, meet a patient's higher-level needs of safety, security, belonging, esteem, and self-actualization.

Nurses prioritize care in different ways. To prioritize your care, evaluate and weigh each competing task or process by asking yourself the following questions (Hansten and Jackson, 2009):

- Is it life threatening or potentially life threatening if the task is not done? Will another patient be endangered if this task is done now or the task is left for later?
- Is this task or process essential to patient or staff safety?
- Is this task or process essential to the medical or nursing plan of care?

When prioritizing care, you need to understand the "big picture" of all your patient's problems and the patient's goals. Once you know all your patient's problems, determine the relationships between the problems. For example, if a patient is not able to walk because of pain from surgery, managing the patient's pain is a priority. Remember that setting priorities is a dynamic process that changes frequently (Alfaro-Lefevre, 2017). Always give high priority to patient and caregiver safety (e.g., fall and injury prevention, safe medication administration, prevention of skin problems, and patient education needs). Use the following steps to classify problems into one of three priority levels, and use this information to help you set priorities (Alfaro-Lefevre, 2017):

1. Assign high priority to first-level problems using *ABC+VL* (*a*irway, *b*reathing, *c*ardiac and circulation problems, *v*ital signs concerns, and life-threatening *l*aboratory values) and attend to these immediately.
2. Next address second-level problems, which are immediately after the first level and include concerns such as mental status changes, untreated medical issues, acute pain, acute elimination problems, abnormal laboratory results, and risks.
3. Then tend to third-level problems, which are health problems other than those at the first two levels, such as more long-term issues in health education, rest, and family coping.

Many patients have all three levels of problems, which requires you to make careful judgments in choosing your course of action. High-priority needs demand your immediate attention. When a patient has diverse priority needs, sometimes it helps to focus on basic needs first. For example, you have a patient in traction who states he is uncomfortable from being in the same position. The dietary assistant arrives in the room to deliver a meal tray. Instead of immediately helping the patient with the meal, you reposition the patient and offer basic hygiene measures. The patient will likely become more interested in eating and more open to your instructions after you make him feel comfortable.

Over time you will prioritize the needs of a group of patients. This requires you to know the priority needs of each patient within the group and assess each patient's needs as soon as possible while addressing high and intermediate needs in a timely manner. Rely on information from the change-of-shift or hand-off report, the patient acuity classification system, and information from each patient's medical record to identify which patients require assessment first. Over time you learn to spontaneously rank patients' needs by priority or urgency. Remember to think about available resources, recognize that priority needs change, and consider how to use your time wisely. The case study provides an example of how to prioritize patient care (Box 13.4).

You also set priorities based on patient expectations. Sometimes you establish an excellent plan of care, but if your patient resists certain therapies or disagrees with your approach, your care will not be safe or effective. Work closely with a patient and family caregiver to include them as you set priorities to establish trust and cooperation.

BOX 13.4   CASE STUDY: PRIORITY SETTING—JENNIFER

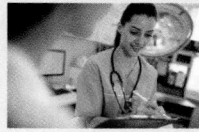

Copyright © wavebreakmedia/ iStock/Thinkstock.

In setting her priorities, Jennifer remembers the categories of priority needs that she learned in class and prioritizes her care according to these. Jennifer asks the unit clerk to send John, another nursing student, to Mr. Timmons' room to check on him and tell him that Jennifer is preparing a patient for surgery and will be with him as soon as she finishes. Jennifer stays with Mrs. Sinclair and begins an assessment to determine the cause of the restlessness. She also asks Mrs. Sinclair if she has any questions or concerns about surgery. Mrs. Sinclair voices her concerns about pain after surgery. Jennifer reinforces the earlier teaching that she did on patient-controlled analgesia pumps. This seems to relax Mrs. Sinclair. Jennifer completes her preoperative preparation and checklist. She tells Mrs. Sinclair that the operating room staff will be here in 15 minutes to get her. Jennifer then goes to assess Mr. Timmons' pain. She prepares and verifies Mr. Timmons' identification using two patient identifiers and administers the prescribed pain medication. Jennifer asks Tina, the nursing assistant, to help him with his walk. Jennifer gathers the supplies for the dressing change. On the way to the room she obtains and verifies the antibiotic for Mr. Dodson. In Mr. Dodson's room, she first verifies Mr. Dodson's identification using two patient identifiers and administers the antibiotic. After Mr. Dodson takes his antibiotic, Jennifer sets up and then completes the dressing change. She finishes caring for Mr. Dodson by documenting the care she performed.

Use of Resources. Appropriate use of resources is another important aspect of clinical care coordination. Resources include members of the health care team. In any setting patient care is more efficient and effective when staff members work together. Never hesitate to ask staff members to help you, especially when there is an opportunity to make a procedure or activity more comfortable and safer for a patient. For example, you will often need help when turning, positioning, and ambulating patients when your patients are immobile. Have a staff member hand equipment and supplies to you during a more complicated procedure such as a blood draw or a dressing change. Asking staff for assistance to make a procedure more efficient is an excellent way for you to learn how to delegate aspects of care activities and work with NAP. Finally, as a student, always look for opportunities to help other staff members. For example, answer the nurse call system, help a staff member make a bed, or offer to sit and talk with another nurse's patient.

In many instances, you recognize personal limitations and use professional resources. For example, while caring for a patient you discover unexpected assessment findings and are unfamiliar with the patient's underlying physical condition. You consult with an experienced RN who confirms your findings and helps you implement an appropriate plan of care. Throughout your professional career you will always have new experiences. A leader knows his or her limitations and seeks professional colleagues for guidance and support.

Time Management. Changes in health care, shorter length of stays, and increasing complexity of patients create stress for nurses as they work to meet patient needs (Huber, 2014). One way to manage this stress is through time-management skills. These skills involve learning how, where, and when to use your time. Managing yourself better leads to better management of your time and a reduced risk of developing burnout (see Chapter 26) (Moss and Good, 2016). Effective time management includes being prepared, being organized, and managing priorities (Mazerolle et al., 2015). Make efficient and effective use of your time by remaining goal oriented and focusing on your patients' priorities. For example, you prioritize care to help you determine which procedures you need to perform first and which patient assessments you will do on an ongoing basis.

One useful time-management skill involves making a to-do list. When you first begin working with a patient or group of patients, make a list of the nursing activities that you need to perform during your shift in the order you need to do them. The hand-off report at the change of shift helps you prioritize activities based on what you learn about your patients' conditions and the care provided before your arrival to the unit.

Consider activities that have specific time limits in terms of meeting patient needs such as administering a pain medication before a scheduled procedure or providing discharge instructions. Analyze the items on your list and identify those scheduled by agency policies or routines. Note which activities need to be done at a specific time and which you are able to do at your discretion. For instance, you need to administer medications within a specific schedule, but you can also perform other activities while you are in a patient's room. Finally, estimate the amount of time needed to complete the various activities. Activities requiring the assistance of other staff members usually take longer because they are more complicated and require you to plan around different staff schedules.

Effective time management also involves setting goals and developing a plan to help you complete one task before starting another. Complete activities with one patient before moving on to the next if possible. Your care is less fragmented, you can better focus on what you are doing for each patient, and you will be less likely to make errors. Other strategies to help you manage your time are keeping a time log to determine where time is currently spent, keeping your work area clean and free of clutter, delegating tasks as possible, and trying to decrease interruptions as you are completing tasks.

Evaluation. One of the most important aspects of clinical care coordination is evaluation (see Chapter 9). A competent nurse constantly evaluates a patient's condition and progress toward an expected patient outcome. Evaluation is an ongoing process. It does not occur only at the end of an activity. Once you assess a patient's needs and implement interventions for a patient's problem, immediately evaluate if the interventions were effective and the patient's response. The process of evaluation compares actual patient outcomes with expected outcomes. When expected outcomes are not met, evaluation reveals the need to continue your current plan for a longer period, revise approaches to care, or introduce new therapies. As you care for a patient, anticipate when you need to return to the bedside to evaluate your care. For example, you decide to return 30 minutes after you administer a pain medication, 15 minutes after an IV line began infusing, or 60 minutes after discussing discharge instructions with a patient and family caregiver.

Team Communication

As a part of an interprofessional health care team, each nurse is responsible for open and professional verbal and electronic communication. Structured communication techniques used by health care teams that improve communication include briefings or short discussions among team members, group rounds on patients, and use of SBAR (Situation-Background-Assessment-Recommendation) when sharing information (see Chapter 11) (Cornell et al., 2014; Clochesy et al., 2015). An enriching, professional environment is one in which staff members respect one another's ideas, share information, and keep one another informed. On a busy nursing unit, this means you keep the nurse in charge of the unit and colleagues informed about patients with emerging problems (Box 13.5). Open communication also promotes safe and effective patient care (Lancaster et al., 2015; Perry, 2016). Strategies to improve your communication with health care providers include addressing a health care provider by name, having the patient

BOX 13.5 SBAR AS COMMUNICATION TOOL

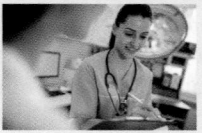

Copyright © wavebreakmedia/ iStock/Thinkstock.

Thirty minutes after Jennifer administered 1 tablet of oxycodone HCl 5 mg/ ibuprofen 400 mg PO to Mr. Timmons she evaluates its effect. Mr. Timmons rates his pain as an 8 on a scale of 0 to 10. Jennifer prepares an SBAR to contact the health care provider.

Situation: Mr. Timmons continues to rate his pain as an 8 on a pain scale of 0 to 10 30 minutes after receiving his pain medication.

Background: Mr. Timmons had abdominal surgery 2 days ago for removal of a colon tumor. He had his patient-controlled analgesia (PCA) pump with IV morphine removed 4 hours ago. He has 1 tablet of oxycodone HCl 5 mg/ ibuprofen 400 mg PO ordered every 6 hours. This is the first dose of the oral medication that was administered.

Assessment: One tablet of oxycodone HCl 5 mg/ibuprofen 400 mg PO is not sufficient to manage Mr. Timmons' pain on the second postoperative day. He does not want to walk with the level of pain he is experiencing.

Recommendation: Request a change of the pain medication order for Mr. Timmons.

chart available when discussing patient issues, focusing on the patient problem, and being professional but not aggressive.

You use open communication when you share unusual diagnostic findings or convey important information regarding a patient's source of family support to other health care providers as needed. One way of fostering good team communication is by setting expectations of one another. An efficient team counts on all members when needs arise. Sharing expectations of what, when, and how to communicate establishes a strong work team (Matzke et al., 2014). Always treat colleagues with respect. Listen to the ideas of other staff members without interruption. Be honest and direct in what you say. Clarify what others are saying and build on the merits of co-workers' ideas (Yoder-Wise, 2015). Be open and courteous, summarize issues, and give only necessary details. When using electronic communication, it is important to communicate the appropriate information to the correct person, always maintaining patient privacy and confidentiality (NCSBN, 2011).

Delegation

The art of effective delegation is a skill that you as a student need to observe and practice to improve your management skills. Delegation is the process of assigning part of one person's responsibility to another qualified person in a specific situation (American Nurses Association [ANA] and NCSBN, 2006; NCSBN, 2016b). The Nurse Practice Act of your state, along with authority, accountability, and responsibility, provide the basis for effective delegation. Delegation results in achievement of quality patient care, improved efficiency, increased productivity, empowerment of staff, and development of others (Yoder-Wise, 2015). For example, asking a staff member to obtain an ordered specimen while you administer a patient's pain medication effectively prevents a delay in a patient gaining pain relief. Delegation also provides job enrichment. A nurse shows trust in colleagues by delegating tasks to them and showing staff members that they are important players in the delivery of care (Lee et al., 2015). Successful delegation is important to the quality of the RN-NAP relationship and their willingness to work together (True et al., 2014). Never delegate a task that you dislike doing or would not do yourself because this creates negative feelings and poor working relationships. Although the delegation of a task transfers the responsibility and authority to another person, remember that you are still accountable for the delegated tasks.

Professional nurses find themselves in situations in which they need more support to do the daily, repetitive tasks of care such as basic hygiene, specimen collection, and feeding patients. An RN needs time to coordinate care delivery for groups of patients, conduct individual assessments, and make professional judgments about a patient's health and therapeutic needs. A nurse also needs time to deliver complex therapies and provide patient counseling and education. An LPN or LVN in acute care benefits from getting support from RNs to deliver care to a group of patients whose needs are complex. In long-term care settings, the LPN or LVN directs care and relies on NAP to provide basic care measures. One nurse is simply not able to do all the work necessary to care for groups of patients.

To be able to perform your professional responsibilities as a nurse, learn how to work effectively with other staff members. Each health care team member has a set of job responsibilities that contribute to the overall care of patients. As a nurse, your job is to help the care team work efficiently. Because you oversee the care of groups of patients, it sometimes is necessary for you to delegate work to others.

As a nurse, you transfer or assign the responsibility to complete a task to others, but you retain accountability for the outcome. For example, you delegate ambulating a patient to a competent and trained NAP after you have assessed the patient's strength, mobility, and ability to walk. However, you are ultimately accountable for ensuring the patient ambulates. As the RN, you remain accountable for the overall nursing care of a patient when you delegate responsibilities to a competent individual (Yoder-Wise, 2015). Because the steps of the nursing process of assessment, diagnosis, planning, implementation, and evaluation require you to use nursing judgment, you do not delegate these activities (ANA and NCSBN, 2006; NCSBN, 2016b). Thus exercise good judgment at all times in deciding which tasks to delegate and in which situations. The NCSBN offers guidelines for delegation of tasks in accordance with an RN's legal scope of practice (Box 13.6).

It is important to recognize that you delegate tasks, not patients. Furthermore, do not automatically delegate a task because it is a task; rather delegate it because it is appropriate for someone else to perform it. For example, as the nurse you

BOX 13.6   THE FIVE RIGHTS OF DELEGATION

RIGHT TASK

The right task is one that you can delegate for a specific patient such as tasks that are repetitive, require little supervision, are relatively noninvasive, have results that are predictable, and have minimal potential risk.

RIGHT CIRCUMSTANCES

Consider the patient setting, available resources, and other relevant factors before delegating. In an acute care setting patients' conditions can change quickly. Good clinical decision making and critical thinking are needed to ensure that the NAP has the appropriate resources, equipment, and supervision to provide safe and effective care.

RIGHT PERSON

The right person is delegating the right tasks to the right person to be performed on the right person.

RIGHT DIRECTION/COMMUNICATION

Give a clear, concise description of the task including its objective, limits, and expectations. Communication must be ongoing between the nurse and NAP during a shift of care.

RIGHT SUPERVISION

Provide appropriate monitoring, evaluation, intervention as needed, and feedback. NAP should feel comfortable asking questions and seeking assistance.

Data from National Council of State Boards of Nursing: *Delegation: concepts and decision-making process,* Chicago, 1995, The Council; National Council of State Boards of Nursing, *The five rights of delegation,* Chicago, 1997, The Council; and American Nurses Association (ANA) and National Council of State Boards of Nursing (NCSBN): *Joint statement on delegation,* 2006. https://www.ncsbn.org/Delegation_joint_statement_NCSBN-ANA.pdf.

are always responsible for the assessment of a patient's ongoing status; however, if a patient is stable, you delegate vital sign monitoring to NAP. It is important for you to collaborate with NAP and ask them to take on tasks that you determine are safe and appropriate for them to provide.

Effective delegation requires constant communication (i.e., sending clear messages and listening so that all participants understand expectations regarding patient care). Know how to give clear instructions, effectively prioritize patient needs and therapies, and give staff members timely and meaningful feedback. Make sure that all participants understand expectations regarding patient care. You need to communicate when and what information to report such as expected observations and specific patient outcomes (NCSBN, 2005). Remember that communication is always a two-way process. Therefore allow NAP the opportunity to ask questions and clarify your expectations during the delegation process (ANA and NCSBN, 2006; NCSBN, 2016b). Conflict occurs between RNs and NAP when there is little or poor communication (Lancaster et al., 2015). Inaccurate hand-off communication, lack of knowledge about the workload of team members, and difficulty dealing with conflict are examples of communication failures that result in ineffective delegation and omissions of nursing care.

The final steps in delegation are evaluation of the staff member's performance, achievement of the patient's outcomes, the communication process used, and any problems or concerns that occurred (NCSBN, 2005, 2016b). Provide praise and recognition when a staff member performs the task correctly and does a good job. If a staff member's performance is not satisfactory, give constructive and appropriate feedback. Give specific feedback when discussing mistakes that staff members make, and explain how to avoid the mistake or a better way to handle the situation. Give feedback in private to preserve the staff member's dignity. When you give feedback, focus on things that are changeable, choose only one issue at a time, and give specific details. When the performance of NAP does not meet expectations, it is often because of inadequate training or assignment of too many tasks. You discover the need to review a procedure with staff and offer demonstration or even recommend that additional training is scheduled with the education department. Nursing practice issues often arise when nurses delegate too many tasks. All staff need to discuss the appropriateness of delegation on their unit. Sometimes NAP need help in learning how to prioritize. In some cases, you may learn that you are overdelegating.

Clear directions and statement of desired outcomes increase the likelihood of successful completion of a task. If you observe a change in patient status, that a task is not being performed as directed or by agency policy and procedures, or that an NAP is having difficulty completing a task, you need to intervene and follow up as needed (ANA and NCSBN, 2006). It is your responsibility to complete documentation of the delegated task. Following are a few tips on appropriate delegation (Yoder-Wise, 2015; NCSBN, 2016b):

- *Assess the knowledge and skills of the person to whom you are delegating:* Determine what an NAP knows and what he or she is able to do by asking open-ended questions that encourage conversation and details. For example, ask, "How do you usually put the cuff on when you measure a blood pressure?" or "Tell me how you prepare the tubing before you give an enema."
- *Match tasks to the assistant's skills:* Know which skills the training program includes for NAP at your organization. Determine if personnel have learned critical thinking skills such as knowing when a patient is in danger or what changes to report.
- *Communicate clearly:* Always provide complete, accurate, and clear directions by describing a task, the desired outcome, and the time period within which a person is to complete the task. Never give instructions through another staff member. Make NAP feel as though they are part of the team. For example, "I'd like you to help me by getting Mr. Floyd up to ambulate before lunch. Please be sure to check his blood pressure before he stands and write it down on the graphic sheet."

- *Listen attentively:* Listen to an NAP's response after you provide directions. Does the NAP feel comfortable in asking questions or requesting clarification? If you encourage a response, listen to what the NAP says. Be especially attentive if a staff member has been given a deadline to meet by another nurse. Help sort out priorities.
- *Provide feedback:* Always give an NAP feedback regarding performance, regardless of outcome. Let the NAP know when a job was well done. If an outcome is undesirable, find a private place to discuss what occurred, any miscommunication, and how to achieve a better outcome in the future.

KEY POINTS

- A manager sets a philosophy for a work unit, ensures appropriate staffing, and mobilizes staff and institutional resources to achieve objectives. A manager also motivates staff members to carry out their work, sets standards of performance, and makes the right decisions to achieve objectives.
- Empowering staff members brings out the best in a manager and allows the manager to concentrate on effective patient care systems, support risk taking and innovation, and focus on results and rewards.
- Nursing care delivery models vary by the responsibility of the RN in coordinating care delivery and the roles that other staff members play in helping with care.
- Critical to the success of decentralized decision making is making staff members aware that they have responsibility, authority, and accountability for the care they give and the decisions they make.
- A nurse manager fosters decentralized decision making by establishing nursing practice committees and supporting interdisciplinary collaboration between nurses and health care providers.
- Clinical care coordination involves accurate clinical decision making, establishing priorities, efficient organizational skills, appropriate use of resources and time-management skills, and an ongoing evaluation of care activities.
- Each member of an interprofessional health care team is responsible for open, professional communication.
- When done correctly, delegation improves job efficiency and job enrichment.
- Exercise good judgment at all times in deciding which tasks to delegate and in which situations.

REFLECTIVE LEARNING

- Reflect on your most recent clinical experience. What nursing care delivery model was used in this health care setting? What made this an effective model for this setting? What potential challenges do you think the team might have experienced with this model?
- Describe how you prioritized care for a recent patient or group of patients you cared for during a recent clinical or simulation experience. Evaluate the effectiveness of your care. Reflecting back on this experience, is there anything you would have done differently? Why or why not?
- Observe two or more different health care team members discussing a patient's care. Reflecting on this experience, what did these team members do to enhance or create a barrier to effective communication and teamwork?

REVIEW QUESTIONS

1. An RN is caring for a patient who has bronchitis. Which of the following tasks can the RN delegate to an NAP? (Select all that apply.)
   1. Teach the patient about ordered medications
   2. Auscultate the patient's lungs
   3. Give the patient a bath
   4. Take the patient's vital signs
   5. Evaluate the patient's temperature to help determine the effectiveness of the patient's antibiotics
   6. Take the patient for a walk down the hall
2. A nurse finished assessing all assigned patients and is discussing with an NAP what needs to be done in the next hour. Which statements require follow-up by the nurse manager? (Select all that apply.)
   1. "Can you please go answer the patient's call light in room 5117 and see what the patient needs?"
   2. "I need to assess this patient's skin. About 5 minutes after you start the bath, I'll come into the room to help you turn her, wash her back, and look at her skin."
   3. "Why did you give that patient his tray? You should have known I needed to talk with him before you let him eat."
   4. "Thank you for helping me get that patient up in the chair. I could not have done it without you."
   5. "Can you please give that patient this medication for me? I have to take a phone call."
3. A nurse is caring for a patient who has type 2 diabetes. Which action shows the nurse is evaluating the effectiveness of the patient's care?
   1. Asking the patient how often he exercises every week
   2. Working with the patient to determine a target range for blood sugar first thing in the morning
   3. Measuring the patient's capillary glucose level before lunch
   4. Asking the patient to explain the side effects of a newly ordered medication
4. A nurse just received hand-off report at the change of shift. Which patient does the nurse need to see first?
   1. A patient who needs to be taught how to change a dressing at home
   2. A patient who is slightly more confused now compared with 4 hours ago
   3. A patient who is ranking incisional pain as a 4 on a 0-to-10 scale
   4. A patient who needs a soapsuds enema

5. A nurse is participating in interdisciplinary team rounds. Which statement made by the nurse reflects appropriate team communication? (Select all that apply.)
   1. "Help me understand what is preventing this patient from being able to walk independently."
   2. "I have a lot of patients to see. Let's get through this as fast as possible."
   3. "You are late. Where have you been?"
   4. "It seems like we need to get another opinion about why the patient isn't gaining weight. Who do you think we should ask to evaluate the patient?"
   5. "Did you hear about what happened between the nurses and doctors last night?"

evolve

Additional Review Questions, as well as rationales for all Review Questions, can be found on the Evolve website.

1, 3, 4, 6; 2, 3, 5; 3, 4, 4, 2; 5, 1, 4.

REFERENCES

Alfaro-Lefevre R: *Critical thinking, clinical reasoning, and clinical judgment: a practical approach*, ed 6, St Louis, 2017, Saunders.

American Nurses Association (ANA) and National Council of State Boards of Nursing (NCSBN): *Joint statement on delegation*, 2006. https://www.ncsbn.org/Delegation_joint_statement_NCSBN-ANA.pdf.

American Nurses Credentialing Center (ANCC): *Magnet recognition program® overview*, 2017. http://www.nursecredentialing.org/Magnet/ProgramOverview.

Benner P, et al: *Educating nurses: a call for radical transformation*, San Francisco, 2010, Jossey-Bass.

Benner P, et al: *Clinical wisdom and interventions in acute and critical care: a thinking-in-action approach*, New York, 2011, Springer Publishing Company.

Brunges M, Foley-Brinza C: Projects for increasing job satisfaction and creating a healthy work environment, *AORN J* 100(6):670, 2014.

Buck S, Doucette J: Transformational leadership practices of CNOs, *Nurs Manage* 46(9):42, 2015.

Case Management Society of America: *What is a case manager?* 2016. http://www.cmsa.org/Home/CMSA/WhatisaCaseManager/tabid/224/Default.aspx.

Clochesy JM, et al: Enhancing communication between patients and healthcare providers: SBAR3, *J Health Hum Serv Adm* 38(2):237, 2015.

Cornell P, et al: Impact of SBAR on nurse shift reports and staff rounding, *Medsurg Nurs* 23(5):334, 2014.

Friese CR, et al: Pod nursing on a medical/surgical unit: implementation and outcomes evaluation, *J Nurs Adm* 44(4):207, 2014.

Fung L, et al: Impact of crisis resource management simulation-based training for interprofessional and interdisciplinary teams: a systematic review, *J Interprof Care* 29(5):433, 2015.

Glymph DC, et al: Healthcare utilizing deliberated discussion linking events (HUDDLE): a systematic review, *AANA J* 83(3):183, 2015.

Hansten R, Jackson M: *Clinical delegation skills: a handbook for professional practice*, ed 4, Sudbury, MA, 2009, Jones & Bartlett.

Hendry C, Walker A: Priority setting in clinical nursing practice: literature review, *J Adv Nurs* 47(4):427, 2004.

Hooper JI, et al: Optimal clinical instruction in nursing education programs: recommendations from the field, *J Nurs Regul* 7(2):53, 2016.

Huber DL: *Leadership and nursing care management*, ed 5, St Louis, 2014, Elsevier.

Institute for Patient- and Family-Centered Care (IPFCC): *Patient- and family-centered care*, n.d. http://www.ipfcc.org/about/pfcc.html.

Institute of Medicine (IOM): *Crossing the quality chasm: a new health system for the twenty-first century*, Washington, DC, 2001, National Academies Press.

Institute of Medicine (IOM): *Keeping patients safe: transforming the work environment*, Washington, DC, 2004, National Academies Press.

Institute of Medicine (IOM): *The future of nursing: leading change, advancing health*, Washington, DC, 2011, National Academies Press.

Interprofessional Education Collaborative (IPEC): *Core competencies for interprofessional collaborative practice: 2016 update*, Washington, DC, 2016, Interprofessional Education Collaborative.

Kear T, Ulrich B: Trends in nursing. The role of interprofessional collaboration in supporting a culture of safety, *Nephrol News Issues* 29(9):21, 2015.

Krautscheid LC: Defining professional nursing accountability: a literature review, *J Prof Nurs* 30(1):43, 2014.

Lancaster G, et al: Interdisciplinary communication and collaboration among physicians, nurses and unlicensed assistive personnel, *J Nurs Scholarsh* 47(3):275, 2015.

Lannin NA, et al: Effects of case management after brain injury: a systematic review, *Neurorehabilitation* 35(4):635, 2014.

LeBlanc P: Leadership by design: creating successful "TEEAMS", *Nurs Manage* 45(3):49, 2014.

Lee CY, et al: Evaluation of a support worker role, within a nurse delegation and supervision model, for provision of medicines support for older people living at home: the Workforce Innovation for Safe and Effective (WISE) medicines care study, *BMC Health Serv Res* 15(1):1, 2015.

Lievens I, Vlerick P: Transformational leadership and safety performance among nurses: the mediating role of knowledge-related job characteristics, *J Adv Nurs* 70(3):651, 2014.

Matzke B, et al: Using a team-centered approach to evaluate effectiveness of nurse-physician communications, *JOGN Nurs* 43(6):684, 2014.

Mazerolle SM, et al: Coping strategies used by athletic training majors to manage clinical and academic responsibilities, *Int J Athl Ther Train* 20(3):4, 2015.

Moss M, Good VS: An official critical care societies collaborative statement: burnout syndrome in critical care health care professionals: a call for action, *Am J Crit Care* 25(4):368, 2016.

National Council of State Boards of Nursing (NCSBN): *Working with others: a position paper*, Chicago, 2005. The Council. https://www.ncsbn.org/Working_with_Others.pdf.

National Council of State Boards of Nursing (NCSBN): *White Paper: a nurse's guide to the use of social media*, Chicago, 2011. National Council of State Boards of Nursing. https://www.ncsbn.org/Social_Media.pdf.

National Council of State Boards of Nursing (NCSBN): *History*, 2016a. https://www.ncsbn.org/history.htm.

National Council of State Boards of Nursing (NCSBN): National guidelines for nursing delegation, *J Nurs Regul* 7(1): 5, 2016b.

Nichols K, et al: Beyond implementation: sustaining family-centered rounds, *MCN Am J Matern Child Nurs* 40(3):145, 2015.

Perry V: CNE series. A daily goals tool to facilitate indirect nurse-physician communication during morning rounds on a medical-surgical unit, *Medsurg Nurs* 25(2):83, 2016.

QSEN Institute: *Pre-licensure KSAs*, 2014. http://qsen.org/competencies/pre-licensure-ksas/#teamwork_collaboration.

Read EA, Laschinger HKS: The influence of authentic leadership and empowerment on nurses' relational social capital, mental health and job satisfaction over the first year of practice, *J Adv Nurs* 71(7):2015, 1611.

Reising DL, et al: Psychometric testing of a simulation rubric for measuring interprofessional communication, *Nurs Educ Perspect* 36(5):311, 2015.

Roberts-Turner R, et al: Effects of leadership characteristics on nurses' job satisfaction, *Pediatr Nurs* 40(5):236, 2014.

Rossler KL, Kimble LP: Capturing readiness to learn and collaboration as explored with an interprofessional simulation scenario: a mixed-methods research study, *Nurse Educ Today* 36:348, 2016.

Shelestak DS, et al: A process to assess clinical decision-making during human patient simulation: a pilot study, *Nurs Educ Perspect* 36(3):185, 2015.

Stelson EA, et al: Perceptions of family participation in intensive care unit rounds and telemedicine: a qualitative assessment, *Am J Crit Care* 25(5):440, 2016.

Sweigart LI, et al: Virtual TeamSTEPPS® simulations produce teamwork attitude changes among health professions students, *J Nurs Educ* 55(1):31, 2016.

True G, et al: Teamwork and delegation in medical homes: primary care staff perspectives in the veterans' health administration, *J Gen Intern Med* 29(2):632, 2014.

Turrentine FE, et al: Interprofessional training enhances collaboration between nursing and medical students: a pilot study, *Nurse Educ Today* 40:33, 2016.

Weiland SA: Understanding nurse practitioner autonomy, *J Am Assoc Nurse Pract* 27(2):95, 2015.

Wilder KA, et al: CLABSI reduction strategy: a systematic central line quality improvement initiative integrating line-rounding principles and a team approach, *Adv Neonatal Care* 16(3): 170, 2016.

Yoder-Wise PS: *Leading and managing in nursing*, ed 6, St Louis, 2015, Elsevier.

Infection Prevention and Control

evolve MEDIA RESOURCES

http://evolve.elsevier.com/Potter/essentials

- Audio Glossary
- Case Study Continuation
- Concept Map
- Nursing Care Plan

- QSEN Activity and Review Questions Answers and Rationales
- Video Clips

OBJECTIVES

- Identify the normal defenses of the body against infection.
- Discuss the development of the inflammatory response.
- Describe the signs and symptoms of a localized infection and a systemic infection.
- Describe characteristics of each link of the infection chain.
- Assess patients at risk for acquiring an infection.
- Explain conditions that promote development of health care–acquired infections (HAIs).

- Describe strategies for standard precautions.
- Identify principles of medical and surgical asepsis.
- Describe nursing interventions designed to break each link in the infection chain.
- Perform proper techniques for transmission-based precautions.
- Describe the Five Moments for Hand Hygiene.
- Perform proper procedures for hand hygiene.
- Describe the steps for applying personal protective equipment.

KEY TERMS

airborne precautions, p. 251
antibody, p. 238
antigen, p. 239
asepsis, p. 239
aseptic technique, p. 239
asymptomatic, p. 236
carriers, p. 237
colonization, p. 236
communicable disease, p. 236
contact precautions, p. 251
disinfection, p. 247
droplet precautions, p. 251

endogenous infection, p. 239
exogenous infection, p. 239
flora, p. 238
health care–acquired infection (HAI), p. 239
immunity, p. 238
infection, p. 236
inflammation, p. 239
inflammatory response, p. 238
medical asepsis, p. 240
microorganisms, p. 236
necrotic, p. 239

pathogenicity, p. 238
pathogens, p. 236
reservoir, p. 236
standard precautions, p. 247
sterilization, p. 240
suprainfection, p. 238
surgical asepsis, p. 240
symptomatic, p. 236
transmission-based precautions, p. 247
virulence, p. 236

Current trends, public awareness, and rising costs of health care have increased the importance of infection prevention and control. Increases in drug-resistant microorganisms and health care–acquired infections (HAIs) and concern about occupational exposure to human immunodeficiency virus (HIV) and hepatitis have increased concern about transmission of infections within health care settings. As a nurse, you will participate in cost-effective, quality health care by using strategies that prevent or reduce the risk for infections. This chapter emphasizes techniques for prevention and

CASE STUDY *Mrs. Eldredge*

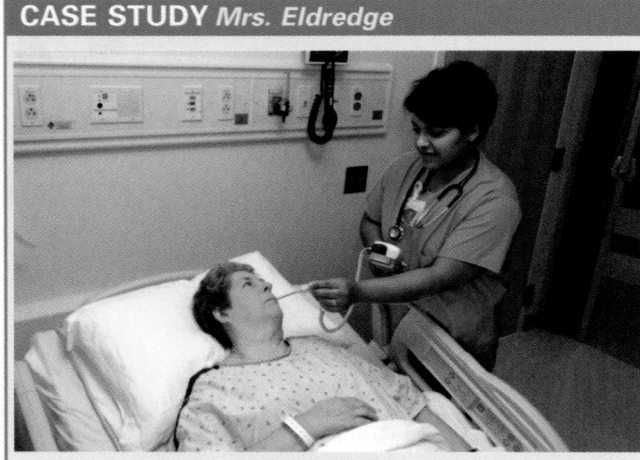

Mrs. Eldredge is a 63-year-old woman who lives alone and enjoys an active social life. She has diabetes that is well controlled with oral hypoglycemic medications and diet. She had a total left hip replacement and went home as expected on the fourth postoperative day. Mrs. Eldredge was readmitted to the hospital 2 weeks after her surgery because she started having increased pain in her left hip.

Kathy Jackson is a nursing student caring for Mrs. Eldredge in the hospital. Kathy assesses Mrs. Eldredge's incision and notes that it is red, swollen, and warm. Mrs. Eldredge has a low-grade fever (37.6°C [99.8°F]). Mrs. Eldredge states, "I am not sure what is wrong with me, but my left hip really hurts." Kathy discusses the situation with Mrs. Eldredge's nurse and orthopedic surgeon. After reviewing x-rays the orthopedic surgeon determines Mrs. Eldredge has an infection. He takes the patient to surgery to perform an incision and drainage and then on return to the orthopedic unit orders wound irrigation with normal saline and dressing changes three times a day. Mrs. Eldredge is to remain on bed rest until tomorrow morning.

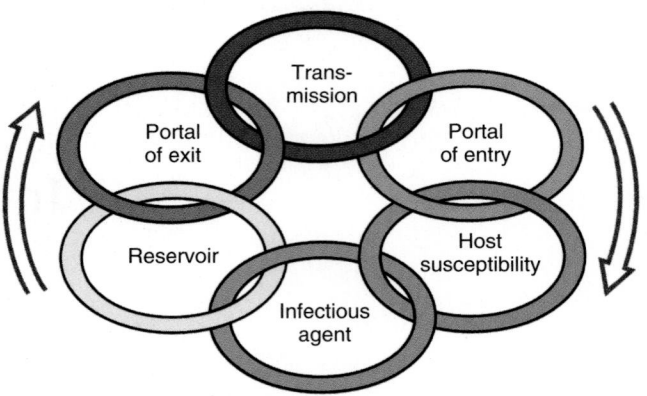

FIG 14.1 Chain of infection.

control of infections and the critical thinking skills necessary to achieve these goals.

SCIENTIFIC KNOWLEDGE BASE

Nature of Infection

An infection is the invasion of a susceptible host (e.g., a patient) by potentially harmful microorganisms (pathogens), resulting in disease. The principal infecting agents are bacteria, viruses, fungi, and protozoa (Table 14.1). It is important to know the difference between an infection and colonization. Colonization is the presence and growth of microorganisms within a host but without tissue invasion or damage (Tweeten, 2015). All people have microorganisms on their skin, but usually no disease or infection develops. Disease or infection results only if the pathogens grow or multiply and alter normal tissue function. An infectious disease transmitted directly from one person to another is considered a contagious or communicable disease (Tweeten, 2015). If the pathogens multiply and cause clinical signs and symptoms, the patient is symptomatic. If the clinical signs and symptoms of the illness are not present, the patient is asymptomatic. For example, hepatitis C is most efficiently transmitted through the direct entry of blood into the skin through a percutaneous exposure, even if the source (patient) is asymptomatic (Centers for Disease Control and Prevention [CDC], 2016a).

Chain of Infection

The presence of a pathogen does not mean that an infection develops. The process resulting in an infection is referred to as the *chain of infection*. Components of the chain of infection include the infectious agent or pathogen, reservoir or place for pathogen growth, portal of exit from the reservoir, mode of transmission or vehicle, portal of entry into the reservoir, and a susceptible host (Fig. 14.1). Infection develops if the links in this chain remain intact. Preventing infections involves breaking the chain of infection.

Infectious Agent. The development of an infection depends on the number of microorganisms present; their virulence, or the ability to produce disease; their ability to enter and survive in a host; and the susceptibility of the host. Resident skin microorganisms are not virulent. However, they can cause serious infection when surgery or an invasive procedure allows them to enter deep inside tissues or when a patient is severely immunocompromised. Patients become immunocompromised when their immune system is impaired. Some factors that increase a patient's risk for being immunocompromised include chemotherapy and organ transplant antirejection medications, or acquired immunodeficiency syndrome (AIDS).

Reservoir. A place where microorganisms survive, multiply, and wait to transfer to a susceptible host is called a reservoir. Common reservoirs are humans and animals (hosts), insects, food, water, and organic matter on inanimate surfaces (fomites). Frequent reservoirs for HAIs include health care workers (especially their hands), body excretions and secretions of patients, equipment, and the health care

TABLE 14.1   COMMON PATHOGENS AND SOME INFECTIONS OR DISEASES THEY PRODUCE

ORGANISM	MAJOR RESERVOIRS	MAJOR DISEASES/INFECTIONS
Bacteria		
Escherichia coli	Colon	Gastroenteritis, urinary tract infection
Staphylococcus aureus	Skin, hair, upper respiratory tract	Wound infection, abscess, cellulitis, osteomyelitis, bacteremia, pneumonia, food poisoning, toxic shock syndrome
Streptococcus (beta-hemolytic group A) organisms	Oropharynx, skin, perianal area	"Strep throat," rheumatic fever, scarlet fever, impetigo, wound infection
Streptococcus (beta-hemolytic group B) organisms	Adult genitalia	Urinary tract infection, wound infection, postpartum sepsis, neonatal sepsis
Mycobacterium tuberculosis	Droplet nuclei from lungs	Tuberculosis
Neisseria gonorrhoeae	Genitourinary tract, rectum, mouth	Sexually transmitted infection, pelvic inflammatory disease, septic arthritis, newborn ophthalmitis
Rickettsia rickettsii	Wood tick	Rocky Mountain spotted fever
Staphylococcus epidermidis	Skin	Wound infection, bacteremia
Viruses		
Hepatitis A virus	Feces	Hepatitis A
Hepatitis B virus	Blood, certain body fluids, tissues involved in sexual contact	Hepatitis B
Hepatitis C virus	Blood, certain body fluids, tissues involved in sexual contact	Hepatitis C
Herpes simplex virus (type I)	Lesions of mouth, skin, genitals	Cold sores, herpetic whitlow, sexually transmitted disease
Human immunodeficiency virus (HIV)	Blood, semen, vaginal secretions via sexual contact	Acquired immunodeficiency syndrome (AIDS)
Fungi		
Aspergillus organisms	Soil, dust, mouth, skin, colon, genital tract	Aspergillosis, pneumonia, sepsis
Candida albicans	Skin, mouth, genital tract	Candidiasis, pneumonia, sepsis
Protozoa		
Plasmodium falciparum	Blood	Malaria

Data from Brown M: Microbiology basics. In Grota P, editor: *APIC text of infection control and epidemiology,* ed 4, Washington, DC, 2015, Association for Professionals in Infection Control and Epidemiology (APIC).

environment. There are two types of human reservoirs: humans with acute or symptomatic disease and humans who show no signs of disease but are carriers of it. Transmission of microorganisms can occur in either case.

Portal of Exit. After microorganisms find a site in which to grow and multiply, they must find a portal of exit if they are to enter another host and cause disease. They exit through a variety of sites such as the skin and mucous membranes, respiratory tract, gastrointestinal (GI) tract, urinary tract, reproductive tract, and blood.

Modes of Transmission. By practicing infection prevention and control techniques such as hand hygiene, you can interrupt the mode of transmission (Box 14.1). The same

microorganism is sometimes transmitted by more than one route. For example, the virus that causes chickenpox spreads by airborne route in droplet nuclei and by direct contact with vesicle fluid. When the hands of a health care worker contacts infectious material directly, the microorganisms will spread to the health care worker. This mode of transmission is called *direct transmission.* Indirect transmission occurs when microorganisms are transferred to a health care worker's hands from contaminated items that are part of patient care such as a stethoscope or a dirty pair of gloves (CDC, 2012).

Portal of Entry. Organisms are able to enter the body through the same routes that they use for exiting. Common portals of entry include broken skin, mucous membranes, genitourinary tract, GI tract, and respiratory tract. For

BOX 14.1   MODES OF TRANSMISSION: ROUTES AND MEANS

CONTACT

- *Direct:* Person-to-person or physical contact between source and susceptible host (e.g., touching patient feces and then touching own face or mouth or consuming contaminated food)
- *Indirect:* Personal contact of susceptible host with contaminated inanimate object (e.g., needles or sharps, dressings)
- *Droplet:* Large particles that travel up to 3 feet and come in contact with susceptible host (e.g., from coughing, sneezing, talking)
- *Airborne:* Droplet nuclei, residue or evaporated droplets suspended in air (e.g., from coughing, sneezing, talking)

VEHICLES

- Contaminated items
- Water
- Drugs, solutions
- Blood
- Food (improperly handled, stored, cooked; fresh or thawed meats)

VECTOR

- External mechanical transfer (flies)
- Internal transmission such as with parasitic conditions between vector and host, for example:
  - Mosquito
  - Louse
  - Tick
  - Flea

Data from Tweeten S: General principles of epidemiology. In Grota P, editor: *APIC text of infection control and epidemiology*, ed 4, Washington, DC, 2015, Association for Professionals in Infection Control and Epidemiology.

example, obstruction to the flow of urine caused by the presence of a blocked urinary catheter allows organisms to go up into the urethra.

Susceptible Host. Susceptibility to an infection depends on an individual's degree of resistance to pathogens. Although everyone is constantly in contact with large numbers of microorganisms, an infection does not develop until an individual becomes susceptible to the strength and numbers of these microorganisms. The amount of pathogen required to cause an infection in the host is defined as the dose. The more virulent an organism, the greater the dose, and the more likely it is that a person will develop an infection. Some factors that influence a person's susceptibility (degree of resistance) to infection include age, nutritional status, presence of chronic disease, trauma, and smoking. Organisms with resistance to key antibiotics are common in all health care settings, but especially acute care. This is associated with the frequent and sometimes inappropriate use of antibiotics over the years in all settings (i.e., acute care, ambulatory care, clinics, and long-term care). A person's natural defenses

against infection and certain risk factors affect susceptibility (see Assessment).

A host is not considered susceptible if it has acquired immunity through either a natural or an artificially induced event. Natural active immunity results from having a certain disease such as measles and mounting an immune response that usually lasts a lifetime. Active immunity also results from the administration of a vaccine. Natural passive immunity is the acquisition of an antibody by one person from another such as an infant born with the mother's antibodies. The infant acquires this short-term immunity from antibodies through the placenta during the last months of pregnancy (Dalal and Rolfman, 2015).

Course of Infection

Infections follow a progressive course (Fig. 14.2). The severity depends on the extent of the infection, the pathogenicity and virulence of the causative microorganism, and the susceptibility of the host. If the infection is localized such as in a wound, antibiotic therapy and proper wound care control the spread of the infection and minimize the illness. The patient usually experiences localized symptoms only such as pain, tenderness, and swelling at the wound site. An infection that affects the entire body instead of just a single organ or part is systemic, characterized by a fever and increase in white blood cells (WBCs). Systemic infections can cause further complications including organ damage and are associated with higher mortality rates.

Defenses Against Infection

The body has normal defenses against infection, including normal flora, body system defenses, and the immune system. Intact skin protects from pathogens, and linings of the nasal passages act to prevent organisms from entering the lungs. Each organ system has defense mechanisms to prevent exposure to infection. In addition, the inflammatory response of the body is a protective reaction that neutralizes pathogens and repairs body cells.

Normal Flora. The normal flora of the body is made up of a large number of microorganisms residing on the surface and deep layers of the skin, in the saliva, and on the oral mucosa and intestinal walls. Normal flora usually does not cause disease but instead maintains health. For example, skin flora reduces multiplication of organisms landing on the skin. The number and variety of flora maintain a sensitive balance with other microorganisms to prevent infection. Any factor that disrupts this balance increases the risk for infection. For example, the use of broad-spectrum antibiotics for the treatment of infection eliminates or changes normal bacterial flora, often leading to suprainfection. Microorganisms resistant to antibiotics cause serious infection (Arnold, 2015).

Body System Defenses. Microorganisms easily enter the skin, respiratory tract, and GI tract. However, these body systems also have unique defenses against infection that are

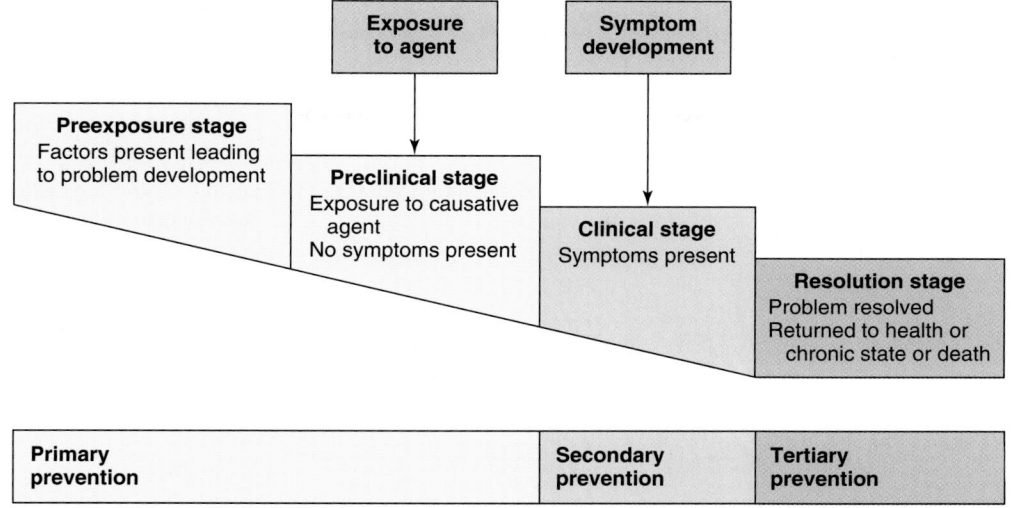

FIG 14.2 Stages of the natural history of a condition and their relationship to primary, secondary, and tertiary levels of prevention. (From Clark MJ: *Community health nursing: caring for populations,* ed 4, Upper Saddle River, NJ, 2003, Pearson Education.)

physiologically suited to their structure and function (Table 14.2). Any condition that impairs the specialized defenses of an organ increases susceptibility to infection.

Inflammation. The cellular responses of the body to injury or infection is **inflammation.** Inflammation is a protective vascular reaction that involves a cascade of physiological responses that neutralize and eliminate pathogens or **necrotic** tissues and establishes a means of repairing body cells and tissues. Acute inflammation is usually a short-lived process, lasting only a few days (e.g., inflammation around a cut or surgical incision). If inflammation lasts longer, it is referred to as chronic inflammation. Chronic inflammation may last weeks, months, or longer. Along with abnormal laboratory values, there are multiple signs and symptoms of inflammation (Table 14.3). Many physical agents (e.g., temperature extremes and radiation), chemical agents (e.g., gastric acid or poisons), and microorganisms trigger inflammation.

Immune Response. When a foreign material (**antigen**) enters the body, a series of responses changes the biological makeup of the body. The next time that the same antigen enters the body, antibodies bind to the antigens they find and neutralize, destroy, or eliminate them.

Health Care–Acquired Infection

Patients in health care settings, especially hospitals and long-term care facilities (LTCFs), are at a higher risk for infection than patients seen in the home. These patients often have multiple illnesses, are older adults, and are poorly nourished. These factors make them more susceptible to infection. In addition, many patients in health care settings have a lowered resistance to infection because of underlying medical conditions (e.g., HIV, diabetes mellitus, autoimmune disorders, malignancies) that impair or damage the immune responses

of the body. Invasive treatment devices such as IV catheters or indwelling urinary catheters impair or bypass the natural defenses of the body against microorganisms. Treatments with multiple antibiotics for long periods of time are also associated with an increased risk for certain infections (Arnold, 2015).

When a patient develops an infection that was not present or incubating at the time of admission to a health care setting, it is called a **health care–acquired infection (HAI).** A community-acquired infection is one that was present at the time of admission to a health care setting. The conscientious practice of hand hygiene and aseptic technique reduces the risk for HAIs. The Joint Commission (TJC) lists prevention of infection as one of its National Patient Safety Goals, with a focus on infections that are difficult to treat and on infections involving central IV access, urinary tract catheterization, and postoperative conditions (TJC, 2018).

HAIs are exogenous or endogenous. An **exogenous infection** comes from microorganisms found outside the individual such as *Salmonella, Clostridium tetani,* and *Aspergillus.* They do not exist as normal flora. An **endogenous infection** occurs when part of a patient's flora becomes altered and overgrowth results (e.g., staphylococci, enterococci, yeasts, streptococci). This often happens when a patient receives broad-spectrum antibiotics that alter normal flora. When sufficient numbers of microorganisms normally found in one body site move to another site, an endogenous infection develops. The number of microorganisms needed to cause an HAI depends on the virulence of the organism, susceptibility of the host, and body site affected (Box 14.2).

Asepsis. Efforts to minimize the onset and spread of infection to patients are based on the principles of **aseptic technique.** The term **asepsis** means the absence of

TABLE 14.2   NORMAL BODY SYSTEM DEFENSE MECHANISMS AGAINST INFECTION

DEFENSE MECHANISMS	ACTION	FACTORS THAT MAY ALTER DEFENSE
Skin		
Intact multilayered surface, first line of defense of body against infection	Provides mechanical barrier to microorganisms and antibacterial activity	Cuts, abrasions, puncture wounds, areas of maceration
Shedding of outer layer of skin cells	Removes organisms that adhere to outer layers of skin	Failure to bathe regularly, improper hand-hygiene techniques
Sebum	Contains fatty acid that kills some bacteria	Excessive bathing
Mouth		
Intact multilayered mucosa	Provides mechanical barrier to microorganisms	Lacerations, trauma, extracted teeth
Saliva	Washes away particles containing microorganisms Contains microbial inhibitors (e.g., lysozyme)	Poor oral hygiene, dehydration
Eye		
Tearing and blinking	Provides mechanisms to reduce entry (blinking) or help wash away (tearing) particles containing pathogens	Injury, exposure-splash, splatter of blood or other potentially infectious material into the eye
Respiratory Tract		
Cilia lining upper airways, coated by mucus	Trap inhaled microbes and sweep them outward in mucus to be expectorated or swallowed	Smoking, high concentration of oxygen and carbon dioxide, decreased humidity, cold air
Macrophages	Engulf and destroy microorganisms that reach alveoli of lung	Smoking, immunosuppression
Urinary Tract		
Flushing action of urine flow	Washes away microorganisms on lining of bladder and urethra	Obstruction to normal flow by indwelling urinary catheter placement, obstruction from growth or tumor, or delayed micturition
Intact multilayered epithelium	Provides barrier to microorganisms	Introduction of urinary catheter, continual movement of catheter in urethra
Gastrointestinal Tract		
Acidity of gastric secretions	Chemically destroys microorganisms incapable of surviving low pH	Administration of antacids, histamine-2 blockers
Rapid peristalsis in small intestine	Prevents retention of bacterial contents	Delayed motility from fecal impaction in large bowel or mechanical obstruction by masses
Vagina		
At puberty normal flora cause vaginal secretions to achieve low pH	Inhibits growth of many microorganisms	Antibiotics and birth control pills that disrupt normal flora

disease-producing microorganisms. The two types of aseptic technique are medical asepsis and surgical asepsis.

Medical asepsis, or clean techniques, includes procedures used to reduce the number and prevent the spread of microorganisms. Hand hygiene, use of barrier techniques such as gloving and gowning, and routine environmental cleaning are examples of medical asepsis.

Surgical asepsis, or sterile technique, includes procedures to eliminate all microorganisms from an area. **Sterilization** destroys all microorganisms and their spores (CDC, 2008).

Nurses in the operating room, in labor and delivery, and at the bedside practice sterile technique when using sterile instruments and supplies for patient care. Surgical asepsis demands the highest level of aseptic technique and requires that all areas be kept free of infectious microorganisms (Association of periOperative Nurses [AORN], 2016).

Health care workers are responsible for providing a safe environment for patients. It is easy to forget key procedural steps or take shortcuts that break aseptic procedures when rushed. For example, here is a common clinical situation: a

TABLE 14.3 INFLAMMATION

PHYSIOLOGICAL RESPONSE	SIGNS AND SYMPTOMS
Vascular and Cellular Response	
Arterioles supplying infected or injured area dilate, delivering blood and leukocytes.	Redness
Tissue necrosis causes release of histamine, bradykinin, prostaglandin, and serotonin, which increase blood vessel permeability.	Warmth, edema
Fluid, protein, and cells enter interstitial spaces to cause swelling.	Pain
WBCs enter tissues and phagocytose microorganisms. More WBCs are released into bloodstream.	WBC count normally 5000–10,000/mm^3; value increased with infection, inflammation, stress, trauma
Phagocytic release of pyrogens from bacteria occurs.	Fever
Inflammatory Exudate	
Fluid, dead cells, and WBCs form exudate at inflammatory site that later clears with lymphatic drainage.	Purulent drainage; serous or sanguineous exudates
Tissue Repair	
Healthy new cells replace damaged cells. Cells mature to take on structural characteristics and appearance of injured cells.	Tissue defects heal and close

WBC, White blood cell.

BOX 14.2 EXAMPLES OF SITES FOR AND CAUSES OF HEALTH CARE–ACQUIRED INFECTIONS

Improperly performing hand hygiene increases patient risk for all types of health care–acquired infections.

URINARY TRACT
- Unsterile insertion of urinary catheter
- Improper positioning of catheter drainage tubing
- Open drainage system
- Disconnection of catheter and tube
- Contact between drainage bag port and contaminated surface
- Improper specimen collection technique
- Obstruction or interference with urinary drainage
- Urine in catheter or drainage tube being allowed to reenter bladder (reflux)
- Repeated catheter irrigations

SURGICAL OR TRAUMATIC WOUNDS
- Improper skin preparation before surgery (i.e., shaving versus clipping hair; not performing a preoperative bath or shower)
- Failure to cleanse skin surface properly
- Failure to use aseptic technique during dressing changes
- Use of contaminated antiseptic solutions

RESPIRATORY TRACT
- Contaminated respiratory therapy equipment
- Failure to use aseptic technique while suctioning airway
- Improper disposal of secretions

BLOODSTREAM
- Contamination of IV fluids by tubing
- Adding medications to IV fluid
- Addition of connecting tube or stopcocks to IV system
- Improper care of needle insertion site
- Contaminated needles or catheters
- Failure to change IV access site when inflammation first appears
- Improper technique during administration of multiple blood products
- Improper care of peritoneal or hemodialysis shunts
- Improperly accessing an IV port

nurse removes a soiled dressing that is considered "dirty," then changes gloves without performing hand hygiene, and then proceeds to place a new sterile dressing over the wound. The shortcut was not performing hand hygiene before changing gloves.

NURSING KNOWLEDGE BASE

Body substances such as feces, urine, and wound drainage contain potentially infectious microorganisms. For this reason, health care workers are at risk for exposure to microorganisms in the hospital, long-term care, and home settings (Fiutem, 2015). Nursing science has contributed to identifying specific infection prevention practices for health care workers. These practices reduce the risk for cross-contamination and transmission to other patients when caring for a patient with a known or suspected infection (CDC, 2012).

The experience of having a serious infection creates feelings of anxiety, frustration, and loneliness in patients and/or their families (Zastrow, 2011). These feelings worsen when patients are isolated to prevent transmission of a microorganism to other patients or health care staff. Isolation disrupts normal social relationships with visitors and caregivers. Patient safety is often an additional risk for the patient on isolation precautions (Zastrow, 2011). For example, a patient with dementia is at increased risk for falling when confined in a room with the door closed. Family members sometimes fear the possibility of developing the infection and avoid contact with the patient. Some patients perceive the simple procedures of proper hand hygiene, masking, and gown and glove use as evidence of rejection. Help patients and families reduce some of these feelings by discussing the disease process and explaining isolation procedures.

Cultural, religious, or social beliefs influence how a patient reacts to an infectious disease and infection prevention. When providing culturally relevant care, increasing information improves patients' health outcomes. Social support for patients promotes their adherence to treatment. How a patient reacts to an infection or infectious disease is important for you to know in establishing a plan of care. The challenge is to identify and support behaviors that maintain human health or prevent infection.

CRITICAL THINKING

Synthesis

Patient care requires you to apply what you know about a patient, your knowledge base, experience, and critical thinking attitudes and standards. Your synthesis of this information allows you to make sound decisions as you apply the nursing process. Critical thinking synthesis involves combining all available information to obtain a clear picture of the approach needed to provide patient-centered care (Box 14.3).

Knowledge. During assessment of your patient, take into consideration your knowledge about infection and principles of infection control. Integrate knowledge from pathophysiology, microbiology, and nursing. Many factors affect the development of an infection such as one involving a surgical site. Conditions such as diabetes and obesity can delay wound healing and increase the risk for infection.

Experience. Reflect on previous clinical experiences with patients to help you recognize signs of infection and determine what interventions are appropriate. Perhaps you cared previously for a patient with diabetes or a patient who had a surgical

---

BOX 14.3 SYNTHESIS IN PRACTICE

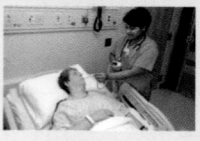

Kathy Jackson, the nursing student caring for Mrs. Eldredge, notes during her initial assessment that Mrs. Eldredge is running a low-grade fever; has a surgical wound that is edematous, warm, and erythematous; and has pain at the surgical site. Kathy remembers from a previous patient experience and her theory course work that the symptoms suggest infection. Kathy has also learned from her course work that a wound infection is not an uncommon complication after hip replacement surgery. Kathy reviews the medical record to find Mrs. Eldredge is diabetic, which Kathy has learned can delay wound healing and increase the risk for infection. After a thorough examination of the patient and medical record, Kathy applies the critical thinking attitudes of discipline and of responsibility and integrity when reporting her findings to her primary nurse. To make sure professional standards are followed, Kathy checks the organization policies and procedures for reportable signs and symptoms of infection and care of postoperative patients.

---

wound infection. Reflection on past experiences prompts you to better recognize any developing problems and to take action earlier.

Attitudes. Application of critical thinking attitudes is an important component of caring for a patient at risk for or known to have an infection. Approach patients with a confident attitude, but at the same time know your limitations and be open to the opinions of other clinicians. Apply a disciplined approach in collecting assessment information so that you can be orderly and systematic. Explore why a particular patient might have developed an infection.

Standards. You will learn to apply intellectual as well as professional standards when you care for patients. In the case of a patient suspected to have an infection, apply intellectual standards such as specificity, accuracy, and logic when assessing a patient's condition. For example, be specific in the criteria you use to assess a wound, be accurate in the way you measure wound size or depth, and use logic when assessing the patient's unique risks for infection. You will also apply professional standards in your care. Use standards of care such as the CDC (2002) guidelines for hand hygiene, the Hospital Infection Control Practices Advisory Committee (HICPAC), or the Society for Healthcare Epidemiology of America (SHEA) and the Infectious Diseases Society of America (IDSA).

NURSING PROCESS

■■■ ASSESSMENT

Nursing History. Your assessment begins with a review of all risk factors or preexisting conditions that affect a patient's susceptibility to infection and his or her current clinical status (Box 14.4). Any risk factors or conditions help you to direct your assessment. Explore these factors with a patient and integrate findings with knowledge of infection control principles. During the interview process, assess the patient's and family's knowledge of a known infection or disease to determine the course of the condition and their level of knowledge of infection control practices.

Medical History. A review of the medical history with a patient and family sometimes reveals a recent exposure to a communicable disease. By assessing existing signs and symptoms (e.g., condition of a wound, presence of fever), you determine whether a patient's clinical condition indicates the onset or extension of an infection.

Diet History. Because a patient's nutritional health directly influences susceptibility to infection, a thorough diet history is necessary. Determine a patient's normal daily nutrient intake by asking him or her to describe a typical daily meal. Also, determine whether preexisting problems such as impaired swallowing or oral pain alter food intake.

BOX 14.4   FACTORS AFFECTING SUSCEPTIBILITY TO INFECTION

AGE
- Infants have immature immune systems.
- Children acquire more immunity but are susceptible to infectious diseases such as mumps and measles if unvaccinated.
- Young and middle-aged adults have refined body system defenses and immunity.
- Older adults experience decline in immune responses, and the structure and function of major organs change (see Box 14.6).

HEREDITY
- Certain congenital and genetic chromosome disorders affect humoral or cellular immunity.
- Patients with diabetes and patients with a hereditary predisposition to diabetes are at increased risk for infections and delayed wound healing.

CULTURAL PRACTICES
- Cultural or religious beliefs or practices influence patients' decisions to seek treatment for an infection or the type of methods used to prevent infections.

NUTRITIONAL STATUS
- A reduction in protein, carbohydrates, and fats as a result of illness, inadequate diet, or debility increases a patient's susceptibility to infection and delays wound repair.

STRESS
- Increased stress elevates cortisol levels, causing decreased resistance to infection.
- Continuous stress exhausts energy stores.

REST AND EXERCISE
- Inadequate rest and exercise increase stress and decrease bodily functions such as elimination and circulation.

INADEQUATE DEFENSES
- Primary and secondary defenses can be altered by broken skin or mucosa, traumatized tissue, or suppressed immune response.

PERSONAL HABITS
- Smoking reduces respiratory ciliary action and decreases resistance to respiratory infections.
- Alcohol ingestion impairs the effect of antibiotics.
- Risky sexual behavior such as multiple sex partners increases the chance for exposure to HIV and agents of other sexually transmitted diseases.

ENVIRONMENTAL FACTORS
- Crowded living conditions and adequacy and safety of water supply influence a patient's susceptibility to infections.
- Inadequate refrigeration and cooking facilities increase a patient's exposure to foodborne illness such as salmonellosis or campylobacteriosis.

IMMUNIZATION/DISEASE HISTORY
- Patients who have not received recommended immunizations are at risk for vaccine-preventable diseases such as measles, mumps, and rubella.
- Older adults with underlying medical conditions decrease their susceptibility to influenza and pneumococcal pneumonia when they receive immunizations.

MEDICAL THERAPIES
- Certain drugs such as cortisone and certain invasive therapies such as IV catheters or surgeries increase the risk for infection.

CLINICAL APPEARANCE AND DATA
- Localized infections usually manifest with redness, swelling, and pain or tenderness. There is sometimes a purulent drainage from wounds or lesions.
- Systemic infections manifest with fever, chills, nausea and vomiting, loss of appetite, or lymph node enlargement.
- Clinical data may show an increase in WBCs, a positive culture, or an abnormal x-ray film examination.

HIV, Human immunodeficiency virus; *WBC*, white blood cell.

Laboratory Data.   Review laboratory data as soon as they are available (Table 14.4). Laboratory values such as increased WBCs and/or a positive blood culture often indicate infection. Consider the patient's age when assessing laboratory data. For example, bacterial growth in urine in an older adult without clinical symptoms does not always indicate the presence of a urinary tract infection (Rowe and Juthani-Mehta, 2013).

Psychosocial Factors.   Assess the effects that an infection has on a patient and family. Often a patient's perceptions will differ based on his or her cultural background. An infection may be perceived as a form of punishment, or it may threaten a patient's sense of remaining a productive family member. Ask a patient how the infection is affecting his or

her ability to maintain relationships and perform activities of daily living. Determine whether chronic infection has drained the patient's financial resources. When a patient is placed on isolation precautions to control the transmission of infection and is restricted to a private room, the patient is limited in being able to interact with others. Research has shown that isolation has a major impact on patients emotionally (Box 14.5). Your assessment must thoroughly examine how a patient is coping with having an infection and the related treatments. Your findings will allow you to provide appropriate supportive care and education specifically related to an infection.

Older Adult Considerations.   When a person ages, normal physiological changes occur that influence susceptibility to infection. These changes include decreased

TABLE 14.4 LABORATORY TESTS TO SCREEN FOR INFECTION

LABORATORY VALUE	NORMAL ADULT VALUES	INDICATION OF INFECTION
WBC count	5000–10,000/mm³	Increased in acute infection; decreased in certain viral or overwhelming infections
Erythrocyte sedimentation rate	Up to 15 mm/hr for men; 20 mm/hr for women	Elevated in presence of inflammatory process
Iron level	80–180 mcg/dL for men; 60–160 mcg/dL for women	Decreased in chronic infection
Blood cultures	Normally sterile, without microorganism growth	Presence of microorganism growth may indicate infection
Wound, sputum, or throat cultures	Possible normal flora	Presence of microorganism growth may indicate infection
Urinalysis	Nitrite and leukocyte negative	Nitrite and leukocyte positive; WBC count greater than 20/mm³
Differential Count (Percentage of Each Type of WBC)		
Neutrophils	55%–70%	Increased in acute infection; may be decreased in overwhelming bacterial infection (older adult)
Lymphocytes	20%–40%	Increased in chronic bacterial and viral infection; decreased in sepsis
Monocytes	2%–8%	Increased in protozoal, rickettsial, and tuberculosis infections
Eosinophils	1%–4%	Increased in parasitic infection
Basophils	0.5%–1%	Normal during infection

WBC, White blood cell.

⊕ BOX 14.5 PATIENT-CENTERED CARE

The use of isolation precautions is not new to health care. The treatment approach can be detrimental to a patient's emotional well-being and sense of identity, regardless of the individual's cultural background. Biagioli et al. (2016) reviewed qualitative studies and found that patients on isolation saw it as a source of suffering. An extensive review of the research has shown that isolation creates a negative impact on a patient's mental well-being and behavior including higher scores for depression, anxiety, and anger among isolated patients (Abad et al., 2010). In the same review of studies it was found that health care workers spend less time with patients in isolation, and patient satisfaction is adversely affected by isolation if patients are kept uninformed of their health care. In addition, isolation can pose a threat to patient safety because of supportive care failures (Abad et al., 2010).

IMPLICATIONS FOR PRACTICE

- Always assess a patient's perceptions about being placed on isolation: "How do you see yourself now that you are on isolation?" "Tell me how being on isolation makes you feel."
- Include family members (when appropriate) to determine their perceptions as well.
- When you provide care for a patient on isolation, maintain interaction as much as possible, and explain the plan of care for the day with a rationale.
- During routine rounding make it a point to ask the patient if he or she has questions about the care to be delivered, the implications, and any discharge plans.
- Encourage family visitation and be sure they understand how to follow isolation precautions (such as hand hygiene and applying gloves) correctly.

---

immunity, dry mucous membranes, decreased secretions, and decreased elasticity in tissues. As a result of these changes, older adults are predisposed to infections (Box 14.6).

Patient Expectations. Identify patients' expectations about their care during your assessment. This is especially important when a patient is placed in isolation. Some patients and their families wish to know more about the disease process, whereas others want to know only the interventions necessary to treat the infection and prevent future infections. If the infection is causing serious or debilitating symptoms, determine what expectations patients and families have

about symptom control. Then establish interventions to meet their expectations.

■ ■ ■ NURSING DIAGNOSIS

After assessment, review all your findings, analyze clusters of defining characteristics and risk factors, and select accurate and relevant nursing diagnoses. For the nursing diagnosis *Risk for Infection,* examples of risk factors include inadequate primary defenses (e.g., broken skin, stasis of body fluids), inadequate secondary defenses (e.g., decreased hemoglobin and WBCs), and chronic disease. Clusters of defining

BOX 14.6 CARE OF THE OLDER ADULT

Infection Control Considerations

- There are fewer tears to flush and remove debris from the eye and a decrease in lysozymes that affect certain microorganisms. A decreased blink reflex leads to corneal dryness. Caution patients and families to observe for eye infections and use artificial tears when necessary.
- Drying of the oral mucosa and recession and weakening of gingival tissues require frequent oral hygiene and regular dental care.
- Increased chest diameter and rigidity, weakened cough, decreased ability to swallow, and decreased elastic tissue surrounding alveoli predispose older adults to ventilatory problems and difficulty handling lung secretions. Good pulmonary hygiene (frequent coughing and deep-breathing exercises, positioning to enhance ventilatory movement, early ambulation, and oral hygiene with chlorhexidine gluconate reduce risk of aspiration and postoperative pneumonia).
- Decreased production of digestive juices and a reduction in intestinal motility affect removal of potential pathogens in the bowel. Patients and families should learn about safe food preparation and eat foods that are nutritionally good and easy to digest. Provide smaller meals more frequently.
- Thinning of the dermal and epidermal skin layers, along with a decrease in skin elasticity, predisposes older adults to skin tearing. Meticulous nursing care is necessary to prevent pressure injuries in bedridden patients (see Chapter 38).
- Production of T and B lymphocytes is decreased. With reduced immunity it is important for older adults to receive regular immunizations and medical checkups.

Data from Roach R: Geriatrics. In Grota P, editor: *APIC text of infection control and epidemiology*, ed 4, Washington, DC, 2015, Association for Professionals in Infection Control and Epidemiology (APIC).

characteristics lead to the selection of a problem-focused nursing diagnosis such as *Impaired Skin Integrity*. The related factors, revealed in the assessment, ensure individualization of the diagnosis.

An accurate related or risk factor ensures a more relevant and thorough care plan. For example, a patient with a decreased WBC count, multiple IV catheters, and inflammation around a single catheter site would have a diagnosis of *Risk for Infection*. The risk factor, *IV catheter placement*, directs you to change the catheter regularly and take measures to minimize microorganism transfer through the IV system such as scrubbing the hub of the catheter before accessing the IV line to give medication (O'Grady et al., 2011).

A number of nursing diagnoses have infection or its associated treatment and/or clinical signs as the related factor. In the case of the problem-focused diagnosis *Social Isolation*, the related factor is sometimes the isolation precautions used for infection control. In this example you would direct nursing interventions at minimizing the effects that isolation has on

the patient's emotional health and ability to socialize. Other nursing diagnoses for patients susceptible to or affected by infection include:

- *Disturbed Body Image*
- *Delayed Surgical Recovery*
- *Risk for Infection*
- *Imbalanced Nutrition: Less Than Body Requirements*
- *Acute Pain*
- *Impaired Skin Integrity*
- *Risk for Impaired Skin Integrity*

Early recognition of infection helps you make the correct nursing diagnoses and establish a treatment plan. In addition, alert other members of the health care team to the need for further investigation of a patient's condition, facilitating initiation of prompt therapy and barrier protection (i.e., use of gloves, masks, and gowns). Because of increased attention to the prevention of infection, the CDC (2007) and Occupational Safety and Health Administration (OSHA, 2003) have stressed the importance of barrier protection.

■ ■ ■ PLANNING

The presence of an actual infection poses a collaborative problem requiring your intervention. Objective data such as an elevated temperature, open draining wound, inflammation of a wound site, and laboratory values revealing an increased WBC count indicate an actual infection. Subjective findings include the patient's complaint of chills, malaise, or tenderness at the wound site. Collaborate with other health care providers and registered dietitians in monitoring the infection and planning therapies such as an increased protein diet, antibiotic administration, and wound care and then implement appropriate infection prevention and control measures.

Develop a plan of care for a patient that incorporates the different nursing diagnoses, with diagnoses prioritized. As you develop goals and outcomes, include a plan for care following discharge.

Goals and Outcomes. Determine goals and outcomes based on the patient's preferences and the identified nursing diagnoses. For example, if your patient has the diagnosis *Risk for Infection*, you set a goal of "Patient will remain free from infection during hospitalization." Related outcomes might include "Wound site will remain closed and without drainage" and "Patient will change own dressing using sterile technique in 2 days." Once goals and outcomes are set, you identify the evidence-based interventions to resolve the nursing diagnoses.

Setting Priorities. Set the priorities for nursing interventions for your patient's plan of care. Give special attention to any urgent needs that an infection creates. For example, if a patient's infection becomes systemic, management of fever and prevention of dehydration are priorities. Once an infection begins to resolve, focus priorities on patient education and emotional support.

Collaborative Care. Collaborate with other members of the health care team such as a wound care nurse, clinical nurse specialist, dietitian, or social worker in your patient's care. Often the health problems associated with infection will require the involvement of different professional disciplines. It is also important that a patient's required level of care be maintained after discharge. Your assessment will determine if the patient, family, and other caregivers are able to provide care at home. Thus during planning, be sure you have arranged for the resources the patient and family will require, such as home care or home durable medical equipment.

■■■ IMPLEMENTATION

The nursing interventions that you select for a patient's plan of care will focus on the control and prevention of infection. Many of the interventions are applicable for all types of health care settings, including a patient's home.

Health Promotion. Prevention is key to reducing infections in all health care settings. Review with and teach patients and their family caregivers measures that strengthen the host's defenses such as nutrition, recommended immunizations, personal hygiene, and regular rest and exercise (Box 14.7). In addition, explain infection prevention and control principles such as hand hygiene and methods for disposing of medical waste that are designed to prevent infections from occurring. Based on your assessment of a patient's cultural views and preferences, integrate infection prevention and control measures into the patient's cultural practices.

Nutrition. Nutrition has a major influence on resistance to infection. Nutritional requirements vary depending on age, health status, and other variables. A proper diet helps the immune system function and consists of a variety of foods from all food groups (see Chapter 35). Provide education strategies specific to a patient's learning needs; for example, have the patient create a meal plan with proper foods high in protein, vitamins C and A, and zinc, and offer a teaching brochure written in plain language. Collaborate with registered dietitians as needed. Cultural considerations such as food selection and method of preparation are critical in influencing a patient's nutritional status. Teach the patient the importance a proper diet plays in maintaining immunity and preventing infection. Incorporate the patient's food preferences when possible.

Hygiene. One infection prevention and control goal of personal hygiene is to reduce microorganisms on the skin and maintain the well-being of mucous membranes such as the mouth and vagina (Fiutem, 2015). Patients need to understand the techniques for cleansing the skin and how to avoid spread of microorganisms in body secretions or excretions. This type of information is easily explained during a bath or when you are assisting with personal hygiene. For example, teach female patients how to wash their perineum from clean to dirty, from the urethra down toward the rectum, using a clean washcloth (see Chapter 31). Also instruct patients on how to perform and maintain good oral hygiene.

BOX 14.7 PATIENT TEACHING
Infection Prevention and Control

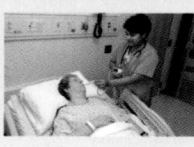 Mrs. Eldredge is nearing discharge. Kathy develops a teaching plan to help Mrs. Eldredge understand how to perform dressing changes, improve resistance to infection, and prevent exposure to further infection at home.

OUTCOME
Mrs. Eldredge changes her dressing using proper infection prevention and control techniques.

TEACHING STRATEGIES
- Demonstrate proper hand hygiene. Instruct Mrs. Eldredge to perform hand hygiene before and after all wound care and after touching infected body fluids.
- Instruct Mrs. Eldredge about the signs and symptoms of wound infection and when to notify the health care provider.
- Instruct Mrs. Eldredge to place contaminated dressings and other disposable items containing infectious body fluids in impervious plastic or brown paper bags.
- Instruct Mrs. Eldredge to clean noticeably soiled linen separate from other laundry. Wash in warm water with detergent. There are no special recommendations for setting dryer temperature.

EVALUATION
- Use the principles of teach-back to evaluate patient/family caregiver learning:
  - "Tell me the signs that we discussed that suggest your infection is spreading."
  - "I want to be sure you understand the steps we reviewed for how to correctly change your dressing. Let's take the time now for you to show me how to change your dressing."

Immunization. Immunization programs for infants and children have decreased the occurrence of many childhood diseases such as diphtheria, whooping cough, and measles. More recently developed vaccines for hepatitis A and chickenpox (varicella) provide immunity to both adults and children for highly communicable diseases (Kak, 2014). In addition, specific vaccines such as influenza and pneumococcal vaccines have decreased the mortality and morbidity previously seen in older adults or patients with underlying medical problems such as chronic lung disease (CLD). Despite the overwhelming evidence of vaccine safety, suspicion and misconception exist in small groups of hesitant or resistant parents, often leading to outbreaks of vaccine-preventable infections (Anderson, 2015). Research supports the concept that primary care providers such as nurse practitioners can promote acceptance of vaccination in most hesitant parents by building trustworthy relationships and being as transparent as possible with information (Dubé et al., 2013; Gowda and Dempsey, 2013). Advise patients about the advantages of immunizations; also make them aware of the contraindications for certain vaccines, especially in pregnant or lactating women. You can access the most current immunization schedule at https://www.cdc.gov/vaccines/acip/index.html.

Adequate Rest and Regular Exercise. Adequate rest (see Chapter 33) and regular exercise (see Chapter 28) help prevent infection. Physical exercise increases lung capacity, circulation, energy, and endurance. It also decreases stress and improves appetite, sleeping, and elimination. Balance the need for regular exercise with the need for rest and sleep. Some patients need education about the importance of sleep and rest for infection prevention.

Acute Care. A patient with an infection has many needs. By monitoring the course of an infection carefully, you can choose the most appropriate measures to maintain or restore a patient's health. Good hand hygiene is one of the best medically aseptic ways to control the spread of microorganisms. Disinfection and sterilization of supplies are examples of sterile aseptic methods used to control the spread of microorganisms.

When a patient develops an infection, continue preventive care to reduce the risk for transmission to health care workers and other patients. Good hand hygiene and use of barriers such as gloves, masks, and gowns minimize exposure to infection. These measures are known as standard precautions, which you use with every patient regardless of diagnosis. Patients with communicable diseases and infections that are easily transmissible to others require special isolation precautions called transmission-based precautions (CDC, 2007). Isolation precautions involve control of a patient's environment by forming barriers against bacterial spread.

Treatment of an infection includes identification and elimination of the organism and support of a patient's defenses. Nurses collect specimens of body fluids or drainage from infected body sites and send the specimens to the laboratory for cultures. When the causative organism is identified, the health care provider usually prescribes an antimicrobial. Administer antibiotics carefully, watching for allergic reactions and assessing the effect on the patient's infection. It is important to teach patients the importance of taking all antibiotics as ordered when discharged home.

Systemic infections (i.e., infections that affect the body as a whole) require measures to manage or prevent the complications of fever (see Chapter 15). Drinking fluids regularly prevents dehydration resulting from diaphoresis. Increased metabolism requires an adequate nutritional intake. Rest preserves energy for the healing process.

Localized infections often require measures to facilitate removal of infectious organisms such as using moist dressings or irrigating wounds (see Chapter 38) to remove infected drainage from wound sites. Applying warm compresses helps blood flow to an infected site, thus delivering components of the blood needed to fight an infection. Use medical and surgical aseptic techniques to manage wounds and handle infected drainage or body fluids correctly.

During any infection, support a patient's body defense mechanisms. For example, when a patient has diarrhea, cleanse and dry the skin promptly to prevent breakdown.

Medical Asepsis. Basic medical aseptic techniques break the infection chain. Use these techniques for all patients, even when no infection is diagnosed. Aggressive preventive measures are highly effective in reducing HAIs.

Control or Elimination of Infectious Agents. With the common use of disposable equipment, nurses are sometimes less aware of disinfection and sterilization procedures. The proper cleaning, disinfection, and sterilization of contaminated objects (e.g., surgical instruments or blood pressure cuffs) significantly reduce and/or eliminate microorganisms (CDC, 2008; Rutala and Weber, 2015).

Cleaning. Cleaning involves removing organic material such as blood or inorganic material such as soil from objects. For example, nurses will often clean the surfaces of bed mattresses when there has been excess soiling. Generally this involves the use of soap and water and proper mechanical scrubbing action. Cleaning occurs before disinfection and sterilization procedures (CDC, 2008; Rutala and Weber, 2015). Best practice recommends that surfaces should be physically clean before disinfection for any disinfectant to be effective (Royal College of Nursing, 2011). Check the policy of the health care agency before cleaning. In most institutions, technicians clean equipment. When cleaning objects soiled with blood or body fluids, use personal protective equipment (PPE) such as gloves, goggles, and mask to protect yourself from splashing fluids.

Disinfection and Sterilization. Disinfection and sterilization use both physical and chemical processes. Both processes disrupt the internal functioning of microorganisms by destroying cell proteins. Disinfection eliminates almost all pathogenic organisms, with the exception of bacterial spores. Nurses commonly use disposable disinfectant cloths (e.g., alcohols and bleach) to wipe off soiled surfaces such as bedside tables and the outer surfaces of equipment. The solutions in these cloths have exposure or dwell times needed for a disinfectant to achieve full efficacy. How well a disinfectant is applied over a surface also affects efficacy (Royal College of Nursing, 2011). There are cloths with solutions specific for destroying certain microorganisms. For example, *Clostridium difficile* is one of the most difficult microorganisms to kill and is becoming a common HAI. The only disinfectants that work against *C. difficile* are accelerated hydrogen peroxide and bleach-based products.

Sterilization eliminates or destroys all forms of microbial life including spores (Rutala and Weber, 2015). Sterilization methods include processing items using steam, dry heat, hydrogen peroxide plasma, or ethylene oxide (ETO). The level of disinfection and sterilization required depends on the type and use of the contaminated item (Box 14.8). Always check package integrity and/or expiration dates before using an object designated as sterile. Dispose of items not meeting the criteria for being sterile or return them to the sterilization-processing department (CDC, 2008).

Control or Elimination of Reservoirs. To control or eliminate infection in reservoir sites, eliminate sources of

BOX 14.8   **CATEGORIES OF ITEMS REQUIRING STERILIZATION, DISINFECTION, AND CLEANING**

CRITICAL ITEMS

Items that enter sterile tissue or the vascular system present a high risk for infection if they are contaminated with microorganisms, especially bacterial spores. *Critical* items must be *sterile.* Some of these items include:

- Surgical instruments
- Cardiac or intravascular catheters
- Surgical implants

SEMICRITICAL ITEMS

Items that come in contact with mucous membranes or nonintact skin also present a risk. These objects must be free of all microorganisms (except bacterial spores). *Semicritical items* must be *high-level disinfected (HLD)* or *sterilized.* Some of these items include:

- Respiratory and anesthesia equipment
- Endoscopes
- Endotracheal tubes
- Gastrointestinal endoscopes
- Diaphragm fitting rings

After rinsing, items must be dried and stored in a manner to protect from damage and contamination.

NONCRITICAL ITEMS

Items that come in contact with intact skin but not mucous membranes must be clean. *Noncritical items* must be *disinfected.* Some of these items include:

- Bedpans
- Blood pressure cuffs
- Bed rails
- Linens
- Stethoscopes
- Bedside trays and patient furniture
- Food utensils

BOX 14.9   **INFECTION PREVENTION AND CONTROL TO REDUCE RESERVOIRS OF INFECTION**

BATHING

- Use soap and water to remove drainage, dried secretions, or excess perspiration.

DRESSING CHANGES

- Change dressings that become wet and/or soiled (see Chapter 38).

CONTAMINATED ARTICLES

- Place tissues, soiled dressings, or soiled linen in fluid-resistant bags for proper disposal.

CONTAMINATED SHARPS

- Place all needles—safety needles and needleless systems—into puncture-proof containers located at the site of use. Federal law requires use of needle safety technology. Blood tube holders are single use only (OSHA, 2015).

BEDSIDE UNIT

- Keep table surfaces clean and dry.

BOTTLED SOLUTIONS

- Do not leave bottled solutions open.
- Keep solutions tightly capped.
- Date bottles when opened and discard in 24 hours.

SURGICAL WOUNDS

- Keep drainage tubes and collection bags patent to prevent accumulation of serous fluid under skin surface.

DRAINAGE BOTTLES AND BAGS

- Wear gloves and protective eyewear if splashing or spraying with contaminated blood or body fluids is anticipated.
- Empty and dispose of drainage suction bottles according to agency policy.
- Empty all drainage systems on each shift unless otherwise ordered by health care provider.
- Never raise drainage system (e.g., urinary drainage bag) above level of site being drained unless it is clamped off.

body fluids, drainage, or solutions that possibly harbor microorganisms. For example, carefully discard disposable articles that become contaminated with infectious material in the proper receptacles (Box 14.9).

Control of Portals of Exit. To control organisms exiting through the respiratory tract, it is important to avoid talking, sneezing, or coughing directly over a surgical wound or sterile dressing field. Also teach patients to protect others when they sneeze or cough and give patients disposable wipes or tissues to control spread of microorganisms. Try not to work with patients who are highly susceptible to infection if you have a cold or other communicable infection.

Another way of controlling the exit of microorganisms is by using standard precautions when handling body fluids such as urine, feces, and wound drainage. Wear clean gloves if there is a chance of contact with any blood or body fluids and perform hand hygiene after providing care. Be sure to bag contaminated items appropriately.

Control of Transmission. Effective infection prevention and control requires knowledge of the modes of transmission of microorganisms and the methods of control. In any health care setting, a patient usually has a personal set of care items. Sharing graduated containers for measuring urine, bath basins, and eating utensils among patients creates routes for transmission of infection. Research supports that the contamination level of a stethoscope is substantial. When using a stethoscope, always wipe off the bell, diaphragm, and ear tips with a disinfectant such as an alcohol wipe before proceeding to the next patient (Longin et al., 2014).

Because certain microorganisms travel easily through the air, do not shake linens or bedclothes. Dust surfaces within a patient's room with a treated or dampened cloth to prevent dust particles from entering the air.

To prevent transmission of microorganisms through indirect contact, do not allow soiled items and equipment to touch your clothing. A common error is to carry dirty linen in the arms against the uniform. Use special linen bags or carry soiled linen with the hands held out from the body. Never put clean or soiled linens on the floor.

Hand Hygiene. The most effective basic technique in preventing and controlling transmission of infection is hand hygiene (Box 14.10). Hand hygiene is a general term that applies to four techniques: handwashing, antiseptic hand wash, antiseptic hand rub, and surgical hand antisepsis. Handwashing is defined by the CDC (2009) as the vigorous, brief rubbing together of all surfaces of lathered hands, followed by rinsing under a stream of warm water. The fundamental principle behind handwashing is removal of microorganisms mechanically from the hands and rinsing with water. Handwashing with soap and water does not kill microorganisms but does remove visible soiling of the hands.

An antiseptic hand wash involves handwashing with warm water and an antiseptic agent. Some antiseptics kill bacteria and some viruses. An antiseptic hand rub involves applying an antiseptic hand-rub product to all surfaces of the hands to reduce the number of microorganisms present. An alcohol-based hand sanitizer is the preferred method for cleaning the hands when working in a health care agency when the hands are not visibly dirty (CDC, 2016b). Ethanol-based hand antiseptics containing 60% to 90% alcohol appear to be the most effective against common pathogens found on the hands (CDC, 2009). Alcohol-based products are more effective for standard handwashing or hand antisepsis (nonsoiled hands) by health care workers than regular soap or antimicrobial soaps (CDC, 2002). Surgical hand antisepsis is an antiseptic hand-wash or hand-rub technique that surgical personnel

---

BOX 14.10 PROCEDURAL GUIDELINES

View Video!

Hand Hygiene

DELEGATION CONSIDERATIONS

The skill of hand hygiene is performed by all caregivers. *Hand hygiene is not optional.*

EQUIPMENT

Alcohol-based waterless antiseptic containing emollients or antimicrobial or nonantimicrobial soap, easy-to-reach sink with warm running water, paper towels or air dryer, and disposable nail cleaner *(optional).*

STEPS

1. Inspect surface of hands for breaks or cuts in skin or cuticles. Cover any skin lesions with a dressing before providing care. If lesions are too large to cover, you may be restricted from direct patient care.
2. Inspect hands for visible soiling.
3. Inspect condition of nails. Natural tips should be no longer than 0.625 cm (¼ inch) long. Be sure that fingernails are short, filed, and smooth. If nails are polished, there should be no chips, and artificial nails or applications are contraindicated.
4. Push wristwatch and long uniform sleeves above wrists. Avoid wearing rings. If worn, remove during hand hygiene.

5. **Antiseptic hand rub**
   a. According to manufacturer directions dispense ample amount of alcohol-based waterless antiseptic product into palm of one hand (usually an amount the size of a dime) (see illustration).
   b. Rub hands together, covering all surfaces of hands and fingers with antiseptic (see illustration).
   c. Rub hands together for 30 seconds to allow your hands to completely absorb the product and the hand sanitizer to completely dry. Allow hands to completely dry before applying gloves. If it takes less than 30 seconds for hands to dry, you likely have not used enough antiseptic.
6. **Handwashing using antimicrobial soap**
   a. Stand in front of sink, keeping hands and uniform away from sink surface. (If hands touch sink during handwashing, repeat sequence.)
   b. Turn on water. Turn faucet on (see illustration) or push knee pedals laterally or press pedals with foot to regulate flow and temperature.
   c. Avoid splashing water against uniform.
   d. Regulate flow of water so that temperature is warm.

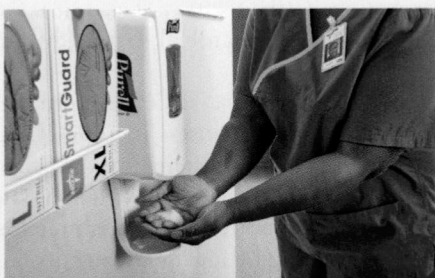

STEP 5a Apply waterless antiseptic to hands.

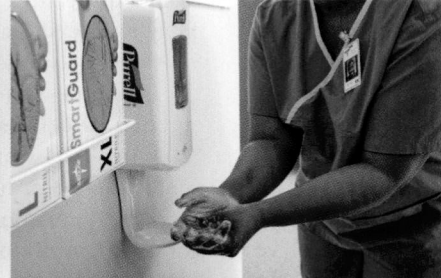

STEP 5b Rub hands thoroughly, making sure to cover all surfaces of the fingers and hands.

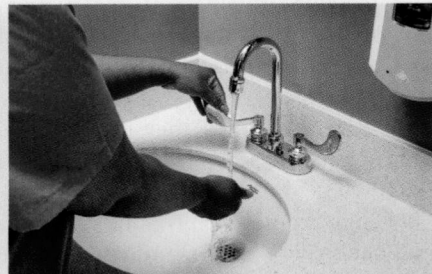

STEP 6b Regulate flow of water.

Continued

BOX 14.10   PROCEDURAL GUIDELINES—cont'd

View Video!

Hand Hygiene

e. Wet hands and wrists thoroughly under running water. Keep hands and forearms lower than elbows during washing.

f. Apply 3 to 5 mL of antiseptic soap and rub hands together (see illustration).

Clinical Decision Point. The most effective basic technique in preventing and controlling transmission of infection is hand hygiene (CDC, 2002).

---

g. Perform hand hygiene using plenty of lather and friction for at least 15 to 20 seconds, making sure you clean all areas of the hands (CDC, 2016b). A tip is to sing the "Happy Birthday" song twice. Interlace fingers and rub palms and back of hands with circular motion at least five times each using friction. Keep fingertips down to facilitate removal of microorganisms.

h. Areas underlying fingernails are often soiled. Clean them with fingernails of other hand and additional soap or with disposable nail cleaner.

i. Rinse hands and wrists thoroughly, keeping hands down and elbows up (see illustration).

j. Dry hands thoroughly from fingers to wrists with paper towel, single-use cloth, or warm air dryer.

k. If used, discard paper towel in proper receptacle.

l. To turn off hand faucet, use clean, dry paper towel; avoid touching handles with hands (see illustration). Turn off water with foot or knee pedals (if applicable).

m. If hands are dry or chapped, use a small amount of lotion or barrier cream dispensed from an individual use container.

7. Inspect surface of hands for obvious signs of dirt or other contaminants.

8. Inspect hands for dermatitis or cracked skin.

9. **Use Teach-Back:** "I want to be sure you remember what we discussed earlier. Explain to me when you and your family should wash your hands at home." Revise your instruction now or develop a plan for revised patient/family caregiver teaching if patient/family caregiver is not able to teach back correctly.

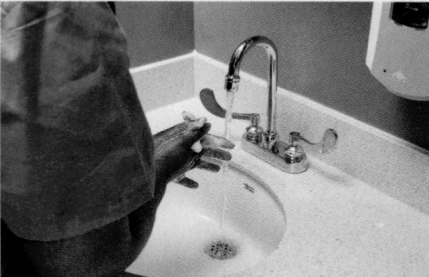

STEP 6f Wet hands; apply soap and lather hands thoroughly.

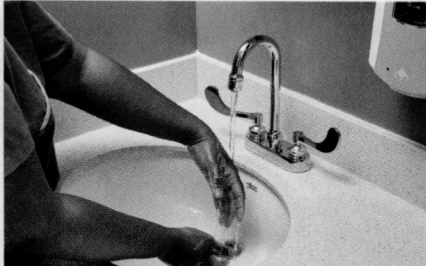

STEP 6i Rinse hands.

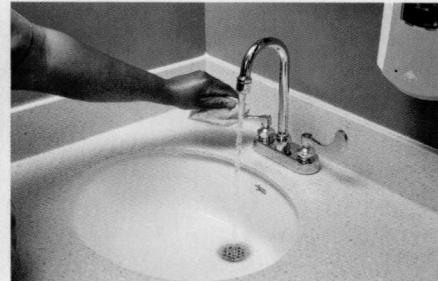

STEP 6l Turn off faucet with clean, dry paper towel.

---

perform before surgery to eliminate transient hand flora and reduce resident flora. Antiseptic detergent preparations have persistent antimicrobial activity (CDC, 2002; World Health Organization [WHO], 2009).

Alcohol-based hand antiseptics are not effective on hands that are visibly dirty or are contaminated with organic materials (Haas, 2015). Thus when hands are visibly dirty or contaminated with proteinaceous material or visibly soiled with blood or other body fluids, wash them with either plain soap or an antimicrobial soap and water. Handwashing is also indicated before eating and after using the toilet. Wash hands with soap and water if they are exposed to spore-forming organisms such as *C. difficile or Bacillus anthracis* (Box 14.11) (CDC, 2008).

If hands are not visibly soiled, you may use an alcohol-based hand rub to decontaminate the hands during the Five Moments for Hand Hygiene (World Health Organization [WHO], 2017):

1. Before touching a patient
2. Before clean/aseptic procedures (e.g., insertion of invasive devices, hygiene care)

3. After body fluid exposure/risk (e.g., contact during bathing, dressing changes, specimen collection)
4. After touching a patient
5. After touching patient surroundings (e.g., overbed table, bed linen, IV pump)

This evidence-based, field-tested, user-centered approach is designed to be easy to learn, logical, and applicable to a wide range of health care settings (WHO, 2017) (Fig. 14.3). You may also wash hands with an antimicrobial soap and water in these situations.

Isolation and Barrier Protection. HICPAC published revised guidelines for isolation precautions in 2007 (CDC, 2007). HICPAC recommends that agencies modify these guidelines according to need and as dictated by federal, state, or local regulations. The guidelines contain recommendations for respiratory hygiene/cough etiquette as part of standard precautions. The CDC recommendations contain two tiers of precautions (Table 14.5). The first and most important tier is called standard precautions; the CDC designed it to be used for care of all patients, in all settings, regardless of risk or presumed infection status. Standard precautions are

BOX 14.11 EVIDENCE-BASED PRACTICE

PICO Question: With hospitalized patients diagnosed with *Clostridium difficile,* does the use of soap and water before and after patient care compared with the use of alcohol-based hand gels before and after patient care decrease the transmission of *C. difficile* to other patients cared for by the same health care personnel?

SUMMARY OF EVIDENCE

Although many types of health care–associated infections (HAIs) are declining, an infection caused by *C. difficile* remains at historically high levels. *C. difficile* is a spore-forming, gram-positive anaerobic bacillus that produces two exotoxins: toxin A and toxin B. It is a common cause of antibiotic-associated diarrhea and is linked to 14,000 deaths in the United States each year (Surawizc et al., 2013). People most at risk are individuals, especially older adults, who take antibiotics and receive medical care. When a person takes antibiotics, normal flora that protect against infection are destroyed for several months. During this time, patients can get sick from *C. difficile* picked up from contaminated surfaces or spread from a health care provider's hands. Evidence shows that alcohol is ineffective in killing *C. difficile* spores. Handwashing with soap and water has the greatest efficacy in removing spores from hands. Thus evidence supports the use of soap and water over the use of alcohol-based hand rubs when contact with *C. difficile* is suspected or likely (Surawizc et al., 2013). The use of gloves by health care workers prevents the contamination of hands with *C. difficile* spores (Edmunds et al., 2013).

APPLICATION TO NURSING PRACTICE

- Use soap and water for hand hygiene when caring for a patient diagnosed with *C. difficile* to remove organisms from the hands.
- Apply gloves before entering the room of a patient with *C. difficile*, and remove gloves properly after care.
- Perform hand hygiene before and after wearing gloves.
- Proper hand hygiene helps to prevent transmission of infections to other patients of health care workers.

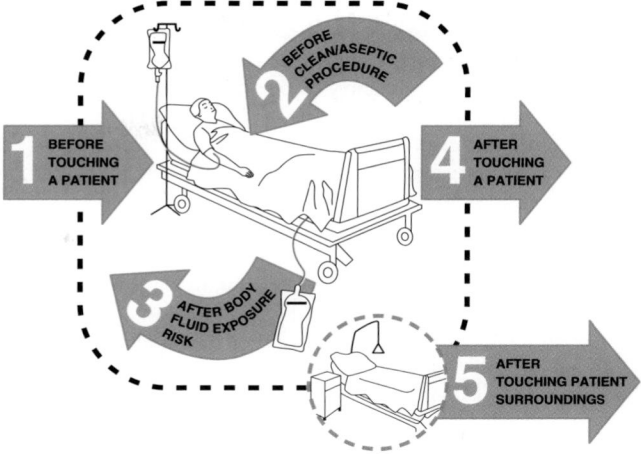

FIG 14.3 Five Moments for Hand Hygiene. (From World Health Organization: *About SAVE Lives: Clean Your Hands: 5 moments for hand hygiene,* 2017, http://www.who.int/gpsc/5may/background/5moments/en/.)

priate protection regardless of the presence of known respiratory infection.

The second tier of precautions (see Table 14.5) includes precautions designed for the care of patients who are known or suspected to be infected or colonized with microorganisms transmitted by the droplet, airborne, or contact route (CDC, 2007; Berends and Walesa, 2015). There are three types of transmission-based precautions: airborne precautions, droplet precautions, and contact precautions. They are used singly or in combination for diseases that have multiple routes of transmission (e.g., chickenpox). Use them in addition to standard precautions.

One important aspect of care for patients on isolation is compliance with hand hygiene and changing gloves between exposure to body sites and patient equipment. Inadequate glove changes and hand hygiene often lead to contamination of previously colonized sites (Haas, 2015). Noncompliance with these practices increases the risk of HAIs.

Because of the resurgence of tuberculosis (TB), the CDC (2005) developed guidelines to prevent its transmission to health care workers and stresses the importance of isolation for patients with known or suspected TB in a special negative-pressure room. Close the doors to the patient's room to control direction of airflow. Wear a special high-filtration particulate respirator on entering a respiratory isolation room. Health care organizations must provide fit-testing to be sure a respirator fits each health care worker with different facial sizes and characteristics (OSHA, n.d.). When worn correctly, particulate respirators and masks (Figs. 14.4 and 14.5) have a tighter face seal and filter at a higher level than routine surgical masks (OSHA, 2009).

Multidrug-resistant organisms (MDROs) such as methicillin-resistant *Staphylococcus aureus* (MRSA) and vancomycin-resistant enterococcus (VRE) have become more common as a cause of colonization and HAIs. MDROs are

the primary strategies for prevention of infection transmission and apply to contact with blood, body fluids, nonintact skin, mucous membranes, and equipment or surfaces contaminated with these potentially infectious materials. The strategy of respiratory hygiene/cough etiquette applies to any person with signs of respiratory infection including cough, congestion, rhinorrhea, or increased production of respiratory secretions when entering a health care site. Educating health care staff, patients, and visitors to cover the mouth and nose with a tissue when coughing, dispose properly of used tissues, and perform hand hygiene is among the elements of respiratory hygiene. These precautions protect patients and health care workers (Box 14.12).

Assess the need for standard precautions based on the potential for transmission of infection, regardless of a patient's diagnosis. For example, when suctioning a patient with a tracheostomy, wearing gloves, eyewear, and a mask is appro-

Text continued on p. 256

TABLE 14.5   CENTERS FOR DISEASE CONTROL AND PREVENTION ISOLATION GUIDELINES

Standard Precautions (Tier 1) for Use With All Patients

- Standard precautions apply to blood, blood products, all body fluids, secretions, excretions (except sweat), nonintact skin, and mucous membranes.
- Perform hand hygiene before, after, and between direct contact with patients. (Examples of between contact: cleaning hands after a patient care activity, moving to a non–patient care activity, then cleaning hands again before returning to perform patient contact.)
- Perform hand hygiene after contact with blood, body fluids, secretions, and excretions; after contact with surfaces or articles in a patient's room; and immediately after gloves are removed.
- When hands are visibly soiled or contaminated with blood or body fluids, wash them with either a nonantimicrobial soap or an antimicrobial soap and water.
- When hands are not visibly soiled or contaminated with blood or body fluids, use an alcohol-based hand rub to perform hand hygiene.
- Wash hands with antimicrobial soap and water if contact with spores (e.g., *Clostridium difficile*) is likely to have occurred.
- Do not wear artificial fingernails or extenders if duties include direct contact with patients at high risk for infection and associated adverse outcomes.
- Wear gloves when touching blood, body fluids, secretions, excretions, nonintact skin, mucous membranes, or contaminated items or surfaces. Remove gloves and perform hand hygiene between patient care encounters and when going from a contaminated to a clean body site.
- Wear PPE when the anticipated patient interaction indicates that contact with blood or body fluids may occur.
- A private room is unnecessary unless the patient's hygiene is unacceptable (e.g., uncontained secretions, excretions, or wound drainage).
- Discard all contaminated sharp instruments and needles in a puncture-resistant container. Health care agencies must make needleless devices available. Any needles should be disposed of uncapped, or a mechanical safety device is activated for recapping.
- Respiratory hygiene/cough etiquette: Have patients cover the nose/mouth when coughing or sneezing; use tissues to contain respiratory secretions, and dispose of in nearest waste container; perform hand hygiene after contacting respiratory secretions and contaminated object/materials; contain respiratory secretions with procedure or surgical masks; sit at least 3 feet away from others if coughing.

Transmission-Based Precautions (Tier 2) for Use With Specific Types of Patients

CATEGORY	DISEASE	BARRIER PROTECTION
Airborne precautions (droplet nuclei smaller than 5 microns)	Measles, chickenpox (varicella), disseminated varicella zoster, pulmonary or laryngeal tuberculosis	Private room, negative-pressure airflow of at least 6–12 exchanges per hour via HEPA filtration Mask or respiratory protection device, n95 respirator (depending on condition)
Droplet precautions (droplets larger than 5 microns; being within 3 feet of the patient)	Examples include *Bordetella pertussis,* influenza virus, adenovirus, rhinovirus, *Neisseria meningitidis,* group A streptococcus (until first 24 h of antimicrobial therapy); refer to agency policy	Private room or cohort patients Mask or respirator required depending on condition (refer to agency policy)
Contact precautions (direct patient or environmental contact)	Colonization or infection with multidrug-resistant organisms such as VRE and MRSA, *Clostridium difficile, Shigella,* and other enteric pathogens; major wound infections; herpes simplex; scabies; varicella zoster (disseminated); respiratory syncytial virus in infants, young children, or immunocompromised adults	Private room or cohort patients (see agency policy), gloves, gowns (patients may leave their room for procedures or therapy if infectious material contained or covered, placed in a clean gown, and if hands are cleaned)
Protective environment	Allogeneic hematopoietic stem cell transplants	Private room; positive-pressure airflow with 12 or more air exchanges per hour; HEPA filtration for incoming air Mask to be worn by patient when out of room during times of construction in area

HEPA, High-efficiency particulate air; *MRSA,* methicillin-resistant *Staphylococcus aureus; PPE,* personal protective equipment; *VRE,* vancomycin-resistant enterococci.
Modified from Centers for Disease Control and Prevention, Hospital Infection Control Practice Advisory Committee: 2007 Guideline for isolation precautions in hospitals, *MMWR Morb Mortal Wkly Rep* 57(RR-16):39, 2007.

BOX 14.12 **PROCEDURAL GUIDELINES**

Caring for a Patient on Isolation Precautions

DELEGATION AND COLLABORATION

The skill of caring for patients on isolation precautions can be delegated to nursing assistive personnel (NAP). However, the nurse must assess the patient's status and the isolation indications. The nurse instructs the NAP about:

- The reason patient is on isolation precautions.
- Precautions for bringing equipment into a patient's room.
- Special precautions regarding individual patient needs such as transportation to diagnostic tests.

EQUIPMENT

Personal protective equipment (PPE) determined by type of isolation required; clean gloves, mask, eyewear or goggles, face shield, and gown (gowns may be disposable or reusable, depending on agency policy); other patient care equipment (as appropriate; e.g., hygiene items, medications, dressing supplies, sharps container, disposable blood pressure cuff); soiled linen bag and trash receptacle, sign for door indicating type of isolation and/or for visitors to come to the nurses' station before entering room. Tuberculosis (TB) isolation: room with negative airflow, N95 or P100 respirator.

STEPS

1. Assess patient's medical history for possible indications for isolation (e.g., risk factors for TB, major draining wound, or purulent productive cough). Review precautions for the specific isolation system, including appropriate barriers to apply (see Table 14.5).
2. Review laboratory test results (e.g., wound culture, acid-fast bacillus [AFB] smears, changes in white blood cell [WBC] count).
3. Review agency policies and isolation precautions necessary for type of isolation ordered, and consider types of care measures that you will perform while in patient's room (e.g., medication administration or dressing change).
4. Review nursing care plan notes or confer with colleagues regarding patient's emotional state and reaction/adjustment to isolation. Also assess patient's understanding of purpose of isolation.
5. Assess whether patient has a known latex allergy. If an allergy is present, refer to agency policy and resources available to provide full latex-free care.
6. Perform hand hygiene (see Box 14.10).
7. Prepare all equipment to be taken into patient's room. In many cases dedicated equipment such as stethoscopes, blood pressure equipment, and thermometers should remain in the room until patient is discharged. If patient is infected or colonized with a resistant organism (e.g., vancomycin-resistant enterococcus [VRE], methicillin-resistant *Staphylococcus aureus* [MRSA]), equipment remains in room and is thoroughly disinfected before removal from room (see agency policy).
8. Prepare for entrance into isolation room. Ideally, before applying PPE, step into patient's room and stay by door. Introduce yourself and explain the care that you are providing. If this is not possible, apply PPE outside of the room.
   a. Apply cover gown, being sure that it covers all outer garments. Pull sleeves down to wrist. Tie securely at neck and waist (see illustration).

   b. Apply either surgical mask or a fitted respirator around mouth and nose (type and fit-testing depend on type of isolation and agency policy). You must have a medical evaluation and be fit-tested before using a respirator mask. You are allowed to pick the most acceptable respirator from a sufficient number of respirator models and sizes so that the respirator is acceptable to you and fits correctly (OSHA, n.d.). Comfort of a respiratory mask includes position of the mask on the nose, room for eye protection, room to talk, and position of mask on the face and cheeks.

   c. If needed, apply protective eyewear or goggles snugly around face and eyes. If you wear prescription glasses, side shields may be used.

   d. Apply clean gloves. (**Note:** Wear unpowdered, latex-free gloves if you, the patient, or another health care worker has a latex allergy.) As of January 19, 2017, the FDA has banned powdered medical gloves (FDA, 2016). If gloves are worn with gown, bring glove cuffs over edge of gown sleeves (see illustration).

9. Enter patient's room and identify patient using at least two personal identifiers, for example, full name and date of birth (TJC, 2018). Then confirm this information with the patient's identification bracelet. Arrange supplies and equipment. (**Note:** If equipment will be reused, place on a clean paper towel.)

10. Explain purpose of isolation and the precautions for the patient and family to follow. Offer opportunity to ask questions and assess for evidence of emotional problems. If the patient is on TB precautions, instruct the patient to cover mouth with tissue when coughing and to wear disposable surgical mask when leaving room.

11. Assess vital signs (see Chapter 15).
   a. If patient is infected or colonized with a resistant organism (e.g., VRE, MRSA), equipment remains in the room including the stethoscope and blood pressure cuff.

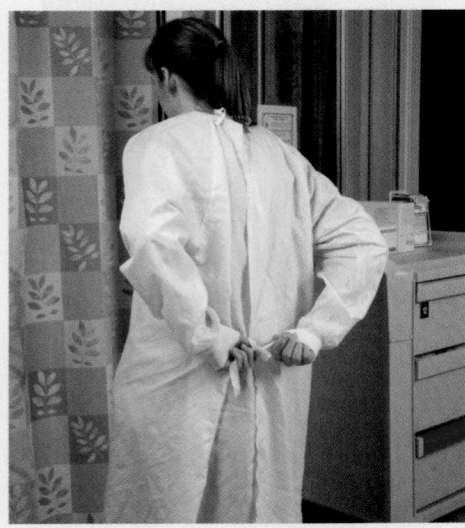

STEP 8a Tie gown at waist and neck.

Continued

BOX 14.12   PROCEDURAL GUIDELINES—cont'd

View Video!

Caring for a Patient on Isolation Precautions

b. If stethoscope is to be reused, clean earpieces and diaphragm or bell with 70% alcohol or agency-approved germicide. Set aside on clean surface.

c. Use individual or disposable thermometers and blood pressure cuffs when available.

Clinical Decision Point. If disposable thermometer indicates a fever, assess for other signs and/or symptoms. Confirm fever using an alternative thermometer. Do not use electronic thermometer if patient is suspected or confirmed to have *Clostridium difficile* infection (Surawizc et al., 2013).

12. Administer medications (see Chapter 17).
    a. Give oral medication in unit dose wrapper or cup.
    b. Dispose of wrapper or cup in plastic-lined receptacle.
    c. Wear gloves when administering an injection.
    d. Discard needleless syringe or safety sheathed needle into designated sharps container.
    e. Place reusable syringe (e.g., Carpujet) on a clean towel for eventual removal and disinfection.

Clinical Decision Point. If gloves are torn and hands come in contact with contaminated article or body fluids, perform hand hygiene as soon as possible and reapply gloves.

13. Administer personal hygiene care, encouraging patient to ask any questions or express concerns about isolation. Provide informal teaching at this time.
    a. Avoid allowing isolation gown to become wet; carry washbasin outward away from gown; avoid leaning against wet tabletop.

Clinical Decision Point. When there is a risk for excess soiling, wear a gown impervious to moisture.

b. Help patient remove own gown; discard in leak-proof linen bag.
c. Remove linen from bed; avoid contact with isolation gown. Place in leak-proof linen bag.

d. Provide clean bed linen.
e. Change gloves. Perform hand hygiene if gloves become excessively soiled and further care is necessary. Reapply gloves.

14. Collect specimens.
    a. Place specimen container on clean paper towel in patient's bathroom and follow procedure for collecting specimen of body fluids.
    b. Follow agency procedure for collecting specimen of body fluids.
    c. Transfer specimen to container without soiling outside of container. Place container in plastic bag, and place label on outside of bag or per agency policy. Label specimen in front of patient (TJC, 2018). Place containers of blood or body fluids in a biohazard bag (see illustration). Perform hand hygiene. Reapply gloves if additional procedures are needed.
    d. Check label on specimen for accuracy. Send to laboratory. (**Note:** Additional warning labels are often used, depending on agency policy.)

15. Dispose of linen, trash, and disposable items.
    a. Use sturdy moisture-impervious bags to contain soiled articles. Use double bag if necessary for heavily soiled linen or heavy wet trash.
    b. Tie bags securely at top in knot (see illustration).

16. Remove all reusable pieces of equipment. Clean any contaminated surfaces with hospital-approved disinfectant (CDC, 2009) (see agency policy).

17. Resupply room as needed. Have staff colleague hand new supplies to you.

18. Leave isolation room. Order of removal of PPE depends on what you wear in room. The following sequence describes steps to take if all barriers were worn. PPE worn in the isolation room must be removed before leaving the room.
    a. Remove gloves. Remove one glove by grasping cuff and pulling glove inside out over hand. Place used glove in gloved hand. With ungloved hand, tuck thumb inside cuff of remaining glove and pull it off, inside out (see illustration).

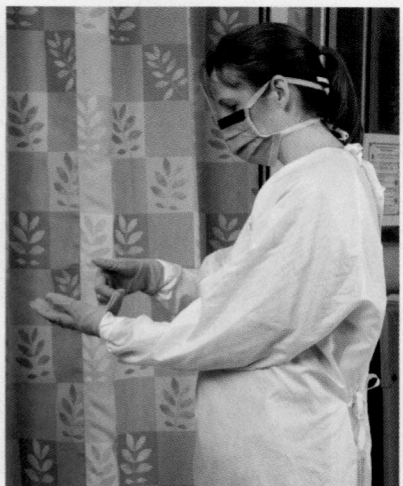

STEP 8d Apply gloves over gown sleeves.

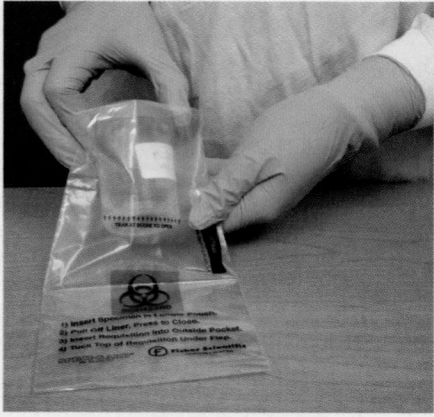

STEP 14c Specimen container placed in biohazard bag and sealed.

BOX 14.12   PROCEDURAL GUIDELINES—cont'd

View Video!

Caring for a Patient on Isolation Precautions

b. Remove eyewear, face shield, or goggles. Handle by headband or earpieces. Discard in proper container.
c. Untie neck strings and then untie back strings of gown. Allow gown to fall from shoulders (see illustration); touch inside of gown only. Remove hands from sleeves without touching outside of gown. Hold gown inside at shoulder seams and fold inside out into a bundle; discard in laundry bag.
d. Remove mask. If mask loops over ears, remove elastic from ears and pull mask away from face. For a tie-on mask, untie *top* mask strings, hold strings, untie *bottom* strings, pull mask away from face (see illustration), and drop into trash receptacle. (Do not touch outer surface of mask.)

Clinical Decision Point. If patient is on TB precautions, place reusable mask in labeled paper bag for storage, being careful not to crush mask (check agency policy for number of times reusable masks can be used).

---

e. Perform hand hygiene.
f. Explain to patient when you plan to return to room. Ask whether patient requires any personal care items. Offer books, magazines, or audiotapes.
g. Leave room and close door if necessary. Close door if patient is on airborne precautions or in negative airflow room.

h. Dispose of all contaminated supplies and equipment in proper manner (see agency policy). Perform hand hygiene.
19. Observe patient and family members' use of isolation precautions when visiting.
20. While in room, ask if patient has had a sufficient opportunity to discuss health problems, course of treatment, or other topics important to him or her.
21. **Use Teach-Back:** "I want to be sure I explained why you need to wear the protective clothing. Tell me why you think you need to wear the gown, gloves, and mask." Revise your instruction now or develop a plan for revised patient/family caregiver teaching if patient/family caregiver is not able to teach back correctly.

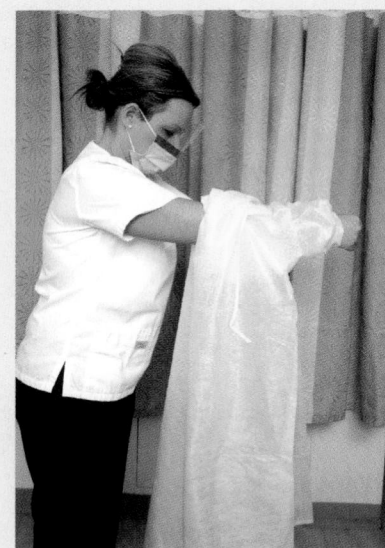

STEP 18c Remove gown by allowing it to fall from shoulders and remove so that outside of gown is now inside.

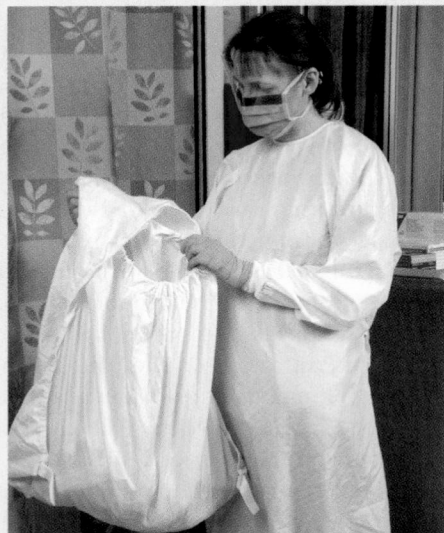

STEP 15b Tie trash bag securely.

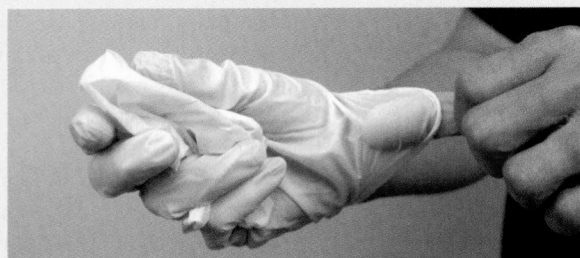

STEP 18a Remove gloves.

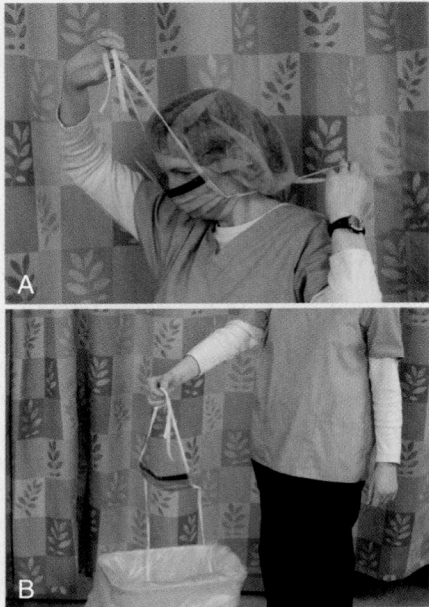

STEP 18d Remove mask.

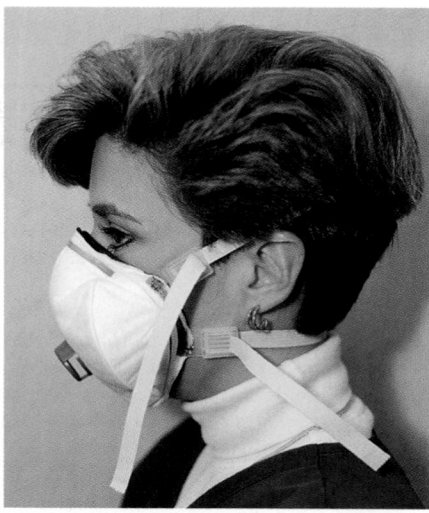

FIG 14.4 Disposable high-efficiency particulate air (HEPA)–purifying respirator.

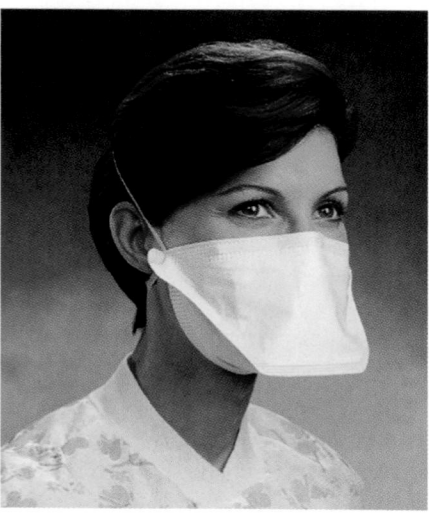

FIG 14.5 N95 respirator mask with protective eyewear. (Courtesy Halyard Health, Inc., Alpharetta, GA.)

organisms that have developed a resistance to one or more broad-spectrum antibiotics, making the organism hard to treat effectively. MRSA is a highly virulent organism that can frequently lead to sepsis and death (Becker and Kock, 2015; CDC, 2016c). VRE poses a risk to patients who are immune-compromised and debilitated (CDC, 2011; Archibald, 2015). *C. difficile* infection is one of the most common and costly HAIs. Patient susceptibility to *C. difficile* usually results from prior treatment with antibiotics (particularly clindamycin). In contrast to MRSA and VRE, *C. difficile* is harder to eliminate from the environment because it is a spore-forming organism, meaning it can remain on surfaces in a dormant state for long periods and is resistant to the contents in commercial hand sanitizers (CDC, 2011). For this reason, when caring for patients with *C. difficile,* it is recommended that vigorous handwashing using soap and water be used to clean hands. To reduce the risk of cross-contamination among patients,

use contact precautions in addition to standard precautions when caring for patients with MDROs.

Regardless of the type of isolation or barrier protection used, follow certain basic principles when delivering care in a patient's room. Understand how certain diseases are transmitted and which barriers you need to prevent transmission. For example, you do not routinely need to wear a gown or gloves when giving oral medications, but you do need these barriers when changing a dressing from a draining wound. Gloves are appropriate when helping a patient with an oral medication if the patient needs assistance putting the medication in the mouth.

Take care to avoid exposing an article brought into a patient's room to any infectious material. Bag or decontaminate any contaminated article (e.g., glucose meter, blood pressure cuff) according to agency policy. Decontaminate equipment that is shared among patients.

Before you institute isolation measures, explain to a patient and family members the nature of the patient's condition, the purpose of the isolation barriers, and ways to carry out specific precautions. Teach them the proper way to perform hand hygiene and apply gloves, masks, or gowns. Demonstrate each procedure, and give the patient and family an opportunity to practice. Always reinforce the specific reasons why these steps are important in the care of the patient. Explain methods of transmission of infectious organisms so they understand the difference between contaminated and clean objects.

Provide for a patient's sensory stimulation during isolation. Encourage the family to bring the patient reading materials, puzzle books, music, and similar items. Take the opportunity to listen to the patient's concerns or interests. If you rush care or show a lack of interest in the patient's needs, he or she will feel rejected and even more isolated. Explain the patient's potential risk for depression or loneliness to family members. Encourage visitors to avoid negative expressions or actions concerning isolation. Advise family members on ways to provide meaningful stimulation.

Protective Environment. In some situations, special isolation rooms are used for highly susceptible patients such as organ transplant recipients and patients with neutropenia (low WBC count). Post a card on the patient's room door with a list of the precautions in use when a private room is recommended (check agency policy). The card is a handy reference for health care workers and visitors and alerts all who enter the room of any special precautions in use. Make sure that you follow agency policies on isolation practice (CDC, 2007).

The isolation room or an adjoining anteroom, if present, needs to contain hand-hygiene supplies, bathing facilities, and toilet facilities. Personnel and visitors need to perform hand hygiene before entering and on exiting a patient's room. Store PPE in an anteroom between the room and hallway or in a location convenient to where the PPE is needed.

Each patient care room, including rooms used for isolation, contains a trash container with plastic liners. Rooms used for isolation also contain a soiled linen hamper. These containers prevent transmission of microorganisms by preventing leakage and waste from contaminating the outside surface. Have a disposable, rigid container available in the room to discard used needles, sharps, and syringes.

Depending on the microorganisms identified and the mode of transmission, critically evaluate which articles or equipment to take into an isolation room. For example, HICPAC recommends taking only dedicated articles into an isolation room when VRE is present (CDC, 2007).

Personal Protective Equipment. Gowns or cover-ups protect health care workers from contacting infected blood and body fluids or materials during procedures or when patients have uncontained secretions. Gowns used for barrier protection are made of a fluid-resistant material. Change a gown immediately if it is damaged or heavily contaminated. Isolation gowns usually open at the back and have ties or snaps at the neck and waist to keep the gown closed and secure. A gown is long enough to cover all outer garments. Long sleeves with tight-fitting cuffs provide added protection.

Wear a mask or respirator if you anticipate splashing or spraying of blood or body fluids. The mask also protects you from inhaling microorganisms from a patient's respiratory tract and prevents the transmission of pathogens from your respiratory tract. Occasionally a patient who is susceptible to infection wears a mask to avoid inhaling pathogens. Patients requiring respiratory precautions wear surgical masks when ambulating or being transported outside of their room to protect other patients and personnel.

Masks prevent the transmission of infections caused by direct contact with mucous membranes. A mask discourages the wearer from touching the nose or mouth. A properly applied mask fits snugly over the mouth and nose so that the pathogens and body fluids cannot enter or escape through the sides (Box 14.13). If a person wears glasses, the top edge of the mask fits below the glasses so that they do not cloud over as the person exhales. Keep talking to a minimum while wearing a mask. Discard a mask that has become moist because it is ineffective. Discard the mask when leaving a patient's room. Warn patients and family members that a mask sometimes causes a sensation of smothering. If family members become uncomfortable, have them leave the room and discard their masks.

Apply disposable gloves when there is a risk for exposing the hands to blood, body fluids, mucous membranes, nonintact skin, or potentially infectious material on objects or surfaces. In addition, use gloves when you have scratches or breaks in your skin and when performing venipuncture, fingersticks, or heelsticks. You wear gloves alone or in combination with other PPE. When other PPE is necessary, first put on a mask and eyewear (if required), apply a gown (if required), and then apply gloves. Pull the glove cuffs up over the wrists or cuffs of a gown.

BOX 14.13　PROCEDURAL GUIDELINES

Applying an Isolation Mask

DELEGATION CONSIDERATIONS
The skill of applying an isolation mask is performed by all caregivers who enter isolation rooms. The RN reinforces with the nursing assistive personnel (NAP) to:
• Change the mask if it becomes moist or contaminated.

EQUIPMENT
Disposable mask

STEPS
1. Find top edge of mask, which usually has thin metal strip along edge.
2. Hold mask by top two strings or loops, keeping top edge above bridge of nose. Tie two top strings at top of back of head, over cap (if worn), with strings above ears (see illustration). Alternatively place loops over ears.
3. Tie two lower ties snugly around neck with mask well under chin (see illustration).
4. Gently pinch upper metal band around bridge of nose.

> **Clinical Decision Point. Change mask if wet, moist, or contaminated.**

5. Remove mask by untying bottom mask strings and then top strings; pull mask away from face and drop into trash receptacle (see illustrations in Box 14.12, Step 18d). (Do not touch outer surface of mask.)

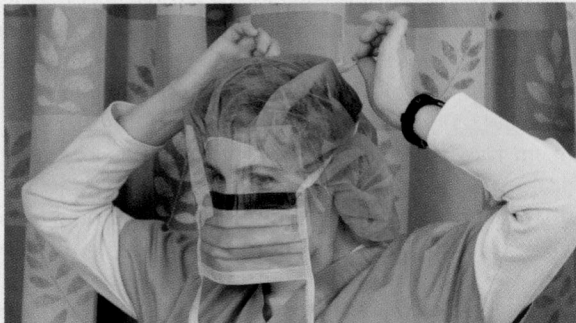

STEP 2 Attaching top two ties of a tie-on mask.

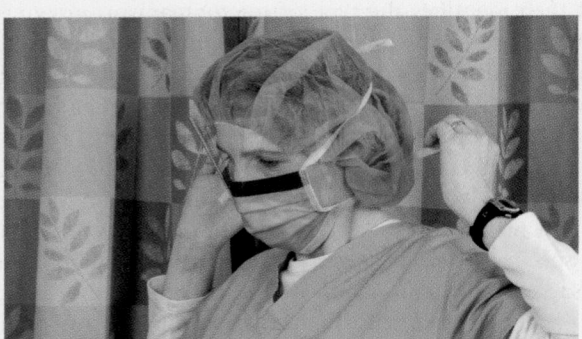

STEP 3 Securing bottom two ties of a tie-on mask.

After contacting infectious material, change gloves and perform hand hygiene even if you have not finished caring for the patient. If your actions do not involve more patient contact, it is not necessary to reapply gloves. Teach patients and their families the reasons for wearing gloves and the correct method for applying them.

Most gloves used for barrier protection or surgical asepsis are latex free. However, when you wear gloves made of latex follow these precautions. Before applying latex gloves, assess a patient's potential for having a latex allergy. Individuals most at risk include individuals with a history of spina bifida, congenital or urogenital defects, indwelling urinary catheterization, use of condom catheters, multiple childhood surgeries, and food allergies. A history of occupational exposure to latex is another risk for a patient. The symptoms of a reaction to latex range from mild dermatitis to severe anaphylactic shock. The Food and Drug Administration (FDA, 2016) has banned the use of powdered gloves. The powder had been a factor in causing latex sensitivity because of repeated contact or by inhaling aerosolized latex allergens. The Association of PeriOperative Registered Nurses (AORN, 2016) provides the following suggestions for nurses to avoid becoming allergic to latex:

1. Wear gloves only when indicated.
2. Wash with a pH-balanced soap immediately after removing gloves.
3. Apply only non–oil-based hand care products (oil-based products break down latex allergens).
4. If a reaction or dermatitis occurs, report to employee health service and/or seek medical treatment immediately.

Wear protective eyewear and face shields properly fitted during procedures in which it is possible to splatter the eyes or face with blood or other infectious material. In many instances caregivers purchase their own eyewear with prescription lenses. Regular glasses are insufficient. Protective eyewear needs to have side shields to prevent material from entering the eye between the glasses and face.

Specimen Collection. A patient with a suspected or actual infectious disease sometimes has many laboratory studies. Body fluids and materials suspected to contain infectious organisms are collected for culture and sensitivity tests. In the laboratory the specimen is placed in a special medium that promotes the growth of organisms. A laboratory technologist then identifies the type of microorganisms growing in the culture and the broad-spectrum antibiotics that may kill those organisms. Additional sensitivity test results indicate the antibiotics to which the organisms are resistant or sensitive. Thus proper medications are ordered.

Obtain all culture specimens with sterile equipment. Collecting fresh material (e.g., wound drainage) from the site of an infection ensures that resident flora do not contaminate the specimen. Seal all specimen containers tightly to prevent spillage and contamination of the outside of the containers (Box 14.14). After you transfer specimens to containers, label each specimen properly with the patient's name, patient identifier, date and time, and type of specimen.

Label specimens in the presence of the patient (TJC, 2018). Place specimen containers in labeled leak-proof biohazard bags before transporting them to the laboratory (see agency policy).

Bagging. In general, bagging articles is the same for all patients regardless of whether they are on isolation or not (see agency policy). Bagging articles prevents accidental exposure of personnel to contaminated articles and contamination of the surrounding environment.

Place all soiled linen in a designated waterproof bag in a patient's room. Do not overfill the bag. Handle, transport, and process linen soiled with blood or body fluids in a way that prevents exposure of skin or mucous membrane and/or contamination of the health care worker's clothing. Some hospitals still require double bagging. A standard-size linen bag, not overfilled, tied securely and intact is adequate to prevent infection transmission. Consult agency policy and any applicable regulations.

Biohazardous waste includes both infectious and medical waste that must be disposed of in special red bags or per agency policy. These disposal procedures are a large expense for health care agencies. Consider the following waste materials to be infectious or medical waste (WHO, 2015):

- Infectious waste such as cultures of infectious organisms or waste from highly infectious patients
- Pathological waste such as discarded human tissue, organs, and body parts
- Blood and blood products
- Sharps, including discarded needles, syringes, scalpels, and blood vials
- Chemicals used for laboratory preparation and disinfectants
- Genotoxic waste from cytotoxic drugs used in cancer treatment
- Radioactive diagnostic material

Removal of Protective Equipment. The method of removing protective clothing, gloves, eyewear, gown, and mask before leaving an isolation room depends on the protective equipment worn at the time. If you wear all four protective items, first remove the gloves because they are most likely to be contaminated. If you untie a gown while wearing gloves, there is a chance of contaminating your hair or a portion of your uniform. See Box 14.12 for steps for removing PPE.

Transporting Patients. Patients infected with highly communicable organisms such as the TB bacillus may leave their rooms only for essential purposes such as diagnostic procedures or surgery. Before transferring a patient to a wheelchair or stretcher, provide the patient with appropriate barrier protection. For example, patients infected by an organism transmitted by the respiratory tract need to wear surgical masks. Personnel transporting patients practice the appropriate precautions while in a patient's room and remove PPE when leaving the room. Notify personnel in diagnostic areas or the operating room that the patient is on isolation precautions. Record the type of isolation on the patient's chart, and explain ways to avoid transmitting infection during transport (CDC, 2007).

BOX 14.14 SPECIMEN COLLECTION TECHNIQUES

Ensure that each specimen container or the bag in which it is placed has a biohazard symbol on the outside. Before collecting specimen, identify patient using at least two identifiers, for example, full name and date of birth (TJC, 2018). Confirm this information on the patient's identification bracelet.

WOUND SPECIMEN

Perform hand hygiene and apply clean gloves. Clean area around wound edges with antiseptic swab. Wipe from edges outward to remove old exudate (see Chapter 38). Remove gloves, perform hand hygiene, and reapply gloves. Use a cotton-tipped swab or syringe to collect as much drainage as possible. Have clean test tube or culture tube ready on clean paper towel. After swabbing center of wound site, grasp collection tube with paper towel. Carefully insert swab without touching outside of tube and secure top of tube. For some specimens you need to crush end of tube and push swab into fluid. Transfer tube into biohazard bag for transport and perform hand hygiene.

BLOOD SPECIMEN CULTURE[a]

Wearing gloves, clean venipuncture site with antiseptic swabs, with first swab moving back and forth on horizontal plane, another swab on vertical plane, and last swab in a circular motion from site outward for 5 cm (2 inches) lasting a total of 30 seconds. Allow to dry. Clean tops of culture bottles for 15 seconds with agency-approved cleansing solution. Use 20-mL needle-safe syringe and collect 10 to 15 mL of blood per culture bottle (check health care agency policy). Perform venipuncture at two different sites to decrease likelihood of both specimens being contaminated with skin flora. Place blood culture bottles on clean paper towel on bedside table or other surface; swab off bottle tops with alcohol. Inject appropriate amount of blood into each bottle. Transfer specimen into clean, labeled biohazard bag for transport. Remove gloves and perform hand hygiene.

STOOL SPECIMEN

Wearing gloves, use clean cup with seal top (need not be sterile) and tongue blade to collect small amount of stool, approximately 2 to 3 cm (approximately 1 inch). Place cup on clean paper towel in patient's bathroom. Using tongue blade, collect needed amount of feces from patient's bedpan. Transfer feces to cup without touching outside surface of cup. Dispose of tongue blade and place seal on cup. Transfer specimen into clean biohazard bag for transport. Remove gloves and perform hand hygiene.

URINE SPECIMEN

Apply gloves; cleanse needleless port on urinary catheter and use needleless syringe to collect 1 to 5 mL of urine. Fill sterile specimen cup or specimen tube, and place on clean towel in patient's bathroom. If the patient is not catheterized, have patient follow procedure to obtain clean voided specimen (see Chapter 36). Secure top of transfer container and place in biohazard bag. Remove gloves and perform hand hygiene.

Note: Health care agency policies may differ on type of containers and amount of specimen material required. For all specimens, label containers for specimens in the presence of the patient (TJC, 2018).
[a]This procedure is usually performed by a laboratory technician.
From Pagana KD, Pagana TJ: *Mosby's diagnostic and laboratory test reference,* ed 11, St Louis, 2012, Mosby.

Control of Portals of Entry. Many measures that control the exit of microorganisms also control the entrance of pathogens. Provide interventions to control and prevent organisms from gaining a portal of entry (Box 14.15).

Protection of the Susceptible Host. A patient's resistance to infection improves by using measures that protect normal body defense mechanisms, including supporting existing body defense mechanisms or controlling exposure to microorganisms. For example, regular bathing removes transient microorganisms from the skin. Bathing with chlorhexidine gluconate has been shown to significantly decrease acquired infection of MRSA or VRE (Donskey and Deshpande, 2016). Lubrication keeps the skin hydrated and intact. Regular oral hygiene removes proteins in the saliva that attract microorganisms. Flossing removes tartar and plaque that cause infection. Adequate fluid intake promotes normal urine formation and a resultant outflow of urine to flush the bladder and urethra of microorganisms. For patients who are immobilized or dependent, regular coughing and deep-breathing exercises remove mucus from lower airways.

Role of the Infection Prevention and Control Department. Most health care agencies employ health professionals who are specially trained in the area of infection prevention and control. Their responsibilities include collection and analysis of data on HAIs, surveillance of MDROs, implementation of evidence-based protocols for infection prevention, and providing consultation and education to staff and others about infection prevention and control.

QSEN **QSEN ACTIVITY** *Quality Improvement*

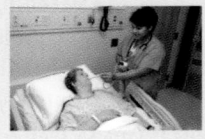

Carman Hernandez, the nurse caring for Mrs. Eldredge, notices that more patients have been readmitted with surgical site infection (SSI) over the past few months. Carman shares her observation with her manager and the infection control and prevention practitioner who covers her surgical nursing unit. After the unit data related to readmissions are reviewed, Carman and her manager put together a quality improvement group with other unit staff and meet with the infection control and prevention practitioner to determine if any variables are common to all the cases and which types of interventions would be appropriate.

• What is a good first step for Carman before attending the meeting?
• What actions might the group take?

evolve   Answers to QSEN Activities can be found on the Evolve website.

BOX 14.15   INFECTION CONTROL OF PORTALS OF ENTRY

INTACT SKIN AND MUCOSA
- Keep skin clean and well lubricated. Use chlorhexidine gluconate for daily bathing of hospitalized patients (Denny and Munro, 2016).
- Avoid positioning patients on tubes or objects that might cause breaks in skin.
- Use dry, wrinkle-free linen.
- Offer frequent oral hygiene (see Chapter 31).
- Provide frequent position changes for patients with impaired mobility.
- Clean skin of patients who are incontinent with nonabrasive agent; avoid drying with abrasive towel or tissue.

URINARY TRACT
- Teach women to clean perineum and rectum by wiping from area of least contamination (urinary meatus) toward area of most contamination (rectum).
- Do not allow urine in drainage bags and tubes to flow back into bladder. Never raise drainage system above level of bladder.
- Keep points of connection between catheter or drain and tubing closed.

INVASIVE TUBES AND LINES
- When obtaining specimens from drainage tubes or inserting safety needles into IV lines, disinfect tube ports by wiping them liberally with disinfectant solution before entering system. **Scrub the hub** before accessing site. Before inserting an IV line, cleanse the skin with antiseptic. Cleansing the skin and tubing removes and, in some cases, kills microorganisms.

WOUND CARE
- Keep draining wounds covered to contain drainage.
- Clean outward from wound site using clean swab for each application (see Chapter 38).

Health Promotion in Health Care Workers and Patients. A health care worker who becomes ill exposes susceptible patients to infectious diseases. Agencies offer employee health services to assist in infection prevention and control such as immunization programs, recommendations for work restrictions, and protocols for management of job-related exposures to infectious diseases (Kak, 2014).

Surgical Asepsis. Surgical asepsis, or aseptic technique, is designed to eliminate all microorganisms including spores and pathogens from an object and to protect an area from these microorganisms. Surgical asepsis requires more precautions than medical asepsis. Breaks in technique result in contamination, increasing a patient's risk for infection (Murphy, 2015).

Surgical asepsis is commonly practiced in the operating room, labor and delivery area, and major diagnostic or procedural areas, but nurses also use surgical aseptic techniques at a patient's bedside (e.g., when inserting IV or urethral

catheters). Use surgical asepsis during procedures that require intentional perforation of a patient's skin (e.g., IV insertion), when the integrity of the skin is broken from trauma or burns, and during procedures that involve insertion of a catheter or surgical instruments into sterile body cavities (AORN, 2016).

Multiple steps involving application of PPE for use of sterile technique are used in the operating room in this order: applying a mask, protective eyewear, and a cap; performing a surgical scrub; and applying a sterile gown and gloves. In contrast, performing a sterile dressing change at a patient's bedside requires only hand hygiene, applying a clean gown if splashing of fluid is likely, and applying sterile gloves (Box 14.16). It is important for you to refer to agency policy and procedure whenever there is a question about a procedure requiring sterile technique. Regardless of the procedures followed in different settings, the use of surgical asepsis depends on developing an aseptic conscience. Always recognize the importance of strict adherence to aseptic principles. In addition, be an excellent role model and patient advocate, reinforcing proper practice for other caregivers (AORN, 2016).

Preparation for Sterile Procedures. In treatment rooms and at the bedside it is important to have a patient's full cooperation in maintaining aseptic technique. Therefore assess the patient's understanding of sterile procedure and the reasons for not moving or interfering with the procedure. Special precautions such as masking the patient or changing his or her position are sometimes necessary to prevent contamination during procedures. Determine whether a patient has undergone a sterile procedure in the past. Explain how you will perform the procedure and what the patient can do to avoid contaminating sterile objects:

1. Avoid sudden movements of body parts covered by sterile drapes.
2. Do not touch sterile supplies, drapes, or your sterile gloves and gown.
3. Avoid coughing, sneezing, or talking over a sterile area.

Certain sterile procedures last for an extended time. Assess each patient's needs (e.g., pain control or elimination) in advance and anticipate factors that will disrupt a procedure. If a patient is in pain, administer prescribed analgesics no more than 30 minutes before a sterile procedure begins. Patients often are placed in relatively uncomfortable positions during sterile procedures. Help the patient assume the most comfortable position possible. Finally, the patient's condition sometimes results in events that contaminate a sterile field. For example, a patient with a respiratory infection coughs, transmitting organisms that contaminate the sterile field. Anticipate such a problem and offer a mask to the patient before the procedure begins.

Principles of Surgical Asepsis. Principles of surgical asepsis include the following:

1. *A sterile object remains sterile only when touched by another sterile object.* The following principles guide you in placement and handling of sterile objects:
   - Sterile touching sterile remains sterile (e.g., wear sterile gloves to handle objects on a sterile field).

- Sterile touching clean becomes contaminated (e.g., if the sterile tip of a syringe touches the surface of a clean disposable glove, the syringe is contaminated).
- Sterile touching contaminated becomes contaminated (e.g., when you touch a sterile object with an ungloved hand, the object is contaminated).
- Sterile touching questionable is contaminated (e.g., when you find a tear or break in the covering of a sterile object, discard or reprocess it, regardless of whether the object appears untouched).

2. *Place only sterile objects on a sterile field.* Be sure the item is sterile before use. The package or container holding a sterile object must be intact and dry. A package that is torn, punctured, wet, or open is unsterile. When placing sterile items on a sterile field (e.g., sterile drape), do not reach over the field (Fig. 14.6).

3. *A sterile object or field out of the range of vision or an object held below a person's waist is contaminated.* Never turn your back on a sterile tray or leave it unattended. Any object held below waist level is considered contaminated because you cannot view it at all times. Keep sterile objects either on or out over the sterile field.

4. *A sterile object or field becomes contaminated by prolonged exposure to the air.* Avoid activities that create air currents such as excessive movements or rearranging linen after a sterile object or field becomes exposed. Minimize the number of individuals walking into an area where sterile packages are being opened or are open.

BOX 14.16 PROCEDURAL GUIDELINES

Putting on Sterile Gloves

View Video!

DELEGATION CONSIDERATIONS

The skill of sterile glove application can be delegated to NAP if NAP are qualified to perform the sterile procedure. The nurse instructs NAP to:

- Stop and reapply gloves if they become contaminated.

EQUIPMENT

Pair of proper-sized sterile gloves (latex or synthetic neolatex)

STEPS

1. Consider the type of procedure to be performed, and consult agency policy on use of sterile gloves.
2. Consider patient's risk for infection (e.g., a preexisting condition and size or extent of area being treated).
3. Select correct size and type of gloves and then examine glove package to determine if it is dry and intact with no water stains.
4. Inspect condition of hands for cuts, hangnails, open lesions, or abrasions. In some settings you are allowed to cover any open lesion with a sterile, impervious transparent dressing (check agency policy). In some cases the presence of such lesions may prevent you from participating in a procedure.
5. Assess patient for the following risk factors before applying latex gloves:
   a. Previous reaction to the following items within hours of exposure: adhesive tape, dental or face mask, golf club grip, ostomy bag, rubber band, balloon, bandage, elastic underwear, IV tubing, rubber gloves, condom
   b. Personal history of asthma, contact dermatitis, eczema, urticaria, or rhinitis
   c. History of food allergies, especially avocado, banana, peach, chestnut, raw potato, kiwi, tomato, or papaya
   d. Previous history of adverse reactions during surgery or dental procedure
   e. Previous reaction to latex product

   Clinical Decision Point. Synthetic nonlatex gloves must be used when patients are at risk or if nurse has sensitivity or allergy to latex.

6. Apply sterile gloves.
   a. Perform thorough hand hygiene. Place glove package near work area.
   b. Remove outer glove package wrapper by carefully separating and peeling apart sides (see illustration).
   c. Grasp inner package and lay on clean, dry, flat surface at waist level. Open package, keeping gloves on inside surface of wrapper.
   d. Identify right and left glove. Each glove has a cuff approximately 5 cm (2 inches) wide. Glove dominant hand first.
   e. With thumb and first two fingers of nondominant hand, grasp glove for dominant hand by touching only inside surface of cuff.
   f. Carefully pull glove over dominant hand, leaving a cuff and being sure that cuff does not roll up wrist. Be sure that thumb and fingers are in proper spaces (see illustration).
   g. With gloved dominant hand, slip fingers underneath cuff of second glove (see illustration).
   h. Carefully pull second glove over fingers of nondominant hand (see illustration).

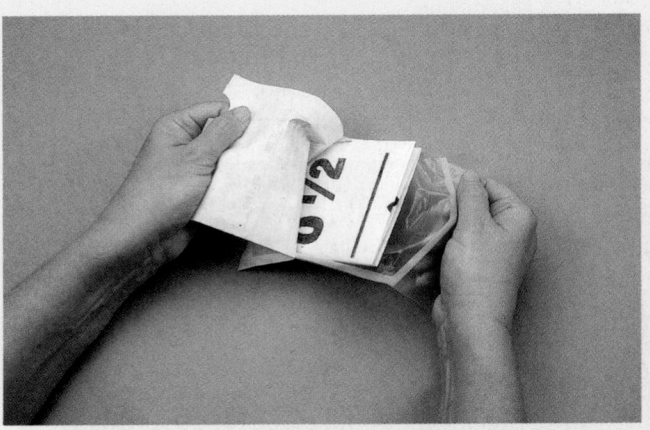

STEP 6b Open outer glove package wrapper.

Continued

BOX 14.16 PROCEDURAL GUIDELINES—cont'd

Putting on Sterile Gloves

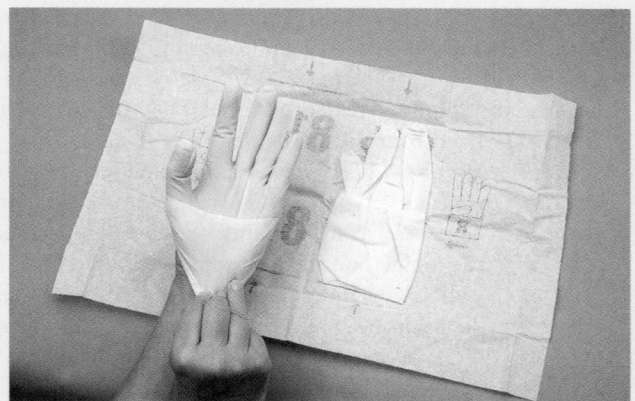

STEP 6f Pick up glove at cuff of dominant hand and insert fingers; pull glove completely over dominant hand (example is for a left-handed person).

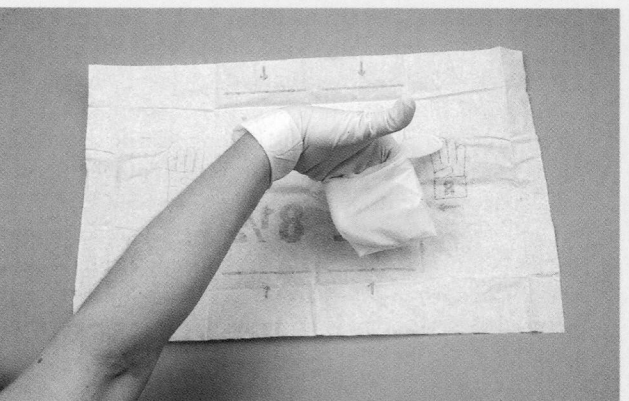

STEP 6g Pick up glove for nondominant hand.

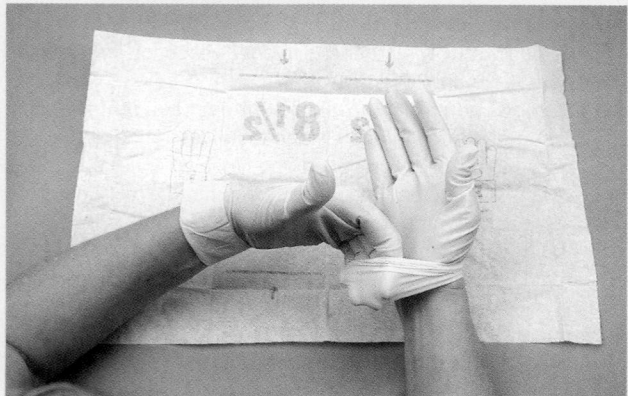

STEP 6h Pull second glove over nondominant hand.

> **Clinical Decision Point. Do not allow fingers and thumb of gloved dominant hand to touch any part of exposed nondominant hand. Keep thumb of dominant hand abducted back.**

   i. After second glove is on, interlock hands and hold away from body above waist level until beginning procedure (see illustration).

7. Remove gloves.

   a. Grasp outside of one cuff with other gloved hand; avoid touching wrist.

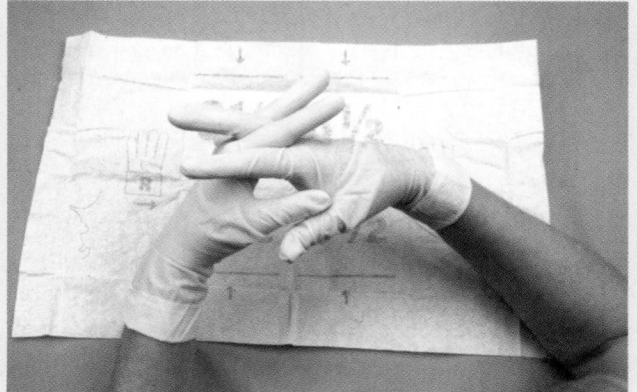

STEP 6i Interlock gloved hands.

   b. Pull glove off, turning it inside out, and place it in gloved hand.

   c. Take fingers of bare hand and tuck inside remaining glove cuff. Peel glove off inside out and over previously removed glove. Discard both gloves in receptacle.

   d. Perform thorough hand hygiene.

8. Assess patient for signs of infection, focusing on area treated.

9. Assess patient for signs of latex allergy.

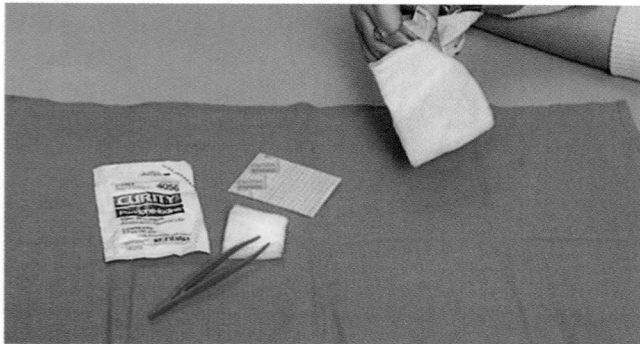

FIG 14.6 Adding item to a sterile field.

Microorganisms also travel by droplet through the air. No one should talk, laugh, sneeze, or cough over a sterile field or when gathering and using sterile equipment. Wear a mask when opening a tray and adding sterile equipment. Microorganisms traveling through the air can fall on sterile items or fields if you reach over the work area (Box 14.17).

5. *A sterile object or field becomes contaminated by capillary action when a sterile surface comes in contact with a wet contaminated surface.* Moisture seeps through the protective covering of a sterile package, allowing microorganisms to travel to the sterile object. When stored sterile packages

BOX 14.17 PROCEDURAL GUIDELINES

Opening Wrapped Sterile Items

DELEGATION CONSIDERATIONS

The skill of opening wrapped sterile items can be delegated to nursing assistive personnel (NAP) if NAP are qualified to perform the procedure. Guide the NAP to:

- Start procedure over with new equipment if contamination occurs at any point.

EQUIPMENT

Sterile kit or package, waist-high countertop or table surface

STEPS

1. Perform hand hygiene (see Box 14.10).
2. Apply PPE as needed (consult agency policy) (see Boxes 14.12 and 14.13).
3. Open sterile commercial kit or pack containing sterile items. Place sterile kit or pack on clean, dry, flat work surface above waist level.
4. Open outside cover (see illustration) and remove package from dust cover. Place on work surface.
5. Grasp outer surface of tip of top outermost flap.
6. Open outermost flap away from body, keeping arm outstretched and away from sterile field (see illustration).
7. Grasp outside surface of edge of first side flap.
8. Open side flap, pulling to side, allowing it to lie flat on table surface. Keep arm to side and not over sterile surface (see illustration).
9. Repeat Steps 7 and 8 for second side flap (see illustration).
10. Grasp outside border of last and innermost flap.
11. Stand away from sterile package and pull flap back, allowing it to fall flat on table (see illustration).
12. Use inner surface of package (except for 1-inch border around edges) as a sterile field to add items because it is sterile. Grasp the 1-inch border to move field over the work surface.

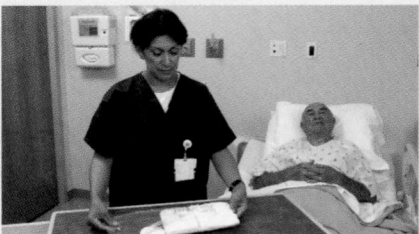

STEP 4 Open outside cover of sterile kit.

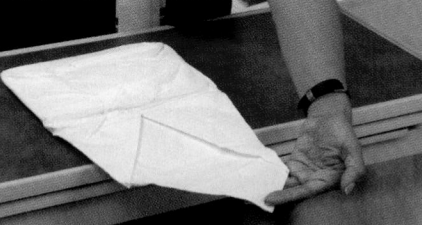

STEP 6 Open outermost flap of sterile kit away from body.

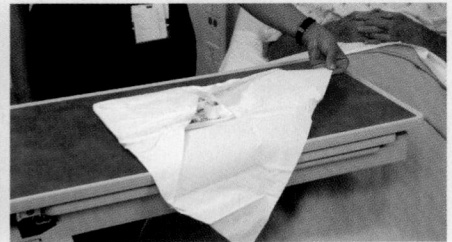

STEP 8 Open first side flap, pulling to side.

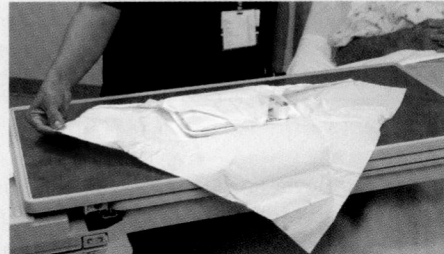

STEP 9 Open second side flap, pulling to side.

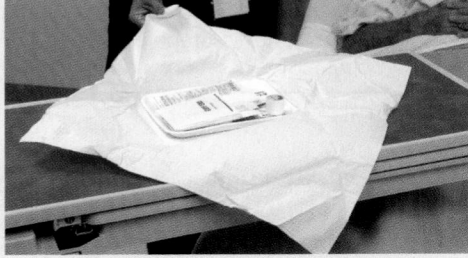

STEP 11 Open last and innermost flap.

become wet, discard the objects immediately or send the equipment to be sterilized again. Spilling solution over a sterile drape contaminates the field unless the drape cannot be penetrated by moisture.

6. *Because fluid flows in the direction of gravity, a sterile object becomes contaminated if gravity causes a contaminated liquid to flow over the surface of an object.* To avoid contamination during a surgical hand scrub, hold your hands above the elbows. This allows water to flow downward without contaminating your hands and fingers. Because gravity makes water flow downward, this is also the reason for drying from fingers to elbows with the hands held up after the scrub.

7. *The edges of a sterile field or container are contaminated.* A 2.5-cm (1-inch) border around a sterile towel or drape is considered contaminated (Box 14.18). The edges of sterile containers become exposed to air after they are open and are thus contaminated. After you remove a sterile needle from its protective cap or after you remove forceps from a container, the objects must not touch the edge of the container. The lip of an opened bottle of solution also becomes contaminated after it is exposed to air. When pouring a sterile liquid, first pour a small amount of solution and discard it. The solution washes away any microorganisms on the bottle lip. Then pour the liquid a second time to fill a sterile container with the amount of solution you need.

Restorative and Continuing Care. The need for infection prevention and control is also present when patients are in the restorative phase of their care. Nurses in LTCFs (nursing homes, skilled nursing facilities, and assisted living)

BOX 14.18   PROCEDURAL GUIDELINES

Preparation of a Sterile Field

DELEGATION CONSIDERATIONS

The skill of preparing a sterile field may be delegated to nursing assistive personnel (NAP) if NAP are qualified to perform the procedure. Guide the NAP to:

- Start procedure over with new equipment if contamination occurs at any point.

EQUIPMENT

Sterile pack, sterile gloves *(optional)*

STEPS

1. Perform hand hygiene.
2. Place pack containing sterile drape on flat, dry surface and open as described in Box 14.17.

3. Apply sterile gloves (*optional*, see agency policy). You may touch outer 2.5-cm (1-inch) border of drape without wearing gloves.
4. Using fingertips of one hand, pick up folded top edge of drape along 1-inch border.
5. Gently lift drape up from its wrapper and let it unfold by itself without touching any object. Discard wrapper with other hand.
6. With other hand, grasp an adjacent corner of drape and hold it straight up and away from body (see illustration).
7. Holding drape, position bottom half over top half of intended work surface (see illustration).
8. Allow top half of drape to be placed over bottom half of work surface (see illustration).
9. Grasp 1-inch border around edge to position drape as needed.

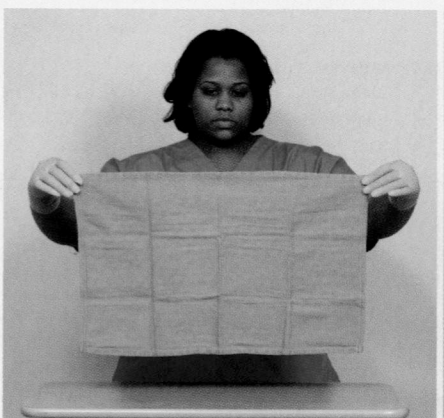 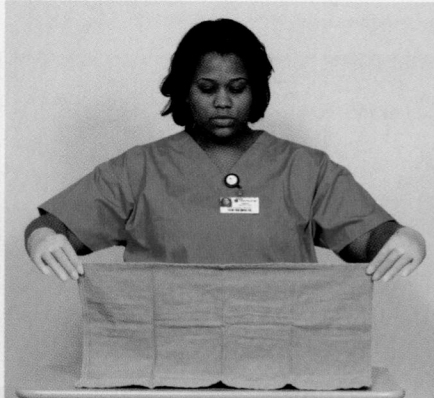 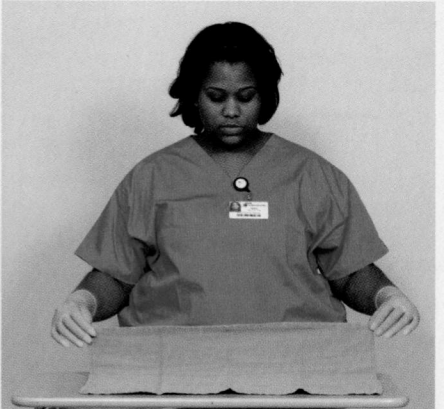

STEP 6 Hold corners of sterile drape up and away from body.   **STEP 7** Position bottom half of sterile drape over top half of work space.   **STEP 8** Allow top half of drape to be placed over bottom half of work surface.

---

contribute to high-quality health care by practicing skills and techniques necessary to prevent infections. Infections commonly found in long-term care include urinary tract infection, respiratory infection, diarrheal diseases, antibiotic-resistant *Staphylococcus* infections, and many others. These types of infections are a major cause of hospitalization and death; 380,000 people die of infections in LTCFs every year (CDC, 2015). Colonization with multidrug-resistant gram-negative bacteria is common among patients in the long-term care setting, especially patients with advanced dementia (Pop-Vicas et al., 2008).

Risks for HAIs in LTCFs increase because most residents are older adults who are dealing with age-associated physical changes that alter the natural barriers to infection (see Box 14.6). In addition, the population in LTCFs requires more complex medical care as a result of increased transitions between health care settings. Infections are among the most frequent causes of transfer from LTCFs to acute care hospitals and 30-day hospital readmissions (Bodily-Bartrum et al., 2016). Increasing the influenza vaccination rates of personnel who work in LTCFs helps reduce this problem.

Nurses play an important role in the control of these infections by using critical thinking skills and knowledge of how to prevent these infections. See Chapters 32, 36, and 37 for more information on infection control.

▪▪▪ EVALUATION

Patient Outcomes. Evaluation of a patient's status is important in determining if an infection has been prevented or controlled. Measure the success of infection prevention and control techniques by determining whether you achieved the goals and outcomes selected in a patient's plan of care. Compare a patient's response such as a decline in fever or decreased wound drainage with the expected outcomes established in the plan of care. For example, when a patient is discharged home with a draining wound, medical asepsis in the home is important. The patient and family members need to practice proper hand-hygiene techniques when interacting with the patient or any care-related equipment. You evaluate their ability to follow medical asepsis through direct observation, and you monitor for patient outcomes such as absence of fever or reduction in wound drainage. Another example is observing if items in the patient's living area (e.g., bed linen or personal bathroom) are properly cleaned.

Patients with surgical or traumatic wounds require extensive management (see Chapter 38). You design infection control practices to either prevent or control spread of wound infection and then evaluate the patient's response to nursing interventions by noting fever, wound pain or drainage, swelling around the wound, decreased energy, and increased fatigue. Evaluation of wound status and patient response to wound healing are priorities. You cannot always use fever as a sole measure because a fever may appear later in the wound infection process, especially with chronic wounds.

Patient Expectations. When providing patient care, routinely review whether you are meeting a patient's expectations. Ask the patient if he or she perceives that the symptoms of an infection are under control (e.g., pain of a healing wound, dysuria of a urinary infection). If your patient is going to be discharged home with an open wound or with a urinary catheter or an IV access device in place, help the patient identify concerns, and determine what he or she needs to ease the transition to care in the home.

Attentive listening to your patients and their families determines their level of satisfaction with care and if the plan of care met their expectations. Maintain open communication and give your patients an opportunity to express new expectations, their satisfaction, and care concerns as they transition from your care to home or other care setting.

KEY POINTS

- Normal body flora help the body resist infection by reducing the reproduction of pathogenic microorganisms.
- Immunity to infection depends on the capacity to produce antibodies in response to exposure to an antigen.
- An infection can develop if the six elements of the infection chain are present and uninterrupted.
- The virulence of a microorganism depends on its ability to resist attack by normal bodily defenses.
- Increasing age, poor nutrition, stress, inherited conditions, chronic disease, and treatments or conditions that compromise the immune response increase susceptibility to infection.
- Wear gloves when in contact with blood or potentially infectious material. Wear a gown and mask in combination with an eye protection device such as goggles or glasses with solid side shields whenever you anticipate splashes or spray of blood or potentially infectious material.
- The main cause of HAIs is nonadherence to hand hygiene.
- Invasive procedures, medical therapies, long hospitalization, and contact with health care personnel increase a hospitalized patient's risk for acquiring an HAI.
- Surgical asepsis requires more stringent techniques than medical asepsis.

- The CDC recommends that all patients be considered as potentially infected with HIV and other bloodborne pathogens; therefore, health care workers reduce the risk for exposure to blood and body fluids by following standard precautions.
- Following aseptic principles is the key to your success in preventing patients from acquiring infections.
- A patient on isolation precautions is subject to sensory deprivation because of the restricted environment.
- If the skin is broken or if you perform an invasive procedure into a body cavity normally free of microorganisms, use surgical aseptic practices.
- A sterile object becomes contaminated by direct contact with a clean or contaminated object, exposure to airborne microorganisms, or contact with a wet surface.

REFLECTIVE LEARNING

- Consider how you would correctly transfer a patient in contact precautions to a diagnostic procedure.
- Describe an action you observed by another health care worker during a recent clinical experience that may have increased a patient's risk for infection.
- Reflect on the infection prevention practices you consistently used during a recent clinical experience when providing direct patient care.

REVIEW QUESTIONS

1. In what order would you prepare to enter the room of a patient in contact and droplet isolation precautions for MRSA?
   1. Put on eyewear
   2. Perform hand hygiene
   3. Put on gloves
   4. Put on mask
   5. Put on gown
2. To decrease the risk of a urinary tract infection while a patient has an indwelling urinary catheter, what should the nurse do? (Select all that apply.)
   1. Encourage fluids before the insertion of the catheter and while the catheter is in place.
   2. Make sure the catheter and insertion supplies remain sterile throughout the insertion procedure.
   3. Place the urine collection bag higher than the bladder to maintain patency of drainage tubing.
   4. Secure the catheter tubing to the patient's thigh.
   5. Assess the patient's history of latex allergy.
3. Which of the steps are designed to control the portal of entry of a microorganism? (Select all that apply.)
   1. Scrub the hub of an IV tubing port before inserting a safety needle
   2. Wearing PPE
   3. Frequent oral hygiene
   4. Daily bathing with chlorhexidine gluconate
   5. Keep point of connection between urinary catheter and drainage tube closed

4. A patient diagnosed with a multidrug-resistant organism in a surgical wound asks the nurse what it means to be placed on isolation. What is the nurse's best response?
   1. The patient must remain in the room at all times so that contact with other patients is avoided.
   2. The organism is easily spread, so family and visitors must be limited to one at a time.
   3. The patient needs to remain in the room at all times and wear gloves when using the restroom.
   4. The patient must remain in the room most of the time to control for transmission of the infection but with proper precautions can leave the room for procedures.

5. Which are the most effective ways to prevent transmission of *C. difficile* between patients? (Select all that apply.)
   1. Place the patient in contact isolation precautions.
   2. Clean hands before and after each patient encounter with soap and water.
   3. Clean hands before and after wearing personal protective equipment such as gloves, gowns, masks, and goggles.
   4. Keep the patient's room door shut at all times.
   5. Use alcohol disinfectant wipes to clean work surfaces.

evolve

Additional Review Questions, as well as rationales for all Review Questions, can be found on the Evolve website.

1, 2, 5, 4, 1, 3; 2, 1, 2, 4; 3, 1, 3, 4, 5; 4, 5; 1, 2, 3.

REFERENCES

Abad C, et al: Adverse effects of isolation in hospitalised patients: a systematic review, *J Hosp Infect* 76:97e102, 2010.

Anderson VL: Promoting childhood immunizations, *J Nurse Pract* 11:1–10, 2015.

Archibald L: Enterococci. In Grota P, et al, editors: *APIC text of infection control and epidemiology*, ed 4, Washington, DC, 2015, Association for Professionals in Infection Control and Epidemiology (APIC).

Arnold F: Antimicrobials and resistance. In Grota P, et al, editors: *APIC text of infection control and epidemiology*, ed 4, Washington, DC, 2015, Association for Professionals in Infection Control and Epidemiology (APIC).

Association of periOperative Nurses (AORN): *2016 guidelines for perioperative practice*, Denver CO, 2016, AORN, Inc.

Becker K, Kock R: Staphylococci. In Grota P, et al, editors: *APIC text of infection control and epidemiology*, ed 4, Washington, DC, 2015, Association for Professionals in Infection Control and Epidemiology (APIC).

Berends C, Walesa B: Isolation precautions (transmission based precautions). In Grota P, et al, editors: *APIC text of infection control and epidemiology*, ed 4, Washington, DC, 2015, Association for Professionals in Infection Control and Epidemiology (APIC).

Biagioli V, et al: The experiences of protective isolation in patients undergoing bone marrow or haematopoietic stem cell transplantation: systematic review and metasynthesis, *Eur J Cancer Care (Engl)* 2016. Feb 19 [e-pub ahead of print].

Bodily-Bartrum M, et al: Long-term care. In Grota P, editor: *APIC text of infection control and epidemiology*, ed 4, Washington, DC, 2016, Association for Professionals in Infection Control and Epidemiology (APIC).

Centers for Disease Control and Prevention (CDC): Guideline for hand hygiene in health-care settings: recommendations of the Healthcare Infection Control Practices Advisory Committee and the HICPAC/SHEA/APIC/IDSA Hand Hygiene Task Force, *MMWR Morb Mortal Wkly Rep* 51(No. RR-16):2002. http://www.cdc.gov/mmwr/PDF/rr/rr5116.pdf.

Centers for Disease Control and Prevention (CDC): Guidelines for preventing the transmission of *Mycobacterium tuberculosis* in health care facilities, *MMWR Recomm Rep* 54:RR–17, 2005.

Centers for Disease Control and Prevention (CDC), Hospital Infection Control Practice Advisory Committee: *2007 Guideline for isolation precautions: preventing transmission of infectious agents in healthcare settings, Healthcare Infection Control Practices Advisory Committee (HICPAC)*, 2007. https://www.cdc.gov/hicpac/2007IP/2007isolationPrecautions.html.

Centers for Disease Control and Prevention (CDC), et al: *Guideline for disinfection and sterilization in healthcare facilities*, 2008.

Centers for Disease Control and Prevention (CDC): *OPRP—general information on hand hygiene*, 2009. http://www.cdc.gov/nceh/vsp/cruiselines/hand_hygiene_general.htm.

Centers for Disease Control and Prevention (CDC): *VRE in healthcare settings*, 2011. http://www.cdc.gov/hai/organisms/vre/vre.html.

Centers for Disease Control and Prevention (CDC): *Principles of epidemiology in public health practice, third edition: an introduction to applied epidemiology and biostatistics*, 2012. http://www.cdc.gov/ophss/csels/dsepd/SS1978/Lesson1/Section10.html.

Centers for Disease Control and Prevention (CDC): *Nursing homes and assisted living (long term care facilities [LTCFs])*, 2015. https://www.cdc.gov/longtermcare/.

Centers for Disease Control and Prevention (CDC): *Viral hepatitis*, 2016a. http://www.cdc.gov/hepatitis/hcv/hcvfaq.htm#b1.

Centers for Disease Control and Prevention (CDC): *Hand hygiene in healthcare settings: show me the science*, 2016b. https://www.cdc.gov/handhygiene/science/index.html.

Centers for Disease Control and Prevention (CDC): *Precautions to prevent the spread of MRSA*, 2016c. https://www.cdc.gov/mrsa/healthcare/clinicians/precautions.html.

Dalal I, Rolfman CM: *Immunity of the newborn*, 2015. http://www.uptodate

.com/contents/immunity-of-the-newborn.

Denny J, Munro CL: Chlorhexidine bathing effects on health-care-associated infections, *Biol Res Nurs* 19(2):123, 2016.

Donskey CJ, Deshpande A: Effect of chlorhexidine bathing in preventing infections and reducing skin burden and environmental contamination: a review of the literature, *Am J Infect Control* 44:e17–e21, 2016.

Dubé E, et al: Vaccine hesitancy an overview, *Hum Vaccin Immunother* 9:1763–1773, 2013.

Edmunds SI, et al: Effectiveness of hand hygiene for removal of *Clostridium difficile* spores from hands, *Infect Control Hosp Epidemiol* 34:302–305, 2013.

Fiutem C: Risk factors facilitating transmission of infectious agents. In Grota P, editor: *APIC text of infection control and epidemiology*, ed 4, Washington, DC, 2015, Association for Professionals in Infection Control and Epidemiology (APIC).

Food and Drug Administration (FDA), Department of Health and Human Services: *Banned Devices; powdered surgeon's gloves, powdered patient examination gloves, and absorbable powder for lubricating a surgeon's glove*, 2016. https://s3.amazonaws.com/public-inspection.federalregister.gov/2016-30382.pdf.

Gowda C, Dempsey A: The rise (and fall?) of parental vaccine hesitancy, *Hum Vaccin Immunother* 9:1755–1762, 2013.

Haas J: Hand hygiene. In Grota P, et al, editors: *APIC text of infection control and epidemiology*, ed 4, Washington, DC, 2015, Association for Professionals in Infection Control and Epidemiology (APIC).

Kak V: Vaccination and infection prevention. In Haiduven D, Poland G, editors: *Hospital infection prevention:*

principles and practices, New York, 2014, Springer India.

Longin Y, et al: Contamination of stethoscopes and physicians' hands after a physical examination, *Mayo Clin Proc* 89:291–299, 2014.

Murphy R: Surgical services. In Grota P, editor: *APIC text of infection control and epidemiology*, ed 4, Washington, DC, 2015, Association for Professionals in Infection Control and Epidemiology (APIC).

Occupational Safety and Health Administration (OSHA): *Personal protective equipment*, OSHA Publication 3151-12R, 2003.

Occupational Safety and Health Administration (OSHA): *Respiratory infection control: respirators versus surgical masks*, OSHA Fact Sheet, 2009. https://www.osha.gov/Publications/respirators-vs-surgicalmasks-factsheet.html.

Occupational Safety and Health Administration (OSHA): *Disposal of contaminated needles and blood tube holders used for phlebotomy*, OSHA Safety and Health Information Bulletin, 2015. https://www.osha.gov/dts/shib/shib101503.html.

Occupational Safety and Health Administration (OSHA): *Fit testing procedures: part I, OSHA-accepted fit test protocols*, n.d., https://www.osha.gov/pls/oshaweb/owadisp.show_document?p_table=standards&p_id=9780.

O'Grady NP, et al: Guidelines for the prevention of intravascular catheter-related infections, *Am J Infect Control* 39(4 Suppl):S1, 2011.

Pop-Vicas A, et al: Multidrug-resistant gram-negative bacteria in a long-term care facility: prevalence and risk factors, *J Am Geriatr Soc* 56:1276–1280, 2008.

Rowe TA, Juthani-Mehta M: Urinary tract infection in older adults, *Aging Health* 9(5):2013.

Royal College of Nursing: *Wipe it out: one chance to get it right*, London, 2011. Royal College of Nursing, https://www.rcn.org.uk/professional-development/publications/pub-004166.

Rutala WA, Weber DJ: Cleaning, disinfection, and sterilization. In Grota P, editor: *APIC text of infection control and epidemiology*, ed 4, Washington, DC, 2015, Association for Professionals in Infection Control and Epidemiology (APIC).

Surawizc C, et al: Guidelines for diagnosis, treatment, and prevention of *Clostridium difficile* infections, *Am J Gastroenterol* 108:478–498, 2013.

The Joint Commission (TJC): *2018 National Patient Safety Goals*, Oakbrook Terrace, IL, 2018. The Commission, https://www.jointcommission.org/hap_2017_npsgs/.

Tweeten S: General principles of epidemiology. In Grota P, editor: *APIC text of infection control and epidemiology*, ed 4, Washington, DC, 2015, Association for Professionals in Infection Control and Epidemiology (APIC).

World Health Organization (WHO): *WHO guidelines on hand hygiene in health care*, Geneva, 2009, WHO.

World Health Organization (WHO): *Health-care waste: fact sheet no 253*, 2015. http://www.who.int/mediacentre/factsheets/fs253/en/.

World Health Organization (WHO): *About SAVE Lives: Clean Your Hands: 5 moments for hand hygiene*, 2017. http://www.who.int/gpsc/5may/background/5moments/en/.

Zastrow RL: Emerging infections: the contact precautions controversy, *Am J Nurs* 111:47, 2011.

evolve MEDIA RESOURCES

http://evolve.elsevier.com/Potter/essentials
- Audio Glossary
- Case Study Continuation

- QSEN Activity and Review Questions Answers and Rationales
- Video Clips

OBJECTIVES

- Explain the principles and mechanisms of thermoregulation.
- Describe nursing interventions that promote heat loss and heat conservation.
- Discuss physiological changes associated with fever.
- Accurately assess body temperature, pulse, respiration, oxygen saturation, and blood pressure.

- Describe factors that cause variations in vital signs.
- Identify ranges of acceptable vital sign values for an infant, child, and adult.
- Explain variations in techniques used to assess vital signs in an infant, child, and adult.
- Correctly delegate vital sign measurement to nursing assistive personnel.

KEY TERMS

afebrile, p. 272
antipyretic, p. 273
apical pulse, p. 279
apnea, p. 289
auscultatory gap, p. 285
bradycardia, p. 279
bradypnea, p. 289
capillary oxygen saturation, p. 289
core temperature, p. 270
diaphoresis, p. 271
diastolic pressure, p. 280
digital thermometer, p. 276
dysrhythmia, p. 279

ETCO$_2$ monitoring, p. 289
eupnea, p. 288
febrile, p. 272
fever, p. 271
heat stroke, p. 273
hypertension, p. 280
hyperthermia, p. 273
hypotension, p. 280
hypothermia, p. 273
infrared thermometer, p. 276
Korotkoff sound, p. 283
nonshivering thermogenesis, p. 271
orthostatic hypotension, p. 280

oxygen saturation, p. 289
perfusion, p. 288
pulse deficit, p. 279
pulse pressure, p. 280
pyrexia, p. 271
sphygmomanometer, p. 282
systolic pressure, p. 280
tachycardia, p. 279
tachypnea, p. 289
vasoconstriction, p. 270
vasodilation, p. 270
ventilation, p. 288
vital signs, p. 268

The cardinal **vital signs** are temperature, pulse, respiration, blood pressure, and oxygen saturation. Another vital sign, pain, is a standard of care for vital signs in many health care settings (see Chapter 34). Frequently pain and discomfort are the problems that lead a patient to seek health care. Therefore assessing your patient for pain helps you understand the patient's clinical status and progress.

Many factors such as the temperature of the environment, physical exertion, medications, and the effects of diagnostic tests and illness cause vital signs to change, sometimes outside

CASE STUDY *Ms. Coburn*

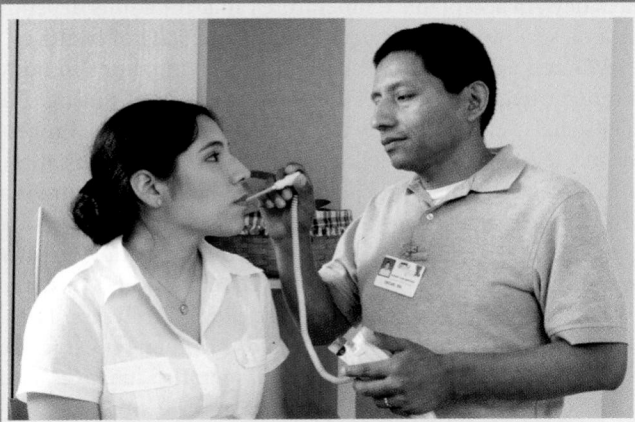

Ms. Coburn is a 26-year-old school teacher who is 20 lb over-weight. Her maternal grandparents immigrated to America from Brazil. She lives alone in an apartment building. She has smoked one pack of cigarettes a day since she was 16 years of age. She reports having two alcoholic drinks each week. Ms. Coburn made an appointment with her health care provider because she started having headaches and frequently felt tired.

Miguel is a 42-year-old nurse who enjoys providing health-related teaching to the patients at the clinic and has provided nursing care for Ms. Coburn for the past 2 years. During Ms. Coburn's visit Miguel assesses her symptoms. He asks her about her headaches and fatigue. After interviewing Ms. Coburn, Miguel takes her vital signs. Her temperature is 36.7° C (98° F), respiratory rate is 14 breaths/min, pulse is 86 beats/min, and blood pressure is 164/98 mm Hg. Ms. Coburn asks Miguel, "So does this mean I'm healthy?" Miguel responds, "Ms. Coburn, your blood pressure is pretty high right now. After you see the nurse practitioner today, I am going to take your blood pressure again. We're also going to talk about the changes you can begin to make to help you be healthier and feel better."

the acceptable range. Accurately measuring vital signs and assessing pain provide data to determine a patient's usual state of health (baseline data), the response to physical and psychological stress, and medical and nursing therapies. A change in vital signs indicates a change in physiological functioning or a change in comfort, signaling the necessity for medical or nursing intervention.

Measuring vital signs is a quick and efficient way of monitoring your patient's condition, identifying problems, and evaluating a patient's response to intervention. You need to take vital signs accurately because they are the backbone for clinical problem solving.

GUIDELINES FOR MEASURING VITAL SIGNS

A complete set of vital signs is included in a complete physical examination (see Chapter 16). Sometimes you take vital signs individually to assess a patient's condition. Likewise, a patient's needs and conditions determine when, where, how,

and by whom vital signs are measured. Correctly obtaining vital signs, interpreting values, implementing interventions, communicating findings to health care team members appropriately, and recognizing the need for reevaluation are essential nursing skills. Use the following guidelines to help incorporate vital sign measurements into your nursing practice:

1. Measuring vital signs is your responsibility. You may delegate this task in certain situations (e.g., stable patients) to nursing assistive personnel (NAP). However, it is your responsibility as the nurse to review vital sign data, interpret their significance, and critically think through decisions regarding implementing appropriate nursing interventions.
2. Assess equipment to ensure that it is working correctly and provides accurate findings.
3. Select equipment based on a patient's condition and physical characteristics (e.g., for a patient who is overweight, use an extra-large size blood pressure cuff rather than an adult size).
4. Vital sign measurements can require removing clothing or exposing areas. Provide patient privacy while being sensitive to cultural norms when measuring vital signs.
5. Know your patient's normal vital signs range. A patient's usual values sometimes differ from the standard range because of age, illness, or physical state. Use a patient's usual values as a baseline comparison.
6. Know a patient's medical history, prescribed medications, therapies, and treatments; these factors can significantly cause vital sign changes.
7. Control or minimize environmental factors that affect vital signs. A patient's respiratory rate taken immediately after exercising does not provide accurate data or a true picture of the patient's condition. Likewise, a patient's temperature taken directly after bathing does not represent an accurate picture of thermoregulation.
8. Use an organized, systematic approach when measuring vital signs.
9. Based on a patient's condition, collaborate with the health care provider to decide the frequency of vital sign assessment. In the hospital the health care provider orders a minimum frequency of vital sign measurements for each patient. After surgery, treatment intervention, or invasive diagnostic procedures you obtain vital signs frequently to detect complications. If a patient's physical condition worsens, it is often necessary to monitor vital signs every 5 to 10 minutes. You also measure vital signs before, during, and after medication administration. For example, a health care provider may order to hold a cardiac medication for a heart rate less than 50 beats/min or a systolic blood pressure less than 100 mm Hg. Vital sign assessment is also done when a patient seeks care from a health care provider in the community. Wherever vital signs are measured you are responsible for judging whether a patient needs more frequent assessments (Box 15.1).

<table>
<tr><td>

BOX 15.1 **WHEN TO MEASURE VITAL SIGNS**

- On admission to a health care agency
- When assessing patients during home care visits
- In a hospital on a routine schedule according to a health care provider's order or standards of practice
- Before, during, and after a surgical procedure or invasive diagnostic procedure
- Before, during, and after transfusion of blood products
- Before, during, and after administration of medications or applications of therapies that affect cardiovascular, respiratory, or temperature-control functions
- When a patient's general physical condition changes (e.g., loss of consciousness or increased intensity of pain)
- Before, during, and after nursing interventions influencing a vital sign (e.g., before and after a patient currently on bed rest ambulates, before and after a patient performs range-of-motion exercises)
- When a patient reports nonspecific symptoms of physical distress (e.g., feeling "funny" or "different")

</td></tr>
</table>

10. Analyze the results of vital sign measurement based on a patient's condition and past medical history (PMH).
11. Verify and communicate significant changes in vital signs. Baseline measurements provide a starting point for identifying and accurately interpreting possible changes. When vital signs appear abnormal, have another nurse repeat the measurement. Inform the charge nurse or health care provider of abnormal vital signs immediately, document findings in your patient's record, and report vital sign changes to nurses during hand-off communications.

BODY TEMPERATURE

Body temperature is the difference between the amount of heat produced by body processes and the amount of heat lost to the external environment.

$$\text{Heat produced} - \text{Heat lost} = \text{Body temperature}$$

Despite environmental temperature extremes and physical activity, temperature-control mechanisms of human beings keep body core temperature, or temperature of deep tissues, relatively constant during sleep, exposure to cold, and strenuous exercise. However, surface temperature fluctuates, depending on blood flow to the skin and the amount of heat lost to the external environment. Bodily tissues and cells function efficiently within a relatively narrow temperature range, from 36° to 38°C (96.8° to 100.4°F), but no single temperature is normal for all people. For healthy young adults the average oral temperature is 37°C (98.6°F). In older adults the average core temperature ranges from 35° to 36.1°C (95° to 97°F) as a result of decreased immunity (Touhy and Jett, 2014). The circadian rhythm also affects body temperature, with the lowest body temperature at 6 a.m. and the highest at 4 p.m. in healthy people. The circadian rhythm

alters body temperature about 0.5°C (0.9°F) throughout each day. An acceptable temperature range for adults depends on age, sex, range of physical activity, and state of health.

Women generally experience greater fluctuations in body temperature than men. Hormonal variations during the menstrual cycle cause body temperature fluctuations. Progesterone levels rise and fall cyclically during menstruation. When progesterone levels are low, the body temperature is a few tenths of a degree below baseline. The lower temperature persists until ovulation occurs. During ovulation greater amounts of progesterone enter the circulation and raise the body temperature to previous baseline levels or higher. These temperature variations help to predict a woman's most fertile time to become pregnant. Body temperature changes also occur during menopause. Women who have stopped menstruating often experience periods of intense body heat and sweating (popularly termed "hot flashes") lasting from 30 seconds to 5 minutes. During these periods there are often intermittent increases in skin temperatures of up to 4°C (7.2°F).

Temperatures vary depending on the measurement site. Sites reflecting core temperature such as the pulmonary artery are more reliable indicators of body temperature than sites reflecting surface temperature such as the armpit or axilla. Pulmonary artery temperature monitoring, used in critically ill patients, offers accurate readings because of the blood mix from all regions of the body.

Body Temperature Regulation

Physiological and behavioral mechanisms precisely regulate and control body temperature mechanisms. For the body temperature to stay constant and within an acceptable range, the body needs to maintain the relationship between heat production and heat loss.

Neural and Vascular Control. The hypothalamus, located between the cerebral hemispheres of the brain and below the thalamus, controls body temperature by attempting to maintain a comfortable temperature or set-point. When the hypothalamus senses an increase in body temperature, it sends out impulses for the release of hormones to reduce body temperature by sweating and vasodilation (widening of blood vessels). Vasodilation increases blood flow to the skin, which enables heat loss through radiation. If the hypothalamus senses that body temperature is lower than the set-point, it triggers hormone release to increase heat production by muscle shivering or heat conservation by vasoconstriction (narrowing of surface blood vessels). Disease or trauma to the hypothalamus or spinal cord, which carries hypothalamic messages, decreases the ability of the body to control body temperature.

Heat Production. Temperature regulation relies on normal heat production processes. Heat is produced as a by-product of metabolism. As metabolism increases the body produces additional heat. When metabolism decreases, the body produces less heat. Heat production occurs during rest, voluntary movement, involuntary shivering, and nonshivering thermogenesis. The voluntary movement of muscular activity during exercise requires additional energy. Metabolism increases during activity, resulting in increased heat production up to 50 times normal. Shivering is an involuntary body response to temperature differences in the body. Shivering can increase heat production four or five times higher than normal. However, in a neonate the immature temperature regulation system does not allow for shivering. Instead a neonate metabolizes vascular brown adipose tissue for heat production until 6 to 12 months of age (Knobel, 2014), a process called *nonshivering thermogenesis*. Premature infants less than 32 weeks of age have insufficient stores of brown fat placing them at highest risk for hypothermia (Knobel, 2014).

Heat Loss. Heat loss and production occur at the same time. The exposure of the skin to the environment results in constant, normal heat loss through radiation, conduction, convection, and evaporation. Infants and young children have a greater ratio of surface area to body weight; thus they lose more heat to the environment than adults.

Radiation is the transfer of heat between two objects without physical contact. Heat radiates from the skin to any surrounding cooler object. Up to 85% of the surface area of the human body radiates heat to the environment. During surgery patients often lose excessive amounts of heat in the cool environment of the operating room; thus you need to closely monitor your patient's temperature during and after surgery.

A small amount of heat loss occurs through conduction, which is the transfer of heat from one object to another with direct contact. When warm skin touches a cooler object, heat transfers from the skin to the object until temperatures equalize. In patients with fevers, heat loss increases with the application of ice packs or bathing with tepid water. Applying several layers of clothing reduces conductive loss. The body gains heat by conduction when it contacts materials warmer than skin temperature such as prewarmed blankets.

Convection is the transfer of heat away from the body by air movement. Fans promote heat loss through convection. The rate of heat loss increases when moist skin comes into contact with slightly moving air. Heat energy transfers from a liquid to a gas state by evaporation. The body continuously loses heat by evaporation; approximately 600 to 900 mL of water evaporates daily from the skin and lungs. The body promotes additional evaporative heat loss through perspiration or sweating. Diaphoresis (i.e., excessive sweating) drastically lowers body temperature and typically manifests on the forehead, upper chest, and arms.

Skin in Temperature Regulation. Skin, subcutaneous tissue, and fat help to maintain body temperature through insulation. Therefore people with more body fat have more natural insulation than slim or muscular individuals. The skin, or integumentary system (along with neural control), regulates body temperature similar to the way a car radiator controls engine temperature. The car engine generates a great deal of heat. Water pumps through the engine to collect the heat and carry it to the radiator, where a fan transfers the heat from the water to the outside air. The internal organs of the body produce heat, and during exercise or increased sympathetic stimulation the amount of heat produced is greater than the usual core temperature. Blood flows from the internal organs, carrying heat to the body surface. At the surface blood passing through the vascular areas of the hands and feet varies from minimal flow to 30% of the blood pumped from the heart. Heat transfers from the blood through vessel walls to the surface of the skin and is lost to the environment through heat loss mechanisms.

Behavioral Control. When the environmental temperature falls, a person adds clothing, moves to a warmer place, raises the thermostat setting on a furnace, increases muscular activity by running in place, or sits with arms and legs tightly wrapped together. In contrast, when the temperature becomes hot, a person removes clothing, stops activity, turns on a fan or lowers the thermostat setting on an air-conditioner, seeks a cooler place, or takes a cool shower.

Considerations for Older Adults. Older adults do not maintain a constant body temperature in stressful situations because of neurosensory changes that occur in their thermoregulation, leaving them sensitive to hyperthermia and hypothermia. Likewise, decreased immune function results in an inability to mount an effective initial response to infection. Consequently older adults often present with a normal to only slightly elevated temperature when an infection is present. Therefore it is important for you to recognize that older adults who have low-grade fevers may be sicker than they appear. Many older adults are on fixed incomes and they decrease their heat or air conditioning to save money, which then places them at high risk for problems with thermoregulation.

Temperature Alterations

Body temperature changes are related to excess heat production, heat loss, too little heat production, or any combination of these alterations. The nature of the change affects the type of clinical problems experienced by a patient.

Fever. The condition of pyrexia or fever occurs because heat loss mechanisms are unable to keep pace with excess heat production, resulting in an abnormal rise in body temperature. A fever is usually not harmful if it stays below 39°C (102.2°F) in adults or 40°C (104°F) in children. A single temperature reading does not always indicate a fever and often results from outside influences such as a recent increase in physical activity or environmental changes. You determine your patient's fever by taking several temperature readings at different times during the day and comparing them with the patient's usual values.

A true fever results from an alteration in the hypothalamic set-point. Substances that trigger the immune system such as bacteria or viruses stimulate the release of hormones in an

BOX 15.2	PATTERNS OF FEVER
Sustained	Constant body temperature continuously above 38°C (100.4°F) that demonstrates little fluctuation
Intermittent	Fever spikes mixed with usual temperature levels; temperature returns to acceptable value at least once in 24 hours
Remittent	Fever spikes and falls without a return to acceptable temperature levels
Relapsing	Periods of febrile episodes mixed with acceptable temperature values; febrile episodes and periods of normothermia sometimes last longer than 24 hours

BOX 15.3   NURSING MANAGEMENT OF PATIENTS WITH A FEVER

ASSESSMENT
- Obtain frequent temperature readings (i.e., tympanic, oral, rectal) during a fever.
- Assess for contributing factors such as dehydration, infection, or environmental temperature.
- Obtain all vital signs.
- Identify physiological response to fever (e.g., diaphoresis, tachycardia, hypotension).
- Assess skin color and temperature and presence of thirst, anorexia, and malaise; observe for shivering and diaphoresis.
- Assess patient comfort and well-being.

INTERVENTIONS (UNLESS CONTRAINDICATED)
- Before antibiotic therapy obtain blood cultures when ordered (see Chapter 14). Obtain blood specimens at the same time as a temperature spike, when the causative organism is most prevalent.
- Minimize heat production: reduce frequency of activities that increase oxygen demand such as excessive turning and ambulation; allow rest periods; limit physical activity.
- Maximize heat loss: reduce external covering on patient's body without causing shivering; keep clothing and bed linen dry.
- Satisfy requirements for increased metabolic rate: provide supplemental oxygen therapy as ordered to improve oxygen delivery to body cells; provide measures to stimulate appetite, and offer well-balanced meals; provide fluids (at least 3 L/day for a patient with normal cardiac and renal function) to replace fluids lost through insensible water loss and sweating.
- Promote patient comfort: encourage oral hygiene because oral mucous membranes dry easily from dehydration and have increased potential for bacterial invasion; control temperature of environment without inducing shivering; apply cool, damp cloth to patient's forehead.
- Identify onset and duration of febrile episode phases: examine previous temperature measurements for trends.
- Initiate health teaching as indicated.
- Maintain environmental temperature at 21°C to 27°C (70°F to 80°F).

effort to promote bodily defense against infection. These hormones also trigger the hypothalamus to raise the set-point, inducing a febrile episode. To reach the new set-point the body produces and conserves heat. The patient experiences chills, shivers, and feels cold, even though the body temperature is rising. If the set-point has been "overshot" or if the immune triggers are removed, the skin becomes warm and flushed because of vasodilation. Diaphoresis results in evaporative heat loss. When a fever "breaks," the temperature returns to an acceptable range, and the patient becomes afebrile. A fever pattern is present when a febrile episode recurs (Box 15.2).

Fever serves as an important defense mechanism. Health care providers are unlikely to treat an adult's fever until it is more than 39°C (102.2°F). Mild temperature elevations enhance the immune system of the body by stimulating white blood cell production. Increased temperature reduces the concentration of iron in the blood plasma, causing bacterial growth to slow. Fever also fights viral infections by stimulating interferon, the natural virus-fighting substance of the body.

Fevers also serve a diagnostic purpose. Fever patterns differ, depending on the causative pyrogen (i.e., the substance such as bacteria that causes the fever). The duration and degree of fever depend on the strength of the pyrogen and the ability of the individual to respond. The term *fever of unknown origin (FUO)* refers to a fever for which the cause cannot be determined.

Treatment for a fever depends on its cause; adverse effects; and strength, intensity, and duration of the elevated temperature. You play a key role in assessing fever and implementing temperature-reducing strategies (Box 15.3). The goal is a "safe" rather than a "low" temperature. Health care providers determine the cause of fever by isolating the causative bacterium or virus by obtaining culture specimens such as urine, blood, sputum, and wound drainage for laboratory analysis. If the culture is bacterial in origin, the health care provider orders antibiotics to be given to effectively destroy bacteria and eliminate the stimulus for fever.

Most fevers in children are of viral origin, last only briefly, and have limited effects. However, children have immature temperature control mechanisms; therefore temperatures sometimes rise rapidly. Dehydration and febrile seizures occur during rising temperatures in children between 6 months and 3 years of age. Febrile seizures are unusual in children older than 5 years of age. The extent of the temperature change, often exceeding 38.8°C (102°F), seems to be a more important factor than the rapidity of the temperature increase. Interventions for children's fevers are based on their response to the illness and not on the temperature level itself.

Sometimes a fever results from a hypersensitivity response to a medication, especially when the medication is taken for the first time. These fevers are often accompanied by other allergy symptoms such as rash, hives, or itching. Treatment involves stopping the medication responsible for the reaction.

The objective of fever therapy is to increase heat loss, reduce heat production, and prevent complications. Nondrug therapies (see Box 15.3) for fever increase heat loss by evaporation, conduction, convection, or radiation. Use caution when implementing nursing interventions and think about heat production and heat loss mechanisms. For example, when using nursing interventions to enhance body cooling, make sure to avoid stimulating shivering. Shivering is counterproductive because of the heat produced by muscle activity. Physical cooling, including regulating room temperature and using fans (as appropriate) and water-cooled blankets, is appropriate when a patient's own thermoregulation fails or in patients with neurological damage (e.g., spinal cord injury).

An **antipyretic** is a medication that reduces fever. Nonsteroidal drugs such as acetaminophen, salicylates, indomethacin, ibuprofen, and ketorolac reduce fever by increasing heat loss. Health care providers order antipyretics if a fever is more than 39°C (102.2°F). Although not used to treat fever, corticosteroids reduce heat production by interfering with the hypothalamic response. It is important to note that these drugs mask signs of infection by suppressing the immune system. Therefore patients on steroids need to be observed closely, especially if they are at risk for infection.

Hyperthermia. Hyperthermia is an elevated body temperature related to the inability of the body to promote heat loss or reduce heat production. Fever is an upward shift in the set-point, whereas hyperthermia is caused by an overload on the temperature release mechanisms. Any injury to the hypothalamus impairs heat loss mechanisms. Educate patients at risk for hyperthermia to:
- Avoid strenuous exercise in hot, humid weather.
- Avoid exercising in areas with poor ventilation.
- Drink fluids such as water and clear fruit juices before, during, and after exercise.
- Wear light, loose-fitting, light-colored clothing.
- Wear a protective covering over the head when outdoors.
- Expose themselves to hot climates gradually.

Prolonged exposure to the sun or high environmental temperatures overwhelms the heat loss mechanisms of the body. Heat also depresses hypothalamic function. These conditions cause **heat stroke**, which is a dangerous heat emergency defined as a body temperature of 40.2°C (104.4°F) or more (Goforth and Kazman, 2015). Exertional heat stroke is a common cause of death in competitive athletes (Sloan et al., 2015). Signs and symptoms of heat stroke include giddiness, confusion, delirium, excess thirst, nausea, muscle cramps, visual disturbances, and incontinence. The most important sign of heat stroke is hot, dry skin. Heat stroke can be fatal. Call 9-1-1 for emergency assistance as you begin cooling the person using the following methods:
- Move the person out of the sun to the shade or a shelter.
- Cool water immersion is the most rapid means (Sloan et al., 2015). Ways to cool include placing wet towels

over the skin, spraying the person with cool water from a garden hose, and placing oscillating fans in the room.
- If the person can drink, give cool nonalcoholic liquids.
- Continue to take the temperature until it drops to 38.3°C to 38.8°C (101°F to 102°F).

Emergency medical treatment includes applying hypothermia blankets, giving IV fluids, and irrigating the stomach and lower bowel with cool solutions.

Hypothermia. Heat loss during prolonged exposure to cold overwhelms the ability of the body to produce heat, causing **hypothermia**. Hypothermia is classified by core temperature measurements as mild, moderate, or severe (Table 15.1). Accidental hypothermia occurs when a person is exposed to a cold environment without protective clothing. Accidental hypothermia usually develops gradually and may go unnoticed for several hours. The patient experiences uncontrolled shivering, loss of memory, depression, and poor judgment. As the body temperature falls below 34°C (93.2°F), heart and respiratory rates and blood pressure decrease. Intentional hypothermia is a therapeutic approach that reduces the body's need for oxygenated blood. Intentional hypothermia can preserve vital organs during prolonged neurological or cardiac surgery and following a cardiac arrest (Perman et al., 2015).

The priority treatment for intentional or accidental hypothermia is prevention of a further decrease in body temperature. Removing wet clothes, replacing them with dry ones, and wrapping the patient in blankets are key nursing interventions. In emergencies, when a patient is not in a health care setting, place the patient under blankets next to a warm person, usually skin to skin, for heat conduction. A conscious patient benefits from drinking hot liquids such as soup while avoiding alcohol and caffeinated fluids. Interventions include keeping the head covered, increasing room temperature, or using forced-air warming systems. The cause and severity of the hypothermia dictate the treatments implemented.

Prevention is the key for patients at risk for hypothermia. Provide education to patients, family caregivers, and friends. People at high risk include the very young; the very old; and people debilitated by trauma, stroke, diabetes, drug or alcohol intoxication, and sepsis. Patients with mental illness or handicaps and older adults are at risk for developing hypothermia because they are unaware of the dangers of cold conditions. People without adequate home heating, shelter, diet, or clothing are also at risk.

TABLE 15.1	CLASSIFICATION OF HYPOTHERMIA	
HYPOTHERMIA	**°C**	**°F**
Mild	34°–36°	93.2°–96.8°
Moderate	30°–34°	86°–93.2°
Severe	Less than 30°	Less than 86°

Measurement of Temperature

Assessment of temperature regulation requires you to make judgments about the site for temperature measurement, type of device, and frequency of measurement.

Sites. Measure body temperature by using core or body surface sites. The core temperatures of the pulmonary artery, esophagus, and urinary bladder are often used in critical care settings and require continuous invasive monitoring devices placed in arteries or internal organs. The most common sites for intermittent temperature measurements are surface sites such as the tympanic membrane, temporal artery, mouth, rectum, and axilla. Skin temperature obtained by applying noninvasive, chemically prepared thermometer patches to the skin are used for screening a patient's temperature. Core temperature measurement sites are more reliable than surface or skin temperature measurement sites (Niven et al., 2016).

To ensure accurate temperature readings, measure each site correctly (see Skill 15.1). Depending on the site used, temperatures normally vary between 36°C (96.8°F) and 38°C (100.4°F). Rectal temperatures are usually 0.5°C (0.9°F) higher than oral temperatures, whereas tympanic and axillary temperatures are usually 0.5°C (0.9°F) lower than oral temperatures. Each temperature measurement site has advantages and disadvantages (Box 15.4). Choose the safest and most accurate site for each patient. Use the same site when repeating measurements.

Thermometers. Four types of thermometers are commonly available for measuring body temperature: electronic, infrared, digital, and disposable chemical dot. Mercury-in-glass

---

BOX 15.4 ADVANTAGES AND LIMITATIONS OF SELECT TEMPERATURE MEASUREMENT SITES

SITE ADVANTAGES	SITE LIMITATIONS
ORAL	
Easily accessible—requires no position change	Causes delay in measurement if patient recently ingested hot/cold fluids or foods, smoked, or chewed gum
Comfortable for patient	
Provides accurate surface temperature reading	Not used with patients who have had oral surgery, trauma, shaking or chills, or history of seizures
Reflects rapid change in core temperature	
Reliable route to measure temperature for intubated patients	Not used with infants; small children; or confused, unconscious, or uncooperative patients
	Risk for body fluid exposure
TYMPANIC MEMBRANE	
Easily accessible site	Susceptible to user error
Obtained without disturbing, waking, or repositioning patient	Has low sensitivity for detecting fever compared with standard core temperature measurement methods (i.e., rectal, bladder)
Used for patients with tachypnea without affecting breathing	
Rapid measurement (2 to 5 seconds)	Requires removal of hearing aids before measurement
Unaffected by oral intake of food or fluids or by smoking	Requires disposable sensor cover with only one size available
Shown to have high precision, sensitivity and specificity (accuracy) in measuring body temperature and a high correlation with nasopharyngeal temperature (Asadian et al., 2016)	Otitis media and cerumen impaction distort readings
	Not used with patients who have had surgery of the ear or tympanic membrane
	Does not accurately measure core temperature changes during and after exercise
	Affected by ambient temperature devices such as incubators, radiant warmers, and facial fans
	Anatomy of ear canal makes it difficult to position correctly in neonates, infants, and children younger than 3 years old
RECTAL	
Considered gold standard for estimating core temperature	Lags behind core temperature during rapid temperature changes
Argued to be more reliable than alternative sites when oral temperature is difficult or impossible to obtain	Not used for patients with diarrhea or patients who have had rectal surgery, rectal disorders, bleeding tendencies, or neutropenia
	Requires positioning and is a source of patient embarrassment and anxiety
	Risk for body fluid exposure; thermometer can serve as reservoir for *Clostridium difficile* (CDC, 2015).
	Requires lubrication
	Not used for routine vital signs in newborns
	Readings sometimes influenced by impacted stool

BOX 15.4 ADVANTAGES AND LIMITATIONS OF SELECT TEMPERATURE MEASUREMENT SITES—cont'd

SITE ADVANTAGES	SITE LIMITATIONS
AXILLA	
Safe and inexpensive	Long measurement time
Recommended only for screening	Requires continuous positioning
Reliable in stable and preterm infants (Charafeddine et al., 2014)	Poorly reflects core temperature (Reynolds et al., 2014)
	Measurement lags behind core temperature during rapid temperature changes
	Not recommended to detect fever in infants and young children
	Requires exposure of thorax, which results in temperature loss, especially in newborns
SKIN	
Inexpensive	Lags behind measurements obtained at other sites during temperature changes, especially during hyperthermia
Provides continuous reading	Diaphoresis or sweat impairs adhesion
Safe and noninvasive	Affected by environmental temperature
Used for neonates	Cannot be used on patients with adhesive allergy
TEMPORAL ARTERY	
Easy to access without position change	Inaccurate with head covering or hair on forehead
Useful for screening body temperature	Affected by skin moisture such as diaphoresis or sweating
Very rapid measurement	Underestimates temperature in patients with fever (Furlong et al., 2015)
No risk for injury to patient or nurse	
Eliminates need to disrobe or unbundle	
Comfortable for patient	
Can be used in premature infants, newborns, and children (Reynolds et al., 2014)	
Reflects rapid change in core temperature	
Sensor cover not required	

thermometers are obsolete in the health care setting because of the environmental hazards of mercury. However, some patients may still use mercury-in-glass thermometers at home. If you find a mercury-in-glass thermometer in the home, teach the patient about safer temperature devices and encourage appropriate disposal of the hazardous device.

Each device measures temperature in either the Celsius or the Fahrenheit scale. Electronic thermometers allow you to convert scales by activating a switch. Use the following formulas for manual conversion:

To convert Fahrenheit to Celsius, subtract 32 from the Fahrenheit reading and multiply the result by $\frac{5}{9}$.

$$\text{Example: } (104°F - 32°F) \times \tfrac{5}{9} = 40°C$$

To convert Celsius to Fahrenheit, multiply the Celsius reading by $\frac{9}{5}$ and add 32 to the product.

$$\text{Example: } (\tfrac{9}{5} \times 40°C) + 32 = 104°F$$

Electronic Thermometers. Electronic thermometers have a rechargeable battery-powered display unit, a thin wire cord, and a temperature-processing probe or sensor covered by a disposable probe cover (Fig. 15.1). Separate probes are available for oral (blue tip) and rectal (red tip) use. You obtain axillary temperatures with the oral probe. Electronic

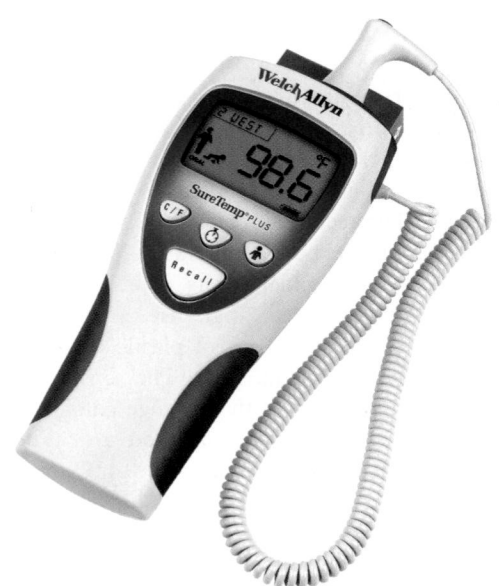

FIG 15.1 Electronic thermometer with disposable plastic probe cover. (Courtesy Welch Allyn.)

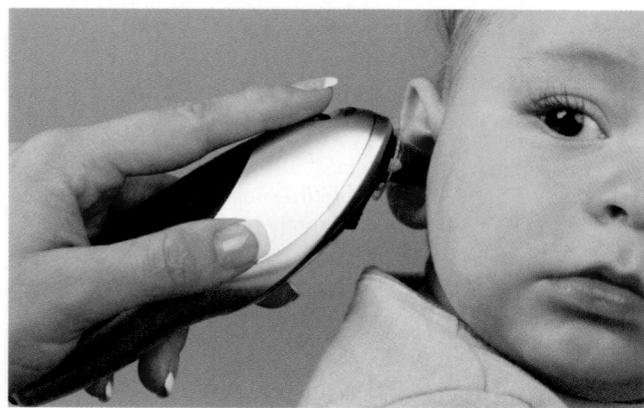

FIG 15.2 Tympanic membrane thermometer. (Courtesy Welch Allyn.)

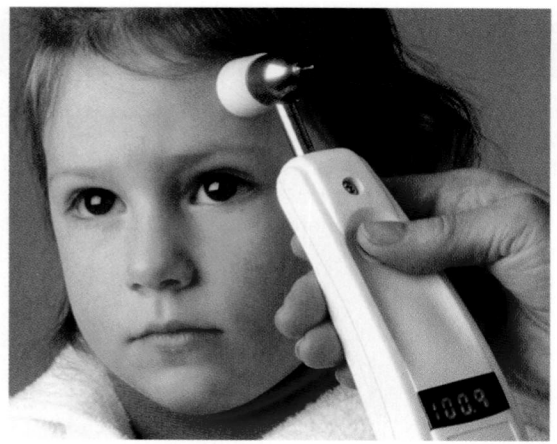

FIG 15.3 Temporal artery thermometer scanning forehead.

thermometers provide two modes of operation, 4-second predictive temperatures and 3-minute standard temperatures. In daily clinical situations the 4-second predictive is more commonly used.

An infrared thermometer relies on thermal radiation to measure body temperature. The tympanic membrane thermometer has an otoscope-like speculum with an infrared sensor tip that detects heat radiated from the tympanic membrane of the ear (Fig. 15.2). Within seconds after placement in the ear canal and pressing the scan button, a sound signals when the peak temperature has been measured, and a reading appears on the display unit. The temporal artery thermometer measures blood flow through the superficial temporal artery. Proper technique involves sweeping an infrared handheld scanner across the forehead then just behind the ear (Fig. 15.3). After scanning is complete, a reading appears on the display unit.

A digital thermometer contains a probe connected to a microprocessor chip, which translates signals into degrees and sends a temperature measurement to a digital display. You use a digital thermometer for oral, rectal, and axillary measurements. The rectal temperature is still the gold standard for estimating core body temperature, but the thermometer is difficult to use in older adults.

Chemical Thermometers. Single-use or reusable chemical thermometers are thin strips of plastic with a temperature sensor on one end (Fig. 15.4). The sensor consists of chemically impregnated dots that change color at different temperatures. In the Celsius version there are 50 dots, each representing temperature increments of 0.1°C over a range of 35.5°C to 40.4°C. The Fahrenheit version has 45 dots with increments of 0.2°F over a range of 96°F to 104.8°F. Chemicals on the thermometer change color to reflect temperature reading, 3 minutes for axilla and 1 minute for oral. Single-use chemical thermometers are useful in caring for patients in emergency departments or in protective isolation (see Chapter 14) and screening temperatures, especially in infants and young children. You need to confirm readings with electronic thermometers when making treatment decisions.

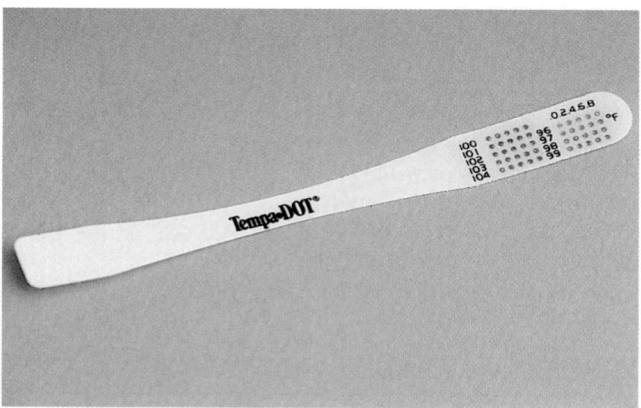

FIG 15.4 Disposable, single-use thermometer strip. (Courtesy Exergen.)

Another form of disposable chemical thermometer is a temperature-sensitive patch or tape. Applied to the forehead or abdomen, temperature-sensitive areas of the patch change color at different temperatures. Home disposable thermometers are useful for temperature screening but are not as accurate as nondisposable electronic thermometers (Counts et al., 2014).

PULSE

The pulse represents the number of cardiac cycles per minute and is the palpable rhythm of blood flow in a peripheral artery. The ejection of blood from the left ventricle during systole enters the aorta after passing through the aortic valve. The ejected blood moves through the major and peripheral arteries (e.g., in the wrist); thus it feels like a tap when you lightly palpate the artery against underlying bone or muscle. The number of pulsing sensations occurring in 1 minute is the pulse rate. An adult's normal heart rate ranges from 60 to 100 beats/min. In children the average heart rate is significantly increased and varies by age.

QSEN ACTIVITY *Evidence-Based Practice*

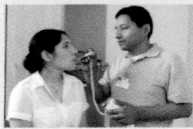

Ms. Coburn has been admitted to the hospital. You are caring for her and decide to verify her temporal temperature reading of 39.2°C (102.6°F) with a tympanic membrane thermometer. Because you are interested in evidence-based practice (see Chapter 7), you recently conducted a literature search pertaining to temperature accuracy in hospitalized patients, and you know that obtaining accurate temperature readings is sometimes problematic. Your literature search showed that nurses who do not use temporal artery thermometers correctly often have inaccurate readings in patients who are febrile. Of the six articles you reviewed, four were randomized controlled trials involving use of the temporal thermometer compared with standard electronic thermometers. Three of the four articles did not recommend the temporal thermometer for definitive temperature determination but stated that it can be used in screening. Two of the articles were systematic reviews. Neither review supported use of the temporal thermometer for anything other than screening. You will present your information at your next unit meeting.
- Regarding the evidence you found, which types of research evidence have greater strength in their findings than others?
- Based on the research articles you collected, do you think you are ready to recommend to your co-workers a change in practice? Explain your answer.

evolve Answers to QSEN Activities can be found on the Evolve website.

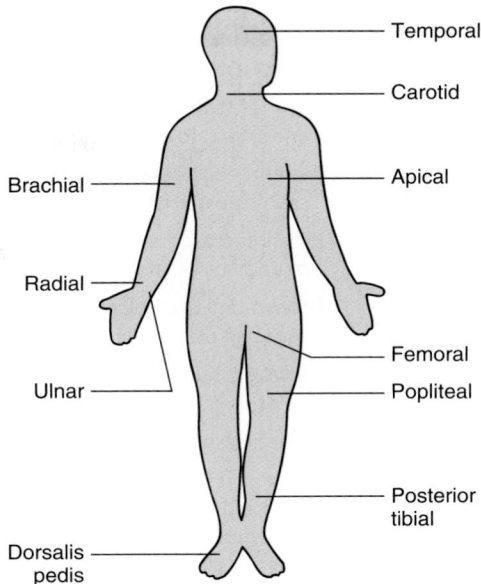

FIG 15.5 Location of peripheral pulses.

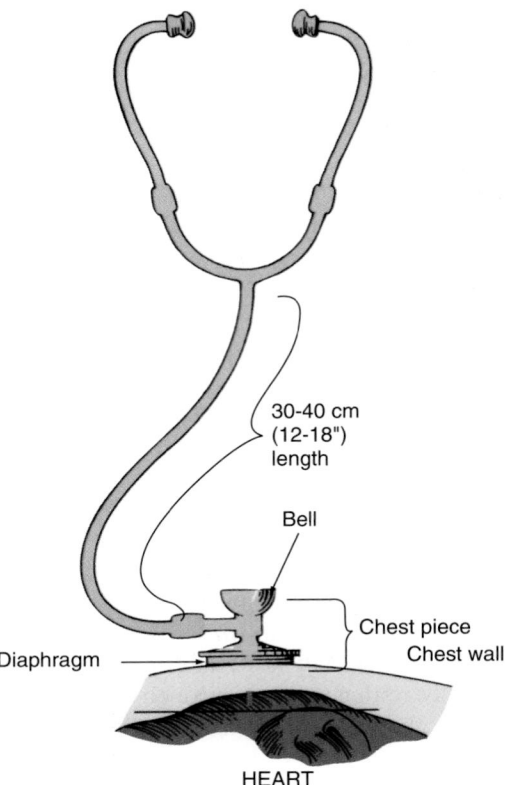

FIG 15.6 Acoustic stethoscope.

Locating a Peripheral Pulse

You assess any accessible artery for pulse rate (Fig. 15.5); however, the radial and apical locations are the most common sites for pulse rate assessment because each is easy to locate and palpate. When a patient's condition deteriorates suddenly, use the carotid site to quickly locate a pulse. Use the radial or carotid pulse when teaching patients how to monitor their own heart rates (e.g., athletes or patients using heart medications). If the radial pulse is abnormal, difficult to palpate, or inaccessible because of a dressing or cast, assess the apical pulse for 1 minute. When a patient takes medication that affects the heart rate, the apical pulse provides a more accurate assessment. Table 15.2 summarizes pulse sites and criteria for measurement. See Skill 15.2, which outlines radial and apical pulse rate assessment.

Using a Stethoscope

You use a stethoscope to auscultate the sound waves created by an apical pulse (Fig. 15.6). The four parts of the stethoscope are the earpieces, binaurals, tubing, and chest piece.

Make sure that the plastic or rubber earpieces fit snugly in the ear canal and that the binaurals are angled and strong enough so that the earpieces stay firmly in place without causing discomfort. The binaurals follow the contour of the ear canal, pointing toward the face when the stethoscope is in place.

The polyvinyl tubing is flexible and 30 to 45 cm (12 to 18 inches) in length. Longer tubing decreases sound-wave transmission. The tubing is thick walled and moderately rigid to eliminate transmission of environmental noise and prevent

TABLE 15.2   PULSE SITES

SITE	LOCATION	ASSESSMENT CRITERIA
Temporal	Over temporal bone of head, above and lateral to eye	Easily accessible site used to assess pulse in children
Carotid	Along medial edge of sternocleidomastoid muscle in neck	Easily accessible site used in patients with physiological shock or during adult CPR when other sites are not palpable
Apical	Fifth intercostal space at left midclavicular line	Site used to auscultate for apical pulse
Brachial	Groove between biceps and triceps muscles at antecubital fossa	Site used to assess upper-extremity blood pressure; used during infant CPR
Radial	Radial or thumb side of forearm at wrist	Common site used to assess character of pulse peripherally; assesses status of circulation to hand
Ulnar	Ulnar side of forearm at wrist	Site used to assess status of circulation to ulnar side of hand; used to perform Allen test
Femoral	Below inguinal ligament, midway between symphysis pubis and anterior superior iliac spine	Site used to assess character of pulse in patients with physiological shock or during CPR when other pulses are not palpable; assesses status of circulation to leg
Popliteal	Behind knee in popliteal fossa	Site used to auscultate lower-extremity blood pressure; assesses status of circulation to lower leg
Posterior tibial	Inner side of ankle, below medial malleolus	Site used to assess status of circulation to foot
Dorsalis pedis	Along top of foot, between extension tendons of great and first toe	Site used to assess status of circulation to foot

CPR, Cardiopulmonary resuscitation.

kinking, which distorts the sound. Stethoscopes have one or two tubes.

The chest piece consists of a bell and diaphragm that rotates into position. Lightly tap each surface to determine which side is functioning. The diaphragm is the circular, flat-surfaced portion of the chest piece covered with a thin plastic disk. It transmits high-pitched sounds created by the high-velocity movement of air and blood. Use the diaphragm to auscultate bowel, lung, and heart sounds. Position the diaphragm of the stethoscope firmly and directly on the patient's skin because clothing can distort the sound (Fig. 15.7).

The bell is the cone-shaped chest piece usually surrounded by a rubber ring to avoid chilling the patient. It transmits low-pitched sounds created by the low-velocity movement of blood. Use it to auscultate heart and vascular sounds. Apply the bell lightly, resting the chest piece on the skin (Fig. 15.8). Compressing the bell against the skin distorts low-pitched sounds.

One type of stethoscope has one chest piece that combines the bell and diaphragm together. When you use light pressure, the chest piece becomes the bell; when you press the chest piece slightly harder, the bell converts to a diaphragm. The size of the stethoscope chest piece varies from small (used for infants and young children) to large. Determine the appropriate chest piece to use by assessing the surface area being auscultated. Either the diaphragm or the bell can be used for blood pressure measurement (Liu et al., 2016).

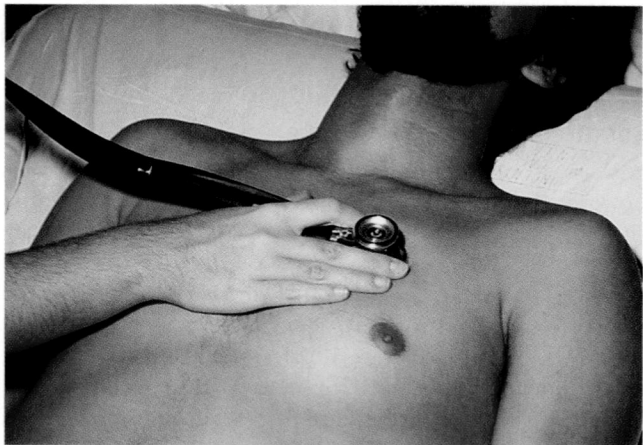

FIG 15.7 Positioning diaphragm of stethoscope.

The stethoscope is a delicate instrument and requires proper care for optimal function. Remove the earpieces regularly and clean them of cerumen (earwax). Inspect the bell and diaphragm for dust, lint, and body oils. Clean with either alcohol or mild soap and water between patients to reduce bacterial contamination and avoid hospital-acquired infections (Longtin et al., 2016). Do not use fabric stethoscope covers. Covers cannot be washed between patients and can be contaminated with bacteria.

Assessment of Pulse

Pulse Rate. Before you measure a pulse, review a patient's medical record to obtain a baseline rate. Remember, pulse rates vary with a patient's age. Compare your patient's actual pulse rate with the expected usual values (Table 15.3). When

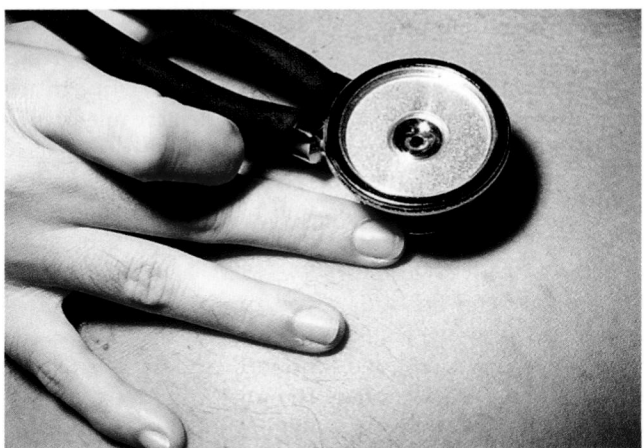

FIG 15.8 Positioning bell of stethoscope.

TABLE 15.3	ACCEPTABLE RANGES OF HEART RATE FOR AGE
AGE-GROUP	**HEART RATE (beats/min)**
Infant	120–160
Toddler	90–140
Preschool child	80–110
School-aged child	75–100
Adolescent	60–90
Adult	60–100

assessing the pulse, consider the variety of factors influencing pulse rate (Table 15.4). A combination of these factors often causes significant changes. If you detect an abnormal rate or rhythm while palpating a peripheral pulse, the next step is to auscultate the apical pulse for 1 minute to obtain a more accurate assessment of cardiac function.

Assess the apical pulse by listening for heart sounds (see Chapter 16). After properly positioning the bell or the diaphragm of the stethoscope on the chest, try to identify the first and second heart sounds (S_1 and S_2). At normal slow rates S_1 is low pitched and dull, sounding like a "lub." S_2 is a higher pitched, shorter sound and creates the sound "dub." Count each set of "lub-dub" as one heartbeat. Count the number of "lub-dubs" occurring in 1 minute.

Pulse rate assessment often reveals variations in heart rate. Two common abnormalities in heart rate are tachycardia and bradycardia. Tachycardia is an abnormally elevated heart rate, more than 100 beats/min in adults. Bradycardia is a slow rate, less than 60 beats/min in adults.

Pulse Rhythm. Normally a regular interval of time occurs between each pulse or heartbeat. A regular interval interrupted by an early beat, late beat, or missed beat indicates an irregular rhythm or dysrhythmia. A dysrhythmia alters cardiac function, particularly if it occurs repetitively. If your patient has a dysrhythmia, assess how often it is occurring. Dysrhythmias are regularly irregular or irregularly irregular. The health care provider sometimes orders additional tests to evaluate the occurrence of dysrhythmias.

An inefficient contraction of the heart that fails to transmit a pulse wave to the peripheral pulse site creates a pulse deficit. To assess a pulse deficit, ask another nurse to assess the radial pulse rate while you assess the apical rate. If you discover a difference between the apical and radial pulse rates, a pulse deficit exists. Pulse deficits are frequently associated with dysrhythmias.

TABLE 15.4	FACTORS INFLUENCING HEART RATES	
FACTOR	**INCREASE HR**	**DECREASE HR**
Exercise	Short-term exercise	Well-conditioned patient may have a slower-than-usual resting HR that returns more quickly to resting rate after exercise
Temperature	Fever, heat, hyperthermia	Hypothermia
Emotions	Emotional stress, anxiety, or fear stimulates sympathetic nervous system	Unrelieved severe pain increases parasympathetic stimulation, affecting HR
Medications	Positive chronotropic medications such as epinephrine; stimulants such as caffeine	Antidysrhythmics and cardiotonics affect rate and rhythm of pulse; large doses of narcotic analgesics; general anesthetics
Hemorrhage	Loss of blood increases sympathetic stimulation	
Postural changes	Standing or sitting	Lying down
Pulmonary conditions	Diseases causing poor oxygenation such as asthma and COPD	

COPD, Chronic obstructive pulmonary disease; *HR,* heart rate.

Strength and Equality. The strength or amplitude of a pulse reflects the volume and pressure of the blood ejected against the arterial wall with each heart contraction and the condition of the arterial vascular system leading to the pulse site. Normally the pulse strength remains the same with each heartbeat. Assess both radial pulses at the same time to compare the characteristics of each. Pulse strength or amplitude is assigned a number grade and described as bounding (+4), full or increased (+3), expected and easily palpable (+2), diminished and barely palpable (+1), or absent (0). Evaluate pulse strength and equality during assessment of the vascular system (see Chapter 16).

BLOOD PRESSURE

Blood pressure is the force exerted on the walls of an artery created by the pulsing blood under pressure from the heart. Blood flows throughout the circulatory system because of pressure changes, moving from an area of high pressure to an area of low pressure. Under high pressure the left ventricle ejects blood into the aorta; the peak pressure is known as **systolic pressure**. When the ventricles relax, the blood remaining in the arteries exerts a minimum or **diastolic pressure**. Diastolic pressure is the minimal pressure exerted against the arterial wall at all times.

The standard unit for measuring blood pressure is millimeters of mercury (mm Hg). The measurement indicates the height to which the blood pressure raises a column of mercury. You record blood pressures as a ratio with the systolic reading before the diastolic (e.g., 120/80 mm Hg). The difference between systolic and diastolic pressure is the **pulse pressure**. For a blood pressure of 120/80 mm Hg, the pulse pressure is 40.

Physiology of Arterial Blood Pressure

Blood pressure depends on the interrelationships of cardiac output, peripheral vascular resistance, blood volume, blood viscosity, and artery elasticity. An increase in cardiac output is usually the result of greater heart muscle contractility, an increase in heart rate, or an increase in blood volume. An increase in cardiac output increases blood pressure. When peripheral arteries constrict such as during periods of stress, peripheral vascular resistance increases, which results in increased blood pressure. As vessels dilate and resistance falls, blood pressure drops. When blood is forced through the rigid arteries, blood pressure rises. If the blood volume decreases, such as during dehydration or hemorrhage, less pressure is exerted against arterial walls, and blood pressure falls. When the percentage of red blood cells increases, the blood viscosity increases, causing the heart to contract more forcefully to move the blood through the circulatory system, resulting in an increased blood pressure.

Blood Pressure Variations

Many factors continually influence blood pressure. A single measurement does not adequately reflect a patient's blood pressure. Blood pressure trends, not individual measurements, guide nursing and medical interventions. Understanding the factors that cause alterations in blood pressure helps to accurately interpret blood pressure measurements. Box 15.5 summarizes factors affecting blood pressure.

Hypertension. The most common alteration in blood pressure is **hypertension**, an often asymptomatic disorder characterized by persistently elevated blood pressure. Hypertension is defined as systolic blood pressure (SBP) greater than 140 mm Hg and diastolic blood pressure (DBP) greater than 90 mm Hg. Patients on antihypertensive medication with acceptable blood pressure measurements are considered to have hypertension. The Joint National Committee on Prevention, Detection, Evaluation, and Treatment of High Blood Pressure (JNC8) (James et al., 2014) published criteria for categories of hypertension (Table 15.5). Hypertension is a known risk factor for cardiovascular morbidity and mortality. Obesity, cigarette smoking, excessive alcohol intake, elevated blood cholesterol, and continued exposure to stress are risk factors for hypertension. The American Heart Association (AHA) recommends maintaining a blood pressure less than 130/80 mm Hg for high-risk groups, and the treatment goal for persons with cardiac dysfunction is blood pressure less than 120/80 mm Hg (James et al., 2014). Normal blood pressure is considered to be less than 120/80 (AHA, 2016).

A diagnosis of hypertension is based on the average of two or more seated blood pressure measurements, properly measured with well-maintained equipment, at each of two or more visits to an office or clinic after an initial screening (James et al., 2014). Thus one blood pressure recording revealing a high SBP or DBP does not qualify as a diagnosis of hypertension. However, if a high reading is obtained (e.g., 150/90 mm Hg), encourage the patient to return for another checkup within 2 months (Table 15.6).

Hypotension. Hypotension is an SBP less than 90 mm Hg. Although some adults have low blood pressure normally, for most individuals hypotension is an abnormal finding associated with an illness (e.g., hemorrhage or myocardial infarction). Hypotension occurs when arteries dilate, the peripheral vascular resistance decreases, the circulating blood volume decreases, or the heart fails to provide adequate cardiac output. Signs and symptoms associated with hypotension include pallor, skin mottling, clamminess, confusion, dizziness, chest pain, increased heart rate, and decreased urine output. Hypotension is usually life threatening and needs to be reported immediately to the patient's health care provider. **Orthostatic hypotension**, also referred to as postural hypotension, is a reduction of SBP of at least 20 mm Hg or a reduction of DBP of at least 10 mm Hg within 3 minutes of quiet standing. It occurs when patients experience a drop in blood pressure on rising to an upright position and is associated with symptoms of light-headedness or dizziness. In severe cases, loss of consciousness occurs. Orthostatic hypotension is a risk factor for falls especially among older adults with hypertension (Angelousi et al., 2014). When a healthy person changes from a lying to sitting to standing

BOX 15.5 FACTORS INFLUENCING BLOOD PRESSURE

AGE

- Blood pressure (BP) tends to rise with advancing age:

AGE	AVERAGE ARTERIAL PRESSURE (mm Hg)
Newborn (3000 g [6.6 lb])	65/41
1 month	85/54
1 year	86/40
6 years	94/56
10–13 years	103/62
14–17 years	110/65
Adult	<120/80*

- Assess the level of BP in a child or adolescent with respect to sex, body size, and age. Larger children have higher BPs than smaller children of the same age (Hockenberry and Wilson, 2015).

GENDER

- There is no clinically significant difference in BP levels between boys and girls before puberty.
- After puberty males have higher BPs.
- During and after menopause women have higher BPs than men of the same age.

ETHNICITY

- The incidence of hypertension is higher in African Americans than in European Americans.
- African Americans tend to develop more severe hypertension at an earlier age and have twice the risk for complications of hypertension such as stroke and heart attack. Hypertension-related deaths are also higher among African Americans.

SYMPATHETIC STIMULATION

- Pain, anxiety, and fear stimulate the sympathetic nervous system, causing BP to rise. A full bladder can increase sympathetic stimulation, elevating BP.

DAILY VARIATION

- BP varies throughout the day with lower BP during sleep, increasing during the day.
- BP can drop 10% to 20% during nighttime sleep.

MEDICATION AND TREATMENT

- Some medications directly or indirectly affect BP. Opioids, sedatives, general anesthetics, antihypertensives, and vasodilators lower BP, whereas vasoconstrictors, blood, and IV fluid infusion raise BP.

ACTIVITY

- Older adults often experience a 5- to 10-mm Hg fall in BP about 1 hour after eating.
- BP falls as a person moves from lying to sitting or standing position; normal postural variations are minimal.
- Increase in oxygen demand by the body during activity increases BP.

WEIGHT

- Obesity is a risk factor for hypertension.
- In school-aged children the higher their body mass index, the greater the risk for developing hypertension at an early age.

DIET

- A diet low in sodium and high in potassium can reduce BP. Vegetarian diets and limited alcohol consumption (fewer than two drinks per day for men and one per day for women) are associated with low BP. BP reductions are greater among older adults implementing dietary modifications.

SMOKING

- Smoking results in vasoconstriction, a narrowing of blood vessels.

*American Heart Association: What is High Blood Pressure, 2016, https://www.heart.org/idc/groups/heart-public/@wcm/@hcm/documents/downloadable/ucm_300310.pdf.

TABLE 15.5 CLASSIFICATION OF BLOOD PRESSURE FOR ADULTS 18 YEARS AND OLDER

CATEGORY	SYSTOLIC (mm Hg)[a]		DIASTOLIC (mm Hg)[a]
Normal	Less than 120		Less than 80
Prehypertension[b]	120–139	or	80–89
Stage 1 hypertension	140–159	or	90–99
Stage 2 hypertension	160 or greater	or	100 or greater

[a]Based on average of two or more readings taken at each of two or more visits after an initial screening. Patient should not be taking antihypertensive drugs and should not be acutely ill. When systolic and diastolic blood pressures fall into different categories, select the higher category to classify the patient's blood pressure status. For example, classify 160/92 mm Hg as stage 2 hypertension.
[b]Based on average of two or more readings.
Data from James P, et al: 2014 evidence-based guideline for the management of high blood pressure in adults report from the panel members appointed to the Eighth Joint National Committee (JNC8), *JAMA* 311:507, 2014.

TABLE 15.6 RECOMMENDATIONS FOR BLOOD PRESSURE FOLLOW-UP

INITIAL BLOOD PRESSURE	FOLLOW-UP RECOMMENDED[a]
Normal	Recheck in 2 years.
Prehypertension	Recheck in 1 year.[b]
Stage 1 hypertension	Evaluate therapy within 1 month
Stage 2 hypertension	Evaluate therapy within 1 month. For patients with higher blood pressure (e.g., greater than 180/110 mm Hg), evaluate and treat immediately or within 1 week, depending on clinical situation and complications.

[a]Modify scheduling of follow-up according to reliable information about past blood pressure measurements, other cardiovascular risk factors, or target organ damage.
[b]Provide advice about lifestyle modifications.
Data from James P, et al: 2014 evidence-based guideline for the management of high blood pressure in adults report from the panel members appointed to the Eighth Joint National Committee (JNC8), *JAMA* 311:507, 2014.

position, the peripheral blood vessels in the legs constrict, preventing the pooling of blood in the legs caused by gravity. Orthostatic hypotension occurs when the peripheral blood vessels in the legs are already constricted or are unable to constrict in response to a change in position. Fluid volume deficit from decreased blood volume, dehydration, or recent blood loss; prolonged bed rest; anemia; and antihypertensive medications place patients at risk for orthostatic hypotension. Assess for orthostatic hypotension by obtaining pulse and blood pressure readings with the patient supine, sitting, and standing (Box 15.6).

Measurement of Blood Pressure

Measure arterial blood pressure either directly (invasively) or indirectly (noninvasively). The direct method requires the insertion of a thin catheter into an artery by a health care provider. Risks, such as sepsis, associated with continuous invasive blood pressure monitoring require the use of an intensive care setting. The more common noninvasive method requires use of the sphygmomanometer and stethoscope. Measure blood pressure indirectly by palpation or auscultation (see Skill 15.3).

Blood Pressure Equipment. Before assessing blood pressure, you need to become comfortable using a sphygmomanometer and stethoscope. A sphygmomanometer includes a pressure manometer, an occlusive cloth or disposable vinyl cuff that encloses an inflatable rubber bladder, and a pressure bulb with a release valve that inflates the bladder. The aneroid manometer has a glass-enclosed circular gauge containing a

BOX 15.6 PROCEDURAL GUIDELINES

Measuring Orthostatic Blood Pressure

DELEGATION CONSIDERATIONS
The skill of measuring orthostatic blood pressure (BP) cannot be delegated to nursing assistive personnel (NAP).

EQUIPMENT
Sphygmomanometer, stethoscope

STEPS
1. Identify patient using at least two identifiers (e.g., name and birthday or name and medical record number) according to agency policy.
2. Determine if it is appropriate to measure patient's orthostatic BP. Orthostatic vital signs are not indicated in patients who:
   • Have supine hypotension.
   • Have a sitting BP 90/60 mm Hg or less.
   • Have acute deep vein thrombosis.
   • Exhibit the clinical syndrome of shock.
   • Have severely altered mental status.
   • Have possible spinal injuries.
   • Have lower extremity or pelvic fractures.
   • Are not mobile enough to get out of bed.
3. Perform hand hygiene.
4. Have patient lie in bed with head of bed flat for a minimum of 3 minutes, preferably 5 minutes. With patient supine, take BP reading in each arm. Select arm with highest systolic reading for subsequent measurements.
5. Leaving BP cuff in place, help patient to sitting position. Take BP at 1 minute. If orthostatic signs or symptoms occur, such as dizziness, weakness, light-headedness, feeling faint, sudden pallor, or sitting BP 90/60 mm Hg or less, put patient back to bed in the supine position.
6. Leaving BP cuff in place, help patient to standing position. Take BP at 1 minute and 3 minutes with patient in standing position. If orthostatic signs or symptoms occur (as previously noted), stop BP measurement, return patient to bed (if possible), and help patient to supine position. In most cases you detect orthostatic hypotension within 1 minute of standing.
7. If patient is unable to stand, take second reading by having patient sit upright with legs dangling over the edge of the bed.
8. Record patient's BP in each position (e.g., "140/80 supine, 132/72 sitting, 108/60 standing"). Note any additional symptoms or complaints. A drop in systolic BP of 20 mm Hg or greater, a drop in diastolic BP of 10 mm Hg or greater, or an experience of light-headedness or dizziness is considered abnormal.
9. Report findings of orthostatic hypotension or orthostatic signs or symptoms to nurse in charge or health care provider. Instruct patient to move slowly when changing from one position to another and to ask for assistance when getting out of bed if orthostatic hypotension is present or orthostatic signs or symptoms occur.
10. Perform hand hygiene.

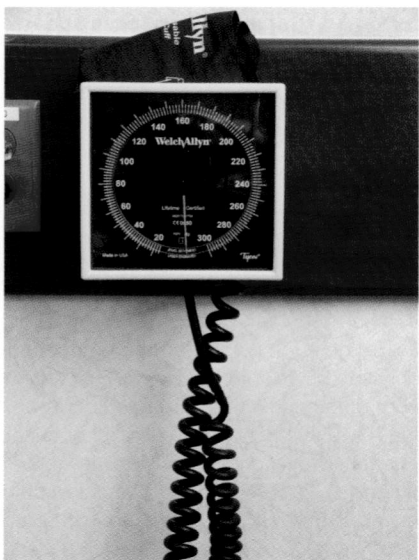

FIG 15.9 Wall-mounted aneroid sphygmomanometer.

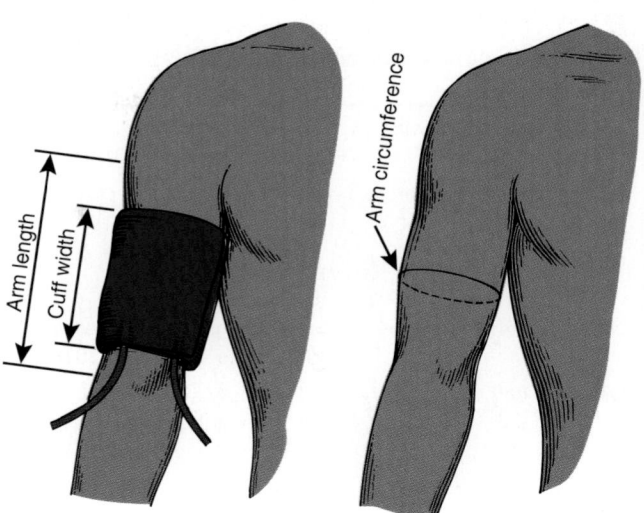

FIG 15.10 Guidelines for proper blood pressure cuff size. Cuff width equals 20% more than upper arm diameter or 40% of circumference around upper arm and two thirds of upper arm length.

needle that registers millimeter calibrations (Fig. 15.9). Aneroid manometers are safe, lightweight, portable, and compact. Before using a manometer, be sure that the needle points to zero. Metal parts in the aneroid manometer are subject to temperature variations and need to be checked every 6 months to verify their accuracy.

The release valves of the sphygmomanometer must be clean and freely movable in either direction. The valve, when closed, should hold the pressure constant. Frequent calibration is necessary to ensure accuracy. A sticky valve makes pressure cuff deflation hard to regulate. The pressure bulb and tubing should be airtight.

Cloth or disposable vinyl compression cuffs contain an inflatable bladder and come in several different sizes. The size selected is proportional to the circumference of the limb being assessed. Select a cuff that is at least 40% greater than the arm circumference (or 20% wider than the diameter) of the midpoint of the limb being used to obtain measurements (Fig. 15.10). The bladder, enclosed by the cuff, encircles at least 80% of the arm of an adult and the entire arm of a child. The lower edge of the cuff is above the antecubital fossa if the arm is being used, allowing room for placement of the stethoscope. An improperly placed or fitted cuff causes inaccurate blood pressure measurements (Table 15.7 and Box 15.7).

Auscultation. The best environment to auscultate blood pressure sounds is a quiet room at a comfortable temperature. Although a patient is able to lie or stand, sitting is the best position. It is also best to have a patient assume the same position during each blood pressure measurement to permit a meaningful comparison of values. Before assessment, control factors responsible for artificially high readings such as pain, anxiety, or exertion. *For example, in the case study, Ms. Coburn was anxious when first entering the examination room. After she sees the nurse practitioner, Miguel retakes her*

blood pressure. Her blood pressure this time is 146/94 mm Hg (first reading was 164/98 mm Hg).

A patient's perception that the physical or interpersonal environment is stressful affects blood pressure. Measurements taken at home are sometimes different from measurements taken at a patient's place of employment or health care provider's office. Home blood pressure devices measuring blood pressure at the wrist lead to falsely elevated values (Casiglia et al., 2016).

During the initial assessment you obtain and record blood pressures in both arms. Normally there is a difference of 5 to 10 mm Hg between the right and left arms. In subsequent assessments measure the blood pressure in the arm with the higher pressure. Pressure differences between extremities greater than 20 mm Hg indicate vascular problems and need to be reported to the charge nurse or health care provider.

Indirect measurement of arterial blood pressure works on a basic principle of pressure. Blood flows freely through an artery until an inflated cuff applies pressure to tissues and causes the artery to collapse. When the cuff slowly deflates, the point at which blood flow returns and sound appears through auscultation is the SBP.

In 1905 Nikolai Korotkoff, a Russian surgeon, first described the sounds heard over an artery during cuff deflation. The first Korotkoff sound is a clear, rhythmic tapping series that corresponds to the pulse rate and gradually increases in intensity. Onset of the sound corresponds to the systolic pressure. A murmur or swishing sound appears as the cuff continues to deflate, which is the second Korotkoff sound. As the artery distends, blood flow becomes turbulent. The third Korotkoff sound is a crisper and more intense

TABLE 15.7   COMMON MISTAKES IN BLOOD PRESSURE ASSESSMENT

ERROR	EFFECT
Bladder or cuff too wide	False-low reading (AACN Practice Alert, 2016)
Bladder or cuff too narrow or too short	False-high reading (AACN Practice Alert, 2016)
Cuff wrapped too loosely or unevenly	False-high reading
Deflating cuff too slowly	False-high diastolic reading (Gunes and Efteli, 2016)
Deflating cuff too quickly	False-low systolic and false-high diastolic reading (Gunes and Efteli, 2016)
Arm below heart level	False-high reading (AACN Practice Alert, 2016)
Arm above heart level	False-low reading (AACN Practice Alert, 2016)
Arm not supported	False-high reading (Gunes and Efteli, 2016)
Stethoscope that fits poorly or impairment of examiner's hearing, causing sounds to be muffled	False-low systolic and false-high diastolic reading
Stethoscope applied too firmly against antecubital fossa	False-low diastolic reading
Inflating too slowly	False-high diastolic reading
Repeating assessments too quickly	False-high systolic reading
Inadequate inflation level	False-low systolic reading
Multiple examiners using different Korotkoff sounds for diastolic readings	False-high systolic and false-low diastolic reading

BOX 15.7   EVIDENCE-BASED PRACTICE

PICO Question: In patients who are obese, which blood pressure cuff measures blood pressure (BP) more accurately, a thigh cuff or a regular cuff?

SUMMARY OF EVIDENCE

Errors in BP measurements result in overdiagnosing or underdiagnosing hypertension. More than one third of adults in the United States are obese. Researchers have found that the upper arm in a person who is obese is conical in shape increasing by as much as 20 cm from distal to proximal circumference. Large adult cuffs are recommended for an arm circumference of 35 to 44 cm. Researchers compared BP measurement obtained using a large adult cuff on the upper arm wrapped evenly, BP measurement obtained using a large cuff wrapped cylindrically, and invasive BP measurements (Anast et al., 2016). Each method of wrapping the cuff underestimated BP. Adult thigh cuffs applied to obese arms have overestimated BP by up to 30 mm Hg because of overcuffing (Halm, 2014). Applying an adult cuff to the forearm and auscultating the radial artery offers an alternative. However, a review of research evidence provided strong evidence that forearm systolic and diastolic BP measurements are greater than measurements in the upper arm (Halm, 2014). Cuff size for thigh BP measurement in patients who are obese can also be a challenge.

APPLICATION TO NURSING PRACTICE

- Assessment of BP in patients who are obese requires consistent use of equipment and methods. Once a method is established, use it consistently.
- Communicate that chosen method to the health care team.
- Recognize that the shape of a patient's arm alters the ability of the BP cuff to fit appropriately.
- Documentation of BP cuff size and location is important when comparing measurements in a patient who is obese.

tapping. The fourth Korotkoff sound becomes muffled and low pitched as the cuff is further deflated. The onset of the fourth Korotkoff sound is the diastolic pressure in infants and children (Basile and Bloch, 2016), pregnant women, and patients with elevated cardiac output or peripheral vasodilation. The fifth Korotkoff sound is the disappearance of sound; in adolescents and most adults this sound corresponds with the DBP (Fig. 15.11) (Basile and Bloch, 2016). In some patients the sounds are clear and distinct, whereas in others only the beginning and the ending sounds are heard. The AHA recommends recording two numbers for a blood pressure measurement: the point on the manometer when the first sound is heard for SBP and the point on the manometer when the fifth sound (disappearance of sound) is heard for DBP (James et al., 2014). Some institutions recommend recording the point when you hear the fourth sound, especially for patients with hypertension. You divide the numbers by slashed lines (e.g., 120/80, 120/100/80), note the arm used to measure the blood pressure, and record the patient's position (e.g., LA 158/78, sitting).

Decisions about patient care and implementing nursing interventions are based on the blood pressure measurements in combination with other findings. Obtaining an accurate blood pressure measurement is critical. There are several possibilities for error if the auscultation procedure is not followed correctly (see Table 15.7). If you are unsure of a reading, ask another nurse to reassess the blood pressure.

Ultrasonic Stethoscope. If you are unable to auscultate Korotkoff sounds because of a weak arterial pulse, use an ultrasonic stethoscope (see Chapter 16). This stethoscope allows you to hear low-frequency systolic sounds and is commonly used in infants and children and for measuring low blood pressure in adults.

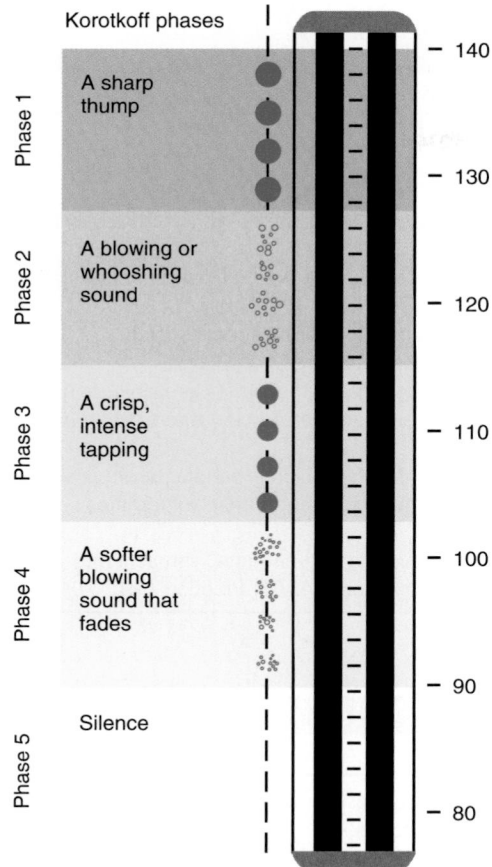

Korotkoff phases

Phase 1	A sharp thump
Phase 2	A blowing or whooshing sound
Phase 3	A crisp, intense tapping
Phase 4	A softer blowing sound that fades
Phase 5	Silence

140

130

120

110

100

90

80

FIG 15.11 Sounds auscultated during blood pressure measurement can be differentiated into five Korotkoff phases. The blood pressure is 140/90 in this example.

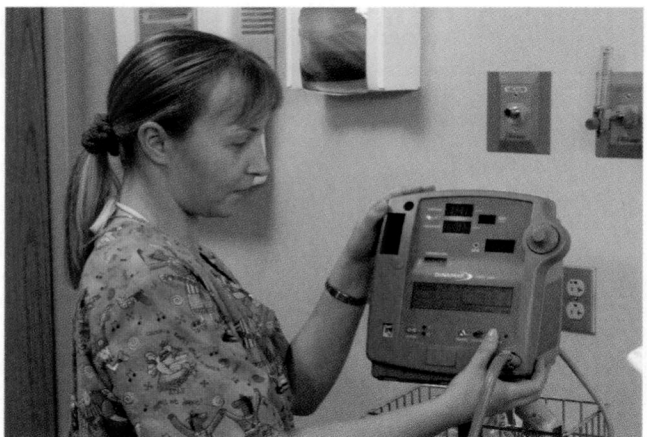

FIG 15.12 Electronic blood pressure machines vary in appearance.

Palpation. Indirect measurement of blood pressure by palpation is useful for patients whose arterial pulsations are too weak to create Korotkoff sounds or when there is excessive environmental noise that cannot be controlled. Severe blood loss and weakened heart contractility are examples of conditions that result in blood pressures too low to auscultate accurately. In this case you assess the SBP by palpation (see Skill 15.3, Step 7). DBP is difficult to determine by palpation. When using the palpation technique, you record the systolic value only and the location and manner in which it was measured (e.g., RA 78/–, palpated).

Sometimes you use palpation techniques with auscultation. In some patients with hypertension the sounds heard over the brachial artery when the cuff pressure is high disappear as pressure is reduced and then reappear at a lower level. This temporary disappearance of sound is the auscultatory gap. It typically occurs between the first and second Korotkoff sounds. The gap in sound can cover a range of 40 mm Hg, possibly causing an underestimation of SBP or an overestimation of DBP. Be certain to inflate the cuff high enough to hear the true SBP before the auscultatory gap. Palpation of the radial artery helps to determine how high to inflate the cuff. Inflate the cuff 30 mm Hg above the pressure at which the palpated radial pulse disappears and slowly release the cuff until the radial pulse returns. The return of the pulse correlates with the systolic pressure. Document the blood pressure reading with an auscultatory gap (e.g., "BP RA 180/94 with an auscultatory gap from 180 to 160").

Electronic Blood Pressure Machines. Many different styles of electronic blood pressure machines are available to determine blood pressure automatically (Fig. 15.12). Electronic blood pressure machines rely on an electronic sensor to detect the vibrations or sounds caused by the rush of blood through an artery. When the cuff deflates, one style of blood pressure machine determines the initial burst of oscillations and translates the information to a systolic pressure reading. The machine records a diastolic measurement when the oscillations are lowest, just before they stop. Although electronic blood pressure machines are fast and free up the care provider for other activities, it is necessary to consider their advantages and limitations (Box 15.8). Use the devices when frequent assessment is necessary, during or after invasive procedures, or when therapies require frequent monitoring (Box 15.9).

Blood Pressure Assessment in Lower Extremities. If your patient has dressings, casts, IV catheters, or an arteriovenous fistula or shunt in one arm, select the other arm for BP assessment. When neither upper extremity is appropriate or available, measure blood pressure in a lower extremity. Comparing upper-extremity blood pressure with the blood pressure in the legs is also necessary for patients with certain cardiac and blood pressure abnormalities. The popliteal artery, palpable behind the knee in the popliteal space, is the site for auscultation. Position the cuff with the bladder over the posterior aspect of the midthigh, 2.5 cm (1 inch) above the popliteal artery. Make sure that the cuff is wide enough and long enough to allow for the larger girth of the thigh. For most measurements place the patient in a prone position. If such a position is impossible, flex the knee slightly for easier access to the artery (Fig. 15.13). The procedure is identical to brachial artery auscultation. SBP in the legs is usually higher

BOX 15.8 ADVANTAGES AND LIMITATIONS OF ASSESSING BLOOD PRESSURE ELECTRONICALLY

ADVANTAGES	LIMITATIONS
• Ease of use • Efficient when frequent repeated blood pressure (BP) measurements are indicated • Stethoscope not required • Allows BP to be recorded more frequently, as often as every 15 seconds, with accuracy	• Expensive • Requires source of electricity • Requires space to position machine • Sensitive to outside motion interference; not used in patients with seizures, tremors, or shivers or patients unable to cooperate • Not accurate for hypotensive patients, hypertensive patients, or patients with cardiac dysrhythmias (AACN Practice Alert, 2016) • Should not be used in patients with rapidly changing BPs (McLean, 2015) • May cause low BP in older adults with arteriosclerosis • Systolic readings by automated wrist manometers are the most unreliable, and automated arm monitors tend to provide higher measures than the mercury standard on average (Casiglia et al., 2016) • Adherence to accuracy standards for electronic BP machine manufacturers is voluntary • Vulnerable to error in patients with irregular heart rate and obese extremities • Systolic BP possibly overestimated • Multiple readings are essential to provide clinicians and patients with accurate information on which to base diagnostic and treatment decisions (AACN Practice Alert, 2016)

BOX 15.9 PROCEDURAL GUIDELINES

Automatic Blood Pressure Measurement

DELEGATION CONSIDERATIONS

The skill of blood pressure (BP) measurement using an electronic BP machine can be delegated to nursing assistive personnel (NAP) unless the patient is considered unstable (i.e., hypotensive). The nurse instructs the NAP by:

• Explaining the frequency and extremity to use for measurement.
• Reviewing how to select appropriate-size BP cuff for designated extremity and appropriate cuff for machine.
• Reviewing patient's usual BP and how to report significant changes or abnormalities to the nurse.

EQUIPMENT

Electronic BP machine, BP cuff of appropriate size as recommended by manufacturer, pen and vital sign flow sheet in chart or electronic health record (EHR)

STEPS

1. Identify patient using at least two identifiers (e.g., name and birthday or name and medical record number) according to agency policy.
2. Assess need to measure BP and determine patient's baseline BP.
3. Determine appropriateness of using electronic BP measurement (see Box 15.8).
4. Perform hand hygiene. Inspect condition of extremities to determine best site for cuff placement.
5. Collect and bring appropriate equipment to patient's bedside. Select appropriate cuff size for patient extremity and appropriate cuff for machine. Electronic BP cuff and machine must be matched by manufacturer and are not interchangeable.
6. Assist patient to comfortable position, either lying or sitting. Plug device into electric outlet and place it near patient, ensuring that connector hose between cuff and machine reaches.
7. Locate on/off switch and turn on machine to enable device to self-test computer systems.
8. Remove constricting clothing to ensure proper cuff application.
9. Prepare BP cuff by manually squeezing all the air out of the cuff and connecting it to connector hose.
10. Wrap flattened cuff snugly around extremity, verifying that only one finger can fit between cuff and patient's skin. Make sure that "artery" arrow marked on outside of cuff is placed correctly (see illustration).

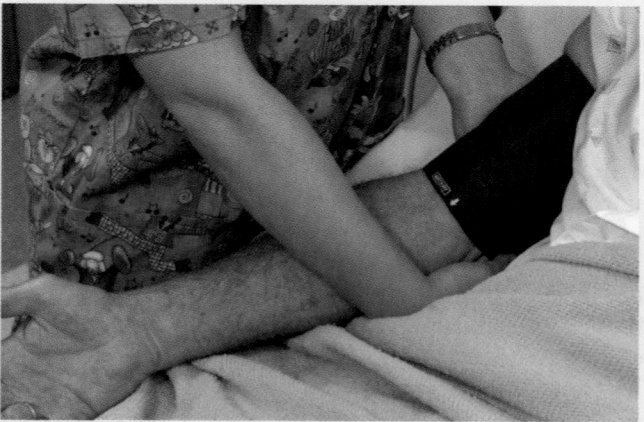

STEP 10 Aligning blood pressure cuff arrow with brachial artery.

11. Verify that connector hose between cuff and machine is not kinked. Kinking prevents proper inflation and deflation of cuff.

BOX 15.9   PROCEDURAL GUIDELINES—cont'd

Automatic Blood Pressure Measurement

12. Following manufacturer directions, set frequency control for automatic or manual, and press start button. The first BP measurement pumps cuff to a peak pressure of approximately 180 mm Hg. After this pressure is reached, the machine begins a deflation sequence that determines the BP. The first reading determines peak pressure inflation for additional measurements.
13. When deflation is complete, digital display provides most recent values and flash time in minutes that has elapsed since the measurement occurred (see illustration).

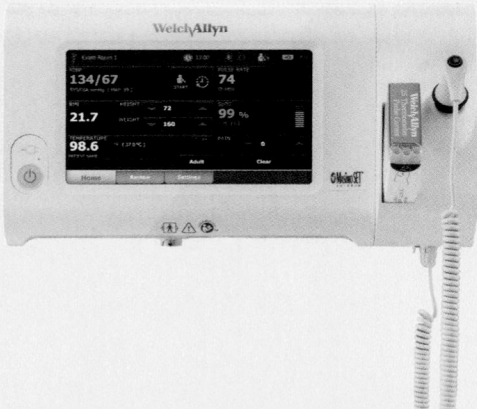

STEP 13 Digital electronic blood pressure display. (Image courtesy Welch Allyn.)

Clinical Decision Point. If unable to obtain BP with electronic device, verify machine connections (e.g., plugged into working electrical outlet, hose-cuff connections tight, machine on, correct cuff). Repeat electronic BP measurement; if unable to obtain, use auscultatory technique.

---

14. Set frequency of measurements and upper and lower alarm limits for systolic, diastolic, and mean BP readings. Intervals between measurements can be set from 1 to 90 minutes. A nurse determines frequency and alarm limits based on patient's acceptable range of BP, nursing judgment, and health care provider order.
15. Obtain additional readings at any time by pressing the start button. Pressing the cancel button immediately deflates the cuff.
16. If frequent measurements are required, the cuff may be left in place. Remove it at least every 2 hours to assess underlying skin integrity and if possible alternate measurement sites. Patients with abnormal bleeding tendencies are at risk for microvascular rupture from repeated inflations. When patient no longer requires frequent BP monitoring, remove and clean cuff according to agency policy to reduce transmission of microorganisms.
17. Discuss findings with patient. Perform hand hygiene.
18. Compare electronic BP readings with auscultatory measurements to verify accuracy of electronic device.
19. Record BP and site assessed on vital sign flow sheet or nurses' notes in chart or EHR; record any signs or symptoms of BP alterations in narrative form in nurses' notes; report abnormal findings to nurse in charge or health care provider.
20. **Use Teach-Back:** "I want to be sure I explained why you need to keep your arm straight while the machine is taking your BP. Tell me why it is important to remain still." Revise your instructions now or develop a plan for revised patient teaching if patient is unable to teach back correctly.

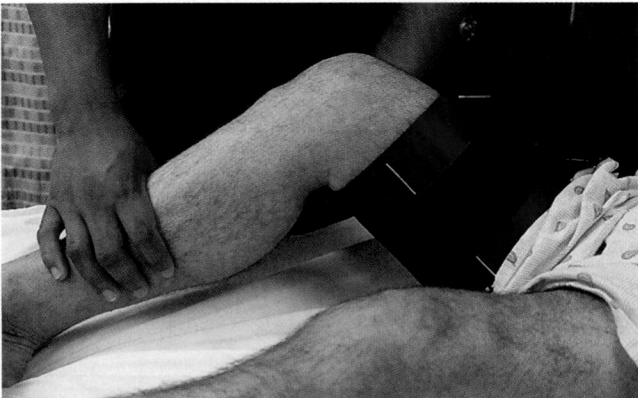

FIG 15.13 Lower-extremity blood pressure cuff positioned above popliteal artery at midthigh with knee flexed.

by 10 to 40 mm Hg than in the brachial artery, with the DBP lower (Halm, 2014).

Assessment of Blood Pressure in Children. All children 3 years of age through adolescence should have blood pressure checked at least annually. Blood pressure values in children change with growth and development. Educate parents about the importance of this routine screening to detect hypertension in children. Measuring blood pressure in infants and children is difficult for several reasons:

1. Smaller cuff size is required.
2. Readings are difficult to obtain in restless or anxious infants and children.
3. Placing stethoscope too firmly on the antecubital fossa causes errors in auscultation.
4. Korotkoff sounds are difficult to hear in children because of low frequency and amplitude; a pediatric stethoscope bell is helpful.

The same auscultation method used with adults is appropriate for children. An infant or child younger than 5 years of age lies supine with the arm supported at heart level. Have older children sit like adults with arm supported at the heart level. It is important for the child to be relaxed and calm. Allow at least 15 minutes for children to recover from recent activity or excitement before taking a reading. It helps to have a parent nearby. Prepare the child for the unusual sensation of the blood pressure cuff during inflation. Most children understand the analogy of a "tight hug on your arm" and will be more cooperative. Do not choose a cuff based on the name of the cuff (e.g., "infant"); rather base it on actual cuff bladder size. Average width of a cuff bladder for an infant is $2\frac{1}{2}$ to $3\frac{1}{4}$ inches; average width of a cuff bladder for a child is $4\frac{3}{4}$ to $5\frac{1}{2}$ inches.

RESPIRATION

Respiration is the mechanism the body uses to exchange gases between the atmosphere, blood, and cells. It involves three processes: ventilation (the mechanical movement of gases into and out of the lungs), diffusion (the movement of oxygen [O_2] and carbon dioxide [CO_2] between the alveoli and the red blood cells), and perfusion (the distribution of red blood cells to and from the pulmonary capillaries). Analyzing a patient's respiratory status requires integrating assessment data from all three processes. Assess ventilation by determining respiratory rate, depth, and rhythm. You assess diffusion and perfusion by evaluating oxygen saturation.

Assessment of Ventilation

Adults normally breathe in a smooth, uninterrupted pattern of 12 to 20 breaths/min. Levels of CO_2 in the arterial blood normally regulate ventilation by stimulation of chemoreceptors in the carotid artery and the heart. The normal rate and depth of ventilation, eupnea, is interrupted by sighing. The sigh, a prolonged deeper breath, is a protective physiological mechanism for expanding small airways and alveoli not ventilated during a normal breath.

Accurate assessment of ventilation depends on recognizing normal thoracic and abdominal movements. During quiet breathing the chest wall gently rises and falls. When breathing requires greater effort, the intercostal and accessory muscles work actively to move air in and out. The shoulders sometimes rise and fall, and the accessory muscles of ventilation in the neck visibly contract. Diaphragmatic movement becomes less noticeable as costal breathing increases.

Measurement of Respiration

Accurate measurement of respiration requires observation and palpation of chest wall movement. A sudden change in the character of respirations is an important assessment finding. Respiratory rate is a strong predictor of acute illness and mortality (Strauss et al., 2014). For example, slow respirations in a patient with head trauma can indicate a brainstem injury. Likewise, increased respirations can be seen in a patient with pneumonia or experiencing pain.

When assessing respiration, keep in mind the patient's usual respiratory rate, breathing pattern, the influence that

---

BOX 15.10 FACTORS INFLUENCING CHARACTER OF RESPIRATIONS

EXERCISE
- Exercise increases respiratory rate and depth to meet the need of the body for additional oxygen and to rid the body of carbon dioxide.

ACUTE PAIN
- Pain alters rate and rhythm of respirations; breathing becomes shallow.
- Patient inhibits or splints chest wall movement when pain is in area of chest or abdomen.

ANXIETY
- Anxiety increases respiratory rate and depth as a result of sympathetic stimulation.

SMOKING
- Chronic smoking changes pulmonary airways, resulting in increased respiratory rate at rest when not smoking.

BODY POSITION
- Standing or sitting erect promotes full ventilatory movement and lung expansion; stooped or slumped position impairs ventilatory movement; lying flat prevents full chest expansion.

MEDICATIONS
- General anesthetics, sedative-hypnotics, and excessive doses of opioid analgesics depress respiratory rate and depth.
- Amphetamines and cocaine may increase rate and depth; bronchodilators cause airway dilation that can ultimately slow respiratory rate.

NEUROLOGICAL INJURY
- Damage to brainstem impairs the respiratory center and inhibits respiratory rate and rhythm.

HEMOGLOBIN FUNCTION
- Decreased hemoglobin levels (anemia) reduce oxygen-carrying capacity of blood, which increases respiratory rate.
- Increased altitude lowers amount of saturated hemoglobin, which increases respiratory rate and depth.
- Abnormal blood cell function (e.g., sickle cell disease) reduces ability of hemoglobin to carry oxygen, which increases respiratory rate and depth.

CHEST WALL MOVEMENT
- Constrictive chest or abdominal dressings limit chest wall movement.
- Presence of abdominal incisions limits chest wall movement.

---

any disease or illness has on respiratory function, and the effect of therapies. Box 15.10 summarizes factors influencing respiration. The objective measurement of respiration includes the rate and depth of breathing and the rhythm of ventilatory movements (see Skill 15.4).

TABLE 15.8	ACCEPTABLE RANGE OF RESPIRATORY RATES FOR AGE
AGE-GROUP	**RATE (breaths/min)**
Newborn	35–40
Infant (6 months)	30–50
Toddler (2 years)	25–32
Child	20–30
Adolescent	16–20
Adult	12–20

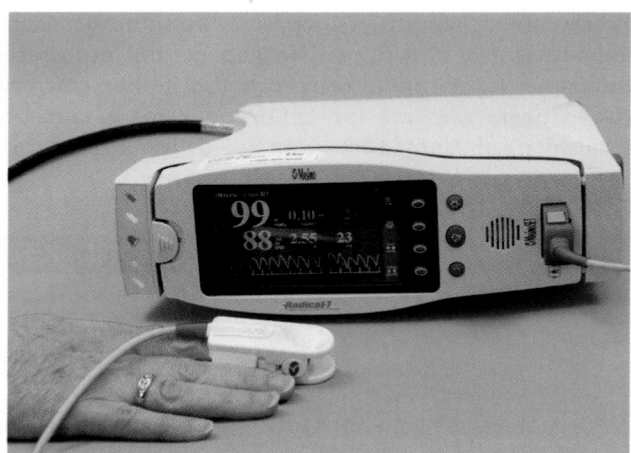

FIG 15.14 Pulse oximeter connected to finger sensor.

Respiratory Rate. Observe a full inspiration and expiration before counting respirations. The respiratory rate varies with age (Table 15.8). Bradypnea is a respiratory rate less than 12 per minute or lower than acceptable limits, whereas tachypnea is a rate more than 20 or greater than the acceptable limits. Apnea is the lack of respiratory movements. The apnea monitor is a respiratory monitoring device that helps assess respiratory rate. This noninvasive device uses electrodes attached to a patient's chest wall to sense movement. An absence of chest wall movement triggers the apnea alarm. Apnea monitoring is used frequently in the hospital and home to observe for prolonged apneic events in infants.

Ventilatory Depth. Assess the depth of respirations by observing the degree of movement in the chest wall. Ventilatory movements are deep, normal, or shallow. A deep respiration involves a full expansion of the lungs with obvious movement of the rib cage and full exhalation. A normal respiration is relaxed, automatic, and silent. Respirations are shallow when only a small quantity of air passes through the lungs and ventilatory movement is difficult to see. When chest wall movement is unusually shallow or not symmetrical, other techniques may be needed (see Chapter 16).

Ventilatory Rhythm. Respiratory rhythm or breathing pattern is either regular or irregular. While assessing respiration, observe the interval between each respiratory cycle. With normal breathing a regular interval occurs between each respiratory cycle. In the presence of irregular breathing pattern such as periods of apnea with shallow or deep breathing, a more detailed physical assessment is imperative (see Chapters 16 and 32). Infants tend to breathe less regularly. Young children sometimes breathe slowly for a few seconds and suddenly breathe more rapidly.

MEASUREMENT OF OXYGEN SATURATION (PULSE OXIMETRY)

Pulse oximetry is the indirect measurement of oxygen saturation and is the fifth vital sign (see Skill 15.5). The pulse oximeter contains a photoelectric sensor with two light-emitting diodes (LEDs) of differing wavelengths that measures the SpO_2 level. SpO_2 stands for peripheral capillary oxygen saturation, an estimate of the amount of oxygen in the blood. More specifically, it is the percentage of oxygenated hemoglobin (hemoglobin containing oxygen) compared with the total amount of hemoglobin in the blood (Fig. 15.14). Normally SpO_2 is between 95% and 100%; however, in patients with extensive respiratory disease such as chronic obstructive pulmonary disease (COPD), SpO_2 greater than 90% may be an acceptable baseline.

The measurement of SpO_2 is simple and painless and carries fewer risks than invasive measurements of oxygen saturation using arterial blood gas sampling. However, the placement of an oximeter forehead sensor can cause a pressure injury, and therefore it requires frequent monitoring of skin condition. A dry, vascular, pulsatile area (e.g., fingertip, earlobe, forehead) is needed to detect the degree of change in the transmitted light from the oximeter. Factors that affect light transmission such as outside light sources or patient motion also affect the measurement of oxygen saturation. Carbon monoxide in the blood, jaundice, and intravascular dyes can influence the light reflected from hemoglobin molecules. An awareness of these factors allows for accurate interpretation of abnormal SpO_2 measurements. Measuring SpO_2 can be conducted intermittently or continuously to assess ongoing therapies.

MEASUREMENT OF END-TIDAL CARBON DIOXIDE

End-tidal carbon dioxide ($ETCO_2$) values are important to assess when monitoring lung ventilation and perfusion. The noninvasive $ETCO_2$ monitor attaches directly to the ventilator system and measures the exhaled carbon dioxide through sensors. $ETCO_2$ monitoring benefits a patient because it is noninvasive and painless and provides an accurate assessment of arterial carbon dioxide retention values. Commonly used in patients on mechanical ventilators, $ETCO_2$ monitoring can also be implemented with patients who are not intubated using a specially designed nasal cannula that can also deliver oxygen (see Chapter 32).

SPECIAL CONSIDERATIONS

Physiological changes caused by aging influence the measurement and interpretation of vital signs in older adults (Box 15.11). You often provide patient teaching to patients of all ages related to vital sign results (Box 15.12). For example,

---

BOX 15.11   CARE OF THE OLDER ADULT

Considerations When Obtaining Vital Sign Measurements

TEMPERATURE
- The normal temperature of older adults is 36°C (96.8°F), which is at the lower end of the acceptable temperature range. Therefore temperatures considered normal for adults may represent fever in older adults.
- Older adults are very sensitive to slight changes in environmental temperature because their thermoregulatory systems are not as efficient (Touhy and Jett, 2014).
- Decreased sweat gland reactivity in older adults results in a higher threshold for sweating at high temperatures, which leads to hyperthermia and heatstroke.
- With aging, loss of subcutaneous fat reduces the insulating capacity of the skin; older men are at especially high risk for hypothermia.

PULSE RATE
- It is often difficult to palpate the pulse of older adults. A Doppler device (see Chapter 16) provides a more accurate reading.
- Older adults typically have a decreased heart rate at rest (Touhy and Jett, 2014).
- It takes longer for the heart rate to rise in older adults to meet sudden increased demands that result from stress, illness, or excitement. Once elevated, the pulse rate of older adults takes longer to return to normal resting rate.
- When assessing apical rate in older women, lift the breast tissue gently and place the stethoscope at the fifth intercostal space (ICS) or the lower edge of the breast.
- Heart sounds are sometimes muffled or difficult to hear in older adults because of an increase in air space in the lungs.

BLOOD PRESSURE
- Older adults often have decreased upper arm mass, which requires special attention to selection of blood pressure (BP) cuff size.
- Skin of older adults is more fragile and susceptible to cuff pressure injury when BP measurements are frequent.
- Older adults sometimes have an increase in systolic BP related to decrease in vessel elasticity, whereas diastolic BP remains the same, resulting in a wider pulse pressure.
- Instruct older adults to change positions slowly and wait after each change to avoid orthostatic hypotension and prevent injuries.

RESPIRATION
- Aging causes ossification of costal cartilage and downward slant of ribs, resulting in a more rigid rib cage, which reduces chest wall expansion. Kyphosis and scoliosis, which may occur in older adults, also restrict chest expansion and decrease tidal volume.
- The respiratory system matures by the time a person reaches 20 years of age and begins to decline in healthy people after the age of 25. Despite this decline, older adults are able to breathe effortlessly as long as they are healthy. However, sudden events that require an increased demand for oxygen (e.g., exercise, stress, illness) can create shortness of breath in older adults (Touhy and Jett, 2014).
- Identifying an acceptable pulse oximeter sensor site is difficult with older adults because of the likelihood of peripheral vascular disease, decreased cardiac output, cold-induced vasoconstriction, and anemia, all of which decrease pulsatile flow.

BOX 15.12   PATIENT TEACHING

Vital Sign Considerations

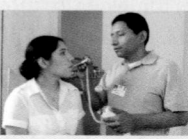

After caring for Ms. Coburn, Miguel sees the need to provide teaching about the different types of vital signs. Based on Ms. Coburn's current problems, Miguel determines that the priority is to focus on hypertension and ways to prevent or control elevated blood pressure (BP). Miguel states, "We need to watch your BP closely over the next few weeks. In the meantime, remember that you decided that you are going to walk for at least 15 minutes 3 days a week, try to eat foods with less salt, and think about not smoking anymore. To maintain your overall health, you also need information about temperature, pulse, respirations, and BP." Miguel then implements a teaching plan.

OUTCOME
Ms. Coburn verbalizes understanding of how temperature, pulse, BP, and respirations relate to her health status.

TEACHING STRATEGIES
When educating Ms. Coburn about vital sign measurement, Miguel considers the following issues and implements appropriate teaching strategies.

Temperature
- Identify Ms. Coburn's ability to initiate preventive health measures and recognize alteration in body temperature. Educate Ms. Coburn and her family about measures to prevent body temperature alterations.

BOX 15.12 PATIENT TEACHING—cont'd

Vital Sign Considerations

- Explain her personal risk factors for hypothermia: fatigue; cold, wet clothing; alcohol intoxication.
- Educate about the risk factors for heat stroke: strenuous exercise in hot, humid weather; tight-fitting clothing in hot environments; exercising in poorly ventilated areas; sudden exposure to hot climates; poor fluid intake before, during, and after exercise.
- Educate Ms. Coburn about the importance of taking and continuing antibiotics as directed until the course of treatment is completed if she ever needs antibiotic therapy.

Pulse Rate

- Teach Ms. Coburn how to take her carotid pulse. Explain which of her medications require her to assess her own pulse rates to detect side effects and the safety of taking these medications.

Blood Pressure

- Educate Ms. Coburn about her risk factors for hypertension. People with family history of hypertension are at significant risk. Obesity, cigarette smoking, heavy alcohol consumption, high blood cholesterol and triglyceride levels, and continued exposure to stress are factors linked to hypertension.
- Ensure that Ms. Coburn understands her own blood BP values, long-term follow-up care and therapy, the usual lack of symptoms, ability of therapy to control but not cure hypertension, and benefits of a consistently followed treatment plan.
- Explain the importance of an appropriate-size BP cuff for home use. Demonstrate how to use the BP cuff, and have Ms. Coburn perform a return demonstration.

- Instruct Ms. Coburn to take BP readings at the same time each day and after she has had a brief rest. Instruct to take measurements while sitting or lying down and to use same position and arm each time BP is taken.
- Describe how to determine the size of BP cuff needed. If the BP is difficult to hear, it is possible that the cuff is too loose, not big enough, or too narrow. Other possible problems include that the stethoscope is not over the arterial pulse, the BP cuff was deflated too quickly or too slowly, or it was not pumped high enough for systolic readings.

Respiration

- Explain the effect of high-risk behaviors such as cigarette smoking on oxygen saturation.
- Instruct Ms. Coburn or her family to contact home care nurse or health care provider if unusual fluctuations in respiratory rate or rhythm occur.
- Educate Ms. Coburn about the signs and symptoms of hypoxemia: headache, somnolence, confusion, shortness of breath, and dyspnea.

EVALUATION

- Use the principles of teach-back to evaluate patient/family caregiver learning:
  - "Describe to me three risk factors for high blood pressure you may be able to alter and how you are making changes."
  - "Show me how you will take your blood pressure at home."
  - "Show me how you will obtain your pulse rate."

patients with hypertension require education on risk-factor modification. Teach patients taking cardiac medications that they affect pulse rate and how to check their own pulse.

DOCUMENTING VITAL SIGNS

Enter vital sign data on graphic flow sheets or directly into the electronic health record (EHR) (see Chapter 10). Record any patient teaching regarding vital signs. When a vital sign is above or below the expected value, enter a note in the patient's record regarding the finding, any interventions taken, and the patient's response.

SAFETY GUIDELINES FOR NURSING SKILLS

Ensuring patient safety is an essential role of the professional nurse. To ensure patient safety, communicate clearly with members of the health care team, assess and incorporate the patient's priorities of care and preferences, and use the best evidence when making decisions about your patient's care. When performing the skills of vital sign measurement, remember the following points to ensure safe, individualized patient care:

- Vital sign measurement devices are often shared among patients. Clean each device carefully between patients to decrease risk for infection.

- Blood pressure cuffs and pulse oximetry sensors can apply excessive pressure on fragile skin. Rotating sites during repeated measurements decreases risk for skin breakdown and subsequent pressure injuries.
- Analyze trends of vital sign measurement and report abnormal findings to the health care provider.
- Determine vital sign frequency based on the patient's condition.

SKILL 15.1 MEASURING BODY TEMPERATURE

DELEGATION CONSIDERATIONS

The skill of temperature measurement can be delegated to nursing assistive personnel (NAP). The nurse instructs the NAP by:

- Communicating the appropriate route, device, and frequency of temperature measurement.
- Explaining any precautions needed in positioning the patient (e.g., for rectal temperature measurement).
- Reviewing the usual temperature values and significant changes to report to the nurse.

EQUIPMENT

- Thermometer (selected based on site used)
- Soft tissue or wipe
- Alcohol swab
- Water-soluble lubricant (for rectal measurements only)
- Pen and vital sign flow sheet, record form, or electronic health record (EHR)
- Clean gloves (optional), plastic thermometer sleeve, disposable probe or sensor cover
- Towel

STEP	RATIONALE

ASSESSMENT

1. Identify patient using at least two identifiers (e.g., name and birthday or name and medical record number) according to agency policy.

2. Determine need to measure patient's body temperature:

   a. Note patient's risks for temperature alterations:
      - Expected or diagnosed infection
      - Open wounds or burns
      - White blood cell count below 5000/mm^3 or above 12,000/mm^3
      - Immunosuppressive drug therapy
      - Injury to hypothalamus
      - Exposure to temperature extremes
      - Blood product infusion
      - Hypothermia or hyperthermia therapy
      - Postoperative status

   b. Assess for other signs and symptoms that accompany temperature alteration:
      - *Hyperthermia:* Decreased skin turgor, dry mucous membranes; tachycardia; hypotension; decreased venous filling; concentrated urine
      - *Heat stroke:* Body temperature 40°C (104°F) or greater (Goforth and Kazman, 2015); hot, dry skin; tachycardia; hypotension; excessive thirst; muscle cramps; visual disturbances; confusion or delirium
      - *Hypothermia:* Pale skin; skin cool or cold to touch; bradycardia and dysrhythmias; uncontrollable shivering; reduced level of consciousness; shallow respirations

   c. Assess for factors that normally influence temperature:

      - Age

Ensures correct patient. Complies with The Joint Commission standards and improves patient safety (TJC, 2018).

Clinical judgment determines need for assessment.

Certain conditions place patients at risk for temperature alterations and require more frequent temperature measurement and nursing assessment.

Physical signs and symptoms alert you to alterations in body temperature.

Allows you to accurately assess for presence and significance of temperature alteration.

Older adults have a narrower range of temperature than younger adults.

Clinical Decision Point. No single temperature is normal for all people. A temperature within an acceptable range in an adult may reflect a fever in an older adult. Undeveloped temperature-control mechanisms in infants and children cause temperature to rise and fall rapidly.

- Exercise

- Hormones

Muscle activity increases metabolism, which increases heat production and raises temperature.

Women have wider temperature fluctuations than men because of menstrual cycle hormonal changes, because body temperature varies during menopause, and because women have a thicker layer of subcutaneous fat.

STEP	RATIONALE
• Stress	Stress elevates temperature by stimulating release of epinephrine.
• Environmental temperature	Infants and older adults are more sensitive to environmental temperature changes.
• Medications	Some drugs impair or promote sweating, vasoconstriction, or vasodilation or interfere with ability of hypothalamus to regulate temperature.
• Daily fluctuations	Body temperature normally changes 0.5°C to 1°C (0.9°F to 1.8°F) during a 24-hour period. Temperature is lowest during early morning. Most patients have maximum temperature elevation between 5 p.m. and 7 p.m.; temperature falls gradually during night.
3. Determine appropriate measurement site and device for patient. Use disposable thermometer for patient on isolation precautions.	Determines if patient's status contraindicates selection of a specific method or site. Eliminates risk of transferring infection to other patients,
4. Determine previous baseline temperature and measurement site (if available) from patient's record.	Allows you to assess for change in the patient's condition and provides comparison with future temperature measurements.
5. Assess patient's knowledge of procedure.	Encourages cooperation, minimizes risks and anxiety, and identifies teaching needs.

PLANNING

1. Provide privacy and prepare bedside environment for patient safety.	Maintains patient comfort and removes barriers that may interfere with procedure.
2. Collect and bring appropriate supplies to patient's bedside.	Ensures an organized approach for body temperature measurement.
3. Verify that patient has not had anything to eat or drink and not has chewed gum or smoked within the past 20 minutes (if having oral temperature measured).	Oral food and fluids, smoking, and gum can alter oral temperature measurement.
4. Explain to patient the way you will measure temperature and the importance of maintaining proper position until reading is complete.	Promotes patient cooperation and increases compliance. Patients are often curious about their temperatures and should be cautioned against prematurely removing thermometer to read results.

IMPLEMENTATION

1. Perform hand hygiene.	Reduces transmission of microorganisms.
2. Assist patient to comfortable position that provides easy access to temperature measurement site.	Ensures patient's comfort and accuracy of temperature reading.
3. Obtain temperature reading.	
a. **Oral temperature (electronic):**	
(1) *Optional:* Apply clean gloves when there is risk for exposure to respiratory secretions or facial or mouth wound drainage.	An oral probe cover is removable without physical contact and thus does not require gloves.
(2) Remove thermometer pack from charging unit. Attach oral thermometer probe stem (blue tip) to thermometer unit. Grasp top of probe stem, being careful not to apply pressure on ejection button.	Charging provides battery power. Ejection button releases plastic cover from probe stem.
(3) Slide disposable plastic probe cover over thermometer probe stem until cover locks in place (see illustration).	Soft plastic cover will not break in patient's mouth and prevents transmission of microorganisms between patients.
(4) Ask patient to open mouth; gently place thermometer probe under tongue in posterior sublingual pocket lateral to center of lower jaw (see illustration).	Heat from superficial blood vessels in sublingual pocket produces temperature reading. With electronic thermometer, temperatures in right and left posterior sublingual pocket are significantly higher than in area under front of tongue.

SKILL 15.1 MEASURING BODY TEMPERATURE—cont'd

View Video!

STEP	RATIONALE
(5) Ask patient to hold thermometer probe with lips closed.	Maintains proper position of thermometer during recording.
(6) Leave thermometer probe in place until audible signal indicates completion and patient's temperature appears on digital display; remove thermometer probe from under patient's tongue.	Probe must stay in place until signal occurs to ensure accurate reading.
(7) Push ejection button on thermometer probe stem to discard plastic probe cover into appropriate receptacle.	Reduces transmission of microorganisms.
(8) If wearing gloves, remove and dispose in appropriate receptacle and perform hand hygiene.	Reduces transmission of microorganisms.
(9) Return thermometer probe stem to storage position of thermometer unit.	Protects probe stem from damage. Returning thermometer probe stem automatically causes digital reading to disappear.

b. Rectal temperature (electronic):

STEP	RATIONALE
(1) Draw curtain around bed and/or close room door. Assist patient to side-lying or Sims position with upper leg flexed. Move aside bed linen to expose only anal area. Keep patient's upper body and lower extremities covered with sheet or blanket.	Maintains patient's privacy, minimizes embarrassment, and promotes comfort.
(2) Apply clean gloves. Cleanse anal region when feces and/or secretions are present. Remove soiled gloves, perform hand hygiene, and reapply clean gloves.	Maintains standard precautions when exposed to items soiled with body fluids (e.g., feces).
(3) Remove thermometer pack from charging unit. Attach rectal thermometer probe stem (red tip) to thermometer unit. Grasp top of probe stem, being careful not to apply pressure on ejection button.	Ejection button releases plastic cover from probe stem.
(4) Slide disposable plastic probe cover over thermometer probe stem until cover locks in place.	Soft plastic probe cover prevents transmission of microorganisms between patients.
(5) Using a single-use package, squeeze a liberal amount of lubricant on tissue. Dip tip of probe cover of thermometer into lubricant, covering 2.5 to 3.5 cm (1 to 1½ inches) for adult.	Lubrication minimizes trauma to rectal mucosa during insertion. Using tissue avoids contamination of remaining lubricant in container.

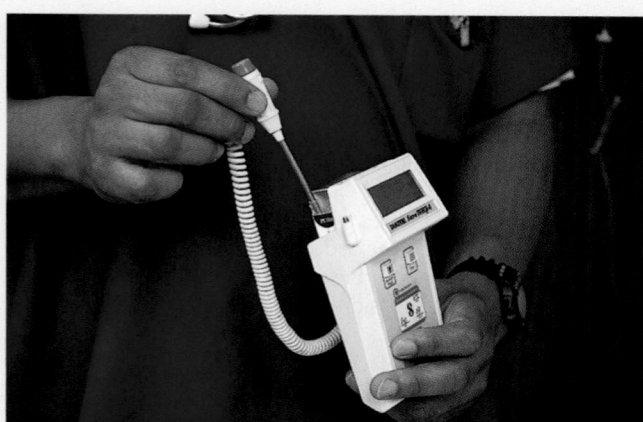

STEP 3a(3) Nurse inserts electronic thermometer probe stem into probe cover. Cover snaps in place.

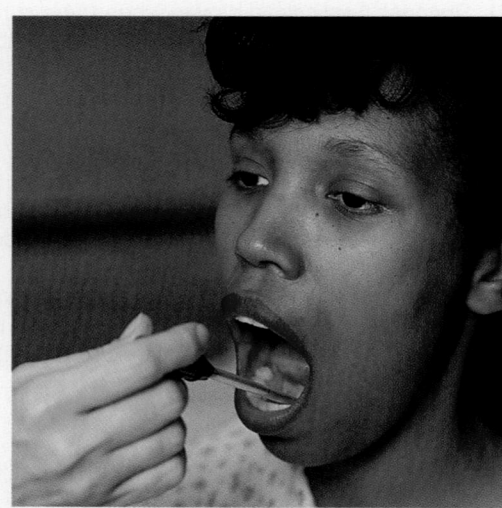

STEP 3a(4) Probe placed under tongue in posterior sublingual pocket.

STEP	RATIONALE
(6) With nondominant hand separate patient's buttocks to expose anus. Ask patient to breathe slowly and relax.	Fully exposes anus and relaxes anal sphincter for easier thermometer insertion.
(7) Gently insert thermometer into anus in direction of umbilicus 3.5 cm (1½ inches) for adult. Do not force thermometer.	Ensures adequate exposure of probe tip against blood vessels in rectal wall.
(8) If you feel resistance during insertion, withdraw immediately. Never force thermometer.	Prevents trauma to mucosa.

Clinical Decision Point. If you cannot adequately insert thermometer into rectum or resistance is felt during insertion, remove thermometer and consider an alternative method for obtaining temperature.

STEP	RATIONALE
(9) Once positioned, hold thermometer probe in place (see illustration) until audible signal indicates completion and patient's temperature appears on digital display; remove thermometer probe from anus.	Keeps probe in place until signal occurs to ensure accurate reading.
(10) Push ejection button on thermometer stem to discard plastic probe cover into appropriate receptacle. Wipe probe stem with alcohol swab, paying particular attention to ridges where probe stem connects to probe.	Reduces transmission of microorganisms. *Clostridium difficile* has been found to reside on thermometer probes if not cleaned properly.
(11) Return thermometer stem to storage position of recording unit.	Protects probe stem from damage. Returning thermometer stem automatically causes digital reading to disappear.
(12) Wipe patient's anal area with soft tissue to remove lubricant or feces and discard tissue. Assist patient in assuming a comfortable position.	Provides for comfort and hygiene.
(13) Remove and dispose of gloves in appropriate receptacle. Perform hand hygiene.	Reduces transmission of microorganisms.

c. Axillary temperature (electronic):

STEP	RATIONALE
(1) Draw curtain around bed and/or close room door. Assist patient to supine or sitting position. Move clothing or gown away from shoulder and arm.	Maintains patient's privacy, minimizes embarrassment, and promotes comfort. Exposes axilla for correct thermometer probe placement.
(2) Remove thermometer pack from charging unit. Attach oral thermometer probe stem (blue tip) to thermometer unit. Grasp top of thermometer probe stem, being careful not to apply pressure on ejection button.	Charging provides battery power. Ejection button releases plastic cover from probe stem.
(3) Slide disposable plastic probe cover over thermometer stem until cover locks in place.	Soft plastic probe cover prevents transmission of microorganisms between patients.

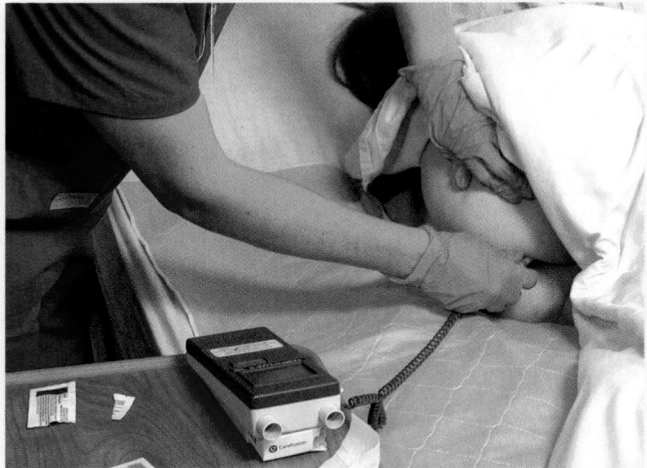

STEP 3b(9) Hold rectal thermometer probe in place in anus until audible signal indicates completion. (Copyright © Mosby's Clinical Skills: Essentials Collection.)

SKILL 15.1   MEASURING BODY TEMPERATURE—cont'd

View Video!

STEP	RATIONALE
(4) Raise patient's arm away from torso. Inspect for skin lesions and excessive perspiration; if needed, dry axilla or select alternative site. Insert thermometer probe into center of axilla (see illustration), lower arm over probe, and place arm across patient's chest.	Maintains proper position of thermometer against blood vessels in axilla.

Clinical Decision Point. Do not use axilla if skin lesions are present because local temperature is sometimes altered and area may be painful to touch.

(5) Once thermometer probe is positioned, hold it in place until audible signal indicates completion and patient's temperature appears on digital display; remove thermometer probe from axilla.	Thermometer probe must stay in place until signal occurs to ensure accurate reading.
(6) Push ejection button on thermometer stem to discard plastic probe cover into appropriate receptacle.	Reduces transmission of microorganisms.
(7) Return thermometer stem to storage position of recording unit.	Returning thermometer stem to storage position automatically causes digital reading to disappear and protects stem from damage.
(8) Assist patient in assuming comfortable position, replacing linen or gown.	Restores comfort and a sense of well-being.
(9) Perform hand hygiene.	Reduces transmission of microorganisms.
d. Tympanic membrane temperature:	
(1) Assist patient in assuming comfortable position with head turned toward side, away from you. If patient has been lying on one side, use upper ear. Obtain temperature from patient's right ear if you are right-handed. Obtain temperature from patient's left ear if you are left-handed.	Ensures comfort and facilitates exposure of auditory canal for accurate temperature measurement. Heat trapped in ear facing down causes false-high temperature reading. The less acute the angle of approach, the better the probe seal.
(2) Note if there is obvious cerumen (earwax) in patient's ear canal.	Cerumen impedes the lens cover of speculum. Switch to other ear, or select alternative measurement site.
(3) Remove thermometer handheld unit from charging base, being careful not to apply pressure to ejection button.	Charging base provides battery power. Removal of handheld unit from base prepares it to measure temperature. Ejection button releases plastic probe cover from thermometer tip.

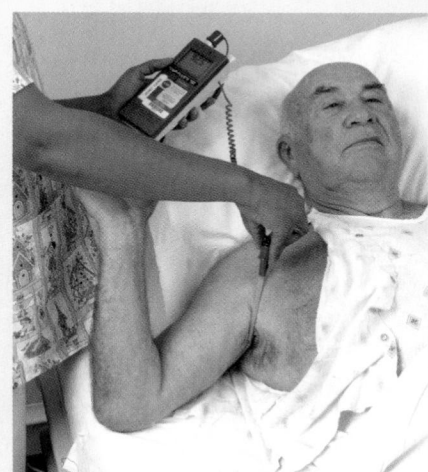

STEP 3c(4) Insert thermometer probe into center of axilla.

STEP	RATIONALE
(4) Slide disposable speculum cover over the otoscope-like lens tip until it locks in place. Be careful not to touch lens cover.	Soft plastic probe cover prevents transmission of microorganisms between patients. Lens cover should not have dust, fingerprints, or cerumen obstructing optical pathway.
(5) Insert speculum into ear canal following manufacturer instructions for tympanic probe positioning (see illustration).	Correct positioning of probe with respect to ear canal allows maximal exposure of tympanic membrane.
(a) Pull ear pinna backward, up, and out for an adult. For children less than 3 years of age, pull pinna down and back, and point covered probe toward midpoint between eyebrow and sideburns. For children older than 3 years, pull pinna up and back (Hockenberry and Wilson, 2015).	The ear tug straightens the external auditory canal, allowing maximum exposure of tympanic membrane and therefore correctly positioning speculum (Hockenberry and Wilson, 2015).
(b) Move thermometer in a figure-eight pattern.	Some manufacturers recommend movement of speculum tip in a figure-eight pattern, which allows sensor to detect maximum tympanic membrane heat radiation.
(c) Fit speculum tip snug in canal, pointing toward the nose.	Gentle pressure seals ear canal from ambient air temperature, which can alter readings 2.8°C (5°F).
(6) Once positioned, press scan button on handheld unit. Leave speculum in place until audible signal indicates completion and patient's temperature appears on digital display.	Pressing scan button causes detection of infrared energy. The speculum probe tip must stay in place until device has detected infrared energy noted by audible signal.
(7) Carefully remove speculum from auditory meatus. Push ejection button on handheld unit to discard speculum cover into appropriate receptacle.	Reduces transmission of microorganisms. Automatically causes digital reading to disappear.
(8) If temperature is abnormal or second reading is necessary, replace probe cover and wait 2 minutes before repeating in same ear, or repeat measurement in other ear. Consider an alternative temperature site or instrument.	Lens cover must be free of cerumen to maintain optical path. Time allows ear canal to regain usual temperature.
(9) Return handheld unit to thermometer base.	Protects sensor tip from damage.
(10) Help patient assume a comfortable position.	Restores comfort and sense of well-being.
(11) Perform hand hygiene.	Reduces transmission of microorganisms.
e. Temporal artery temperature:	
(1) Ensure that forehead is dry; dry with a towel if needed.	Moisture interferes with thermometer sensor.
(2) Place sensor firmly on patient's forehead.	Flush contact avoids measurement of ambient temperature.

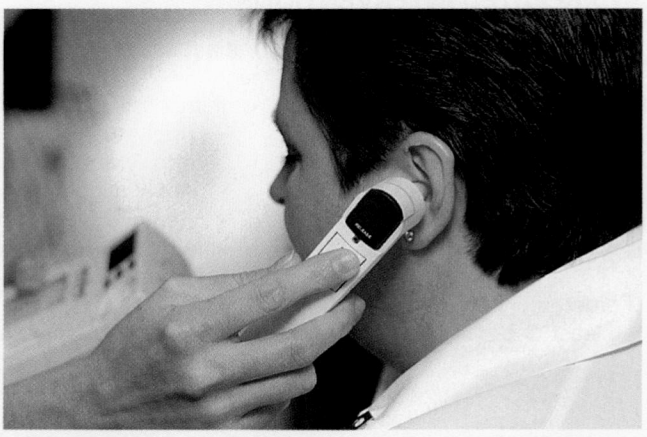

STEP 3d(5) Tympanic membrane thermometer with probe cover placed in patient's ear.

SKILL 15.1   MEASURING BODY TEMPERATURE—cont'd

STEP	RATIONALE
(3) Press red scan button with your thumb. Slowly slide thermometer straight across forehead while keeping sensor flat and firmly on skin. Keeping scan button depressed, lift sensor after sweeping forehead and touch sensor on neck just behind earlobe. Read temperature when clicking sound during scanning stops. Release scan button.	Thermometer continuously scans for highest temperature when scan button is depressed. Area behind earlobe is less affected by diaphoresis and verifies temperature.
(4) Gently clean sensor with alcohol swab, return to storage unit, and perform hand hygiene.	Prevents transmission of microorganisms.
4. Inform patient of temperature reading, determine if the patient has questions, and record measurement.	Promotes participation in care and understanding of health status.
5. Return thermometer to charger.	Maintains battery charge of thermometer unit.

EVALUATION

1. If you are assessing temperature for the first time, establish it as baseline if it is within acceptable range.	Used to compare future temperature measurements.
2. Compare temperature reading with patient's previous baseline and acceptable temperature range for patient's age group.	Body temperature fluctuates within narrow range; comparison reveals the presence of abnormality. Improper placement or movement of thermometer can cause inaccuracies. Second measurement confirms initial findings of abnormal body temperature.
3. If patient has fever, take temperature approximately 30 minutes after administering antipyretics and every 4 hours until temperature stabilizes.	Determines if temperature begins to fall in response to therapy.
4. **Use Teach-Back:** "I want to be sure I explained how to check your child's temperature at home. Show me how to swipe his forehead using the thermometer." Revise your instruction now or develop a plan for revised patient/family caregiver teaching if patient/family caregiver is unable to teach back correctly.	Evaluates what the patient is able to demonstrate and explain.

RECORDING AND REPORTING

- Record temperature and route on vital sign flow sheet or nurses' notes in EHR or chart.
- Record patient's knowledge following evaluation of teach-back in nurses' notes.

- Report abnormal findings to nurse in charge or health care provider.

UNEXPECTED OUTCOMES AND RELATED INTERVENTIONS

- Patient has temperature 1°C (1.8°F) or more above usual range.
  - Initiate measures to lower body temperature.
    - Cool room environment.
    - Reduce external covering on patient's body to promote heat loss, but do not induce shivering.
    - Keep clothing and bed linen dry.
    - Limit physical activity and sources of emotional stress.
    - Administer antipyretics as ordered.
    - Increase fluid intake to at least 3 L daily (unless contraindicated).

- Patient has temperature 1°C (1.8°F) or more below usual range.
  - Initiate measures to raise body temperature.
    - Apply warm blankets and, unless contraindicated, offer warm liquids.
    - Apply hyperthermia blankets if ordered.
    - Remove wet clothing or linen.
- Unable to obtain temperature.
  - Reassess correct placement of temperature probe or sensor.
  - Choose alternative temperature measurement site.
  - Obtain alternative temperature measurement device.

SKILL 15.2 ASSESSING RADIAL AND APICAL PULSES

View Video!

DELEGATION CONSIDERATIONS

The skill of radial pulse measurement can be delegated to nursing assistive personnel (NAP) if a patient's condition is stable. The skill cannot be delegated when a patient's condition is unstable, as the patient is at high risk for acute or serious cardiac problems, or when the nurse is evaluating a patient's response to a treatment or medication. The skill of measuring the apical pulse (or heart rate [HR]) cannot be delegated to NAP. Often you measure the apical pulse when you suspect an irregularity in the radial pulse or when a patient's condition requires a more accurate assessment. The nurse instructs the NAP by:

- Indicating the appropriate site for measuring pulse rate; frequency of measurement; and factors related to the patient history such as risk for abnormally slow, rapid, or irregular pulse.
- Reviewing patient's usual pulse rate and significant changes to report to the nurse.

EQUIPMENT

- Wristwatch with second hand or digital display
- Stethoscope
- Alcohol swab
- Pen and vital sign flow sheet in chart or electronic health record (EHR)

STEP	RATIONALE

ASSESSMENT

1. Identify patient using at least two identifiers (e.g., name and birthday or name and medical record number) according to agency policy.

   Ensures correct patient. Complies with The Joint Commission standards and improves patient safety (TJC, 2018).

2. Determine need to assess radial or apical pulse rate:

   Clinical judgment determines need for assessment.

   a. Assess for risk factors for pulse alterations such as history of heart disease, cardiac dysrhythmia, onset of sudden chest pain or acute pain from any site, surgery, sudden infusion of large volume of IV fluid, hemorrhage, and medications that alter cardiac function.

   Certain conditions place patients at risk for pulse alterations. A history of peripheral vascular disease often alters pulse rate and quality.

   b. Assess for signs and symptoms of altered cardiac function such as presence of dyspnea, fatigue, chest pain, orthopnea, syncope, palpitations, edema of dependent body parts, cyanosis, or pallor of skin.

   Physical signs and symptoms often indicate alteration in cardiac function, which affects radial pulse rate and rhythm.

   c. Assess for signs and symptoms of peripheral vascular disease such as pale, cool extremities; thin, shiny skin with decreased hair growth; and thickened nails.

   Physical signs and symptoms indicate alteration in local arterial blood flow.

   d. Assess for factors that influence pulse rate and rhythm (see Table 15.4).

   Allows you to anticipate factors that alter apical pulse rate, ensuring an accurate interpretation.

3. Determine patient's previous baseline pulse rate (if available) from patient's record.

   Allows you to assess for change in condition and provides comparison with future pulse measurements.

4. Determine any report of latex allergy. If patient has latex allergy, ensure that stethoscope is latex free.

   Reduces risk of allergic reaction to stethoscope.

5. If you anticipate need for patient or family caregiver to monitor HR at home, assess their knowledge of the procedure and rationale for measurement.

   Determines need for patient or family caregiver instruction.

PLANNING

1. Provide privacy for patient; if necessary, draw curtain around bed and/or close door.

   Maintains privacy and minimizes embarrassment, helping patient relax.

2. Collect appropriate equipment and bring to patient's bedside.

   Ensures an organized approach for assessing a radial pulse.

3. Explain to patient that you will assess radial pulse rate or apical pulse rate (HR). Encourage patient to relax as much as possible. If patient has been active, wait 5 to 10 minutes before assessing pulse. If patient has been smoking or ingesting caffeine, wait 15 minutes before assessing pulse.

   Anxiety, activity, caffeine, and smoking elevate heart rate.

View Video!

SKILL 15.2 ASSESSING RADIAL AND APICAL PULSES—cont'd

STEP	RATIONALE

IMPLEMENTATION

1. Perform hand hygiene.
2. Assist patient with assuming a supine or sitting position.

   a. **Radial pulse:**

      (1) If patient is supine, place his or her forearm straight alongside or across lower chest or upper abdomen (see illustration A). If sitting, bend patient's elbow 90 degrees and support lower arm on chair or on your arm. Place tips of first two or middle three fingers of hand over groove along radial or thumb side of patient's inner wrist (see illustration B). Slightly extend or flex wrist with palm down until you note strongest pulse.

      (2) Lightly compress pulse against radius, losing the pulse initially, and then relax pressure so that pulse becomes easily palpable.

      (3) Determine strength of pulse. Note whether thrust of vessel against fingertips is bounding (4+); full increased, strong (3+); expected (2+); barely palpable, diminished (1+); or absent, not palpable (0).

      (4) After palpating a regular pulse, look at watch second hand and begin to count rate. Count the first beat after the second hand hits the number on the dial; count as one, then two, and so on.

      (5) If pulse is regular, count rate for 30 seconds and multiply total by 2.

      (6) If pulse is irregular, count rate for a full 60 seconds. Assess frequency and pattern of irregularity.

      (7) When pulse is irregular, compare radial pulses bilaterally.

   b. **Apical pulse:**

      (1) Draw curtain around bed and/or close door. Assist patient to supine or sitting position. Move aside bed linen and gown to expose sternum and left side of chest.

RATIONALE (right column):

Reduces transmission of microorganisms.
Provides easy access to pulse sites and chest wall.

Fingertips are most sensitive parts of hand to palpate arterial pulsation. Your thumb has pulsation that interferes with accuracy.

Pulse assessment is more accurate when using moderate pressure. Too much pressure occludes pulse and impairs blood flow.

Accurate description of strength improves communication among nurses and other health care providers and ensures appropriate treatment.

Rate is determined accurately only after pulse has been palpated. Timing begins with zero. Count of one is first beat palpated after timing begins.

A 30-second count is accurate for rapid, slow, or regular pulse rates.

Inefficient contraction of heart fails to transmit pulse wave, resulting in irregular pulse. Longer time ensures accurate count.

A marked difference between pulses indicates that arterial flow is compromised to one extremity, and as a nurse you need to take action.

Maintains privacy. Exposes portion of chest wall for selection of auscultatory site. Stethoscope diaphragm must touch skin for best sounds.

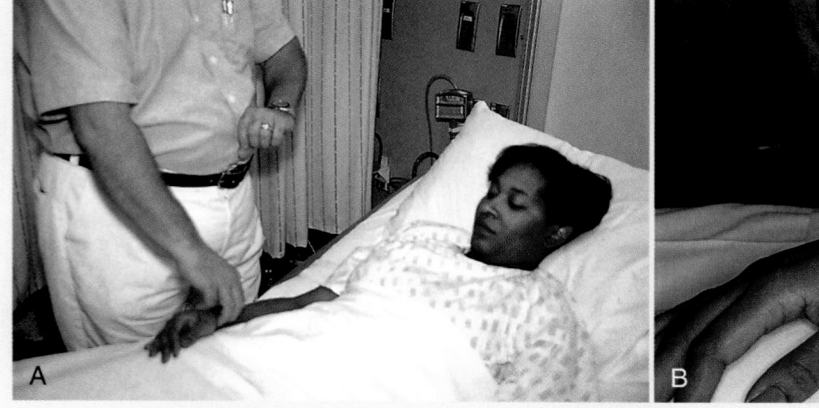
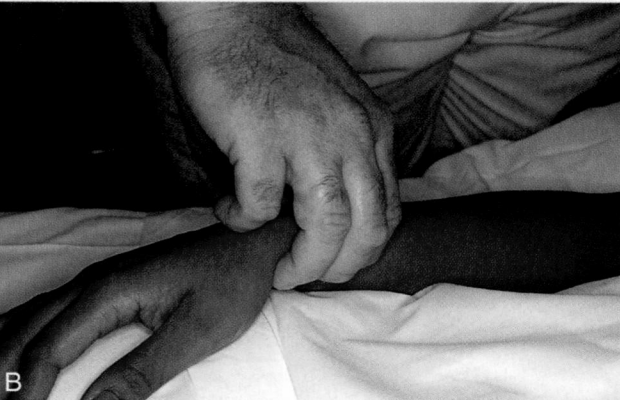

STEP 2a(1) A, Pulse check with patient's forearm at side with wrist extended. **B,** Hand placement for pulse check.

STEP	RATIONALE

(2) Locate anatomical landmarks to identify point of maximal impulse (PMI), also called apical *impulse*. The heart is located behind and to the left of sternum with base at top and apex at bottom. Find angle of Louis just below suprasternal notch between the sternal body and manubrium; it feels like a bony prominence (see illustration A). Slip fingers down each side of angle to find second intercostal space (ICS) (see illustration B). Carefully move fingers down left side of sternum to fifth ICS and laterally to left midclavicular line (MCL) (see illustration C). A light tap felt within area 1 to 2.5 cm ($\frac{1}{2}$ to 1 inch) of PMI is reflected from apex of heart (see illustration D).

Use of anatomical landmarks allows correct placement of stethoscope over apex of heart. This position enhances ability to hear heart sounds clearly. If unable to palpate PMI, reposition patient on left side. In the presence of serious heart disease, you may locate PMI to the left of the MCL or at the sixth ICS. The PMI may not be palpated in obese adults or patients with severe pulmonary disease that has changed the shape of the thorax.

(3) Place diaphragm of stethoscope in palm of hand for 5 to 10 seconds.

Warming of metal or plastic diaphragm prevents patient from being startled and promotes comfort.

(4) Place diaphragm of stethoscope over PMI at fifth ICS, at left MCL, and auscultate for normal S_1 and S_2 heart sounds (heard as "lub-dub") (see illustrations).

Allow stethoscope tubing to extend straight without kinks that would distort sound transmission. Normal sounds S_1 and S_2 are high-pitched and best heard with diaphragm.

(5) When you hear S_1 and S_2 with regularity, use second hand of watch and begin to count rate: when sweep hand hits number on dial; start counting with zero, then one, two, and so on.

Apical rate is determined accurately only after you are able to auscultate sounds clearly. Timing begins with zero. Count of one is first sound auscultated after timing begins.

(6) If apical rate is regular, count for 30 seconds and multiply by 2.

The first time the apical rate is measured, it should be counted for 60 seconds. If the rate is regular, subsequent measurements will be accurate for 30 seconds.

(7) If HR is irregular or patient is receiving cardiovascular medication, count for a full 1 minute (60 seconds).

Irregular rate is more accurately assessed when measured over longer interval.

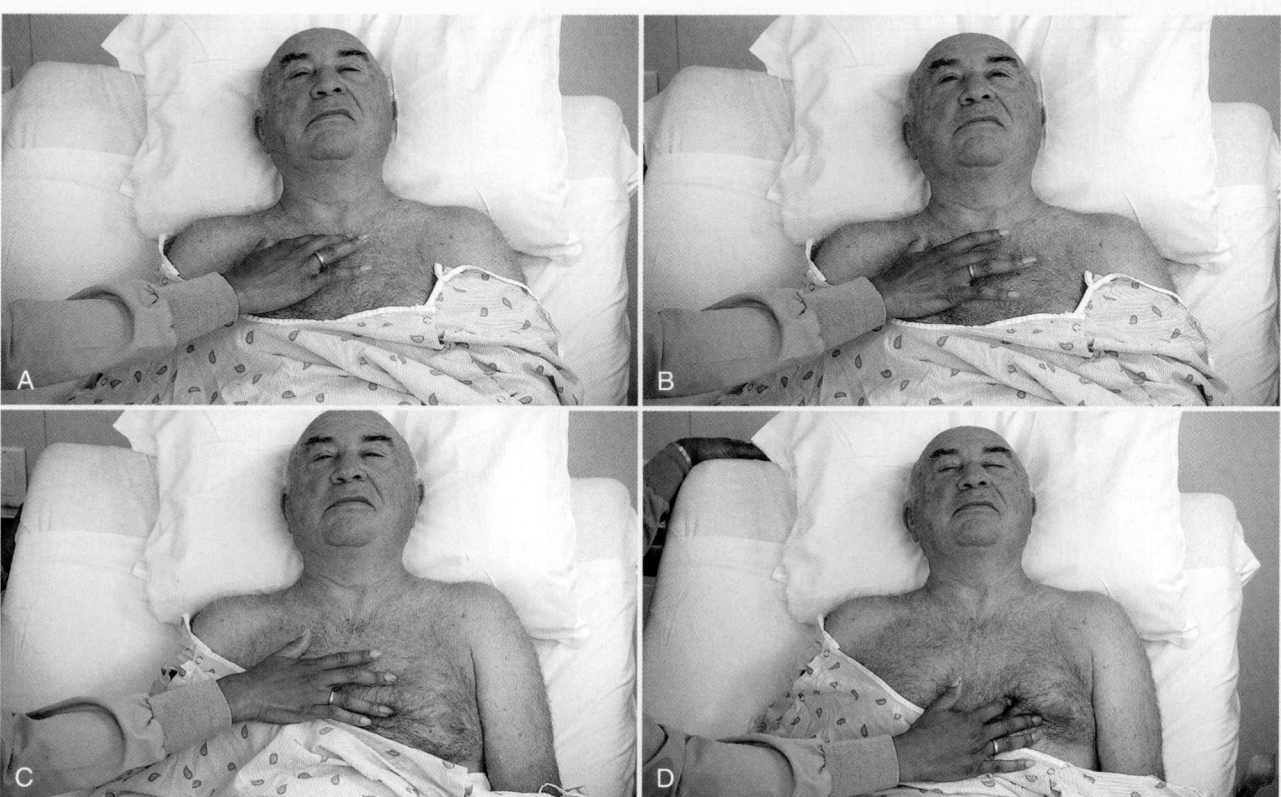

STEP 2b(2) **A,** Nurse locates sternal notch. **B,** Nurse locates second intercostal space. **C,** Nurse locates fifth intercostal space. **D,** Nurse locates point of maximal impulse at fifth intercostal space at left midclavicular line.

SKILL 15.2 ASSESSING RADIAL AND APICAL PULSES—cont'd

STEP	RATIONALE
(8) Note regularity of any dysrhythmia (S_1 and S_2 occurring early or late after previous sequence of sounds) (e.g., every third or every fourth beat is skipped).	Regular occurrence of dysrhythmia within 1 minute indicates inefficient contraction of heart and potential alteration in cardiac output.

Clinical Decision Point. If apical rate is abnormal or irregular, repeat measurement or have another nurse conduct measurement. Original measurement may be incorrect. Second measurement confirms initial findings of an abnormal HR.

3. Replace patient's gown and bed linen; assist patient to return to comfortable position.	Restores comfort and promotes sense of well-being.
4. Discuss findings with patient.	Promotes patient's participation in care and understanding of health status.
5. Perform hand hygiene.	Reduces transmission of microorganisms.

EVALUATION

1. If assessing pulse for first time, establish baseline if it is within acceptable range.	Used to compare future HR assessments.
2. Compare HR and pulse character with patient's previous baseline and acceptable range for patient's age.	Allows for assessment of change in patient's condition and presence of cardiac alteration.
3. **Use Teach-Back:** "I want to be sure I explained why it is important to check your pulse at home. Tell me what medication you are taking that would decrease your heart rate." Revise your instruction now or develop a plan for revised patient/family caregiver teaching if patient/family caregiver is unable to teach back correctly.	Evaluates what the patient understands and is able to explain.

RECORDING AND REPORTING

- Record pulse site, pulse rate, pulse strength, and apical rate on vital sign flow sheet or nurses' notes in EHR or chart.
- Record patient's knowledge following evaluation of teach-back in nurses' notes.

- Document measurement of HR after administration of specific therapies in nurses' notes in EHR or chart.
- Report abnormal findings to nurse in charge or health care provider.

UNEXPECTED OUTCOMES AND RELATED INTERVENTIONS

- Patient has weak, thready, or difficult-to-palpate radial pulse.
  - Assess both radial pulses and compare findings.

- Observe for symptoms associated with ineffective tissue perfusion, including pallor and cool skin distal to weak pulse.

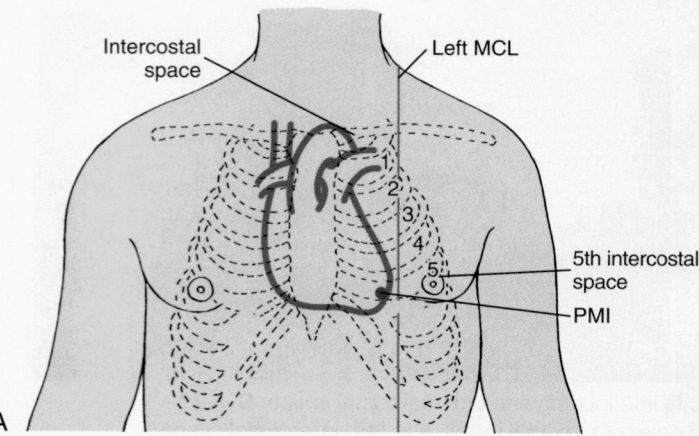

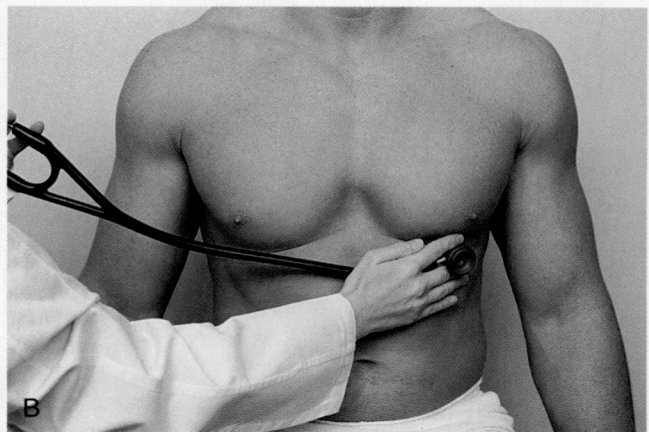

STEP 2b(4) A, Location of point of maximal impulse *(PMI)* in adult. **B,** Listening to PMI in an adult. *MCL,* Midclavicular line.

- Assess for swelling in surrounding tissues or any encumbrance (e.g., dressing or cast) that may impede blood flow.
- Obtain Doppler or ultrasound stethoscope to detect low-velocity blood flow.
- Obtain apical pulse.
- An adult patient's HR is less than 60 beats/min (bradycardia) or more than 100 beats/min (tachycardia).
  - Identify related data, including fever, pain, fear or anxiety, recent exercise, low blood pressure, blood loss, or inadequate oxygenation.
  - Observe for signs and symptoms associated with abnormal cardiac function including dyspnea, fatigue, chest pain, orthopnea, syncope, palpitations, edema of body parts, cyanosis, or pallor of the skin.
  - Report findings to nurse in charge and/or health care provider. It may be necessary to withhold prescribed

medications that alter HR until health care provider can evaluate need to alter dosage.
  - Be prepared to order and/or obtain an electrocardiogram.
- Patient has an irregular HR.
  - **Assess for pulse deficit:** (a) nurse auscultates apical pulse while a second provider palpates radial pulse; (b) nurse begins 60-second pulse count by calling out loud when to begin counting pulses; (c) the two pulse rates are compared. If pulse count differs by more than 2, a deficit exists; assess for other signs and symptoms of decreased cardiac output.
  - Report findings to nurse in charge and/or health care provider, who may order an electrocardiogram to detect cardiac conduction alteration.

SKILL 15.3 BLOOD PRESSURE MEASUREMENT

DELEGATION CONSIDERATIONS

The skill of blood pressure (BP) measurement can be delegated to nursing assistive personnel (NAP) unless the patient is considered unstable (i.e., hypotensive). The nurse instructs the NAP by:

- Explaining the appropriate limb to use for measurement, BP cuff size, and equipment (manual or electronic) to be used.
- Communicating the frequency of measurement and factors related to the patient's history such as risk for orthostatic hypotension.

- Reviewing the patient's usual BP values and significant changes or abnormalities to report to the nurse.

EQUIPMENT
- Aneroid sphygmomanometer
- Cloth or disposable vinyl BP cuff of appropriate size for patient's extremity
- Stethoscope
- Alcohol swab
- Pen and vital sign flow sheet in chart or electronic health record (EHR)

STEP	RATIONALE

ASSESSMENT

1. Identify patient using at least two identifiers (e.g., name and birthday or name and medical record number) according to agency policy.

2. Determine need to assess patient's BP:
   a. Assess risk factors for BP alterations:
      - History of cardiovascular disease
      - Renal disease
      - Diabetes mellitus
      - Circulatory shock (hypovolemic, septic, cardiogenic, or neurogenic)
      - Acute or chronic pain
      - Rapid IV infusion of fluids or blood products
      - Increased intracranial pressure
      - Postoperative status
      - Toxemia of pregnancy
   b. Assess for signs and symptoms of BP alterations. In patients at risk for hypertension; assess for headache (usually occipital), flushing of face, nosebleed, and fatigue in older adults. In patients at risk for hypotension; assess for dizziness; mental confusion; restlessness; pale, dusky, or cyanotic skin and mucous membranes; and cool, mottled skin over extremities.

Ensures correct patient. Complies with The Joint Commission standards and improves patient safety (TJC, 2018).
Clinical judgment determines need for assessment.
Certain conditions place patients at risk for BP alteration.

Physical signs and symptoms indicate alterations in BP. Hypertension is often asymptomatic until BP is very high.

SKILL 15.3 BLOOD PRESSURE MEASUREMENT—cont'd

STEP	RATIONALE
c. Assess for factors that influence BP:	Allows you to anticipate factors that influence blood pressure, ensuring a more accurate interpretation.
• Age	Acceptable values for BP vary throughout life.
• Gender	During and after menopause women often have higher BP values than men of same age.
• Daily (diurnal) variation	BP varies throughout day; BP is highest during the day between 10:00 a.m. and 6:00 p.m. and lowest in early morning.
• Position	BP falls as person moves from lying to sitting or standing position; normally postural variations are minimal.
• Exercise	Increases in oxygen demand by the body during activity increase BP.
• Weight	Obesity is an independent predictor of hypertension.
• Sympathetic stimulation	Pain, anxiety, or fear stimulates the sympathetic nervous system, causing BP to rise.
• Medications	Antihypertensives, diuretics, beta-adrenergic blockers, vasodilators, calcium channel blockers, angiotensin-converting enzyme (ACE) inhibitors, angiotensin receptor blockers (ARBs), and antidysrhythmics lower BP; opioids and general anesthetics also cause a drop in BP.
• Smoking	Smoking results in vasoconstriction, a narrowing of blood vessels. BP rises acutely and returns to baseline approximately 30 minutes after stopping smoking (James et al., 2014).
• Ethnicity	Incidence of hypertension is higher in African Americans than in European Americans. African Americans tend to develop more severe hypertension at an earlier age and have twice the risk for complications of hypertension (i.e., stroke, heart attack). Hypertension-related deaths are also higher among African Americans.
3. Determine best site for BP assessment. Avoid applying cuff to extremity when IV fluids are infusing, an arteriovenous shunt or fistula is present, or breast or axillary surgery has been performed on that side. Also avoid applying cuff to traumatized or diseased extremity or one that has a cast or bulky bandage. Use lower extremities when brachial arteries are inaccessible.	Inappropriate site selection may result in poor amplification of sounds, causing inaccurate readings. Application of pressure from inflated bladder temporarily impairs blood flow and can further compromise circulation in extremity that already has impaired blood flow.
4. Determine previous baseline BP and site (if available) from patient's record. Determine any report of latex allergy.	Assesses for change in condition and provides comparison with future blood pressure measurements. If patient has latex allergy, verify that stethoscope and BP cuff are latex free.
5. Assess patient's knowledge of procedure and any BP alteration that exists.	Encourages cooperation, minimizes risks and anxiety, and identifies teaching needs.

PLANNING

1. Provide privacy and prepare bedside environment for patient safety.	Providing privacy and preparing the environment early helps you to think about the steps in the procedure and removes clutter from the over-bed or bedside table.
2. Select appropriate cuff size (see Fig. 15.10) and ensure that other equipment is in the patient's room.	Use of improper-size cuff causes false-low or false-high reading (Gunes and Efteli, 2016).
3. Explain to patient that you will assess BP. Have patient rest at least 5 minutes before measuring lying or sitting BP and 1 minute before measuring standing BP. Ask patient not to speak while you are measuring BP.	Reduces anxiety that falsely elevates readings. Exercise causes false elevations in BP. Deep breathing lowers systolic BP (SBP) and diastolic BP (DBP) up to 5 mm Hg (Zheng et al., 2014). Talking with a patient during assessment increases BP (AACN Practice Alert, 2016).

STEP	RATIONALE

4. Be sure that patient has not exercised, ingested caffeine, or smoked for 30 minutes before assessment of BP.

Smoking increases BP immediately, and increase lasts up to 15 minutes. The effects of coffee or caffeine increase BP for up to 3 hours (James et al., 2014).

IMPLEMENTATION

1. Perform hand hygiene

Reduces transmission of microorganisms.

2. Have patient assume sitting or lying position. Be sure that room is warm, quiet, and relaxing.

Maintains patient's comfort during measurement. Patient's perceptions that the physical or interpersonal environment is stressful affect BP.

3. Assess BP by auscultation:

   a. *Upper extremity:* With patient sitting or lying, position patient's forearm at heart level with palm turned up (see illustration). If sitting, instruct patient to keep feet flat on floor without legs crossed. If supine, patient should not have legs crossed. If the patient cannot be placed in the prone position, position patient supine with knee slightly bent.
   Lower extremity: With patient prone, position patient so that knee is slightly flexed.

If arm is extended and not supported, patient will perform isometric exercise that can increase SBP (Gunes and Efteli, 2016). Placement of arm above level of heart causes false-low reading, 2 mm Hg for each 1 inch above heart level. Leg crossing can falsely increase BP.

   b. Expose extremity (arm or leg) fully by removing constricting clothing. Cuff may be placed over a sleeve of thin clothing as long as stethoscope rests on the skin.

Ensures proper cuff application. Placing a cuff over rolled-up or thick clothing, especially in older adults, can increase BP (Ozone et al., 2016)

   c. Palpate brachial artery (arm; see illustration A) or popliteal artery (leg). With cuff fully deflated, apply bladder of cuff above artery by centering arrows marked on cuff over artery (see illustration B). If cuff does not have any center arrows, estimate center of bladder and place this center over artery. Position cuff 2.5 cm (1 inch) above site of pulsation (antecubital or popliteal space). With cuff fully deflated, wrap it evenly and snugly around upper arm (see illustration C) or leg (see illustration D).

Brachial artery is along groove between biceps and triceps muscles above elbow at antecubital fossa. Popliteal artery is just below patient's thigh, behind knee.
Placing bladder directly over artery ensures that you apply proper pressure during inflation. Loose-fitting cuff causes false-high readings.

   d. Position manometer gauge vertically at eye level. You should be no farther than 1 meter (approximately 1 yard) away.

Looking up or down at scale can result in distorted readings.

   e. **Measure BP using two-step method:**

   (1) Palpate brachial or popliteal pulse. Palpate artery distal to cuff with fingertips of nondominant hand while inflating cuff rapidly to pressure 30 mm Hg above point at which pulse disappears. Slowly deflate cuff and note point when pulse reappears. Deflate cuff fully and wait 30 seconds.

Estimating prevents false-low readings. Determine maximal inflation point for accurate reading by palpation. If unable to palpate artery because of weakened pulse, use an ultrasonic stethoscope. Completely deflating cuff prevents venous congestion and false-high readings.

   (2) Place stethoscope earpieces in ears and be sure that sounds are clear, not muffled.

Ensure that each earpiece follows angle of ear canal to facilitate hearing.

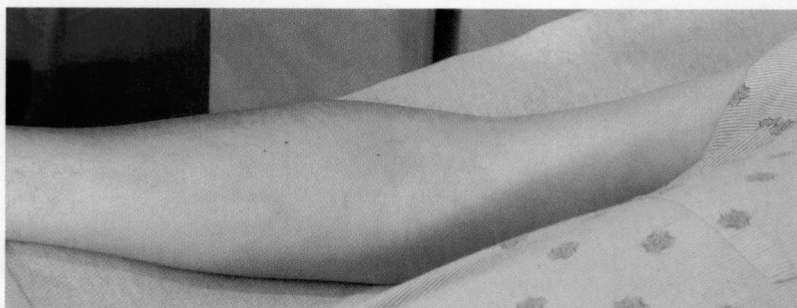

STEP 3a Patient's forearm supported on bed. (Copyright © Mosby's Clinical Skills: Essentials Collection.)

SKILL 15.3 BLOOD PRESSURE MEASUREMENT—cont'd

STEP	RATIONALE
(3) Palpate artery and place bell or diaphragm chest piece of stethoscope over it. Do not allow chest piece to touch cuff or clothing.	Proper stethoscope placement ensures best sound reception. Stethoscope improperly positioned causes muffled sounds that often result in false-low systolic and false-high diastolic readings. The bell provides better sound reproduction, whereas the diaphragm is easier to secure with fingers and covers a larger area.
(4) Close valve of pressure bulb clockwise until tight. Quickly inflate cuff to 30 mm Hg above patient's estimated SBP.	Tightening valve prevents air leak during inflation. Rapid inflation ensures accurate measurement of SBP.
(5) Slowly release pressure bulb valve and allow manometer needle to fall at rate of 2 to 3 mm Hg/sec.	Too-rapid or too-slow decline causes inaccurate readings (Gunes and Efteli, 2016).
(6) Note point on manometer when you hear first clear sound. The sound will slowly increase in intensity.	First sound reflects SBP.
(7) Continue to deflate cuff gradually, noting point at which sound disappears in adults. Note pressure to nearest 2 mm Hg. Listen for 20 to 30 mm Hg after last sound and allow remaining air to escape quickly.	Beginning of the last or fifth sound is indication of DBP in adults (Basile and Bloch, 2016). In children the distinct muffling of sounds indicates DBP (Basile and Bloch, 2016).

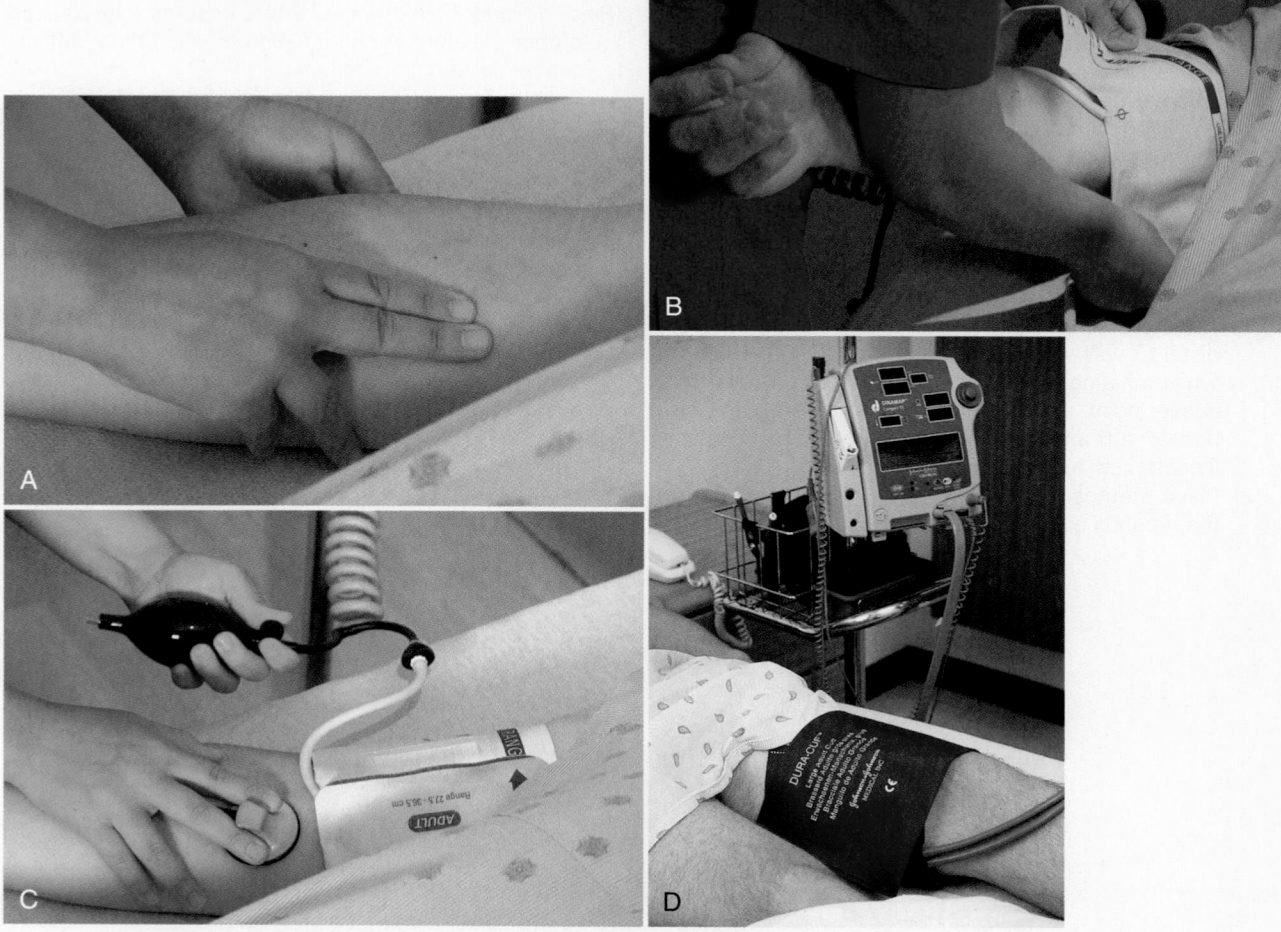

STEP 3c A, Palpating brachial artery. **B,** Aligning blood pressure cuff arrow with brachial artery. **C,** Blood pressure cuff wrapped around upper arm. **D,** Blood pressure cuff applied around thigh. (**A** to **C** copyright © Mosby's Clinical Skills: Essentials Collection.)

STEP	RATIONALE
f. Measure BP using one-step method:	
(1) Place stethoscope earpieces in ears and be sure that sounds are clear, not muffled.	Earpieces should follow angle of ear canal to facilitate hearing.
(2) Palpate brachial or popliteal artery and place bell or diaphragm chest piece of stethoscope over it. Do not allow chest piece to touch cuff or clothing.	Proper stethoscope placement ensures optimal sound reception. Improperly positioned stethoscope causes muffled sounds that often result in false readings. Bell provides better sound reproduction, whereas diaphragm is easier to secure with fingers and covers larger area.
(3) Close valve of pressure bulb clockwise until tight. Quickly inflate cuff to 30 mm Hg above patient's usual SBP.	Tightening valve prevents air leak during inflation. Inflation above systolic level ensures accurate measurement of systolic pressure.
(4) Slowly release pressure bulb valve and allow manometer needle to fall at rate of 2 to 3 mm Hg/ sec. Note point on manometer when you hear first clear sound. Sound will slowly increase in intensity.	Too-rapid or too-slow a decline in mercury level causes inaccurate readings (Gunes and Efteli, 2016). First sound reflects SBP.
(5) Continue to deflate cuff gradually, noting point at which sound disappears in adults. Note pressure to nearest 2 mm Hg. Listen for 10 to 20 mm Hg after last sound and allow remaining air to escape quickly.	Beginning of fifth sound is indication of DBP in adults (Basile and Bloch, 2016). In children the distinct muffling of sounds indicates DBP (Basile and Bloch, 2016).
4. American Heart Association recommends average of two sets of BP measurement, 2 minutes apart. Use second set of BP measurements as baseline. If readings are different by more than 5 mm Hg, additional readings are necessary.	Prevents false-positive readings based on patient's sympathetic response (alert reaction). Repeating measurements too soon creates venous congestion, which makes sounds difficult to hear (Dokoohaki et al., 2015). Averaging minimizes effect of anxiety, which often causes first reading to be higher than subsequent measures (Basile and Bloch, 2016).
5. Remove cuff from patient's arm/leg unless you need to repeat measurement.	Continuous cuff inflation causes arterial occlusion, resulting in numbness and tingling of patient's arm/leg.
6. If this is first assessment of patient, repeat procedure on other arm/leg.	Comparison of blood pressure in both arms/legs detects circulatory problems. (Normal difference of 5 to 10 mm Hg exists between arms.) Use arm with the higher pressure for subsequent measurements (AACN Practice Alert, 2016).
7. Assess SBP by palpation:	
a. Follow Steps 3a through 3d of auscultation method.	
b. Locate and then continually palpate brachial, radial, or popliteal artery with fingertips of one hand. Inflate cuff to pressure 30 mm Hg above point at which you can no longer palpate pulse.	Ensures accurate detection of true SBP once pressure valve is released.

Clinical Decision Point. If unable to palpate artery because of weakened pulse, use a Doppler device (Fig. 15.15).

c. Slowly release valve and deflate cuff, allowing manometer needle to fall at rate of 2 mm Hg/sec. Note point on manometer when pulse is again palpable. First palpable pulse reflects SBP.	Too-rapid or too-slow a decline results in inaccurate readings (Gunes and Efteli, 2016). Palpation helps identify SBP only.
d. Deflate cuff rapidly and completely. Remove cuff from patient's extremity unless you need to repeat measurement.	Continuous cuff inflation causes arterial occlusion, resulting in numbness and tingling of extremity.
8. Help patient return to comfortable position and cover upper arm/leg if previously clothed.	Restores comfort and provides a sense of well-being.
9. Discuss findings with patient.	Promotes participation in care and understanding of health status and makes patient accountable for follow-up assessment. SBP in leg is 10 to 40 mm Hg higher.
10. Clean earpieces and diaphragm of stethoscope with alcohol swab as needed. Wipe cuff with agency-approved disinfectant if used between patients. Perform hand hygiene.	Reduces transmission of microorganisms. Controls transmission of microorganisms when nurses share stethoscope.

SKILL 15.3 BLOOD PRESSURE MEASUREMENT—cont'd

STEP	RATIONALE

EVALUATION

1. If assessing BP for the first time, establish baseline BP if it is within acceptable range.
2. Compare BP reading with patient's previous baseline and usual BP for patient's age.
3. **Use Teach-Back:** "I want to be sure I explained why it is important to stand up slowly since you have a high blood pressure. Tell me which of your medications might make you dizzy if you stand up too fast, and tell me what should you do if you suddenly feel dizzy." Revise your instruction now or develop a plan for revised patient/family caregiver teaching if patient/family caregiver is unable to teach back correctly.

Used to compare future BP measurements.

Allows you to assess for change in condition and provides comparison with future BP measurements.
Evaluates what the patient is able to explain.

RECORDING AND REPORTING

- Record BP and site assessed on vital sign flow sheet or nurses' notes in EHR or chart.
- Record patient's knowledge following evaluation of teach-back in nurses' notes.

- Document measurement of BP and any signs or symptoms of BP alterations after administration of specific therapies in nurses' notes in EHR or chart.
- Report abnormal findings to nurse in charge or health care provider.

UNEXPECTED OUTCOMES AND RELATED INTERVENTIONS

- Patient's BP is above acceptable range.
  - Repeat measurement in other extremity and compare findings.
  - Verify correct size and placement of BP cuff.
  - Have another nurse repeat measurement in 1 to 2 minutes.

- Observe for related symptoms that are not apparent unless BP is extremely high including headache, facial flushing, nosebleed, and fatigue in older patient.
- Report BP to nurse in charge or health care provider to initiate appropriate evaluation and treatment.
- Administer antihypertensive medications as ordered.

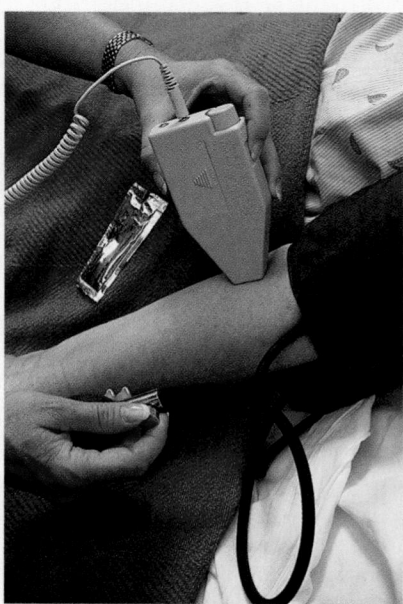

FIG 15.15 Doppler ultrasonic stethoscope over brachial artery to measure blood pressure.

- Patient's BP is not sufficient for adequate perfusion and oxygenation of tissues.
  - Compare BP value with baseline.
  - Position patient in supine position to enhance circulation and restrict activity that decreases BP further.
  - Assess for signs and symptoms associated with hypotension including tachycardia; diminished, barely palpable pulse; weakness; dizziness; confusion; and cool, pale, dusky, or cyanotic skin.
  - Assess for factors that contribute to low BP including hemorrhage, dilation of blood vessels resulting from hyperthermia, anesthesia, or medication side effects.
  - Report BP to nurse in charge or health care provider to initiate appropriate evaluation and treatment.
  - Increase rate of IV infusion or administer vasoconstriction drugs if ordered.

- Unable to obtain BP reading.
  - Determine that no immediate crisis is present by obtaining pulse and respiratory rates.
  - Assess for signs and symptoms of decreased cardiac output; if present, notify nurse in charge or health care provider immediately.
  - Use alternative sites or procedures to obtain BP: use Doppler or ultrasonic stethoscope; palpate SBP.
- Patient experiences orthostatic hypotension.
  - Maintain patient safety.
  - Return patient to safe position in bed or chair.

SKILL 15.4   ASSESSING RESPIRATION

View Video!

DELEGATION CONSIDERATIONS

The skill of counting respirations can be delegated to nursing assistive personnel (NAP) unless the patient is considered unstable (i.e., complaints of dyspnea). The nurse instructs the NAP by:

- Communicating the frequency of measurement and factors related to patient history or risk for increased or decreased respiratory rate or irregular respirations.

- Reviewing any unusual respiratory values and significant changes to report to the nurse.

EQUIPMENT

- Wristwatch with second hand or digital display
- Pen and vital sign flow sheet in chart or electronic health record (EHR)

STEP	RATIONALE

ASSESSMENT

1. Identify patient using at least two identifiers (e.g., name and birthday or name and medical record number) according to agency policy.
2. Determine need to assess patient's respirations:
   a. Assess for risk factors of respiratory alterations:
      - Fever
      - Pain and anxiety
      - Diseases of chest wall or muscles
      - Constrictive chest or abdominal dressings
      - Presence of abdominal incisions
      - Gastric distention
      - Chronic pulmonary disease (emphysema, bronchitis, asthma)
      - Traumatic injury to chest wall with or without collapse of underlying lung tissue
      - Presence of a chest tube
      - Respiratory infection (pneumonia, acute bronchitis)
      - Pulmonary edema and emboli
      - Head injury with damage to brainstem
      - Anemia

Ensures correct patient. Complies with The Joint Commission standards and improves patient safety (TJC, 2018).

Clinical judgment determines need for assessment.

Certain conditions place patients at risk for ventilatory alterations detected by changes in respiratory rate, depth, and rhythm.

SKILL 15.4   ASSESSING RESPIRATION—cont'd

View Video!

STEP	RATIONALE
b. Assess for signs and symptoms of respiratory alterations: • Bluish or cyanotic appearance of nail beds, lips, mucous membranes, and skin • Restlessness, irritability, confusion, reduced level of consciousness • Pain during inspiration • Labored or difficult breathing • Orthopnea • Use of accessory muscles • Adventitious breath sounds • Inability to breathe spontaneously • Thick, frothy, blood-tinged, or copious sputum production	Physical signs and symptoms indicate alterations in respiratory status.
c. Assess for factors that influence the character of respirations:	Allows you to anticipate factors that influence respirations, ensuring a more accurate interpretation.
• Exercise	Respirations increase in rate and depth to meet need for additional oxygen and rid body of carbon dioxide.
• Anxiety	Anxiety causes increase in respiration rate and depth because of sympathetic nervous system stimulation.
• Acute pain	Pain alters rate and rhythm of respirations; breathing becomes shallow. Patient inhibits or splints chest wall movement when pain is in area of chest or abdomen.
• Smoking	Chronic smoking changes pulmonary airways, resulting in increased respiratory rate at rest when not smoking.
• Medications	Narcotic analgesics, general anesthetics, and sedative-hypnotics depress rate and depth; amphetamines and cocaine increase rate and depth; bronchodilators cause dilation of airways, which ultimately slows respiratory rate.
• Body position	Standing or sitting erect promotes full ventilatory movement and lung expansion; stooped or slumped posture impairs ventilatory movement; lying flat prevents full chest expansion.
• Neurological injury	Damage to brainstem impairs the respiratory center and inhibits rate and rhythm.
• Hemoglobin function	Decreased hemoglobin levels lower amount of oxygen carried in blood, which results in increased respiratory rate to increase oxygen delivery. An increase in altitude lowers amount of saturated hemoglobin, which increases respiratory rate and depth.
3. Assess pertinent laboratory/clinical values: **a.** *Arterial blood gases (ABGs):* Normal ranges (values vary slightly among agencies): • pH, 7.35 to 7.45 • $PaCO_2$, 35 to 45 mm Hg • HCO_3, 22 to 28 mEq/L • PaO_2, 80 to 100 mm Hg • SaO_2, 95% to 100%	Measure arterial blood pH, partial pressure of oxygen and carbon dioxide, and arterial oxygen saturation, which reflect patient's ventilation and oxygenation status.
b. *Pulse oximetry (SpO_2):* Normal SpO_2 95%-100% or greater; less than 90% is a clinical emergency (WHO, 2011).	SpO_2 less than 90% is often accompanied by changes in respiratory rate, depth, and rhythm.
c. *Complete blood count (CBC):* Normal CBC for adults (values vary within agencies): • Hemoglobin: 14 to 18 g/100 mL, male patients; 12 to 16 g/100 mL, female patients • Hematocrit: 42% to 52%, male patients; 37% to 47%, female patients • Red blood cell count: 4.7 million to 6.1 million/mm³, male patients; 4.2 million to 5.4 million/mm³, female patients	Measures red blood cell count; volume of red blood cells; and concentration of hemoglobin, which reflects patient's capacity to carry oxygen.

STEP	RATIONALE
4. Determine previous baseline respiratory rate (if available) from patient's record.	Assesses for change in condition and provides comparison with future respiratory measurements.
5. Assess patient's knowledge of procedure and any respiratory alteration that exists.	Encourages cooperation, minimizes risks and anxiety, and identifies teaching needs.

PLANNING

1. Provide privacy.	
2. If patient has been active, wait 5 to 10 minutes before assessing respirations.	Exercise increases respiratory rate and depth. Assessing respirations while patient is at rest allows for objective comparison of values.
3. Assess respirations after pulse measurement in an adult.	Inconspicuous assessment of respirations immediately after pulse assessment prevents patient from consciously or unintentionally altering rate and depth of breathing.
4. Be sure that patient is in comfortable position, preferably sitting or lying with the head of the bed elevated 45 to 60 degrees.	Sitting erect promotes full ventilatory movement. A position of discomfort causes patient to breathe more rapidly.
5. Explain to patient that you will assess respirations or rate of breathing.	Helps to decrease patient anxiety during measurement.

Clinical Decision Point. Assess patients with difficulty breathing (dyspnea) such as patients with heart failure or abdominal ascites or in late stages of pregnancy in the position of greatest comfort. Repositioning may increase the work of breathing, which increases respiratory rate.

IMPLEMENTATION

1. Perform hand hygiene.	Prevents transmission of microorganisms.
2. Draw curtain around bed and/or close door.	Maintains privacy.
3. Be sure that patient's chest is visible. If necessary, move bed linen or gown.	Ensures clear view of chest wall and abdominal movements.
4. Place patient's arm in relaxed position across abdomen or lower chest, or place your hand directly over patient's upper abdomen.	A similar position used during pulse assessment allows respiratory rate assessment to be inconspicuous. Patient's hand or your hand rises and falls during respiratory cycle.
5. Observe complete respiratory cycle (one inspiration and one expiration) (see illustration).	On inspiration, the diaphragm normally contracts, and the abdominal organs move down to increase the size of the chest cavity. At the same time the ribs and sternum lift outward. On expiration, the diaphragm relaxes upward, and the ribs and sternum return to their relaxed position (see illustration). Rate is accurately determined only after viewing a complete respiratory cycle.
6. After observing a cycle, look at second hand of watch and begin to count rate: when sweep hand hits number on dial, begin time frame, counting one with first full respiratory cycle.	Timing begins with count of one. Respirations occur more slowly than pulse; thus timing does not begin with zero.
7. If rhythm is regular, count number of respirations in 30 seconds and multiply by 2. If rhythm is irregular, less than 12, or greater than 20, count for 1 full minute.	Respiratory rate is equivalent to number of respirations per minute. Suspected irregularities require assessment for at least 1 minute.

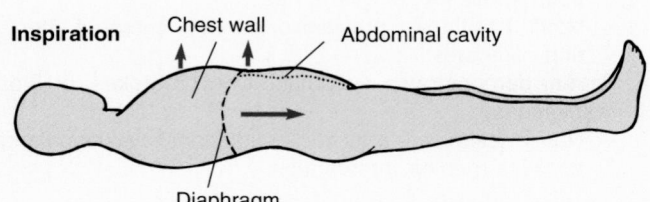
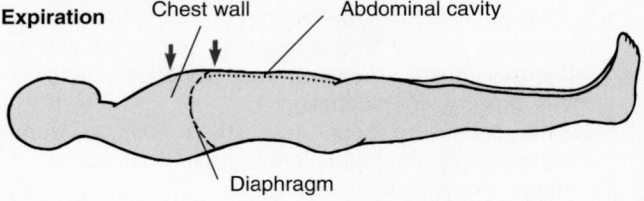

STEP 5 Diaphragmatic and chest wall movement during inspiration and expiration.

SKILL 15.4 ASSESSING RESPIRATION—cont'd

View Video!

STEP	RATIONALE
8. Note depth of respirations by observing degree of chest wall movement while counting rate. Assess depth by palpating chest wall excursion or auscultating posterior thorax after you have counted rate. Describe depth as shallow, normal, or deep.	Character of ventilatory movement reveals specific disease states restricting volume of air from moving into and out of lungs.
9. Note rhythm of ventilatory cycle. Normal breathing is regular and uninterrupted. Do not confuse sighing with abnormal rhythm.	Character of ventilations reveals specific types of alterations. Periodically people unconsciously take single deep breaths or sighs to expand small airways prone to collapse.

Clinical Decision Point. Any irregular respiratory pattern or periods of apnea (cessation of respiration for several seconds) are symptoms of underlying disease in an adult patient, and you need to report this to the health care provider or nurse in charge. Further assessment and immediate intervention are often necessary.

10. Replace bed linen and patient's gown.	Restores comfort and promotes a sense of well-being.
11. Discuss findings with patient.	Promotes participation in care and understanding of health status.
12. Perform hand hygiene.	Reduces transmission of microorganisms.

EVALUATION

1. If assessing respirations for first time, establish rate, rhythm, and depth as baseline if within acceptable range.	Used to compare future respiratory assessment.
2. Compare respirations with patient's previous baseline and usual rate, rhythm, and depth.	Allows you to assess for changes in patient's condition and presence of respiratory alterations.
3. Correlate respiratory rate, depth, and rhythm with data obtained from pulse oximetry and ABG measurements if available.	Evaluation of ventilation, perfusion, and diffusion is interrelated.
4. **Use Teach-Back:** "I want to be sure I explained why you will be reminded to take deep breaths after surgery. Tell me why deep breathing is important." Revise your instruction now or develop a plan for revised patient/family caregiver teaching if patient/family caregiver is unable to teach back correctly.	Evaluates what the patient is able to explain.

RECORDING AND REPORTING

- Record respiratory rate, depth, and rhythm on vital sign flow sheet or nurses' notes in EHR or chart.
- Record patient knowledge following evaluation of teach-back in nurses' notes.
- Document measurement of respiratory rate after administration of specific therapies in nurses' notes in EHR or chart.

- Record type and amount of oxygen therapy, if used, in nurses' notes.
- Report abnormal findings to nurse in charge or health care provider.

UNEXPECTED OUTCOMES AND RELATED INTERVENTIONS

- Adult patient's respiratory rate is below 12 breaths/min (bradypnea) or above 20 breaths/min (tachypnea). Breathing pattern is sometimes irregular. Depth of respirations is increased or decreased. Patient complains of dyspnea.
  - Assess for related factors including obstructed airway, abnormal breath sounds, productive cough, restlessness, anxiety, and confusion.
  - Assist patient to supported sitting position (semi-Fowler or high-Fowler) unless contraindicated.
  - Provide oxygen as ordered.

- Assess for environmental factors that influence patient's respiratory rate such as secondhand smoke, poor ventilation, or gas fumes.
  - Notify health care provider or nurse in charge if alteration continues.
- Patient demonstrates Kussmaul, Cheyne-Stokes, or Biot respirations.
  - Notify health care provider for additional evaluation and possible medical intervention.

SKILL 15.5 MEASURING OXYGEN SATURATION (PULSE OXIMETRY)

DELEGATION CONSIDERATIONS

The skill of oxygen saturation measurement can be delegated to nursing assistive personnel (NAP) unless patient is unstable. The nurse instructs the NAP by:

- Communicating specific factors related to the patient that can falsely lower oxygen saturation.
- Informing NAP about appropriate sensor site and probe and the need to assess condition of site routinely.
- Notifying frequency of oxygen saturation measurements for specific patient.
- Instructing to notify nurse immediately of any reading lower than SpO_2 of 95% or value for specific patient.

- Instructing to refrain from using pulse oximetry to obtain heart rate because oximeter will not detect an irregular pulse.

EQUIPMENT

- Oximeter
- Oximeter probe appropriate for patient and recommended by manufacturer (single use or reusable are available)
- Acetone or nail polish remover if needed for fingertip sensor
- Pen, vital sign flow sheet or record form, or electronic health record (EHR)

STEP	RATIONALE
ASSESSMENT	
1. Identify patient using at least two identifiers (e.g., name and birthday or name and medical record number) according to agency policy.	Ensures correct patient. Complies with The Joint Commission standards and improves patient safety (TJC, 2018).
2. Determine need to assess patient's oxygen saturation:	Clinical judgment determines need for assessment.
a. Identify risk factors of decreased oxygen saturation including acute or chronic compromised respiratory function, recovery from general anesthesia or conscious sedation, traumatic injury to chest wall with or without collapse of underlying lung tissue, ventilator dependence, and changes in supplemental oxygen therapy.	Certain conditions place patients at risk for decreased oxygen saturation.
b. Assess for signs and symptoms of alterations in oxygen saturation such as altered respiratory rate, depth, or rhythm; adventitious breath sounds (see Chapter 16); cyanotic appearance of nail beds, lips, mucous membranes, and skin; restlessness, irritability, confusion; reduced level of consciousness; and labored or difficult breathing.	Physical signs and symptoms often indicate abnormal oxygen saturation.
3. Assess for factors that normally influence measurement of SpO_2 in addition to oxygen therapy, hemoglobin level, body temperature, and medications such as bronchodilators.	Allows you to accurately assess oxygen saturation variations.
4. Determine previous baseline SpO_2 (if available) from patient's record.	Baseline information provides basis for comparison and assists in assessment of current status and evaluation of interventions.
5. Determine most appropriate patient-specific site (e.g., finger, toe, earlobe, forehead, nose) for sensor probe placement by measuring capillary refill (see Chapter 16). If capillary refill is greater than 2 seconds, select alternative site other than digit.	Sensor requires pulsating vascular bed to identify hemoglobin molecules that absorb emitted light. Changes in SpO_2 are reflected in circulation of finger capillary bed within 30 seconds and capillary bed of earlobe within 5 to 10 seconds. Forehead sensors are preferred for critically ill patients requiring vasopressors.
a. Site must have adequate local circulation and be free of moisture and skin breakdown.	Moisture prevents sensor from detecting SpO_2 levels.
b. Place probe on finger free of polish or artificial nail.	Black or brown nail polish colors alter readings.
c. If tremors are present, use earlobe as site.	Motion artifact is most common cause of inaccurate readings.
d. If patient is obese, clip-on probe may not fit properly; obtain a single-use (tape-on) probe.	
6. Determine if patient has a latex allergy.	Do not use adhesive sensors if patient has a latex allergy.
7. Assess patient's knowledge of measurement of oxygen saturation and pulse oximetry.	Encourages cooperation, minimizes risks and anxiety, and identifies teaching needs.

SKILL 15.5 MEASURING OXYGEN SATURATION (PULSE OXIMETRY)—cont'd

View Video!

STEP	RATIONALE

PLANNING

1. Provide privacy and prepare environment for patient safety.

2. Prepare and organize pulse oximetry equipment.
3. Explain purpose of procedure and how you measure oxygen saturation to patient. Instruct patient to breathe normally.

Providing privacy and preparing the environment helps you to think about the steps needed and removes clutter from over-bed or bedside table.
Ensures organized procedure.
Promotes patient cooperation and increases compliance. Prevents large fluctuations in minute ventilation and possible error in SpO_2 readings.

IMPLEMENTATION

1. Perform hand hygiene.
2. Position patient comfortably. When using finger as monitoring site, support lower arm.
3. Instruct patient to breathe normally and relax.

4. When using finger as monitoring site, consider removing any fingernail polish with acetone or polish remover. Acrylic nails without polish do not interfere with SpO_2 determination.
5. Attach transmittance sensor probe following manufacturer directions. In most sensors involving finger, toe, or ear, the LEDs and the photodector must be aligned directly across from one another.
   a. Instruct patient that clip-on probe feels like a clothespin but will not hurt.
6. Attach reflectance sensor to forehead following manufacturer's directions. LEDs are already aligned as part of sensor design. Remove cover over adhesive to apply to forehead or use a Velcro band/device to apply.

Reduces transmission of microorganisms.
Ensures probe positioning and decreases motion artifact that interferes with SpO_2 determination.
Prevents large fluctuations in respiratory rate and depth and possible changes in SpO_2.
Ensures accurate readings. Nail polish may falsely alter saturation.

Ensures transmission of light between emitter and detector through the digit or ear across the arteriolar bed (Nellcor, n.d.).

Pressure spring tension of sensor probe on peripheral digit or earlobe is unexpected.
Reflects light from the emitter/detector across the skin surface. Forehead site is preferred if patient has poor circulation (Nellcor, n.d.).

Clinical Decision Point. Do not attach sensor to finger, ear, forehead, or bridge of nose if area is edematous or skin integrity is compromised. Do not attach sensor to fingers that are hypothermic. Select forehead, ear, or bridge of nose if adult patient has history of peripheral vascular disease. Do not use earlobe and bridge of nose sensors for infants and toddlers because of skin fragility. Do not use disposable adhesive sensors if patient has latex allergy. Do not place sensor on same extremity as electronic blood pressure cuff because blood flow to finger is temporarily interrupted when cuff inflates and causes inaccurate readings that trigger alarms.

---

7. Once sensor is in place, turn on oximeter by activating power. Observe pulse waveform/intensity display and audible beep. Correlate oximeter pulse rate with patient's radial pulse. Differences require reevaluation of oximeter sensor placement and may require reassessment of pulse rates.

8. Leave sensor in place until oximeter readout reaches constant value and pulse display reaches full strength during each cardiac cycle. Inform patient that oximeter alarm will sound if sensor falls off or patient moves sensor. Read SpO_2 on digital display.
9. If continuous SpO_2 monitoring is necessary, verify SpO_2 alarm limits and volume, which are preset by the manufacturer at a low of 85% and a high of 100%. Determine limits for SpO_2 and pulse rate alarms based on each patient's condition. Verify that alarms are on.
10. Assess skin integrity every 2 hours under sensor. Routinely relocate sensor at least every 24 hours or more frequently (see manufacturer's recommendations). This is especially important if skin integrity is altered or tissue perfusion is compromised. Use care during removal to avoid damage to skin.

Pulse waveform/intensity display enables detection of valid pulse or presence of interfering signal. Pitch of audible beep is proportional to SpO_2 value. Double-checking pulse rate ensures oximeter accuracy. Oximeter pulse rate, patient's radial pulse, and apical pulse rate should be the same. Any difference requires reevaluation of oximeter sensor placement and reassessment of pulse rates.
Reading takes 10 to 30 seconds, depending on site selected.

Alarms are set at appropriate limits and volumes to avoid frightening patients and visitors.

Sensor tension and sensitivity to disposable sensor adhesive cause skin irritation and lead to disruption of skin integrity. There have been reports of forehead and nasal pressure injuries (Schallom et al., 2016).

STEP	RATIONALE
11. Help patient return to comfortable position.	Restores comfort and promotes a sense of well-being.
12. Clean the surface of a reusable sensor between patients with 70% Isopropyl alcohol solution or solution recommended by manufacturer.	Reduces transmission of infection.
13. Discuss findings with patient as needed.	Promotes participation in care and understanding of health status.
14. Perform hand hygiene.	Reduces transmission of microorganisms.
15. If planning intermittent or spot-checking SpO_2 measurements, remove sensor and turn oximeter power off. Store reusable sensor in appropriate location.	Batteries will run out if oximeter is left on. Sensor probes are expensive and vulnerable to damage.

EVALUATION

1. If you are assessing SpO_2 for the first time, establish it as baseline if it is within acceptable range.	Used to compare future SpO_2 measurements.
2. Compare SpO_2 readings with patient's previous baseline and acceptable values. Note use of oxygen therapy, which can effect SpO_2.	Comparison reveals presence of abnormality.
3. Correlate SpO_2 with SaO_2 obtained from arterial blood gas measurements (see Chapter 32) if available.	Documents reliability of noninvasive assessment.
4. Correlate SpO_2 reading with data obtained from respiratory rate, depth, and rhythm assessment (see Skill 15.4).	Measurements assessing ventilation, perfusion, and diffusion are interrelated.
5. During continuous monitoring assess skin integrity underneath probe at least every 2 hours.	Prevents tissue ischemia.
6. **Use Teach-Back:** "I want to be sure I explained why you need to keep the sensor on your finger. Tell me why this measurement is important and how moving your finger affects the reading." Revise your instruction now or develop a plan for revised patient teaching if patient/family caregiver is unable to teach back correctly.	Evaluates what the patient is able to demonstrate and explain.

RECORDING AND REPORTING

- Record SpO_2 on vital sign flow sheet or nurses' notes in EHR or chart.
- Indicate type and amount of oxygen therapy used by patient during assessment.
- Record signs and symptoms of oxygen desaturation in nurses' notes.
- Document oxygen saturation after administration of specific therapies in narrative form in nurses' notes.

- Record patient's knowledge following evaluation of teach-back in nurses' notes.
- Record in nurses' notes patient's use of continuous or intermittent pulse oximetry. Document use of equipment for third-party payers.
- Report abnormal findings to nurse in charge or health care provider.

UNEXPECTED OUTCOMES AND RELATED INTERVENTIONS

- SpO_2 is less than 90%.
  - Verify that oximeter sensor is intact and properly applied.
  - Observe for signs and symptoms of decreased oxygenation such as anxiety, restlessness, tachycardia, and cyanosis.
  - Verify that supplemental oxygen is delivered as ordered and system is functioning properly.
  - Observe for and minimize factors that decrease SpO_2 such as lung secretions, increased activity, and hyperthermia.
  - Assist patient to a position that maximizes ventilatory effort (e.g., place an obese patient in a high-Fowler position).

- Pulse rate indicated on the oximeter is less than patient's radial or apical pulse.
  - Reposition sensor probe to an alternative site with increased blood flow.
  - Assess patient for signs of altered cardiac output (e.g., decreased blood pressure, cool skin, confusion).
- Pressure injury develops under sensor site.
  - Remove and relocate sensor.
  - Provide appropriate skin care (see Chapter 38).
  - Inform health care provider.

KEY POINTS

- Vital sign measurement includes the physiological measurements of temperature, pulse, blood pressure, respiration, and oxygen saturation.
- You measure vital signs as part of a complete physical examination or in an episodic review of a patient's condition.
- Measure vital signs when your patient is at rest and the environment is controlled for comfort.
- Evaluate vital sign changes with other physical assessment findings using clinical judgment to determine measurement frequency.
- Knowledge of the factors influencing vital signs helps to determine and evaluate abnormal values.
- Changes related to aging influence vital sign measurement and nursing interventions for older adults.
- Vital signs provide a basis for evaluating response to nursing interventions.
- Changes in one vital sign often influence characteristics of the other vital signs.
- Maintain a patient's body temperature by initiating interventions that promote heat loss, production, or conservation.
- Respiratory assessment includes determining the effectiveness of ventilation, perfusion, and diffusion.
- Assessment of respiration involves observing ventilatory movements throughout the respiratory cycle.
- Hypertension is diagnosed only after an average of readings made during two or more subsequent visits reveals an elevated blood pressure.
- Selecting and applying the blood pressure measurement cuff improperly results in errors in blood pressure measurement.
- Routinely assess the condition of the skin underlying an oximeter sensor.

REFLECTIVE LEARNING

- Consider your experience with vital sign delegation and how you met the rights of delegation.
- Consider the vital sign measurement equipment you used and describe how you prevented the spread of infection.
- Consider a patient you cared for today and provide your rationale for the frequency and order of the vital sign measurements you completed.

REVIEW QUESTIONS

1. A 16-year-old girl with a history of poorly controlled asthma is admitted with dyspnea and fatigue. Her vital signs on admission are HR 118, BP 108/82 mm Hg, RR 28, tympanic temperature 37°C (98.6°F), and oxygen saturation 92%. She is receiving oxygen via nasal cannula at 2 L. Which of the following vital signs indicate the patient is improving following treatment for her asthma? (Select all that apply.)
   1. Temperature 36.8°C (98.2°F)
   2. Radial pulse 124
   3. Respiratory rate 22
   4. Oxygen saturation 94%
   5. Blood pressure 112/80 mm Hg

2. A nurse observes a nursing assistive personnel (NAP) obtaining a blood pressure on a patient. The patient's blood pressure range over the past 2 hours has been 118/72 to 112/68 mm Hg. Which of the following blood pressure readings obtained by the NAP is most likely caused by the NAP deflating the cuff too fast?
   1. 132/52 mm Hg
   2. 124/88 mm Hg
   3. 106/48 mm Hg
   4. 102/80 mm Hg

3. A nursing assistive personnel (NAP) reports to the charge nurse that a patient's pulse oximeter machine continues to alarm with a reading of 88%. The charge nurse enters the room and assesses for signs and symptoms of alterations in oxygen saturation and finds none. What action does the nurse take next?
   1. Remove the current machine from service and ask the NAP to use another pulse oximeter device
   2. Verify that the patient's oxygen device and flow are correct
   3. Verify that the oximeter sensor is intact and the skin under the sensor is dry
   4. Notify the health care provider immediately

4. The nurse is explaining to a student nurse how to use the two-step method of blood pressure assessment to obtain accurate measurements. Place the steps in correct order:
   1. Place stethoscope in ears.
   2. Palpate brachial artery while inflating blood pressure cuff 30 mm Hg over the pulse disappearance.
   3. Note point where you hear first Korotkoff sound.
   4. Wait 30 seconds.
   5. Apply blood pressure cuff 1 inch above brachial artery.
   6. Continue to deflate cuff until sound disappears.

5. A patient with a body mass index of 45 is being admitted for bariatric surgery. The nursing assistive personnel (NAP) obtains the admission vital signs and reports that she had to use a thigh cuff to obtain the patient's blood pressure on the left arm. The blood pressure was 180/100 mm Hg. What action should the nurse take?
1. Instruct the NAP to obtain a blood pressure on the right arm for comparison
2. Obtain a blood pressure using a large adult cuff on the forearm
3. Instruct the NAP to use the thigh cuff to obtain a popliteal blood pressure
4. Notify the nurse in charge or health care provider

evolve

Additional Review Questions, as well as rationales for all Review Questions, can be found on the Evolve website.

1, 3, 4; 2, 4, 3; 3, 4, 5; 4, 5, 2, 4, 1, 3, 6; 5, 2.

REFERENCES

AACN Practice Alert: Obtaining accurate noninvasive blood pressure measurements in adults, *Crit Care Nurse* 36(3):e12, 2016.

American Heart Association: *What is high blood pressure*, 2016. https://www.heart.org/idc/groups/heart-public/@wcm/@hcm/documents/downloadable/ucm_300310.pdf.

Anast N, et al: Impact of blood pressure cuff location on the accuracy of noninvasive blood pressure measurement in obese patients: an observational study, *Can J Anaesth* 63(3):298, 2016.

Angelousi A, et al: Association between orthostatic hypotension and cardiovascular risk, cerebrovascular risk, cognitive decline and falls as well as overall mortality: a systematic review and meta-analysis, *J Hypertens* 32:1562, 2014.

Asadian S, et al: Accuracy and precision of four common peripheral temperature measurement methods in intensive care patients, *Med Devices (Auckl)* 9:301–308, 2016.

Basile J, Bloch MJ: Overview of hypertension in adults, *UpToDate* 2016. http://www.uptodate.com/contents/overview-of-hypertension-in-adults.

Casiglia E, et al: Poor reliability of wrist blood pressure self-measurement at home, *Hypertension* 68:896, 2016.

Centers for Disease Control and Prevention (CDC): *Healthcare-associated infections: Clostridium difficile infection information for patients*, 2015. https://www.cdc.gov/hai/organisms/cdiff/cdiff-patient.html.

Charafeddine L, et al: Axillary and rectal thermometry in the newborn: do they agree? *BMC Res Notes* 31(7):584, 2014.

Counts D, et al: Evaluation of temporal artery and disposable digital oral thermometers in acutely ill patients, *Medsurg Nurs* 23(4):239, 2014.

Dokoohaki R, et al: Frequency of errors of blood pressure measurement among nurses, *Int Cardiovasc Res J* 9(1):41, 2015.

Furlong D, et al: Comparison of temporal to pulmonary artery temperature in febrile patients, *Dimens Crit Care Nurs* 34(1):47, 2015.

Goforth CW, Kazman JB: Exertional heat stroke in Navy and Marine personnel, *Crit Care Nurs* 35(1):52, 2015.

Gunes UY, Efteli EU: Does errors made during indirect blood pressure measurement affect the results? *Int J Caring Sci* 9(2):520, 2016.

Halm MA: Arm circumference, shape and length: how interplaying variables affect blood pressure measurement in obese persons, *Am J Crit Care* 23(2):166, 2014.

Hockenberry MJ, Wilson D: *Wong's nursing care of infants and children*, ed 10, St Louis, 2015, Mosby.

James P, et al: 2014 evidence-based guideline for the management of high blood pressure in adults report from the panel members appointed to the Eighth Joint National Committee (JNC8), *JAMA* 311:507, 2014.

Knobel R: Fetal and neonatal thermal physiology, *Newborn Infant Nurs Rev* 14:45, 2014.

Liu C, et al: Comparison of stethoscope bell and diaphragm and of stethoscope tube length for clinical blood pressure measurement, *Blood Press Monit* 21(3):178, 2016.

Longtin Y, et al: Contamination of stethoscopes and physicians' hands after a physical examination, *Mayo Clin Proc* 89(3):291, 2016.

McLean B: Comparing blood pressure measures: does one measurement equal another? *Crit Care Nurs* 35(1):75, 2015.

Nellcor: *Clinicians' guide to Nellcor sensors*, n.d., http://nbninfusions.com/wp-content/uploads/nbnmanuals/Ventilator%20Manuals/Nellcor%20Sensors%20Clinician%27s%20Manual.pdf.

Niven DJ, et al: Accuracy of peripheral thermometers for estimating temperature, *Ann Intern Med* 163(10):768, 2016.

Ozone S, et al: Comparison of blood pressure measurements on the bare arm, over a sleeve and over a rolled-up sleeve in the elderly, *Fam Pract* 33(5):517, 2016.

Perman SM, et al: The utility of therapeutic hypothermia for post-cardiac arrest syndrome patients with initial nonshockable rhythm, *Circulation* 132:2146, 2015.

Reynolds M, et al: Are temporal artery temperatures accurate enough to replace rectal temperature measurement in pediatric ED patients? *J Emerg Nurs* 40:46, 2014.

Schallom M, et al: Comparison of nasal and forehead oximetry accuracy and pressure injury in critically ill patients, *Crit Care Med* 44(12) (Suppl.):121, 2016.

Sloan BK, et al: On-site treatment of exertional heat stroke, *Am J Sports Med* 43:823, 2015.

Strauss R, et al: Prognostic significance of respiratory rate in patients with pneumonia, *Dtsch Arztebl Int* 111:503, 2014.

The Joint Commission (TJC): *2018 National Patient Safety Goals*, Oakbrook Terrace, IL, 2018, The Commission. https://www.jointcommission.org/assets/1/6/NPSG_Chapter_HAP_Jan2017.pdf.

Touhy TA, Jett KF: *Ebersole and Hess' gerontological nursing & healthy aging*, ed 4, St Louis, 2014, Mosby.

World Health Organization (WHO): *Pulse Oximetry Training Manual*, 2011. http://www.who.int/patientsafety/safesurgery/pulse_oximetry/who_ps_pulse_oxymetry_training_manual_en.pdf.

Zheng D, et al: Effect of respiration on Korotkoff sounds and oscillometric cuff pressure points during blood pressure measurement, *Med Biol Eng Comput* 52:467, 2014.

16

Health Assessment and Physical Examination

evolve MEDIA RESOURCES

http://evolve.elsevier.com/Potter/essentials

- Audio Glossary
- QSEN Activity and Review Questions Answers and Rationales
- Video Clip

OBJECTIVES

- Discuss the purposes of health assessment.
- Describe the techniques used with each physical assessment skill.
- Discuss how cultural awareness influences health assessment.
- Describe proper patient positioning during each phase of the examination.
- List techniques to promote a patient's physical and psychological comfort during an examination.
- Demonstrate preparation of a therapeutic environment before the physical examination.
- Identify data to collect from the nursing history before an examination.

- Discuss ways to incorporate health promotion and health teaching into an assessment.
- Discuss normal physical findings for patients across the life span.
- Identify self-screening assessments commonly performed by patients.
- Use physical-assessment techniques and skills during routine nursing care.
- Document assessment findings on appropriate forms.
- Communicate abnormal findings to appropriate personnel.

KEY TERMS

adventitious sounds, p. 346

arcus senilis, p. 336

atrophy, p. 365

auscultation, p. 321

bruit, p. 352

cerumen, p. 337

costovertebral angle, p. 360

crackles, p. 347

cyanosis, p. 328

dorsum, p. 331

dyspnea, p. 345

dysrhythmia, p. 350

edema, p. 328

erythema, p. 330

indurated, p. 331

inspection, p. 320

integument, p. 328

intercostal spaces, p. 344

jaundice, p. 329

olfaction, p. 321

orthopnea, p. 345

pallor, p. 329

palpation, p. 320

percussion, p. 321

petechiae, p. 331

phlebitis, p. 355

thrill, p. 352

turgor, p. 331

CASE STUDY *Mr. Neal*

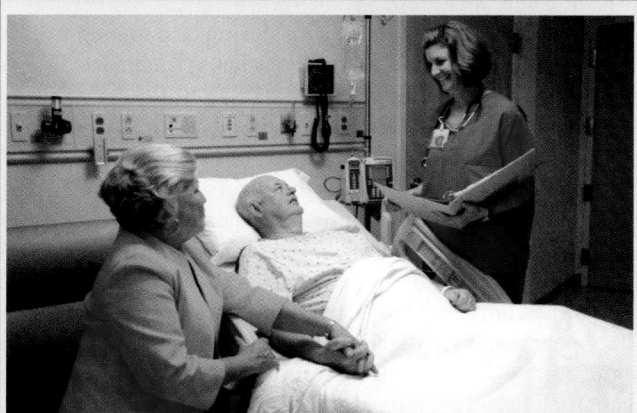

Mr. Neal, a 76-year-old retired college professor, has a history of rectal bleeding and change in bowel habits. He reports worsening constipation over the last few months. He has a history of mild hypertension and a high-fat dietary intake and has smoked two packs of cigarettes a day for 60 years. He denies any family history of colon cancer or colonoscopy screening. Mr. Neal is being admitted to the surgical floor for bowel surgery to remove a mass. His wife is present and actively involved in his care at home.

Jane is assigned to care for Mr. Neal during the day shift. She begins her assessments with a review of the patient's medical record and the health care provider's orders.

Nurses conduct health assessments to obtain information important to planning patient care. Health assessments are conducted in a variety of settings such as health fairs, screening clinics, health care providers' offices, patients' homes, or acute care settings. You conduct either a complete or a focused health assessment to gather patient information. A complete health assessment involves a nursing history, behavioral assessment, and physical examination. Focused health assessments gather information related to a specific body system or problem such as when a patient first presents to the hospital or comes for cholesterol and blood glucose screening.

PURPOSES OF HEALTH ASSESSMENT AND PHYSICAL EXAMINATION

A health assessment and physical examination are conducted as an initial evaluation in triage for emergency care; for routine health screening; to determine eligibility for health insurance, military service, or a new job; or to admit a patient to a hospital or other health care setting. As a nurse you may focus an initial assessment on a patient's chief concern—the reason the patient is seeking health care. For example, in the case of a patient who presents with abdominal pain, your assessment and examination will focus on gastrointestinal function and condition of the abdomen and underlying structures. When a patient is not at risk and is relatively stable

clinically, you can take the time needed to perform a more comprehensive assessment of all body systems.

During a health assessment, think critically about the information the patient provides, apply knowledge, and then methodically conduct the examination to create a clear picture of the patient's status. Complete a thorough assessment to accurately identify nursing diagnoses and construct a plan of care. Learn to group significant findings into patterns of data that reveal problem-focused, health promotion, or "risk for" nursing diagnoses (see Chapter 9). Gather information obtained during the initial physical examination to provide a baseline of the patient's functional abilities. Use this baseline as a comparison for future assessment findings. Subsequent physical examinations reveal information that confirms, refutes, or adds to the history and demonstrates the patient's progress.

A physical examination is patient centered. Apply what you are able to learn from the patient, the nature of the problem, and how it is affecting the ability to function. Include family caregiver input when available. In an acutely ill patient, the assessment is focused on the involved body systems. Once the patient is stable, a more comprehensive examination is conducted to learn more about the patient's total health status. Use a health assessment and physical examination to:

1. Gather baseline information about a patient's health status.
2. Supplement, confirm, or refute information learned during the health history.
3. Identify or confirm actual or at-risk nursing diagnoses.
4. Make clinical judgments about a patient's current or changing health status and ability to manage it.
5. Evaluate the outcomes of care.

CULTURAL SENSITIVITY

Respect the cultural differences of patients when completing an examination (see Chapter 21). Remember that cultural differences influence a patient's behavior. Consider the patient's health beliefs, use of alternative therapies, nutritional habits, relationships with family, and comfort with your physical closeness during the examination and history taking. If the patient does not speak English, obtain a medical translator who can interpret questions and patient's responses correctly. Consider cultural or social norms when performing an examination of the opposite gender; another person of the patient's gender or a culturally approved family member needs to be in the room when this situation occurs.

Recognition of and respect for cultural differences is an important aspect of patient care. Avoid stereotyping based on ethnicity, gender, or race. There are differences between cultural and physical characteristics. Learn to recognize common disorders for ethnic populations within the local community. A patient's attitude, feelings, and beliefs may guide the clinical decision making process (Ball et al., 2015). Recognition of cultural differences helps you provide high-quality care.

INTEGRATION OF PHYSICAL ASSESSMENT WITH NURSING CARE

Learn to integrate an examination during routine patient care. For example, assess the condition of the skin during a bed bath or observe a patient's gait, range of motion (ROM), or muscle strength as the patient ambulates. This practice makes efficient use of time, provides ongoing data collection, and conserves a patient's energy.

SKILLS OF PHYSICAL EXAMINATION

A comprehensive physical examination involves the use of five skills: inspection, palpation, percussion, auscultation, and olfaction.

Inspection

Inspection is the use of vision to distinguish normal from abnormal findings. It is important to know what to consider normal for patients of different age, gender, or cultural group. With experience you are better able to recognize normal variations among patients. Inspection is a simple technique, and the quality of an inspection depends on your willingness to be thorough and systematic. To inspect body parts accurately follow these principles:

1. Make sure that adequate lighting is available.
2. Position and expose body parts so that you can view all surfaces.
3. Inspect each area for size, shape, color, symmetry, position, and abnormalities.
4. When possible compare each area inspected with the same area on the opposite side of the body.
5. Use additional light (e.g., a penlight) to inspect skin surfaces or body cavities.
6. Do not hurry inspection. Pay attention to detail.

After inspection of a body part, findings may indicate the need for further examination. Use palpation with or after visual inspection.

Palpation

Palpation involves the use of the hands to touch body parts and make sensitive assessments. It typically occurs right after inspection. However, when examining the abdomen, palpation occurs after auscultation. Use palpation to examine all accessible parts of the body. For example, palpate the skin for temperature, moisture, texture, turgor, tenderness, and thickness. Palpate the abdomen for tenderness, distention, or masses. Use different parts of the hand to detect characteristics such as texture, temperature, and perception of movement. Use standard precautions (see Chapter 14) if any body fluids are present or could become present during palpation.

Assist the patient with relaxing and positioning comfortably because muscle tension during palpation impairs your ability to interpret physical findings. Asking the patient to take slow, deep breaths enhances muscle relaxation. Be sure to instruct the patient to point out more sensitive or tender areas and observe for any nonverbal signs of discomfort. *Palpate tender areas last.*

Do not palpate without considering a patient's overall condition. For example, if a patient has a fractured rib, use extra care to locate the painful area. Do not palpate a vital artery with pressure that obstructs blood flow. Patient safety and doing no harm are top priorities.

To palpate you need warm hands and short fingernails, and you need to be conscious of a gentle approach. After washing hands, perform palpation slowly, gently, and deliberately. Light palpation of structures such as the abdomen determines areas of irregularity or tenderness (Fig. 16.1A). Place your hand on the area you are examining and depress about 1 cm ($\frac{1}{2}$ inch). Light intermittent pressure is best when palpating; heavy prolonged pressure causes loss of sensitivity in the hand. If a patient reports pain, do not proceed to deep palpation in the area of concern.

After light palpation use deeper palpation to examine the condition of organs (Fig. 16.1B) if appropriate. To avoid injuring a patient do not try deep palpation without clinical supervision. Depress the area that you are examining deeply and evenly (Ball et al., 2015). Caution is the rule. Apply deep palpation with one or both hands (bimanually). Bimanual palpation involves one hand placed over the other while applying pressure. The upper hand exerts downward pressure as the other hand feels the subtle characteristics of underlying organs and masses.

Use the most sensitive parts of the hand (i.e., the palmar surface of the fingers and finger pads) to determine position, texture, size, consistency, masses, fluid, and pulsation (Fig. 16.2A). Assess temperature with the dorsal surface, or back, of the hand (Fig. 16.2B). The palm of the hand is more

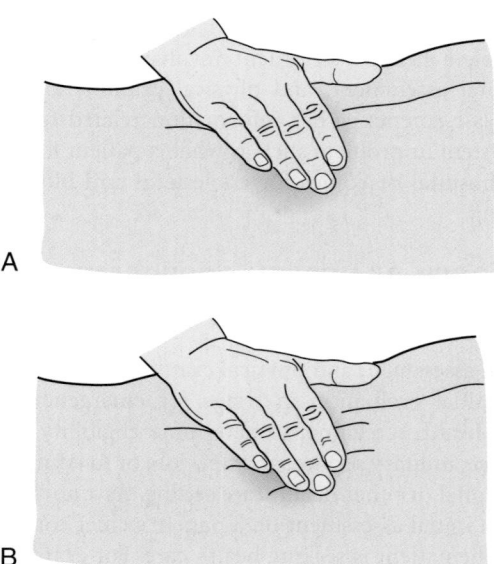

FIG 16.1 A, During light palpation gentle pressure against underlying skin and tissues can detect areas of irregularity and tenderness. **B,** During deep palpation depress tissue to assess condition of underlying organs.

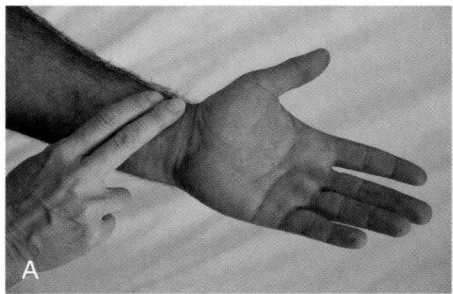 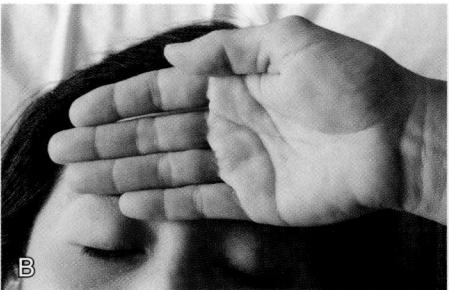 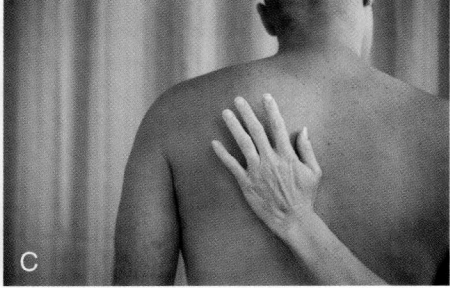

FIG 16.2 A, Radial pulse is detected with pads of fingertips, the most sensitive part of the hand. **B,** Dorsum of hand detects temperature variations in skin. **C,** Bony part of the palm at base of fingers detects vibrations.

sensitive to vibration (Fig. 16.2C). Measure position, consistency, and turgor by lightly grasping the body part with the fingertips (see Fig. 16.4).

Percussion

Percussion involves tapping the body with the fingertips to produce a vibration that travels through body tissues. This vibration is transmitted through the body tissues, and the character of the sound heard depends on the density of the underlying tissue. The resulting sounds determine the location, size, and density of underlying structures and help verify abnormalities assessed by palpation and auscultation. The skill of percussion is used more often by advanced practice nurses than by nurses in daily practice at the bedside.

Auscultation

Auscultation is listening for sounds produced by the body. Some sounds such as voice sounds are audible to the human ear. Other sounds such as those made by the cardiovascular, respiratory, and gastrointestinal (GI) systems require use of a stethoscope. Recognize abnormal sounds after learning normal variations. Become more proficient at auscultation by learning the type of sounds that each body structure makes and the location in which you hear the sounds best. Also learn which areas do not normally produce sounds.

To auscultate you need good hearing acuity, a good stethoscope, and knowledge of how to use the stethoscope properly. Individuals with a hearing impairment can use a stethoscope with additional sound amplification. Chapter 15 describes the parts of the stethoscope and its general use. The bell is best for low-pitched sounds such as vascular and certain heart sounds, and the diaphragm is best for high-pitched sounds such as bowel and lung sounds. Practice using the stethoscope (Box 16.1). Placing the bell or diaphragm under the gown or clothing, directly on the skin, aids in accurate assessment. Extraneous sounds created by movement of the tubing or chest piece interfere with auscultation of body organ sounds. By deliberately producing these sounds, you learn to recognize and disregard them during the actual examination. Learn to recognize the following characteristics of sounds:

- *Frequency:* The number of sound waves generated per second by a vibrating object. The higher the frequency, the higher the pitch of a sound and vice versa.

- *Intensity:* Amplitude of a sound wave. Auscultated sounds are described as loud or soft.
- *Quality:* Sounds of similar frequency and loudness from different sources. Terms such as *blowing* or *gurgling* describe quality of sound.
- *Duration:* Length of time that sound vibrations last. Duration of sound is short, medium, or long. Layers of soft tissue dampen the duration of sounds from deep internal organs.

Auscultation requires concentration and practice. Always consider the part of the body auscultated and the cause of the sounds. For example, the sounds heard over the abdomen are caused by intestinal peristalsis and are heard over all four abdominal quadrants as intermittent "tinkling" sounds. After understanding the cause and character of normal auscultated sounds, it becomes easier to recognize abnormal sounds and their origins.

Olfaction

While assessing a patient become familiar with the nature and source of body odors (Table 16.1). Olfaction, or smelling, helps to detect abnormalities not recognized by other means. Unusual smells lead to detection of serious abnormalities.

PREPARATION FOR EXAMINATION

Preparation of the environment, equipment, and patient ensures a smooth examination. A disorganized approach when preparing for a physical examination causes errors and incomplete findings. Use standard precautions during an examination (see Chapter 14). It is necessary to wear gloves during palpation and percussion when there is a possibility of coming in contact with body fluids to reduce contact with microorganisms. Perform hand hygiene before and after an examination.

Environment

A physical examination requires privacy. An examination room is preferable, but often the examination occurs in the patient's room. In a patient's home, the examination could possibly be done in the patient's bedroom. Adequate lighting is necessary to perform inspection. Ideally

BOX 16.1 USING A STETHOSCOPE

1. Ensure that earpiece follows the contour of the ear canals. Learn which fit is best for you by comparing the amplification of sounds with the earpieces in both directions.
2. Place earpieces in both ears with tips of earpieces turned toward the face. *Lightly* blow into the diaphragm. Again place earpieces in your ears, this time with ends turned toward the back of the head. *Lightly* blow into the stethoscope diaphragm. You find that you hear clearer sounds with the earpiece turned toward the face. After you have learned the right fit for the loudest sound, wear the stethoscope the same way each time.
3. Put the stethoscope on and *lightly* blow into the diaphragm. If sound is barely audible, *lightly* blow into the bell. Sound is carried through only one part of the chest piece at a time. If the sound is greatly amplified through the diaphragm, the diaphragm is in position for use. If sound is barely audible through the diaphragm, the bell is in position for use.
4. Place the diaphragm over the anterior part of your chest. Ask a friend to speak in a normal conversational tone. Environmental noise seriously detracts from hearing the noise created by body organs. When using a stethoscope, the patient and the examiner need to remain quiet.
5. Put the stethoscope on and gently tap the tubing. It is often difficult to avoid stretching or moving the stethoscope tubing. Position yourself so that the tubing hangs free. Moving or touching the tubing creates extraneous sounds.
6. *Care of the stethoscope:* Remove earpieces regularly and clean or remove cerumen (earwax). Keep the bell and diaphragm free of dust, lint, and body oils. Keep the tubing away from your body oils. Avoid draping the stethoscope around the neck next to the skin. To clean, wipe the entire stethoscope (e.g., diaphragm, tubing) with alcohol or soapy water. Be sure to dry all parts thoroughly. Follow manufacturer recommendations.
7. *Infection control:* Harmful bacteria, even antibiotic-resitant microorganisms, transfer from patient to patient when using portable equipment such as stethoscopes. Follow institution infection control guidelines, especially contact precautions, to decrease this risk. Clean the stethoscope (diaphragm/bell) with a disinfectant before reuse on another patient. Using a disinfectant such as isopropyl alcohol (with or without chlorhexidine), benzalkonium, or sodium hypochlorite is effective in reducing the number of bacterial colonies. Earpieces of stethoscopes are sources of transferable bacteria as well when you inadvertently touch your ears and then care for the patient. Potential pathogens could contaminate earpieces. Using hand hygiene before and after patient contact decreases the risk for transmitting microorganisms from your ear to your patient. Do not use cloth stethoscope covers because these have been shown to easily become contaminated.

BOX 16.2 EQUIPMENT AND SUPPLIES FOR PHYSICAL ASSESSMENT

- Cervical brush or broom (if needed)
- Cotton applicators
- Disposable pad/paper towels
- Drapes
- Eye chart (e.g., Snellen chart)
- Flashlight and spotlight
- Forms (e.g., physical, laboratory)
- Gloves (sterile or clean)
- Gown for patient
- Ophthalmoscope
- Otoscope
- Papanicolaou (Pap) liquid preparation (if needed)
- Percussion (reflex) hammer
- Pulse oximeter
- Ruler
- Scale with height measurement rod
- Specimen containers, slides, wooden or plastic spatula, and cytological fixative (if needed)
- Sphygmomanometer and cuff
- Sterile swabs
- Stethoscope
- Tape measure
- Thermometer
- Tissues
- Tongue depressors
- Tuning fork
- Vaginal speculum (if needed)
- Water-soluble lubricant
- Wristwatch with second hand or digital display

Sometimes it is difficult to perform a complete examination when patients are in beds or on stretchers. A special examination table makes it easier for you to reach the patient and eases patient movement into specific positions. Patients with mobility impairments require safe transfer to an examination table; assist the patient as needed on and off the table. The patient is the expert; thus you need to ask for the patient's input when moving him or her from the bed to the table safely, either with a standing assisted transfer or by being lifted, as with a child or small adult.

Consider patient comfort while on the examination table. When a patient lies supine, raise the head of the table about 30 degrees, using a small pillow if needed. When examining a patient in bed, raise the bed to reach the patient's body parts more easily. Do not leave a confused, combative, or uncooperative patient unsupervised on an examination table.

Equipment

Perform hand hygiene before equipment preparation and the examination. Have equipment readily available and arranged in order for easy use (Box 16.2). Prepare equipment as needed (e.g., warm diaphragm of stethoscope between the hands; be sure to have a proper size ear piece for an otoscope). Check all equipment to ensure that it functions properly. The ophthalmoscope and otoscope require batteries and light bulbs.

Physical Preparation of a Patient

A patient's physical comfort is vital for a successful examination. Before starting ask if the patient needs to use the restroom. An empty bladder and bowel make examination of the abdomen, genitalia, and rectum easier. If needed, collect urine or fecal specimens at this time. Be sure to explain the

an examination room is soundproof so that patients feel comfortable discussing their conditions. Be sure to eliminate other sources of noise, take precautions to prevent interruptions, and ensure that the room is warm enough to maintain comfort.

TABLE 16.1	ASSESSMENT OF CHARACTERISTIC ODORS	
ODOR	**SITE OR SOURCE**	**POTENTIAL CAUSES**
Alcohol	Oral cavity	Ingestion of alcohol, diabetes
Ammonia	Urine	Urinary tract infection, renal failure
Body odor	Skin, particularly in areas where body parts rub together (e.g., under arms and breasts)	Poor hygiene, excess perspiration (hyperhidrosis), foul-smelling perspiration (bromhidrosis)
	Wound site	Wound abscess
	Vomitus	Abdominal irritation, contaminated food
Feces	Vomitus/oral cavity (fecal odor)	Bowel obstruction
	Rectal area	Fecal incontinence
Foul-smelling stools in infant	Stool	Malabsorption syndrome
Halitosis	Oral cavity	Poor dental and oral hygiene, gum disease
Sweet, fruity ketones	Oral cavity	Diabetic ketoacidosis
Stale urine	Skin	Uremic acidosis
Sweet, heavy, thick odor	Draining wound	*Pseudomonas* (bacterial) infection
Musty odor	Casted body part	Infection inside cast
Fetid, sweet odor	Tracheostomy or mucus secretions	Infection of bronchial tree (*Pseudomonas* bacteria)

proper method for collecting specimens, and make sure to label each specimen properly.

Physical preparation involves ensuring that a patient is dressed or covered properly. A patient in the hospital wears a simple gown. A patient at an office visit or screening event might have to undress and wear a light cover, depending on the body part involved. Cover sheets and gowns are made of disposable paper, cotton, or linen. Provide a patient privacy and plenty of time during undressing, avoiding unnecessary embarrassment. After patients have undressed and put on a gown, they sit or lie down on the examination table with a sheet over the lap or lower trunk. Make sure that the patient stays warm by eliminating drafts, controlling room temperature, and providing warm blankets. Routinely ask if the patient is comfortable.

Positioning. During the examination ask the patient to assume proper positions so that body parts are accessible and the patient stays comfortable. Table 16.2 lists and shows the preferred positions for each part of the examination. A patient's ability to assume positions depends on the patient's physical strength, mobility, ease of breathing, age, and degree of wellness. Explain the positions and help patients assume them. Adjust the sheets or drapes so that the area examined is accessible, making sure not to unnecessarily expose a body part. A patient may need to assume more than one position during the examination. To decrease the number of times a patient changes positions, organize the examination so that you perform all techniques requiring a sitting position first, those that require a supine position next, and so forth. Use extra care when positioning older adults or patients with weak muscles because they are more prone to having limitations.

Psychological Preparation of a Patient

Many patients find an examination tiring or stressful, or they experience anxiety about possible findings. A thorough, simple, and clear explanation of the purpose and steps of each assessment lets patients know what to expect and helps them cooperate with each step. Give a detailed explanation as you examine each body system. Convey an open, professional, and relaxed approach. A stiff, formal approach inhibits a patient's ability to communicate, but being too casual does not give the patient confidence in your ability (Ball et al., 2015).

Use a medical interpreter for patients who do not speak or understand English. If a patient has a hearing or speech impairment, identify the communication system that will be used (sign language interpreter, word board, or talk box). If necessary, use Braille, audiotaped information, or three-dimensional anatomical models to help a patient with visual impairments understand information (Ball et al., 2015).

When a patient and nurse are of opposite gender, it helps to have a third person of the patient's gender in the room. The presence of a third person assures the patient that you will behave ethically. This person is also a witness to the conduct of the examiner and the patient. In addition, some cultures may require a gender-congruent health care provider to conduct the physical examination.

During the examination watch the patient's emotional responses. Observe whether the patient's facial expression shows fear or concern. Watch if body movements appear stiff from anxiety. Remain calm and explain each step clearly. It is sometimes necessary to stop the examination and ask how the patient feels. Do not force a patient to continue. Findings are more accurate if you postpone until the patient can cooperate and relax.

TABLE 16.2 POSITIONS FOR EXAMINATION

POSITION	AREAS ASSESSED	RATIONALE	LIMITATIONS
Sitting	Head and neck, back, posterior thorax and lungs, anterior thorax and lungs, breasts, axillae, heart, vital signs, upper extremities	Sitting upright provides full expansion of lungs and better visualization of symmetry of upper body parts.	Physically weakened patient is sometimes unable to sit. Use supine position with head of bed elevated instead.
Supine	Head and neck, anterior thorax and lungs, breasts, axillae, heart, abdomen, extremities, pulses	This is most normally relaxed position. It provides easy access to pulse sites.	If patient becomes short of breath easily, raise head of bed.
Dorsal recumbent	Head and neck, anterior thorax and lungs, breasts, axillae, heart, abdomen	This position is for abdominal assessment because it promotes relaxation of abdominal muscles.	Patients with painful disorders are more comfortable with knees flexed.
Lithotomy[a]	Female genitalia and genital tract	This position provides maximal exposure of genitalia and facilitates insertion of vaginal speculum.	Lithotomy position is embarrassing and uncomfortable; examiner minimizes time that patient spends in it. Keep patient well draped.
Sims[a]	Rectum and vagina	Flexion of hip and knee improves exposure of rectal area.	Joint deformities hinder patient's ability to bend hip and knee.
Prone	Musculoskeletal system	This position is only for assessing extension of hip joint, skin, and buttocks.	Patients with respiratory difficulties do not tolerate this position well.
Lateral recumbent	Heart	This position helps to detect murmurs.	Patients with respiratory difficulties do not tolerate this position well.
Knee-chest[a]	Rectum	This position provides maximal exposure of rectal area.	This position is embarrassing and uncomfortable.

[a]Patients with arthritis or other joint deformities may be unable to assume this position.

Assessment of Different Age-Groups

Different interview styles and approaches are needed to perform a health history and examine patients of different age-groups. When assessing children be sensitive and anticipate a child's reaction to the examination as a strange and unfamiliar experience. Routine pediatric examinations focus on health promotion and illness prevention, particularly for the care of well children who receive competent parenting and have no serious health problems (Hockenberry et al., 2017). The examination focuses on growth and development, sensory screening, dental examination, and behavioral assessment. Children who are chronically ill or disabled, foster children, foreign born, or adopted sometimes require additional assessments because of their unique health risks. When examining children the following tips help in data collection:

1. Gain a child's trust before doing any type of an examination. Talk and play with the child first. It also helps to perform parts of the examination that you can do visually before actually touching the child.
2. Children feel safer during an examination if it is initiated from the periphery and then moves to the center. For example, examine the extremities before moving to the chest.

3. When obtaining histories of infants and children gather all or part of the information from parents or guardians.

4. Because parents sometimes think they are being tested or judged by the examiner, offer support during examination and do not pass judgment.

5. Call children by their preferred name and address parents formally (e.g., as "Mr. and Mrs. Brown") rather than by first names.

6. Open-ended questions often allow parents to share more information and describe more of the child's problems.

7. Older children and adolescents tend to respond best when treated as adults and individuals and often can provide details about their health history and severity of symptoms.

8. Remember an adolescent has a right to confidentiality. After talking with parents about historical information, arrange to speak privately with the adolescent.

A comprehensive health assessment and examination of older adults includes physical data, developmental stage, family relationships, group involvement, and religious and occupational pursuits. An important part of health assessment involves analysis of basic activities of daily living (ADLs) (e.g., dressing, bathing, toileting, feeding, continence) that are fundamental to independent living. In addition, assess the more complex instrumental ADLs (e.g., using the telephone, preparing meals, managing money). Any examination of an older adult also includes an evaluation of mental status.

During the examination recognize that with advancing age the body does not respond vigorously to injury or disease. Therefore older people do not always exhibit the expected signs and symptoms. Characteristically older adults have blunted or atypical signs and symptoms. Follow these principles described by Touhy and Jett (2018) during examination of an older adult:

1. Do not assume that aging is always accompanied by illness or disability. Older adults are able to adapt to change and maintain functional independence.

2. Allow extra time; be patient, relaxed, and unhurried with older adults.

3. Provide adequate space for an examination, particularly if a patient uses a mobility aid.

4. Plan the history and examination, taking into account an older adult's energy level, physical limitations, pace, and adaptability. More than one session is sometimes necessary to complete the assessment.

5. Measure performance under the most favorable conditions. Take advantage of natural opportunities for assessment (e.g., during bathing, grooming, mealtime).

6. Sequence an examination to keep position changes to a minimum. Be efficient throughout the examination to limit patient movement.

7. Be sure that an examination of an older adult includes review of mental status.

ORGANIZATION OF THE EXAMINATION

A physical examination follows the completion of the health history (see Chapter 9). Health assessment documentation needs to include each body system, including subjective data collected. Electronic or paper physical examination documentation forms allow you to record objective and subjective data in the same sequence that it was gathered. Use common and accepted medical abbreviations to keep documentation accurate and concise. Information from the health history focuses your attention on specific parts of the examination. For example, if a patient with asthma shares recent experiences of coughing with difficulty in breathing, conduct a careful examination of the thorax and lungs. New objective data from the examination supplement information from the history to confirm or refute the data.

Be systematic and well organized about the examination so that you do not miss important assessments. A complete head-to-toe approach includes all body systems and helps you anticipate each step. In an adult begin by assessing the head and neck, progressing methodically down the body to include all body systems. Compare both sides of the body for symmetry. If a patient is seriously ill, examine the body system most at risk for being abnormal. Provide rest periods if a patient becomes fatigued. Perform any painful procedures near the end of the examination.

General Survey

Before meeting a patient review the health record to determine his or her primary health problems or concerns and the reason the patient is seeking health care. Begin your assessment with a general survey when you first meet your patient. Make mental notes of your patient's behavior, physical appearance, body structure, and mobility. The survey includes assessments about characteristics of an illness; a patient's hygiene, skin condition, and body image; emotional state; recent changes in weight; and developmental status. Be alert for any signs of physical or psychological abuse. The survey reveals important information about the patient's behavior that influences how you communicate instructions to the patient and continue on to the examination.

General Appearance and Behavior

Assess appearance and behavior while preparing the patient for the examination. The review of general appearance and behavior includes the following:

1. *Gender and race:* A person's gender affects the type of examination necessary. Note that different physical features are related to gender and race.

2. *Age:* A person's ability to participate in some parts of the examination may be influenced by age-related physical characteristics.

3. *Signs of distress:* Sometimes there are obvious signs or symptoms indicating pain (grimacing, splinting painful area), difficulty in breathing (increased work of breathing or shortness of breath), or anxiety. These signs help you determine the order of the examination.

4. *Body type:* Observe if a patient appears trim and muscular, obese, or excessively thin. Body type reflects level of health, age, and lifestyle.

5. *Posture:* Normal standing posture is an upright stance with parallel alignment of hips and shoulders. Normal sitting posture involves some degree of rounding of the shoulders. Older adults often have a stooped, forward-bent posture, with the hips and knees flexed and arms bent at the elbows.

6. *Gait:* Observe the patient walking into the room or along the bedside (if ambulatory). Note whether movements are coordinated or uncoordinated. A person normally walks with arms swinging freely at the sides, with the head and face leading the body. Note how well a patient who uses a wheelchair, cane, or walker is able to move.

7. *Body movements:* Observe whether movements are purposeful. Note any tremors involving the extremities. Determine if any body parts are immobile.

8. *Hygiene and grooming:* Note the patient's level of cleanliness by observing the appearance of the hair, skin, and fingernails. Note if the patient's clothes are clean. Grooming depends on both the activities being performed just before the examination and the patient's occupation or socioeconomic level. Note the use of hygiene products or excessive use of cosmetics.

9. *Dress:* Culture, lifestyle, socioeconomic level, and personal preference affect clothing choices. Note whether clothing is appropriate for temperature and weather conditions. Depressed or mentally ill people may be unable to choose proper clothing. Some older adults wear extra clothing because of sensitivity to cold.

10. *Body or breath odor:* Unpleasant odors result from physical exercise, poor hygiene, or certain disease states.

11. *Affect, mood, and behavior:* Affect is a person's feelings as they appear to others. Patients express mood or emotional state verbally and nonverbally. Note if verbal expressions match nonverbal behavior and whether or not mood is appropriate for the situation. Observe facial expressions while asking questions.

12. *Speech:* Normal speech is understandable and moderately paced; speech patterns are associated with the patient's thoughts. Note if the patient talks rapidly or slowly. Emotions or neurological impairment may cause an abnormal speech pace. Observe if the patient speaks in a normal tone with clear inflection of words.

13. *Patient abuse:* Child maltreatment, intimate partner violence, and elder abuse are growing health problems. Elder abuse is a major public problem and often goes undetected in emergency room visits (Evans et al., 2017). The World Health Organization (WHO) has a plan to ensure healthy lives and promote well-being for people of all ages (WHO, 2017). Assess for abuse and if found, find a way to interview the patient privately. If you are inexperienced, seek another health care provider's assistance. Patients are more likely to reveal problems when the suspected abuser is not present. Assess for the patient's fear of the spouse or partner, caregiver, parent, or adult child. Note if the partner or caregiver has a history of violence, alcoholism, or drug abuse. Identify if the partner or caregiver is unemployed, ill, or frustrated in caring for the patient. *If you assess a pattern of findings indicating abuse, most states mandate a report to a social service center (refer to state guidelines). Obtain immediate consultation with a health care provider, social worker, and other support staff to facilitate placement of the patient in a safer environment.* Table 16.3 summarizes clinical indicators of abuse.

14. *Drug use:* Drug abuse and addiction result from excessive use of alcohol, nicotine, illegal substances, or prescription drugs used for nonmedical reasons. Drug abuse and addiction affect all socioeconomic groups. A single visit with a health care provider does not always reveal the problem, but after several visits one may be able to confirm signs or behaviors with a well-focused history and physical examination. Establish trust with the patient, remaining nonjudgmental, because substance abuse involves both emotional and lifestyle issues. Box 16.3 lists indicators that should lead to further assessment for alcohol abuse. When you suspect abuse or addiction among adults 18 years of age or older, a tool such as the

---

BOX 16.3   RED FLAGS FOR SUSPICION OF SUBSTANCE ABUSE

- Patients who frequently miss appointments
- Patients who frequently request written excuses for absence from work
- Patients who have chief complaints of insomnia, "bad nerves," or pain that does not fit a particular pattern
- Patients who often report lost prescriptions (e.g., tranquilizers, pain medications) or ask for frequent refills
- Patients who make frequent emergency department visits
- Patients who have a history of changing health care providers or bring in medication bottles prescribed by several different providers
- Patients with histories of gastrointestinal bleeds, peptic ulcers, pancreatitis, cellulitis, or frequent pulmonary infections
- Patients with frequent sexually transmitted diseases, complicated pregnancies, multiple abortions, or sexual dysfunction
- Patients who complain of chest pains or palpitations or who have a history of admissions to rule out myocardial infarctions
- Patients who give histories of activities that place them at risk for human immunodeficiency virus (HIV) infections (e.g., multiple partners, multiple rapes)
- Patients with family history of addiction; history of childhood sexual, physical, or emotional abuse or social and financial or marital problems

Data from American Psychiatric Association: *Diagnostic and statistical manual of mental disorders*, ed 5, Washington, DC, 2013, The Association; Ries R, Wilford B: *Principles of addiction medicine*, ed 5, Chevy Chase, MD, 2014, Lippincott Williams & Wilkins.

TABLE 16.3 CLINICAL INDICATORS OF ABUSE

PHYSICAL FINDINGS	BEHAVIORAL FINDINGS
Child Sexual Abuse • Vaginal or penile discharge • Blood on underclothing • Pain, itching, or unusual odor in genital area • Genital injuries • Difficulty sitting or walking • Pain while urinating; recurrent urinary tract infections • Foreign bodies in rectum, urethra, or vagina • Sexually transmitted diseases • Pregnancy in young adolescent	• Problems with sleeping or eating, anxiety, depression • Fear of certain people or places • Play activities recreate abuse situation • Regressed behavior • Sexual acting out or knowledge of explicit sexual matters • Preoccupation with others' or own genitals • Profound and rapid personality changes • Poor school performance • Poor relationship with peers
Intimate Partner Violence • Injuries and trauma inconsistent with reported cause • Multiple injuries involving head, face, neck, breasts, abdomen, and genitalia (black eyes, orbital fractures, broken nose, fractured skull, lip lacerations, broken teeth, strangulation marks) • X-ray films show old and new fractures in different stages of healing • Abrasions, lacerations, bruises, welts • Burns • Human bites • Stress-related disorders such as irritable bowel syndrome, exacerbation of asthma, or chronic pain	• Attempted or thoughts of suicide • Emotional distress • Anxiety and phobias • Posttraumatic stress disorder • Pattern of substance abuse (follows physical abuse) • Low self-esteem • Depression and problems with eating or sleeping • Physical inactivity • Smoking • Unsafe sexual behavior • Stress-related complaints (headache, anxiety)
Older Adult Abuse • Injuries and trauma inconsistent with reported cause (e.g., cigarette burn, scratch, bruise, bite) • Hematomas • Bruises at various stages of resolution • Bruises, chafing, excoriation on wrist or legs (restraints) • Burns • Frequent fractures or fractures inconsistent with cause described • Dried blood	• Dependent on caregiver • Physically and/or cognitively impaired • Combative • Wandering • Verbally belligerent • Minimal social support • Prolonged interval between injury and medical treatment

Data from Cooper C, et al: The prevalence of elder abuse and neglect: a systematic review, *Age Aging* 37(2):151, 2008; Hockenberry MJ, et al: *Essentials of pediatric nursing*, ed 10, St Louis, 2017, Mosby; and WHO, *Brief sexually-related communication; recommended for a public health approach*, 2016, http://www.who.int/reproductivehealth/publications/sexual_health/sexuality-related-communication/en/.

National Institute on Drug Abuse (NIDA) Quick Screen V1.0 helps to identify the level of risks associated with substance abuse (NIDA, 2014).

Vital Signs

Assessment of vital signs (see Chapter 15) is the first part of the physical examination. Positioning or moving a patient excessively can result in inaccurate values. Be sure to recheck and report any vital signs outside of normal ranges.

Height and Weight

Height and weight reflect a patient's general level of health. This information may also be important for diagnostic testing and dosing of medications. Weight is routinely measured during health screenings and visits to health care providers' offices or clinics and when patients are admitted to a health care setting. Measuring an infant's or child's height and weight provides data about his or her growth and development. In older adults, height and weight coupled with a nutritional assessment help to identify dietary problems or dental or other functional deficits. Be sure to recognize overall trends in height and weight changes. Frequently adults become shorter with vertebral changes related to aging.

Daily variation in a patient's weight normally occurs as a result of fluid loss or retention. Health assessments screen for abnormal weight changes, using the nursing history data to focus on possible causes for weight changes. Determine the patient's current height and weight, noting weight gains or losses. Assess changes in diet habits, appetite, use of prescription or over-the-counter drugs, or physical symptoms. Standardized tables provide normal expected weights for a patient at a given height.

Several types of scales are available including built-in hospital bed scales, wheelchair scales, and digital or mechanical standing scales. Mechanical scales need to be calibrated regularly. To accurately weigh a patient, use the same scale and weigh the patient at about the same time each day (Ball et al., 2015). Patients capable of bearing their own weight use a

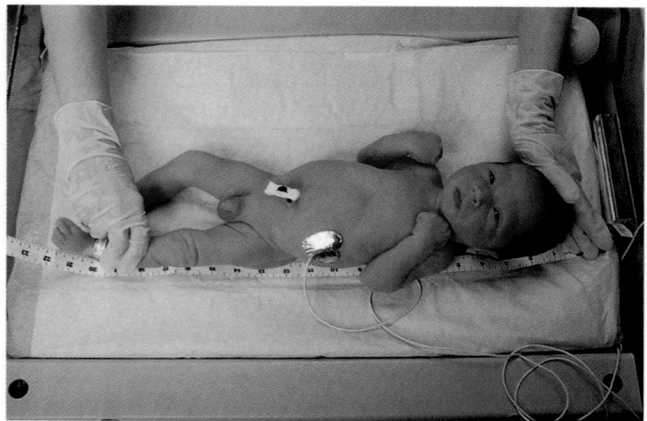

FIG 16.3 Measuring infant length. (From Murray SS, McKinney ES: *Foundations of maternal-newborn and women's health nursing,* ed 5, St Louis, 2014, Saunders.)

standing scale. The scale measures in weight increments to the nearest 0.1 kg or 0.1 lb depending on how the scale is set (Ball et al., 2015). The patient stands on the scale platform and remains still. Electronic scales automatically display weight within seconds. Electronic scales are automatically calibrated each time they are used.

Weigh infants in baskets or on platform scales. Remove the infant's clothing, keeping the room warm to reduce heat loss. A light cloth or paper placed on the scale prevents surface contamination from urine or feces. Hold a hand lightly above the infant to prevent falls. Measure the weight of an infant in ounces, grams, and kilograms.

To measure the height of a weight-bearing patient, have the patient remove his or her shoes. When needed place a paper towel on the scale platform so that the patient's feet remain clean. The platform scale has a metal rod attached to the back of the scale; this swings out and over the crown of the patient's head. Have the patient stand erect. Measure his or her height in centimeters or inches.

Place an infant in the supine position on a firm surface with shoes removed (Fig. 16.3). Portable devices are available that provide a reliable means to measure height. While the caregiver holds the infant's head against the headboard, straighten the legs at the knees and place the footboard against the bottom of the infant's feet. Record the infant's length to the nearest 0.5 cm or $\frac{1}{8}$ inch (Hockenberry et al., 2017).

SKIN, HAIR, AND NAILS

The integument consists of the skin, hair, scalp, and nails. First inspect all skin surfaces or assess the skin gradually while examining other body systems. Use the skills of inspection, palpation, and olfaction to assess the function and integrity of the integument.

Skin

Skin assessment reveals changes in oxygenation, circulation, nutrition, local tissue damage, and hydration. In a hospital setting many patients are older adults, debilitated patients, or

young but seriously ill patients. Such patients may be at risk for skin lesions resulting from trauma to the skin during administration of care, prolonged pressure during immobilization, or reactions to medications. Patients at high risk include neurologically impaired, chronically ill, and orthopedic patients. Others at risk include patients with diminished mental status, poor tissue oxygenation, low cardiac output, or inadequate nutrition. In nursing homes and extended care facilities some patients are at risk for many of the same problems, depending on their level of mobility and the presence of chronic illness. Routinely assess the skin to look for primary or initial lesions that develop. Without proper care primary lesions often deteriorate to become secondary lesions that require more extensive nursing care.

Be alert for any lesions that show evidence of cancer. Melanoma, an aggressive form of skin cancer, is the cause of most skin cancer deaths (American Cancer Society [ACS], 2016a). Cutaneous malignancies are the most common neoplasms seen in patients. Although it is important to perform a thorough skin assessment for all patients, research demonstrates the effectiveness of patient education and self-examination for prevention and early detection of skin cancers (Box 16.4).

The condition of the patient's skin reveals the need for nursing intervention. Use assessment findings to determine the type of hygiene measures required to maintain integrity of the integument (see Chapter 31). Adequate nutrition and hydration become goals of therapy if an alteration in the status of the integument is identified.

Provide adequate lighting and comfortable temperatures when assessing the skin. The recommended light is natural sunlight; halogen lighting is another option. A room that is too warm causes superficial vasodilation, resulting in increased skin redness. Patients who are sensitive to cold develop cyanosis (bluish color) around the lips and nail beds.

You inspect all skin surfaces during an examination; begin with a brief overall visual review of the entire body. The examination includes inspecting skin color, moisture, temperature, texture, and turgor; vascular changes; edema; phlebitis; and lesions. Wear clean gloves when any moisture is present. Carefully palpate any abnormalities. Skin odors are usually noted in skinfolds such as the axillae or under the breasts in female patients.

Nursing History. Ask the patient about history of skin changes including dryness, pruritus, sores, rashes, lumps, color, odor, and nonhealing lesions. Localized changes in skin color are sometimes the first indicators of skin cancer. Inquire about the patient's history of sun exposure, use of sunscreen, and predisposition to develop skin cancer (fair, freckled, light-colored hair or eyes, family history). Assess for use of topical medications, sun lamps, or tanning beds and exposure to creosote, coal, tar, or radium. Ask if the patient has noticed any changes in skin coloring; then proceed with inspection.

Color. Skin color varies by body part and person. Despite individual variations, skin color is usually uniform over

BOX 16.4 EVIDENCE-BASED PRACTICE

PICO Question: In individuals who practice high-risk behaviors or have a familial tendency for skin cancers, does monthly systematic skin inspection result in earlier diagnosis of skin cancers than annual examinations with the health provider?

SUMMARY OF EVIDENCE

The American Cancer Society (ACS) estimated that 83,510 new cases and 13,650 deaths would result from skin cancers in 2016 (ACS, 2016a). These numbers are not including the most common types of cancer—basal cell and squamous cell skin cancer (also referred to as nonmelanoma). A melanoma is a cancerous (malignant) tumor that begins in the cells that produce the skin coloring (melanocytes). There are several risk factors for melanoma. Major risk factors are positive family history of melanoma, a prior melanoma, and multiple or unusual moles (nevi). Other risk factors include fair skin, freckling, and light hair; immune suppression; age younger than 30 years; and excessive exposure to the sun and ultraviolet light (especially before 18 years of age) (ACS, 2016b).

Research has indicated that when detected early and treated properly skin cancer is highly curable. Overall survival rates for melanoma at 5 and 10 years are 92% and 89% (ACS, 2016a). Therefore early intervention is of utmost importance. In July 2014, a call to action to prevent skin cancer by the surgeon general increased awareness and encouraged all Americans to initiate a reduction in skin cancer (USPHS, 2014).

The Skin Cancer Foundation (2015) emphasizes the importance of skin self-examination from the crown of your head to the soles of your feet. Familiarize yourself with all moles on your body; have a loved one help if needed. The deadliest melanomas do not appear in preexisting moles; 70% to 80% develop in previously normal skin. Any new or changing lesion needs to be reported to a health care provider.

The current evidence does not demonstrate a benefit for health care providers to complete a visual skin examination to screen for skin cancer (U.S. Preventive Services Task Force [USPSTF], 2016). This does not mean that health care providers should not complete a visual assessment at this time, as it is a screening tool; there is not sufficient evidence to support the benefit. A new publication by the U.S. Preventive Services Task Force, *Skin Cancer Prevention: Behavioral Counseling,* is currently in progress and is due for release in 2018 (USPSTF, 2017).

APPLICATION TO NURSING PRACTICE

- Use a well-lit room and mirrors to examine all skin surfaces. If necessary have the patient ask a family member and/or significant other to aid in the examination.
- Use visual images to teach patients how to routinely assess their skin and the importance of contacting their health care provider if a skin lesion or mole starts to change, bleed, or ooze or feels different (swollen, hard, lumpy, itchy, or tender to the touch) (McWhirter and Hoffman-Gomez, 2013; Skin Cancer Foundation, 2015). Especially instruct older adults, who tend to have delayed wound healing.
- For adolescents and young adult patients, online programs to teach how to identify and reduce risks for skin cancers are effective (Heckman et al, 2016).
- Inform patients of ways to prevent skin cancer by avoiding overexposure to the sun:
  - Wear sunglasses, wide-brimmed hats, and long sleeves and long pants.
  - Apply broad-spectrum sunscreens with sun protection factor (SPF) 15 or greater to protect against ultraviolet B (UVB) and ultraviolet A (UVA) rays approximately 15 minutes before going into the sun and after swimming, perspiring, or bathing.
  - Avoid tanning under the direct sun at midday (10 a.m. to 4 p.m.).
  - Do not use indoor sunlamps, tanning parlors, or tanning pills.
  - Inform patients who are on medications that make the skin more sensitive to the sun (e.g., oral contraceptives, statins, antiinflammatories, antihypertensives, immunosuppressives) to take extra precautions when spending time in the sun.
  - Inform patients to protect their children from the sun. Severe sunburns in childhood greatly increase melanoma risk later in life (ACS, 2016b).

the body. Table 16.4 lists common variations in skin color. Normal skin pigmentation ranges from ivory or light pink to ruddy pink in light skin and from light to deep brown or olive in dark skin. In older adults the pigmentation increases unevenly, causing discolored skin. While inspecting the skin, be aware that cosmetics or tanning agents sometimes mask color.

Assessment of skin color first involves areas of the skin not exposed to the sun. Usually you see color hues best on the palms of the hands, soles of the feet, lips, tongue, and nail beds. Note if the skin is unusually pale or dark. Areas of increased color (hyperpigmentation) and decreased color (hypopigmentation) are common. Skin creases and folds are darker than the rest of the body.

Inspect sites where you can more easily identify abnormalities. For example, you can see **pallor** (unusual paleness) more easily in the face, buccal mucosa (mouth), conjunctivae, and nail beds. Observe for cyanosis (bluish discoloration) in the lips, nail beds, palpebral conjunctivae, and palms. To recognize pallor in a dark-skinned patient observe that normal brown skin appears to be yellow-brown, and normal black skin appears to be ashen gray. Also assess the lips, nail beds, and mucous membranes for generalized pallor that causes them to appear ashen gray. Assessment of cyanosis in dark-skinned patients requires that you observe areas where pigmentation occurs the least (conjunctivae, sclera, buccal mucosa, tongue, lips, nail beds, and palms and soles). A bluish tint of the lips and gums may be a normal finding in dark-skinned patients (Ball et al., 2015).

The best site to inspect for **jaundice** (yellow-orange discoloration) is the patient's sclera. You can see normal reactive hyperemia, or redness, most often in regions exposed

TABLE 16.4 SKIN COLOR VARIATIONS

COLOR	CONDITION	CAUSES	ASSESSMENT LOCATIONS
Bluish (cyanosis)	Increased amount of deoxygenated hemoglobin (associated with hypoxia)	Heart or lung disease, cold environment	Nail beds, lips, base of tongue, skin (severe cases)
Pallor (decrease in color)	Reduced amount of oxyhemoglobin	Anemia	Face, conjunctivae, nail beds, palms of hands
	Reduced visibility of oxyhemoglobin resulting from decreased blood flow	Shock	Skin, nail beds, conjunctivae, lips
Loss of pigmentation	Vitiligo	Congenital or autoimmune condition causing lack of pigment	Patchy areas on skin over face, hands, arms
Yellow-orange (jaundice)	Increased deposit of bilirubin in tissues	Liver disease, destruction of red blood cells	Sclerae, mucous membranes, skin
Red (erythema)	Increased visibility of oxyhemoglobin caused by dilation or increased blood flow	Fever, direct trauma, blushing, alcohol intake	Face, area of trauma, sacrum, shoulders, other common sites for pressure injuries
Tan-brown	Increased amount of melanin	Suntan, pregnancy	Areas exposed to sun (face, arms), areolae, nipples

to pressure such as the sacrum, heels, and greater trochanter (see Chapter 38). Inspect for any patches or areas of skin color variation. Localized skin changes such as pallor or erythema (red discoloration) often indicate circulatory changes or are caused by localized vasodilation resulting from sunburn or fever. To help identify erythema in a dark-skinned patient, palpate the area for heat and warmth to note the presence of skin inflammation. An area of an extremity that appears unusually pale results from an arterial occlusion or edema.

There is a pattern of findings associated with patients who are chemically dependent and IV drug abusers (Table 16.5). It is sometimes difficult to recognize signs and symptoms with just one examination. Edematous, reddened, and warm areas along the arms and legs suggest a pattern of recent repeated IV injections. Evidence of old injection sites appears as hyperpigmented and shiny or scarred areas.

Moisture. The hydration of skin and mucous membranes helps to reveal body fluid imbalances, changes in skin environment, and regulation of body temperature. Moisture refers to wetness and oiliness. The skin is normally smooth and dry, whereas areas such as the axillae are normally moist; minimal perspiration or oiliness is present (Ball et al., 2015). Increased perspiration is associated with activity, warm environments, obesity, anxiety, or excitement. Diaphoresis could also occur in patients with certain conditions such as diabetes, fever, menopause, and hyperthyroidism. Use ungloved fingertips to palpate skin surfaces and observe for dullness, dryness, crusting, and flaking. Flaking is the appearance of dandruff when the skin surface is rubbed lightly. Scaling involves fishlike scales that are easily rubbed off the surface of the skin. Both flaking and scaling indicate abnormally dry skin. Other factors causing dry skin include lack of humidity, exposure to sun, smoking, stress, excessive perspiration, and

TABLE 16.5 PHYSICAL FINDINGS OF THE SKIN INDICATIVE OF SUBSTANCE ABUSE

PHYSICAL FINDING	COMMONLY ASSOCIATED DRUG
Diaphoresis	Sedative-hypnotic (including alcohol)
Spider angiomas	Alcohol, stimulants
Burns (especially fingers)	Alcohol
Needle marks	Opioids
Contusions, abrasions, cuts, scars	Alcohol, other sedative-hypnotics
"Homemade" tattoos	Cocaine, IV opioids (prevents detection of injection sites)
Increased vascularity of face	Alcohol
Red, dry skin	Phencyclidine (PCP)

Modified from Burchum JR, Rosenthal LD: *Lehne's pharmacology for nursing care*, ed 9, St Louis, 2016, Elsevier; Ries R, Wilford B: *Principles of addiction medicine*, ed 5, Chevy Chase, MD, 2014, Lippincott Williams & Wilkins.

dehydration. Excessive dryness worsens existing skin conditions. In bariatric patients pay close attention to the areas with minimal airflow such as folds of large breasts, abdomen, and inguinal areas (Ball et al., 2015).

Temperature. The temperature of the skin depends on the amount of blood circulating through the dermis. Increased or decreased skin temperature reflects an increase or decrease in blood flow. An increase in skin temperature often accompanies localized erythema or redness of the skin. A reduction in skin temperature reflects a decrease in blood flow. Remember that a cold examination room affects the patient's skin temperature and color.

Accurately assess temperature by palpating the skin with the dorsum or back of the hand. Compare symmetrical body parts. Normally the skin temperature is warm and consistent throughout the body. Always assess skin temperature for patients at risk for impaired circulation, such as when skin temperature varies in one area or after a cast application or vascular surgery. A stage 1 pressure injury can be identified early by noting warmth and erythema on an area of the skin (see Chapter 38).

Texture.   The character of the surface of the skin and the feel of deeper portions are its texture. Determine whether the patient's skin is smooth or rough, thin or thick, tight or supple, or indurated (hardened) or soft by stroking it lightly with the fingertips. The texture of the skin is normally smooth, soft, and flexible in children and adults. However, it is usually not uniform. The palms of the hands and soles of the feet tend to be thicker. In older adults the skin becomes wrinkled and leathery because of a decrease in collagen, subcutaneous fat, and sweat glands.

Localized changes result from trauma, surgical wounds, or lesions. If you find irregularities in texture such as scars or induration, ask the patient if there has been recent skin injury. Deeper palpation sometimes reveals irregularities such as tenderness or localized areas of induration commonly caused by repeated injections.

Turgor.   Turgor is the elasticity of the skin. Normally the skin loses its elasticity with age. Edema or dehydration diminishes turgor. To assess skin turgor grasp a fold of skin on the back of the forearm or sternal area with the fingertips and release (Fig. 16.4). Normally the skin lifts easily and snaps back immediately to its resting position. It stays pinched or tented when turgor is poor. A decrease in turgor predisposes a patient to skin breakdown. When assessing an older adult,

skin may hang loosely because of loss of elasticity and loss of adipose tissue. In this case, tenting may be a normal finding when evaluating for skin turgor (Ball et al., 2015).

Vascularity.   Skin circulation affects color in localized areas and the appearance of superficial blood vessels. Capillaries become fragile with aging. Localized pressure areas, found after a patient has remained in one position, appear reddened, pink, or pale (see Chapter 38). Petechiae are pinpoint-size red or purple spots on the skin caused by small hemorrhages in the skin layers. They do not blanch and may indicate serious blood-clotting disorders, drug reactions, or liver disease.

Edema.   Areas of the skin become swollen or edematous from fluid buildup in the tissues. Direct trauma and impairment of venous return are two common causes of edema. Inspect edematous areas for location, color, and shape. The formation of edema separates the surface of the skin from the pigmented and vascular layers, masking skin color. Edematous skin also appears stretched and shiny. Palpate edematous areas to determine mobility, consistency, and tenderness. When pressure from your finger leaves an indentation in the edematous area, it is called *pitting edema*. To assess pitting edema press the edematous area firmly with the thumb for several seconds and release. The depth of pitting, recorded in millimeters, determines the degree of edema (Ball et al., 2015). For example, +1 edema equals 2 mm depth, and +2 edema equals 4 mm (see Fig. 16.32).

Lesions.   The skin is normally free of lesions except for common freckles or age-related changes such as skin tags or senile keratosis (thickening of skin), cherry angiomas (ruby red papules), and atrophic warts. Primary lesions occur as initial spontaneous manifestations of a pathological process such as an insect bite or are secondary and result from later formation of trauma to a primary lesion such as a pressure injury. When you detect a lesion inspect it for color, location, texture, size, shape, type (Box 16.5), grouping (e.g., clustered or linear), and distribution (localized or generalized). Observe any exudate for color, odor, amount, and consistency. Measure the size of the lesion by using a small, clear, flexible ruler divided in centimeters. Measure lesions in height, width, and depth.

Palpation determines the mobility, contour (flat, raised, or depressed), and consistency (soft or indurated) of the lesion. Palpate gently, covering the entire area of the lesion. If the lesion is moist or has draining fluid, wear clean gloves during palpation. Note if the patient complains of tenderness during palpation. Cancerous lesions frequently undergo changes in color and size. Report abnormal lesions that have changed in character (e.g., color or size) to a health care provider for further examination.

Hair and Scalp

Inspecting the condition and distribution of body hair and integrity of the scalp requires good lighting. Hair assessment

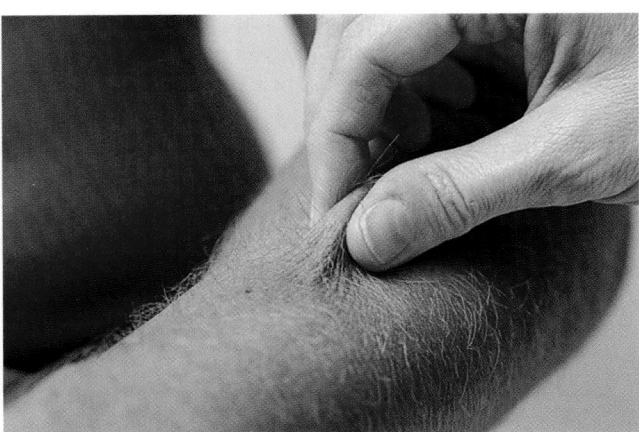

FIG 16.4 Assessment of skin turgor.

BOX 16.5   TYPES OF PRIMARY SKIN LESIONS

Macule: Flat, nonpalpable change in skin color, smaller than 1 cm (e.g., freckle, petechia)

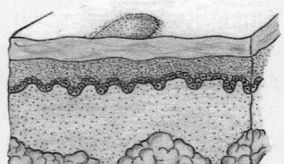

Papule: Palpable, circumscribed, solid elevation in skin, smaller than 0.5 cm (e.g., elevated nevus)

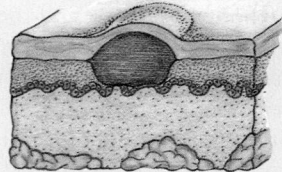

Nodule: Elevated solid mass, deeper and firmer than papule, 0.5 to 2 cm (e.g., wart)

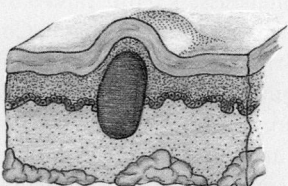

Tumor: Solid mass that extends deep through subcutaneous tissue, larger than 1 to 2 cm (e.g., epithelioma)

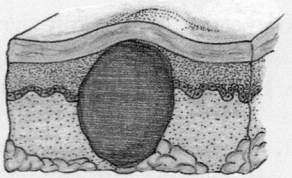

Wheal: Irregularly shaped, elevated area or superficial localized edema, varies in size (e.g., hive, mosquito bite)

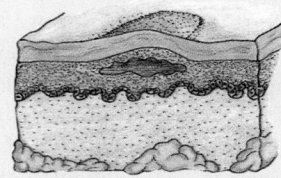

Vesicle: Circumscribed elevation of skin filled with serous fluid, smaller than 1 cm (e.g., herpes simplex, chickenpox)

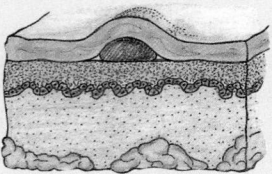

Pustule: Circumscribed elevation of skin similar to vesicle but filled with pus; varies in size (e.g., acne, staphylococcal infection)

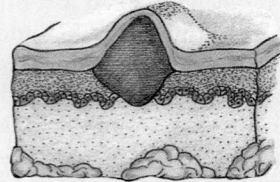

Ulcer: Deep loss of skin surface that sometimes extends to dermis and frequently bleeds and scars; varies in size (e.g., venous stasis ulcer)

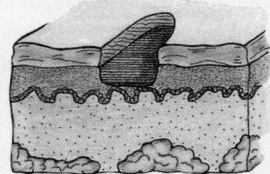

Atrophy: Thinning of skin with loss of normal skin furrow with skin appearing shiny and translucent; varies in size (e.g., arterial insufficiency)

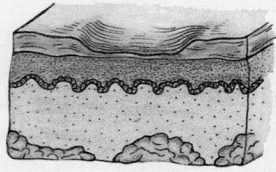

occurs during all portions of the examination. Assess its distribution, thickness, texture, lubrication, and grooming.

Nursing History. Assess if the patient has noticed a change in growth or loss of hair or change in texture. Determine if the patient wears a wig or hairpiece, and ask if he or she is comfortable with it being removed briefly to examine the skin underneath. Determine if the patient is on a medication or has any medical conditions that possibly alter hair texture or growth (e.g., chemotherapy or vasodilator).

During inspection explain that it is necessary to separate parts of the hair to detect abnormalities. Wear clean gloves to avoid possible infection from lesions or lice. First inspect the color, distribution, quantity, thickness, texture, and lubrication of body hair. Hair is normally distributed evenly, is neither excessively dry nor oily, and is pliant or flexible. While separating sections of scalp hair, observe for characteristics of color and coarseness. Normal terminal hair (long, coarse, thick hair on the scalp, axillae, and pubic areas) varies in color from light blond to black to gray. In older adults the hair becomes dull gray, white, or yellow. It also thins over the scalp, axillae, and pubic areas. Older men lose facial hair, whereas older women sometimes develop hair on the chin and upper lip.

Changes occur in the thickness, texture, and lubrication of scalp hair. Disturbances such as a febrile illness or scalp disease sometimes result in hair loss. Conditions such as thyroid disease alter the condition of the hair, making it fine and brittle. Hair loss (alopecia) or thinning of the hair is usually related to genetic tendencies and endocrine disorders such as diabetes and menopause. Poor nutrition causes stringy, dull, dry, and thin hair. The hair is lubricated from the oil of sebaceous glands. Excessively oily hair is associated with androgen hormone stimulation. Dry, brittle hair occurs with aging and excessive use of chemical agents.

The amount of hair covering the extremities is sometimes reduced as a result of aging or a disease process such as arterial insufficiency most commonly over the lower extremities. In women do not confuse a loss of hair with shaved legs.

Inspect the scalp for lesions, which are not easily noticed in thick hair. The scalp is normally smooth and inelastic with even coloration. Thoroughly examine the scalp for lesions by carefully separating strands of hair,. Note the characteristics of any scalp lesions. If you find lumps or bruises, ask if the patient has experienced recent head trauma. Moles on the scalp are common. Warn the patient that combing or brushing sometimes causes a mole to bleed. Dandruff or psoriasis frequently causes scaliness or dryness.

Careful inspection of hair follicles on the scalp and pubic areas may reveal lice or other parasites. There are head lice, body lice, and crab lice. Head and crab lice attach their eggs

BOX 16.6 PATIENT TEACHING

Hair and Scalp Assessment

OUTCOME
Patient performs proper hygiene practices for care of the hair and scalp.

TEACHING STRATEGIES
- Instruct in basic hygiene practices for care of the hair and scalp (see Chapter 31).
- Instruct patients who have head lice to shampoo thoroughly with pediculicide (shampoo available at drug stores) in cold water, comb thoroughly with fine-tooth comb (following product directions), and discard comb. *Caution against the use of products containing lindane, a toxic ingredient known to cause adverse reactions.* Repeat shampoo treatment 12 to 24 hours later.
- After combing remove any detachable nits or nit cases with tweezers or between the fingernails. A dilute solution of vinegar and water helps loosen nits.
- Instruct patients and parents about ways to reduce transmission of lice:
  - Do not share personal-care items with others.
  - Vacuum all rugs, car seats, pillows, furniture, and flooring thoroughly and discard vacuum bag.
  - Seal nonwashable items in plastic bags for 14 days if unable to dry-clean or vacuum.
  - Use thorough hand-hygiene practices.
  - Launder all clothing, linen, and bedding in hot soap and water and dry in a hot dryer for at least 20 minutes. Dry-clean nonwashable items.
  - Do not use insecticide.
  - Instruct patient to notify partner if lice were sexually transmitted.
  - Avoid physical contact with individuals who are infested and their belongings, especially clothing and bedding.
  - Soak combs, brushes, and hair accessories in lice-killing products for 1 hour or in boiling water for 10 minutes.

EVALUATION
- Use the principles of teach-back to evaluate patient/family caregiver learning:
  - "Describe for me the methods you use to care for your hair and scalp."
  - "Tell me the steps we discussed to reduce lice transmission."

to hair. Lice eggs look like oval particles of dandruff. The lice themselves are difficult to see. Observe for bites or pustular eruptions in the follicles and areas where skin surfaces meet such as behind the ears and in the groin. The discovery of lice requires immediate treatment and family education (Box 16.6).

Nails

The condition of the nails reflects general health, state of nutrition, a person's occupation, and level of self-care. The most visible portion of the nails is the nail plate, the transparent layer of epithelial cells covering the nail bed. The vascularity of the nail bed creates the underlying color of the nail. The semilunar, whitish area at the base of the nail bed is called the *lunula,* from which the nail plate develops.

Nursing History. Ask the patient if there have been any recent changes in the nails (e.g., splitting, breaking, or thickening) or recent trauma. Determine the patient's nail care practices such as use of acrylic nails or risk for exposure to fungi at nail salons. Determine any physiological risk factors for nail problems (e.g., diabetes mellitus, peripheral vascular disease, older age).

Inspect the nail bed color, cleanliness, and length; the thickness and shape of the nail; the texture of the nail; the angle between the nail and the nail bed; and the condition of tissue around the nail. The nails are normally transparent, smooth, well rounded, and convex, with surrounding cuticles smooth, intact, and without inflammation. In light-skinned patients nail beds are pink with translucent white nail tips. In dark-skinned patients nail beds are darkly pigmented, have a blue or reddish hue, and have yellow-tinged nail tips. A brown or black pigmentation is normal with longitudinal streaks. Trauma, cirrhosis, diabetes mellitus, and hypertension cause splinter hemorrhages. Vitamin, protein, and electrolyte changes cause various lines or bands to form on nail beds.

Nails normally grow at a constant rate, but direct injury or generalized disease impairs growth. With aging the nails of the fingers and toes become harder and thicker. Longitudinal striations develop, and the rate of nail growth slows. Nails become more brittle, dull, and opaque and turn yellow in older adults because of insufficient calcium. Also with age the cuticle becomes less thick and wide.

Inspection of the angle between the nail and nail bed normally reveals an angle of 160 degrees (Box 16.7). A larger angle and softening of the nail bed indicate clubbing resulting from chronic oxygenation problems.

Palpate the nail base to determine firmness and condition of circulation. It is normally firm. To palpate gently grasp the patient's finger and observe its color. An ongoing bluish or purplish cast to the nail bed occurs with cyanosis. A white cast or pallor can result from anemia and/or liver disease. Observe for jaundice (yellow/orange), which can also indicate liver disease.

Calluses and corns often occur on the toes or fingers. A callus is flat and painless, resulting from thickening of the epidermis such as on the finger that supports a pencil or pen or on the bottom of the feet. Friction and pressure from shoes cause corns, usually over bony prominences. During the examination instruct the patient in proper nail care (Box 16.8).

HEAD AND NECK

An examination of the head and neck includes assessment of the head, eyes, ears, nose, mouth, pharynx, and neck (lymph nodes, carotid arteries, thyroid gland, and trachea). You may defer assessment of the carotid arteries until the vascular

BOX 16.7 ABNORMALITIES OF THE NAIL BED

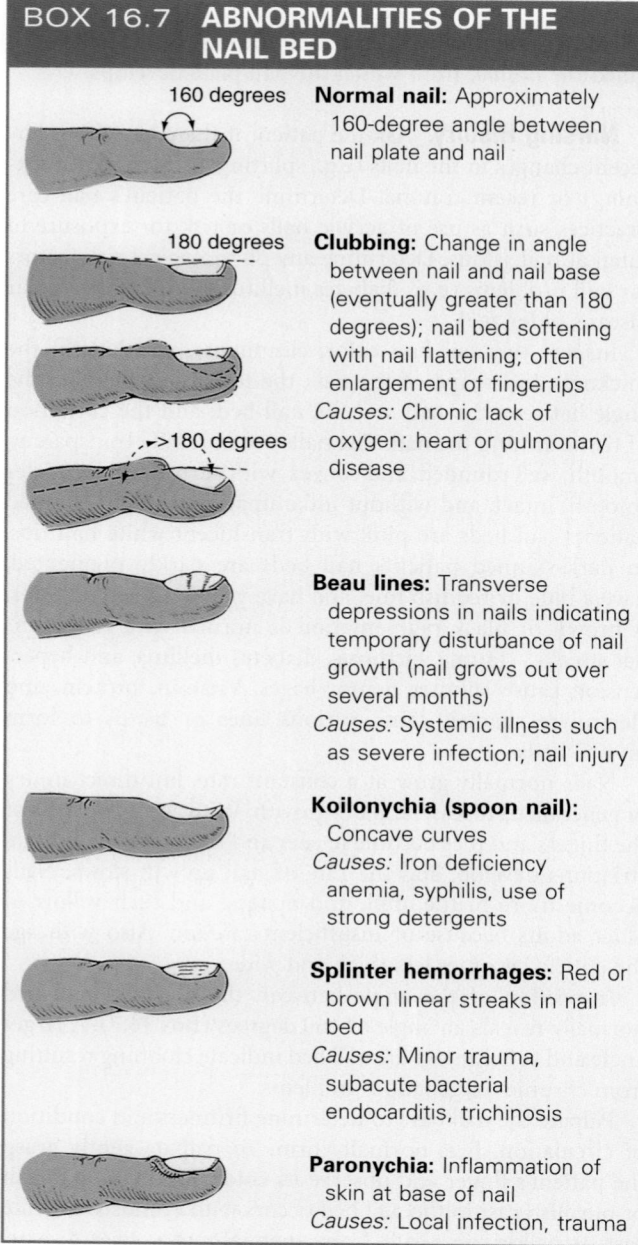

Normal nail: Approximately 160-degree angle between nail plate and nail

160 degrees

180 degrees

>180 degrees

Clubbing: Change in angle between nail and nail base (eventually greater than 180 degrees); nail bed softening with nail flattening; often enlargement of fingertips
Causes: Chronic lack of oxygen: heart or pulmonary disease

Beau lines: Transverse depressions in nails indicating temporary disturbance of nail growth (nail grows out over several months)
Causes: Systemic illness such as severe infection; nail injury

Koilonychia (spoon nail): Concave curves
Causes: Iron deficiency anemia, syphilis, use of strong detergents

Splinter hemorrhages: Red or brown linear streaks in nail bed
Causes: Minor trauma, subacute bacterial endocarditis, trichinosis

Paronychia: Inflammation of skin at base of nail
Causes: Local infection, trauma

BOX 16.8 PATIENT TEACHING

Nail Assessment

OUTCOME
Patient properly cares for fingernails, feet, and toenails.

TEACHING STRATEGIES
- Instruct patient to cut nails only after soaking them about 10 minutes in warm water. (Exception: Patients with diabetes are warned against soaking nails because this dries the hands and feet; dry skin leads to infection.)
- Caution patient to avoid using over-the-counter preparations to treat corns, calluses, or ingrown toenails.
- Tell patient to cut nails straight across and even with tops of fingers or toes. If patient has diabetes, tell him or her to file rather than cut nails (see Chapter 31).
- Instruct patient to shape nails with file or emery board.
- If patient has diabetes (ADA, 2014):
  - Set a time to inspect feet each day in good lighting, looking for dry places and cracks in skin.
  - Wash feet daily in warm water and carefully dry them, especially between toes.
  - Soften dry feet. Rub a thin coat of skin lotion over the tops and bottoms of feet.
  - Do not put lotion between toes; moisture between toes promotes growth of microorganisms, leading to infection.
  - Caution patient against using sharp objects to poke or dig under toenail or around cuticle.
  - Wear shoes and socks and don't go barefoot.
  - Protect feet from extreme heat and cold.
  - Keep blood flowing to feet. Elevate feet when sitting, and wiggle toes and move ankles periodically. Don't cross legs for long periods of time.
  - Have patient see a podiatrist for treatment of ingrown toenails and nails that are thick or tend to split.

EVALUATION
- Use the principles of teach-back to evaluate patient/family caregiver learning:
  - "Describe to me how you regularly check your nails for problems."
  - "List for me the steps to you take to avoid injury to your fingernails, feet, and toenails."

examination. Assessment of the head and neck uses inspection, palpation, and auscultation.

Head

Nursing History. Determine if your patient has a recent history of head trauma or neurological symptoms such as headache, dizziness, seizures, poor vision, or loss of consciousness. Review the patient's occupation, participation in contact sports, and use of protective head gear.

Inspect the patient's head, noting the position, size, shape, and contour. The head is normally held upright and midline to the trunk. Holding the head tilted to one side is an indication of unilateral hearing or visual loss. A horizontal jerking or bobbing indicates a tremor.

Note facial features looking at the eyelids, eyebrows, nasolabial folds, and mouth for shape and symmetry. It is normal for slight asymmetry to exist. If there is facial asymmetry, note if all features on one side of the face are affected or if only part of the face is involved. Various neurological disorders such as a facial nerve paralysis affect different nerves that innervate muscles of the face.

Examine the size, shape, and contour of the skull. Generally it is round with prominences in the frontal area anteriorly and the occipital area posteriorly. Trauma typically causes local skull deformities. Palpate the skull for nodules or masses. Gently rotate the fingertips down the midline of the scalp and then along the sides of the head to identify abnormalities.

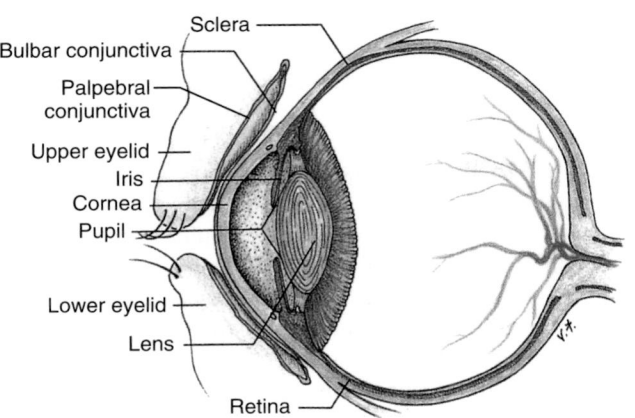

FIG 16.5 Cross section of eye.

In infants a large head results from congenital anomalies or the accumulation of cerebrospinal fluid in the ventricles (hydrocephalus). Acromegaly causes an enlarged jaw and facial bones in affected adults.

Eyes

Examination of the eye includes assessment of visual acuity, visual fields, and external and internal eye structures. Fig. 16.5 shows a cross section of the eye. The assessment detects visual alterations and determines the level of assistance that patients require when ambulating or performing self-care activities. Patients with visual problems need special aids for reading educational materials or instructions.

Nursing History. Review with the patient any history of partial or complete vision loss from eye disease (e.g., glaucoma, cataracts), eye trauma, diabetes, hypertension, or eye surgery. Assess for common symptoms of eye disease such as eye pain, photophobia (sensitivity to light), burning, itching, excessive tearing, diplopia (double vision), blurred vision, or visual disturbances (e.g., flashing lights, halos, "film" over vision field). Review the patient's occupational history, use of glasses or contact lenses, use of safety glasses, and visits to an optometrist (Box 16.9). Determine the patient's current medication use including any eye medication.

Visual Acuity. The assessment of visual acuity (i.e., the ability to see small details) tests central vision. The easiest way to assess visual acuity is to ask the patient to read printed material or a Snellen chart under adequate lighting. Patients need to wear prescription glasses or contact lenses during the assessment. Identify the language the patient speaks and reading ability. Asking the patient to read aloud helps determine literacy. Position the patient 6 m (20 feet) away from the chart. Test each eye separately by covering one eye with a card or gauze square, avoiding pressure on the eye. A patient who has difficulty reading related to vision needs to consult an ophthalmologist or optometrist for further evaluation.

BOX 16.9 PATIENT TEACHING

Eye Assessment

OUTCOME

Patient follows recommendations for preventive eye care, including regular eye care examinations and protection from injury.

TEACHING STRATEGIES

- Tell patient that people younger than 40 years of age need to have a complete eye examination every 3 to 5 years (or more often if family histories reveal risks such as diabetes or hypertension).
- Teach patients that people older than 40 years of age need to have a complete eye examination every 2 years to screen for conditions that may develop without patient awareness (e.g., glaucoma); this increases to annual examinations after 65 years of age.
- Describe the typical symptoms of eye disease (see Chapter 39).
- Instruct older adults to take the following precautions because of normal vision changes: avoid or use caution while driving at night, increase lighting in the home to reduce risk for falls, and paint the first and last steps of a staircase and the edge of each step in between a bright color to aid in depth perception.

EVALUATION

- Use the principles of teach-back to evaluate patient/family caregiver learning:
  - "Please describe to me when your most recent ophthalmologist visit was and what plans you have for future visits."
  - "Describe to me the common symptoms of eye disease that we discussed."
  - "Describe for me the safety measures for eye protection you take when working at home or with tools and equipment."

Visual Fields. Objects in the periphery can normally be seen when a person looks straight ahead. To assess visual fields, remove the patient's eyeglasses. Have the patient stand or sit 60 cm (2 feet) away facing you at eye level. He or she gently closes or covers one eye (e.g., the left) and looks at your eye directly opposite. Close the opposite eye as the field of vision is superimposed on that of the patient. Move a finger equidistant at arm's length from you and the patient outside the field of vision and then slowly bring it back into the visual field. Ask the patient to tell you when the finger is visible. If you see the finger before the patient does, this reveals that a portion of the patient's visual field is reduced.

External Eye Structures. To inspect external eye structures stand directly in front of the patient at eye level and ask him or her to look at your face. Ask patients to remove glasses or contacts for the remainder of the examination.

Position and Alignment. Assess the position of the eyes in relation to one another. Normally they are parallel to one another. Bulging eyes (exophthalmos) usually indicate hyperthyroidism. Crossed eyes (strabismus) result from neuromuscular injury or inherited abnormalities. A tumor or inflammation of the orbit may cause abnormal eye protrusion.

Eyebrows. Inspect the eyebrows for size, extension, texture of hair, alignment, and movement. Coarseness of hair and failure to extend beyond the temporal canthus may reveal hypothyroidism. If the brows are thinned, identify if the patient plucks or waxes the hair. Aging causes loss of the lateral third of the eyebrows. Have the patient raise and lower the eyebrows. They normally raise and lower symmetrically. An inability to move them indicates a facial nerve (cranial nerve VII) paralysis.

Eyelids. Inspect the eyelids for position, color, condition, and direction of lashes; assess the patient's ability to open, close, and blink. When the eyes are open in a normal position, the lids do not cover the pupil, and you cannot see the sclera above the iris. The lids are also close to the eyeball. An abnormal drooping of the lid over the pupil is called *ptosis,* which is caused by edema or impairment of the third cranial nerve. In older adults ptosis results from a loss of elasticity that accompanies aging. An older adult frequently has lid margins that turn out (ectropion) or in (entropion). An entropion sometimes leads to the lashes of the lid irritating the conjunctiva and cornea, increasing risk for infection. Normally the eyelashes are distributed evenly and curved outward away from the eye.

The lids close symmetrically. Ask the patient to open the eyes, and observe the blink reflex, during which the cornea is lubricated. Normally a patient blinks involuntarily and bilaterally up to 20 times a minute. Report absent, infrequent, rapid, or monocular (one-eyed) blinking. Failure of lids to close exposes the cornea to drying. This condition happens in unconscious patients or patients with facial nerve paralysis.

Lacrimal Apparatus. The lacrimal gland (Fig. 16.6), located in the upper, outer wall of the anterior part of the orbit, is responsible for tear production. Tears flow from the gland across the surface of the eye to the lacrimal duct, which is in the nasal corner or inner canthus of the eye. Inspect the lacrimal gland for edema and redness. Palpate the gland area gently to detect tenderness. Normally the gland cannot be felt. The nasolacrimal duct may become obstructed, blocking the flow of tears. Observe for evidence of excess tearing or edema in the inner canthus. Gentle palpation of the duct at the lower eyelid just inside the orbital rim causes a regurgitation of tears.

Conjunctivae and Sclerae. The bulbar conjunctiva covers the exposed surface of the eyeball up to the outer edge of the cornea. Observe the sclera under the bulbar conjunctiva; it normally has the color of white porcelain in Caucasians and light yellow in dark-skinned patients. To view both structures gently retract both lids simultaneously with thumb and index finger pressed against the lower and upper bony orbits. For adequate exposure retract the eyelids without placing pressure directly on the eyeball. Ask the patient to look up, down, and side to side. Inspect for color, texture, and the presence of edema or lesions.

Normally the conjunctivae are free of erythema. The presence of redness indicates traumatic, allergic, or infectious conjunctivitis. Conjunctivitis is a highly contagious infection, and the crusty drainage that collects on eyelid margins easily spreads from one eye to the other. Perform proper hand hygiene (see Chapter 14) before and after the examination. Wear clean gloves during the examination.

Corneas. The cornea is the transparent, colorless portion of the eye covering the pupil and iris. From a side view it looks like the crystal of a wristwatch. While the patient looks straight ahead, inspect the cornea for clarity and texture while shining a penlight obliquely across its surface. Normally the cornea is shiny, transparent, and smooth. In older adults it loses its luster. Any irregularity in the surface indicates an abrasion or tear that requires further examination by a health care provider. Both conditions are very painful. To test for the corneal blink reflex, see the cranial nerve function section of this chapter.

Pupils and Irises. Observe the pupils for size, shape, equality, accommodation, and reaction to light. They are normally black, round, regular, and equal in size (2 to 6 mm in diameter) (Fig. 16.7). The iris should be clearly visible. Note the color and details of the iris. In an older adult it becomes faded. A thin white ring along the margin of the iris, called an arcus senilis, is common with aging but abnormal in anyone younger than 40 years of age.

Cloudy pupils indicate cataracts. Continuous dilation of pupils results from neurological disorders, glaucoma, trauma, eye medication, or withdrawal from opioids. Pinpoint pupils are a common sign of opioid intoxication. When shining a beam of light through the pupil and onto the retina, the third cranial nerve is stimulated, causing the muscles of the iris to constrict. Any abnormality along the nerve pathways from the retina to the iris alters the ability of the pupils to react to light. Changes in intracranial pressure, lesions along the nerve pathways, locally applied ophthalmic medications, and direct trauma to the eye alter pupillary reaction.

Test pupillary reflexes (to light and accommodation) in a dimly lit room. Instruct the patient to look straight ahead, bring a penlight from the side of the patient's face, and direct the light onto the pupil (Fig. 16.8A–B). A directly illuminated

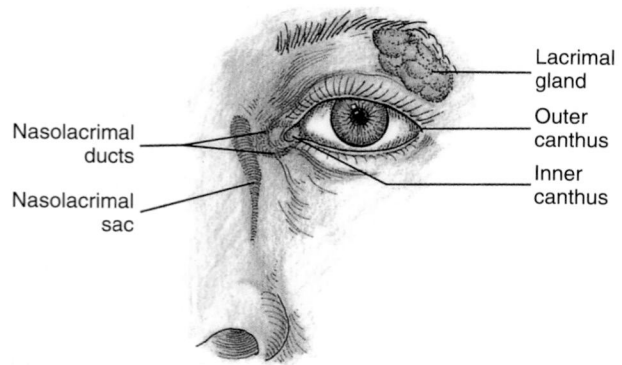

FIG 16.6 Lacrimal apparatus.

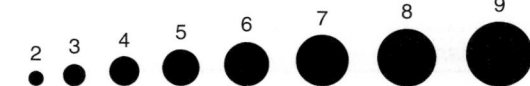

FIG 16.7 Chart depicting pupillary size in millimeters.

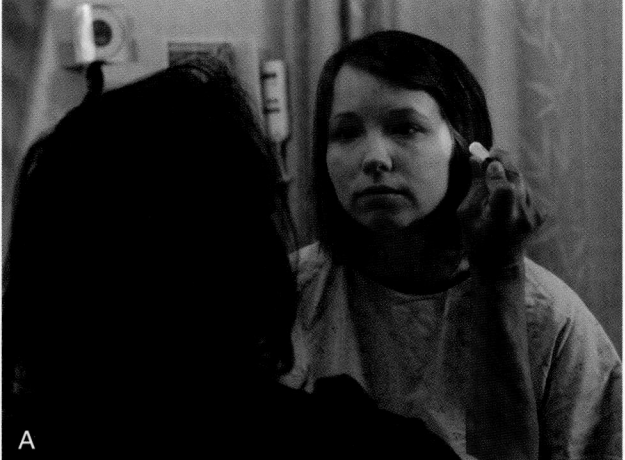

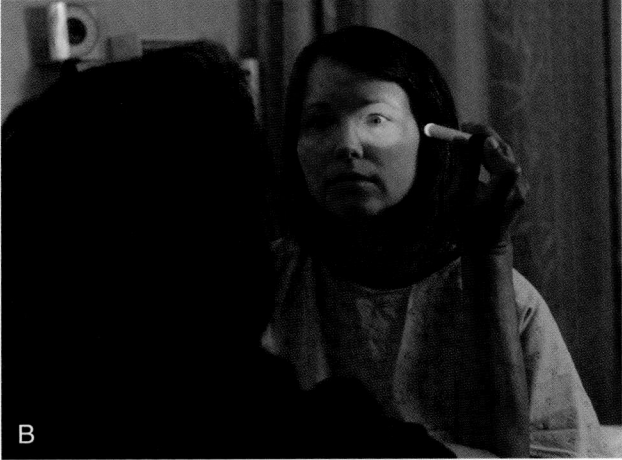

FIG 16.8 **A,** To check pupillary reflexes the nurse first holds the penlight to the side of the patient's face. **B,** Illumination of pupil causes pupillary constriction.

pupil constricts, and the opposite pupil constricts consensually. Observe the quickness and equality of the reflex. Repeat the examination for the opposite eye.

To test accommodation ask the patient to gaze at a distant object (the far wall) and then at a test object (finger or pencil) held approximately 10 cm (4 inches) from the bridge of the patient's nose. The pupils normally converge and accommodate by constricting when looking at close objects. The responses of the pupils are equal. If assessment of pupillary reaction is normal in all tests, record the abbreviation PERRLA (pupils equal, round, reactive to light and accommodation).

Internal Eye Structures. An advanced nurse practitioner or other health care provider usually performs examination of the internal eye structures through the use of an ophthalmoscope.

Ears

The ear assessment determines the integrity of ear structures and hearing acuity. Inspect and palpate external ear structures, inspect middle ear structures with the otoscope, and test the inner ear by measuring the patient's hearing acuity. Assessment of patients with hearing impairment provides useful data in planning effective communication techniques.

Nursing History. Review risk factors for hearing problems with the patient (e.g., intake of aspirin or noise exposure) and assess for history of ear trauma or surgery. Determine if the patient has ear pain, itching, discharge, tinnitus (ringing in ears), vertigo (loss of balance), or change in hearing. Note behavior that indicates hearing loss such as leaning forward to hear, inattentiveness to speech, and requests to repeat comments. Determine the onset and contributing factors to any hearing problem. Assess if the patient wears a hearing aid and how he or she normally cleans it and the ears.

Auricles. With the patient sitting inspect the size, shape, symmetry, flexibility, landmarks, position, and color of the auricle. The auricles are normally of equal size and level with one another. The upper point of attachment to the head is normally in a straight line with the outer canthus, or corner of the eye. Ears that are low set or at an unusual angle may indicate a chromosome abnormality or renal disorders. Ear color is the same as the face without moles, cysts, deformities, or nodules. Redness is a sign of inflammation or fever.

Palpate the auricles for texture, tenderness, swelling, and skin lesions. Auricles are normally smooth, firm, mobile, and without lesions. If the patient complains of pain, gently pull the auricle, press on the tragus, and palpate behind the ear over the mastoid process. If palpating the tragus increases the pain, an external ear canal infection is likely. If palpating the auricle and tragus does not influence the pain, the patient may have a middle ear infection. Tenderness in the mastoid area indicates mastoiditis.

Inspect the opening of the ear canal for size and presence of discharge. If discharge is present, wear clean gloves during the examination. A swollen or occluded meatus is not normal. A yellow, waxy substance called cerumen is common. Yellow or green foul-smelling discharge indicates infection or a foreign body in the canal. The color of cerumen is darker in dark-skinned patients.

Ear Canals and Eardrums. Observe the deeper structures of the external and middle ear with the use of an otoscope. A special ear speculum attaches to the handle of the ophthalmoscope. For best visualization select the largest speculum that fits comfortably in the patient's ear. Before inserting it, check for foreign bodies in the opening of the auditory canal.

Make sure that the patient avoids moving the head during the examination to avoid damage to the canal and tympanic membrane. Hold the head of moving infants and young

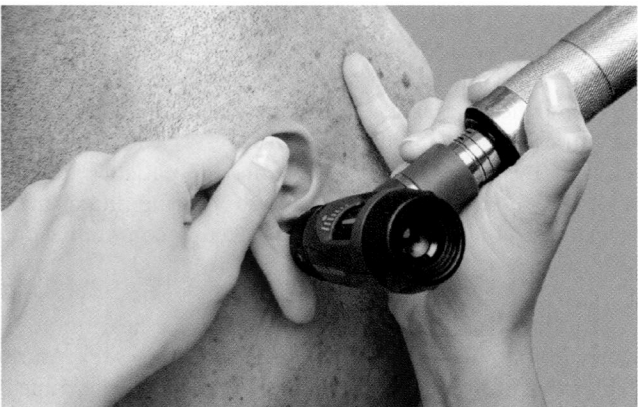

FIG 16.9 Otoscopic examination. (From Wilson S, Gidden J: *Health assessment for nursing practice,* ed 6, St Louis, 2016, Elsevier.)

children. Lie infants supine with their heads turned to one side and their arms held securely at their sides or wrap them snugly in a blanket. Have young children sit on their parents' laps with their legs held between the parents' knees.

Turn on the otoscope by rotating the dial at the top of the handle. To insert the speculum properly, ask the patient to tip the head slightly to the opposite shoulder. Hold the handle of the otoscope in the space between the thumb and index finger, supported on the middle finger. This leaves the ulnar side of your hand to rest against the patient's head, stabilizing the otoscope as it is inserted into the canal (Ball et al., 2015). Insert the scope while pulling the auricle upward and backward in adults and older children (Fig. 16.9). This maneuver straightens the ear canal. In children younger than 3 years of age, pull the auricle down and back.

Insert the speculum slightly down and forward, 1 to 1.5 cm (¼ to ¾ inch) into the ear canal. Take care not to scrape the sensitive lining of the ear canal, which is painful. The ear canal normally has little cerumen and is uniformly colored with tiny hairs in the outer third of the canal. Observe for color, discharge, scaling, lesions, foreign bodies, and cerumen. Normally cerumen is dry (light brown to gray and flaky) or moist (dark yellow or brown) and sticky. Dry cerumen occurs more often in Asians and Native Americans (Ball et al., 2015). A reddened canal with discharge is a sign of inflammation or infection. In older adults accumulated cerumen is a common cause of mild hearing loss. During the examination ask the patient how he or she normally cleans the ear canal (Box 16.10). Caution the patient on the danger of inserting pointed objects into the canal. Avoid the use of cotton-tipped applicators to clean the ears because this causes impaction of cerumen deep in the ear canal.

The light from the otoscope allows visualization of the eardrum (tympanic membrane). Know the common anatomical landmarks and their appearance (Fig. 16.10). Move the auricle to see the entire drum and its periphery. Because the eardrum is angled away from the ear canal, the light from the otoscope appears as a cone shape rather than a circle. The umbo is near the center of the drum, behind

BOX 16.10 PATIENT TEACHING
Ear Assessment

OUTCOME
Patient follows preventive guidelines for screening hearing loss of voice and environmental sounds.

TEACHING STRATEGIES
- Encourage patients older than 65 years of age or with noticeable change in hearing to have regular hearing checks. Explain that a reduction in hearing is a normal part of aging (see Chapter 39).
- Instruct family members of patients with hearing losses to avoid shouting, speaking instead with low tones while directly facing the patient.

EVALUATION
- Use the principles of teach-back to evaluate patient/family caregiver learning:
  - "Tell me how often you have your hearing checked."
  - "Explain how you adjust with your hearing loss when you interact with family members."

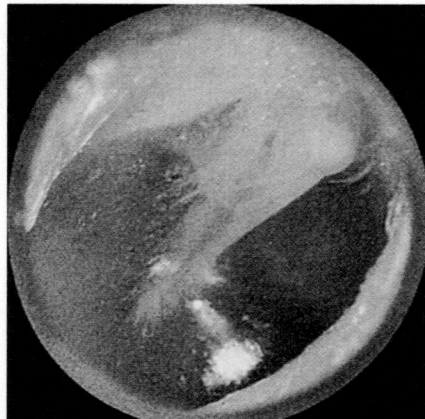

FIG 16.10 Normal tympanic membrane. (Courtesy Dr. Richard A. Buckingham, Abraham Lincoln School of Medicine, University of Illinois, Chicago.)

which is the attachment of the malleus. The underlying short process of the malleus creates a knoblike structure at the top of the drum. Check carefully to be sure that there are no tears or breaks in the membrane of the eardrum. The normal eardrum is taut, translucent, shiny, and pearly gray. It is free from tears or breaks. A pink or red bulging membrane indicates inflammation. A white color reveals pus behind it. If cerumen is blocking the tympanic membrane, warm water irrigation safely removes the wax.

Hearing Acuity. A patient with hearing loss often fails to respond to conversation. The three types of hearing loss are conduction, sensorineural, and mixed. A conduction loss interrupts sound waves as they travel from the outer ear to the cochlea of the inner ear because they are not transmitted through the outer and middle ear structures. A sensorineural loss involves the inner ear, auditory nerve, or hearing center of the brain. In this instance sound is conducted through the outer and middle ear structures, but the continued transmission of sound becomes interrupted at some point beyond the bony ossicles. A mixed loss involves a combination of conduction and sensorineural loss.

Patients working or living around loud noises are at risk for hearing loss. Adolescents are at risk for premature hearing loss from continued exposure to loud music through earbuds connected to electronic music devices or loud concerts. Deterioration of the cochlea and thickening of the tympanic membrane cause older adults to gradually lose hearing acuity. Older adults experience an inability to hear high-frequency sounds and consonants (e.g., *s, z, t, g*). Hearing loss can be caused by ototoxicity resulting from high maintenance doses of antibiotics (e.g., aminoglycosides).

To conduct a hearing assessment have the patient remove any hearing aid, if worn. Note the patient's response to questions. Normally the patient responds without excess requests to have the questions repeated. If you suspect a hearing loss, check the patient's response to the whispered voice. Test one ear at a time while the patient occludes the other ear with a finger. Ask the patient to gently move the finger up and down during the test. While standing 30 to 60 cm (1 to 2 feet) from the testing ear, cover your mouth so the patient is unable to read lips. After exhaling fully, whisper softly toward the non-occluded ear, reciting random numbers with equally accented syllables such as *nine-four-ten*. Ask the patient to repeat what was heard. If necessary gradually increase voice intensity until the patient repeats the numbers correctly. Then test the other ear for comparison. If a hearing loss is present, further testing should be recommended with experienced practitioners using a tuning fork or audiometry.

Nose and Sinuses

Assess the integrity of the nose and sinuses by inspection and palpation. The patient sits during the examination. A penlight allows for gross examination of each naris. A more detailed examination requires using a nasal speculum to inspect deeper nasal turbinates. Do not use a speculum unless a qualified practitioner is present.

Nursing History. Determine if the patient has a history of exposure to dust or pollutants, allergies, nasal obstruction, recent nasal trauma or discharge, frequent infections, headaches, or postnasal drip. Assess for a history of nosebleed (epistaxis) or use of nasal sprays, including frequency and duration (Box 16.11). Ask about breathing difficulties or snoring.

Nose. When inspecting the external nose, observe the shape, size, skin color, and presence of deformity or inflammation. The nose is normally smooth and symmetrical and is the same color as the face (Fig. 16.11). Recent trauma causes edema and discoloration. If swelling or deformities exist, gently palpate the ridge and soft tissue of the nose by placing one finger on each side of the nasal arch and gently

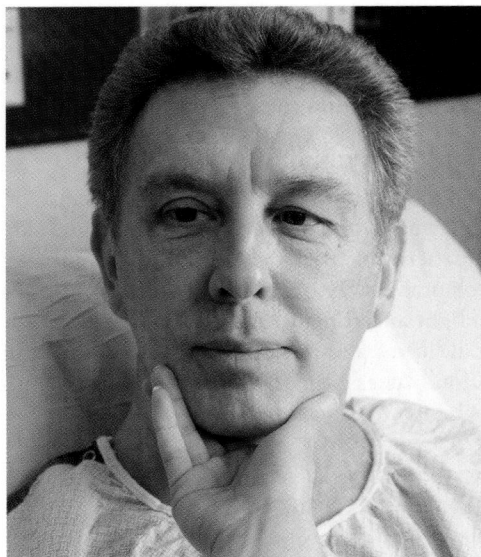

FIG 16.11 Inspection of nose and facial features for symmetry.

moving fingers from the nasal bridge to the tip. Note any tenderness, masses, and underlying deviations. Nasal structures are usually firm and stable.

When a person breathes, air normally passes freely and noiselessly through the nose. To assess patency of the nares, place a finger on the side of the patient's nose and occlude one naris. Ask the patient to breathe with the mouth closed. Repeat the procedure for the other naris.

While illuminating the anterior nares, inspect the mucosa for color, lesions, discharge, swelling, and evidence of bleeding. If discharge is present apply clean gloves. Normal mucosa is pink and moist without lesions. Pale mucosa with clear

---

BOX 16.11 PATIENT TEACHING

Nose and Sinus Assessment

OUTCOME

Patient follows good preventive practices to ensure against injury to olfactory organs, or maintenance of safety when there is decreased olfaction.

TEACHING STRATEGIES

- Caution patients against overuse of over-the-counter nasal sprays, which can injure nasal olfactory organs.
- Instruct older adults to install smoke detectors on each floor of their home.
- Instruct older adults to always check dated labels on food to ensure against spoilage.

EVALUATION

- Use the principles of teach-back to evaluate patient/family caregiver learning:
  - "I want you to show me how to use your over-the-counter nasal spray."
  - "Describe the safety practices you use in your home."
  - "Show me how you check whether the foods in your refrigerator are safe to eat."

discharge indicates allergy. A mucoid discharge indicates rhinitis. A sinus infection results in yellowish or greenish discharge. Habitual use of intranasal cocaine and opioids causes puffiness and increased vascularity of the nasal mucosa. For a patient with a nasogastric tube check for local skin breakdown (excoriation) of the naris, characterized by redness and skin sloughing.

To view the septum and turbinates have the patient tip the head back slightly to provide a clear view. Illuminate the septum and look for alignment, perforation, or bleeding. Normally it is close to the midline and thicker anteriorly than posteriorly. Normal mucosa is pink and moist without lesions. A deviated septum obstructs breathing and interferes with passage of an enteral nasal tube. Perforation of the septum often occurs after repeated use of intranasal cocaine. Note any polyps (tumorlike growths) or purulent drainage.

Sinuses. Examination of the sinuses involves palpation. In cases of allergies or infection the interior of the sinuses becomes inflamed and swollen. The most effective way to assess for tenderness is by externally palpating the frontal and maxillary facial areas. Palpate the frontal sinus by exerting pressure with the thumb up and under the patient's eyebrow. Gentle, upward pressure easily elicits tenderness if sinus irritation is present. Do not apply pressure to the eyes. If tenderness of sinuses is present, ask a nurse or health care provider with advanced experience to transilluminate the sinuses to monitor for fluid within the sinus cavity.

Mouth and Pharynx

Assess the mouth and pharynx to detect signs of overall health; determine oral hygiene needs; and develop therapies for patients with dehydration, restricted intake, oral trauma, or oral airway obstruction. To assess the oral cavity use a penlight and tongue depressor or single gauze square. Wear clean gloves and have the patient sit or lie during the examination. Assess the oral cavity while administering oral hygiene.

Nursing History. Determine if the patient wears dentures or retainers and how they fit. Assess for any recent changes in appetite or weight, which indicate problems with chewing and swallowing. Assess the patient's dental hygiene practices. To identify cancer risks determine if the patient smokes, chews tobacco, or consumes alcohol. Identify if he or she still has his or her tonsils and adenoids.

Lips. Inspect the lips for color, texture, hydration, contour, and lesions. With the patient's mouth closed, view the lips from end to end. Normally they are pink, moist, symmetrical, smooth, and without lesions. Lip color in dark-skinned patients varies from pink to plum. Have female patients remove their lipstick before the examination. Anemia causes pallor of the lips, with cyanosis caused by respiratory or cardiovascular problems. Any lesions such as nodules or ulcerations can be related to infection, irritation, or skin cancer.

BOX 16.12 PATIENT TEACHING

Mouth and Pharyngeal Assessment

OUTCOME

Patient follows good preventive practices to ensure oral and dental health.

TEACHING STRATEGIES

- Discuss proper techniques for oral hygiene, including brushing and flossing (see Chapter 31).
- Explain the early warning signs of oral cavity and pharynx cancer, including a sore that bleeds easily and does not heel, a lump or thickening in the throat, red or white patch on the mucosa that persists, ear pain, a neck mass, and coughing up blood. Difficulty chewing, swallowing, and moving the tongue or jaw are late symptoms (ACS, 2016a).
- Encourage regular dental examinations every 6 months for children, adults, and older adults.
- Identify older patients who have difficulty chewing and changes in the teeth. Teach patients to eat soft foods; cut food into small pieces; and eat more frequent, smaller meals.

EVALUATION

- Use the principles of teach-back to evaluate patient/family caregiver learning:
  - "Show me the proper way to brush your teeth."
  - "Explain to me how often you should visit your dentist each year."
  - "Describe to me the warning signs of oral and throat cancer."

Buccal Mucosa, Gums, and Teeth. Ask the patient to clench the teeth and smile to observe teeth occlusion. The upper molars normally rest directly on the lower molars, and the upper incisors slightly override the lower incisors. Assess for symmetry.

Inspect the teeth to determine the quality of a patient's dental hygiene (Box 16.12). Note the position and alignment of the teeth. To examine the posterior surface of the teeth have the patient open the mouth with lips relaxed. Use a tongue depressor to retract the lips and cheeks, especially when viewing the molars. Note the color of teeth and the presence of dental caries, tartar, and extraction sites. Normal healthy teeth are smooth, white, and shiny. A chalky white discoloration of the enamel is an early sign of caries formation. Brown or black discolorations indicate the formation of caries. An older adult's teeth often feel rough when tooth enamel calcifies, and there may be loose or missing teeth because of increased bone resorption. Yellow and darkened teeth are also common in older adults because of general wear and tear that exposes the darker, underlying dentin.

To view the inner oral mucosa ask the patient to remove any dental appliance. View the inner oral mucosa by having the patient open the mouth slightly and gently pull the lower lip away from the teeth (Fig. 16.12A). Repeat this process for the upper lip. Inspect the mucosa for color; hydration; texture; and lesions such as ulcers, abrasions, or cysts. Normally the mucosa

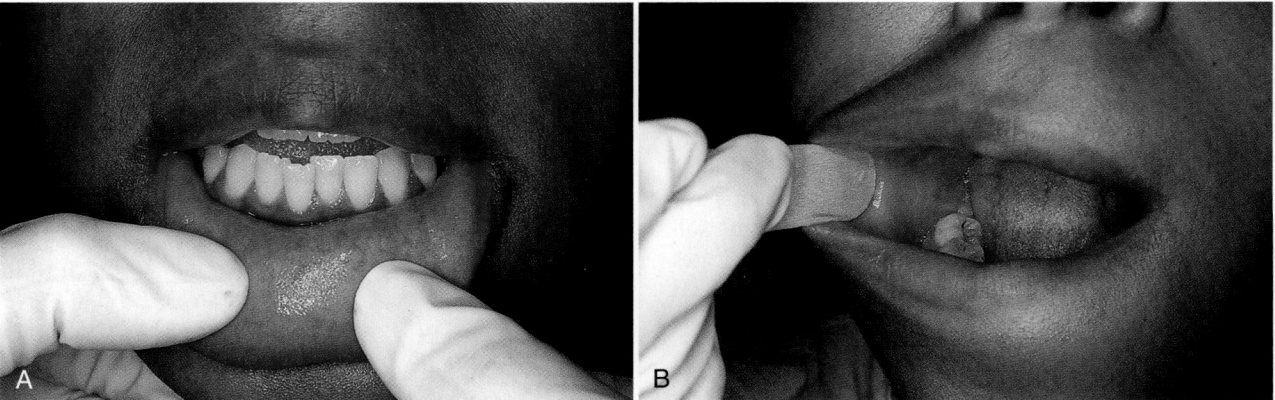

FIG 16.12 **A,** Inspection of inner oral mucosa of lower lip. **B,** Retraction of buccal mucosa allows for clear visualization.

is a glistening pink, smooth, and moist. Palpate any lesions with a gloved hand for tenderness, size, and consistency.

To inspect the buccal mucosa ask the patient to open the mouth, and gently retract the cheeks with a tongue depressor or gloved finger covered with gauze (Fig. 16.12B). View the surface of the mucosa from right to left and top to bottom. A penlight illuminates the most posterior portion of the mucosa. For patients with normal pigmentation the buccal mucosa is a good site to inspect for jaundice and pallor. In older adults it is normally dry because of reduced salivation. Thick white patches (leukoplakia) are often a precancerous lesion seen in heavy smokers and alcoholics. Palpate for any buccal lesions by placing the gloved index finger within the buccal cavity and the thumb on the outer surface of the cheek.

Examine the gums (gingivae) for color, edema, retraction, bleeding, and lesions while retracting the cheeks. Healthy gums are pink, moist, and smooth and fit tightly around each tooth. Dark-skinned patients often have patchy pigmentation. In older adults the gums are usually pale. With clean gloves palpate the gums to assess for lesions, thickening, or masses. Normally there is no tenderness. Spongy gums that bleed easily indicate periodontal disease or vitamin C deficiency.

Tongue and Floor of Mouth. Carefully inspect the tongue on all sides and the floor of the mouth. Have the patient relax the mouth and stick the tongue out halfway. The gag reflex is elicited if the patient protrudes the tongue too far. Using the penlight examine the tongue for color, size, position, texture, movement, and coating or lesions. A normal tongue appears medium or dull red in color, moist, slightly rough on the top surface, and smooth along the lateral margins. When the tongue protrudes it remains at midline. To test the tongue for mobility, ask the patient to raise it and move it from side to side. It should move freely.

The undersurface of the tongue and floor of the mouth are highly vascular. Take extra care to inspect this area, a common site of origin for oral cancer lesions. The patient lifts the tongue by placing its tip on the palate behind the upper incisors. Inspect for color, swelling, and lesions such as cysts.

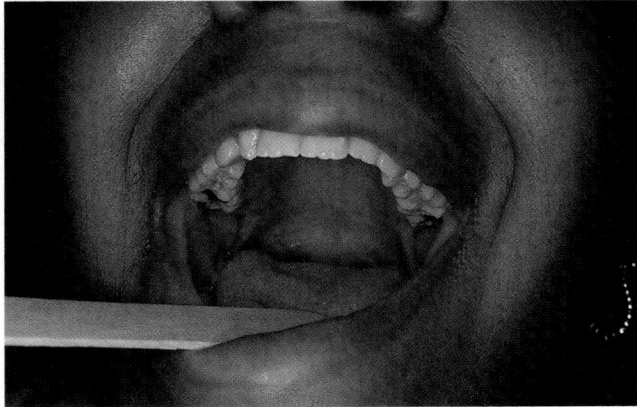

FIG 16.13 Penlight and tongue depressor allow visualization of uvula and posterior soft palate.

The ventral surface of the tongue is pink and smooth, with large veins between the frenulum folds.

Palate. Have the patient extend the head backward, holding the mouth open to allow you to inspect the hard and soft palates. The hard palate, or roof of the mouth, is located anteriorly. The whitish hard palate is dome shaped. The soft palate extends posteriorly toward the pharynx. It is normally light pink and smooth. Observe the palates for color, shape, texture, and extra bony prominences or defects.

Pharynx. Perform an examination of the pharyngeal structures to rule out infection, inflammation, or lesions. Have the patient tip the head back slightly, open the mouth wide, and say "Ah" while the tip of a tongue depressor is placed on the middle third of the tongue. Take care not to press the lower lip against the teeth (Fig. 16.13). By placing the tongue depressor too far anteriorly, the posterior part of the tongue mounds up, obstructing the view. Placing the tongue depressor on the posterior tongue elicits the gag reflex.

With a penlight first inspect the uvula and soft palate. Both structures, which are innervated by the tenth cranial nerve (vagus), rise centrally as the patient says "Ah." Examine the anterior and posterior tonsillar pillars and note the presence or absence of tonsillar tissue. The posterior pharynx is behind the pillars. Normally pharyngeal structures are smooth, pink, and well hydrated. Small irregular spots of lymphatic tissue and small blood vessels are normal. Note edema, petechiae, lesions, or exudate. Patients with chronic sinus problems frequently exhibit a clear exudate that drains along the wall of the posterior pharynx. Yellow or green exudate indicates infection. A patient with a typical sore throat has a reddened and edematous uvula and tonsillar pillars with possible presence of yellow exudate.

Neck

Assessment of the neck includes assessing the neck muscles, lymph nodes of the head and neck, carotid arteries, jugular veins, thyroid gland, and trachea (Fig. 16.14). Examination of the carotid arteries and jugular veins is addressed as part of the vascular system assessment. Inspect and palpate the neck to determine the integrity of neck structures, and examine the lymphatic system. An abnormality of superficial lymph nodes sometimes reveals the presence of infection or malignancy. Examination of the thyroid gland and trachea also helps to rule out malignancies. Perform this examination with the patient sitting.

Nursing History. Determine if the patient has a history of a recent cold or infection, enlarged lymph nodes, or exposure to radiation or toxic chemicals. If there is a history of enlarged lymph nodes, inquire about any past history of IV drug use, hemophilia, and risk factors for human immunodeficiency virus (HIV) infection. Learn if the patient takes thyroid medication for a history of hypothyroidism or hyperthyroidism; ask about a family history of thyroid disease. Ask the patient to describe any head or neck injury or pain of head and neck structures.

Neck Muscles. First inspect the gross neck structures with the neck in the usual anatomical position. Observe for symmetry of neck muscles. Ask the patient to flex the neck with the chin to the chest, hyperextend the neck backward, and move the head laterally to each side and then sideways with the ear moving toward the shoulder. This tests the sternocleidomastoid and trapezius muscles. The neck normally moves freely without discomfort.

Lymph Nodes. An extensive system of lymph nodes collects lymph from the head, ears, nose, cheeks, and lips (Fig. 16.15). With the patient's chin raised and head tilted slightly back, first inspect the area where lymph nodes are distributed and compare both sides. This position stretches the skin slightly over any possible enlarged nodes. Inspect visible nodes for edema, erythema, or red streaks. Nodes are not normally visible.

Use a methodical approach to palpate the lymph nodes to avoid overlooking any single node or chain. The patient relaxes with the neck flexed slightly forward. Inspect and

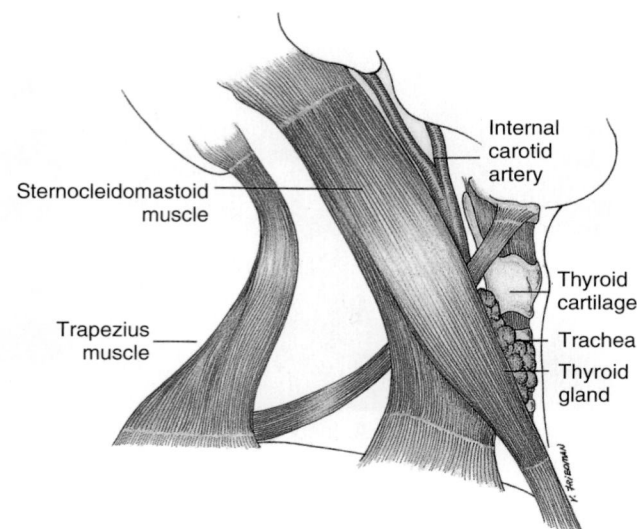

FIG 16.14 Anatomical position of major neck structures. Note triangles formed by muscles.

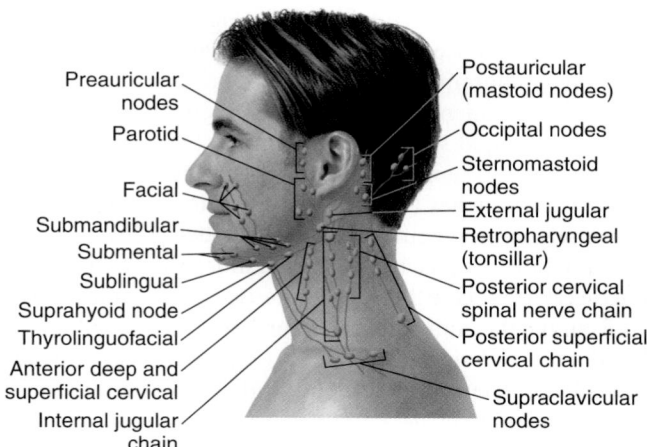

FIG 16.15 Palpable lymph nodes in head and neck. (From Ball JW, et al: *Seidel's guide to physical examination*, ed 8, St Louis, 2015, Elsevier.)

palpate both sides of the neck for comparison. During palpation either face or stand to the side of the patient for easy access to all nodes. Using the pads of the middle three fingers of each hand, gently palpate in a rotary motion over the nodes. Check each node methodically in the following sequence: occipital nodes at the base of the skull, postauricular nodes over the mastoid, preauricular nodes just in front of the ear, retropharyngeal nodes at the angle of the mandible, submandibular nodes, and submental nodes in the midline behind the mandibular tip. Try to detect enlargement and note the location, size, shape, surface characteristics, consistency, mobility, tenderness, and warmth of the nodes. If the skin is mobile, move it over the area of the nodes (Fig. 16.16). It is important to press underlying tissue in each area and not simply move the fingers over the skin.

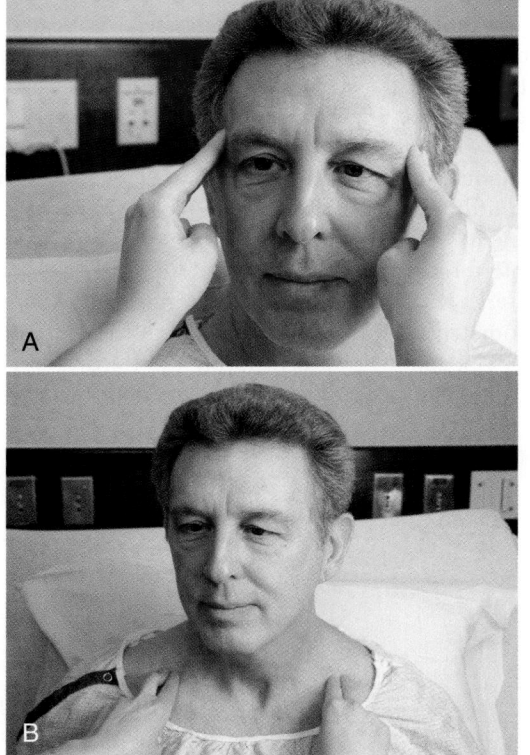

FIG 16.16 A, Palpation of preauricular lymph nodes. **B,** Palpation for supraclavicular lymph nodes.

To palpate supraclavicular nodes ask the patient to bend the head forward and relax the shoulders. Palpate these nodes by hooking the index and third finger over the clavicle, lateral to the sternocleidomastoid muscle. Palpate the deep cervical nodes only with the fingers hooked around the sternocleidomastoid muscle.

Normally lymph nodes are not easily palpable. Lymph nodes that are large, fixed, inflamed, or tender indicate a problem such as local infection, systemic disease, or neoplasm (Ball et al., 2015). Tenderness almost always indicates inflammation (Box 16.13). A problem involving a lymph node of the head and neck means an abnormality in the mouth, throat, abdomen, breasts, thorax, or arms. These are the areas drained by the head and neck nodes.

Thyroid Gland. The thyroid gland lies in the anterior lower neck, in front of and to both sides of the trachea. The gland is fixed to the trachea with the isthmus overlying the trachea and connecting the two irregular, cone-shaped lobes (Fig. 16.17). Inspect the lower neck overlying the thyroid gland for obvious masses, symmetry, and any subtle fullness at the base of the neck. Give the patient a glass of water and observe the neck as the patient swallows. This maneuver helps to visualize an abnormally enlarged thyroid gland. More experienced nurses examine the thyroid by palpating for more subtle masses.

Carotid Artery and Jugular Vein. Examination of these vessels is discussed under examination of the vascular system.

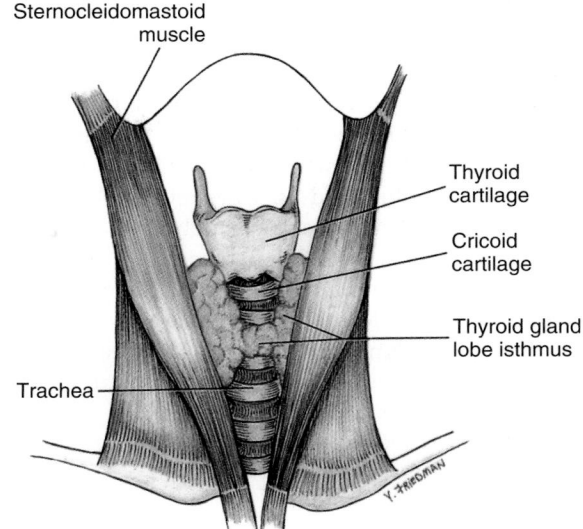

FIG 16.17 Anatomical position of the thyroid gland.

BOX 16.13 PATIENT TEACHING

Neck Assessment

OUTCOME
Patient takes proper preventive action if a mass is noticed in the neck.

TEACHING STRATEGIES
- Stress the importance of regular compliance with medication schedule to patients with thyroid disease.
- Instruct patients about the lymph nodes and how infection commonly causes node tenderness.
- Instruct patients to call a health care provider when they notice a lump or mass in the neck.

EVALUATION
- Use the principles of teach-back to evaluate patient/family caregiver learning:
  - "Explain to me when you would notify your health care provider about a neck mass."

Trachea. The trachea is a part of the upper respiratory system that requires direct palpation. It is normally located in the midline above the suprasternal notch. Masses in the neck or mediastinum and pulmonary abnormalities cause lateral displacement. Have the patient sit or lie down during palpation. Determine the position of the trachea by palpating at the suprasternal notch, slipping the thumb and index fingers to each side. Note if your finger and thumb shift laterally. Do not apply forceful pressure to the trachea because this elicits coughing.

THORAX AND LUNGS

Physical assessment of the thorax and lungs requires an in-depth review of the ventilatory and respiratory functions of the lungs. If disease is affecting the lungs, it affects other body systems as well. For example, reduced oxygenation causes changes in mental alertness because of the sensitivity of the brain to lowered oxygen levels. Use data from all body systems to determine the nature of pulmonary alterations.

Before assessing the thorax and lungs, be familiar with the landmarks of the chest (Fig. 16.18). These landmarks help you locate findings and use assessment skills correctly. The patient's suprasternal notch, manubrium, costal angle, clavicles, angle of Louis, and vertebrae are key landmarks that provide a series of imaginary lines for identification of signs and symptoms. Keep a mental image of the location of the lobes of the lung and the position of each rib (Fig. 16.19A). The proper orientation to anatomical structures ensures a thorough assessment of the anterior, lateral, and posterior thorax.

Locating the position of each rib is critical to visualizing the lobe of the lung being assessed. To begin, locate the angle of Louis at the junction between the manubrium and the body of the sternum. Knowing that the second rib extends from the angle makes it easy to locate and palpate the intercostal spaces (between the ribs) in succession. The spinous process of the third thoracic vertebra and the fourth, fifth, and sixth ribs serves to locate the lobes of the lung laterally (Fig. 16.19B). The lower lobes project laterally and anteriorly.

Posteriorly the tip or inferior margin of the scapula lies approximately at the level of the seventh rib. Identify the seventh rib, count upward to locate the third thoracic vertebra, and align it with the inner borders of the scapula to locate the posterior lobes (Fig. 16.19C).

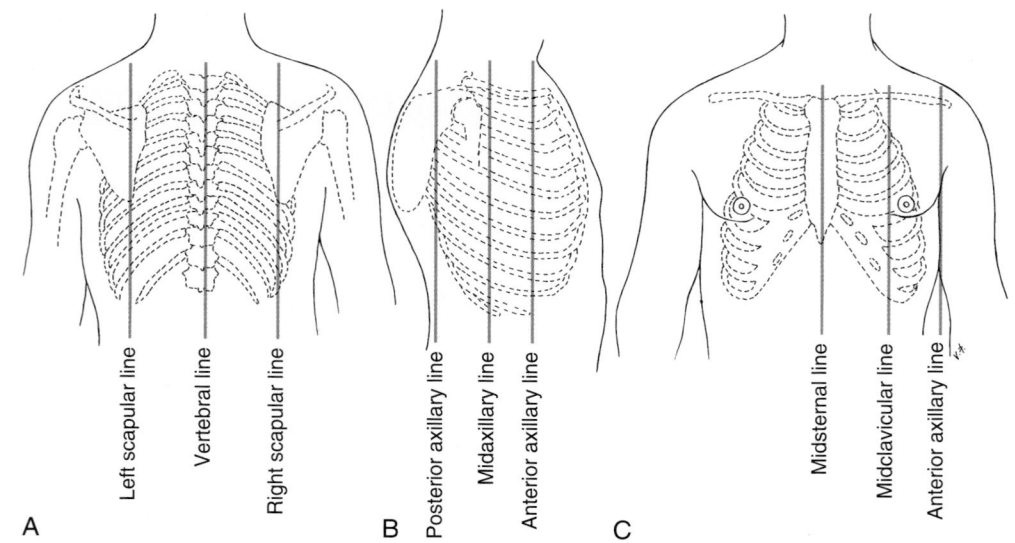

FIG 16.18 Anatomical chest wall landmarks. **A,** Posterior chest. **B,** Lateral chest. **C,** Anterior chest.

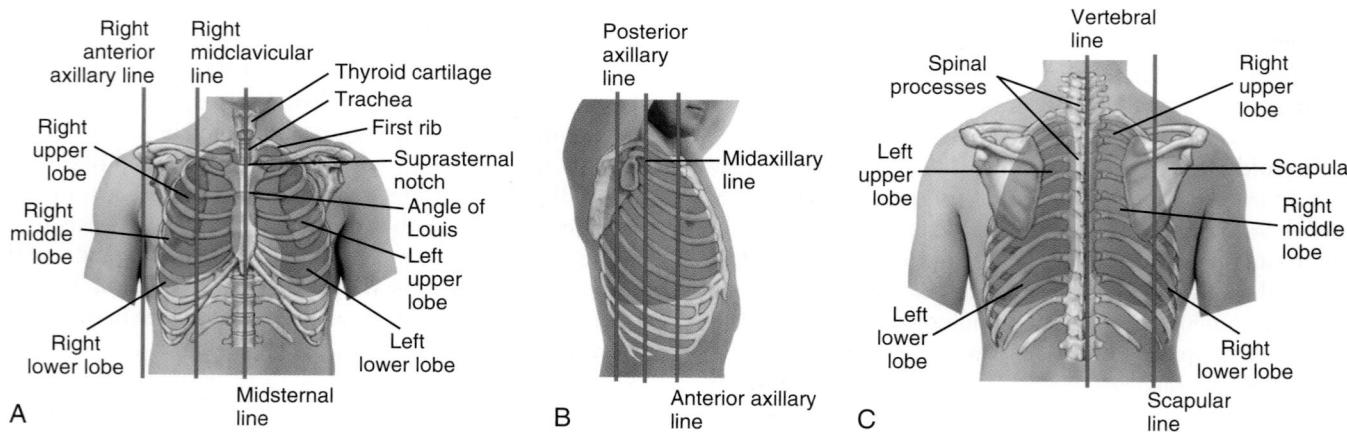

FIG 16.19 A, Anterior position of lung lobes in relation to anatomical landmarks. **B,** Lateral position of lung lobes in relation to anatomical landmarks. **C,** Posterior position of lung lobes in relation to anatomical landmarks. (From Ball JW, et al: *Seidel's guide to physical examination,* ed 8, St Louis, 2015, Elsevier.)

Examination of the lungs and thorax is most effective when the patient is undressed to the waist. Begin with the patient sitting for assessment of the posterior and lateral chest and sitting or lying down for examination of the anterior chest. Have a female patient keep a gown draped loosely over her chest while you examine the posterior chest.

Nursing History

First interview the patient for any recent problems of increased work of breathing. Ask the patient about *persistent cough* (productive or nonproductive), *blood-streaked sputum, voice change, chest pain*, shortness of breath, orthopnea (must be in upright position to breathe), dyspnea (breathlessness) during exertion or at rest, poor activity tolerance, or *recurrent pneumonia or bronchitis*. These reveal cardiopulmonary problems or warning signs for lung cancer (symptoms in italics). Assess for a history of tobacco or marijuana use, including type of tobacco, duration and amount (pack-years = number of years smoking × number of packs per day), age started, efforts to quit, and length of time since smoking stopped. Determine if your patient works in an environment containing pollutants (e.g., asbestos, coal dust), is exposed to radiation, or resides in an area with high levels of particulate air contaminants. Teach the patient about warning signs of lung disease (Box 16.14).

Review risk factors for tuberculosis (TB) and/or HIV infection, and assess for symptoms including persistent cough, hemoptysis, unexplained weight loss, fatigue, anorexia, night sweats, and fever. Assess history of allergies to airborne irritants, foods, drugs, or chemical substances. Ask if the patient has had pneumonia or influenza vaccine and a TB test. Review the patient's family history for cancer, TB, allergies, or chronic obstructive pulmonary disease.

Posterior Thorax

Begin examination of the posterior thorax by observing for any signs or symptoms in other body systems that indicate pulmonary problems. Reduced mental alertness, nasal flaring, somnolence (sleepiness), and cyanosis are examples of symptoms or findings that indicate oxygenation problems. Inspect the posterior thorax by observing the shape and symmetry of the chest from the patient's back and sides. Pay close attention to the position of the scapula bilaterally. Note the anteroposterior (AP) diameter. Body shape or posture significantly affects ventilatory movement. Normally the chest contour is symmetrical, with the AP diameter $\frac{1}{3}$ to $\frac{1}{2}$ the size of the transverse or side-to-side diameter. Infants have an almost round shape with a 1:1 ratio between the AP and transverse diameters. In adults a barrel-shaped chest (AP diameter = transverse) characterizes chronic lung disease. A more rounded chest is also associated with older age. Congenital and postural alterations cause abnormal contours. Patients with breathing problems may lean over a table or splint the side of the chest. Splinting or holding the chest wall because of pain causes a patient to bend toward the affected side, which impairs ventilatory movement.

With the patient sitting or standing position yourself at a midline position behind the patient, and look for deformities,

BOX 16.14 PATIENT TEACHING

Lung Assessment

OUTCOME

Patient follows recommendations that improve and protect pulmonary health.

TEACHING STRATEGIES

- Explain risk factors for chronic lung disease and lung cancer, including cigarette smoking (most important factor); history of smoking for more than 20 years; exposure to environmental pollution; and radiation exposure from occupational, medical, and environmental sources. Exposure to residential radon and asbestos also increases risk, especially for cigarette smokers. Other risk factors include certain metals (arsenic, cadmium), some organic chemicals, and personal history of tuberculosis. Genetics plays a role as well, especially in patients who develop disease at a young age (ACS, 2016a).
- Share brochures on lung cancer from the American Cancer Society with patient and family caregiver before discharge from the hospital.
- Discuss with patient the warning signs of lung cancer such as a persistent cough, blood-streaked sputum, chest pains, and recurrent attacks of pneumonia or bronchitis.
- Counsel patients on the benefits of receiving appropriate vaccines. Pneumonia vaccines are recommended for all adults 65 years of age or older, and for adults 19 to 64 years of age who smoke (CDC, 2016). Annual influenza vaccinations are recommended for all individuals 6 months of age and older (Grohskopf et al., 2016).
- Instruct patients with chronic obstructive pulmonary disease (COPD) or other respiratory illnesses in coughing and pursed lip–breathing exercises (see Chapter 32).
- Refer people at risk for tuberculosis for skin testing.

EVALUATION

- Use the principles of teach-back to evaluate patient/family caregiver learning:
  - "Describe for me the risk factors for lung disease and lung cancer and tell me which risk factors that you have."
  - "List for me the warning signs for lung cancer."
  - "Tell me how often you should have a vaccination for the flu and for pneumonia. Tell me when you were last tested for tuberculosis."
  - "Show me how to do the breathing and coughing exercises that we reviewed."

position of the spine, slope of the ribs, retraction of the intercostal spaces during inspiration, and bulging of the intercostal spaces during expiration. The scapulae are normally symmetrical and closely attached to the thoracic wall. The normal spine is straight without lateral deviation. Posteriorly the ribs tend to slope across and down. The ribs and intercostal spaces are easier to see in a thin person. Normally no bulging or active movement occurs within the intercostal spaces during breathing. Bulging or retraction indicates that the patient is using great effort to breathe.

Also assess the rate and rhythm of breathing at this time (see Chapter 15). Observe the thorax as a whole. It normally expands and relaxes with equality (symmetry) of movement bilaterally. In healthy adults the normal respiratory rate varies from 12 to 20 respirations/min.

Palpate the posterior thorax beginning with the thoracic muscles and skeleton for lumps, masses, pulsations, and unusual movement. Use caution if you note pain or tenderness. Fractured rib fragments could be displaced against vital organs. If you find a suspicious mass or swollen area, lightly palpate it for size, shape, and typical qualities of a lesion.

To measure chest excursion or depth of breathing stand behind the patient and place the thumbs along the spinal processes at the tenth rib, with the palms lightly contacting the posterior lateral surfaces. Place thumbs about 5 cm (2 inches) apart pointing toward the spine and fingers pointing laterally (Fig. 16.20). Press the hands toward the spine so that a small skinfold appears between the thumbs. Do not slide the hands over the skin. Instruct the patient to take a deep breath after exhaling. Note movement of the thumbs. Expect chest excursion to be symmetrical, separating the thumbs 3 to 5 cm (1¼ to 2 inches). Reduced chest excursion is caused by pain, postural deformity, or fatigue. In older adults chest

excursion normally declines because of costal cartilage calcification and respiratory muscle atrophy.

Auscultation assesses the movement of air through the tracheobronchial tree and detects mucus or obstructed airways. Normally air flows through the airways in an unobstructed pattern. Recognizing the sounds created by normal airflow allows for detection of sounds caused by airway obstruction. The patient sits during auscultation of the lungs.

Place the diaphragm of the stethoscope firmly on the skin, over the posterior chest wall between the ribs. Ask the patient to take slow, deep breaths with the mouth slightly open. Listen to an entire inspiration and expiration at each position of the stethoscope (Fig. 16.21A). If sounds are faint or distant, as in an obese patient, ask the patient to temporarily breathe harder and faster. Breath sounds are much louder in children because of their thin chest walls. In small children listen through the bell of a pediatric stethoscope because of their small chest. Use a systematic pattern comparing the sounds in one region on one side of the body with sounds in the same region on the opposite side.

Auscultate for normal breath sounds and abnormal or adventitious sounds. Normal breath sounds differ in character depending on the area you auscultate. Bronchovesicular

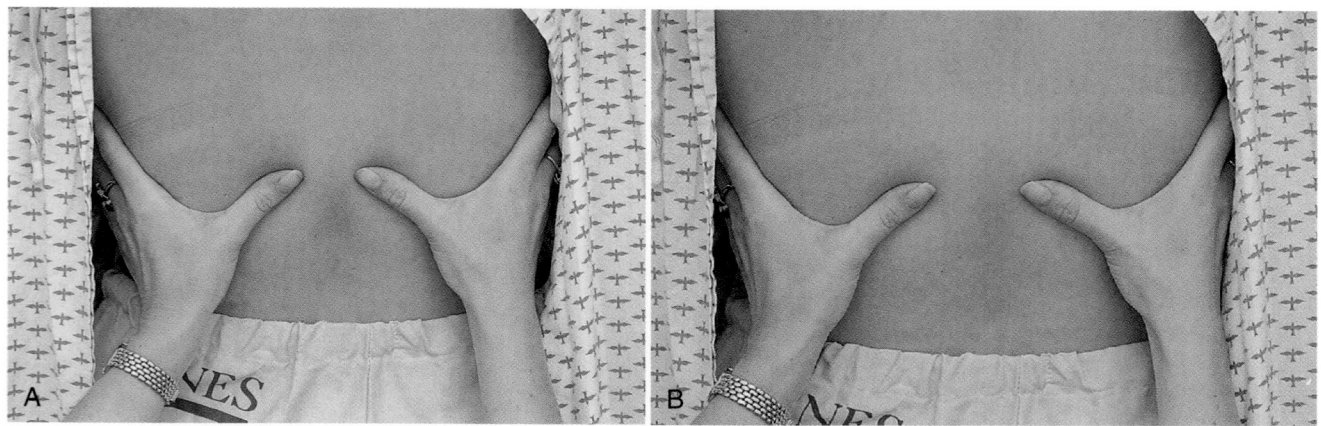

FIG 16.20 A, Palpating thoracic expansion by placing thumbs at the level of the tenth rib. **B,** As patient inhales, movement of chest excursion separates thumbs.

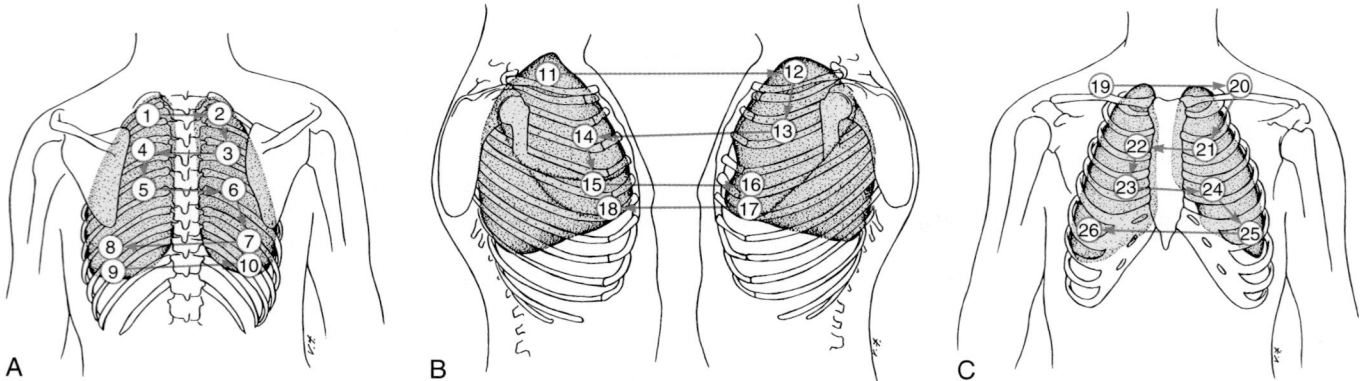

FIG 16.21 A to C, A systematic pattern (posterior-lateral-anterior) is followed for palpating and auscultating the thorax.

and vesicular sounds normally are heard over the posterior thorax. Bronchovesicular sounds are medium-pitched blowing sounds normally heard between the scapulae. The sounds have equal inspiratory and expiratory phases. The character of bronchovesicular sounds is created by air moving through large airways. Vesicular sounds are normally heard over the periphery of the lungs. Air moving through the smaller airways creates these sounds. Vesicular sounds are soft, breezy, and low pitched; the inspiratory phase is about 3 times longer than the expiratory phase.

Abnormal sounds result from air passing through moisture, mucus, or narrowed airways. They also result from alveoli suddenly reinflating or from an inflammation between the pleural linings of the lung. Adventitious sounds often occur superimposed over normal sounds. The four types of adventitious sounds are **crackles**, rhonchi, wheezes, and pleural friction rub. Each sound has its own cause and is characterized by typical auditory features (Table 16.6 and Fig. 16.22). During auscultation note whether the sound is on inspiration, expiration, or both and the location and characteristics of the sounds. Listen for the absence of breath sounds (found in patients with collapsed or surgically removed lobes).

Lateral Thorax

Extend the assessment of the posterior thorax to the lateral sides of the chest (see Fig. 16.21B). Have the patient raise

TABLE 16.6	ADVENTITIOUS BREATH SOUNDS		
SOUND	**SITE AUSCULTATED**	**CAUSE**	**CHARACTER**
Crackles	Most common in dependent lobes: right and left lung bases	Random, sudden reinflation of groups of alveoli; disruptive passage of air through small airways	Fine crackles: High-pitched fine, short, interrupted crackling sounds heard during end of inspiration; usually not cleared with coughing Moist crackles: Lower, more moist sounds heard during middle of inspiration; not cleared with coughing Coarse crackles: Loud, bubbly sounds heard during inspiration; not cleared with coughing
Rhonchi (sonorous wheeze)	Primarily heard over trachea and bronchi; if loud enough, can be heard over most lung fields	Muscular spasm, fluid, or mucus in larger airways, new growth or external pressure causing turbulence	Loud, low-pitched, rumbling coarse sounds heard during either inspiration or expiration; may be cleared by coughing
Wheezes (sibilant wheeze)	Heard over all lung fields	High-velocity airflow through severely narrowed or obstructed airway	High-pitched, continuous musical sounds such as a squeak heard continuously during inspiration or expiration; usually louder on expiration
Pleural friction rub	Heard over anterior lateral lung field (if patient is sitting upright)	Inflamed pleura, parietal pleura rubbing against visceral pleura	Has dry, grating quality heard during inspiration; does not clear with coughing; heard loudest over lower lateral anterior surface

Data from Ball JW, et al: *Seidel's guide to physical examination*, ed 8, St Louis, 2015, Elsevier.

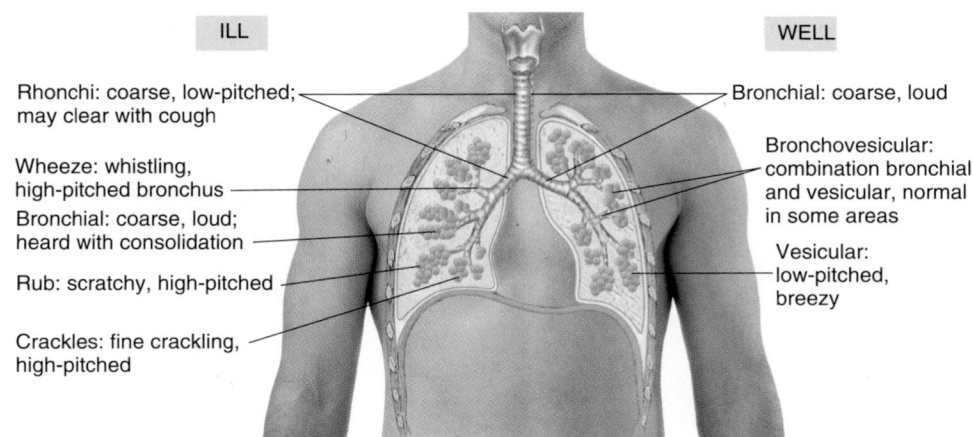

FIG 16.22 Schema of breath sounds in the ill and well patient. (From Ball JW, et al: *Seidel's guide to physical examination*, ed 8, St Louis, 2015, Elsevier.)

the arms to improve access to lateral thoracic structures. Use inspection, palpation, and auscultation skills to examine the lateral thorax. Normally the breath sounds you hear are vesicular.

Anterior Thorax

Inspect the anterior thorax for the same features as the posterior thorax. Have the patient sit upright if possible to maximize chest expansion. Observe the accessory muscles of breathing: sternocleidomastoid, trapezius, and abdominal muscles. The accessory muscles move minimally with normal passive breathing. The accessory and abdominal muscles contract when a patient requires effort to breathe as a result of strenuous exercise or disease.

Observe the width of the costal angle. It is usually larger than 90 degrees between the two costal margins. Observe the breathing pattern. Assess respiratory rate and rhythm anteriorly (see Chapter 15). The male patient's respirations in male patients are usually diaphragmatic, whereas the respirations in female patients are more costal.

Auscultation of the anterior thorax follows a systematic pattern (see Fig. 16.21C). Pay special attention to the lower lobes, where mucus secretions commonly gather. Listen for bronchovesicular and vesicular sounds above and below the clavicles and along the lung periphery. Auscultate for bronchial sounds, which are loud, high pitched, and hollow sounding with expiration lasting longer than inspiration (3:2 ratio). You normally hear this sound over the trachea.

HEART

Compare your assessment of heart function with findings from the vascular assessment. Alterations in either system sometimes manifest as changes in the other. Some patients with signs and symptoms of heart (cardiac) problems have a life-threatening condition requiring immediate attention. In this case act quickly and conduct only the parts of the examination that are absolutely necessary. When a patient is more stable, conduct a more thorough assessment.

Assess cardiac function through the anterior thorax. Form a mental image of the exact location of the heart (Fig. 16.23). In the adult the heart is located in the center of the chest (precordium) behind and to the left of the sternum, with a

small section of the right atrium extending to the right of the sternum. The base of the heart is the upper portion, and the apex is the bottom tip. The surface of the right ventricle constitutes most of the anterior surface of the heart. A section of the left ventricle shapes the left anterior side of the apex. The point of maximal impulse (PMI) is palpable at the fifth intercostal space at the left midclavicular line in adults and children older than 7 years of age. In children younger than 7 years of age the PMI is at the fourth intercostal space at the left midclavicular line (Hockenberry et al., 2017).

To assess heart function you need to understand the cardiac cycle and associated physiological events (Fig. 16.24). The heart normally pumps blood through its four chambers in a methodical, even sequence. Events on the left side occur just before events on the right. As the blood flows through each chamber, valves open and close, pressures within chambers rise and fall, and chambers contract. Each event creates a physiological sign. Both sides of the heart function in a coordinated fashion.

There are two phases to the cardiac cycle: systole and diastole. During systole the ventricles contract and eject blood from the left ventricle into the aorta and from the right ventricle into the pulmonary artery. During diastole the ventricles relax, and the atria contract to move blood into the ventricles and fill the coronary arteries.

Heart sounds occur in relation to physiological events in the cardiac cycle. As systole begins, ventricular pressure rises and closes the mitral and tricuspid valves. Valve closure causes the first heart sound (S_1), often described as "lub." The ventricles then contract, and blood flows through the aorta and pulmonary circulation. After the ventricles empty ventricular pressure falls below the pressure in the aorta and pulmonary artery. This allows the aortic and pulmonic valves to close, causing the second heart sound (S_2), described as "dub." As ventricular pressure continues to fall, it drops below that

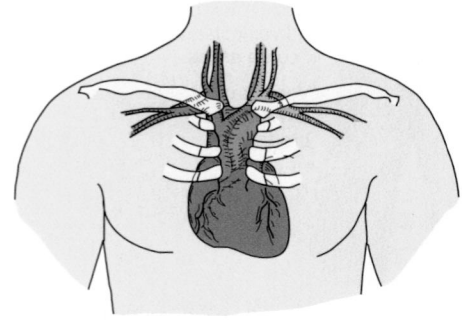

FIG 16.23 Anatomical position of the heart.

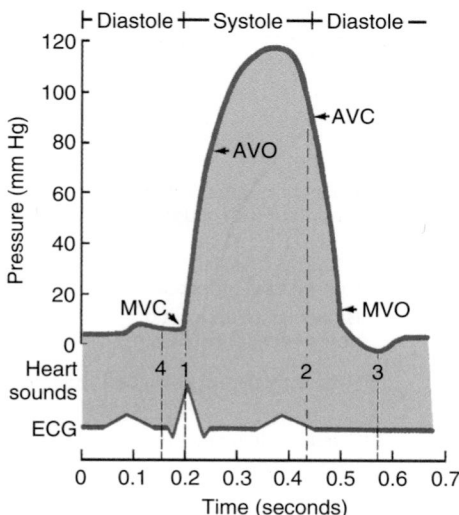

FIG 16.24 Cardiac cycle. *MVC*, Mitral valve closes; *AVO*, aortic valve opens; *AVC*, aortic valve closes; *ECG*, electrocardiogram; *MVO*, mitral valve opens.

of the atria. The mitral and tricuspid valves reopen to allow ventricular filling. Rapid ventricular filling may create a third heart sound (S_3), which is heard more often in children and young adults. S_3 is an abnormal finding in adults older than 30 years of age and is heard after S_2. A fourth heart sound (S_4) occurs when the atria contract to enhance ventricular filling and is heard before S_1. S_4 may be heard in healthy older adults, children, and athletes; but it is not normal in adults. S_4 needs to be reported to a health care provider.

Nursing History

The nursing history focuses on risk factors for cardiovascular disease (Box 16.15). Determine the patient's history

BOX 16.15 PATIENT TEACHING

Heart Assessment

OUTCOME

Patient chooses healthy heart practices, noting personal risk factors for heart disease.

TEACHING STRATEGIES

- Explain risk factors for heart disease including high dietary intake of saturated fat or cholesterol, lack of regular aerobic exercise, smoking, excess weight, stressful lifestyle, hypertension, and family history of heart disease.
- Refer patient to appropriate available resources for controlling or reducing risks (e.g., nutritional counseling, smoking cessation, exercise class, stress-reduction programs).
- Explain that research shows clinical benefit from reducing dietary intake of cholesterol and saturated fats. Teach patient that approximately 70% to 75% of saturated fatty acids come from meats, poultry, fish, and dairy products. The American Heart Association (AHA, 2015) recommends a diet that includes a variety of fruits and vegetables, whole grains, low-fat dairy products, skinless poultry and fish, nuts and legumes, and nontropical vegetable oils.
- Encourage regular measurement of total blood cholesterol levels and triglycerides. Desirable levels of total cholesterol are less than 170 mg/dL. More than one cholesterol measurement is needed to assess the blood cholesterol level accurately. Because low-density lipoprotein (LDL) cholesterol is the major component of atherosclerotic plaques, tests should include separate measurement of LDL cholesterol. An LDL cholesterol level of 130 mg/dL or higher indicates high risk for heart disease (Ball et al., 2015).
- Advise patients to minimize alcohol, quit smoking, and avoid secondhand cigarette smoke (AHA, 2015).
- Have patient consult with health care provider regarding the benefit of taking a daily low dose of aspirin.

EVALUATION

- Use the principles of teach-back to evaluate patient/family caregiver learning:
  - "Tell me the risk factors for heart disease that we discussed."
  - "Show me the meal plan low in saturated fat and cholesterol that you developed for yourself."
  - "Review with me your most recent cholesterol level from your follow-up appointment."

of smoking, alcohol intake, caffeine intake, use of prescription and recreational drugs, exercise habits, and dietary patterns including fat and sodium intake. Ask if the patient is taking medications for cardiovascular function (e.g., antidysrhythmics or antihypertensives) and if he or she knows their purpose, dosage, and side effects. Assess for chest pain or discomfort, palpitations, excess fatigue, cough, dyspnea, edema of the feet, cyanosis, fainting, or orthopnea. These are key symptoms of heart disease. If the patient reports chest pain, determine if it is cardiac in nature; anginal pain is usually a deep pressure or ache that is substernal and diffuse radiating to one or both arms, the neck, or the jaw. Determine if the patient has a stressful lifestyle. Assess for personal or family history of heart disease, diabetes, high cholesterol, hypertension, stroke, or rheumatic heart disease.

Inspection and Palpation

Ensure that the patient is comfortable and not anxious. Anxiety and discomfort may cause tachycardia, which produces inaccurate findings. Use the skills of inspection and palpation simultaneously. The examination begins with the patient supine and the upper body elevated 45 degrees because patients with heart disease frequently experience shortness of breath while lying flat. Stand at the patient's right side. Discourage the patient from talking, especially when auscultating heart sounds. Good lighting in the room is essential.

Direct your attention to the anatomical sites best suited for assessment of cardiac function. Inspect the angle of Louis; feel the ridge in the sternum approximately 5 cm (2 inches) below the sternal notch. Slip the fingers along the angle on each side of the sternum to feel the adjacent ribs. The intercostal spaces are just below each rib. The second intercostal space allows for identification of each of the six anatomical landmarks (Fig. 16.25). The second intercostal space on the right is the aortic area, and the second intercostal space on the left is the pulmonic area. You need deeper palpation to feel the spaces in obese or heavily muscled patients. After locating the pulmonic area, move the fingers down the patient's left

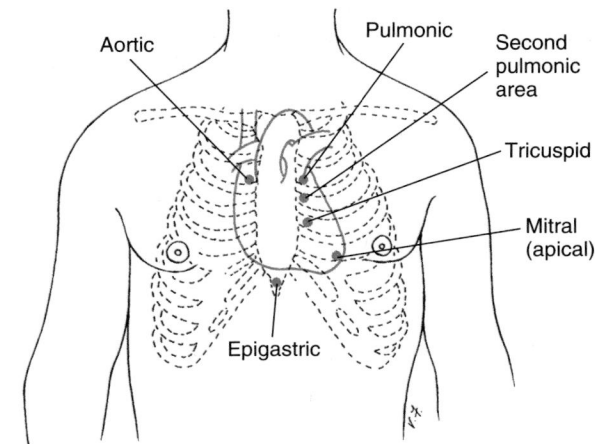

FIG 16.25 Anatomical sites for assessment of cardiac function.

sternal border to the third intercostal space, called the *second pulmonic area*. The tricuspid area is located at the fourth or fifth intercostal space along the sternum. To find the apical or mitral area, locate the fifth intercostal space just to the left of the sternum and move the fingers laterally to the left midclavicular line. Locate the apical area with the palm of the hand or the fingertips. Normally you feel the apical impulse as a light tap in an area 1 to 2 cm (¼ to ¾ inch) in diameter at the apex. Another landmark is the epigastric area at the tip of the sternum where you palpate for aortic abnormalities.

Locate the six anatomical landmarks of the heart; inspect and palpate each area. Look for the appearance of pulsations, viewing each area over the chest at an angle to the side. Normally you do not see pulsations except perhaps at the PMI in thin patients or the epigastric area as a result of abdominal aortic pulsation. Use the proximal halves of the four fingers together and alternate with the ball of the hand to palpate for pulsations. Touch the areas gently to allow movements to lift the hand. Normally you do not feel any pulsations or vibrations in the second, third, or fourth intercostal spaces. Loud murmurs cause a vibration. Time palpated pulsations or vibrations and their occurrence in relation to systole or diastole by auscultating heart sounds simultaneously.

The apical impulse or PMI should be felt easily. If not, have the patient turn onto the left side, moving the heart closer to the chest wall. Estimate the size of the heart by noting the diameter of the PMI and its position relative to the midclavicular line. In cases of serious heart disease the cardiac muscle enlarges, with the PMI found to the left of the midclavicular line. The PMI is sometimes difficult to find in older adults because the chest deepens in its AP diameter. It is also difficult to find in muscular or overweight patients. You usually find an infant's PMI at the third or fourth intercostal space more easily because of the infant's thin chest wall.

Auscultation

Auscultation of the heart detects normal heart sounds, extra heart sounds, and murmurs. Concentrate on detecting low-intensity sounds caused by valve closure. To begin auscultation eliminate all sources of room noise and explain the procedure to reduce the patient's anxiety. Follow a systematic pattern beginning at the aortic area and inching the stethoscope across each of the anatomical sites. Listen for the complete cycle ("lub-dub") of heart sounds clearly at each location. If you suspect a problem, repeat the sequence using the bell of the stethoscope. Sometimes the patient assumes three different positions during the examination (Fig. 16.26):

- Sitting up and leaning forward—good for all areas and to hear high-pitched murmurs
- Supine—good for all areas
- Left lateral recumbent—good for all areas and best position to hear low-pitched sounds in diastole

Learn to identify S₁ and S₂ heart sounds. At normal rates S₁ occurs after the long diastolic pause and before the short systolic pause. S₁ is high pitched, is dull in quality, and is heard best at the apex. If it is difficult to hear S₁, time it in relation to the carotid pulse. S₂ follows the short systolic

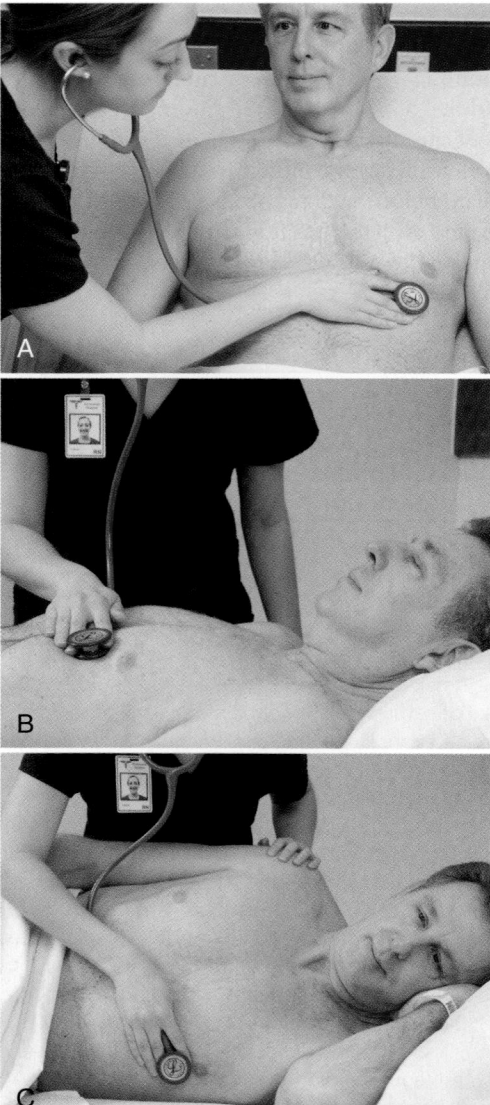

FIG 16.26 Sequence of patient positions for heart auscultation. **A,** Sitting. **B,** Supine. **C,** Left lateral recumbent.

pause and precedes the long diastolic pause; you hear it best at the aortic area.

Auscultate for rate and rhythm after hearing both sounds clearly. Each combination of S₁ and S₂ or "lub-dub" counts as one heartbeat. Count the rate for 1 minute and listen for the interval between S₁ and S₂ and then the time between S₂ and the next S₁. A regular rhythm involves regular intervals of time between each sequence of beats. There is a distinct silent pause between S₁ and S₂. Failure of the heart to beat at regular successive intervals is a dysrhythmia. Some dysrhythmias are life threatening.

When assessing an irregular heart rhythm, compare apical and radial pulse rates simultaneously to determine if a pulse deficit exists. Auscultate the apical pulse first and then immediately assess the radial pulse (one-examiner technique). Assess the apical and radial rates at the same time when two examiners are present. When a patient has a pulse deficit, the radial pulse is slower than the apical pulse because ineffective contractions fail to send pulse waves to the periphery. Report a difference in pulse rates to the health care provider immediately.

Assess extra heart sounds and murmurs at each auscultatory site. Use the bell of the stethoscope and listen for low-pitched extra sounds such as S_3 and S_4 gallops, clicks, murmurs, and rubs. Clicks can occur when a device such as a prosthetic valve is present. A pericardial friction rub resembles a scratching or raspy sound. If a swooshing sound is heard, this is a murmur that usually represents turbulent blood flow. The presence of extra heart sounds sometimes indicates a pathological condition; therefore such sounds should be reported to the health care provider immediately. Typically advanced practice nurses perform this part of the examination.

VASCULAR SYSTEM

Examination of the vascular system includes measuring the blood pressure (see Chapter 15) and assessing the integrity of the peripheral vascular system. Use the skills of inspection, palpation, and auscultation. You may perform portions of the vascular examination during other body system assessments. For example, check the carotid pulse after palpating the cervical lymph nodes.

Health History

Determine if the patient has leg cramps; numbness or tingling in the extremities; sensation of cold hands or feet; pain in the legs; or swelling or cyanosis of the feet, ankles, or hands. These signs and symptoms may indicate vascular disease. If the patient has leg pain or cramping in the lower extremities, ask if walking or standing for long periods or sleep aggravates or relieves the symptoms. This question helps to clarify if the problem is musculoskeletal or vascular. Ask patients if they wear tight-fitting garters or hosiery and if they sit or lie in bed with legs crossed. These activities impair venous return. Consider previous cardiac risk factors that may predispose to vascular disease (e.g., smoking, nutritional problems). Assess the patient's medical history for heart disease, hypertension, phlebitis, diabetes, or varicose veins.

Carotid Arteries

When the left ventricle pumps blood into the aorta, the arterial system transmits pressure waves. The carotid artery reflects heart function better than peripheral arteries because their pressure correlates with the pressure of the aorta. The carotid artery supplies oxygenated blood to the head and neck (Fig. 16.27). The overlying sternocleidomastoid muscle protects it.

To examine the carotid arteries have the patient sit or lie supine with the head of the bed elevated 30 degrees. Examine one carotid artery at a time. If both arteries are simultaneously occluded during palpation, the patient loses consciousness as a result of inadequate circulation to the brain. Do not palpate or massage the carotid arteries vigorously because the

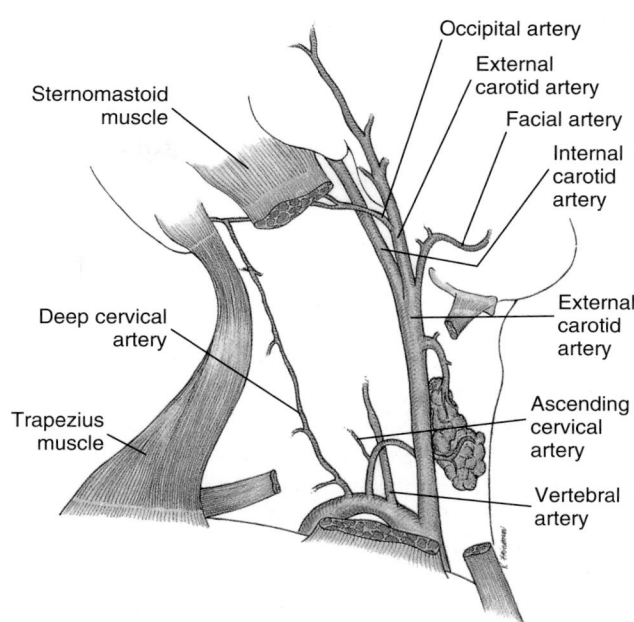

FIG 16.27 Anatomical position of carotid artery.

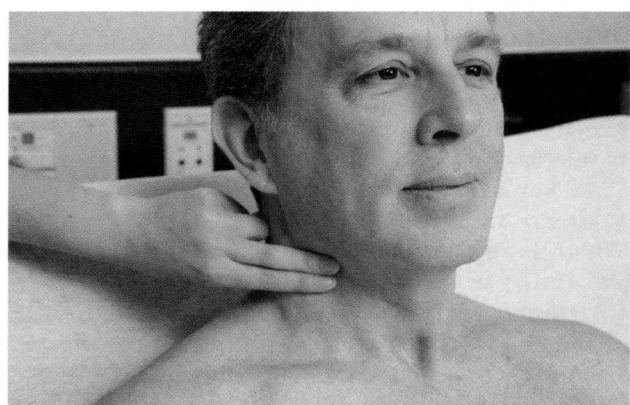

FIG 16.28 Palpation of internal carotid artery along margin of sternocleidomastoid muscle.

carotid sinus is in the upper third of the neck. The sinus sends impulses along the vagus nerve. Stimulating the vagus nerve causes a reflex drop in heart rate and blood pressure, which causes syncope (light-headedness) or circulatory arrest. This is a particular problem for older adults.

Begin inspection of the neck for obvious pulsation of the artery. Have the patient turn the head slightly away from the artery being examined. Sometimes the wave of the pulse is visible. Absence of a pulse wave may indicate arterial occlusion (blockage) or stenosis (narrowing).

To palpate the pulse ask the patient to look straight ahead or turn the head slightly toward the side being examined. Turning relaxes the sternocleidomastoid muscle. Slide the tips of your index and middle fingers around the medial edge of the sternocleidomastoid muscle. Gently palpate to avoid occlusion of circulation (Fig. 16.28).

The normal carotid pulse is localized rather than diffuse. As a strong pulse the carotid has a thrusting quality. As the patient breathes no change occurs. Rotation of the neck or a shift from a sitting to a supine position does not change the quality of the carotid artery. Both carotid arteries normally are equal in pulse rate, rhythm, and strength and are equally elastic. Diminished or unequal carotid pulsations indicate atherosclerosis (plaque buildup in arteries) or other forms of arterial disease.

The carotid is the most commonly auscultated pulse. Auscultation is especially important for middle-aged or older adults or patients suspected to have cerebrovascular disease. When the lumen of a blood vessel is narrowed, blood flow is disturbed. As blood passes through the narrowed section, this creates turbulence, causing a blowing or swishing sound. The blowing sound is called a **bruit** (pronounced "brew-ee"). Place the bell of the stethoscope over the carotid artery at the base of the neck and move it gradually toward the jaw. Ask the patient to hold his or her breath for a few heartbeats so that respiratory sounds do not interfere with auscultation. Normally you do not hear any sound during carotid auscultation. Palpate the artery lightly for a **thrill** (palpable bruit) if you hear a bruit.

Jugular Veins

The most accessible veins for examination are the internal and external jugular veins in the neck. Both veins drain bilaterally from the head and neck into the superior vena cava. The external jugular lies superficially and is just above the clavicle. The internal jugular lies deeper, along the carotid artery (Fig. 16.29). Normally when a patient lies in the supine position, the external jugular distends and becomes easily visible. In contrast the jugular veins normally flatten when the patient is in a sitting or standing position. However, some patients with heart disease have distended jugular veins when sitting.

To measure venous pressure inspect the jugular veins with the patient in the supine position (normally veins protrude), when standing (normally veins are flat), and when sitting at a 45-degree angle (jugular veins are distended only if

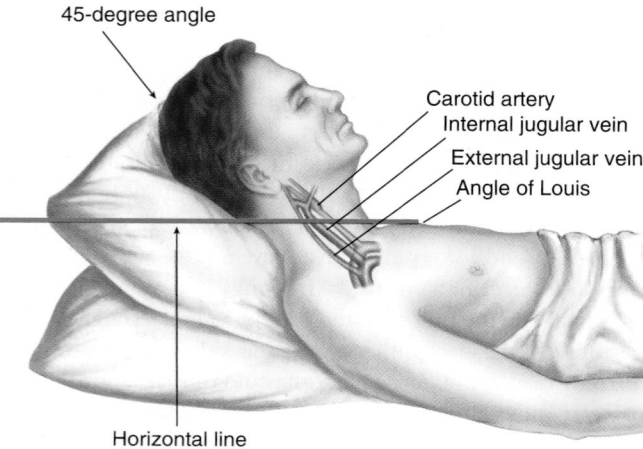

FIG 16.29 Position of patient to assess jugular vein distention. (From Thompson JM, et al: *Mosby's clinical nursing*, ed 4, St Louis, 1997, Mosby.)

patient has right-sided heart failure). An advanced practice nurse completes the specific measurement of jugular venous pressure.

Peripheral Arteries and Veins

To examine the peripheral vascular system, begin by assessing the adequacy of blood flow to the extremities by measuring arterial pulses and inspecting the skin and nails. Then assess the integrity of the venous system. Assess the arterial pulses in the extremities to determine sufficiency of the entire arterial circulation. Factors such as coagulation disorders, local trauma or surgery, constricting casts or bandages, and systemic diseases impair circulation to the extremities. Discuss risk factors for circulatory problems with the patient (Box 16.16).

Peripheral Arteries. Examine each peripheral artery using the distal pads of the second and third fingers. The thumb helps anchor the brachial and femoral arteries. Apply firm pressure, but avoid occluding a pulse. When a pulse is difficult to find, it helps to vary pressure and feel all around the pulse site.

Routine vital signs usually include assessment of the rate and rhythm of the radial artery because it is easily accessible (see Chapter 15). Count the pulse for either 30 or 60 seconds depending on the character of the pulse. Always count an

---

BOX 16.16 PATIENT TEACHING

Vascular Assessment

OUTCOME
Patient chooses activities that maintain or improve peripheral vascular status.

TEACHING STRATEGIES
- Explain the effects of high-fat diet choices, discussing how cholesterol and *trans* fats contribute to the development of atherosclerosis and lead to hypertension.
- Explain high risks for peripheral artery disease including smoking, hypertension, diabetes, stroke, kidney disease with hemodialysis, and heart disease.
- Explain the benefit of regular monitoring of blood pressure (daily, weekly, or monthly) with available home blood pressure monitors.
- Instruct patients with risk or evidence of vascular insufficiency in the lower extremities to avoid tight clothing over the lower body or legs, avoid sitting or standing for long periods, walk regularly, and elevate the feet when sitting.

EVALUATION
- Use the principles of teach-back to evaluate patient/family caregiver learning:
  - "Explain to me what is the normal blood pressure for your age."
  - "Show me how you take your blood pressure with your home equipment."
  - "Describe to me how you have progressed with smoking cessation practices, worked at controlling your diabetes, and followed treatment for your other health problems."

irregular pulse for 60 seconds. With palpation you normally feel the pulse wave at regular intervals. When an interval is interrupted by an early, late, or missed beat, the pulse rhythm is irregular. In emergencies health care providers usually assess the carotid artery because it is accessible and most useful in evaluating heart activity. To check local circulatory status of tissues, palpate the peripheral arteries long enough to note that a pulse is present.

Assess each peripheral artery for elasticity of the vessel wall, strength, and equality. Normally the arterial wall is elastic, making it easily palpable. Depress the artery; it springs back to shape when pressure is released. An abnormal artery is described as hard, inelastic, or calcified.

The strength of a pulse is a measurement of the force with which blood is ejected against the arterial wall. Some examiners use a rating from 0 (absent, not palpable) to 4 (bounding) (Ball et al., 2015).

Measure all peripheral pulses for equality and symmetry. Compare pulses on each side of the body. Lack of symmetry indicates impaired circulation such as a localized obstruction or an abnormally positioned artery.

In the upper extremities the brachial artery channels blood to the radial and ulnar arteries of the forearm and hand. If circulation in this artery becomes blocked, the hands do not receive adequate blood flow. If circulation in the radial or ulnar artery becomes impaired, the hand still receives adequate perfusion. An interconnection between the radial and ulnar arteries guards against arterial occlusion (Fig. 16.30A).

To locate pulses in the arm have the patient sit or lie down. Find the radial pulse along the radial side of the forearm at the wrist. Thin individuals have a groove lateral to the flexor

tendon of the wrist. Feel the radial pulse with light palpation in the groove (Fig. 16.30B). The ulnar pulse is on the opposite side of the wrist and feels less prominent (Fig. 16.30C). Palpate the ulnar pulse only when evaluating arterial insufficiency to the hand.

To palpate the brachial pulse find the groove between the biceps and triceps muscle above the elbow at the antecubital fossa (Fig. 16.30D). The artery runs along the medial side of the extended arm. Palpate the artery with the fingertips of the first three fingers in the muscle groove.

The femoral artery is the primary artery in the leg, delivering blood to the popliteal, posterior tibial, and dorsalis pedis arteries (Fig. 16.31A). An interconnection between the posterior tibial and dorsalis pedis arteries guards against local arterial occlusion. Wearing disposable gloves, find the femoral pulse with the patient lying down with the inguinal area exposed (Fig. 16.31B). The femoral artery runs below the inguinal ligament, midway between the symphysis pubis and the anterior superior iliac spine. Sometimes you use deep palpation to feel the pulse. Bimanual palpation is effective in obese patients. Place the fingertips of both hands on opposite sides of the pulse site. Feel a pulsatile sensation when the arterial pulsation pushes the fingertips apart.

The popliteal pulse runs behind the knee (Fig. 16.31C). Have the patient slightly flex the knee with the foot resting on the examination table or assume a prone position with the knee slightly flexed. Instruct the patient to keep leg muscles relaxed. Palpate with the fingers of both hands deeply into the popliteal fossa, just lateral to the midline. The popliteal pulse is difficult to locate.

With the patient's foot relaxed locate the dorsalis pedis pulse. The artery runs along the top of the foot in a line with the groove between the extensor tendons of the great and first toes (Fig. 16.31D). To find the pulse place the fingertips between the great and first toe and slowly move up the dorsum of the foot. This pulse is sometimes congenitally absent.

Find the posterior tibial pulse on the inner side of each ankle (Fig. 16.31E). Place the fingers behind and below the patient's medial malleolus (ankle bone). With the patient's foot relaxed and slightly extended, palpate the artery.

Ultrasound Stethoscopes. If a pulse is difficult to palpate, an ultrasound (Doppler) stethoscope is a useful tool that amplifies sounds of a pulse wave. Apply a thin layer of transmission gel to the patient's skin at the pulse site or directly onto the transducer tip of the probe. Turn on the volume control and place the tip of the probe at a 45- to 90-degree angle on the skin. Move the transducer until you hear a pulsating "whooshing" sound, which indicates that arterial blood flow is present. Document in the patient's record that the recorded pulse was obtained by Doppler and at what location.

Tissue Perfusion. The condition of the skin, mucosa, and nail beds offers useful data about the status of circulatory blood flow. Examine the face and upper extremities, looking at the color of skin, mucosa, and nail beds. The presence

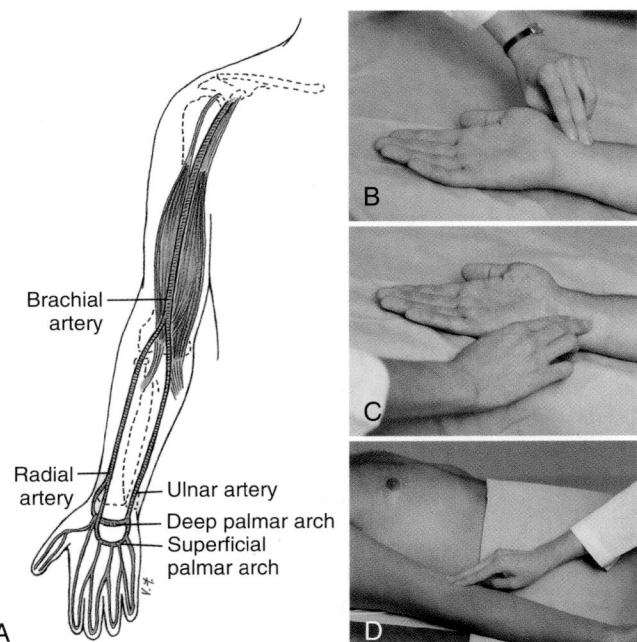

FIG 16.30 A, Anatomical positions of brachial, radial, and ulnar arteries. **B,** Palpation of radial pulse. **C,** Palpation of ulnar pulse. **D,** Palpation of brachial pulse.

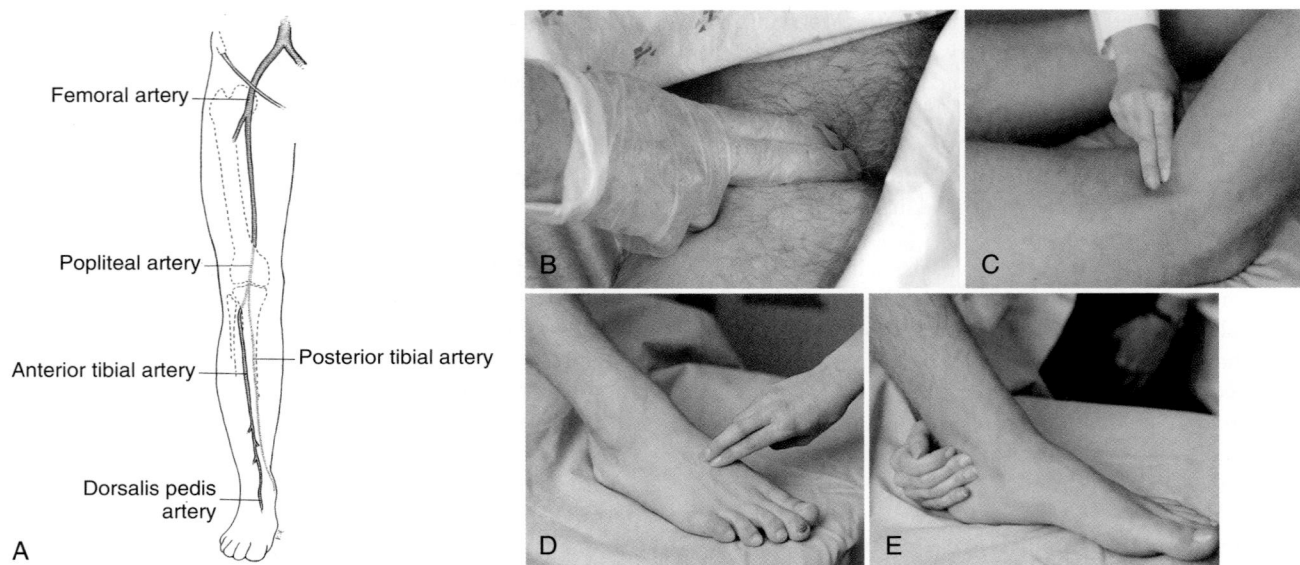

FIG 16.31 A, Anatomical position of femoral, popliteal, dorsalis pedis, anterior tibial, and posterior tibial arteries. **B,** Palpation of femoral pulse. **C,** Palpation of popliteal pulse. **D,** Palpation of dorsalis pedis pulse. **E,** Palpation of posterior tibial pulse.

of cyanosis requires special attention. Heart disease sometimes causes central cyanosis (bluish discoloration of the lips, mouth, and conjunctivae), indicating poor arterial oxygenation. Blue lips, earlobes, and nail beds are signs of peripheral cyanosis, which indicates peripheral vasoconstriction. When cyanosis is present, consult with a health care provider to have laboratory testing of oxygen saturation to determine the severity of the problem. Examination of the nails involves inspection for clubbing (a bulging of the tissues at the nail base), resulting from insufficient oxygenation at the periphery.

Inspect the lower extremities for changes in color, temperature, and condition of the skin indicating either arterial or venous alterations (Table 16.7). This is a good time to ask the patient about history of pain in the legs. If an arterial occlusion is present, the patient has signs resulting from absence of blood flow. Pain is distal to the occlusion. The *5 Ps* characterize an occlusion: *p*ain, *p*allor, *p*ulselessness, *p*aresthesias, and *p*aralysis. Venous congestion causes tissue changes indicating inadequate circulatory flow back to the heart.

During examination of the lower extremities also inspect skin and nail texture; hair distribution on the lower legs, feet, and toes; venous pattern; and scars, pigmentation, or ulcers. Palpate the legs for color and temperature. Assess for capillary refill.

The absence of hair growth over the legs indicates circulatory insufficiency. Do not confuse an absence of hair on the legs with shaved legs. Many men have less hair around the calves because of tight-fitting dress socks or jeans. Chronic recurring ulcers of the feet or lower legs are a serious sign of circulatory insufficiency and require a health care provider's intervention.

Peripheral Veins. Assess the status of the peripheral veins by asking the patient to assume sitting and standing

TABLE 16.7	SIGNS OF VENOUS AND ARTERIAL INSUFFICIENCY	
ASSESSMENT CRITERION	**VENOUS**	**ARTERIAL**
Color	Normal or cyanotic	Pale; worsened by elevation of extremity; dusky red when extremity lowered
Temperature	Normal	Cool (blood flow blocked to extremity)
Pulse	Normal	Decreased or absent
Edema	Often marked	Absent or mild
Skin changes	Brown pigmentation around ankles	Thin, shiny skin; decreased hair growth; thickened nails

positions. Assessment includes inspection and palpation for varicosities, peripheral edema, and phlebitis. Varicosities are superficial veins that become dilated, especially when legs are in a dependent position. They are common in older adults because the veins normally fibrose, dilate, and stretch. They are also common in people who stand for prolonged periods. Varicosities in the anterior or medial part of the thigh and the posterolateral part of the calf are abnormal.

Dependent edema around the feet and ankles is a sign of venous insufficiency or right-sided heart failure. It is common in older adults and people who spend a lot of time standing (e.g., nurses, waitresses, security guards). To assess for pitting edema, use your thumb to press firmly for several seconds over the medial malleolus or the shins and then release. A depression left in the skin indicates edema.

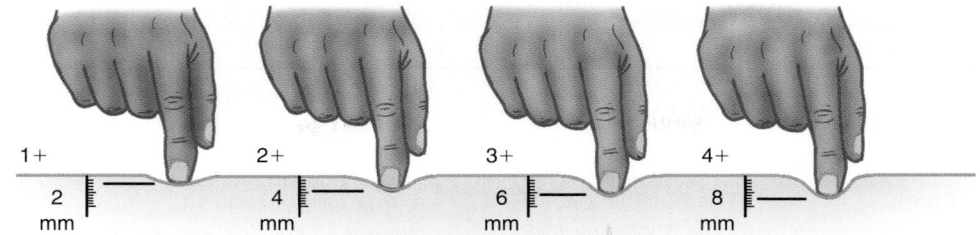

FIG 16.32 Assessing for pitting edema. (From Ball JW, et al: *Seidel's guide to physical examination*, ed 8, St Louis, 2015, Elsevier.)

Grading +1 through +4 characterizes the severity of the edema (Fig. 16.32).

Phlebitis (inflammation of a vein) occurs commonly after trauma to the vessel wall, infection, immobilization, or prolonged insertion of IV catheters (see Chapter 18). To assess for phlebitis inspect the calves for localized redness, tenderness, and swelling over vein sites. Gentle palpation of calf muscles reveals warmth, tenderness, and firmness of the muscle. Unilateral edema of the affected leg is one of the most reliable findings of phlebitis. A Doppler study is a noninvasive test that examines venous blood flow and is commonly done if deep vein thrombosis is suspected. The Homan's sign is no longer a reliable indicator of phlebitis or deep vein thrombosis (DVT), and it can be present in other conditions (Ball et al., 2015). The Homan's sign test is contraindicated in patients with DVT. If a clot is in the leg, it may dislodge from its original site during a Homan's sign test, resulting in a pulmonary embolus.

Lymphatic System

Assess the lymphatic drainage of the lower extremities during examination of the vascular system or during the female or male genital examination. Superficial and deep lymph nodes drain the legs, but only two groups of superficial nodes are palpable. With the patient supine palpate the area of the superior superficial inguinal nodes in the groin area (Fig. 16.33). Then move your fingertips toward the inner thigh, feeling for any palpable inferior nodes. Use a firm but gentle pressure when palpating over each lymphatic chain. Multiple nodes are not normally palpable, although a few soft, non-tender nodes are not unusual. Enlarged, hardened, tender nodes reveal potential sites of infection or metastatic disease.

BREASTS

It is important to examine the breasts of female and male patients. Men have a small amount of glandular tissue, a potential site for the growth of cancer cells, in the breast. In contrast most of the female breast is glandular tissue.

Female Breasts

An estimated 246,660 new cases of invasive breast cancer in women and 2600 new cases in men in the United States were predicted by the American Cancer society in 2016 (ACS,

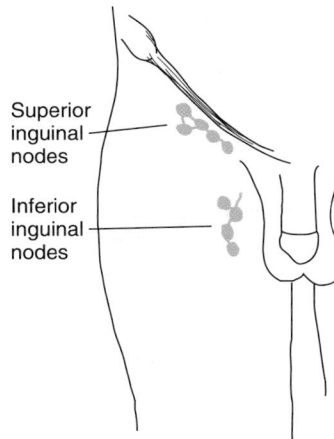

FIG 16.33 Inguinal lymph nodes.

2016a). Because of this, it is important to know the recommended breast cancer screening guidelines. According to the ACS (2015, 2016c), screening tests and examinations are used to find cancer in people who do not have any symptoms. Although research does not support the clear benefit of regular breast self-examination (BSE), it is important for all women to be familiar with how their breasts look and feel. Experts have concluded that knowing how one's own breasts look and feel is as effective for detecting breast cancer as a structured BSE (ACS, 2015). A BSE is optional for women starting in their 20s (ACS, 2016c). Women should be told about the benefits and limitations of BSE and to report any breast changes to the health care provider right away (Box 16.17).

BSE plays a small role in finding breast cancer compared with finding a breast lump by chance or simply being aware of what is normal for each woman. Some women feel very comfortable doing BSE regularly (usually monthly after their period), using a systematic step-by-step approach to examine the look and feel of their breasts. Other women are more comfortable simply looking at and feeling their breasts in a less systematic approach (e.g., while showering or getting dressed) (ACS, 2016c). Familiarity makes it easier to notice any changes in the breast from one month to another. Early discovery of a change from "normal" is the idea behind regular BSE.

For women who menstruate, the best time to do BSE is 2 or 3 days after the period ends when breasts are least likely to

BOX 16.17 PATIENT TEACHING

Female Breast Assessment

OUTCOME

Patient performs activities to ensure breast health or provide early identification of breast disease.

TEACHING STRATEGIES

- Women who are 20 years of age and older should be told about the benefits of knowing one's own breasts and to evaluate for any changes (Siu, 2016). The more familiar women are with the usual appearance and feel of their breasts, the more likely they are to notice changes that would require a visit to a health care provider. Prompt reporting of any new breast symptoms to a health care professional is important. Provide the following information about breast self-examination (BSE) (ACS, 2015):
  1. BSE should be done once a month so that the woman becomes familiar with the usual appearance and feel of her breasts.
  2. For women who menstruate, the best time to do BSE is between the fourth and the seventh day of the menstrual cycle or right after the menstrual cycle ends, when the breasts are least likely to be tender or swollen. Women who no longer menstruate should pick a day such as the first day of the month to remind them to do BSE.
  3. Men should also examine their breasts, areolas, nipples, and axillae for any swelling, nodules, or ulcerations.
  4. When implants are present, help the patient determine the edges of each implant and demonstrate how to evaluate each breast. At the time of implant, the surgeon usually shows the patient how to identify the edges of the implant. However, it is important to verify that the patient is able to palpate the edges of the implant.
- Teach the steps for performing BSE (ACS, 2015):
  1. Lie down on your back and place your right arm behind your head. This position is recommended because when you lie down the breast tissue spreads evenly over the chest wall and is as thin as possible, making it much easier to feel all the breast tissue.
  2. Use the finger pads of the three middle fingers on your left hand to feel for lumps in the right breast. Use overlapping, dime-sized, circular motions of the finger pads to feel the breast tissue. Use three different levels of pressure to feel all of the breast tissue. Light pressure is needed to feel the tissue closest to the skin, medium pressure is needed to feel a little deeper, and firm pressure is needed to feel the tissue closest to the chest and ribs. It is normal to feel a firm ridge in the lower curve of each breast, but you should tell your health care provider if you feel anything else out of the ordinary. If you are not sure how hard to press, discuss this with your health care provider. Use each pressure level to feel the breast tissue before moving on to the next spot.
  3. Move around the breast in an up-and-down pattern starting at an imaginary line drawn straight down your side from the underarm and moving across the breast to the middle of the chest (sternum, or breastbone). Be sure to check the entire breast area going down until you feel only ribs and up to the neck or collarbone (clavicle).
  4. Repeat the self-examination in the left breast, putting your left arm behind your head and examining the breast as noted in Steps 1 to 3.
  5. While standing in front of a mirror with your hands pressing firmly down on your hips, look at your breasts, observing for any changes in size, shape, contour, dimpling, or redness or scaliness of the nipple or breast tissue. Pressing down on your hips contracts the chest wall muscles and enhances any breast changes.
  6. Examine each underarm while sitting or standing and with your arm only slightly raised so that you can easily feel in this area for any lumps or changes. Raising your arm straight tightens the tissue in this area, making it harder to examine.
  7. Call your health care provider if you find a lump or other abnormality.
- If the patient is obese, has a family history of breast cancer, or has a history of chest radiation at a young age, she is at higher risk for the disease (Siu, 2016). Diet recommendations are to follow a low-fat diet including limiting meat consumption to well-trimmed, lean beef, pork, or lamb; removing skin from cooked chicken before eating it; selecting tuna and salmon packed in water and not oil; and using low-fat dairy products. Additionally, encourage the patient to reduce intake of caffeine. Although this is controversial, many believe that decreasing caffeine intake reduces symptoms of benign (fibrocystic) breast disease.

EVALUATION

- Use the principles of teach-back to evaluate patient/family caregiver learning:
  - "Tell me when you had your last screening mammogram and how often you should have one."
  - "Describe for me the signs and symptoms of breast cancer compared with benign (fibrocystic) breast disease."
  - "Show me how you would perform BSE."
  - "Describe for me changes that you could make in your diet to reduce the risk of breast disease and cancer."

be tender or swollen. A pregnant woman should also check her breasts on a monthly basis. Women who no longer menstruate should pick a day such as the first of the month to remind themselves to do BSE. A clinical breast examination should be part of a regular health examination by a health care provider.

Older women require special attention when reviewing the need for BSE. Fixed incomes limit many older women; thus they often do not have regular clinical breast examination and mammography. Older women often ignore changes in their breasts, assuming that they are part of aging. Review the patient's history for normal developmental changes and signs of breast disease. Because of the glandular structure, the breast undergoes changes during a woman's life. Knowledge of these changes (Box 16.18) allows you to complete an accurate assessment.

BOX 16.18 NORMAL CHANGES IN THE BREAST DURING A WOMAN'S LIFE SPAN

PUBERTY (8 TO 20 YEARS)
Breasts mature in five stages. One breast may grow more rapidly than the other. The ages at which changes occur and rate of developmental progression vary.

Stage 1 (Preadolescent)
This stage involves elevation of the nipple only.

Stage 2
The breast and nipple elevate as a small mound, and the areolar diameters enlarge.

Stage 3
There is further enlargement and elevation of the breast and areola, with no separation of contour.

Stage 4
The areola and nipple project into the secondary mound above the level of the breast (does not occur in all girls).

Stage 5 (Mature Breast)
Only the nipple projects, and the areola recedes (varies in some women).

YOUNG ADULTHOOD (20 TO 31 YEARS)
Breasts reach full (nonpregnant) size. Shape is generally symmetrical. Breasts are sometimes unequal in size.

PREGNANCY
Breast size gradually enlarges to two to three times the previous size. Nipples enlarge and become erect. Areolae darken, and diameters increase. Superficial veins become prominent. The nipples expel a yellowish fluid (colostrum).

MENOPAUSE
Breasts shrink. Tissue becomes softer, sometimes flabby.

OLDER ADULTHOOD
Breasts become elongated, pendulous, and flaccid as a result of glandular tissue atrophy. The skin of the breasts tends to wrinkle, appearing loose and flabby.
Nipples become smaller and flatter and lose erectile ability. Nipples invert because of shrinkage and fibrotic changes.

Data from Hockenberry MJ et al. *Essentials of pediatric nursing,* ed 10, St Louis, 2017, Mosby; Ball JW, et al: *Seidel's guide to physical examination,* ed 8, St Louis, 2015, Elsevier; and Touhy TA, Jett KF: *Ebersole and Hess' gerontological nursing and healthy aging,* ed 5, St Louis, 2018, Mosby.

The American Cancer Society (ACS, 2015) and U.S. Preventive Services Task Force (Siu, 2016) recommend the following guidelines for the detection of breast cancer in women who are at average risk (i.e., no personal or strong family history of breast cancer, no genetic mutation such as the *BRCA* gene, or no chest irradiation before 30 years of age):

1. Monthly BSE is an option for women starting in their 20s.

2. Women 20 years of age and older need to report any breast changes to a health care provider immediately.
3. Health care providers may perform a clinical breast examination every 3 years in women 20 to 40 years of age and annually in women older than 40 years of age.
4. Women 40 to 49 years of age may begin screening mammograms. Women should discuss options with their health care provider.
5. Screening mammograms should take place every 2 years for women 50 to 74 years of age.
6. For women of any age with an increased risk the ACS recommends discussion of screening options and additional testing with a health care provider.

For women with a high risk for breast cancer, the ACS (2016c) recommends an MRI and mammogram every year. This includes women who:

- Have a lifetime risk of breast cancer of about 20% to 25% or greater, according to risk assessment tools that are based mainly on family history
- Have a known *BRCA1* or *BRCA2* gene mutation
- Have a first-degree relative (parent, brother, sister, or child) with a *BRCA1* or *BRCA2* gene mutation and have not had genetic testing themselves
- Had radiation therapy to the chest when they were between the ages of 10 and 30 years of age

The patient's history may reveal an increased risk for breast cancer, normal developmental changes, or signs of breast disease, and these should be addressed on an individual basis. Knowledge of these risk factors and changes (see Boxes 16.17 and 16.18) are an important aspect of breast health.

Nursing History. The nursing history should explore risk factors for breast cancer such as being a woman older than 40 years of age or a personal or family history of breast cancer, especially with the *BRCA1* and *BRCA2* inherited gene mutations (ACS, 2015). Early-onset menarche (before 12 years of age) and late-age menopause (after 55 years of age) also affect risk. Other risk factors include never having children, giving birth to the first child after 30 years of age, recent use of oral contraceptives, previous chest radiation, alcohol use, and being overweight. Ask if the patient (both male and female) has noticed a lump, thickening, pain, or tenderness of the breast; discharge, distortion, retraction, or scaling of the nipple; or change in breast size. Determine the patient's use of medications that increase risk (oral contraceptives, steroids).

Inspection. Research does not show benefit of physical breast examinations done by a patient or a health care provider in relation to breast cancer screening (ACS, 2015). A full examination needs to be conducted when a patient identifies a change. At that time it is appropriate to inspect the breasts for size and symmetry. It is common for one breast to be smaller. However, inflammation or a mass can cause a difference in size. With age the ligaments supporting the breast tissue weaken, causing the breasts to sag and the nipples to lower. To be able to recognize abnormalities the patient needs

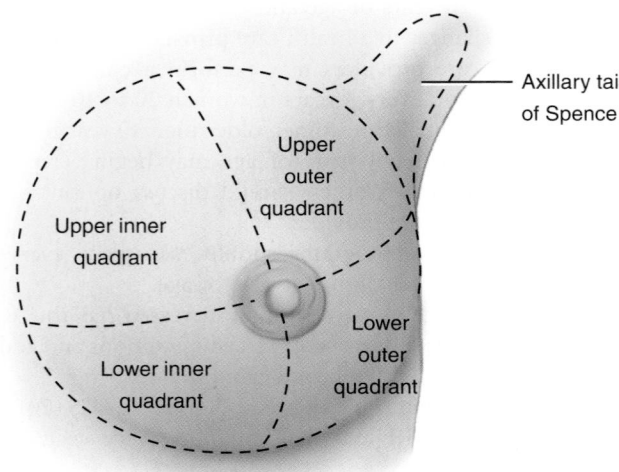

FIG 16.34 Quadrants of the left breast and axillary tail of Spence. (From Shiland BJ: *Medical terminology and anatomy for coding*, ed 3, St Louis, 2017, Mosby.)

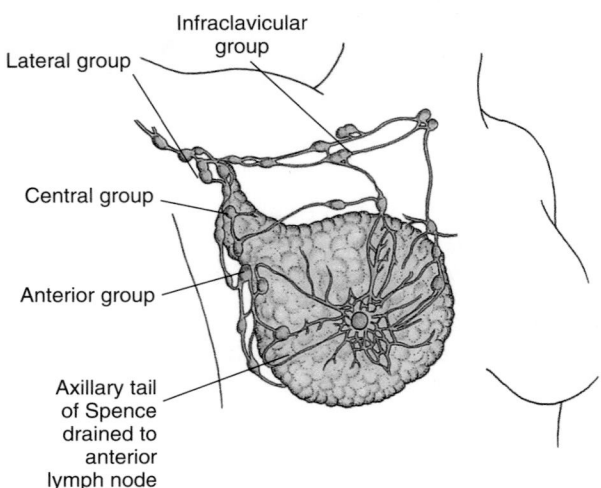

FIG 16.35 Anatomical position of axillary and clavicular lymph nodes.

to be familiar with the normal appearance of her breasts (Fig. 16.34).

Observe the contour or shape of the breasts and note masses, flattening, retraction, or dimpling. Breasts vary in shape from convex to pendulous or conical. Retraction or dimpling results from invasion of underlying ligaments by tumors. Edema also changes the contour of the breasts. To detect the presence of retraction or changes in the shape of the breasts, ask the patient to assume three positions: raise arms above the head, press hands against the hips, and extend arms straight ahead while sitting and leaning forward. Each maneuver causes a contraction of the pectoral muscles, which accentuates the presence of any retraction.

Carefully inspect the skin for color; venous pattern; and presence of edema, lesions, or inflammation. Lift each breast when necessary to observe lower and lateral aspects for color and texture changes. The breasts are the color of neighboring skin, and venous patterns are the same bilaterally. Venous patterns are easily visible in thin or pregnant women. Women with large breasts often have redness and excoriation of the undersurface caused by rubbing of skin surfaces.

Inspect the nipple and areola for size, color, shape, discharge, and the direction the nipples point. The normal areolae are round or oval and nearly equal bilaterally. Color ranges from pink to brown. In light-skinned women the areola turns brown during pregnancy and remains dark. In dark-skinned women the areola is brown before pregnancy (Ball et al., 2015). Normally the nipples point in symmetrical directions, are everted, and have no drainage. If the nipples are inverted, ask if this has been present since birth. A recent inversion or inward turning of the nipple indicates an underlying growth. Rashes or ulcerations are not normal on the breast or nipples. Note any bleeding or discharge from the nipple. Clear yellow discharge 2 days after childbirth is common. While inspecting the breasts, explain the

characteristics you see. Teach the patient the significance of abnormal signs or symptoms.

Palpation. Once again, palpation is not part of the general assessment process, but further assessment is required if abnormalities are identified by the patient. Palpation assesses the condition of underlying breast tissue and lymph nodes. Breast tissue consists of glandular tissue, fibrous supportive ligaments, and fat. Glandular tissue is organized into lobes that end in ducts opening onto the surface of the nipple. The largest portion of glandular tissue is in the upper outer quadrant and tail of each breast. Suspensory ligaments connect to skin and fascia underlying the breast to support the breast and maintain its upright position. Fatty tissue is located superficially and to the sides of the breast.

A large proportion of lymph from the breasts drains into axillary lymph nodes. Learn the location of supraclavicular, infraclavicular, and axillary nodes (Fig. 16.35). The axillary nodes drain lymph from the chest wall, breasts, arms, and hands. A tumor of one breast sometimes involves nodes on both sides of the body.

To palpate lymph nodes, have the patient sit with arms at her sides and muscles relaxed. While facing the patient and standing on the side you are examining, support her arm in a flexed position and abduct the arm from the chest wall. Place the free hand against her chest wall and high in the axillary hollow (Fig. 16.36). With your fingertips press gently down over the surface of the ribs and muscles. Palpate the axillary nodes with the fingertips gently rolling soft tissue. Palpate four areas of the axilla: the edge of the pectoralis major muscle along the anterior axillary line, the chest wall in the midaxillary area, the upper part of the humerus, and the anterior edge of the latissimus dorsi muscle along the posterior axillary line. Normally lymph nodes are not palpable. Note the number, consistency, mobility, and size of

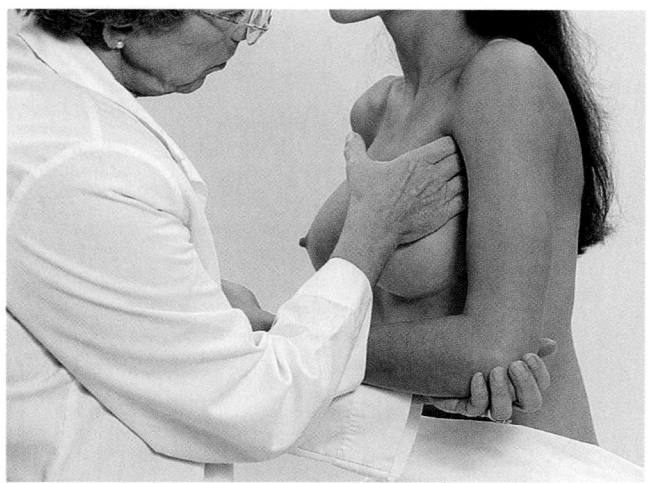

FIG 16.36 Support patient's arm and palpate axillary lymph nodes. (From Wilson S, Gidden J: *Health assessment for nursing practice*, ed 6, St Louis, 2016, Elsevier.)

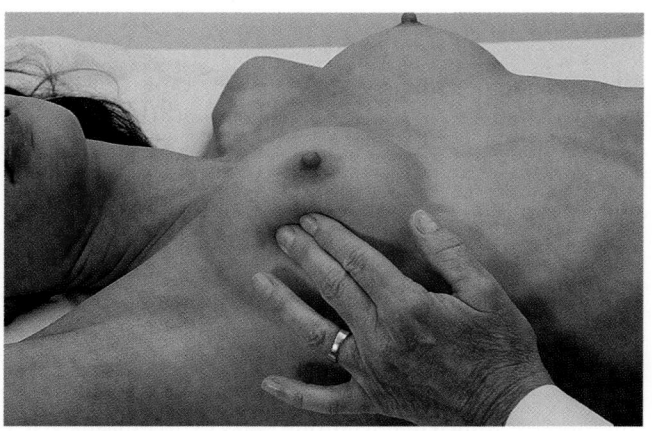

FIG 16.37 Patient lies flat with arm abducted and hand under head to help flatten breast tissue evenly over the chest wall. (From Wilson S, Gidden J: *Health assessment for nursing practice*, ed 6, St Louis, 2016, Elsevier.)

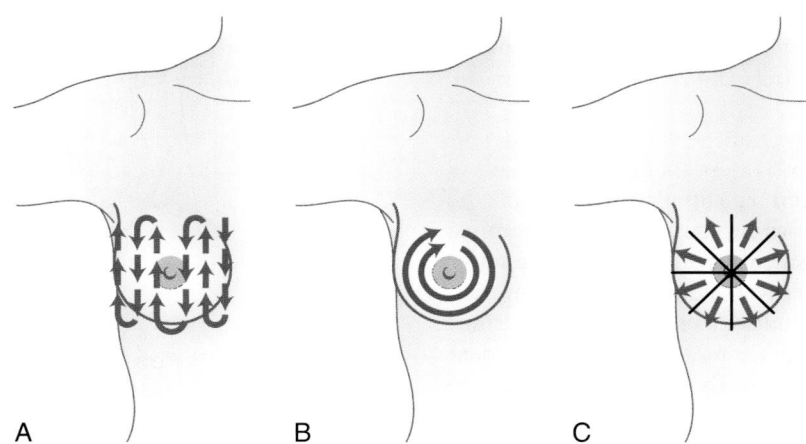

FIG 16.38 Various methods for breast palpation. **A,** Palpate from top to bottom in vertical strips. **B,** Palpate in concentric circles. **C,** Palpate out from the center in wedge sections.

palpable nodes. A palpable node feels like a small mass that is hard, tender, and immobile. Also palpate along the upper and lower clavicular ridges. Repeat the procedure for the patient's other side.

Perform palpation of breast tissue with the patient lying supine. This position allows the breast tissue to flatten evenly against the chest wall. The patient raises her hand and places it behind the neck to further stretch and position breast tissue evenly. Place a small pillow or towel under her shoulder blade to further position breast tissue (Fig. 16.37).

If the patient complains of a mass, examine the opposite breast first to ensure an objective comparison of normal and abnormal tissue. Use the pads of the first three fingers to compress breast tissue gently against the chest wall, noting tissue consistency. During a clinical breast examination perform palpation systematically in one of three ways: (1) using a vertical technique with the fingers moving up and down each quadrant; (2) clockwise or counterclockwise, forming small circles with the fingers along each quadrant

and the tail; or (3) palpating from center of the breast in a radial fashion, returning to the areola to begin each spoke (Fig. 16.38). Whatever approach you use, be sure to cover the entire breast and tail, directing attention to any areas of tenderness. When palpating large, pendulous breasts, use a bimanual technique. Support the inferior portion of the breast in one hand while using the other hand to palpate breast tissue against the supporting hand.

During palpation note the consistency of breast tissue. The breasts of a young patient are firm and elastic. In an older patient the tissue may feel stringy and nodular. The patient's familiarity with the texture of her own breasts is most important. The lobular feel of glandular tissue is normal. The lower edge of each breast feels firm and hard and indicates the normal inframammary ridge, not a tumor. It helps to move the patient's hand so that she feels normal tissue variations. Palpate abnormal masses to determine location in relation to quadrants, diameter in centimeters, shape (e.g., round or discoid), consistency (soft, firm, or hard), tenderness, mobility, and discreteness (clear or unclear borders). Cancerous lesions are hard, fixed, nontender, irregular in shape, and usually unilateral.

Pay special attention when palpating the nipple and areola. Palpate the entire surface gently. Use the thumb and index finger to compress the nipple and note any discharge. During the examination of the nipple and areola the nipple may become erect with wrinkling of the areola. These changes are normal.

Male Breasts

Inspect the nipple and areola for nodules, edema, and ulceration. An enlarged male breast results from obesity or glandular enlargement. Steroid use contributes to breast enlargement in young men. Male breast cancer is associated with obesity, Klinefelter syndrome, and gynecomastia (NCI, 2014). Fatty tissue feels soft. Glandular tissue is firm. Use the same techniques to palpate for masses used in examination of the female breast. Because male breast cancer is relatively rare, routine self-examinations are unnecessary. However, men with a first-degree relative (e.g., mother) with breast cancer are at increased risk and should perform regular breast self-examinations.

ABDOMEN

The abdominal examination is complex because of the number of organs located within and near the abdominal cavity. It includes an assessment of structures of the lower GI tract in addition to the liver, stomach, uterus, ovaries, kidneys, and bladder. Abdominal pain is a common complaint of patients seeking health care. An accurate assessment requires matching patient history data with an assessment of the location of physical symptoms.

Assess the organs anteriorly and posteriorly. A system of landmarks helps to map out the abdominal region. The xiphoid process (tip of the sternum) is the upper boundary of the anterior abdominal region. The symphysis pubis is the lower boundary. Divide the abdomen into four imaginary quadrants to refer to assessment findings (Fig. 16.39A) and record them in relation to each quadrant. Posteriorly the lower ribs and heavy back muscles protect the kidneys, which are located from the T12 to L3 vertebrae (Fig. 16.39B). The costovertebral angle formed by the last rib and vertebral column is a landmark used during palpation of the kidney.

During the abdominal examination, use interventions that help the patient to relax. Tight abdominal muscles make palpation difficult. Ask the patient to void before beginning. Be sure that the room is warm and cover the patient's upper chest and legs. The patient lies supine or in a dorsal recumbent position with the arms at the sides and knees slightly bent. Place small pillows beneath the knees. If the patient places the arms under the head, the abdominal muscles tighten. Proceed calmly and slowly, being sure that there is adequate lighting. Expose the abdomen from just above the xiphoid process down to the symphysis pubis. Warm hands and stethoscope

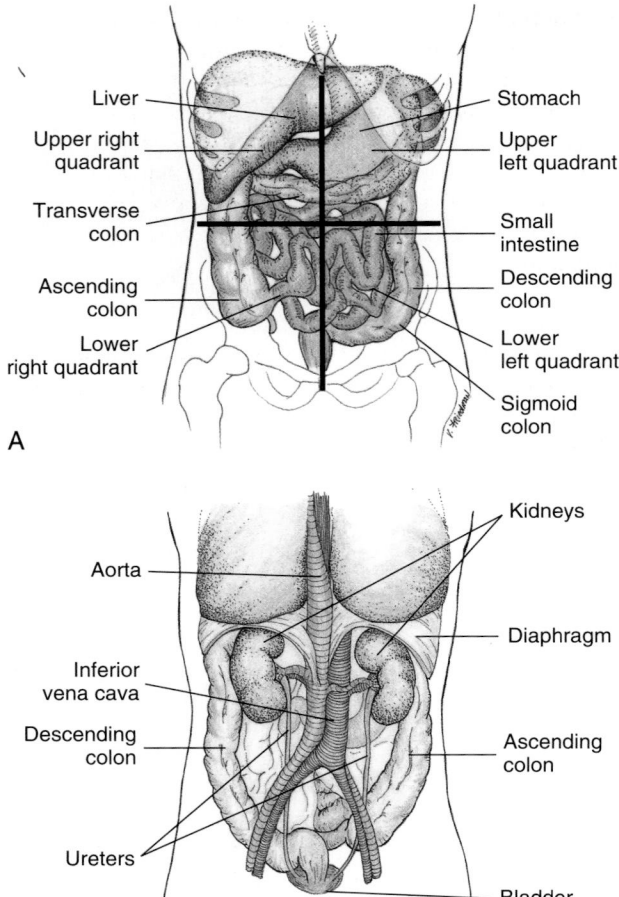

FIG 16.39 A, Anterior view of abdomen divided by quadrants. **B,** Posterior view of abdominal sections.

promote relaxation. Ask the patient to report pain and point out areas of tenderness. Assess tender areas last.

The order for an abdominal examination differs slightly from that for previous assessments. Begin with inspection and then auscultation. By using auscultation before palpation there is less chance of altering the frequency and character of bowel sounds. Palpation could falsely increase peristalsis. Have a tape measure and marking pen available during the examination.

Nursing History

Ask whether the patient has abdominal or low back pain, and assess the character of the pain in detail (see Chapter 34). Also review the patient's normal bowel habits and stool character, including use of laxatives. Determine if the patient has had abdominal surgery, trauma, or diagnostic tests of the GI tract. Assess for difficulty swallowing, belching, flatulence (gas), bloody emesis (hematemesis), black or tarry stools (melena), heartburn, diarrhea, or constipation. Assess if the patient has had a recent weight change or intolerance to diet (e.g., nausea, vomiting, or cramping). If the patient takes antiinflammatory drugs (e.g., aspirin, ibuprofen, or steroids) and antibiotics, there is risk for GI upset or bleeding. Inquire about a family history of cancer, kidney disease, alcoholism, hypertension, or heart disease. Assess the patient's usual intake of alcohol. Also determine if a female patient is pregnant and note the date of her last menstrual period. Review the patient's history for risk factors for hepatitis B virus (HBV) exposure (e.g., hemodialysis or IV drug use). Finally ask the patient to locate any tender areas before beginning the examination.

Inspection

Always observe the patient during routine care activities. Note the patient's posture and look for evidence of abdominal splinting, lying with the knees drawn up, or moving restlessly in bed. A patient free from abdominal pain does not guard or splint the abdomen. To inspect the abdomen for abnormal movement or shadows, stand on the patient's right side and inspect the abdomen from above. By sitting down to look across the abdomen, you assess abdominal contour. Direct the examination light over the abdomen. Inspect it for continuity, any retractions, bulging, and symmetry.

Skin. Inspect the skin over the abdomen for color, scars, venous patterns, lesions, and striae (stretch marks). The skin is subject to the same color variations as the rest of the body. Venous patterns are normally faint except in thin patients. Artificial openings indicate drainage sites resulting from surgery (see Chapter 40) or an ostomy (see Chapters 36 and 37). Scars reveal evidence of past trauma or surgery that created permanent changes in underlying organ anatomy. Bruising indicates accidental injury, physical abuse, or a type of bleeding disorder. Ask if the patient self-administers injections (e.g., insulin or anticoagulants). Unexpected findings include generalized skin color changes such as jaundice or cyanosis. A glistening taut (tight) appearance indicates ascites.

Umbilicus. Note the position; shape; color; and presence of inflammation, discharge, or protruding masses. A normal umbilicus is flat or concave with the color the same as surrounding skin. Underlying masses (e.g., hernias) cause displacement of the umbilicus.

Contour and Symmetry. Inspect for contour, symmetry, and surface motion of the abdomen, noting any masses, bulging, or distention. A flat abdomen forms a horizontal plane from the xiphoid process to the symphysis pubis. A round abdomen protrudes in a convex sphere from a horizontal plane. A concave abdomen appears to sink into the muscular wall. Each of these findings is normal if the shape of the abdomen is symmetrical. In older adults there is often an overall increased distribution of adipose tissue. The presence of masses on only one side, or asymmetry, indicates an underlying pathological condition.

Intestinal gas, tumor, or fluid in the abdominal cavity causes distention (swelling). When distention is generalized, the entire abdomen protrudes. The skin often appears taut, as if it were stretched over the abdomen. When gas causes distention, the flanks do not bulge. However, if fluid is the source of the problem such as in ascites, the flanks bulge. Ask the patient to roll onto one side. A protuberance forms on the dependent side if fluid is the cause of the distention. Ask the patient if the abdomen feels unusually tight. Be careful not to confuse distention with obesity. In obesity the abdomen is large, rolls of adipose tissue are often present along the flanks, and the patient does not complain of tightness in the abdomen. If abdominal distention is expected, measure the abdomen by placing a tape measure around it at the level of the umbilicus. Consecutive measurements show any increase or decrease in distention. Use a marking pen to indicate where you applied the tape measure.

Enlarged Organs or Masses. Observe the contour of the abdomen while asking the patient to take a deep breath and hold it. Normally the contour remains smooth and symmetrical. To evaluate abdominal musculature, have the patient raise his or her head. This position causes superficial abdominal wall masses, hernias, and muscle separations to become more apparent.

Movement or Pulsations. Inspect for movement. A patient with severe pain has diminished respiratory movement and tightens abdominal muscles to guard against the pain. Observe for peristaltic movement and aortic pulsation by looking across the abdomen from side to side. These movements are visible in thin patients; otherwise no movement is present.

Auscultation

In an abdominal examination, always auscultate before you palpate to reduce the risk of altering the frequency and intensity of bowel sounds. Ask the patient not to speak when you auscultate. Patients with GI tubes connected to suction need them temporarily turned off before beginning the examination.

Bowel Motility. Bowel sounds are the audible passage of air and fluid that normal intestinal contractions (peristalsis) create. Place the warmed diaphragm of the stethoscope lightly over each of the four quadrants (Fig. 16.40). Normally air and fluid move through the intestines, creating soft gurgling or clicking sounds that occur irregularly 5 to 35 times per minute (Ball et al., 2015). Sounds may last $\frac{1}{2}$ second to several seconds. It normally takes 5 to 20 seconds to hear a bowel sound. However, it takes 5 minutes of continuous listening before determining that bowel sounds are absent. Auscultate all four quadrants, starting in the right lower quadrant, to be sure that you do not miss any sounds. The best time to auscultate is between meals. Sounds are generally described as normal, audible, absent, hyperactive, or hypoactive.

Absent sounds indicate a lack of peristalsis, possibly caused by bowel obstruction, paralytic ileus (decreased or

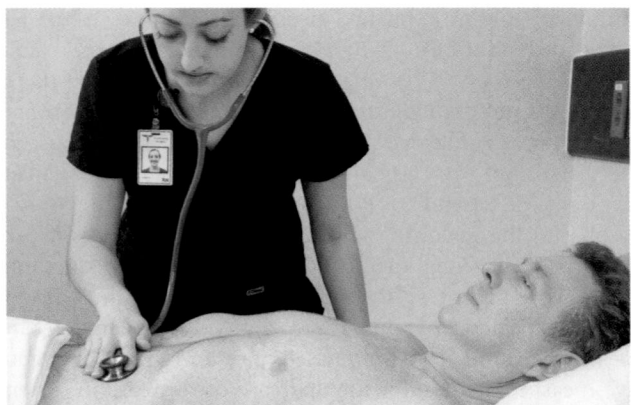

FIG 16.40 Auscultation of abdomen using diaphragm of stethoscope.

absent peristalsis), or peritonitis (inflammation of the peritoneum). Hyperactive sounds are loud, "growling" sounds (borborygmi) that indicate increased GI motility. Inflammation of the bowel, anxiety, bleeding, excess ingestion of laxatives, and reaction of the intestines to certain foods cause increased motility (Box 16.19).

Vascular Sounds. Bruits auscultated in affected blood vessels indicate narrowing of the blood vessels and turbulent disrupted blood flow. The presence of bruits in the abdominal area reveals aneurysms or stenotic vessels. Use the bell of the stethoscope to auscultate in the epigastric region and each of the four quadrants. Normally there are no vascular sounds over the aorta (midline through the abdomen) or femoral arteries (lower quadrants). Report a bruit immediately to a health care provider.

Palpation

Palpation primarily detects areas of abdominal tenderness, distention, or masses. As assessment skills improve, learn to palpate for specific organs such as the liver using light and deep palpation.

Use light palpation over each abdominal quadrant. Initially avoid areas previously identified as problem spots. Lay the palm of the hand with fingers extended and approximated lightly on the abdomen. Explain the maneuver to the patient; with the palmar surface of the fingers depress 1.3 cm ($\frac{1}{2}$ inch) in a gentle dipping motion (Fig. 16.41A). Avoid quick jabs and use smooth, coordinated movements. For ticklish patients first place the patient's hand on the abdomen with your hand on the patient's hand; continue until the patient tolerates palpation. Assess for muscular resistance, tenderness, distention, and superficial organs or masses. Observe for signs of discomfort. The abdomen is normally smooth with consistent softness and nontender without masses. Older adults often lack abdominal tone.

With experience perform deep palpation (Fig. 16.41B–C) to assess abdominal organs and detect less obvious masses. You need short fingernails. It is important for the patient to be relaxed while the hands depress approximately 2.5 to

BOX 16.19 **PATIENT TEACHING**

Abdominal Assessment

OUTCOME

Patient experiences improved digestion and elimination health.

TEACHING STRATEGIES

- Explain factors that promote normal bowel elimination such as diet, regular exercise, limited use of over-the-counter drugs causing constipation, establishment of a regular elimination schedule, and adequate fluid intake (see Chapter 37).
- Caution patient about dangers of excessive use of laxatives or enemas.
- Instruct patient with new onset of abdominal pain or discomfort to be evaluated by a health care provider.
- If patient has chronic pain, explain measures used for pain relief (e.g., relaxation exercises, positioning) (see Chapter 34).
- Instruct patient about warning signs of colon cancer including rectal bleeding, cramping pain in lower abdomen, black or tarry stools, blood in the stool, and a change in bowel habits (constipation or diarrhea).
- Instruct patient to report any noticeable yellowing of eyes, mucous membranes, or skin.
- If patient is a health care worker or has contact with blood or body fluids of affected people, encourage the patient to receive series of three hepatitis B virus (HBV) vaccine doses.

EVALUATION

- Use the principles of teach-back to evaluate patient/family caregiver learning:
  - "Describe for me a meal plan that includes foods that will improve your bowel habits."
  - "Show me how to perform the relaxation exercise we reviewed to help reduce your abdominal pain."
  - "Explain to me the signs and symptoms of bowel problems that you should report to your doctor."
  - "Tell me the dates that you have had your HBV vaccine."
  - "Describe to me the signs and symptoms of colon cancer."

7.5 cm (1 to 3 inches) into the abdomen. Never use deep palpation over a surgical incision or over extremely tender organs. It is also unwise to use deep palpation on abnormal masses. Deep pressure causes tenderness in the healthy patient over the cecum, sigmoid colon, and aorta and in the midline near the xiphoid process (Ball et al., 2015).

Assess each quadrant systematically. Palpate masses for size, location, shape, consistency, tenderness, pulsation, and mobility. Test for rebound tenderness by pressing a hand slowly and deeply into the involved area and then letting go quickly. The test is positive if the patient feels pain when the hand is released. Rebound tenderness occurs in patients with peritoneal irritation such as in appendicitis; pancreatitis; or any peritoneal injury causing bile, blood, or enzymes to enter the peritoneal cavity.

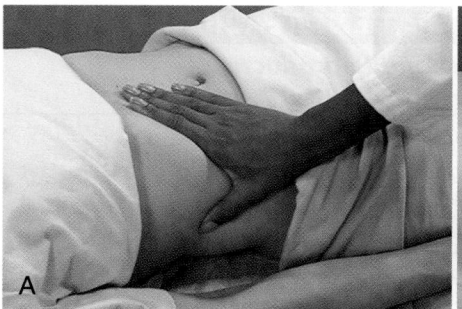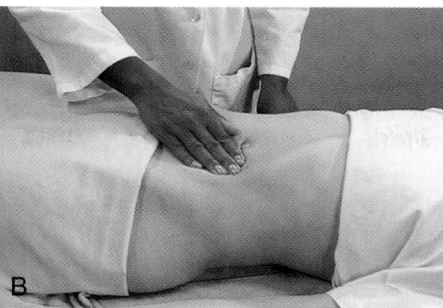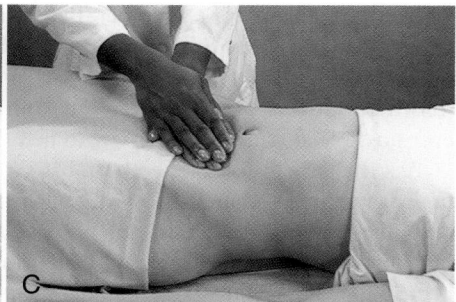

FIG 16.41 A, Light palpation of abdomen. **B,** Deep palpation of abdomen. **C,** Deep bimanual palpation. (From Ball JW, et al: *Seidel's guide to physical examination,* ed 8, St Louis, 2015, Elsevier.)

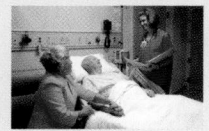 **QSEN ACTIVITY** *Patient-Centered Care*

After surgery the surgeon informs Mr. Neal of the diagnosis of bowel cancer. As she plans discharge teaching, Jane considers Mr. Neal's habits and current health practices that are high risk not only for bowel cancer but also for lung and heart disease. Mrs. Neal stated that she was primarily responsible for menu planning and food preparation. Jane considers which information to emphasize, while recognizing the importance of teaching both Mr. Neal and his wife.

- Which patient-centered approach should Jane use when selecting teaching materials? Give examples of effective questions that can be used to learn more about the Neals' current knowledge and preferences. Identify which level of evidence provides the strongest background information and teaching resources on which to base teaching plans.

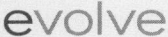 Answers to QSEN Activities can be found on the Evolve website.

Aortic Pulsation. To assess aortic pulsation palpate with the thumb and forefinger of one hand deeply into the upper abdomen just left of the midline. Normally a pulsation is transmitted forward. If the aorta is enlarged from an aneurysm (localized dilation of a vessel wall), the pulsation expands laterally. Do not palpate a pulsating abdominal mass. In obese patients it is often necessary to palpate with both hands, one on each side of the aorta.

FEMALE GENITALIA AND REPRODUCTIVE TRACT

Examination of the female genitalia requires a calm, relaxed approach. The gynecological examination is one of the most difficult experiences for adolescents. Cultural background further adds to apprehension. For example, in some cultural groups women allow only a female health care provider to perform a physical assessment. Other cultures have a strong social value for modesty. Provide a thorough explanation of the reason for the procedures used in the examination, and ask the patient if there is a need for a chaperone during the examination. The lithotomy position assumed during the examination is often a source of embarrassment. Make the patient feel comfortable by correctly positioning and draping her. Be sure to explain each portion of the examination in advance so that the patient anticipates each action. Adolescents sometimes choose to have a female parent present in the examination room.

Sometimes a patient requires a complete examination, including assessing external genitalia and performing a vaginal examination. As a nurse, you can examine external genitalia while performing routine hygiene measures or inserting a urinary catheter. An examination is a part of each woman's preventive health care because ovarian cancer was estimated to cause 14,240 deaths in 2016 and accounts for 5% of cancer deaths among women, more than any other gynecological cancer (ACS, 2016a).

Adolescents and young adults are examined because of the growing incidence of sexually transmitted infections (STIs). The average age of menarche among girls has declined, and most male and female teenagers are sexually active by 19 years of age (Hockenberry et al., 2017). Because the patient assumes a lithotomy or dorsal recumbent position, rectal and anal assessments are combined with this examination.

Nursing History

Begin by asking what the patient hopes to learn or do as a result of the examination. Establish rapport with her to increase her comfort level, focusing on her feelings about exposing herself to a health care provider. Next the nursing history reviews the patient's previous illnesses or surgeries involving reproductive organs, including STIs. A review of the menstrual history includes age at menarche, frequency and duration of menstrual cycle, character of flow, presence of dysmenorrhea (painful menstruation), pelvic pain, dates of last two menstrual periods, and premenstrual symptoms. Ask if the patient has had signs of bleeding, vaginal discharge, or pain outside the normal menstrual period or after menopause. Ask if she has symptoms or history of genitourinary problems such as burning during urination, frequency, urgency, nocturia, hematuria, incontinence, or stress incontinence.

It is important to remember that this nursing history usually contains sensitive information. The adolescent may be uncomfortable sharing symptoms and other valuable information if a parent or guardian is in the room. Whenever possible, obtain the history with just the patient present.

Ask the patient to describe her obstetrical history, including each pregnancy and history of abortions or miscarriages. Also question her about current and past contraceptive practices and problems encountered. It is important to determine if the patient uses safe sex practices. Discuss risks of STIs and HIV infection. Also review a patient's risk for developing cervical, endometrial, or ovarian cancer (Box 16.20).

Preparation of the Patient

It is your responsibility to assist the patient's primary health care provider with the examination. For a complete examination you need the following special equipment: examination table with stirrups, vaginal speculum of correct size, adjustable light source, sink, clean gloves, plastic or wooden spatula, cervical brush or broom device, glass slides and cytological fixative, culture plates or media, and deoxyribonucleic acid (DNA) probe kits for chlamydia and gonorrhea (Ball et al., 2015).

Make sure that equipment is ready before the examination begins. Ask the patient to empty her bladder; often it is necessary to collect a urine specimen. For an external genitalia assessment, help the patient to the lithotomy position in bed or on an examination table. On the table place and stabilize her feet into stirrups for a speculum examination and have her slide the buttocks down to the edge of the table. Place a hand at the edge of the table and instruct the patient to move until touching the hand. Her arms should be at her sides or folded across the chest to prevent tightening of abdominal muscles.

Provide a drape or sheet for the patient. A good method is to cover the knees and symphysis, depressing the drape between her knees (Ball et al., 2015). After the examination begins, lift the drape over the perineum. A male examiner always needs to have a female attendant during the examination. A female examiner may prefer to work alone but should have a female attendant if the patient is particularly anxious, is emotionally unsteady, or has requested one.

External Genitalia

Make sure that the perineal area is well illuminated. Apply clean gloves on both hands. The perineum is extremely sensitive and tender; do not touch the area suddenly without warning the patient. It is best to touch the neighboring thigh first before advancing to the perineum.

While sitting at the end of the examination table or bed, inspect the quantity and distribution of hair growth. Preadolescents have no pubic hair. During adolescence hair grows along the labia, becoming darker, coarser, and curlier. In an adult hair grows in a triangle over the female perineum and along the medial surface of the thighs. Normally it is free of nits and lice.

Inspect surface characteristics of the labia majora. The skin of the perineum is smooth, clean, and slightly darker

---

BOX 16.20 PATIENT TEACHING

Female Genital and Reproductive Tract Assessment

OUTCOME
Patient follows routine preventive and safety measures for gynecological health.

TEACHING STRATEGIES
- Instruct patient in the purpose and recommended frequency of Papanicolaou (Pap) tests and gynecological examinations. Explain that the Pap test is needed annually for women who are sexually active or older than 21 years of age. Patients are screened more often if certain risk factors exist such as a weak immune system, multiple sex partners, smoking, and a history of infections (e.g., human papillomavirus [HPV]).
- Counsel women and men about genital HPV infection and the need to receive the HPV vaccine. The vaccine is ideally recommended at age 11 or 12 years (ACS, 2016a).
- Counsel patients with sexually transmitted infections (STIs) about diagnosis and treatment.
- Instruct in genital self-examination: Using a mirror, position self to examine the area covered by the pubic hair. Spread the hair apart, looking for bumps, sores, or blisters, Also look for any warts, which appear as small, bumpy spots and enlarge to fleshy, cauliflower-like lesions. Next spread the outer vaginal lips apart and look at the clitoris for bumps, blisters, sores, or warts. Also look at both sides of the inner vaginal lips. Inspect the area around the urinary and vaginal openings for bumps, blisters, sores, or warts.
- Explain warning signs of STIs: pain or burning on urination, pain during sex, pain in the pelvic area, bleeding between menstrual periods, itchy rash around the vagina, and vaginal discharge.
- Teach measures to prevent STIs: male partner's use of condoms, restricting number of sexual partners, avoiding sex with people who have several other partners, and perineal hygiene measures.
- Tell patients with STIs to inform their sexual partner or partners of the need for an examination.
- Reinforce the importance of perineal hygiene (as appropriate).

EVALUATION
- Use the principles of teach-back to evaluate patient/family caregiver learning:
  - "Explain to me why routine gynecological examination and Pap test are important."
  - "Describe to me ways to prevent transmission of STIs."
  - "Tell me how you will use safe sex practices."

---

than other skin. The mucous membranes appear dark pink and moist. The labia majora are gaping or closed and appear dry or moist. They are usually symmetrical. After childbirth the labia majora separate, causing the labia minora to become more prominent. When a woman reaches menopause, the labia majora become thinned. With advancing age they become atrophied (decrease in size). The labia majora are normally without inflammation, edema, lesions, or lacerations.

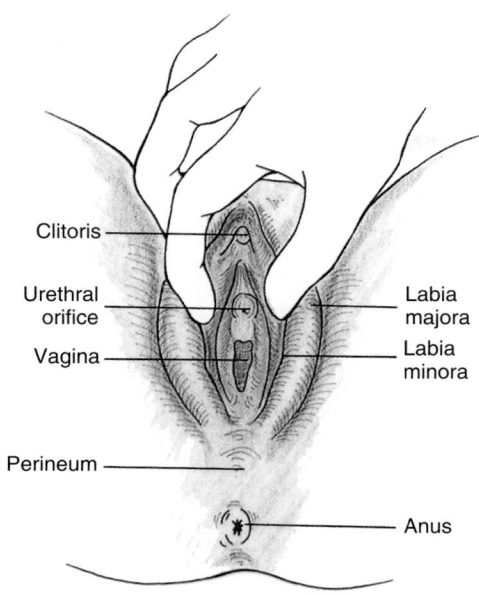

Clitoris

Urethral orifice

Vagina

Labia majora

Labia minora

Perineum

Anus

FIG 16.42 Female external genitalia.

To inspect the remaining external structures, use your nondominant hand and gently place the thumb and index finger inside the labia minora and retract the tissues outward (Fig. 16.42). Be sure to have a firm hold to avoid repeated retraction against the sensitive tissues. Use the other hand to palpate the labia minora between the thumb and second finger. On inspection the labia minora are normally thinner than the labia majora, and one side is sometimes larger. The tissue feels soft on palpation and without tenderness. The size of the clitoris varies, but it normally does not exceed 2 cm (¾ inch) in length and 0.5 cm (¼ inch) in diameter. Look for **atrophy**, inflammation, or adhesions. If inflamed the clitoris is a bright cherry red. In young women the clitoris is a common site for syphilitic lesions or chancres, which appear as small open ulcers that drain serous material. Some older women have malignant changes that result in dry, scaly, nodular lesions.

Inspect the urethral orifice carefully for color and position. Normally it is intact and without inflammation. The urethral meatus is anterior to the vaginal orifice and pink. It appears as a small slit or pinhole opening just above the vaginal canal. Note any discharge, polyps, or fistulas.

Inspect the vaginal orifice (introitus) for inflammation, edema, discoloration, discharge, and lesions. Normally the introitus is a thin vertical slit or large orifice. The tissue is moist. While inspecting the vaginal orifice or introitus, note the condition of the hymen, which is just inside the introitus. In the virgin female the hymen restricts the opening of the vagina. Only remnants of the hymen remain after sexual intercourse.

Inspect the anus looking for lesions and hemorrhoids (see rectal examination). After completion of the external examination, dispose of examination gloves, offer the patient perineal hygiene, and perform hand hygiene.

Patients who are at risk for contracting STIs need to learn to perform a genital self-examination (see Box 16.20). The purpose of the examination is to detect signs or symptoms of STIs. Many people do not know that they have an STI (e.g., chlamydial infection), and some STIs (e.g., syphilis) can remain undetected for years. Therefore it is essential to stress the importance of regular screening for STIs in sexually active individuals.

Speculum Examination of Internal Genitalia

An examination of internal genitalia requires much skill and practice. Advanced practice nurses and primary care providers perform this examination. Beginning students more than likely only observe the procedure or assist the examiner by helping the patient with positioning, handing off specimen supplies, and comforting the patient.

The examination involves use of a plastic or metal speculum consisting of two blades and an adjustable thumbscrew. The examiner inserts the speculum into the vagina to assess the vaginal walls and cervix for cancerous lesions and other abnormalities. During the examination the examiner collects a sample for a Papanicolaou (Pap) test for cervical and vaginal cancer.

MALE GENITALIA

An examination of the male genitalia assesses the integrity of the external genitalia, inguinal ring, and canal. Because the incidence of STIs in adolescents and young adults is high, an assessment of the genitalia needs to be a routine part of any health maintenance examination for this age-group. Use a calm, gentle approach to lessen the patient's anxiety. Offer the patient the option of having a companion or parent available during the examination. Have him void and then lie supine with the chest, abdomen, and lower legs draped or stand during the examination. Apply clean gloves.

Nursing History

Begin by explaining the purpose of the genital examination. Especially for adolescents, discuss the components of the male examination. Review the patient's normal urinary elimination pattern, including frequency of voiding; history of nocturia; character and volume of urine; daily fluid intake; and symptoms of burning, urgency and frequency, difficulty starting stream, and hematuria. The history also includes a review of previous surgery or illness involving urinary or reproductive organs including STIs. The patient's sexual history and use of safe sex habits identifies any risks for HIV infection or other STIs. Patients at risk require extensive education. Ask if the patient has difficulty achieving erection or ejaculation, and review medications that influence sexual performance including diuretics, sedatives, antihypertensives, and tranquilizers. Ask if the patient has noted penile pain or swelling, genital lesions, or urethral discharge, which indicate signs and symptoms of STIs. The patient's knowledge of testicular self-examination provides a guide for health teaching (Box 16.21). Determine if the patient has noticed heaviness or painless enlargement of a testis or irregular lumps (warning signs of testicular cancer). If he reports an enlargement in

BOX 16.21 PATIENT TEACHING

Male Genitalia Assessment

OUTCOME

Patient follows routine preventive and safety measures for genital and testicular health.

TEACHING STRATEGIES

- Provide the following information about genital self-examination to all male patients 15 years and older:
  - Perform examination monthly after a warm bath or shower when the scrotal sac is relaxed and less thick.
  - Stand naked in front of a mirror, hold the penis in your hand, and examine the head. Pull back the foreskin if uncircumcised to expose the glans (see illustration A).
  - Inspect and palpate the entire head of the penis in a clockwise motion, looking carefully for any bumps, sores, blisters, or unusual discharge. Blisters and bumps may be light colored or red and resemble pimples.
  - Look for genital warts.
  - Look at the opening (urethral meatus) at the end of the penis for discharge.
  - Look along the entire shaft of the penis for the same signs.
  - Be sure to separate pubic hair at the base of the penis and carefully examine the skin underneath.
- Provide the following information about testicular self-examination (TSE) to all men 15 years and older:
  - Look for swelling or lumps in the skin of the scrotum while looking in the mirror.
  - Use both hands, placing the index and middle fingers under the testicles and the thumb on top (see illustration B).
  - Gently roll the testicle, feeling for lumps, swelling, soreness, or change in consistency (hardening).
  - Find the epididymis (a cordlike structure on the top and back of the testicle; it is not a lump).
  - Feel for small, pea-size lumps on the front and side of the testicle. The lumps are usually painless and are abnormal.
  - Call your health care provider about abnormal findings.
  - Counsel patients with sexually transmitted infections (STIs) about diagnosis and treatment.
  - Explain warning signs of STIs: pain on urination and during sex, abnormal penile discharge (different from usual), swollen lymph nodes, or rash or ulcer on skin or genitalia.
  - Teach measures to prevent STIs: use of condoms, avoiding sex with infected partners, restricting number of

sexual partners, avoiding sex with people who have multiple partners, using regular perineal hygiene.
- Tell patients with an STI to inform sexual partner or partners of the need to have an examination.
- Instruct patient to seek treatment as soon as possible if partner becomes infected with an STI.

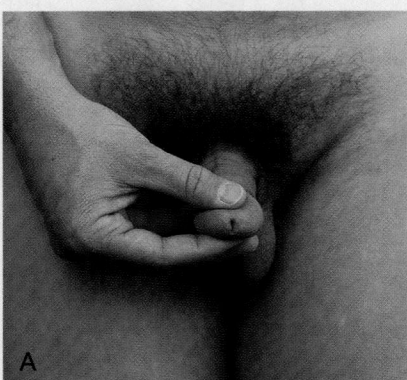

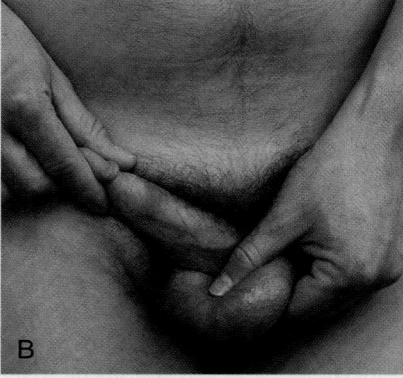

EVALUATION

- Use the principles of teach-back to evaluate patient/family caregiver learning:
  - "Demonstrate to me how you perform genital self-examination and testicular self-examination."
  - "Describe for me ways you can prevent getting a sexually transmitted disease."

Illustrations from Ball JW, et al: *Seidel's guide to physical examination,* ed 8, St Louis, 2015, Elsevier.

the inguinal area, assess if it is intermittent or constant; if it is associated with straining or lifting; if it is painful; and whether coughing, lifting, or straining at stool increases the pain. These are all signs and symptoms that indicate an inguinal hernia.

Sexual Maturity

First note the sexual maturity of the patient by observing the size and shape of the penis and testes; the size, color, and texture of scrotal skin; and the character and distribution of pubic hair. The testes first increase in size in preadolescence.

By the end of puberty the testes and penis enlarge to adult size and shape, and scrotal skin darkens and becomes wrinkled. Hair growth occurs with puberty, and hair is coarse and abundant in the pubic area. The penis has no hair, and the scrotum has very little hair. Also inspect the skin covering the genitalia for lice, rashes, excoriations, or lesions. Normally the skin is clear, without lesions.

Penis

To inspect penile surfaces thoroughly, manipulate the genitalia or have the patient help. Inspect the corona, prepuce

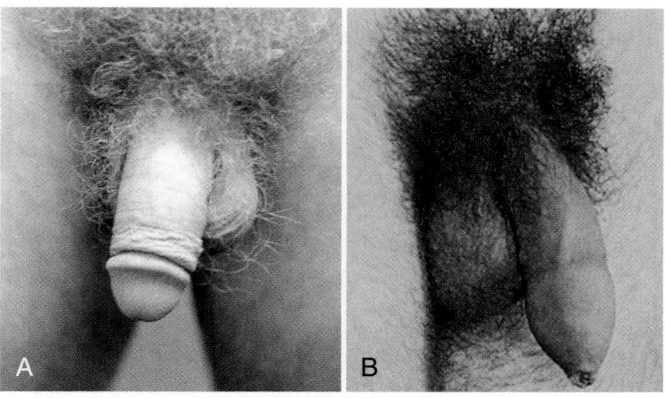

FIG 16.43 Normal male genitalia. **A,** Circumcised. **B,** Uncircumcised. (From Ball JW, et al: *Seidel's guide to physical examination,* ed 8, St Louis, 2015, Elsevier.)

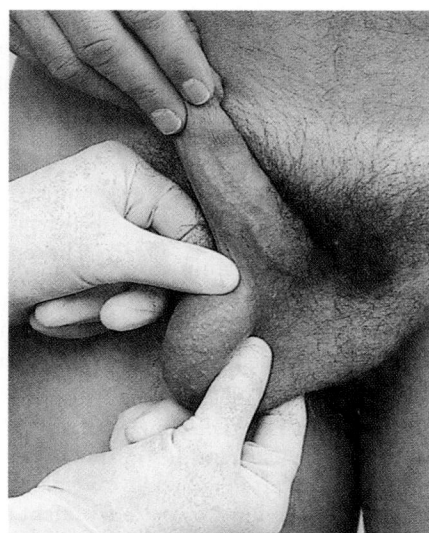

FIG 16.44 Palpating contents of scrotal sac. (From Ball JW, et al: *Seidel's guide to physical examination,* ed 8, St Louis, 2015, Elsevier.)

(foreskin), glans, urethral meatus, and shaft (Fig. 16.43). In uncircumcised patients, retract the foreskin to reveal the glans and urethral meatus. The foreskin usually retracts easily. A small amount of white, thick smegma sometimes collects under this foreskin. In the circumcised male patient, the glans is exposed. It should look smooth and pink along all surfaces. The urethral meatus is slitlike and normally positioned at the tip of the glans. In some congenital conditions the meatus is displaced along the penile shaft. The area between the foreskin and glans is a common site for venereal lesions.

Gently compress the glans between your thumb and index finger; this opens the urethral meatus for inspection of discharge, lesions, and edema. Normally the opening is glistening and pink without discharge. Palpate any lesion gently to note tenderness, size, consistency, and shape. When inspection and palpation of the glans are complete, pull the foreskin down to its original position. Continue by inspecting the entire shaft of the penis including the undersurface looking for any lesions, scars, or edema. Palpate the shaft between the thumb and first two fingers to detect localized areas of hardness or tenderness. A patient who has lain in bed for a prolonged time may develop dependent edema in the penile shaft.

It is important for all male patients to learn to perform a genital self-examination to detect signs and symptoms of STIs. Many people who have an STI do not know it. Self-examination is a routine part of self-care (see Box 16.21).

Scrotum

Be especially cautious while inspecting and palpating the scrotum because the structures that lie within the scrotal sac are very sensitive. The scrotum is divided internally into two halves. Each half contains a testicle, epididymis, and the vas deferens, which travels upward into the inguinal ring. Normally the left testicle is lower than the right. Inspect the size, color, shape, and symmetry of the scrotum while observing for lesions or edema.

Gently lift the scrotum to view the posterior surface. The scrotal skin is usually loose, and the surface is coarse. The skin color is often more deeply pigmented than body skin. Tightening or loss of wrinkling reveals edema. The size of the scrotum normally changes with temperature variations, contracting in cold and relaxing in warm temperature. Lumps in the scrotal skin are commonly sebaceous cysts.

Testicular cancer is a solid tumor commonly found in young men 18 to 34 years of age. Early detection is critical. Explain testicular self-examination while examining the patient. The testes are normally sensitive but not tender. The underlying testicles are normally ovoid and approximately 2×4 cm ($\frac{3}{4} \times 1\frac{5}{8}$ inches) in size. While the patient retracts the penis upward, gently palpate the testes and epididymis between the thumb and first two fingers (Fig. 16.44). Note the size, shape, and consistency of tissue and ask if the patient feels any tenderness. The testes feel smooth and rubbery and are free from nodules. The epididymis is resilient. In the older adult the testicles decrease in size and are less firm during palpation. The most common symptoms of testicular cancer are a painless enlargement of one testis and appearance of a palpable small, hard lump about the size of a pea on the front or side of the testicle. Continue to palpate the vas deferens separately as it forms the spermatic cord toward the inguinal ring, noting nodules or swelling. It normally feels smooth and discrete.

Inguinal Ring and Canal

The external inguinal ring provides the opening for the spermatic cord to pass into the inguinal canal. The canal forms a passage through the abdominal wall, a potential site for hernia formation. A hernia is a protrusion of a portion of intestine through the inguinal wall or canal. Sometimes an intestinal loop enters the scrotum. The patient stands during this portion of the examination.

During inspection ask the patient to strain or bear down. The maneuver helps to make a hernia more visible. Look for obvious bulging in the inguinal area. Complete the examination by palpating for inguinal lymph nodes. Normally small, nontender, mobile horizontal nodes are palpable. Any abnormality indicates local or systemic infection or malignant disease.

RECTUM AND ANUS

A good time to perform the rectal examination is after the genital examination. This examination is not performed in the examination in children or adolescents. The examination can detect colorectal cancer in its early stages. In men the rectal examination also detects prostatic enlargement and tumors. The rectal examination is uncomfortable; thus explaining all steps helps the patient relax.

Nursing History

The nursing history reviews a patient's risk factors for colorectal cancer including personal and family history of colorectal cancer, polyps, obesity, physical inactivity, long-term smoking, moderate to heavy alcohol consumption, and diet (ACS, 2016a). Determine if the patient has experienced bleeding from the rectum, black or tarry stools (melena), rectal pain, or change in bowel habits, all of which are warning signs of colorectal cancer (ACS, 2017). Assess dietary habits including intake of high-fat foods, diet high in processed or red meats, or deficient fiber content, which are linked to colon cancer. Determine whether the patient has undergone screening for colorectal cancer (digital examination, fecal occult blood test, flexible sigmoidoscopy, and colonoscopy). Ask male patients if they have experienced weak or interrupted urine flow, an inability to urinate, or difficulty starting or stopping the urine flow. In addition, ask if they have had polyuria; nocturia; hematuria; dysuria; or continuing pain in the lower back, pelvis, or upper thighs. These all are warning signs of prostate cancer. Finally, review the patient's use of laxatives, cathartics, codeine, or iron preparations, which can cause elimination problems (Box 16.22).

Inspection

Female patients remain in the dorsal recumbent position after the genitalia examination, or they assume a side-lying (Sims) position. The best way to examine male patients is to have the patients stand and bend over forward with the hips flexed and upper body resting across the examination table. Examine a nonambulatory patient in Sims position.

Using the nondominant hand gently retract the buttocks to view the perianal and sacrococcygeal areas. Perianal skin is smooth and more pigmented and coarser than skin overlying the buttocks. Inspect anal tissue for skin characteristics, lesions, external hemorrhoids (dilated veins that appear as reddened skin protrusions), ulcers, inflammation, rashes, or excoriation. Anal tissues are moist and hairless, and the anus is held closed by the voluntary external sphincter. Next ask the patient to bear down as though having a bowel movement. Any internal hemorrhoids or fissures appear at this time. Use clock referents (e.g., 12 o'clock or 5 o'clock) to

BOX 16.22   PATIENT TEACHING

Rectal and Anal Assessment

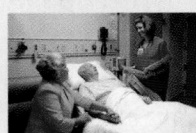

OUTCOME
Mr. Neal follows recommended guidelines for early detection of colorectal cancer and prostate screenings.

TEACHING STRATEGIES
- Discuss the ACS guidelines (ACS, 2017; 2016a) for early detection of colorectal cancer. Beginning at 50 years of age both men and women at average risk should use one of these screening tests (ACS, 2017):
  - Fecal occult blood test (FOBT) or fecal immunochemical test (FIT) annually *or*
  - Flexible sigmoidoscopy (FSIG): visual inspection of the rectum and lower colon with a hollow, lighted tube performed by a health care provider every 5 years *or*
  - Double-contrast barium enema every 5 years *or*
  - Colonoscopy every 10 years *or*
  - Computed tomography (CT) colonoscopy every 5 years
- Individuals at increased risk need to discuss options with their health care provider.
- Discuss warning signs of colorectal cancer.
- Discuss dietary planning and healthy lifestyle choices to maintain or improve colon health.
- Warn patients about problems caused by overuse of laxatives, cathartic medications, codeine, or enemas.
- Discuss with male patients the ACS guidelines (ACS, 2016a) for early detection of prostatic cancer:
  - Discuss with male patients the warning signs of prostate cancer.
  - Beginning at 50 years of age patients should have a conversation with their health care provider discussing risks and screen opportunities.
  - This discussion should start at 45 years of age for men at high risk including African American men and men who have a first-degree relative diagnosed with prostate cancer at an early age (before 65 years of age).
  - The discussion starts at 40 years of age for patients at even higher risk (history of several relatives positive for prostate cancer).

EVALUATION
- Use the principles of teach-back to evaluate patient/family caregiver learning:
  - "Tell me when you should have your next rectal examination."
  - "Explain to me the warning signs of colorectal and prostate cancer."
  - "Describe to me a meal that would contain the right types of food choices to maintain your colon health."

describe the location of findings. There normally is no protrusion of tissue.

Digital Palpation

Examine the anal canal and sphincters with digital palpation. In male patients palpate the prostate gland to rule out enlargement. Usually advanced practitioners perform this part of the examination.

MUSCULOSKELETAL SYSTEM

The assessment of the musculoskeletal system focuses on determining ROM, muscle strength and tone, and joint and muscle condition. The examination is conducted as a separate examination as for a sports physical or integrated into other parts of the total physical examination. Assess this system while performing other nursing care measures such as bathing or positioning. Muscular disorders often result from neurological disease. For this reason health care providers often conduct a neurological assessment simultaneously.

While examining the patient's musculoskeletal function, visualize the anatomy of bone and muscle placement and joint structure (see Chapter 28). Joints vary in their degree of mobility. Some such as joints in the knee are freely movable. The spinal vertebrae are examples of slightly movable joints. For a complete examination you uncover the limb or area being examined so that the muscles and joints are free to move. Have the patient sit, lie supine or prone, or stand while assessing muscle groups.

Nursing History

Determine the patient's history of musculoskeletal injury or trauma resulting from sports, employment, exercise, or chronic illnesses. Assess for osteoporosis risk factors including use of alcohol and/or caffeine; cigarette smoking; constant dieting; poor calcium or vitamin D intake; thin and light body frame; nulliparous status; menopause before 45 years of age; estrogen deficiency; postmenopause status; family history of osteoporosis; Caucasian, Asian, Native American, or Northern European ancestry; advanced age; history of fractures and/or falls; sedentary lifestyle; chronic diseases (e.g., Cushing disease, hyperthyroidism and hypothyroidism, malabsorption and/or malnutrition disorders, neoplasms); long-term use of corticosteroids, methotrexate, phenytoin, and aluminum-containing antacids; and lack of exposure to sunlight.

The nursing history includes a patient's description of problems with bone, muscle, or joint function including history of recent falls, trauma, lifting heavy objects, fractures, and bone or joint disease. It is useful to assess a patient's normal activity pattern including the type of exercise routinely performed (Box 16.23). Also assess the nature and extent of pain or stiffness and determine if alterations affect the patient's ability to perform ADLs, sleep, and participate in social activities.

General Inspection

Observe the patient's gait and posture when entering the examination room. The gait is more natural when a patient is unaware of being observed. Later a more formal test has the patient walk in a straight line away, turn, and return to the origin point. Note how the patient walks, sits, and rises from a sitting position. Normally patients walk with arms swinging

---

BOX 16.23 PATIENT TEACHING

Musculoskeletal Assessment

OUTCOME

Patient follows measures to prevent or minimize osteoporosis.

TEACHING STRATEGIES

- Instruct patient in correct postural alignment. Consult with a physical therapist to provide patient with exercises for improving posture.
- Explain that the risk for osteoporosis increases after 50 years of age; women and men should have screening completed by health care providers (NIH, 2015).
- Instruct patients to reduce the risk of fractures by increasing bone density and reducing the risk of falls (NIH, 2015):
  - Building and maintaining bone density: Perform weight-bearing exercises (e.g., walking, climbing stairs, dancing). Perform resistance exercises, such as weight training with free weights or weight machines.
  - Reducing risk of falls: Perform activities to improve balance (yoga, tai chi), flexibility (yoga, tai chi, swimming, stretching exercises), and strength (resistance exercises).
- Encourage intake of calcium and vitamin D to meet the recommended daily allowance. Increased vitamin D aids calcium absorption.
  - Recommendation for calcium supplements is 1000 mg/day for men and women up to the age of 50 and 1200 mg/

day for women over 50 and men over 70 years of age (NIH, 2015).
  - Recommendation for vitamin D supplement is 600 mg/day for men and women up to 70 years of age and increased to 800 mg/day after age 70 (NIH, 2015).
- Explain to patients with low back pain that they will benefit from modification of worker risk factors (e.g., lifting heavy weights, use of protective equipment), regular aerobic exercise, exercises that strengthen the back and increase trunk flexibility, and learning how to lift properly.
- Instruct older adults and adults with osteoporosis in proper body mechanics and ROM and moderate weight-bearing exercises (e.g., swimming, walking) to minimize trauma and subsequent bone fractures.
- Instruct older patients to pace activities to compensate for loss in muscle strength (Touhy and Jett, 2018).

EVALUATION

- Use the principles of teach-back to evaluate patient/family caregiver learning:
  - "Describe for me the types of exercises you can begin to do that will lessen the risks related to osteoporosis."
  - "Show me how you perform range-of-motion exercises."
  - "Let's review what we discussed about calcium and vitamin D. What are the doses to take each day?"

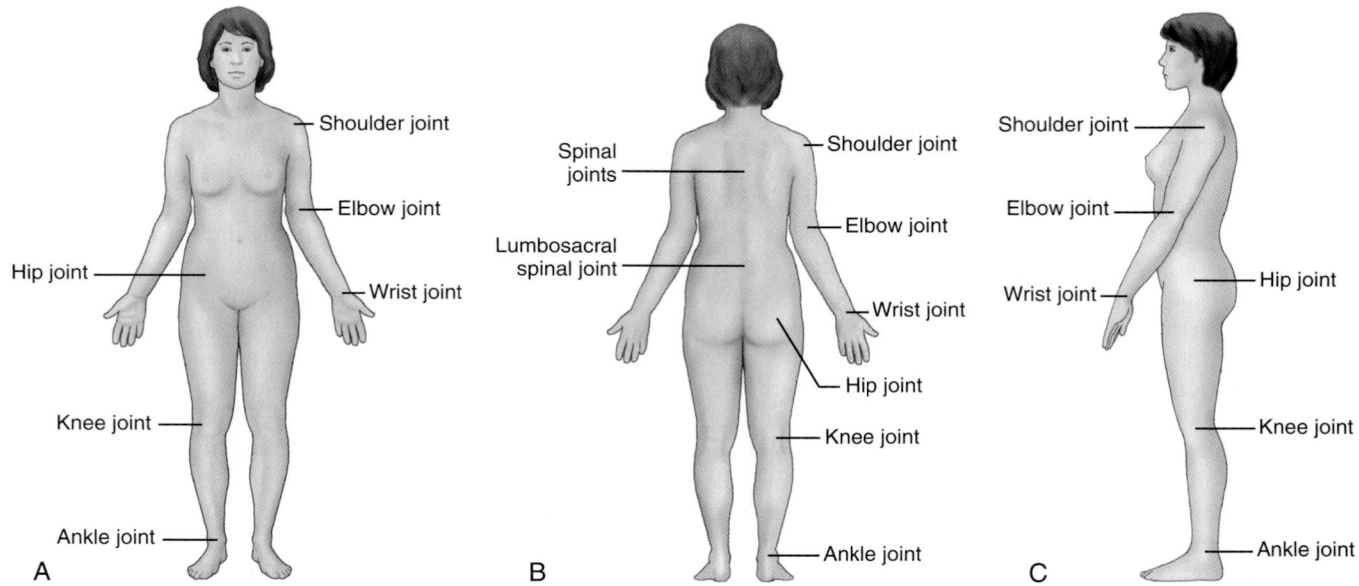

FIG 16.45 Inspection of overall body posture. **A,** Anterior view. **B,** Posterior view. **C,** Lateral view. (From Muscolino JE: *Kinesiology: the skeletal system and muscle function,* ed 2, St Louis, 2011, Elsevier.)

freely at the sides and the head leading the body. Older adults walk with smaller steps and a wider base of support. Note foot dragging, limping, shuffling, and the position of the trunk in relation to the legs. Compare extremities bilaterally. Patients in wheelchairs or who use walking assistance are assessed for smooth movements and stability.

Observe the patient from the side in a standing position. The normal standing posture is an upright stance with parallel alignment of the hips and shoulders (Fig. 16.45). There should be an even contour of the shoulders, level scapulae and iliac crests, alignment of the head over the gluteal folds, and symmetry of extremities. With the patient standing sideways note the normal cervical, thoracic, and lumbar curves. Holding the head erect is normal. As the patient sits, some degree of rounding of the shoulders is normal. Older adults tend to assume a stooped, forward-bent posture, with hips and knees somewhat flexed and arms bent at the elbows, raising the level of the arms.

Common postural abnormalities include lordosis, kyphosis, and scoliosis (Fig. 16.46). Lordosis, or swayback, is an increased lumbar curvature. Kyphosis, or hunchback, is an exaggeration of the posterior curvature of the thoracic spine. This postural abnormality is common in older adults. Scoliosis is a lateral spinal curvature. Loss of height is frequently the first clinical sign of osteoporosis, in which height loss occurs in the trunk as a result of vertebral fracture and collapse. Osteoporosis is a metabolic bone disease that causes a decrease in quality and quantity of bone. The National Institutes of Health (NIH) reports that 53 million Americans already have or are at risk for developing osteoporosis secondary to low bone mass (NIH, 2015). Although a small amount of height loss is expected with aging, if the amount of loss is great, osteoporosis is likely. As men and women

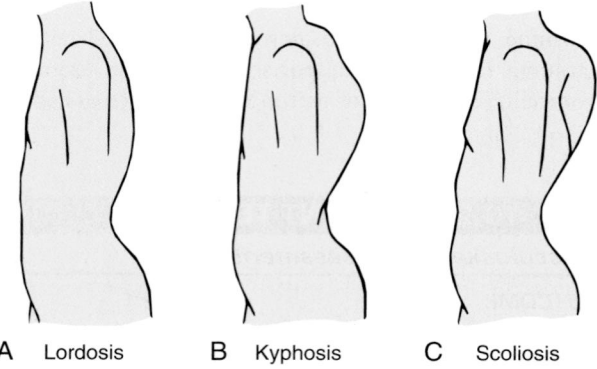

A   Lordosis   B   Kyphosis   C   Scoliosis

FIG 16.46 Common postural abnormalities. **A,** Lordosis. **B,** Kyphosis. **C,** Scoliosis.

age, they are more likely to have osteoporotic fractures of the forearm and/or wrists, hips, and vertebrae.

During general inspection look at the extremities for overall size, gross deformity, bony enlargement, alignment, and symmetry. Normally there is bilateral symmetry in length, circumference, alignment, and position and number of skinfolds (Ball et al., 2015). A general review pinpoints areas requiring specialized assessment.

Palpation

During a complete examination apply gentle palpation to all bones, joints, and surrounding muscles. In the case of a focused assessment, examine only the involved area. Note any warmth, tenderness, edema, or resistance to pressure. The patient should feel no discomfort when you apply palpation. Muscles should be firm. When assessing the vertebrae, ask the patient to bend at the waist, arms hanging down. Bimanually

TABLE 16.8 TERMINOLOGY FOR NORMAL RANGE-OF-MOTION POSITIONS

TERM	RANGE OF MOTION	EXAMPLES OF JOINTS
Flexion	Movement decreasing angle between two adjoining bones; bending of limb	Elbow, fingers, knee
Extension	Movement increasing angle between two adjoining bones	Elbow, fingers, knee
Hyperextension	Movement of body part beyond normal resting extended position	Head
Pronation	Movement of body part so that front or ventral surface faces downward	Hand, forearm
Supination	Movement of body part so that front or ventral surface faces upward	Hand, forearm
Abduction	Movement of extremity away from midline of body	Leg, arm, fingers
Adduction	Movement of extremity toward midline of body	Leg, arm, fingers
Internal rotation	Rotation of joint inward	Knee, hip
External rotation	Rotation of joint outward	Knee, hip
Eversion	Turning of body part away from midline	Foot
Inversion	Turning of body part toward midline	Foot
Dorsiflexion	Flexion of toes and foot upward	Foot
Plantar flexion	Bending of toes and foot downward	Foot

palpate either side of the spinal column to note any deviations or curvatures.

Range of Joint Motion

The examination includes comparison of both active and passive full ROM. Ask the patient to put each major joint and its muscle groups through full ROM. Learn the terminology for each joint movement (Table 16.8), and teach the patient how to move each joint through ROM. To assess passive ROM ask the patient to relax, and you then passively move the joints through their ROM. Compare the same body parts for equality in movement. Do not force a joint into a painful position. Know the normal range of each joint and the extent to which you can move the patient's joints. Ideally assess the patient's normal range to determine a baseline for assessing later change. Joints are typically free from stiffness, instability, swelling, or inflammation. There normally is no discomfort when applying pressure to bones and joints. In older adults joints often become swollen and stiff, with reduced ROM resulting from cartilage erosion and fibrosis of synovial membranes. If a joint appears swollen and inflamed, palpate it for warmth.

Muscle Tone and Strength

Assess muscle strength and tone during ROM measurement. Note muscle tone (i.e., the slight muscular resistance felt as you move the relaxed extremity passively through its ROM). Ask the patient to allow an extremity to relax or hang limp, which is sometimes difficult if the patient feels pain in the extremity. Support the extremity and grasp each limb, moving it through the normal ROM. Normal tone causes a mild, even resistance to passive movement through the entire range.

If a muscle has increased tone, or hypertonicity, you meet considerable resistance with sudden passive movement of a joint. Continued movement eventually causes the muscle to relax. A muscle that has little tone (hypotonicity) feels flabby.

The involved extremity hangs loosely in a position determined by gravity.

For assessment of muscle strength the patient assumes a stable position. The patient performs maneuvers demonstrating strength of major muscle groups (Table 16.9). Compare symmetrical muscle pairs for strength based on a grading scale of 0 to 5 (Table 16.10). The arm on the dominant side is normally stronger than the arm on the nondominant side. In the older adult a loss of muscle mass causes bilateral weakness, but muscle strength remains greater in the dominant arm or leg.

Examine each muscle group. Ask the patient first to flex the muscle to be examined and then to resist when you apply opposing force against that flexion (Fig. 16.47). It is important to not allow the patient to move the joint. Gradually increase pressure to a muscle group (e.g., elbow extension). Have the patient resist the pressure applied by attempting to move against resistance (e.g., elbow flexion). The patient resists until instructed to stop. Vary the amount of pressure applied and observe the joint move. If you identify a weakness, compare the size of the muscle with its opposite counterpart by measuring the circumference of the muscle body with a tape measure. A muscle that has atrophied (reduced in size) feels soft and baggy when palpated.

NEUROLOGICAL SYSTEM

An assessment of neurological function alone is quite time-consuming. For efficiency integrate neurological measurements with other parts of the physical examination. For example, test cranial nerve function while assessing the head and neck. Observe mental and emotional status during the initial interview.

Consider many variables when deciding the extent of the examination. A patient's level of consciousness influences the ability to follow directions. General physical status influences

TABLE 16.9	MANEUVERS TO ASSESS MUSCLE STRENGTH
MUSCLE GROUP	**MANEUVER**
Neck (sternocleidomastoid)	Place hand firmly against patient's upper jaw. Ask patient to turn head laterally against resistance.
Shoulder (trapezius)	Place hand over midline of patient's shoulder, exerting firm pressure. Have patient raise shoulder against resistance.
Elbow	
Biceps	Pull down on forearm as patient attempts to flex arm.
Triceps	Apply pressure against forearm as you flex patient's arm. Ask patient to straighten arm.
Hip	
Quadriceps	When patient is sitting, apply downward pressure to thigh. Ask patient to raise leg up from table.
Gastrocnemius	Patient sits while examiner holds shin of flexed leg. Ask patient to straighten leg against resistance.

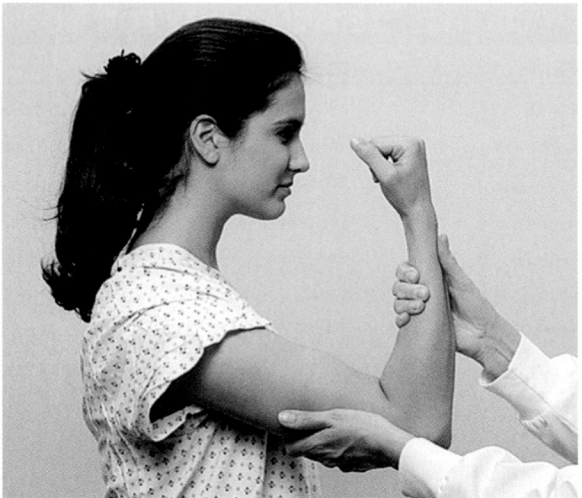

FIG 16.47 Assess muscle strength: flexion of elbow against opposing force. (From Wilson S, Gidden J: *Health assessment for nursing practice*, ed 6, St Louis, 2016, Elsevier.)

TABLE 16.10	MUSCLE STRENGTH
MUSCLE FUNCTION LEVEL	**GRADE**
No evidence of contractility	0
Trace of movement	1
Full ROM, not against gravity[a]	2
Full ROM against·gravity but not against resistance	3
Full ROM against gravity; some resistance but weak	4
Full ROM against gravity; full resistance	5

ROM, Range of motion.
[a]Passive movement.
From Ball JW, et al: *Seidel's guide to physical examination*, ed 8, St Louis, 2015, Elsevier.

tolerance to assessment. A patient's description of signs and symptoms helps to determine the need for a thorough neurological assessment. If a patient complains of headache or a recent loss of function in an extremity, he or she needs a complete neurological assessment. For a complete examination you need the following special equipment:

- Reading material
- Vials of aromatic substances (e.g., orange, peppermint extract, coffee)
- Opposite tip of cotton swab broken in half or paper clip for testing ability to distinguish sharp from dull
- Snellen eye chart
- Penlight
- Vials containing sugar, salt, and lemon with applicators
- Tongue blade
- Two test tubes containing hot and cold water for temperature sensation testing
- Cotton balls or cotton-tipped applicators
- Tuning fork
- Reflex hammer
- Familiar objects such as coins, keys, or paperclips

Nursing History

Review the patient's use of analgesics, alcohol, sedative-hypnotics, antipsychotics, antidepressants, nervous system stimulants, or recreational drugs. In addition, review the patient's use of over-the-counter sleeping aids. Determine if the patient has a recent history of seizures and/or convulsions and screen for symptoms of headache, tremors, dizziness, vertigo, numbness or tingling of body parts, visual changes, weakness, pain, or changes in speech. The presence of any symptom requires a more detailed review (e.g., onset, severity, precipitating factors, sequence of events). Discuss with the patient's family any recent changes in the patient's behavior (e.g., increased irritability, mood swings, memory loss, change in energy level). Ask the patient for a history of changes in vision, hearing, smell, taste, and touch. A history of head or spinal cord trauma, meningitis, congenital anomalies, neurological disease, or psychiatric counseling focuses your assessment of select findings. If an older adult patient displays sudden acute confusion (delirium), review history for drug toxicity, serious infections, metabolic disturbances, heart failure, and severe anemia.

Mental and Emotional Status

You learn about mental capacities and emotional state by interacting with a patient. Ask questions during an examination to gather data and observe the appropriateness of emotions and thoughts. Special assessment tools designed to assess a patient's mental status are available. For example, the Mini-Mental State Examination (MMSE) measures a patient's orientation and cognitive function. It asks questions such as "What is the date?" and "Tell me where you are now."

To ensure an objective assessment consider a patient's cultural and educational background, values, beliefs, and previous experiences. An alteration in mental or emotional status reflects a disturbance in cerebral functioning. The cerebral cortex controls and integrates intellectual and emotional functioning. Primary brain disorders, medications, and metabolic changes are examples of factors that change cerebral function.

Level of Consciousness

A person's level of consciousness exists along a continuum from being fully awake, alert, and cooperative to unresponsiveness to any form of external stimuli. Talk with the patient, asking questions about events involving him or her or concerns about health problems. A fully conscious patient responds to questions quickly and expresses ideas logically. As a patient's consciousness lowers, use the Glasgow Coma Scale (GCS) for an objective measurement of consciousness on a numerical scale (Table 16.11). The patient needs to be as alert as possible before testing. Use caution when using the GCS if a patient has sensory losses (e.g., vision or hearing) or is intubated with mechanical ventilation. The GCS allows evaluation of a patient's neurological status over time. The higher the score, the better the patient's neurological function. Ask short, simple questions such as "What is your name?" or "Where are you?" Also ask the patient to follow simple commands such as "Move your toes."

If a patient is not conscious enough to follow commands, try to elicit a pain response. Apply firm pressure with the thumb over the root of the patient's fingernail. The normal response to painful stimuli is withdrawal of the body part from the stimulus.

Behavior and Appearance

Behaviors, moods, hygiene, grooming, and choice of dress reveal pertinent information about mental status. Assess the patient's mannerisms and actions during the entire physical assessment. Note both nonverbal and verbal behaviors. Does the patient respond appropriately to directions? Does his or her mood vary with no apparent cause? Does he or she show concern about appearance? Is the patient's hair clean and neatly groomed, and are the nails trimmed and clean? The patient should behave in a manner expressing concern and interest in the examination. He or she should make eye contact and express appropriate feelings that correspond to the situation. Normally a patient's appearance shows some degree of personal hygiene.

Choice and fit of clothing reflect socioeconomic background or personal taste rather than deficiency in self-concept or self-care. Avoid being judgmental and focus assessments on the appropriateness of clothing for the weather. Older adults sometimes neglect their appearance because of a lack of energy, finances, or reduced vision.

Language

Normal cerebral function allows a person to understand spoken or written words and express himself or herself through written words or gestures. Assess the patient's voice inflection, tone, and manner of speech. Normally a patient's voice has inflections, is clear and strong, and increases in volume appropriately. Speech is fluent. When communication is clearly ineffective (e.g., omission or addition of letters and words, misuse of words, hesitations), assess the patient for aphasia.

Injury to the cerebral cortex results in aphasia. The two types of aphasia are sensory (or receptive) and motor (or expressive). With receptive aphasia a person cannot understand written or verbal speech. With expressive aphasia a person understands written and verbal speech but cannot write or speak appropriately when attempting to communicate. A patient sometimes suffers from a combination of receptive and expressive aphasia. When communication is ineffective, assess language capabilities with simple assessment techniques. Ask the patient to name familiar objects when pointing at them. Ask him or her to respond to simple verbal commands such as "Stand up." Finally ask the patient to read a simple sentence out loud. Normally a patient names objects correctly, follows commands, and reads sentences correctly.

Intellectual Function

Intellectual function includes memory, knowledge, abstract thinking, and judgment. Testing each aspect of function involves a specific technique. However, because cultural and educational background influences the ability to respond to test questions, do not ask questions related to concepts or ideas with which the patient is unfamiliar. Validate information with a family member if appropriate.

TABLE 16.11 GLASGOW COMA SCALE

ACTION*	RESPONSE	SCORE
Eyes open	Spontaneous opening	4
	To verbal stimuli	3
	To pain	2
	No response	1
Verbal response	Oriented to appropriate stimulation	5
	Confused	4
	Inappropriate words	3
	Incoherent	2
	No response	1
Motor response	Obeys commands	6
	Localizes pain	5
	Withdraws from pain	4
	Flexion to pain (decorticate)	3
	Extension to pain (decerebrate) extension	2
	None	1

Patient's total score ranges from 3 to 15.
The patient's best response is matched to the criteria for scoring.

Memory. Assess immediate recall and recent and remote memory. Patients demonstrate immediate recall by repeating a series of numbers in the order they are presented or reverse order. Patients normally recall five to eight digits forward or four to six digits backward.

First explain that you will test the patient's memory. Then state clearly and slowly the names of three unrelated objects. After stating all three, ask the patient to repeat each. Continue until the patient is successful. Later in the assessment ask the patient to repeat the three words again. The patient should be able to identify the three words. Another test for recent memory involves asking the patient to recall events occurring during the same day (e.g., what was eaten for breakfast).

To assess past memory ask the patient to recall the maiden name of the patient's mother, a birthday, or a special date in history. Compare the response with recorded data from the health record. It is best to ask open-ended questions rather than simple yes/no questions. A patient usually has immediate recall of such information. With older adults do not interpret a hearing loss as confusion.

Knowledge. Assess knowledge by asking how much the patient knows about his or her illness or the reason for seeking health care. You can also ask questions about basic facts (e.g., who is the president?). By assessing a patient's knowledge you can determine his or her ability to learn or understand. If there is an opportunity to teach, test the patient's mental status by asking for feedback during a follow-up visit.

Abstract Thinking. Interpreting abstract ideas or concepts reflects the capacity for abstract thinking. For an individual to explain common sayings such as "A stitch in time saves nine" or "Don't count your chickens before they're hatched" requires a higher level of intellectual functioning. Note whether the patient's explanations are relevant and concrete. A patient with altered mental state would probably interpret the phrase literally or merely rephrase the words.

Judgment. Judgment requires a comparison and evaluation of facts and ideas to understand their relationships and form appropriate conclusions. Attempt to measure the patient's ability to make logical decisions with questions such as "Why did you decide to seek health care?" or "What would you do if you suddenly became ill at home?" Normally a patient makes logical decisions.

Cranial Nerve Function

Although cranial nerve function is not commonly completed as part of the bedside assessment, you may test all 12 cranial nerves or a single nerve or related group of nerves to determine function. A dysfunction in one nerve reflects an alteration at some point along the distribution of the cranial nerve. Measurements used to assess the integrity of organs within the head and neck also assess cranial nerve function. A complete assessment involves testing the 12 cranial nerves in order of their numbers. To remember the order of the nerves, using a simple phrase is helpful. One example is: "On old Olympus' towering tops a Finn and German viewed some hops." The first letter of each word in the phrase is the same as the first letter of the names of the cranial nerves listed in order (Table 16.12).

Sensory Function

The sensory pathways of the central nervous system conduct the sensations of pain, temperature, position, vibration, and crude and finely localized touch. Different nerve pathways relay the sensations. Most patients require only a quick screening of sensory function unless there are symptoms of reduced sensation, motor impairment, or paralysis.

Normally a patient has sensory responses to all stimuli tested. The patient feels sensations equally on both sides of the body in all areas. Perform all sensory testing with the patient's eyes closed so that the patient is unable to see when or where a stimulus strikes the skin (Table 16.13). Then apply stimuli in a random, unpredictable order to maintain the patient's attention and prevent detection of a predictable pattern. Ask the patient to describe when, what, and where each stimulus is felt. Compare symmetrical areas of the body while applying stimuli to the arms, trunk, and legs.

Motor Function

An assessment of motor function includes measurements made during the musculoskeletal examination. In addition, you assess cerebellar function. The cerebellum coordinates muscular activity, maintains balance and equilibrium, and helps to control posture. Patients with any degree of motor dysfunction are at risk for injury (Box 16.24).

Coordination. To avoid confusion, demonstrate each maneuver and have the patient repeat it while you observe for smoothness and balance in the patient's movement. In older adults normally slow reaction time causes movements to be less rhythmical.

To assess fine-motor function, have the patient extend the arms out to the sides and touch each forefinger alternately to the nose, first with eyes open, then with eyes closed (Fig. 16.48). Performing rapid, rhythmical, alternating movements demonstrates coordination in the upper extremities. While sitting, the patient begins by patting the knees with both hands. Then he or she alternately turns up the palm and back of the hands while continuously patting the knees (Fig. 16.49). Test lower extremity coordination with the patient lying supine, legs extended. Place your hand at the ball of the patient's foot. The patient taps the hand with the foot as quickly as possible, alternating feet. The feet do not normally move as rapidly or evenly as the hands.

Balance. Assess balance and gross-motor function by asking the patient to stand with feet together, arms at the sides, both with eyes open and with eyes closed. Protect the patient's safety by standing at the side and observe for swaying. Expect slight swaying of the body in the Romberg test. A loss of balance (positive Romberg) causes a patient to fall to the side.

TABLE 16.12 CRANIAL NERVE FUNCTION AND ASSESSMENT

CRANIAL NERVE	NAME	TYPE	FUNCTION	ASSESSMENT METHOD
I	Olfactory	Sensory	Sense of smell	Ask patient to identify different aromas in each nostril such as coffee and vanilla.
II	Optic	Sensory	Visual acuity and visual fields	Use Snellen chart or ask patient to read printed material while wearing glasses.
III	Oculomotor	Motor	Pupil constriction and dilation	Measure pupil reaction to light reflex and accommodation.
			Extraocular eye movement	Assess directions of gaze.
IV	Trochlear	Motor	Upward and inward eye movement	Assess directions of gaze.
V	Trigeminal	Sensory	Sensory nerve to cornea, eyelids, forehead, skin of face	Lightly touch cornea with wisp of cotton. Assess corneal reflex. Measure sensation of light pain and touch across skin of face.
		Motor	Motor nerve to muscles of jaw	Palpate temples as patient clenches teeth; observe chewing.
VI	Abducens	Motor	Lateral eye movement	Assess directions of gaze.
VII	Facial	Sensory	Taste	Have patient identify salty or sweet taste on front of tongue.
		Motor	Facial expression	Look for asymmetry as patient smiles, frowns, puffs out cheeks, and raises and lowers eyebrows.
VIII	Auditory	Sensory	Hearing and equilibrium	Assess ability to hear spoken word.
IX	Glossopharyngeal	Sensory	Taste	Ask patient to identify sour or sweet taste on back of tongue.
		Motor	Ability to swallow and speak	Use tongue blade to elicit gag reflex; have person swallow.
X	Vagus	Sensory	Sensation of pharynx and behind ear	Ask patient to say "Ah." Observe movement of palate and pharynx.
		Motor	Movement of vocal cords	Assess speech for hoarseness.
XI	Spinal accessory	Motor	Movement of shoulders and head	Ask patient to shrug shoulders and turn head against passive resistance.
XII	Hypoglossal	Motor	Position of tongue	Ask patient to stick out tongue to midline and move it from side to side.

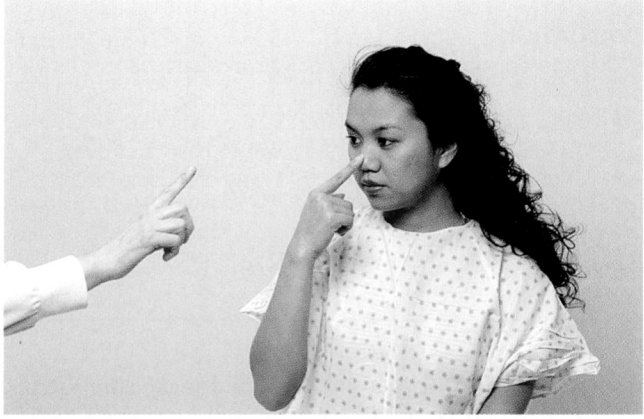

FIG 16.48 Examination of fine motor function. (From Wilson S, Gidden J: *Health assessment for nursing practice*, ed 6, St Louis, 2016, Elsevier.)

Reflexes. Eliciting reflexes, usually performed by an advanced practice nurse, assesses integrity of sensory and motor pathways. Deep tendon reflexes are elicited by mildly stretching a muscle and tapping a tendon with a reflex hammer. Cutaneous reflexes are tested by stimulating the skin superficially.

AFTER THE EXAMINATION

Record the physical assessment findings during the examination or at the end. Specific forms are available to record data. Review all findings before helping the patient dress in case of a need to recheck any information or gather additional data. Integrate physical assessment findings into the plan of care.

Give the patient time to dress after completing the assessment. A hospitalized patient often needs help with hygiene and returning to bed. When the patient is comfortable, share a summary of the assessment findings. If the findings show serious abnormalities such as an irregular heart rate, consult the patient's health care provider before revealing any

TABLE 16.13 ASSESSMENT OF SENSORY NERVE FUNCTION

FUNCTION	EQUIPMENT	METHOD	PRECAUTIONS
Pain	End of paper clip or wooden end of cotton applicator	Ask patient to say when he or she feels dull or sharp sensation. Alternately apply sharp and blunt ends of paper clip or broken cotton swab to surface of skin. Note areas of numbness or increased sensitivity.	Remember that areas where skin is thickened such as heel or sole of foot are less sensitive to pain.
Temperature	Two test tubes, one filled with hot water, one filled with cold water	Touch skin with tube. Ask patient to identify hot or cold sensation.	Omit test if pain sensation is normal.
Light touch	Cotton ball or cotton-tipped applicator	Apply light wisp of cotton to different points along surface of skin. Ask patient to say when he or she feels sensation.	Apply at areas where skin is thin or more sensitive (e.g., face, neck, inner aspect of arms, top of feet and hands).
Vibration	Tuning fork	Apply stem of vibrating fork to distal interphalangeal joint of fingers and interphalangeal joint of great toe, elbow, and wrist. Have patient say when and where he or she feels vibration.	Be sure that patient feels vibration and not merely pressure.
Position		Grasp finger or toe, holding it by its sides with thumb and index finger. Alternate moving finger or toe up and down. Ask patient to say when finger is up or down. Repeat with toes.	Avoid rubbing adjacent appendages as you move finger or toe. Do not move joint laterally; return to neutral position before moving again.
Two-point discrimination	Two ends of paper clip	Lightly apply one or both ends of paper clip simultaneously to surface of skin. Ask patient whether he or she feels one or two pricks. Find the distance at which patient can no longer distinguish two points.	Apply paper clip tips to same anatomical site (e.g., fingertips, palm of hand, upper arms). Minimum distance at which patient discriminates two points varies (2–8 mm on fingertips).

BOX 16.24 PATIENT TEACHING

Neurological Assessment

OUTCOME

Patient and family caregiver learn the warning signs of stroke and follow safety measures needed for reduced neurologic function.

TEACHING STRATEGIES

- Teach patient and family caregiver to seek emergency care to rule out stroke with any of these symptoms: any sudden visual changes; sudden confusion; change in speech; weakness, sudden numbness, tingling, or loss of movement, especially on one side of the body.
- Teach patient and family caregiver to immediately seek emergency treatment for a sudden, severe headache that is different from past headaches.
- Explain to family or friends the implications of any behavioral or mental impairment shown by the patient.

- If patient has sensory or motor impairments, explain measures to ensure safety (e.g., use of ambulation aids, use of safety bars in bathrooms or on stairways).
- Teach older adults to plan enough time to complete tasks because their reaction time is slow.

EVALUATION

- Use the principles of teach-back to evaluate patient/family caregiver learning:
  - "As a family member, describe the patient's behaviors that you would observe if he were to have a stroke."
  - "Explain safety measures that you are using at home to prevent injury from the weakness you have in your left leg."

findings. It is the health care provider's responsibility to make definitive medical diagnoses. Explain the type of abnormality found and the need for the health care provider to conduct an additional examination.

The examination space needs to be cleaned when you are finished. Use infection control practices to remove materials or instruments soiled with potentially infectious wastes. If the patient's bedside was the site for the examination, clear away soiled items from the bedside table and make sure the bed linen is dry and clean. The patient will appreciate a clean gown and the opportunity to wash the face and hands. Afterward be sure to perform hand hygiene.

Arrange for ordered ancillary examinations after a physical examination if needed such as x-ray film examinations, laboratory tests, or ultrasonography. These tests provide additional screening information to rule out and help diagnose

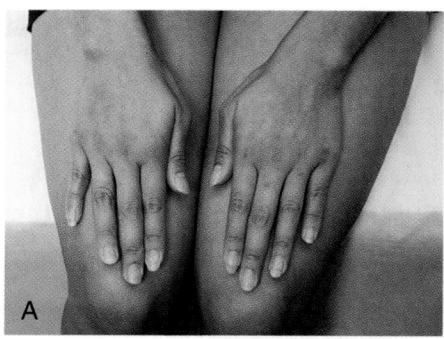 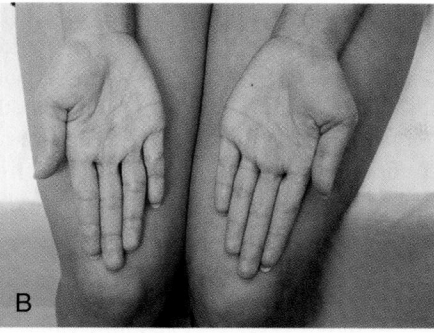 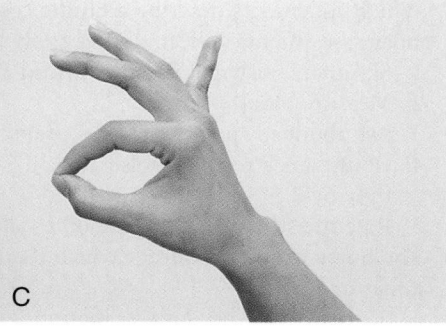

FIG 16.49 Examination of coordination with rapid alternating movements. **A** and **B,** Alternatively pat knees with back and then palm of both hands. **C,** Touch thumb to each finger in sequence, increasing in speed. (From Wilson S, Gidden J: *Health assessment for nursing practice,* ed 6, St Louis, 2016, Elsevier.)

specific abnormalities found during the examination. Explain the purpose of these tests and the sensations that the patient will experience.

KEY POINTS

- Baseline assessment findings reflect a patient's functional abilities and serve as the basis for comparison with subsequent assessment findings.
- Physical assessment of a child or infant requires application of the principles of growth and development.
- The normal process of aging affects physical findings collected from an older adult.
- If you suspect substance abuse, conduct a NIDA Quick Screen to determine the patient's need for further intervention.
- Integrate patient teaching throughout the examination to help patients learn about health promotion and disease prevention.
- Inspection requires good lighting, full exposure of the body part, and a careful comparison of the part with its counterpart on the opposite side of the body.
- Palpation involves the use of parts of the hand to detect different types of physical characteristics.
- Use auscultation to assess the character of sounds created in various body organs.
- Perform a physical examination only after properly preparing the environment and equipment and preparing the patient physically and psychologically.
- Keep the patient warm, comfortable, and informed of each step of an examination. Ensure confidentiality.
- Be systematic while combining assessments of different body systems simultaneously.
- Information from the history helps to focus on body systems likely to be affected.
- Creating a mental image of internal organs in relation to external anatomical landmarks enhances accuracy in assessing the thorax, heart, and abdomen.
- When assessing heart sounds, imagine events occurring during the cardiac cycle.
- Never palpate the carotid arteries simultaneously.

- When examining a woman's breasts, explain the techniques for BSE.
- The abdominal assessment differs from other parts of the examination in that auscultation follows inspection.
- During assessment of the genitalia explain the technique for genital self-examination.
- Assess musculoskeletal function when observing a patient ambulate or participate in other active movements.
- Assess mental and emotional status by interacting with the patient throughout the examination.
- At the end of the examination provide for the patient's comfort and document a detailed summary of physical assessment findings.

REFLECTIVE LEARNING

- How did you practice cultural awareness when completing the health assessment on a patient you recently cared for?
- How did you prepare a patient mentally and physically for their health assessment examination today?
- When using your stethoscope to assess heart, lungs and abdomen, how did you differentiate between the various sounds heard?

REVIEW QUESTIONS

1. The nurse is conducting a skin assessment on a newly admitted patient. Which finding is consistent with the presence of edema?
   1. Bluish color around lips and nail beds
   2. Dandruff present when the skin is rubbed gently
   3. Hypopigmentation on the palms of bilateral hands
   4. Swollen bilateral lower extremities
2. When completing an abdominal assessment, which action should the nurse perform first?
   1. Palpate the large and small intestines.
   2. Assess for bowel sounds.
   3. Percuss gas within the four quadrants of the abdominal cavity.
   4. Focus on areas of pain.

3. Which statements describe accurate completion of a vascular assessment? (Select all that apply.)
   1. Simultaneously palpate the carotid arteries.
   2. Measure blood pressure.
   3. Ask about any pain, cramping, or discomfort in the legs.
   4. Count an irregular pulse for 30 seconds and multiply by 2.
   5. Rate the strength of a pulse of a scale of 0 to 4.
4. The nurse would encourage which female patient to have a mammogram?
   1. 53-year-old who had a mammogram completed 6 months ago
   2. 20-year-old with a positive family history of breast disease
   3. 41-year-old at an annual visit who has no complaints
   4. 32-year-old with no family history of breast cancer

5. A patient who has heart failure is complaining of shortness of breath. Which assessment finding is the nurse most concerned about?
   1. Moist crackles in the base of bilateral lungs
   2. Respiratory rate of 20
   3. 1+ edema in lower extremities
   4. Bronchovesicular sounds over posterior thorax

evolve

Additional Review Questions, as well as rationales for all Review Questions, can be found on the Evolve website.

1. 4; 2, 3; 3, 5; 4, 3; 5, 1.

REFERENCES

American Cancer Society (ACS): *Breast cancer early detection and diagnosis*, 2015. http://www.cancer.org/cancer/breastcancer/moreinformation/breastcancerearlydetection/breast-cancer-early-detection-acs-recs.

American Cancer Society (ACS): *Cancer facts and figures 2016*, 2016a. https://www.cancer.org/research/cancer-facts-statistics/all-cancer-facts-figures/cancer-facts-figures-2016.html.

American Cancer Society (ACS): *Risk factors for melanoma skin cancer*, 2016b. http://www.cancer.org/cancer/skincancer-melanoma/detailedguide/melanoma-skin-cancer-risk-factors.

American Cancer Society(ACS): *American Cancer Society recommendations for the early detection of breast cancer*, 2016c. https://www.cancer.org/cancer/breast-cancer/screening-tests-and-early-detection/american-cancer-society-recommendations-for-the-early-detection-of-breast-cancer.html.

American Cancer Society (ACS): *Recommendations for colorectal early detection: people at average risk*, 2017. https://www.cancer.org/cancer/colon-rectal-cancer/detection-diagnosis-staging/acs-recommendations.html.

American Diabetes Association: *Foot Care*, 2014. http://www.diabetes.org/living-with-diabetes/complications/foot-complications/foot-care.html.

American Heart Association (AHA): *The American Heart Association's diet and lifestyle recommendations*, 2015. http://www.heart.org/HEARTORG/HealthyLiving/HealthyEating/Nutrition/The-American-Heart-Associations-Diet-and-Lifestyle-Recommendations

_UCM_305855_Article.jsp#.WU0yoGjyuUk.

Ball JW, et al: *Seidel's guide to physical examination*, ed 8, St Louis, 2015, Elsevier.

Centers for Disease Control and Prevention: *Pneumococcal vaccines*, 2016. https://www.cdc.gov/vaccines/vpd/pneumo/index.html.

Evans C, et al: Diagnosis of elder abuse in U.S. emergency departments, *J Am Geriatr Soc* 65(1):91, 2017.

Grohskopf LA, et al: Prevention and control of seasonal influenza with vaccines: recommendations of the advisory committee on immunization practices—United States, 2016-2017, *MMWR Morb Mortal Wkly Rep* 65(5):1, 2016. https://www.cdc.gov/mmwr/volumes/65/rr/rr6505a1.htm.

Heckman CH, et al: An online skin cancer risk-reduction intervention for young adults: mechanisms of effects, *Health Psychol* 36(3):215, 2016.

Hockenberry MJ, et al: *Essentials of pediatric nursing*, ed 10, St Louis, 2017, Mosby.

McWhirter JE, Hoffman-Gomez L: Visual images for patient skin self-examination and melanoma detection: a systematic review of published studies, *J Am Acad Dermatol* 69(1):47, 2013.

National Cancer Institute (NCI): *NIH study confirms risk factors for male breast cancer*, 2014. https://www.cancer.gov/news-events/press-releases/2014/BreastCancerMalePoolingStudy.

National Institute on Drug Abuse (NIDA): *Screening, assessment, and drug testing resources*, 2014. https://www.drugabuse.gov/nidamed-medical-health-professionals/tool-resources-your-practice/additional-screening-resources.

National Institutes of Health (NIH): *Once is enough: a guide to preventing future fractures*, 2015. http://www.niams.nih.gov/Health_Info/bone/Osteoporosis/Fracture/default.asp.

Siu A, U.S. Preventive Services Task Force: Screening for breast cancer: U.S. Preventive Services Task Force Recommendation Statement, *Ann Intern Med* 164(4):279, 2016.

Skin Cancer Foundation: *Know your skin, save your life*, 2015, http://www.skincancer.org/publications/sun-and-skin-news/fall-2015-32-4/know.

Touhy T, Jett K: *Ebersole and Hess' gerontological nursing & healthy aging*, ed 5, St Louis, 2018, Mosby.

U.S. Preventive Services Task Force (USPSTF): Screening for skin cancer. U.S. Preventive Services Task Force Recommendation statement, *JAMA* 316(4):429, 2016.

U.S. Preventive Services Task Force (USPSTF): *Skin cancer prevention: behavioral counseling*, 2017. https://www.uspreventiveservicestaskforce.org/Page/Document/UpdateSummaryDraft/skin-cancer-counseling2?ds=1&s=counseling%20to%20prevent%20skin%20cancer.

U.S. Public Health Service (USPHS): *Surgeon general call to action to prevent skin cancer*, 2014. http://www.surgeongeneral.gov/library/calls/prevent-skin-cancer/call-to-action-prevent-skin-cancer.pdf.

World Health Organization (WHO): *The World Health Assembly endorses the global plan of action on violence against women and girls, and also against children*, 2017. http://www.who.int/reproductivehealth/topics/violence/action-plan-endorsement/en/.

Medication Administration

evolve MEDIA RESOURCES

http://evolve.elsevier.com/Potter/essentials

- Audio Glossary
- QSEN Activity and Review Questions Answers and Rationales
- Video Clips

OBJECTIVES

- Identify the characteristics of adverse drug events.
- Discuss nursing roles and responsibilities in medication administration.
- Compare and contrast the roles of the health care provider, pharmacist, and nurse in medication administration.
- Discuss legal responsibilities in medication administration.
- Compare and contrast the different types of medication effects and reactions.
- Discuss factors that influence medication actions.

- Discuss factors to include in assessing a patient's needs for and response to medication therapy.
- Implement nursing actions to prevent medication errors.
- Describe factors to consider when choosing routes of medication administration.
- Calculate prescribed medication doses correctly.
- List the six rights of medication administration and apply them in clinical practice.
- Discuss methods used to educate patients and family caregivers about prescribed medications.
- Correctly and safely prepare and administer medications.

KEY TERMS

absorption, p. 383

adverse drug effects (ADEs), p. 384

anaphylactic reactions, p. 385

biotransformation, p. 383

buccal, p. 387

detoxify, p. 383

idiosyncratic reaction, p. 385

infusions, p. 390

injection, p. 383

instillation, p. 389

intradermal (ID), p. 387

intramuscular (IM), p. 389

intraocular, p. 389

intravenous (IV), p. 389

irrigations, p. 390

medication error, p. 398

medication interaction, p. 386

medication reconciliation, p. 399

medication tolerance, p. 385

metric system, p. 389

minimum effective concentration (MEC), p. 386

motivational interviewing (MI), p. 408

Nurse Practice Acts (NPAs), p. 380

ophthalmic medications, p. 416

parenteral administration, p. 387

peak, p. 386

pharmacokinetics, p. 383

polypharmacy, p. 410

prescriptions, p. 389

pressurized metered-dose inhalers (pMDIs), p. 421

side effects, p. 384

six rights of medication administration, p. 401

solution, p. 390

subcutaneous, p. 387

sublingual, p. 387

synergistic effect, p. 386

therapeutic effect, p. 384

therapeutic range, p. 386

toxic effects, p. 385

transdermal disk, p. 389

trough, p. 386

verbal order, p. 394

Z-track method, p. 432

CASE STUDY *Esther Simmons*

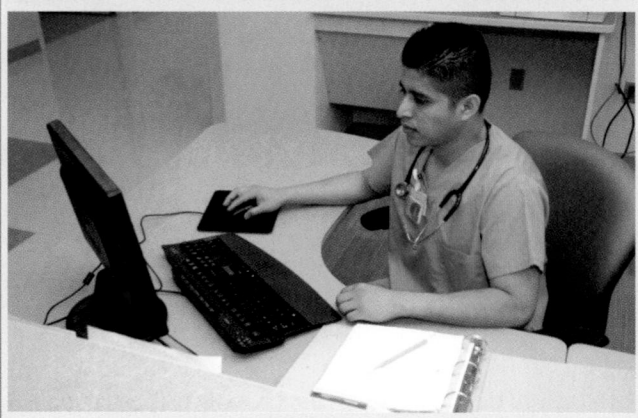

Esther Simmons is an 85-year-old woman who lives in her home. She is on a skilled care floor in a hospital following hip replacement surgery. Esther's strength and mobility are improving, and she is planning to return home with home care nursing within the week.

Emilio Fernandez is a 31-year-old nursing student who is assigned to care for Esther today. While reviewing the medical record, Emilio finds that Ms. Simmons has several chronic illnesses including diabetes mellitus, heart disease, hypertension, and arthritis. To manage these illnesses successfully, Esther needs to take several different medications on a routine basis. Several of her medications have changed, and several have been added since she was admitted. Based on this assessment, Emilio determines that it will be important to provide instruction and support so that Ms. Simmons can administer her medications safely at home.

Patients with health problems use a variety of methods to restore or maintain their health. One method is the use of medication, a substance used in the diagnosis, treatment, cure, relief, or prevention of health problems. Regardless of where patients receive health care (e.g., hospitals, clinics, home), nurses play an essential role in assessing for factors that place patients at risk when receiving medications and in preparing, administering, and evaluating the effects of medications. Family caregivers, friends, or home care personnel often administer medications when patients cannot perform this task at home. Nurses are also responsible for teaching a patient and family caregiver about medications and their side effects, helping patients adopt practices for adhering to their medication regimen, and evaluating the ability of a patient and family caregiver to administer medications.

SCIENTIFIC KNOWLEDGE BASE

Medication administration and evaluation are critical nursing responsibilities, so nurses must understand the actions and effects of all medications they give their patients. To safely and accurately administer medications, you need to have an understanding of the legal aspects of medication administration, pharmacokinetics (the movement of drugs in the human body), life sciences, anatomy, pathophysiology, and mathematics.

Medication Legislation and Standards

Federal Regulations. The U.S. government protects the health of citizens by ensuring that medications are safe and effective. The first Pure Food and Drug Act required that all medications be free of impure products. Later legislation set standards for safety, potency, and efficacy of medications. The Food and Drug Administration (FDA) currently enforces medication laws. These laws ensure that all medications undergo vigorous testing before they are sold to the public. Federal laws also control medication sales and distribution, testing, naming, labeling, and use of controlled substances.

Official publications such as the *United States Pharmacopeia* (USP) and the *National Formulary* set standards for medication strength, quality, purity, packaging, safety, labeling, and dose form. In 1993 the FDA instituted the MedWatch program. This voluntary program encourages nurses and other health care professionals to report any incident in which a medication, product, or medical event causes serious harm to a patient. Health care professionals report the incident by completing the MedWatch form. This form is available on the MedWatch website (FDA, 2016).

State and Local Regulation of Medication. State and local medication laws must conform to federal laws. States often have more laws including control of substances not regulated by the federal government. Local governmental bodies regulate the use of alcohol and tobacco.

Health Care Agencies and Medication Laws. Health care agencies set individual policies to meet federal, state, and local regulations. The size of the agency, the services it provides, and the professional personnel it employs affect these policies. Agency policies often are more restrictive than governmental controls. For example, a common agency policy is the automatic discontinuation of narcotics after a set number of days. A health care provider can reorder the narcotic if necessary. This policy helps to prevent unnecessarily prolonged medication therapy because it requires the health care provider to regularly review the need for the medication.

Medication Regulations and Nursing Practice. State Nurse Practice Acts (NPAs) define the scope of nurses' professional functions and responsibilities. The primary intent of NPAs is to protect the public from unskilled, undereducated, and unlicensed nurses. Most NPAs are intentionally broad to avoid limiting nurses' professional responsibilities. Health care agencies can interpret specific actions allowed under NPAs, but they cannot modify, expand, or restrict the intent of an act.

You are responsible as a nurse for following legal provisions when administering controlled substances such as opioids, which are controlled by federal and state guidelines. Nurses who violate the Controlled Substances Act face fines,

| BOX 17.1 | GUIDELINES FOR SAFE OPIOID (NARCOTIC) ADMINISTRATION AND CONTROL |

- Store all narcotics in a locked, secure cabinet or container (e.g., computerized locked cabinets are preferred).
- Maintain a running count of opioids by counting them whenever dispensing them. If you find a discrepancy, correct the error if possible and report it immediately.
- Use a special inventory record each time a narcotic is dispensed. Records are often kept electronically and provide an accurate ongoing count of narcotics used, wasted, and remaining.
- Use the record to document the patient's name, date, time of medication administration, name of medication, and dosage. Documentation also includes the name of the nurse dispensing and administering the medication.
- A second nurse witnesses disposal of the unused part if a nurse gives only part of a dose of a controlled substance. Ensure documentation includes the names of the nurses wasting the unused portion of the medication.
- Follow agency policy for appropriate waste of controlled substances. Do not place wasted parts of medications in sharps containers.

imprisonment, and loss of licensure. Hospitals and other health care agencies have policies for the proper storage and distribution of controlled substances (Box 17.1).

Nontherapeutic Medication Use

Medication misuse includes overuse, underuse, erratic use, and contraindicated use of medications. Patients of all ages misuse medications. Some people use them for purposes other than their intended effect. Factors such as peer pressure, curiosity, and the pursuit of pleasure are some motivators for nontherapeutic medication use. Results from the 2014 National Survey on Drug Use and Health indicated that approximately 15 million people 12 years of age or older were using prescription drugs nonmedically (Substance Abuse and Mental Health Services Administration [SAMSHA], 2015a). This issue is a growing national problem in the United States. Prescription drugs are misused and abused more often than any other drug except marijuana and alcohol (SAMSHA, 2015b). This growth is fueled by misperceptions about prescription drug safety and increasing availability. Medication misuse is not limited to heroin, cocaine, and other illegal drugs. The most commonly abused prescription medications include opioids such as hydrocodone (Vicodin) and oxycodone hydrochloride (Oxycontin), stimulants for treating attention-deficit/hyperactivity disorder (ADHD) such as amphetamine and dextroamphetamine (Adderall) and methylphenidate (Ritalin), and central nervous system (CNS) depressants for relieving anxiety such as diazepam (Valium) or alprazolam (Xanax) (National Institutes of Health National Institute on Drug Abuse [NIH NIDA], 2015). Common

over-the-counter (OTC) medications that patients misuse or abuse include cough syrup and cold medication containing dextromethorphan (NIH NIDA, 2015).

Pharmacological Concepts

Medication Names. Some medications have three different names: chemical, generic, and trade. The chemical name of a medication gives an exact description of its chemical composition and molecular structure. Nurses rarely use chemical names in clinical practice. The manufacturer who creates the medication gives the generic or nonproprietary name. However, the name requires United States Adopted Names (USAN) Council approval (American Medical Association [AMA], 2016). Each drug has only one generic name. The generic name is not as complex as a chemical name, and it becomes the official name listed in publications such as the *United States Pharmacopeia* (USP). The trade name, brand name, or proprietary name is the name under which a manufacturer markets a medication. The trade name has the trademark symbol (™) at the upper right of the name, indicating that the manufacturer has trademarked the name of the medication. The following is an example of the different names of a common medication:

- Chemical name: *N*-acetyl-para-aminophenol
- Generic name: Acetaminophen
- Trade names: Panadol™, Tempra™, Tylenol™

Manufacturers create trade names that are easy to pronounce, spell, and remember. Trade names are approved by the FDA so that no two trade names are too similar. However, because many companies produce the same medication, similarities in trade names are still often confusing and can result in a medication error. For example, confusing names include Adderall versus Inderal and clonazepam versus lorazepam. Therefore, obtain the exact name and spelling for each medication you administer to your patients. For a full list of medications that are often confused with one another go to the Institute for Safe Medication Practices (ISMP) website at https://www.ismp.org/tools/confuseddrugnames.pdf (ISMP, 2015a). The ISMP (2016a) has posted the use of FDA-approved tall man (upper case) or mixed-case letters when possible (e.g., aMILoride versus amLODIPine). The recommended, **bolded** tall man (uppercase) letters help nurses recognize the dissimilarities in look-alike drug names.

Classification. Medications with similar characteristics are grouped into classifications. Medication classifications identify the effect a medication has on a body system, the symptoms a medication relieves, or the desired effect of a medication. Sometimes the last syllables of a generic name indicate the medication classification. For example, the syllables *-olol* at the end of *propranolol* tell you that this medication is in the beta-adrenergic blocker classification. Usually each class contains more than one medication that health care providers can prescribe for a type of health problem. For example, patients who have asthma often take a variety of medications from the class of beta$_2$-adrenergic agonists. Other medications are sometimes found in more than one

TABLE 17.1 FORMS OF MEDICATION

FORM	DESCRIPTION
Medication Forms Commonly Prepared for Administration by Oral Route	
Solid Forms	
Caplet	Solid dosage form for oral use; shaped like capsule and coated for ease of swallowing
Capsule	Medication encased in gelatin shell
Tablet	Powdered medication compressed into hard disk or cylinder; in addition to primary medication, contains binders (adhesive to allow powder to stick together), disintegrators (to promote tablet dissolution), lubricants (for ease of manufacturing), and fillers (for convenient tablet size)
Enteric-coated tablet	Coated tablet that does not dissolve in stomach; coatings dissolve in intestine, where medication is absorbed
Liquid Forms	
Elixir	Clear fluid containing water and/or alcohol; often sweetened
Extract	Concentrated medication form made by removing the active part of medication from its other components
Aqueous solution	Substance dissolved in water and syrups
Aqueous suspension	Finely dissolved drug particles dispersed in liquid medium; when suspension is left standing, particles settle to bottom of container
Syrup	Medication dissolved in concentrated sugar solution
Other Oral Forms and Terms Associated With Oral Preparations	
Troche (lozenge)	Flat, round tablets that dissolve in the mouth to release medication; not meant for ingestion
Aerosol	Aqueous medication sprayed and absorbed in the mouth and upper airway; not meant for ingestion
Sustained release	Tablet or capsule that contains small particles of a medication coated with material that requires a varying amount of time to dissolve
Medication Forms Commonly Prepared for Administration by Topical Route	
Ointment (salve or cream)	Semisolid, externally applied preparation, usually containing one or more medications
Liniment	Usually contains alcohol, oil, or soapy emollient applied to skin
Lotion	Semiliquid suspension that usually protects, cools, or cleanses skin
Paste	Thick ointment; absorbed through skin more slowly than ointment; often used for skin protection
Transdermal disk or patch	Medicated disk or patch absorbed through skin slowly over long period of time (e.g., 24 hours)
Medication Forms Commonly Prepared for Administration by Parenteral Route	
Solution	Sterile preparation that contains water with one or more dissolved compounds
Powder	Sterile particles of medication that are dissolved in a sterile liquid (e.g., water, normal saline) before administration
Medication Forms Commonly Prepared for Instillation Into Body Cavities	
Intraocular disk	Small, flexible oval (similar to contact lens) consisting of two soft, outer layers and a middle layer containing medication; slowly releases medication when moistened by ocular fluid
Suppository	Solid dosage form mixed with gelatin and shaped in form of pellet for insertion into body cavity (rectum or vagina); melts when it reaches body temperature, releasing medication for absorption

class. For example, aspirin is an analgesic, an antipyretic, and an antiinflammatory medication.

Medication Forms. Medications come in a variety of forms or preparations. The form of the medication determines its route of administration. The form of a medication is intended to improve its absorption and metabolism. Many medications come in several forms such as tablets, capsules, elixirs, and suppositories. When you administer a medication, be certain to use the proper form (Table 17.1).

Pharmacokinetics as the Basis of Medication Actions

For a medication to be therapeutically useful, it is taken into a patient's body; is absorbed and distributed to cells, tissues, or a specific organ; and alters physiological functions.

Pharmacokinetics is the study of four major processes: medication absorption, distribution, metabolism, and excretion. You use knowledge of pharmacokinetics when you time medication administration, select the route of administration, and evaluate a patient's response.

Absorption.
Absorption is the movement of medication molecules into the blood from the site of medication administration. Factors that affect absorption are the route of administration, ability of the medication to dissolve, blood flow to the site of administration, body surface area (BSA), and lipid solubility of medication.

Route of Administration. Each route of medication administration has a different rate of absorption. The routes of administration, ranked in order from slowest to fastest, are:

- Topical application to the skin has slow absorption because of the physical makeup of the skin.
- Orally administered medications pass through the gastrointestinal (GI) tract, so the rate of absorption is slow.
- Medications placed on the mucous membranes and respiratory airways are absorbed quickly because these tissues contain many blood vessels.
- Intramuscular (IM) and subcutaneous medications absorb more quickly than oral medications, with medications in IM injections entering the bloodstream more quickly than medications in subcutaneous injections.
- Intravenous (IV) injection produces the most rapid absorption because medications are available immediately when they enter the systemic circulation.

Ability of a Medication to Dissolve. The ability of an oral medication to dissolve depends mostly on its form or preparation. The body absorbs solutions and suspensions more readily than tablets or capsules. Acidic medications pass through the gastric mucosa rapidly. Medications that are basic are not absorbed before reaching the small intestine.

Blood Flow to the Site of Administration. The blood supply at the site of administration determines how quickly the body absorbs a drug. Medications are absorbed as blood comes into contact with the site of administration. The richer the blood supply at the site of administration, the faster a medication is absorbed.

Body Surface Area. The size of the surface that a medication comes in contact with affects how quickly the body absorbs the medication. When a medication comes in contact with a large surface area, it is absorbed at a faster rate. This explains why most oral medications are absorbed in the small intestine and not in the stomach (Burchum and Rosenthal, 2016).

Lipid Solubility. Because the cell membrane has a lipid layer, highly lipid-soluble medications cross cell membranes easily and are absorbed quickly. Another factor that often affects medication absorption is whether the stomach contains food. Some oral medications are absorbed more easily when administered between meals. This is because food changes the structure of a medication and sometimes impairs its absorption. When some medications are administered together, they interfere with one another, impairing the absorption of both medications.

To safely administer medications, you need to know the factors that alter or impair absorption of prescribed medications. Use your knowledge and confer with a pharmacist to choose medication administration times that will promote optimal absorption. For example, administer medications as prescribed before or after meals so that the medications will not interact with food. When medications interact with one another, make sure that you avoid giving them at the same time.

Distribution.
After a medication is absorbed, it is distributed within the body to tissues and organs and ultimately to its specific site of action. The rate and extent of distribution depend on the physical and chemical properties of the medication and the physiology of the person taking it.

Circulation. Once a medication enters the bloodstream, the blood carries it throughout the tissues and organs of the body. How fast it reaches the intended site depends on the vascularity of the various tissues and organs. Conditions that limit blood flow or blood perfusion inhibit the distribution of a medication. For example, patients with heart failure have impaired circulation, which slows medication delivery to the intended site of action.

Membrane Permeability. Membrane permeability is the ability of tissues and membranes to allow a medication to pass through and enter target cells. To be distributed to an organ, a medication must pass through all of the tissues and biological membranes of that organ. Some membranes serve as barriers to the passage of medications. For example, the blood–brain barrier allows only fat-soluble medications to pass into the brain and cerebrospinal fluid. Thus CNS infections often require antibiotics to be injected directly into the subarachnoid space in the spinal cord. Some older adults experience adverse effects as a result of the change in the permeability of the blood–brain barrier, with easier passage of fat-soluble medications.

Protein Binding. The degree to which medications bind to serum proteins such as albumin reduces their distribution. Most medications partially bind to albumin, reducing the drug's pharmacological activity. The unbound or "free" medication is its active form. Older adults and patients with liver disease or malnutrition have decreased albumin in the bloodstream. Because more medication is unbound in these patients, they are at risk for an increase in medication activity, toxicity, or both.

Metabolism.
After a medication reaches its site of action, it becomes metabolized into a less active or an inactive form that is easier to excrete. Biotransformation occurs under the influence of enzymes that detoxify, break down, and remove biologically active chemicals. Most biotransformation occurs within the liver, although the lungs, kidneys, blood, and intestines also metabolize medications. The liver is especially important because it oxidizes and transforms many toxic substances. The liver degrades many harmful chemicals before

they become distributed to the tissues. If a decrease in liver function occurs such as with aging or liver disease, a medication is usually eliminated more slowly, resulting in its accumulation. Patients are at risk for medication toxicity if organs that metabolize medications are not functioning correctly.

Excretion. After medications are metabolized, they exit the body through the kidneys, liver, bowel, lungs, and exocrine glands. The chemical makeup of a medication determines the organ of excretion. The kidneys are the main organs that excrete medications. Some medications escape metabolism and exit unchanged in the urine. Others undergo biotransformation in the liver before the kidneys excrete them. If renal function declines, a patient is at risk for medication toxicity. If the kidney cannot adequately excrete a medication, it becomes necessary for the health care provider to reduce the dose. Maintaining an adequate fluid intake (50 mL/kg/day) promotes proper medication elimination for an average adult.

Gaseous and volatile compounds such as nitrous oxide and alcohol exit through the lungs. Deep breathing and coughing (see Chapter 40) help patients eliminate anesthetic gases more rapidly after surgery. The exocrine glands excrete lipid-soluble medications. When medications exit through sweat glands, the skin often becomes irritated, requiring you to teach patients good hygiene practices (see Chapter 31).

The GI tract is another route for medication excretion. The liver breaks down medications that enter the hepatic circulation and excretes them into the bile. After chemicals enter the intestines through the biliary tract, the intestines reabsorb them. Factors that increase peristalsis (e.g., laxatives and enemas) accelerate medication excretion through the feces, whereas factors that slow peristalsis (e.g., inactivity and improper diet) often prolong the effects of a medication.

Types of Medication Action

A variety of factors affect medication actions (Box 17.2). Understand that patients do not always respond in the same way to each successive dose of a medication. Sometimes the same medication causes very different responses in different patients.

Therapeutic Effects. Each medication has a **therapeutic effect**, the intended or desired physiological response of a medication. For example, you administer morphine sulfate, an analgesic, to relieve a patient's pain. Sometimes a single medication has many therapeutic effects. For example, prednisone, a steroid, decreases swelling, inhibits inflammation, reduces allergic responses, and prevents rejection of transplanted organs. Knowing the desired therapeutic effect for each medication allows you to accurately evaluate its desired effect.

Adverse Drug Effects. **Adverse drug effects (ADEs)** are unintended, undesirable, and often unpredictable responses to medication. Although ADEs are sometimes seen immediately, they often take weeks or months to develop. Early

> ### BOX 17.2   FACTORS INFLUENCING MEDICATION ACTIONS
>
> **GENETIC DIFFERENCES**
> - A person's genetic makeup influences drug metabolism. Family members may have similar reactions to the same medication.
>
> **PHYSIOLOGICAL VARIABLES**
> - Gender, age, body weight, nutritional status, and illnesses influence drug effects.
> - Hormonal differences between men and women affect drug metabolism.
> - Children usually require lower drug doses than adults.
> - Changes accompanying aging influence drug effects.
> - There is a direct relationship between the concentration of a medication administered and how quickly it is absorbed by tissues.
>
> **ENVIRONMENTAL CONDITIONS**
> - Stress and exposure to heat and cold affect drug actions.
> - The setting in which a person takes a drug influences a patient's reaction. For example, when patients are alone or isolated, they may need more pain medication than if they were in a room with other patients.
>
> **PSYCHOLOGICAL FACTORS**
> - Attitudes, beliefs about the meaning of a drug, and perceptions of a nurse's behaviors can affect drug actions. Assess these factors in each patient. While administering drugs demonstrate supportive behaviors and provide relevant instruction.
>
> **DIET**
> - Medication and nutrient interactions alter the action of a drug. For example, mineral oil decreases absorption of fat-soluble vitamins.
> - Proper drug metabolism requires healthy nutritional levels.

clinical recognition of ADEs is the important first step in identification. ADEs range from mild (e.g., rashes or photosensitivity to light) to potentially fatal (anaphylaxis). Prompt recognition and reporting of ADEs prevents serious injury to patients. Although some patients such as pregnant women, very young patients, and patients with chronic disorders (e.g., hypertension, epilepsy, heart disease, psychoses) are at a higher risk, assess all your patients for ADEs (Burchum and Rosenthal, 2016). Health care providers report adverse effects to the FDA using the MedWatch program (FDA, 2016).

Side Effects. Every medication has the potential for harm. No medication is totally safe and absolutely free of nontherapeutic effects. **Side effects** are predictable and often unavoidable secondary effects produced at a usual therapeutic drug dose. Side effects either are harmless or cause injury. The intensity of side effects is often dose dependent. If the side effects are serious enough to outweigh the benefits of the therapeutic action of a medication, the health care provider will likely discontinue the medication. Patients

TABLE 17.2 MILD ALLERGIC REACTIONS

SYMPTOM	DESCRIPTION
Urticaria (hives)	Raised, irregularly shaped skin eruptions with varying sizes and shapes; eruptions have reddened margins and pale centers
Rash	Small, raised vesicles that are usually reddened; often distributed over entire body
Pruritus	Itching of skin; accompanies most rashes
Rhinitis	Inflammation of mucous membranes lining nose; causes swelling and clear, watery discharge

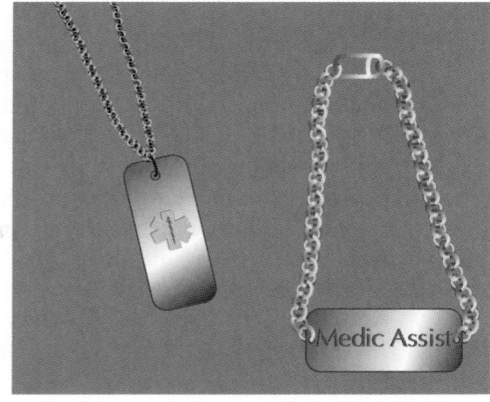

FIG 17.1 Identification bracelet and medal.

commonly stop taking medications because of side effects such as anorexia, nausea, vomiting, dizziness, drowsiness, dry mouth, constipation, and diarrhea. Report any side effect to the health care provider to ensure that it is not incorrectly interpreted as a more serious adverse medication reaction.

Toxic Effects. Toxic effects develop after prolonged intake of a medication or when a medication accumulates in the blood because of impaired metabolism or excretion. Excess amounts of a medication within the body can have lethal effects, depending on the action of the medication. For example, a toxic level of morphine, an opioid, causes severe respiratory depression and death. Antidotes are available to treat specific types of medication toxicity. For example, naloxone, an opioid antagonist, reverses the effects of opioid toxicity.

Idiosyncratic Reactions. An idiosyncratic reaction is an unpredictable effect, in which a patient overreacts or under-reacts to a medication or has a reaction different from normal. Predicting which patients will have an idiosyncratic response is impossible. For example, lorazepam is an antianxiety medication that may cause agitation and delirium when given to an older adult.

Allergic Reactions. Allergic reactions also are adverse unpredictable responses to a medication. Exposure to an initial dose of a medication causes a patient to become sensitized immunologically. The medication acts as an antigen, which causes antibodies to be produced. With repeated administration a patient develops an allergic response to the drug, its chemical preservatives, or a metabolite. An allergic reaction ranges from mild to severe, depending on the patient and the medication (Table 17.2). Among the different classes of medications, antibiotics cause a high incidence of allergic reactions. Severe or anaphylactic reactions, which are life threatening, are characterized by sudden constriction of bronchiolar muscles, edema of the pharynx and larynx, severe wheezing, and shortness of breath. Some patients become severely hypotensive, necessitating emergency measures.

Hospitalized patients with known drug allergies commonly have their allergy information recorded in a clearly identifiable place. This allows all caregivers to be aware of each patient's allergies. In many health care agencies this information is recorded in a special section of the electronic health record (EHR), on the front of a patient's hard-copy medical record or chart, in the medication administration record (MAR), or on a specially designed label that is applied to the front of a patient's chart. Patients also receive color-coded allergy identification bands to wear around the wrist. *Always record a patient's allergies in the MAR.* Patients who are cared for in other settings (e.g., home or community clinics) and have a known history of an allergy to a medication or substance should wear an identification bracelet or medal, which alerts all health care providers to the allergies in case a patient is found unconscious or is unable to communicate (Fig. 17.1). Patients commonly list having an allergy to a drug when it is not a true allergy but rather a side effect or ADE. For example, nausea is most often a side effect, whereas hives is a common allergic reaction. It is important to be aware of the difference between a true allergy and a side effect. Ask a patient to describe in detail what type of reactions he or she has experienced.

Medication Tolerance and Dependence. Medication tolerance occurs over time. It is usually noted clinically when patients receive more and more medication (higher doses) to achieve the same therapeutic effect (Bartlett et al., 2013). Medications that produce tolerance include opium alkaloids (e.g., morphine), nitrates, and ethyl alcohol. Patients hospitalized for acute illnesses usually do not develop tolerance. It may take a month or longer for tolerance to occur.

Medication tolerance is not the same as medication dependence. Two types of medication dependence (addiction) exist: physical or psychological. In psychological dependence a patient desires the medication for benefit other than the intended effect. Physical dependence is a physiological adaptation to a medication that manifests by intense physical disturbance when the medication is withdrawn. Dependence is rare when patients receive medications for a short time such as for postoperative pain. If a patient is dependent on alcohol, a higher-than-usual medication dose is necessary for the desired effect of the medication.

Nurses and other health care providers play an important role in the care of patients with drug addictions. When patients with addiction are approached by health care providers with disdain and rejection, no matter how subtly, they may reject the care offered. Negative behaviors such as these may result in a missed opportunity for a person who is addicted to learn about important treatments. Incorporating harm reduction strategies and evidence-based interventions in the care of patients with addiction can help them get the care and treatment they need (Bartlett et al., 2013).

Medication Interactions. In a medication interaction, one medication modifies the action of another. Medication interactions are common in individuals who take several medications. Some medications increase or reduce the action of others or alter the way another medication is absorbed, metabolized, or eliminated from the body. In a synergistic effect, the combined effect of two medications is greater than the effects when given separately. For example, alcohol is a CNS depressant that has a synergistic effect on antihistamines, antidepressants, barbiturates, and narcotic analgesics.

Sometimes a medication interaction is desirable. Health care providers order a combination of medications to create an interaction beneficial for the patient. For example, a patient with high blood pressure might take several medications such as diuretics and vasodilators that act together to reduce blood pressure when one medication is not effective.

Medication Dose Responses

A medication undergoes absorption, distribution, metabolism, and excretion after administration. Medications take time to enter the bloodstream except when administered intravenously. When a medication is prescribed, the goal is a constant blood level within a safe therapeutic range. The minimum effective concentration (MEC) is the plasma level of a medication below which the effect of the medication does not occur. The toxic concentration is the level at which toxic effects occur. The safe therapeutic range is between the MEC and the toxic concentration (Fig. 17.2). When a medication is administered repeatedly, its serum level fluctuates between doses. The highest level is called the *peak concentration,* and the lowest level is called the *trough concentration.* After peaking, the serum concentration falls progressively. With IV infusions, the peak concentration occurs quickly, but the serum level also begins to fall immediately. Some antibiotic doses (e.g., vancomycin or gentamicin) are based on peak and trough serum levels. To determine a peak and trough level, a blood sample is collected 30 minutes before administering the drug (trough) and at the time when the drug is expected to reach its peak concentration (peak). The results of the blood test reveal if the drug is reaching its therapeutic blood level.

All medications have a biological half-life, which is the time it takes for excretion processes to lower the serum medication concentration by half. To maintain a therapeutic plateau, a patient needs to receive regular fixed doses. For example,

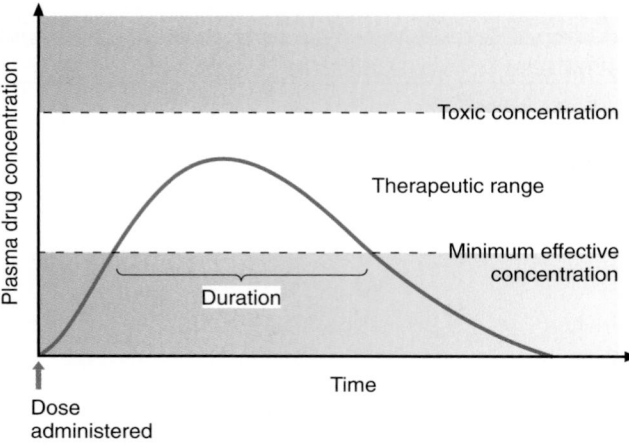

FIG 17.2 Single-dose time course for an oral medication.

pain medications are most effective for some patients with cancer when they are given around the clock rather than when a patient intermittently complains of pain because the body maintains an almost constant level of pain medication (Burchum and Rosenthal, 2016). After an initial medication dose, the patient receives each successive dose when the previous dose reaches its half-life. The patient and nurse need to follow regular dosage schedules and administer prescribed doses at correct intervals. Know the following time intervals of medication action to anticipate the effect of a medication:

- *Onset of medication action:* Period of time it takes after you administer a medication for it to produce a therapeutic effect.
- *Peak action:* Time it takes for a medication to reach its highest effective peak concentration.
- *Trough:* Minimum blood serum concentration of medication reached just before the next scheduled dose.
- *Duration of action:* Length of time during which a medication is present in a concentration great enough to produce a therapeutic effect.
- *Plateau:* Blood serum concentration reached and maintained after repeated, fixed doses.

You and your patient follow prescribed doses and dosage intervals (Table 17.3). Health care agencies usually set schedules for medication administration. However, you can change this schedule based on your knowledge about a medication. For example, you work at an agency where medications ordered once a day are given at 0800. Your patient has a medication ordered once a day that works better when given before bedtime; therefore you adjust the time to give the medication accordingly. Acute care agencies also follow guidelines from the ISMP to determine safe, effective, and timely administration of medications (Centers for Medicare and Medicaid Services [CMS], 2011; ISMP, 2011a). According to the guidelines, hospitals determine if medications are time-critical. Medications that are time-critical most likely cause harm or have subtherapeutic effects if they are not administered on time (usually 30 minutes before or after the

TABLE 17.3	COMMON DOSAGE ADMINISTRATION SCHEDULES
DOSAGE SCHEDULE	**ABBREVIATION**
Before meals	AC, ac
Twice each day	BID, bid
After meals	PC, pc
Whenever there is a need	prn
Every morning, every a.m.	q am
Every hour	qh
Every day	Daily
Every 4 hours	Q4h
4 times per day	QID, qid
Give immediately	STAT, stat
3 times per day	TID, tid

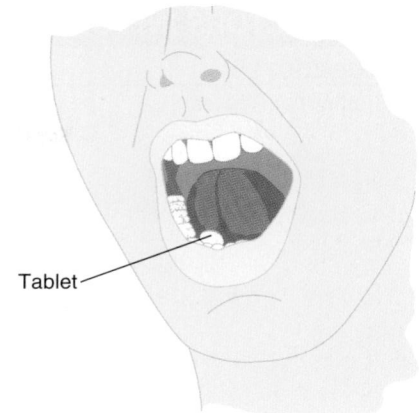

FIG 17.3 Sublingual administration of tablet.

QSEN QSEN ACTIVITY *Evidence-Based Practice*

You are a member of the shared governance practice council in your hospital. The practice council is investigating evidence-based practices to reduce medication errors. The chairperson explains to the committee that evidence-based practice changes are based on the current best evidence, resources, nursing expertise, and patient preferences. One of the nurses asks, "How can we ensure that patient preferences are respected when we administer medications?"
• How would you respond?

evolve Answers to QSEN Activities can be found on the Evolve website.

scheduled dose). Non–time-critical medications most likely do not cause harm if they are given within 1 to 2 hours before or after the scheduled time. Thus you need to administer time-critical medications at a precise time, within 30 minutes before or after their scheduled time. You administer non–time-critical medications within 1 to 2 hours of their scheduled time. Ensure that you follow your agency medication policies about the timing of medications to ensure that your patients receive their medications at the right time (CMS, 2011; ISMP, 2011a).

When you teach patients about dosage schedules, use familiar language. For example, when teaching a patient about twice-daily medication dosing, instruct him or her to take the medication in the morning and again in the evening.

Routes of Administration

The route prescribed for administering a medication depends on its properties and desired effect and on a patient's physical and mental condition. Because of what you know about each patient, you need to collaborate with a health care provider in determining the best route for a patient's medical condition. Table 17.4 summarizes the factors that influence the choice of administration routes.

Oral Routes. The oral route is the easiest and the most frequent route of medication administration. Medications are given by mouth and swallowed with fluid. Oral medications have a slower onset of action and a more prolonged effect than parenteral medications. Patients generally prefer the oral route.

Sublingual Administration. Sublingual medications (e.g., nitroglycerin, certain enzymes) are readily absorbed when placed under the tongue to dissolve (Fig. 17.3). The area under the tongue is highly vascular, making absorption rapid. Instruct patients not to swallow a **sublingual** medication or

drink anything until the medication is completely dissolved to ensure that the medication will produce the desired effect. A sublingual medication may also be ordered if the effects will be lessened during the digestion process. The drug is not metabolized through the liver, and thus a lower dose can be used.

Buccal Administration. A medication is administered by the **buccal** route by placing the solid medication in the mouth against the mucous membranes of the cheek until it dissolves. The cheek is very vascular. Teach patients to alternate cheeks with each subsequent dose to avoid mucosal irritation. Warn patients not to chew or swallow the medication or to take any liquids with it. A buccal medication acts locally on the mucosa or systemically as it is swallowed in a person's saliva.

Parenteral Routes. In **parenteral administration,** you inject a medication into body tissues and not by the GI tract. The four major sites of injection are as follows:
• **Intradermal (ID):** Injection into the dermis just under the epidermis.
• **Subcutaneous:** Injection into tissues just below the dermis of the skin.

TABLE 17.4   FACTORS INFLUENCING CHOICE OF ADMINISTRATION ROUTES

ADVANTAGES OF ROUTE	DISADVANTAGES/CONTRAINDICATIONS
Oral, Buccal, Sublingual Routes	
Convenient and comfortable	Oral route is avoided when patient has alterations in GI function (e.g.,
Economical	nausea, vomiting), reduced GI motility (after general anesthesia or
Easy to administer	bowel inflammation), and surgical resection of GI tract.
Often produce local or systemic effects	Oral route is contraindicated in patients unable to swallow (e.g.,
Rarely cause anxiety for patient	patients with neuromuscular disorders, esophageal strictures, mouth
	lesions) and patients who are unconscious, confused, or unable or
	unwilling to swallow or hold medication under tongue.
	Oral medications cannot be administered when patients have gastric
	suction and are contraindicated before some tests or surgery.
	Oral medications sometimes irritate lining of GI tract, discolor teeth, or
	have unpleasant taste.
	Gastric secretions destroy some medications.
Parenteral Routes (Subcutaneous, IM, IV, ID)	
Can be used when oral medications are	There is risk of introducing infection.
contraindicated	Some parenteral medications are expensive.
More rapid absorption than with topical or oral	Some patients experience pain from repeated needlesticks.
routes	Subcutaneous, IM, and ID routes are avoided in patients with bleeding
IV infusion provides medication delivery when	tendencies.
patient is critically ill or long-term therapy is	There is risk of tissue damage.
necessary; if peripheral perfusion is poor	IM and IV routes have higher absorption rates, placing patient at higher
IV route preferred over injections	risk for reactions.
	They often cause considerable anxiety in many patients, especially
	children.
Topical Routes	
Skin	
Primarily provides local effect	Patients with skin abrasions are at risk for rapid medication absorption
Painless	and systemic effects.
Limited side effects	Medications are absorbed through skin slowly.
Transdermal	
Prolonged systemic effects with limited side	Medication leaves oily or pasty substance on skin and sometimes soils
effects	clothing.
Mucous Membranes[a]	
Therapeutic effects provided by local application	Mucous membranes are highly sensitive to some medication
to involved sites	concentrations.
Aqueous solutions readily absorbed and capable	Patients with ruptured eardrum cannot receive ear irrigations.
of causing systemic effects	Insertion of rectal and vaginal medication often causes embarrassment.
Potential route of administration when oral	Rectal suppositories are contraindicated if patient has had rectal
medications are contraindicated	surgery or if active rectal bleeding is present.
Other Routes	
Inhalation	
Provides rapid relief for local respiratory problems	Some local agents cause serious systemic effects.
Used for introduction of general anesthetic gases	
Intraocular Disk	
Route advantageous because it does not require	Local reactions are possible.
frequent administration such as with eye drops	Medication is expensive.
	Patients must be taught to insert and remove disk.
	Intraocular disks are contraindicated with eye infections.

GI, Gastrointestinal; *ID*, intradermal; *IM*, intramuscular; *IV*, intravenous.
[a]Includes eyes, ears, nose, vagina, rectum, and ostomy.

- **Intramuscular (IM):** Injection into a muscle.
- **Intravenous (IV):** Injection into a vein.

Health care providers administer some medications into body cavities through other parenteral routes including epidural, intrathecal, intraperitoneal, intrapleural, and intraarterial. Nurses usually do not administer medications through these routes. Whether or not you actually administer a medication by these less common routes, you remain responsible for the following:

- Monitoring the integrity of the medication delivery system
- Understanding the therapeutic value of the medication
- Evaluating a patient's response to the therapy

Topical Administration. Medications applied to the skin and mucous membranes generally have local effects. You apply topical medications to the skin through one of the following methods:

- Painting or spreading the medication over an area
- Applying moist dressings
- Soaking body parts in a solution
- Giving medicated baths

Systemic effects often occur if a patient's skin is thin or has broken down, the medication concentration is high, or contact with the skin is prolonged. A transdermal disk or patch (e.g., nitroglycerin, scopolamine, and estrogens) has systemic effects. The disk secures the medicated ointment to the skin. The nurse may leave a topical application in place for 12 hours to 7 days.

You apply topical medications to mucous membranes by:

- Direct application of a liquid or ointment (e.g., instilling eyedrops, gargling, or swabbing the throat).
- Insertion of a medication into a body cavity (e.g., placing a suppository in the rectum or vagina or inserting medicated packing into the vagina).
- Instillation of fluid into a body cavity (e.g., eardrops, nose drops, or bladder and rectal instillation). The fluid is retained.
- Irrigation of a body cavity (e.g., flushing eye, ear, vagina, bladder, or rectum) with medicated fluid. The fluid is not retained.
- Spraying a medication into a body cavity (e.g., instillation into nose and throat).

Inhalation Route. The deeper passages of the respiratory tract provide a large surface area for inhaled medications to be absorbed, resulting in local or systemic effects. You administer inhaled medications into the pulmonary airways via the nasal and oral passages, where medication passes from the pharynx and larynx into the trachea. Medications given by the inhalation route are readily absorbed and work quickly because of the rich vascular alveolar-capillary network in the pulmonary tissue.

Intraocular Route. Intraocular medication delivery involves administering medication into the eye by drops, ointment, or disk. As a patient blinks, eye drops clear rapidly through the tear ducts. To manage this, the drugs used to treat glaucoma, eye injuries, and other conditions come in

very high drug concentrations (Bourzac, 2015). These high drug levels increase the chances of systemic side effects once the drops are absorbed. One intraocular route involves inserting a medication disk into a patient's eye. The eye medication disk has two soft outer layers that have medication enclosed in them. You insert the disk into the patient's eye, much like a contact lens. The disk remains in the patient's eye for up to 1 week (Lavik et al., 2011). Research is investigating the development of dissolvable optic disks (Bourzac, 2015).

Systems of Medication Measurement

Safely administering medications requires the ability to compute medication doses accurately and measure medications correctly. A careless mistake in placing a decimal point or adding a zero to a dose can lead to a fatal error. Check every dose carefully before giving a medication.

The health care industry in the United States and internationally uses primarily the metric system as the standard measurement system for medication therapy. Recently the ISMP recommended that health care providers, pharmacists, and other health care professionals as well as pharmacy computer system and e-prescribing system vendors use only metric measurements in prescription directions (ISMP, 2011b). However, the household system (e.g., cups, teaspoons) may still be used in medication orders, particularly when health care providers write prescriptions or orders for medications that are to be taken at home by patients or administered by family caregivers. The ISMP (2011b) recommends that a household measure can be listed in parentheses in an order immediately following the metric measure, as follows: 5 mL (1 teaspoonful). It is also no longer recommended that the apothecary system be used as a system of medication measurement (ISMP, 2011b).

Metric System. As a decimal system the metric system is the most logically organized and safest to use. Metric units are easy to convert and calculate using simple multiplication and division. Each basic unit of measurement is organized into units of 10. Multiplying or dividing by 10 forms secondary units. In multiplication the decimal point moves to the right; in division the decimal moves to the left. For example:

$$10\,mg \times 10 = 100\,mg$$
$$10\,mg \div 10 = 1\,mg$$

The basic units of measurement in the metric system are the meter (length), liter (volume), and gram (weight). For medication calculations only the volume and weight units are used, and lowercase or uppercase letters are used to designate units:

$$gram = g \text{ or } gm$$
$$liter = l \text{ or } L$$
$$milligram = mg$$
$$milliliter = mL$$

A system of Latin prefixes designates subdivision of the basic units: deci- ($\frac{1}{10}$ or 0.1), centi- ($\frac{1}{100}$ or 0.01), and milli- ($\frac{1}{1000}$ or 0.001). Greek prefixes designate multiples of the basic units: deka- (10), hecto- (100), and kilo- (1000). Use fractions or multiples of a unit when writing medication doses in metric units. Always give fractions in decimal form:

$$500 \text{ mg or } 0.5 \text{ g, not } \frac{1}{2} \text{ g}$$

$$10 \text{ mL or } 0.01 \text{ L, not } \frac{1}{100} \text{ L}$$

Many actual and potential medication errors occur with the use of fractions. For example, $\frac{1}{4}$ can look like 14. Follow practice standards when medications are ordered in fractions to prevent medication errors. For example, to make the decimal point more visible, a leading zero is always placed in front of a decimal (e.g., use 0.5, not .5). Do not use a trailing zero (i.e., a zero after a decimal point) because if a health care worker does not see the decimal point, the patient may end up receiving 10 times more medication than that which is prescribed (e.g., use 5 not 5.0) (The Joint Commission [TJC], 2014a). Fractions used to express the number of tablets should appear in the font used for fractions (i.e., $\frac{1}{2}$), with a redundant statement in parentheses (one-half) (ISMP, 2010).

Household Measurements. Most people are familiar with household measures, which include liquid measures such as drops, teaspoons, tablespoons, cups, pints, and quarts. Although household measurements are convenient and familiar, they are inaccurate. Dose errors have occurred when household measures are used (ConsumerMedSafety, 2015; ISMP, 2016b). As a result, the ISMP recommends a best practice for all oral liquids that are not commercially available as unit dose products. The liquids should be dispensed by the pharmacy in an oral syringe using metric measurement (ISMP, 2016b). The ISMP also recommends that patients or family caregivers purchase oral liquid dosing devices (oral syringes, cups, droppers) that display the metric scale only. Encourage patients to never use household measuring devices with liquid medicines. OTC liquid medicines currently available almost always come with their own measuring devices (ConsumerMedSafety, 2015).

Solutions. Nurses use solutions of various concentrations for injections, irrigations, and infusions. A solution can be:

- A mass of solid substance dissolved in a known volume of fluid.
- A given volume of fluid dissolved in a known volume of another fluid.

When a solid is dissolved in a fluid, the concentration is in units of mass per units of volume (e.g., g/L, mg/mL). You also can express a concentration of a solution as a percentage. For example, a 10% solution is 10 g of solid dissolved in 100 mL of solution. A proportion also expresses concentrations. A $\frac{1}{1000}$ solution represents a solution containing 1 g of solid in 1000 mL of liquid or 1 mL of liquid mixed with 1000 mL of another liquid.

NURSING KNOWLEDGE BASE

In 1999 the Institute of Medicine (IOM) published the book *To Err Is Human: Building a Safer Health System.* This book created national awareness about the effect of medical errors within the health care system. Researchers from Johns Hopkins more recently estimated that more than 250,000 Americans die each year as a result of medical errors (Makary and Daniel, 2016). According to the Centers for Disease Control and Prevention (CDC, 2016a), more people die as a result of medical errors (e.g., surgical complications, health care acquired infections, and medication errors) than from chronic lower respiratory diseases, accidents, stroke, Alzheimer disease, and diabetes mellitus.

Nurses play an important role in patient safety, especially when it comes to medication administration. The safe administration of medications and prevention of medication errors are national patient safety concerns (Agency for Healthcare Research and Quality [AHRQ], 2015; National Quality Forum [NQF], 2016; TJC, 2018). To safely administer medications to patients, it is essential that you calculate dosages accurately. You also need to understand the roles that different health care providers play in prescribing and administering medications. Your previous learning is important. Apply what you know, and do not be afraid to ask questions when administering medications. Use the nursing process as a framework to organize your thoughts and actions.

Clinical Calculations

Often you will not prepare a medication for administration in the unit of measure in which it is ordered and delivered. Pharmaceutical companies package and bottle medications in standard dosages. However, a patient's order may be for a different dosage. For example, a patient is ordered to receive a 2-mg dose of a drug, but the drug is dispensed in 4-mg amounts. Another patient has an order for 1 g of a medication that is available only in milligrams. Accurate drug calculation is essential to administer medications safely. Use your mathematics skills to calculate dosages and mix solutions. You are responsible for converting available units of volume and weight to the desired doses. Know the approximate equivalents in all major measurement systems.

Conversions Within One System. When converting measurements within the metric system, you use division or multiplication. For example, to change milligrams to grams, divide by 1000 or move the decimal three points to the left:

$$1000 \text{ mg} = 1 \text{ g}$$

$$350 \text{ mg} = 0.35 \text{ g}$$

To convert liters to milliliters, multiply by 1000 or move the decimal three points to the right:

$$1 \text{ L} = 1000 \text{ mL}$$

$$0.25 \text{ L} = 250 \text{ mL}$$

To convert units of measurement within the household system, you need to know the equivalent. For example, when converting fluid ounces to quarts, you know that 32 ounces is the equivalent of 1 quart. To convert 8 ounces to a quart measurement, divide 8 by 32 to get the equivalent, $\frac{1}{4}$ or 0.25 quart.

Conversion Between Systems. The conversion between measurement systems is becoming less common because of the recommendations for use of the metric system for liquid medication dosing (ISMP, 2011b). Although health care providers are encouraged to order using the metric system, you may encounter a situation when you calculate the correct dose of a medication by converting weights or volumes from one system of measurement to another. For example, metric units are sometimes converted to equivalent household measures for medication administration at home. To convert from one measurement system to another, always use equivalent measurements. Tables of equivalent measurements are available in all health care agencies. The pharmacist is also a good resource.

Before making a conversion, compare the measurement system available with what was ordered. For example, a health care provider orders 10 mL of guaifenesin for your patient. To provide proper instruction to the patient, you convert "mL" to a common household measurement. By referring to an equivalents table you determine that 10 mL = 2 tsp. Therefore you instruct the patient to take 2 tsp of Robitussin.

Dosage Calculations. Dosage calculation methods include the ratio and proportion method, the formula method, and dimensional analysis. Use the method that is the most logical and comfortable for you. Use this same method consistently. Before you begin any calculation, make a mental estimate of the approximate and reasonable dosage. If your estimate does not closely match the answer you calculate, you need to recheck your math before preparing and administering the medication. Many nursing students feel uncomfortable or anxious when they have to do medication calculations. To enhance accuracy and decrease your anxiety, think critically about the steps you go through in calculating medications and practice doing calculations to feel more confident about your math skills.

Most health care agencies require a nurse to double-check calculations with another nurse when high-risk medications are prepared (e.g., heparin, chemotherapeutic drug, or insulin). The ISMP (2013c) recommends that the most effective double check is conducted independently by a second person to reduce the risk of bias that occurs when the person preparing and checking the medication is likely to see what they expect to see, even if an error has occurred. Because double checks take considerable time and have not consistently been found to prevent errors, independent double checks should be used only for very selective high-alert medications that most warrant their use (ISMP, 2013c). Consult agency policy regarding double checks of medications. *Always* have another nurse or health care professional double-check your work if the answer to a medication calculation seems unreasonable or inappropriate.

The Ratio and Proportion Method. A ratio indicates the relationship between two numbers. The numbers in a ratio are separated by a colon (:). The colon in the ratio indicates that you need to use division. Think of a ratio as a fraction; the number to the left is the numerator and the number to the right is the denominator. For example, the ratio 1:2 is the same as $\frac{1}{2}$. A proportion is an equation that has two ratios of equal value. Write a proportion in one of three ways:

$$\text{Example 1: } 1:2 = 5:10$$
$$\text{Example 2: } 1:2 :: 5:10$$
$$\text{Example 3: } \frac{1}{2} = \frac{5}{10}$$

In a proportion the first and last numbers are called the *extremes,* and the second and third numbers are called the *means.* If you multiply the extremes, you get the same result as if you multiplied the means. For example, in the preceding proportions, if you multiply the means and extremes, you end up with the following equations: $1 \times 10 = 10$ and $2 \times 5 = 10$. Because the numbers in a proportion are in a specific relationship with one another, if you know three of the numbers in the proportion, it is easy to calculate the unknown number. To use this method, you first need to make sure that all terms are in the same unit and system of measurement. After estimating the correct dose in your mind, set up the proportion, labeling all terms in the proportion. Place the ratio that you know (e.g., information on the drug label) first. Put the terms of the ratio in the same sequence (e.g., mg:mL = mg:mL). Cross multiply the means and the extremes, and then divide both sides by the number before the $\times$ to obtain the dosage. Always remember to label your answer. If your answer is not close to your estimate, recheck your math.

Example: A health care provider ordered 100 mg of phenytoin to be administered to a patient in a gastric tube. The solution comes in a bottle labeled phenytoin 125 mg/5 mL. Use the following steps to calculate how many milliliters to give:

1. Estimate the answer: The amount you have to give is a little less than the amount that is provided in the solution. Therefore the patient needs a little less than 5 mL of medication.

2. Set up the proportion:

$$\frac{125\,\text{mg}}{5\,\text{mL}} = \frac{100\,\text{mg}}{x\,\text{mL}}$$

3. Cross multiply the means and the extremes:

$$125x = 100 \times 5$$
$$125x = 500$$

4. Divide both sides by the number before x:

$$\frac{125x}{125} = \frac{500}{125}$$

$$x = \frac{500}{125}$$

$$x = 4\,mL$$

5. Compare your estimate from Step 1 with your answer in Step 4: The answer (4 mL) is close to the estimated amount (a little less than 5 mL). Therefore your answer is correct; prepare and administer 4 mL in the patient's gastric tube.

The Formula Method. When using the formula method to calculate medication dosages, you memorize the formula and substitute information from the medication order into the formula. Estimate what you think the answer should be; then place and label all the information from the medication order into the formula. Ensure that all measures in the formula are in the same units and system of measurement before calculating the dosage. If the measures are not in the same measurement system, convert the numbers to the same system before calculating the dosage. Calculate and label your answer. Compare your answer with your estimated answer; if your estimate is not similar to your answer, recheck your math. Use the following basic formula when using the formula method:

$$\frac{\text{Dose ordered}}{\text{Dose on hand}} \times \text{Amount on hand} = \frac{\text{Amount to}}{\text{administer}}$$

The dose ordered is the amount of medication prescribed. The dose on hand is the weight or volume of medication available in units supplied by the pharmacy. It is expressed on the medication label as the contents of a tablet or capsule or as the amount of medication dissolved per unit volume of liquid. The amount on hand is the basic unit or quantity of the medication that contains the dose on hand. For solid medications the amount on hand is usually one capsule or tablet. The amount of liquid on hand depends on the container (e.g., 1 mL or 1 L). The amount to administer is the actual amount of available medication that you will administer. You always express your answer in the same unit as the amount on hand.

Example: Your patient needs to receive meperidine, 50 mg IM (dose ordered). The medication is available only in ampules containing 100 mg (dose on hand) in 1 mL (amount on hand). You apply the formula method as follows:

1. Estimate the answer: The medication is a liquid; thus you need to figure out the answer in milliliters. The amount that you need to give is ½ of what the dose is, so your answer is going to be about a ½ mL.

2. Set up the formula:

$$\frac{\text{Dose ordered}}{\text{Dose on hand}} \times \text{Amount on hand} = \frac{\text{Amount to}}{\text{administer}}$$

$$\frac{50\,mg}{100\,mg} \times 1\,mL = \text{Amount to administer}$$

3. Calculate your answer:

$$\frac{50\,mg}{100\,mg} \times 1\,mL = 0.5\,mL$$

4. Compare your estimate from Step 1 with your answer in Step 3: both your estimate and your answer are the same; prepare 0.5 mL in a syringe and administer it to your patient.

Dimensional Analysis. Dimensional analysis is also known as the factor-label method or the unit factor method. Because only one equation is needed and the same steps are used in solving every medication problem, you do not have to memorize formulas. Dimensional analysis requires you to use your critical thinking skills. Some nursing students who use dimensional analysis calculate medications more accurately than when they use the formula method (Koohestani and Baghcheghi, 2010). Use the following steps to solve medication problems using dimensional analysis:

1. Identify the unit of measure that you need to administer. For example, if you are giving a pill, you are usually giving a tablet or a capsule; for parenteral or liquid oral medications the unit is milliliters.
2. Estimate the answer in your mind.
3. Place the name or appropriate abbreviation for x on the left side of the equation (e.g., x tab, x mL).
4. Place available information from the problem in a fraction format on the right side of the equation. Place the abbreviation or unit that matches what you are going to administer (determined in Step 1) in the numerator.
5. Look at the medication order and add other factors into the problem. Set up the numerator so that it matches the unit in the previous denominator.
6. Cancel out like units of measurement on the right side of the equation. You should end up with only one unit left in the equation, and it should match the unit on the left side of the equation.
7. Reduce to the lowest terms if possible and solve the problem or solve for x. Label your answer.
8. Compare your estimate from Step 1 with your answer in Step 2.

Example: A patient's health care provider orders 0.5 g of ampicillin to be given IM q8h. You have a vial of ampicillin that says 250 mg/mL. Calculate the dose to administer using dimensional analysis by following these steps:

1. *Identify the unit of measure that you need to administer:* This medication is given intramuscularly, which is a parenteral medication. Therefore, your answer will be in milliliters (mL).

2. *Estimate the answer in your mind:* The medication order of 0.5 g is larger than 250 mg. Because the medication is in a vial of 250 mg in 1 mL, you will need to give more than 1 mL. Based on your knowledge about converting in the metric system, you convert 0.5 g to milligrams by moving the decimal point three places to the right. Therefore 0.5 g is the same as 500 mg. The number 500 is 2 × 250; thus the answer is about 2 mL.

3. *Place the name or appropriate abbreviation for x on the left side of the equation:*

$$x \text{ mL} =$$

4. *Place available information from the problem in a fraction format on the right side of the equation:* You are going to administer the medication in milliliters, so place the milliliter in the numerator.

$$x \text{ mL} = \frac{1 \text{ mL}}{250 \text{ mg}}$$

5. Look at the medication order and add other factors into the problem. Set up the numerator so that it matches the unit in the previous denominator: The order is for 0.5 g, and the medication is available in 250-mg vials. You know that 1 g = 1000 mg; add this conversion to your calculation.

$$x \text{ mL} = \frac{1 \text{ mL}}{250 \text{ mg}} \times \frac{1000 \text{ mg}}{1 \text{ g}} \times \frac{0.5 \text{ g}}{1}$$

6. Cancel out like units of measurement on the right side of the equation.

$$x \text{ mL} = \frac{1 \text{ mL}}{250 \, \cancel{\text{mg}}} \times \frac{1000 \, \cancel{\text{mg}}}{1 \, \cancel{\text{g}}} \times \frac{0.5 \, \cancel{\text{g}}}{1}$$

7. Reduce to the lowest terms if possible and solve the problem or solve for x. Label your answer.

$$x = \frac{1000 \times 0.5}{250}$$

$$x = \frac{500}{250}$$

$$x = 2 \text{ mL}$$

8. *Compare your estimate from Step 1 with your answer in Step 2:* Your answer is 2 mL, which matches the estimate you made in Step 2. Prepare and administer 2 mL of the medication as calculated.

Pediatric Calculations. Children are at high risk for experiencing medication errors. The ISMP (2015d) reported that children are three times more likely than adults to have a harmful medication error or adverse drug reaction because of their size, immature renal and hepatic functions, and inability to communicate symptoms of adverse effects. It is not unusual for a child to receive either the wrong dose or the wrong amount of medication. The risk for medication errors is especially high because medication dosages are often weight-based, and many medications are packaged for adults.

Calculating children's medications dosages requires caution (Hockenberry and Wilson, 2015). Even small discrepancies or errors in medication amounts can negatively affect a child's health status. A child's age, weight, and maturity of body systems affect the ability to metabolize and excrete medications. For example, premature infants have underdeveloped livers and kidneys, which make them especially susceptible to the harmful effects of medications. As children develop out of the newborn period, they metabolize medications more quickly, resulting in the need for more frequent dosing of medications to achieve the desired effect of the medication. It is difficult to evaluate a child's response to medications, especially when he or she cannot communicate with you verbally. For example, a side effect of vancomycin, an antibiotic, is ototoxicity. If a child taking vancomycin cannot talk yet, assessing for ototoxicity is challenging.

Different methods are used to calculate medication dosages for children. Most of the time you use a child's weight to calculate the medication dose. You can use the ratio and proportion method, the formula method, or dimensional analysis to calculate a pediatric dose using body weight. Body surface area (BSA) is used in rare situations (e.g., determining chemotherapy doses). If you have to calculate medication doses for a child, refer to a pediatric or pharmacology resource and consult with a patient's health care provider or pharmacist.

Administering Medications

In addition to nurses, a health care provider and pharmacist also help ensure that the right medication gets to the right patient. You are responsible to know which health care providers are able to prescribe medications. Health care providers who can prescribe medications include physicians, advanced practice nurses, and physician assistants. Practice acts vary by state, and policies vary by agency. Know your Nurse Practice Act and agency policies when taking prescriptions and administering medications to protect your patient and yourself. In addition, you are accountable for knowing which medications are prescribed, their therapeutic and nontherapeutic effects, and a patient's needs and abilities related to medication administration. You also are responsible for evaluating the desired effects of a patient's medications.

Health Care Provider's Role. A health care provider prescribes a patient's medications by writing an order on a form in the patient's medical record, in an order book, or on a legal prescription pad. Medications may also be ordered through computers or handheld electronic devices (e.g., smartphones, tablets). Many health care settings use computerized physician order entry (CPOE) to enter medication orders. CPOE requires a health care provider to enter essential information about the medication order, preventing incomplete and illegible orders, enhancing communication, and decreasing medication errors. In a systematic review of

BOX 17.3   GUIDELINES FOR TELEPHONE AND VERBAL ORDERS

- Only authorized staff members receive and record telephone or verbal orders. Institutional policies identify which members are authorized.
- Clearly identify patient's name, room number, and diagnosis.
- Read back all orders to health care provider (TJC, 2018).
- Use clarification questions to avoid misunderstandings.
- Write "TO" (telephone order) or "VO" (verbal order) and include date and time, name of patient, and complete order; sign the name of the health care provider and nurse.
- Follow agency policies; some require documentation of the "read-back" or require two nurses to review and sign telephone or verbal orders.
- Health care provider co-signs the order within the time frame required by the agency (usually 24 hours; verify agency policy).

the literature, Radley et al. (2013) found that processing a prescription drug order through a CPOE system decreases the likelihood of error on that order by 48%. The researchers also estimated a 12.5% reduction in medication errors, or approximately 17.4 million medication errors averted in the United States in 1 year, up to 2008.

In some situations, a health care provider talks directly with a nurse and gives a **verbal order.** Other times the health care provider gives the nurse an order over the phone; this is known as a *telephone order.* To ensure safety, telephone and verbal orders are given only when written or electronic communication between a health care provider and nurse is not possible (Box 17.3). The National Coordinating Council for Medication Error Reporting and Prevention (NCCMERP, 2015) recommends the following to reduce confusion pertaining to verbal orders and to minimize medication errors:

1. Limit verbal communication of prescription or medication orders to urgent situations where immediate written or electronic communication is not feasible.
2. Health care organizations should establish policies and procedures that do the following:
   - Describe limitations or prohibitions on use of verbal orders.
   - Provide a mechanism to ensure validity/authenticity of the health care provider.
   - List the elements required for inclusion in a complete verbal order.
   - Describe situations in which verbal orders may be used.
   - List and define the individuals who may send and receive verbal orders.
   - Provide guidelines for clear and effective communication of verbal orders.

A nurse writes an order and the name of the health care provider, signs the order, and follows agency policy to indicate that the order was verified by reading the order back to the health care provider. The health care provider countersigns the order at a later time, usually within 24 hours after

making it. Generally nursing students cannot take medication orders, and verbal orders should be taken only in emergency situations. You cannot give any medication without an order.

Health care providers often use abbreviations when writing orders. The abbreviations indicate dosage frequencies or times, routes of administration, and special information for giving medications (see Table 17.3). Many medication errors occur because of the use of abbreviations. The ISMP maintains a list of abbreviations that are associated with a high incidence of medication errors (ISMP, 2015b) (Table 17.5). *Do not use these abbreviations* when documenting medication orders or other information about medications (TJC, 2016). Abbreviations often vary; check agency policy to determine which abbreviations you can use and what they mean.

Some conditions change the status of a patient's medication orders. For example, surgery automatically cancels all of a patient's preoperative medications (see Chapter 40). A transfer from a general medical unit to an intensive care unit also cancels all of a patient's medication orders, requiring the health care provider to write new orders. When a patient is transferred to another health care agency or to a different unit within a hospital or is discharged, the health care provider reviews the medications, reconciles the list, and writes new orders as indicated.

Types of Orders in Acute Care Agencies. Health care providers make five common types of medication orders, based on the frequency and/or urgency of medication administration. As a nurse it is important to understand the policies and procedures of your agency.

Standing Orders. You carry out a standing order until the health care provider cancels it by another order or until a prescribed number of days elapses. A standing order will sometimes indicate a final date or number of dosages. Many agencies have policies for automatically discontinuing standing orders. The following are examples of standing orders:

quinapril 20 mg PO q12h

azithromycin, 500 mg PO daily for 2 days,
then 500 mg PO daily for 7 days

prn Orders. A health care provider sometimes orders a medication to be given only when a patient requires it for a specific situation, such as pain, nausea, or constipation. This is a prn order. The collection of objective and subjective assessment data and your nursing judgment determine whether a patient needs the medication. Often the health care provider sets minimum intervals for the time of administration. This means that you cannot give the medication any more frequently than when it is prescribed. An example of a prn order is:

magnesium hydroxide 30 mL PO prn for constipation

After administering a prn medication, document the assessment data you used to decide to give the medication and the time of medication administration. Frequently evaluate the effectiveness of the medication and record findings in the appropriate record. A prn medication order that includes a range (e.g., morphine sulfate 2–4 mg IV push q2–4h prn for pain) is unclear and frequently causes a medication error. If a health care provider writes an order with a range, ensure that the order follows agency policies. An example of a safer range order is: increase morphine dosage 50% to 100% if pain is moderate to severe.

When a provider orders multiple prn medications with the same action, the orders must identify the time each medication is to be used and how to use the medications in relation

---

TABLE 17.5 PROHIBITED AND ERROR-PRONE ABBREVIATIONS[a]

The abbreviations, symbols, and dose designations found in this table have been reported to ISMP through the USP-ISMP Medication Error Reporting Program as being frequently misinterpreted and involved in harmful medication errors. They should NEVER be used when communicating medical information. This includes internal communications, telephone/verbal prescriptions, computer-generated labels, labels for drug storage bins, medication administration records, and pharmacy and health care provider computer order entry screens. The Joint Commission (TJC) has established a National Patient Safety Goal that specifies that certain abbreviations must appear on the do-not-use list of the accredited organization; they are highlighted with a double asterisk (**). However, we hope that you will consider others beyond the minimum TJC requirements. By using and promoting safe practices and educating one another about hazards, we can better protect our patients.

ABBREVIATIONS	INTENDED MEANING	MISINTERPRETATION	CORRECTION
μg	Microgram	Mistaken as "mg"	Use "mcg"
AD, AS, AU	Right ear, left ear, each ear	Mistaken as OD, OS, OU (right eye, left eye, each eye)	Use "right ear," "left ear," or "each ear"
OD, OS, OU	Right eye, left eye, each eye	Mistaken as AD, AS, AU (right ear, left ear, each ear)	Use "right eye," "left eye," or "each eye"
BT	Bedtime	Mistaken as "BID" (twice daily)	Use "bedtime"
HS	Half-strength	Mistaken as bedtime	Use "half-strength" or "bedtime"
hs	At bedtime, hours of sleep	Mistaken as half-strength	Use "bedtime" or "half-strength"
IU**	International unit	Mistaken as IV (intravenous) or 10 (ten)	Use "units"
o.d. or OD	Once daily	Mistaken as "right eye" (OD—oculus dexter), leading to oral liquid medications administered in the eye	Use "daily"
Per os	By mouth, orally	The "os" can be mistaken as "left eye" (OS—oculus sinister)	Use "PO," "by mouth," or "orally"
q.d. or QD**	Every day	Mistaken as q.i.d., especially if the period after the "q" or the tail of the "q" is misunderstood as an "I"	Use "daily"
qhs	Nightly at bedtime	Mistaken as "qhr" or every hour	Use "nightly"
SC, SQ, sub q	Subcutaneous	SC mistaken as SL (sublingual); SQ mistaken as "5 every"; the "q" in "sub q" has been mistaken as "every" (such as a heparin dose ordered "sub q 2 hours before surgery" misunderstood as every 2 hours before surgery)	Use "subcut" or "subcutaneously"
TIW or tiw	3 times a week	Mistaken as "3 times a day" or "twice in a week"	Use "3 times weekly"
U or u**	Unit	Mistaken as the number 0 or 4, causing a 10-fold overdose or greater (for example, 4 U seen as "40" or 4 u seen as "44"); mistaken as "cc" so dose given in volume instead of units (e.g., 4 u seen as 4 cc)	Use "unit"

Continued

TABLE 17.5   PROHIBITED AND ERROR-PRONE ABBREVIATIONS[a]—cont'd

DOSE DESIGNATIONS AND OTHER INFORMATION	INTENDED MEANING	MISINTERPRETATION	CORRECTION
Trailing zero after decimal point (e.g., 1.0 mg)[b]	1 mg	Mistaken as 10 mg if the decimal point is not seen	Do not use trailing zeros for doses expressed in whole numbers
"Naked" decimal point (e.g., 0.5 mg)**	0.5 mg	Mistaken as 5 mg if the decimal point is not seen	Use zero before a decimal point when the dose is less than a whole unit
Abbreviations such as mg. or mL. with a period following the abbreviation	mg, mL	The period is unnecessary and could be mistaken as the number 1 if written poorly	Use mg, mL, etc., without a terminal period

DRUG NAME ABBREVIATIONS	INTENDED MEANING	MISINTERPRETATION	CORRECTION
HCl	Hydrochloric acid or hydrochloride	Mistaken as potassium chloride (The "H" is misinterpreted as "K")	Use complete drug name unless expressed as a salt of a drug
HCT	Hydrocortisone	Mistaken as hydrochlorothiazide	Use complete drug name
HCTZ	Hydrochlorothiazide	Mistaken as hydrocortisone (seen as HCT250 mg)	Use complete drug name
MgSO4**	Magnesium sulfate	Mistaken as morphine sulfate	Use complete drug name
MS, MSO4**	Morphine sulfate	Mistaken as magnesium sulfate	Use complete drug name
PCA	Procainamide	Mistaken as patient-controlled analgesia	Use complete drug name

STEMMED DRUG NAMES	INTENDED MEANING	MISINTERPRETATION	CORRECTION
"Nitro" drip	Nitroglycerin infusion	Mistaken as sodium nitroprusside infusion	Use complete drug name

SYMBOLS	INTENDED MEANING	MISINTERPRETATION	CORRECTION
ʒ	Dram	Symbol for dram mistaken as "3"	Use metric system
×3d	For three days	Mistaken as "3 doses"	Use "for three days"
> and <	Greater than and less than	Mistaken as opposite of intended; mistakenly use incorrect symbol; "<10" mistaken as "40"	Use "greater than" or "less than"
@	At	Mistaken as "2"	Use "at"
&	And	Mistaken as "2"	Use "and"
+	Plus or and	Mistaken as "4"	Use "and"
°	Hour	Mistaken as a zero (e.g., q2° seen as q20)	Use "hr," "h," or "hour"

ISMP, Institute for Safe Medication Practices; *USP,* United States Pharmacopeia.
**These abbreviations are included on The Joint Commission "minimum list" of dangerous abbreviations, acronyms, and symbols that must be included on the "Do Not Use" list of an organization, effective January 1, 2004.
[a]Applies to all orders and medication-related documentation that is handwritten (including free-text computer entry or on preprinted forms).
[b]Exception: A "trailing zero" may be used only where required to show precision of a reported value (such as laboratory test results), in studies that report the size of lesions, or for catheter and tube sizes. A "trailing zero" cannot be used in medication orders or medication-related documentation (Institute for Safe Medication Practices [ISMP], 2013a).
From The Joint Commission (TJC): *Facts About the Official "Do Not Use" List of Abbreviations,* 2016, https://www.jointcommission.org/facts_about_do_not_use_list/. Reprinted with permission.

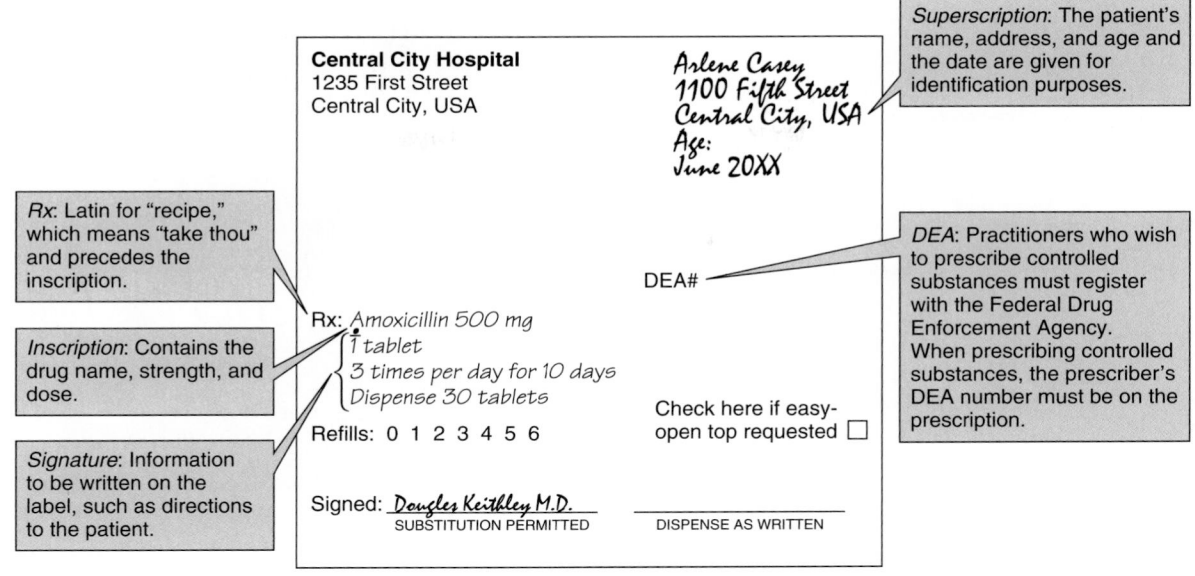

Superscription: The patient's name, address, and age and the date are given for identification purposes.

Rx: Latin for "recipe," which means "take thou" and precedes the inscription.

DEA: Practitioners who wish to prescribe controlled substances must register with the Federal Drug Enforcement Agency. When prescribing controlled substances, the prescriber's DEA number must be on the prescription.

Inscription: Contains the drug name, strength, and dose.

Signature: Information to be written on the label, such as directions to the patient.

Central City Hospital
1235 First Street
Central City, USA

Arlene Casey
1100 Fifth Street
Central City, USA
Age:
June 20XX

DEA#

Rx: Amoxicillin 500 mg
1 tablet
3 times per day for 10 days
Dispense 30 tablets

Refills: 0 1 2 3 4 5 6

Check here if easy-open top requested ☐

Signed: *Douglas Keithley M.D.*
SUBSTITUTION PERMITTED   DISPENSE AS WRITTEN

FIG 17.4 Example of medication prescription.

to each other. The following order is an example of a safe prn order for two medications used for treating constipation:

Docusate 100 mg PO tid prn for constipation

Bisacodyl 10 mg suppository rectally daily prn for constipation in addition to docusate if no bowel movement in 2 days

Single (One-Time) Orders. A health care provider often orders a medication to be given only once at a specified time. This is common for preoperative medications or medications given before diagnostic examinations. For example:

Versed 6 mg IM on call to OR

STAT Orders. A STAT order means that you give a single dose of a medication immediately and only once. Health care providers usually write STAT orders for emergencies when a patient's condition changes suddenly. For example:

Apresoline 10 mg IV push STAT

NOW Orders. A NOW order is more specific than a one-time order and is used when a patient needs a medication quickly but not right away, as in a STAT order. Verify your agency policy to determine how much time you have to administer a NOW medication after it is ordered. Only administer medications ordered NOW one time. For example:

Give vancomycin 1 g IV piggyback NOW

Prescriptions. Prescriptions are written for patients who are to take medications at home. The prescription includes more detailed information than a regular hospital medication order because the patient needs to understand how to take a medication and when to refill the prescription if necessary. The parts of a prescription are included in Fig. 17.4.

Pharmacist's Role. Pharmacists prepare and distribute prescribed medications. They work with nurses and other health care providers to evaluate the effectiveness of medication therapy. Pharmacists assess the medication plan, make recommendations for revisions, and evaluate a patient's medication-related needs. Pharmacists are responsible for filling prescriptions accurately and for being sure that prescriptions are valid. They rarely mix compounds or solutions except in the case of IV medications because most pharmaceutical companies deliver medications in a form ready for use. Pharmacists are responsible for ensuring the dispensation of the right medication, in the right dosage and amount, and with an accurate label. Pharmacists also act as resources and provide information to nurses and health care providers about appropriateness of a medication for a patient's condition and characteristics of medications including actions, side effects, interactions, and incompatibilities.

Distribution Systems. Systems for storing and distributing medications vary. Pharmacists provide the medications, but nurses distribute them to patients. Agencies providing nursing care have special areas for stocking and dispensing medications such as special medication rooms, portable locked carts, computerized medication cabinets, and individual storage units in patients' rooms. Medication storage areas need to be locked when unattended.

Unit Dose. The unit-dose system uses portable carts containing a drawer with a 24-hour supply of medications for

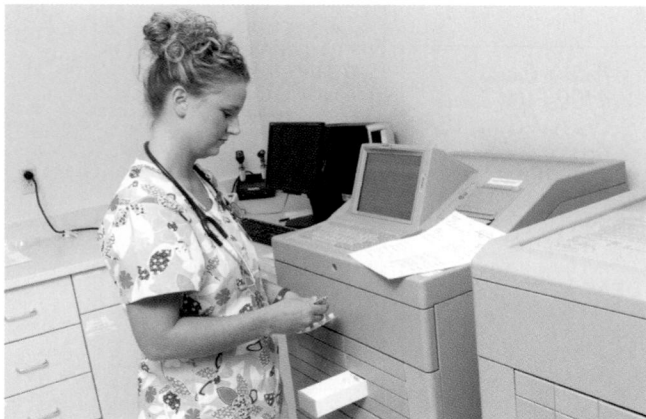

FIG 17.5 Computer-controlled medication dispensing system.

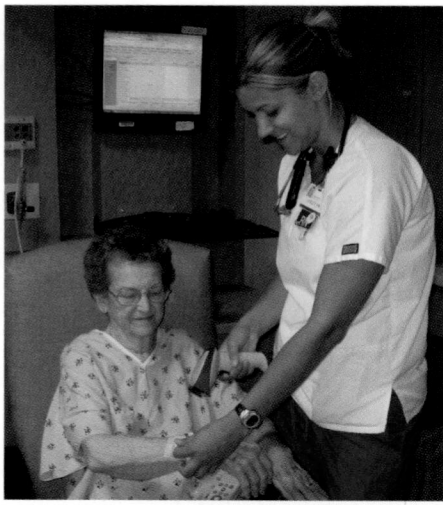

FIG 17.6 Nurse using bar-code scanner during medication administration.

each patient. The unit dose is the ordered dose of medication that a patient receives at one time. Each tablet or capsule is wrapped separately. At a designated time each day, the drawers in the cart are refilled by a pharmacy technician. The cart also contains limited amounts of prn and stock medications for special situations. The unit-dose system is designed to reduce the number of medication errors and saves steps in dispensing medications.

Automated Medication Dispensing Systems. Automated medication dispensing systems (AMDSs) are used successfully throughout the United States (Fig. 17.5). The systems within a health care agency are networked with one another and with other computer systems in the agency (e.g., the computerized medical record). Research suggests that AMDSs have the potential for reducing nursing time, dispensing and medication errors, and costs in hospital units (Mandrack et al., 2012; Chapuis et al., 2015). AMDSs control the dispensing of all medications including opioids and other controlled substances. Each nurse has a security code that allows access to the system. If your agency uses a system that requires biometric identification, you have to place your finger on a screen to confirm your fingerprint so that you can access the computer. Once logged onto the AMDS, you select the patient's name and medication profile. Then you select the medication, dosage, and route from a list on the computer screen. The system opens the medication drawer or dispenses the medication, records the event, and charges it to the patient. If the system is connected to the patient's medical record, it records information about the medication (e.g., name, dose, and time) and the name of the nurse who retrieved the medication from the AMDS in the patient's medical record. Some systems require nurses to scan bar codes before recording this information in the patient's computerized medical record (Fig. 17.6).

Nurse's Role. When you administer medications to patients, you need knowledge and a set of skills that are unique to nursing. Responsibilities of medication administration include knowing medication therapeutics, assessing a patient for administration, administering medications correctly at the right time, monitoring and evaluating their effects, and assessing a patient's ability to self-administer medications. Patient and family caregiver education about proper medication administration and monitoring is an integral part of your role. Never delegate this to nursing assistive personnel (NAP). Use the nursing process to integrate medication therapy into care.

Medication Errors

A medication error can cause or lead to inappropriate medication use or patient harm. Medication errors include inaccurate prescribing; administering the wrong medication, dose, route, and time interval; administering to the wrong patient; and administering extra doses or failing to administer a medication. A patient death or serious injury because of a medication administration error is a serious reportable event (NQF, 2016), which makes the prevention of medication errors a national priority (see Chapter 30). The process of administering medications is very complex; thus it is highly prone to errors. As a nurse, it is essential to be vigilant in prevention of medication errors during preparation and administration (Box 17.4). Advances in technology and informatics help decrease the occurrence of medication errors (Box 17.5).

Medication errors are often related to miscommunication among the members of the health care team, product design, or procedures and systems such as product labeling and distribution. When an error occurs, a patient's safety and well-being become the top priority. As a nurse, assess and examine a patient's condition and notify the health care provider of an incident as soon as possible. Report the incident to the appropriate person in the institution (e.g., manager or supervisor) once the patient is stable.

When a medication error occurs and you are involved, you are responsible for preparing a written occurrence or adverse event report within 24 hours of the incident. The report includes patient identification information; the location and time of the incident; an accurate, factual description of what

BOX 17.4   STEPS TO TAKE TO PREVENT MEDICATION ERRORS

- Prepare medications for only one patient at a time.
- Follow the six rights of medication administration.
- Be sure to read labels at least three times (comparing medication administration record [MAR] with label) before administering medication.
- Use at least two patient identifiers.
- Review a patient's allergies whenever administering a medication.
- Do not allow any other activity to interrupt administration of medication to a patient (such as a telephone call, pager, or a discussion with other staff) (Hopkinson and Jennings, 2013).
- Double-check all calculations and other high-risk medication administration processes (such as patient-controlled analgesia) and verify with another nurse.
- Do not interpret illegible handwriting; clarify with health care provider.
- Question unusually large or small doses or any dose outside of the recommended dosage range (or typically prescribed dose).
- Document all medications as soon as they are given.
- When you have made an error, reflect on what went wrong and ask how you could have prevented the error. Complete an adverse event report per institution policy.
- Evaluate the context or situation in which the medication error occurred. This helps to determine whether nurses have the necessary resources for safe medication administration.
- Attend in-service programs that focus on the medications commonly administered.
- Ensure that you are well rested when caring for patients. Nurses make more errors when they are tired (Murphy and While, 2012).
- Involve and educate patients when administering medications. Address patients' concerns about medications before administering them (such as concerns about appearance of medication or side effects).
- Follow established institution policies and procedures when using technology to administer medications (such as automated medication dispensing systems [AMDSs] and bar-code scanning). Medication errors occur when nurses "work around" the technology (that is, override alerts without thinking about them) (Voshall et al., 2013).

BOX 17.5   INFORMATICS AND MEDICATION SAFETY

Medication errors frequently occur when a nurse incorrectly administers medications at a patient's bedside. Innovations in technology and informatics have reduced the number of medication errors in nursing practice:

- Networked computers allow health care providers to see a current list of ordered and discontinued medications.
- Internet and intranet access allows nurses and other health care providers to access current information about medications (e.g., indications, desired effects, adverse effects) and specific agency policies that address medication administration (e.g., how fast to administer an intravenous push [IVP] medication).
- Automated medication dispensing systems (AMDSs), bar-coding technology, and electronic medication administration records (MARs) help with medication reconciliation, administration, and documentation.

APPLICATION TO NURSING PRACTICE

- Actively participate in the evaluation and selection of advanced technologies. Also participate in the development of nursing policies and protocols used for medication administration.
- Always follow agency policies when administering medications.
- Implement agency policies when technology cannot be used (e.g., during downtime or power outages).
- Follow manufacturer guidelines for care of electronic equipment and report problems with technology immediately.

occurred and what was done; and your signature. The report is not a permanent part of the medical record and should not be referred to in the patient's medical record (see Chapter 5). This legally protects the health care professional and agency. Agencies use occurrence reports to track incident patterns and initiate quality improvement programs as needed.

Report all medication errors including mistakes that do not cause obvious or immediate harm or near misses. You need to feel comfortable in reporting an error and not fear repercussions from managerial staff (NCCMERP, 2015). Many hospitals have adopted "just culture" environments. A just culture is a learning culture within a health care

organization that is constantly improving and oriented toward patient safety and ensures balanced accountability for individuals and the organization responsible for designing and improving systems in the workplace (Boysen, 2013). These organizations create an open, fair, and just culture to learn from errors and then adopt improved systems and processes that minimize risk of human error. Even if patients suffer no harm from medication errors, agencies benefit from learning why mistakes occurred and what can be done to avoid similar errors in the future.

Medication errors frequently occur when a patient is transferred (e.g., to another health care agency or another unit within the hospital) or discharged. Therefore reconciling a patient's list of medications during the transfer or discharge process is a National Patient Safety Goal (TJC, 2018). You play an important role in medication reconciliation (Box 17.6). It is a process in which you compare the medications that your patient took in the previous setting (e.g., home or another nursing unit) with the current medication orders whenever there is a transition in care (e.g., discharge or transfer) and when a new medication is ordered (Alexander et al., 2012; Infusion Nurses Society [INS], 2016). When a patient leaves that setting for another setting (e.g., skilled care facility or intensive care unit), you communicate the patient's current medications with the health care providers in the new setting. Most health care agencies have computerized or written forms

BOX 17.6	PROCESS FOR MEDICATION RECONCILIATION

1. **Obtain, Verify, Document:** Obtain a current comprehensive list of a patient's medications whenever he or she experiences a change in health care setting (e.g., during admission, transfer, discharge). Include all current prescription and over-the-counter (OTC) medications.
2. **Consider and Compare:** Review what the patient was taking at home or preadmission and make sure that the list of medications, dosages, and frequencies is accurate. Compare this list with the current ordered medications and treatment plan to ensure accuracy. Include family caregivers in this discussion when appropriate.
3. **Reconcile:** Compare new medication orders with the current list; investigate any discrepancies with the patient's health care provider and document changes.
4. **Communicate:** Ensure that all the patient's health care providers have the most updated list of medications. Communicate and verify changes in medications with the patient.

Data from Gleason KM, et al: *Medications at transitions and clinical handoffs (MATCH) toolkit for medication reconciliation,* Agency for Healthcare Research and Quality, AHRQ Publication No. 11(12)-0059, 2012, http://www.ahrq.gov/professionals/quality-patient-safety/patient-safety-resources/resources/match/match.pdf.

used to facilitate medication reconciliation. Reconciling medications is challenging and requires a great deal of concentration and time. Eliminate distractions and take your time when reconciling your patient's medications. Always clarify information whenever needed by consulting with your patient, the patient's family caregivers, and the interprofessional health care team (e.g., physicians, advanced practice nurses, pharmacists) when reconciling a patient's medications.

CRITICAL THINKING

Synthesis

Patient care requires you to apply what you know about a patient, your knowledge base, experience, and critical thinking attitudes and standards. Your synthesis of this information allows you to make sound decisions as you apply the nursing process. Critical thinking synthesis involves combining all available information to obtain a clear picture of the approach needed to provide patient-centered care.

Knowledge. You use knowledge from many disciplines when administering medications. Knowledge of physiology and pathophysiology helps you understand why a particular medication has been prescribed for a patient and how it will alter the patient's physiology as it exerts its therapeutic effect. *For example, in the case study, Emilio knows that Esther Simmons has type 2 diabetes and why an oral hypoglycemic agent is necessary to maintain a normal blood sugar. His knowledge of heart disease and hypertension helps him to understand why Esther is receiving a diuretic and beta blocker. Knowledge about the actions and potential side effects of the medications*

enables Emilio to anticipate the types of problems Esther might develop. He is also familiar with developmental and patient education concepts, knowing that he will have to apply this knowledge to develop a teaching plan for Esther that will likely prove beneficial.

Patients take a variety of medications, and new medications are constantly approved. As a result, you will not always understand all the medications ordered for a patient. As a critical thinker, you must admit what you do not know and acquire the knowledge to safely administer unfamiliar medications. This means that you will consult a reliable source (such as a more experienced nurse, pharmacist, health care provider, or a reference book) *before* administering a medication you do not completely understand.

Experience. Nursing students have limited experience with medication administration as it applies to professional practice. However, clinical experiences give you the chance to use the nursing process as it applies to medication administration. As you gain experience in medication administration, cognitive skills (e.g., medication calculations and recognizing side effects) and psychomotor skills (e.g., preparing a syringe or giving a medication IV push) become more refined. As you continue to observe patients' responses to medications, you increase your ability to anticipate and evaluate the effects of medications.

Attitudes. To administer medications safely to patients, several critical thinking attitudes are essential. For example, be disciplined and take adequate time to prepare and administer medications. Take the time to read your patient's medical record before administering medications. Carefully review the patient's history, physical examination, and health care provider's orders. Look up unfamiliar medications in a medication reference and determine why the patient is taking each of the medications. Every step of safe medication administration requires a disciplined attitude and a comprehensive, systematic approach. Follow the same procedure each time you administer medications to ensure safe administration.

Responsibility and accountability are examples of other critical thinking attitudes essential to safe medication administration. Accept the responsibility that the nursing actions in administering a medication will not harm the patient in any way. You are also responsible for knowing that the medication that is ordered for a patient is the correct medication and the correct dose. You are ultimately accountable for administering an ordered medication that is obviously inappropriate for a patient. For example, you are accountable if you give a medication to a patient who is known to be allergic to the medication.

Perseverance is another critical thinking attitude for finding solutions to patient care problems. *In the case study, Emilio recognizes that Esther Simmons will need to manage a number of medications in the home and will likely require a family caregiver, if possible. Emilio decides to further assess Esther's social support network to identify who might be available to assist her with medication administration.*

Standards. Standards define the actions that ensure safe nursing practice. Health care agencies and the nursing profession set standards for medication administration. Agency policy sets limits on a nurse's ability to administer medications in certain units of the acute care setting. For example, nurses who work on general medical surgical units cannot administer IV chemotherapy without having received specialized training. Most agencies have nursing procedure manuals that define the types of medications nurses can and cannot administer. These types and dosages of medications vary from unit to unit within the same institution. For example, phenytoin, a medication used for treating seizures, may be administered by mouth or IV push. In large dosages, phenytoin affects heart rhythm. Therefore, some agencies limit the dosage nurses can administer on a nursing unit that does not have the ability to monitor a patient's heart rate and rhythm.

Professional standards such as *Nursing: Scope and Standards of Practice* (American Nurses Association [ANA], 2015) (see Chapters 1 and 5) apply to medication administration. To prevent medication errors, follow the six rights of medication administration consistently every time you administer medications. Many medication errors can be linked in some way to an inconsistency in adhering to these six rights:

1. The right medication
2. The right dose
3. The right patient
4. The right route
5. The right time
6. The right documentation

Right Medication. A medication order is required for every medication that you administer to a patient. Health care providers sometimes write orders in patients' medical records by hand. However, most hospitals and outpatient practices now use some form of CPOE (AHRQ, 2016). CPOE systems were originally developed to improve the safety of medication orders, but modern systems now allow electronic ordering of tests, procedures, and consultations. CPOE allows a health care provider to order medications electronically, eliminating the need for written orders and improving medication safety (Radley et al., 2013). Regardless of the way a nurse receives a medication order, the most important step of this first right involves the nurse comparing the health care provider's written orders with the MAR or electronic MAR (eMAR) when it is first ordered. Nurses also verify medication information whenever MARs are created or distributed or when patients transfer from one nursing unit or health care setting to another.

When you have determined that information in a patient's MAR is accurate, use the MAR to prepare and administer medications. When you prepare medications compare the label of the medication container with the MAR *three times:*

1. Before removing the container from the drawer, compartment, or shelf
2. As the amount of medication ordered is removed from the container
3. At the patient's bedside before administering the medication to the patient

Never prepare medications from unmarked containers or containers with illegible labels (TJC, 2018). When taking unit-dose packaged medications out of the medication dispensing system, compare the label of the medication with the MAR. Finally, compare all medications at the patient's bedside with the patient's MAR, and use at least two identifiers (patient's name verbally or on ID band, patient's date of birth, or medical record number) before giving the patient any medications (TJC, 2018).

Patients who self-administer medications must keep them in their original labeled containers, separate from other medications, to avoid confusion. Many agencies require that nurses administer all medications rather than letting patients self-administer to maintain accuracy and patient safety. Because the nurse who administers the medication is responsible for any related errors, nurses administer only the medications they prepare. You cannot delegate preparation of medication to another person and then administer the medication to the patient. If a patient questions the medication, do not ignore this concern. A patient or a family caregiver familiar with a patient's medications often knows whether a medication differs from those received previously. In most such cases, the patient's medication order has changed. In some cases, however, patient questions reveal an error.

When a patient questions a medication, withhold the medication and recheck it against the health care provider's orders. If a patient refuses a medication, discard it rather than returning it to the original container. Unit-dose medications can be saved if they are not opened. If a patient refuses narcotics, follow proper institution procedure by having someone else witness the "wasted" medication.

Right Dose. The unit-dose system is designed to minimize errors. When you withdraw a medication from a larger volume or strength than needed, or when the health care provider orders a system of measurement that differs from the pharmacy system of measurement, the risk of error increases. When you calculate medication dosages or conversions, you must have another qualified nurse check the calculation. Prepare medications accurately by using standard measurement devices such as graduated cups, syringes, and scaled droppers. Educate patients to use similar measurement devices at home such as measuring spoons with metric calibrations rather than household teaspoons and tablespoons, which are inaccurate.

Splitting pills often leads to medication errors. To ensure patient safety in inpatient settings, pharmacists split the medications, label them, package them, and then send them to the nurse for administration. Because pill splitting is particularly risky in the home care setting, the FDA (2013) developed suggestions to help patients split pills. These suggestions include ensuring that the tablet is designed to be split, using a tablet splitter, not splitting the entire prescription at one time, and determining if the patient has the motor dexterity or visual acuity to split tablets. If possible, health care providers should avoid ordering medications that require splitting.

Tablets are sometimes crushed and mixed with food. Always clean a crushing device thoroughly before crushing a new tablet. Remnants of previously crushed medications increase the concentration of a medication or cause a patient to receive part of a medication that was not prescribed. Mix crushed medications with very small amounts of food or liquid (such as a single tablespoon). Do not use a patient's favorite foods or liquids because medications alter their taste and reduce the patient's desire for the medication. This is especially a concern for pediatric patients. Not all medications are suitable for crushing. Some medications (such as extended-release capsules) have special coatings to prevent them from being absorbed too quickly. These medications should not be crushed. Refer to the ISMP "Do Not Crush List" available at http://www.ismp.org/tools/donotcrush.pdf (ISMP, 2015c) to ensure that a medication is safe to crush.

Right Patient. A patient getting a drug intended for another patient is a common medication error. There are often two or more patients with the same last name on a patient care unit. Thus you must be sure that you give the right medication to the right patient. Remembering every patient's name and face is impossible. Before you administer a medication, use at least two patient identifiers (TJC, 2018). Acceptable patient identifiers include:

1. A patient's name on an armband.
2. A patient stating his or her name or an identification number assigned by a health care agency.
3. A patient's date of birth on an armband.
4. A patient's social security number.
5. A patient's phone number (note phone numbers can change at any time).

Do not use a patient's room number as an identifier. To identify a patient correctly in an acute care setting, compare the patient identifiers on the MAR with the patient's identification bracelet while at his or her bedside. If an identification bracelet becomes illegible or is missing, get a new one for the patient. Health care settings that are not acute care settings do not require the use of armbands for identification. However, you still need to use a system that verifies the patient's identification with at least two identifiers before administering medications.

Implementing the required identification process requires you to collect patient identifiers reliably when the patient is admitted to a health care agency. Once the identifiers are assigned to a patient (e.g., putting identifiers on an armband and placing the armband on the patient), you use them to match the patient with the MAR, which lists the correct medications.

In addition to using two identifiers, some agencies use bar-code medication administration (BCMA) to identify a patient (see Fig. 17.6). This system requires nurses to first scan a personal bar code that is commonly placed on the patient's armband. The nurse then scans a bar code on the single-dose medication package. Finally, the nurse scans the patient's armband again. All this information is stored in a computer for documentation. This system is designed to be in compliance with the six rights of medication administration and to prevent adverse drug events. Safe use of BCMA requires proper organizational policies, and nurses need to be educated in best practices for BCMA to be most effective.

Right Route. Always consult the health care provider if an order does not include a route of administration. Likewise alert the health care provider immediately if the specified route is not the recommended route. A patient's condition might have changed since the order was written, as in the case of a patient developing nausea and no longer being able to take an oral medication. Medication errors result from use of the wrong route (Teunissen et al., 2013). For example, when nurses prepare an oral medication in a syringe, the risk of administering the medication via the wrong route (such as intravenously) is very high. The ISMP (2011b) recommends that pharmacists, *not nurses,* prepare all oral medications as a unit product to ensure patient safety. Medications prepared commercially are an exception.

The accidental IV injection of a liquid designed for oral use produces local complications, such as sterile skin abscess, or systemic effects, such as a fatality. If you work in a setting that requires you to prepare oral medications, use only enteral syringes (e.g., ENFit) when you prepare oral medications. The new ENFit low-dose syringe has a male design feature within the ENFit female connector (syringe tip) that fits inside the fluid lumen of the ENFit male connector on the feeding tube (ISMP, 2015g). Enteral syringes often use a color different from the parenteral syringes and are clearly labeled for oral or enteral use. The ENFit syringe tips will not connect with parenteral medication administration systems (ISMP, 2017). Needles do not attach to enteral syringes, and the syringes cannot be inserted into any type of IV line. Label the syringe after preparing the medication and be sure to remove any caps from the tip of an oral syringe before administering the medication. Failure to remove the cap can result in the patient aspirating it, thereby blocking the trachea.

Right Time. To administer medications safely, know why a medication is ordered for certain times of day and whether you are allowed to alter the schedule. For example, two medications are ordered, one q8h (every 8 hours) and the other tid (3 times a day). Both medications are scheduled to be administered three times within 24 hours. The health care provider intends for you to give the q8h medication every 8 hours around the clock to maintain therapeutic blood levels of the medication. In contrast, you give the tid medication at three different times during waking hours. Each agency has a recommended time schedule for medications ordered at frequent intervals. Use your nursing judgment to alter the recommended times if necessary or appropriate.

A health care provider often gives specific instructions for the timing of medication administration. A preoperative medication to be given "on call" means that you give the medication when the operating room staff members notify you that they are coming to pick up a patient for surgery. Give a medication ordered PC (after meals) within half an hour of a meal, when a patient has a full stomach. Give a STAT medication immediately.

Give priority to time-critical medications that must act at certain times and thus must be given at certain times. Hospitals designate medications that are time-critical and medications that are non–time-critical (CMS, 2011; ISMP, 2011a).

You administer time-critical medications within 30 minutes before or after their scheduled time around the clock to maintain therapeutic blood levels. Examples of time-critical medications include antibiotics, anticoagulants, insulin, anticonvulsants, and immunosuppressive agents. Give all routinely ordered non–time-critical medications (e.g., laxatives, antihypertensives, vitamin supplements) within 1 to 2 hours before or after the scheduled time or per agency policy (CMS, 2011; ISMP, 2011a). Researchers found that medication administration time errors are the most common medication error (Teunissen et al., 2013).

Your clinical judgment is required when determining the proper time for administration of some medications. For example, administer a prn sleeping medication when a patient is prepared for bed. In addition, use your judgment when administering prn analgesics. For example, you may need to obtain a STAT order from the health care provider if a patient requires a medication before the prn interval has elapsed. Always document your call to a patient's health care provider to change a medication order.

Before a patient's discharge from a health care agency, evaluate a patient's eligibility for home care, especially if the patient was admitted because of problems with medication self-administration. At home patients often have to take multiple medications throughout the day. Help plan schedules based on recommended medication intervals and a patient's daily schedule. Use calendars, daily dosage containers, or timers. Involve family caregivers in monitoring medication adherence. In addition, determine whether the medications are adequate or prescribed at therapeutic levels.

Right Documentation. Nurses and other health care providers use documentation to communicate with one another. Many medication errors result from inaccurate documentation. Therefore always document medications accurately at the time of administration and identify any inaccurate documentation before you give medications.

Before you administer a medication, ensure that the MAR clearly shows:
- The patient's full name.
- The full name of the ordered medication (without abbreviations of medication names).
- The time the medication is to be administered.
- The dosage, route, and frequency of administration.

Common problems with medication orders include incomplete information, inaccurate dosage form or strength, illegible order or signature, incorrect placement of decimals, and nonstandard terminology. If you ever have any question about a medication order because it is incomplete, illegible, vague, or not understood, contact the health care provider before you administer the medication. The health care provider is responsible for providing accurate, complete, and understandable medication orders. If you are unable to contact the health care provider or resolve confusion about the medication, follow your agency policy. There is usually a chain-of-command call policy to determine who you need to contact next. Follow this policy until you resolve issues related to your patient's medication orders.

Some medications require you to assess a patient before administration (e.g., taking a blood pressure before administering an antihypertensive medication). Ensure that you document all preassessment data in a patient's medical record before administering the medication. *Record the administration of each medication on the MAR immediately after administration.* Never document that you have given a medication until you have actually given it. Inaccurate documentation, such as forgetting to document giving a medication or documenting an incorrect dose, leads to errors in subsequent decisions about patient care. Consider the following situation: A patient is to receive an antihypertensive medication at 1600, but the nurse who gives the medication fails to document it. The nurse caring for the patient goes home, and you are the patient's new nurse for the day. You notice that the antihypertensive is not documented, so you assume that the previous nurse did not give the medication. You give the patient another dose of the medication. About 2 hours later, the patient develops hypotension, causing him to fall and break a hip when getting out of bed. Accurate documentation and follow-up with the nurse from the previous shift could have confirmed that the antihypertensive was given as ordered and could have prevented this situation.

Document the name of the medication, the dose, the time of administration, and the route in the MAR. Also document the site of any injections you give and the patient's responses to medications, whether positive or negative. Notify the patient's health care provider of any negative responses to medications, and document the time, date, and name of the health care provider who was notified in the patient's medical record. The efforts you make to ensure proper documentation help ensure safe care.

Maintaining Patients' Rights. Another important standard to apply in critically thinking about your approach to medication administration involves patients' rights. In accordance with *The Patient Care Partnership* (American Hospital Association [AHA], 2003) and because of the potential risks related to medication administration, a patient has the following rights:
- To be informed of the name, purpose, action, and potential undesired effects of a medication
- To refuse a medication regardless of the consequences
- To have qualified nurses or physicians assess a medication history including allergies and use of herbals
- To be properly advised of the experimental nature of medication therapy and give written consent for its use
- To receive labeled medications safely without discomfort in accordance with the six rights of medication administration
- To receive appropriate supportive therapy in relation to medication therapy
- To not receive unnecessary medications
- To be informed if medications are a part of a research study

Know these rights and answer all patient and family questions courteously and professionally. Do not become defensive if a patient refuses medication therapy. Remember that every person of consenting age has a right to refusal.

NURSING PROCESS

You assess many factors to determine a patient's need for and potential response to medication therapy. Perform a thorough assessment on all your patients to help ensure safe medication administration.

■■■ ASSESSMENT

History. Before administering medications, obtain or review a patient's medical history, which provides indications or contraindications for medication therapy. Disease or illness places patients at risk for adverse medication effects. For example, if a patient has a gastric ulcer, compounds containing aspirin increase the likelihood of bleeding. Long-term health problems such as arthritis or chronic lung disease require specific medications. This knowledge helps you anticipate the medications that your patient requires. A patient's surgical history sometimes indicates use of medications also. For example, after a thyroidectomy a patient requires thyroid hormone replacement.

Allergies. All members of the health care team need to know a patient's history of allergies to medications, foods, and latex. Many medications have ingredients found in food sources. For example, propofol, which is used for anesthesia and sedation, contains inactive ingredients of egg lecithin and soybean oil. Therefore patients who have an egg or soy allergy should not receive propofol (Skidmore-Roth, 2016). If a patient has a latex allergy, latex-free gloves are applied when administering parenteral or topical medications. In an acute care setting patients wear allergy identification bands that list medication allergies. All allergies and the types of reactions are noted on the patient's admission notes and history and physical examination. List patient's food and drug allergies on each page of the MAR.

Medication History. When taking a medication history, assess which medications a patient takes, including prescription and nonprescription drugs and herbal supplements. Include the length of time the patient has taken each drug, current dosage schedule, and whether the patient has experienced adverse effects to any of the medications. Assess the patient's level of understanding about any medication he or she is currently taking. If it is possible, assess if the patient takes medications correctly (e.g., count doses or have the patient keep a diary to track when medications are taken). Review information about the medications including action, purpose, normal dosages, routes, side effects, and nursing implications for administration and monitoring.

Be sure that the health care provider has ordered a safe dose, especially in the case of older adults or children. In addition, be aware of medication interactions and special nursing interventions needed for medication administration. Often you need to consult several references. Valuable resources are pharmacology textbooks and handbooks; electronic medication manuals available on a desktop, laptop, or handheld computer; nursing journals; the *Physicians' Desk Reference* (PDR); medication package inserts; and pharmacists. You are responsible for knowing as much as possible about each medication that your patients receive.

Diet History. Collect a diet history (see Chapter 35) of a patient's normal eating patterns and food preferences so that you can plan an effective dosage schedule (e.g., important when patients take medications around meal times). Some medications interact with food (e.g., green leafy vegetables and warfarin, grapefruit juice and statins). In these cases, assess when patients take these medications to determine if they avoid foods that interact with their medications.

Physical Examination. Before administering medications, perform a physical assessment (see Chapter 16) of the body systems likely to reveal physical findings that will indicate or contraindicate the medications you are administering. For example, observe the integrity of skin and mucous membranes for patients who are to receive topical medications; assess lung sounds and heart status if you are to give a medication influencing cardiopulmonary function. Be sure to also assess a patient's sensory, motor, and cognitive functions to determine if the patient can prepare and administer medications at home. For example, if a patient is wheelchair bound, is he or she able to self-administer the medications or is a family caregiver needed? Is a patient with poor visual acuity able to read labels on a medication bottle? Assess a patient's ability to prepare doses (e.g., open containers or fill syringes), remember a dosage schedule, and take medications (e.g., perform self-injection or instill eye drops) correctly. If a patient is unable to self-administer medications, assess whether a family caregiver or friend is available to assist.

Patient's Health Literacy Level. Health literacy has been defined by the CDC (2016b) and in the Patient Protection and Affordable Care Act of 2010 as the degree to which an individual has the capacity to obtain, communicate, process, and understand basic health information and services to make appropriate health decisions, which includes self-administering medications. A common measure for defining adherence is taking at least 90% of one's prescribed doses (Sawkin et al., 2015). If a patient has low health literacy, he or she will have difficulty reading prescriptions, preparing doses that require even simple calculation (e.g., number of tablets), and reading drug information. Use available literacy assessment tools such as the Rapid Estimate of Adult Literacy in Medicine (REALM) which is often chosen for its ease of use and short administration and scoring time. Ask patients to read their prescription labels to you and discuss what times they are to take their medications to assess their understanding of medication regimens. Perform the same assessments with family caregivers if they are administering medications to patients in the home.

Patient's Current Condition. The ongoing physical or mental status of a patient affects whether you give a medication and how you administer it. Assess a patient carefully before giving any medication. For example, check the patient's blood pressure before giving an antihypertensive. If the blood pressure is unusually low (e.g., systolic pressure below 100 mm Hg), hold the medication and notify the patient's health care provider. Assessment findings serve as a baseline in evaluating the effects of medication therapy.

Patient's Attitude About Medication Use. Patients' attitudes about medications affect their willingness to take medication therapy. Sometimes their attitudes reveal medication dependence or avoidance. Patients do not usually express their feelings about taking a medication especially if dependence is a problem. Include a family caregiver in your assessment if appropriate. In the home setting observe a patient's behavior for evidence of medication dependence or avoidance. Also assess a patient's cultural and personal beliefs about Western medicine to determine if his or her beliefs interfere with medication compliance (Box 17.7) (see Chapter 21).

Older Adult Considerations. When assessing an older adult, consider factors that can affect his or her ability to self-administer medications when you conduct the physical assessment. Also assess if a family caregiver commonly assists the patient, and if so, assess his or her knowledge of the medications and how to administer each. Include an assessment of the patient's adherence to medication therapy. Adherence is the extent to which a person's behavior agrees with the medication regimen from a health care provider with respect to the timing, dosage, and frequency of therapies (Leporini et al., 2014). Nonadherence with medications affects the health and safety of all patients and is common in older adults because they often take many medications and have complex medication administration schedules (Touhy and Jett, 2014).

Medication adherence rates among patients varies widely, depending on the type of therapy, patient condition, and how adherence is measured (Foulon et al., 2011; Sawkin et al., 2015). A patient's risk for nonadherence increases with the number of medications that the patient takes and the amount of times in a day that he or she has to take them (Bae et al., 2012). Poor patient education, fear of addiction, or the perception that a medication is not needed also cause nonadherence. Other factors contributing to nonadherence in older adult populations include depression, cognitive or functional disabilities, dislike for medication side effects, a busy and active lifestyle, and inability to afford or easily obtain medications. Carefully assess all the medications that your patients take and compare what your patients tell you they take with what their health care provider prescribed. If you suspect nonadherence, assess for contributing factors and work with a patient to develop a medication schedule that the patient will follow.

⊕ BOX 17.7 PATIENT-CENTERED CARE

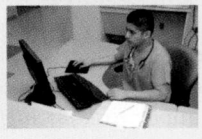

Emilio is worried that Ms. Simmons will have trouble managing her medications at home because she takes so many. Emilio asks Ms. Simmons her feelings about taking multiple medications. She tells Emilio that she gets easily confused and states, "I am not sure that all these medicines really help me." He asks if anyone helps her at home and learns that Esther has a granddaughter who visits her weekly. Emilio also asks, "Tell me how you keep track of what medicines you take each day." Ms. Simmons hesitates and says, "Well I have a container for all medicines I take in the morning and all I take in the afternoon and evening. There are so many." Emilio decides to ask if the granddaughter could perhaps come to visit and that the two of them might discuss how to help Ms. Simmons with her medicines. Ms. Simmons agrees.

Compared with the general population, African Americans have a greater chance of dying as a result of diabetes, heart disease, cancer, and stroke. African American patients have reported that self-efficacy, patient-provider communication, and social support contribute to their ability to comply with a hypertension regimen (Rimando, 2013). It is important for Emilio to assess Esther's socioeconomic status and social support resources she has to take her medicines. Is the granddaughter willing to offer more assistance? Does the granddaughter have transportation to get to Esther's home regularly? Are there individuals in Esther's church who can help? Many African Americans have large social networks and a strong religious faith, both of which can be helpful in managing illness (Giger, 2017).

Elderly patients often have many chronic illnesses. Patients with chronic illnesses often take multiple medications multiple times of the day, placing them at a greater risk for having problems with adherence. The more medications a patient takes, the greater the risk of having drug interactions and side effects.

IMPLICATIONS FOR PRACTICE

- Emilio will use the patient's social support network to identify individuals who can assist in monitoring and even administering medications in the home.
- Motivational interviewing, reminder devices, community health worker (CHW)–delivered interventions, and pharmacist-delivered interventions have shown some benefit in improving medication adherence in African American patients (Hu et al., 2014).
- Education and counseling that is provided only once or very briefly may be insufficient to influence a patient's values and behaviors (Hu et al., 2014).
- Interventions that work for individuals of one ethnicity may not be as effective for individuals of a different background. Culturally sensitive interventions can more effectively address patient beliefs regarding their conditions, therapy, and values while appropriately encouraging better adherence (Hu et al., 2014).

TABLE 17.6 FOCUSED PATIENT ASSESSMENT

FACTORS TO ASSESS	QUESTIONS	PHYSICAL ASSESSMENT
Understanding of medication	Explain which medications you are taking and why you are taking them. Tell me how frequently and what times of the day you take each of your medications.	Assess nonverbal communication to determine if patient's response matches his or her explanation. Assess content of answers for accuracy in response.
Medication side effects	How do you feel after you take your medication? (Discuss each.) Describe for me any symptoms that bother you.	Assess for side effects based on medications the patient is taking (e.g., if patient is on antihypertensive medication, measure blood pressure)
Medication adherence	Tell me about times when you have not taken your medication as it is prescribed. Do you have difficulties paying for your medications? Which pharmacy fills your prescriptions; how do you get there?	Assess for expected desired effects when medications taken regularly (e.g., if patient is on antidepressant, assess for signs and symptoms of depression)

Patient's Knowledge and Understanding of Medication Therapy. Ask questions to assess your patient's knowledge and understanding of medications (Table 17.6). A patient's knowledge and understanding influence his or her willingness and ability to take medications safely and correctly. Unless a patient understands the purpose of a medication, the importance of regular dosage schedules, proper administration methods, and the possible side effects, adherence is difficult. If a patient is having trouble adhering to medication therapy, be sure to discuss financial resources and transportation issues as well. Can the patient get to a pharmacy regularly? Is mail order service for medications an option? During assessment you will discover that some patients do not understand their medications, and assessment of literacy level becomes a priority. Also determine your patient's readiness and ability to learn. Is the patient experiencing symptoms of a condition or side effects of medications that affect his or her ability to attend to or understand any discussion you have about medications? If so you might have to return later for a more thorough assessment.

Patient Expectations. When assessing patients' expectations about medication administration, determine their perceptions about their illnesses, how they believe their medications will help them, and when they expect to receive the medications. For example, in an acute care setting, when patients have pain, they will expect to receive their analgesics when they perceive they need them. This is a time to clarify medication schedules, for example, when prn medications can next be given. Assess whether patients believe that their medications will be helpful. How does a patient feel about having adverse effects? Do your patients believe that they will be able to afford their medications? It is your responsibility to monitor your patients' expectations and corresponding medication adherence, especially if you choose to work in settings where you will see patients repeatedly.

■ ■ ■ NURSING DIAGNOSIS

Assessment produces data about a patient's condition, risks for medication-related problems, ability to self-administer medications, knowledge about medications, and medication adherence. Use these data to identify the patient's appropriate nursing diagnoses that apply to medication therapy. Certain data are defining characteristics that, when clustered together, reveal problem-focused nursing diagnoses. For example, *Ineffective Health Management related to complexity of treatment regimen* is indicated when patients have a complex medication schedule and admit to difficulty integrating their medications into their daily routine. Risk factors enable you to identify a risk nursing diagnosis. For example, *Risk for Ineffective Peripheral Tissue Perfusion* may be a diagnosis in a patient with diabetes who is to receive a topical skin ointment. This list of nursing diagnoses frequently applies during medication administration in a variety of settings:

- *Anxiety*
- *Ineffective Health Maintenance*
- *Deficient Knowledge (Medication Self-administration)*
- *Noncompliance (Medications)*
- *Impaired Swallowing*
- *Impaired Memory*

After selecting the diagnosis, identify the related factor or risk factor that drives the selection of nursing interventions. In the example of *Noncompliance,* the related factors of *financial barriers* and *insufficient knowledge about the regimen* require different interventions. If a patient's problem-focused nursing diagnosis is related to inadequate finances, you can collaborate with family members, social workers, case managers, or community agencies to connect the patient with the necessary financial resources and develop a medication regimen the patient can afford. If the related factor is *insufficient knowledge,* you implement a culturally appropriate teaching plan with appropriate follow-up.

PLANNING

Always organize your care activities to ensure that you administer medications safely. Rushing to give medications to patients leads to errors. Minimize distractions or interruptions when preparing and administering medications (Ching et al., 2013; Donaldson et al., 2014). No-interruption zones (NIZs) have been recommended to reduce distractions and interruptions during medication administration (Yoder et al., 2015). Be diligent in planning and following a safe routine every time you prepare and administer medications.

Goals and Outcomes. Goals of medication administration include better control of a patient's disease, improved health function, and adherence to a medication regimen. Work closely with your patients to set goals and outcomes and to select appropriate interventions. This is especially important in the home setting where you establish time schedules that meet the aim of medication orders and adapt to a patient's lifestyle or you help a patient who has limited facilities to prepare medicines correctly. Whether a patient self-administers medications or you assume responsibility for administering medications, set goals and expected outcomes to use time wisely during medication administration. For example, if you are caring for a patient with newly diagnosed heart failure, you establish the following goal and expected outcomes:

Goal: The patient will verbalize a plan to safely
   self-administer all ordered medications before discharge.
Outcomes:

- The patient verbalizes understanding of desired and adverse effects of medications.
- The patient states signs and symptoms of heart failure.
- The patient prepares a dose of ordered medication correctly.
- The patient describes a daily routine that integrates timing of medication with daily activities.

Setting Priorities. It is important to set your priorities during medication administration, especially when you care for multiple patients. Assess your patients' clinical conditions on an ongoing basis to determine their status and the nursing diagnoses that take the greatest priority. An initial review of medication orders at the beginning of a work shift allows you to prioritize when to administer medications versus providing other interventions. Use patient assessment data to identify the medications to give first, whether it is time to evaluate a patient's response to a medication, or when it is appropriate to administer prn medications. For example, if one of your patients is in pain, you must give pain medication as soon as possible. If a patient's blood pressure is elevated, administer the blood pressure medication before other medications.

In addition to administering medications, teaching patients about their medications is another priority. Plan to teach patients about their medications while you administer them. This efficient use of time makes the teaching more relevant.

When teaching about medications, if you know a family caregiver is involved, plan teaching sessions accordingly.

Collaborative Care. Collaboration with patients and their family caregivers is essential, particularly if patients will require assistance with self-administration and if medication regimens are complicated. A family caregiver can assist with helping a patient stay on daily medication schedules, prepare doses correctly, store medications, and monitor ongoing patient responses to medications. Partner together so that the patient's medication plan is easy to follow.

You will often collaborate with patients' health care providers, pharmacists, and case managers to ensure that patients can afford their medications and are able to reach a pharmacy. In some cases, having a pharmacy mail drugs to patients' homes is more convenient.

Some patients also need to be able to calculate dosages and prepare complex medication regimens. Collaborate with community resources (e.g., agency on aging, public health department, medical interpreters) when patients have significant health literacy issues or difficulty understanding medication instructions (see Chapter 12).

IMPLEMENTATION

Health Promotion. In promoting or maintaining patients' health, remember that health beliefs, illness characteristics, personal motivation, and personal habits (e.g., excessive alcohol intake, busy work schedules) influence their adherence with medication schedules (Jimmy and Jose, 2011). Factors including belonging to an ethnic minority, unemployment, and cost of a patient's medications consistently showed a negative effect on adherence, which indicates a strong socioeconomic impact (Mathes et al., 2014). Several nursing interventions such as patient education (see Chapter 12) and motivational interviewing promote adherence. Always integrate a patient's health beliefs and cultural practices into the treatment plan. Make referrals to community resources if a patient is unable to afford or cannot arrange transportation to obtain needed medications.

Patient Education and Behavioral Support. The following guidelines will allow you to prepare patients to be more adherent to medication regimens (Jimmy and Jose, 2011):

- **Explain key information when administering a medication.** Address key information about the drugs (e.g., what the medication is; why is it prescribed; and when, how, and how long to take it) during administration. Inform patients and family caregivers about the common side effects to expect. Being informed about side effects can lessen the worry that occurs when a side effect does develop. Knowing how to respond to and manage a side effect will lessen the likelihood of nonadherence to the medication.

   Adapt your approaches so that patients understand all medication instructions. Many health care agencies offer easy-to-read patient education sheets on specific types of medications. A patient needs to know how to take a medication properly and what will happen if he or she fails to do so. For example, after receiving a prescription for an antibiotic, a patient needs to understand the importance of taking the full prescription. Failure to do this can lead to a worsening of the condition and the development of bacteria resistant to the medication. Also teach patients ways to change medication schedules to fit into their lifestyles. Patients who are placed on newly prescribed medications may need more involved instruction (Box 17.8).

- **Use medication adherence–improving aids.** Provide medication calendars, timers, or schedules that specify the time to take medications. Use drug cards, medication charts, or medicine-related information sheets as resources for essential information. Use pill boxes, unit-dose packaging, and special containers indicating the time of dose to help organize a patient's medication routine. Provide specially designed equipment such as syringes with enlarged calibrated scales for easier reading or Braille-labeled medication vials for patients with visual alterations.
- **Provide behavioral support.** Motivational interviewing (MI) is a direct, patient-centered counseling approach that aims to help people change problem behaviors (such as medication nonadherence, smoking, weight gain) by helping patients explore and resolve ambivalence to change

(Ingersoll et al., 2016). A review of research shows that MI also outperforms traditional advice giving (Rubak et al., 2005). MI is very collaborative because it supports patient autonomy and helps patients discuss their thoughts, feelings, and memories that influence a behavior. By using MI clinicians seek to understand patients' perspectives, while directing them toward considering changing one or more behaviors (such as adherence) by building awareness of a discrepancy between the patient's current and hoped-for self, avoiding confrontation, and supporting patients' optimism about the possibility and methods for change (Ingersoll et al., 2016). Motivation to change comes from the patient and is not imposed by the health care provider. The motivational interview is designed to elicit, clarify, and resolve a patient's ambivalence and to perceive benefits and costs associated with taking medications routinely on time. Readiness to change is not a patient trait, but readiness will fluctuate during interpersonal interaction between a patient and health care provider.

An important resource for behavioral support is a well-trained and informed family caregiver. When you know that a family member or friend is going to assume responsibility for either directly administering or assisting

---

BOX 17.8 PATIENT TEACHING

Preparing for Home Medication Administration

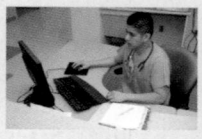 Emilio partners with Ms. Simmons and her granddaughter in developing a teaching plan before Ms. Simmons goes home at the end of the week. Emilio wants Esther to be able to self-administer her medications at home with a family caregiver's supervision for the first 4 weeks. The granddaughter and a close friend from Esther's church set up a schedule to check on Esther daily. Older adult patients often have difficulty taking medications out of their normal containers, have difficulties opening medication packages, and have problems related to health literacy. Based on this information, Emilio develops the following teaching plan for Esther.

OUTCOME
- At the end of the teaching session, Esther is able to self-administer her medications safely and correctly.

TEACHING STRATEGIES
- Sit with Esther at a table in a room that is well lit and has limited distractions (e.g., television off).
- Include Esther's granddaughter in educational sessions (Ownby et al., 2012).
- Have Esther's granddaughter bring all of Esther's medications from home to the hospital. Compare the medications Esther currently has at home with the medications that she is going to take at home. Determine which medications she understands.
- Assess Esther's health literacy by determining her ability to understand what she reads and do simple medication

calculations. If she has poor health literacy, ensure that information is presented at a level that she can understand. Be sure the granddaughter is able to perform the calculations.
- Review information about medications including desired effect, dose, frequency, and side effects with Esther and her granddaughter.
- Show Esther and her granddaughter how to fill a medication organizer correctly.
- Provide patient teaching materials that include helpful pictures to enhance Esther's understanding of prescribed medications. Ensure that the print and pictures on the teaching sheets are large enough for her to see.

EVALUATION
- Use the principles of teach-back to evaluate patient/family caregiver learning:
  - "In your own words, tell me why you are taking these medications."
  - "Write out a medication schedule that includes how much of each medication you should take and when you should take it."
  - "What are the symptoms related to the possible side effects of medications that you are taking? What should you report to your health care provider?"
  - "Have your granddaughter review the doses removed from the medication organizer 1 week after you have been home and record the results in a diary to take to your next physician visit."

patients with administering medications, you are responsible for preparing that individual. This means that the family caregiver needs to learn the same information about medication pharmacology, storage and preparation, administration, and monitoring that you provide patients.

Emilio is able to arrange to have Esther's granddaughter come to the skilled care floor to learn about her grandmother's medications. The granddaughter agrees to come to Esther's home 3 mornings a week to check on her. The granddaughter will help set up Esther's weekly doses in a medication organizer, check the organizer with each visit, and regularly check Esther for any common side effects.

- **Schedule appropriate follow-up.** Do not wait until your last contact with a patient to provide information about a medication. In the acute care setting schedule time for follow-up so that patients can ask questions and you can perform teach-back. In the home setting monitoring for medication adherence (e.g., checking total doses taken over a week, having family caregiver report on doses given) should also be a follow-up criterion. Follow-up includes ensuring patients understand what to observe for and how and when to act so that they are better able to cope with problems caused by medications. Safety guidelines should be included in your instruction and teach-back to ensure the proper use and storage of medications in the home.

Acute Care. In the acute care setting expert nursing interventions, timely observation, and documentation of patient responses to medications are essential. Several nursing interventions are critical to providing safe and effective medication administration.

Receiving, Transcribing, and Communicating Medication Orders. A medication order is required to administer any medication to a patient. The medication order needs to contain all the elements listed in Box 17.9. The process of verification of medications varies among health care agencies. During the transcription process a nurse and pharmacist check all medication orders for accuracy and thoroughness several times. They also verify that a patient's ordered medications are appropriate, taking into consideration the patient's current health problems, treatments, laboratory values, and other prescribed medications. Once the nurse and pharmacist determine that the medication is appropriate, it is added to the MAR. The MAR either is printed on paper or is available electronically. When it is electronic, it is called an *eMAR*. Regardless of the type of MAR your agency uses, it includes a patient's name, medical record number, room, and bed number; medical and food allergies; other patient identifiers (e.g., birth date); and name, dosage, frequency, time, and route of administration for each medication.

For patient safety it is essential that you refer to the MAR each time you prepare a medication and have it available at the patient's bedside when administering medications. Verify the accuracy of every medication you give to a patient with the patient's orders. If the medication order is incomplete, incorrect, or inappropriate or if there is a discrepancy between the written order and what is on the MAR, consult with the

---

BOX 17.9 COMPONENTS OF MEDICATION ORDERS

A medication order needs to have all the following parts:

Patient's full name: A patient's full name distinguishes the patient from other people with the same last name. In the acute care setting patients are sometimes assigned special identification numbers (such as medical record number) to help distinguish patients with the same names. This number is often included with the order.

Date and time that order is written: The day, month, year, and time must be included. Designating the time that an order is written clarifies when certain orders are to start and stop. If a medication error occurs, it is easier to document the incident when this information is available.

Medication name: A health care provider orders a medication by its generic or trade name. Correct spelling is essential to prevent confusion with medications with similar spelling.

Dosage: The amount or strength of the medication is included.

Route of administration: A health care provider uses only accepted abbreviations for medication routes. Accuracy is important to ensure that patients receive medications by the intended route.

Time and frequency of administration: An order will also include the time and frequency of medication administration, which is essential information for anyone filling the order (prescription) or administering the medication including family caregivers. Orders for multiple doses establish a routine schedule for medication administration.

Signature of health care provider: The signature makes an order a legal request.

---

health care provider. Do not give a medication until you are certain that you are able to follow the six rights of medication administration. When you give the wrong medication or an incorrect dose, you are legally responsible for the error.

Accurate Dosage Calculation and Measurement. You calculate each dose when preparing medications. To avoid calculation errors, pay close attention to the process of calculation and avoid interruptions from other people or nursing activities. Ask another nurse to double-check your calculations against the health care provider's order if you are in doubt about the accuracy of your calculation or if you are calculating a new or unusual dose.

Correct Administration. Before administering a medication, verify the patient's identity by using at least two patient identifiers (TJC, 2018). Identifiers are usually on a patient's armband. Compare at least two identifiers with the MAR to ensure that you are giving the medication to the correct patient. Use aseptic technique and proper procedures when handling and giving medications. Some medications require an assessment before administration (e.g., assessing heart rate before giving a cardiac glycoside).

Avoidance of Distractions. Research shows that distractions lead to medication errors. Each interruption was associated with a 12.1% increase in procedural failures (medication preparation) and a 12.7% increase in clinical errors (medication administration) (Westbrook et al., 2010). Error severity increased with interruption frequency; without interruption, the estimated risk of a major error was 2.3%; four interruptions doubled the risk to 4.7% (Westbrook et al., 2010). Distraction comes from a variety of sources such as a page, phone call, or request from a colleague that disturbs or diverts attention from a current desired task or forces attention on a new task at least temporarily. Follow these approaches to reduce distractions (Yoder et al., 2015): (1) establish no interrupt zone (NIZ) with signage; (2) ensure colleagues do not disturb you when you prepare medications (wear a visual signal such as a colored vest); (3) provide staff education about risks of interruptions; (4) determine the best time for necessary interruptions; (5) create checklists for critical procedures requiring medication administration; (6) turn off or manage mobile devices; and (7) gather supplies before prescribing, preparing, or administering medication.

Recording Medication Administration. After administering a medication, record it immediately on the appropriate record form. Never chart a medication before administering it. Recording immediately after administration prevents errors. Documentation of medication administration includes the name of the medication, dosage, route, and exact time of administration. Some agency policies require that you record the location of an injection.

Restorative and Continuing Care. Medication administration practices vary in the many restorative settings where you will care for patients. Patients with functional limitations often require a nurse to administer all medications. In long-term care settings trained nurse assistants and licensed practical nurses administer certain medications. In the home care setting patients usually administer their own medications or receive assistance from family caregivers.

Regardless of the type of medication activity, you are responsible for supervising any staff colleagues involved in medication administration and for instructing patients and family caregivers in medication storage, preparation, administration, and how to monitor for actions and side effects. As a nurse you are also responsible for monitoring patient adherence with the medication regimen and determining the effectiveness of medications.

Special Considerations for Administering Medications to Specific Age-Groups. A patient's developmental level is a factor in the administration of medications. Your knowledge of developmental needs helps you anticipate responses to medication therapy.

Infants and Children. The standard of practice in many pediatric settings is to have a second nurse verify all pediatric dose calculations before administration. All children require special psychological preparation before receiving medications. A child's parents often are valuable resources for determining the best way to give the child a medication. Having the parent give the medication while the nurse supervises might be less traumatic for a child.

BOX 17.10　TIPS FOR ADMINISTERING MEDICATIONS TO CHILDREN

ORAL MEDICATIONS
- Liquids are safer to swallow than pills to avoid aspiration.
- Use calibrated droppers for administering liquids to infants.
- Offer juice, a soft drink, or frozen juice bar, if allowed, after the child swallows a drug.
- When mixing medications in other foods or liquids, use only a small amount. The child may refuse to take all of a larger mixture.
- Avoid mixing a medication in a child's favorite foods or liquids because the child may later refuse them.
- A plastic, disposable oral syringe is the most accurate device for preparing liquid doses, especially doses less than 10 mL (cups, teaspoons, and droppers are inaccurate).

INJECTIONS
- Use caution when selecting intramuscular (IM) injection sites. Infants and small children have underdeveloped muscles. Follow agency policy.
- Children are sometimes unpredictable and uncooperative. Make sure that someone (preferably another nurse) is available to restrain a child if needed. If restraint is necessary, have the parent act as a comforter, not restrainer.
- Always awaken a sleeping child before giving an injection.
- Distracting a child with conversation, bubbles, or a toy reduces pain perception.
- If time allows, apply a lidocaine ointment to an injection site before the injection to reduce pain perception during the injection.

Supportive care is necessary to gain a child's cooperation. Explain the procedure to the child, using words appropriate to the child's level of comprehension. Long explanations increase a child's anxiety, especially for painful procedures such as an injection. Giving the child choices whenever possible can produce greater success. For example, say, "It's time to take your pill now. Do you want it with water or juice?" Do not give the child the option of not taking a medication. After taking a medication, praise the child and offer a simple reward such as a star or token. Box 17.10 offers suggestions for administering medication to children.

Older Adults. ADEs occur in 15% or more of older adult patients who come to medical offices, hospitals, and extended care facilities (Pretorius et al., 2013). The most common serious effects of ADEs include falls, orthostatic hypotension, heart failure, and delirium. Older adults require special nursing considerations during medication administration (Box 17.11). Be vigilant when administering medications and know the physiological changes of aging (Fig. 17.7) so that you can anticipate adverse reactions. Collaborate with health care providers to minimize ADEs in older adults by discontinuing medications, prescribing new medications sparingly, reducing the number of health care providers, and frequently reconciling medications (Pretorius et al., 2013).

Polypharmacy. Polypharmacy is the use of multiple medications, the use of potentially inappropriate or unnecessary

BOX 17.11   CARE OF THE OLDER ADULT

Safety in Medication Administration

- Frequently review a patient's medication history including use of over-the-counter medications, and consult with the health care provider to simplify the drug therapy plan whenever possible (Pasina et al., 2014).
- Keep instructions clear and simple, provide memory aids (e.g., calendar, medication schedule), and ensure that written information about medications is in print large enough for a patient to see (Touhy and Jett, 2014).
- Assess functional status (including vision, hand grasp, fine motor skills) to determine whether a patient will require assistance in taking medications (Touhy and Jett, 2014).
- Some older adults have a greater sensitivity to drugs, especially drugs that act on the central nervous system. Therefore carefully monitor patients' responses to medications and anticipate dosage adjustments as needed (Touhy and Jett, 2014).
- If a patient has difficulty swallowing a capsule or tablet, ask the health care provider to substitute a liquid medication. If you must give an oral tablet or capsule, instruct the patient to place medication on the front of the tongue and then swallow fluid to help wash it to the back of the throat. If the patient continues to have problems, have him or her try taking medication with a very small amount of semisolid food (e.g., applesauce) (Touhy and Jett, 2014).

medications, or the use of a medication that does not match a diagnosis (Touhy and Jett, 2014). An example of polypharmacy is the use of two medications from the same chemical class to treat the same illness in a patient. You suspect polypharmacy if your patient uses two or more medications with the same or similar actions to treat several illnesses simultaneously or mixes nutritional supplements or herbal products with medications. Older adults often practice polypharmacy when they seek relief from a variety of symptoms (e.g., pain, constipation, insomnia, and indigestion) by using OTC preparations.

Polypharmacy is unavoidable at times. For example, some patients need to take more than one medication to control high blood pressure. When the patient experiences polypharmacy, the risk of adverse reactions and medication interactions with other medications and food is increased. Because many older adults have chronic health problems, polypharmacy is common. Polypharmacy also is becoming more common in children and patients with mental illnesses. The risk for polypharmacy increases with:

- Frequent use of OTC medications.
- Lack of knowledge about medications.
- Incorrect beliefs about medications.
- Visits to several health care providers for different illnesses.

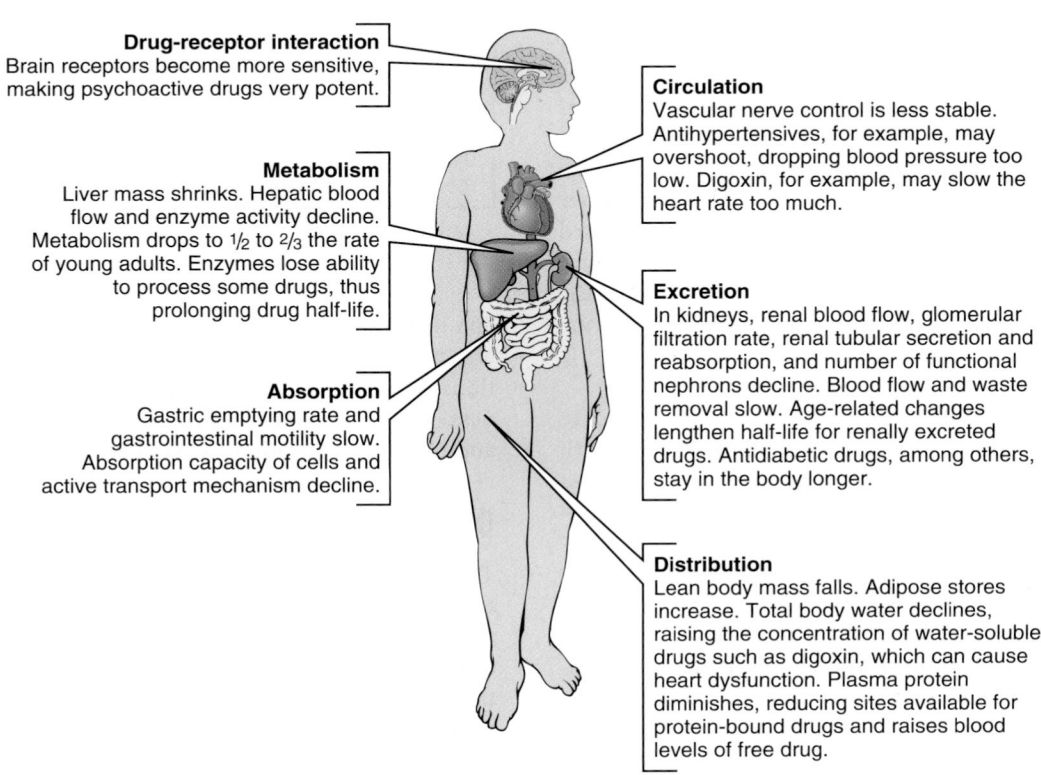

Drug-receptor interaction
Brain receptors become more sensitive, making psychoactive drugs very potent.

Metabolism
Liver mass shrinks. Hepatic blood flow and enzyme activity decline. Metabolism drops to ½ to ⅔ the rate of young adults. Enzymes lose ability to process some drugs, thus prolonging drug half-life.

Absorption
Gastric emptying rate and gastrointestinal motility slow. Absorption capacity of cells and active transport mechanism decline.

Circulation
Vascular nerve control is less stable. Antihypertensives, for example, may overshoot, dropping blood pressure too low. Digoxin, for example, may slow the heart rate too much.

Excretion
In kidneys, renal blood flow, glomerular filtration rate, renal tubular secretion and reabsorption, and number of functional nephrons decline. Blood flow and waste removal slow. Age-related changes lengthen half-life for renally excreted drugs. Antidiabetic drugs, among others, stay in the body longer.

Distribution
Lean body mass falls. Adipose stores increase. Total body water declines, raising the concentration of water-soluble drugs such as digoxin, which can cause heart dysfunction. Plasma protein diminishes, reducing sites available for protein-bound drugs and raises blood levels of free drug.

FIG 17.7 Effects of aging on drug metabolism. (From Lewis SL, et al: *Medical-surgical nursing: assessment and management of clinical problems,* ed 8, St Louis, 2011, Mosby.)

Frequent communication among health care providers is essential to minimize risks associated with polypharmacy and to ensure that patients' medication regimens are as simple as possible (Pasina et al., 2014).

■ ■ ■ EVALUATION

You evaluate the effects of a medication after administering a dose. You are responsible for monitoring and conducting the necessary assessments to determine how a medication affects a patient. This often involves immediately evaluating a patient's response at the peak onset of a medication (e.g., 30 to 60 minutes after a dose is administered) or evaluating a patient weekly or monthly when you follow the patient in a clinic or home health setting. Evaluation of medication administration is an essential role of professional nursing that requires:

- Assessment skills.
- Knowledge of medications, physiology, and pathophysiology.
- Analysis and synthesis of data.
- Critical judgment and decision making.

Patient Outcomes. The goal of safe and effective medication administration is met when a patient responds appropriately to medication therapy and is able to self-administer a medication safely and correctly. Because time is limited in acute care, your aim will be to ensure that the patient can assume responsibility for self-administration. Constantly ask questions and use your knowledge of each of a patient's medications to evaluate his or her responses. You use many different measures to evaluate patient responses to medication including direct observation of physiological measures (e.g., blood pressure or laboratory values), behavioral responses (e.g., level of agitation, cognition), and rating scales (e.g., pain rating scale). Also use patients' statements and responses to questions you ask as evaluation measures (e.g., "I slept better last night"). When a patient does not experience expected outcomes of medication therapy, investigate possible reasons, revise any relevant nursing diagnoses, collaborate with the health care provider, and choose appropriate revisions to the plan of care.

Patient Expectations. Evaluation is more effective when you value your patients' participation. Partner with your patients and include them in the evaluation process (Box 17.12). Evaluate the results of instruction by determining if they understand and can safely administer their medications. For example, if you are caring for a child who needs an inhaler, be sure to watch the child use the inhaler. To determine whether patients understand their medication schedules, ask them to explain when they take their medications and whether they can take them as prescribed.

When patients struggle with their medication schedule, identify what they see as barriers to medication adherence (e.g., cost and lack of knowledge), and remove these barriers if possible. Also remember that patients have differing values

---

BOX 17.12 EVALUATION

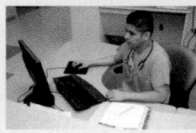

Emilio prepares for Esther's discharge home. He knows from the preparation that he did before caring for Esther that older adult African American women often have trouble adhering to their medications when they are discharged from the hospital. He knows that issues related to poor knowledge about the medications, transportation, and cost often prohibit patients from taking their medications. The day before discharge he has a final session with Esther and her granddaughter. He asks Esther to explain the purpose, dosage, and adverse effects of each medication. As Esther describes her medications, Emilio reinforces information as needed and gives her medication teaching sheets. He asks her if she thinks she is going to have any difficulty getting her medications. Esther tells Emilio that she knows she will be able to afford her medications and that her granddaughter will be able to pick up her medicines most of the time. She does worry that there may be times her granddaughter is not available. Together they decide that Emilio will call her pastor to see if there is anyone in her church who can help her get to the pharmacy if necessary.

DOCUMENTATION NOTE

"Provided patient education and teaching sheets for all medications to patient and granddaughter. Both able to give teach-back, describing medications, potential side effects, and what to do if problems develop. Patient and granddaughter were not able to explain treatment of hypoglycemia related to glyburide. Reinforcement and teaching sheets about hypoglycemia treatment provided. Plan to recommend reinforcement by home health nurse. Patient states she does not anticipate financial difficulties in paying for medications. Granddaughter agrees to pick up medicines at local pharmacy. Will contact church pastor to determine if a friend from church might also be able to help as a backup. Patient and granddaughter were able to demonstrate setting up doses in medication organizer for 1 week."

---

and define health in different ways. These values and beliefs affect their perception of the effectiveness of their medications. Thus, you should ask patients to describe this effectiveness. Ask whether they are satisfied with their medications and how the medications make them feel.

ORAL ADMINISTRATION

The easiest and best route for administering medications is by mouth (see Skill 17.1). Patients usually can self-administer oral medications. Food sometimes affects absorption. Give medications on an empty stomach if this improves absorption. Likewise give medications with meals if absorption is improved by food (Burchum and Rosenthal, 2016). Most tablets and capsules must be swallowed and administered with about 60 to 240 mL of fluid (as allowed).

BOX 17.13 PROTECTING A PATIENT FROM ASPIRATION

- Allow patients to self-administer medications if possible.
- Know and assess for signs of dysphagia (difficulty swallowing): cough, change in voice tone or quality after swallowing, delayed swallowing, incomplete oral clearance or pocketing of food, regurgitation.
- Assess patient's ability to swallow and cough by checking for presence of gag reflex and then offering 50 mL of water in 5-mL allotments. Stop if patient begins to cough.
- Position patient in an upright seated position at a 90-degree angle with feet on the floor, hips and knees at 90 degrees, head midline, and back erect if possible and if not contraindicated by his or her condition.
- Usually having the patient slightly flex the head in a chin-down position before swallowing helps prevent aspiration.
- Prepare oral medications in the form that is easiest to swallow.
- If patient has unilateral weakness, place the medication in the stronger side of the mouth. Turning the head toward the weaker side helps the medication move down the stronger side of the esophagus.
- Give pills one at a time, ensuring that each pill is swallowed properly before the next one is introduced.
- Thicken regular liquids or offer fruit nectars if a patient cannot tolerate thin liquids.
- Some medications can be crushed and mixed with pureed foods if necessary. Refer to a medication reference to identify medications that are safe to crush.
- Avoid straws because they reduce the control a patient has over volume intake, which increases the risk of aspiration.
- Have a patient hold and drink from a cup if possible.
- Time medications to coincide with mealtimes or when a patient is well rested and awake.
- Administer medications using another route if risk of aspiration is severe.

The oral route is contraindicated in some situations (see Table 17.4). Many medications interact with nutritional and herbal supplements. Learn about these interactions to determine the best time to give oral medications.

An important precaution with any oral preparation is to protect patients from aspiration. Aspiration is the inadvertent entry of food, fluid, or medication into the respiratory tract when it is intended for GI administration. Protect a patient from aspiration by assessing his or her ability to swallow. Box 17.13 presents techniques to protect patients from aspiration. Use an interprofessional approach (such as with a speech therapist, dietitian, and occupational therapist) to determine the best techniques for patients who have difficulty swallowing (see Chapter 35).

Give special consideration when administering oral medications to patients with enteral or small-bore feeding tubes (Box 17.14). Failing to follow current evidence-based recommendations from the American Society for Parenteral and Enteral Nutrition (ASPEN) can result in tube obstruction, reduced medication effectiveness, and increased risk of medication toxicity (Malone, 2014). Tube misconnections continue to cause patient injury because tubes with different functions can be connected with Luer connectors. In response to this issue, the International Organization for Standardization (ISO) (TJC, 2014b) has developed tube connector standards in which the enteral connector will no longer be Luer compatible. A new ISO enteral-only connector (ENFit) is now available to health care agencies, resulting in changes to enteral nutrition practices, policies, procedures, and processes per the new guidelines (ISMP, 2017; TJC, 2014b) (Box 17.15). Before giving a medication by the enteral route, verify that the location of the feeding tube (e.g., stomach or jejunum) is compatible with medication absorption. For example, iron dissolves in the stomach and is mostly absorbed in the duodenum. If it is administered through a jejunal tube, it bypasses the stomach and thus has poor bioavailability. Use only oral syringes, not parenteral syringes, when preparing oral medications for the enteral route to prevent accidental parenteral administration into an IV line. In prior adverse events, the inadvertent IV administration of an oral product has led to patient harm, including sepsis, emboli, or diffuse intravascular coagulation when injecting an unsterile solution with particulates into a patient's vein (ISMP, 2015f). ENFit connectors are engineered to make it nearly impossible to connect one delivery system to another delivery system that serves a completely different function—for example, accidentally connecting a feeding administration set to a tracheostomy tube, an IV tube to an epidural site, or a tube feeding administration to an IV line (ISMP, 2017; TJC, 2014b).

When giving oral medications enterally, flush feeding tubes with at least 30 mL of water before and after giving medications. When administering more than one medication, give each medication separately and flush the tube with 15 to 30 mL of water between medications.

Determine whether you need to give medications on an empty stomach or if they are compatible with the patient's enteral feeding. If you need to give a medication on an empty stomach or it is not compatible with the feeding (e.g., phenytoin, carbamazepine, warfarin, fluoroquinolones, proton pump inhibitors), give the feeding at least 30 minutes before or 30 minutes after medication administration. Some medications require up to 120 minutes to be absorbed (Guenther and Boullatta, 2013). Verify the time with a drug reference or consult with a pharmacist. Monitor the patient closely for adverse reactions. The risk for drug-drug interactions is high when two or more medications are given via this route because they can interact as soon as they are administered.

TOPICAL MEDICATION APPLICATIONS

Topical medications are applied locally, most often to intact skin. They come in many forms (see Table 17.1). They are also applied to mucous membranes.

BOX 17.14 PROCEDURAL GUIDELINES

Administering Medications Through a Small-Bore Feeding Tube, Gastrostomy Tube, or Jejunostomy Tube

DELEGATION CONSIDERATIONS

The skill of administering medications by enteral feeding tubes cannot be delegated to nursing assistive personnel (NAP). The nurse instructs the NAP to:

- Keep the head of the bed elevated a minimum of 30 degrees (preferably 45 degrees) for 1 hour after medication administration; follow agency policy.
- Report immediately to the nurse coughing, choking, gagging, or drooling of liquid or dissolved pills.
- Report to the nurse occurrence of possible medication side effects (specific to medication).

EQUIPMENT

Medication administration record (MAR) (electronic or printed); appropriate medication syringe or 60-mL Asepto syringe for large-bore tubes only; enteral-only connector (ENFit) designed to fit the specific enteral tube (TJC, 2014b) (see illustration); gastric pH test strip (scale of 1 to 11); graduated container; medication to be administered; pill crusher if medication in tablet form; water or sterile water for immunocompromised patients; clean gloves; stethoscope and pulse oximeter (for evaluation)

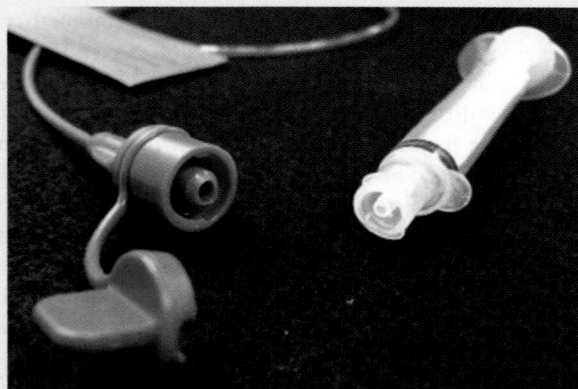

STEPS

1. Check accuracy and completeness of each MAR with health care provider's medication order. Check patient's name, drug name and dosage, route of administration, and time for administration. Clarify incomplete or unclear orders with health care provider before administration.
2. Review pertinent information related to medication including action, purpose, normal dose and route, side effects, time of onset and peak action, and nursing implications.
3. Assess for any contraindications to receiving enteral medications including presence of bowel inflammation, reduced peristalsis, recent gastrointestinal (GI) surgery, and gastric suction that cannot be turned off.
4. Avoid complicated medication schedules that often interrupt enteral feedings. Use alternative routes of medication administration if possible (e.g., transdermal, rectal, IV).
   a. Determine where medication is absorbed and ensure that point of absorption is not bypassed by feeding tube. For example, some medications such as antacids are absorbed in stomach, not jejunum.

b. Determine if medication interacts with enteral feeding. If so, hold feeding for at least 30 minutes before giving medication (see agency policy or consult pharmacist).

5. Assess patient's medical, medication, and diet history and history of allergies. List drug allergies on each page of MAR and prominently display allergies on patient's medical record per agency policy. When patient has allergy, provide allergy bracelet.
6. For postoperative patient review postoperative orders for type of enteral tube care.
7. Perform hand hygiene. Gather and review physical assessment data (e.g., bowel sounds, abdominal distention) and laboratory data (e.g., renal and liver function) that may influence drug administration.
8. Check with pharmacy for availability of liquid preparation for patient's medications. Health care provider may need to change dosage form.
9. Before administration of enteral medications, verify placement of feeding tube (see Chapter 35), and determine that tube is placed in stomach or small intestine correctly.
10. Perform hand hygiene. Collect appropriate equipment and MAR.
11. Prepare medications for instillation into feeding tube (see Skill 17.1). Attend to procedure and avoid distraction. Check label of medication against MAR two times, when removing medication from unit dose or automated medication dispensing system (AMDS) and before leaving medication preparation area. *These are the first and second checks for accuracy.* Fill graduated container with 50 to 100 mL of tepid water. Use sterile water for immunocompromised or critically ill patients (Malone, 2014; Allen, 2015).

Clinical Decision Point. Make sure that concentrated liquid medications are thoroughly diluted. Never add crushed medications directly to tube feeding (Guenther and Boullatta, 2013).

---

a. *Tablets:* Crush each tablet into a fine powder, using pill-crushing device or two medication cups (see Skill 17.1). Dissolve each tablet in separate cup of 30 mL of warm water.

b. *Capsules:* Apply clean gloves. Ensure that contents of capsule (granules or gelatin) can be expressed from covering (consult with pharmacist). Open capsule or pierce gel cap with sterile needle and empty contents into 30 mL of warm water (or solution designated by drug company). Gel caps dissolve in warm water, but this may take 15 to 20 minutes. Remove and dispose of gloves.

c. Prepare liquid medication (prepared by pharmacy in appropriate syringe).

d. Perform hand hygiene.

12. Take medications to patient at correct time (see agency policy). Consider if medication is time critical. During administration, apply six rights of medication administration.
13. Identify patient using at least two identifiers (e.g., name and birthday or name and medical record number) according to

BOX 17.14 PROCEDURAL GUIDELINES—cont'd

Administering Medications Through a Small-Bore Feeding Tube, Gastrostomy Tube, or Jejunostomy Tube

agency policy. Compare identifiers with information on patient's MAR or medical record.

14. At patient's bedside again compare MAR or computer printout with names of medications on medication labels and patient name. Ask patient if he or she has allergies. *This is the third check for accuracy.*

15. Explain procedure to patient and discuss purpose of each medication, action, and possible adverse effects. Allow patient to ask any questions about medications.

16. Assist patient to sitting position. Elevate head of bed to minimum of 30 degrees and preferably 45 degrees (unless contraindicated) or sit patient up in a chair (Malone, 2014).

17. If continuous enteral tube feeding is infusing, adjust infusion pump setting to hold tube feeding.

18. Perform hand hygiene. Apply clean gloves. Check placement of feeding tube (see Chapter 35) by observing gastric contents and checking pH of aspirate contents. *Gastric pH less than 5.0 is a good indicator that tip of tube is correctly placed in stomach.*

19. Check for gastric residual volume (GRV) (see Chapter 35).

20. Irrigate tubing.
    a. Pinch or clamp enteral tube. Draw up 30 mL of water into irrigation syringe. Reinsert tip of syringe into tube, release clamp, and flush tubing. Clamp tube again and remove syringe.
    b. Using appropriate enteral connector, attach to enteral tube.

> **Clinical Decision Point. Verify that connector meets the ISO tubing connector standards (TJC, 2014b). Do not attach enteral tubing to a standardized Luer syringe or needleless device (TJC, 2014b; Guenther, 2015).**

21. Remove bulb or plunger of syringe and reinsert syringe into tip of feeding tube.

22. Administer dose of first liquid or dissolved medication by pouring into syringe. Allow to flow by gravity.

> **Clinical Decision Point. If medication does not flow freely, raise the height of the syringe to increase the rate of flow or try having the patient change position slightly because the end of the feeding tube may be**

against the gastric mucosa. If these measures do not improve the flow, a gentle push with bulb of Asepto syringe or plunger of the syringe may facilitate flow of fluid.

a. If giving only one dose of medication, flush tubing with 30 to 60 mL of water after administration.
b. To administer more than one medication, give each separately, and flush between medications with 15 to 30 mL of water.
c. Follow last dose of medication with 30 to 60 mL of water.

23. Clamp proximal end of feeding tube if tube feeding is not being administered, and cap end of tube.

24. When continuous tube feeding is being administered by infusion pump, if medications are not compatible with feeding solution, hold feeding for additional 30 to 60 minutes (Klang et al., 2013).

25. Help patient to comfortable position and keep head of bed elevated for 1 hour (see agency policy).

26. Dispose of soiled supplies, rinse graduated container and syringe with tap water, remove and dispose of gloves, and perform hand hygiene.

27. Document name of medication, dose, route, and time administered on MAR. Document patient's response in nurses' notes of MAR in electronic health record (EHR) or chart.

28. Record patient teaching and validation of patient's understanding on flow sheet or nurses' notes in EHR or chart.

29. Observe patient for signs of aspiration such as choking, gurgling, gurgling speech, breath sounds, and difficulty breathing.

30. Return within 30 minutes to evaluate patient's response to medications.

31. **Use Teach-Back:** "I want to be sure I explained clearly why your father must take his medications through his feeding tube. Tell me why he is receiving his medications through his feeding tube." Revise your instruction now or develop a plan for revised patient/family caregiver teaching if patient/family caregiver is not able to teach back correctly. Determines patient's/family caregiver's level of understanding of instructional topic.

Skin Applications

Because many locally applied medications (e.g., lotions, pastes, and ointments) produce systemic and local effects, apply these medications with gloves and applicators. Use sterile technique if a patient has an open wound. Skin encrustation and dead tissues harbor microorganisms and block contact of medications with the tissues to be treated. Before applying medications, clean the skin thoroughly by washing the area gently with soap and water, soaking the intended site, or locally debriding tissue.

Apply each type of medication according to directions to ensure proper penetration and absorption. When applying ointments or pastes, spread the medication evenly over the involved surface and cover the area well without applying an overly thick layer. Health care providers sometimes order a gauze dressing to be applied over a topical medication to prevent soiling of clothes and accidental wiping away of the medication. Lightly spread lotions and creams onto the surface of the skin. Rubbing often causes irritation. Apply a liniment by rubbing it gently but firmly into the skin. Dust a thin layer of powder over the affected area.

You apply some topical medications in the form of a transdermal patch that remains in place for a longer time (e.g., 12 hours or 7 days). Before applying a new patch, put on

| BOX 17.15 | THE JOINT COMMISSION RECOMMENDATIONS FOR ENFIT ENTERAL TUBE CONNECTORS |

- Trace tubing from the patient to the point of origin:
  - Before connecting or reconnecting any device or infusion.
  - At any care transition such as to a new setting or service.
  - As part of a hand-off process with another health care provider.
- Route tubes and catheters with different purposes in standard directions (e.g., toward the head, toward the feet), and label proximal and distal ends of tubes.
- Use tubing and related equipment only for their intended use.
  - Never use standard Luer syringes for oral medications or enteral feedings.
  - Do not use IV tubing or IV pumps for enteral feedings.
  - Use distinctly dedicated pumps for IV applications.
  - Eliminate the use of temporary adapters on tubing.
  - Do not force a connection and avoid workarounds.
- Use safe practices for high-alert medications.
  - Label the tubing.
  - Do not use tubing with injection port.
  - Use an independent double-check procedure.
- Create a culture of safety and report adverse events.

Adapted from The Joint Commission (TJC): *Sentinel alert event: managing risk during transition to new ISO connector standards,* 2014, https://www.jointcommission.org/sea_issue_53/.

disposable clean gloves and remove the old patch. Medication remains on a patch even after it has been used for the recommended time. Nurses and patients have inadvertently left old transdermal patches in place, resulting in a patient receiving an overdose of the medication. For example, patients who use fentanyl transdermal patches for pain management can experience respiratory depression, coma, and death when the patches are not removed. In addition, some people, especially children, have experienced life-threatening harm from accidental exposure to fentanyl patches that were not disposed of properly (FDA, 2012). Many patches are clear, which makes them difficult to see. Therefore carefully assess a patient's skin and be sure to remove an existing patch before applying a new one. Follow these guidelines to ensure safe administration of transdermal or topical medications:

- When taking a medication history or reconciling medications, specifically ask patients whether they take any medications in the forms of patches, topical creams, or any route other than the oral route.
- When applying a transdermal patch, ask the patient whether he or she currently uses a patch.
- Wear disposable clean gloves when removing and applying transdermal patches.
- If the dressing or patch is difficult to see (e.g., clear), apply a noticeable label to the patch.
- Use the MAR to document the location on the patient's body where the medication was placed.

- Use the MAR to document removal of the patch or medication.
- In most cases, dispose of patches by folding sticky sides of the patch together and disposing in a child-proof container. There are exceptions; a fentanyl patch, an adhesive patch that delivers a potent pain medicine through the skin, comes with instructions to flush used or leftover patches (FDA, 2012). Always read package directions.

Mucous Membrane Applications

Nasal Instillation. Patients with nasal sinus alterations sometimes receive medications by spray, drops, or tampons (Box 17.16). The most common form of nasal instillation is decongestant spray or drops. These are used to relieve symptoms of sinus congestion and colds. Caution patients to avoid abuse of nasal medications because overuse leads to a rebound effect in which the nasal congestion worsens. When a patient swallows excess decongestant solution, serious systemic effects can develop, especially in children. Saline drops are safer as a decongestant for children than nasal preparations that contain sympathomimetics (such as Afrin or Neo-Synephrine).

Patients can more easily self-administer sprays because they can control the spray and inhale as the medication enters the nasal passages. Always check the nares for irritation in patients who use nasal sprays repeatedly. When a spray is prescribed for a sinus infection, position patients to permit the nasal medication to reach the affected sinus. Severe nosebleeds are usually treated with packing or nasal tampons and are treated with epinephrine to reduce blood flow. A health care provider usually places nasal tampons.

Eye Instillation. Ophthalmic medications in the form of eyedrops and ointments are given for eye conditions such as glaucoma and conjunctivitis. Some eyedrops are prescribed, and others are available OTC (e.g., Visine or Murine). Many patients who receive eye medications are older adults. Age-related problems including poor vision, hand tremors, and difficulty grasping or manipulating small containers affect the ability of older adults to self-administer eye medications. Educate your patients and family caregivers about the proper techniques for administering eye medications (see Skill 17.2). Evaluate the patient's and family caregiver's ability to self-administer through a return demonstration of the procedure. Showing patients each step of the procedure for instilling eyedrops improves their adherence. Apply the following principles when administering eye medications:

1. Avoid instilling any form of eye medication directly onto the cornea. The cornea of the eye has many pain fibers and is very sensitive to anything applied to it.
2. Avoid touching the eyelids or other eye structures with eyedroppers or ointment tubes. The risk for transmitting infection from one eye to the other is high.
3. Use eye medication only for a patient's affected eye.
4. Never allow a patient to use another patient's eye medications.

BOX 17.16 PROCEDURAL GUIDELINES

Administering Nasal Instillations

DELEGATION CONSIDERATIONS

The skill of administering nasal instillations cannot be delegated to nursing assistive personnel (NAP). The nurse instructs the NAP about:

- Potential side effects of medications and to report their occurrence to the nurse.
- Reporting any bloody nasal drainage to the nurse.

EQUIPMENT

Medication administration record (MAR) (electronic or printed); prepared medication with clean dropper or spray container; facial tissue; small pillow *(optional)*; washcloth *(optional)*; clean gloves

STEPS

1. Check accuracy and completeness of each MAR with health care provider's medication order. Check patient's name, drug name and dosage, route (which sinus), and time for administration. Clarify incomplete or unclear orders with health care provider before administration.
2. Review pertinent information related to medication including action, purpose, normal dose and route, side effects, time of onset and peak action, and nursing implications.
3. Assess patient's medical and medication history and history of allergies. List drug allergies on each page of MAR and prominently display allergies on patient's medical record per agency policy. When patient has allergy, provide allergy bracelet.
4. Perform hand hygiene. Use penlight and inspect condition of nose and sinuses (see Chapter 16). Palpate sinuses for pain or tenderness. Note type of drainage if present.
5. Assess patient's knowledge regarding use of nasal instillations, technique for instillation, and willingness to learn self-administration.
6. Perform hand hygiene. Collect appropriate equipment and MAR.
7. Prepare medications for instillation. Attend to procedure and avoid distraction. Check label of medication against MAR two times (see Skill 17.1). Preparation usually involves checking label when removing nasal drops or sprays out of storage and before leaving preparation area. Check expiration date on container. *These are the first and second checks for accuracy.* Perform hand hygiene.
8. Take medications to patient at correct time (see agency policy). Consider if medication is time critical. During administration, apply six rights of medication administration.
9. Identify patient using at least two identifiers (e.g., name and birthday or name and medical record number) according to agency policy. Compare identifiers with information on patient's MAR or medical record.
10. At patient's bedside again compare MAR or computer printout with names of medications on medication labels and patient name. Ask patient if he or she has allergies. *This is the third check for accuracy.*
11. Explain procedure to patient and sensations to expect. Discuss purpose of each medication, action, and possible adverse effects. Allow patient to ask any questions about medications. Patients who self-instill medications may be allowed to give drops under nurse's supervision (check

agency policy). Tell patients receiving nasal instillation that they may experience burning or stinging of mucosa or choking sensation as medication trickles into throat.
12. Arrange supplies and medications at bedside. Perform hand hygiene and apply clean gloves (if drainage is present).
13. Gently roll or shake container. Instruct patient to clear or blow nose gently unless contraindicated (e.g., risk of increased intracranial pressure or nosebleed).
14. Administer nose drops.
    a. Help patient to supine position and position head properly (American Society of Health-System Pharmacists [ASHP], 2013b).
       (1) For access to posterior pharynx, tilt patient's head backward.
       (2) For access to ethmoid or sphenoid sinus, tilt head back over edge of bed, or place small pillow under patient's shoulder and tilt head back (see illustration).
       (3) For access to frontal or maxillary sinus, tilt head back over edge of bed or pillow with head turned toward side to be treated (see illustration).
    b. Support patient's head with nondominant hand.
    c. Instruct patient to breathe through mouth.
    d. Hold dropper 1 cm (½ inch) above nares and instill prescribed number of drops toward midline of ethmoid bone.
    e. Have patient remain in supine position 5 minutes.
    f. Offer facial tissue to blot runny nose, but caution patient against blowing nose for several minutes.

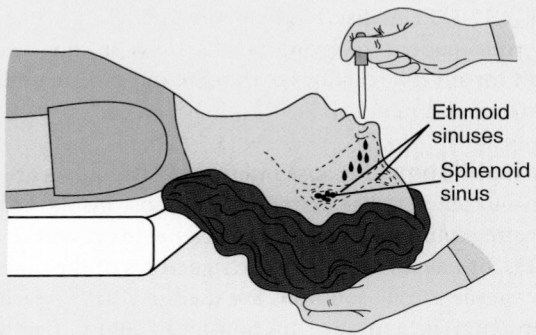

STEP 14a(2) Position for instilling nose drops into ethmoid and sphenoid sinus.

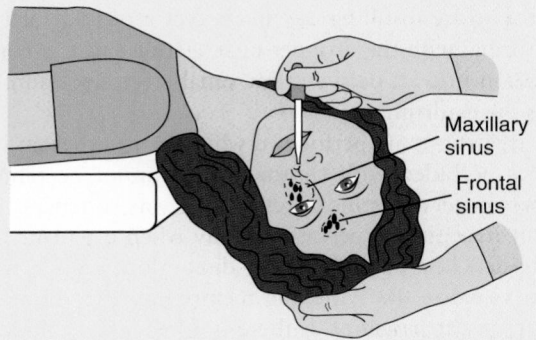

STEP 14a(3) Position for instilling nose drops into frontal and maxillary sinus.

Continued

BOX 17.16 PROCEDURAL GUIDELINES—cont'd

Administering Nasal Instillations

15. Administer nasal spray.
    a. Help patient into upright position with head tilted slightly forward.
    b. Instruct or assist patient to insert tip of nasal spray into appropriate nares and occlude other nostril with finger. Point spray tip toward side and away from center of nose (ASHP, 2013b).
    c. Have patient spray medication into nose while inhaling. Help patient remove nozzle from nose and instruct to breathe out through mouth.
    d. Offer facial tissue to blot runny nose, but caution patient against blowing nose for several minutes.

Clinical Decision Point. Some medications are designed for one spray per dose. Examples include calcitonin, desmopressin (DDAVP, Stimate), and sumatriptan. It is essential to ensure that the patient understands the correct number of sprays to use per dose to prevent overdosing.

---

16. Help patient to comfortable position after medication is absorbed.
17. Dispose of soiled supplies, remove and dispose of gloves, and perform hand hygiene.

18. Document name of medication, dose, route, and time administered on MAR.
19. Observe patient for onset of side effects 15 to 30 minutes after administration.
20. Ask if patient is able to breathe through nose after decongestant administration. It may be necessary to have patient occlude one nostril at a time and breathe deeply.
21. Reinspect condition of nasal passages between instillations.
22. Ask patient to describe risks of overuse of decongestants and methods for administration. Feedback ensures that patient can self-administer medications properly.
23. Have patient demonstrate self-medication.
24. Record patient response to medication, patient teaching, and validation of patient understanding and self-administration on flow sheet or nurses' notes in electronic health record (EHR) or chart.
25. **Use Teach-Back:** "I want to be sure I explained the importance to not overuse your nasal spray. Explain to me why it is important not to overuse nasal sprays." Revise your instruction now or develop a plan for revised patient/family caregiver teaching if patient/family caregiver not able to teach back correctly. Determines patient's/family caregiver's level of understanding of instructional topic.

You administer some medications using an intraocular disk (see Skill 17.2). The disk remains in place for up to 1 week. Teach your patient receiving medications in this way to monitor for adverse reactions to the disk and explain methods of insertion and removal.

Ear Instillation. Because internal ear structures are very sensitive to temperature extremes, you must instill eardrops or irrigating solutions at room temperature to prevent vertigo, dizziness, or nausea. Although the structures of the outer ear are not sterile, sterile solutions are used in case the eardrum is ruptured. The entrance of nonsterile solution into the middle ear often results in infection.

If a patient has ear drainage, check with the health care provider to ensure that the patient does not have a ruptured eardrum before instilling the drops. Never occlude or block the ear canal with the dropper or irrigating syringe. Forcing medication into an occluded ear canal creates pressure that injures the eardrum.

Ear irrigations are performed when the external ear canal becomes occluded with cerumen and cannot be removed by more conservative measures such as wax softeners. Typically, an irrigation is performed only when a patient has a hearing deficit, a patient has ear discomfort, or it is necessary to visualize the tympanic membrane. You should not perform an ear irrigation if there is a history of middle ear infection in the last 6 weeks, if the patient has undergone *any* form of ear surgery, or if the patient has a perforation or there is a history of a mucus discharge in the last year. Box 17.17 provides guidelines for administering eardrops and ear irrigations.

Vaginal Instillation. Vaginal medications are available as suppositories, foam, jellies, and creams. Solid, oval-shaped suppositories are packaged individually in foil wrappers and are sometimes stored in the refrigerator to prevent them from melting. After a suppository is inserted into the vaginal cavity, body temperature causes it to melt and be distributed and absorbed. Foam, jellies, and creams are administered with an applicator inserter (Box 17.18).

Give a suppository with a gloved hand in accordance with standard precautions (see Chapter 14). Patients often prefer to administer their own vaginal medications and need privacy. Vaginal medications are often given to treat infection, and vaginal discharge in patients who need vaginal medications usually smells foul. Follow aseptic technique, and offer the patient frequent opportunities to maintain perineal hygiene (see Chapter 31).

Rectal Instillation. Rectal suppositories are thinner and more bullet shaped than vaginal suppositories. The rounded end prevents anal trauma during insertion. Rectal suppositories contain medications that exert local effects, such as promoting defecation, or systemic effects, such as reducing nausea. They are stored in a refrigerator until administered. Sometimes the rectum must be cleared with a small cleansing

BOX 17.17 PROCEDURAL GUIDELINES

Administering Ear Medications

DELEGATION CONSIDERATIONS

The skill of administering ear medications cannot be delegated to nursing assistive personnel (NAP). The nurse instructs the NAP about:

- Potential side effects of medications and to report their occurrence.
- Potential for dizziness or irritation after administration of ear medications.

EQUIPMENT

Medication administration record (MAR) (electronic or printed)
Drops: Medication bottle with dropper; cotton-tipped applicator; cotton balls; clean gloves if drainage is present
Irrigation: Irrigating solution and syringe; kidney basin; towel

STEPS

1. Check accuracy and completeness of each MAR with health care provider's medication order. Check patient's name, drug name and dosage, route, and time for administration. Clarify incomplete or unclear orders with health care provider before administration.
2. Review pertinent information related to medication including action, purpose, normal dose and route (one or both ears), side effects, time of onset and peak action, and nursing implications.
3. Assess patient's medical and medication history and history of allergies (including latex). List drug allergies on each page of MAR and prominently display allergies on patient's medical record per agency policy. When patient has allergy, provide allergy bracelet.
4. Perform hand hygiene. Assess condition of external ear structures (see Chapter 16). This may be done just before drug instillation (apply clean gloves if drainage is present).
5. Determine whether patient has any symptoms of ear discomfort or hearing impairment.
6. Assess patient's level of consciousness (LOC) and ability to follow directions.
7. Assess patient's knowledge regarding drug therapy and desire to self-administer medication.
8. Assess patient's ability to manipulate and hold ear dropper.
9. Perform hand hygiene. Collect appropriate equipment and MAR.
10. Prepare medications for instillation. Attend to procedure and avoid distraction. Check label of medication against MAR two times (see Skill 17.1). Preparation usually involves checking label when removing ear drops out of storage and before leaving preparation area. Preparation usually involves taking eardrops out of refrigerator and rewarming to room temperature before administering to patient. Check expiration date on container. *These are the first and second checks for accuracy.* Perform hand hygiene.
11. Take medications to patient at correct time (see agency policy). Consider if medication is time critical. During administration, apply six rights of medication administration.
12. Arrange supplies at bedside.

13. Identify patient using at least two identifiers (e.g., name and birthday or name and medical record number) according to agency policy. Compare identifiers with information on patient's MAR or medical record.
14. At patient's bedside again compare MAR or computer printout with names of medications on medication labels and patient name. Ask patient if he or she has allergies. *This is the third check for accuracy.*
15. Explain procedure to patient and sensations to expect. Discuss purpose of each medication, action, and possible adverse effects. Allow patient to ask any questions about the medications. Patients who self-instill medications may be allowed to give drops under nurse's supervision (check agency policy).
16. Perform hand hygiene (apply clean gloves if drainage present).
17. Administer eardrops.
    a. Position patient on side (if not contraindicated) with ear to be treated facing up, or patient may sit in chair or at bedside.
    b. If cerumen or drainage occludes outermost part of ear canal, wipe out gently with cotton-tipped applicator or washcloth. Take care not to force cerumen into canal.
    c. Hold container in the palm of your hands for a few minutes to warm the contents to body temperature. If eardrops are in a cloudy suspension, shake bottle for about 10 seconds.
    d. Straighten ear canal by pulling pinna up and back to 10 o'clock position (adult or child older than 3 years of age) or down and back to 6 to 9 o'clock position (child younger than 3 years of age).
    e. Instill prescribed drops holding dropper 1 cm ($\frac{1}{2}$ inch) above ear canal. Avoid contact of dropper tip against external ear canal (see illustration).

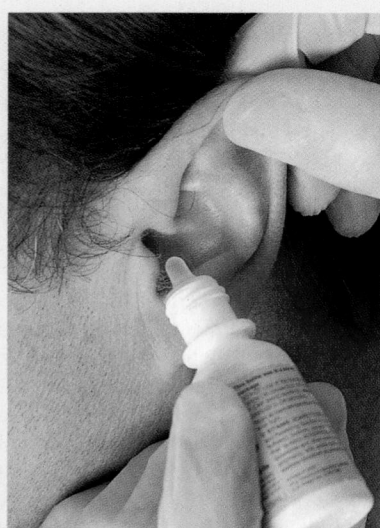

STEP 17e Instill prescribed drops holding dropper above ear canal.

Continued

BOX 17.17 **PROCEDURAL GUIDELINES—cont'd**

Administering Ear Medications

f. Ask patient to remain in side-lying position for a few minutes. Apply gentle massage or pressure to tragus of ear with finger.

g. If ordered, gently insert part of cotton ball into outermost part of canal. Do not press cotton into canal.

h. Remove cotton after 15 minutes. Help patient to comfortable position after drops are absorbed.

18. Administer ear irrigations.

a. Assess tympanic membrane or review medication record for history of eardrum perforation, which contraindicates ear irrigation.

b. Help patient into sitting position or lying position with head tilted or turned toward affected ear. Place towel under patient's head and shoulder and have patient hold basin under affected ear.

c. Fill irrigating syringe with solution (approximately 50 mL) at room temperature.

d. Gently grasp auricle and straighten ear by pulling pinna down and back for children younger than 3 years of age or upward and outward for adults and children 3 years of age and older.

e. Slowly instill irrigating solution by holding tip of syringe 1 cm (½ inch) above opening of ear canal. Allow fluid

to drain out during instillation. Continue until you use all solution.

19. Clean area and put supplies away.

20. Remove gloves and perform hand hygiene.

21. Record drug, concentration, dose or strength, number of drops, site of application (left, right, or both ears), and time of administration on MAR immediately after administration.

22. Observe response to medication by assessing hearing changes, asking if symptoms are relieved, and noting any side effects or discomfort felt.

23. Ask patient to discuss purpose of drug, action, side effects, and technique of administration.

24. Record patient response to medication, patient teaching, and validation of patient understanding and self-administration on flow sheet or nurses' notes in electronic health record (EHR) or chart.

25. **Use Teach-Back:** "I want to be sure I clearly showed you how to give yourself eardrops. Show me how to place eardrops in your ear." Revise your instruction now or develop a plan for revised patient/family caregiver teaching if patient/family caregiver is not able to teach back correctly.

BOX 17.18 **PROCEDURAL GUIDELINES**

Administering Vaginal Medications

DELEGATION CONSIDERATIONS

The skill of administering vaginal medications cannot be delegated to nursing assistive personnel (NAP). The nurse instructs the NAP about:

• Potential side effects of medications and to report their occurrence to the nurse.

• Reporting any change in comfort level or new or increased vaginal discharge or bleeding to the nurse.

EQUIPMENT

Medication administration record (MAR) (electronic or printed); vaginal cream, foam, jelly, tablet, suppository, or irrigating solution; applicators (if needed); clean gloves; tissues; towels and/or washcloths; perineal pad; drape or sheet; water-soluble lubricants; bedpan; irrigation or douche container (if needed); gooseneck lamp (optional)

STEPS

1. Review pertinent information related to medication including action, purpose, normal dose and route, side effects, time of onset and peak action, and nursing implications.

2. Assess patient's medical and medication history and history of allergies. List drug allergies on each page of MAR and prominently display allergies on the patient's medical record per agency policy. When patient has allergy, provide allergy bracelet.

3. Perform hand hygiene and apply clean gloves. During perineal care inspect condition of vaginal tissues; note if drainage is present. Remove gloves and perform hand hygiene.

4. Ask if patient is experiencing any symptoms of pruritus, burning, or discomfort.

5. Review patient's knowledge of medication and readiness to learn (e.g., asks questions about medication, requests education in use of suppository).

6. Assess patient's ability to manipulate applicator, suppository, or irrigation equipment and to properly position self to insert medication (may be done just before insertion).

7. Perform hand hygiene. Collect appropriate equipment and MAR.

8. Prepare suppository for administration. Attend to procedure and avoid distraction. Check label of medication against MAR two times (see Skill 17.1). Preparation usually involves checking label when removing suppository from refrigerator and before leaving preparation area. Check expiration date on container. *These are the first and second checks for accuracy.* Perform hand hygiene.

9. Take medications to patient at correct time (see agency policy). Consider if medication is time critical. During administration, apply six rights of medication administration.

10. Identify patient using at least two identifiers (e.g., name and birthday or name and medical record number) according to agency policy. Compare identifiers with information on patient's MAR or medical record.

11. At patient's bedside again compare MAR or computer printout with names of medications on medication labels and patient name. Ask patient if he or she has allergies. *This is the third check for accuracy.*

12. Explain procedure to patient. Be specific if patient plans to self-administer medication. Discuss purpose of each

BOX 17.18 PROCEDURAL GUIDELINES—cont'd

Administering Vaginal Medications

medication, action, and possible adverse effects. Allow patient to ask any questions about the medications.

13. Perform hand hygiene. Arrange supplies at bedside and apply clean gloves. Close door or pull curtain.

14. Help patient lie in dorsal recumbent position. Patients with restricted mobility in knees or hips may lie supine with legs abducted.

15. Keep abdomen and lower extremities draped.

16. Be sure that vaginal orifice is well illuminated by room light. Otherwise position portable gooseneck lamp.

17. Insert vaginal suppository.
    a. Remove suppository from wrapper and apply liberal amount of water-soluble lubricant to smooth or rounded end. Be sure that suppository is at room temperature. Lubricate gloved index finger of dominant hand.
    b. With nondominant gloved hand gently separate labial folds in front-to-back direction to expose vaginal orifice.
    c. With dominant gloved hand insert rounded end of suppository along posterior wall of vaginal canal the entire length of finger (7.5 to 10 cm [3 to 4 inches]) (see illustration).
    d. Withdraw finger and wipe away remaining lubricant from around orifice and labia with tissue or cloth.

18. Apply cream or foam.
    a. Fill cream or foam applicator following package directions.
    b. With nondominant gloved hand gently separate labial folds.
    c. With dominant gloved hand gently insert applicator approximately 5 to 7.5 cm (2 to 3 inches). Push applicator plunger to deposit medication into vagina (see illustration).

d. Withdraw applicator and place on paper towel. Wipe off residual cream from labia or vaginal orifice with tissue or cloth.

19. Instruct patient to remain on her back for at least 10 minutes to prevent loss through vaginal orifice.

20. If using an applicator, wash with soap and warm water, rinse, air dry, and then store for future use.

21. Offer perineal pad when patient resumes ambulation.

22. Dispose of supplies, remove and dispose of gloves, and perform hand hygiene.

23. Record drug, dosage, route, and actual time and date of administration on MAR immediately after administration, not before. Include initials or signature.

24. Wait 30 minutes after administration and then perform hand hygiene and apply clean gloves. Inspect condition of vaginal canal and external genitalia. Assess vaginal discharge if present. Remove gloves and perform hand hygiene.

25. Question patient regarding continued pruritus, burning, discomfort, or discharge.

26. Ask patient to discuss purpose, action, and side effects of medication.

27. Record patient response to medication, patient teaching, and validation of patient understanding and self-administration of suppository on flow sheet or nurses' notes in electronic health record (EHR) or chart.

28. **Use Teach-Back:** "I want to be sure I explained how to use the vaginal cream applicator. Tell me how you will draw the correct amount of cream into the applicator." Revise your instruction now or develop a plan for revised patient teaching if patient is not able to teach back correctly.

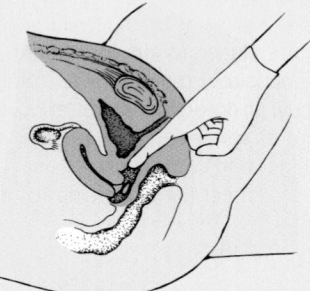

STEP 17c Insertion of suppository into vaginal canal.

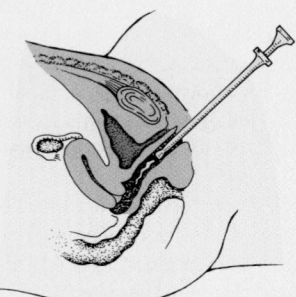

STEP 18c Instillation of medication in vaginal canal.

enema (see Chapter 37) before a suppository is inserted (Box 17.19).

Administering Medications by Inhalation

Medications administered with handheld inhalers are dispersed through an aerosol spray, mist, or powder that penetrates lung airways. The alveolar-capillary network absorbs medications rapidly. **Pressurized metered-dose inhalers (pMDIs)**, breath-actuated metered-dose inhalers (BAIs), and dry powder inhalers (DPIs) deliver inhaled medications that produce local effects in the airway such as bronchodilation. Some medications create serious systemic side effects.

pMDIs use a chemical propellant to push the medication out of the inhaler, requiring a patient to apply about 5 to 10 lb of pressure to the top of the canister to administer the medication. Children and older adults with chronic lung diseases often use pMDIs. Because of their diminished hand strength, be sure to assess if patients have enough strength to use pMDIs.

Sometimes patients use a spacer with the pMDI. A spacer is a tube 10.16 to 20.32 cm (4 to 8 inches) long that attaches

BOX 17.19   PROCEDURAL GUIDELINES

Administering Rectal Suppositories

DELEGATION CONSIDERATIONS

The skill of rectal medication administration cannot be delegated to nursing assistive personnel (NAP). The nurse instructs the NAP about:

- Reporting expected fecal discharge or bowel movement to the nurse.
- Potential side effects of medications and to report their occurrence to the nurse.
- Informing nurse of any rectal pain or bleeding.

EQUIPMENT

Medication administration record (MAR) (electronic or printed); rectal suppository; water-soluble lubricating jelly; clean gloves; tissue; drape

STEPS

1. Check accuracy and completeness of each MAR with health care provider's medication order. Check patient's name, drug name and dosage, route, and time for administration. Clarify incomplete or unclear orders with health care provider before administration.
2. Review pertinent information related to medication, including action, purpose, normal dose and route, side effects, time of onset and peak action, and nursing implications.
3. Review patient's medical history (e.g., history of rectal surgery or bleeding, cardiac problems), medication history, and history of allergies. List drug allergies on each page of MAR and prominently display allergies on patient's medical record per agency policy. When patient has allergy, provide allergy bracelet.
4. Review any presenting signs and symptoms of GI alterations (e.g., constipation or diarrhea).
5. Assess patient's ability to hold suppository and position self to insert medication.
6. Review patient's knowledge of purpose of drug therapy and interest in self-administering suppository.
7. Perform hand hygiene. Collect appropriate equipment and MAR.
8. Prepare suppository for administration. Attend to procedure and avoid distraction. Check label of medication against MAR two times (see Skill 17.1). Preparation usually involves checking label when removing suppository out of refrigerator and before leaving preparation area. Check expiration date on container. *These are the first and second checks for accuracy.* Perform hand hygiene.
9. Take medications to patient at correct time (see agency policy). Consider if medication is time critical. During administration, apply six rights of medication administration.
10. Identify patient using at least two identifiers (e.g., name and birthday or name and medical record number) according to agency policy. Compare identifiers with information on patient's MAR or medical record.
11. At patient's bedside again compare MAR or computer printout with names of medications on medication labels and patient name. Ask patient if he or she has allergies. *This is the third check for accuracy.*
12. Explain procedure to patient. Be specific if patient wishes to self-administer drug. Discuss purpose of each medication, action, and possible adverse effects. Allow patient to ask any questions about the medications. Explain procedure if patient plans to self-administer medication.
13. Perform hand hygiene. Arrange supplies at bedside, and apply clean gloves. Close room curtain or door.
14. Help patient assume left side-lying Sims position with upper leg flexed upward.
15. If patient has impairment of mobility, help into lateral position. Obtain help to turn patient, and use pillows under upper arm and leg.
16. Keep patient draped with only anal area exposed.
17. Examine condition of anus externally. *Option:* Palpate rectal walls as needed (e.g., if impaction is suspected) (see Chapter 16). If you palpate rectal walls, dispose of gloves by turning them inside out and placing them in proper receptacle if they become soiled. Otherwise keep gloves on your hands (proceed to Step 19).
18. Perform hand hygiene and apply new pair of clean gloves (if previous gloves were soiled and discarded).
19. Remove suppository from foil wrapper and lubricate rounded end with water-soluble lubricant (see illustration). Lubricate gloved index finger of dominant hand. If patient has hemorrhoids, use liberal amount of lubricant and touch area gently.
20. Ask patient to take slow, deep breaths through mouth and relax anal sphincter.
21. Retract patient's buttocks with nondominant hand. With gloved index finger of dominant hand, insert suppository gently through anus, past internal sphincter, and against rectal wall, 10 cm (4 inches) in adults (see illustration) or 5 cm (2 inches) in infants and children. You should feel rectal sphincter close around your finger.
22. *Option:* A suppository may be given through a colostomy (not ileostomy) if ordered. Patient should lie supine. Use small amount of water-soluble lubricant for insertion.
23. Withdraw finger and wipe patient's anal area.
24. Ask patient to remain flat or on side for 5 minutes.

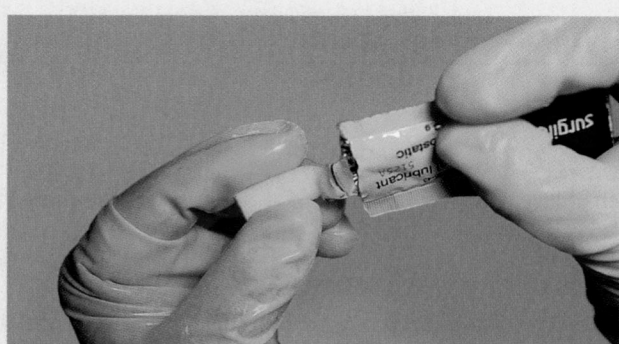

STEP 19 Lubricate tip of rectal suppository with water-soluble jelly.

BOX 17.19 PROCEDURAL GUIDELINES—cont'd

Administering Rectal Suppositories

25. Discard gloves by turning them inside out and dispose of them and used supplies in appropriate receptacle. Perform hand hygiene.

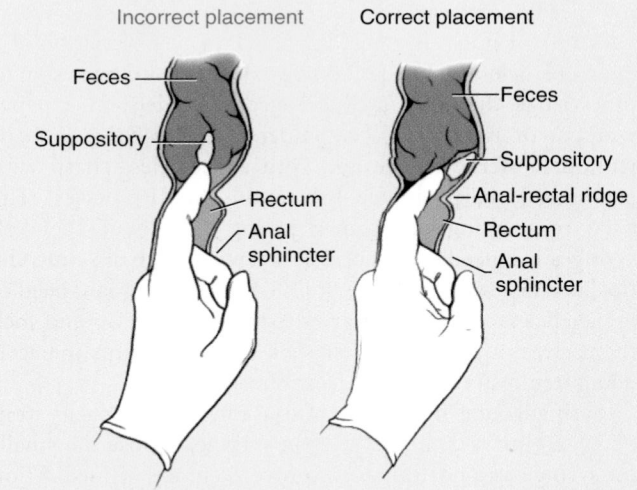

Incorrect placement   Correct placement

Feces — Suppository — Rectum — Anal sphincter

Feces — Suppository — Anal-rectal ridge — Rectum — Anal sphincter

STEP 21 Inserting rectal suppository. (From DeWit S: *Fundamental concepts and skills for nursing*, ed 3, Philadelphia, 2009, Saunders.)

26. If suppository contains laxative or fecal softener, be sure nurse call system is in an accessible location so patient can obtain help to reach bedpan or toilet.
27. If suppository was given for constipation, remind patient *not* to flush commode after bowel movement so that you can observe characteristics of stool.
28. Record drug, dosage, route, and actual time and date of administration on MAR immediately after administration, not before. Include initials or signature.
29. Return to bedside within 5 minutes to determine if suppository was expelled.
30. Ask if patient experienced localized anal or rectal discomfort during insertion.
31. Evaluate patient at time of peak drug effect for relief of symptoms for which medication was prescribed.
32. Record patient response to medication, patient teaching, and validation of patient understanding and self-administration of suppository on flow sheet or nurses' notes in electronic health record (EHR) or chart.
33. **Use Teach-Back:** "I want to be sure I explained clearly to you how to insert a rectal suppository. Describe the steps you will follow to insert the suppository." Revise your instruction now or develop a plan for revised patient/family caregiver teaching if patient/family caregiver is not able to teach back correctly.

to the pMDI and allows the particles of medication to slow down and break into smaller pieces. This helps the medication get deeper into the lungs and enhances absorption. Spacers are helpful when a patient has difficulty coordinating the steps or coordinating inhalation with the steps involved in self-administering inhaled medications. Patients who do not use their spacers correctly do not receive the full effect of the medication. BAIs and DPIs do not use spacers. BAIs release medication when a patient raises a lever and inhales. A BAI is a good choice for patients who have difficulty using pMDIs because the BAI eliminates the need for hand-breath coordination (Ari and Restrepo, 2012).

DPIs hold dry powder medication and create an aerosol when a patient inhales through a reservoir. The reservoir holds a dose of the medication. Compared with MDIs, DPIs deliver more medication to the lungs (Burchum and Rosenthal, 2016). When DPIs are unit dosed, a patient loads a single dose of medication into the inhaler with each use. Other DPIs hold enough medication to last for a month. DPIs require less manual dexterity. There is no need to coordinate puffs with inhalation because the device is activated when a patient breathes. However, the medication sometimes clumps when a patient is in a humid environment, and some patients cannot inspire fast enough to administer the entire medication dosage.

Patients who receive medications by inhalation frequently have a chronic respiratory disease such as chronic asthma, emphysema, or bronchitis. Some inhaled medications are described as *rescue* medications, whereas others are called *maintenance* medications. Rescue medications are short-acting; patients take them to relieve acute respiratory distress immediately. Patients need to be cautioned not to overuse rescue medications. If respiratory distress increases, instruct the patient to contact his or her health care provider and not to overuse the rescue mediations. The patient may need an adjustment of the maintenance medication.

Patients take maintenance medications on a daily schedule to prevent acute respiratory distress; their effects start within hours of administration and last for a longer period of time than rescue inhalers. Some inhalers combine rescue and maintenance medications. Proper use of inhalers improves patient outcomes and decreases mortality associated with chronic airway diseases. However, current evidence shows that many patients do not use their inhalers correctly. Thus teach your patients about safe and effective use of these inhalers and verify they can use an inhaler even if they have been using one for a long time (see Skill 17.3) (Ari and Restrepo, 2012).

Help your patients determine when inhalers are empty and need to be replaced. Do not float the pMDI in water to determine how much medication is left because the container floats even if it is empty. Devices that attach onto the MDI and count down the number of remaining doses are available for MDIs. Some DPIs have an indicator that shows how many doses are left. However, these are not always accurate. Therefore the best way to calculate how long medication in an inhaler will last is to divide the number of doses in the container by the number of doses that your patient takes per day. For example, your patient is to take albuterol, a beta-adrenergic agonist bronchodilator. The ordered dose is 2 puffs 4 times a day (qid). The canister has 200 puffs. You complete the following calculations to determine how long the MDI will last:

$$2 \text{ puffs} \times 4 \text{ times a day} = 8 \text{ puffs per day}$$

$$200 \text{ puffs} \div 8 \text{ puffs per day} = 25 \text{ days}$$

Therefore the canister will last 25 days. To ensure that the patient does not run out of medication, teach the patient to refill the medication at least 7 to 10 days before it runs out.

Administering Medications by Irrigations

Some medications irrigate or wash a body cavity and are delivered through a stream of solution. Irrigations most often use sterile water, saline, or antiseptic solutions on the eye, ear, throat, vagina, and urinary tract. Use aseptic technique if there is a break in the skin or mucosa. Use clean technique when the cavity to be irrigated is not sterile, as in the case of the ear canal or vagina. Irrigations are used to:
- Cleanse an area.
- Instill a medication.
- Apply heat or cold to injured tissue (see Chapter 38).

PARENTERAL ADMINISTRATION OF MEDICATIONS

Parenteral administration of medications involves the injection of a medication into body tissues. A needle piercing the skin carries a risk of infection. This is an invasive procedure that is performed with the following aseptic techniques:
- Draw up medication quickly to avoid contaminating solutions. Do not allow ampules to stand open.
- Avoid letting a needle touch contaminated surfaces (e.g., outer edges of ampule or vial, outer surface of needle cap).
- Avoid touching length of plunger or inner part of barrel. Keep tip of syringe covered with cap or needle.
- Prepare skin by washing with soap and water if soiled. Use friction and a circular motion when cleaning with an antiseptic swab. Swab from center of site and move outward in a 5-cm (2-inch) radius.

Each type of injection requires certain skills to ensure that the medication reaches the proper location. The effects of a parenteral medication occur rapidly, depending on the rate of medication absorption. You must closely observe a patient's response to parenteral medications.

Equipment

You will administer parenteral medications by using a needle and a syringe, available in a variety of sizes. Each size is designed to deliver a certain volume of a medication to a specific type of tissue. Determine the appropriate size of syringe, length and gauge of needle, volume of solution, and

medication route based on the quantity and type of medication prescribed and the body size of a patient. Most syringes come with needleless systems or safety needles that help prevent needlestick injuries.

Syringes. A syringe has a cylindrical barrel with a close-fitting plunger and a tip designed to fit the hub of a hypodermic needle. Syringes are single use, disposable, and either Luer-Lok or non–Luer-Lok (Fig. 17.8). The designation of a Luer-Lok or non–Luer-Lok syringe depends on the design of the syringe tip. They are packaged separately, in a paper wrapper or rigid plastic container. Syringes come with or without a sterile needle and with a needleless sharp with engineered sharps injury protection (SESIP) device. The parts of a syringe are shown in Fig. 17.9. Non–Luer-Lok syringes use needles or needleless devices that slip onto the tip. Luer-Lok syringes (see Fig. 17.8 A–B) use standard needles or needleless devices that are twisted onto the tip and lock themselves in place. The Luer-Lok design prevents the accidental removal of a needle from the syringe.

Syringes come in a variety of sizes ranging in capacity from 0.5 to 60 mL. When you select a syringe, choose the smallest syringe size possible to improve accuracy of medication preparation. In addition, avoid injecting a large volume of fluid into tissues. A 1- to 3-mL syringe is usually adequate for

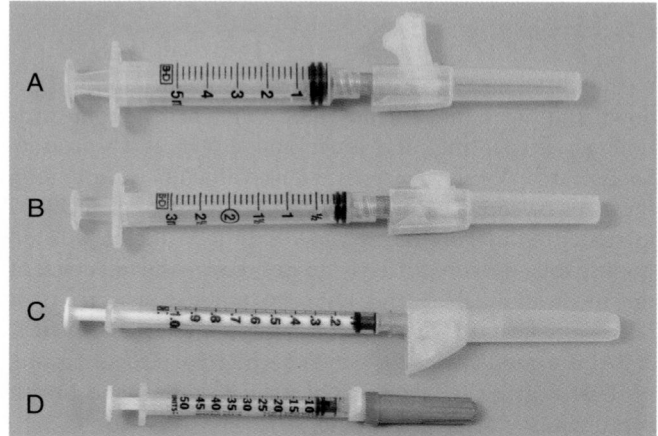

FIG 17.8 Types of syringes. **A,** 5-mL syringe. **B,** 3-mL syringe. **C,** Tuberculin syringe marked in 0.01 (hundredths) for doses less than 1 mL. **D,** Insulin syringe marked in units (50).

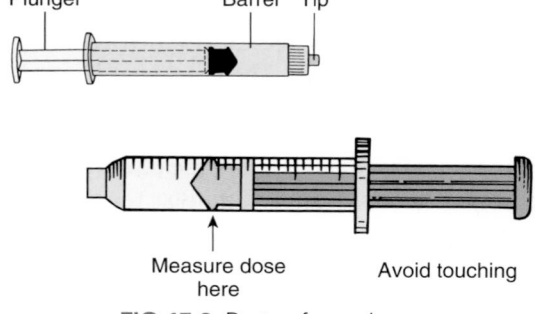

FIG 17.9 Parts of a syringe.

a subcutaneous or IM injection. Larger volumes result in pain and discomfort for a patient. Syringes are most commonly marked in a scale of tenths of a milliliter. You use tuberculin (TB) syringes to prepare small amounts of medications for ID and subcutaneous injections (see Fig. 17.8C). Insulin syringes (see Fig. 17.8D) hold 0.3 to 1 mL; low-dose insulin syringes (30 units per 0.3 mL or 50 units per 0.5 mL) hold 0.3 to 0.5 mL. All insulin syringes come with preattached needles and are calibrated in units. Most insulin syringes are U-100s, designed for use with U-100–strength insulin. Each 1 mL of solution contains 100 units of insulin.

To fill a syringe, pull the plunger outward while the needle tip remains immersed in the prepared solution. To maintain sterility, touch the outside of the syringe barrel and the handle of the plunger only.

Use larger syringes to administer some IV medications and irrigate drainage tubes. Some syringes are packaged with their needle attached, and some syringes require you to change the needle based on the viscosity of the medication, route of administration, and size of the patient. Before use carefully examine the syringe to determine the measurement scale and ensure that you use the correct syringe for preparing the ordered medication.

Needles. Some needles come attached to syringes. Others come packaged individually to allow flexibility in selecting the right needle for a patient. Needles are disposable, and most are made of stainless steel. A needle has three parts: the hub, which fits onto the tip of a syringe; the shaft, which connects to the hub; and the bevel, or slanted tip (Fig. 17.10). When injected into tissue, the bevel creates a narrow slit that quickly closes when you remove the needle. This prevents leakage of medication, blood, or serum. Long, beveled tips are sharp and narrow, which minimizes discomfort when entering tissue used for subcutaneous and IM injections. The needle hub, shaft, and bevel must remain sterile at all times. To prevent contamination, use gentle force to place the needle onto the syringe with the cap intact. Some needles come with filters for preparation of medications. Never use a filter to administer a medication.

Needles vary in length from $\frac{1}{4}$ to 3 inches (Fig. 17.11). Choose the needle length according to a patient's size and weight and the type of tissue into which the medication is to be injected. Current evidence suggests that IM needle length should be based on the patient's weight (Davidson and Rourke, 2013). There should be a 5-mm depth of muscle penetration to achieve an IM injection (Hibbard et al., 2015). A child or slender adult generally requires a shorter needle. Use longer needles (1 to $1\frac{1}{2}$ inches) (25 to 38 mm) for IM injections and a shorter needle ($\frac{3}{8}$ to $\frac{5}{8}$ inch) (9 to 16 mm) for subcutaneous injections. Needles also vary in gauge or circumference. As the needle gauge becomes smaller, the needle diameter becomes larger. The selection of a gauge depends on the viscosity of fluid to be injected or infused.

Disposable Injection Units. Single-dose, prefilled, disposable syringes are available for some medications. You do

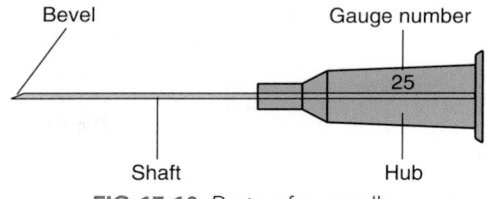

FIG 17.10 Parts of a needle.

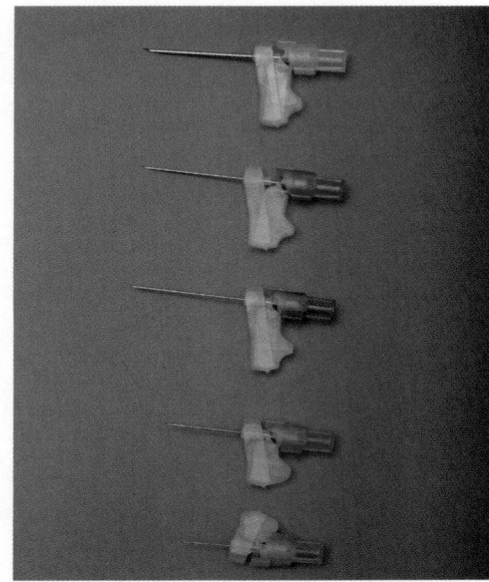

FIG 17.11 Hypodermic needles (top to bottom): 18 gauge, $1\frac{1}{2}$-inch length; 21 gauge, $1\frac{1}{2}$-inch length; 22 gauge, $1\frac{1}{2}$-inch length; 23 gauge, 1-inch length; and 25 gauge, $\frac{5}{8}$-inch length.

not need to prepare the medication dose except perhaps to expel unneeded portions of medication or air. However, it is important to check the medication and concentration carefully because prefilled syringes appear very similar. Prefilled unit-dose systems such as Tubex and Carpuject injection systems include reusable plastic syringe holders and disposable, prefilled, sterile, glass cartridge units (Fig. 17.12A). To assemble a prefilled system, place the cartridge, barrel first, into the plastic syringe holder (Fig. 17.12B). Following manufacturer instructions, turn the plunger rod to the left (counterclockwise) (see Fig. 17.12C) and then lock to the right (clockwise) until it "clicks." Finally remove the needle guard and advance the plunger (see Fig. 17.12D) to expel air and excess medication as with a regular syringe. The cartridge may be used with SESIP needles. After giving the medication dispose of the glass cartridge safely in a puncture-proof and leak-proof container. This design reduces the risk for needlestick injury.

Preparing an Injection From an Ampule

Ampules contain single doses of medication in a liquid. They are available in several sizes, from 1 mL to 10 mL or more (Fig. 17.13A). An ampule consists of glass with a constricted neck that you snap off to access the medication. A colored

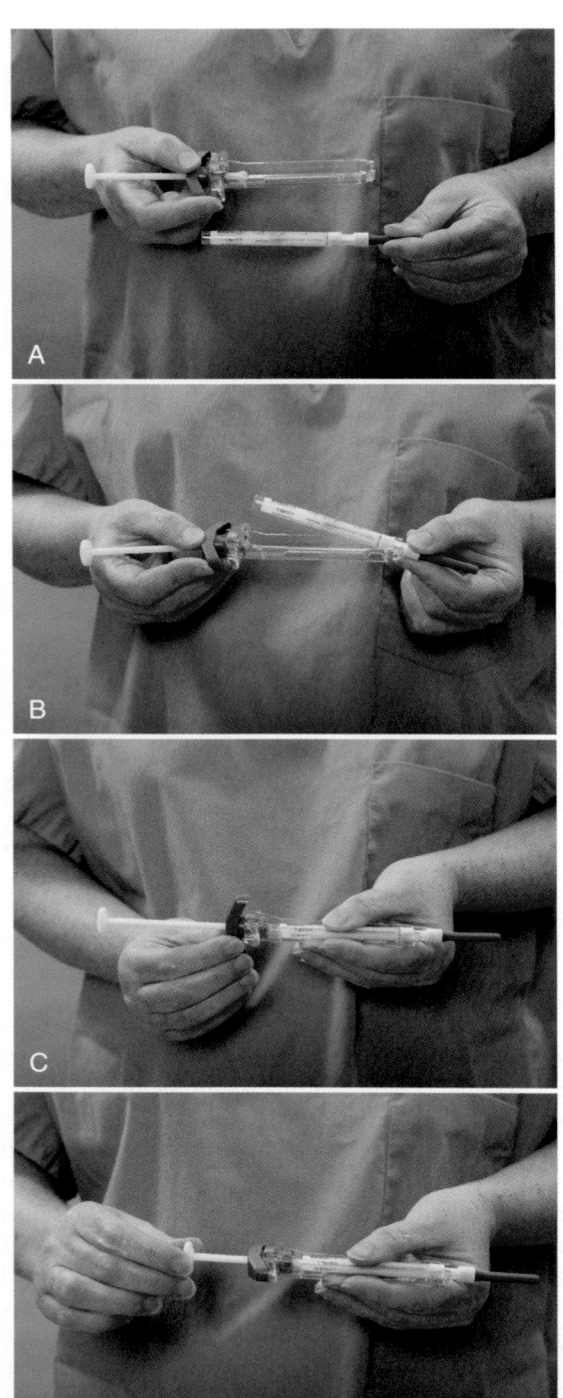

FIG 17.12 A, Carpuject syringe and prefilled sterile cartridge with needle. **B,** Assembling Carpuject. **C,** Cartridge slides into syringe barrel, turns, and locks at needle end. **D,** Plunger screws into cartridge end. Expel excess medication to obtain accurate dose (not pictured).

ring around the neck indicates where the ampule is scored so that you can break it easily. Carefully aspirate the medication into a syringe (see Skill 17.4) with a filter needle. Use a filter needle to prevent particulate matter such as small glass fragments from entering the syringe (Alexander et al., 2014).

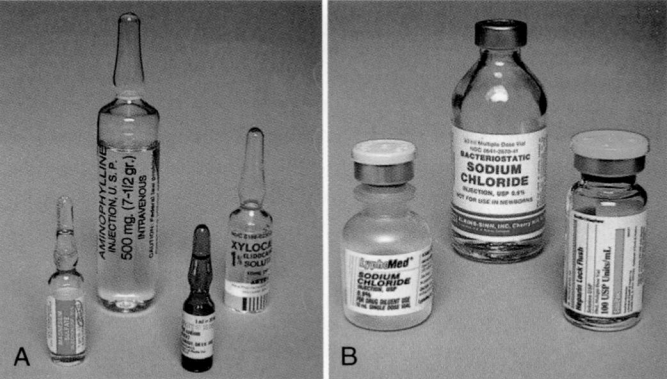

FIG 17.13 A, Medication in ampules. **B,** Medication in vials. Rubber top must be cleansed with alcohol when vial is opened or reused.

Replace the filter needle with an appropriate-size needle or a needleless access device before administering the injection.

Preparing an Injection From a Vial

A vial is a single-dose or multidose container with a rubber seal at the top (see Fig. 17.13B). A metal cap protects the seal until it is ready for use. Vials contain liquid or dry forms of medications. Medications that are unstable in solution are packaged dry. The vial label specifies the solvent or diluent, usually sterile normal saline or sterile distilled water, used to dissolve the medication and the amount of diluent needed to prepare a desired concentration.

In contrast to the ampule, the vial is a closed system, and air must be injected into the vial to permit easy withdrawal of the solution. Failure to inject air when withdrawing creates a vacuum within the vial that makes withdrawal difficult. If you are concerned about drawing up parts of the rubber stopper or other particles into the syringe, use a filter needle when preparing medications from vials (Alexander et al., 2014).

Some vials contain powder, which is mixed with a diluent during preparation and before injection (see Skill 17.4). After you mix multidose vials, make a label that includes the date and time of mixing and the concentration of medication per milliliter. Some multidose vials require refrigeration after the contents have been reconstituted.

Mixing Medications

If two medications are compatible, you may mix them in one injection if the total dose is within accepted limits. This prevents a patient from having to receive more than one injection at a time. Most patient care units have charts that list common compatible medications. If you have any doubts about medication compatibilities, consult a pharmacist or a medication reference.

Mixing Medications From a Vial and an Ampule.

When you mix medication from both a vial and an ampule, prepare the medication from the vial first. Using the same syringe and filter needle, next withdraw medication from

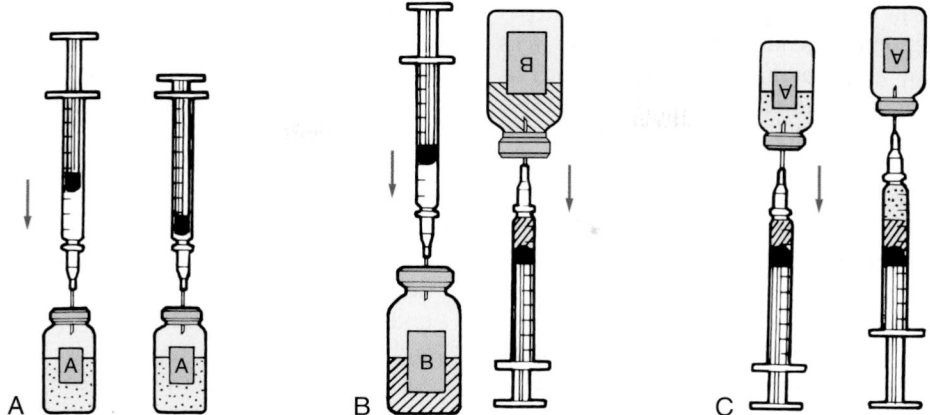

FIG 17.14 Steps in mixing medications from two vials.

the ampule. This technique prepares the medications in this order so it is not necessary to add air to withdraw medication from an ampule.

Mixing Medications From Two Vials. Apply these principles when mixing medications from two vials:

1. Do not contaminate one medication with another.
2. Ensure that the final dose is accurate.
3. Maintain aseptic technique.

Use only one syringe with an attached needle or needleless access device to mix medications from two vials. Aspirate the volume of air equivalent to the first medication dose (vial A) into the syringe. Then inject the air into vial A (Fig. 17.14A), making sure that the needle does not touch the solution. Withdraw the needle and aspirate air equivalent to the dose of the second medication (vial B). Inject the volume of air into vial B (Fig. 17.14B). Immediately withdraw the medication from vial B into the syringe and insert the needle back into vial A, being careful not to push the plunger and expel the medication within the syringe into the vial. Withdraw the desired amount of medication from vial A into the syringe (Fig. 17.14C). After you withdraw the necessary amount, withdraw the needle and apply a new safety needle or needleless access device suitable for injection.

Insulin Preparation

Insulin is the hormone used to treat diabetes mellitus. You must administer it by subcutaneous injection because the GI tract breaks down and destroys an oral form of insulin. Most patients with diabetes mellitus who require insulin injections learn to administer their own injections. In the United States and Canada, health care providers usually prescribe insulin in concentrations of 100 units per milliliter of solution. This is called *U-100 insulin.* Insulin is also commercially available in concentrations of 50 and 500 units per milliliter of solution, or *U-50* and *U-500 insulin.* U-500 insulin is 5 times as strong as U-100 insulin and is used only in rare cases in which patients are very resistant to insulin.

When preparing insulin use the correct syringe that corresponds to the unit concentration ordered. For example, use a 100-unit insulin syringe or insulin pen to prepare U-100 insulin. Because no syringe is currently available for preparing U-500 insulin, many medication errors result with this kind of insulin. To prevent errors, ensure that the order for U-500 specifies units and volume (e.g., 150 units, 0.3 mL of U-500 insulin), and use tuberculin syringes to draw up the doses (ISMP, 2013a). Verify every injection you prepare with another nurse before administering it. Additional safety measures common with U-500 insulin include:

- Listing the insulin as being concentrated in computerized medication dispensing systems.
- Making health care providers and pharmacists verify that a patient is to receive U-500 insulin when it is ordered.
- Stocking only U-500 insulin on patient care units when it is ordered for a specific patient (ISMP, 2013a).

Insulin is classified by rate of action including rapid-acting, short-acting, intermediate-acting, and long-acting. To provide safe and effective care, you must know the onset, peak, and duration for your patients' ordered insulin doses. Refer to a medication reference or consult with a pharmacist if you are unsure of this information. Regular insulin is the only type of insulin that can be given intravenously.

A patient with diabetes mellitus sometimes requires more than one type of insulin. For example, a patient receiving a short-acting (regular) and an intermediate-acting (NPH) insulin receives greater sustained control of blood glucose levels over 24 hours. The timing of insulin injections attempts to imitate the normal pattern of insulin release from the pancreas. Some insulins come in a stable premixed solution (e.g., 70/30 insulin is 70% NPH [intermediate] and 30% regular), eliminating the need to mix the insulins in a syringe. Other patients use an insulin pen. The insulin pen contains multiple doses and enables a patient to select the dose, avoiding the need to use a syringe.

Research shows that various types of a patient's blood cells can enter an insulin pen after an injection. Several U.S. health care organizations recently reported that the same insulin pen was inadvertently used on multiple patients. This exposed the patients to bloodborne illnesses (such as human immunodeficiency virus [HIV], hepatitis B virus, and hepatitis C virus). Thus the ISMP recommends that insulin pens be used only at home and that inpatient settings such as hospitals stop using them whenever possible (ISMP, 2013b).

Insulin is ordered as a specific dose at specific times of the day. Thus timely administration is critical. Correction insulin, also known as sliding-scale insulin, is a dose of insulin based on a patient's blood glucose level. The term *correction insulin* is preferred because it indicates that small doses of rapid-acting or short-acting insulin are used to correct a patient's elevated blood sugar. Reliance on correction insulin is unlikely to achieve long-term glucose control. Thus it should be ordered only temporarily (American Diabetes Association [ADA], 2015). An example of a correction insulin order follows:

Give regular U-100 insulin subcutaneously

2 units for glucose 150 to 200 mg/dL

4 units for glucose 201 to 275 mg/dL

Call for dosage for glucose greater than 275 mg/dL

In the case of a patient's blood glucose being 201 mg/dL following lunch, the nurse would refer to the correction insulin order and administer 4 units of regular insulin to the patient.

Before preparing an insulin dose, gently roll all cloudy insulin preparations between the palms of your hands to resuspend the insulin (Diggle, 2014). Do not shake insulin vials. Shaking causes bubbles to form. Bubbles take up space in the syringe and alter the dose. If the patient requires more than one type of insulin to manage his or her diabetes, you may mix two different types of insulin into one syringe *if* they are compatible (Box 17.20). If regular and intermediate-acting insulins are ordered, prepare the regular insulin first to prevent it from becoming contaminated with the intermediate-acting insulin (Diggle, 2014). Use the following principles when mixing insulins (Diggle, 2014; McCulloch, 2015; Novo Nordisk, 2015):

- Patients whose blood glucose levels are well controlled on a mixed-insulin dose need to maintain their individual routine when preparing and administering their insulin.
- Do not mix insulin with any other medications or diluents unless approved by the health care provider.
- Never mix insulin glargine (Lantus) or insulin detemir (Levemir) with other types of insulin.
- Inject rapid-acting insulins mixed with NPH insulin within 15 minutes before a meal.
- Verify insulin doses with another nurse while you are preparing the injection.

Administering Injections

Each injection route differs with the type of tissues the medication enters. The characteristics of the tissues affect the rate of medication absorption, affecting the onset of medication action. Before injecting a medication, know the volume of the medication to administer, the characteristics and viscosity of the medication, and the location of anatomical structures underlying injection sites (see Skill 17.5).

If you administer injections incorrectly, negative patient outcomes result. For example, the American Pharmacists' Association (APhA, 2015) reported a rare condition that results from an incorrect injection technique into the deltoid muscle, shoulder injury related to vaccine administration (SIRVA). SIRVA is thought to occur as a result of unintentional injection of a vaccine antigen into tissues and structures underlying the deltoid muscle or trauma from the needle into and around the underlying shoulder bursa. Failure to consider anatomical landmarks when selecting an injection may result in nerve or bone damage during needle insertion. Inability to maintain stability of the needle and syringe unit can result in pain and tissue damage. If you fail to aspirate the syringe before injecting an IM medication, the medication may be accidentally injected directly into an artery or vein. Injecting too large a volume of medication for the site selected causes extreme pain and results in local tissue damage.

Many patients, particularly children, fear injections. Patients with serious or chronic illness often are given several injections daily. Minimize discomfort in the following ways:

- Use a sharp-beveled needle in the smallest suitable length and gauge.
- Position a patient comfortably to reduce muscular tension.
- Use anatomical landmarks to select the proper injection site.
- Apply a vapocoolant spray (e.g., Fluori-Methane spray or ethyl chloride) or topical anesthetic (e.g., eutectic mixture of local anesthetics [EMLA] cream) to the injection site before giving the medication when possible.
- Divert the patient's attention from the injection by asking open-ended questions.
- Insert the needle quickly and smoothly to minimize tissue pulling.
- Hold the syringe steady while the needle remains in tissues.
- Inject the medication slowly and steadily.

Subcutaneous Injections. Subcutaneous injections involve injecting medication into the loose connective tissue underlying the dermis. Subcutaneous tissue does not contain as many blood vessels as muscles, and thus medications are absorbed more slowly than with IM injections. Physical exercise or application of hot or cold compresses influences the rate of drug absorption by altering local blood flow to tissues. Any condition that impairs blood flow is a contraindication for subcutaneous injections.

Because subcutaneous tissue contains pain receptors, patients often experience slight discomfort. Injection into blood vessels is rare; thus you do not need to aspirate when giving subcutaneous injections (Lilley et al., 2016). Subcutaneous tissue is sensitive to irritating solutions and large volumes of medications. Thus you administer only small volumes (0.5 to 1.5 mL) of water-soluble medications

BOX 17.20 PROCEDURAL GUIDELINES

Mixing Two Types of Insulin in One Syringe

DELEGATION CONSIDERATIONS

The skill of mixing two kinds of insulin in one syringe cannot be delegated to nursing assistive personnel (NAP).

EQUIPMENT

Medication administration record (MAR) (electronic or printed); insulin vials; insulin syringe; antiseptic swab

STEPS

1. Check accuracy and completeness of each MAR with health care provider's medication order. Check patient's name, drug name and dosage, route of administration, and time for administration. Clarify incomplete or unclear orders with health care provider before administration.
2. Review medication and medical history (e.g., type of diabetes, reason for elevated blood sugars) and allergies to medications, food, and latex.
3. Verify insulin labels carefully against MAR before preparing the dose to ensure that you give the correct type of insulin. *This is the first accuracy check.*
4. Perform hand hygiene.
5. If patient takes insulin that is cloudy, roll the bottle of insulin between the hands to resuspend the insulin preparation.
6. Wipe off tops of both insulin vials with alcohol swabs and allow to dry.
7. Verify insulin dosages against MAR a second time. *This is the second accuracy check.*
8. If mixing rapid-acting or short-acting insulin with intermediate-acting insulin, take insulin syringe and aspirate volume of air equivalent to dose to be withdrawn from intermediate-acting insulin first. If two intermediate-acting insulins are mixed, it makes no difference which vial you prepare first.

9. Insert needle and inject air into vial of intermediate-acting insulin. Do not let the tip of the needle touch the insulin.
10. Remove the syringe from the vial of intermediate-acting insulin without aspirating medication.
11. With the same syringe, inject air equal to the dose of rapid-acting or short-acting insulin into the vial and withdraw the correct dose into the syringe.
12. Remove the syringe from the rapid-acting or short-acting insulin and get rid of air bubbles to ensure accurate dosing.
13. After verifying insulin dosages with MAR a third time, show insulin prepared in syringe to another nurse to verify that you prepared correct dosage of insulin. *This is the third accuracy check.* Determine which point on syringe scale combined units of insulin measure by adding the number of units of both insulins together (e.g., 5 units regular + 10 units NPH = 15 units total).
14. Place the needle of the syringe back into the vial of intermediate-acting insulin. Be careful not to push plunger and inject insulin in syringe into the vial.
15. Invert the vial and carefully withdraw the desired amount of insulin into syringe.
16. Withdraw needle and check fluid level in syringe. Keep needle of prepared syringe sheathed or capped until ready to administer medication. Show another nurse the syringe to verify that you prepared the correct dose.
17. Dispose of soiled supplies in proper receptacle. Place empty vials in puncture-proof and leak-proof container and perform hand hygiene.
18. Because rapid-acting or short-acting insulin binds with intermediate-acting insulin, which reduces the action of the faster-acting insulin, administer mixture within 5 minutes of preparing it.

Modified from American Diabetes Association (ADA): *Insulin and other injectables*, 2013, http://www.diabetes.org/living-with-diabetes/treatment-and-care/medication/insulin; and Dunning T: *Care of people with diabetes: a manual of nursing practice*, ed 4, Hoboken, NJ, 2013, Wiley-Blackwell.

subcutaneously to adults. In children, you give smaller volumes up to 0.5 mL (Hockenberry and Wilson, 2015). Examples of subcutaneous medications include epinephrine, insulin, allergy medications, opioids, and heparin.

The best subcutaneous injection sites include the outer posterior aspect of the upper arms, the abdomen from below the costal margins to the iliac crests, and the anterior aspects of the thighs (Fig. 17.15). These areas are easily accessible and are large enough to allow rotating multiple injections within each anatomic location. Site rotation prevents the formation of lipohypertrophy or lipoatrophy in the skin. Choose an injection site that is free of skin lesions, bony prominences, and large underlying muscles or nerves.

The site most frequently recommended for heparin injections is the right or left side of the abdomen, at least 5 cm (2 inches) away from the umbilicus (Fig. 17.16). The administration of low-molecular-weight heparin (LMWH) (e.g., enoxaparin) requires special considerations. Administer LMWH in its prefilled syringe with the attached needle, and do not expel the air bubble in the syringe before giving the medication. Some evidence supports a slower injection rate of 30 seconds to reduce bruising and pain (Akbari Sari et al., 2014; Sanofi-Aventis, 2014).

Recommended sites for insulin injection include the abdomen, upper arm, anterior and lateral parts of the thigh, and buttocks. Rotating injections within the same body part (intrasite rotation) produces consistency in the absorption of the insulin. For example, if a patient receives morning insulin in the right arm, give the next injection in a different place in the same arm, at least 2.5 cm (1 inch) away from the previous site (Frid et al., 2016). Do not reuse injection sites for at least 1 month. The rate of insulin absorption varies based on the site. The abdomen has the fastest absorption, followed by the arms, thighs, and buttocks (McCulloch, 2015).

A patient's body weight and adipose tissue indicate the depth of the subcutaneous layer. Therefore choose the needle

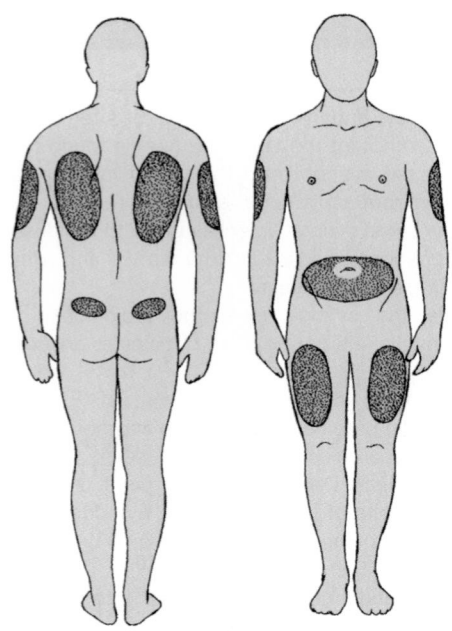

FIG 17.15 Sites recommended for subcutaneous injections.

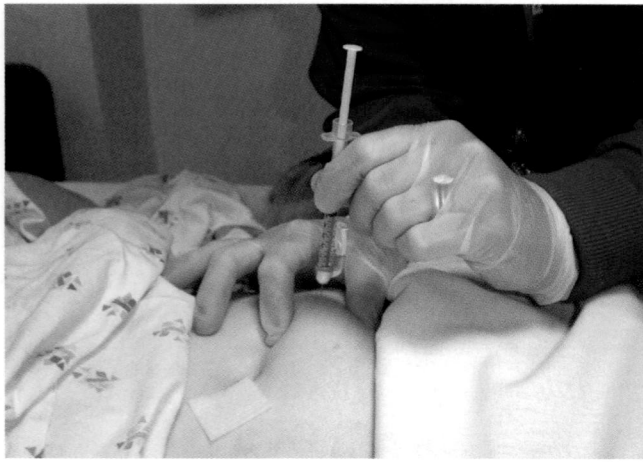

FIG 17.16 Giving subcutaneous heparin in abdomen.

length and angle of insertion on the basis of a patient's weight and an estimation of the amount of subcutaneous tissue (Ogston-Tuck, 2014a). Nurses typically use a 25-gauge, 16-mm (⅝-inch) needle inserted at a 45-degree angle for injections (Fig. 17.17) or a 12-mm (½-inch) needle inserted at a 90-degree angle to administer subcutaneous medications to a normal-size adult patient (except with insulin; see next paragraph). Some children require only a 12-mm (½-inch) needle. If the patient is obese, pinch the tissue and use a needle long enough to insert through fatty tissue at the base of the skinfold. Thin patients often do not have sufficient tissue for subcutaneous injections; the upper abdomen is usually the best site in this case. To ensure that a subcutaneous medication reaches the subcutaneous tissue, follow this rule: If you can grasp 5 cm (2 inches) of tissue, insert the needle at a 90-degree angle; if you can grasp only 2.5 cm (1 inch) of tissue, insert the needle at a 45-degree angle.

Research in insulin administration now shows that insulin needles that are ⁵⁄₁₆ inch (8 mm) or longer often enter the muscles of men and people with a body mass index (BMI) of 25 or less. Shorter (³⁄₁₆-inch or 4- to 5-mm) needles were associated with less pain, adequate control of blood sugars, and minimal leakage of medication (Hirsch et al., 2012; Diggle, 2014). Thus when administering insulin, you should use ³⁄₁₆-inch (4- to 5-mm) needles administered at a 90-degree angle to reduce pain and achieve adequate control of blood sugars with minimal adverse effects for people of all body mass indices including children (American Association of Diabetes Educators [AADE], 2013).

Frequently patients who self-administer insulin at home reuse needles because of financial limitations. In a systematic review of the current scientific literature there is no clear evidence to suggest for or against reuse of needles in the home setting for subcutaneous insulin injection (Zabaleta-Del-Olmo et al., 2016; Frid et al., 2016) with regard to patient safety. A few studies have found that reused needles cause more discomfort. The practice of reusing needles is very common among people with diabetes mellitus; thus the researchers recommend further research.

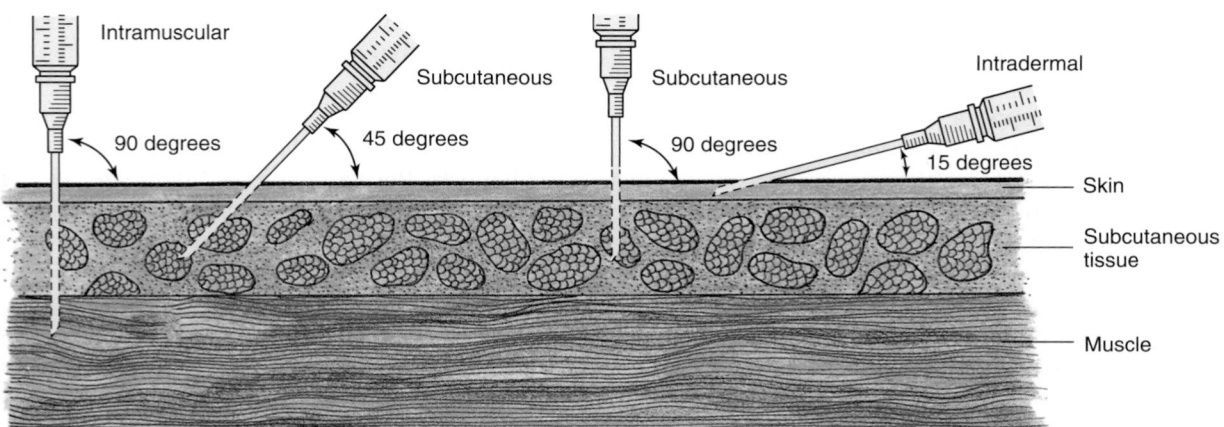

FIG 17.17 Comparison of angles of insertion for intramuscular (90 degrees), subcutaneous (45 and 90 degrees), and intradermal (15 degrees) injections.

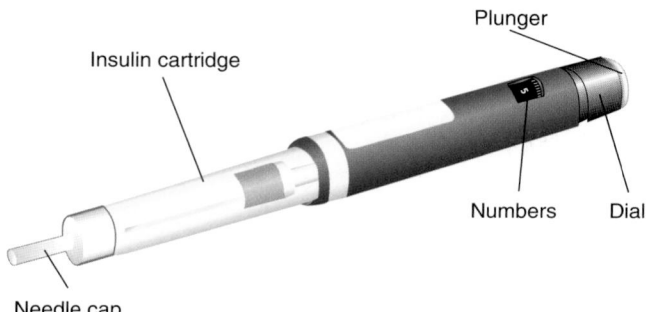

FIG 17.18 Insulin injection pen. (From Lewis SL, et al: *Medical-surgical nursing: assessment and management of clinical problems,* ed 8, St Louis, 2011, Mosby.)

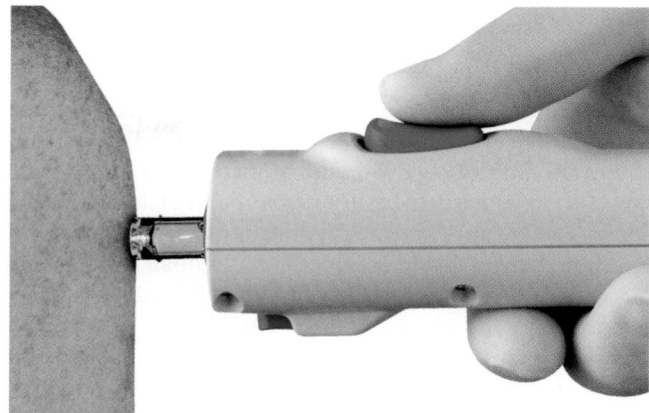

FIG 17.19 Jet injection system is held perpendicular to skin. (Image courtesy Pharmajet. All rights reserved.)

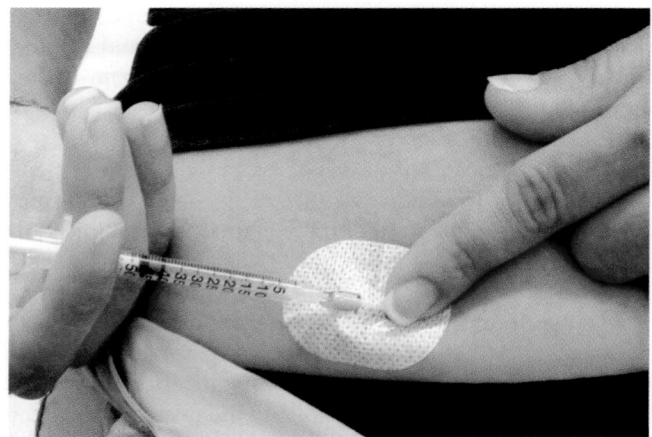

FIG 17.20 Subcutaneous device. (Image courtesy IntraPump Infusion Systems. All rights reserved.)

Several different devices are available for administration of subcutaneous injections. *Injection pens* allow patients to self-administer medications (e.g., epinephrine, insulin, or interferon) subcutaneously (Fig. 17.18). Injection pens are a convenient delivery method using prefilled, disposable cartridges. The patient pinches the skin, inserts the needle, and injects a predetermined medication dose. Teaching is essential to ensure that patients use the correct injection technique and deliver the correct dose of medication. Reinforce to patients and family caregivers that insulin pens are used by only one patient and are not shared (Frid et al., 2016). In addition, teach patients the importance of priming the pen before use. Priming involves pointing the pen needle up in the air, dialing one or two units (see package directions) on the pen and then pressing the plunger fully with the thumb repeatedly until a drop appears. This clears the needle of air and ensures a full dose is ready. The disadvantages to this device include increased risk for needlestick injury and user's lack of knowledge and skill in administration technique (Ogston-Tuck, 2014a). The *needleless jet injection system* administers subcutaneous medications without the use of needles. Needle-free injections use high pressure to penetrate the skin with the medication into the subcutaneous tissue (Fig. 17.19). Another option for subcutaneous injection is the *subcutaneous injection device* (e.g., insuflon) (Fig. 17.20). You insert the device into the subcutaneous tissue. You then remove the needle, leaving the cannula in the tissue to provide an avenue for administering medications for up to 3 days without having to puncture the skin with each injection.

Intramuscular Injections. The IM injection route deposits medication into deep muscle tissue, which has a rich blood supply, allowing medication to absorb faster than by the subcutaneous route. However, there is a risk for injecting drugs directly into blood vessels. Any factor that interferes with local tissue blood flow affects the rate and extent of IM drug absorption. In addition, if a medication is not injected correctly into a muscle, complications can arise such as abscess, hematoma, ecchymosis, pain, and vascular and nerve injury (Nicoll and Hesby, 2002; Kara et al., 2015; Kaya et al., 2015). Therefore whenever administering a medication by the IM route, first verify that the injection is justified (Nicoll and Hesby, 2002; World Health Organization [WHO], 2015). Some medications such as hepatitis B and tetanus, diphtheria, and pertussis (Tdap) immunizations are given only intramuscularly.

The viscosity of a medication, injection site, patient's weight, and amount of adipose tissue influence needle gauge and length selection. Use a longer and heavier-gauge needle to pass through subcutaneous tissue and penetrate deep muscle tissue (see Skill 17.5). A patient's body mass index and the amount of adipose tissue affect the choice of needle. Many needles available in health care settings are not long enough to reach the muscle, especially in female patients and patients who are obese (Bhalla et al., 2013; Palma and Strohfus, 2013; Dayananda et al., 2014). Because most health care agencies have needles that range in length from only $\frac{3}{8}$ to $1\frac{1}{2}$ inches (9 to 38 mm), investigate other medication routes, especially when IM injections are ordered for female patients who are obese.

The angle of insertion for an IM injection is 90 degrees (see Fig. 17.17). Muscle is less sensitive to irritating and viscous medications. An adult patient who is well developed tolerates 2 to 5 mL of medication in a larger muscle without severe muscle discomfort (Nicoll and Hesby, 2002; Hopkins and Arias, 2013). Larger volumes of medication (4 to 5 mL), however, are unlikely to be absorbed properly. Children, older adults, and patients who are thin tolerate only 2 mL of an IM injection. Do not give more than 1 mL to small children and older infants, and do not give more than 0.5 mL to younger infants (Hockenberry and Wilson, 2015).

Assess a muscle before giving an injection. Properly identify the site for the IM injection by palpating bony landmarks, and be aware of the potential complications associated with each site. The site needs to be free of tenderness because repeated injections in the same muscle cause severe discomfort. With the patient relaxed, palpate the muscle to rule out hardened lesions. Minimize discomfort during an injection by helping a patient assume a position that reduces muscle strain. Other interventions such as distraction and application of ice or pressure to an IM site reduce pain during an injection.

Rotate IM injection sites to decrease the risk for tissue hypertrophy. Emaciated or atrophied muscles absorb medication poorly; avoid their use when possible. The **Z-track method,** a technique for pulling the skin during an injection, is recommended for IM injections (Nicoll and Hesby, 2002). It prevents leakage of medication into subcutaneous tissues, seals medication in the muscle, and minimizes irritation. To use the Z-track method, attach the appropriate-size needle to the syringe and select an IM site, preferably in a large, deep muscle such as the ventrogluteal. Pull the overlying skin and subcutaneous tissues approximately 2.5 to 3.5 cm (1 to 1½ inches) laterally to the side with the ulnar side of the nondominant hand. Hold the skin in this position until you have administered the injection (Fig. 17.21A). After cleaning a site, inject the needle deeply into the muscle. Aspirate the injection and if no blood is returned on aspiration, inject the medication slowly into the muscle. To reduce injection site discomfort, there is no longer any need to aspirate after the needle is injected when *administering vaccines* (CDC, 2015). It is the nurses' responsibility to follow agency policy for aspiration when giving vaccines. Keep the needle inserted for 10 seconds to allow the medication to disperse evenly. Release the skin after withdrawing the needle. This leaves a zigzag path that seals the needle track wherever tissue planes slide across one another see (Fig. 17.21B). The medication is sealed in the muscle tissue.

Injection Sites. When selecting an IM site, consider the following:
- Is the area free of infection or necrosis?
- Are there local areas of bruising or abrasions?
- What are the locations of underlying bones, nerves, and major blood vessels?
- What volume of medication is to be administered?
- Can you position a patient anatomically and comfortably so as to access the site?

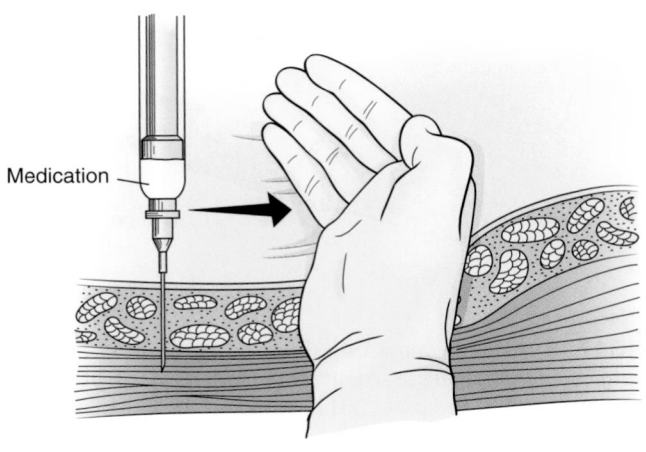

Medication

A   During injection

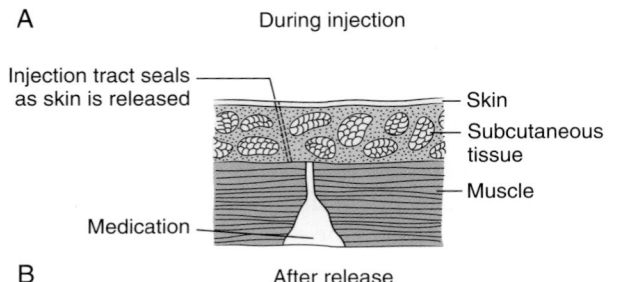

Injection tract seals as skin is released

Skin

Subcutaneous tissue

Muscle

Medication

B   After release

FIG 17.21 Z-track method of injection prevents deposit of medication into sensitive tissues.

Ventrogluteal Muscle. The ventrogluteal muscle is the preferred and safest site for all adults, children, and infants, especially for large volume, viscous and irritating medications (Hopkins and Arias, 2013; Hockenberry and Wilson, 2015; Kara et al., 2015; Gūnes et al., 2016). The site involves the gluteus medius where the thickness of subcutaneous tissue is less than other injection sites and there are relatively fewer nerves and blood vessels (Kara et al., 2015). Furthermore, in this site the muscles are large and well established, and it is easy to find the muscle limit points (Kara et al., 2015).

The ventrogluteal site is recommended for volumes greater than 2 mL (Nicoll and Hesby, 2002; Hopkins and Arias, 2013). Research shows that injuries such as fibrosis, nerve damage, abscess, tissue necrosis, muscle contraction, gangrene, and pain are associated with all the common IM sites *except* the ventrogluteal site (Hopkins and Arias, 2013).

One way to locate the ventrogluteal muscle is to use the "V" method (Kara et al., 2015). You position a patient in a supine or lateral position with the knee and hip flexed to relax the muscle. Use your right hand for the left hip and your left hand for the right hip. For example, if you are administering the injection into the patient's left hip, place the palm of your right hand over the greater trochanter of the patient's hip with your wrist perpendicular to the femur. Then move your thumb toward the patient's groin and your index finger toward the anterior superior iliac spine. Extend or open your middle finger back along the iliac crest toward the patient's buttock. The index finger, middle finger and the

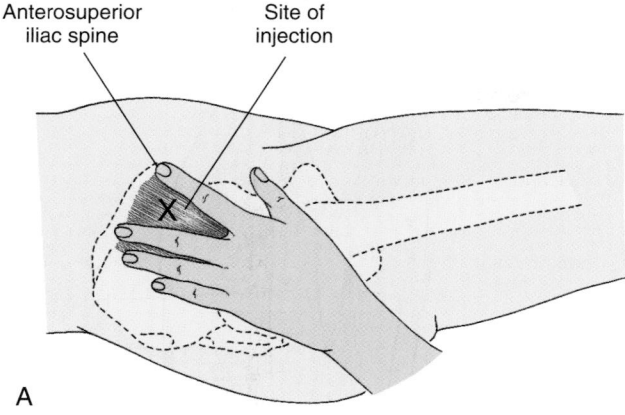

Anterosuperior
iliac spine

Site of
injection

A

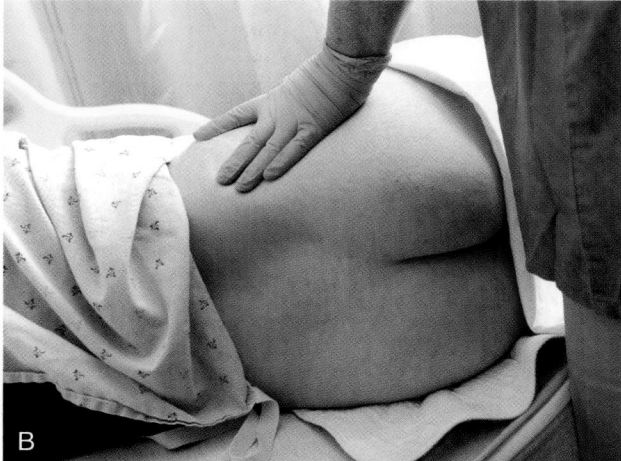

B

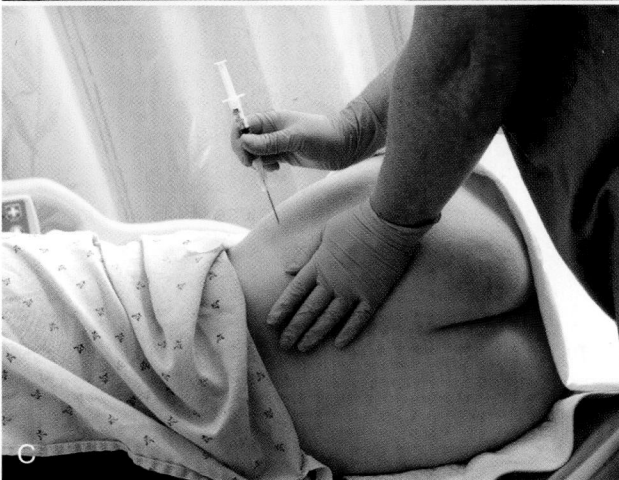

C

FIG 17.22 **A,** Landmarks for "V" ventrogluteal injection site. **B,** Locating ventrogluteal site in patient. **C,** Giving intramuscular injection in ventrogluteal muscle using Z-track method.

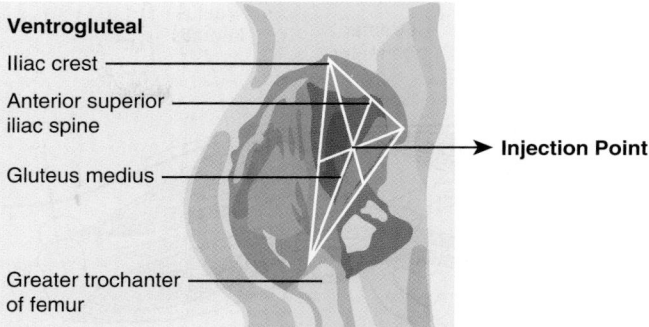

Ventrogluteal

Iliac crest

Anterior superior
iliac spine

Gluteus medius

Greater trochanter
of femur

Injection Point

FIG 17.23 Determination of intramuscular injection site according to the G method. (From Kaya N, et al: The reliability of site determination methods in ventrogluteal area injection: a cross-sectional study, *Int J Nurs Stud* 52:355, 2015.)

iliac crest form a V-shaped triangle with the injection site in the center of the triangle (Fig. 17.22) (Kilic et al., 2014; Kara et al., 2015).

There has been some evidence to suggest that the "V" technique is not always reliable because of differences in hand structure of nurses and body structure of patients, especially when a patient is obese (Kara et al., 2015). Thus the "G"

method or geometric method is another option for selecting the correct ventrogluteal site. With a patient in the side-lying position you reference three bone prominences and draw imaginary lines between the ends of the bones (Kara et al., 2015). You imagine lines drawn from the patient's greater trochanter to the iliac crest and then to the anterior superior iliac spine and from the greater trochanter to the anterior superior iliac spine. Thus a triangle is created by the imaginary lines. After that, draw median lines from every corner of the triangle to the opposite side. As shown in Fig. 17.23, the convergence point of the three median lines is the center for the triangle, the needle entry point for IM injections (deMeneses and Marques, 2007; Kaya et al., 2015). In a study by deMeneses and Marques (2007), the G method was found to be 100% reliable in determining the ventrogluteal site in IM injections.

Vastus Lateralis Muscle. The vastus lateralis muscle is another injection site for adults and children. The muscle is thick and well developed, is located on the anterior lateral aspect of the thigh, and extends in an adult from a hand breadth above the knee to a hand breadth below the greater trochanter of the femur (Fig. 17.24A–B). Use the middle third of the muscle for injection. The width of the muscle usually extends from the midline of the thigh to the midline of the outer side of the thigh. With young children or cachectic patients, grasping the body of the muscle during injection helps to ensure that the medication is deposited in muscle tissue. To help relax the muscle, ask the patient to lie flat with the knee slightly flexed or in a sitting position. The vastus lateralis site is often used for infants, toddlers, and children receiving biologicals (such as immunoglobulins, vaccines, or toxoids) (Nicoll and Hesby, 2002).

Deltoid Muscle. Although the deltoid site is easily accessible, this muscle is not well developed in many adults. This site has a potential for injury because the axillary, radial, brachial, and ulnar nerves and the brachial artery lie within the upper arm under the triceps and along the humerus (Barnes et al., 2012; Imran and Hayley, 2013). Use this site for small

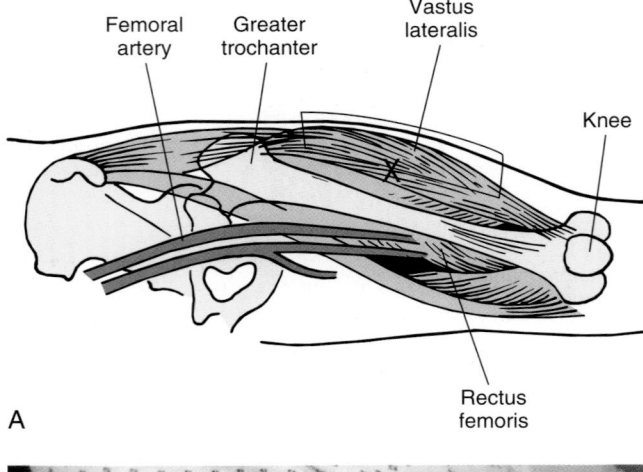

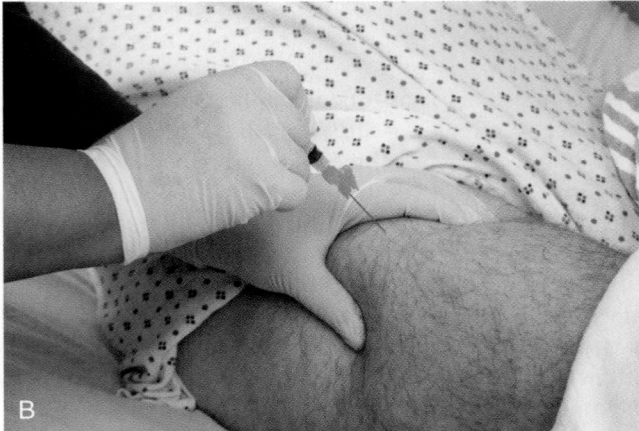

FIG 17.24 **A,** Landmarks for vastus lateralis site. **B,** Giving intramuscular injection in vastus lateralis muscle.

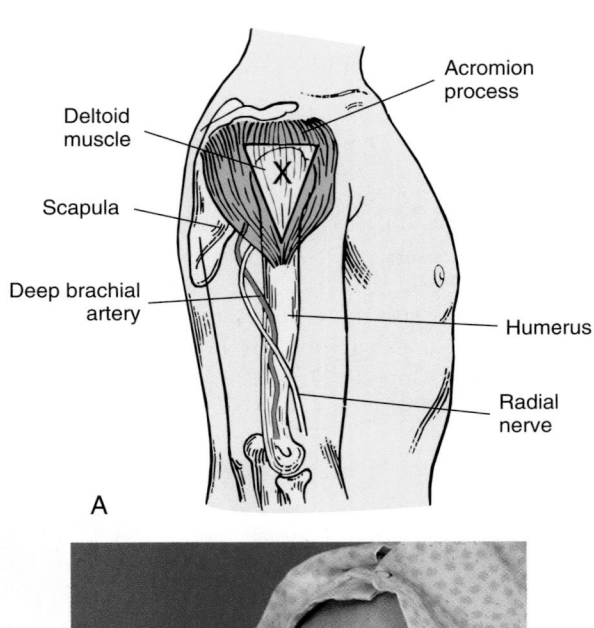

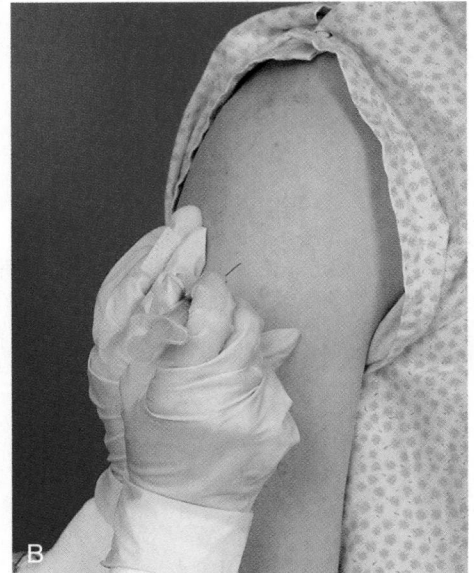

FIG 17.25 **A,** Landmarks for deltoid site. **B,** Giving intramuscular injection in deltoid muscle.

medication volumes (2 mL or less), as in the case of immunizations (e.g., hepatitis B, flu shot) or when other sites are inaccessible because of dressings or casts (Nicoll and Hesby, 2002; Davidson and Rourke, 2013; Hopkins and Arias, 2013).

Carefully assess the condition of the deltoid muscle, consult medication references for suitability of the medication, and carefully locate the injection site using anatomical landmarks (Fig. 17.25A). To locate the muscle, fully expose the patient's upper arm and shoulder. Do not roll up a tight-fitting sleeve. Have the patient relax the arm at the side and flex the elbow. The patient may sit, stand, or lie down (Fig. 17.25B). Palpate the lower edge of the acromion process, which forms the base of a triangle in line with the midpoint of the lateral aspect of the upper arm. The injection site is in the center of the triangle, about 3 to 5 cm (1 to 2 inches) below the acromion process. You also can locate the site by placing four fingers across the deltoid muscle, with the top finger along the acromion process. The injection site is then three finger widths below the acromion process.

Intradermal Injections. ID injections are used for skin testing (e.g., tuberculosis screening and allergy tests). Because

such medications are potent, you inject them into the dermis, where blood supply is reduced and drug absorption occurs slowly. A patient may have an anaphylactic reaction if the medication enters the circulation too rapidly. For patients with a history of multiple allergies, a health care provider will perform skin testing using ID injections. Skin testing often requires you to visually inspect the test site. Therefore make sure that the ID site is free of lesions and injuries and is relatively hairless. The inner forearm and upper back are ideal locations.

To administer an ID injection, use a TB or small syringe with a short ($\frac{3}{8}$ - to $\frac{5}{8}$ -inch) (3 to 16 mm), fine-gauge (25 to 27) needle. The angle of insertion for an ID injection is 5 to 15 degrees (see Fig. 17.17). Inject only small amounts of medication (0.01 to 0.1 mL) intradermally. Administer amounts only up to 0.1 mL to children (Hockenberry and Wilson, 2015). If a bleb does not appear or if the site bleeds after needle withdrawal, the medication may have entered subcutaneous tissues. In this situation, skin test results will not be valid.

Safety in Administering Medications by Injection

Needleless Devices. Approximately 5.6 million health care workers in the United States are at risk of occupational exposure to bloodborne pathogens such as HIV and hepatitis B virus (Occupational Safety and Health Administration [OSHA], n.d.). In the case of parenteral injections, an exposure is defined as a percutaneous injury (e.g., needlestick or cut with a sharp object) (CDC, 2013). Needlestick injuries often occur when health care workers do the following:

- Recap needles
- Mishandle IV lines and needles
- Leave needles at a patient's bedside

Exposure to bloodborne pathogens is one of the deadliest daily hazards to which nurses are exposed. Most needlestick injuries can be prevented with the use of safe engineering controls such as sharps disposal containers, rubber dams, self-sheathing needles, and needleless devices (CDC, 2013).

Safety syringes have a sheath or guard that covers a needle immediately after it is withdrawn from the skin (Fig. 17.26). This feature eliminates the chance for a needlestick injury. The syringe and sheath are discarded together in a sharps container. Needleless devices used for injections include a blunt cannula attached to a syringe. Use needleless devices for injections when available. Always dispose of needles and other instruments considered sharps into clearly marked appropriate containers (Fig. 17.27). Containers must be clearly visible to health care workers in the area where sharps are used. Additionally, they need to be puncture-proof, leak-proof, durable during installation and transport, and an appropriate size and shape. The closure should be secure and minimize exposure during use (CDC, 2010). Never force a needle into a full needle disposal receptacle. Receptacles should be emptied when they are two-thirds full. Never place used needles and syringes in a wastebasket, in your pocket, on a patient's meal tray, or at the patient's bedside. Box 17.21 summarizes the recommendations for the prevention of needlestick injuries.

Intravenous Administration. Nurses administer medications intravenously by:

1. Infusion of large volume IV fluid containers that contain medications mixed by the pharmacy.
2. Injection of a bolus or small volume of medication through an existing IV infusion line or intermittent venous access (heparin or saline lock).
3. "Piggyback" infusion of a solution containing the prescribed medication and a small volume of IV fluid through an existing IV line.

In all three methods, the patient has either an existing IV infusion running continuously or an IV access site for intermittent infusions. Most policies and procedures list the people who may give IV medications, the types of medications, and the patient care units in which they can be given. These policies are based on the medication, capability, and availability of staff and the type of monitoring equipment available. Chapter 18 describes the technique for performing venipuncture and establishing continuous IV fluid infusions.

When you administer IV medications, observe patients closely for symptoms of adverse reactions. After a medication enters the bloodstream, it begins to act immediately, and

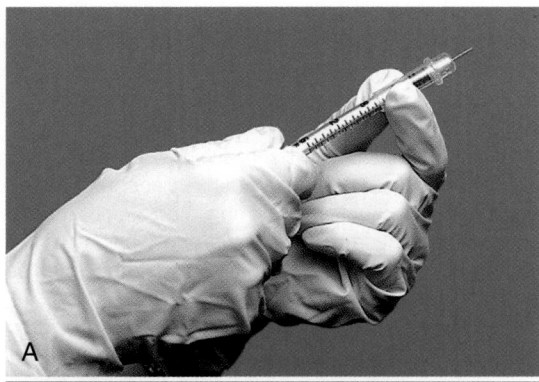

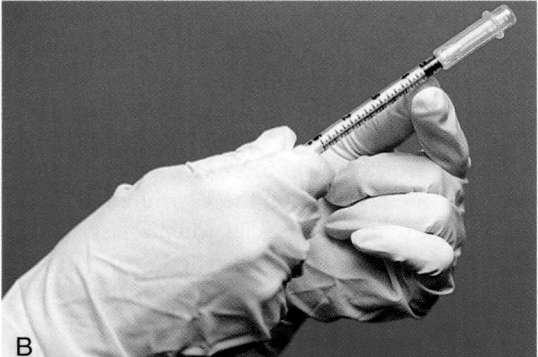

FIG 17.26 Needle with plastic guard to prevent needlesticks. **A,** Position of guard before injection. **B,** After injection a nurse locks guard in place, covering needle.

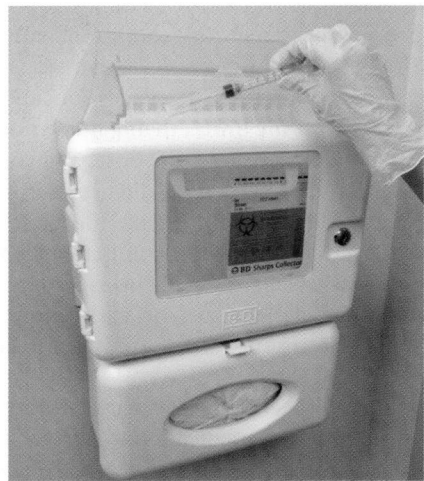

FIG 17.27 Sharps disposal using only one hand.

BOX 17.21   RECOMMENDATIONS FOR PREVENTION OF NEEDLESTICK INJURIES

- Avoid using needles when effective needleless systems or sharps with engineered sharps injury protection (SESIP) safety devices are available.
- Do not recap any needle after medication administration.
- Plan safe handling and disposal of needles before beginning a procedure.
- Immediately dispose of needles, needleless systems, and SESIP devices into puncture-proof, leak-proof sharps disposal containers.
- Maintain a sharps injury log that includes the following: type and brand of device involved in incident, location of incident (e.g., department or work area), description of incident, and a way to protect privacy of the employees who have had sharps injuries.
- Attend educational programs on bloodborne pathogens and follow recommendations for infection prevention, including receiving the hepatitis B vaccine.
- Participate in the selection and evaluation of SESIP devices with safety features within your institution whenever possible.

Data from Occupational Safety and Health Administration (OSHA): Bloodborne pathogens and needlestick injuries, *Fed Reg* 77(64):19934, 2012, https://www.osha.gov/FedReg_osha_pdf/FED20120403.pdf.

there is no way to stop its action. Thus take special care to avoid errors in dose calculation and preparation. Carefully follow the six rights of safe medication administration and know the desired action and side effects of every medication you give. If the medication has an antidote, make sure that it is available during administration. There are situations where it is recommended to do an independent double check of a medication dosage, especially high-risk medications given intravenously. The ISMP (2013c) describes how to do an independent double check:

- A double check must be conducted independently by a second person.
- Two people must *separately* check each component of the work process. For example, a pharmacist calculates a dose, prepares a syringe of medication, and compares the product with the order; then a nurse *independently* checks the order, calculates the dose, and compares the results with the dispensed product for verification.
- Two people are unlikely to make the same mistake if they work independently. It is not effective to hold up a syringe and a vial and say, "This is 5 units of insulin, can you check it?" The person asking for the double check must not influence the individual checking the product in any way.
- Use a double check only for very selective high-risk tasks or high-alert medications *(not all)* that most warrant their use (see agency policy) (Box 17.22). High-alert medications are defined as medications that

BOX 17.22   EVIDENCE-BASED PRACTICE

PICO Question: What guidelines should RNs follow in the safe administration of high-alert medications?

SUMMARY OF EVIDENCE

High-alert medications (e.g., insulin, anticoagulants, opioids) are medications that are the most likely to cause significant patient harm, even when used correctly (Pfoh et al., 2013). These medications are more likely to be associated with harm because of narrow therapeutic ranges (increasing the potential for a prescribing error). Drugs with a narrow therapeutic range are dangerous because small changes in dosage or blood drug levels can lead to dose-dependent or blood concentration–dependent critical therapeutic failures or adverse drug events (Anderson and Townsend, 2015). High-alert medications also cause more significant harm when an error does occur because of the significant nature of the potential adverse effects such as bleeding or hypoglycemia (Pfoh et al., 2013). The Joint Commission (2014a) requires hospitals to develop an up-to-date list of high-alert medications, to have a process for managing high-alert medications, and to implement that process. The Institute for Safe Medication Practices (2014) routinely updates a list of high-alert medications (https://www.ismp.org/tools/institutionalhighAlert.asp).

APPLICATION TO NURSING PRACTICE

- Hospitals should form multidisciplinary pharmacy and therapeutics committee teams with nurses and pharmacists working together to identify issues contributing to high-alert medication errors.
- Nurses should perform independent double checks for high-alert medications (ISMP, 2014).
- Other strategies include improving access to information about high-alert drugs; limiting physical access to high-alert medications; using auxiliary labels and automated alerts; and standardizing ordering, storage, preparation, and administration of these drugs (ISMP, 2014).
- Errors may be avoided by reducing interruptions from patients' families, transporters, physicians, and telephone calls. Limit communication during medication administration by screening telephone calls and placing removable warning signs on medication carts during medication administration (Pfoh et al., 2013).

are the most likely to cause significant patient harm, even when used correctly.

- Fewer double checks performed strategically at the most vulnerable points of the medication use process are more effective than too many.

Administering medications by the IV route has advantages. It is the best route in emergencies when a fast-acting medication must be delivered quickly. The IV route is also best when the patient needs medications at constant therapeutic blood levels.

Some medications are highly alkaline and irritating to muscle and subcutaneous tissue. These medications cause less discomfort when given intravenously. Because IV medications are immediately available to the bloodstream after they are

BOX 17.23 BEST PRACTICES FOR ADMINISTRATION OF INTRAVENOUS SOLUTIONS AND MEDICATIONS

- Use standardized concentrations and dosages of medication.
- Use standardized procedures for ordering, preparing, and administering IV medications.
- Use technology (e.g., bar code, smart pump with dose-error reduction software), when available, to verify medications before administration.
- Administer solutions and medications prepared and dispensed from the pharmacy or as commercially prepared solutions and medications in accordance with the United States Pharmacopeia (USP).
- Never prepare high-alert medications (e.g., heparin, dopamine, dobutamine, nitroglycerin, potassium, antibiotics, or magnesium) on a patient care unit.
- Use standardized infusion concentrations of high-alert medications.
- Standardize storage of IV medications.
- Use the mnemonic CATS PRRR to help remember safety checks for administering IV medications: *C*, compatibilities; *A*, allergies; *T*, tubing correct; *S*, site checked; *P*, pump safety checked; *R*, right rate; *R*, release clamps; *R*, return and reassess the patient.
- Use standardized label practices: Patient name in bold, generic drug name, and patient-specific dose.

Adapted from Infusion Nurses Society: Infusion nursing standards of practice, *J Intraven Nurs* 39(1S), 2016; Institute for Safe Medication Practices (ISMP): *Guidelines for standard order sets*, 2010, available at http://www.ismp.org/tools/guidelines/StandardOrderSets.pdf; Institute for Safe Medication Practices (ISMP): *Principles of designing a medication label for intravenous piggyback medication for patient specific, inpatient use*, 2015, http://www.ismp.org/Tools/guidelines/labelFormats/Piggyback.asp; and The Joint Commission: *2017 National Patient Safety Goals hospital program*, 2017, http://www.jointcommission.org/standards_information/npsgs.aspx.

administered, you must verify the rate of administration with a medication reference or a pharmacist before giving these medications to ensure that you give them safely over the appropriate amount of time. Patients experience severe adverse reactions if IV medications are administered too quickly.

Large-Volume Infusions. In the past nurses often mixed medications into large volumes of IV fluids (500 to 1000 mL). However, safety standards and scientific evidence no longer support this practice (INS, 2016). Many patient safety risks such as incorrect calculation, poor aseptic technique, incorrect labeling, pump programming errors, lack of medication knowledge, and mix-up with another medication occur when nurses have to prepare medications in IV containers on patient care units. Box 17.23 summarizes current best practices for preparation and administration of IV medications.

Pharmacies prepare medications in large volumes (500 or 1000 mL) of compatible IV fluids such as normal saline or lactated Ringer solution. Vitamins and potassium chloride are two types of medications often added to IV fluids. Continuous infusion carries a risk: If the IV fluid is infused too rapidly, the patient is at risk for medication overdose and circulatory fluid overload.

Nurses mix medications into IV fluids *only* in emergencies. A nurse *never* prepares high-alert medications (such as heparin, dopamine, dobutamine, nitroglycerin, potassium, antibiotics, or magnesium) on a patient care unit. Check with a pharmacist to confirm medication and dose before mixing a medication in an IV container. If a pharmacist confirms that you need to prepare the medication, ask another nurse to verify your medication calculations and add medications *only* to new IV bags. *Do not* add medications to IV bags that are already hanging because you have no way to know the exact concentration of the medication. Always have an experienced nurse watch you during the entire procedure to ensure that you prepare the medication safely.

Administer the medication to the patient at the prescribed rate (see Chapter 18). When you administer medications in large IV infusions, regulate the IV rate according to the health care provider's order. Monitor patients closely for adverse reactions to the medication and fluid volume overload. Also check the site often for infiltration and phlebitis.

Intravenous Bolus. An IV bolus introduces a concentrated dose of a medication directly into the systemic circulation (see Skill 17.6). Because a bolus requires only a small amount of fluid to deliver a medication, it is especially useful in patients who have fluid restrictions. The IV bolus, or "push," is the most dangerous method for administering medications because there is no time to correct errors. A bolus may cause irritation to the lining of blood vessels.

Before you administer a bolus, confirm placement of the IV line. Never give a medication intravenously if the insertion site appears swollen or edematous or the IV fluid cannot flow at the proper rate. Accidental injection of a medication into the tissues around a vein causes pain, sloughing of tissues, and abscesses, depending on the composition of the medication. Medications that carry a risk of adverse effects if administered too quickly into a vein should be diluted and administered as a piggyback or via an infusion pump.

Determine the rate of administration of an IV bolus medication by the amount of medication that can be given each minute. For example, if a patient is to receive 4 mL of a medication over 2 minutes, give 2 mL of the IV bolus medication every minute. Refer to a pharmacy reference to look up each medication to determine its recommended concentration and rate of administration. The ISMP (2015e) recommends avoiding terms such as "IV push," "IVP," or "bolus" in orders with drugs that require administration over 1 minute or longer. Use more descriptive terms such as "IV over 5 minutes." Consider the purpose for which a medication is prescribed and any potential adverse effects related to the rate or route of administration.

Volume-Controlled Infusions. Another method of administering IV medications is through small amounts (50 to

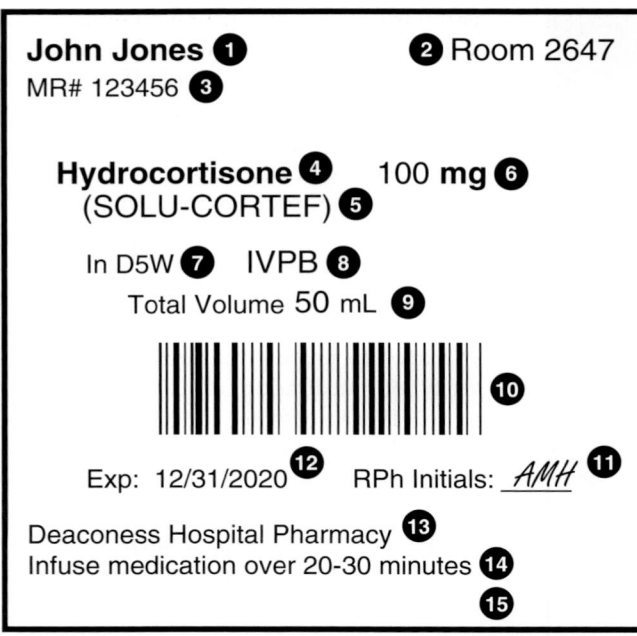

John Jones ❶   ❷ Room 2647
MR# 123456 ❸

Hydrocortisone ❹   100 mg ❻
(SOLU-CORTEF) ❺

In D5W ❼   IVPB ❽
Total Volume 50 mL ❾

‖‖‖‖‖‖‖‖‖‖ ❿

Exp: 12/31/2020 ⓬   RPh Initials: _AMH_ ⓫

Deaconess Hospital Pharmacy ⓭
Infuse medication over 20-30 minutes ⓮
                    ⓯

1. **Patient name**
2. Location
3. Second identifier
   (Date of birth, financial #,
   Encounter #, Medical Record #)
4. **Generic name**
5. BRAND name
6. **Patient dose**
7. Diluent
8. Route
9. Total volume
10. Bar code
11. Initials as needed
12. Expiration Date as needed in a
    MM/DD/YYYY format
13. Pharmacy information if required
14. Comments
15. Other information as required
    by state or federal law

FIG 17.28 IV piggyback medication label following Institute for Safe Medication Practices safe labeling guidelines.

100 mL) of compatible IV fluids. The fluid is within a secondary fluid container separate from the primary fluid bag. The container connects directly to the primary IV line or to separate tubing that inserts into the primary line (see Skill 17.7). There are three types of containers: piggyback sets, volume-control administration sets (such as Volutrol or Pediatrol), and syringe pumps. Volume-controlled infusion has several advantages:

- It reduces the risk of rapid-dose infusion by IV push. Medications are diluted and infused over longer time intervals (e.g., 30 to 60 minutes).
- It allows for administration of medications (such as antibiotics) that are stable for a limited time in solution.
- It allows for control of IV fluid intake.

A piggyback is a small (25- to 250-mL) IV bag or bottle connected to a short tubing line that connects to the *upper* Y-port of a primary infusion line or to an intermittent venous access device such as a saline lock. The label on the medication follows the ISMP IV piggyback medication label format (Fig. 17.28) (ISMP, 2016c).

The piggyback tubing is a microdrip or macrodrip system (see Chapter 18). The set is called a *piggyback* because the small bag or bottle is set *higher* than the primary infusion bag or bottle. In the piggyback setup the main line does not infuse when a compatible piggybacked medication is infusing. The port of the primary IV line contains a back-check valve that automatically stops the flow of the primary infusion once the piggyback infusion flows. After the piggyback solution infuses and the solution within the tubing falls below the level of the primary infusion drip chamber, the back-check valve opens, and the primary infusion starts to flow again.

Volume-control administration (such as with Buretrol) sets are small (150-mL) containers that attach just below the primary infusion bag or bottle. The set is attached and filled in a manner similar to that used with a regular IV infusion. Follow package directions for priming sets.

A syringe pump is battery operated and allows medications to be given in very small amounts of fluid (5 to 60 mL) within controlled infusion times using standard syringes.

Intermittent Venous Access. An intermittent venous access (commonly called a *saline lock*) is an IV catheter capped off on the end with a small chamber covered by a rubber diaphragm or a specially designed cap. Special rubber-seal injection caps usually accept needleless safety devices (see Chapter 18). The advantages of intermittent venous access include cost savings resulting from the omission of continuous IV therapy and saving a nurse's time by eliminating constant monitoring of flow rates. Intermittent venous access allows increased patient mobility, safety, and comfort.

Before you administer an IV bolus or volume-controlled medications, assess the patency of the line and placement of the IV catheter. After the medication has been administered through an intermittent venous access, the access must be flushed with a solution to keep it patent. Normal saline generally is an effective flush solution for peripheral catheters. Some agencies require the use of heparin. Follow agency policies for the care and maintenance of the IV site.

Administration of Intravenous Therapy in the Home. Patients sometimes need IV medication therapy at home. Common infusions that patients receive include antibiotics, chemotherapy, total parenteral nutrition, and analgesics. Most patients receive home IV therapy through a long-term central venous catheter (CVC) (see Chapter 18). Home health nurses assess patients' responses to the medication, monitor the CVC site, and teach patients and family caregivers how to administer infusions and medications and maintain the CVC.

Carefully assess patients and family caregivers to determine their ability to manage IV therapy at home. Begin instruction on IV care as soon as you know that a patient will have IV therapy at home. Patients and families must learn to recognize problems such as signs of infections related to IV therapy, symptoms of ADEs and steps to take when these problems occur. Patients also need to know when to notify the home care nurse or health care provider. Plan to teach patients and family caregivers how to maintain IV administration equipment including the infusion pump.

SAFETY GUIDELINES FOR NURSING SKILLS

Ensuring patient safety is an essential role of the professional nurse. To ensure patient safety, communicate clearly with members of the health care team, assess and incorporate the patient's priorities of care and preferences, and use the best evidence when making decisions about your patient's care. When you perform the skills covered in this chapter, remember the following points to ensure safe, individualized patient care:

- Be vigilant during the entire process of medication preparation and administration, and make sure that your patients receive the appropriate medications. Know why your patient is receiving each medication; know what you need to do before, during, and after medication administration; and evaluate the effectiveness of the medication and assess for adverse effects.
- Use strict aseptic technique during medication preparation and administration.
- Take care of yourself. Ensure that you are as healthy as possible to enable yourself to think as clearly and critically as possible. Healthy behaviors help you better process information and make safe decisions during medication administration.
- Prepare medications in areas that are free from distractions. No-interruption zones (NIZs) are recommended (Yoder et al., 2015). NIZs are created by placing red tape or tile borders on the floor around medication carts. Nurses standing in these zones are not to be interrupted.

- Always verify that medications have not expired.
- Use at least two patient identifiers before administering medications to your patients.
- Clarify unclear orders and ask for help whenever you are uncertain about a medication order or calculation. Consult with your peers, pharmacists, and other health care providers.
- Use technology (e.g., bar scanning, electronic MARs) that your institution uses when preparing and giving medications. Follow all policies related to use of the technology and do not use work-arounds. Nurses who use work-arounds fail to follow institution protocols, policies, or procedures during medication administration in an attempt to administer medications to patients more quickly.
- Follow standards set by your state's Nurse Practice Act and guidelines established by your health care agency before delegating medication administration. Licensed practical nurses (LPNs) or licensed vocational nurses (LVNs) usually can administer medications via the oral (PO), subcutaneous, IM, and ID routes. Some states also allow certified medical assistants (CMAs) to administer some types of medications (e.g., oral medications) in some health care settings (e.g., long-term care facilities).
- Follow safety guidelines to prevent needlestick injuries. Use engineering devices, and dispose of all sharps in safety containers.

SKILL 17.1 ADMINISTERING ORAL MEDICATIONS

View Video!

DELEGATION CONSIDERATIONS
The skill of administering oral medications cannot be delegated to nursing assistive personnel (NAP). The nurse instructs the NAP about:

- Potential side effects of medications and to report their occurrence.
- Informing the nurse if the patient's condition changes or worsens (e.g., pain, itching, or rash) after medication administration.

EQUIPMENT
- Automated, computer-controlled drug dispensing system or medication cart

- Oral syringe dispensed by pharmacy (liquid medications only)
- Disposable medication cups (for holding tablets and/or capsules)
- Glass of water, juice, or preferred liquid and drinking straw
- Device for crushing or splitting tablets (optional)
- Paper towels
- Medication administration record (MAR) (electronic or printed)
- Clean gloves (if handling an oral medication)

SKILL 17.1 ADMINISTERING ORAL MEDICATIONS—cont'd

View Video!

STEP	RATIONALE

ASSESSMENT

1. Check accuracy and completeness of each MAR with health care provider's medication order. Check patient's name and drug name, dosage, and route and time of administration Clarify incomplete or unclear orders with health care provider before administration.

The order sheet is the most reliable source and only legal record of medications that patient is to receive. Ensures that patient receives correct medications (Mandrack et al., 2012). Illegible MARs are a source of medication errors (Alassaad et al., 2013).

2. Review pertinent information related to medication including action, purpose, normal dose and route, side effects, time of onset and peak action, and nursing implications.

Allows you to anticipate effects of drug while observing patient's response.

3. Assess for any contraindications to patient receiving oral medication including being on NPO status, inability to swallow, nausea/vomiting, bowel inflammation, reduced peristalsis, recent gastrointestinal (GI) surgery, gastric suction, and decreased level of consciousness (LOC). Notify health care provider if any contraindications are present.

Alterations in GI function can interfere with drug absorption, distribution, and excretion. Giving oral medications to patients with impaired swallowing or decreased LOC increases their risk for aspiration (Park et al., 2013). Patients with GI suction do not experience actions of oral medications because the medications are suctioned from the GI tract before they are absorbed.

4. Assess patient's medical, medication, and diet history and history of allergies. List any drug allergies on each page of the MAR and prominently display on patient's medical record. When allergies are present, patient should wear an allergy bracelet.

These factors influence how certain drugs act. Information reveals previous problems with medication administration. Allergy alert helps prevent adverse events.

5. Perform hand hygiene. Gather and review physical assessment findings including patient's weight (in metric units), vital signs, and laboratory data that influence drug administration such as results of renal and liver function studies.

Many medication doses are based on a patient's weight (ISMP, 2016b). Physical examination findings or laboratory data may contraindicate drug administration. Renal and liver function status affects metabolism and excretion (Burchum and Rosenthal, 2016).

6. Assess risk for aspiration using a dysphagia screening tool if available (see Chapter 35). Protect patient from aspiration by assessing swallowing ability.

Aspiration occurs when food, fluid, or medication intended for GI administration is inadvertently administered into the respiratory tract. Patients with altered ability to swallow are at higher risk for aspiration (Park et al., 2013).

7. Assess patient's symptoms before initiating medication therapy.

Provides information to evaluate desired effect of medication.

8. Assess patient's and family caregiver's knowledge regarding health and medication use, medication schedule, and ability to prepare medications.

Determines patient's and caregiver's need for medication education and guidance to achieve drug adherence.

9. Assess patient's preference for fluids and determine if medications can be given with these fluids. Maintain fluid restrictions as prescribed.

Some fluids interfere with medication absorption (e.g., dairy products affect tetracycline). Offering fluids during drug administration is an excellent way to increase patient's fluid intake. Fluids ease swallowing and facilitate absorption from the GI tract. However, if fluid restrictions exist, skillful planning of fluid intake must coordinate with medication times and type of medications.

PLANNING

1. Perform hand hygiene. Collect appropriate equipment and MAR.

Promotes time management and efficiency when preparing medications for all patients.

2. Plan preparation to avoid interruptions. Create a quiet environment. Do not take phone calls or talk with others. Follow agency no-interruption zone policy.

Interruptions contribute to medication errors (see Box 17.4) (Beyea, 2014; Yoder et al., 2015).

IMPLEMENTATION

1. Prepare medications.

   a. Perform hand hygiene.

   Reduces transfer of microorganisms.

   b. Arrange medication tray and cups in medication preparation area or move medication cart to position outside patient's room.

   Organization of equipment saves time and reduces error.

STEP	RATIONALE
c. Log on to automated dispensing system (ADS) or unlock medicine drawer or cart.	Medications are safeguarded when locked in cabinet, cart, or ADS.
d. Prepare medications for *one patient at a time*. Follow the six rights of medication administration. Keep all pages of MARs or computer printouts for one patient together or look at only one patient's medication administration computer screen.	Prevents preparation errors.
e. Select correct medication from ADS, unit-dose drawer, or stock supply. Compare name of medication on label with MAR or computer printout (see illustration). Exit ADS after removing drug.	Reading label and comparing it against transcribed order reduces errors. Exiting ADS ensures that no one else can remove medications using your identity. *This is the first check for accuracy.*
f. Check or calculate drug dose as necessary. Double-check any calculation. Check expiration date on all medications and return outdated medication to pharmacy.	Double-checking pharmacy calculations reduces risk for error. Agency policy may require you to check calculations of certain medications such as insulin with another nurse (Kim and Bates, 2013). Expired medications may be inactive or harmful to patient.
g. If preparing a controlled substance, check record for previous medication count and compare current count with supply available. Controlled drugs may be stored in computerized locked cart.	Controlled substance laws require nurses to carefully monitor and count dispensed controlled drugs (e.g., opioids).
h. Prepare solid forms of oral medications.	
(1) To prepare unit-dose tablets or capsules, place packaged tablet or capsule directly into medication cup without removing wrapper. Administer medications only from containers with labels that are clearly marked.	Wrappers maintain cleanliness and identify drug name and dose, which can facilitate teaching.
(2) When using a blister pack, "pop" medications through foil or paper backing into a medication cup (see illustration).	Packs provide a 1-month supply, with each "blister" usually containing a single dose.
(3) If it is necessary to give half the dose of medication, pharmacy should split, label, package, and send medication to unit. If you must split medication, use clean, gloved hand to cut with clean pill-cutting device. Only cut tablets that are prescored by the manufacturer (line traverses the center of the tablet).	Reduces contamination of tablet. In health care agencies, only pharmacy should split tablets to ensure patient safety (FDA, 2013). If a tablet is FDA-approved to be split, this information will be printed in the "HOW SUPPLIED" section of the professional label insert.
(4) Place all tablets or capsules that patient will receive in one medicine cup except for those requiring preadministration assessments (e.g., pulse rate or blood pressure). Place these in separate additional cup with wrapper intact.	Keeping medications that require preadministration assessments separate from others serves as a reminder and makes it easier to withhold drugs as necessary.

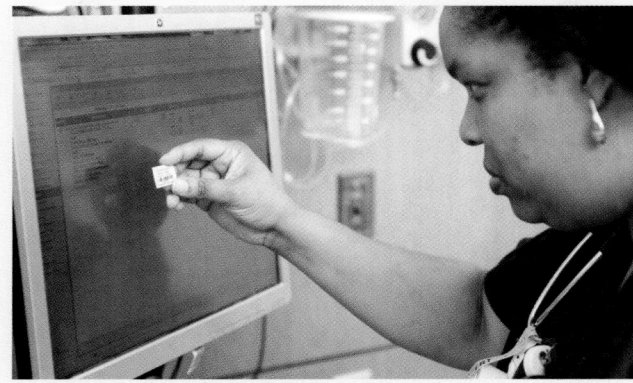

STEP 1e Check label of medication with patient's MAR.

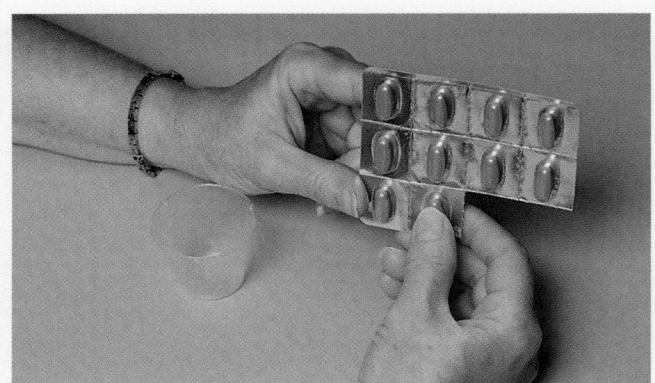

STEP 1h(2) Place tablet from blister pack into medicine cup without removing wrapper.

SKILL 17.1   ADMINISTERING ORAL MEDICATIONS—cont'd

View Video!

STEP	RATIONALE
(5) If patient has difficulty swallowing and liquid medications are not an option, use a pill-crushing device (see illustration). Clean device before using. If a device is not available, place medicine in between two cups, and grind and crush. Mix ground tablet in small amount (teaspoon) of soft food (custard or applesauce).	Large tablets are often difficult to swallow. Ground tablet mixed with palatable soft food is usually easier to swallow.

Clinical Decision Point. Not all medications can be safely crushed. Consult with a pharmacist or the ISMP Do Not Crush List (ISMP, 2015c).

STEP	RATIONALE
i. Prepare liquids.	
(1) Unit-dose container with correct amount of medication: Gently shake the container. Administer medication packaged in a single-dose cup directly from the single-dose cup. Do not pour medicine into another cup.	Using unit-dose container with correct dosage of medication provides most accurate dose of medication (ISMP, 2016b). Shaking container ensures that medication is mixed before administration.
(2) Unit-dose oral syringe (see illustration): Be sure to use only oral syringes marked "Oral Use Only" dispensed by the pharmacy.	Ensure that all oral liquids that are not commercially available as unit-dose products are dispensed by the pharmacy in an oral syringe (ISMP, 2016b).

Clinical Decision Point. Based on current best practice (Paparella, 2014; ISMP, 2016b), liquid medications that are not available or are not in correct dose in a unit-dose container should be dispensed by the pharmacy in special oral syringes marked "Oral Use Only." These syringes do not connect to any type of parenteral (e.g., IV) tubing. Additionally, current evidence shows that liquid measuring devices on patient care units result in inaccurate dosing. Having oral medications prepared in the pharmacy ensures accurate dosing and prevents parenteral administration of oral medications.

STEP	RATIONALE
j. Return stock containers or unused unit-dose medications to shelf or drawer. Label medication cups and poured medications with patient's name before leaving medication preparation area. Do not leave drugs unattended. Perform hand hygiene.	Ensures that correct medications are prepared for correct patient.
k. Before going to patient's room, compare patient's name and name of medication on label of prepared drugs with MAR.	Reading labels a second time reduces errors. *This is the second check for accuracy.*

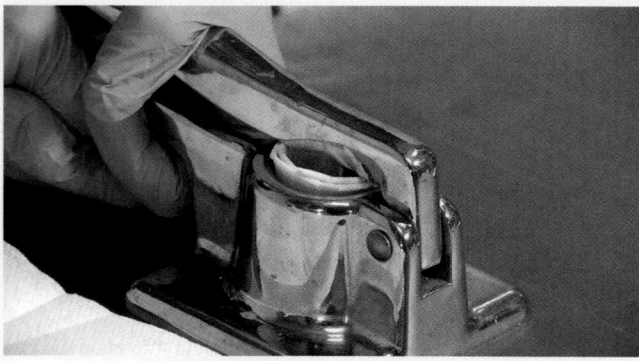

STEP 1h(5) Pill-crushing device.

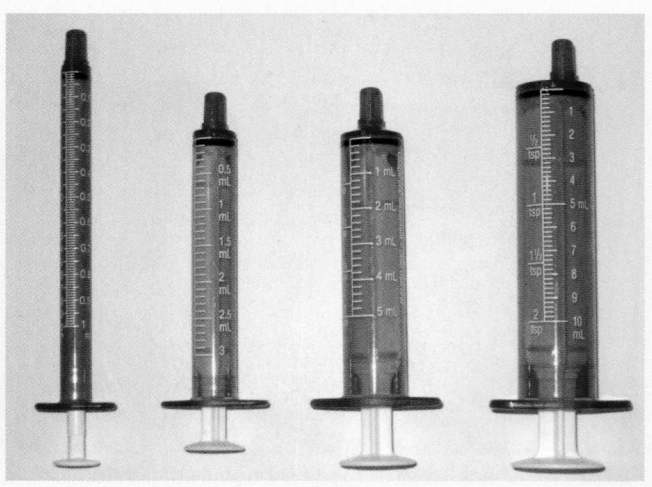

STEP 1i(2) Unit dose oral syringe.

STEP	RATIONALE
2. Administer medications.	
a. Take medication to patient at correct time (see agency policy). Medications that require exact timing include STAT doses, first-time or loading doses, and one-time doses. Give time-critical scheduled medications at exact time ordered (no later than 30 minutes before or after scheduled dose). Given non–time-critical scheduled medications within a range of 1 or 2 hours of scheduled dose (ISMP, 2011a). During administration, apply six rights of medication administration.	Hospitals must adopt medication administration policy and procedure for timing of medication administration that considers the nature of prescribed medication, specific clinical application, and patient needs (CMS, 2011; ISMP, 2011a). Time-critical scheduled medications are those for which early or delayed administration of maintenance doses may cause harm or result in substantial suboptimal therapy or pharmacological effect. Non–time-critical medications are those for which early or delayed administration should not cause harm or result in substantial suboptimal therapy or pharmacological effect (ISMP, 2011a; CMS, 2011).
b. Identify patient using at least two identifiers (e.g., name and birthday or name and medical record number) according to agency policy. Compare identifiers with information on patient's MAR or medical record.	Ensures correct patient. Complies with The Joint Commission Standards and improves patient safety (TJC, 2018).
c. At patient's bedside, again compare MAR or computer printout with name of medication on medication label and patient name. Ask patient if he or she has allergies.	*This is the third check for accuracy* and ensures that patient receives correct medication. Confirms patient's allergy history.
d. Explain the purpose of each medication, action, and most common possible adverse effects. Allow sufficient time for patient to ask questions. Include family caregiver if appropriate.	Patient has the right to be informed, and patient and family caregiver understanding of each medication improves adherence with drug therapy.
e. Perform hand hygiene. Perform necessary preadministration assessment (e.g., blood pressure, pulse) for specific medications. Ask patient again if he or she has allergies.	Reduces transmission of microorganisms. Determines whether specific medications should be withheld at that time. Confirms patient's allergy history.

Clinical Decision Point. If patient expresses concern regarding accuracy of a medication, do not give the medication. Explore patient's concern and verify health care provider's order before administering. Listening to patient's concerns may prevent a medication error.

STEP	RATIONALE
f. Assist patient to sitting or Fowler's position. Use side-lying position if patient is unable to sit. Have patient stay in this position for 30 minutes after administration.	Decreases risk for aspiration during swallowing.
g. For tablets: Patient may wish to hold solid medication in hand or cup before placing in mouth. Offer water or preferred liquid to help patient swallow medication.	Patient can become familiar with medications by seeing each drug. Choice of fluid can improve fluid intake.
h. For orally disintegrating formulations (tablets or strips): Remove medication from packet just before use. Do not push tablet through foil. Place medication on top of patient's tongue. Caution against chewing it.	Orally disintegrating formulations begin to dissolve when placed on tongue. Water is not needed. Careful removal from packaging is necessary because tablets and strips are thin and fragile.
i. For sublingually administered medications: Have patient place medication under tongue and allow it to dissolve completely. Caution patient against swallowing tablet or saliva.	Drug is absorbed through blood vessels of undersurface of tongue. If swallowed, drug is destroyed by gastric juices or rapidly detoxified by liver, preventing therapeutic blood level.
j. For buccal administered medications: Have patient place medication in mouth against mucous membranes of cheek and gums until it dissolves.	Buccal medications act locally or systemically as they are swallowed in saliva.

Clinical Decision Point. Avoid administering anything by mouth until orally disintegrating buccal or sublingual medication is completely dissolved.

STEP	RATIONALE
k. For powdered medications: Mix with liquids at bedside and give to patient to drink.	When prepared in advance, powdered drugs thicken and some even harden, making swallowing difficult.
l. For crushed medications mixed with food: Give each medication separately in teaspoon of food.	Ensures that patient swallows all of medicine. *Never mix medication in a meal serving of food.*

SKILL 17.1   ADMINISTERING ORAL MEDICATIONS—cont'd

View Video!

STEP	RATIONALE
m. For lozenges: Caution patient against chewing or swallowing lozenges.	Lozenges act through slow absorption through oral mucosa, not gastric mucosa.
n. For effervescent medications: Add tablet or powder to a glass of water. Administer immediately after dissolving.	Effervescence improves unpleasant taste and often relieves GI problems.
o. If patient is unable to hold medications, place medication cup or oral syringe to lips and gently introduce each drug into mouth. Give a tablet or capsule one at a time. Inject a liquid slowly. A spoon can also be used to place a pill in patient's mouth. Do not rush or force medications.	Administering a single-dose tablet, capsule, or oral syringe dose eases swallowing and decreases risk for aspiration.

Clinical Decision Point. If tablet or capsule falls to the floor, it becomes contaminated; discard it and repeat preparation.

STEP	RATIONALE
p. Stay until patient swallows each medication completely or takes it by the prescribed route. Ask patient to open mouth if uncertain whether medication has been swallowed.	Ensures that patient receives ordered dose. If left unattended, patient may not take dose or may save drugs, causing health risks.
q. For highly acidic medications (e.g., aspirin), offer patient a nonfat snack (e.g., crackers) if not contraindicated by his or her condition.	Reduces gastric irritation. Fat content of foods may delay drug absorption.
r. Help patient return to position of comfort.	Maintains patient's comfort.
s. Dispose of soiled supplies and perform hand hygiene. Return cart to medication room if used. Clean work area.	Reduces spread of microorganisms.
3. Replenish stock such as cups and straws, and return cart to medication room and clean work area.	Enhances efficiency and reduces transfer of microorganisms.

EVALUATION

1. Return within an appropriate time to evaluate patient's response to medications including therapeutic effects, side effects or allergy, and adverse reactions.	Evaluates therapeutic benefit of drug and helps to detect onset of side effects or allergic reactions. Sublingual medications act in 15 minutes; most oral medications act in 30 to 60 minutes.
2. Ask patient or family caregiver to identify drug name and explain purpose, action, dose schedule, and potential side effects.	Determines level of knowledge gained by patient and family caregiver.
3. **Use Teach-Back:** "I want to be sure I showed you how to use your sublingual nitroglycerin. For this dose, show me where you will place the tablet in your mouth." Revise your instruction now or develop a plan for revised patient/family caregiver teaching if patient/family caregiver is not able to teach back correctly.	Determines patient's/family caregiver's level of understanding of instructional topic.

RECORDING AND REPORTING

- Record drug, dose, route, and time administered on patient's MAR immediately after administration, not before. Include initials or signature.
- Record patient response to medication, instruction (including teach-back), and validation of understanding on flow sheet or nurses' notes in electronic health record (EHR) or chart.
- If you do not give the drug, record reason on flow sheet or nurses' notes in EHR or chart, and follow agency policy for noting withheld doses.
- Report adverse effects and patient response and/or withheld drugs to nurse in charge or health care provider. Depending on medication, immediate notification of health care provider may be required.

UNEXPECTED OUTCOMES AND RELATED INTERVENTIONS

- Patient exhibits adverse effects (e.g., side effect, toxic effect, allergic reaction).
  - Notify health care provider and pharmacy.
  - Withhold further doses.
  - Assess vital signs.
- Symptoms such as urticaria, rash, pruritus, rhinitis, and wheezing may indicate an allergic reaction and need for emergency medications.
  - Add allergy information to patient's medical record.

- Patient refuses medication.
  - Assess reason for patient refusing medication.
  - Provide further instruction.
  - Do not force patient to take medications.
  - Notify health care provider.

- Patient is unable to explain drug information.
  - Further assess patient's or family caregiver's knowledge of medications and guidelines for drug safety.
  - Further instruction or different approach to instruction is necessary.

SKILL 17.2   ADMINISTERING EYE (OPHTHALMIC) MEDICATIONS

DELEGATION AND COLLABORATION

The skill of administering eye medications cannot be delegated to nursing assistive personnel (NAP). The nurse instructs the NAP about:
- Potential side effects of medications and to report their occurrence.
- The potential for temporary burning or blurring of vision after administration of eye medications.

EQUIPMENT
- Appropriate medication (eyedrops with sterile eyedropper, ointment tube)

- Clean gloves
- Medication administration record (MAR) (electronic or printed)

Eyedrops/Ointment Only
- Cotton ball or tissue
- Washbasin filled with warm water and washcloth
- Eye patch and tape *(optional)*

STEP	RATIONALE

ASSESSMENT

1. Check accuracy and completeness of each MAR with health care provider's medication order. Check patient's name, drug name and dosage, route, and time for administration. Clarify incomplete or unclear orders with health care provider before administration.

2. Review pertinent information related to medication including action, purpose, normal dose and route, side effects, time of onset and peak action, and nursing implications.

3. Assess patient's medical and medication history and history of allergies. List any drug allergies on each page of the MAR and prominently display on patient's medical record. When allergies are present, patient should wear an allergy bracelet.

4. Perform hand hygiene. Assess condition of external eye structures (see Chapter 16). This may be done just before drug instillation (if drainage is present, apply clean gloves).

5. Determine whether patient has any symptoms of eye discomfort or visual impairment.

6. Assess patient's level of consciousness (LOC) and ability to follow directions.

7. Assess patient's and family caregiver's knowledge regarding drug therapy and patient's desire to self-administer medication.

8. Assess patient's ability to manipulate and hold dropper or ocular disk.

PLANNING

1. Perform hand hygiene. Collect appropriate equipment and MAR.

2. Plan preparation to avoid interruptions. Create a quiet environment. Do not take phone calls or talk with others. Follow agency no-interruption zone policy.

The order sheet is the most reliable source and only legal record of medications that patient is to receive. Ensures that patient receives correct medications (Mandrack et al., 2012). Illegible MARs are a source of medication errors (Alassaad et al., 2013).

Allows you to anticipate effects of drug while observing patient's response.

Factors influence how certain drugs act. Reveals patient's need for medication. Allergy alert prevents adverse event.

Provides baseline to determine if local response to medications occurs. Also indicates need to clean eye before drug application.

Certain eye medications act to either lessen or increase these symptoms. Provides baseline for evaluation of medication effect.

If patient becomes restless or combative during procedure, greater risk for accidental eye injury exists.

Indicates need for health teaching. Motivation influences teaching approach.

Reflects patient's ability to learn to self-administer drug.

Reduces transmission of microorganisms. Promotes time management and efficiency when preparing medications for all patients.

Distractions and interruptions contribute to medication errors (see Box 17.4) (Beyea, 2014; Yoder et al., 2015).

SKILL 17.2   ADMINISTERING EYE (OPHTHALMIC) MEDICATIONS—cont'd

View Video!

STEP	RATIONALE

IMPLEMENTATION

1. Prepare medications for one patient at a time. Attend to procedure and avoid distraction. Check label of medication against MAR two times, when removing medication from unit dose or AMDS and before leaving medication preparation area (see Skill 17.1). Prepare eyedrops by taking container out of refrigerator and rewarming to room temperature before administering to patient. Check expiration date on container. Perform hand hygiene.

Warming eyedrops reduces eye irritation. *These are the first and second checks for accuracy.* Process ensures that right patient receives right medication.

2. Take medication to patient at correct time (see agency policy). Medications that require exact timing include STAT doses, first-time or loading doses, and one-time doses. Give time-critical scheduled medications at exact time ordered (no later than 30 minutes before or after scheduled dose). Give non–time-critical scheduled medications within a range of 1 or 2 hours of scheduled dose (ISMP, 2011a). During administration, apply six rights of medication administration.

Hospitals must adopt medication administration policy and procedure for timing of medication administration that considers nature of prescribed medication, specific clinical application, and patient needs (CMS, 2011; ISMP, 2011a). Time-critical scheduled medications are those for which early or delayed administration of maintenance doses may cause harm or result in substantial suboptimal therapy or pharmacological effect. Non–time-critical medications are those for which early or delayed administration should not cause harm or result in substantial suboptimal therapy or pharmacological effect (CMS, 2011; ISMP, 2011a).

3. Identify patient using at least two identifiers (e.g., name and birthday or name and medical record number) according to agency policy. Compare identifiers with information on patient's MAR or medical record.

Ensures correct patient. Complies with The Joint Commission Standards and improves patient safety (TJC, 2018).

4. At patient's bedside again compare MAR or computer printout with names of medications on medication labels and patient name. Ask patient if he or she has allergies.

This is the third check for accuracy and ensures that patient receives correct medication. Confirms patient's allergy history.

5. Discuss purpose of each medication, action, and possible adverse effects. Allow patient to ask any questions about the drugs. Patients who self-instill medications may be allowed to give drops under nurse's supervision (check agency policy).

Patient has right to be informed, and patient's understanding of each medication improves adherence to drug therapy.

6. Tell patients receiving eyedrops (e.g., mydriatics) that vision will be blurred temporarily and sensitivity to light may occur.

May relieve anxiety.

Clinical Decision Point. Instruct and reinforce that patient should not drive or operate machinery or perform any activity that requires clear vision until vision and sensitivity to light return to normal.

---

7. Instill eye medications.

   a. Apply clean gloves. Ask patient to lie supine or sit back in chair with head slightly hyperextended, looking up.

   Position provides easy access to eye for medication instillation and minimizes drainage of medication into tear duct.

Clinical Decision Point. Do not hyperextend the neck of a patient with cervical spine injury.

---

   b. If drainage or crusting is present along eyelid margins or inner canthus, gently wash away. Soak any dried crusts with warm, damp washcloth or cotton ball over eye for several minutes. Always wipe clean from inner to outer canthus. Remove gloves and perform hand hygiene.

   Soaking allows easy removal of crusts without applying pressure to eye. Cleaning from inner to outer canthus avoids entrance of microorganisms into lacrimal duct (Burchum and Rosenthal, 2016).

   c. Explain there might be temporary burning sensation from drops.

   Corneas are highly sensitive.

STEP	RATIONALE

d. Instill eyedrops.

    (1) Hold clean cotton ball or tissue in nondominant hand on patient's cheekbone just below lower eyelid.

Cotton or tissue absorbs medication that escapes eye.

    (2) With tissue or cotton ball resting below lower lid, gently press downward with thumb or forefinger against bony orbit, exposing conjunctival sac. Never press directly against patient's eyeball.

Prevents pressure and trauma to eyeball and prevents fingers from touching eye.

    (3) Ask patient to look at ceiling. Rest dominant hand on patient's forehead; hold filled medication eyedropper approximately 1 to 2 cm (0.5 to 1.0 inch) above conjunctival sac (see illustration).

Action moves cornea up and away from conjunctival sac and reduces blink reflex. Prevents accidental contact of eyedropper with eye and reduces risk of injury and transfer of microorganisms to dropper (ophthalmic medications are sterile).

    (4) Drop prescribed number of drops into conjunctival sac.

Conjunctival sac normally holds 1 or 2 drops. Provides even distribution of medication across eye.

    (5) If patient blinks or closes eye, causing drops to land on outer lid margins, repeat procedure.

Drops must enter conjunctival sac to achieve therapeutic effect.

    (6) When administering drops that have systemic effects, apply gentle pressure to patient's nasolacrimal duct with clean tissue for 30 to 60 seconds over each eye, one at a time. Avoid pressure directly against patient's eyeball.

Prevents overflow of medication into nasal and pharyngeal passages. Prevents absorption into systemic circulation (American Society of Health-System Pharmacists [ASHP], 2013a).

    (7) After instilling drops, ask patient to close eyes gently.

Helps distribute medication. Squinting or squeezing eyelids forces medication from conjunctival sac (ASHP, 2013a).

e. Instill ophthalmic ointment.

    (1) Holding applicator above lower lid margin, apply thin ribbon of ointment evenly along inner edge of lower eyelid on conjunctiva (see illustration) from inner to outer canthus.

Distributes medication evenly across eye and lid margin.

    (2) Have patient close eye and rub lid lightly in circular motion with cotton ball if not contraindicated. Avoid placing pressure directly against patient's eyeball.

Further distributes medication without traumatizing eye.

    (3) If excess medication is on eyelid, gently wipe it from inner to outer canthus.

Promotes comfort and prevents trauma to eye.

    (4) If patient needs an eye patch, place it over affected eye so that entire eye is covered. Tape securely without applying pressure to eye.

Clean eye patch reduces risk of infection.

8. After administering eye medications remove and dispose of gloves and soiled supplies, perform hand hygiene.

Reduces spread of microorganisms.

EVALUATION

1. Observe response to medication by assessing visual changes, asking if symptoms are relieved, and noting any side effects or discomfort felt.

Evaluates effects of medication.

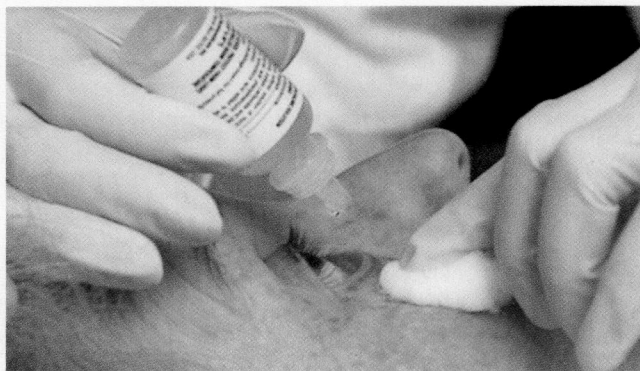

STEP 7d(3) Hold eyedropper above conjunctival sac.

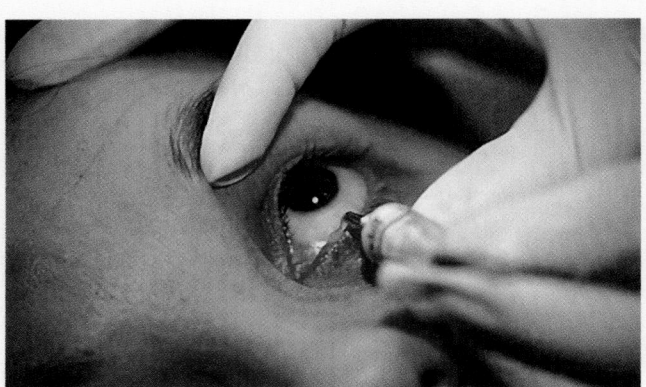

STEP 7e(1) Apply ointment along lower eyelid.

SKILL 17.2 ADMINISTERING EYE (OPHTHALMIC) MEDICATIONS—cont'd

View Video!

STEP	RATIONALE
2. Ask patient to discuss purpose of drug, action, side effects, and technique of administration.	Determines patient's level of understanding.
3. **Use Teach-Back:** "I want to be sure I explained to you clearly how to give yourself eyedrops. Show me how to insert your drops into your left eye." Revise your instruction now or develop a plan for revised patient/family caregiver teaching if patient/family caregiver is not able to teach back correctly.	Determines patient's/family caregiver's level of understanding of instructional topic.

RECORDING AND REPORTING

- Record drug, concentration, dose or strength, number of drops, site of application (left, right, or both eyes), and time of administration on MAR immediately after administration, not before. Include initials or signature.
- Record objective data related to tissues involved (e.g., redness, drainage, irritation), any subjective data (e.g., pain, itching, altered vision), and patient's response to medications. Note any side effects experienced on flow sheet or nurses' notes in electronic health record (EHR) or chart.
- Record patient teaching and validation of understanding on flow sheet or nurses' notes in EHR or chart. Report adverse effects and patient response and/or withheld drugs to nurse in charge or health care provider.

UNEXPECTED OUTCOMES AND RELATED INTERVENTIONS

- Patient complains of burning or pain or experiences local side effects (e.g., headache, bloodshot eyes, local eye irritation). Drug concentration and patient's sensitivity both influence chances of side effects developing.
  - Notify health care provider for possible adjustment in medication type and dosage.
- Patient experiences systemic effects from drops (e.g., increased heart rate and blood pressure from epinephrine, decreased heart rate and blood pressure from timolol).
- Notify health care provider immediately.
- Remain with patient. Assess vital signs.
- Withhold further doses.
- Patient is unable to explain drug information or steps for taking eyedrops and/or has trouble manipulating dropper.
  - Repeat instructions and include family caregiver as appropriate. Include return demonstration.

SKILL 17.3 USING METERED-DOSE OR DRY POWDER INHALERS

DELEGATION AND COLLABORATION

The skill of administering inhaled medications cannot be delegated to nursing assistive personnel (NAP). The nurse instructs the NAP about:
- Potential side effects of medications and to report their occurrence to the nurse.
- Reporting breathing difficulty (e.g., paroxysmal or sustained coughing, audible wheezing).

EQUIPMENT

- Inhaler device with medication canister (metered-dose inhaler [MDI] or dry powder inhaler [DPI])

- Spacer device, such as AeroChamber or InspirEase *(optional for MDI)*
- Facial tissues *(optional)*
- Stethoscope
- Medication administration record (MAR) (electronic or printed)
- Peak flowmeter *(optional)*

STEP	RATIONALE
ASSESSMENT	
1. Check accuracy and completeness of each MAR with health care provider's medication order. Check patient's name, drug name and dosage, route, and time for administration. Clarify incomplete or unclear orders with health care provider before administration.	The order sheet is the most reliable source and only legal record of medications that patient is to receive. Ensures that patient receives correct medications (Mandrack et al., 2012). Illegible MARs are a source of medication errors (Alassaad et al., 2013).
2. Review pertinent information related to medication including action, purpose, normal dose and route, side effects, time of onset and peak action, and nursing implications.	Allows you to anticipate effects of drug while observing patient's response.

STEP	RATIONALE
3. Assess patient's medical and medication history and history of allergies. List any drug allergies on each page of MAR and prominently display on patient's medical record. When allergies are present, patient should wear an allergy bracelet.	Factors influence how certain drugs act. Reveals patient's need for medication. Allergy alert helps prevent adverse events.
4. Perform hand hygiene. Assess patient's respiratory pattern and auscultate breath sounds.	Reduces transmission of infection. Establishes baseline of airway status for comparison during and after treatment.
5. Measure the patient's peak expiratory flow rate using a peak flowmeter. Have patient measure if patient does so at home. Use patient's peak flowmeter if available (see Chapter 32).	A peak flowmeter is used to measure air flow or peak expiratory flow rate and aids in monitoring airway status of patients with chronic asthma (American Academy of Allergy, Asthma and Immunology [AAAAI], 2016).
6. Assess patient's symptoms before initiating medication therapy.	Provides information to evaluate desired effect of medication.
7. Assess patient's ability to hold, manipulate, and depress canister and inhaler.	Any impairment of grasp or presence of hand tremors interferes with patient's ability to depress canister within inhaler. Spacer device is often necessary with an MDI.
8. If patient was previously instructed in self-administration, have patient demonstrate how to use the device.	Patients who have adequate understanding of how to use an inhaler often forget the procedure. Ongoing assessment of inhaler technique identifies areas for further education and reinforcement (Ari and Restrepo, 2012).
9. Assess patient's readiness and ability to learn and use inhaler. Determine type of device patient prefers, considering portability, access to obtain, and cost. Ask questions about medication and its availability; is patient alert and participative in own care; is patient fatigued, in pain, or in respiratory distress?	When selecting an aerosol delivery device, consider several factors such as drug availability and administration time, patient age and ability to use device correctly, portability of device, convenience in both outpatient and inpatient settings, costs, and physician and patient preference (Barrons et al., 2015; Bonini and Usmani, 2015). In some situations, mental or physical limitations affect patient's ability to learn and methods used for instruction.
10. Assess patient's knowledge and understanding of disease and purpose and action of prescribed medications.	Knowledge of disease is essential for patient to realistically understand when to use inhaler.

PLANNING

1. Perform hand hygiene. Collect appropriate equipment and MAR.	Reduces transmission of microorganisms. Promotes time management and efficiency when preparing medications for all patients.
2. Plan preparation to avoid interruptions. Create a quiet environment. Do not take phone calls or talk with others. Follow agency no-interruption zone policy.	Interruptions contribute to medication errors (see Box 17.4) (Beyea, 2014; Yoder et al., 2015).

IMPLEMENTATION

1. Prepare medications for inhalation. Attend to procedure and avoid distraction. Check label of medication against MAR two times, when removing inhaler from unit dose or AMDS and before leaving medication preparation area (see Skill 17.1). Preparation usually involves taking inhaler device out of storage and into patient room. Check expiration date on container. Perform hand hygiene.	*These are the first and second checks for accuracy.* Process ensures that right patient receives right medication.
2. Take medication to patient at correct time (see agency policy). Medications that require exact timing include STAT doses, first-time or loading doses, and one-time doses. Give time-critical scheduled medications at exact time ordered (no later than 30 minutes before or after scheduled dose). Give non–time-critical scheduled medications within a range of 1 or 2 hours of scheduled dose (ISMP, 2011a). During administration, apply six rights of medication administration.	Hospitals must adopt medication administration policy and procedure for timing of medication administration that considers nature of prescribed medication, specific clinical application, and patient needs (CMS, 2011; ISMP, 2011a). Time-critical scheduled medications are those for which early or delayed administration of maintenance doses may cause harm or result in substantial suboptimal therapy or pharmacological effect. Non–time-critical medications are those for which early or delayed administration should not cause harm or result in substantial suboptimal therapy or pharmacological effect (CMS, 2011; ISMP, 2011a).

SKILL 17.3   USING METERED-DOSE OR DRY POWDER INHALERS—cont'd

STEP	RATIONALE
3. Identify patient using at least two identifiers (e.g., name and birthday or name and medical record number) according to agency policy. Compare identifiers with information on patient's MAR or medical record.	Ensures correct patient. Complies with The Joint Commission Standards and improves patient safety (TJC, 2018).
4. At patient's bedside again compare MAR or computer printout with names of medications on medication labels and patient name. Ask patient if he or she has allergies.	*This is the third check for accuracy* and ensures that patient receives correct medication. Confirms patient's allergy history.
5. Help patient sit comfortably in chair.	Patient is more likely to remain receptive to nurse's explanations in a comfortable position, and it is easier to use inhaler.
6. Discuss purpose of each medication, action, and possible adverse effects. Allow patient to ask any questions about the drugs. Warn about overuse of inhaler and side effects.	Patient has right to be informed, and patient's understanding of each medication improves adherence to drug therapy.
7. Explain procedure to patient. Be specific if patient wishes to self-administer drug. Allow adequate time for patient to manipulate inhaler, canister, or spacer device (if appropriate). Explain where and how to set up at home.	Patient must be familiar with how to use equipment.
8. Explain and demonstrate steps for administering MDI without spacer.	Simple one-on-one instruction and demonstration of step-by-step administration allows patient to ask questions at any point during procedure and increases patient adherence to inhaler use (Ari and Restrepo, 2012).
a. Insert MDI canister into holder. Then remove mouthpiece cover from inhaler.	

Clinical Decision Point. If dirt or foreign objects are in mouthpiece, clean before using inhaler to avoid inhalation of unwanted material.

Clinical Decision Point. If MDI is new or has not been used for several days, push a "test spray" into the air to prime the device before using. This ensures that the MDI is patent and the metal canister is positioned properly.

STEP	RATIONALE
b. Shake inhaler well 5 or 6 times.	Aerosolizes fine particles of medication.
c. Have patient hold inhaler in dominant hand.	Easier position to activate device.
d. Instruct patient to position inhaler in one of two ways:	
(1) Have patient close mouth around mouthpiece with opening toward back of throat, closing lips tightly around it (see illustration). This is most common method.	Proper positioning of inhaler is essential to administering medication correctly.
(2) Position mouthpiece 2 to 4 cm (about 1 to 2 inches) in front of widely opened mouth (see illustration), with opening of inhaler toward back of throat. Lips should not touch inhaler.	Directs aerosol spray toward airway. This is best way to deliver medication without a spacer.
e. With inhaler positioned correctly, be sure patient holds inhaler with thumb at mouthpiece and index finger and middle finger at the top. *This is a three-point or lateral hand position.*	MDIs are easier to activate when patients use a three-point or lateral hand position to activate canister (Burchum and Rosenthal, 2016).
f. Instruct patient to tilt head back slightly and inhale slowly and deeply through mouth for 3 to 5 seconds while depressing canister fully.	Medication is distributed to airways during inhalation.
g. Have patient hold breath for as long as comfortable, up to 10 seconds.	Allows aerosol spray droplets to reach deeper branches of airways.
h. Have patient remove MDI from mouth and then exhale slowly through nose or pursed lips.	Keeps small airways open during exhalation.
9. Explain and demonstrate steps to administer MDI using spacer device.	Simple one-on-one instruction and demonstration of step-by-step administration allows patient to ask questions at any point during procedure and increases patient adherence to inhaler use (Ari and Restrepo, 2012).
a. Remove mouthpiece cover from MDI and mouthpiece of spacer device.	Inhaler fits into end of spacer device.
b. Shake inhaler well 5 or 6 times.	Aerosolizes fine particles of medication.

STEP	RATIONALE
c. Insert MDI into end of spacer device.	Spacer device traps medication released from MDI; patient then inhales drug from device. Spacer reduces hand-breath coordination difficulty, thus improving delivery of correct dose of inhaled medication (Barrons et al., 2015).
d. Instruct patient to place spacer device mouthpiece in mouth and close lips. Do not insert beyond raised lip on mouthpiece. Avoid covering small exhalation slots with the lips.	Medication should not escape through mouth.
e. Have patient take a deep breath, exhale, and then breathe normally through spacer device mouthpiece (see illustration).	Allows patient to empty lungs and relax before delivering medication.
f. Instruct patient to depress medication canister 1 time, spraying one puff into spacer device.	Spacer contains fine spray and allows patient to inhale more medication. This increases drug delivery and deposition of medication on oropharyngeal mucosa (Burchum and Rosenthal, 2016).
g. Have patient breathe slowly and fully through mouth for 5 seconds.	Ensures that particles of medication are distributed to deeper airways.
h. Instruct patient to hold full breath for 10 seconds.	Ensures full drug distribution through airways.
i. Have patient remove MDI and spacer and then exhale.	
10. Explain steps to administer DPI or breath-activated MDI.	
a. If DPI has an external counter, note number indicated.	Determines doses remaining.
b. Remove mouthpiece cover. *Do not shake* inhaler.	
c. Prepare medication. Some DPIs require loading medication before administration, some require rotation of a lever to load medication or insertion of a capsule, and some require insertion of a disk into inhaler device. Follow manufacturer's specific instructions.	Primes inhaler, ensuring that medication is delivered to patient effectively.
d. Have patient take a breath and exhale away from the inhaler.	Prevents loss of powder.
e. Have patient position mouthpiece of DPI between lips and inhale quickly and deeply through mouth (see illustration).	Keeps medication from escaping through mouth. Forceful inhalation creates an aerosol.

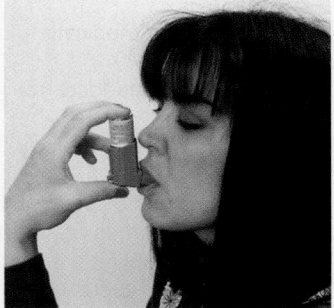

STEP 8d(1) One technique for use of inhaler. Patient opens lips and places inhaler in mouth with opening aimed toward back of throat.

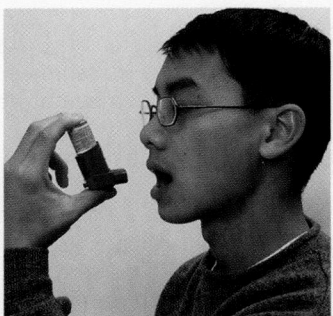

STEP 8d(2) One technique for use of inhaler. Patient positions mouthpiece 1 to 2 inches from mouth.

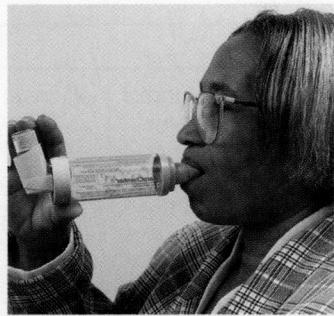

STEP 9e Have patient place mouthpiece in mouth and close lips, being careful to keep exhalation slots exposed.

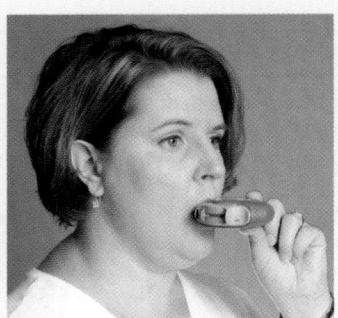

STEP 10e Have patient place mouthpiece of dry powder inhaler between lips.

SKILL 17.3 USING METERED-DOSE OR DRY POWDER INHALERS—cont'd

STEP	RATIONALE
f. Have patient hold breath for 5 to 10 seconds and then exhale.	Distributes medication.
11. Instruct patient to wait 20 to 30 seconds between inhalations (if same medication) or 2 to 5 minutes between inhalations (if different medications). Be sure patient inhales correct number of prescribed puffs.	Drugs must be inhaled sequentially. Always administer bronchodilators before steroids so that dilators can open airway passages (Burchum and Rosenthal, 2016).
12. Instruct patient to not repeat inhalations before next scheduled dose.	Drugs are prescribed at intervals during day to provide constant drug levels and minimize side effects. Beta-adrenergic MDIs are ordered on an "as needed" basis or regularly every 4 to 6 hours.
13. Warn patients that they may feel gagging sensation in throat caused by droplets of medication on pharynx or tongue.	This occurs when medication is sprayed and inhaled incorrectly.
14. About 2 minutes after last dose, instruct patient to rinse mouth with warm water and spit water out.	Steroids may alter normal flora of oral mucosa and lead to development of fungal infection. Rinsing out the mouth reduces the risk of fungal infection and risk (Ari and Restrepo, 2012).
15. Instruct patient on how to clean the inhaler.	Removes residual medication and reduces spread of microorganisms.
a. Once a day remove MDI canister and cap from the mouthpiece. Do not wash the canister or immerse it in water. Run warm tap water through the top and bottom of the plastic mouthpiece for 30 to 60 seconds. Make sure that inhaler is completely dry before reusing. Do not get valve mechanism of canister wet.	Water damages valve mechanism of canister. Accumulation of medication around mouthpiece interferes with proper drug distribution during use.
b. Instruct patient to clean the mouthpiece of MDI and spacer twice a week with a mild dishwashing soap, rinse thoroughly, and dry completely before storage.	Provides better antimicrobial removal. Pressurized MDIs are potential reservoirs for bacteria (Borovina et al., 2012).
16. Help patient to comfortable position, and perform hand hygiene.	Reduces spread of microorganisms and promotes patient comfort.

EVALUATION

1. Auscultate patient lungs, listen for abnormal breath sounds, and obtain peak flow measures if ordered.	Determines patient response to medication.
2. Have patient explain and demonstrate steps in use and cleaning of inhaler.	Return demonstration provides feedback for measuring patient's learning.
3. Ask patient to explain drug schedule and dose of medication.	Improves likelihood of adherence to therapy.
4. Ask patient to describe side effects of medication and criteria for calling health care provider.	Allows patient to recognize signs of overuse and need to seek medical support when drugs are ineffective.
5. Use Teach Back: "I want to be sure I showed you how to use your inhaler. For this dose, show me how you take a dose of your medicine." Revise your instruction now or develop a plan for revised patient/family caregiver teaching if patient/family caregiver is not able to teach back correctly.	Determines patient's/family caregiver's level of understanding of instructional topic.

RECORDING AND REPORTING

- Record drug administered, dose or strength, route, number of inhalations, and actual time administered on MAR immediately after administration, not before. Include initials or signature.
- Record on flow sheet or nurses' notes in electronic health record (her) or chart the patient's response to inhaled medication (e.g., breath sounds, peak flow rate), evidence of side effects (e.g., arrhythmia, feelings of anxiety), and patient's ability to use inhaler.
- Record patient teaching and validation of understanding on flow sheet or nurses' notes in EHR or chart.
- Report adverse effects and patient response and/or withheld drugs to nurse in charge or health care provider.

UNEXPECTED OUTCOMES AND RELATED INTERVENTIONS

- Patient's respirations are rapid and shallow; breath sounds indicate wheezing.
  - Evaluate vital signs and respiratory status.
  - Notify health care provider.
  - Reassess type of medication and/or delivery method.
- Patient needs bronchodilator more than every 4 hours (may indicate respiratory problem).
  - Reassess type of medication and delivery methods needed with health care provider.

- Patient experiences cardiac dysrhythmias (light-headedness, syncope), especially if receiving beta-adrenergic medications.
  - Withhold all further doses of medication.
  - Evaluate cardiac and pulmonary status (see Chapter 16).
  - Notify health care provider for reassessment of type of medication and delivery method.

SKILL 17.4 PREPARING INJECTIONS FROM VIALS AND AMPULES

DELEGATION CONSIDERATIONS
The skill of preparing injections from ampules and vials cannot be delegated to nursing assistive personnel (NAP).

EQUIPMENT
Medication in an Ampule
- Syringe, needle, and filter needle
- Small sterile gauze pad or unopened alcohol swab

MEDICATION IN A VIAL
- Syringe and two needles
- Needles:
  - Needleless blunt-tip vial access cannula or needle (with safety sheath) for drawing up medication (if needed)
  - Filter needle if indicated

- Small, sterile gauze pad or alcohol swab
- Diluent (e.g., 0.9% sodium chloride or sterile water if indicated)

BOTH
- Medication administration record (MAR) or computer printout
- Sharps with engineered sharps injury protection (SESIP) safety needle for injection
- Medication in vial or ampule
- Puncture-proof container for disposal of syringes, needles, and glass

STEP	RATIONALE
ASSESSMENT	
1. Check accuracy and completeness of each MAR or computer printout with health care provider's written medication order. Check patient's name, medication name and dosage, route of administration, and time of administration. Recopy or reprint any part of MAR that is difficult to read.	The order sheet is the most reliable source and only legal record of medications that patient is to receive. Ensures that patient receives correct medications (Mandrack et al., 2012). Illegible MARs are a source of medication errors (Alassaad et al., 2013).
2. Assess patient's medical and medication history and history of allergies. List any drug allergies on each page of MAR and prominently display on patient's medical record. When allergies are present, patient should wear an allergy bracelet.	Determines need for medication or possible contraindications for medication administration. Allergy alert helps prevent adverse events.
3. Review medication reference information for action, purpose, side effects, and nursing implications.	Allows you to administer drug properly and monitor patient's response.
4. Assess patient's body build, muscle size, and weight if giving subcutaneous or IM medication.	Determines type and size of syringe and needle for injection.
PLANNING	
1. Perform hand hygiene. Collect appropriate equipment and MAR.	Reduces transmission of microorganisms. Ensures organized procedure.
2. Follow agency's no-interruption zone (NIZ) policy. Prepare medications for one patient at a time. Keep all pages of MARs or computer printouts for one patient together or look at only one patient's electronic MAR at a time.	Preventing distractions reduces medication preparation errors. Use NIZ when possible (Beyea, 2014; Yoder et al., 2015).
IMPLEMENTATION	
1. Prepare medication.	
a. If using a medication cart, move it outside patient's room.	Organization of equipment saves time and reduces error.
b. Unlock medication drawer or cart or log onto computerized medication dispensing system.	Medications are safeguarded when locked in cabinet, cart, or computerized medication dispensing system.

SKILL 17.4 PREPARING INJECTIONS FROM VIALS AND AMPULES—cont'd

STEP	RATIONALE
c. Select correct drug from stock supply or unit-dose drawer. Compare label of medication with MAR computer printout or computer screen.	Reading label and comparing it with transcribed order reduces errors. *This is the first check for accuracy.*
d. Check expiration date on each vial or ampule, one at a time.	Medications used past their expiration date are sometimes inactive, less effective, or harmful to patients.
e. Calculate drug dose as necessary. Double-check calculation. Ask another nurse to check calculations if needed.	Double-checking may help reduce error especially for high-risk medications.
f. If preparing a controlled substance, check record for previous drug count and compare with supply available.	Controlled substance laws require careful monitoring of dispensed narcotics.
g. Do not leave drugs unattended.	Nurse is responsible for safekeeping of drugs.
2. Prepare ampule.	
a. Tap top of ampule lightly and quickly with finger until fluid moves from its neck (see illustration).	Dislodges any fluid that collects above neck of ampule. All solution moves into lower chamber.
b. Place small gauze pad around neck of ampule (see illustration).	Protects fingers from trauma as glass tip is broken off. Do not use opened alcohol swab to wrap around top of ampule because alcohol may leak into ampule.
c. Snap neck of ampule quickly and firmly away from hands (see illustration).	Protects your fingers and face from shattering glass.
d. Draw up medication quickly, using filter needle long enough to reach bottom of ampule to access medication.	System is open to airborne contaminants. Filter needles filter out any fragments of glass (Alexander et al., 2014).
e. Hold ampule upside down or set it on flat surface. Insert filter needle into center of ampule opening. Do not allow needle tip or shaft to touch rim of ampule.	Broken rim of ampule is considered contaminated. When ampule is inverted, solution dribbles out if needle tip or shaft touches rim of ampule.
f. Aspirate medication into syringe by gently pulling back on plunger (see illustrations).	Withdrawal of plunger creates negative pressure within syringe barrel, which pulls fluid into syringe.
g. Keep needle tip under surface of liquid. Tip ampule to bring all fluid within reach of needle.	Prevents aspiration of air bubbles.
h. If you aspirate air bubbles, do not expel air into ampule.	Air pressure forces fluid out of ampule, and medication will be lost.
i. To expel excess air bubbles, remove needle from ampule. Hold syringe vertically with needle pointing up. Tap side of syringe to cause bubbles to rise toward needle. Draw back slightly on plunger and push plunger upward to eject air. Do not eject fluid.	Withdrawing plunger too far removes it from barrel. Holding syringe vertically allows fluid to settle in bottom of barrel. Pulling back on plunger allows fluid within needle to enter barrel so that fluid is not expelled. You then expel air at top of barrel and within needle.
j. If syringe contains excess fluid, use sink for disposal. Hold syringe vertically with needle tip up and slanted slightly toward sink. Slowly eject excess fluid into sink. Recheck fluid level in syringe by holding it vertically.	Safely disperses excess medication into sink. Position of needle allows you to expel medication without having it flow down needle shaft. Rechecking fluid level ensures proper dose.
k. Cover needle with its safety sheath or cap. Replace filter needle with regular SESIP needle.	Minimizes needlesticks. Filter needles cannot be used for injection.
3. Prepare vial containing a solution.	
a. Remove cap covering top of unused vial to expose sterile rubber seal. If a multidose vial has been used before, the cap is already removed and does not require cleansing. Firmly and briskly wipe surface of rubber seal with alcohol swab. Allow it to dry.	Vial comes packaged with cap that cannot be replaced after seal removal. Not all drug manufacturers guarantee that rubber seals of unused vials are sterile. Swabbing with alcohol reduces transmission of microorganisms. Allowing alcohol to dry prevents alcohol from coating needle and mixing with medication.
b. Pick up syringe and remove needle cap or cap covering the needleless vial access device (see illustration). Pull back on plunger to draw amount of air into syringe equivalent to volume of medication to be aspirated from vial.	Injecting air into vial prevents buildup of negative pressure in vial when aspirating medication.

Clinical Decision Point. Some medications and agencies require use of a filter needle when preparing medications from vials. Check agency policy or medication reference. If you use a filter needle to aspirate medication, you need to change it to a regular SESIP needle of the appropriate size to administer medication (Alexander et al., 2014).

STEP	RATIONALE

c. With vial on flat surface, insert tip of needle or needleless vial access device through center of rubber seal (see illustration). Apply pressure to tip of needle during insertion.

Center of seal is thinner and easier to penetrate. Using firm pressure prevents dislodging rubber particles that could enter vial or needle.

d. Inject air into air space of vial, holding on to plunger. Hold plunger firmly; plunger is sometimes forced backward by air pressure within vial.

Injection of air creates vacuum needed to get medication to flow into syringe. Injecting into air space of vial prevents formation of bubbles and an inaccurate dose.

e. Invert vial while keeping firm hold on syringe and plunger. Hold vial between thumb and middle fingers of nondominant hand. Grasp end of syringe barrel and plunger with thumb and forefinger of dominant hand to counteract pressure in vial.

Inverting vial allows fluid to settle in lower half of container. Position of hands prevents forceful movement of plunger and permits easy manipulation of syringe.

f. Keep tip of needle or needleless device below fluid level.

Prevents aspiration of air.

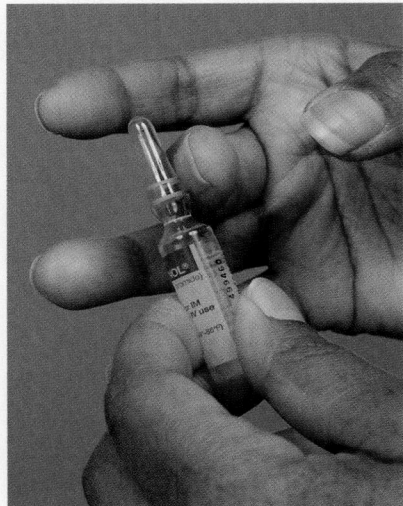

STEP 2a Tapping ampule moves fluid down ampule neck.

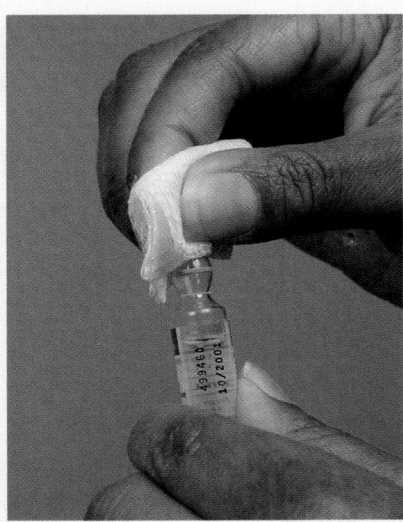

STEP 2b Gauze pad placed around neck of ampule protects fingers.

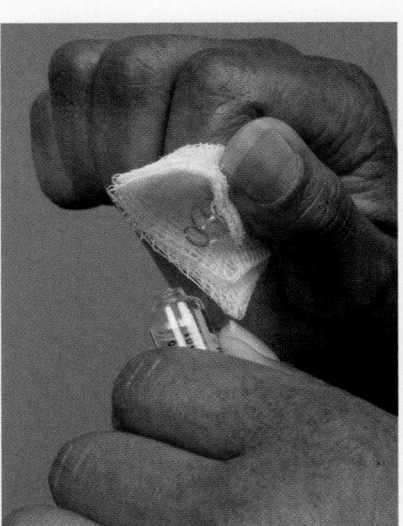

STEP 2c Snapping neck away from hands.

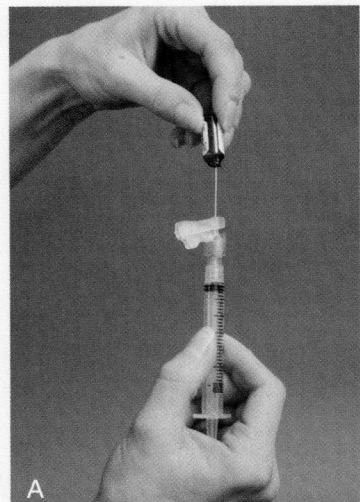 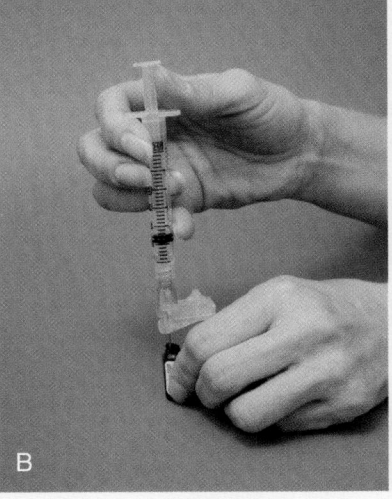

STEP 2f A, Medication aspirated with ampule inverted. **B,** Medication aspirated with ampule on flat surface.

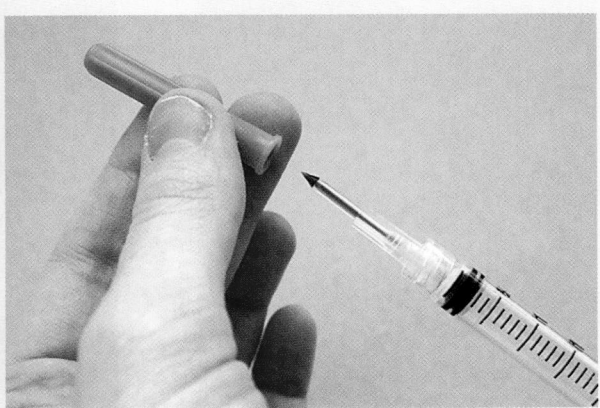

STEP 3b Syringe with needless vial adapter.

SKILL 17.4   PREPARING INJECTIONS FROM VIALS AND AMPULES—cont'd

STEP	RATIONALE
g. Allow air pressure from vial to fill syringe gradually with medication. If necessary, pull back slightly on plunger to obtain correct amount of medication (see illustration).	Positive pressure within vial forces fluid into syringe.
h. When you obtain desired volume, position needle or needleless device into air space of vial; tap side of syringe barrel gently to dislodge any air bubbles (see illustration). Eject any air remaining at top of syringe into vial.	Forcefully striking barrel while needle is inserted in vial may bend needle. Accumulation of air displaces medication and causes dose errors.
i. Remove needle or needleless access device from vial by pulling back on barrel of syringe.	Pulling plunger rather than barrel causes plunger to separate from barrel, resulting in loss of medication.
j. Hold syringe at eye level at 90-degree angle to ensure correct volume and absence of air bubbles. Remove any remaining air by tapping barrel to dislodge any air bubbles. Draw back slightly on plunger; then push it upward to eject air. Do not eject fluid. Recheck volume of medication.	Holding syringe vertically allows fluid to settle in bottom of barrel. Tapping dislodges air to top of barrel. Pulling back on plunger allows fluid within needle to enter barrel so that you do not expel fluid. You then expel air at top of barrel and within needle.

Clinical Decision Point. When preparing medication from single-dose vial, do not assume that volume listed on label is total volume in vial. Some manufacturers provide small amount of extra liquid, expecting loss during preparation. Be sure to draw up only desired volume.

k. If you need to inject medication into patient's tissue, change needle with regular SESIP to appropriate gauge and length according to route of medication administration.	Inserting needle through rubber stopper dulls beveled tip. New needle is sharper and, because no fluid is along shaft, does not track medication through tissues. Filter needles cannot be used for injection.
l. Cover needle with its safety sheath or cap.	Minimizes needlesticks.
m. For multidose vial, make label that includes date of opening, concentration of drug (per milliliter), and your initials.	Ensures that nurses will prepare future doses correctly. You discard some drugs within a certain time frame after mixing.
4. Prepare vial containing powder (reconstituting medications).	
a. Remove cap covering vial of powdered medication and cap covering vial of proper diluent. Firmly swab both rubber seals with alcohol swab and allow alcohol to dry.	Allowing alcohol to dry prevents it from coating needle and mixing with medication.
b. Draw up manufacturer's suggestion for volume and type of diluent into syringe following Steps 3b through 3j.	Prepares diluent for injection into vial containing powdered medication.

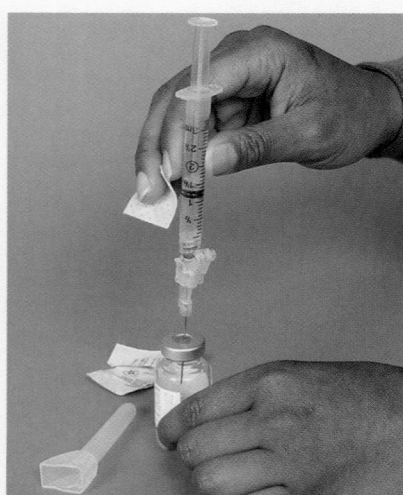

STEP 3c Insert safety needle through center of vial diaphragm (with vial setting flat on table).

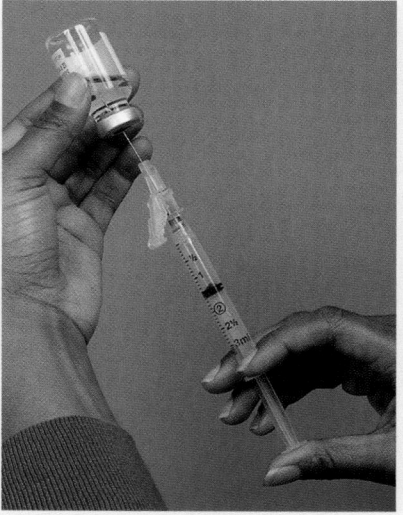

STEP 3g Fluid withdrawn from vial.

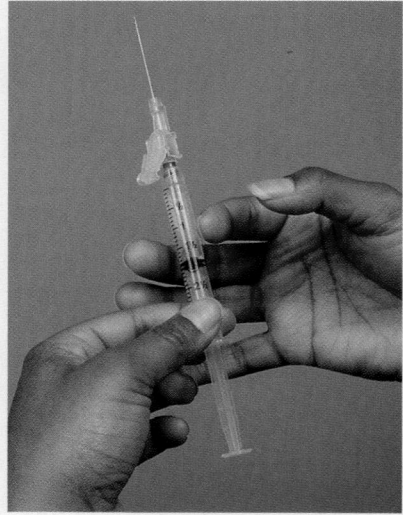

STEP 3h Hold syringe upright; tap barrel to dislodge air bubbles.

STEP	RATIONALE
c. Insert tip of needle or needleless device through center of rubber seal of vial of powdered medication. Inject diluent into vial. Remove needle.	Diluent begins to dissolve and reconstitute medication.
d. Mix medication thoroughly. Roll in palms. Do not shake.	Ensures proper dispersal of medication throughout solution and prevents formation of air bubbles.
e. Reconstituted medication in vial is ready to be drawn into new syringe. Read label carefully to determine dose after reconstitution.	Once you add diluent, concentration of medication (mg/mL) determines dose you give. Reading medication label carefully decreases medication errors.
f. Draw up reconstituted medication into syringe. Insert needleless device/needle into vial. Do not add air. Then follow Steps 3e through 3l.	Prepares medication for administration.

Clinical Decision Point. Some agencies require that you verify dose of certain medications (e.g., insulin and heparin) for accuracy with another nurse. Check guidelines before administering medication.

5. Compare label of medication with MAR, computer screen, or computer printout.	*This is the second check for accuracy.*
6. Dispose of soiled supplies. Place broken ampule and/or used vials and used needle or needleless device in puncture-proof and leak-proof container. Clean work area, and perform hand hygiene.	Proper disposal of glass and needle prevents accidental injury to staff. Controls transmission of infection.

EVALUATION

1. Just before administering drug to patient, compare MAR with label of prepared drug and compare dose in syringe with desired dose.	Ensures that dose is accurate. *This is the third check for accuracy.*

UNEXPECTED OUTCOMES AND RELATED INTERVENTIONS

- Air bubbles remain in syringe.
  - Expel air from syringe and add medication to it until you prepare correct dose.

- Incorrect dose of medication is prepared.
  - Discard prepared dose.
  - Prepare correct new dose.

SKILL 17.5 ADMINISTERING INJECTIONS

View Video!

DELEGATION AND COLLABORATION

The skill of administering injections cannot be delegated to nursing assistive personnel (NAP). The nurse instructs the NAP about:

- Potential medication side effects and allergic responses and to report their occurrence along with any changes in vital signs or level of consciousness immediately to the nurse.

EQUIPMENT

Proper size syringe and sharps with engineered sharps injury protection (SESIP) needle:

- Subcutaneous: syringe (1- to 3-mL) and needle (25- to 27-gauge, $\frac{1}{8}$- to $\frac{5}{8}$-inch)
  - Immunizations: 23- to 25-gauge, $\frac{5}{8}$-inch needle (CDC, 2015)
  - Subcutaneous U-100 insulin: insulin syringe (1 mL) with preattached needle (28- to 31-gauge, $\frac{5}{16}$- to $\frac{3}{16}$-inch)
  - Subcutaneous U-500 insulin: 1 mL tuberculin (TB) syringe with needle (25- to 27-gauge, $\frac{1}{2}$- to $\frac{5}{8}$-inch)
- Intramuscular (IM): syringe 2 to 3 mL for adult, 0.5 to 1 mL for infants and small children (21- to 23-gauge, 1- to 1$\frac{1}{2}$-inch needle).

- Needle length corresponding to site of injection, age, gender, and size of patient. Refer to following guidelines; length needed may vary outside of these guidelines for patients who are smaller or larger than average.

Needle Length for Immunizations[a]

Site	Child	Adult
Ventrogluteal	$\frac{1}{2}$–1 inch	1$\frac{1}{2}$ inches
Vastus lateralis	$\frac{5}{8}$–1 inch	$\frac{5}{8}$–1 inch
Deltoid	$\frac{1}{2}$–1 inch	1–1$\frac{1}{2}$ inches

Male Gender	Female Gender	Needle Length
Less than 130 lb	Less than 130 lb	$\frac{5}{8}$–1 inch
130–152 lb	130–152 lb	1 inch
153–260 lb	153–200 lb	1–1$\frac{1}{2}$ inches
Greater than 260 lb	Greater than 200 lb	1$\frac{1}{2}$ inches

[a]Based on CDC (2015) guidelines.

- Needle gauge often depends on length of needle; administer biologicals and medication in aqueous

SKILL 17.5   ADMINISTERING INJECTIONS—cont'd

solution with a 20- to 25-gauge needle. Use 18- to 21-gauge needles for medications in oil-based solutions.

- Intradermal (ID): 1-mL TB syringe with preattached 25- or 27-gauge needle, $\frac{1}{8}$- to $\frac{5}{8}$-inch
- All injections
  - Small gauze pad *(optional)*

- Alcohol swab
- Medication vial or ampule
- Clean gloves
- Medication administration record (MAR) or computer printout
- Puncture-proof container for sharps

STEP	RATIONALE

ASSESSMENT

1. Check accuracy and completeness of MAR or computer printout with health care provider's original medication order. Check patient's name, medication name and dosage, route of administration, and time of administration. Recopy or reprint any part of MAR that is difficult to read.

2. Assess patient's medical and medication history and history of allergies. List any drug allergies on each page of the MAR and prominently display on patient's medical record. When allergies are present, patient should wear an allergy bracelet.

3. Review medication reference information for medication action, purpose, normal dose, side effects, time and peak of onset, and nursing implications. In the case of an ID injection, review expected reaction and/or anticipated effects when testing skin with specific allergen and appropriate time to read site.

4. Assess for contraindication to injections:
   - ID injections—reduced local tissue perfusion. Assess for history of severe adverse reactions or necrosis that occurred after previous ID injection.
   - Subcutaneous injection—circulatory shock or reduced local tissue perfusion.
   - IM injection—muscle atrophy, reduced blood flow, or circulatory shock.

5. Assess patient's knowledge of purpose and expected response to medication or skin testing.

6. Assess patient's symptoms before initiating medication therapy.

7. For subcutaneous insulin or heparin, assess relevant laboratory results (e.g., blood glucose, partial thromboplastin time).

8. Observe patient's previous verbal and nonverbal responses to injection.

9. Check date of expiration for medication.

The order sheet is the most reliable source and only legal record of medications that patient is to receive. Ensures that patient receives correct medications (Mandrack et al., 2012). Illegible MARs are a source of medication errors (Alassaad et al., 2013).

Determines need for medication or possible contraindications for medication administration. Allergy alert helps prevent adverse events.

Allows you to administer medication safely and monitor patient's response to therapy. Type of reaction to an immunization depends on patient's ability to mount a cell-mediated immune response. Knowledge of expected and adverse reactions to skin testing helps you determine for which symptoms to monitor, how frequently, and when to reassess patient.

Decreased tissue perfusion reduces absorption of subcutaneous and ID medications and affects drug distribution of subcutaneous medication. Prior history of severe reactions increases risk for future severe reactions. Factors interfering with blood flow to muscles impair IM drug absorption.

Patients need to know when to return for follow-up reading of skin test and when and how to report any reaction. Poses implications for patient education.

Provides information to evaluate desired effect of medication.

Provides baseline for measuring drug response.

Anticipating patient's anxiety allows you to use distraction to reduce pain awareness.

Dose potency increases or decreases when outdated.

PLANNING

1. Perform hand hygiene. Collect appropriate equipment and MAR.

2. Follow agency no-interruption zone (NIZ) policy. Prepare medications for one patient at a time. Keep all pages of MARs or computer printouts for one patient together or look at only one patient's electronic MAR at a time.

Reduces transmission of microorganisms. Ensures organized procedure.

Preventing distractions reduces medication preparation errors. Use NIZ when possible (Beyea, 2014; Yoder et al., 2015).

IMPLEMENTATION

1. Prepare medication for one patient at a time using aseptic technique. Attend to preparation and avoid distraction. Check label of medication carefully with MAR or computer printout 2 times, when removing medication from unit dose or AMDS and before leaving medication preparation area (see Skill 17.4). Perform hand hygiene.

Reduces transmission of microorganisms. Ensures that medication is sterile. *These are the first and second checks for accuracy* and ensure that correct medication is administered.

STEP	RATIONALE
2. Take medication to patient at correct time (see agency policy). Medications that require exact timing include STAT doses, first-time or loading doses, and one-time doses. Give time-critical scheduled medications at exact time ordered (no later than 30 minutes before or after scheduled dose). Give non–time-critical scheduled medications within a range of 1 or 2 hours of scheduled dose (ISMP, 2011a). During administration apply six rights of medication administration.	Hospitals must adopt medication administration policy and procedure for timing of medication administration that considers nature of the prescribed medication, specific clinical application, and patient needs (CMS, 2011; ISMP, 2011a). Time-critical scheduled medications are those for which early or delayed administration of maintenance doses may cause harm or result in substantial suboptimal therapy or pharmacological effect. Non–time-critical medications are those for which early or delayed administration should not cause harm or result in substantial suboptimal therapy or pharmacological effect (CMS, 2011; ISMP, 2011a).
3. Close room curtain or door.	Provides privacy.
4. Identify patient using at least two identifiers (e.g., name and birthday or name and medical record number) according to agency policy. Compare identifiers with information on patient's MAR or medical record.	Ensures correct patient. Complies with The Joint Commission standards and improves patient safety (TJC, 2018).
5. At patient's bedside again compare MAR or computer printout with names of medications on medication labels and patient name. Ask patient if he or she has allergies.	*This is the third check for accuracy* and ensures that patient receives correct medication. Confirms patient's allergy history.
6. Discuss purpose of each medication and/or skin test, action, and possible adverse effects. Allow patient to ask any questions. Tell patient that injection will cause slight burning or sting. An ID injection will create a small bleb on the skin.	Patient has right to be informed, and patient's understanding of each medication improves adherence to drug therapy. Helps minimize patient's anxiety.
7. Perform hand hygiene and apply clean gloves. Keep sheet or gown draped over body parts not requiring exposure.	Reduces transmission of infection.
8. Select appropriate injection site. Inspect skin surface over sites for bruises, inflammation, or edema. • ID: Note lesions or discolorations of skin. If possible, select site three to four finger widths below antecubital space and one hand width above wrist. If you cannot use forearm, inspect upper back. If necessary, use sites appropriate for subcutaneous injections. • Subcutaneous: Do not use an area that is bruised or has signs associated with infection. Palpate sites and avoid those with masses or tenderness. Be sure that needle is correct size by grasping skinfold at site with thumb and forefinger. Measure fold from top to bottom. Make sure that needle is one-half length of fold. When administering insulin or heparin, use abdominal injection sites first, followed by thigh injection site. Choose site on right or left side of abdomen at least 5 cm (2 inches) away from umbilicus. • IM: Note integrity and size of muscle. Palpate for tenderness or hardness. Avoid these areas. If patient receives frequent injections, rotate sites. Use ventrogluteal if possible.	Injection sites need to be free of abnormalities that interfere with medication absorption. An ID injection site is free of discoloration or hair so that you can see results of skin test and interpret them correctly (WHO, 2015). Injection sites are free of abnormalities that interfere with drug absorption. Subcutaneous sites used repeatedly become hardened from lipohypertrophy (increased growth in fatty tissue). You can mistakenly give subcutaneous injections in muscle, especially in abdomen and thigh sites. Appropriate size of needle ensures that you inject medication into subcutaneous tissue (Hirsch et al., 2012; Ogston-Tuck, 2014a). Injecting low-molecular-weight heparin on side of abdomen helps decrease pain and bruising at injection site (Sanofi-Aventis, 2014).
9. Help patient into comfortable position. • ID: Have patient extend elbow and support it and forearm on flat surface. • Subcutaneous: Have patient relax arm, leg, or abdomen, depending on site selection. • IM: Position patient depending on chosen site (e.g., sit, lie flat, on side, or prone).	Stabilizes injection site for easy accessibility. Relaxation of site minimizes discomfort. Reduces strain on muscle and minimizes injection discomfort.
10. Relocate site using anatomical landmarks. For subcutaneous insulin, rotate site within an anatomical area (e.g., abdomen) and systematically rotate sites within that area.	Injection into correct anatomical site prevents injury to nerves, bone, and blood vessels. Rotating injection sites within an anatomical site maintains consistency in day-to-day insulin absorption.

View Video!

SKILL 17.5   ADMINISTERING INJECTIONS—cont'd

STEP	RATIONALE
11. Clean site with antiseptic swab. Apply swab at center of site and rotate outward in circular direction for about 5 cm (2 inches) (see illustration).	Mechanical action of swab removes secretions containing microorganisms.
• *Option for IM injection:* Apply eutectic mixture of local anesthetics (EMLA) cream on injection site at least 1 hour before IM injection or use vapocoolant spray (e.g., ethyl chloride) just before injection.	Decreases pain at injection site.
12. Hold swab or gauze between third and fourth fingers of nondominant hand.	Swab or gauze remains readily accessible for use when withdrawing needle after injection.
13. Remove needle cap from needle by pulling it straight off.	Preventing needle from touching sides of cap prevents contamination.
14. Hold syringe between thumb and forefinger of dominant hand:	Smooth injection requires proper manipulation of syringe parts. With bevel up, you are less likely to deposit medication into ID tissues below dermis.
• ID: Hold syringe with bevel of needle pointing up.	
• Subcutaneous and IM: Hold as dart, palm down (see illustration).	
15. Administer injection.	
a. **ID:**	
(1) With nondominant hand stretch skin over site with forefinger or thumb.	Needle pierces tight skin more easily.
(2) With needle almost against patient's skin, insert it slowly at 5- to 15-degree angle until resistance is felt. Advance needle through epidermis to approximately 3 mm ($\frac{1}{8}$ inch) below skin surface. You will see bulge of needle tip through skin.	Ensures that needle tip is in dermis. You obtain inaccurate results if you do not inject needle at correct angle and depth (WHO, 2015).
(3) Inject medication slowly. Normally you feel resistance. If not, needle is too deep; remove and begin again.	Slow injection minimizes discomfort at site. Dermal layer is tight and does not expand easily when you inject solution.

Clinical Decision Point. It is not necessary to aspirate an ID injection because dermis is relatively avascular.

(4) While injecting medication, note that small bleb (approximately 6 mm [$\frac{1}{4}$ inch]) resembling mosquito bite appears on skin surface (see illustration).	Bleb indicates that you deposited medication in dermis.
b. **Subcutaneous:**	
(1) For average-size patient, hold skin across injection site or pinch skin with nondominant hand.	Needle penetrates tight skin more easily than loose skin. Pinching elevates subcutaneous tissue and desensitizes area.

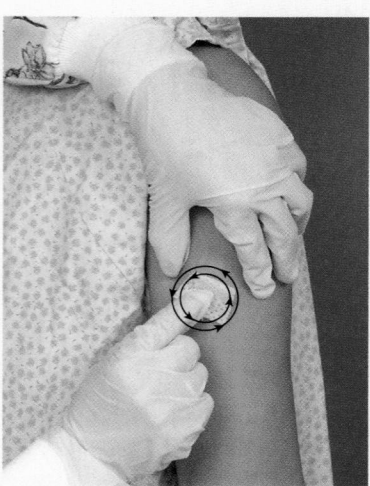

STEP 11 Clean site using circular motion.

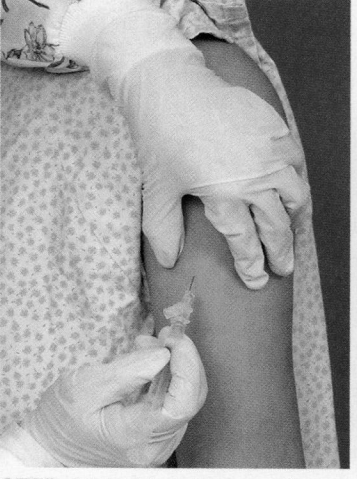

STEP 14 Hold syringe as if grasping a dart.

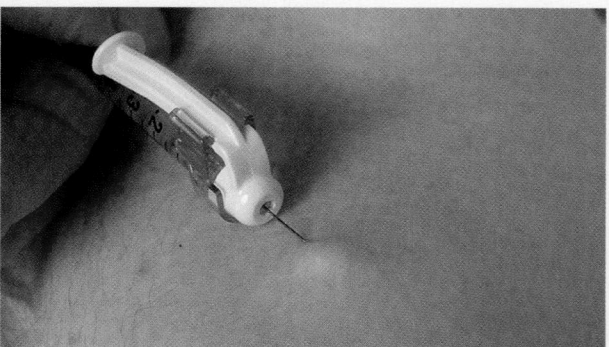

STEP 15a(4) Intradermal injection creates small bleb.

STEP	RATIONALE
(2) Inject needle quickly and firmly at 45- to 90-degree angle (see illustration). Release skin if pinched. *Option:* When using injection pen or giving heparin, continue to pinch skin while injecting medicine.	Quick, firm insertion minimizes discomfort. (Injecting medication into compressed tissue irritates nerve fibers.) Correct angle prevents accidental injection into muscle.
(3) For obese patient pinch skin at site and inject needle at 90-degree angle below tissue fold.	Obese patients have fatty layer of tissue above subcutaneous layer.
(4) After needle enters site, grasp lower end of syringe barrel with nondominant hand to stabilize it. Move dominant hand to end of plunger and slowly inject medication over several seconds (see illustration). When giving heparin, inject over 30 seconds (Akbari Sari et al., 2014; Sanofi-Aventis, 2014). Avoid moving syringe.	Movement of syringe may displace needle and cause discomfort. Slow injection of medication minimizes discomfort.

Clinical Decision Point. Aspiration after injecting a subcutaneous medication is not necessary. Piercing a blood vessel in a subcutaneous injection is very rare. Aspiration after injecting heparin and insulin is not recommended (Lilley et al., 2016).

---

c. **IM:**

(1) Position ulnar side of nondominant hand just below site and pull skin laterally approximately 2.5 to 3.5 cm (1 to 1½ inches) (see Fig. 17.21). Hold position until medication is injected. With dominant hand inject needle quickly at 90-degree angle into muscle (see Fig. 17.17).	Z-track creates zigzag path through tissues that seals needle track to avoid tracking medication. A quick dartlike injection reduces discomfort. Use Z-track for all IM injections (Nicoll and Hesby, 2002; Hopkins and Arias, 2013; Ogston-Tuck, 2014b).
(2) *Option:* If patient's muscle mass is small, grasp body of muscle between thumb and forefingers.	Ensures that medication reaches muscle mass (CDC, 2015; Hockenberry and Wilson, 2015).
(3) After needle pierces skin, while still pulling on skin with nondominant hand, grasp lower end of syringe barrel with fingers of nondominant hand to stabilize it. Move dominant hand to end of plunger. Avoid moving syringe.	Smooth manipulation of syringe reduces discomfort from needle movement. Skin remains pulled until after medication is injected to ensure Z-track administration.
(4) Pull back on plunger 5 to 10 seconds. If no blood appears, inject medication slowly at rate of 1 mL/10 sec (Nicoll and Hesby, 2002).	Aspiration of blood into syringe indicates possible placement into a vein. Aspiration of blood into syringe indicates IV placement of needle. Slow injection rate reduces pain and tissue trauma and reduces chance of leakage of medication back through needle track (Nicoll and Hesby, 2002; Hockenberry and Wilson, 2015).

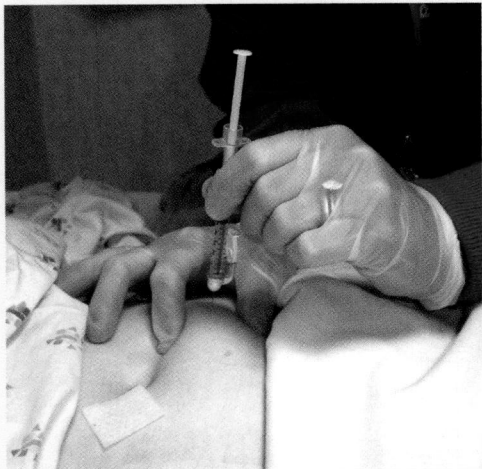

STEP 15b(2) Subcutaneous injection. Angle and needle length depend on thickness of skinfold.

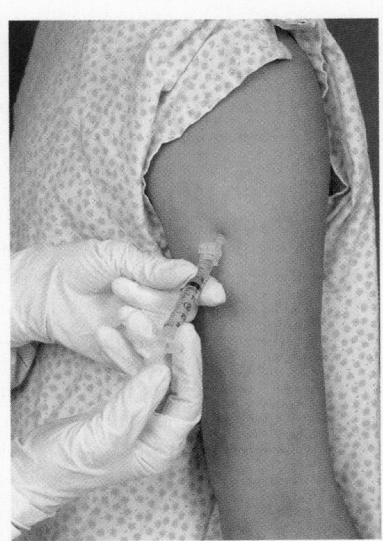

STEP 15b(4) Inject medication slowly.

SKILL 17.5 ADMINISTERING INJECTIONS—cont'd

View Video!

STEP	RATIONALE

Clinical Decision Point. The Centers for Disease Control and Prevention (CDC, 2015) no longer recommends aspiration when administering an immunization. For all other IM injections, if blood appears in syringe, remove needle, dispose of medication and syringe properly, and prepare another dose of medication for injection to prevent injection of medication directly into the bloodstream.

(5) Once medication is injected, wait 10 seconds, then smoothly and steadily withdraw needle, release skin, and apply gauze gently over site.	Allows time for medication to absorb into muscle before removing syringe. Dry gauze minimizes discomfort associated with alcohol on nonintact skin.
16. Apply gentle pressure to site. Do not massage site. Apply bandage if needed.	Massage damages underlying tissue.
17. Help patient to comfortable position.	Gives patient sense of well-being.
18. Discard uncapped needle or needle enclosed in safety shield and attached syringe into puncture-proof and leak-proof receptacle (see Fig. 17.27).	Prevents injury to patients and health care personnel. Recapping needles increases risk for needlestick injury (OSHA, n.d.).
19. Remove gloves and perform hand hygiene.	Reduces transmission of microorganisms.
20. Stay with patient for several minutes and observe for any allergic reactions.	Dyspnea, wheezing, and circulatory collapse are signs of severe anaphylactic reaction and are likely to occur immediately after injection.

EVALUATION

1. Return to room in 15 to 30 minutes and ask if patient feels any acute pain, burning, numbness, or tingling at injection site.	After an ID injection continued discomfort could indicate injury to underlying tissues. Continued discomfort after a subcutaneous or IM injection may indicate injury to underlying bones or nerves.
2. After an ID injection ask patient to discuss implications of skin testing and signs of hypersensitivity.	Patient's ability to recognize signs of skin testing helps to ensure timely reporting of results.
3. Inspect ID bleb. *Optional:* Use skin pencil and draw circle around perimeter of injection site. Read TB test site at 48 to 72 hours; look for induration (hard, dense, raised area) of skin around injection site of:	Determines if reaction to antigen occurs; indication positive for tuberculosis or tested allergens. Site must be read at various intervals to determine test results. Pencil marks make site easy to find. You determine results of skin testing at various times, based on type of medication used or type of skin testing completed. Manufacturer directions determine when to read test results.
• 15 mm or more in patients with no known risk factors for tuberculosis.	
• 10 mm or more in patients who are recent immigrants; injection drug users; residents and employees of high-risk settings; patients with certain chronic illnesses; children younger than 4 years of age; and infants, children, and adolescents exposed to high-risk adults.	
• 5 mm or more in patients who are human immunodeficiency virus (HIV) positive, have fibrotic changes on chest x-ray film consistent with previous tuberculosis infection, have had organ transplants, or are immunosuppressed.	
4. Inspect subcutaneous or IM site; note any bruising or induration. Apply warm compress to site if bruising or induration noted.	Bruising or induration indicates complication associated with injection. Document findings and notify health care provider.
5. Observe patient's response to medication at times that correlate with onset, peak, and duration of medication. Review laboratory results as appropriate (e.g., blood glucose, partial thromboplastin time).	Adverse effects of parenteral medications develop rapidly. Evaluate effect of medication on basis of onset, peak, and duration of action.
6. **Use Teach-Back:** "I want to be sure I explained to you the purpose of your TB injection. Explain for me why you are receiving the injection and what to look for on your skin tomorrow." Revise your instruction now or develop a plan for revised patient/family caregiver teaching if patient/family caregiver is not unable to teach back correctly.	Determines patient's/family caregiver's level of understanding of instructional topic.

RECORDING AND REPORTING

- Record drug, dose, route, site, time, and date on MAR in electronic health record (EHR) or chart immediately after administration, not before. Correctly sign MAR according to agency policy.
- Record area of ID injection and appearance of skin in EHR or chart.
- Record patient teaching, validation of understanding, and patient's response to medication in EHR or chart.
- Report any undesirable effects from medication to patient's health care provider, and document adverse effects in record.

UNEXPECTED OUTCOMES AND RELATED INTERVENTIONS

- Patient complains of localized pain or continued burning at injection site, indicating potential injury to nerve or vessels.
  - Assess injection site.
  - Notify patient's health care provider.
- Raised, reddened, or hard zone (induration) forms around ID test site.
  - Notify patient's health care provider.
  - Document sensitivity to injected allergen or positive test if tuberculin skin testing was completed.
- During IM injection blood is aspirated.
  - Immediately stop injection and remove needle.
  - Prepare new syringe of medication for administration.
- Patient displays adverse reaction with signs of urticaria, eczema, pruritus, wheezing, and dyspnea.
  - Follow agency policy or guidelines for appropriate response to allergic reactions (e.g., administration of antihistamine such as diphenhydramine or epinephrine).
  - Notify patient's health care provider immediately.
  - Add allergy information to patient's record.

SKILL 17.6 ADMINISTERING MEDICATIONS BY INTRAVENOUS BOLUS

DELEGATION CONSIDERATIONS

The skill of administering medications by IV bolus cannot be delegated to nursing assistive personnel (NAP). The nurse instructs the NAP about:
- Potential medication actions and side effects of the medications and immediately reporting their occurrence to the nurse.
- Reporting any patient complaints of moisture or discomfort around IV insertion site.
- Obtaining any required vital signs and reporting them to the nurse.

EQUIPMENT
- Watch with second hand
- Clean gloves

- Antiseptic swab
- Medication in vial or ampule
- Proper-size syringes for medication and saline flush with needleless device or sharps with engineered sharps injury protection (SESIP) needle (21- to 25-gauge)
- IV lock: Vial of normal saline flush solution (saline recommended [Alexander et al., 2014]); if institution continues to use heparin flush, the most common concentration is 10 units/mL; check institution policy
- Medication administration record (MAR) or computer printout
- Puncture-proof container for sharps

STEP	RATIONALE

ASSESSMENT

1. Compare accuracy and completeness of each MAR or computer printout with health care provider's written medication order. Check patient's name, medication name and dosage, route of administration, and time of administration. Recopy or reprint any portion of MAR that is difficult to read.

The order sheet is the most reliable source and only legal record of medications that patient is to receive. Ensures that patient receives correct medications (Mandrack et al., 2012). Illegible MARs are a source of medication errors (Alassaad et al., 2013).

Clinical Decision Point. Some IV medications can be pushed safely only when monitoring a patient continuously for dysrhythmias, blood pressure changes, or other adverse effects. Therefore, some medications can be pushed only in specific patient care units. Confirm agency guidelines.

2. Assess patient's medical and medication history and history of allergies. List any drug allergies on each page of the MAR and prominently display on patient's medical record. When allergies are present, patient should wear an allergy bracelet.

Determines need for medication or possible contraindications for medication administration. IV bolus delivers medication rapidly. Allergic response is immediate.

SKILL 17.6   ADMINISTERING MEDICATIONS BY INTRAVENOUS BOLUS—cont'd

STEP	RATIONALE
3. Review medication reference information for medication action, purpose, side effects, normal dose, time of peak onset, how slowly to give medication, and nursing implications such as need to dilute medication or administer it through a filter.	Knowledge of medication allows you to give it safely and monitor patient's response to therapy.
4. If you give medication through an existing IV line, determine compatibility of medication with IV fluids and any additives within IV solution.	IV medication is not always compatible with IV solution and/or additives, and a new site may be needed.
5. Assess patient's symptoms before initiating medication therapy.	Provides information to evaluate desired effects of medication.
6. Perform hand hygiene. (Apply clean gloves if risk of contacting body fluids.) Assess condition of IV needle insertion site for signs of infiltration or phlebitis.	Reduces transmission of microorganisms. Do not administer medication if site is edematous or inflamed.
7. Assess patency of patient's existing IV infusion line or saline lock.	For medication to reach venous circulation effectively, IV line must be patent, and fluids must infuse easily.
8. Assess patient's understanding of purpose of drug therapy.	Poses implications for education.

PLANNING

1. Perform hand hygiene. Collect appropriate equipment and MAR.	Reduces transmission of microorganisms. Ensures organized procedure.
2. Follow agency's no-interruption zone (NIZ) policy. Prepare medications for one patient at a time. Keep all pages of MARs or computer printouts for one patient together or look at only one patient's electronic MAR at a time.	Preventing distractions reduces medication preparation errors. Use NIZ when possible (Beyea, 2014; Yoder et al., 2015).

IMPLEMENTATION

1. Prepare medication for one patient at a time using aseptic technique. Attend to preparation and avoid distraction. Keep all pages of MARs or computer printouts for one patient together or look at only one patient's electronic MAR at a time. Check label of medication against MAR two times, when removing medication from unit dose or AMDS and before leaving medication preparation area (see Skill 17.4 when preparing IV medication). Perform hand hygiene.	Reduces transmission of microorganisms. Ensures that medication is sterile. *These are the first and second checks for accuracy* and ensure that correct medication is administered.

Clinical Decision Point. Some IV medications require dilution before administration. Verify with agency policy or pharmacy if dilution is permitted. If a small amount of medication is given (e.g., less than 1 mL), dilute medication in small amount (e.g., 5 mL) of normal saline or sterile water so the medication does not collect in the "dead spaces" (e.g., Y-site injection port, IV cap) of the IV delivery system.

---

2. Take medication to patient at correct time (see institution policy). Medications that require exact timing include STAT doses, first-time or loading doses, and one-time doses. Give time-critical scheduled medications at exact time ordered (no more than 30 minutes before or after scheduled dose). Give non–time-critical scheduled medications within a range of 1 or 2 hours of scheduled dose (ISMP, 2011a). During administration, apply six rights of medication administration.	Hospitals must adopt medication administration policy and procedure for timing of medication administration that considers nature of the prescribed medication, specific clinical application, and patient needs (CMS, 2011; ISMP, 2011a). Time-critical scheduled medications are those for which administration of maintenance doses more than 30 minutes before or after the scheduled dose may cause harm or result in substantial suboptimal therapy or pharmacological effect. Non–time-critical medications are those for which early or delayed administration within a specified range of either 1 or 2 hours should not cause harm or result in substantial suboptimal therapy or pharmacological effect (CMS, 2011; ISMP, 2011a).
3. Close room curtain or door.	Provides privacy.
4. Identify patient using at least two identifiers (e.g., name and birthday or name and medical record number) according to agency policy. Compare identifiers with information on patient's MAR or medical record.	Ensures correct patient. Complies with The Joint Commission standards and improves patient safety (TJC, 2018).

STEP	RATIONALE
5. At patient's bedside again compare MAR or computer printout with names of medications on medication labels and patient name. Ask patient if he or she has allergies.	*This is the third check for accuracy* and ensures that patient receives correct medication. Confirms patient's allergy history.
6. Discuss purpose of each medication, action, and possible adverse effects. Allow patient to ask questions. Explain that you will give medication through existing IV line. Encourage patient to report any discomfort at IV site.	Keep patient informed of planned therapies, minimizing anxiety. Patients who report pain at IV site help detect IV infiltrations early, lessening damage to surrounding tissues.
7. Perform hand hygiene and apply clean gloves.	Reduces transmission of infection.
8. IV push (existing IV line):	
a. Select injection port of IV tubing closest to patient. Use needleless injection port.	Follows provisions of Needle Safety and Prevention Act of 2001 (OSHA, n.d.).

Clinical Decision Point. Never administer IV medications through tubing that is infusing blood, blood products, or parenteral nutrition solutions.

STEP	RATIONALE
b. Clean injection port with antiseptic swab. Allow to dry.	Prevents transfer of microorganisms during blunt cannula insertion.
c. Connect syringe to IV line: Insert needleless tip of syringe containing drug through center of port (see illustration).	Prevents introduction of microorganisms. Prevents damage to port diaphragm and possible leakage from site.
d. Occlude IV line by pinching tubing just above injection port (see illustration). Pull back gently on plunger of syringe to aspirate for blood return.	Final check ensures that medication is being delivered into bloodstream.

Clinical Decision Point. In some cases, especially with smaller-gauge IV needles, blood return is not aspirated even if IV line is patent. If IV site does not show signs of infiltration and IV fluid is infusing without difficulty, give IV push.

STEP	RATIONALE
e. Release tubing and inject medication within amount of time recommended by institution policy, pharmacist, or medication reference manual. Use watch to time administrations (see illustration). You can pinch IV line while pushing medication and release it when not pushing medication. Allow IV fluids to infuse when not pushing medication.	Ensures safe medication infusion. Rapid injection of IV drug can be fatal. Allowing IV fluids to infuse while pushing IV drug enables medication to be delivered to patient at prescribed rate.
f. After injecting medication, withdraw syringe and recheck IV fluid infusion rate.	Injection of bolus may alter rate of fluid infusion. Rapid fluid infusion can cause circulatory fluid overload.

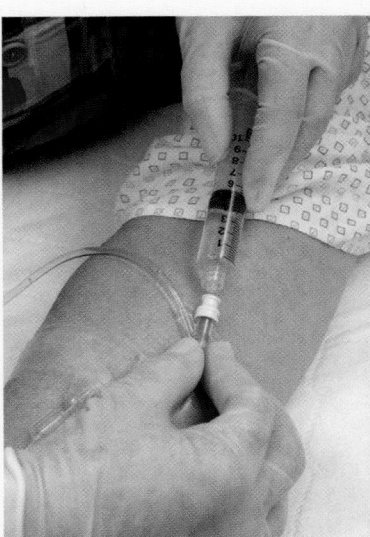
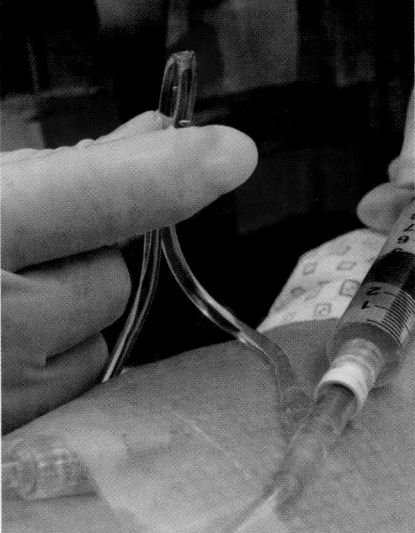
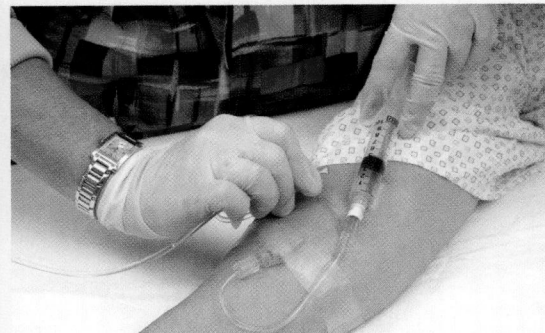

STEP 8c Connecting syringe to IV line with blunt needleless cannula tip.

STEP 8d IV line pinched above injection port allowing to aspirate for blood return.

STEP 8e Using watch to time an IV push medication.

SKILL 17.6   ADMINISTERING MEDICATIONS BY INTRAVENOUS BOLUS—cont'd

STEP	RATIONALE
g. If IV medication is incompatible with IV fluids, stop IV fluids, clamp IV line, and flush with 10 mL of normal saline or sterile water (see institution policy). Then give IV bolus over appropriate amount of time and flush with another 10 mL of normal saline or sterile water at *same rate* as medication was administered. Restart IV fluids at prescribed rate.	Allows IV bolus to be administered without risks associated with IV incompatibilities. Ensure that institution guidelines permit flushing lines with incompatible medications. A new site may be needed.
h. If IV line that is currently hanging is a medication, disconnect it and administer IV push medication as outlined in Step 9. Verify institution policy for stopping IV fluids or continuous IV medications. If unable to stop IV infusion, start new IV site and administer medication using IV push (IV lock) method.	Avoids giving patient sudden bolus of medication in existing IV line.
9. IV push (IV lock):	
a. Prepare two syringes filled with 2 to 3 mL of normal saline (0.9%).	Normal saline is effective in keeping IV locks patent, is compatible with wide range of medications (Patidar et al., 2014), and does not carry risk of thrombocytopenia with heparin.
b. Administer medication:	
(1) Clean lock injection port with antiseptic swab.	Prevents transfer of microorganisms during needle insertion.
(2) Insert needleless tip of syringe with normal saline 0.9% through center of injection port of IV lock (see illustrations).	
(3) Pull back gently on syringe plunger and check for blood return.	Indicates whether needle or catheter is in vein.
(4) Flush IV site with normal saline by pushing slowly on plunger.	Clears needle and reservoir of blood. Flushing without difficulty indicates patent IV line.

Clinical Decision Point. Carefully observe the area of skin above the IV catheter. Note any puffiness or swelling as IV site is flushed, which could indicate infiltration into the vein, requiring removal of catheter.

---

(5) Remove saline-filled syringe.	
(6) Clean injection port with antiseptic swab.	Prevents transmission of microorganisms.
(7) Insert needleless tip of syringe containing prepared Gmedication through injection port of IV lock.	Allows administration of medication.
(8) Inject medication within amount of time recommended by institution policy, pharmacist, or medication reference manual. Use watch to time administration.	Many medication errors are associated with IV pushes that are administered too quickly. Following guidelines for IV push rates promotes patient safety.
(9) After administering bolus, withdraw syringe.	

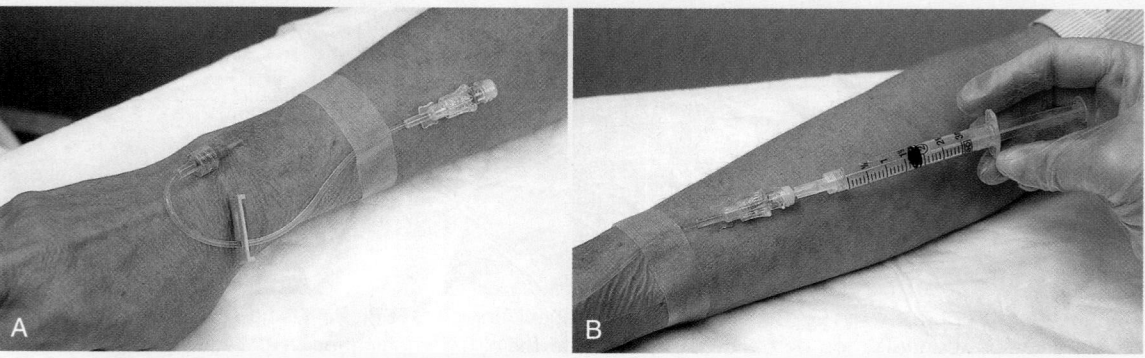

STEP 9b(2) A, IV catheter with saline lock adapter. **B,** Syringe inserted into injection port.

STEP	RATIONALE
(10) Clean injection port with antiseptic swab.	Prevents transmission of microorganisms.
(11) Flush injection port by attaching syringe with normal saline and inject flush at same rate that medication was delivered. Remove syringe.	Flushing IV line with saline prevents occlusion of IV access device and ensures that all medication is delivered. Flushing IV site at same rate as medication ensures that any medication remaining within IV needle is delivered at the correct rate.
10. Dispose of SESIP-covered needles and syringes in puncture-proof and leak-proof container.	Prevents accidental needlestick injuries and follows CDC guidelines for disposal of sharps (OSHA, n.d.).
11. Stay with patient for several minutes and observe for any allergic reactions.	Dyspnea, wheezing, and circulatory collapse are signs of anaphylactic reaction.
12. Remove gloves and perform hand hygiene.	Reduces transmission of microorganisms.

EVALUATION

1. Observe patient closely for adverse reactions during administration and for several minutes thereafter.	IV medications act rapidly.
2. Observe IV site during injection for sudden swelling and for 48 hours after IV push.	Swelling indicates infiltration into tissues surrounding vein. Signs of infiltration may not occur for 48 hours.
3. Evaluate patient's status after giving medication to evaluate effectiveness of the medication.	Some IV bolus medications can cause rapid changes in patient's physiological status. Some medications require careful monitoring and assessment and possibly future laboratory testing (such as vasopressors and antiarrhythmics, which require blood pressure and heart rate monitoring, and heparin, which requires laboratory studies after administration to determine therapeutic levels).
4. **Use Teach-Back:** "I want to be sure I explained to you why you are receiving this medication I am giving you in your IV. Tell me in your own words what this medication is for and what we expect it will do for you." Revise your instruction now or develop a plan for revised patient/family caregiver teaching if patient/family caregiver is not able to teach back correctly	Determines patient's/family caregiver's level of understanding of instructional topic.

RECORDING AND REPORTING

- Immediately record medication administration including drug, dose, route, time instilled, and date and time administered on MAR in electronic health record (EHR) or chart. Include initials or signature.
- Record patient teaching and validation of understanding on flow sheet or nurses' notes in EHR or chart.
- Record patient's medication response in nurses' notes.
- Report any adverse reactions to patient's health care provider. Patient's response sometimes indicates need for additional medical therapy.

UNEXPECTED OUTCOMES AND RELATED INTERVENTIONS

- Patient develops adverse reaction to medication.
  - Stop delivering medication immediately and follow institution policy or guidelines for appropriate response to allergic reaction and reporting of adverse drug reactions.
  - Notify patient's health care provider of adverse effects immediately. Add allergy information to patient's record.
- IV site shows symptoms of infiltration or phlebitis.
  - Stop IV infusion immediately or discontinue access device and restart in another site.
  - Determine how much damage IV medication can produce in subcutaneous tissue.
  - Provide IV extravasation care as indicated by institution policy.

SKILL 17.7 ADMINISTERING INTRAVENOUS MEDICATIONS BY PIGGYBACK, INTERMITTENT INFUSION SETS, AND MINI-INFUSION PUMPS

DELEGATION AND COLLABORATION

The skill of administering IV medications by piggyback, intermittent infusion sets, and mini-infusion pumps cannot be delegated to nursing assistive personnel (NAP). The nurse instructs the NAP about:

- Potential medication actions and side effects and immediately reporting their occurrence to the nurse.
- Reporting any patient complaints of moisture or discomfort around IV insertion site.
- Reporting any change in patient's condition or vital signs to the nurse.

EQUIPMENT

- Adhesive tape *(optional)*
- Antiseptic swab
- Clean gloves
- IV pole

- Medication administration record (MAR) or computer printout
- Puncture-proof container for sharps

Piggyback or Mini-Infusion Pump

- Medication prepared in 50- to 250-mL labeled infusion bag or syringe
- Prefilled syringe of normal saline flush solution (for saline lock only)
- Short microdrip, macrodrip, or mini-infusion IV tubing set with blunt-ended (needleless) cannula attachment
- Needleless device
- Mini-infusion pump if indicated

Volume-Control Administration Set

- Volutrol or Buretrol
- Infusion tubing with needleless system attachment
- Syringe (1 to 20 mL)
- Vial or ampule of ordered medication

STEP	RATIONALE

ASSESSMENT

1. Check accuracy and completeness of each MAR or computer printout with health care provider's written medication order. Check patient's name, medication name and dosage, route of administration, and time of administration. Recopy or reprint any portion of MAR that is difficult to read.

2. Assess patient's medical and medication history and history of allergies. List any drug allergies on each page of the MAR and prominently display on patient's medical record. When allergies are present, patient should wear an allergy bracelet.

3. Review medication reference information for medication action, purpose, normal dose, side effects, time and peak of onset, how slowly to give medication, and nursing implications (e.g., need to dilute medication, administer through filter).

4. If you give medication through existing IV line, determine compatibility of medication with IV fluids and any additional additives within IV solution.

The order sheet is the most reliable source and only legal record of medications that patient is to receive. Ensures that patient receives correct medications (Mandrack et al., 2012). Illegible MARs are a source of medication errors (Alassaad et al., 2013).

Determines need for medication or possible contraindications for medication administration. IV administration delivers medication rapidly and can cause rapid allergic response.

Allows you to administer medication safely and monitor patient's response to therapy.

IV medication is sometimes not compatible with IV solution and/or additives.

Clinical Decision Point. Never administer IV medications through tubing that is infusing blood, blood products, or parenteral nutrition solutions.

---

5. Perform hand hygiene. Assess condition of IV needle insertion site for signs of infiltration or phlebitis.

6. Assess patency and placement of patient's existing IV infusion line or saline lock (see Chapter 18).

Do not administer medication if site is edematous or inflamed.

For medication to reach venous circulation effectively, IV line must be patent, and fluids must infuse easily.

Clinical Decision Point. If patient's IV site is saline locked, clean the port with alcohol and assess the patency of the IV line by flushing it with 2 to 3 mL of sterile sodium chloride.

---

7. Assess patient's symptoms before initiating medication therapy.

8. Assess patient's knowledge of medication.

Provides information to evaluate desired effects of medication.

Poses implications for education.

STEP	RATIONALE

PLANNING

1. Perform hand hygiene. Collect appropriate equipment and MAR.

   Reduces transmission of microorganisms. Ensures organized procedure.

2. Follow agency's no-interruption zone (NIZ) policy. Prepare medications for one patient at a time. Keep all pages of MARs or computer printouts for one patient together or look at only one patient's electronic MAR at a time.

   Preventing distractions reduces medication preparation errors. Use NIZ when possible (Beyea, 2014; Yoder et al., 2015).

IMPLEMENTATION

1. Prepare medications for one patient at a time using aseptic technique. Attend to the procedure and avoid distraction. Check label of medication against MAR two times, when removing medication from unit dose or AMDS and before leaving medication preparation area (see Skill 17.4). Pharmacy prepares piggyback and prefilled syringes. You will prepare medication for a volume administration set. Perform hand hygiene.

   Reduces transmission of microorganisms. Ensures that medication is sterile. *These are the first and second checks for accuracy* and ensure that correct medication is administered.

2. Take medication to patient at correct time (see agency policy). Medications that require exact timing include STAT doses, first-time or loading doses, and one time doses. Give time-critical scheduled medications at exact time ordered (no later than 30 minutes before or after scheduled dose). Give non–time-critical scheduled medications within a range of 1 or 2 hours of scheduled dose (ISMP, 2011a). During administration, apply six rights of medication administration.

   Hospitals must adopt medication administration policy and procedure for timing of medication administration that considers nature of the prescribed medication, specific clinical application, and patient needs (CMS, 2011; ISMP, 2011a). Time-critical scheduled medications are those for which early or delayed administration of maintenance doses may cause harm or result in substantial suboptimal therapy or pharmacological effect. Non–time-critical medications are those for which early or delayed administration should not cause harm or result in substantial suboptimal therapy or pharmacological effect (CMS, 2011; ISMP, 2011a).

3. Close room curtain or door.

   Provides privacy.

4. Identify patient using at least two identifiers (e.g., name and birthday or name and medical record number) according to agency policy. Compare identifiers with information on patient's MAR or medical record.

   Ensures correct patient. Complies with The Joint Commission standards and improves patient safety (TJC, 2018).

5. At patient's bedside again compare MAR or computer printout with names of medications on medication labels and patient name. Ask patient if he or she has allergies.

   This is the third check for accuracy and ensures that patient receives correct medication. Confirms patient's allergy history.

6. Discuss purpose of each medication, action, and possible adverse effects. Allow patient to ask any questions. Explain that you will give medication through existing IV line. Encourage patient to report symptoms of discomfort at site.

   Keeping patient informed of planned therapies minimizes anxiety. Patients who report pain at IV site help detect IV infiltrations early, lessening damage to surrounding tissues.

7. Perform hand hygiene and apply clean gloves. Administer drug infusion.

   Reduces transmission of infection.

   a. **Piggyback infusion:**

      (1) Connect infusion tubing to medication bag (see Chapter 18). Fill tubing by opening regulator flow clamp. Once tubing is full, close clamp and cap end of tubing.

      Filling infusion tubing with solution and freeing air bubbles prevent air embolus.

SKILL 17.7   ADMINISTERING INTRAVENOUS MEDICATIONS BY PIGGYBACK, INTERMITTENT INFUSION SETS, AND MINI-INFUSION PUMPS—cont'd

STEP	RATIONALE
(2) Hang piggyback (see illustration) medication bag above level of primary fluid bag. (Use hook to lower main bag.)	Height of fluid bag affects rate of flow to patient.
(3) Connect tubing of piggyback infusion to appropriate connector on upper Y-port of primary infusion line:	Connection allows IV medication to enter main IV line.
(a) Needleless system: Wipe off needleless port of main IV line with alcohol swab, allow to dry, and insert cannula tip of piggyback infusion tubing (see illustrations).	Use needleless connections to prevent accidental needlestick injuries (INS, 2016; OSHA, n.d.).
(4) *Option:* Normal saline lock: Follow steps to flush and prepare a saline lock (see Chapter 18). Wipe off port with alcohol swab, let dry, and insert tip of piggyback infusion tubing via needleless access.	Flushing of lock ensures patency.
(5) Regulate flow rate of medication solution by adjusting regulator clamp or IV pump infusion rate. Infusion times vary. Refer to medication reference or agency policy for safe flow rate.	Provides slow, safe, intermittent infusion of medication and maintains therapeutic blood levels.

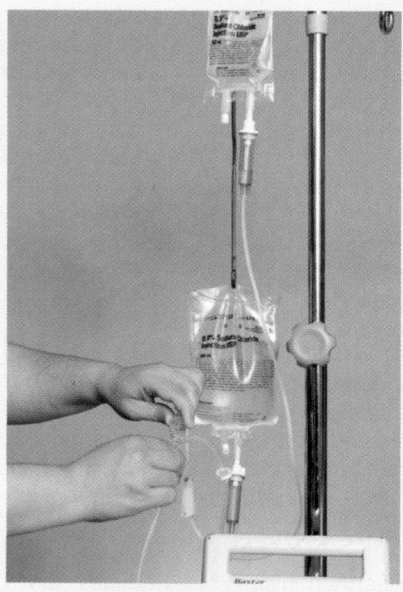

STEP 7a(2) Small-volume minibag for piggyback infusion.

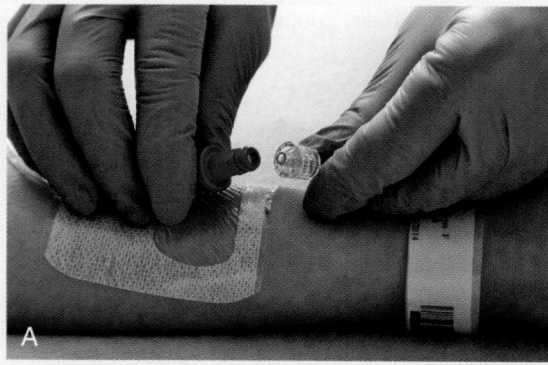
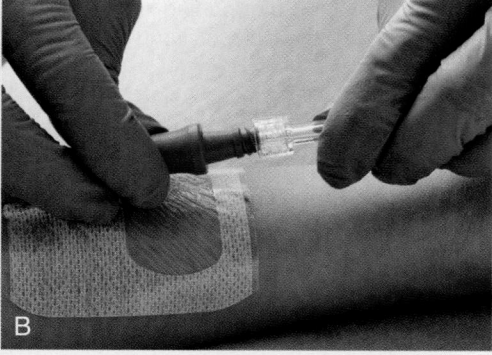

STEP 7a(3)(a) A, Needless lock cannula system. **B,** Blunt-ended cannula inserts into port and locks.

STEP	RATIONALE
(6) Once medication has infused:	
(a) Continuous infusion: Check flow rate of primary infusion. Primary infusion automatically begins after piggyback solution is empty.	Back-check valve on piggyback prevents flow of primary infusion until medication infuses. Checking flow rate ensures proper administration of IV fluids.
(b) Normal saline lock: Disconnect tubing, clean port with alcohol, and flush IV line with 2 to 3 mL of sterile 0.9% sodium chloride. Maintain sterility of IV tubing between intermittent infusions.	
(7) Regulate continuous main infusion line to ordered rate.	Infusion of piggyback sometimes interferes with main line infusion rate.
(8) Leave IV piggyback and tubing in place for future drug administration (see agency policy) or discard in puncture-proof and leak-proof container.	Establishment of secondary line produces route for microorganisms to enter main line. Repeated changes in tubing increase risk for infection transmission.
b. Volume-control administration set (e.g., Volutrol):	
(1) Fill Volutrol with desired amount of IV fluid (50 to 100 mL) by opening clamp between Volutrol and main IV bag (see illustration).	Small volume of fluid dilutes IV medication and reduces risk of fluid infusing too rapidly.
(2) Close clamp and check to be sure that clamp on air vent Volutrol chamber is open.	Prevents additional leakage of fluid into Volutrol. Air vent allows fluid in Volutrol to exit at regulated rate.
(3) Clean injection port on top of Volutrol with antiseptic swab.	Prevents introduction of microorganisms during needle insertion.
(4) Remove needle cap or sheath and insert needleless syringe or syringe needle through port and inject medication (see illustration). Gently rotate Volutrol between hands.	Rotating mixes medication with solution to ensure equal distribution in Volutrol.
(5) Regulate IV infusion rate to allow medication to infuse in time recommended by agency policy, pharmacist, or medication reference manual.	For optimal therapeutic effect, medication should infuse in prescribed time interval.
(6) Label Volutrol with name of medication, dosage, total volume including diluent, and time of administration following ISMP (2015h) safe medication label format.	Alerts nurses to medication being infused. Prevents other medications from being added to Volutrol.
(7) If patient is receiving continuous IV infusion, check infusion rate after Volutrol infusion is complete.	Ensures appropriate rate of administration.
(8) Dispose of uncapped needle or needle enclosed in safety shield and syringe in puncture-proof and leak-proof container. Discard supplies in appropriate container. Perform hand hygiene.	Prevents accidental needlesticks (OSHA, n.d.). Reduces transmission of microorganisms.

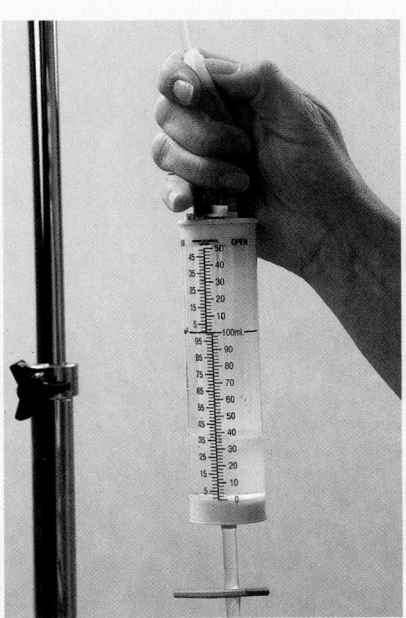

STEP 7b(1) Fill volume-control administration device.

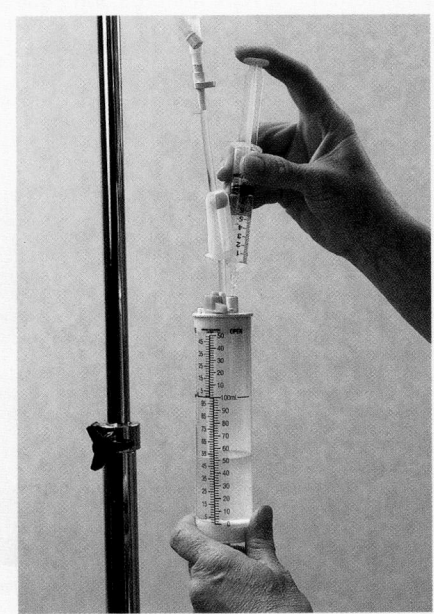

STEP 7b(4) Medication injected into device.

SKILL 17.7   ADMINISTERING INTRAVENOUS MEDICATIONS BY PIGGYBACK, INTERMITTENT INFUSION SETS, AND MINI-INFUSION PUMPS—cont'd

STEP	RATIONALE
c. Mini-infusion pump administration:	
(1) Connect prefilled syringe to mini-infusion pump tubing; remove end cap of tubing.	Special tubing designed to fit syringe delivers medication to main IV line.
(2) Carefully apply pressure to syringe plunger, allowing tubing to fill with medication.	Ensures that tubing is free of air bubbles to prevent air embolus.
(3) Place syringe into mini-infusion pump (follow product directions) and hang on IV pole. Be sure that syringe is secured (see illustration).	Secure placement is needed for proper infusion.
(4) Connect end of mini-infusion pump tubing to main IV line or saline lock:	Establishes route for IV medication to enter main IV line.
(a) Existing IV line: Wipe off needleless port on main IV line with alcohol swab, allow to dry, and insert tip of mini-infusion pump tubing through center of port.	Needleless connections reduce risk for accidental needlestick injuries (OSHA, n.d.).
(b) Normal saline lock: Follow steps to flush and prepare saline lock (see Chapter 18). Wipe off port with alcohol swab, allow to dry, and insert tip of mini-infusion tubing.	Flushing of lock ensures patency.
(5) Set pump to deliver medication within time recommended by agency policy, pharmacist, or medication reference manual. Press button on pump to begin infusion.	Pump automatically delivers medication at safe, constant rate based on volume in syringe.
(6) Once medication has infused:	
(a) Main IV infusion: Check flow rate. Infusion automatically begins to flow once pump stops. Regulate infusion to desired rate as needed.	Maintains patent primary IV fluids.
(b) Normal saline lock: Disconnect tubing, clean port with alcohol, and flush IV line with 2 to 3 mL of sterile 0.9% sodium chloride. Maintain sterility of IV tubing between intermittent infusions.	
8. Dispose of uncapped needles or needle enclosed in safety shield and syringes in puncture-proof and leak-proof container. Discard supplies in appropriate container. Remove and dispose of gloves, and perform hand hygiene.	Prevents accidental needlesticks (OSHA, n.d.). Reduces transmission of microorganisms.
9. Stay with patient for several minutes and observe for any allergic reactions.	Dyspnea, wheezing, and circulatory collapse are signs of severe anaphylactic reaction.

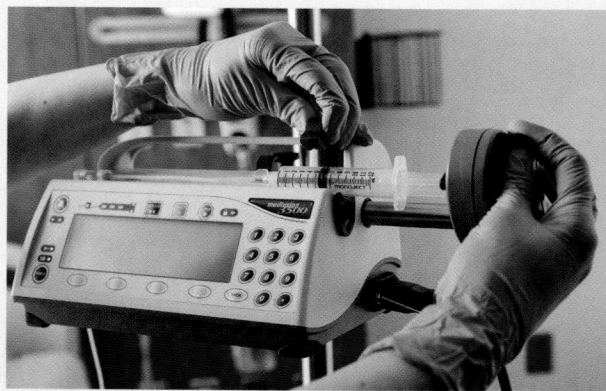

STEP 7c(3) Ensure that syringe is secure after placing it into mini-infusion pump.

STEP	RATIONALE

EVALUATION

1. Observe patient for signs or symptoms of adverse reaction.
2. During infusion periodically check infusion rate and condition of IV site.
3. Ask patient to explain purpose and side effects of medication.
4. **Use Teach-Back:** "I want to be sure I explained to you the reason for this IV medication. Can you explain to me why you are receiving the medication and what to report to the nurse?" Revise your instruction now or develop a plan for revised patient/family caregiver teaching if patient/family caregiver is not able to teach back correctly.

IV medications act rapidly.

IV must remain patent for proper drug administration. Infiltration of IV site requires discontinuing infusion.

Evaluates patient's understanding of instruction.

Determines patient's/family caregiver's level of understanding of instructional topic.

RECORDING AND REPORTING

- Immediately record medication, dose, route, infusion rate, and date and time administered on MAR in electronic health record (EHR) or chart. Include initials or signature.
- Record volume of fluid in medication bag or Volutrol on intake and output (I&O) form.

- Record patient teaching and validation of understanding on flow sheet or nurses' notes in EHR or chart.
- Report any adverse reactions to patient's health care provider.

UNEXPECTED OUTCOMES AND RELATED INTERVENTIONS

- Patient develops adverse or allergic reaction to medication.
  - Stop medication infusion immediately.
  - Follow agency policy or guidelines for appropriate response to allergic reaction (e.g., administration of antihistamine such as diphenhydramine or epinephrine) and reporting of adverse medication reactions.
  - Notify patient's health care provider of adverse effects immediately.
  - Add allergy information to patient record per agency policy.
- Medication does not infuse over established time frame.
  - Determine reason (e.g., improper calculation of flow rate, poor positioning of IV needle at insertion site, infiltration).
  - Take corrective action as indicated.

- IV site shows signs of infiltration or phlebitis (see Chapter 18).
  - Stop IV infusion and discontinue access device.
  - Treat IV site as indicated by agency policy.
  - Insert new IV catheter if therapy continues.
  - For infiltration determine how harmful IV medication is to subcutaneous tissue. Provide IV extravasation care (e.g., injecting phentolamine around IV infiltration site) as indicated by agency policy or consult pharmacist to determine appropriate follow-up care.

▌ KEY POINTS

- Application of knowledge about the four major pharmacokinetic processes—medication absorption, distribution, metabolism, and excretion—allows you to better time medication administration, select the route of administration, and evaluate a patient's response.
- Prompt recognition and reporting of adverse drug events prevents serious patient injury.
- Hospitalized patients with known drug allergies have their allergy information recorded in a clearly identifiable place to inform all caregivers.
- When a medication is prescribed, the goal is a constant blood level within a safe therapeutic range.

- Medications that are time-critical most likely cause harm or have subtherapeutic effects if they are not administered on time (usually 30 minutes before or after scheduled dose).
- The route prescribed for administering a medication depends on its properties and desired effect and on a patient's physical and mental condition.
- Metric units are easy to convert and calculate using simple multiplication and division with each basic unit of measurement organized into units of 10.
- Responsibilities of medication administration include knowing medication therapeutics, assessing a patient for administration, calculating doses, administering medications using the six rights of medication administration,

monitoring and evaluating medication effects, and assessing a patient's ability to self-administer medications.

- The six rights of medication administration are the right medication, right dose, right patient, right route, right time, and right documentation.
- Before administering medications, perform a physical assessment to reveal physical findings for any indications or contraindications for medication therapy.
- Factors contributing to medication nonadherence in older adults include depression, problems with cognitive or functional abilities, dislike for medication side effects, a busy and active lifestyle, and inability to afford medications.
- Collaboration with patients and family caregivers is essential, particularly if patients will require assistance with self-administration and if medication regimens are complicated.
- For patient safety it is essential that you refer to the MAR each time you prepare a medication and have it available at the patient's bedside when administering medications.
- Distractions may cause a medication error. Distractions include a page, phone call, request from a colleague or patient that draws away, disturbs, or diverts attention from a current desired task or forces attention on a new task at least temporarily.
- An important precaution with any oral preparation is to protect patients from aspiration.
- Rotate IM injection sites to decrease the risk for tissue hypertrophy, and use the Z-track method for administration.

REFLECTIVE LEARNING

- At the end of a clinical day when you have administered medications, describe how you incorporated patient teaching into the procedure.
- After being assigned a patient to whom you administered an oral medication, consider how you would administer a tablet differently for a patient with difficulty swallowing compared with a patient with normal swallowing.
- Consider a patient to whom you are assigned. Identify three risks specific for that patient to receive an IV bolus medication.

REVIEW QUESTIONS

1. A patient who had a stroke 3 days ago is still hospitalized and receiving oral medications. Which of the following techniques reduce the patient's risk of aspiration? (Select all that apply.)
   1. Do not allow patient to self-administer medication.
   2. Assess patient for cough or change in voice tone or quality after swallowing.
   3. Assess patient's gag reflex by offering 50 mL of water in 5-mL allotments.
   4. Position the patient laying on the side with head tilted backward.
   5. Give medication either as a liquid or as a solid based on patient's swallowing ability.

2. A nurse is administering an oral tablet to a patient. Which of the following steps is the *second check* for accuracy in determining the patient is receiving the right medication?
   1. Logging on to ADS or unlocking medicine drawer or cart.
   2. Before going to patient's room, comparing patient's name and name of medication on label of prepared drugs with MAR.
   3. Selecting correct medication from ADS, unit-dose drawer, or stock supply and comparing name of medication on label with MAR or computer printout.
   4. Comparing MAR or computer printout with names of medications on medication labels and patient name at patient's bedside.

3. The nurse is preparing to administer medications to an 80-year-old patient who had a total hip replacement 12 hours ago. The patient has a history of heart failure, diabetes, and glaucoma. The nurse will administer furosemide 40 mg PO, a subcutaneous injection of 20 units NPH insulin, pilocarpine gtts 1 in both eyes, and 1.0 mL of hydromorphone IV push. Which of the medications is most dangerous to administer to this patient?
   1. Furosemide 40 mg PO
   2. Pilocarpine gtts 1 in both eyes
   3. Hydromorphone 1.0 mL IV push
   4. NPH insulin 20 units subcutaneous

4. The nurse is preparing a heparin injection for a patient who has a recent history of a deep vein thrombosis. The patient's height and weight are 172 cm (5 feet 9 inches) and 102 kg (225 lb). Place the steps for administering the injection in the correct order:
   1. Cleanse site with antiseptic swab.
   2. Hold syringe between thumb and forefinger of dominant hand like a dart, with palm down.
   3. Choose an injection site on the abdomen.
   4. Assist patient to lie in a supine position, relaxing abdomen.
   5. Pinch skin with nondominant hand and insert needle quickly at 90-degree angle.
   6. While holding antiseptic swab between third and fourth finger of dominant hand, remove needle cap from syringe

5. A young adult patient tells her nurse that she is afraid of injections. The nurse is preparing to administer the patient a flu vaccine. Which of the following techniques can the nurse use to reduce the patient's discomfort? (Select all that apply.)
   1. Ask the patient to think about why the injection is necessary
   2. Position the patient comfortably
   3. Apply a vapocoolant to the skin before giving the injection
   4. Use a large gauge needle
   5. Carefully use anatomical landmarks to select injection site

evolve

Additional Review Questions, as well as rationales for all Review Questions, can be found on the Evolve website.

1, 2, 3, 5; 2, 3; 3, 4, 3, 4, 1, 6, 2, 5; 5, 2, 3, 5.

REFERENCES

Agency for Healthcare Research and Quality (AHRQ): *Medication errors*, 2015. https://psnet.ahrq.gov/primers/primer/23/medication-errors.

Agency for Healthcare Research and Quality (AHRQ): *Computerized physician order entry*, 2016. https://psnet.ahrq.gov/primers/primer/6/computerized-provider-order-entry.

Akbari Sari A, et al: Slow versus fast subcutaneous heparin injections for preventing bruising and site-pain intensity, *Cochrane Database Syst Rev* (7):CD008077, 2014.

Alassaad A, et al: Prescription and transcription errors in multidose-dispensed medication on discharge from hospital: an observational and interventional study, *J Eval Clin Pract* 19(1):185, 2013.

Alexander AJ, et al: Medication reconciliation campaign in a clinic for homeless patients, *Am J Health Syst Pharm* 69(7):558, 2012.

Alexander M, et al: *Core curriculum for infusion nursing*, ed 4, Philadelphia, 2014, Williams & Wilkins.

Allen SM: As a flushing agent for enteral nutrition, does sterile water compared with tap water affect associated risk of infection in critically ill patients, *Ala Nurse*, March-April-May:5, 2015.

American Academy of Allergy, Asthma and Immunology (AAAAI): *Peak flow meter*, 2016. https://www.aaaai.org/conditions-and-treatments/library/at-a-glance/peak-flow-meter.

American Association of Diabetes Educators (AADE): *Teaching injection technique to people with diabetes*, 2013. https://www.diabeteseducator.org/docs/default-source/legacy-docs/_resources/pdf/research/injectioneducationpracticeguide.pdf?sfvrsn=2.

American Diabetes Association (ADA): Diabetes care in the hospital, nursing home, and skilled nursing facility, *Diabetes Care* 38(S1):S80, 2015. http://care.diabetesjournals.org/content/38/Supplement_1/S80.full.

American Hospital Association (AHA): *The patient care partnership*, 2003. http://www.aha.org/advocacy-issues/communicatingpts/pt-care-partnership.shtml.

American Medical Association (AMA): *Procedure for USAN name selection*, 2016. http://www.ama-assn.org/ama/pub/physician-resources/medical-science/united-states-adopted-names-council/generic-drug-naming-explained.page.

American Nurses Association (ANA): *Nursing: scope and standards of practice*, ed 3, Silver Spring, MD, 2015, The Association.

American Pharmacists' Association (APhA): *Incorrect injection technique can result in serious shoulder injuries*, 2015. https://www.pharmacist.com/incorrect-injection-technique-can-result-serious-shoulder-injuries-0.

American Society of Health-System Pharmacists (ASHP): *How to use eye drops properly*, 2013a. http://www.safemedication.com/safemed/MedicationTipsTools/HowtoAdminister/HowtoUseEyeDropsProperly.aspx.

American Society of Health-System Pharmacists (ASHP): *How to use nose drops properly*, 2013b. http://www.safemedication.com/safemed/MedicationTipsTools/HowtoAdminister/HowtoUseNoseDropsProperly.aspx.

Anderson P, Townsend T: Preventing high-alert medication errors in hospital patients, *Am Nurse Today* 10(5):2015. https://www.americannursetoday.com/preventing-high-alert-medication-errors.

Ari A, Restrepo RD: Aerosol delivery device selection for spontaneously breathing patients, *Respir Care* 57(4):613, 2012.

Bae JP, et al: Adherence and dosing frequency of common medications for cardiovascular patients, *Am J Manag Care* 18(3):139, 2012.

Barnes MG, et al: A "needling" problem: shoulder injury related to vaccine administration, *J Am Board Fam Med* 25:919, 2012.

Barrons R, et al: Opportunities for inhaler device selection in elderly patients with asthma or COPD, *Patient Intell* 7:53, 2015. https://www.dovepress.com/opportunities-for-inhaler-device-selection-in-elderly-patients-with-as-peer-reviewed-article-PI.

Bartlett R, et al: Harm reduction: compassionate care of persons with addictions, *Medsurg Nurs* 22(6):349, 2013.

Beyea S: *Interruptions and distractions in health care: improved safety with mindfulness*, Agency for Healthcare Research and Quality, 2014. https://psnet.ahrq.gov/perspectives/perspective/152/interruptions-and-distractions-in-health-care-improved-safety-with-mindfulness.

Bhalla MC, et al: Predictors of epinephrine autoinjector needle length inadequacy, *Am J Emerg Med* 31(12):1671, 2013.

Bonini M, Usmani OS: The importance of inhaler devices in the treatment of COPD, *COPD Res Pract* 1:9, 2015. https://copdrp.biomedcentral.com/articles/10.1186/s40749-015-0011-0.

Borovina LR, et al: The microbial contamination of pressurised metered-dose inhalers anonymously sourced from the South-East Queensland Australia community population, *Int J Pharm Pract* 20(2):129, 2012.

Bourzac K: Dissolving disks deliver drugs to the eye, *Chemical and Engineering News*, February 5, 2015. http://cen.acs.org/articles/93/web/2015/02/Dissolving-Disks-Deliver-Drugs-Eye.html.

Boysen PG: Just culture: a foundation for balanced accountability and patient safety, *Ochsner J* 13(3):400, 2013.

Burchum J, Rosenthal L: *Lehne's pharmacology for nursing care*, ed 9, St Louis, 2016, Saunders.

Centers for Disease Control and Prevention (CDC): *Stop sticks campaign*, 2010. http://www.cdc.gov/niosh/stopsticks/sharpsdisposal.html.

Centers for Disease Control and Prevention (CDC): *Bloodborne pathogens—occupational exposure*, 2013. https://www.cdc.gov/oralhealth/infectioncontrol/bloodborne_exposures.htm.

Centers for Disease Control and Prevention (CDC): *Vaccine administration*, 2015. http://www.cdc.gov/vaccines/pubs/pinkbook/vac-admin.html.

Centers for Disease Control and Prevention (CDC): *Deaths and mortality: numbers of deaths for leading cause of death*, 2016a. https://www.cdc.gov/nchs/fastats/deaths.htm.

Centers for Disease Control and Prevention (CDC): *What is health literacy?* 2016b. http://www.cdc.gov/healthliteracy/learn/index.html.

Centers for Medicare and Medicaid Services (CMS): *Updated guidance on medication administration, Hospital Appendix A of the State Operations Manual (SOM)*, 2011. http://www.ismp.org/download/files/Updated_IGs_Medication_Adminis_Nov-18-11.pdf.

Chapuis C, et al: Automated drug dispensing systems in the intensive care unit: a financial analysis, *Crit Care* 19:318, 2015.

Ching JM, et al: Using lean "automation with a human touch" to improve medication safety: a step closer to the "perfect dose", *Jt Comm J Qual Patient Saf* 40(8):342, 2013.

ConsumerMedSafety: *Tips for measuring liquid medicines safely*, 2015. http://www.consumermedsafety.org/tools-and-resources/medication-safety-tools-and-resources/taking-your-medicine-safely/measure-liquid-medications.

Davidson K, Rourke L: Teaching best evidence: deltoid intramuscular injection technique, *J Nurs Educ Pract* 3(7):122, 2013.

Dayananda L, et al: Intended intramuscular gluteal injections: are they truly intramuscular? *J Postgrad Med* 60(2):175, 2014.

deMeneses AS, Marques IR: A proposal for a geometrical delimitation model for ventro-gluteal injection, *Rev Bras Enferm* 60(5):552, 2007.

Diggle D: Are you FIT for purpose? The importance of getting injection technique right, *J Diabetes Nurs* 18:50, 2014.

Donaldson N, et al: Improving medication administration safety: using naïve observation to assess practice and guide improvements in process and outcomes, *J Healthc Qual* 36(6):58, 2014.

Food and Drug Administration (FDA): *FDA reminds the public about the potential for life-threatening harm from accidental exposure to fentanyl transdermal systems ("patches")*, 2012. http://www.fda.gov/Drugs/DrugSafety/ucm300747.htm.

Food and Drug Administration (FDA): *Best practices for tablet splitting*, 2013. http://www.fda.gov/Drugs/ResourcesForYou/Consumers/BuyingUsingMedicineSafely/EnsuringSafeUseofMedicine/ucm184666.htm.

Food and Drug Administration (FDA): *MedWatch: the FDA safety information and adverse event reporting program*, 2016. http://www.fda.gov/Safety/MedWatch/.

Foulon V, et al: Patient adherence to oral anti-cancer drugs: an emerging issue in modern oncology, *Acta Clin Belg* 66(2):85, 2011.

Frid AH, et al: New insulin delivery recommendations, *Mayo Clin Proc* 91(19):1231, 2016.

Giger JN: *Transcultural nursing: assessment and intervention*, ed 7, St Louis, 2017, Elsevier.

Guenther P: New enteral connectors: raising awareness, *Nutr Clin Pract* 29:612, 2015.

Guenther P, Boullatta J: Drug administration by enteral feeding tube, *Nursing* 43(12):26, 2013.

Gūnes Y, et al: Is the ventrogluteal site suitable for intramuscular injections in children under the age of three? *J Adv Nurs* 72(1):127, 2016.

Hibbard P, et al: Approach to immunizations in healthy adults, *UpToDate*, 2015. http://www.uptodate.com/contents/approach-to-immunizations-in-healthy-adults.

Hirsch LJ, et al: Glycemic control, reported pain and leakage with a 4 mm × 32 G pen needle in obese and nonobese adults

with diabetes: a post hoc analysis, *Curr Med Res Opin* 28(8):1305, 2012.

Hockenberry MJ, Wilson D: *Wong's nursing care of infants and children*, ed 10, St Louis, 2015, Mosby.

Hopkins U, Arias CY: Large-volume IM injections: a review of best practices, *Oncol Nurse Advis* 32, 2013. http://www.oncologynurseadvisor.com/chemotherapy/large-volume-im-injections-a-review-of-best-practices/article/281208/.

Hopkinson SG, Jennings BM: Interruptions during nurses' work: a state-of-the-science review, *Res Nurs Health* 36(1):38, 2013.

Hu D, et al: Interventions to increase medication adherence in African-American and Latino populations: a literature review, *Hawaii J Med Public Health* 73(1):11, 2014.

Imran M, Hayley D: Injection-induced axillary nerve injury after a drive-through flu shot, *Clin Geriatr* 21(12):2013.

Infusion Nurses Society (INS): Infusion therapy standards of practice, *J Infus Nurs* 39(1 Suppl):S1, 2016.

Ingersoll K, et al: Motivational interviewing for substance use disorders, *UpToDate*, 2016. http://www.uptodate.com/contents/motivational-interviewing-for-substance-use-disorders.

Institute for Safe Medication Practices (ISMP): *ISMP's guidelines for standard order sets*, 2010. http://www.ismp.org/tools/guidelines/standardordersets.pdf.

Institute for Safe Medication Practices (ISMP): *Acute care guidelines for timely administration of scheduled medications*, 2011a. http://www.ismp.org/Tools/guidelines/acutecare/tasm.pdf.

Institute for Safe Medication Practices (ISMP): *ISMP statement on use of metric measurements to prevent errors with oral liquids*, 2011b. https://www.ismp.org/pressroom/PR20110808.pdf.

Institute for Safe Medication Practices (ISMP): *As U-500 insulin safety concerns mount, it's time to rethink safe use of strengths above U-100*, 2013a. https://www.ismp.org/newsletters/acutecare/showarticle.aspx?id=62.

Institute for Safe Medication Practices (ISMP): *Ongoing concern about insulin pen reuse shows hospitals need to consider transitioning away from them*, 2013b. http://www.ismp.org/newsletters/acutecare/showarticle.aspx?id=41.

Institute for Safe Medication Practices (ISMP): *Independent double checks: undervalued and misused: selective use of this strategy can play an important role in medication safety*, 2013c. https://www.ismp.org/newsletters/acutecare/showarticle.aspx?id=51.

Institute for Safe Medication Practices (ISMP): *List of high-alert medications in acute care settings*, 2014. https://www.ismp.org/tools/institutionalhighAlert.asp.

Institute for Safe Medication Practices (ISMP): *ISMP's list of confused drug names*, 2015a. https://www.ismp.org/tools/confuseddrugnames.pdf.

Institute for Safe Medication Practices (ISMP): *ISMP's list of error-prone abbreviations, symbols, and dose designations*, 2015b. https://www.ismp.org/tools/errorproneabbreviations.pdf.

Institute for Safe Medication Practices (ISMP): *Oral dosage forms that should not be crushed*, 2015c. http://www.ismp.org/tools/donotcrush.pdf.

Institute for Safe Medication Practices (ISMP): *Results of pediatric medication safety survey (part 2): comparing data subsets points out areas for improvement*, 2015d. https://www.ismp.org/newsletters/acutecare/showarticle.aspx?id=112.

Institute for Safe Medication Practices (ISMP): *ISMP safe practice guidelines for adult IV push medications*, 2015e. http://www.ismp.org/Tools/guidelines/IVSummitPush/IVPushMedGuidelines.Pdf.

Institute for Safe Medication Practices (ISMP): *Acute Care: ISMP Medication safety alert, A successful ENFit launch still won't stop all incidents of oral medications given intravenously* 20(16):1-4, 2015f. http://www.ismp.org/newsletters/acutecare/showarticle.aspx?id=115.

Institute for Safe Medication Practices (ISMP): *ENFit update*, 2015g. https://www.ismp.org/newsletters/acutecare/showarticle.aspx?id=1127.

Institute for Safe Medication Practices (ISMP): *Principles of designing a medication label for intravenous piggyback medication for patient-specific inpatient use*, 2015h. http://www.ismp.org/Tools/guidelines/labelFormats/Piggyback.asp.

Institute for Safe Medication Practices (ISMP): *FDA and ISMP lists of look-alike drug names with recommended tall man letters*, 2016a. https://www.ismp.org/tools/tallmanletters.pdf.

Institute for Safe Medication Practices (ISMP): *2016-2017 targeted medication safety best practices for hospitals*, 2016b. http://www.ismp.org/tools/bestpractices/TMSBP-for-hospitals.pdf.

Institute for Safe Medication Practices (ISMP): *Principles of designing a medication label for intravenous piggyback medication for patient specific inpatient use*, 2016c. https://www.ismp.org/tools/guidelines/labelFormats/IVPB.asp.

Institute for Safe Medication Practices (ISMP): *Acute Care ISMP Medication Safety Alert. Transition adapters for ENFit syringes can defeat the purpose of ENFit itself*, ISMP 22(19):1, 2017. https://www.ismp.org/newsletters/acutecare/currentissue.aspx.

Institute of Medicine (IOM): *Report brief, to err is human: building a safer health system*, 1999. http://www.nationalacademies.org/hmd/~/media/Files/Report%20Files/1999/To-Err-is-Human/To%20Err%20is%20Human%201999%20%20report%20brief.pdf.

Jimmy B, Jose J: Patient medication adherence: measures in daily practice, *Oman Med J* 26(3):155, 2011.

Kara D, et al: Using ventrogluteal site in intramuscular injections is a priority or an alternative? *Int J Caring Sciences* 8(2):507, 2015.

Kaya N, et al: The reliability of site determination methods in ventrogluteal area injection: a cross-sectional study, *Int J Nurs Stud* 52:355, 2015.

Kilic E, et al: Comparing applications of intramuscular injections to dorsogluteal or ventrogluteal regions, *J Exp Integr Med* 4(3):171, 2014.

Kim J, Bates DW: Medication administration errors by nurses: adherence to guidelines, *J Clin Nurs* 22(3/4):590, 2013.

Klang M, et al: Osmolality, pH, and compatibility of selected oral liquid medication with an enteral nutrition product, *JPEN J Parenter Enteral Nutr* 37:869, 2013.

Koohestani H, Baghcheghi N: Comparing the effects of two educational methods of intravenous drug rate calculations on rapid and sustained learning of nursing students: formula method and dimensional analysis method, *Nurse Educ Pract* 10(4):233, 2010.

Lavik E, et al: Novel drug delivery systems for glaucoma, *Eye (Lond)* 25(5):578, 2011.

Leporini C, et al: Adherence to therapy and adverse drug reactions: is there a link? *Expert Opin Drug Saf* 13(Suppl 1):S41, 2014.

Lilley LL, et al: *Pharmacology and the nursing process*, ed 8, St Louis, 2016, Mosby.

Makary MA, Daniel M: Medical error—the third leading cause of death in the US, *BMJ* 353:i2139, 2016.

Malone A: Clinical guidelines from the American Society for Parenteral and Enteral Nutrition: best practices recommendations for patient care, *J Infus Nurs* 37(3):179, 2014.

Mandrack M, et al: Nursing best practices using automated dispensing cabinets: nurses' key role in improving medication safety, *Medsurg Nurs* 21(3):134, 2012.

Mathes T, et al: Adherence influencing factors—a systematic review of systematic reviews, *Arch Public Health* 72:37, 2014.

McCulloch D: General principles of insulin therapy in diabetes mellitus, *UpToDate*, 2015. http://www.uptodate.com/contents/general-principles-of-insulin-therapy-in-diabetes-mellitus.

Murphy M, While A: Medication administration practices among children's nurses: a survey, *Br J Nurs* 21(15):928, 2012.

National Coordinating Council for Medication Error Reporting and Prevention (NCCMERP): *Recommendations to reduce medication errors associated with verbal medication orders and prescriptions*, 2015. http://www.nccmerp.org/recommendations-reduce-medication-errors-associated-verbal-medication-orders-and-prescriptions.

National Institutes of Health National Institute on Drug Abuse (NIH NIDA): *Prescription and over-the-counter medications*, 2015. https://www.drugabuse.gov/publications/drugfacts/prescription-over-counter-medications.

National Quality Forum (NQF): *Serious reportable events*, 2016. http://www.qualityforum.org/Topics/SREs/Serious_Reportable_Events.aspx.

Nicoll L, Hesby A: Intramuscular injection: an integrative research review and guideline for evidence-based practice, *Appl Nurs Res* 16(2):159, 2002.

Novo Nordisk: *Levemir*, 2015. http://www.levemir.com/.

Occupational Safety and Health Administration (OSHA): *Bloodborne pathogens and needlestick prevention*, n.d. https://www.osha.gov/SLTC/bloodbornepathogens/index.html.

Ogston-Tuck S: Subcutaneous injection technique: an evidence based approach, *Nurs Stand* 29(3):53, 2014a.

Ogston-Tuck S: Intramuscular injection technique: an evidence based approach, *Nurs Stand* 29(4):55, 2014b.

Ownby RL, et al: Tailored information and automated reminding to improve medication adherence in Spanish- and English-speaking elders treated for memory impairment, *Clin Gerontol* 35(3):221, 2012.

Palma S, Strohfus P: Are IM injections IM in obese and overweight females? A study in injection technique, *Appl Nurs Res* 26(4):e1, 2013.

Paparella S: Adopt the 2014-2015 targeted best practices for medication safety, *J Emerg Nurs* 40(3):263, 2014.

Park YH, et al: Prevalence and associated factors of dysphagia in nursing home residents, *Geriatr Nurs* 34(3):212, 2013.

Pasina L, et al: Medication non-adherence among elderly patients newly discharged and receiving polypharmacy, *Drugs Aging* 31(4):283, 2014.

Patidar AB, et al: Comparative efficacy of heparin saline and normal saline flush for maintaining patency of peripheral intravenous lines: a randomized control trial, *Int J Health Sci Res* 4(3):159, 2014.

Pfoh E, et al: High-alert drugs: patient safety practices for intravenous anticoagulants. In *Making health care safer II: an updated critical analysis of the evidence for patient safety practices*, Rockville, MD, 2013, Agency for Healthcare Research and Quality.

Pretorius RW, et al: Reducing the risk of adverse drug events in older adults, *Am Fam Physician* 87(5):331, 2013.

Radley DC, et al: Reduction in medication errors in hospitals due to adoption of computerized provider order entry systems, *J Am Med Inform Assoc* 20(3):470, 2013.

Rimando M: Factors influencing medication compliance among hypertensive older African American adults, *Ethn Dis* 23(4):469, 2013.

Rubak S, et al: Motivational interviewing: a systematic review and meta-analysis, *Br J Gen Pract* 55:305, 2005.

Sanofi-Aventis: *Lovenox subcutaneous injection*, 2014. http://www.lovenox.com/hcp_default.aspx.

Sawkin MT, et al: Health literacy and medication adherence among patients treated in a free health clinic: a pilot study, *Health Serv Res Manag Epidemiol* 2:2015. https://www.ncbi.nlm.nih.gov/pmc/articles/PMC5266426/.

Skidmore-Roth L: *Mosby's 2016 nursing drug reference*, ed 29, St Louis, 2016, Mosby.

Substance Abuse and Mental Health Services Administration (SAMHSA): *Behavioral health trends in the United States: results from the 2014 National Survey on Drug Use and Health*, 2015a. http://www.samhsa.gov/data/sites/default/files/NSDUH-FRR1-2014/NSDUH-FRR1-2014.pdf.

Substance Abuse and Mental Health Services Administration (SAMHSA): *Prescription drug misuse and abuse*, 2015b. http://www.samhsa.gov/prescription-drug-misuse-abuse.

Teunissen R, et al: Clinical relevance of and risk factors associated with medication administration time errors, *Am J Health Syst Pharm* 70(12):1052, 2013.

The Joint Commission (TJC): *Revisions to the medication management standards regarding sample medications*, July 2014a.

http://www.jointcommission.org/assets/1/6/SampleMedications_HAP.pdf.

The Joint Commission (TJC): *Sentinel alert event 53: managing risk during transition to new ISO connector standards*, 2014b. https://www.jointcommission.org/sea_issue_53/.

The Joint Commission (TJC): *Facts about the official "do not use" list of abbreviations*, 2016. https://www.jointcommission.org/facts_about_do_not_use_list/.

The Joint Commission (TJC): *2018 National Patient Safety Goals*, Oakbrook Terrace, IL, 2018, The Commission. http://www.jointcommission.org/standards_information/npsgs.aspx.

Touhy TA, Jett KF: *Ebersole and Hess' gerontological nursing and healthy aging*, ed 4, St Louis, 2014, Elsevier.

Voshall B, et al: Barcode medication administration work-arounds, *J Nurs Adm* 43(10):530, 2013.

Westbrook JI, et al: Association of interruptions with and increased risk and severity of medication administration errors, *Arch Intern Med* 170:683, 2010.

World Health Organization (WHO): *Injection safety*, 2015. http://www.who.int/injection_safety/en/.

Yoder M, et al: The effect of a safe zone on nurse interruptions, distractions, and medication administration errors, *J Infus Nurs* 38(2):140, 2015.

Zabaleta-Del-Olmo E, et al: Safety of the reuse of needles for subcutaneous insulin injection: a systematic review and meta-analysis, *Int J Nurs Stud* 60:121, 2016.

Fluid, Electrolyte, and Acid-Base Balances

evolve MEDIA RESOURCES

http://evolve.elsevier.com/Potter/essentials

- Audio Glossary
- Butterfield's Fluids and Electrolytes Tutorial
- QSEN Activity and Review Questions Answers and Rationales
- Video Clips
- Case Study Continuation

OBJECTIVES

- Describe physiological mechanisms that maintain fluid, electrolyte, and acid-base balances.
- Discuss risk factors for fluid, electrolyte, and acid-base imbalances.
- Describe different fluid, electrolyte, and acid-base imbalances.
- Identify appropriate clinical assessments for specific fluid, electrolyte, and acid-base imbalances.
- Discuss appropriate nursing interventions for patients with fluid, electrolyte, and acid-base imbalances.

- Describe purpose and procedures for initiation and maintenance of IV therapy.
- Calculate an IV flow rate.
- Discuss complications of IV therapy and what to do if they occur.
- Describe how to change IV solutions, tubing, and dressings.
- Describe the procedure for initiating a blood transfusion and complications of blood therapy.

KEY TERMS

acidosis, p. 486
active transport, p. 481
ADH, p. 483
aldosterone, p. 483
allogeneic transfusion, p. 506
alkalosis, p. 486
angiotensin, p. 483
anion gap, p. 486
anions, p. 481
arterial blood gas (ABG), p. 486
autologous transfusion, p. 506
buffers, p. 484
cations, p. 480
clinical dehydration, p. 484
colloid osmotic pressure, p. 482
colloids, p. 499
concentration, p. 484
crystalloids, p. 499

diffusion, p. 481
electrolyte, p. 480
electronic infusion devices (EIDs), p. 500
extracellular fluid volume (ECV) deficit, p. 490
extracellular fluid volume (ECV) excess, p. 484
filtration, p. 481
fluid, p. 480
fluid homeostasis, p. 482
hemolysis, p. 505
hydrostatic pressure, p. 482
hypercalcemia, p. 486
hyperchloremia, p. 486
hyperkalemia, p. 486
hypermagnesemia, p. 486
hypernatremia, p. 484

hypertonic, p. 481
hypocalcemia, p. 486
hypochloremia, p. 486
hypokalemia, p. 484
hypomagnesemia, p. 486
hyponatremia, p. 484
hypotonic, p. 481
hypovolemia, p. 484
infiltration, p. 504
insensible water loss, p. 482
ions, p. 480
isotonic, p. 481
metabolic acidosis, p. 486
metabolic alkalosis, p. 486
oncotic pressure, p. 482
osmolality, p. 481
osmoreceptors, p. 482
osmosis, p. 481

CASE STUDY *Mrs. Reynolds*

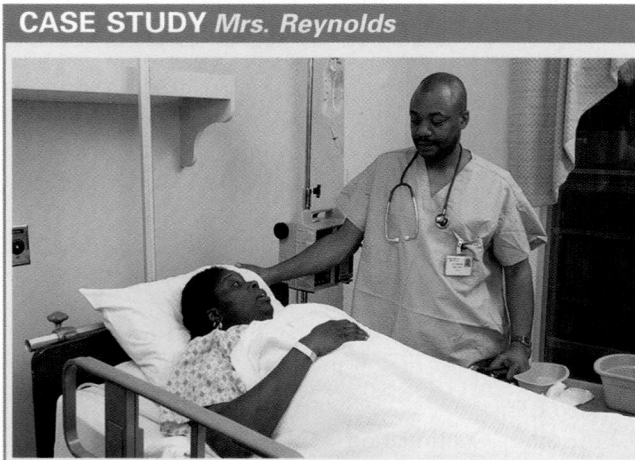

Susan Reynolds, a 42-year-old married accountant, was admitted yesterday to an acute care unit with a history of nausea, loss of appetite, and diarrhea for 7 days. She believes that her symptoms are related to "bad food" that she had on her recent business trip. Past medical history includes hypertension controlled by hydrochlorothiazide 25 mg by mouth once daily and a no added–salt diet.

Robert is a nursing student assigned to Mrs. Reynolds. He has cared for other patients with gastrointestinal (GI) disorders but none with fluid and electrolyte imbalances. Robert plans his care by reviewing Mrs. Reynolds' electronic health record (EHR) and health care provider's orders.

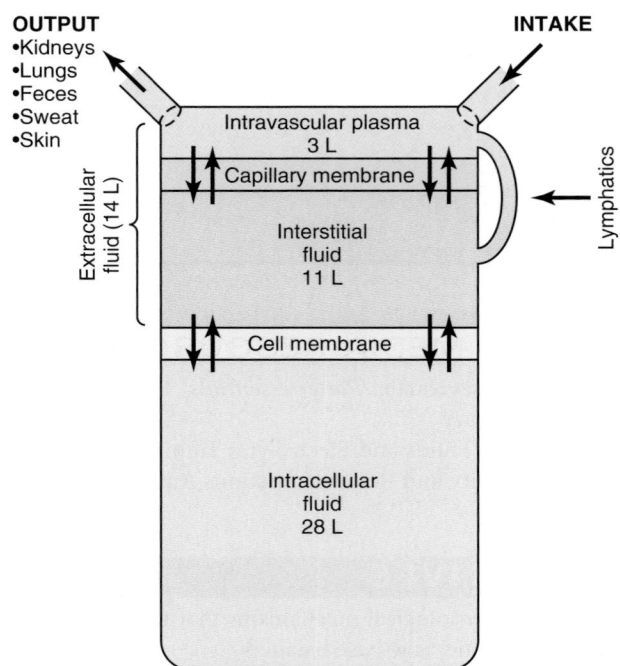

FIG 18.1 Body fluid compartments. (From Hall JE: *Guyton and Hall textbook of medical physiology,* ed 13, Philadelphia, 2016, Elsevier.)

Fluid, electrolyte, and acid-base balances within the body maintain health and function of all body cells, organs, and systems. The body maintains fluid and electrolyte balance by adjusting the intake and output (I&O) of water and electrolytes and their distribution in the body. The body maintains acid-base balance by buffering and excreting acid. Factors that alter these normal processes can cause fluid, electrolyte, or acid-base imbalances. This chapter discusses how the body maintains balance; how imbalances develop and affect patients; and nursing interventions that help patients maintain or restore fluid, electrolyte, and acid-base balance.

SCIENTIFIC KNOWLEDGE BASE

Water is the largest single component of the body; 60% of the average man's weight is fluid. The proportion of water is lower in women and older adults and higher in infants (Hall, 2016). The term **fluid** means water that contains dissolved or suspended substances such as glucose, mineral salts, and proteins.

Distribution of Body Fluids

Body fluids are distributed in two major compartments, one containing intracellular fluid (ICF), and the other containing extracellular fluid (ECF) (Fig. 18.1). ICF is inside cells. In adults the ICF is approximately two-thirds of total body water (Hall, 2016).

ECF is all the fluid outside the cells, approximately one-third of total body water. The ECF is divided into two major compartments plus a minor compartment: intravascular (within blood vessels), interstitial (within tissues), and transcellular (minor). Intravascular fluid is the liquid portion of the blood, the plasma. Interstitial fluid is located between cells and outside the blood vessels. Transcellular fluid is secreted by epithelial cells and includes cerebrospinal, GI, peritoneal, and synovial fluids (Hall, 2016).

Composition of Body Fluids

Body fluid contains mineral salts that are called electrolytes. An **electrolyte** is a compound that separates into **ions** (charged particles) when dissolved in water. Positively charged ions are **cations**. Major cations within body fluids include sodium (Na^+), potassium (K^+), calcium (Ca^{2+}), and magnesium (Mg^{2+}). Negatively charged ions are **anions**. The three major body fluid anions are chloride (Cl^-), bicarbonate (HCO_3^-), and phosphate (PO_4^{3-} and other forms). Electrolyte concentration is measured in milliequivalents per liter (mEq/L), millimoles per liter (mmol/L), or milligrams per deciliter (mg/dL).

Movement of Water and Electrolytes

Cell membranes and capillary walls separate the body compartments. Water and electrolytes move between body compartments by processes that allow the compartments to have different electrolyte concentrations while keeping the overall particle concentration (osmolality) equal in all compartments. They move across cell membranes by four processes: active transport, diffusion, osmosis, and filtration.

Active transport moves electrolytes or other substances across cell membranes against a concentration gradient (from an area of low concentration to one of higher concentration). This process requires energy, usually in the form of adenosine triphosphate (ATP). An example of active transport is the sodium-potassium pump that moves sodium ions out of a cell and potassium ions into it, thus keeping the ICF lower in sodium and higher in potassium than the ECF.

Diffusion is passive movement of electrolytes or other particles from an area of higher concentration to one of lower concentration. In other words, the electrolytes move down their concentration gradient until the electrolyte concentration is equal in all areas. Electrolytes cannot diffuse across cell membranes unless the membranes have proteins that serve as ion channels. When ion channels are open, an electrolyte can diffuse across a membrane; when they are closed, no electrolytes pass. Opening and closing of ion channels play an important role in nerve and muscle function.

Osmosis moves water across a semipermeable membrane from a compartment of lower particle concentration to one that has a higher particle concentration (Fig. 18.2). Osmosis equalizes the concentration of particles on each side of a membrane. Cell membranes are known as semipermeable membranes because water crosses them easily but electrolytes do not. The particles in any fluid compartment exert an inward-pulling force called **osmotic pressure**. If a semipermeable membrane separates two fluid compartments with different particle concentrations, water is drawn through the membrane to the more concentrated side because it has higher osmotic pressure (inward-pulling force). Osmosis continues until the particle concentration is equal in both fluid compartments. This process controls movement of water between interstitial fluid and the intracellular compartment. The **osmolality** of a fluid is a measure of the number of particles per kilogram of water, reported in milliosmoles per kilogram (mOsm/kg). Changes in extracellular osmolality cause rapid shifts of water into or out of cells to equalize the osmolality. Osmosis is a passive process that does not require energy from cells.

IV solutions are hypertonic, isotonic, or hypotonic (Fig. 18.3). Infusion of **hypertonic** IV solutions (more concentrated than normal blood) such as 3% sodium chloride pulls fluid from cells by osmosis, causing them to shrink. **Isotonic** solutions such as 0.9% sodium chloride (same osmolality as normal blood) expand the extracellular fluid volume (ECV) of the body without causing water to shift in or out of cells. Physiologically **hypotonic** solutions (less concentrated than normal blood after they are infused) such as dextrose 5% in water (D_5W) move water from the extracellular compartment into the cells by osmosis causing them to swell. When health care providers write fluid orders for an IV, they prescribe the type of IV fluid that will distribute to specific fluid compartments as needed by each patient's condition.

Filtration is the net effect of several forces that move fluid across a membrane. Fluid moves into and out of capillaries

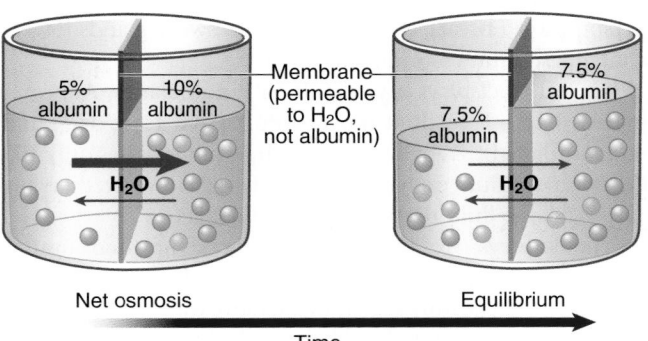

FIG 18.2 Osmosis moves water through a semipermeable membrane. (From Patton KT, Thibodeau GA: *Anatomy and physiology*, ed 9, St Louis, 2016, Elsevier.)

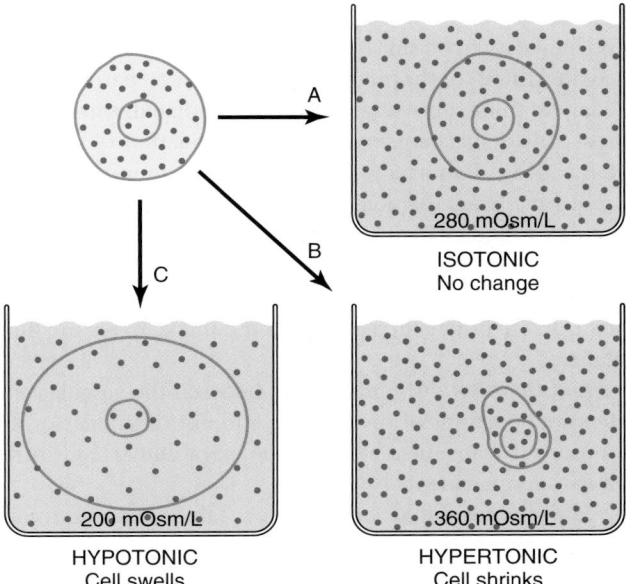

FIG 18.3 Effects of isotonic, hypotonic, and hypertonic solutions. (From Hall JE: *Guyton and Hall textbook of medical physiology*, ed 13, Philadelphia, 2016, Elsevier.)

(between the vascular and interstitial spaces) by filtration. Hydrostatic pressure is the force of a fluid pressing outward against the walls of its container. Thus capillary hydrostatic pressure is an outward-pushing force. Capillary hydrostatic pressure is greater at the arterial end of a capillary. Colloid osmotic pressure, also known as oncotic pressure, is an inward-pulling force caused by the presence of protein molecules. Blood colloid osmotic pressure is greater at the venous end of a capillary. Normally fluid leaves a capillary at the arterial end (high outward-pushing capillary hydrostatic pressure) carrying oxygen and nutrients to cells; fluid enters the capillary at the venous end (high inward-pulling colloid osmotic pressure) carrying carbon dioxide and other waste products into the blood for disposal. The lymph channels return excess fluid and a few small proteins that entered the interstitial space to the intravascular compartment. Edema occurs when changes in these forces cause fluid to accumulate in the interstitial space.

Fluid Balance. Fluid homeostasis is the dynamic interaction between fluid intake and absorption, fluid distribution, and fluid output (Felver, 2017b). Our daily fluid output consists of hypotonic sodium-containing fluid. To maintain fluid balance we must have an intake of an equivalent amount of hypotonic sodium-containing fluid (water plus foods with some salt).

Fluid Intake. Fluid intake occurs orally through drinking and eating. Food metabolism creates additional water. Average fluid intake for healthy adults is approximately 2200 to 2700 mL (Table 18.1), although it varies widely. Other routes of fluid intake that nurses encounter include IV, GI (tube feedings), rectal (e.g., enemas), and irrigation of body cavities that results in fluid absorption.

Although many people believe thirst regulates oral fluid intake, habit and social reasons actually account for most fluid intake. Thirst, a conscious desire for water, regulates fluid intake when plasma osmolality increases (osmoreceptor-mediated thirst) or the blood volume decreases (baroreceptor-mediated thirst and angiotensin II–mediated thirst). The thirst-control mechanism is in the hypothalamus of the brain (Hall, 2016). Osmoreceptors continually monitor plasma osmolality; when osmolality increases, the hypothalamus stimulates thirst. This thirst mechanism becomes less active in older adults. Dryness of oral mucous membranes also causes thirst. People who can obtain fluid or communicate their thirst to others increase their fluid intake to restore fluid balance.

Fluid Distribution. Fluid moves between the vascular and interstitial portions of the ECF (in and out of capillaries) by filtration. It distributes between the extracellular and intracellular compartments by osmosis.

Fluid Output. Fluid output (see Table 18.1) normally occurs through four organs: the skin, lungs, GI tract, and kidneys. When patients are seriously ill, output also occurs abnormally such as through vomiting, wound drainage, and hemorrhage (Felver, 2017b). Insensible water loss is not visible; it is continuous and occurs through the skin and

TABLE 18.1	HEALTHY ADULT AVERAGE DAILY FLUID INTAKE AND OUTPUT	
	NORMAL (mL/day)	**PROLONGED, HEAVY EXERCISE (mL/h)**
Intake		
Fluids ingested		
Oral	1100–1400 mL	280–1100 mL/hr
Foods	800–1000 mL	Highly variable
From metabolism	300 mL	16–50 mL/hr
Total intake	2200–2700 mL/day	300–1150 mL/hr
Output		
Skin (insensible and sweat)	500–600 mL	300–2100 mL/hr
Insensible: lungs	400 mL	20 mL/hr
Feces	100–200 mL	Negligible, unless diarrhea during exercise
Urine	1200–1500 mL	20–1000 mL/hr depending on hydration status
Total output	2200–2700 mL/day	340–3120 mL/hr Rehydration with Na⁺-containing fluid necessary after prolonged vigorous exercise

Data from Hall JE: *Guyton and Hall textbook of medical physiology,* ed 13, Philadelphia, 2016, Elsevier; American College of Sports Medicine (ACSM): Position stand on exercise and fluid replacement, *Med Sci Sports Exerc* 39(2):377, 2007.

lungs. Insensible water output from the lungs changes in response to respiratory rate and depth. Administration of nonhumidified supplemental oxygen increases insensible water loss from the lungs. Output of insensible water also increases with fever (Kamel and Halperin, 2017). Visible perspiration (sweat) is secreted by the sweat glands. Sweat contains sodium chloride and water.

The GI tract plays a vital role in fluid balance. Approximately 3 to 6 L of fluid moves into the GI tract daily and returns to the ECF. An average healthy adult excretes only 100 to 200 mL of fluid each day through feces. However, diarrhea causes a large fluid output from the GI tract.

The kidneys are the major regulator of fluid output because they respond to hormones that influence urine production. When healthy people drink more water, they produce more urine to maintain fluid balance. If they drink less water, sweat a lot, or lose fluid by vomiting, their urine volume decreases to maintain fluid balance. These adjustments primarily are the result of the actions of antidiuretic hormone

(ADH), aldosterone, and atrial natriuretic peptides (Kamel and Halperin, 2017).

Antidiuretic Hormone. ADH regulates osmolality of body fluids by influencing how much water is excreted in urine. The hypothalamus controls release of ADH from the posterior pituitary gland. It circulates to the kidneys where it acts on the collecting ducts causing them to resorb water (Hall, 2016). This antidiuretic effect removes water from the renal tubules and returns it to the blood, diluting the blood. More ADH is released when plasma osmolality increases; increased ADH causes more water resorption and dilutes the plasma back to normal. Conversely less ADH is released when plasma osmolality decreases; less water is resorbed, so it leaves the body in the urine and plasma osmolality returns to normal. Pain, nausea, stressors, some medications, and severely decreased blood volume increase the secretion of ADH and thus can cause plasma to become more dilute than normal. Ethyl alcohol decreases ADH release, which is why people urinate frequently when they drink alcoholic beverages.

Aldosterone. Aldosterone regulates ECV by influencing how much sodium and water are excreted in urine. The adrenal cortex releases aldosterone in response to increased plasma potassium concentration or as the end product of the renin-angiotensin-aldosterone system (RAAS). Renin released by the kidneys acts on the inactive protein angiotensinogen to produce angiotensin I, which other enzymes in the lung capillaries convert to angiotensin II. Angiotensin II causes vasoconstriction, which helps regulate blood pressure, and it stimulates the release of aldosterone, which assists fluid homeostasis. Aldosterone circulates to the kidneys where it acts on the distal tubules causing them to resorb sodium and water in isotonic proportions. Removing sodium and water from the renal tubules and returning them to the blood increases ECV. If ECV decreases such as through vomiting and diarrhea, the kidneys release more renin and the RAAS produces more aldosterone to increase sodium and water resorption and restore the ECV. Aldosterone also contributes to electrolyte and acid-base balance by increasing urinary excretion of K^+ and H^+.

Atrial Natriuretic Peptide. Atrial natriuretic peptide (ANP) is a hormone that opposes the action of aldosterone and promotes vasodilation. It is secreted from the cells of the heart in response to atrial stretching and an increased circulating blood volume. ANP causes sodium and water to be excreted in the urine, decreasing ECV slightly (Hall, 2016).

Electrolyte Balance. Electrolyte homeostasis refers to the relationship between electrolyte intake and absorption, electrolyte distribution, and electrolyte output (Felver, 2017b). To maintain electrolyte balance, electrolyte intake must equal electrolyte output and the electrolyte distribution must be normal.

Sodium Regulation. Normal serum Na^+ concentration ranges from 135 to 145 mEq/L. Sodium is the most abundant cation in ECF but has a smaller concentration inside cells.

This unequal distribution is maintained by the Na^+-K^+ pump in cell membranes, which also maintains an unequal K^+ distribution. The concentration of Na^+ in ECF is greatly influenced by the relative amount of water and reflects the osmolality (concentration) of the ECF. Sodium concentration imbalances are water imbalances and are discussed under Fluid Imbalances.

Potassium Balance. The normal range for serum K^+ concentration is 3.5 to 5 mEq/L. In contrast to this small concentration of K^+ in the ECF, K^+ has a high intracellular concentration (Hall, 2016). This maintains the resting membrane potential of cardiac, skeletal, and smooth muscle contraction, allowing for normal muscle function (Kamel and Halperin, 2017). K^+ absorbs easily with dietary intake of food sources such as bananas, spinach, and apricots. Insulin, epinephrine, and alkalosis shift K^+ into cells. Acute and chronic diarrhea increase output of K^+ from the GI tract. Aldosterone facilitates K^+ renal excretion, as does polyuria.

Calcium Balance. Ca^{2+} in blood has two major forms: bound and free. Ca^{2+} bound to albumin and other blood components is inactive. Free (ionized) Ca^{2+} is available for physiological actions. Normal serum total Ca^{2+} levels (bound plus free) are 8.4 to 10.5 mg/dL. Normal serum ionized Ca^{2+} levels range from 4.5 to 5.3 mg/dL. Most of the calcium in the body is in bone, although intracellular Ca^{2+} has important functions. Ca^{2+} influences the excitability of nerve and muscle cells and is necessary for muscle contraction and blood clotting. Plasma Ca^{2+} concentration is regulated primarily by the actions of parathyroid hormone (shifts Ca^{2+} out of cells) and calcitonin (shifts Ca^{2+} into cells). Vitamin D is necessary to make proteins responsible for dietary Ca^{2+} absorption in the duodenum. Chronic diarrhea and undigested fat increase output of Ca^{2+} in the feces.

Magnesium Balance. Normal plasma concentration of Mg^{2+} ranges from 1.5 to 2.5 mEq/L. Similar to Ca^{2+}, some Mg^{2+} in the blood is bound and inactive. Most of the Mg^{2+} in the body is in bones and inside cells. Mg^{2+} is essential for action of many enzymes and for normal action at neuromuscular junctions. Absorption of dietary Mg^{2+} occurs primarily in the terminal ileum. Chronic diarrhea and undigested fat increase output of Mg^{2+} in the feces. Renal Mg^{2+} excretion increases with a rising blood alcohol.

Chloride Regulation. Normal serum Cl^- concentration ranges from 95 to 105 mEq/L. Cl^- is the major anion in ECF and an important part of gastric hydrochloric acid.

Bicarbonate Regulation. Normal arterial bicarbonate level ranges between 22 and 26 mEq/L; normal venous bicarbonate is 24 to 30 mEq/L. Bicarbonate is a base and a key component of the bicarbonate buffering system essential to acid-base balance. The kidneys assist with regulating bicarbonate levels.

Phosphate Balance. Normal serum phosphate level ranges from 2.7 to 4.5 mg/dL. Phosphate exists in three forms ($H_2PO_4^-$, HPO_4^{2-}, and PO_4^{3-}), which are added together in any standard laboratory measurement. Most phosphate in the body is in bone and inside cells. Insulin and epinephrine shift phosphate into cells. Phosphate is needed to produce ATP, the energy source for cellular metabolism. Ca^{2+} and phosphate blood levels are inversely proportional; if one rises, the other falls, except during end-stage renal disease. The GI tract absorbs dietary phosphate easily except in the presence of aluminum or magnesium antacids. Renal excretion is the largest route of phosphate output and decreases greatly with oliguria.

Acid-Base Balance. Optimal cell function requires a balance between acids and bases. Acids release H^+; bases (alkaline substances) take up H^+. Acid-base homeostasis balances acid production, acid buffering, and acid excretion (Felver, 2017a). Acid-base balance requires acid excretion to be equal to acid production, with acid buffering in blood and renal tubular fluid.

The pH is a measure of fluid acidity or alkalinity. A pH value of 7.0 is neutral; below 7.0 is acid, and above 7.0 is alkaline. The greater the concentration of H^+, the more acidic the solution and the lower the pH; the lower the concentration of H^+ ions, the more alkaline the solution and the higher the pH. Normal pH range of arterial blood is 7.35 to 7.45.

Acid Production. Cellular metabolism constantly produces two kinds of acid: carbonic and metabolic. Carbonic acid (H_2CO_3) arises from the carbon dioxide (CO_2) that cells produce. Metabolic acids are all other acids produced by cells that are not carbonic acid such as lactic acid and citric acid.

Acid Buffering. Buffers are pairs of chemicals that work together to maintain normal pH of body fluids. If there are too many free H^+ ions, a buffer can take them up so that they no longer are free and cannot decrease the pH. If there are not enough free H^+ ions, a buffer can release H^+ to restore a normal pH. All body fluids contain buffers. The major buffer in ECF is the bicarbonate buffer system, which buffers metabolic acids. Other buffers include hemoglobin, protein buffers, and phosphate buffers. Buffers normally keep the blood from becoming too acidic when acids produced by cells are circulating to lungs and kidneys for excretion.

Acid Excretion. The body has two acid excretion mechanisms: lungs (excrete carbonic acid) and kidneys (excrete metabolic acids). The lungs excrete carbonic acid in the form of CO_2 and water. The chemoreceptors regulate this excretion by altering respiratory rate and depth. Respirations increase when more carbonic acid needs to be excreted, and they decrease (within limits) when the body needs to excrete less carbonic acid. The kidneys excrete all acids except carbonic acid by adjusting the amount of H^+ excreted in the urine to maintain acid-base homeostasis (Kamel and Halperin, 2017).

Disturbances in Fluid, Electrolyte, and Acid-Base Balances

Disturbances in fluid, electrolyte, and acid-base balances disrupt normal body processes and often occur together. As a nurse, you need to be familiar with these imbalances and their effects on body functioning.

Fluid Imbalances. Fluid imbalances are isotonic (volume) and/or osmolality (concentration) imbalances (Table 18.2 and Fig. 18.4). An isotonic deficit or excess exists when water and sodium are lost or gained in equal proportions, affecting the volume of the ECF. In contrast, an osmolality imbalance is a loss or excess of only water, which affects the concentration (osmolality) of the body fluids.

Extracellular Fluid Volume Imbalances. Extracellular fluid volume (ECV) excess is too much isotonic fluid in the extracellular compartment (see Table 18.2). Signs and symptoms come from too much vascular volume and interstitial volume. ECV deficit, as the name indicates, is too small a volume of isotonic fluid in the vascular and interstitial areas. The term hypovolemia refers to the decreased vascular volume in ECV deficit.

Osmolality Imbalances. Hypernatremia is abnormally high Na^+ concentration in ECF caused by loss of relatively more water than salt or gain of relatively more salt than water (see Table 18.2) (Felver, 2018). Water leaves cells by osmosis, and they shrivel. Signs of cerebral dysfunction occur when brain cells shrivel. Hypernatremia often occurs in combination with ECV deficit; the two together are clinical dehydration.

Hyponatremia is abnormally low Na^+ concentration in the ECF, which occurs from gaining relatively more water than salt or losing relatively more salt than water (see Table 18.2) (Felver, 2018). Water enters cells by osmosis, causing them to swell. Signs of cerebral dysfunction occur when brain cells swell.

Electrolyte Imbalances

Potassium Imbalances. Hypokalemia, a common electrolyte imbalance, is an inadequate level of K^+ in the blood. Common causes of hypokalemia involve increased K^+ output

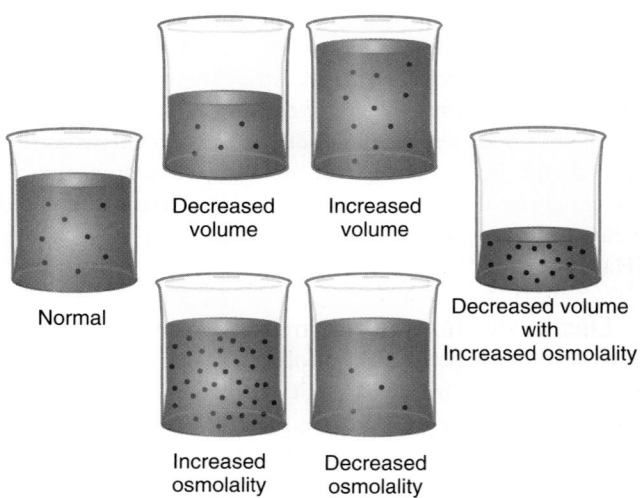

FIG 18.4 Fluid volume and osmolality imbalances. (From Copstead LC, Banasik JL: *Pathophysiology*, ed 6, St Louis, 2018, Elsevier.)

TABLE 18.2   FLUID IMBALANCES

IMBALANCE AND RELATED CAUSES	SIGNS AND SYMPTOMS
Isotonic Imbalances—Water and Sodium Lost or Gained in Equal or Isotonic Proportions	
Extracellular Fluid Volume Deficit—Body Fluids Have Decreased Volume but Normal Osmolality	
Sodium and Water Intake Less Than Output, Causing Isotonic Loss: Severely decreased oral intake of water and salt Increased GI output: vomiting, diarrhea, laxative overuse, drainage from fistulas or GI drainage tubes Increased renal output: use of diuretics, adrenal insufficiency Loss of blood or plasma: hemorrhage, burns Massive sweating without water and salt intake	*Physical examination:* sudden weight loss (overnight), postural hypotension, tachycardia, thready pulse, dry mucous membranes, poor skin turgor, slow vein filling, flat neck veins when supine, dark yellow urine *If severe:* thirst; restlessness; confusion; hypotension; oliguria (urine output **below** 30 mL/hr); cold, clammy skin; hypovolemic shock *Laboratory findings:* increased hematocrit, increased BUN **above** 25 mg/dL (hemoconcentration); urine specific gravity usually **above** 1.030, unless renal cause
Extracellular Fluid Volume Excess—Body Fluids Have Increased Volume but Normal Osmolality	
Sodium and Water Intake Greater Than Output, Causing Isotonic Gain: Excessive intake of Na⁺-containing isotonic IV fluids or oral intake of salty foods and water Renal retention of Na⁺ and water: heart failure, cirrhosis, aldosterone or glucocorticoid excess, acute or chronic oliguric renal disease	*Physical examination:* sudden weight gain (overnight), edema (especially in dependent areas), full neck veins when upright or semi-upright, crackles in lungs *If severe:* confusion, pulmonary edema *Laboratory findings:* decreased hematocrit, decreased BUN **below** 10 mg/dL (hemodilution)
Osmolality Imbalances	
Hypernatremia (Water Deficit; Hyperosmolar Imbalance)—Body Fluids Too Concentrated	
Loss of Relatively More Water Than Salt: ADH deficiency (diabetes insipidus) Osmotic diuresis Large insensible perspiration and respiratory water output without increased water intake **Gain of Relatively More Salt Than Water:** Administration of salt tablets, tube feedings, or hypertonic parenteral fluids Lack of access to water, deliberate water deprivation, inability to respond to thirst (e.g., immobility, aphasia) Dysfunction of osmoreceptor-driven thirst drive	*Physical examination:* decreased level of consciousness (confusion, lethargy, coma), perhaps thirst; seizures if develops rapidly or is very severe *Laboratory findings:* serum sodium level **above** 145 mEq/L, serum osmolality **above** 300 mOsm/kg
Hyponatremia (Water Excess; Hypoosmolar Imbalance)—Body Fluids Too Dilute	
Gain of Relatively More Water Than Salt: Excessive ADH (SIADH) Psychogenic polydipsia or forced excessive water intake Excessive IV administration of D₅W Use of hypotonic irrigating solutions Tap water enemas **Loss of Relatively More Salt Than Water:** Replacement of large body fluid output (diarrhea, vomiting) with water but no salt	*Physical examination:* decreased level of consciousness (confusion, lethargy, coma); seizures if develops rapidly or is very severe *Laboratory findings:* serum sodium level **below** 135 mEq/L, serum osmolality **below** 280 mOsm/kg
Combined Isotonic and Osmolality Imbalance	
Clinical Dehydration (ECV Deficit Plus Hypernatremia)—Body Fluids Have Decreased Volume and Are Too Concentrated	
Sodium and Water Intake Less Than Output, With Loss of Relatively More Water Than Salt: Most of the causes of ECV deficit (see previous causes) plus poor or no water intake; often with fever causing increased insensible water output	*Physical examination and laboratory findings:* combination of findings for ECV deficit plus findings for hypernatremia (see previous signs)

ADH, Antidiuretic hormone; *BUN,* blood urea nitrogen; *ECV,* extracellular fluid volume; *GI,* gastrointestinal; *D₅W,* dextrose 5% in water; *SIADH,* syndrome of inappropriate secretion of ADH.

not balanced by K^+ intake: diarrhea and use of K^+-wasting diuretics (Table 18.3) (Felver, 2018). Hypokalemia causes muscle weakness and, if severe, cardiac dysrhythmias.

Hyperkalemia is abnormally high blood K^+ concentration. Its causes are increased K^+ intake, shift of K^+ out of cells, and decreased K^+ output. Hyperkalemia produces muscle weakness and dangerous dysrhythmias.

Calcium Imbalances. **Hypocalcemia** is abnormally low blood concentration of total Ca^{2+} or ionized Ca^{2+}. It usually results from decreased Ca^{2+} intake and absorption or shift of Ca^{2+} into bones or unavailable forms (see Table 18.3) (Felver, 2018). Signs and symptoms are caused by increased neuromuscular excitability.

Hypercalcemia is abnormally high Ca^{2+} concentration in the blood. Hypercalcemia often occurs from an underlying disease such as cancer or hyperparathyroidism that causes bone resorption, shifting Ca^{2+} from bones into the ECF. The person may develop pathological fractures from the weak bones that result.

Magnesium Imbalances. **Hypomagnesemia**, abnormally low blood Mg^{2+} level, often occurs with chronic alcoholism and causes increased neuromuscular excitability (see Table 18.3). **Hypermagnesemia**, abnormally high blood Mg^{2+} level, is the result of excess Mg^{2+} intake or decreased Mg^{2+} excretion with oliguric renal disease. It causes decreased neuromuscular excitability.

Chloride Imbalances. **Hypochloremia** is abnormally low blood chloride level. It frequently is associated with alkalosis and conditions that cause loss of hydrochloric acid (vomiting, nasogastric suction, and gastric fistula drainage). It always occurs with other imbalances and has no unique signs and symptoms.

Hyperchloremia is abnormally high blood chloride level, which occurs with some types of acidosis, some renal conditions, and other electrolyte imbalances. It also has no unique signs and symptoms.

Acid-Base Imbalances.
Acid-base imbalances disrupt cell function and can be fatal if untreated. **Arterial blood gas (ABG)** analysis evaluates acid-base balance and oxygenation. Interpreting ABG levels involves understanding the physiology of six components: pH, $PaCO_2$, PaO_2, SaO_2, base excess, and HCO_3^-. Deviation from normal values indicates that a patient has an acid-base imbalance.

pH. The pH measures H^+ concentration in body fluids. Even a slight change is potentially life threatening. An increase in concentration of H^+ makes a solution more acidic; a decrease makes a solution more alkaline. Normal arterial blood pH value is 7.35 to 7.45 (acidic is less than 7.35, and alkalotic is greater than 7.45).

$PaCO_2$. $PaCO_2$ is the partial pressure of carbon dioxide in arterial blood and reflects the amount of H_2CO_3 in the blood. Normal range is 35 to 45 mm Hg. Hyperventilation produces a $PaCO_2$ less than 35 mm Hg. As rate and depth of respiration increase, more CO_2 is exhaled, decreasing the $PaCO_2$. Conversely, hypoventilation produces a $PaCO_2$ greater than 45 mm Hg. As rate and depth of respiration decrease, less

CO_2 is exhaled while cells continue to produce it, which increases the $PaCO_2$.

PaO_2. PaO_2 is the partial pressure of oxygen in arterial blood. Normal range is 80 to 100 mm Hg. When PaO_2 is within normal range, it has no primary role in acid-base regulation. A PaO_2 less than 60 mm Hg leads to anaerobic metabolism, causing lactic acid production and metabolic acidosis. Hypoxemia can cause hyperventilation leading to respiratory alkalosis.

SaO_2. SaO_2 (oxygen saturation) is the percentage of hemoglobin molecules that are carrying as much oxygen as is possible (saturated). Normal range is 95% to 100%. Changes in temperature, pH, and $PaCO_2$ affect SaO_2 levels.

Base Excess. Base excess (or deficit) is the amount of blood buffer (hemoglobin and bicarbonate) present in the blood. The normal range is ± 2 mmol/L. A higher positive value indicates **alkalosis**, and a lower negative value indicates **acidosis**.

Bicarbonate. Normal range of bicarbonate (HCO_3^-) is 22 to 26 mEq/L. HCO_3^- is the principal buffer in the ECF. HCO_3^- levels reflect the action of the kidneys in managing metabolic acid. A level less than 22 mEq/L usually indicates metabolic acidosis; a level greater than 26 mEq/L indicates metabolic alkalosis.

Types of Acid-Base Imbalances. Acid-base imbalances are either respiratory or metabolic. The four primary types of acid-base imbalance are respiratory acidosis, respiratory alkalosis, metabolic acidosis, and metabolic alkalosis (Table 18.4). It is possible to have two primary (mixed) acid-base imbalances.

Respiratory acidosis is an increased $PaCO_2$ and an increased hydrogen ion concentration (pH less than 7.35) that reflect the excess carbonic acid (H_2CO_3) in the blood. Hypoventilation produces respiratory acidosis, which causes cerebrospinal fluid and brain cells to become acidic, decreasing the level of consciousness (see Table 18.4).

Respiratory alkalosis is a decreased $PaCO_2$ and increased pH (greater than 7.45) that reflect the deficit of carbonic acid (H_2CO_3) in the blood. Hyperventilation produces respiratory alkalosis, which causes cerebrospinal fluid and brain cells to become alkalotic, decreasing the level of consciousness (see Table 18.4).

Metabolic acidosis results from conditions that increase metabolic acids in the body or decrease the amount of base (HCO_3^-) (Felver, 2018). The HCO_3^- level always is low because the bicarbonate system buffers metabolic acids. Diabetic ketoacidosis is a common cause of metabolic acidosis (see Table 18.4). Calculation of the anion gap is useful for identifying the cause of metabolic acidosis. An **anion gap** reflects unmeasurable anions present in plasma. One way of calculating anion gap is by adding the Cl^- and HCO_3^- levels and subtracting this number from the Na^+ concentration (Kamel and Halperin, 2017).

Metabolic alkalosis results from a gain of HCO_3^- or from excessive excretion of metabolic acid (Felver, 2018). The most common causes are vomiting and gastric suction (see Table 18.4).

TABLE 18.3 ELECTROLYTE IMBALANCES

IMBALANCE AND RELATED CAUSES	SIGNS AND SYMPTOMS
Hypokalemia—Low Serum Potassium (K⁺) Concentration **Decreased K⁺ Intake:** excessive use of K⁺-free IV solutions **Shift of K⁺ into Cells:** alkalosis; treatment of diabetic ketoacidosis with insulin **Increased K⁺ Output:** acute or chronic diarrhea, vomiting, or other GI losses; use of potassium-wasting diuretics; aldosterone excess; polyuria; glucocorticoid therapy	*Physical examination:* bilateral muscle weakness, abdominal distention, decreased bowel sounds, constipation, dysrhythmias *Laboratory findings:* serum K⁺ level **below** 3.5 mEq/L *ECG abnormalities:* U waves, flattened or inverted T waves; ST segment depression
Hyperkalemia—High Serum Potassium (K⁺) Concentration **Increased K⁺ Intake:** iatrogenic administration of large amounts of IV K⁺; rapid infusion of stored blood; excess ingestion of K⁺ salt substitutes **Shift of K⁺ out of Cells:** massive cellular damage (e.g., crushing trauma, cytotoxic chemotherapy); insufficient insulin (e.g., diabetic ketoacidosis); some types of acidosis **Decreased K⁺ Output:** acute or chronic oliguria (e.g., severe ECV deficit, end-stage renal disease); use of potassium-sparing diuretics; adrenal insufficiency	*Physical examination:* bilateral muscle weakness, transient abdominal cramps, diarrhea, dysrhythmias; cardiac arrest if severe *Laboratory findings:* serum potassium level **above** 5 mEq/L *ECG abnormalities:* peaked T waves; widened QRS complex; PR prolongation; terminal sine-wave pattern
Hypocalcemia—Low Serum Calcium (Ca²⁺) Concentration **Decreased Ca²⁺ Intake and Absorption:** calcium-deficient diet; vitamin D deficiency (includes end-stage renal disease); chronic diarrhea, laxative misuse; steatorrhea **Shift of Ca²⁺ Into Bone or Inactive Form:** hypoparathyroidism; rapid administration of citrated blood; hypoalbuminemia; alkalosis; pancreatitis **Increased Ca²⁺ Output:** chronic diarrhea; steatorrhea	*Physical examination:* numbness and tingling of fingers and circumoral (around mouth) region, positive Chvostek sign (contraction of facial muscles when facial nerve is tapped), hyperactive reflexes, muscle twitching and cramping, carpal and pedal spasms, tetany, seizures, laryngospasm, dysrhythmias *Laboratory findings:* total serum calcium **below** 8.4 mg/dL or serum ionized calcium level **below** 4.5 mg/dL *ECG abnormalities:* prolonged ST segments
Hypercalcemia—High Serum Calcium (Ca²⁺) Concentration **Increased Ca²⁺ Intake and Absorption:** milk-alkali syndrome **Shift of Ca²⁺ out of Bone:** prolonged immobilization; hyperparathyroidism; bone tumors; nonosseous cancers that secrete bone-resorbing factors **Decreased Ca²⁺ Output:** use of thiazide diuretics	*Physical examination:* anorexia, nausea and vomiting, constipation, diminished reflexes, lethargy, decreased level of consciousness, personality change; cardiac arrest if severe *Laboratory findings:* total serum calcium level **above** 10.5 mg/dL or serum ionized calcium level **above** 5.3 mg/dL *ECG abnormalities:* heart block, shortened ST segments
Hypomagnesemia—Low Serum Magnesium (Mg²⁺) Concentration **Decreased Mg²⁺ Intake and Absorption:** malnutrition; chronic alcoholism; chronic diarrhea, laxative misuse; steatorrhea **Shift of Mg²⁺ Into Inactive Form:** rapid administration of citrated blood **Increased Mg²⁺ Output:** chronic diarrhea; steatorrhea; other GI losses (e.g., vomiting, nasogastric or fistula drainage); use of thiazide or loop diuretics; aldosterone excess	*Physical examination:* positive Chvostek sign, hyperactive deep tendon reflexes, muscle twitching and cramping, grimacing, dysphagia, tetany, seizures, insomnia, tachycardia, hypertension, dysrhythmias *Laboratory findings:* serum magnesium level **below** 1.5 mEq/L *ECG abnormalities:* prolonged Q–T interval
Hypermagnesemia—High Serum Magnesium (Mg²⁺) Concentration **Increased Mg²⁺ Intake and Absorption:** excessive use of Mg²⁺-containing laxatives and antacids; parenteral overload of Mg²⁺ **Decreased Mg²⁺ Output:** oliguric end-stage renal disease; adrenal insufficiency	*Physical examination:* lethargy, hypoactive deep tendon reflexes, bradycardia, hypotension *Acute elevation in Mg²⁺ levels:* flushing, sensation of warmth *Severe acute hypermagnesemia:* decreased rate and depth of respirations, dysrhythmias, cardiac arrest *Laboratory findings:* Serum magnesium level **above** 2.5 mEq/L *ECG abnormalities:* prolonged P–R interval

ECG, Electrocardiogram; *ECV,* extracellular fluid volume; *GI,* gastrointestinal.

TABLE 18.4 ACID-BASE IMBALANCES

IMBALANCE AND RELATED CAUSES	SIGNS AND SYMPTOMS
Respiratory Acidosis—Excessive Carbonic Acid Resulting From Alveolar Hypoventilation	
Impaired Gas Exchange: Type B COPD (chronic bronchitis) or end-stage type A COPD (emphysema) Bacterial pneumonia Airway obstruction Extensive atelectasis (obstruction of small airways often caused by retained mucus) Severe acute asthma episode **Impaired Neuromuscular Function:** Respiratory muscle weakness or paralysis from hypokalemia or neurological dysfunction Respiratory muscle fatigue, respiratory failure Chest wall injury or surgery causing pain with respiration **Dysfunction of Brainstem Respiratory Control:** Drug overdose with a respiratory depressant Some types of head injury	*Physical examination:* headache, light-headedness, decreased level of consciousness (confusion, lethargy, coma), dysrhythmias *Laboratory findings:* arterial blood gas alterations: pH **below** 7.35, PaCO$_2$ **above** 45 mm Hg, bicarbonate level normal (if uncompensated) or **above** 26 mEq/L (if compensated)
Respiratory Alkalosis—Deficient Carbonic Acid Resulting From Alveolar Hyperventilation	
Hypoxemia from any cause (e.g., initial portion of asthma episode, pneumonia) Acute pain Anxiety, psychological distress, sobbing Inappropriate mechanical ventilator settings Stimulation of brainstem respiratory control (meningitis, gram-negative sepsis, head injury, salicylate overdose)	*Physical examination:* light-headedness; numbness and tingling of fingers, toes, and circumoral region; tachypnea; excitement and confusion possibly followed by decreased level of consciousness; dysrhythmias *Laboratory findings:* arterial blood gas alterations: pH **above** 7.45, PaCO$_2$ **below** 35 mm Hg, bicarbonate level normal (if short lived or uncompensated) or **below** 22 mEq/L (if compensated)
Metabolic Acidosis—Excessive Metabolic Acids	
Increase of Metabolic Acids (High Anion Gap): Ketoacidosis (diabetes, starvation, alcoholism) Hypermetabolic state (severe hyperthyroidism, burns, severe infection) Oliguric renal disease (acute kidney injury, end-stage renal disease) Circulatory shock (lactic acidosis) Ingestion of acid or acid precursors (e.g., methanol, ethylene glycol, boric acid, aspirin overdose) **Loss of Bicarbonate (Normal Anion Gap):** Diarrhea Pancreatic fistula or intestinal decompression Renal tubular acidosis	*Physical examination:* decreased level of consciousness (confusion, lethargy, coma), abdominal pain, dysrhythmias, increased rate and depth of respirations (compensatory hyperventilation) *Laboratory findings:* arterial blood gas alterations: pH **below** 7.35, PaCO$_2$ normal (if uncompensated) or **below** 35 mm Hg (if compensated), bicarbonate level **below** 22 mEq/L
Metabolic Alkalosis—Deficient Metabolic Acids	
Increase of Bicarbonate: Excessive administration of sodium bicarbonate Massive blood transfusion (liver converts citrate to bicarbonate) Mild or moderate ECV deficit **Loss of Metabolic Acid:** Excessive vomiting or gastric suctioning Hypokalemia Excess aldosterone	*Physical examination:* light-headedness; numbness and tingling of fingers, toes, and circumoral region; muscle cramps; possible excitement and confusion followed by decreased level of consciousness; dysrhythmias (may be caused by concurrent hypokalemia) *Laboratory findings:* arterial blood gas alterations: pH **above** 7.45, PaCO$_2$ normal (if uncompensated) or **above** 45 mm Hg (if compensated), bicarbonate level **above** 26 mEq/L; K$^+$ level often decreased (below 3.5 mEq/L)

COPD, Chronic obstructive pulmonary disease; *ECV,* extracellular fluid volume.
Data from Felver L: Fluid and electrolyte homeostasis and imbalances. In Copstead LC, Banasik JL, editors: *Pathophysiology,* ed 6, St Louis, 2018, Elsevier.

NURSING KNOWLEDGE BASE

Fluid and electrolyte imbalances occur in all patients, regardless of age, gender, or race and other cultural variables. Your nursing knowledge base helps you understand how fluid and electrolyte imbalances affect patients. For example, you apply knowledge of growth and development when managing patients with fluid and electrolyte imbalances. Infants are at significant risk because of their limited ability to respond independently to early warnings of a problem (Hockenberry et al., 2017). Similarly, adults who are severely ill, disoriented, and immobile have difficulty expressing symptoms when fluid and electrolyte imbalances develop. A nursing knowledge base regarding communication and health assessment techniques is invaluable in detecting problems early. In addition, a nursing knowledge base has contributed to the science of intravenous therapy, which is discussed later in this text.

CRITICAL THINKING

Synthesis

Patient care requires you to apply what you know about a patient, your knowledge base, experience, and critical thinking attitudes and standards. Your synthesis of this information allows you to make sound decisions as you apply the nursing process. Critical thinking synthesis involves combining all available information to obtain a clear picture of the approach needed to provide patient-centered care (Box 18.1). Patients' conditions often change quickly during fluid and electrolyte imbalances. Use clinical decision making and judgment to analyze clinical data and make decisions regarding patient care. Professional standards guide your assessment.

Knowledge

To provide care for patients with alterations in fluid and electrolyte or acid-base imbalance, use previously learned nursing knowledge and related knowledge acquired in anatomy, physiology, pharmacology, or chemistry courses. Consider all factors contributing to a patient's health problem. *In the case study, synthesizing previously learned knowledge about ECV deficit and orthostatic hypotension helps Robert plan and provide appropriate patient care. Mrs. Reynolds is at high risk for ECV deficit from her diarrhea, diuretic use, and decreased fluid intake. Robert knows that she has a risk for falls because she is at risk for becoming light-headed as a result of orthostatic hypotension when she changes position such as when getting out of bed.*

Experience

Professional experience helps you when caring for patients with fluid, electrolyte, or acid-base imbalances. Understanding patients' clinical signs and symptoms helps you identify and make appropriate clinical decisions when presented with a similar assessment. Prior patient care experiences make you more adept at future problem solving and decision making.

BOX 18.1   SYNTHESIS IN PRACTICE

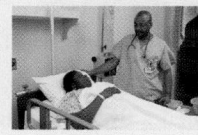

Robert reviews Mrs. Reynolds' clinical condition. Her history reveals that Mrs. Reynolds has loss of appetite, episodes of diarrhea, and continued use of hydrochlorothiazide (a potassium-wasting diuretic) for hypertension. She is at risk for fluid and electrolyte imbalances from gastrointestinal (GI) disturbance and continued use of a diuretic. The cause of her GI symptoms is unclear; therefore her health care provider plans further diagnostic tests. Robert reviews the physiology of fluid and potassium balance and studies the signs and symptoms of extracellular fluid volume (ECV) deficit and hypokalemia. He also reads recommendations in a pharmacology text on how to minimize the risk for hypokalemia when taking diuretics. Robert anticipates the need to perform a focused physical assessment and manage and monitor Mrs. Reynolds' IV therapy. He knows that patient education eventually will be important for Mrs. Reynolds because her therapy for hypertension will continue after discharge.

Just a few weeks ago Robert cared for a patient with ulcerative colitis. Although Mrs. Reynolds' condition is different, both patients had diarrhea. Robert knows that Mrs. Reynolds will require careful monitoring of intake and output (I&O) and stabilization of GI function. The lessons learned from his previous patient will help Robert to be more alert if Mrs. Reynolds' clinical condition changes during his care.

Robert applies the critical thinking attitude of discipline by completing a thorough examination and assessment. The attitude of curiosity is important when a clinical sign or symptom may be unclear and further information is needed.

When Robert checks the policy and procedures at his institution for an IV therapy protocol, he applies professional standards in practice. He reviews the standards for initiating and maintaining IV sites to be familiar with the procedures.

Attitudes

Accountability and discipline are essential when caring for patients with fluid, electrolyte, and acid-base imbalances. Be accountable by reporting changes in patient behavior or physical assessment findings immediately and follow standards of practice. Patients with fluid and electrolyte imbalances often present with a group of signs and symptoms; therefore use discipline in conducting a thorough and comprehensive assessment.

Standards

Apply intellectual standards of accuracy, relevancy, and significance in obtaining a health history for a patient with fluid and electrolyte imbalances. Apply Infusion Nurses Society (INS) standards of care for establishing, maintaining, monitoring, and discontinuing IV therapy (Gorski et al., 2016). Also apply the Centers for Disease Control and Prevention (CDC) standards of infection control for invasive procedures such as IV therapy (CDC, 2015). Laboratory standards provide normal electrolyte ranges.

NURSING PROCESS

ASSESSMENT

It is important to use knowledge of fluid, electrolyte, and acid-base balance to guide your assessment. By gathering assessment data and using critical thinking skills, nurses identify patients at risk for and patients with imbalances. Thorough assessment enables identification of appropriate nursing diagnoses.

Nursing History. Assessment begins with a patient history, which may reveal risk factors or preexisting conditions that cause or contribute to fluid, electrolyte, and acid-base imbalances. For example, explore a patient's diet history, including normal fluid intake. Determine if the patient is taking medications that can create electrolyte alterations. Explore these factors with the patient and integrate the information with knowledge of regulation of fluid, electrolyte, and acid-base balances.

Age. Age is an important assessment consideration. Infants and very young children have relatively more body water than older children and adults. They have greater water needs and immature kidneys (Hockenberry et al., 2017). They are at greater risk for **extracellular fluid volume (ECV) deficit** and hypernatremia because their body water loss is proportionately greater per kilogram of weight. Children ages 2 through 12 have less stable regulatory responses to imbalances; therefore they have a narrow range of tolerance for severe fluid or electrolyte imbalances. Adolescent girls have greater ECV fluctuations because of hormonal changes associated with the menstrual cycle.

Older Adult Considerations. Older adults experience age-related changes that can affect fluid, electrolyte, and acid-base balances. These changes include a reduction in lean muscle mass resulting in a reduction of body water, diminished thirst sensation, and decreased ability to concentrate urine and increase the risk of ECV deficit and hypernatremia (Touhy and Jett, 2014; Felver, 2017b). Kidney changes of normal aging make it more difficult to excrete a large metabolic acid load, increasing the risk for metabolic acidosis. Normal aging changes, chronic diseases, and multiple medications often make maintaining fluid and electrolyte balance a challenge.

Environment. Hot environments increase fluid output through sweating. Sweat is a hypotonic Na^+-containing fluid. Ask patients whether they engage in vigorous physical work or exercise in hot environments. If so, are Na^+-containing fluid replacements available during activity?

Dietary Intake. Assess a patient's normal 24-hour dietary intake of food and fluids. Determine the intake of salt and foods rich in K^+, Ca^{2+}, and Mg^{2+}. Assess recent changes in appetite and ability to chew and swallow, which affect nutritional status and fluid hydration. Also consider a patient's economic situation. Does he or she have the resources to prepare food? Assess if the patient is on a self-imposed type of diet. Starvation diets or high-fat, no-carbohydrate diets can cause metabolic acidosis.

Lifestyle. Take an alcohol intake history. Ask the patient the number of alcoholic drinks he or she normally consumes in a week. Is the patient a binge drinker? Binge drinking typically occurs after 4 drinks for women and 5 drinks for men in about 2 hours (NIAAA, n.d.). Chronic alcohol abuse commonly causes hypomagnesemia, in part because it increases renal Mg^{2+} excretion.

Medications. Obtain a complete list of current medications including over-the-counter (OTC) and herbal preparations to assess risk for fluid, electrolyte, and acid-base imbalances. Box 18.2 lists medications that often cause these imbalances. If your patient takes a medication that causes an electrolyte or acid-base imbalance, assess pertinent laboratory values.

BOX 18.2 COMMONLY USED MEDICATIONS THAT CAUSE FLUID, ELECTROLYTE, AND ACID-BASE IMBALANCES

- **ACE inhibitors** (e.g., captopril), **angiotensin II receptor antagonists** (e.g., losartan), **aldosterone antagonists** (e.g., eplerenone), and **direct renin inhibitors** (e.g., aliskiren): hyperkalemia
- **Antidepressants,** SSRI (e.g., fluoxetine): hyponatremia
- **Calcium carbonate antacids:** hypercalcemia, mild metabolic alkalosis
- **Corticosteroids** (e.g., prednisone): hypokalemia, metabolic alkalosis
- **Diuretics, potassium-wasting** (e.g., furosemide, thiazides): ECV deficit, hypokalemia, hypomagnesemia, mild metabolic alkalosis
- **Diuretics, potassium-sparing** (e.g., spironolactone): hyperkalemia, mild metabolic acidosis
- Effervescent (fizzy) antacids and cold medications (high Na^+ content): ECV excess
- **Laxatives** (overuse): ECV deficit, hypokalemia, hypocalcemia, hypomagnesemia, metabolic acidosis
- **Magnesium hydroxide** (e.g., Milk of Magnesia): hypermagnesemia
- **Nonsteroidal antiinflammatory drugs** (NSAIDs [e.g., ibuprofen]): mild ECV excess, hyponatremia
- **Opioid analgesics, overdose** (e.g., morphine): respiratory acidosis
- **Penicillin G, IV** medication (contains K^+): hyperkalemia

ACE, Angiotensin-converting enzyme; *ECV,* extracellular fluid volume; *NSAIDs,* nonsteroidal antiinflammatory drugs; *SSRI,* selective serotonin reuptake inhibitor.
Data from Burchum JR, Rosenthal LD: *Lehne's pharmacology for nursing care,* ed 9, St Louis, 2016, Elsevier.

Medical History. A patient's prior medical history provides valuable data about fluid, electrolyte, and acid-base imbalances. When patients have chronic diseases (e.g., cancer, heart failure, oliguric renal disease), review these conditions to understand how they affect fluid, electrolyte, and acid-base balance. Assess duration of the disease and treatment regimens. In addition to chronic health problems, determine if a patient has a history of recent GI alterations (e.g., diarrhea or vomiting), nasogastric suctioning, or intestinal drainage. Loss of GI fluids predisposes patients to ECV deficit, hypokalemia, and other electrolyte imbalances.

Recent surgery, head injury, respiratory disorders, and burns place patients at high risk for fluid and electrolyte imbalances. The physiological stress response to surgery causes increased secretion of aldosterone, cortisol, and ADH in the first few postoperative days. These changes cause increased ECV, decreased osmolality, and increased K^+ excretion. In otherwise healthy patients these imbalances resolve without difficulty, but patients with preexisting imbalances or additional risk factors may need treatment.

Physical Assessment. Data gathered through a focused physical assessment validate and extend information gathered in the patient history. Table 18.5 summarizes assessments for patients with fluid, electrolyte, and acid-base imbalances. Focus your assessment on the areas pertinent to each patient situation. For example, for patients at risk for ECV imbalances, focus your assessment on body weight changes and clinical markers of vascular and interstitial volume. Carefully assess patients' cardiac, respiratory, neuromuscular, and GI status when they are at high risk for electrolyte and acid-base imbalances. Grouping your assessments under these categories helps you know which assessments to prioritize and enables you to assess effectively. Table 18.6 provides a focused assessment of fluid status for Mrs. Reynolds.

TABLE 18.5 PHYSICAL AND BEHAVIORAL NURSING ASSESSMENT FOR FLUID, ELECTROLYTE, AND ACID-BASE IMBALANCES

ASSESSMENT	IMBALANCES
Body Weight Changes From Previous Day	
Loss of 2.2 lb (1 kg) or more in 24 hours for adults	ECV deficit
Gain of 2.2 lb (1 kg) or more in 24 hours for adults	ECV excess
Clinical Markers of Vascular Volume	
Blood Pressure	
Hypotension or orthostatic hypotension	ECV deficit
Light-headedness on sitting upright or standing	ECV deficit
Pulse Rate and Character	
Rapid, thready	ECV excess
Bounding	ECV excess
Fullness of Neck Veins	
Flat or collapsing with inspiration when supine	ECV deficit
Full or distended when upright or semi-upright	ECV excess
Other Assessments of Vascular Volume	
Capillary refill: sluggish	ECV deficit
Lung auscultation, dependent portions: crackles or rhonchi with progressive dyspnea	ECV excess
Urine output: small volume of dark yellow urine	ECV deficit
Clinical Markers of Interstitial Volume	
Edema: present in dependent areas (ankles or sacrum) and possibly fingers or around eyes	ECV excess
Mucous membranes: dry between cheek and gum, tears decreased or absent	ECV deficit
Skin turgor: pinched skin fails to return to normal position within 3 seconds	ECV deficit
Thirst	
Thirst present	Hypernatremia, severe ECV deficit

Continued

TABLE 18.5 PHYSICAL AND BEHAVIORAL NURSING ASSESSMENT FOR FLUID, ELECTROLYTE, AND ACID-BASE IMBALANCES—cont'd

ASSESSMENT	IMBALANCES
Behavior and Level of Consciousness	
Restlessness and mild confusion	Severe ECV deficit
Decreased level of consciousness (confusion, lethargy, coma)	Hyponatremia, hypernatremia, hypercalcemia, acid-base imbalances
Cardiac and Respiratory Signs of Electrolyte or Acid-Base Imbalances	
Pulse rhythm and ECG abnormalities	K^+, Ca^{2+}, Mg^{2+}, or acid-base imbalances
Rate and Depth of Respirations	
Increased rate and depth	Metabolic acidosis (compensatory mechanism); respiratory alkalosis (cause)
Decreased rate and depth	Metabolic alkalosis (compensatory mechanism); respiratory acidosis (cause)
Neuromuscular Markers of Electrolyte or Acid-Base Imbalances	
Muscle Strength	
Muscle weakness, bilateral, especially quadriceps	Hypokalemia, hyperkalemia
Reflexes and Sensations	
Decreased deep tendon reflexes	Hypercalcemia, hypermagnesemia
Hyperactive reflexes, positive Chvostek sign	Hypocalcemia, hypomagnesemia
Muscle twitching and cramping	Hypocalcemia, hypomagnesemia, respiratory alkalosis
Numbness; tingling in fingertips, around mouth	Hypocalcemia, hypomagnesemia, respiratory alkalosis
Tremor	Hypomagnesemia
Gastrointestinal Signs of Electrolyte Imbalances	
Inspection and Auscultation	
Abdominal distention	Hypokalemia
Decreased bowel sounds	Hypokalemia
Motility	
Constipation	Hypokalemia, hypercalcemia

ECG, Electrocardiogram; *ECV,* extracellular fluid volume.

TABLE 18.6 FOCUSED PATIENT ASSESSMENT

FACTORS TO ASSESS	QUESTIONS	PHYSICAL ASSESSMENT
Vital signs and neck veins	Tell me how you feel when you stand up? Do you ever feel light-headed?	Palpate patient's pulse and auscultate heart rate. Monitor patient's blood pressure and pulse when supine and then at 1 minute after sitting with legs dependent or at 1 minute after standing. Observe patient for light-headedness (unsteady gait). Inspect neck veins when patient is supine to see if they are flat or collapsing with inspiration.
I&O	Describe for me how often you are thirsty? How often do you usually urinate?	Monitor patient's 24-hour I&O; note if having diarrhea fluid. Inspect urine (expect dark yellow color).
Skin, mucous membranes, and daily weight	Is your mouth dry? Has your skin recently been more dry than usual?	Check dryness of mucous membranes between cheek and gum. Inspect patient's skin; test for turgor over sternum. Obtain a baseline weight and monitor daily.

ECV, Extracellular fluid volume; *I&O,* intake and output.

Daily Weights and Fluid Intake and Output Measurement. Daily weights are an important indicator of fluid status (Felver, 2017b). Each kilogram (2.2 lb) of weight gained or lost overnight is equal to 1 L of fluid gained or lost. Weigh patients with heart failure or patients who are at high risk for or have ECV excess daily. In a hospital or nursing home setting, obtain the weight at the same time each day with the same calibrated scale after a patient voids, if possible. Also have patients wear a gown that weighs the same each time they weigh. In medical clinics and other outpatient centers, use the same scale each time and have patients void beforehand. If you are using a bed scale, always use the same number of linens. Teach patients with heart failure to take and record daily weights at home and to contact their health care provider if weight increases suddenly according to parameters their providers set. Recognizing trends in daily weights is important. Patients who are hospitalized for decompensated heart failure often experience significant increases in daily weights during the week before hospitalization (Wang et al., 2014).

Measuring and recording all liquid I&O during a 24-hour period is an important aspect of fluid balance assessment. Compare 24-hour intake with 24-hour output. The two measures should be approximately equal if the person has normal fluid balance. Recognizing I&O trends is important (e.g., a gradually decreasing fluid output with increased intake may indicate a developing ECV excess).

In most health care settings, I&O measurement is a nursing assessment. Some agencies require a health care provider's order for I&O. Check your agency policies if you want to measure I&O for a patient with compromised fluid status. Fluid intake includes all liquids that a person eats (e.g., gelatin, ice cream, broth), drinks (e.g., juice, coffee, tea, water), or receives through nasogastric or jejunostomy feeding tubes (see Chapter 35). IV fluids (continuous and intermittent) and blood components also count as intake. A patient receiving tube feedings may receive numerous liquid medications; water is used to flush the tube before and/or after the medications. During a 24-hour period these liquids can amount to significant intake; always record them on the I&O record. Patient and family caregiver cooperation is essential for maintaining accurate I&O measurements. Ask alert patients to help measure their oral intake and explain to family members why they should not eat or drink from the patient's meal tray or water pitcher.

Liquid output includes urine, diarrhea, vomitus, gastric suction, and blood and drainage from postsurgical wounds, burns, or other tubes (see Chapters 36, 37, 38). Record urinary output after each voiding. Instruct patients who are alert and ambulatory to save their urine in a calibrated (graduated) insert that attaches to the rim of a toilet bowl (Fig. 18.5). Teach patients and families the purpose of I&O; tell them to notify a nurse or nursing assistive personnel (NAP) to empty the container with voided fluid, or teach them how to measure and record the result themselves. Patients need good vision and motor skills to perform these assessments. When a patient has an indwelling urinary catheter, drainage tube, or suction,

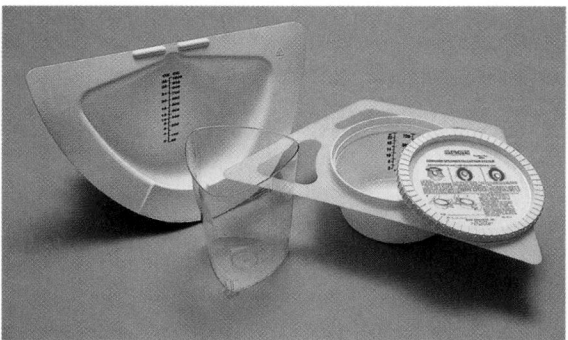

FIG 18.5 Graduated measuring containers. *Clockwise from top left:* "Hat" receptacle, specimen, and measurement container.

record that output (e.g., at the end of each nursing shift or every hour) as the patient's condition requires.

You can delegate portions of I&O measurement to NAP. Emphasize the importance of accurate measurements, even when available time is limited (McGloin, 2015). In many agencies NAP can record oral intake but not intake through tubes or IV lines; they can record urine, diarrhea, and vomitus output but not drainage through tubes. Work as a team with the NAP to record measurements in the designated location in the electronic health record (EHR) or appropriate paper forms. Accurate I&O evaluates a patient's hydration status.

Laboratory Studies. Review a patient's laboratory test results and compare them with normal ranges to obtain additional data about fluid, electrolyte, and acid-base balances. Box 18.3 and Table 18.7 summarize laboratory data useful for this purpose. The frequency of measurement of electrolyte levels depends on the severity of a patient's illness. Serum electrolyte tests are performed routinely on patients entering a hospital to screen for imbalances and serve as a baseline for future comparisons.

Patient Expectations. Fluid, electrolyte, and acid-base imbalances often accompany serious illness that prevents a review of patient expectations. Reviewing expectations with patients who are alert may reveal short-term (e.g., provision of comfort from nausea) or long-term (e.g., understanding how to prevent imbalances in the future) needs. Strengthen a patient's trust through competent responses to sudden changes in condition and by keeping patients and/or family caregivers informed so that they become active participants in care.

■■■■ NURSING DIAGNOSIS

When caring for patients with potential fluid, electrolyte, or acid-base imbalances, use critical thinking to formulate nursing diagnoses. The assessment data that establish the risk for or the actual presence of a nursing diagnosis may be subtle, but patterns and trends emerge after astute assessment.

BOX 18.3 LABORATORY DATA REFLECTING FLUID, ELECTROLYTE, AND ACID-BASE IMBALANCES

FLUID AND ELECTROLYTES
- Alterations in serum sodium, osmolality, potassium, magnesium, calcium, phosphate, and chloride
- Alterations in hematocrit and BUN
- Alterations in urine specific gravity

METABOLIC ALKALOSIS
- pH more than 7.45
- $PaCO_2$ normal or more than 45 mm Hg if lungs are compensating
- HCO_3^- more than 26 mEq/L
- Ionized calcium less than 4.5 mg/dL
- K^+ less than 3.5 mEq/L

METABOLIC ACIDOSIS
- pH less than 7.35
- $PaCO_2$ normal or less than 35 mm Hg if lungs are compensating
- HCO_3^- less than 22 mEq/L
- K^+ more than 5 mEq/L

RESPIRATORY ALKALOSIS
- pH more than 7.45
- $PaCO_2$ less than 35 mm Hg
- HCO_3^- less than 22 mEq/L if kidneys are compensating
- Ionized calcium less than 4.5 mg/dL
- K^+ less than 3.5 mEq/L

RESPIRATORY ACIDOSIS
- pH less than 7.35
- $PaCO_2$ more than 45 mm Hg
- HCO_3^- normal if early respiratory acidosis or more than 26 mEq/L if kidneys are compensating
- K^+ more than 5 mEq/L

BUN, Blood urea nitrogen.

Multiple body systems may be involved, so carefully analyze the defining characteristics or risk factors in clusters. For example, relevant assessment data for the problem-focused nursing diagnosis *Deficient Fluid Volume* include defining characteristics such as insufficient oral intake, sudden weight loss, dry oral mucous membranes, decreased skin turgor, decreased blood pressure, and increased heart rate.

In addition to accurate clustering of assessment data, another part of developing nursing diagnoses is identifying the relevant and accurate causes or related factors for problem-focused and health promotion nursing diagnoses. For example, *Deficient Fluid Volume related to loss of GI fluids from vomiting* requires interventions to manage the patient's vomiting and restore fluid volume (e.g., administer antiemetics, remove sights and odors that induce nausea, and provide IV fluid replacement). The same nursing diagnosis with a different related factor such as *Deficient Fluid Volume related to elevated body temperature* requires different interventions (e.g., administer antipyretics and provide oral fluids).

Possible nursing diagnoses for patients with fluid, electrolyte, and acid-base alterations include:
- *Decreased Cardiac Output*
- *Acute Confusion*
- *Risk for Electrolyte Imbalance*
- *Deficient Fluid Volume*
- *Excess Fluid Volume*
- *Risk for Imbalanced Fluid Volume*
- *Impaired Gas Exchange*
- *Risk for Injury*

■■■ PLANNING

Goals and Outcomes. During the planning phase collaborate with each patient to establish goals and expected outcomes for each nursing diagnosis (see Care Plan). Make sure that goals are individualized and realistic with measurable outcomes. *In the case study, Robert sets goals in the*

TABLE 18.7 ARTERIAL BLOOD GAS ASSESSMENT

TEST	NORMAL RANGE FOR ADULTS	SIGNIFICANCE OF ABNORMAL FINDINGS
pH	7.35–7.45	Increased: metabolic or respiratory alkalosis Decreased: metabolic or respiratory acidosis Small changes in pH indicate large changes in H^+ concentration and are clinically important.
PaO_2 (mm Hg)	80–100	Decreased: poor oxygenation of the blood
SaO_2 (%)	95–100	Decreased: poor oxygenation of the blood
$PaCO_2$ (mm Hg)	35–45	Increased: respiratory acidosis or compensation for metabolic alkalosis (differentiate with pH) Decreased: respiratory alkalosis or compensation for metabolic acidosis (differentiate with pH)
Bicarbonate (mEq/L or mmol/L)	22–26	Increased: metabolic alkalosis or compensation for respiratory acidosis (differentiate with pH) Decreased: metabolic acidosis or compensation for respiratory alkalosis (differentiate with pH)

◎ CARE PLAN

Extracellular Fluid Volume Deficit

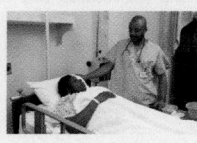

ASSESSMENT

Mrs. Susan Reynolds, a 42-year-old married accountant, was admitted yesterday to an acute care unit with a history of nausea, loss of appetite, and diarrhea for 7 days. After obtaining a blood sample for electrolyte levels, complete blood count, and an electrocardiogram (ECG), her health care provider admitted her for observation. Orders include intravenous (IV) infusion of 0.9% saline at 125 mL/h, intake and output (I&O) recordings, vital signs every 4 hours, and daily weights.

ASSESSMENT ACTIVITIES	FINDINGS[a]
Ask Mrs. Reynolds to describe when her nausea began.	Mrs. Reynolds states that she became nauseous after a short business trip, has no appetite, is nauseous, and has had diarrhea for 7 days.
Assess vital signs.	Vital signs: temperature 99.6° F (37.6° C); **pulse, 100 beats/min** and regular; supine **blood pressure (BP), 105/60 mm Hg** with no changes when standing; respirations 18/min and nonlabored; lung sounds clear to auscultation bilaterally.
Assess abdomen and I&O.	Bowel sounds present and hyperactive in all four quadrants. Abdomen soft to palpation. Her 24-hour intake was 1850 mL, with output of 2200 mL **(urine output accounted for only 1000 mL).** She has **dark yellow urine.**
Assess skin, mucous membranes, and daily weight for indicators of extracellular fluid volume (ECV) deficit.	Skin is **dry,** without discoloration, but **turgor is decreased.** Neck veins barely visible when supine. **Dry mucous membranes** between cheek and gum. **Weight of 143 lb (65 kg) is decreased 1 lb** (0.45 kg) since her admission yesterday.
Evaluate laboratory values.	Laboratory result: hematocrit 44% (suggesting hypovolemia); serum K^+ 3.5 mEq/L (low normal because of diarrhea) and Na^+ 140 mEq/L.

[a]**Defining characteristics/risk factors** are shown in **bold** type.

NURSING DIAGNOSIS: Deficient Fluid Volume related to increased fluid output from diarrhea and diuretic

---

PLANNING

GOAL	EXPECTED OUTCOMES (NOC)[b]
	Fluid Balance
Mrs. Reynolds' fluid volume will return to normal by time of discharge.	Urine output equals at least 1400 mL/day in 2 days.
	Urine color becomes light yellow within 24 hours.
	Heart rate (HR) and BP return to normal in 24 hours.
	Mucous membranes are moist in 24 hours.
	Skin turgor returns to normal within 24 hours.
	Daily weights do not decrease over next 2 days.
Mrs. Reynolds will describe how to manage fluid balance at home before hospital discharge.	Mrs. Reynolds describes how to replace diarrhea fluid loss.
	She describes signs and symptoms that indicate the need to increase fluid and sodium intake.
	Electrolyte and Acid-Base Balance
Mrs. Reynolds' electrolyte balance will be within normal limits by discharge.	Serum electrolyte levels are within normal limits within 48 hours.

[b]Outcomes classification labels from Moorhead S, et al, editors: *Nursing outcomes classification (NOC)*, ed 5, St Louis, 2013, Mosby.

INTERVENTIONS (NIC)[c]	RATIONALE
Fluid/Electrolyte Management	
Administer IV fluids (0.9% sodium chloride) at 125 mL/hr as prescribed.	Replacement of isotonic fluid restores blood volume; isotonic solutions expand ECV without causing fluid shift into cells.
Provide patient with additional 480 mL of her favorite noncaffeinated oral fluids at her preferred temperature during every 8 hours.	Patient-centered care takes individual preferences into account. Cultural preferences regarding temperature of oral fluid when ill influence fluid intake (Abitz, 2016).
Administer bismuth subsalicylate (Pepto-Bismol) as ordered for diarrhea.	Pepto-Bismol is an antidiarrheal that inhibits gastrointestinal secretions, stimulates absorption of fluid and electrolytes, and inhibits intestinal inflammation (Burchum and Rosenthal, 2016).
Maintain accurate I&O measurements.	Documents hydration and fluid balance for directing therapy.
Weigh Mrs. Reynolds daily and monitor trends.	Daily weights provide an indication of fluid balance (Felver, 2017b).

[c]Interventions classification labels from Bulechek GM, et al, editors: *Nursing interventions classification (NIC)*, ed 6, St Louis, 2013, Mosby.

Continued

◎ CARE PLAN—cont'd

Extracellular Fluid Volume Deficit

EVALUATION

NURSING ACTIONS	PATIENT RESPONSE/FINDING	ACHIEVEMENT OF OUTCOME
Monitor electrolyte levels, daily weights, and I&O trends.	Serum electrolyte levels: K⁺ 3.7 mEq/L and Na⁺ 140 mEq/L; weight, 143 lb (65 kg). Mrs. Reynolds' 24-hour intake is 2800 mL, and output is 2200 mL with 1800 mL urine. Urine is light yellow.	Electrolyte levels within normal range. Daily weight stable. Fluid balance is improving with urine output exceeding stool output.
Assess oral mucous membranes, neck vein fullness, skin turgor, HR, and BP.	Mucous membranes remain dry. Neck veins full when supine. Skin turgor normal. Heart rate 80 beats/min, BP 126/78 mm Hg.	ECV is returning to normal.
Evaluate effectiveness of teaching regarding maintaining fluid and electrolyte balance at home.	Identifies foods and fluids she can eat and drink at home to maintain electrolyte balance.	Mrs. Reynolds describes effective home management of fluid and electrolyte balance.

nursing care plan for improving Mrs. Reynolds' fluid status. Later Robert determines if these goals are met (e.g., by monitoring the outcome of focused assessments and I&O). Each goal and outcome needs a time frame for achievement. For Mrs. Reynolds this time frame is for her goals to be met before hospital discharge.

In the acute care setting a long-term goal is to anticipate the needs of a patient and family to ease the transition to home or long-term care. *For example, Mrs. Reynolds likely will be discharged home with new medications or recommendations for a diet that causes less GI upset.* When creating a patient care plan, remember to take into consideration the patient's personal preferences, knowledge and skills of the patient and family caregiver, and available resources.

Setting Priorities. A patient's clinical condition determines which diagnosis takes the greatest priority. Many nursing diagnoses in the area of fluid, electrolyte, and acid-base balance are of highest priority because the consequences for the patient can be serious or life threatening. *For example, in the concept map (Fig. 18.6) Mrs. Reynolds has diarrhea, which has created ECV deficit. The nursing diagnosis Deficient Fluid Volume ranks highest priority, requiring intervention to stabilize her status and prevent further complications.* As a patient's status changes, the priority nursing diagnoses also change. For example, the priority nursing diagnosis changes to *Deficient Knowledge* once a patient is well enough to be discharged home. The priority at this time is to ensure that the patient returns safely to the home, which often requires extensive patient and family caregiver education (see Chapter 12).

Collaborative Care. Consult with the patient's health care provider to identify realistic time frames for the goals of care, particularly when a patient's physiological status is unstable. Planning care for a patient requires collaboration

with other members of the health care team such as the dietitian or pharmacist. You cannot delegate administration of IV medications and/or oxygen therapy to NAP. When a patient is stable, you can delegate daily weights, I&O measurement, and direct physical patient care. Establish a rapport of open communication and teamwork with NAP, as with any member of the interdisciplinary team, to ensure timely and effective administration of care.

Continuity of care is essential as a patient moves from one health care setting to another or to home. Therapeutic regimens established in one setting continue until completed in the next setting. For example, a patient who will continue to monitor I&O at home needs to know how to measure and document fluid I&O. When the patient's discharge has been ordered, it is important to identify which resources are available to promote positive outcomes. Dietitians are a valuable resource for recommending food sources to increase or reduce intake of specific electrolytes. Chapter 35 describes various therapeutic diets (e.g., low Na⁺). Pharmacists can provide information about a patient's prescription and OTC medications that may cause electrolyte or acid-base imbalances. The health care provider directs the treatment of any fluid, electrolyte, or acid-base imbalance. Be sure that a patient who will be discharged has the resources for continuing therapeutic regimens to return to a state of optimal functioning. A case manager or social worker might be able to connect patients with those resources.

■■■ IMPLEMENTATION

Health Promotion. Health promotion activities focus primarily on patient education. Teach patients and family caregivers how to recognize risk factors for development of imbalances and implement appropriate preventive measures. For example, parents of infants need to understand that GI losses lead quickly to serious fluid imbalances; therefore when

CONCEPT MAP

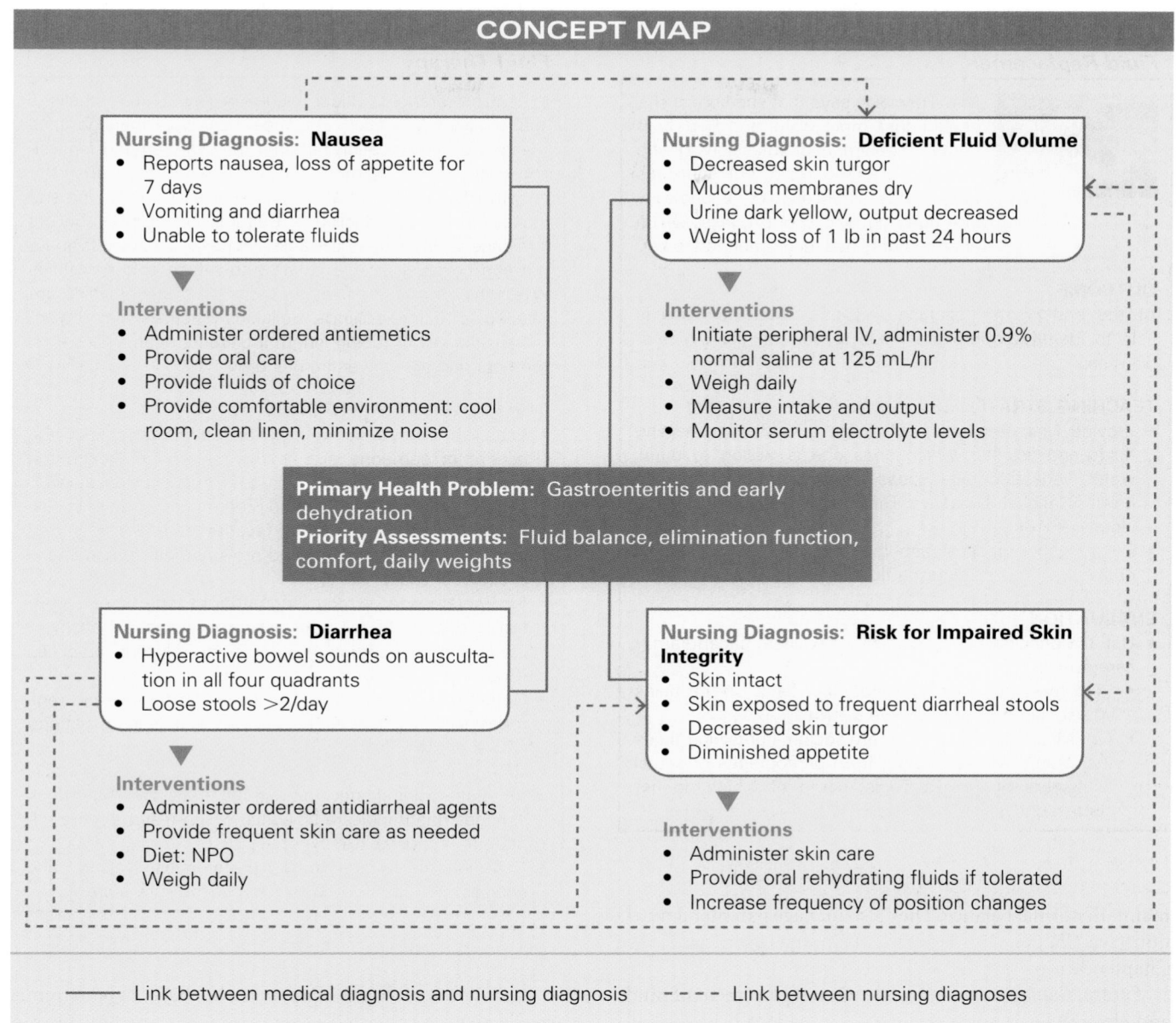

Nursing Diagnosis: Nausea
- Reports nausea, loss of appetite for 7 days
- Vomiting and diarrhea
- Unable to tolerate fluids

Interventions
- Administer ordered antiemetics
- Provide oral care
- Provide fluids of choice
- Provide comfortable environment: cool room, clean linen, minimize noise

Nursing Diagnosis: Deficient Fluid Volume
- Decreased skin turgor
- Mucous membranes dry
- Urine dark yellow, output decreased
- Weight loss of 1 lb in past 24 hours

Interventions
- Initiate peripheral IV, administer 0.9% normal saline at 125 mL/hr
- Weigh daily
- Measure intake and output
- Monitor serum electrolyte levels

Primary Health Problem: Gastroenteritis and early dehydration
Priority Assessments: Fluid balance, elimination function, comfort, daily weights

Nursing Diagnosis: Diarrhea
- Hyperactive bowel sounds on auscultation in all four quadrants
- Loose stools >2/day

Interventions
- Administer ordered antidiarrheal agents
- Provide frequent skin care as needed
- Diet: NPO
- Weigh daily

Nursing Diagnosis: Risk for Impaired Skin Integrity
- Skin intact
- Skin exposed to frequent diarrheal stools
- Decreased skin turgor
- Diminished appetite

Interventions
- Administer skin care
- Provide oral rehydrating fluids if tolerated
- Increase frequency of position changes

——— Link between medical diagnosis and nursing diagnosis   - - - - Link between nursing diagnoses

FIG 18.6 Concept map.

vomiting or diarrhea occurs, they should immediately begin rehydrating with Na^+-containing fluid. People of all ages need to learn to replace body fluid losses with Na^+-containing fluid and water (Box 18.4). Encourage patients who have low calcium or vitamin D levels to take daily supplements.

Patients with chronic health alterations need to understand their own risk factors and how to avoid imbalances. For example, patients with oliguric end-stage renal disease often need to restrict intake of fluid, Na^+, K^+, Mg^{2+}, and phosphate. Patients with severe heart failure must limit their intake of liquids and high-sodium foods to prevent fluid retention. Through diet education patients learn the types of foods to avoid and the daily volume of fluid they are permitted. Know that patients from different cultures may have difficulty with food selection. Be sure to know their likes and dislikes, and

try to match appropriate foods with their dietary preferences. Teach patients with chronic diseases and their family caregivers the early signs and symptoms of fluid, electrolyte, and acid-base imbalances for which they are at risk and what to do about them. For example, teach patients with heart failure to measure body weight each day at the same time and inform their health care provider of significant changes in weight from one day to another.

Acute Care. Although patients with fluid, electrolyte, and acid-base imbalances are in all health care settings, it is common to manage them in acute care settings. Acute care nurses conduct frequent and often complex monitoring (e.g., ABG measurement) and administer oral and IV fluids and medications to replace fluid and electrolyte deficits or

BOX 18.4 PATIENT TEACHING

Fluid Replacement

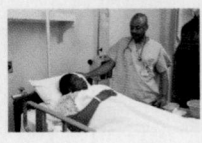

Mrs. Reynolds says that she knows she should drink more water and fluids that contain sodium and potassium if she develops diarrhea again, but she does not know which fluids to drink. She says she does not like sports drinks, which another nurse had recommended to her.

OUTCOME

At the end of the teaching sessions, Mrs. Reynolds is able to identify appropriate fluids to drink in the event of diarrhea

TEACHING STRATEGIES

- Provide Mrs. Reynolds with a list of sodium-containing fluids and ask her which ones she is willing to drink: water, vegetable juice, sodas without caffeine, and salty broth (National Digestive Disease Information Clearing House, 2016).
- Discuss the practical aspects (e.g., access, costs) of obtaining and preparing the fluids she has chosen.

EVALUATION

- Use the principles of teach-back to evaluate patient/family caregiver learning:
  - "Tell me what we discussed about what kind of fluids you should drink if you have diarrhea."
  - Ask Mrs. Reynolds to identify sodium-containing fluids that she is willing to drink from photographs or actual containers of various fluids, some of which do not contain sodium and some that do.

BOX 18.5 PATIENT-CENTERED CARE

Fluid Therapy

Patient preferences, values, economic resources, ethnicity, and religious practices influence how you manage fluid therapy. Communication patterns may vary among families and cultures. For example, the family elder rather than the patient may be the person who receives explanations and makes health care decisions. Cultural and religious beliefs influence acceptance of therapies. For example, beliefs about hot and cold may cause patients to refuse cold oral fluids when they are ill because they believe that hot fluids are needed to restore balance. Religious practices may require modification of IV tubing length if patients need to kneel on the floor and pray several times daily.

IMPLICATIONS FOR PRACTICE

- Establish trusted communication and determine if the patient or someone else is the decision maker in the family. Explain fluid restriction or IV therapy procedures.
- Elicit patient/family values and preferences in your assessment. Ask specifically about favorite fluids and preferred temperature of oral fluids and provide them (if oral intake is allowed) (Abitz, 2016).
- Incorporate one or more segments of long IV extension tubing into the IV setup for patient to increase mobility or participate in appropriate cultural or religious practices (Gorski et al., 2016).
- Determine acceptance or avoidance of therapeutic regimens including blood transfusions, and respect patient/family choices regarding therapy.
- When a patient's natural skin color is dark, assess carefully for subtle color changes around the IV insertion site. Such changes might indicate phlebitis, which may be more difficult to recognize (Gorski et al., 2016).
- Communicate patient/family preferences, values, and choices to other members of the health care team.

maintain normal balance. They also manage parenteral nutrition (see Chapter 35) and patients' oxygenation needs (see Chapter 32).

Enteral Replacement of Fluids. Oral replacement of fluids and electrolytes is appropriate when a patient is physiologically stable enough for oral fluids to be replaced rapidly. Oral replacement is contraindicated when a patient has a mechanical obstruction of the GI tract, is at high risk for aspiration, or has impaired swallowing. Patients unable to tolerate solid foods may still be able to ingest fluids. Strategies to encourage fluid intake include offering small sips of fluid frequently, popsicles, and ice chips. If possible, provide each patient's preferred fluids at the preferred temperature (Box 18.5). Cultural beliefs regarding appropriate fluid temperature can interfere with fluid intake unless fluid at the preferred temperature is available (Abitz, 2016).

When replacing fluids by mouth in a patient with ECV deficit, choose fluids that contain Na^+ (e.g., Gatorade, salty broth, Pedialyte). Liquids containing lactose or low-Na^+ content are not appropriate when a patient has diarrhea. A feeding tube is used for fluid replacement when a patient's GI tract is healthy but the patient cannot ingest fluids (e.g., after oral surgery or with impaired swallowing) (see Chapter 35).

Restriction of Fluids. Patients who have hyponatremia usually require restricted water intake so their kidneys can resolve the imbalance. Patients who have very severe ECV excess may have both sodium and fluid restrictions. Fluid restriction is difficult for patients, particularly if they take medications that dry the oral mucous membranes or if they breathe through their mouth. Explain why fluids are restricted and ensure that the patient and any family visitors know the amount of fluid permitted orally and understand that ice chips, gelatin, and ice cream are fluids. Allow patients to decide the amount of fluid to drink with each meal, between meals, before bed, and with medications. Unless contraindicated, encourage patients to choose their preferred fluids. Frequently patients on fluid restriction can swallow multiple pills with 30 mL of liquid.

In acute care settings fluid restrictions often allot half the oral fluids between 7 a.m. and 3 p.m., the period when patients usually are more active, receive two meals, and take most of their oral medications. Offer the remainder of the fluid allowance during the evening and night shifts. Patients on fluid restriction need frequent mouth care to moisten mucous membranes, decrease mucosal drying and cracking, and maintain comfort (see Chapter 31).

Parenteral Replacement of Fluids and Electrolytes. Fluid and electrolytes may be replaced through infusion of fluids intravenously (i.e., directly into veins). Parenteral replacement includes **parenteral nutrition (PN)**, IV fluid and electrolyte therapy (**crystalloids**), and blood product (**colloids**) administration. Practice standard body fluid precautions (see Chapter 14) when administering parenteral fluids to minimize your own risk for exposure to bloodborne pathogens. Understand and follow the policy and procedures for parenteral infusions at the agency for which you work.

Parenteral Nutrition. PN is a nutritionally adequate solution consisting of glucose, other nutrients, and electrolytes administered through a central venous catheter. It is the nutritional therapy of choice when a patient's GI tract is nonfunctional (Winkler and Guenter, 2014) (see Chapter 35).

Intravenous Therapy. The goal of IV fluid administration is to deliver continuous or intermittent infusion of fluids and medications via the vascular system to correct or prevent fluid and electrolyte imbalances. IV fluid therapy requires frequent monitoring to detect ongoing changes in a patient's fluid and electrolyte balance. To provide safe care to patients who require IV fluid administration, you need knowledge of the correct solution ordered, the reason it was ordered, the equipment needed, evidence-based procedures required to initiate an infusion, how to regulate the infusion rate and maintain the system, how to identify and correct problems, and how to discontinue the infusion. Whenever you care for a patient who requires IV therapy, you need to follow specific standards to decrease the incidence of infection related to the therapy (Box 18.6).

Vascular Access Devices. **Vascular access devices (VADs)** are catheters or infusion ports designed for repeated access to the vascular system. Peripheral catheters are for short-term use (e.g., to restore fluid volume). Devices for long-term use include central lines, peripherally inserted central catheters (PICCs), and implanted ports. These devices are more effective than peripheral catheters for administering PN, medications, and solutions that are irritating to veins. Nurses need specialized education in the use of these central devices to provide safe care (Wallace and Macy, 2016).

Types of Solutions. Many prepared IV solutions are available for use. An IV solution is isotonic, hypotonic, or hypertonic. Solutions that contain glucose have a greater tonicity in the IV container than their effective concentration in the body because the glucose enters cells rapidly; thus the rest of the infused fluid determines the effective physiological concentration (Table 18.8). Sodium-containing isotonic solutions are used for ECV replacement (e.g., ECV deficit after prolonged vomiting). A health care provider bases the decision to use a physiologically hypotonic or hypertonic solution on a patient's specific fluid and electrolyte imbalance. For example, a patient with hypernatremia that cannot be treated with oral water generally receives a hypotonic solution to dilute the ECF and rehydrate the cells. Administer all IV fluids

---

BOX 18.6 **INFUSION NURSES SOCIETY STANDARDS TO DECREASE INTRAVASCULAR INFECTION RELATED TO IV THERAPY**

- Palpate catheter insertion site for tenderness daily through the intact dressing.
- Directly inspect a catheter site if patient develops tenderness at site, fever without obvious source, or symptoms of local or bloodstream infection.
- Perform hand hygiene before and after palpating, inserting, replacing, or dressing any intravascular device.
- Clean skin site vigorously before venipuncture with an appropriate single-use antiseptic solution.
- Allow site to air-dry before proceeding with procedure: 2% chlorhexidine for 30 seconds, povidone-iodine for at least 2 minutes.
- Do not palpate insertion site after skin has been cleaned with single-use antiseptic solution.
- Use a catheter stabilization device that allows visual inspection of access site.
- Change gauze dressings that cover a catheter site every 48 hours.
- Leave transparent dressings in place until IV tubing is replaced.
- IV tubing administration sets can remain sterile for 96 hours.
- Replace dressing over peripheral venous catheters when replacing catheter or when dressing becomes damp, loosened, or soiled.
- Clean injection ports with single-use antiseptic solution before accessing system.
- Replace short-peripheral catheters and rotate sites based on clinical assessment indicating signs or symptoms of IV-related complications.

Modified from Gorski L, et al: Infusion therapy standards of practice, *J Infus Nurs* 39(suppl 1):S1, 2016.

---

carefully because too-rapid or excessive infusion of any IV fluid can cause serious patient problems.

Additives such as potassium chloride (KCl) are common in IV solutions. An IV therapy order includes the IV solution and any additives plus the volume and prescribed infusion time or rate. Usually a pharmacist prepares the solution. An example of an order follows:

Infusion No. 1: 1000 mL D$_5$NS
with 20 mEq KCl at 125 mL/hr.

Patients with normal renal function who do not have oral intake need to have potassium added to IV solutions. The body does not store potassium, and the kidneys continue to excrete potassium even when plasma levels fall. Hypokalemia develops quickly without potassium intake. Remember that failure to verify that a patient has adequate renal function and urine output before administering an IV solution containing potassium could cause hyperkalemia. *Under no circumstances should you give KCl by IV push (directly through a port in IV*

TABLE 18.8 INTRAVENOUS SOLUTIONS

SOLUTION	CONCENTRATION IN IV CONTAINER AND AT TIP OF VAD	EFFECTIVE CONCENTRATION IN BODY	COMMENTS
Dextrose (Glucose) in Water Solutions			
Dextrose 5% in water (D₅W)	Isotonic	Hypotonic	Isotonic when first enters vein; dextrose enters cells rapidly, leaving free water, which dilutes ECF; most of the water then enters cells by osmosis.
Dextrose 10% in water (D₁₀W)	Hypertonic	Hypotonic	Hypertonic when first enters vein; dextrose enters cells rapidly, leaving free water, which dilutes ECF; most of the water then enters cells by osmosis.
Saline (Sodium Chloride [NaCl] in Water) Solutions			
0.225% NaCl (quarter NS; ¼ NS)	Hypotonic	Hypotonic	Expands ECV (vascular and interstitial) and rehydrates cells.
0.45% NaCl (half NS; ½ NS)	Hypotonic	Hypotonic	Expands ECV (vascular and interstitial) and rehydrates cells.
0.9% NaCl (NS)	Isotonic	Isotonic	Expands ECV (vascular and interstitial); does not enter cells.
3% or 5% NaCl (hypertonic saline; 3% or 5% NaCl)	Hypertonic	Hypertonic	Draws water from cells into ECF by osmosis.
Dextrose in Saline Solutions			
Dextrose 5% in 0.45% NaCl (½ NS; D₅0.45% NaCl)	Hypertonic	Hypotonic	Dextrose enters cells rapidly, leaving 0.45% NaCl.
Dextrose 5% in 0.9% NaCl (D₅NS; D₅0.9% NaCl)	Hypertonic	Isotonic	Dextrose enters cells rapidly, leaving 0.9% NaCl.
Multiple Electrolyte Solutions			
Lactated Ringer (LR) solution	Isotonic	Isotonic	LR contains Na⁺, K⁺, Ca²⁺, Cl⁻, and lactate, which liver metabolizes to HCO₃⁻; expands ECV (vascular and interstitial); does not enter cells.
Dextrose 5% in LR (D₅LR)	Hypertonic	Isotonic	Dextrose enters cells rapidly, leaving LR.

ECF, Extracellular fluid; *ECV*, extracellular fluid volume; *NS*, normal saline; *VAD*, vascular access device.

tubing). A direct IV infusion of KCl is fatal. IV administration of KCl requires dilution in solution and infusion with an IV pump over a period of time.

Equipment. Correct selection and preparation of IV equipment ensures safe and quick placement of an IV line. Because IV fluids infuse directly into the bloodstream, sterile technique is necessary. Organize all equipment at the bedside for efficient insertion. IV equipment includes VADs, tourniquet, clean gloves, dressings, IV fluid containers, various types of tubing, and electronic infusion devices (EIDs), also called *IV pumps*. Peripheral IV catheters are available in a variety of gauges (e.g., 20 gauge, 22 gauge). The gauge indicates the diameter of the catheter. A larger gauge indicates a smaller-diameter catheter.

You use different types of infusion tubing to administer medications or IV fluids. EIDs are commonly used in acute and critical care settings and in some care settings outside of hospitals to ensure a constant, regulated rate. Use the tubing that is designated for the particular EID that you are using,

typically a macrodrip tubing. Macrodrip tubing delivers large drops (standard drop size is 10 or 15 gtt/mL depending on the manufacturer). In contrast, microdrip tubing provides a standard drop size of 60 gtt/mL, which facilitates precise regulation of IV fluids at slow rates. Add IV extension tubing to increase patient mobility and decrease manipulation and potential contamination of the insertion site.

Initiating Peripheral Intravenous Access. After organizing collected equipment at the bedside, prepare to insert the IV catheter by assessing the patient for a venipuncture site. The most common IV sites are on the inner arm (Fig. 18.7). You may insert an IV in a foot vein in children, but avoid this site in adults because of the danger of thrombophlebitis (Gorski et al., 2016). When assessing patients for potential venipuncture sites, consider conditions that exclude certain sites. For example, because older adults and patients receiving corticosteroids have fragile veins, avoid sites that are easily bumped or moved such as the dorsal surface of the hand (Box 18.7).

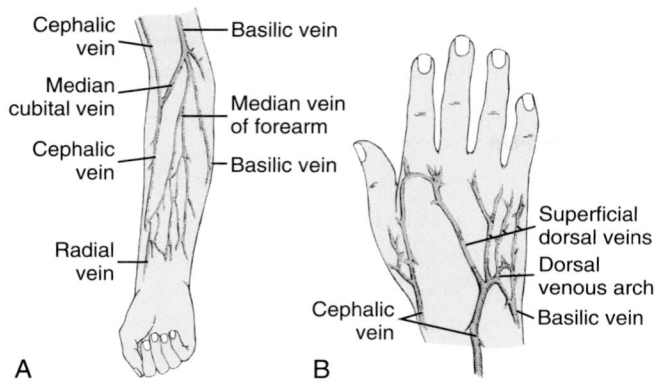

FIG 18.7 Common IV sites. **A,** Inner arm. **B,** Dorsal surface of hand.

BOX 18.7 CARE OF THE OLDER ADULT

Protection of Skin and Veins During IV Therapy

- Avoid using a tourniquet when selecting a vein. Position the arm in a dependent position to fill the veins sufficiently for a venipuncture or use a blood pressure cuff for better protection of the older adult's skin. If using a tourniquet, place it over the patient's sleeve.
- Use the smallest-gauge IV catheter or needle possible such as 22 or 24 gauge to protect fragile veins. A smaller gauge allows better blood flow to provide increased hemodilution of IV fluids or medications (Phillips and Gorski, 2014).
- Avoid placing IV in veins that are easily bumped because older adults have less subcutaneous support tissue.
- Avoid the back of the hand, which may compromise a patient's need for independence and mobility.
- Use strict aseptic technique because an older adult patient is more likely to be immunocompromised.
- Do not slap the arm to visualize the patient's veins or use vigorous friction while cleansing the site to prevent tearing fragile skin.
- Decrease the venipuncture insertion angle because of decreased supportive tissue (Phillips and Gorski, 2014).
- Veins roll away from the needle easily as a result of loss of subcutaneous tissue. To stabilize the vein, apply traction to the skin below the projected insertion site (Phillips and Gorski, 2014).
- Secure IV site with a catheter stabilization device and a mesh dressing for protection, avoiding excessive use of tape on fragile skin (Touhy and Jett, 2014).
- Use electronic infusion devices or controllers to titrate infusion volume and rate.

Venipuncture is contraindicated in a site that has signs of inflammation, infiltration, or thrombosis. An infected site is red, tender, swollen, and possibly warm to the touch. Avoid using an extremity with a vascular (dialysis) graft or fistula or on the same side as a mastectomy (breast surgery). Initially place IV catheters at the most distal point, which allows for the use of proximal sites later if the patient needs a venipuncture site change (Gorski et al., 2016).

Venipuncture accesses a vein by puncture through the skin using a sharp rigid stylet (e.g., metal needle). To collect a blood specimen, the needle has an attached syringe or collection tube. To start an IV infusion you use a stylet partially covered with a plastic catheter (over-the-needle catheter [ONC]). You use aseptic technique to prepare the skin. Only experienced practitioners perform venipuncture on patients with fragile veins (e.g., infants or older adults).

You will use venipuncture to collect a blood specimen, start an IV fluid infusion, instill a medication, or inject a tracer for diagnostic examinations. Use intermittent infusion when a patient requires medications only at certain times, in an emergency situation, and to avoid the discomfort of repeated injections. An intermittent infusion involves the same techniques as a continuous IV drip, but after you give the complete dose of medication, you disconnect the tubing from the IV access device and leave it in place. A continuous infusion of fluids, with or without medications, is achieved over a 24-hour period through use of a VAD. Skill 18.1 describes the technique for initiating peripheral IV fluid infusion and incorporates INS standards of practice (Box 18.8) (Gorski et al., 2016).

Regulating Infusion Flow Rate. After initiating an IV infusion and checking it for patency, regulate the rate of infusion according to the health care provider's orders (see Skill 18.2). An infusion rate that is too slow fails to reverse cardiovascular and circulatory collapse in a critically ill patient who has severe ECV deficit or is in shock. An infusion rate that is too rapid can cause fluid and electrolyte overload.

Calculate IV infusion rates to maintain a consistent flow at the ordered rate (e.g., 125 mL/h). EIDs deliver an accurate hourly IV infusion rate. Familiarize yourself with the brand of EID in use at your institution so that you can set the flow rate accurately. Safeguards prevent free flow of infusion and sudden volume infusion when regulators are removed from the tubing housing. However, if you open a clamp on an infusion tubing that is not yet properly inserted in an EID or gravity-flow IV system, the IV fluid may infuse very rapidly.

Nonelectronic volume-control devices are used occasionally above an EID to prevent accidental infusion of a large fluid volume, especially in pediatrics. These devices hold small amounts of fluid and hang between the IV fluid container and the EID. They also may be used with gravity-flow infusions. The rate of infusion with an IV gravity controller depends on the height of the IV fluid container, IV tubing size, and fluid viscosity. Regardless of the device in use, monitor the patient regularly to verify correct infusion of IV fluid and detect complications.

Patency of an IV catheter means that fluid flows easily through it. To be patent, the catheter tip needs to be free from clots and be away from the vein wall. A blocked catheter slows or stops the infusion of IV fluids. Infiltration (fluid leaking into tissues), a knot or kink in the tubing, external pressure on the tubing, and patient position changes decrease IV flow rates. If the IV flow decreases or stops, assess the system until you locate the problem. Start your assessment at the catheter insertion site for signs and symptoms of infiltration

BOX 18.8 EVIDENCE-BASED PRACTICE

PICO Question: In patients with peripheral IV catheters, does vascular access device (VAD) insertion on the dorsum of the hand increase the complication rate compared with VAD insertion on the forearm?

SUMMARY OF EVIDENCE

Complications of peripheral IV catheters such as phlebitis, infiltration, extravasation, catheter occlusion, nerve damage, and accidental removal impair patient safety and comfort and increase the cost of care (Helm et al., 2015; Gorski et al., 2016). Research indicates that the site chosen for peripheral VAD insertion can influence the rate of complications. A large study of adult medical-surgical patients in three hospitals found increased rates of catheter occlusion and of accidental removal for VADs inserted in the dorsum of the hand compared with VADs inserted in the forearm (Wallis et al., 2014). Another large multisite study of hospitalized older adults found increased rates of phlebitis in VADs inserted in the dorsum of the hand compared with VADs inserted in the forearm (Cicolini et al., 2014). A small study of hospitalized older adults found no statistical difference in phlebitis rates between the two sites, although the researchers indicated that the small number of subjects limited any conclusions (Benaya et al., 2015). The Infusion Nursing Standards of Practice (Gorski et al., 2016) indicate increased risk of infiltration, extravasation, and sensory nerve damage with VAD insertion in the dorsum of the hand compared with forearm insertion.

APPLICATION TO NURSING PRACTICE

- Consider the potential rate of complications, among the other considerations, when selecting a site for VAD insertion (Helm et al., 2015; Gorski et al., 2016).
- If possible, avoid VAD insertion in the dorsum of the hand of older adults (Cicolini et al., 2014).
- If infusing an IV solution that is known to be irritating to veins, avoid using the dorsum of the hand because that site has increased risk of extravasation (Gorski et al., 2016).

VAD, Vascular access device.

TABLE 18.9 INFUSION NURSES SOCIETY PHLEBITIS SCALE

GRADE	CLINICAL CRITERIA
0	No symptoms
1	Erythema at access site with or without pain
2	Pain at access site with erythema and/or edema
3	Pain at access site with erythema, streak formation, palpable venous cord
4	Pain at access site with erythema, streak formation, palpable venous cord greater than 2.5 cm (1 inch) in length, purulent drainage

From Gorski L, et al: Infusion therapy standards of practice, *J Infus Nurs* 39(suppl 1):S1, 2016.

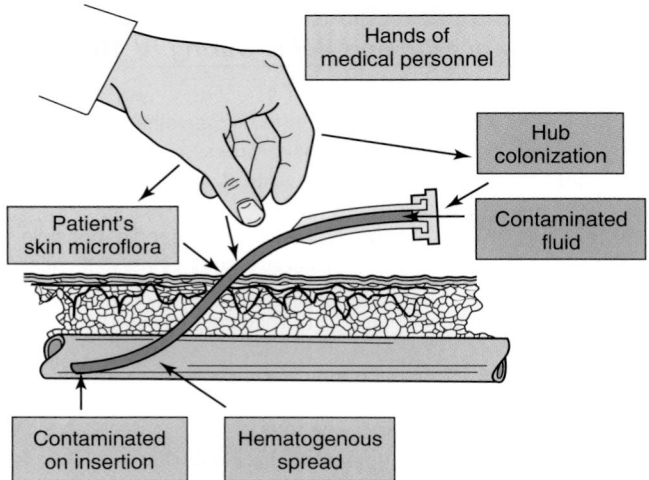

FIG 18.8 Potential sites for contamination of an intravascular device.

and phlebitis (Table 18.9). The clinical presentation of infiltration is easily confused with phlebitis or irritant reactions (Gorski et al., 2016). Systematically continue your assessment by inspecting the area around the insertion site and the tubing for anything blocking the flow of IV fluids, such as a patient lying or sitting on the tubing. Frequently the flow rate resumes after you remove the tubing obstruction. Check for proper function of the EID. For gravity-flow systems the height of an IV container affects flow rates. Raising the container usually increases the rate because of increased driving pressure.

Flexion of an extremity, particularly at the wrist or elbow, often decreases the IV flow rate by pushing the tip of the catheter against the vein wall or compressing the vein. Although VAD placement in areas of flexion is discouraged, occasionally it is necessary. In that case INS standards specify use of an arm board or other joint stabilization device to

protect the IV site by keeping the joint extended (Gorski et al., 2016). Use padding with arm boards to reduce the risk for skin or nerve damage from pressure. Sometimes it is more comfortable for a patient to have an infusion started in a new location rather than relying on a site that causes problems. Before discontinuing the current infusion, choose another site and start the infusion to verify that the patient has other accessible veins.

Maintaining the System. Once a catheter is in place, maintain the integrity of the site and regulate the flow rate accurately to maintain the IV system. Agency policies regulate the maintenance of IV lines. IV line maintenance includes (1) keeping the system sterile and intact; (2) changing IV fluid containers, tubing, and contaminated site dressings; (3) assisting a patient with self-care activities (e.g., bathing) so that the IV system is not disrupted; and (4) monitoring for complications of IV therapy.

Patient safety requires maintaining the integrity of an IV line to prevent introduction of microorganisms that can cause infection (Vizcarra et al., 2014). Fig. 18.8 shows potential sites for contamination of a VAD. The procedure for IV insertion minimizes contamination during catheter insertion. After insertion, prevent infection through conscientious use of infection control principles, including thorough hand hygiene before and after handling any part of the IV system and maintaining sterility of the system during tubing and fluid container changes.

Always maintain the integrity of an IV system. Never disconnect tubing because it becomes tangled or because it is more convenient to position or move a patient or apply a gown. If a patient needs more room to maneuver, add extension tubing to an IV line using aseptic technique. *Never let IV tubing touch the floor.* Do not use stopcocks for connecting multiple solutions to a single IV site because they are sources of contamination (Gorski et al., 2016). IV tubing contains injection ports through which you can insert needleless syringes or other adapters for medication administration. Clean an injection port thoroughly with 2% chlorhexidine (preferred), 70% alcohol, or povidone-iodine, and let it dry before accessing the system (Gorski et al., 2016).

Changing IV Fluid Containers, Tubing, and Dressings. Patients receiving IV therapy over several days require periodic changing of IV fluid containers. Organize your tasks so that you can change solutions before a clot forms in a catheter. Recommended frequency of IV tubing change depends on whether it is used for continuous or intermittent infusion. INS standards (Gorski et al., 2016) specify that *continuous* infusion tubing changes should occur *no more frequently than every 96 hours* unless the tubing has been compromised or contaminated, which requires immediate tubing change. In contrast, you should change tubing for *intermittent* infusion every 24 hours because of the increased risk of contamination from opening the IV system (Gorski et al., 2016). Blood products and lipids easily promote bacterial growth in tubing. Therefore change tubing containing blood products every 4 hours and tubing for continuous IV lipids every 24 hours (Gorski et al., 2016). Whenever possible, schedule tubing changes when it is time to hang a new IV container to decrease risk of infection (see Skill 18.3) (Gorski et al., 2016). To prevent entry of microorganisms into the bloodstream, maintain sterility during tubing and IV fluid container changes (Gorski et al., 2016).

A sterile dressing over an IV site reduces the entrance of bacteria into the insertion site. Transparent dressings, the most common type, help secure the VAD, allow continuous visual inspection of the IV site, and stay cleaner and drier than gauze dressings. Leave transparent dressings in place until the IV tubing is replaced (Gorski et al., 2016). If a gauze dressing is used, change it every 48 hours (Gorski et al., 2016). You change either form of dressing when the IV device is removed or when the dressing becomes damp, loosened, or soiled (see Skill 18.4) (Gorski et al., 2016). Agency policy may require routine dressing changes in different time frames.

Helping Patients Protect IV Integrity. To prevent accidental disruption of an IV system, patients often need assistance with hygiene, comfort measures, meals, and ambulation. Bathing and changing gowns are difficult for a patient with an IV line in the arm. Teach NAP and patients that they must

not disconnect tubing of an IV line because this leads to contamination. If available, use a gown with snaps along the top sleeve seam to facilitate gown changes without disturbing the venipuncture site. Change regular gowns by following these steps:

1. Remove the sleeve of the gown from the arm without the IV line, maintaining the patient's privacy.
2. Remove the sleeve of the gown from the arm with the IV line.
3. Remove the IV solution container from its stand and pass it and the tubing through the sleeve. If this involves removing the tubing from an EID, use the roller clamp to slow the infusion to prevent accidental infusion of a large volume of fluid.
4. To apply a gown, place the IV solution container and tubing through the sleeve of the clean gown and hang it back on the stand. If the IV infusion is controlled by an EID, reassemble, turn on the pump, and open the roller clamp.
5. Place the arm with the IV line through the new gown sleeve.
6. Place the arm without the IV line through the new gown sleeve.

Mechanical catheter securement devices extend the time that a VAD can be used. Commercial protective devices also prevent accidental dislodgment of an IV catheter (Fig. 18.9).

A patient with an arm or a hand infusion is able to walk unless contraindicated. Offer a rolling IV pole on wheels. See that the patient has help to get out of bed, if needed, and place the pole next to the involved arm. Teach the patient to hold on to the pole with the involved hand and push it while walking. Check that the IV container is at the proper height, there is no tension on the tubing, and the flow rate is correct. Instruct the patient to report any blood in the tubing, stoppage in flow, an EID alarm, or increased discomfort.

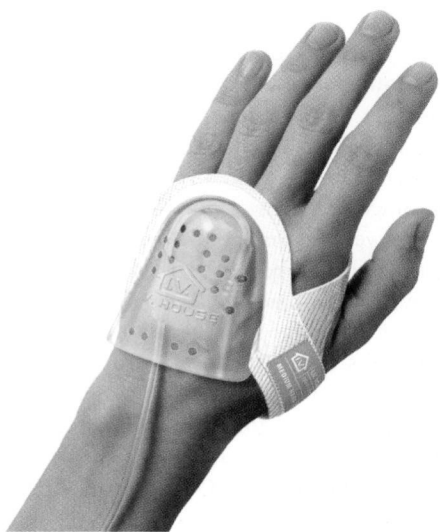

FIG 18.9 I.V. House protective device. (Courtesy I.V. House, St Louis, MO.)

Complications of IV Therapy. An infiltration occurs when IV fluids leak into the subcutaneous tissue around the venipuncture site because the catheter tip no longer is in the vein. When the leakage of IV fluids is harmful, causing damage to extravascular tissue, the injury is called an extravasation. Infiltration causes swelling (from increased interstitial fluid), paleness, and coolness (from decreased circulation) around the venipuncture site. The IV infusion may slow or stop. Pain may occur, increasing as the infiltration progresses. The INS recommends using an infiltration scale for assessment (Gorski et al., 2016).

If extravasation occurs, discontinue the infusion and medication immediately. Disconnect the IV tubing from the VAD but do not remove the VAD (ONS, 2016) (see agency policy). Certified nurses or a health care provider may attempt to aspirate the residual drug from the IV device using a syringe. Later, you will likely remove the VAD. Depending on the solution that extravasates, you may need to administer an antidote. If IV therapy still is necessary, insert a new VAD in a vein at a new location. To reduce discomfort, elevate the extremity to promote venous drainage and decrease edema. Apply a warm, moist compress to the site for 15 to 20 minutes at a time at least four times a day to promote venous return and reduce pain and edema (ONS, 2016).

Certain IV medications, especially potassium and some antibiotics, can cause discomfort and burning sensations at the IV site. Evaluate the source of discomfort, decrease the infusion rate if allowed, or start a new IV line in a larger vein if needed.

Phlebitis is inflammation of a vein. Risk factors include acidic or hypertonic IV solutions; rapid IV rate; irritating IV drugs such as potassium chloride (KCl) and vancomycin; VAD in area of flexion; poorly secured catheter; poor hand hygiene; and lack of aseptic technique (Helm et al., 2015). Signs and symptoms include redness, tenderness, and warmth along the course of the vein starting at the access site, with possibly a red streak and/or palpable cord along the vein (Gorski et al., 2016). The INS Phlebitis Scale (see Table 18.9) is easy to use, valid, and reliable (Gorski et al., 2016).

If phlebitis develops, discontinue the IV line and insert a new line in another vein. Warm, moist compresses on the site of phlebitis offer some relief to patients (see Chapter 38). Phlebitis is dangerous because blood clots (thrombi) can form, increasing the risk for an embolus (i.e., a clot that becomes dislodged and travels to the lungs). Phlebitis sometimes damages veins permanently. Although some agencies require routine removal of VADs and site rotation to prevent phlebitis, the INS Standards of Practice (Gorski et al., 2016) recommend replacing a peripheral VAD only if clinically indicated in adults. Assess the VAD site at least every 4 hours and more frequently with critically ill patients, children, and patients receiving IV solutions containing irritating drugs or vasoconstrictors. Avoid routine replacement of peripheral VADs in infants and children (Gorski et al., 2016).

Local infection at a VAD insertion site is possible, showing redness and/or edema and exudate. Before removing a VAD, immediately notify the health care provider to find out if you need to send the exudate of the catheter tip for a culture. After you take the culture sample, remove the VAD and insert a new one in another site if continued IV therapy is necessary. If the health care provider orders antibiotics, do not start them until a blood culture is taken if ordered.

Another complication of IV therapy is fluid overload from a too-rapid infusion. Assessment findings depend on the type of solution. Excessive infusion of a sodium-containing isotonic solution causes ECV excess, with shortness of breath and crackles in the lungs. If these clinical signs are present, slow the rate of IV infusion, notify the health care provider, raise the head of the bed, provide supplemental oxygen and diuretics as ordered, and monitor the patient's vital signs. Excessive infusion of D_5W causes hyponatremia with confusion, lethargy, and possibly seizures. Whenever your patient has an IV running, monitor for the effects of overload of the IV fluid.

QSEN **QSEN ACTIVITY** *Quality Improvement*

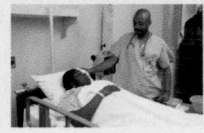

Nurses on the unit where Mrs. Reynolds is a patient are performing a quality improvement project to decrease the complications of IV therapy on their unit. They formed a day-shift IV team that performs all IV starts and coaches nurses on IV maintenance and monitoring on day shift. Evening and night shifts do not yet have IV teams.

- List at least four outcomes that the nurses could measure to determine the effectiveness of this quality improvement project.

evolve   Answers to QSEN Activities can be found on the Evolve website.

Discontinuing Peripheral IV Access. You discontinue a VAD after the prescribed amount of fluid is infused, when infiltration occurs, if phlebitis is present, or if a clot develops in the catheter. Review the health care provider's order before discontinuing a VAD. Explain to patients the reason for discontinuing an IV infusion and that they might feel a burning sensation when the catheter is removed. Perform hand hygiene and apply clean gloves. Close the IV tubing roller clamp and turn off the EID (if your patient has one) to prevent spilling IV fluid. Remove the IV site dressing and any catheter stabilization device. Then remove any tape securing the catheter without using scissors (Gorski et al., 2016). Remove secretions around the skin puncture site by holding the catheter hub and using an antiseptic swab. Allow skin to dry completely. Place sterile gauze over the venipuncture site and apply light pressure while withdrawing the catheter by pulling away from the insertion site in a slow, steady motion (Fig. 18.10). Keep the catheter hub parallel to the skin during withdrawal. Inspect the catheter end for intactness after removal. Keep gauze in place and apply continuous pressure to the site for 2 to 3 minutes to control bleeding

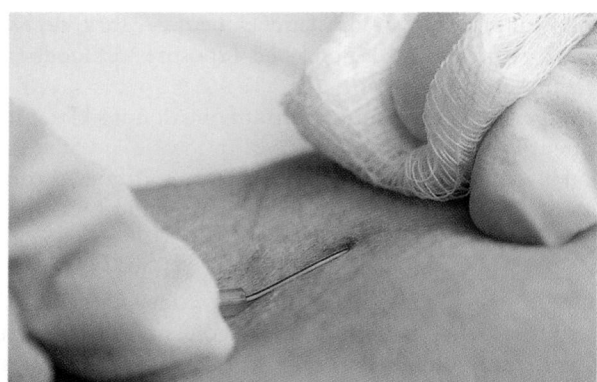

FIG 18.10 Withdraw IV catheter slowly, keeping catheter parallel to vein.

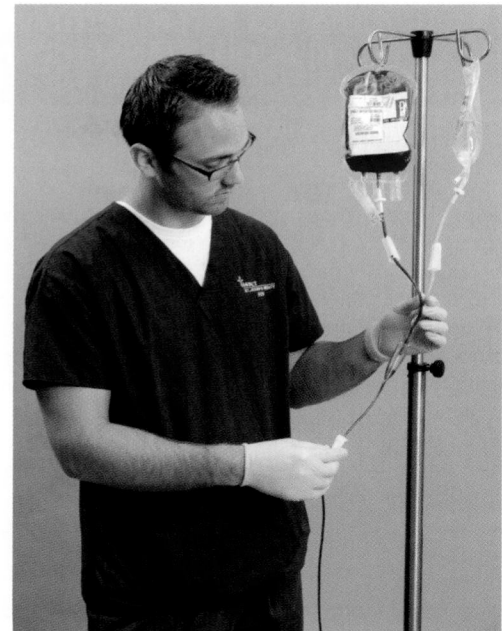

FIG 18.11 Filling tubing for blood administration.

and minimize hematoma formation (Gorski et al., 2016). If a patient receives anticoagulants or platelet inhibitors, apply steady pressure for 5 to 10 minutes and assess bleeding. Apply a sterile folded gauze dressing over the removal site and secure it with tape. Then perform hand hygiene. Record the amount of fluid infused and the time the IV infusion was discontinued in the medical record. Routinely inspect the site for redness, edema, and tenderness for 48 hours. In some settings licensed practical nurses (LPNs) discontinue peripheral IV infusions (consult agency policy or state Nurse Practice Act).

Blood Replacement. Blood replacement or transfusion is the IV administration of whole blood or a blood component such as plasma, packed red blood cells (RBCs), or platelets. Blood transfusions (1) increase circulating blood volume after surgery, trauma, or hemorrhage; (2) increase the number of RBCs to maintain hemoglobin levels in patients with severe anemia; and (3) provide selected cellular components as replacement therapy (e.g., clotting factors, platelets, albumin).

Transfusing blood or blood components is a nursing procedure requiring an order from a health care provider. Perform thorough patient assessment before, during, and after a transfusion. Adverse blood transfusion events are included in the public reporting of safety events of a health care institution (NQF, 2016). Before a transfusion assess the patient to determine if he or she knows the reason for the blood transfusion and whether he or she has had a previous transfusion or transfusion reaction. Patients who have had a transfusion reaction usually are not at greater risk for a reaction with a subsequent transfusion. However, they usually are anxious about the transfusion, requiring nursing intervention. Before starting a transfusion explain the procedure and instruct the patient to report any side effects (e.g., chills, light-headedness, or fever) once transfusion begins. Ensure that the patient or representative has signed an informed consent. People from certain cultural backgrounds may refuse blood transfusions or seek alternatives to it (Guinn et al., 2015). Be sensitive to patient preferences.

Because of the danger of transfusion reactions, your pretransfusion assessment includes baseline vital signs

(Crookston et al., 2015). These data allow you to determine when changes in vital signs occur as a result of a transfusion reaction. ABO incompatibility is a serious error with transfusions. This error commonly involves misidentification of the patient, unit of blood, or label on the pretransfusion blood sample. For patient safety follow agency procedure to verify three things: that blood components delivered are the ones that were ordered, that blood delivered is compatible with the patient's blood type listed in the medical record, and that the right patient receives the blood. Many hospitals use bar-code technology to identify patients and verify compatible blood before beginning transfusions. Nurses are responsible for determining that the blood delivered to a patient corresponds to the patient's blood type documented in the medical record. Together two RNs or one RN and one LPN (check agency policy and procedures) must check the label on the blood product against the medical record and the patient's identification number, blood group, and complete name. *If even a minor discrepancy exists, do not give the blood. Notify the blood bank immediately.*

When administering a transfusion, you need an appropriately sized IV catheter and special tubing with a 20-μm in-line filter (Fig. 18.11). Adults require a large catheter such as 18 or 20 gauge because blood is more viscous than crystalloid IV fluids. Prime the tubing with 0.9% sodium chloride to reduce hemolysis (breakdown of RBCs). Start a transfusion slowly to allow for early detection of a transfusion reaction. Maintain the ordered infusion rate, monitor for side effects, assess vital signs, and promptly record all findings. Stay with the patient during the first 15 minutes, the time when a reaction is most likely to occur. After that time period continue to monitor the patient and obtain vital signs periodically during the transfusion as directed by agency policy. If you

BOX 18.9 NURSING INTERVENTIONS FOR BLOOD TRANSFUSION REACTION

- *STOP the transfusion immediately,* even when you just suspect a reaction.
- Remove blood component and tubing containing blood product. Replace them with new primed tubing with a container of 0.9% sodium chloride (normal saline). Connect tubing to hub of IV catheter.
- **Caution:** Do not turn off the blood and simply turn on the 0.9% (normal saline) that is connected to the Y-tubing infusion set. This would cause blood remaining in the Y-tubing to infuse into the patient. Even a small amount of mismatched blood can cause a major reaction.
- Maintain patent IV line using 0.9% normal saline.
- Remain with the patient, observing signs and symptoms and monitoring vital signs every 5 minutes.
- Immediately notify the health care provider or emergency response team.
- Notify blood bank.
- Prepare to perform CPR and administer emergency drugs such as antihistamines, vasopressors, fluids, and corticosteroids per health care provider's order or protocol.
- Save the blood container, tubing, attached labels, and transfusion record for return to the blood bank.
- Obtain blood and first voided urine specimens per health care provider's order or protocol. **Note:** If patient is unable to void, insert a catheter to obtain urine specimen.
- Document the transfusion reaction, description, treatment, and outcome.

CPR, Cardiopulmonary resuscitation; *NS,* normal saline.

suspect a transfusion reaction, *stop* the transfusion immediately and follow the guidelines in Box 18.9.

The transfusion rate usually is specified in the health care provider's orders. Ideally 1 unit of whole blood or packed RBCs is transfused in 2 hours. Lengthen the time to 4 hours if a patient is at risk for ECV excess. Beyond 4 hours there is an increased risk for bacterial contamination of the blood.

When patients have a severe blood loss such as with hemorrhage, they often receive rapid transfusions through a central venous catheter. A blood-warming device is necessary because the tip of the central venous catheter lies in the superior vena cava, above the right atrium. Rapid administration of cold blood can cause cardiac dysrhythmias. Patients who receive large-volume transfusion of citrated blood have high risk of hyperkalemia, hypocalcemia, hypomagnesemia, and metabolic alkalosis (Crookston et al., 2015).

Autologous Transfusion. Autologous transfusion (autotransfusion) is the collection and reinfusion of a patient's own blood. Blood for an autologous transfusion usually is obtained by preoperative donation up to 6 weeks before the scheduled surgery, depending on the type of surgery and ability of the patient to maintain an acceptable hematocrit. Blood for autologous transfusion also can be obtained at the time of surgery. After surgery blood can be salvaged from drainage from chest tubes or joint cavities. Autologous

transfusions are safer for patients because they decrease the risk of mismatched blood and exposure to bloodborne infectious agents.

Allogeneic Transfusion. Infusion of a donor's blood into a patient is allogeneic transfusion. In the United States the blood is collected in a donation center and goes through numerous tests to ensure that it is free from infectious agents such as human immunodeficiency virus (HIV) and hepatitis B virus (HBV) and hepatitis C virus (HCV) before it is infused. Blood testing positive for infectious agents is discarded; the donor is notified and placed on a list (deferral registry) that prohibits the donor from donating blood again (AABB, 2016).

ABO System. A blood transfusion must be matched to each patient to avoid dangerous incompatibility. Blood-typing systems are used to ensure a close match between transfused products and a patient's blood. The presence or absence of specific antigens on the surface of RBCs determines blood type in the ABO system. When the type A antigen is present, the blood group is type A. When the type B antigen is present, the blood group is type B. When both A and B antigens are present, the blood group is type AB; and, when neither A nor B antigens are present, the blood group is type O (Simmons and Savage, 2015).

Antibodies that react against the A and B antigens naturally are present in the plasma of people whose RBCs do not carry the antigen. These antibodies react against the foreign antigens from mismatched transfusions. For example, if a person who is type A accidentally receives type B blood, antibodies in the person's blood attack the type B antigens. Incompatible RBCs agglutinate (clump together), causing a potentially life-threatening immune response known as a hemolytic transfusion reaction. People with type A blood have anti-B antibodies; people with type B blood have anti-A antibodies. People with type AB blood have neither antibody and can receive all blood types. People with type O blood have both A and B antibodies and can receive only type O blood.

Rh System. Another consideration for matching blood for transfusion is presence of Rh factor, an antigenic substance on RBCs in most people. A person with Rh factor is Rh positive, whereas a person without it is Rh negative. In contrast to ABO antigens, there are no naturally occurring antibodies to the Rh antigen. A person with Rh-negative blood must first be exposed to Rh-positive blood before developing antibodies. People who are Rh negative should receive only Rh-negative blood components.

Transfusion Reactions and Other Adverse Effects. A transfusion reaction is an immune system response to a transfusion that ranges from a mild response to severe anaphylactic shock, acute intravascular hemolysis, or acute lung injury, all of which are life threatening. Prompt nursing intervention is essential to maintain a patient's physiological stability (see Box 18.9).

Circulatory overload is a risk when a patient receives massive transfusions for hemorrhagic shock or when a patient with normal intravascular volume receives blood. Older adults and patients with cardiopulmonary diseases have high risk for circulatory overload and need careful monitoring during transfusion.

Another category of adverse transfusion effects is diseases transmitted by blood from infected donors who are asymptomatic. Symptoms of these diseases often arise long after the transfusion. Diseases transmitted through transfusions include malaria, HBV and HCV, HIV infection and acquired immunodeficiency syndrome (AIDS), Chagas disease, West Nile virus infection, and cytomegalovirus infection (Crookston et al., 2015; Custer et al., 2015). Blood collected for blood banks in developed countries undergoes screening for at least HIV, HBV, HCV, and syphilis, which reduces the risk for acquiring these bloodborne infections (AABB, 2016).

Interventions for Acid-Base Imbalances. Nursing interventions to promote acid-base balance support prescribed medical therapies and aim at reversing the underlying disorder causing the acid-base imbalance while providing for patient safety. Acid-base imbalances often are life threatening and require a rapid nursing response to deliver treatment. Maintain a patent IV line and check for changes in prescribed therapies. Give fluid and electrolyte replacements and prescribed drugs promptly. In addition, monitor patients closely for changes in their status. Use protective measures such as bedrails for patients with decreased level of consciousness.

Arterial Blood Gas Measurement. Patients with serious fluid and electrolyte imbalance often require frequent ABG monitoring. ABG analysis reveals a patient's acid-base status and the adequacy of ventilation and oxygenation. The analysis involves removing a blood sample from an artery. A qualified RN, respiratory therapist, or other personnel draws arterial blood from a peripheral artery (usually the radial) or from an arterial line (see agency policy and procedures). Before an arterial blood draw, ensure that the patient has an ulnar pulse to prevent loss of blood flow to the hand in the event of radial artery damage. After the arterial puncture, apply pressure to the puncture site for at least 5 minutes to reduce risk of hematoma (bleeding under skin) formation. Apply pressure for a longer period if the patient takes anticoagulant medications or has a clotting disorder. Reassess the radial pulse after removing pressure. After obtaining the specimen, prevent air from entering the syringe because this alters the blood gas results. To reduce oxygen use by RBCs, submerge the syringe in crushed ice and transport it immediately to the laboratory.

Restorative and Continuing Care. After experiencing acute fluid, electrolyte, or acid-base imbalances, patients often require ongoing maintenance to prevent recurrence. Older adults require special considerations to prevent complications from developing.

Home Intravenous Therapy. IV therapy often continues at home for patients requiring long-term hydration, parenteral nutrition, or long-term medication administration. A home IV therapy nurse works closely with a patient and family caregivers to ensure that they know how to maintain a sterile IV system; how to dispose of sharps and materials exposed to blood safely; techniques for ambulation, hygiene, and other activities of daily living without dislodging the IV catheter or disconnecting the system; and how to avoid complications or recognize and report them promptly.

Nutritional Support. Most patients who have electrolyte or acid-base imbalances require ongoing nutritional support. Depending on the type of disorder, you encourage or restrict certain fluids or food. Teach patients or family caregivers who are responsible for meal preparation the nutritional content of foods and how to read the labels of commercially prepared foods.

Medication Safety. Numerous prescription and OTC drugs and supplements contain components or create side effects that alter fluid and electrolyte balance. Patients with chronic disease who receive multiple medications and patients with renal disorders have high risk for fluid and electrolyte imbalances. Apply literacy principles (see Chapter 12), and teach patients and families regarding potential side effects and drug interactions that alter fluid, electrolyte, or acid-base balance. Review all medications with patients and family caregivers, confirm the correct schedule for administering each medication, and encourage the patient to consult the local pharmacist before using an OTC drug or supplement.

■ ■ ■ EVALUATION

Patient Outcomes. Evaluation of a patient's clinical status is important when an acute fluid, electrolyte, or acid-base imbalance exists. You need to recognize the signs and symptoms of impending problems by considering a patient's presenting risk factors and clinical status, effects of the present treatment regimen, and the potential causative agent. Perform an evaluation to determine if changes have occurred from the patient's baseline or previous patient assessment.

For example, if a patient's hypokalemia is improving, you expect the signs and symptoms of hypokalemia to diminish. The patient's heart rhythm becomes more regular, muscle strength improves, and bowel function returns. The serum potassium level returns to normal levels. If the hypokalemia is not improving, the signs and symptoms continue, and the serum potassium level remains below normal.

For patients with less acute imbalances, evaluation occurs over a longer period of time. In these situations, focus your evaluation more on behavioral changes (e.g., the patient's adherence to dietary restrictions and medication schedules). Also evaluate the family caregiver's ability to anticipate imbalances and prevent problems from recurring.

A patient's level of progress determines whether you continue or revise the plan of care. If goals are not met, consult with other members of the health care team to discuss additional methods such as increasing the frequency of an intervention (e.g., provide more fluids to a dehydrated patient), introducing a new therapy (e.g., initiate insertion of an IV), or discontinuing a particular therapy. Once a patient meets the outcomes of care, the nursing diagnosis is resolved, and you can focus on other priorities including maintaining

BOX 18.10 EVALUATION

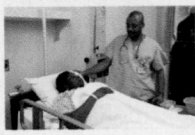

Robert continues to care for Mrs. Reynolds 2 days after her admission. He asks her how she feels and prepares to conduct a brief physical assessment. Mrs. Reynolds remarks, "I feel much better. I have had no nausea since early yesterday and no diarrhea since late yesterday afternoon." The IV infusion of 0.9% sodium chloride (normal saline) still is in place, infusing now at 100 mL/h. However, because Mrs. Reynolds is tolerating oral fluids, the health care provider just ordered to reduce the rate to 40 mL/h.

During examination Robert notices that her skin turgor has returned to normal, but her oral mucosa are still slightly dry. Mrs. Reynolds' vital signs are blood pressure, 126/78 mm Hg; pulse, 80 beats/min; and respirations, 18 breaths/min. She is afebrile. The serum potassium level drawn at 7 a.m. was 4 mEq/L.

Robert is encouraged by Mrs. Reynolds' progress. He brings her breakfast meal tray, which includes the first soft food that she has had since being hospitalized. Robert sits down and discusses with Mrs. Reynolds what she has learned from their discussion about food sources for potassium. Robert asks, "Now that we've discussed the importance of potassium in your diet, tell me which foods you would select that are high in potassium." Mrs. Reynolds identifies five different sources of potassium among foods that she enjoys and can routinely include in her diet.

DOCUMENTATION NOTE

"Denies nausea and reports feeling better. No diarrheal stool since yesterday afternoon around 4 p.m. On inspection oral mucosa remains dry without lesions or inflammation. Skin turgor is normal. Bowel sounds are normal in all four quadrants, abdomen soft to palpation. IV of 0.9% sodium chloride is infusing in left cephalic vein in forearm at 40 mL/h per MD order. No tenderness or inflammation at IV site. Is able to identify five food sources for potassium to include in diet. Is resting comfortably, out of bed in a chair, and ate all of breakfast. Will continue to monitor."

normal fluid, electrolyte, and acid-base balance. If an outcome is not met, revise the plan of care as needed.

Patient Expectations. Review with patients how well their major concerns regarding fluid, electrolyte, or acid-base situations were alleviated or addressed. For example, if a patient's concern was feeling uncomfortable with very dry mouth, ask, "How does your mouth feel now?" (Box 18.10).

If a patient's concerns involve having a better understanding of a newly diagnosed problem, evaluate the patient's satisfaction with the education provided. Often a patient's level of satisfaction with care also depends on success in involving family caregivers and friends. If patients have concerns about returning home or to a different care setting, it is important to evaluate how well prepared they feel for the transition from acute care.

SAFETY GUIDELINES FOR NURSING SKILLS

Ensuring patient safety is an essential role of a professional nurse. To ensure patient safety, communicate clearly with members of the health care team, assess and incorporate the patient's priorities of care and preferences, and use the best evidence when making decisions about your patient's care. When performing the skills in this chapter, remember the following points to ensure safe, individualized care:

- Check that you have the necessary information, an order if required, and equipment available for the procedure before beginning.
- Determine if the patient has latex allergy and use nonlatex items if allergy is present (Gorski et al., 2016).
- Conduct a complete history and physical assessment including vital signs, and review laboratory findings before initiating any solutions or medications. Consider prolonged environmental conditions that affect a patient's fluid status (e.g., exposure to hot, humid weather) leading to fluid and electrolyte imbalances, particularly in infants, older adults, and patients with chronic illnesses.
- Know the indications for prescribed therapy before initiating IV therapy. Obtain and review the health care practitioner's order to ensure appropriateness of the prescribed solution or medication for patient's age, health status, medical diagnosis, allergy status, acuity, VAD type and tip location, dose, frequency, and route of administration (Gorski et al., 2016).
- Use special designated tubing for the specific brand of EID and for blood transfusions and some medications.
- Review the steps of the procedure before entering a patient's room, considering modifications that you may need to make for each specific patient and verifying that the type of IV solution is appropriate for the patient.
- Maintain strict aseptic and sterile techniques when manipulating the IV system to prevent development of bloodstream infections (Gorski et al., 2016).
- If you contaminate a sterile object during the procedure, do not use it. Use a new sterile one.
- Know and implement the standard precautions for infection control and the Occupational Safety and Health Administration (OSHA) standards for occupational exposure to bloodborne pathogens. Place all disposable blood-contaminated and sharp items in designated puncture-resistant biohazard containers (Gorski et al., 2016).

SKILL 18.1 INITIATING INTRAVENOUS THERAPY

DELEGATION CONSIDERATIONS

The skill of inserting a short-peripheral IV access device cannot be delegated to nursing assistive personnel (NAP). Delegation to licensed practical nurses (LPNs) varies by state Nurse Practice Act. The nurse instructs the NAP to:

- Notify the nurse if the patient complains of any IV site–related complications such as redness, pain, tenderness, swelling, bleeding, drainage, or leaking from under dressing.
- Notify the nurse if the patient's IV dressing becomes wet.
- Notify the nurse if the level of fluid in the IV bag is low or the electronic infusion device (EID) is alarming.

EQUIPMENT

- Short-peripheral IV start kit supplies (available in some agencies): single-use tourniquet, tape, transparent semipermeable membrane (TSM) dressing or sterile gauze and sterile tape, antiseptic solution (chlorhexidine solution preferred, povidone-iodine, or 70% alcohol), 2 × 2–inch gauze pads, and label. **Note:** If kit is not available, gather all equipment separately.
- Appropriate short-peripheral IV catheter with safety mechanism for venipuncture (Fig. 18.12) (see Table 29.3) (Gorski et al., 2016)
- Clean gloves (latex free for patients with latex allergy); sterile gloves are recommended if palpating the site after skin antisepsis (Gorski et al., 2016)
- Single-use hair clippers or scissors for hair removal if indicated
- Short extension tubing with fused needleless connector or separate needleless connector (also called *injection cap, saline lock, heparin lock, IV plug, buff cap, buffalo cap,* or *PRN adapter*)
- 5-mL prefilled syringe with preservative-free 0.9% sodium chloride (normal saline [NS]) (Gorski et al., 2016)
- Antiseptic swabs and pads

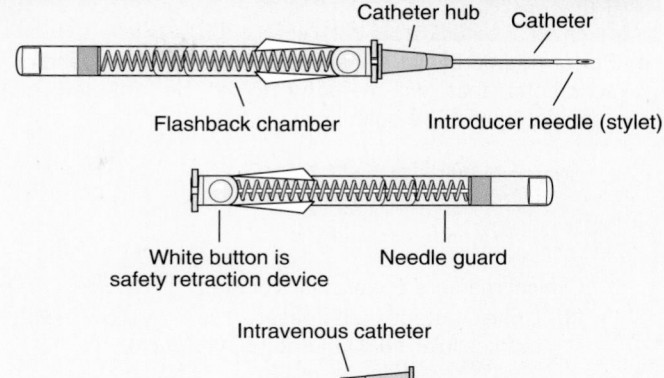

FIG 18.12 Intravenous access device options.

- Manufactured catheter stabilization device (if available) and skin protectant swab
- Prescribed IV solution or medication
- Electronic infusion device (EID) (if indicated) and IV pole
- IV administration set (IV tubing), either macrodrip or microdrip, depending on prescribed rate; if using EID, appropriate administration set
- 0.2-micron filter for parenteral nutrition solutions that do not contain lipids (fats) (may be incorporated into the infusion set)
- Protective equipment: Goggles and mask (optional based on agency policy)
- Vein visualization device (optional based on agency policy)
- Watch with second hand to calculate drip rate
- Special patient gown with snaps at shoulder seams if available (makes removal with IV tubing easier)
- Needle disposal container (*sharps container* or *biohazard container*)
- Stethoscope

STEP	RATIONALE

ASSESSMENT

1. Identify patient using at least two identifiers (e.g., name and birthday or name and medical record number) according to agency policy. Compare identifiers with information on patient's MAR or medical record.

    Ensures correct patient. Complies with The Joint Commission standards and improves patient safety (TJC, 2018).

2. Review accuracy of health care provider's order: date and time, IV solution, route of administration, volume, rate, duration, and signature of ordering health care practitioner (Phillips and Gorski, 2014). Follow the rights of medication administration (see Chapter 17).

    Before administering IV therapy, a complete order from a health care provider is needed (Gorski et al., 2016).

   a. Check approved online database, drug reference book, or pharmacist about IV solution composition, purpose, potential incompatibilities, adverse reactions, and side effects.

    Ensures safe and correct administration of IV therapy and appropriate selection of vascular access device (VAD).

3. Review medical record for patient's history of allergies, especially to iodine, adhesive, or latex. Confirm with patient.

    Equipment used during VAD insertion may contain substances to which patient is allergic.

SKILL 18.1   INITIATING INTRAVENOUS THERAPY—cont'd

View Video!

STEP	RATIONALE
4. Perform hand hygiene. Assess for clinical factors and/or conditions that will respond to or be affected by administration of IV solutions.	Provides baseline to determine effectiveness of prescribed therapy. A systems approach is recommended to assess for fluid and electrolyte imbalances (Phillips and Gorski, 2014).
a. Body weight	Rapid changes in body weight can indicate fluid loss or gain (Alexander et al., 2014). A rapid weight gain or loss of 2.2 lb (1 kg) is equivalent to the gain or loss of 1 L of body water.
b. Clinical markers of vascular volume:	
(1) Urine output (decreased, dark yellow with extracellular fluid volume [ECV] deficit).	Kidneys respond to ECV deficit by reducing urine production and concentrating urine. Kidney disease can also cause oliguria.
(2) Vital signs: blood pressure, respirations, pulse, temperature.	Changes in blood pressure may be associated with fluid volume status (e.g., postural hypotension or hypotension seen in ECV deficit). Respirations can be altered in presence of acid-base imbalances. Temperature elevations increase fluid requirements (temperature of 101° F [38.3° C] to 103° F [39.4° C] requires at least 500 mL of fluid replacement within a 24-hour period) (Weinstein and Hagle, 2014).
(3) Fullness of neck veins. (Normally veins are distended when person is supine and flat when person is upright.)	Indicator of fluid volume status: flat or collapsing with inhalation when supine with ECV deficit; full when upright or semi-upright with ECV excess.
(4) Auscultation of lungs.	Crackles or rhonchi in dependent portions of lung may signal fluid buildup caused by ECV excess.
(5) Capillary refill.	Indirect measure of tissue perfusion (sluggish with ECV deficit).
c. Clinical markers of interstitial volume:	
(1) Skin turgor. (Pinch skin over sternum or inside of forearm.)	Failure of skin to return to normal position after several seconds indicates ECV deficit (Alexander et al., 2014). Not a reliable indicator for older adults (Touhy and Jett, 2014).
(2) Dependent edema (pitting or nonpitting).	Edema is not usually apparent until 4.4 to 8.8 lb (2 to 4 kg) of fluid is retained (Phillips and Gorski, 2014).
(3) Oral mucous membrane between cheek and gum.	More reliable indicator than dry lips or skin. Dry between cheek and gums indicates ECV deficit.
d. Thirst	Occurs with hypernatremia and severe ECV deficit. Not a reliable indicator for older adults (Phillips and Gorski, 2014).
e. Behavior and level of consciousness:	
(1) Restlessness and mild confusion	Occurs with ECV deficit or acid-base imbalance.
(2) Decreased level of consciousness (lethargy, confusion, coma)	Occurs with severe ECV deficit, osmolality imbalances, and acid-base imbalances.
5. Determine if patient is to undergo any planned surgeries or procedures.	Allows anticipation and placement of appropriate VAD for infusion and avoids placement in an area that will interfere with medical procedures (Gorski et al., 2016).
6. Assess available laboratory data (e.g., hematocrit, serum electrolytes, arterial blood gases, kidney function [blood urea nitrogen, urine specific gravity, urine osmolality]).	Helps determine priority assessments and establishes baseline for determining if therapy is effective. Laboratory values are an assessment of hydration status (Alexander et al., 2014).
7. Assess patient's knowledge of procedure, reason for prescribed therapy, and arm placement preference.	Provides patient-centered care by determining level of emotional support and instruction needed.

PLANNING

1. Perform hand hygiene. Collect and organize equipment on clean, clutter-free bedside stand or over-bed table.	Reduces transmission of infection. Provides for an organized procedure and reduces contamination of equipment (Gorski et al., 2016).

STEP	RATIONALE
a. Be sure you have correct infusion set for EID if being used.	Ensures patient receives infusion therapy as prescribed (Gorski et al., 2016).
2. Provide privacy and prepare bedside environment for patient safety.	Providing privacy and preparing the environment before the procedure helps to ensure a clean and distraction-free area.

IMPLEMENTATION

STEP	RATIONALE
1. Instruct patient about rationale for infusion including solution and medications ordered, procedure for initiating an IV, and signs and symptoms of complications (e.g., redness, pain, tenderness, swelling, bleeding, drainage or leaking from under dressing). Also explain sensation associated with needlestick.	Provides patient with information about procedure and promotes compliance (Gorski et al., 2016). May help to lessen patient anxiety.
2. Help patient to comfortable sitting or supine position. Provide adequate lighting.	Promotes comfort and relaxation of patient. Aids in successful vein location.
3. Perform hand hygiene.	Reduces transmission of infection and contamination of equipment (Gorski et al., 2016).
4. *Option:* Change patient's gown to more easily removed gown with snaps at shoulder if available.	Use of this gown decreases risk of inadvertently dislodging VAD or administration set when changing gown.
5. Select appropriate size catheter, and open and prepare sterile packages.	Use the smallest gauge peripheral catheter that will accommodate the prescribed therapy and patient need (Gorski et al., 2016).
6. Prepare short extension tubing with fused needleless connector or separate needleless connector (injection cap) to attach to catheter hub after VAD insertion.	Needleless connectors protect health care workers by eliminating needles and the potential for needlestick injuries when accessing VAD (Gorski et al., 2016).
a. Remove protective cap from needleless connector and attach syringe with 1- to 3-mL 0.9% sodium chloride (NS), maintaining sterility. Slowly inject enough NS to prime (fill) short extension tubing and connector, removing all air. Leave syringe attached to tubing.	Replaces air with NS, preventing air from entering patient's vein later during VAD insertion.
b. Maintain sterility of end of connector by reapplying end caps, and set aside for attaching to catheter hub after successful venipuncture.	Prevents touch contamination, which allows microorganisms to enter infusion equipment and bloodstream.

Clinical Decision Point. Short extension sets may be used on short-peripheral catheters to reduce catheter manipulation. For patient safety, all connections should be of Luer-Lok type (Gorski et al., 2016). Many agencies use short extension tubing for continuous infusions and stand-alone saline locks (capped catheters).

STEP	RATIONALE
7. Prepare IV tubing and solution for continuous infusion.	
a. Check IV solution using rights of medication administration and review the label for name, dosage and concentration, volume, beyond-use and expiration dates, sterility state, and route, rate, and frequency of administration as well as any other special instructions or considerations. If using bar code, scan code on patient's wristband and then on IV fluid container. Be sure that prescribed additives such as potassium and vitamins have been added. Check solution for color, clarity, and expiration date. Check bag for leaks.	Reviewing the label for accuracy reduces the risk for medication errors (Gorski et al., 2016).
	Bar code system reduces human error (Gorski et al., 2016).
	Risk for medication errors can be reduced with safe medication practices including:
	• Do not use unlabeled medication syringes unless prepared at the bedside and immediately administered (Gorski et al., 2016).
	• Do not add medications to infusing containers of IV solutions (Gorski et al., 2016).
	• Do not use solutions that are discolored, contain precipitates, or are expired.
	Risk for transmission of infection can be reduced with safe medication practices including:
	• Do not use leaking bags because the integrity has been compromised.
	• Begin administration of any medications compounded outside the pharmacy within 1 hour after the start of its preparation (Gorski et al., 2016).

SKILL 18.1 INITIATING INTRAVENOUS THERAPY—cont'd

STEP	RATIONALE
b. Open IV infusion set, maintaining sterility. EIDs sometimes have a dedicated administration set.	Prevents touch contamination, which allows microorganisms to enter infusion equipment and bloodstream.
c. Place roller clamp (see illustration A) about 2 to 5 cm (1 to 2 inches) below drip chamber of tubing and move roller clamp to "off" position (see illustration B).	Close proximity of roller clamp to drip chamber allows more accurate regulation of flow rate. Moving clamp to "off" prevents accidental spillage of IV solution during priming.
d. Remove protective sheath over IV tubing port on plastic IV solution bag (see illustration) or top of bottle, while maintaining sterility of port.	Provides access for insertion of IV tubing spike into solution using sterile technique.
e. Remove protective cover from IV tubing spike while maintaining sterility of spike. Insert spike into port of IV bag (see illustration). If solution container is a glass bottle, clean rubber stopper on glass-bottled solution with antiseptic swab and insert spike into rubber stopper of IV bottle. Bottles require vented tubing.	Flat surface on top of bottled solution may contain contaminants, whereas opening to plastic bag is recessed. Prevents contamination of bottled solution during insertion of spike. If sterility of spike is compromised, discard IV tubing and obtain a new one.
f. Compress drip chamber and release, allowing it to fill one-third to one-half full (see illustration).	Creates suction effect; fluid enters drip chamber to prevent air from entering tubing.

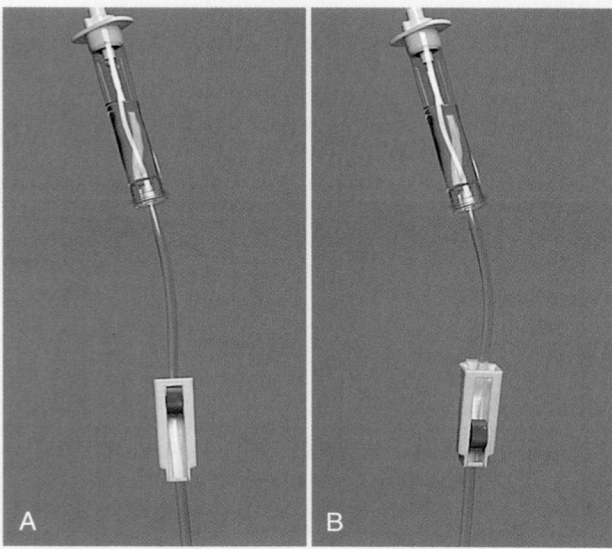

STEP 7c A, Roller clamp in open position. **B,** Roller clamp in closed position.

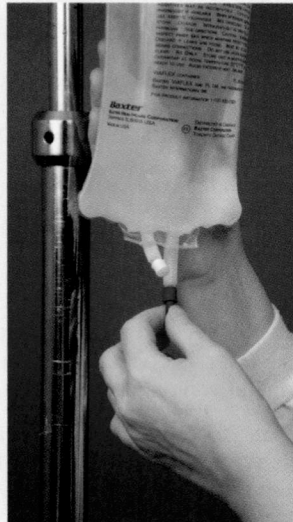

STEP 7d Removing protective sheath from IV tubing port.

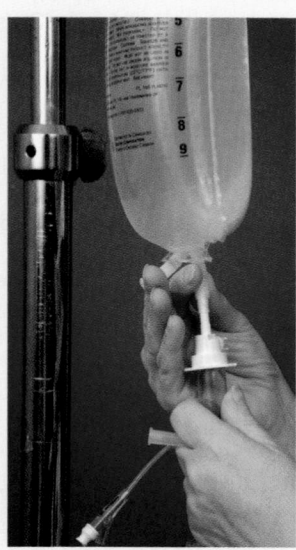

STEP 7e Inserting spike into IV bag.

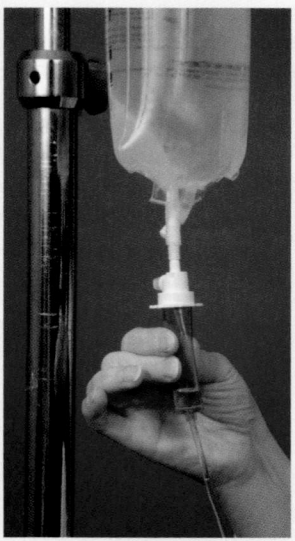

STEP 7f Squeezing drip chamber to fill with fluid.

STEP	RATIONALE
g. Prime air out of IV tubing by filling with IV solution: Remove protective cover on end of IV tubing (some tubing can be primed without removing the protective cover), and slowly open roller clamp to allow fluid to flow from drip chamber to distal end of IV tubing. If tubing has a Y connector, invert Y connector when fluid reaches it to displace air. Return roller clamp to "off" position after priming tubing (filled with IV fluid). Replace protective cover on distal end of tubing. Label IV tubing with date according to agency policy and procedure.	Priming ensures that IV tubing is clear of air and filled with IV solution before connecting to VAD. Slowly filling tubing decreases turbulence and chance of bubble formation. Closing clamp prevents accidental loss of fluid. Maintains sterility. Labeling IV tubing allows for recognition of length of time that tubing has been in use and when to change it.
h. Be certain that IV tubing is clear of air and air bubbles. To remove small air bubbles, firmly tap tubing where air bubbles are located. Check entire length of tubing to ensure that all air bubbles are removed (see illustration).	Large air bubbles act as emboli (Cook, 2013).
i. If using optional long extension tubing (not short tubing in Step 6), remove protective cover and attach it to distal end of IV tubing, maintaining sterility. Then prime long extension tubing.	Priming removes air from long extension tubing so that it does not enter patient's vascular system.
j. Insert tubing into EID with power off (if using).	Prepares for administration of infusion.
8. Perform hand hygiene.	Decreases potential risk of microbial contamination and cross-contamination (Gorski et al., 2016).

Clinical Decision Point. Clean gloves are not necessary to locate vein but must be applied for VAD insertion (Gorski et al., 2016; INS, 2016).

STEP	RATIONALE
9. Apply tourniquet around upper arm about 10 to 15 cm (4 to 6 inches) above proposed insertion site (see illustration). Do not apply tourniquet too tightly. Check for presence of pulse distal to the tourniquet.	Tourniquet should be tight enough to impede venous flow while maintaining arterial circulation (Gorski et al., 2016; INS, 2016). If patient has fragile veins or bruises easily, tourniquet should be applied loosely or not at all to prevent damage to veins and bruising (Gorski et al., 2016).
a. *Option A:* Apply tourniquet on top of a thin layer of clothing such as a gown sleeve to protect fragile or hairy skin.	

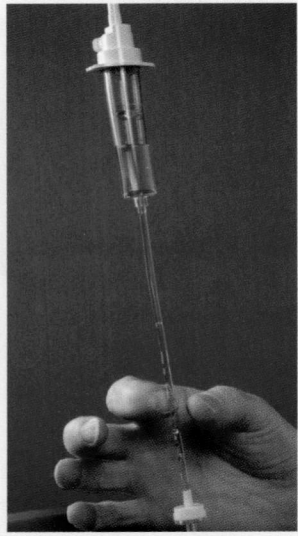

STEP 7h Removing air bubbles from tubing.

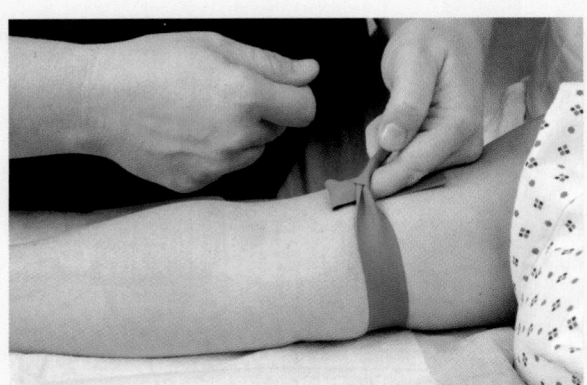

STEP 9 Tourniquet placed on arm for initial vein selection.

STEP	RATIONALE
b. *Option B:* Blood pressure cuff may be used in place of tourniquet: activate cuff and hold at approximately 50 mm Hg.	Reduces trauma to the skin.
10. Select vein for VAD insertion (see illustration). Veins on dorsal and ventral surfaces of arms (e.g., metacarpal, cephalic, basilic, median) are preferred in adults.	Ensures adequate vein that is easy to puncture and less likely to rupture.
a. Use most distal site in nondominant arm if possible.	Patients with VAD placement in their dominant hand have decreased ability to perform self-care.
b. With your fingertip, palpate vein at the intended insertion site by pressing downward. Note resilient, soft, bouncy feeling while releasing pressure (see illustration).	Fingertip is more sensitive and better for assessing vein location and condition.
c. Select a well-dilated vein. Methods to improve vascular distention:	Increased volume of blood in vein at venipuncture site makes vein more visible.
(1) Position extremity lower than heart, have patient slowly open and close fist, and lightly stroke the vein downward.	Use of gravity promotes vascular distention (Gorski et al., 2016).
(2) Apply dry heat to extremity for several minutes.	Dry heat increases successful peripheral catheter insertion (Gorski et al., 2016).

Clinical Decision Point. Slapping or hard tapping of a vein, especially in older adults, can cause venous constriction and/or bruising and hematoma (Phillips and Gorski, 2014).

11. When selecting a vein:	
a. Avoid vein selection in:	
(1) Areas with pain on palpation, compromised areas, sites distal to compromised areas (e.g., open wounds, bruising, infection, infiltration, extravasation) (Gorski et al., 2016).	It is difficult to assess for any signs or symptoms of complications if an IV device is inserted in an area already compromised.
(2) Upper extremity on the side of breast surgery with axillary node dissection, lymphedema, or after radiation; arteriovenous fistulas or grafts; or affected extremity from a cerebrovascular accident (Gorski et al., 2016).	Increases risk for complications such as infection, lymphedema, or vessel damage.
(3) Site distal to previous venipuncture site, sclerosed or hardened veins, previous infiltrations or extravasations, areas of venous valves, or phlebitic vessels.	Such sites cause infiltration around newly placed VAD site and vessel damage.

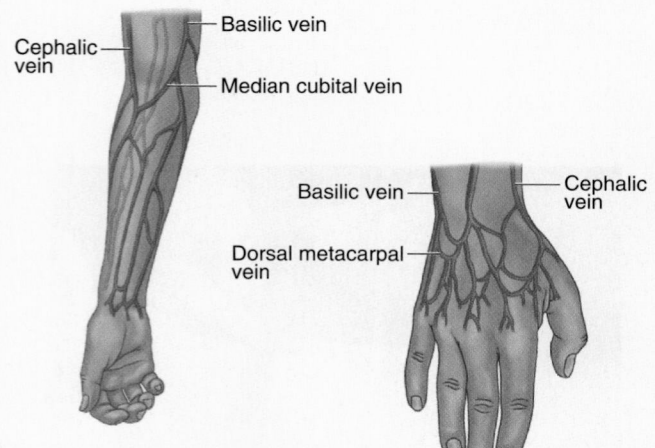

STEP 10 Cephalic, basilic, and median cubital veins are best for IV placement in adults.

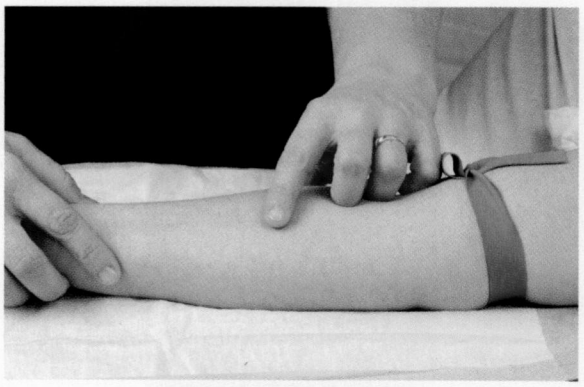

STEP 10b Palpate vein.

STEP	RATIONALE
(4) Fragile dorsal hand veins in older adults. Do not use veins in lower extremities for routine IV therapy in adults because of risk of tissue damage and thrombophlebitis (Gorski et al., 2016).	Veins have increased risk for infiltration.
(5) Areas of flexion such as wrist or antecubital area (Gorski et al., 2016).	Veins have increased risk for infiltration, phlebitis, or dislodgment.
(6) Ventral surface of wrist (10 to 12.5 cm [4 to 5 inches]).	Venipuncture in the ventral surface of wrist is painful and has potential for nerve damage (Gorski et al., 2016).
b. Choose site that will not interfere with patient's activities of daily living, use of assist devices, or planned procedures.	Keeps patient as mobile as possible.
12. Release tourniquet temporarily.	Restores blood flow and prevents venospasm when preparing for venipuncture.

Clinical Decision Point. If hair removal is needed, do not shave area with a razor. Shaving may increase risk of infection (Gorski et al., 2016). Clip hair with scissors or hair clippers if necessary (explain to patient).

Clinical Decision Point. Local anesthetic reduces discomfort associated with placement of a VAD. Topical, transdermal, injectable, or pressure-accelerated local anesthetics can be used to reduce pain and require a health care provider's order. You may apply topical local anesthetic to intended IV site 30 minutes before insertion. Follow manufacturer's recommendations and monitor for allergic reaction (Gorski et al., 2016).

STEP	RATIONALE
13. Perform hand hygiene and apply clean gloves. Wear eye protection and mask (see agency policy) if splash or spray of blood is possible.	Decreases potential risk of microbial contamination and cross-contamination (Gorski et al., 2016).
14. Place adapter end of short extension set (prepared in Step 6) or needleless connector (injection cap) for saline lock nearby in sterile package.	Permits smooth, quick connection of infusion to short-peripheral catheter once vein is accessed.
15. If area of insertion is visibly soiled, clean site with antiseptic soap and water and dry. Perform skin antisepsis with chlorhexidine solution using friction in a back-and-forth motion (see illustration) for 30 seconds and allow to dry completely. If using alcohol or povidone-iodine, clean in concentric circle moving from insertion site outward with the swab. Allow drying time between agents if agents are used in combination (alcohol and povidone-iodine).	Mechanical friction in this pattern allows penetration of antiseptic solution to epidermal layer of the skin (Alexander et al., 2014). Reduces the incidence of catheter-related infections (Alexander et al., 2014). Allow any skin antiseptic agent to fully dry for complete antisepsis; alcoholic chlorhexidine solutions, for at least 30 seconds; iodophors, for at least 1.5 to 2 minutes (Gorski et al., 2016).

Clinical Decision Point. If you need to palpate the vein after performing skin antisepsis, use sterile gloves for palpation, or perform skin antisepsis again, as touching cleaned area introduces microorganisms from your finger to site (Gorski et al., 2016; INS, 2016).

STEP	RATIONALE
16. Reapply tourniquet 10 to 15 cm (4 to 6 inches) above anticipated insertion site. Check for presence of pulse distal to the tourniquet.	Pressure of tourniquet promotes vein distention. Diminished arterial flow prevents venous filling.

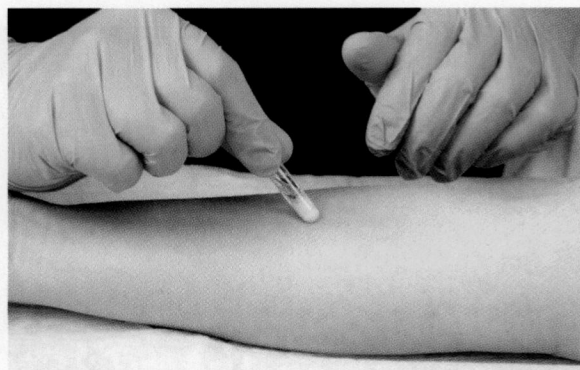

STEP 15 Clean site with greater than 0.5% chlorhexidine alcoholic solution.

SKILL 18.1   INITIATING INTRAVENOUS THERAPY—cont'd

View Video!

STEP	RATIONALE
17. Perform venipuncture. Anchor vein below anticipated insertion site by placing thumb over vein 4 to 5 cm (1½ to 2 inches) distal to site (see illustration) and gently stretching skin against direction of insertion. Instruct patient to relax hand.	Stabilizes vein for needle insertion, prevents vein from rolling, and stretches skin taut decreasing drag during insertion.
	Some devices require loosening the needle (stylet) from the catheter before venipuncture. Follow manufacturer's directions for use.
a. Warn patient of a sharp stick. Hold VAD with the needle bevel up. Align catheter on top of vein at a 10- to 30-degree angle. Puncture skin and anterior vein wall (see illustration) (Gorski et al., 2016).	Accessing vein at an angle reduces risk for puncturing posterior vein wall. Superficial veins require smaller angle. Deeper veins require a greater angle.

Clinical Decision Point. Use each VAD only once for each insertion attempt.

STEP	RATIONALE
18. Observe for blood return in the catheter or flashback chamber of catheter, indicating that bevel of needle has entered vein (see illustration A). Advance VAD approximately 0.6 cm (¼ inch) into vein and loosen stylet (needle) of over-the-needle catheter. Continue to hold skin taut while stabilizing VAD, and with the index finger on the push-off tab of the VAD advance the catheter off needle into the vein until hub rests at venipuncture site (see illustration B). Do not push from open catheter hub. *Do not reinsert stylet into catheter once catheter has been advanced into vein.*	Increased venous pressure from tourniquet causes backflow of blood into catheter and/or flashback chamber. Some VADs have a notch in the stylet allowing flash of blood into the catheter. Stabilizing VAD allows for placement of catheter into vein and advancement of catheter off stylet.
	Advancing entire stylet into vein may penetrate wall of vein, resulting in hematoma.
	Advancing the catheter with finger on open hub will cause contamination (Gorski et al., 2016).
	Reinsertion of stylet can cause catheter to shear off with embolization into vein.

Clinical Decision Point. A single clinician should not make more than two attempts at initiating IV access, and total attempts should be limited to no more than four (Gorski et al., 2016).

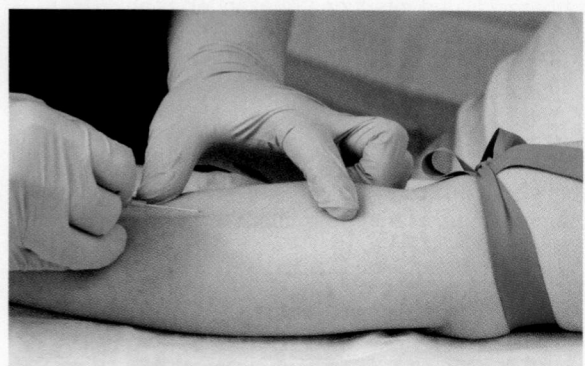

STEP 17 Stabilize vein below insertion site.

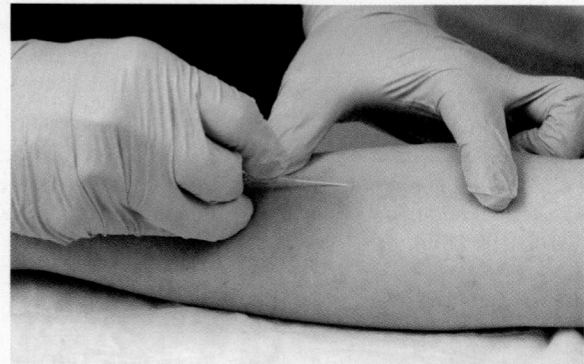

STEP 17a Puncture skin with catheter at 10- to 30-degree angle.

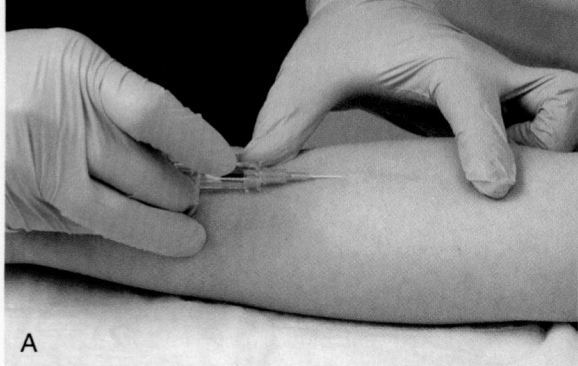

A

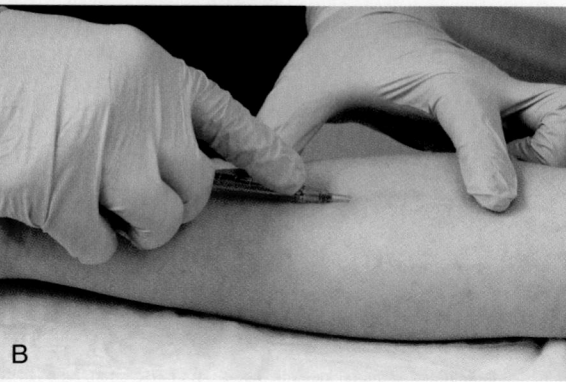

B

STEP 18 A, Observe for blood return in catheter and/or flashback chamber. **B,** Advance catheter into vein until hub rests at venipuncture site.

STEP	RATIONALE
19. Stabilize VAD with nondominant hand and release tourniquet or blood pressure cuff with other hand. While keeping the VAD stable with the index finger, apply gentle but firm pressure with middle finger of nondominant hand 3 cm (1¼ inches) above insertion site. Withdraw stylet from catheter or activate safety device to retract stylet (technique varies by product type; follow manufacturer guidelines).	Permits venous flow and reduces backflow of blood. Digital pressure minimizes blood loss and allows attachment of extension set or needleless connector (INS, 2016).
20. Quickly connect Luer-Lok end of short extension tubing with needleless connector to end of catheter hub. Secure connection. Avoid touching sterile connection ends. a. *Option:* IV tubing can be attached directly to catheter hub in place of short extension tubing or needleless connector.	Prompt connection maintains patency of vein, minimizes blood loss, and prevents risk of exposure to blood. Maintains sterility.
21. Attach prefilled flush syringe of 0.9% sodium chloride to short extension set and aspirate to remove any air and assess blood return. Slowly inject NS from prefilled syringe into VAD (see illustration A). Remove syringe and discard. **Note:** Minimal amount of air should be aspirated if tubing prepared correctly.	Blood return that is the color and consistency of whole blood confirms placement of catheter in vein (Gorski et al., 2016). Flushing prevents reflux of blood into catheter and occlusion (INS, 2016). Initiates flow of fluid through IV catheter, preventing clotting of device. Swelling indicates infiltration, and catheter would need to be removed. Aspirating air prevents air embolism.
a. *Option:* To begin a primary infusion, swab the needleless connector with antiseptic swab and attach the Luer-Lok end of the IV tubing to the needleless connector (see illustration B). Fully open roller clamp of IV tubing, turn on EID, and begin infusion at correct rate. If using gravity flow instead of EID, adjust roller clamp slowly to regulate rate.	Prevents infusion of large volume of fluid.

Clinical Decision Point. Needleless connectors protect health care workers and decrease risk for needlestick injuries. They have different internal mechanisms for fluid displacement and vary in the flush-clamp-disconnect sequence to prevent reflux of blood into catheter on disconnection (Gorski et al., 2016). The sequence depends on the type of internal mechanism (Phillips and Gorski, 2014):

- Neutral displacement devices do not have a specified flush-clamp-disconnect sequence.
- For negative pressure displacement devices, flush, clamp catheter, then disconnect syringe.
- For positive pressure displacement, flush, disconnect syringe, then clamp catheter.

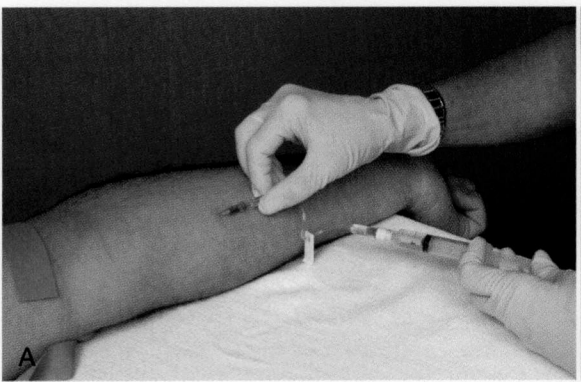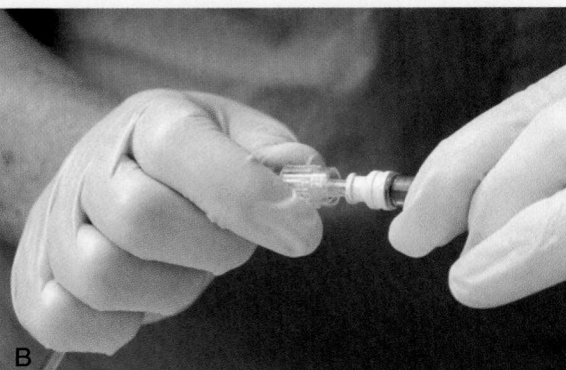

STEP 21 A, Flush short extension set after aspirating air and assessing blood return. **B,** Connect IV tubing to the short extension set that is attached to the catheter.

View Video!

STEP	RATIONALE
22. Observe site for swelling.	Swelling indicates infiltration, which requires immediate removal of catheter.
23. Apply sterile dressing over site.	
a. TSM dressing:	
(1) Continue to secure catheter with nondominant hand. Remove adherent backing. Apply one edge of dressing and gently smooth remaining dressing over IV insertion site, leaving Luer-Lok connection between tubing and catheter hub uncovered. Gently press dressing to adhere to skin. Remove outer covering and smooth dressing gently over site (see illustration).	Transparent membrane protects catheter insertion site and minimizes risk for infection (Phillips and Gorski, 2014). Allows visualization of insertion site and surrounding area for complications (Gorski et al., 2016). Access to Luer-Lok connection between tubing and catheter hub facilitates changing tubing if necessary.
(2) Place a 2.5-cm (2-inch) piece of tape over Luer-Lok connection (see illustration). **Do not apply tape on top of TSM dressing.**	Removal of tape from TSM dressing can tear dressing and cause catheter dislodgment. Tape on top of TSM dressing prevents moisture from being carried away from skin.
b. Sterile gauze dressing:	
(1) Place 5-cm (2-inch) piece of sterile tape over catheter hub (see illustration).	Stabilizes catheter under gauze dressing.
(2) Place a 2 × 2–inch gauze pad over insertion site and edge of catheter hub. Secure all edges with tape. Do not place tape over insertion site. Do not cover connection between IV tubing and catheter hub (see illustration).	Use gauze dressings for site drainage, excessive perspiration, or sensitivity and/or allergic reactions to TSM dressings (Phillips and Gorski, 2014; Gorski et al., 2016).

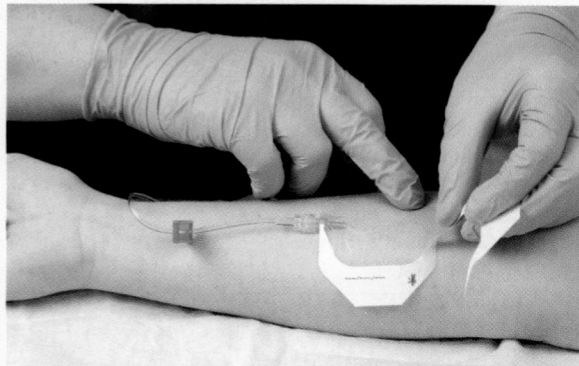
STEP 23a(1) Apply transparent semipermeable membrane (TSM) dressing.

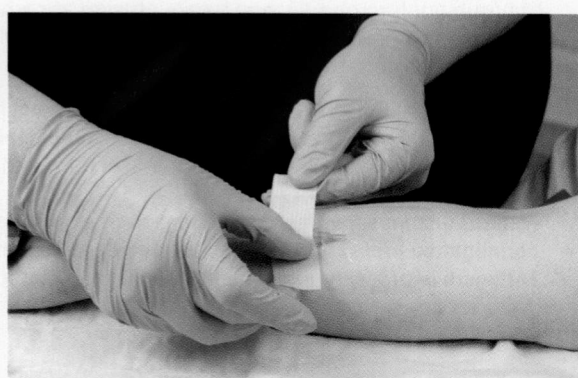
STEP 23a(2) Place tape over administration set tubing.

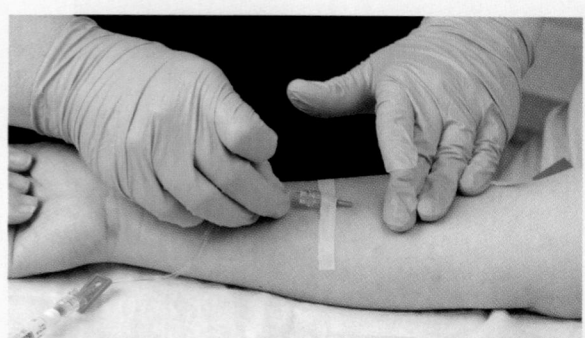
STEP 23b(1) Sterile tape over catheter hub.

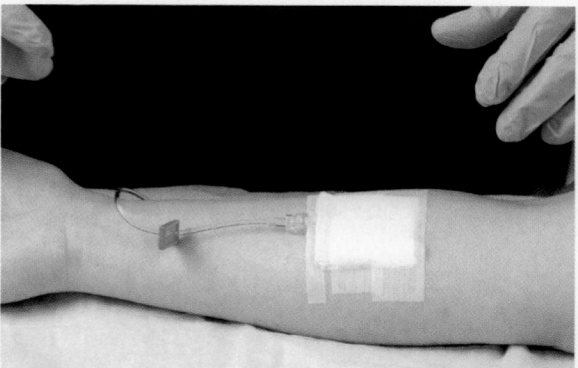
STEP 23b(2) Place 2 × 2–inch gauze over insertion site and edge of catheter hub.

STEP	RATIONALE
(3) Fold 2 × 2–inch gauze in half and cover with 1-inch-wide (2.5 cm) tape so that about 1 inch will extend on each side of dressing. Place under Luer-Lok connection (see illustration). Secure Luer-Lok connection and tubing to tape on the folded gauze with a 2.5-cm (1-inch) piece of tape. Avoid applying tape or gauze around arm. Do not use rolled bandages with or without elastic to secure VAD. Taping Luer-Lok connection can be eliminated if an engineered stabilization device is to be used.	Tape on top of gauze makes it easier to access hub and/or tubing junction. Gauze pad elevates hub off skin to prevent pressure area. Prevents back-and-forth motion of catheter. Rolled bandages do not adequately secure VAD, can impair circulation or flow of infusion, and obscure visualization for complications (Gorski et al., 2016).
24. *Option:* Secure IV catheter using engineered stabilization device (follow manufacturer's directions; follow agency policy).	Use of engineered stabilization devices that allow visual inspection of an insertion site can reduce risk for VAD complications (i.e., phlebitis, infection, migration) and unintentional loss of access (Gorski et al., 2016).
a. Apply skin protectant to stabilization site and allow to dry completely.	Risk for medical adhesive–related skin injury (MARSI) is increased secondary to age, joint movement, and edema; use of skin protectant can decrease risk (Gorski et al., 2016).
(1) Align anchoring pads with directional arrow pointing to insertion site. Press device retainer over top of Luer-Lok connection while supporting underneath the connection.	
(2) Stabilize catheter and peel off one side of liner and press to adhere to skin. Repeat on other side (see illustration).	
(3) Monitor for MARSI.	Early detection of MARSI is key.
25. Loop extension or IV tubing alongside dressing on arm and secure with second piece of tape directly over tubing (see illustration).	Securing tubing reduces risk for dislodging catheter if IV tubing is pulled (i.e., loop comes apart before catheter dislodges).
26. For continuous infusion, verify ordered rate of infusion, and be sure EID is programmed correctly. If infusing by gravity drip, adjust flow rate to correct drops per minute.	EID maintains correct rate of flow for IV solution. Gravity flow fluctuates; thus it must be checked at intervals for accuracy.

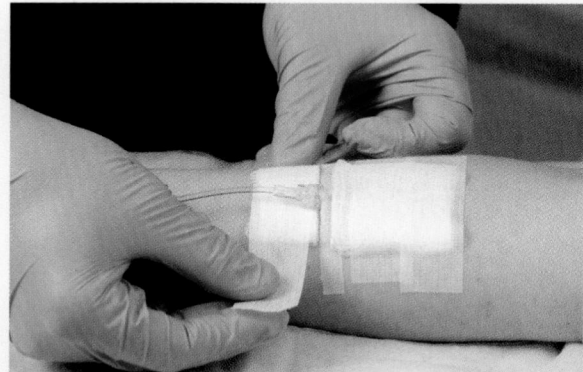

STEP 23b(3) Apply folded 2 × 2–inch gauze dressing under tubing junction.

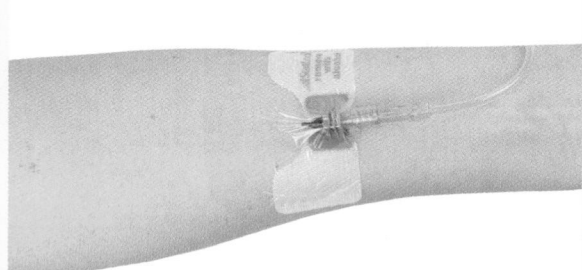

STEP 24a(2) Catheter stabilization device in place. (Image courtesy CR Bard, Inc. All rights reserved.)

SKILL 18.1 INITIATING INTRAVENOUS THERAPY—cont'd

View Video!

STEP	RATIONALE
27. Label dressing per agency policy. Include date and time of IV insertion, VAD gauge size and length, and your initials (see illustration).	Allows for recognition of type of device and length of time that device has been in place.
28. Dispose of used stylet or other sharps in appropriate sharps container. Discard supplies. Remove gloves and perform hand hygiene.	Reduces transmission of microorganisms; prevents accidental needlestick injuries.
29. Instruct patient in how to move or turn without dislodging VAD.	Prevents accidental dislodgment of catheter.

EVALUATION

1. Observe patient every 1 to 2 hours or at established intervals per agency policy and procedure for function, intactness, and patency of IV system and for correct infusion rate and accurate type and amount of IV solution infused by observing level in IV container.	Ensures delivery of prescribed volume over prescribed time and decreases risk for fluid and electrolyte imbalance.
2. Monitor patient to determine response to therapy (e.g., laboratory values, intake and output [I&O], weights, vital signs, postprocedure assessments).	Early recognition of complications leads to prompt treatment.
3. Observe patient at established intervals per agency policy and procedure for signs and symptoms of IV-related complications by inspecting and gently palpating skin around and above IV site over the dressing.	Identifies complications that compromise integrity of VAD or cause inaccurate IV solution flow rate.

Clinical Decision Point. If IV is positional, fluid will run slowly or stop, depending on position of patient's arm; if this continues, you may have to restart IV.

4. **Use Teach-Back:** "I want to make sure that I explained problems that can happen with your IV site. Tell me what you might feel or observe about the IV site that can mean a problem has developed and that you would report." Revise your instruction now or develop a plan for revised patient/family teaching if patient/family caregiver is unable to teach back correctly.	Determines patient's and family caregiver's level of understanding of instructional topic.

RECORDING AND REPORTING

- Record in nurses' notes in electronic health record (EHR) or chart the number of attempts (successful and unsuccessful) and sites of insertion; precise description of insertion site (e.g., cephalic vein on dorsal surface of right lower arm, 2.5 cm [1 inch] above wrist); flow rate; method of infusion (gravity or EID), size and type, length, and brand

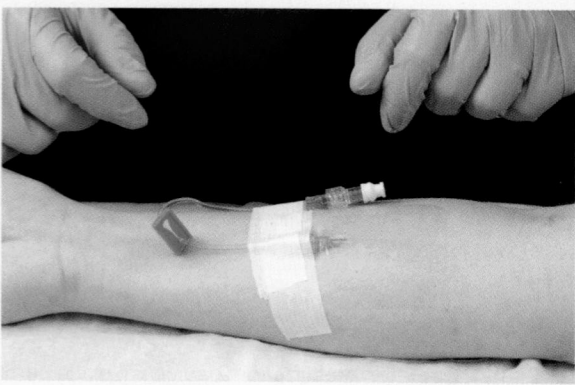

STEP 25 Loop and secure tubing.

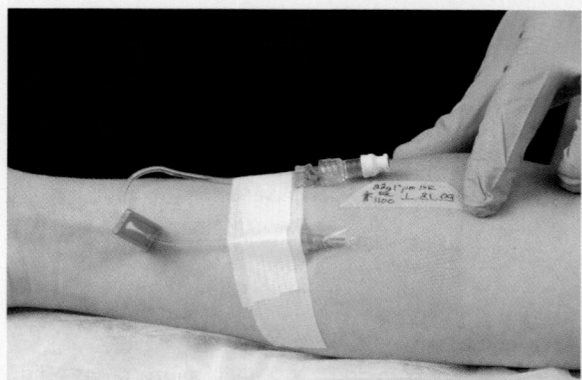

STEP 27 Label IV dressing.

of catheter; time infusion started; and patient's response to insertion. Use an infusion therapy flow sheet when available.

- If using an EID, document type and rate of infusion and device identification number.
- Record patient's status, IV fluid, amount infused, and integrity and patency of system according to agency policy.
- Record patient's/family caregiver's knowledge following evaluation of teach-back in nurses' notes.

- Report to oncoming nursing staff type of fluid, flow rate, status of VAD, amount of fluid remaining in present solution, expected time to hang subsequent IV container, and patient condition.
- Report to health care provider any signs and symptoms of IV-related complications.
- Record signs and symptoms of IV-related complications including interventions and patient response to treatments.

UNEXPECTED OUTCOMES AND RELATED INTERVENTIONS

- Fluid and electrolyte imbalances develop (Table 18.5):
  - Notify health care provider.
  - Readjust infusion rate as ordered.
  - Adjust additives in IV or type of IV fluid as ordered; contact pharmacy
  - Continue monitoring signs and symptoms of imbalances.
- IV-related complications:
  - Infiltration develops at IV site.
    - Avoid applying pressure, which can force solution into contact with more tissue causing tissue damage (INS, 2016).
    - Stop infusion and remove IV catheter at first sign of infiltration and elevate affected extremity.
    - Use a standard scale for assessing and documenting infiltration (Gorski et al., 2016).
  - Catheter occlusion develops.
    - Determine cause and consider catheter removal.
    - Positional or kinked catheters can be repositioned/readjusted to improve IV flow.
    - Remove occluded IV catheter. Do not flush occluded catheters, because an embolus can result from dislodging a clot (Alexander et al., 2014).
  - Phlebitis, or vein inflammation, develops. Rate of infusion may be altered.
    - Notify health care provider.
    - Determine cause (i.e., chemical, mechanical, bacterial) and consider removal or replacement of VAD.
      - Chemical phlebitis: apply heat, elevate limb, consider slowing infusion rate, and determine if catheter removal is necessary (Gorski et al., 2016).
      - Mechanical phlebitis: apply heat, elevate limb, monitor for 24 to 48 hours, consider catheter

removal if signs and symptoms persist (Gorski et al., 2016).
      - Bacterial phlebitis: remove IV catheter (Gorski et al., 2016).
    - Document phlebitis using a standardized scale including nursing interventions per agency policy and procedure (see Table 18.9).
  - Catheter-related infection with redness, swelling around or above IV site, pain, purulent drainage at insertion site, and body temperature elevations (Gorski et al., 2016).
    - Notify health care provider. Obtain order to culture drainage (Gorski et al., 2016).
    - Remove IV catheter and culture purulent drainage from around IV site (Gorski et al., 2016).
  - Hematoma (bleeding under skin) at IV site develops.
    - Remove IV catheter immediately and apply pressure and a dry sterile dressing.
    - Monitor for additional bleeding.
    - Elevate extremity and monitor for circulatory, neurological, or motor dysfunction (Phillips and Gorski, 2014).
  - Nerve injury develops with patient complaints of paresthesia including shocklike pain, tingling or "pins and needles," burning, or numbness on insertion.
    - Notify health care provider of any signs and symptoms of nerve injury (INS, 2016).
    - Immediately stop VAD insertion and remove device if patient complains of symptoms of paresthesia (Gorski et al., 2016).
    - Continue to monitor neurovascular status (INS, 2016).

SKILL 18.2 REGULATING INTRAVENOUS FLOW RATE

DELEGATION CONSIDERATIONS

The skill of regulating IV flow rates cannot be delegated to nursing assistive personnel (NAP). Delegation to licensed practical nurses (LPNs) varies by state Nurse Practice Act. The nurse instructs the NAP to:

- Inform the nurse when the electronic infusion device (EID) alarm signals.
- Inform the nurse when the fluid container is empty.
- Report any patient complaints of discomfort related to infusion such as pain, burning, bleeding, or swelling.

EQUIPMENT

- Watch with second hand
- Calculator, paper, and pencil
- Tape
- Label
- IV solution bag and appropriate administration set
- IV administration set: EID *(optional)*
- Clean gloves

SKILL 18.2   REGULATING INTRAVENOUS FLOW RATE—cont'd

STEP	RATIONALE

ASSESSMENT

1. Review accuracy and completeness of health care provider order in patient's medical record for patient name and correct solution: type, volume, additives, infusion rate, and duration of IV therapy. Follow rights of drug administration (see Chapter 17).

Ensures delivery of correct IV solution and prescribed volume over prescribed time.

2. Identify patient using at least two identifiers (e.g., name and birthday or name and medical record number) according to agency policy. Compare identifiers with information on patient's MAR or medical record.

Ensures correct patient. Complies with The Joint Commission standards and improves patient safety (TJC, 2018).

3. Identify patient risk for fluid and electrolyte imbalance, given type of IV solution (e.g., neonate, older adult, history of cardiac or renal disease).

Helps prioritize assessments. Volume control needs to be strict. Guides choice of infusion device.

4. Perform hand hygiene and apply clean gloves. Inspect and gently palpate skin around and above IV site over dressing. Ask patient how IV site feels. Assess vascular access device (VAD) for patency and signs and symptoms of IV-related complications (e.g., infiltration, occlusion of VAD, phlebitis, infection, patient complaints of pain, or leaking under dressing). Remove gloves and perform hand hygiene.

Identifies complications that compromise integrity of VAD and may necessitate replacement of VAD. Reduces transmission of infection.

5. Assess IV system for patency from IV container to insertion site.

Ensures delivery of prescribed volume over prescribed time.

6. Assess patient's knowledge of purpose of maintaining prescribed flow rate and how positioning of IV site affects flow rate.

Fosters patient participation in maintaining most effective position of arm for optimal flow rate.

PLANNING

1. Provide privacy and prepare bedside environment for patient safety.

Providing privacy and preparing the environment before the procedure helps to ensure a clean and distraction-free area for organizing procedure-related equipment.

2. Have paper and pencil or calculator to calculate flow rate.

Use mathematical calculations to obtain correct rate.

3. Verify with health care provider's order regarding how long each liter of fluid should infuse. If hourly rate (mL/hr) is not provided in order, calculate it by dividing volume by hours (see Step 7).

Basis of calculation to ensure infusion of solution over prescribed hourly rate. A volume of 1 L = 1000 mL.

Clinical Decision Point. It is common for health care providers to write an abbreviated IV order such as: "D$_5$W with 20 mEq KCl 125 mL/hr continuous." This order implies that the IV should be maintained at this rate until an order has been written for the IV to be discontinued or changed to another order.

---

4. If keep vein open (KVO) rate is ordered, check agency policy regarding flow rate of KVO.

Prevents catheter clotting, preserving venous access while infusing a minimal amount of fluid. An order for KVO rate must specify an infusion rate as required by the rights of medication administration. Rates may vary from 0.5 mL/hr to 30 mL/hr based on type of VAD, patient-specific therapy, and method of infusion (gravity or EID).

5. Use hourly rate to program EID or, if gravity-flow infusion, calculate drops per minute (gtt/min).

EID automatically delivers correct minute flow rate. Gravity infusion requires calculation of gtt/min.

6. *For gravity-flow infusion:* Know calibration (drop factor) in drops per milliliter (gtt/mL) of infusion set by agency:

   a. Microdrip: 60 gtt/mL: used to deliver rates less than 100 mL/hr.

   Microdrip tubing universally delivers 60 gtt/mL. Used when small or very precise volumes are to be infused.

   b. Macrodrip: 10 to 15 gtt/mL (depending on manufacturer): used to deliver rates greater than 100 mL/hr

   There are different commercial parenteral administration sets for macrodrip tubing. Used when large volumes or fast rates are necessary. Know drop factor for tubing being used.

STEP	RATIONALE

7. Select one of the following formulas to calculate minute flow rate (drops per minute) based on drop factor of infusion set:
  a. Milliliters per hour/60 min = mL/min
      Drop factor × mL/min = Drops/min
      OR
  b. mL/hr × Drop factor/60 min = Drops/min
  Example: Calculate minute flow rate for a bag 1000 mL with 20 mEq KCl at 125 mL/h.
  Microdrip:
      125 mL/hr × 60 gtt/mL = 7500 gtt/hr
      7500 gtt ÷ 60 min = 125 gtt/min
  Macrodrip:
      125 mL/hr × 15 gtt/mL = 1875 gtt/hr
      1875 gtt ÷ 60 min = 31–32 gtt/min
	Once you determine hourly rate, these formulas compute the correct flow rate.
	
	When using microdrip, milliliters per hour (mL/hr) always equals drops per minute (gtt/min).
	
	Multiply volume by drop factor and divide product by time (in minutes).

8. Explain to patient and family caregiver the purpose of the procedure, what is expected of patient, and when the patient or family caregiver should alert the nurse about problems with flow rate.	Decreases anxiety and promotes cooperation and compliance with therapy.

IMPLEMENTATION

1. Perform hand hygiene.	Reduces transmission of microorganisms.
2. Gravity infusions: Confirm hourly rate and minute rate based on drop factor of infusion set. Use formula in Planning Step 7 to calculate flow rate.	Confirms calculation of minute flow rate for regulation of gravity infusion.
a. Ensure that IV container is at least 76.2 cm (30 inches) above IV site for adults. Increase height for more viscous fluids (Alexander et al., 2014).	Pressure caused by gravity is necessary to overcome venous pressure and resistance from tubing and catheter.
b. Slowly open roller clamp on tubing until you can see drops in drip chamber. Hold a watch with second hand at same level as drip chamber and count drip rate for 1 minute (see illustration). Adjust roller clamp to increase or decrease rate of infusion.	Regulates flow to prescribed rate.

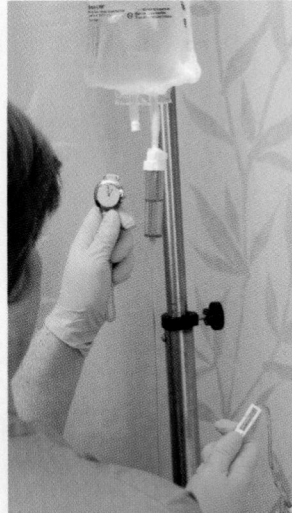

STEP 2b Nurse counting drip rate on gravity flow.

SKILL 18.2 REGULATING INTRAVENOUS FLOW RATE—cont'd

View Video!

STEP	RATIONALE
c. Monitor drip rate at least hourly.	Many factors influence drip rate; frequent monitoring ensures IV fluid administration as prescribed.
3. **EID (infusion pump or smart pump):** Follow manufacturer guidelines for setup of EID. Be sure you are using infusion tubing compatible with EID.	Smart pumps with medication safety software are designed for administration of IV fluids that contain medications.
a. Close roller clamp on primed IV infusion tubing.	Prevents fluid leakage.
b. Insert compatible infusion tubing into chamber of control mechanism (see manufacturer directions) (see illustration). Roller clamp on IV tubing goes between EID and patient.	Most EIDs use positive pressure to infuse. Infusion pumps propel fluid through tubing by compressing and milking IV tubing.
c. Secure portion of IV tubing through "air in line" alarm system. Close door (see illustration A) and turn on power button, select required drops per minute or volume per hour, close door to control chamber, and press start button (see illustration B). If infusing a medication, access the EID library of medications and set the appropriate rate and dose limits. If smart pump alarms immediately and shuts down, your settings were outside unit parameters.	Ensures safe administration of ordered flow rate or medication dose. Smart pumps require additional information such as patient unit and medication. Computer matches pump setting against a drug database.

Clinical Decision Point. An anti–free flow safeguard (preventing bolus infusion in the event of machine malfunction or when tubing is removed from machine) is an important element of an EID and is required. Always check and follow manufacturer recommendations for specific device features.

STEP	RATIONALE
d. Open infusion tubing drip regulator completely while EID is in use.	Ensures that pump freely regulates infusion rate.
e. Monitor infusion rate and IV site for complications according to agency policy. Use watch to verify rate of infusion, even when using EID.	Flow controllers and pumps do not replace frequent, accurate nursing evaluation. EIDs can continue to infuse IV solutions after a complication has developed (Gorski et al., 2016).
f. Assess IV system from container to VAD insertion site when alarm signals.	Alarm indicates a situation that requires attention. Empty solution container, tubing kinks, closed clamp, infiltration, clotted catheter, air in the tubing, or low battery can trigger EID alarm.
4. Attach label to IV solution container with date and time container was changed (check agency policy).	Provides reference to determine next time for container change.

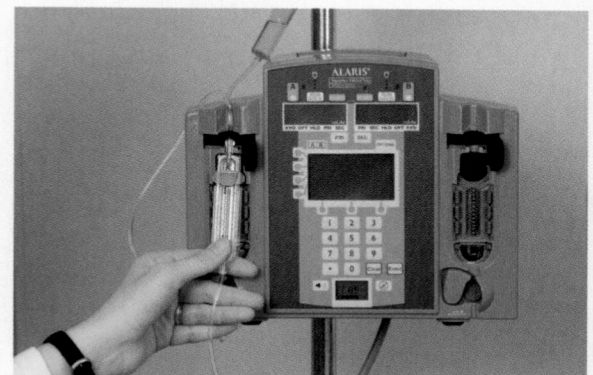

STEP 3b Insert IV tubing into chamber of control mechanism.

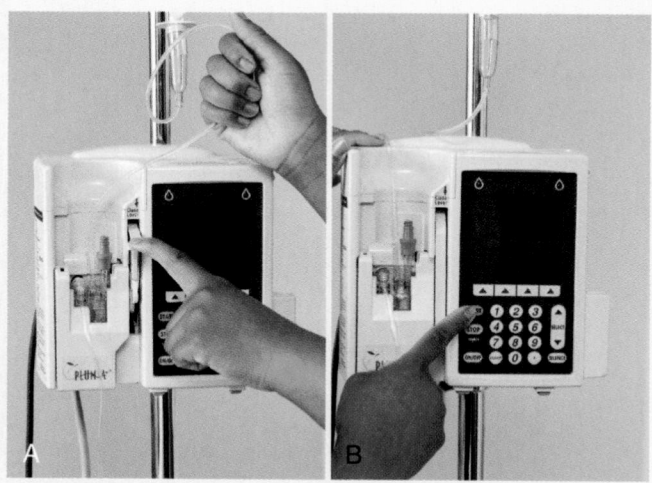

STEP 3c A and **B,** Select rate and volume to be infused and press start button.

STEP	RATIONALE
5. Instruct patient and family caregiver about the purpose of EID if infusion therapy is delivered by EID; about purpose of alarms; to avoid raising hand or arm, which affects flow rate; and to avoid touching control clamp.	Information allows patient to protect IV site and informs patient about rationale for not altering control rate.
6. Remove and dispose of any used supplies. Perform hand hygiene.	Prevents transmission of infection.

EVALUATION

STEP	RATIONALE
1. Observe patient every 1 to 2 hours or at established intervals per agency policy and procedure for function, intactness, and patency of IV system and for correct infusion rate and type and amount of IV solution infused.	Ensures delivery of prescribed volume over prescribed time and decreases risk for fluid and electrolyte imbalance.
2. Monitor patient's response to therapy (e.g., laboratory values, intake and output [I&O], weights, vital signs, postprocedure assessments).	Provides ongoing evaluation of patient's fluid status including monitoring for extracellular fluid volume (ECV) excess, ECV deficit, or electrolyte imbalances. Early recognition of complications leads to prompt treatment.
3. Observe patient at established intervals per agency policy and procedure for signs and symptoms of IV-related complications.	Prevents complications that compromise integrity of VAD or cause inaccurate IV solution flow rate.
4. **Use Teach-Back:** "I want to be sure that I explained the importance that your IV fluids run on time at the rate ordered. Tell me reasons that may cause the pump to alarm to sound and what you would do." Revise your instruction now or develop a plan for revised patient/family caregiver teaching if patient/family caregiver is unable to teach back correctly.	Determines patient's/family caregiver's level of understanding of instructional topic.

RECORDING AND REPORTING

- Record IV solution, rate of infusion in drops per minute (gtt/min) or milliliters per hour (mL/hr), and integrity and patency of system in nurses' notes in electronic health record (EHR) or chart and on infusion therapy flow sheet according to agency policy.
- Record use of any EID or control device and identification number on that device.
- Record patient response (e.g., laboratory values, intake and output [I&O], weights, vital signs, postprocedure assessments) to therapy and unexpected outcomes (e.g., signs and symptoms of ECV excess, ECV deficit, or IV-related complications).
- Record patient's/family caregiver's knowledge following evaluation of teach-back in nurses' notes.
- At change of shift or when leaving on break, report rate of and volume left in infusion to nurse in charge or next nurse assigned to care for patient.

UNEXPECTED OUTCOMES AND RELATED INTERVENTIONS

- Solution does not infuse at prescribed rate.
  - Sudden infusion of large volume of solution occurs and patient develops dyspnea; crackles in lung; distended neck veins when upright; and edema, indicating fluid overload (ECV excess).
    - Slow infusion rate: KVO rates must have specific rate ordered by health care provider.
    - Notify health care provider immediately.
    - Place patient in high-Fowler position.
    - Anticipate new IV orders.
    - Anticipate administration of oxygen per order.
    - Administer diuretics if ordered.
- IV solution runs slower than ordered.
  - Check for positional change that affects rate, height of IV container, kinking of tubing, or obstruction.
  - Check VAD site for complications.
  - Consult health care provider for new order to provide necessary fluid volume.
- IV patency is lost subsequent to IV solution container running empty.
  - Discontinue present IV, and restart new short-peripheral catheter in new site.

SKILL 18.3 CHANGING INTRAVENOUS SOLUTION AND TUBING

DELEGATION CONSIDERATIONS

The skill of changing an IV solution or tubing cannot be delegated to nursing assistive personnel (NAP). Delegation to licensed practical nurses (LPNs) varies by state Nurse Practice Act. The nurse instructs the NAP to:

- Inform the nurse when an IV container is near completion.
- Report any cloudiness or precipitate in the IV solution.
- Report to the nurse any leakage from or around IV site or the IV tubing.
- Report if tubing has become disconnected and contaminated (lying on the floor).
- Report alarm sounding on electronic infusion device (EID).
- Report any patient complaints of discomfort related to infusion such as pain, burning, bleeding, or swelling.

EQUIPMENT

- IV solution as ordered by health care provider
- Clean gloves
- Antiseptic swabs (chlorhexidine solution [preferred], povidone-iodine, or 70% alcohol)
- Label

Continuous IV Infusion

- Microdrip or macrodrip administration set IV tubing as appropriate
- Add-on device as necessary (e.g., filters, extension set, needleless connector)
- Tubing label

Intermittent Extension Set

- 3- to 5-mL syringe filled with preservative-free 0.9% sodium chloride (normal saline [NS])
- Short extension tubing (if necessary), injection cap

STEP	RATIONALE

ASSESSMENT

1. Review accuracy and completeness of health care provider's order in patient's medical record for patient name and correct solution: type, volume, additives, rate, and duration of IV therapy. Follow rights of drug administration.

Ensures delivery of correct IV solution and prescribed volume over prescribed time (Gorski et al., 2016).

2. Identify patient using at least two identifiers (e.g., name and birthday or name and medical record number) according to agency policy. Compare identifiers with information on patient's MAR or medical record.

Ensures correct patient. Complies with The Joint Commission standards and improves patient safety (TJC, 2018).

3. Note date and time when IV tubing and solution were last changed.

Ensures correct timing of tubing changes.

4. Perform hand hygiene and apply clean gloves. Gently palpate skin around and above IV site over the dressing. Inspect vascular access site and device (VAD) for patency and signs and symptoms of IV-related complications (e.g., infiltration, occlusion of VAD, phlebitis, infection, patient complaints of pain, leaking under dressing).

Identifies complications that compromise integrity of VAD and necessitate replacement of VAD.

5. Check infusion system from the solution container down to the VAD insertion site for integrity including, but not limited to, discoloration, cloudiness, leakage, expiration date, tubing puncture, contamination, or occlusion. Determine compatibility of all IV solutions and additives by consulting approved online database, drug reference, or pharmacist. Remove and discard gloves. Perform hand hygiene.

If there has been a break in integrity of the solution container, a new container is needed (Alexander et al., 2014).
May indicate need for IV tubing change.
Incompatibilities cause physical, chemical, and therapeutic changes with adverse patient outcomes (Alexander et al., 2014).

6. Check medical record for pertinent laboratory data such as potassium level.

Compare data with baseline to determine ongoing response to IV solution administration.

7. Determine patient's understanding of need for continued IV therapy.

Indicates need for any patient education.

PLANNING

1. Perform hand hygiene. Collect equipment and assemble at bedside. Have next IV solution prepared at least 1 hour before needed. If solution is prepared in pharmacy, ensure that it has been delivered to patient care unit. Allow solution to warm to room temperature if it has been refrigerated. Check that solution is correct and properly labeled. Check solution expiration date. Ensure that any light sensitivity restrictions are followed.

Reduces transmission of infection and contamination of equipment (INS, 2016). Proper handling of solutions prevents IV-related complications such as occlusion. Checking that solution is correct prevents medication error.

STEP	RATIONALE
2. Provide privacy and prepare bedside environment for patient safety	Providing privacy and preparing the environment before the procedure helps to ensure a clean and distraction-free area for organizing procedure-related equipment.
3. Prepare patient and family caregiver by explaining procedure, its purpose, and what is expected of patient.	Decreases anxiety and promotes cooperation and compliance with therapy.

IMPLEMENTATION

1. *Changing IV fluid container with existing tubing or continuous IV infusion:*

a. Change solution when fluid remains only in neck of container (approximately 50 mL) or when new type of solution has been ordered.	Prevents waste of solution.
b. Perform hand hygiene.	Reduces transmission of microorganisms.
c. Prepare new solution for changing. If using plastic bag, hang on IV pole and remove protective cover from IV tubing port. If using glass bottle, remove metal cap and metal and rubber disks.	Permits quick, smooth, and organized change from old to new container.
d. Close roller clamp on existing solution to stop flow rate. Remove IV tubing from EID (if used). Then remove old IV solution container from IV pole. Hold container with tubing port pointing upward.	Prevents solution remaining in drip chamber from emptying while changing solutions. Prevents any solution left in bag from spilling.
e. Quickly remove spike from old solution container and, without touching tip, insert spike into new container (see illustration).	Reduces risk for solution in drip chamber becoming empty and maintains sterility.

Clinical Decision Point. If spike is contaminated, you will need a new IV tubing set. See Step 2

---

f. Check for air in IV tubing. If air bubbles have formed, remove them by closing roller clamp, stretching tubing downward, and tapping tubing with finger (bubbles rise in fluid to drip chamber) (see Skill 18.1, Step 7h).	Reduces risk for air entering tubing. Use of an air-eliminating filter also reduces risk.
g. Make sure drip chamber is one-third to one-half full. If drip chamber is too full, level can be decreased by removing bag from IV pole, pinching off IV tubing below drip chamber, inverting container, squeezing drip chamber (see illustration), releasing and turning solution container upright, and releasing pinch on tubing.	Reduces risk for air entering IV tubing. If chamber is completely filled, you cannot observe or regulate drip rate.

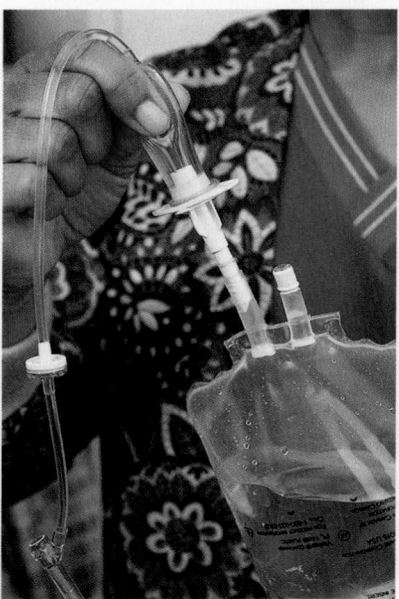

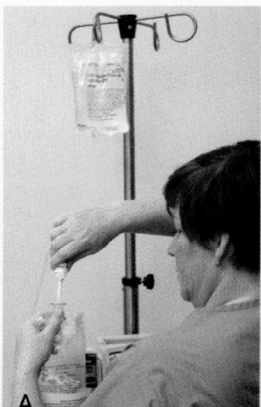 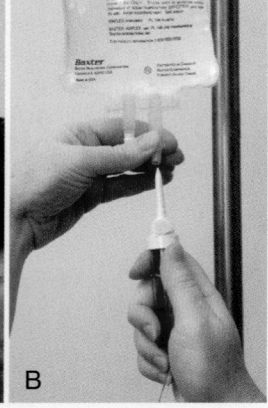

STEP 1e A, Quickly remove spike from old solution container. **B,** Without touching tip, insert spike into new container.

STEP 1g Squeeze drip chamber to fill with fluid. Be sure to leave chamber one-third to one-half full.

SKILL 18.3 CHANGING INTRAVENOUS SOLUTION AND TUBING—cont'd

STEP	RATIONALE
h. Reinsert tube into EID if being used. Regulate flow to ordered rate by using roller clamp on IV tubing or by programming EID.	Maintains measures to restore fluid balance and deliver IV solution as ordered.
i. Place time label on side of container and label with time hung, time of completion, and appropriate hourly intervals. If using plastic bags, mark only on label and not container.	Provides visual comparison of volume infused compared with prescribed rate of infusion.
j. Instruct patient in purpose of new IV solution, additives, flow rate, potential side effects and what to report.	Informs patient about purpose for continued IV therapy and what to report and protects VAD patency.
k. Discard old IV container in appropriate receptacle. Perform hand hygiene.	Reduces transmission of microorganisms.
2. *Changing IV tubing:*	
a. Coordinate IV tubing changes with solution changes when possible.	Reduces risk of infection by decreasing number of times system is open.
b. Perform hand hygiene.	Reduces transmission of infection and contamination of equipment (Gorski et al., 2016).
c. Open new infusion set and connect add-on pieces (e.g., filters, extension tubing). Keep protective coverings over infusion spike and distal adapter. Place roller clamp about 2 to 2.5 cm (1 to 2 inches) below drip chamber and move roller clamp to "off" position. Secure all connections using sterile technique.	Close proximity of roller clamp to drip chamber allows more accurate regulation of flow rate. Securing connections reduces risk later of air emboli and infection. Protective covers reduce entrance of microorganisms. All connections should be of Luer-Lok type (Gorski et al., 2016).
d. Apply clean gloves. If patient's IV cannula hub is not visible, remove IV dressing. Do not remove tape securing cannula to skin.	Cannula hub must be visible to provide smooth transition when removing old and inserting new tubing.
e. Prepare IV tubing with new IV container. (See Skill 18.1, Steps 7a-j.)	Process ensures sterility of system and filling of tubing.
f. *Prepare IV tubing with existing continuous IV infusion container:*	
(1) Move roller clamp on new IV tubing to "off" position.	Prevents fluid spillage.
(2) Slow rate of infusion through old tubing to keep vein open (KVO) rate, using EID or roller clamp.	Prevents occlusion of VAD.
(3) Compress and fill drip chamber of old tubing.	Ensures that drip chamber remains full until new tubing is changed.
(4) Invert container and remove old tubing. Keep spike sterile and upright.	Solution in drip chamber will continue to run and maintain catheter patency.
(5) Insert spike of new infusion tubing into existing solution container. Hang solution bag on IV pole, and compress drip chamber on new tubing and release allowing it to fill one-third to one-half full.	Permits drip chamber to fill and promotes rapid, smooth flow of solution through tubing.
(6) Prime air out of IV tubing by filling with IV solution. Remove protective cover on end of tubing and slowly open roller clamp to allow solution to flow from drip chamber to distal end of IV tubing. If tubing has a Y connector, invert Y connector when solution reaches it to displace air. Return roller clamp to "off" position after priming tubing (filled with IV solution). Replace protective cover on end of IV tubing. Place end of adapter near patient's IV site.	Priming ensures that IV tubing is clear of air before connection with VAD and filled with IV solution. Slow fill of tubing decreases turbulence and chance of bubble formation. Closing clamp prevents accidental loss of fluid. Maintains sterility. Equipment is positioned for a quick connection of new tubing.
(7) Stop EID or turn roller clamp on old tubing to "off" position.	Prevents fluid spillage.
g. *Prepare extension set or saline lock:*	
(1) If short extension tubing is needed, use sterile technique to connect new injection cap to new extension set or IV tubing.	Prepares extension set for connecting with IV.

STEP	RATIONALE
(2) Scrub injection cap with antiseptic swab for at least 15 seconds and allow to dry completely. Attach syringe containing 3 to 5 mL of NS flush solution and inject through injection cap into extension set.	Ensures effective disinfection (Phillips and Gorski, 2014). Maintains patency of catheter.
h. *Reestablish infusion:*	
(1) Gently disconnect old tubing from extension tubing (or from IV catheter hub) and quickly insert Luer-Lok end of new tubing or saline lock into extension tubing connection (or IV catheter hub) (see illustrations for example of connecting tubing to short extension set).	Allows smooth transition from old to new tubing, minimizing time system is open.
(2) For continuous infusion, open roller clamp on new tubing and regulate drip rate of gravity infusion by adjusting roller clamp, or remove old tubing from EID, insert new tubing, then open clamp fully and restart EID at prescribed rate.	Ensures catheter patency and prevents occlusion.
(3) Attach piece of tape or preprinted label with date and time of IV tubing change onto tubing below drip chamber.	Provides reference to determine next time for tubing change.
(4) Form loop of tubing and secure it to patient's arm with strip of tape.	Avoids accidental pulling against site and stabilizes catheter.
i. Remove and discard old IV tubing with roller clamp closed. If necessary, apply new IV dressing. Remove and dispose of gloves. Perform hand hygiene.	Reduces transmission of microorganisms.
j. Instruct patient and family caregiver on purpose of new solution, additives, flow rate, potential side effects, how to avoid occluding the tubing, and how move and turn to prevent contamination of IV tubing.	Informs patient about purpose for continued IV therapy and what to report and protects VAD patency. Prevents accidental contamination of IV tubing.

EVALUATION

1. Observe patient every 1 to 2 hours or at established intervals per agency policy and procedure for function, intactness, and patency of IV system; for leaking at connection sites; and for correct infusion rate and type and amount of IV solution infused.	Ensures delivery of prescribed volume over prescribed time and decreases risk for fluid and electrolyte imbalance. Ensures that IV system is functioning appropriately and minimizes risk of infection secondary to breach in system integrity.
2. Evaluate patient to determine response to therapy (e.g., laboratory values, intake and output [I&O], weights, vital signs, postprocedure assessments).	Provides ongoing evaluation of patient's fluid status.
3. Monitor patient for signs of extracellular fluid volume (ECV) excess, ECV deficit, or signs and symptoms of electrolyte imbalances.	Early recognition of complications leads to prompt treatment.
4. Evaluate patient at established intervals per agency policy and procedure for signs and symptoms of IV-related complications.	Prevents complications that compromise integrity of VAD or cause inaccurate IV solution flow rate.

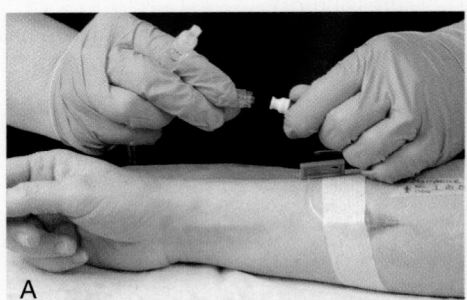 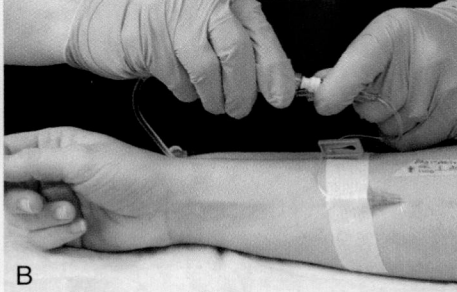

STEP 2h(1) **A,** Disconnect old tubing. **B,** Insert adapter of new tubing.

SKILL 18.3 CHANGING INTRAVENOUS SOLUTION AND TUBING—cont'd

STEP	RATIONALE
5. **Use Teach-Back:** "I want to be sure that I explained the problems that can occur with your IV. Can you tell me what signs and symptoms you would report?" Revise your instruction now or develop a plan for revised patient/family caregiver teaching if patient/family caregiver is unable to teach back correctly.	Determines patient's/family caregiver's level of understanding of instructional topic.

RECORDING AND REPORTING

- Record on nurse's notes in electronic health record (EHR) or chart IV solution, rate of infusion, and integrity and patency according to agency policy and procedure.
- Record use of any EID or control device and identification number on that device.
- Record solution and tubing change, type of solution, and volume and rate of infusion on patient's record. Use infusion therapy flow sheet for parenteral solutions per agency policy.

- Record patient response to therapy and unexpected outcomes (e.g., causes of flow rate inaccuracy).
- Record patient's/family caregiver's knowledge following evaluation of teach-back in nurses' notes.
- At change of shift or when leaving on break, report changes of solution, infusion rate, and volume left in infusion to nurse in charge or next nurse assigned to care for patient.

UNEXPECTED OUTCOMES AND RELATED INTERVENTIONS

- IV fluid infusing slower than ordered.
  - Check for positional change that affects rate, height of IV container, kinking of tubing, or obstruction.
  - Check for patency by opening roller clamp.
  - Check VAD site for complications.
  - Consult health care provider for new order to provide necessary fluid volume.
- Flow rate is incorrect; patient receives too little or too much solution.
  - Notify health care provider if patient's anticipated infusion is 100 to 200 mL less than or greater than anticipated (as per agency policy and procedure).

- Evaluate patient for adverse effects of infusion (e.g., ECV excess or ECV deficit).
- Determine and correct the cause of incorrect flow rate (e.g., change in position, tubing kink, loss of IV patency or intactness).
- Use EID when accurate flow rate is critical.
- Fluid and/or electrolyte imbalances (see Table 18.5)
  - Notify health care provider.
  - Anticipate orders for changes in IV solution or additives.

SKILL 18.4 CHANGING A PERIPHERAL INTRAVENOUS DRESSING

DELEGATION CONSIDERATIONS

The skill of changing a peripheral intravenous (IV) dressing cannot be delegated to nursing assistive personnel (NAP). The nurse instructs NAP to:

- Report to the nurse if a patient mentions moistness or loosening of IV dressing.
- Protect the IV dressing during hygiene and activities of daily living.

EQUIPMENT

- Antiseptic swabs (2% chlorhexidine [preferred], povidone-iodine, or 70% alcohol)

- Skin protectant swab *(optional)*
- Adhesive remover *(optional)*
- Clean gloves
- Strips of nonallergenic tape
- Engineered catheter stabilization device or precut strips of sterile tape
- Commercially available IV site protection device *(optional)*
- Sterile transparent semipermeable membrane (TSM) dressing *or*
- Sterile 2 × 2– or 4 × 4–inch gauze pad

STEP	RATIONALE

ASSESSMENT

1. Identify patient using at least two identifiers (e.g., name and birthday or name and medical record number) according to agency policy. Compare identifiers with information on patient's MAR or medical record.

   Ensures correct patient. Complies with The Joint Commission standards and improves patient safety (TJC, 2018).

2. Determine when dressing was last changed. Dressing should be labeled to include date and time applied, size and type of vascular access device (VAD), and insertion date.

   Provides information regarding length of time that present dressing has been in place and allows planning for dressing change.

3. Perform hand hygiene and apply gloves. Observe present dressing for moisture and intactness. Determine if moisture is from site leakage or external source.

   Nonadhering dressing increases risk for insertion site infection or dislodgment of VAD.

4. Inspect and gently palpate skin around and above IV site over dressing. Assess VAD for patency and signs and symptoms of IV-related complications (e.g., infiltration, occlusion of VAD, phlebitis, infection, patient complaints of pain, leaking under dressing). Remove and discard gloves, and perform hand hygiene.

   Identifies complications that compromise integrity of VAD and may necessitate replacement of VAD.

5. Assess patient's understanding of need for continued IV infusion.

   Reveals need for patient instruction.

PLANNING

1. Provide privacy and prepare bedside environment for patient safety.

   Providing privacy and preparing the environment before the procedure helps to ensure a clean and distraction-free area for organizing procedure-related equipment.

2. Perform hand hygiene. Collect equipment and organize on clean, clutter-free bedside stand or over-bed table. Apply clean gloves.

   Reduces transmission of infection and contamination of equipment (Gorski et al., 2016).

3. Explain procedure and purpose to patient and family caregiver. Explain that patient will need to hold affected extremity still.

   Decreases anxiety, promotes cooperation, and gives patient time frame around which to plan personal activities.

IMPLEMENTATION

1. Perform hand hygiene and apply clean gloves. Remove dressing.

   Technique minimizes discomfort during removal. Use alcohol swab on TSM dressing next to patient's skin to loosen dressing.

   a. *For TSM dressing:* Stabilize catheter with nondominant hand (see illustration) and remove dressing by pulling up one corner and gently pulling straight out and parallel to skin. Repeat on all sides until dressing has been removed.

   b. *For gauze dressing:* Stabilize catheter hub while loosening tape and removing old dressing one layer at a time by pulling toward insertion site. Be cautious if tubing becomes tangled between two layers of dressing.

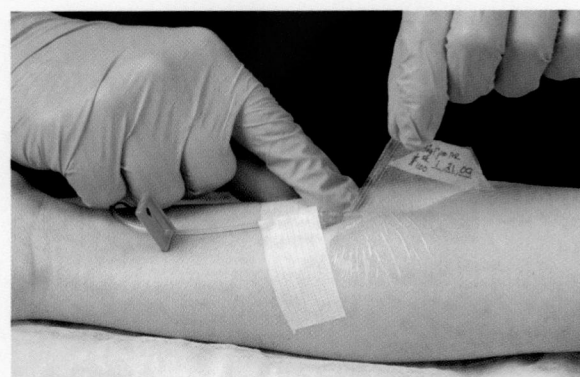

STEP 1a Remove transparent semipermeable membrane (TSM) dressing by pulling side laterally.

SKILL 18.4 CHANGING A PERIPHERAL INTRAVENOUS DRESSING—cont'd

STEP	RATIONALE
2. Assess VAD insertion site for signs and symptoms of IV-related complications. If complication exists, determine if VAD requires removal. Remove catheter if ordered by health care provider.	Presence of complication may necessitate VAD removal.
3. If catheter is to remain in place, assess integrity of engineered stabilization device if used. Continue to stabilize catheter and remove as recommended by manufacturer's directions for use.	Removing stabilization device allows for appropriate skin antisepsis before applying dressing and new stabilization device (Gorski et al., 2016). Stabilization prevents accidental dislodgment of VAD.
Note: Some stabilization devices are designed to remain in place for the length of time VAD is in as long as adequate stabilization is evident.	

Clinical Decision Point. Keep one finger over catheter at all times until dressing secures catheter hub. If patient is restless or uncooperative, it is helpful to have another staff member help with procedure.

---

4. While stabilizing IV, perform skin antisepsis to insertion site with chlorhexidine solution using friction in a back-and-forth motion for 30 seconds and allow to dry completely. If using alcohol or povidone-iodine, clean in concentric circle moving from insertion site outward with swab (see Illustration). Allow antiseptic solution to dry completely.	Reduces incidence of catheter-related infections (Alexander et al., 2014). Allow any skin antiseptic agent to fully dry for complete antisepsis (Gorski et al., 2016).
5. *Optional:* Apply skin protectant to area where you will apply tape or dressing. Allow to dry.	Coats skin with protective solution to maintain skin integrity, prevents irritation from adhesive, and promotes adhesion of dressing.
6. While stabilizing catheter, apply a sterile dressing over site (procedures differ; follow agency policy).	
a. *TSM dressing:* Apply TSM dressing. See Skill 18.1, Step 23a.	Protects catheter insertion site and minimizes risk for infection (Phillips and Gorski, 2014). Allows visualization of insertion site and surrounding area for complications (Gorski et al., 2016).
b. *Sterile gauze dressing:* Apply sterile gauze dressing. See Skill 18.1, Step 23b.	Use only sterile tape under sterile dressing to prevent site contamination. Gauze dressing obscures observation of insertion site and is changed every 2 days (Gorski et al., 2016).
c. *Engineered catheter stabilization device:* Apply catheter stabilization device.	Use of engineered stabilization devices that allow visual inspection of an insertion site can reduce risk for VAD complications (i.e., phlebitis, infection, migration) and unintentional loss of access (Gorski et al., 2016).

Clinical Decision Point. Because Band-Aids are not occlusive and nonsterile tape increases the risk for insertion site infection, do not use either type over catheter insertion points.

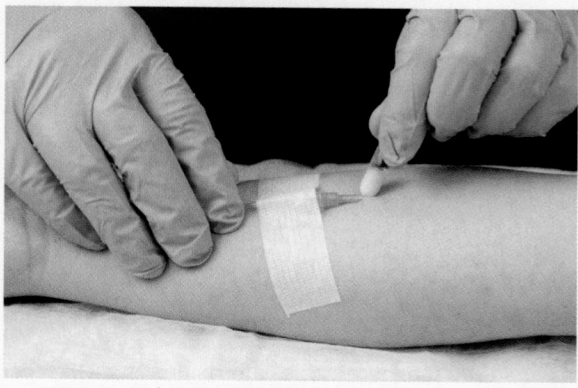

STEP 4 Cleanse peripheral site with antiseptic.

STEP	RATIONALE
7. Remove and discard gloves. Perform hand hygiene.	Prevents transmission of microorganisms.
8. *Optional:* Apply site protection device (e.g., I.V. House Ultra Protective Dressing).	Reduces risk of VAD dislodgment (Gorski et al., 2016).
9. Anchor extension tubing or IV tubing alongside dressing on arm and secure with tape directly over tubing. When using TSM dressing, avoid placing tape over the dressing.	Prevents accidental dislodgment of VAD if tubing is pulled.
10. Label dressing per agency policy. Information on label includes date and time of IV insertion, VAD gauge size and length, and your initials.	Communicates type of device and time interval for dressing change and site rotation.
11. Discard equipment and perform hand hygiene.	Reduces transmission of microorganisms.

EVALUATION

1. Evaluate function, patency of IV system, and flow rate after changing dressing.	Validates that IV is patent and functioning correctly. Manipulation of catheter and tubing will affect rate of infusion.
2. Evaluate patient at established intervals per agency policy and procedure for signs and symptoms of IV-related complications.	Identifies complications that compromise integrity of VAD or cause inaccurate IV solution flow rate.
3. **Use Teach-Back:** "I want to be sure that I explained reasons that the IV dressing may need to be changed. Tell me the problems you would report to the nurse that would require a dressing change." Revise your instruction now or develop a plan for revised patient/family caregiver teaching if patient/family caregiver is unable to teach back correctly.	Determines patient's/family caregiver's level of understanding of instructional topic.

RECORDING AND REPORTING

- Record in nurse's notes in electronic health record (EHR) or chart the time short-peripheral dressing was changed, reason for change, type of dressing material used, patency of system, and description of VAD site.
- Record patient's/family caregiver's knowledge following evaluation of teach-back in nurses' notes.

- Report to nurse in charge or oncoming shift nurse that dressing was changed and any significant information about integrity of system.
- Report to health care provider and document any complications, interventions, and patient response to treatment.

UNEXPECTED OUTCOMES AND RELATED INTERVENTIONS

- IV catheter is accidentally removed or dislodged.
  - Restart new short-peripheral IV in other extremity or above previous insertion site if continued therapy is necessary.
- IV solution is not infusing or runs slower than ordered.
  - Check IV catheter for bending, kinking, or dislodgment, as catheter may require replacement.

- Check for positional IV site and reposition catheter, applying new dressing if necessary.
- Check and adjust height of IV container, kinking, or obstruction of IV tubing.

KEY POINTS

- Body fluids, consisting of water and the substances dissolved or suspended in it, are distributed in ECF (vascular plus interstitial) and ICF compartments.
- To maintain normal fluid and electrolyte balance, daily intake must equal output, and the fluid and electrolytes must be distributed normally between body fluid compartments.
- Fluid output normally occurs through skin, lungs, GI tract, and kidneys and may occur through abnormal routes in patient populations.
- Patients who are very young or very old; patients whose I&O of fluid and/or electrolytes are not equal; and patients who have various hormone imbalances, chronic diseases, or trauma are at greatest risk for fluid, electrolyte, and acid-base imbalances.
- ECV excess and deficit are abnormal volumes of isotonic sodium-containing fluid, which manifest as sudden changes in body weight and changes in markers of vascular and interstitial volume.
- Osmolality imbalances are abnormal concentrations of body fluids, which manifest as altered serum sodium concentration and altered level of consciousness.
- Treatment for ECV excess is sodium restriction plus fluid restriction if severe; treatment for hyponatremia usually is water restriction.
- Enteral or parenteral administration of appropriate fluids prevents or treats ECV deficit, hypernatremia, and electrolyte deficits.
- Cellular metabolism constantly produces carbonic and metabolic acids; to maintain normal acid-base balance, carbonic acid must be excreted through the lungs, and metabolic acid must be buffered and then excreted through the kidneys.
- Acid-base imbalances are respiratory (excess or deficit of carbonic acid) or metabolic (excess or deficit of metabolic acids), manifested as changes in pH, $PaCO_2$, HCO_3^-, and level of consciousness.
- Initiation and maintenance of IV therapy require clinical decision making, skill, and organized procedures to maintain sterility and patency of the system.
- Nurses monitor for complications of IV therapy including infiltration, phlebitis, infection, and overload of the specific IV fluid.
- Administration of blood products entails a specific procedure for identification of the patient and the blood product and frequent monitoring during the transfusion for patient safety.
- Risks of blood transfusion include transfusion reactions, circulatory overload, infection, hyperkalemia, hypocalcemia, and hypomagnesemia from rapid administration of blood.
- Nursing interventions for acid-base imbalances support prescribed medical therapies and treat the underlying disorder while providing for patient safety.

REFLECTIVE LEARNING

- Consider a patient you encountered today and list that patient's risk factors for fluid and electrolyte imbalances.
- Think about a patient you encountered today and describe aspects of patient-centered care related to fluid intake.
- What patient safety protections related to fluid therapy did you encounter today?

REVIEW QUESTIONS

1. Your patient is at risk for an ECV deficit. Which assessment is a priority to report to the patient's health care provider?
   1. Weight loss of 1 kg in 24 hours
   2. Dry oral mucous membranes and thirst
   3. Skin tenting over sternum when pinched
   4. Hypotension and oliguria
2. Your patient has a severe acute asthma episode. Which set of arterial blood gas values is consistent with that diagnosis?
   1. pH, 7.52; PaO_2, 90 mm Hg; $PaCO_2$, 42 mm Hg; HCO_3^-, 36 mEq/L
   2. pH, 7.52; PaO_2, 80 mm Hg; $PaCO_2$, 28 mm Hg; HCO_3^-, 24 mEq/L
   3. pH, 7.22; PaO_2, 90 mm Hg; $PaCO_2$, 30 mm Hg; HCO_3^-, 12 mEq/L
   4. pH, 7.26; PaO_2, 70 mm Hg; $PaCO_2$, 55 mm Hg; HCO_3^-, 24 mEq/L
3. You need to discontinue a VAD. Place the steps in the correct order:
   1. Turn off the roller clamp on the IV tubing.
   2. Place sterile gauze over the VAD insertion site and apply light pressure while removing the catheter.
   3. Document VAD removal.
   4. Review the health care provider's order for discontinuing the VAD.
   5. Perform hand hygiene and apply clean gloves.
   6. Inspect the catheter end for intactness while applying firm pressure with the gauze.
   7. Explain to the patient the reason for discontinuing the VAD.
   8. Maintain continuous firm pressure with the gauze for 2 to 3 minutes or longer if needed.
   9. Remove IV site dressings and tape, and clean any secretions.
4. Your patient is receiving an IV infusion of 0.9% NaCl and develops crackles in the lung bases and shortness of breath. What is the priority nursing action?
   1. Contact the health care provider.
   2. Stop the infusion and remove the VAD.
   3. Slow the IV infusion rate.
   4. Replace the IV tubing.

5. To prevent fluid and electrolyte imbalance, what should you teach patients with normal renal function to do if they develop diarrhea? (Select all that apply.)
   1. Remember to replace the fluid loss with a lot of water.
   2. Stop oral intake of food and fluid until the diarrhea has stopped.
   3. Take in banana, orange juice, or other source of potassium.
   4. Replace the fluid loss with fluid that contains some sodium.
   5. Avoid milk, cheese, and other sources of calcium.

evolve

Additional Review Questions, as well as rationales for all Review Questions, can be found on the Evolve website.

1. 4; 2. 4; 3. 4, 7, 5, 1, 9, 2, 6, 8, 3; 4. 3; 5. 3, 4.

REFERENCES

AABB: *Blood donation FAQs*, 2016. http://www.aabb.org/tm/donation/Pages/donatefaqs.aspx.

Abitz T: Cultural congruence and infusion nursing practice, *J Infus Nurs* 39(2):77, 2016.

Alexander M, et al: *Core curriculum for infusion nursing*, ed 4, Philadelphia, 2014, Lippincott Williams & Wilkins.

Benaya A, et al: Relative incidence of phlebitis associated with peripheral intravenous catheters in the lower versus upper extremities, *Eur J Clin Microbiol Infect Dis* 34(5):913, 2015.

Burchum JR, Rosenthal LD: *Lehne's pharmacology for nursing care*, ed 9, St Louis, 2016, Elsevier.

Centers for Disease Control and Prevention (CDC): *Guidelines for the prevention of intravascular catheter-related infections*, 2015. https://www.cdc.gov/infectioncontrol/guidelines/bsi/index.html.

Cicolini G, et al: Phlebitis risk varies by peripheral venous catheter site and increases after 96 hours: a large multi-centre prospective study, *J Adv Nurs* 70(11):2539, 2014.

Cook LS: Infusion-related air embolism, *J Infus Nurs* 36(1):26, 2013.

Crookston KP, Koenig SC, et al: Transfusion reaction identification and management at the bedside, *J Infus Nurs* 38(2):105, 2015.

Custer B, et al: Risk factors for retrovirus and hepatitis virus infections in accepted blood donors, *Transfusion* 55(5):1098, 2015.

Felver L: Acid-base balance. In Giddens JF, editor: *Concepts for nursing practice*, ed 2, St Louis, 2017a, Elsevier.

Felver L: Fluid and electrolytes. In Giddens JF, editor: *Concepts for nursing practice*, ed 2, St Louis, 2017b, Elsevier.

Felver L: Fluid and electrolyte homeostasis and imbalances. In Copstead LC, Banasik JL, editors: *Pathophysiology*, ed 6, St Louis, 2018, Elsevier.

Gorski L, et al: Infusion therapy standards of practice, *J Infus Nurs* 39(Suppl 1):S1, 2016.

Guinn NR, et al: Costs and outcomes after cardiac surgery in patients refusing transfusion compared with those who do not: a case-matched study, *Transfusion* 55(12):279, 2015.

Hall JE: *Guyton and Hall textbook of medical physiology*, ed 13, Philadelphia, 2016, Elsevier.

Helm RE, et al: Accepted but unacceptable: peripheral IV catheter failure, *J Infus Nurs* 38(3):189, 2015.

Hockenberry MJ, et al: *Essentials of pediatric nursing*, ed 10, St Louis, 2017, Mosby.

Infusion Nurses Society (INS): *Policies and procedures for infusion nursing*, ed 5, Norwood, MA, 2016, Infusion Nurses Society.

Kamel KS, Halperin ML: *Fluid, electrolyte, and acid-base physiology: a problem-based approach*, ed 5, St Louis, 2017, Elsevier.

McGloin S: The ins and outs of fluid balance in the acutely ill patient, *Br J Nurs* 24(1):14, 2015.

National Digestive Disease Information Clearing House: *Diarrhea*, 2016. https://www.niddk.nih.gov/health-information/digestive-diseases/diarrhea/all-content.

National Institute on Alcohol Abuse and Alcoholism (NIAAA): *Drinking levels defined*, n.d. https://www.niaaa.nih.gov/alcohol-health/overview-alcohol-consumption/moderate-binge-drinking.

National Quality Forum (NQF): *Field guide to NQF resources*, Washington, DC, 2016. http://www.qualityforum.org/Field_Guide/List_of_Measures.aspx.

Oncology Nursing Society: *Extravasation precautions crucial when administering Vincristine*, 2016. https://www.ons.org/practice-resources/clinical-practice/extravasation-precautions-crucial-when-administering.

Phillips LD, Gorski L: *Manual of I.V. therapeutics: evidence-based practice for infusion therapy*, ed 6, Philadelphia, 2014, F.A. Davis.

Simmons DP, Savage WJ: Hemolysis from ABO incompatibility, *Hematol Oncol Clin North Am* 29(3):429, 2015.

The Joint Commission (TJC): *2018 National Patient Safety Goals*, Oakbrook Terrace, IL, 2018. The Commission. https://www.jointcommission.org/standards_information/npsgs.aspx.

Touhy TA, Jett KF: *Ebersole and Hess' gerontological nursing and healthy aging*, St Louis, 2014, Elsevier.

Vizcarra C, et al: Recommendations for improving safety practices with short peripheral catheters, *J Infus Nurs* 37(2):121, 2014.

Wallace MC, Macy DL: Reduction of central line-associated bloodstream infection rates in patients in the adult intensive care unit, *J Infus Nurs* 39(1):47, 2016.

Wallis MC, et al: Risk factors for peripheral intravenous catheter failure: a multivariate analysis of data from a randomized controlled trial, *Infect Control Hosp Epidemiol* 35(1):63, 2014.

Wang XH, et al: Reduction of heart failure rehospitalization using a weight management education intervention, *J Cardiovasc Nurs* 29(6):528, 2014.

Weinstein SM, Hagle SM: *Plumer's principles and practice of infusion therapy*, ed 9, Philadelphia, 2014, Lippincott Williams & Wilkins.

Winkler M, Guenter P: Long-term home parenteral nutrition: it takes an interdisciplinary approach, *J Infus Nurs* 37(5):389, 2014.

Complementary, Alternative, and Integrative Therapies

evolve MEDIA RESOURCES

http://evolve.elsevier.com/Potter/essentials
- Audio Glossary
- QSEN Activity and Review Questions Answers and Rationales

OBJECTIVES

- Describe complementary, alternative, and integrative therapies.
- Describe clinical applications for use of relaxation therapies.
- Discuss the relaxation response and its effect on somatic ailments.
- Identify the principles and effectiveness of imagery, meditation, breathwork and animal-assisted therapy.
- Describe the purpose and principles of biofeedback.
- Describe the methods of and the psychophysiological responses to therapeutic touch.
- Describe safe and unsafe herbal therapies.

KEY TERMS

acupoints, p. 545

acupuncture, p. 544

allopathic medicine or biomedicine, p. 536

alternative therapies, p. 537

animal-assisted therapy, p. 543

biofeedback, p. 544

chiropractic therapy, p. 537

complementary therapies, p. 537

creative visualization, p. 542

cupping, p. 546

imagery, p. 542

integrative health care, p. 549

integrative nursing, p. 537

meditation, p. 542

moxibustion, p. 546

passive relaxation, p. 541

progressive relaxation, p. 541

qi gong, p. 546

relaxation response, p. 540

stress response, p. 540

tai chi, p. 546

therapeutic touch (TT), p. 545

traditional Chinese medicine (TCM), p. 537

vital energy (qi), p. 544

whole medical systems, p. 537

yin and yang, p. 546

Heart disease and cancer are the top two causes of death in the United States (Xu et al., 2016). Changes in knowledge, technology, science, and health care have successfully altered the course of many of these illnesses. However, there is more work to be done. Despite the success of allopathic medicine or biomedicine (conventional western medicine), many conditions such as chronic back and neck pain, arthritis, gastrointestinal problems, allergies, headache, and anxiety continue to be difficult to treat. As a result, more patients are exploring alternative methods to relieve their symptoms.

The number of patients seeking unconventional treatments has increased considerably over the past decade. The 2012 National Health Interview Survey (NHIS) reported that the top five most common complementary health approaches used by adults were natural products such as herbs, vitamins and minerals, and probiotics; deep breathing; yoga, tai chi or qi

CASE STUDY *James*

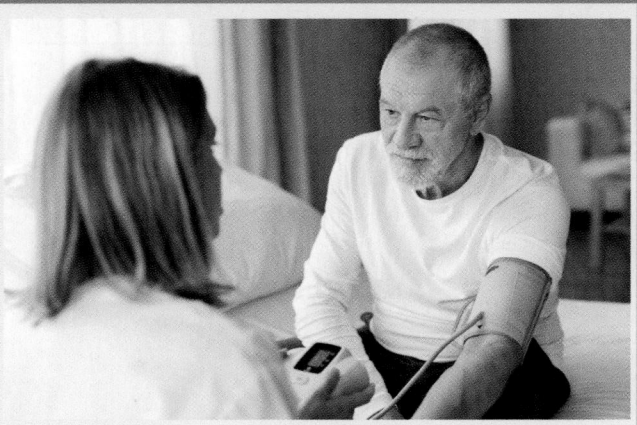

Copyright © Halfpoint/iStock/Thinkstock.

James is a 59-year-old man who has had several heart attacks over the past few months. Because of changes in his health, he needed to retire from work. Kathryn, a public health nurse, visits James in his home for a follow-up check after the most recent heart attack and talks with him about how he is adjusting to being retired. James tells the nurse he physically feels good and has not had any chest pain, but he is having a lot of difficulty sleeping at night. He has feelings of anxiety about having another heart attack. James does not want to take any more medication than he needs to and has resisted taking antianxiety medication or medication at night to help him fall asleep. The nurse talks with James about his feelings and explores alternative methods that can help James deal with his anxiety and fall asleep.

gong; chiropractic or osteopathic manipulation; and meditation (National Institutes of Health/National Center for Complementary and Integrative Health [NIH/NCCIH], 2016a). These data highlight the variety of approaches adult patients are using and the growing acceptance of these approaches.

COMPLEMENTARY, ALTERNATIVE, AND INTEGRATIVE APPROACHES TO HEALTH

The NIH/NCCIH (2016a) distinguishes between complementary, alternative, and integrative approaches to health. NCCIH identifies approaches as complementary when a nonmainstream practice is used together with conventional medicine. Alternative approaches are when a nonmainstream approach replaces conventional medicine. When conventional and complementary approaches are brought together in a coordinated way, this is referred to as an integrative approach. In general, NCCIH uses the term "complementary health approaches" when discussing practices and products of nonmainstream origin and "integrative health" when discussing incorporating complementary approaches into mainstream health care. These approaches can also be referred to as therapies (such as massage therapy) or techniques (such as relaxation techniques).

Many approaches such as therapeutic touch contain diagnostic and therapeutic methods that require special training.

Others such as guided imagery and breathwork are easily learned and applied. Complementary therapies include relaxation; exercise; massage; reflexology; prayer; biofeedback; hypnotherapy; creative therapies such as art, music, or dance therapy; meditation; chiropractic therapy; and herbs and supplements (Lindquist et al., 2014).

Alternative therapies sometimes include the same interventions as complementary therapies, but they become the primary treatment (Table 19.1). For example, a person with chronic pain uses yoga to encourage flexibility and relaxation to augment the effects of prescribed nonsteroidal antiinflammatory or opioid medications. Both sets of interventions are based on conventional pathophysiology and anatomy, while acknowledging the mind-body connection that contributes to the physiological pain response. In this case yoga is used as a complementary intervention. In contrast, another patient decides that a meditative practice that includes yoga and other lifestyle changes is more helpful than an allopathic approach to chronic pain. This patient studies these practices more deeply, adhering to one of the many schools or traditions, and decides to use them as the primary approach to manage chronic pain. In this case yoga is an alternative treatment. Several therapies are always considered alternative because they are based on completely different philosophies and life systems than those used by allopathic medicine. These are identified by the NIH/NCCIH as whole medical systems and include practices such as traditional Chinese medicine (TCM), Ayurveda, and naturopathy (see Table 19.1).

Because of the increased interest in complementary therapies, many health care programs including medical and nursing schools have integrated conventional "biomedical" education with programs that incorporate complementary and alternative therapy content. Integrative health care practitioners recommend that patients receive a full spectrum of possible biomedical and complementary treatments.

Historically nurses practiced in an integrative fashion; a review of nursing theories reveals the values of holism, relational care, and informed practice. Holistic nursing focuses on the body-mind-spirit of patients. Holistic nurses use interventions such as relaxation therapy, music therapy, touch therapies, and guided imagery (Dossey and Keegan, 2015). The American Holistic Nurses Association maintains standards of holistic nursing practice, which define and establish the scope of holistic practice and describe the level of care expected from a holistic nurse (American Holistic Nursing Association/American Nurses Association [AHNA/ANA], 2015).

In 2014, Kreitzer and Koithan challenged the nursing profession to embrace its long-standing roots of integrative care and to stand alongside physician colleagues to transform the current health care system and offer whole-person care that is patient centered, relationship based, and supported by evidence, incorporating the best of all possible interventions. Grounded in six principles, integrative nursing is defined as "a way of being-knowing-doing that advances the health and well-being of people, families, and communities through caring-healing relationships. Integrative nurses use

TABLE 19.1 COMPLEMENTARY AND INTEGRATIVE THERAPIES

TYPES	DEFINITIONS
Biologically Based Therapies	
Natural Products	
Dietary supplements	Defined by the Dietary Supplement Health and Education Act of 1994 and used to supplement dietary/nutritional intake by mouth; contain one or more dietary ingredients including vitamins, minerals, herbs, or other botanical products.
Herbal medicines	Plant-based therapies used in whole systems of medicine or as individual preparations by allopathic providers and consumers for specific symptoms or issues.
Mycotherapies	Fungi-based (mushroom) products.
Probiotics	Live microorganisms (in most cases, bacteria) that are similar to beneficial microorganisms found in the human gastrointestinal system; also called good bacteria.
Energy Therapies	
Use or Manipulation of Energy Fields	
Healing touch	Biofield therapy; uses gentle touch directly on or close to body to influence and support the human energy system and bring balance to the whole body (physical, spiritual, emotional, and mental); a formal educational and certification system provides credentials for practitioners.
Reiki therapy	Biofield therapy derived from ancient Buddhist rituals; practitioner places hands on or above a body area and transfers "universal life energy" providing strength, harmony, and balance to treat a patient's health disturbances.
Therapeutic touch	Biofield therapy involving direction of a practitioner's balanced energies in an intentional manner toward those of a patient; practitioner's hands lay on or close to a patient's body.
Manipulative and Body-Based Methods	
Involve Movement of Body With Focus on Body Structures and Systems	
Acupressure	Applying digital pressure in a specified way on designated points on the body to relieve pain, produce analgesia, or regulate a body function.
Chiropractic medicine	Manipulating the spinal column; includes physiotherapy and diet therapy.
Craniosacral therapy	Assessing the craniosacral motion for rate, amplitude, symmetry, and quality and attuning/aligning the spinal column, cerebrospinal fluid, and rhythmic processes, releasing restrictions or abnormal barriers to motion.
Massage therapy	Manipulating soft tissue through stroking, rubbing, or kneading to increase circulation, improve muscle tone, and provide relaxation.
Mind-Body Interventions	
Honor Connections Between Thoughts and Physiological Functioning Using Emotion to Influence Health and Well-Being	
Animal-assisted therapy	Process using trained animals by trained health care professionals to assist with an individualized patient need (e.g., pain control, managing attention-deficit/hyper activity [ADHD] in children).
Biofeedback	Process providing a person with visual or auditory information about autonomic physiological functions of the body such as muscle tension, skin temperature, and brain wave activity using instruments.
Breathwork	Using a variety of breathing patterns to relax, invigorate, or open emotional channels.
Guided imagery	Concentrating on an image or series of images to treat pathological conditions.
Meditation	Self-directed practice for relaxing the body and calming the mind with focused rhythmic breathing.
Music therapy	Using music to address physical, psychological, cognitive, and social needs of individuals with disabilities and illnesses; improves physical movement and/or communication, develops emotional expression, evokes memories, and distracts individuals who are in pain.
Tai chi	Incorporating breath, movement, and meditation to cleanse, strengthen, and circulate vital life energy and blood; stimulate the immune system; and maintain external and internal balance.
Yoga	Focuses on body musculature, posture, breathing mechanisms, and consciousness; goal is attainment of physical and mental well-being through mastery of body achieved through exercise, holding of postures, proper breathing, and meditation.

TABLE 19.1 COMPLEMENTARY AND INTEGRATIVE THERAPIES—cont'd

TYPES	DEFINITIONS
Movement Therapies *Eastern or Western Approaches to Promote Well-Being*	
Dance therapy	Intimate and powerful medium because it is a direct expression of the mind and body; treats people with social, emotional, cognitive, or physical problems.
Pilates	Method of body movement used to strengthen, lengthen, and improve the voluntary control of muscles and muscle groups, especially muscles used for posture and core strengthening.
Whole Medical Systems *Complete Systems of Theory and Practice That Have Evolved Independently From or Parallel to Allopathic (Conventional) Medicine*	
Ayurvedic medicine	One of the oldest systems of medicine practiced in India since the 1st century. Treatments balance the doshas with a combination of dietary and lifestyle changes, herbal remedies and purgatives, massage, meditation, and exercise.
Homeopathic medicine	Developed in Germany and practiced in the United States since the mid-1800s. A system of medical treatments based on the theory that certain diseases can be cured by giving small, highly diluted doses of substances made from naturally occurring plant, animal, or mineral substances that stimulate the vital force of the body so that it can heal itself.
Latin American traditional healing	Curanderismo is a Latin American traditional healing system that includes a humoral model for classifying food, activity, drugs, and illnesses and a series of folk illnesses. The goal is to create a balance between the patient and his or her environment, thereby sustaining health.
Native American traditional healing	Tribal traditions are individualistic, but similarities across traditions include the use of sweating and purging, herbal remedies, and ceremonies in which a shaman (a spiritual healer) contacts spirits to ask their direction in bringing healing to people to promote wholeness and healing.
Naturopathic medicine	A system of therapeutics focused on treating the whole person and promoting health and well-being rather than treating an individual disease. Therapeutics include herbal medicine, nutritional supplementation, physical medicine, homeopathy, lifestyle counseling, and mind-body therapies with an orientation toward assisting the person's internal capacity for self-healing (vitalism).
Traditional Chinese medicine (TCM)	An ancient healing tradition identified in the 1st century focused on balancing yin/yang energies. It is a set of systematic techniques and methods including acupuncture, herbal medicines, massage, acupressure, moxibustion (use of heat from burning herbs), qi gong (balancing energy flow through body movement), and cupping. Fundamental concepts are from Taoism, Confucianism, and Buddhism.

evidence to inform traditional and emerging interventions that support whole person/whole systems healing" (Kreitzer and Koithan, 2014).

Increasing interest in complementary and integrative health approaches is evident in the increased number of publications in respected health care journals and continued support of research and discovery. The mission of the NIH/NCCIH (2016b) is to "define, through rigorous scientific investigation, the usefulness and safety of complementary and integrative health interventions and their roles in improving health and health care." Although research in this area continues to advance, you need to weigh the risks and benefits of each intervention and consider the following when recommending complementary and integrative health approaches: (1) the history of each therapy (many have been used by cultures for thousands of years to support health and reduce suffering), (2) the history and experience of nursing with a particular therapy, (3) outcomes and safety data, (4) research results, and (5) cultural influences and context for certain patient populations (Box 19.1).

Open communication ensures safe and effective use of any approach or therapy. People choose these therapies based on many reasons including personal preference, experience of a family or friend, desire for a more holistic approach to their care, or a feeling that traditional medicine alone is not effective. It is important to first assess why a person chose the therapy and his or her understanding of it. For example, if a patient uses an herbal therapy, it is important to determine if the patient is taking it correctly and that the side effects or potential interaction with other medicine is known. Often patients do not realize that herbal supplements may interfere with other medications they are taking. Therefore patient education is key.

This chapter describes several types of complementary and alternative therapies, the clinical applications of each, and the limitations of each therapy. The therapies are organized into two categories. The first are nursing-accessible therapies that you can learn and implement in patient care. The second category includes training-specific therapies such as therapeutic touch or acupressure that a

BOX 19.1 EVIDENCE-BASED PRACTICE

PICO Question: In children with chronic illnesses, are complementary and alternative therapies effective in relieving pain and anxiety?

SUMMARY OF EVIDENCE

Pain is a complex phenomenon involving psychological, biological, and sociological factors. Hospitalization and pain are often linked in the minds of children, and for children with chronic conditions pain significantly impacts their quality of life. One group of researchers found that adolescents who had scoliosis and used guided imagery to control pain following spinal fusion surgery experienced significantly less overall pain and improvements in eating and sleeping (Charette et al., 2015). Guided imagery also helped children with sickle cell disease improve their self-efficacy and better control their pain (Dobson, 2015).

APPLICATION TO NURSING PRACTICE

- Children who are hospitalized often respond positively to complementary therapies, such as relaxation and guided imagery. Use of these therapies often leads to reduced pain and the need for fewer medications for pain control (Charette et al., 2015).
- Children and adolescents with chronic conditions often experience pain. Use complementary and alternative therapies, such as guided imagery, to help alleviate pain and assist these patients to feel more in control of their lives (Dobson, 2015).
- Nurses need to learn about complementary and alternative therapies so that they can offer children with chronic illnesses a variety of approaches that can assist in alleviating the pain and anxiety associated with their disease and/or procedures.

nurse cannot perform without additional training and/or certification.

NURSING-ACCESSIBLE THERAPIES

Some complementary therapies and techniques are general in nature and use natural processes (e.g., breathing, thinking and concentration, presence, movement) to help people feel better and cope with both acute and chronic conditions. Ongoing assessment and evaluation of your patient's responses to these interventions determine both the appropriateness and the usefulness of these complementary therapies. Sometimes changes to therapies prescribed by a health care provider (e.g., medication doses) are needed when complementary therapies alter physiological responses and lead to improved therapeutic responses (Kreitzer and Koithan, 2014).

Complementary therapies teach behavioral modifications that often alter physical responses to stress and improve symptoms such as anxiety, muscle tension, gastrointestinal discomfort, pain, or sleep disturbances. Active involvement is a primary principle for these therapies; individuals achieve better responses if they practice the techniques or exercises daily. Therefore to achieve effective outcomes, match therapeutic strategies with an individual's lifestyle, beliefs and values, and treatment preferences.

All therapies have the potential to interact with medication or other therapies currently in use. Patients need to understand what the therapy is; how it is used; and what benefits, contraindications, and side effects can occur. In addition, patients and family caregivers need to understand any medication interactions. For example, when pain is controlled with relaxation, the patient's type and dose of analgesia may require changing. Informed consent is needed for many therapies, and you need to ensure that institutional policy is followed. Although a therapy may not be invasive, such as an injection of medication, all therapies have potential side effects.

Relaxation Therapy

People face situations in everyday life that evoke the **stress response** (see Chapter 26). The mind varies the biochemical functions of the major organ systems in response to feedback. Thoughts and feelings influence the production of chemicals (i.e., neurotransmitters, neurohormones, peptides) that circulate throughout the body and convey messages via cells to various systems within the body. The stress response is a good example of the way in which systems cooperate to protect an individual from harm. Physiologically the cascade of changes associated with the stress response causes increased heart and respiratory rates; tightened muscles; increased metabolic rate; and a general sense of foreboding, fear, nervousness, irritability, and negative mood. Other physiological responses include elevated blood pressure; dilated pupils; stronger cardiac contractions; and increased levels of blood glucose, cortisol, serum cholesterol, and triglycerides. Although these responses prepare a person for short-term stress, the effects on the body of long-term stress sometimes create structural damage and chronic illness such as angina, tension headaches, cardiac arrhythmias, pain, ulcers, and atrophy of the immune system organs (Kreitzer and Koithan, 2014).

The **relaxation response** is a state of generalized decreased cognitive, physiological, or behavioral arousal. Relaxation also involves arousal reduction through parasympathetic activity. The process of relaxation elongates the muscle fibers and reduces the neural impulses sent to the brain, thus decreasing the activity of the brain and other body systems. Decreased heart and respiratory rates, blood pressure, and oxygen consumption and increased alpha brain activity and peripheral skin temperature characterize relaxation. It occurs using techniques that incorporate a repetitive mental focus and the adoption of a calm, peaceful attitude (Lindquist et al., 2014).

Relaxation helps individuals develop cognitive skills to reduce the negative ways in which they respond to situations within their environment. Cognitive skills include the following:

- Focusing—the ability to identify, differentiate, maintain attention on, and return attention to simple stimuli for an extended period

- Passivity—the ability to stop unnecessary goal-directed and analytic activity
- Receptivity—the ability to tolerate and accept experiences that are uncertain, unfamiliar, or paradoxical

The long-term goal of relaxation therapy is for people to continually monitor themselves for indicators of tension and consciously let go and release the tension contained in various body parts.

Progressive relaxation training teaches an individual how to effectively rest and reduce tension in the body. The person learns to detect subtle localized muscle tension sequentially, one muscle group at a time (e.g., upper arm muscles, forearm muscles). In doing so, an individual learns to differentiate between high-intensity tension, subtle tension, and relaxation by practicing with different muscle groups (Dossey and Keegan, 2015). One active progressive relaxation technique involves the use of slow, deep abdominal breathing while tightening and relaxing an ordered succession of muscle groups, focusing on the associated bodily sensations while letting go of extraneous thoughts. Choose a logical order when guiding a patient through progressive relaxation. For example, begin with the muscles in the face, followed by muscles in the arms, hands, abdomen, legs, and feet, or begin with the feet and work up the body.

Another deep breathing exercise you can teach your patient was developed by Weil (2017a). This exercise, known as "4-7-8 breath," does not require special equipment and can be done anywhere (Box 19.2).

The goal of passive relaxation is to still the mind and body intentionally without the need to tighten and relax a specific body part. One effective passive relaxation technique incorporates slow, abdominal breathing exercises while imagining warmth and relaxation flowing through specific body parts such as the lungs or hands.

Clinical Applications of Relaxation Therapy. Relaxation techniques are associated with numerous benefits. Research shows that relaxation techniques slow the heart rate, lower blood pressure, slow respiratory rate, reduce release of stress hormones, increase blood flow to major muscles, reduce muscle tension and chronic pain, improve concentration and mood, decrease fatigue, reduce anger and frustration, and boost confidence to handle problems (Mayo Clinic, 2017). Relaxation also reduces hypertension (Nagele et al., 2014). The Mayo Clinic reports that greater benefits are seen in patients who incorporate several relaxation techniques in their lives such as positive coping methods (e.g., finding humor and thinking positively) and relaxation exercises (e.g., yoga or tai chi) (Fig. 19.1).

Relaxation enables individuals to exert control over their lives. Some experience a decreased feeling of helplessness and a more positive psychological state overall. *Consider the case study with James at the beginning of this chapter. Relaxation therapy is one therapy that the nurse could help him learn to calm his mind, relieve his anxiety, and help him to sleep.*

Limitations of Relaxation Therapy. During relaxation training individuals learn to differentiate between low and high levels of muscle tension. During the first months of training sessions, when the person is learning how to focus on body sensations and tensions, there are reports of increased sensitivity in detecting muscle tension. Usually these feelings are minor and resolve as the person continues with the training. However, be aware that occasionally some relaxation techniques can either intensify symptoms or create new ones (Dossey and Keegan, 2015).

An important consideration when choosing a relaxation technique is the physiological and psychological status of the individual. Some patients with a chronic illness such as cancer seek relaxation training to reduce their stress response.

BOX 19.2 TEACHING YOUR PATIENT HOW TO IMPLEMENT THE 4-7-8 BREATH

Instruct your patient to place the tip of the tongue against the ridge of tissue just behind the upper front teeth, and keep it there through the entire exercise. Explain the patient will inhale quietly through the nose and exhale through the mouth around the tongue. Instruct the patient to try pursing lips slightly if this seems awkward. Teach your patient the following steps to use this technique:

1. Exhale completely through your mouth, making a whoosh sound.
2. Close your mouth and inhale quietly through your nose to a mental count of four.
3. Hold your breath for a count of seven.
4. Exhale completely through your mouth, making a whoosh sound to a count of eight. (**Note:** exhaling takes twice as long as inhaling.)
5. This is one breath. Now inhale again and repeat the cycle three more times for a total of four breaths.

Data from Weil A: *The art and science of breathing,* 2017, https://www.drweil.com/health-wellness/balanced-living/meditation-inspiration/the-art-and-science-of-breathing/.

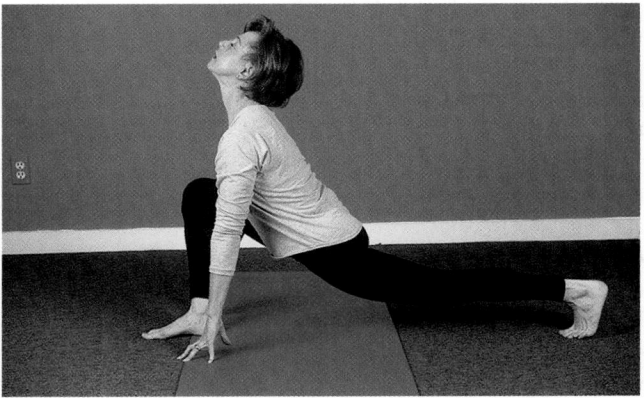

FIG 19.1 Yoga is a discipline that focuses on muscles, posture, breathing, and consciousness.

However, techniques such as active progressive relaxation require a moderate expenditure of energy, which often increases fatigue and limits an individual's ability to complete relaxation sessions and practice. Therefore active progressive relaxation is not appropriate for patients with advanced disease or decreased energy reserves. Passive relaxation or guided imagery is more appropriate for these individuals because it requires less energy.

Meditation and Breathing

Meditation is any activity that limits stimulus input by directing attention to a single unchanging or repetitive stimulus so the person becomes more aware of self (Lindquist et al., 2014). Meditation is a general term for a wide range of practices that involve relaxing the body and stilling the mind. The root word, *meditari,* means to consider or pay attention to something. Although meditation has its roots in eastern religious practices (Hindu, Buddhism, and Taoism), conventional health care practitioners began to recognize its healing potential in the early 1970s (Lindquist et al., 2014). The four components of meditation were identified by Benson (1975) as (1) a quiet space, (2) a comfortable position, (3) a receptive attitude, and (4) a focus of attention. Meditation is a process that anyone can use to calm down; cope with stress; and, for individuals with spiritual inclinations, feel one with God or the universe.

Meditation is different from relaxation; its purpose is to become "mindful," increasing the ability to live freely and escape destructive patterns of negativity. Meditation allows a patient to focus attention inward to induce a state of deep relaxation (Harvard Health Publications, 2014). People practice meditation in many ways including walking meditation, concentration meditation, and mindfulness meditation. Some patients meditate on their own or in a group. A benefit of meditation is that it does not require equipment, making it a practice that can be done almost anywhere and is cost-effective.

Clinical Applications of Meditation.
Numerous studies have focused on meditation to determine its benefits and usefulness for different patients. Wells et al. (2014) found that meditation helped reduce stress and headache duration in patients with migraines. In another study, regular practice of transcendental meditation decreased the need for psychotropic medications in men with anxiety and posttraumatic stress disorder (PTSD) following service in the military (Barnes et al., 2016).

In addition, meditation increases productivity, improves mood, increases sense of identity, and decreases irritability (Dossey and Keegan, 2015). Considerations for the appropriateness of meditation include a person's degree of self-discipline. Meditation requires ongoing practice to achieve lasting results. Most meditation activities are easy to learn and do not require memorization or procedures. Patients typically find mindfulness and meditation self-reinforcing. The peaceful, positive mental state is usually pleasurable and provides an incentive for individuals to continue meditating.

Limitations of Meditation.
Although meditation contributes to improvement in a variety of physiological and psychological ailments, it is contraindicated for some people. Therefore consult with a health care provider before a patient begins to meditate. For example, a person who has a strong fear of losing control can perceive it as a form of mind control and thus will be resistant to learning the technique. Some individuals also become hypertensive during meditation and require a much shorter session than the average 15- to 20-minute session.

Meditation sometimes increases the effects of certain drugs. Therefore monitor individuals learning meditation closely for physiological changes with respect to their medications. Prolonged practice of meditation techniques sometimes reduces the need for antihypertensive, thyroid-regulating, and psychotropic medications (e.g., antidepressants and antianxiety agents). In these cases, adjustment of the medication is necessary.

Imagery

Imagery or visualization is a mind-body therapy that uses the conscious mind to create mental images to stimulate physical changes in the body, improve perceived well-being, and enhance self-awareness. Frequently imagery combined with some form of relaxation training facilitates relaxation. Imagery is sometimes self-directed, in which individuals create their mental images. Other times it is guided, during which a practitioner leads an individual through a scenario (Lindquist et al., 2014). When guiding an imagery exercise, direct a patient to begin slow abdominal breathing while focusing on the rhythm of breathing. Then direct the patient to visualize a specific image such as ocean waves coming to shore, walking along a country road with birds chirping, or sitting by a running stream with each inspiration. Then direct the patient to allow the image to recede with each exhalation. Next instruct the patient to take notice of the smells, sounds, and temperatures that he or she is experiencing. As the imagery session progresses, instruct the patient to visualize warmth entering the body during inspiration and tension leaving the body during exhalation.

There is insufficient evidence to support that imagery alters disease progression. However, evidence supports its usefulness in reducing patient's pain and anxiety and improving their quality of life (Kubes, 2015). Imagery evokes different responses, from fear to relaxation, depending on the image. However, imagery is commonly used to evoke relaxation. When the relaxation response occurs, a patient's blood pressure decreases, and respiratory rate and anxiety levels lessen (Kubes, 2015). Creative visualization is self-directed imagery based on the principle of mind-body connectivity (i.e., every mental image leads to physical or emotional changes) (Gawain, 2016). Box 19.3 lists teaching strategies for helping patients use creative visualization. People typically respond to their environment based on their perceptions, visualizations, and expectancies. Therefore it is necessary to individualize imagery for each patient (Lindquist et al., 2014).

Copyright © Halfpoint/
iStock/Thinkstock.

BOX 19.3 PATIENT TEACHING

Creative Visualization

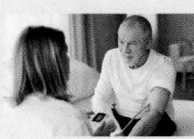

OUTCOME

The patient will demonstrate skills in creative visualization.

TEACHING STRATEGIES

- Set goals the patient can meet. Success increases confidence and self-esteem.
- Teach patient how to create a clear image. Although it is sometimes difficult to develop a visual image, if a patient views the goals of the imagery with clear thoughts and in the present tense, he or she will be more successful in creating an effective image.
- Have the patient frequently visualize the image during relaxing states and throughout the day but particularly before bedtime or on wakening, when the mind usually is more relaxed.
- Have the patient repeat encouraging statements while focusing on the image. This alleviates any doubts about his or her ability to achieve established goals.
- Encourage family caregiver to remind patient to perform visualization exercise and to participate in the exercise itself.

EVALUATION

- Use the principles of teach-back to evaluate patient/family caregiver learning:
  - Ask patient or family caregiver to discuss ways visualization can be helpful to reduce conditions such as anxiety and pain.
  - Ask patient, "How are you coping with daily stressors?"

this intervention. In the study by Burhenn et al. (2014), only three of seven nurses completed the training sessions to learn how to use guided imagery in the study. Barriers to the use of imagery included lack of time, difficulty in contacting a nurse trained in guided imagery, refusal of the intervention by some patients, and some physicians requiring notification before a nurse offered guided imagery to a patient, which created a delay or prevented the intervention being offered in some cases.

QSEN QSEN ACTIVITY *Patient-Centered Care*

You are caring for Carmen, a 48-year-old woman with stage 3 breast cancer who has returned to the hospital after being discharged following a mastectomy. She developed an infection in her suture line and around her drain site. Just before changing her dressings, you notice that she is withdrawn and unwilling to speak more than one or two words and only to answer direct questions. When you question her further, she states that she cannot stop thinking about her future and fears that "this will be how it's going to be … one hospital visit after another." She also says that she is concerned about the amount of pain medication she is taking and that she is "tired of feeling drowsy and out-of-it" when her family comes to visit but does not know how else to manage her fear and pain.

- Which techniques could you offer Carmen to alleviate her suffering and help control her pain?
- What strategies would help her cope with future hospital visits and potentially painful procedures?

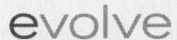 Answers to QSEN Activities can be found on the Evolve website.

Clinical Applications of Imagery. You can use imagery in patients across the life span. When using guided imagery in children, be sure the child understands the process and exercises. Older adults will also benefit, but be sure their primary illness does not affect their ability to follow instruction. Imagery is frequently used with patients who have cancer. In one study, Burhenn et al. (2014) found that most patients experienced less cancer-related pain immediately after using guided imagery, and for some patients, this effect lasted for an hour. Many of the patients in the study recommended guided imagery be offered more often and for longer periods. Guided imagery also helps treat other chronic conditions such as asthma, sickle cell anemia, migraines, autoimmune disorders, atrial fibrillation, functional urinary disorders, menstrual and premenstrual syndromes, irritable bowel syndrome, ulcerative colitis, and rheumatoid arthritis (Lindquist et al., 2014).

Limitations of Imagery. As with all therapies, you need to monitor patients closely when beginning this therapy. Images can evoke positive or negative feelings in patients. Another issue is the time it takes for you to learn how to use

TRAINING-SPECIFIC THERAPIES

Training-specific therapies are complementary treatments that nurses or other health care providers administer only after completing a specific course of study and training. These therapies require postgraduate certificates or degrees indicating completion of additional education and training, national certification, or additional licensure beyond the RN to practice and administer them. Many of these therapies have positive effects but carry some risk, particularly when used along with conventional medical therapies. You need knowledge to talk about them effectively with patients and provide education about their safe use.

Animal-Assisted Therapy

Pet therapy, also referred to as animal-assisted therapy (AAT), has gained in popularity as a complementary and alternative therapy. Although some may refer to service animals as pet therapy animals, the two are not the same. Therapy animals are not owned by the patient but rather are brought to a therapy session by a handler (Goddard and Gilmer, 2015). Animal-assisted therapy is defined as "the use of trained animals by trained health professionals to facilitate specific, measurable goals for individual patients for whom there is documented progress" (Calcaterra et al., 2015).

Historically there have always been examples of the human-animal connection, with Florence Nightingale reportedly practicing what she called "animal-companion therapy" for her patients who were sick or disabled (Goddard and Gilmer, 2015). Nightingale found the pets to be an essential part of healing for her patients. Sigmund Freud was reported to have said his dog had a special sense. Psychiatrist Boris Levinson began incorporating his dog, Jingles, into his child therapy sessions in 1969; this is credited as the birth of modern practice in AAT (Goddard and Gilmer, 2015).

There are numerous documented benefits of AAT for patients of all ages and with all conditions. However, remember to take into consideration the patient's comfort with animals and potential allergy issues before attempting to include AAT in your plan of care. A recent study examined postoperative benefits for children who received AAT. The children in the study who received a 20-minute session with an AAT dog 2 hours after surgery experienced a more rapid recovery and improved pain control (Calcaterra et al., 2015). AAT holds many possibilities for application to different age-groups; therefore research in this area continues to be a popular focus.

More research is needed to further link the benefits of AAT directly to its outcomes. For children, parents may be fearful of this therapy if they are not comfortable with animals, or the child may have fears. There are also some contraindications to AAT such as conditions that could be aggravated by pet dander (e.g., allergies, asthma). AAT is also sometimes contraindicated in patients who are immunocompromised (e.g., patients with human immunodeficiency virus [HIV]/acquired immunodeficiency syndrome [AIDS], patients receiving high-dose steroids, patients receiving chemotherapy or radiation) and patients with methicillin-resistant *Staphyloccocus aureus* owing to the possibility of spreading the infection (Goddard and Gilmer, 2015; Weil, 2017b).

Biofeedback

Biofeedback is a mind-body technique that uses instruments to teach self-regulation and voluntary self-control over specific physiological responses. Electronic or electromechanical instruments measure, process, and provide information to patients about their muscle tension, cardiac activity, respiratory rates, brain-wave patterns, and autonomic nervous system activity. This feedback is given in physical, physiological, auditory, or visual feedback signals that increase a person's awareness of internal processes that are linked to illness and distress. Several biofeedback therapies can change thinking, emotions, and behaviors, which support beneficial physiological changes, resulting in improved health and well-being. For example, patients connected to a biofeedback device sometimes hear a sound if their pulse rate or blood pressure increases out of their therapeutic zone. Practitioners then help patients interpret these sounds and use a variety of breathing, relaxation, and imaging exercises to gain voluntary

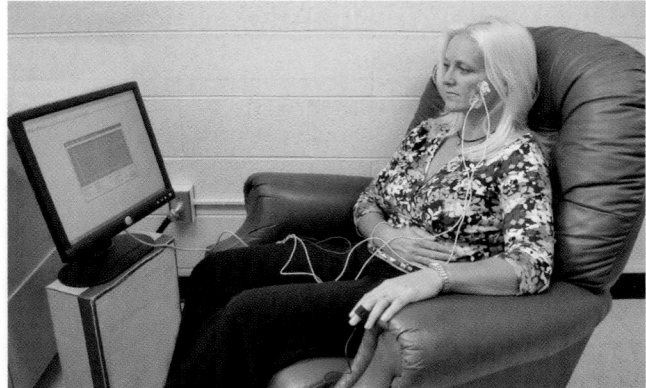

FIG 19.2 A patient using biofeedback can visually see how relaxation affects physiological functions. (From Okeson JP: *Management of temporomandibular disorders and occlusion,* ed 7, St Louis, 2013, Elsevier.)

control over their racing heart or their increasing systolic blood pressure (Lindquist et al., 2014).

Biofeedback is an effective addition to more traditional relaxation programs because it immediately demonstrates to patients their ability to control some physiological responses and the relationship among thoughts, feelings, and physiological responses. It helps individuals focus on and monitor specific body parts by providing immediate feedback about which stress-relaxation behaviors work most effectively. Eventually patients notice positive physiological changes without the need for instrument feedback. One of the most critical components of any behavioral program is adherence to a treatment regimen. Patients who follow their treatment plans have more positive results.

Biofeedback is a noninvasive intervention used in numerous situations (Fig. 19.2). Although biofeedback produces effective outcomes in many patients, there are several precautions to consider. During biofeedback sessions repressed emotions or feelings sometimes surface. For this reason, practitioners who offer biofeedback need to be trained in more traditional psychological methods or have qualified professionals available for referral. In addition, long-term use of biofeedback sometimes lowers blood pressure, heart rates, and other physiological parameters. As with other biobehavioral interventions, monitor patients closely to determine the need for medication adjustments.

Acupuncture

As a key component of TCM, **acupuncture** is one of the oldest practices in the world. When used outside of TCM, it is viewed as a mind-body therapy and is called *medical acupuncture*. In the United States, medical acupuncture is often provided by specially trained health care providers.

Acupuncture regulates or realigns the **vital energy (qi)**, which flows like a river through the body in channels that form a system of 20 pathways called meridians. An obstruction in these channels blocks energy flow in other parts of the body. Acupuncturists insert needles into the skin in specific areas along the channels called acupoints, through which the qi can be influenced and flow reestablished.

Current evidence shows that acupuncture modifies the response of the body to pain and how pain is processed by central neural pathways and cerebral function (NIH/NCCIH, 2016c). Acupuncture has helped control symptoms related to PTSD and to manage tinnitus symptoms in war veterans (Arhin et al., 2016).

Acupuncture is a safe therapy when the practitioner has the appropriate education and training. Therapists should use sterilized needles. Although needle complications occur (e.g., infection, fainting), they are rare if the practitioner takes appropriate precautions. In addition, caution pregnant patients and patients with a history of seizures or immunosuppression about the use of acupuncture. Treatment is contraindicated in people who have bleeding disorders and skin infections.

Therapeutic Touch

Therapeutic touch (TT), developed in the 1970s, is one of the "touch therapies" identified by NCCIH. TT affects the energy fields that surround and penetrate the human body with the conscious intent to help or heal (Dossey and Keegan, 2015). Blending ancient eastern traditions with modern nursing theory, TT uses the energy of the provider to positively influence a patient's energy field.

TT consists of placing a practitioner's open palms either on or close to the body of a person (Fig. 19.3). It occurs in five phases: centering, assessing, unruffling, treating, and evaluating. To begin, the practitioner centers physically and psychologically, becoming fully present in the moment and quieting outside distractions. Then he or she scans the body of the patient with the palms (roughly 5 to 15 cm [2 to 6 inches] from the body) from head to toe. While assessing a patient's energetic biofield, the practitioner focuses on the quality of the qi and areas of energy obstructions, redirecting the energy to harmonize and move. Using long, downward strokes over the energy fields of the body, the practitioner touches the body or maintains the hands in a position a few inches away from the body. The final phase consists of evaluating the patient, ensuring that energy is flowing freely, and determining additional outcomes and responses to the treatment.

Biofield therapies, including TT, were the focus of a recent review to determine their effectiveness for symptom management for palliative and end-of-life care (Henneghan and Schnyer, 2015). Patients at this stage of illness often report difficulty in managing symptoms of pain and stress and need support to maintain quality of life and well-being. TT was found to be cost-effective, did not require special equipment, and could be taught to family caregivers to assist patients in dealing with symptoms (Henneghan and Schnyer, 2015). Although the use of TT causes very few complications or side effects, it is contraindicated in situations when patients are sensitive to human interaction and touch (e.g., patients who have been physically abused or have psychiatric disorders).

Box 19.4 summarizes the importance of touch in older adults.

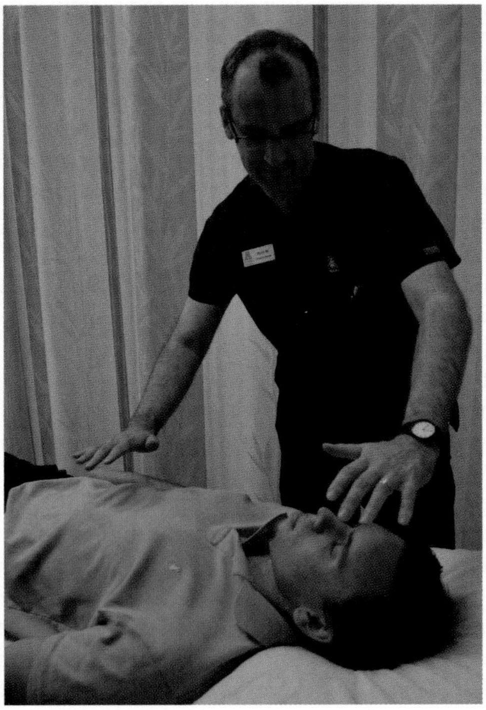

FIG 19.3 During a therapeutic touch session, the practitioner intentionally directs energy to facilitate the patient's healing process.

BOX 19.4 CARE OF THE OLDER ADULT

The Importance of Touch

- Touch is a primal need, as necessary as food, growth, or shelter. It is like a nutrient transmitted through the skin "Skin hunger" is like a form of malnutrition that has reached epidemic proportions in the United States, especially among older adults (Fontaine, 2014).
- Touch enhances self-esteem and a sense of worth.
- Older adults need touch as much as or more than any other age-group. However, older adults often experience "skin hunger."
- Older adults often have fewer family members or friends to touch them, especially when other senses are reduced (Dossey and Keegan, 2015).
- Simple touch helps older adults feel more connected to and accepted by people around them and more in tune with their environment. Touch enhances self-esteem and sense of worth.
  - Nurses who react adversely to skin changes caused by aging often find it difficult to touch older adults. This reluctance communicates a negative message to older adults (Dossey and Keegan, 2015).
  - Be aware of your own reactions to touch when caring for older adults to ensure a therapeutic approach to patient-centered care.

Traditional Chinese Medicine

TCM is a whole system of medicine that began approximately 3600 years ago. Chinese medicine views health as "life in balance," which manifests as lustrous hair, a radiant complexion, engaged interactions, a body that functions without limitations, and emotional balance. Health promotion encourages healthy diet, moderate regular exercise, regular meditation/introspection, healthy family and social relationships, and avoidance of environmental toxins such as cigarette smoke.

Several concepts and principles guide the TCM system of assessment, diagnosis, and intervention. The most important of these is the concept of yin and yang, which represent opposing yet complementary phenomena that exist in a state of dynamic equilibrium. Examples are night and day, hot and cold, and shady and sunny. Yin represents shade, cold, and inhibition, whereas yang represents light, fire, and excitement. Yin also represents the inner part of the body, specifically the viscera, liver, heart, spleen, lung, and kidney, whereas yang represents the outer part, specifically the bowels, stomach, and bladder. Harmony and balance in every aspect of life are the keys to health, including yin and yang balance. Practitioners believe that disease occurs when there is an imbalance in these two paired opposites.

TCM practitioners use four methods to assess and evaluate a patient's condition: observing, hearing and smelling, asking and interviewing, and touching and palpating. In Chinese medicine, outward manifestations reflect the internal environment. For example, the color, shape, and coating of the tongue reflect the general condition of the internal organs. The pulses provide information about the condition and balance of qi, blood, yin and yang, and internal organs. Therapeutic modalities include acupuncture, Chinese herbs, tui na massage, moxibustion (burning moxa, a cone or stick of dried herbs that has healing properties, on or near the skin) cupping (placing a heated cup on the skin to create a slight suction), tai chi (originally a martial art that is now viewed as a moving meditation in which patients move their bodies slowly, gently, and with awareness while breathing deeply), qi gong (originally a martial art, now viewed as a series of carefully choreographed movements or gestures that are designed to promote and manipulate the flow of qi within the body), lifestyle modifications, and dietary changes.

Despite widespread use of TCM in Asia, evidence about its effectiveness is limited. Most research in this field focuses on the study of individual treatment components of TCM such as acupuncture and herbal therapies. However, some evidence shows that TCM is helpful in addressing symptoms associated with menopause (Taylor-Swanson et al., 2014).

There is some concern about the safety of Chinese herbal treatments that are used in teas, remedies, and supplements. The U.S. Food and Drug Administration does not regulate, inspect, or ensure that the ingredients of these herbs are safe and without toxins. Recent reports about these products suggest that many Chinese herbs are contaminated with drugs, toxins, or heavy metals or that many ingredients may not be clearly listed or labeled. Furthermore, these herbs can be very powerful, interact with medications, and cause serious complications. When assessing a patient using TCM, you need to ask the patient about the therapies he or she receives, including the types of herbs that he or she uses. Some patients consider these herbs as teas or dietary additives, powders, or supplements and not as over-the-counter medications. Explain to the patient and family caregiver why informing health care providers about the use of herbal teas and supplements is an important component of their medical history.

Natural Products and Herbal Therapies

Researchers estimate that approximately 25,000 plant species are used medicinally throughout the world. Herbal medicine is the oldest form of medicine known to man. Archeological evidence suggests that people have used herbal remedies for more than 60,000 years. Herbal medicines are a prominent part of health care worldwide.

A natural product is a chemical compound or substance produced by a living organism and includes herbal medicines (also known as botanicals), dietary supplements, vitamins, minerals, mycotherapies (fungi-based products), essential oils (aromatherapy), and probiotics. Many are sold over the counter as dietary supplements. The most frequently used products are garlic, echinacea, saw palmetto, ginkgo biloba, cranberry, soy, ginseng, black cohosh, St. John's wort, glucosamine, peppermint, fish oil/omega 3, soy, and milk thistle. In the United States, St. John's wort is the most popular complementary and alternative therapy for the treatment of depression (Davis et al., 2014).

Herbal medicines are not approved for use as drugs and are not regulated by the Food and Drug Administration. For this reason, many are sold as food or food supplements. The Dietary Supplement Health and Education Act of 1994 allows companies to sell herbs as dietary supplements if their labels do not contain health claims. Natural products in the United States are prepared primarily from plant materials. They are provided as tinctures or extracts, elixirs, syrups, capsules, pills, tablets, lozenges, powders, ointments or creams, drops, and suppositories.

Many herbs are safe and effective for a variety of conditions (Table 19.2). For example, ginger therapy, applied as a warm compress over the kidney region, was recently used to treat a patient with osteoarthritis (Therkleson, 2014). The patient reported the positive effects of a warm feeling throughout his body and increased hip flexibility. However, as noted in Table 19.2, some of these herbs have potential drug interactions. It is important that the patient and family caregiver know about potential drug interactions and always inform the health care provider about the use of herbs and supplements.

A product that is "natural" is not necessarily "safe." Although herbal medicines provide beneficial effects for a variety of conditions, they are not regulated. Thus concentrations of the active ingredients vary considerably. Contamination with other herbs or chemicals, including pesticides and heavy metals, is problematic. Not all companies follow strict quality control and manufacturing guidelines that set

TABLE 19.2 SELECT HERBS AND CORRESPONDING EFFECTS

COMMON NAME AND USES	EFFECTS	POTENTIAL DRUG INTERACTIONS
Aloe Vera		
Skin disorders including inflammation and acute injuries (used topically)	Acceleration of wound healing	Furosemide (Lasix) and loop diuretics
GI ulcerations including Crohn's disease and ulcerative colitis (taken orally)	Unknown mechanism, although there is a known laxative effect	May enhance effects of laxatives when taken orally
Chamomile		
Inflammatory diseases of GI and upper respiratory tracts	Antiinflammatory	Drugs that cause drowsiness (alcohol, barbiturates, benzodiazepines, narcotics, antidepressants)
Generalized anxiety disorder	Calming agent	
Echinacea		
Upper respiratory tract infections	Stimulant of immune system	Antirejection and other drugs that weaken immune system; may interact with antiretrovirals and other drugs used in treatment of HIV/AIDS
Feverfew		
Wound healing	Antiinflammatory	Warfarin (Coumadin) and anticoagulants
Arthritis	Inhibition of serotonin and prostaglandins	Aspirin and ibuprofen
Garlic		
Elevated cholesterol levels	Inhibition of platelet aggregation	Warfarin and anticoagulants
Hypertension		Saquinavir (Fortovase) and other anti-HIV drugs
Ginger		
Nausea and vomiting	Antiemetic	Warfarin and anticoagulants, aspirin and NSAIDs
Gingko Biloba		
Forgetfulness	Memory improvement, although these effects are in question given inconclusive research results	Warfarin and anticoagulants, aspirin and NSAIDs
Ginseng		
Age-related diseases	Increased physical endurance, improved immune function	Warfarin and anticoagulants, aspirin and NSAIDs, and MAO inhibitors
Licorice		
GI disorders including gastric ulcers and hepatitis C	Unknown	Corticosteroids and other immunosuppressive drugs, digoxin, and antihypertensive drugs
Saw Palmetto		
Benign prostatic hyperplasia	Prevention of conversion of testosterone to dihydrotestosterone (needed for prostate cell multiplication)	Finasteride (Propecia) and antiandrogen drugs
Chronic pelvic pain	Unknown mechanism	None known
St. John's Wort (SJW)		
Depression and related psychiatric disorders (Davis et al., 2014). Antiinflammatory and wound-healing properties (Saper, 2015).	A number of compounds isolated from St. John's wort have pharmacological activity (e.g., amino acids, flavonoids); neuropsychiatric activity (hyperforin and related compounds are mostly responsible for effect of St. John's wort on mood) (Saper, 2015).	Oral contraceptives, anticoagulants, benzodiazepines, cancer chemotherapy medications, digoxin, HIV medications, statins, immunosuppressants, SSRIs, and verapamil (Davis et al., 2014)
Valerian		
Sleep disorders, mild anxiety, and restlessness	Central nervous system depression	Barbiturates and other sleep medications, alcohol, and antihistamines

AIDS, Acquired immunodeficiency disease; *GI,* gastrointestinal; *HIV,* human immunodeficiency virus; *MAO,* monoamine oxidase; *NSAID,* nonsteroidal antiinflammatory drug; *SSRI,* selective serotonin reuptake inhibitor.
Data from National Institutes of Health/National Center for Complementary and Integrative Health: *Herbs at a glance,* 2016, https://nccih.nih.gov/health/herbsataglance.htm.

TABLE 19.3   UNSAFE HERBS

COMMON NAME	EFFECTS	COMMENTS
Calamus (Indian type most toxic)	Fever Digestive aid	Contains varying amounts of carcinogenic *cis*-isoasarone Documented cases of kidney damage and seizures with oral preparations
Chaparral	Anticancer Used for bronchitis in traditional healing systems (Native American and Hispanic folk medicine) Found in "natural" weight-loss products	No proven efficacy Induces severe liver toxicity in some cases and severe uterine contractions
Coltsfoot	Antitussive	Contains carcinogenic pyrrolizidine alkaloids Hepatotoxic
Comfrey	Wound healing and acute injuries Used for antiinflammatory effects in osteoarthritis and rheumatoid arthritis	Contains carcinogenic pyrrolizidine alkaloids May induce venoocclusive disease Hepatotoxic
Ephedra (ma huang)	Central nervous system stimulant Bronchodilator Cardiac stimulation Weight loss	Unsafe for people with hypertension, diabetes, or thyroid disease Avoid consumption with caffeine
Life root	Menstrual flow stimulant	Hepatotoxic
Pokeweed	Antirheumatic Anticancer	Do not use with children, but many websites state that it is safe with observation, monitoring, and proper dosing; often used with folk remedies and in Native American healing

Data from National Institutes of Health/National Center for Complementary and Integrative Health: *Herbs at a glance*, 2016, https://nccih.nih.gov/health/herbsataglance.htm; Natural Medicines, *Food, herbs & supplements*, 2017, https://naturalmedicines.therapeuticresearch.com/databases/food,-herbs-supplements.aspx; US Pharmacopeia, 2017, http://www.usp.org/.

standards for acceptable levels of pesticides, residual solvents, bacterial levels, and heavy metals. For this reason, teach patients to purchase herbal medicines only from reputable manufacturers. Labels on herbal products need to contain the scientific name of the botanical, the name and address of the actual manufacturer, a batch or lot number, the date of manufacture, and the expiration date. Using natural products that have been verified by the U.S. Pharmacopeia (USP) is another way to ensure product safety, quality, and purity. Look for the USP Verified Dietary Supplement mark on product labels when buying or recommending natural products.

Some herbs also contain toxic products that have been linked to cancer. Table 19.3 lists several unsafe herbs. Some herbal substances contain powerful chemicals. As with any other medication, examine herbs for interaction and compatibility with other prescribed or over-the-counter substances that are being used simultaneously.

INTEGRATIVE NURSING ROLE

Interest in complementary/integrative therapies continues to increase. Most people using and seeking information about these therapies are well educated and have a strong desire to actively participate in decision making about their health care. This increased interest comes not only from health care consumers but also from health care providers, who have increasing concerns that current conventional medicine is not meeting the needs of their patients. While many health care providers are not referring their patients for complementary therapies because they are not familiar with them or their advantages, other providers are beginning to recognize their benefits.

These complimentary therapies need future testing and research to fully understand the benefits and risks. In North America and Europe professional groups support the use of complementary and alternative therapies and monitor research in this area. Health care providers need to assess the use of complementary therapies, teach the principles of integrative health care across all professional educational programs, teach the public to inform health care providers when using various therapeutics as self-care and health promotion strategies, improve public education about complementary therapies, and support studies that examine the safety and effectiveness of these therapies in a way that ensures improved quality of care.

Complementary therapy providers need to participate in the research process, working with scientists to demonstrate the effectiveness of these therapies on patient outcomes within the more rigorous framework of western science. All providers including nurses need to encourage open, honest dialogue about the use of complementary therapies by patients and better understand the benefits of therapies that encourage active participation by their patients in preventing or managing illness rather than relying solely on surgery or drugs.

Integrative health care, a strategy that is gaining popularity, involves interprofessional group practices in which patients receive care simultaneously from more than one type of practitioner. Patients have the option to choose the type of practitioner that they believe is beneficial for their health problem. Patients with the most to gain are patients who have chronic health problems (e.g., fibromyalgia, chronic fatigue syndrome, chronic pain) that have historically been difficult to treat with traditional biomedical approaches. An interprofessional group practice represents a truly integrated system in which all practitioners work side by side to improve the well-being of their patients.

This integrative approach is patient centered and focuses on the whole person's well-being and health. Nurses are essential participants in this type of health care delivery system because many already practice the use of touch, relaxation techniques, imagery, and breathwork using the principles of integrative nursing (Kreitzer and Koithan, 2014). Familiarize yourself with the evidence in each modality that you use in your practice. Know which patient is most likely to benefit from each therapy, when to use the various therapies, which complications might occur, and which precautions are needed when using these therapies.

In addition, you need enough knowledge to discuss the full range of possible therapeutic options, both biomedical and complementary, so that you can help patients make informed health care decisions. Always ask patients directly about their use of complementary therapies including self-care activities such as yoga, meditation, or dietary supplements. Be knowledgeable about the evidence for different complementary therapies so that you can make appropriate therapy recommendations for patients. Know about the different credentialing processes and how to refer patients to competent providers. Understand thoroughly the potential benefits and risks so that you can clearly and fully disclose information. Be knowledgeable so that you can give advice to patients about when to seek conventional care and when it is safe to consider complementary care services. For example, if a patient complains of right lower abdominal pain, nausea, and vomiting, be suspicious of appendicitis and recommend the patient seek medical care immediately. However, if the patient has a chronic gastrointestinal disorder and has a diagnosis of irritable bowel syndrome, he or she may benefit from relaxation and herbal therapy. Be aware of the safety precautions for each complementary therapy and incorporate them in your teaching plans. Finally understand your state Nurse Practice Act regarding complementary therapies and practice only within the scope of these laws.

Nurses work very closely with their patients and are in the unique position of becoming familiar with a patient's spiritual and cultural viewpoints. They are often able to determine which complementary therapies are more appropriately aligned with these beliefs and offer recommendations accordingly. Being knowledgeable about complementary therapies will help you provide accurate information to patients and other health care professionals.

KEY POINTS

- Integrative health care programs use the full complement of treatment approaches (biomedical and complementary) when providing patient-centered care to patients.
- Complementary therapies such as therapeutic touch require commitment and regular involvement by a patient and family caregiver to be most effective and have prolonged beneficial outcomes.
- Choose complementary therapies appropriately, considering a patient's overall health status, severity of presenting symptoms and distress, beliefs and cultural values, access to health care options, and insurance coverage and/or ability to pay.
- Continuously evaluate a patient's response to complementary therapies because medication doses may need to change based on physiological responses.
- Complementary therapies accessible to nursing include relaxation, meditation and mindfulness techniques, and imagery.
- Many complementary therapies require additional education and certification, including animal-assisted therapy, biofeedback, touch therapies, and acupuncture.
- Although there is increasing evidence to support the use of complementary therapies, additional research of sufficient quality and rigor is needed.

REFLECTIVE LEARNING

- Describe how your thoughts, beliefs, feelings, and attitudes influence your perception and acceptance of complementary, alternative, and integrative therapies. How could your personal opinions influence the care of a patient who uses one or more of these therapies?
- How would you respond if you had a patient who refused to allow an AAT dog into the room?
- Think about the patients you cared for recently; would any of them have benefited from the use of a complementary, alternative, or integrative therapy? If so, which therapy and why?

REVIEW QUESTIONS

1. Which of the following is a contraindication to using animal-assisted therapy with young children?
   1. Asthma
   2. Anxiety
   3. Attention-deficit disorder
   4. Diabetes
2. What is the focus of a nurse who practices in an integrative manner when caring for patients?
   1. Disease, spirit, and family interactions
   2. Desires and emotions of the patient
   3. Mind-body-spirit of the patient and family
   4. A patient's muscle, nerve, and spine disorders

3. A 20-year-old patient tells a nurse she has severe menstrual cramps and has begun to take life root to help alleviate the pain. What is the nurse's best response?
   1. "You should try coltsfoot instead of life root."
   2. "Congratulations on taking control of your life."
   3. "Vomiting may occur when taking life root."
   4. "This herb is unsafe and you should stop taking it immediately."

4. Which cognitive skills can a patient develop while practicing relaxation? (Select all that apply.)
   1. Ability to focus attention for an extended time
   2. Limiting stimuli that come into one's field of vision
   3. Stopping a focus on unnecessary goal-directed activity
   4. Being able to tolerate experiences that are uncertain
   5. Building relationships with significant others

5. Which teaching strategy does a nurse use in creative visualization?
   1. Incorporating yoga poses in practice
   2. Creating a clear image
   3. Having the patient remain quiet
   4. Not picturing the image before bedtime

evolve

Additional Review Questions, as well as rationales for all Review Questions, can be found on the Evolve website.

1. 1; 2. 3; 3. 4; 4. 1, 3, 4; 5. 2.

REFERENCES

American Holistic Nursing Association/ American Nurses Association (AHNA/ANA): *Holistic nursing: scope and standards of practice*, ed 3, Silver Spring, MD, 2015, American Nurses Publishing.

Arhin AO, et al: Acupuncture as a treatment option in treating posttraumatic stress disorder-related tinnitus in war veterans, *J Holist Nurs* 34(1):56, 2016.

Barnes VA, et al: Impact of transcendental meditation on psychotropic medication use among active duty military service members with anxiety and PTSD, *Mil Med* 181(1):56, 2016.

Benson H: *The relaxation response*, New York, 1975, Avon.

Burhenn P, et al: Guided imagery for pain control, *Clin J Oncol Nurs* 18(5):501, 2014.

Calcaterra V, et al: Post-operative benefits of animal-assisted therapy in pediatric surgery: a randomised study, *PLoS ONE* 10(6):e0125813, 2015.

Charette S, et al: Guided imagery for adolescent post-spinal fusion pain management: a pilot study, *Pain Manag Nurs* 16(3):211, 2015.

Davis SA, et al: Use of St. John's wort in potentially dangerous combinations, *J Altern Complement Med* 20(7):578, 2014.

Dobson C: Outcome results of self-efficacy in children with sickle disease pain who were trained to use guided imagery, *Appl Nurs Res* 28(4):384, 2015.

Dossey B, Keegan L: *Holistic nursing: a handbook for practice*, ed 7, Burlington, MA, 2015, Jones & Bartlett.

Fontaine K: *Complementary and alternative therapies for nursing practice, healing practices: alternative therapies for nursing*, ed 4, Upper Saddle River, NJ, 2014, Prentice Hall.

Gawain S: *Creative visualization: use the power of your imagination to create what you want in your life (40th anniversary edition)*, Novato, CA, 2016, New World Library.

Giggins OM, et al: Biofeedback in rehabilitation, *J Neuroeng Rehabil* 10:60, 2013.

Goddard AT, Gilmer MJ: The role and impact of animals with pediatric patients, *Pediatr Nurs* 41(2):65, 2015.

Harvard Health Publications: What meditation can do for your mind, mood, and health, *Harv Womens Health Watch* 2014. http://www.health.harvard.edu/staying-healthy/what-meditation-can-do-for-your-mind-mood-and-health-.

Henneghan AM, Schnyer RN: Biofield therapies for symptom management in palliative and end-of-life care, *Am J Hosp Palliat Care* 32(1):90, 2015.

Kreitzer MJ, Koithan M: *Integrative Nursing*, New York, 2014, Oxford Press.

Kubes LF: Imagery for self-healing and integrative nursing practice, *Am J Nurs* 115(11):36, 2015.

Lindquist R, et al: *Complementary and alternative therapies in nursing*, ed 7, New York, 2014, Springer.

Mayo Clinic: *Types of relaxation techniques*, 2017, http://www.mayoclinic.org/healthy-lifestyle/stress-management/in-depth/relaxation-technique/art-20045368?pg=2.

Nagele E, et al: Clinical effectiveness of stress-reduction techniques in patients with hypertension: systematic review and meta-analysis, *J Hypertens* 32(10):1936, 2014.

National Institutes of Health/National Center for Complementary and Integrative Health (NIH/NCCIH): *Complementary, alternative, or integrative health: what's in a name?* 2016a. https://nccih.nih.gov/health/integrative-health/.

National Institutes of Health/National Center for Complementary and Integrative Health (NIH/NCCIH): *NCCIH facts-at-a-glance and mission*, 2016b. https://nccih.nih.gov/about/ataglance.

National Institutes of Health/National Center for Complementary and Integrative Health (NIH/NCCIH): *Acupuncture: in depth*, 2016c. https://nccih.nih.gov/health/acupuncture/introduction.

Saper R: *Clinical use of St John's wort*, 2015. http://www.uptodate.com/contents/clinical-use-of-st-johns-wort#H5.

Taylor-Swanson L, et al: Effects of traditional Chinese medicine on symptom clusters during the menopausal transition, *Climacteric* 18(2):1, 2014.

Therkleson T: Ginger therapy for osteoarthritis, *J Holist Nurs* 32(3):232, 2014.

Weil A: *The art and science of breathing*, 2017a. https://www.drweil.com/health-wellness/balanced-living/meditation-inspiration/the-art-and-science-of-breathing/.

Weil A: *Animal-assisted therapy*, 2017b. https://www.drweil.com/health-wellness/balanced-living/wellness-therapies/animal-assisted-therapy/.

Wells RE, et al: Meditation for migraines: a pilot randomized controlled trial, *Headache* 54:1484, 2014.

Xu J, et al: *Mortality in the United States, 2015*, 2016. https://www.cdc.gov/nchs/data/databriefs/db267.pdf.

Caring in Nursing Practice

evolve MEDIA RESOURCES

http://evolve.elsevier.com/Potter/essentials
- Audio Glossary
- QSEN Activity and Review Questions Answers and Rationales

OBJECTIVES

- Discuss the role that caring plays in building nurse-patient relationships.
- Describe the commonalities among theories of caring.
- Discuss the evidence about patients' perceptions of caring.
- Explain how caring principles influence nurses' decision making.
- Describe ways to express caring through presence and touch.
- Describe the therapeutic benefit of listening to patients.
- Describe how health care agencies stress the importance of caring practices in achieving patient satisfaction.
- Explain the relationship between knowing a patient and clinical decision making.

KEY TERMS

caring, p. 552   presence, p. 557   transcultural, p. 553

In the case study on the next page, Sue displays caring through her words and actions. Her calm presence, eye contact, touch, and attention to the patient's concerns all convey a relationship-centered, caring approach to meeting a patient's needs (Ray and Turkel, 2014). Nursing, as a humanistic profession, is closely related to the core of caring in both illness and health (Theofanidis and Sapountzi-Krepia, 2015). Caring is central to the foundational values of nursing practice. In today's fast-paced and complex health care environment, financial pressures, technological advances, increasing patient acuity, and fewer resources threaten nurses' opportunities to establish interpersonal connections that are important components of caring practice (Adams, 2016).

Despite these challenges, more professional organizations are emphasizing the importance of nurse caring in health care. The American Nurses Association (ANA) states in *Nursing's Agenda for the Future,* "Nursing is *the* pivotal health care profession highly valued for its specialized knowledge, skill, and *caring* in improving the health status of the public...." (ANA, 2002). The American Organization of Nurse Executives (AONE) (2010) describes caring and knowledge as the core of nursing, with caring being a key component of the nurse's contribution to the patient experience (Fig. 20.1).

Now is the time to value and embrace the caring practices and expert knowledge that are the heart of competent nursing practice (Benner et al., 2010). Caring relationships require sincerity, presence, availability, and engagement (Martin, 2015).

You learn that engaging patients in a caring and compassionate way contributes to their health and well-being. In addition, when you show care as you administer nursing interventions (such as providing personal hygiene, starting an IV line, or changing a patient's dressing), you engage the patient in the care. This enables the patient to state his or her care preferences. As a result, the patient is usually more satisfied with care.

CASE STUDY *Mrs. Levine*

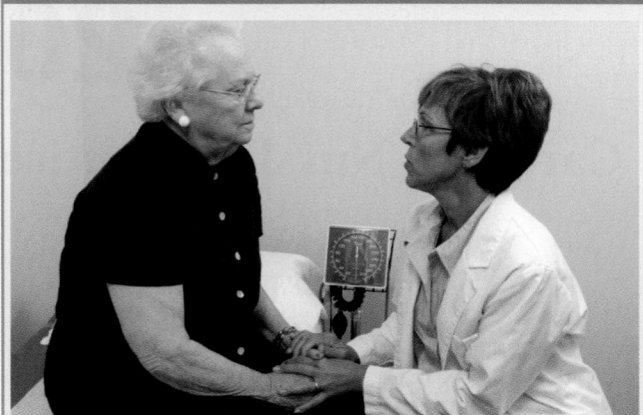

Mrs. Levine is a 76-year-old woman who was diagnosed 6 months ago with lymphoma, a cancer of the lymph tissue. She is experiencing weakness and fatigue. Over the last 4 weeks she lost 8 lb. She was relatively independent before her diagnosis, playing bridge each week with friends and going to lunch with fellow church members. But now she has much less energy to do the things she enjoys. Her son, Jim, lives only a few miles away and is consistently available when she needs transportation to the health care provider, trips to the grocery store, or assistance with other activities. She will begin another round of chemotherapy treatments this week at the oncology clinic.

Sue is an oncology nurse. She enters the examination room where Mrs. Levine is waiting, introduces herself, sits down near Mrs. Levine, and holds her hands. Sue says, "Mrs. Levine, I am here to listen to your story. I want to understand and learn how I can best help you." Sue uses eye contact while talking and leans toward Mrs. Levine to establish a physical presence.

Mrs. Levine nods, smiles, and begins her story. "I've had a good life. I just don't know what's going to happen." Sue replies, "Go on." Mrs. Levine explains, "The doctor tells me the cancer is serious, and I need more chemotherapy. I worry about what's going to happen to me and how it will affect my son, Jim. I don't want to become a burden to him." Sue responds in a calm, soothing tone, "Mrs. Levine, your concerns are very normal. I understand that it is important for you to remain as independent as possible. Let's talk about ways to help you retain your independence."

THEORETICAL VIEWS ON CARING

Caring is a universal phenomenon influencing the ways we think, feel, and behave with one another. Since the time of Florence Nightingale, nurses have studied caring from a variety of philosophical and ethical perspectives. Caring is also very personal. One challenge is to find ways to communicate with patients to learn their cultural behaviors and words that show human caring (Box 20.1) (see Chapter 21).

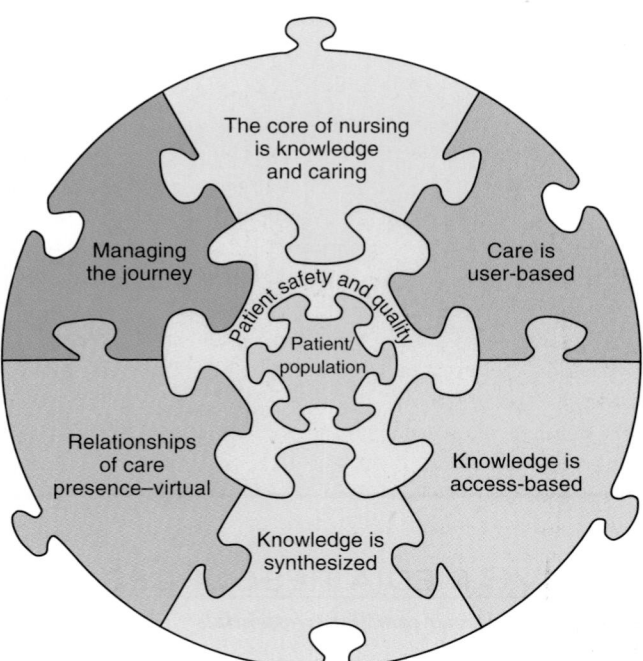

FIG 20.1 AONE guiding principles for the role of the nurse in future patient care delivery. (Copyright 2015 by the American Organization of Nurse Executives (AONE). All rights reserved.)

BOX 20.1 PATIENT-CENTERED CARE

As a nurse, you show caring through communicating and connecting with a patient. Caring includes knowing your patient's cultural values and beliefs; respecting privacy, diversity, and individual needs; and interacting and listening to the patient and his or her family (Darnell and Hickson, 2015). To provide culturally sensitive patient-centered care, you must understand how patients' cultural beliefs and values affect their responses to illness and treatments.

IMPLICATIONS FOR PRACTICE

- Take time to know and clarify patients' values and beliefs regarding health care and caring practices (Zolnierek, 2014; Darnell and Hickson, 2014).
- Determine if a member of a patient's family or cultural group is the best resource to guide caring practices (e.g., presence, use of touch) (Lusk and Fater, 2013).
- Allow patients to share their own perspective of the impact of their illness/trauma (Palos, 2014).
- Know patients' cultural practices regarding end-of-life care. In some cultures it is considered insensitive to tell a patient that he or she is dying (Maroon, 2012).
- Understand how patients choose to communicate their feelings. For example, in some cultures it is considered unwise or even dangerous to express one's opinion.

Some nursing scholars have developed theories of caring. This chapter does not cover all the theories of caring, but it provides theoretical information to help you understand how caring is at the heart of a nurse's ability to work with all patients in a respectful and therapeutic way.

Caring Is Primary

A caring relationship between nurse and patient is dynamic and includes respect for person, love of humanity, and freedom of choice (Watson, 2012). The nurse-patient relationship is a caring process that changes and grows (Martin, 2015). After spending time studying and analyzing the clinical stories of expert nurses, Benner (2010) describes caring as the essence of excellent nursing practice. The stories revealed the many behaviors and decisions that express nurses' caring. Caring means that people, events, projects, and things matter to people. The word *caring* means being connected; that is, "caring creates possibility" (Benner and Wrubel, 1989; Benner, 2010). Caring shows what matters to a person. It describes a range of involvement, from parental love to friendship, from caring about one's work to caring for one's pet to caring for and about one's patients.

Understanding how to provide humanistic caring and compassion begins early in nursing education and continues to mature through experiential practice. Nursing care and caring are crucial in making positive differences in a patient's health and well-being (Palese et al., 2011). *In the case study, Sue's concern for Mrs. Levine provides Sue motivation and direction to better understand the meaning that cancer has for Mrs. Levine and how it affects her life. Sue's concern also helps her identify the best approach to help Mrs. Levine cope with her cancer.*

Patients are not all the same. Each person brings a unique background of experiences, values, and cultural perspectives to a health care encounter. Caring is always specific, and its meaning is unique for each nurse-patient encounter. As nurses acquire more experience, they learn that caring helps them focus on their patients (Porter et al., 2014). Caring improves a nurse's ability to know a patient, recognize the patient's problems, and find and implement individualized solutions.

Because illness is the human experience of loss or dysfunction, any treatment or intervention given without consideration of its meaning to an individual is unlikely to be effective. Expert nurses understand the differences between health, illness, and disease. Through caring relationships nurses listen to patients' stories to understand the meaning of their illness. With this understanding, nurses provide therapeutic, patient-centered care.

When Mrs. Levine first began to feel fatigued 6 months ago, she thought it was just a part of being older. When the fatigue began to threaten her ability to manage her home and care for herself, she sought medical care. By listening to Mrs. Levine's story, Sue begins to understand Mrs. Levine's illness within the context of her life.

Leininger's Transcultural Caring

Leininger (1991) offers a transcultural view of caring. She describes the concept of care as the domain that sets nursing apart from other health care disciplines. Care is an essential human need. Care, in contrast to cure, helps an individual or group improve a human condition. Acts of caring are nurturing and skillful activities, processes, and decisions that help people in empathetic, compassionate, and supportive ways. A caring act depends on the needs, problems, and values of a patient. Leininger's studies found that care protects, develops, nurtures, and provides survival to people. It is universal and vital to recovery from illness and the maintenance of healthy life practices in all cultures.

Watson's Transpersonal Theory of Caring

Caring is a central focus of nursing. It is basic to maintaining the ethical and philosophical roots of the profession (Lusk and Fater, 2013; Porter et al., 2014). Patients and their family members expect high-quality human interaction from nurses. Unfortunately, many conversations between patients and their nurses are very brief and shallow. Workload demands and lack of personnel limit opportunities to develop a close relationship with a patient (Flagg, 2015).

Watson's transpersonal theory of caring (2010, 2012) is a holistic model that describes a conscious recognition that caring for a person involves sensitivity, respect, and a high moral and ethical commitment. The emphasis is on the nurse-patient relationship. How a nurse chooses to be with a patient and family in any given moment influences the caring-healing relationship. Watson identified 10 carative factors that serve as tools for establishing the nurse-patient caring relationship (Table 20.1).

Watson's theory integrates human caring processes with healing environments. The theory incorporates the life-generating and life-receiving processes of caring with the healing process of nurses and their patients (Watson Caring Science Institute [WCSI], 2017). The transpersonal caring theory rejects the disease orientation of health care and places care before cure (Watson, 2010). Transpersonal caring seeks deeper sources of inner healing to protect, improve, and preserve a person's dignity and harmony.

Caring becomes almost spiritual because it preserves human dignity in a cure-dominated health care system (Watson, 2009). Nurses connect with patients at a deep spiritual level, sometimes for only a moment, and that connectedness allows both a nurse and a patient to collaborate on a patient's health care needs and expectations. The theory emphasizes the care of the whole patient rather than treatment of the pathological condition.

Watson's theory supports a holistic approach that enables a caring nurse to gain a unique level of understanding about a patient. Consider the example of a nurse who is performing a nursing assessment. When applying the transpersonal theory of caring, the nurse accurately assesses a patient's physical needs along with the patient's preferences, social environment, and emotional needs.

For example, Sue wants to assess Mrs. Levine's nutritional status to ensure that she takes a holistic approach to her patient's nutritional needs. Her assessment goes beyond what Mrs. Levine eats, her weight, and her sense of an appetite. To gain a deeper understanding of Mrs. Levine's nutritional status Sue also considers her food preferences, availability of food, social environment, and emotional attachment to food. A nurse who applies

TABLE 20.1 WATSON'S 10 CARATIVE FACTORS

CARATIVE FACTOR	EXAMPLE IN PRACTICE
Forming a human-altruistic value system	Use loving kindness to extend yourself. Use self-disclosure appropriately to promote a therapeutic alliance with your patient.
Instilling faith-hope	Provide a connection with the patient that offers purpose and direction when trying to find the meaning of an illness.
Cultivating a sensitivity to one's self and others	Learn to accept yourself and others for their full potential. A caring nurse matures into becoming a self-actualized nurse.
Developing a helping-trusting, human, caring relationship	Learn to develop and sustain helping-trusting, authentic caring relationships through effective communication with your patients.
Promoting and accepting the expression of positive and negative feelings	Support and accept your patients' feelings. In connecting with your patients, show a willingness to take risks in what you share with one another.
Using creative problem-solving, caring processes	Apply the nursing process in a systematic way to provide patient-centered care.
Promoting transpersonal teaching-learning	Learn together while educating the patient to acquire self-care skills. The patient assumes responsibility for learning.
Providing for a supportive, protective, and/or corrective mental, physical, societal, and spiritual environment	Create a healing environment at all levels, physical and nonphysical. This promotes wholeness, beauty, comfort, dignity, and peace.
Meeting human needs	Assist patients with basic needs with an intentional care and caring consciousness.
Allowing for existential-phenomenological-spiritual forces	Allow spiritual forces to provide a better understanding of yourself and your patient.

Data from Watson J: *The philosophy and science of caring*, Boulder, CO, 2008, University Press of Colorado.

TABLE 20.2 SWANSON'S THEORY OF CARING

CARING PROCESS	DEFINITIONS	SUBDIMENSIONS
Knowing	Striving to understand an event as it has meaning in the life of the other	Avoiding assumptions Centering on the one cared for Assessing thoroughly Seeking cues Engaging the self or both
Being with	Being emotionally present to the other	Being there Conveying ability Sharing feelings Not burdening
Doing for	Doing for the other as he or she would do for self if it were at all possible	Comforting Anticipating Performing skillfully Protecting Preserving dignity
Enabling	Facilitating the other's passage through life transitions (e.g., birth, death) and unfamiliar events	Informing/explaining Supporting/allowing Focusing Generating alternatives Validating/giving feedback
Maintaining belief	Sustaining faith in the other's capacity to get through an event or transition and face a future with meaning	Believing in/holding in esteem Maintaining a hope-filled attitude Offering realistic optimism "Going the distance"

Data from Swanson KM: Empirical development of a middle-range theory of caring, *Nurs Res* 40(3):161, 1991.

Watson's theory during an assessment collects accurate data to plan care in a way that goes beyond the physical aspect of a patient's disease.

Swanson's Theory of Caring

Swanson's studies of patients and professional caregivers (1991) led to the development of a theory of caring for nursing practice. Three perinatal studies involved interviews with women who miscarried, parents and health professionals in a newborn intensive care unit, and socially at-risk mothers who received long-term public health intervention (Swanson, 1991). The researchers asked each group questions about how they experienced or expressed caring in their situation. After analyzing the stories, Swanson developed a theory of caring that consists of five categories or processes (Table 20.2). She defines caring as a nurturing way of relating to a valued other, toward whom one feels a personal sense of commitment and responsibility (Swanson, 1991). The theory supports caring as a central nursing phenomenon that is useful and effective for multiple age-group and health care settings. Teaching students and new nurses how to use Swanson's five caring processes helps new nurses gain confidence when providing patient-centered care (Moffa, 2015).

An example of caring is the way Sue administers chemotherapy. Knowing that the medications are toxic and can cause adverse reactions, Sue first gathers necessary equipment in case of a reaction. Then she begins the administration slowly as ordered, and she explains to Mrs. Levine the reasons for each step of the administration.

Summary of Theoretical Views

There are common themes among the theoretical view of caring. Porter et al. (2014) support earlier findings and identify these commonalities as human interaction or communication, mutuality, appreciating the uniqueness of individuals, and improving the welfare of patients and families. Caring is relational, and in a health care setting, a nurse and patient enter into a relationship that is much more than one person simply doing tasks for another. In a caring relationship, a mutual give-and-take develops as nurse and patient begin to know and care for one another (Martin, 2015; Turpin, 2014).

Caring seems invisible at times when a nurse and patient enter a relationship of respect, concern, and support. A nurse's empathy and compassion become a natural part of each patient encounter. However, when caring is absent, it becomes very obvious. For example, if a nurse is disinterested or avoids a patient's request for help, the nurse's inaction quickly conveys an uncaring attitude. Patients and family caregivers are perceptive, and they can recognize nurses' behaviors that demonstrate an uncaring approach (Adams, 2016).

As you practice caring, your patients will sense your commitment and willingness to enter into a relationship. This will help you understand their illness experience and the impact of the illness on the family caregiver (Porter et al., 2014). Patients particularly sense caring when nurses are accessible and compassionate. As a nurse-patient relationship forms, a nurse becomes a coach and partner rather than a detached provider of care (Porter et al., 2014; Adams, 2016).

Sue works with Mrs. Levine to help her remain independent. By considering Mrs. Levine's relationship with her son as well as the effects of her cancer and treatment, Sue's caring behavior becomes enabling. When the nurse practices enabling, the patient and nurse work together to identify alternatives and resources. For example, Sue helps Mrs. Levine to organize her day so that she can take frequent rest periods and still complete her daily tasks. Sue also explains the effects of cancer and chemotherapy and helps Mrs. Levine identify ways to perform self-care activities. By understanding Mrs. Levine's unique needs, Sue increases Mrs. Levine's sense of well-being.

PATIENT SATISFACTION

Caring is a moral imperative, not a commodity to be bought and sold. Caring for other human beings protects, enhances, and preserves human dignity. It is a professional, ethical covenant that nursing has with its patients (Watson, 2010).

BOX 20.2   EVIDENCE-BASED PRACTICE

PICO Question: Do patient satisfaction rates among hospitalized adults improve when carative nursing practices are used?

SUMMARY OF EVIDENCE

Researchers identify a strong, positive relationship between nurse caring behaviors and patient satisfaction. Patients feel their care is more individualized and report higher satisfaction when nurses listen to their stories and concerns (Brewer and Watson, 2015). Evidence shows that patient satisfaction is more likely to improve if nurses adapt their work to accommodate patients' specific requests or communicate the reasons why these requests cannot be met immediately (Lusk and Fater, 2013; Duffy et al., 2014). Promotion of caring, compassionate, supportive, and therapeutic environments for patients not only increases patient satisfaction but also increases job satisfaction of nurses (Kramer et al., 2014). Caring nursing practices also improve functional status, self-efficacy, coping, and self-care of patients (Arslan-Ozkan et al., 2013). Finally, patient-centered care models emphasize that caring interventions are an influential dimension of patient advocacy and are predictive of patient satisfaction (Porter et al., 2014).

APPLICATION TO NURSING PRACTICE

- Respond promptly to a patient request, either personally or by directing unlicensed nursing assistive personnel (NAP) to respond (Duffy et al., 2014).
- Speedy response of staff to requests, the condition of the hospital environment, and patient perception of nurses' intent to provide pain control strongly predict patient satisfaction (Kahn et al., 2015).
- Advocate for your patient (e.g., initiating a change in pain-control measures or changing the timing of physical therapy) (Porter et al., 2014).
- Use principles of presence, "being with" and "being there," to dedicate time to interact one-on-one with your patient or just to sit quietly with your patient (Yagasaki and Komatsu, 2011).
- Use knowing to connect with your patient, discuss all aspects of care, and learn the patient's personal preferences. Explain how you will include or adapt personal preferences to your patient (Zolnierek, 2014).

Evidence shows a connection between patient satisfaction and nurse caring (Box 20.2). When the nurses within a health care agency successfully demonstrate caring, nursing care improves, and more patients are satisfied and more likely to return when they need further care. Nurses also benefit when they integrate caring processes into their nursing actions. Nurses not only improve patient satisfaction, but they also improve their own job performance and satisfaction. This helps to reduce nurse turnover rates (Martin, 2015). When patients sense that their health care providers are sensitive, sympathetic, compassionate, and interested in them as people, they usually become active partners in the plan of care (Palese et al., 2011; Papastavrou et al., 2011).

More institutions are adopting patient-centered care models that incorporate relationship-centered caring approaches. An organization must measure caring from a patient's point of view to document the value of nursing. Duffy et al. (2007, 2014) developed and refined the Caring Assessment Tool (CAT) to assess quality of nurse-patient relationships, assess effectiveness of professional practice models, and provide support for professional advancement. The CAT measures caring from the patient perspective, rating nurses' attitudes, skills, and behaviors. As a beginning nurse, you can use this tool to help you identify and appreciate the types of behaviors that hospitalized patients identify as caring. The CAT includes eight major factors, with three to six items that describe nursing behaviors for each factor (Box 20.3).

Mutual Problem Solving

A caring nurse helps patients understand their health and illness and form questions to ask their health care providers. In addition, a caring nurse helps patients explore different ways to resolve their health problems (Duffy et al., 2007, 2014). Using evidence in practice is an aspect of mutual problem solving, with nurses continuously learning about their patients and engaging patients and families in discussions about their health issues (Winsett and Hauck, 2011).

Attentive Reassurance

Patients perceive nurses to be caring when they are accessible and show interest in their well-being. Nurses who look toward a better future and confidently express optimism and new realistic possibilities often give patients hope (Duffy et al., 2007; Palese et al., 2011). Attentive reassurance is consistent with Watson's faith-hope, sensitivity, and helping-trust relationship factors. Attentive reassurance is also consistent with Swanson's principle of maintaining belief.

Human Respect

Respect for patients is integral to care. Human respect in nursing means appreciating the value of human beings. Respect also means that nurses display behaviors that value the patient such as accepting or paying attention to a patient's fears and concerns (Duffy et al., 2007, 2014). A nurse who shows respect is honoring the worth of individuals (Watson, 2010).

Encouraging Manner

Patients face very difficult situations involving anxiety and fear of an unknown future, family role changes, and many diagnostic tests and physical ailments when they are hospitalized. Patients perceive nurses as caring when nurses behave professionally such as by staying calm, anticipating patient needs, and helping patients to see positive aspects in their situation (Duffy et al., 2007, 2014). Encouraging a patient also helps the patient handle negative feelings.

Appreciation of Unique Meanings

In Swanson's theory of caring (1991), nurses attempt to know patients by understanding the patients' experiences. Duffy

---

BOX 20.3   FACTORS AND ITEMS CONSTITUTING THE CARING ASSESSMENT TOOL (CAT)

Each item begins with the stem: "Since I have been a patient here, the nurses…"

MUTUAL PROBLEM SOLVING
- Help me understand how I am thinking.
- Ask me how I think treatment is going.
- Help me explore alternative ways of dealing.
- Ask me what I know.
- Help me figure out questions to ask.

ATTENTIVE REASSURANCE
- Are available.
- Seem interested.
- Support a sense of hope.
- Help me believe in myself.
- Anticipate my needs.

HUMAN RESPECT
- Listen to me.
- Accept me.
- Treat me kindly.
- Respect me.
- Pay attention to me.

ENCOURAGING MANNER
- Support my beliefs.
- Encourage me to ask questions.
- Help me to see some good.
- Encourage me to go on.
- Help me deal with bad feelings.

APPRECIATION OF UNIQUE MEANINGS
- Are concerned with how I view things.
- Know what is important to me.
- Acknowledge my inner feelings.
- Show respect for things having meaning to me.

HEALING ENVIRONMENT
- Check up on me.
- Pay attention to me when I am talking.
- Make me feel comfortable.
- Respect my privacy.
- Treat my body carefully.

AFFILIATION NEEDS
- Are responsive to my family.
- Talk openly with my family.
- Allow my family to be involved.

BASIC HUMAN NEEDS
- Make sure I get food.
- Help me with routine needs for sleep.
- Help me feel less worried.

Modified from Duffy JR, et al: Dimensions of caring: psychometric evaluation of the Caring Assessment Tool, *Adv Nurs Sci* 30(3):235, 2007.

---

et al. (2007, 2014) reported that patients who are hospitalized can perceive if nurses value the priorities of the patients and their families. This is especially important, as nurses care for patients from many cultures (see Chapter 21). This aspect of caring is challenging because a nurse needs time to develop a relationship with a patient that enables the nurse to appreciate the patient's feelings (Winsett and Hauck, 2011).

Healing Environment

Florence Nightingale was the first nurse to understand how improving the patient's environment (e.g., providing nutrition, hygiene, and comfort) promotes healing. In a healing environment nurses check patients frequently, respect patient privacy, reduce noise, treat patients carefully, and provide comfort. Such an environment gives patients the sense of security and protection from harm (Duffy et al., 2014).

Affiliation Needs

Including family members in a patient's care is basic nursing practice. Involving family caregivers is a key element in discharge planning (see Chapter 3). Patients who are hospitalized perceive nurses who are responsive to family caregivers and allow them to be involved in the patient's care as caring (Duffy et al., 2007, 2014). Thus actively engage families in conversation and explain (when appropriate) the care that a patient is receiving. Family caregivers help determine how a patient will manage health care needs in the home. A caring nurse engages the family in such decisions.

Basic Human Needs

All humans have basic needs (Maslow, 1987). Unfortunately, these needs are not readily met when nurses focus on managing technological demands and complex therapies. Often RNs delegate basic care to unlicensed nursing assistive personnel (NAP) (see Chapter 13). However, patients perceive nurses as caring when they take patients' basic needs into account and treat their body carefully (Duffy et al., 2007, 2014).

CARING IN NURSING PRACTICE

As you begin clinical practice, consider how patients perceive you; are you able to display caring? Find the best way to individualize your patient's care. Always focus on building a patient-centered relationship that directs you to learn a patient's priorities. For those who find caring a normal part of their life, it is a product of their culture, values, experiences, and relationships with others. People who do not experience care in their lives often find it difficult to act in caring ways. As you deal with health and illness in your practice, you grow in your ability to care and develop caring behaviors. When you use a caring approach with each patient encounter you develop a caring presence in your professional practice.

Providing Presence

In providing **presence** you develop a person-to-person relationship that conveys a closeness and sense of caring. In today's high-tech and fast-paced health care environments, nursing presence is essential. Presence establishes the nurse-patient relationship and is linked to positive patient outcomes (Yagasaki and Komatsu, 2013; Turpin, 2014).

Nursing presence occurs when a nurse and a patient are mutually open to one another, and the nurse acts toward the patient in such a way to meet the patient's needs (Turpin, 2014). Presence involves "being there" and "being with." "Being there" is more than a physical presence; it also includes

communication and understanding. Nursing presence makes time for the patient and family caregiver. In the interpersonal relationship of being there the nurse is attentive and receptive to a patient (Penque and Kearney, 2015).

For example, Sue decides that it is important to be with Mrs. Levine during her chemotherapy treatment. Sue tells her patient, "You know, I want to be the one who gives you this chemotherapy treatment. I know it's an anxious moment for you." Sue sits down next to Mrs. Levine and carefully prepares the infusion supplies while continuing their conversation. When Sue sees Mrs. Levine's son at the doorway, she invites him in to sit with his mother.

Nursing requires being present with patients at a moment of crisis or need. Eye contact, body language, expressions, listening, and a positive and encouraging manner act together to create openness and understanding (Fig. 20.2). Presence conveys a message that the other's experience matters to the one caring (Swanson, 1991). Establishing presence strengthens your ability to provide effective patient-centered care. Presence is also valuable during patient- and family-centered rounds, during which nurses offer their presence to help patients achieve positive outcomes, reduce the intensity of unwanted feelings, promote reassurance, and guide family caregivers (Yagasaki and Komatsu, 2013; Sharma et al., 2014). As a result patients often are more satisfied with the nursing care and the health care system in general (Penque and Kearney, 2015).

"Being with" is also interpersonal. A nurse is purposefully attentive to a patient and family caregiver when present (Fahlberg and Roush, 2016). A nurse gives himself or herself, which means being available and open to a patient. Patients who accept their nurse invite the nurse to see, share, and touch their vulnerability and suffering. Through presence a nurse enters a patient's world. A patient is able to put words to feelings and understand himself or herself in a way that leads to identifying solutions, seeing new directions, and making choices.

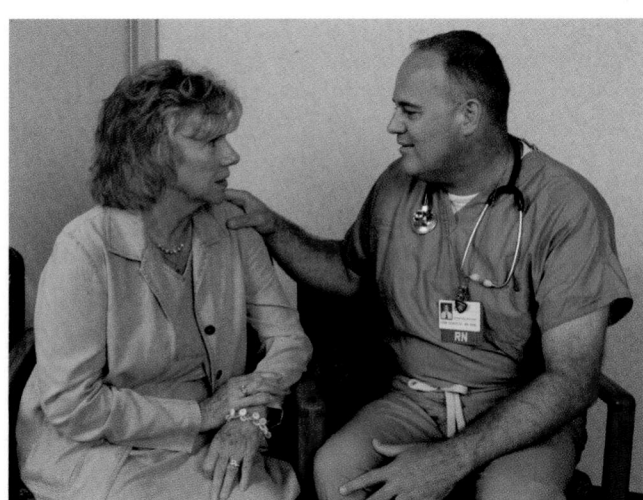

FIG 20.2 A nurse conveying presence to a patient.

Nursing presence reduces anxiety and fear when patients are experiencing stressful events or situations. Awaiting a doctor's report of test results, preparing for an unfamiliar procedure, and planning for a return home after serious illness are just a few examples of stressful situations that create unpredictability. Reassuring a patient, explaining a procedure, remaining at the patient's side, and coaching the patient through the experience convey a presence that promotes the patient's well-being.

Touch

Patients face embarrassing, frightening, and painful situations. Whatever the feeling or symptom, patients look to nurses for comfort. Nurses use appropriate touch to comfort and communicate concern and support (Love and Femia, 2014). You must remember, however, that the simple gesture of touching a patient on the arm either can be consoling and sympathetic or can be invasive and offensive depending on the patient's culture (Winsett and Hauck, 2011).

Touch is relational and often leads to a connection between nurse and patient. Touch is task-oriented, caring, and protective. Nurses use task-oriented touch when performing a task or procedure. The skillful and gentle performance of a nursing procedure conveys security and competence. When you use gentle touch as an intervention in combination with a specific nursing skill such as inserting a nasogastric tube, you convey to a patient that you will perform the procedure safely, skillfully, and successfully. You demonstrate this by the gentle way you position the patient and gently manipulate and insert the nasogastric tube. Talk quietly with a patient throughout a procedure to provide reassurance and support.

Expert nurses learn that any procedure is more effective when they administer it carefully and in consideration of any patient concern. For example, therapeutic touch is effective in controlling pain in some patients with cancer. The use of touch helps a patient relax and focus on relaxation response (Kiefer, 2016). Caring touch is a form of nonverbal communication. Caring touch influences a patient's comfort and security, enhances self-esteem, increases confidence of caregivers, and improves mental well-being (Love and Femia, 2014). You perform caring touch in the way you hold a patient's hand, give a back massage, gently position a patient, or participate in a conversation. When you use caring touch, you connect with the patient and show acceptance of the individual.

Protective touch is a form of touch that protects a nurse and/or a patient. A patient views it either positively or negatively. The most obvious form of protective touch is preventing an accident (e.g., holding and bracing a patient to avoid a fall). Protective touch also protects the nurse emotionally. For example, the nurse may withdraw from a patient when he or she is unable to tolerate suffering or needs to escape from a situation that is causing tension. When protective touch is used in this way, it elicits negative feelings in a patient.

Because touch can convey many messages, use it with discretion. Touch can be a concern when it crosses the cultural boundaries of the patient or nurse (Benner et al., 2010). Most patients allow task-oriented touch because they give nurses and physicians an unwritten license to enter their personal space to provide care. Know and understand whether patients accept touch and how they interpret your intentions before providing hands-on care.

Listening

Caring is an interpersonal interaction that is much more than two people simply talking back and forth (Watson, 2012; Martin, 2015). In a caring relationship a nurse establishes trust, opens lines of communication, and listens to what a patient has to say. Listening is critical because it shows that the patient has the nurse's full attention and interest. Listening includes hearing what a patient says, interpreting it, understanding it, and reflecting that understanding back to the patient (Porter et al., 2014). Listening to the meaning in a patient's words creates mutual communication. Listening to a patient enables the nurse to know and respond to the real priorities of a patient and family.

People usually have a story to tell about the meaning of their illness when they become ill. Any critical or chronic illness affects all the life choices and decisions of a patient, and sometimes even his or her identity. Telling that story helps a patient break the distress of illness. A story needs a listener. In the following example a patient described his own feelings during his experience with cancer: "I needed a [health care professional's] gift of listening in order to make my suffering a relationship between *us,* instead of an iron cage around *me.*" The patient needed to be able to express what he needed when he was ill (Frank, 1998). The personal concerns that are part of a patient's illness story determine what is at stake for a patient. Caring through listening enables you to participate in a patient's life.

Through active listening you begin to know your patients and what is important to them. Learning to listen to a patient can be difficult. You can easily become distracted by tasks at hand, colleagues interrupting, or other patients waiting to have their own needs met. However, the time you take to listen effectively is worthwhile both in the information gained and the strengthening of the nurse-patient relationship. Listening enables you to help patients find meaning, release fears, and answer their own questions.

Knowing the Patient

One of the five caring processes described by Swanson (1991) is knowing the patient. Knowing the patient is a complex process that occurs within the context of the nurse-patient relationship (Zolnierek, 2014). It is an essential element of nursing practice and is linked to patient satisfaction (Kelley et al., 2013). Knowing develops over time. Knowing helps you respond to what really matters to a patient. To know a patient means that you avoid assumptions, focus on the patient, and engage in a caring relationship that reveals information and cues that facilitate critical thinking and clinical judgments (see Chapter 8).

Knowing the patient is at the core of clinical decision making. Through caring you develop an understanding that helps you to better know the patient as a unique individual and choose the most appropriate and effective nursing therapies (Potter and Savette, 2014). Knowing the patient helps you understand how the uncertainties related to illness, treatment, or rehabilitation affect the patient and family caregiver (Tyreman, 2015).

The caring relationships that a nurse develops over time, as well as the nurse's growing knowledge and experience with multiple patients, create a rich source of meaning that allows a nurse to recognize changes in a patient's clinical status (Nielsen et al., 2015). Expert nurses are able to detect changes in patients' conditions almost effortlessly.

Clinical decision making uses several aspects of knowing the patient, including responses to therapies, routines and habits, coping resources, physical capacities and endurance, and body typology and characteristics. The experienced nurse knows additional facts about his or her patients such as their experiences, behaviors, feelings, and perceptions. When you make clinical decisions based on your knowledge of a patient, the patient's outcomes improve. The following can help you develop your skill in knowing patients:

- Routinely make patient rounds at the beginning of a work shift and continuously as appropriate.
- Do not depend on another's observations. Be thorough and make your own assessment.
- Go back and evaluate the patient's response to your interventions.
- Reflect on what you have learned with each patient encounter.

Success in knowing a patient depends on the relationship that you form together. To know a patient is to enter into a caring, social process, which results in a nurse-patient relationship; the patient comes to feel known by the nurse (Zolnierek, 2014). When patient care is fragmented, patient-centered care is compromised (Lusk and Fater, 2013; Zolnierek, 2014).

Spiritual Caring

Spiritual caring is about fostering connections with patients by promoting spiritual comfort and well-being (see Chapter 22). Research shows a link between mind, body, and spirit. An individual's beliefs and expectations affect the person's physical well-being.

Establishing a caring relationship means a nurse and patient become interconnected. This interconnectedness is why Watson (2010, 2012) describes the caring relationship in a spiritual sense. Spirituality offers intrapersonal (connected with oneself), interpersonal (connected with others and the environment), and transpersonal (connected with the unseen, God, or a higher power) connectedness. In a caring relationship the patient and the nurse come to know one another, and both move toward a healing relationship by doing the following (WCSI, 2017; Watson and Brewer, 2015):

- Mobilizing hope for the patient and the nurse
- Finding an understanding of illness, symptoms, or emotions that is acceptable to the patient
- Assisting the patient in using social, emotional, or spiritual resources

QSEN QSEN ACTIVITY *Patient-Centered Care*

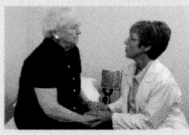

Mrs. Levine and her son Jim want to "look down the road" as her treatments continue and her disease progresses. They ask Sue to help guide them in this journey. Mrs. Levine is happy with her life and wants to remain independent. When Mrs. Levine and her son talked, they identified symptom management issues of pain control, fatigue management, nausea, and poor nutritional intake. Jim clearly states his desire to help his mother through her illness and end-of-life care. He told her that being with her and helping her is just as important to him as her desire to maintain her independence. Jim wants to care for his mom but not make her an invalid.

They want Sue to give them strategies that they can use to care for one another. Mrs. Levine tells her son that, as his mother, she worries and cares for him and wants to help him through this process.

- What caring strategies can Sue teach each of them as Mrs. Levine transitions back to her home?

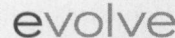 Answers to QSEN Activities can be found on the Evolve website.

- Recognizing that caring relationships connect us human to human

Relieving Symptoms and Suffering

Relieving symptoms such as pain and nausea is more than giving pain medications, repositioning a patient, or cleaning a wound. The relief of symptoms and suffering includes implementing caring nursing actions that give a patient comfort, dignity, respect, and peace (Michael et al., 2014). By ensuring that a patient care environment is clean, reasonably quiet, and pleasant and includes personal items, you make the physical environment a place that soothes and heals the mind, body, and spirit (Fahlberg and Roush, 2016).

Skillful and accurate assessment helps you identify the level, type, and frequency of a patient's pain or other symptoms and their impact on the patient's lifestyle (see Chapter 34). This accurate assessment allows you to design a patient-centered plan of care to provide symptom relief. The skills previously discussed of presence, touching, listening, and knowing your patient help you and your patient build a relationship so you can develop goals for symptom relief.

Human suffering is multifaceted and affects patients physically, emotionally, socially, and spiritually. In addition, suffering affects a patient's family and friends. Their emotional suffering can include anger, guilt, fear, or grief. Although you cannot fix their suffering, you can provide comfort by being a listening, nonjudgmental caring presence. Patients and their families feel comforted by a caring listener.

Mrs. Levine has multiple pain-control challenges. In addition, she is trying to maintain independence as long as her illness allows. Her son wants to help but also respects his mother's needs and concerns. Both Mrs. Levine and her son experience emotional suffering.

BOX 20.4   NURSE CARING BEHAVIORS AS PERCEIVED BY FAMILIES

- Being honest
- Advocating for patient's care preferences
- Giving clear explanations
- Keeping family members informed
- Asking permission before doing something to a patient
- Providing comfort: offering a warm blanket, finding food a patient can swallow, rubbing a patient's back
- Reading to patient passages from religious texts, a favorite book, cards, or mail
- Providing for and maintaining patient privacy
- Assuring the patient that nursing services will be available
- Helping patient to do as much for self as possible
- Teaching the family caregiver how to keep the patient physically comfortable

---

Family Care

Everyone experiences life through their relationships with others. You must include the patient's family and friends when appropriate in your delivery of patient-centered care. The family is an important resource (see Chapter 25). Your success with nursing interventions often depends on the family's willingness to share information about the patient, their acceptance and understanding of therapies, whether the interventions fit with the family's daily practices and values, and whether the family is willing to provide the therapies recommended and assume a family caregiving role. It is critically important to know who the primary family caregiver is. In some cases it may be more than one individual. Ensuring a patient's well-being and being able to be active participants in care are critical for some family members.

Sue spends time with Mrs. Levine's son discussing how he can help his mother manage the side effects of her chemotherapy. Sue prepares him to deal with the nausea or loss of appetite that his mother may experience.

The behaviors listed in Box 20.4 offer useful guidelines for developing a caring relationship with all families. Begin a relationship by learning who makes up a patient's family and what their roles are in the patient's life. Showing the family care and concern for the patient creates an openness that then enables you to form a relationship with them. Caring for the family considers the context of the patient's illness and the stress it imposes on all members (see Chapter 25).

THE CHALLENGE OF CARING

Many students enter nursing to help patients during their time of need. When nurses commit themselves to be caring individuals, they achieve a meaning and purpose in their lives (Benner et al., 2010). The concept of caring motivates people to become nurses. Nurses gain a sense of satisfaction when they know they have made a difference in their patients' lives.

Today's health care system presents many challenges to providing a patient-centered plan of care (Porter et al., 2014).

Nurses are torn between the human caring model and the task-oriented biomedical model and institutional demands that consume their time (Winsett and Hauck, 2011; Adams, 2016). Nurses have less time to spend with patients, making it much harder to know who they are. Our reliance on technology and cost-effective health care strategies and efforts to standardize and refine work processes all undermine the nature of caring. Too often patients become just a number, with their real needs either overlooked or ignored. In addition, nurses, especially nurses practicing in inpatient settings, deal with multiple stressors (e.g., interdepartmental, technology, paperwork stressors, high patient acuity rates, and multiple patient care interruptions). As a result nurses are at risk for compassion fatigue and burnout (Mason, 2014; Hunsaker et al., 2015).

The Robert Wood Johnson Foundation (RWJF) "Future of Nursing: Campaign for Action" is identifying methods to improve both patient care and satisfaction and nurse job satisfaction. This campaign focuses on increasing the amount of time nurses actually spend with their patients and families. This initiative also includes environmental factors so that care environments are designed to facilitate care activities, offers a way for staff to discuss problems and concerns about being able to provide care, and has adequate resources (RWJF, 2014). To create environments conducive to caring, health care organizations must introduce greater flexibility into the work environment structure, reward experienced nurse mentors, offer programs for compassion fatigue, improve nurse staffing, and provide nurses with autonomy over their practice.

If health care is to make a positive difference, it must become more compassionate. Nurses play an important role in making care an integral part of health care delivery. This begins when institutions make caring a part of the philosophy and environment of the workplace and incorporate care concepts into standards of nursing care and guidelines for professional conduct.

■ KEY POINTS

- Human caring is the essence of clinical nursing practice; it is a foundational component of the nurse-patient relationship.
- The theories of caring have common themes including the ideas that caring is highly relational, involves communication and mutual respect, has an appreciation for the uniqueness of individuals, and improves the welfare of patients and families.
- Caring theories note that human caring is universal and that the expressions, processes, and patterns of caring vary among cultures.
- When nurses within an organization successfully demonstrate caring, positive patient outcomes occur, and patient satisfaction improves.
- Understanding the behaviors that patients associate with caring allows you to establish caring practices.

- Caring nursing practices help patients explore options for resolving health problems and setting priorities of care.
- A nurse conveys openness and understanding to a patient when the nurse establishes presence, maintains eye contact, uses appropriate body language and voice tone, listens actively, and has a positive attitude.
- Touch is an effective caring intervention; however, touch conveys many messages and should be used with discretion in selected patients.
- Listening includes "taking in" what a patient says, interpreting and understanding a patient's words, and giving back that understanding to the patient.
- Showing a family your care and concern for the patient creates an openness that enables you to form a relationship with the family.
- Through caring you understand and know a patient better as a unique individual, which enables you to identify the most effective nursing therapies.

■ REFLECTIVE LEARNING

- Think of a past personal or clinical situation when you needed to use caring principles to help a friend, family member, or patient. Write down some of the caring principles you used.
- Reflect on your previous answer. Knowing what you have learned in this chapter, ask yourself:
  - How would I change my approach?
  - What new caring interventions would I use?
  - Why did I select these interventions?
- Comfort and expertise in using caring practices will come with experience. Before your next clinical assignment, take an inventory of caring practices and rate your expertise. Look at this inventory after the next few clinical experiences and your previous rating, and describe any changes in your caring practices.

■ REVIEW QUESTIONS

1. Touch is a caring intervention. Before implementing touch, what does the nurse need to know about touch? (Select all that apply.)
   1. Some cultures may have specific restrictions about non–skill-based touch.
   2. Touch is a type of verbal communication.
   3. Touch forms a connection between nurse and patient.
   4. There is never a problem with using touch at any time.
   5. Touch reduces physical pain only.

2. A young woman comes to a clinic for the first time for a gynecological examination. Which nursing behavior applies Swanson's caring process of "knowing" the patient?
   1. Sharing feelings about the importance of having regular gynecological examinations
   2. Explaining risk factors for cervical cancer
   3. Recognizing that the patient is modest and maintaining her privacy during the examination
   4. Asking the patient what it means to have a vaginal examination

3. Which of the following are strategies for creating work environments that support nurse caring interventions? (Select all that apply.)
   1. Increasing technological support
   2. Improving flexibility for scheduling
   3. Providing opportunities to discuss care
   4. Promoting autonomy of practice
   5. Encouraging increased input concerning nursing functions from health care providers

4. Which of the following is an example of a nurse caring behavior that families perceive to be important to a patient's well-being?
   1. Making health care decisions for the patient
   2. Having family members provide a patient's total personal hygiene
   3. Injecting the nurse's personal views about death into a patient's story
   4. Asking permission before performing a procedure on a patient

5. A nurse is caring for an older man who is going to an assisted-living facility after discharge. Which description is an example of listening that displays caring?
   1. The nurse encourages the patient to talk about his concerns while reviewing a computer screen at the patient's bedside.
   2. The nurse sits at the patient's bedside, listens as he relays his fear of never seeing his home again, and then asks if he needs anything for pain.
   3. The nurse listens to the patient's story while sitting on the side of the bed and summarizes an interpretation of the patient's story.
   4. The nurse enters the patient's room, listens as he talks about his fears of not returning home, and tells the patient to think positively.

evolve

Additional Review Questions, as well as rationales for all Review Questions, can be found on the Evolve website.

1. 1,3; 2. 3; 3. 2, 3, 4; 4. 4; 5. 3.

REFERENCES

Adams LY: The conundrum of caring in nursing, *Int J Caring Sci* 9(1):1, 2016.

American Nurses Association (ANA): *Nursing's agenda for the future: a call to the nation*, Washington, DC, 2002, The Association.

American Organization of Nurse Executives (AONE): *Guiding principles for the role of the nurse in future health care delivery*, 2010. http://www.aone.org/resources/role-nurse-future-patient-care.pdf.

Arslan-Ozkan I, et al: A randomized controlled trial of the effects of nursing care based on Watson's Theory of Human Caring on distress, self-efficacy and adjustment in infertile women, *J Adv Nurs* 70(8):1801, 2013.

Benner P, Wrubel J: *The primacy of caring: stress and coping in health and illness*, Menlo Park, CA, 1989, Addison Wesley.

Benner P, et al: *Educating nurses: a call for radical transformation*, Stanford, CA, 2010, Carnegie Foundation for the Advancement of Teaching.

Brewer BB, Watson J: Evaluation of authentic human caring professional practices, *J Nurs Adm* 45(12):622, 2015.

Darnell L, Hickson S: Cultural competent patient-centered nursing care, *Nurs Clin North Am* 50(1):99, 2015.

Duffy JR, et al: Dimensions of caring: psychometric evaluation of the caring assessment tool, *ANS Adv Nurs Sci* 30(3):235, 2007.

Duffy JR, et al: Revision and psychometric properties of the Caring Assessment Tool, *Clin Nurs Res* 23(1):80, 2014.

Fahlberg B, Roush T: Mindful presence: being "with" in our nursing care, *Nursing* 46(3):14, 2016.

Flagg A: The role of patient-centered care in nursing, *Nurs Clin North Am* 50(1):75, 2015.

Frank AW: Just listening: narrative and deep illness, *Fam Syst Health* 16(3):197, 1998.

Hunsaker S, et al: Factors that influence the development of compassion fatigue, burnout, and compassion satisfaction in emergency department nurses, *J Nurs Scholarsh* 47(2):186, 2015.

Kahn S, et al: Measuring satisfaction: factors that drive hospital consumer assessment of healthcare providers and systems survey responses in a trauma and acute care surgery population, *Am Surgeon* May(61):537, 2015.

Kelley T, et al: Information needed to support knowing the patient, *ANS Adv Nurs Sci* 36(4):351, 2013.

Kiefer D: Therapeutic touch for cancer pain: an RCT, *Integr Med* 19(10):109, 2016.

Kramer M, et al: The evolution and development of an instrument to measure essential professional nursing practices, *J Nurs Adm* 44(11):569, 2014.

Leininger M: *Culture and care diversity and universality: a theory of nursing*, Pub No 15-2402, New York, 1991, National League for Nursing.

Love K, Femia E: Touch therapy, *Health Prog* 95(6):28, 2014.

Lusk JM, Fater K: A concept analysis of patient-centered care, *Nurs Forum* 48(2):89, 2013.

Maroon AM: Ethical palliative family nursing care: a new concept of caring for patients and families, *JONAS Healthc Law Ethics Regul* 14(4):115, 2012.

Martin MB: Caring in nursing professional development, *J Nurses Prof Dev* 31(5):271, 2015.

Maslow AH: *Motivation and personality*, ed 3, Upper Saddle River, NJ, 1987, Prentice Hall.

Mason VM: Compassion fatigue, moral distress, and work engagement in surgical intensive care unit trauma nurses, *Dimens Crit Care Nurs* 33(4):215, 2014.

Michael N, et al: Cancer caregivers advocate a patient- and family-centered approach to advance care planning, *J Pain Symptom Manage* 47(6):1064, 2014.

Moffa C: Caring for novice nurses applying Swanson's Theory of Caring, *Int J Human Caring* 19(1):63, 2015.

Nielsen LS, et al: Patient-centered care or cultural competence: negotiating palliative care at home for Chinese Canadian immigrants, *Am J Hosp Palliat Care* 32(4):372, 2015.

Palese A, et al: Surgical patient satisfaction as an outcome of nurses' caring behaviours: a descriptive correlational study in six European countries, *J Nurs Scholarsh* 43(4):341, 2011.

Palos GR: Care, compassion, and communication in professional nursing: art, science, or both, *Clin J Oncol Nurs* 18(2):247, 2014.

Papastavrou E, et al: Nurses' and patients' perceptions of caring behaviours: quantitative systematic review of comparative studies, *J Adv Nurs* 67(6):1191, 2011.

Penque S, Kearney G: The effect of nursing presence on patient satisfaction, *Nurs Manage* 46(4):38, 2015.

Porter CA, et al: Nurse caring behaviors following implementation of a relationship centered care professional practice model, *Int J Caring Sci* 7(3):818, 2014.

Potter TM, Savette LA: Ways of knowing: a nurse and physician discuss clinical decisions, actions, and lessons, *Creat Nurs* 20(1):59, 2014.

Ray MA, Turkel MC: Caring as emancipatory nursing praxis: the theory of relational caring complexity, *ANS Adv Nurs Sci* 37(2):123, 2014.

Robert Wood Johnson Foundation (RWJF): *Campaign for action is chalking up successes that will improve patient care*, 2014, http://www.rwjf.org/en/library/articles-and-news/2014/06/campaign-for-action-is-chalking-up-successes-that-will-improve-p.html.

Sharma A, et al: A quality improvement initiative to achieve high nursing presence during patient- and family-centered rounds, *Hosp Pediatr* 4(1):1, 2014.

Swanson KM: Empirical development of a middle-range theory of caring, *Nurs Res* 40(3):161, 1991.

Theofanidis D, Sapountzi-Krepia D: Nursing and caring: an historical overview from ancient Greek tradition to modern times, *Int J Caring Sci* 8(3):791, 2015.

Turpin RL: State of the science of nursing presence revisited: knowledge for preserving nursing presence capability, *Int J Human Caring* 18(4):14, 2014.

Tyreman S: Trust and truth: uncertainty in health care practices, *J Eval Clin Pract* 21:470, 2015.

Watson Caring Science Institute (WCSI): *Caring science theory*, 2017, https://www.watsoncaringscience.org/jean-bio/caring-science-theory/.

Watson J: Caring science and human caring theory: transforming personal and professional practices of nursing and health care, *J Health Hum Serv Adm* 31(4):466, 2009.

Watson J: Caring science and the next decade of holistic healing: transforming self and system from the inside out, *Beginnings* 30(2):14, 2010.

Watson J: *Human caring science: a theory of nursing*, Sudbury, MA, 2012, Jones & Bartlett.

Watson J, Brewer BB: Caring science research, *J Nurs Adm* 45(5):235, 2015.

Winsett RP, Hauck S: Implementing relationship-based care, *J Nurs Adm* 41(6):285, 2011.

Yagasaki K, Komatsu H: The need for a nursing presence in oral chemotherapy, *Clin J Oncol Nurs* 17(5):512, 2013.

Zolnierek CD: An integrative review of knowing the patient, *J Nurs Scholarsh* 46(1):3, 2014.

Cultural Competence

evolve MEDIA RESOURCES

http://evolve.elsevier.com/Potter/essentials

- Audio Glossary

- QSEN Activity and Review Questions Answers and Rationales

OBJECTIVES

- Explain the concepts of cultural awareness, cultural knowledge, cultural skill, cultural encounters, and cultural desire in the cultural competence model.
- Describe social and cultural influences in health and illness.
- Describe health disparity and the social determinants that affect it.

- Describe the role communication plays in developing cultural competence.
- Explain the approaches to use in conducting a cultural nursing history and physical assessment.
- Describe how teach-back helps a patient with limited health literacy.
- Explain the principles to apply when using an interpreter.

KEY TERMS

core measures, p. 567
cultural assessment, p. 570
cultural awareness, p. 568
cultural competence, p. 563
cultural desire, p. 568
cultural encounter, p. 568

cultural knowledge, p. 568
cultural skill, p. 568
culturally congruent, p. 568
culture, p. 563
explanatory model, p. 570
health disparity, p. 564

intersectionality, p. 565
linguistic competence, p. 571
marginalized groups, p. 565
oppression, p. 565
social determinants of health, p. 564
world view, p. 566

Culture, in its broadest sense, reflects the whole of human behavior including ideas, beliefs, and values; ways of relating to one another; language and manners of speaking; and work and lifestyle practices (Ball et al., 2015). Every one of us has some type of bias that is culturally driven. A bias is an inclination or the holding of a partial perspective, often accompanied by a refusal to consider a different point of view. One might have a bias toward or against an individual based on his or her culture such as a bias toward an ethnic group, a race, gender, a nation, a religion, a social class, or a political party. When you as a nurse hold a bias toward an individual patient or group of patients, it is very difficult to provide patient-centered care. A patient-centered approach

to providing care requires you to be respectful of and responsive to individual patient preferences, needs, and values and to ensure that patient values guide all clinical care decisions (Institute of Medicine [IOM], 2001). This chapter explains the importance of cultural competence and its relationship to patient-centered care. Cultural beliefs, values, and practices are learned from birth, first in the home, then in the church or other places where people congregate, and then in educational and other social settings (Purnell, 2013). This cultural learning applies to both you and your patients. The process of cultural competence in delivering health care services is "a culturally conscious model of care in which a healthcare professional continually strives to achieve the ability and

564   UNIT 4   Promoting Psychosocial Health

CASE STUDY *Ms. Tatum*

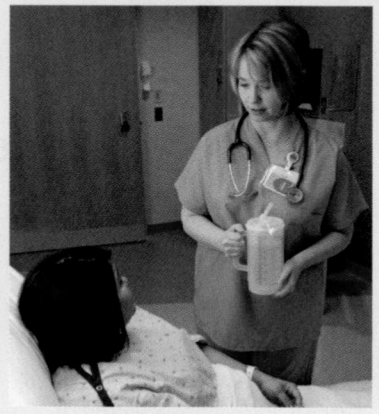

Ms. Tatum is a 27-year-old African American woman. She is overweight and was diagnosed with diabetes 2 years ago and now requires insulin to control her blood sugar. She became homeless after losing her job and health insurance. She currently lives in housing provided through a neighborhood shelter. Ms. Tatum was admitted to the hospital with a blood sugar of 322 mg/dL (her normal targeted range is 80 to 130 mg/dL) and a hemoglobin A$_{1c}$ of 11% (target for Ms. Tatum is 7% or less). Marina, a 23-year-old nursing student, is assigned to care for Ms. Tatum. After reading her medical record, Marina notices that Ms. Tatum has come to the emergency department 3 times during the past 6 months for the same reason. Ms. Tatum's previous health care providers documented that she verbalized an understanding of how to manage her diabetes but has difficulty following her treatment plan. Marina teaches Ms. Tatum that it is important to take her insulin as prescribed. She also explains how to make healthy food choices. As Marina provides patient education, Ms. Tatum nods. Marina gives Ms. Tatum a chance to ask questions, but Ms. Tatum says she has none.

availability to effectively work within the cultural context of a client" (family, individual, or community) (Transcultural C.A.R.E. Associates, 2015). It is a process of becoming culturally competent, not being culturally competent (Transcultural C.A.R.E. Associates, 2015).

The United States is a complex multicultural society. The changing demographics of the U.S. population create challenges for the health care system and health care providers. By 2030, one in five Americans is projected to be age 65 and older according to the U.S. Census bureau; more than half of all Americans are projected to belong to a minority group (any group other than non-Hispanic White alone) by 2044; and nearly one in five of the total U.S. population is projected to be foreign born by 2060 (Colby and Ortman, 2015). The wealth gap between blacks and whites is demonstrated in the fact that blacks lag behind whites in homeownership, household wealth, and median income. These differences remain even when controlling for levels of education (Pew Research Center, 2016). According to the 2003 National Adult Assessment of Literacy (NAAL) (the only national data on health literacy skills), only 12% of U.S. adults are proficient in

obtaining, processing, and understanding basic health information and services needed to make appropriate health decisions (National Center for Education Statistics [NCES], 2006). Additionally, the Centers for Disease Control and Prevention (CDC) (2015) reports that studies show adults who self-report the worst health also have the most limited literacy, numeracy, and health literacy skills. Although death rates have declined overall in the United States over the past 50 years, people who are poorly educated and people living in poverty still die at higher rates from the same conditions than people who are better educated and economically advantaged (Ball et al., 2015). These statistics reveal examples of cultural factors that are influencing the health care system and why issues such as health care resource accessibility, patient adherence to medical therapies, patient satisfaction, and health care outcomes are so difficult to manage.

The Joint Commission (TJC), the National Quality Forum (NFQ), and the National Commission on Quality Assurance (NCQA) are a few of the influential organizations that have responded to these complexities in health care by implementing new standards focused on cultural competency, health literacy, and patient-centered and family-centered care. These standards recognize that valuing each patient's unique needs improves the overall safety and quality of the patient's care.

HEALTH DISPARITIES

What is quality health care? More than a decade ago, a report by the Institute of Medicine (IOM, 2001) defined it as health care that is safe, effective, patient centered, timely, efficient, and equitable or fair. Although the U.S. health care system has improved in most of those areas since the IOM report was published, the system still does not emphasize equality of care (Mutha et al., 2012). As a result, many health disparities remain.

Healthy People 2020 defines a health disparity as "a particular type of health difference that is closely linked with social, economic, and/or environmental disadvantage" (Office of Disease Prevention and Health Promotion [ODPHP], 2016) (Box 21.1). Poor health status, disease risk factors, poor health outcomes, and limited access to health care are types of disparities often interrelated and influenced by the conditions and social context in which people live (CDC, 2013).

The World Health Organization (WHO) defines social determinants of health as the conditions in which people are born, grow, live, work, and age (WHO, 2016). This includes conditions within a health care system. According to the WHO, social determinants of health are mostly responsible for health disparities seen within and between countries (WHO, 2016). Social determinants of health include factors such as age, race and ethnicity, socioeconomic status, access to nutritious food, transportation resources, religion, sexual orientation, age, level of education, literacy level, disability (physical and cognitive), and geographical location (e.g., access to health care) (CDC, 2013). As a nurse, you will care for patients in a variety of health care settings. It is

BOX 21.1 EXAMPLES OF HEALTH DISPARITIES IDENTIFIED BY THE CENTERS FOR DISEASE CONTROL AND PREVENTION

- Among adults aged 25 years and older in 2011, noncompletion of high school was generally more common among adults who were foreign born than adults born in the United States.
- In 2011, 30.3% of U.S. census tracts did not have at least one healthier food retailer (supermarkets, large grocery stores, supercenters and warehouse clubs, and fruit and vegetable specialty stores) within the tract or within $\frac{1}{2}$ mile of tract boundaries. This represents 83.6 million people, representing approximately 27% of the 2010 continental U.S. population.
- Non-Hispanic black adults were at least 50% more likely to die of heart disease or stroke prematurely (i.e., before age 75 years) than their non-Hispanic white counterparts.
- Colorectal cancer incidence and mortality increased with advancing age. Incidence and death rates were highest among people aged 75 years and older. Non-Hispanic blacks had higher colorectal cancer incidence and death rates than non-Hispanic whites, Asians/Pacific Islanders, and American Indians/Alaska Natives.
- The number of individuals who had colorectal cancer screening (any of the test options) was greater among people aged 65 to 75 years compared with people aged 50 to 64 years, among non-Hispanics compared with Hispanics, among people with a disability compared with people with no disability, and among people with health insurance compared with people with no health insurance.

Adapted from Centers for Disease Control and Prevention (CDC): CDC health disparities and inequalities report—United States, 2013, *MMWR Morb Mortal Wkly Rep* 62(Suppl 3):1, 2013, http://www.cdc.gov/mmwr/pdf/other/su6203.pdf.

important that you understand how patients' cultural factors and their social determinants of health influence their health disparities. You also need to understand the implications this has on how you provide patient-centered care.

The 2015 National Healthcare Disparities Report (Agency for Healthcare Research and Quality [AHRQ], 2016b) offers some promise regarding health care access and quality. The report noted that access to health care has improved dramatically, led by sustained reductions in the number of Americans without health insurance and increases in the number of Americans with a usual source of medical care; however, blacks and Hispanics are still less likely than whites to have a usual place to go for medical care. In addition, the quality of health care improved generally through 2013 based on quality measures such as patient safety, healthy living, and effective treatment. However, the AHRQ (2016b) also reported that people in poor households received worse care than people in high-income households for approximately 60% of the same quality measures.

People who are in marginalized groups are more likely to have poor health outcomes and die earlier because of a complex interaction between their individual behaviors, the

environment of the communities in which they live, the policies and practices of health care and government systems, and the clinical care they receive (United Health Foundation, 2015). Examples of marginalized groups include people who are gay, lesbian, bisexual, or transgender; people of color; people who are physically and/or mentally challenged; and people who are not college educated. Marginalization places or keeps someone in a powerless or an unimportant position within a society or group. Poor access to health care is one social determinant of health that contributes to health disparities. Access to primary care is an important indicator of broader access to health care services. A patient who regularly visits a primary care provider is more likely to receive adequate preventive care than a patient who lacks such access.

Research shows that health care systems and health care providers sometimes contribute significantly to the problem of health care disparities. Disparities have been linked to inadequate resources, poor patient-provider communication, a lack of culturally competent care, and inadequate access to language services (National Quality Forum [NQF], 2016).

In the case study, Ms. Tatum has a number of social determinants that affect her health status and ability to manage her diabetes: socioeconomic status (no employment or health insurance, no home, limited financial resources if any), no access to primary care (uses the emergency department), being female, and a questionable literacy problem indicated by her neutral reaction to Marina's instruction. Marina needs to consider all these factors to provide Ms Tatum a more culturally competent health care plan.

Intersectionality

Intersectionality is a research and policy model used to study the complexities of people's lives and experiences (Institute for Intersectionality Research and Policy, 2016). The model looks at how being marginalized affects people's health and access to care. It serves to describe the forces, factors, and power structures that shape and influence life. Each of us is at the intersection of two categories: privilege and oppression. Oppression is a formal and informal system of advantages and disadvantages tied to membership in social groups (Adams et al., 2007). Oppression occurs at individual, cultural, and institutional levels, affecting individual and group experiences. For example, a patient experiencing oppression has limited access to resources such as health care, housing, education, employment, and legal services. In contrast, a patient experiencing privilege has no difficulty accessing these resources. Individuals who support the theory of intersectionality believe that we must each determine how privileged and how oppressed we are to understand ourselves, the people around us, and the choices we make. Then as health care providers, we are better able to identify the nature or source of patients' health care problems and how best to find solutions. Social groups affect our daily lives, shape our world view, control our access to resources, and ultimately determine our health outcomes. Whether we live in a disadvantaged community or in a community with access to social power and resources, we all are affected by the system of

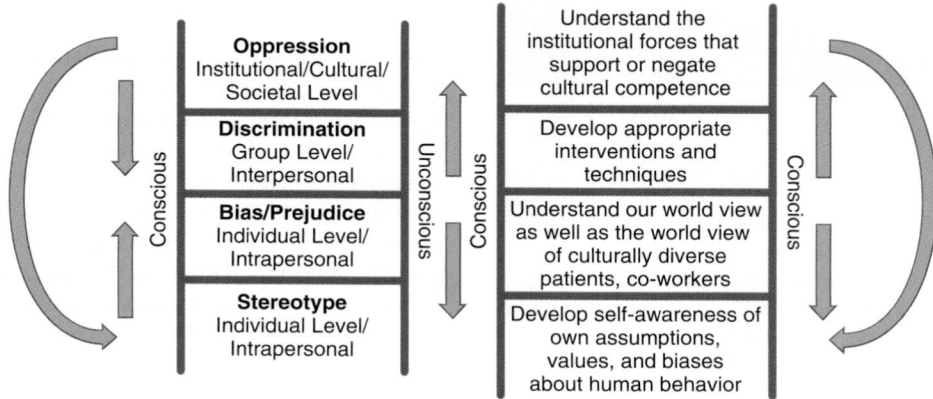

FIG 21.1 Ladders of oppression and cultural competence. Each level of the ladder of cultural competence offers a response to the ladder of oppression. Because of the extensiveness and complexity of the systems of oppression, individuals and organizations move up and down both ladders simultaneously. (©2011 BJH Center for Diversity and Cultural Competence.)

oppression. Understanding the different levels of oppression and where you stand helps you develop cultural competence (Fig. 21.1).

To apply the intersectionality model to daily nursing practice, think about the following patients: Ms. Tatum, a 27-year-old homeless woman with diabetes; an 85-year-old African American woman who is a retired nurse from rural Alabama; a 32-year-old Latina lesbian executive in San Francisco who is Catholic; and a woman who is an undocumented immigrant from Eastern Europe and has a 3-year-old child with a developmental disability. How might the experiences of each of these women compare with the experiences of other Americans? How do their experiences with the health care system differ? How does age affect their perspective? How would these answers change if you looked at their lives 15 years ago or 35 years ago? These scenarios are likely to draw a wide range of responses. The idea of intersectionality supports a broad view of culture by allowing consideration of a multitude of experiences within the context of power, privilege, and oppression.

RACIAL, ETHNIC, AND CULTURAL IDENTITY

Cultural competence is challenging to achieve, but it begins with gaining an awareness of your own racial, ethnic, and cultural identity. That awareness prepares you to better understand patients within the context of their own racial, ethnic, and cultural identity. As a nurse, you will counsel and comfort patients to help them to better understand their health issues (e.g., medication adherence, ability to follow diet restrictions, knowledge of risk factors) and to be willing to partner with you in making important necessary behavioral changes when necessary. Reflect on your own sense of how you identify with race and ethnicity within the context of your family, community, society, and cultural history (Substance Abuse and Mental Health Services Administration [SAMHSA], 2014). Here are two classic definitions. Racial

identity "refers to a sense of group or collective identity based on one's perception that he or she shares a common heritage with a particular racial group" (Helms, 1990, p. 3). Ethnic and cultural identity are "the frame in which individuals identify consciously or unconsciously with those with whom they feel a common bond because of similar traditions, behaviors, values, and beliefs" (Chavez and Guido-DiBrito, 1999, p. 41). These definitions help us to understand how individuals negotiate their own and other cultures in life (SAMHSA, 2014). It is important for you to examine your own racial, ethnic, and cultural identity to better recognize and understand normal and abnormal behavior. If you fail to do this self-examination, you will be more likely to prejudge patients and not accurately assess their health care problems. A self-examination allows you to understand the cultural factors that shape a patient's life experiences, a patient's health care problems, and how a patient might perceive those problems.

WORLD VIEW

Historical and social realities shape an individual's or group's world view, which determines how people perceive others, how they interact and relate to reality, and how they process information (Walker et al., 2010). World view is a set of assumptions that begin to develop during childhood and guide how one sees, thinks about, experiences, and interprets the world (SAMHSA, 2014). It creates a lens through which we view all of life's experiences through our own uniquely tinted view. Our world view evolves during a lifetime process of interacting with family, peers, communities, organizations, media, and institutions (Fig. 21.2). It is important for you to advocate for patients based on their world views. This requires a thorough ongoing assessment and planning in partnership with each patient to ensure that your care is safe, effective, and culturally sensitive.

In any intercultural encounter there is an insider perspective (emic world view) and an outsider perspective (etic world

How We Develop Our World View

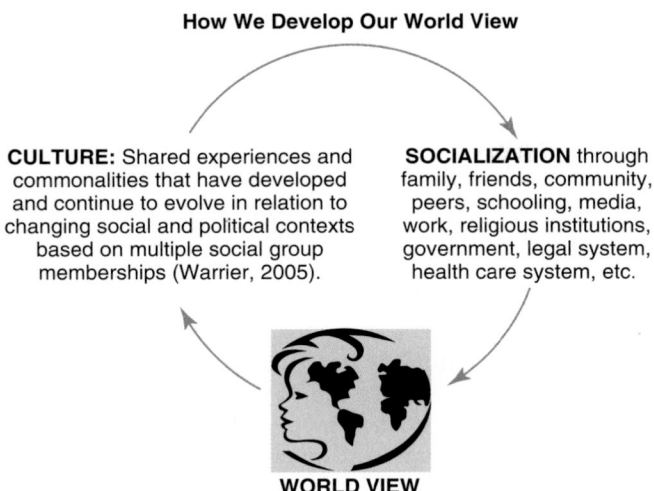

CULTURE: Shared experiences and commonalities that have developed and continue to evolve in relation to changing social and political contexts based on multiple social group memberships (Warrier, 2005).

SOCIALIZATION through family, friends, community, peers, schooling, media, work, religious institutions, government, legal system, health care system, etc.

WORLD VIEW

FIG 21.2 How we develop our world view. (©2011 BJH Center for Diversity and Cultural Competence.)

view). For example, a Korean woman requests seaweed soup for her first meal after giving birth. This request puzzles her nurse. The nurse has an insider's view of professional postpartum care but is an outsider to the Korean culture. As such, the nurse is not aware of the meal's significance to the patient. Conversely, the Korean patient has an outsider's view of American professional postpartum care and assumes that seaweed soup is available in the hospital because, according to her cultural beliefs, the soup cleanses the blood and promotes healing and lactation (Edelstein, 2011). Conflict arises when health care providers interpret the behaviors of patients through their own world view lens instead of trying to uncover the world view that guides the behavior of their patients.

It is easy to stereotype various cultural groups after reading general information about their ethnic values, practices, and beliefs. Avoid stereotypes or unwarranted generalizations about any particular group that prevents an accurate assessment of an individual's unique characteristics and world view. Instead approach each person individually and ask questions to gain a better understanding of a patient's perspective and needs. *In the case study, Ms. Tatum has limited access to healthy foods in her neighborhood. She often eats foods high in fat and sodium because that is all that is available at her local convenience store. The shelter provides dinner that includes healthier food choices. Marina has an insider's or emic view of dietary standards for diabetes and is unaware of her patient's inability to obtain healthy food options. Ms. Tatum has an outsider's view of the types of food to include in a diabetic diet. She assumes that the foods she buys locally or eats at the shelter are suitable to eat (e.g., frozen meals, packaged lunch meat, mashed potatoes and gravy). Marina realizes after her interaction with Ms. Tatum that she needs to ask Ms. Tatum what she typically eats during a day. She needs to reassess Ms. Tatum to better understand how her patient relates to the need to eat healthy foods and her understanding of previous instruction.*

DISEASE AND ILLNESS

Culture affects how an individual defines the meaning of illness (see Chapter 2). Some illnesses (e.g., human immunodeficiency virus [HIV] and manic depression) are embedded with meaning that is not always based on the physical nature of the condition but is culturally interpreted, which affects how society responds to afflicted individuals and influences the experience of that illness (Conrad and Barker, 2010). All illnesses are socially constructed through experiences of people, specifically, how individuals come to understand and live with their illness (Conrad and Barker, 2010). This is particularly true with chronic disease. Patients learn the effects of their disease and how to adapt to live as normal a life as possible.

Culture also provides the context in which a person interacts with family members, peers, community members, and institutions (e.g., educational, religious, media, health care, legal). Therefore culture and life experiences shape a person's world view about health, illness, and health care.

An understanding of the difference between disease and illness allows you to become culturally competent in providing patient care. Illness is the way that individuals and families react to disease, whereas disease is a malfunctioning of biological or psychological processes. People react differently to disease based on their unique cultural perspective. Most health care providers in the United States are primarily educated to treat disease, whereas most individuals seek health care because of their experience with illness. As an example, a patient may have a combination of symptoms that, based on previous experiences with family members and beliefs about illness, the patient believes are untreatable, whereas the patient's physician believes aggressive therapy might offer a cure. Such different perspectives between patients and their health care providers often frustrate patients and providers, fostering a lack of trust, lack of patient adherence to treatment plans, and poor health outcomes. Providing safe, quality care to all patients means taking into consideration both disease and illness.

Core Measures

The Centers for Medicare and Medicaid Services (CMS), commercial insurance plans, The Joint Commission (TJC), Medicare and Medicaid managed care plans, physician and other care provider organizations, and consumers worked together through the Core Quality Measures Collaborative to identify a set of core measures (CMS, 2016). An aim of the collaborative is to hold health care providers accountable for considering patients' unique cultural perspectives to provide safe quality care. The core measure sets need to be meaningful to patients, consumers, and physicians, while reducing variability in outcome measure selection, financial collection burden, and cost (CMS, 2016).

The core measures are a set of evidence-based, scientifically researched standards of care (CMS, 2016; TJC, 2016). The **core measures** are key quality indicators that help health care institutions improve performance, increase accountability, and reduce costs. The measures apply to all patients. All the core measures are consistent with national health priorities and are in the following seven sets (CMS, 2016):

- Accountable Care Organizations (ACOs), Patient Centered Medical Homes (PCMH), and Primary Care
- Cardiology
- Gastroenterology
- HIV and Hepatitis C
- Medical Oncology
- Obstetrics and Gynecology
- Orthopedics

In addition to improving the standard of care, the core measures are intended to reduce health disparities. When hospitals are held accountable to meet the core quality measures, all patients regardless of cultural and socioeconomic status are to be treated equally because the standard of care applies to all. For example, one Obstetrics and Gynecology core measure is women are to receive breast cancer screening (CMS, 2016). In another example, patients who present with heart failure are to receive beta blocker therapy for left ventricular systolic dysfunction.

A MODEL OF CULTURAL COMPETENCE

Cultural competence is the ongoing process in which a health care professional tries to achieve the ability and availability to effectively work within the cultural context of a patient (individual, family, or community) (Transcultural C.A.R.E. Associates, 2015). Cultural competence is a developmental process that evolves over a lifetime as individuals engage with others and learn from their experiences. Campinha-Bacote's model of cultural competency has five interrelated constructs (Transcultural C.A.R.E. Associates, 2015): cultural awareness, cultural knowledge, cultural skill, cultural encounters, and cultural desire. The five constructs provide a framework for you to practice in a culturally competent manner.

- **Cultural awareness** is the process of conducting a self-examination of one's own biases toward other cultures and the in-depth exploration of one's cultural and professional background. It also involves being aware of the existence of documented racism and other "isms" in health care delivery.
- **Cultural knowledge** is the process in which a health care professional seeks and obtains a sound educational base about culturally diverse groups. In acquiring this knowledge, health care professionals must focus on the integration of three specific issues: health-related beliefs and cultural values, care practices, and disease incidence and prevalence.
- **Cultural skill** is the ability to conduct a cultural assessment of a patient to collect relevant cultural data about a patient's presenting problem as well as accurately conducting a culturally based physical assessment.
- **Cultural encounter** is a process that encourages health care professionals to directly engage in face-to-face cultural interactions and other types of encounters with

patients from culturally diverse backgrounds. A cultural encounter aims to modify a health care provider's existing beliefs about a cultural group and to prevent possible stereotyping.
- **Cultural desire** is the motivation of a health care professional to "want to" (and not "have to") engage in the process of becoming culturally aware, culturally knowledgeable, and culturally skillful and seeking cultural encounters.

When you provide culturally competent care, you bridge cultural gaps to provide meaningful and supportive care for all patients. Care is culturally congruent when it fits a person's life patterns, values, and system of meaning. These patterns and meaning are generated by people themselves and not from biased, predetermined criteria. For example, during nursing school you are assigned to care for a female patient who observes Muslim beliefs. You notice the woman's discomfort with several of the male health care providers. You wonder if this discomfort is related to your patient's religious beliefs. While preparing for clinical, you learn that Muslims differ in their adherence to tradition, but that modesty is an important Islamic ethic that pertains to interaction between the sexes. Thus you say to the patient, "I know that for many of our Muslim patients, modesty is very important. I want to respect your beliefs; is there some way I can make you more comfortable?" You do not assume that the information will automatically apply to this patient. Instead you combine your knowledge about a cultural group with an attitude of helpfulness and flexibility to provide quality, patient-centered, culturally congruent care.

Cultural Awareness and Knowledge

Cultural awareness requires a self-examination of one's own biases toward other cultures and an in-depth exploration of one's own cultural and professional background (SAMHSA, 2014). A self-examination helps you to understand your own world view of how you perceive and engage patients. Before you begin to assess the cultures, races, and ethnicities of your patients and use this information to improve their care, first examine and understand your own cultural history, racial and ethnic heritage, and cultural values and beliefs (SAMHSA, 2014). Nurses who understand themselves and their own cultural groups and perceptions are better equipped to respect patients with diverse belief systems. Being open to understanding a patient's beliefs and forming a partnership is more important than knowing everything about a patient's specific culture (Ball et al., 2015).

Campinha-Bacote recommends that you begin to gain cultural awareness by not only asking yourself if you hold any biases but also questioning if there are any "isms" that exist where you work (Transcultural C.A.R.E. Associates, 2015). For example, are there ageism practices in how older adults have their pain treated (e.g., undertreatment)? Be mindful of such practices so that you can adopt care approaches that minimize biases.

Health care providers gain cultural knowledge by taking time to better understand the populations that they serve and obtaining specific cultural knowledge as it relates to help seeking, treatment, and recovery (SAMHSA, 2014). As an example, certain cultures believe in the importance of balance and harmony to stay healthy. Aspects of this concept are evident among the beliefs of many Hispanics, Native Americans, Asians, and Middle Eastern groups (Ball et al., 2015). Box 21.2 summarizes the naturalistic or holistic balance that many people believe they can achieve by using "hot" and "cold" foods and medicines. People from different cultures define "hot" and "cold" differently. For example, people who are of Chinese heritage often uphold the philosophical concept of yin (cold) and yang (hot). To restore (treat) a disturbed balance requires the use of opposites (e.g., a "hot" remedy for a "cold" problem and vice versa). Remember, every patient is unique. However, if you know about a particular culture's risks for disease, for example, you can focus your nursing history more appropriately during your assessment. If you learn that an individual believes in a "hot" and "cold" balance when choosing certain foods to eat, support your patient's practices and adapt this information into the patient's dietary plan.

Do not form inappropriate biases or stereotypes when you assess a patient's culture. Stereotyping occurs in two cognitive phases. In the first phase there is an activation of a stereotype when an individual is categorized into a social group. When this occurs, the beliefs and prejudices come to mind about what members of that particular group are like (Ball et al., 2015). Stereotypical views eventually occur without awareness automatically. In the second phase, people use these activated beliefs and feelings when they interact with the individual (Ball et al., 2015). Studies have shown that health care providers activate these stereotypes or nonconscious bias routinely when communicating with and providing care to minority individuals (Moskowitz et al., 2012). As a result, diagnoses and treatments of patients may be biased even in the absence of the practitioner's intent or awareness.

Storytelling. One way to begin to understand a patient's cultural perspective is storytelling. Storytelling conveys culture, combining personal experience with the commonalities of all human experiences (Wilson et al., 2015). When you encourage a patient to tell a story or when you tell your own story, you frame important messages in ways that make them memorable for you and your patient. Telling stories engages a nurse and patient in a way that broadens their relational understanding. Use storytelling to explore pertinent health care issues; for example, have patients describe previous surgical experiences, problems with childrearing, or approaches used with self-administration of medications. A story helps you identify the real problems affecting a patient's health status and find culturally appropriate ways to intervene (Box 21.3).

World View of Providers and Patients. Health care has its own culture of hierarchies, power, values, beliefs, and practices. Most health care providers educated in Western traditions are immersed in the culture of science and biomedicine through their coursework and professional experience. Consequently, they often have a world view that differs from that of their patients. As a nurse, you need to assume that every patient encounter will be a cross-cultural one.

When patients and health care providers interact there are always two different perspectives. When patients access the health care system they want to (1) see their health care provider and (2) feel better. In return health care providers expect patients to (1) make and keep appointments; (2) give a medication history; (3) give informed consent; (4) follow (discharge) instructions; (5) read, understand, and use health

BOX 21.2 **BALANCE OF "HOT" AND "COLD"**			
COLD CONDITIONS	**HOT TREATMENTS**	**HOT CONDITIONS**	**COLD TREATMENTS**
Cancer	Foods	Constipation	Foods
Cold, flu	Beef	Diarrhea	Barley water
Earaches	Cereals	Fever	Chicken
Headaches	Chili peppers	Infection	Dairy products
Joint pain	Chocolate	Kidney problems	Fresh vegetables
Menses	Eggs	Rash	Fruits
Pneumonia	Liquor	Sore throat	Honey
Stomach cramps	Onions		Medicines and herbs
	Medicines and herbs		Bicarbonate of soda
	Anise		Milk of Magnesia
	Aspirin		Sage
	Castor oil		
	Cinnamon		
	Garlic		
	Ginger root		
	Iron		
	Penicillin		

Adapted from Ball JW, et al: *Seidel's guide to physical examination*, ed 8, St Louis, 2015, Elsevier; and Purnell LD: *Transcultural health care: A culturally competent approach*, ed 4, Philadelphia, 2013, FA Davis.

BOX 21.3 EVIDENCE-BASED PRACTICE

PICO Question: Does the use of storytelling compared with standard assessment approaches among adult and pediatric patients affect patient involvement in selecting health care interventions?

SUMMARY OF EVIDENCE

A patient's ability to understand the complexities of many health issues and to be able to become engaged in decision making requires the ability to discuss and clarify confusing issues. Storytelling allows participants to reflect on their illness experience and create meaning from it (Gucciardi et al., 2016). Storytelling has thus been shown to enhance self-management of chronic disease (e.g., cancer, diabetes). A recent study involved patients telling stories about their aspirations for the future (Terkildsen and Wittrup, 2015). The information that was shared then allowed clinicians to initiate interventions based on patient experiences of health problems. When patients are able to express their experiences, there is a negotiation with health care providers that leads to a mutual plan of care.

Digital storytelling is being widely used especially in pediatric patients. In a study by Wilson et al. (2015), digital storytelling gave children and adolescents with cancer a platform for making sense of and sharing their cancer experience. Houston et al. (2011) used DVDs to deliver stories of real patients with hypertension to patients being treated for hypertension. Patients with baseline uncontrolled hypertension who watched the storytelling DVDs experienced a greater reduction in systolic and diastolic blood pressure at 3 months compared with patients watching an attention DVD (a DVD on general health topics unrelated to hypertension). The act of telling a story is valuable, allowing a patient to initiate the process of reflection to gain understanding of the self and his or her disease process (Gucciardi et al., 2016).

APPLICATION TO NURSING PRACTICE

* Create a safe, caring, and nonjudgmental environment when using storytelling (Gucciardi et al., 2016).
* Storytelling should be participant-centered; give patients substantial control over when and how to tell a story (Gucciardi et al., 2016).
* Use storytelling to clarify issues when performing a cultural assessment.
* When asking a patient to describe his or her major concerns about a health problem, try to use storytelling to frame the context of those concerns.
* Tell your own stories about patient experiences (respecting confidentiality) to help explain procedures or treatment plans.

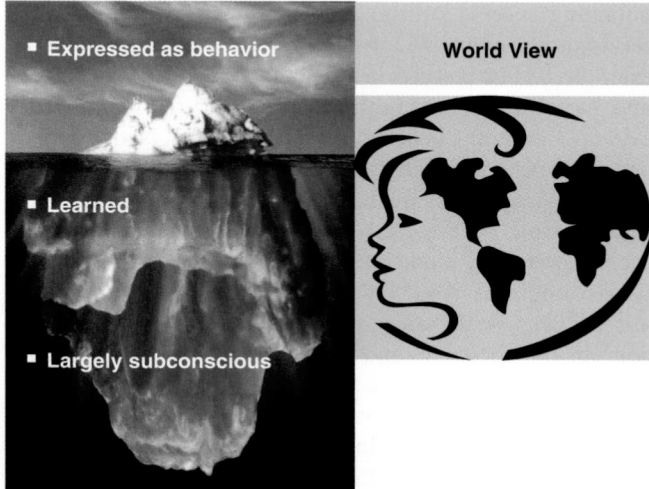

FIG 21.3 This model has been adapted from Campinha-Bacote et al. (2005) Iceberg analogy. It incorporates the Kleinman (1980) **explanatory model** to emphasize that both the nurse and the patient act in accordance with their own world views. (©2011 BJH Center for Diversity and Cultural Competence.)

Patients and all their health care providers bring each of their world views into the care process. The iceberg analogy (Fig. 21.3) is a tool that helps you visualize the visible and invisible aspects of your own world view. Just as most of an iceberg lies beneath the surface of the water, most aspects of a person's world view lie outside of his or her awareness and are invisible to those around the person. For example, a patient who has willingly agreed to be admitted to the hospital for a serious medical condition requiring surgery may refuse the surgery for religious reasons. In the patient's view, she came to the hospital for help to eliminate the pain and infection from her illness. At the same time, she believes that she needs to seek God for a decision that entails removing a body part. The patient's health care provider assumes the patient is in the hospital to receive care for a serious illness and is willing to accept any and all treatments to cure the illness. The patient's deeply held religious beliefs about removing a body part are not obvious by assessing for a religious preference. Thus the nurse needs to conduct a comprehensive **cultural assessment** to understand how the patient's religious values will affect her willingness to receive care. These deeply held values reside underneath the iceberg. The observed behavior (in this case, coming to the hospital) is a visible sign of a person's world view, but the beliefs, attitudes, knowledge, and experiences that guide the behavior are not visible to others. Conflict arises when health care providers interpret the behaviors of patients through their own world view lens instead of trying to uncover the world view that guides the behavior of their patients.

CULTURAL SKILL

Collecting a culturally based nursing history, performing a culturally based physical assessment, and using teach-back

education materials; (6) correctly complete insurance forms; (7) pay their bills; and (8) go home and manage their care by taking their medication the right way, eating the right foods, and stopping, starting, or changing a variety of behaviors (American Medical Association [AMA], 2007, p. 11). This list shows how complex each patient interaction is even before the interaction begins. The complexity increases depending on the cultural background of a patient and health care provider.

BOX 21.4 THE TWELVE DOMAINS OF CULTURE

- Overview, inhabited localities—country of origin and current residence
- Communication—interrelationship of verbal language skills including dominant language, dialects, touch, contextual use of language, and willingness to share information
- Family roles and organization—defines relationship of insiders and outsiders; includes concepts related to head of household, gender roles, family goals and priorities, and developmental goals of family members
- Workforce issues—type of employment, location, autonomy, language barriers
- Biocultural ecology—skin color, heredity, genetics, drug metabolism
- High-risk behaviors—tobacco, alcohol, recreational drugs, physical activity, safety
- Nutrition—meaning of foods, common foods, deficiencies, rituals, limitations
- Pregnancy and childbearing practices—fertility practices, views toward pregnancy, birthing, postpartum
- Death rituals—bereavement, ceremonies
- Spirituality—religious practices, use of prayer, meaning of life
- Health care practices—focus of health care, traditional practices, responsibility for health, self-medication, pain, sick role, barriers
- Health care providers—perceptions of providers, folk practitioners, gender, and health care status

Adapted from Purnell LD: *Transcultural health care: a culturally competent approach*, ed 4, Philadelphia, 2013, FA Davis.

with plain language are cultural skills that take practice and require you to apply your cultural awareness and knowledge. The summary of the domains of culture in Box 21.4 is a framework for the information you might choose to include in a nursing history (Purnell, 2013). It takes time to gather a comprehensive culturally based nursing history. If you work in a setting such as home health, school nursing, or a health clinic, you will be able to gather more information with each patient visit. When you are in an acute setting, you must focus your assessment on the domains most relevant to a patient's condition and the impending treatment plan. For example, if you know a patient will require extensive postoperative education, it will be important to assess the patient's and family's language, family roles, and health care practices.

Collecting a Nursing History

You begin a patient assessment by being mindful that cultural differences will exist. It is important to grasp exactly what the patient means and know exactly what the patient thinks you mean in words and actions (Ball et al., 2015). Do not make assumptions. Listen carefully, let patients tell their stories, rephrase statements for clarity, and validate any assumptions you make about the patient's condition or needs with the patient. As you perform an assessment, the patient may hesitate to offer his or her beliefs and fears, which can

be overcome through respectful, nonjudgmental questioning (Box 21.5). Have a patient help set the agenda for the visit to help you better understand the patient's needs.

A cultural assessment is intrusive and time consuming and requires a trusting relationship between participants. Miscommunication commonly occurs in intercultural transactions. This is because of language communication differences between and among participants and differences in interpreting one another's behaviors. Linguistic competence is the ability to communicate effectively and convey information in a manner that is easily understood by diverse audiences. You use transcultural communication skills to interpret a patient's behavior and to behave in a culturally congruent way. Effective communication is a critical skill in culturally competent care and helps you engage a patient and family in respectful, patient-centered dialogue.

The National Culturally and Linguistically Appropriate Services (CLAS) Standards are intended to advance health equity, improve quality, and help eliminate health care disparities by establishing a blueprint to help individuals and health care organizations implement culturally and linguistically appropriate services (Office of Minority Health [OMH], n.d.). The CLAS standards include standards for communication and language assistance. The standards apply when you are caring for patients who have limited English proficiency and/or other communication needs. All health care organizations must provide the following:

- Language assistance resources (e.g., trained medical interpreters, qualified translators, telecommunication devices for the deaf) for individuals who have limited English proficiency and/or other communication needs, at no cost to them, to facilitate timely access to all health care and services.
- Inform all individuals of the availability of language assistance services clearly and in their preferred language verbally and in writing.
- Ensure the competence of individuals providing language assistance. Do not use untrained individuals and/or minors as interpreters.
- Provide easy-to-understand print and multimedia materials and signage in the languages commonly used by the populations in the service area.

When you begin a cultural assessment there are some basic questions that can help you explore a patient's culture (Ball et al., 2015):

- What do you call your problem?
- What do you think caused it?
- Why do you think it started when it did?
- What does your sickness do to you?
- How long do you think it will last?
- How different is this problem from the one you had a month ago?
- What is the difference between what we are doing and what you think we should be doing for you?
- Why did you come to us for treatment?
- What benefit will you get from the treatment?
- How do you typically deal with a problem with your health?

BOX 21.5 CULTURAL ASSESSMENT GUIDE: ASPECTS OF UNDERSTANDING

HEALTH BELIEFS AND PRACTICES

- How does the patient define health and illness? How are feelings concerning pain, fatigue, and illness in general expressed?
- Are particular methods used for treatment of illness?
- What is the attitude toward preventive health measures such as immunizations?
- Are there restrictions imposed by modesty that must be respected (e.g., constraints related to exposure of parts of the body, discussion of sexual health)?
- What are attitudes toward mental illness, pain, chronic disease, being handicapped, and death and dying?
- Is there a person in the family responsible for health-related decisions?
- Does the patient prefer a health professional of the same gender, age, and ethnic and racial background?

FAITH-BASED INFLUENCES AND SPECIAL RITUALS

- Is there a religion or faith to which the patient adheres?
- Is there a significant person to whom the patient looks for guidance?
- What events, rituals, and ceremonies are important within the life cycle of birth, puberty, marriage, and death?

LANGUAGE AND COMMUNICATION

- What language is spoken in the home?
- How well does the patient understand spoken and written English?
- Are there special signs of demonstrating respect or disrespect?
- Is touch an acceptable form of communication?

PARENTING STYLES AND FAMILY ROLES

- Who makes the decisions in the family?
- What is the composition of the family? How many generations are considered to be a single family?
- What is the role of and attitude toward children in the family?
- When do children need to be disciplined or punished, and how is this done?
- Do family members show physical affection toward each other and their children?
- What major events are important to the family, and how do they celebrate?

SOURCES OF SUPPORT BEYOND THE FAMILY

- Are there ethnic organizations that may influence the patient's approach to health care?
- Are there individuals in the patient's social network that influence perception of health and illness?
- Is there a particular cultural group with which the patient identifies?

DIETARY PRACTICES

- What does the family like to eat? Does everyone in the family have similar tastes in food?
- Who is responsible for food preparation?
- Are any foods forbidden by the culture, or are some foods a cultural requirement in observance of a rite or ceremony?
- How is food prepared and eaten?
- Are there periods of required fasting?

Adapted from Ball JW, et al: *Seidel's guide to physical examination*, ed 8, St Louis, 2015, Elsevier.

Each question requires an open ended response, enabling you to gain important details about a patient's perceptions, values, and attitudes. A patient's answer to a question may allow you to explore his or her cultural background more thoroughly.

After realizing that Ms. Tatum needs help to better understand the types of foods that are appropriate for a diabetic diet, Marina refocuses her assessment on some basic questions. How do you think the foods that you eat affect your diabetes? What does diabetes do to you if your blood sugar becomes too high? What benefit will you get from eating healthy foods? Tell me what you eat during a typical day.

Culture influences how feelings are expressed verbally and nonverbally. Touch, facial expressions, eye contact, and movement and body posture all have varying significance. The questions in Box 21.5 can help provide further insight to particular situations and help avoid misunderstanding and miscommunication (Ball et al., 2015).

Assessing Health Literacy

Health literacy is the degree to which individuals have the capacity to obtain, process, and understand basic health information and the services needed to make appropriate health decisions (AHRQ, 2016a). Limited health literacy can be a problem for anyone. It is important to understand that

even people with good literacy skills find that understanding health care information is a challenge. Patients and family members often do not understand medical vocabulary and the basic concepts in health and medicine, such as how the body works or how to navigate the health care system. During your assessment, be alert for patient behaviors that might reflect a literacy deficit such as having difficulty completing registration forms or health histories, failing to make follow-up appointments, asking few questions during a physical examination, and responding simply "yes" when asked if explanations are understood.

Assessment tools to determine the level of a patient's health literacy include the following:

- The Short Assessment of Health Literacy–Spanish and English (SAHL-S&E) is a new instrument consisting of comparable tests in English and Spanish, with good reliability and validity in both languages (Lee et al., 2010).
- The Rapid Estimate of Adult Literacy in Medicine–Short Form (REALM-SF) is a seven-item word recognition test to provide clinicians with a valid quick assessment of patient health literacy (Arozullah et al., 2007). The REALM-SF has been validated and field tested in diverse research settings.

QSEN **QSEN ACTIVITY** *Safety*

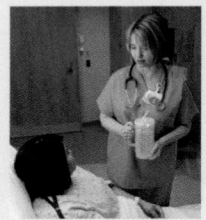

After teaching Ms. Tatum further about diabetes management, Marina finishes the conversation by asking, "Do you have any questions?" Ms. Tatum states that she does not.

- What is a more effective way to end this conversation to ensure that Ms. Tatum understands how to manage her disease with minimal complications? How could thinking about the impact of health literacy on patient safety allow Marina to provide the highest quality of care to Ms. Tatum?

evolve   Answers to QSEN Activities can be found on the Evolve website.

Assessing a patient's health literacy level is very important in planning appropriate patient education approaches (see Chapter 12).

Culturally Based Physical Assessment

In Chapter 16 you learned about the skills and techniques to use when performing a physical assessment. Knowledge about a patient directs your physical assessment. For example, if you know a patient has had diabetes for many years, you focus on the peripheral vascular examination because of the common incidence of circulatory problems in patients with diabetes. If a patient uses an asthma inhaler, you perform a more detailed assessment of the lungs compared with what you might do for a healthy patient you see during a routine checkup.

Similarly, you learn to anticipate physical findings based on a patient's cultural health practices and distinguish physical characteristics of an ethnic or racial group. For example, the practices of "coining" and "cupping" are commonly used by some Asian subcultures to release excess force from the body and restore balance (Ball et al., 2015). The practices leave imprints and markings on the skin that can be wrongly interpreted as signs of abuse or disease. Thus it is always important to ask patients about their home remedies and practices. Another example of anticipating findings is to consider sickle cell anemia when blood tests reveal laboratory values that show anemia in a patient of African descent. As you practice and become more knowledgeable of different ethnic groups in your practice, you will more readily recognize physical characteristics of conditions unique to those groups.

Teach-Back and Plain Language

Linguistic competence requires the application of health literacy principles in providing readily available, culturally appropriate oral and written language services to patients and families with limited English proficiency (AHRQ, 2013). The dual challenges of caring for patients with limited health literacy and cultural differences are likely to increase with an expanding, increasingly diverse, and older population. Evidence suggests that health care providers who attend to both issues help reduce medical errors and improve adherence, communication between provider and patient and family, and outcomes of care at both individual and population levels (Lie et al., 2012). Clear communication is essential for effective delivery of quality and safe health care, but most patients experience significant challenges when communicating with their health care providers. Studies have shown that 40% to 80% of the medical information given to patients during medical office visits is immediately forgotten, and nearly half of the information retained is incorrect (AHRQ, 2015).

The use of plain language in communicating with patients makes any information you are providing easy to read, understand, and use. Plain language is grammatically correct language that includes complete sentence structure and accurate word usage (National Institutes of Health [NIH], n.d.). It is not unprofessional writing or a method of "dumbing down" or "talking down" to a reader. You can find the following tips for writing in plain language on the website PlainLanguage.gov (http://www.plainlanguage.gov/index.cfm):

- "You" and other pronouns
- Active voice
- Short sentences
- Common, everyday words
- Easy-to-read design features

Offering patients clear instructions and using educational materials written in plain language tells a learner exactly what to know without using unnecessary words or expressions.

Use the teach-back method following any patient instruction to confirm that you have explained what a patient needs to know in a manner that the patient understands. The teach-back technique is an ongoing process of asking patients for feedback through explanation or demonstration and of presenting information in a new way until you feel confident that you communicated clearly and that your patient has a full understanding of the information presented (Fig. 21.4). When a family caregiver is the recipient of your instruction, use teach-back to confirm his or her learning. You also use teach-back to identify explanations and communication strategies your patients most commonly understand (AHRQ, 2015).

When using the teach-back technique do not ask a patient, "Do you understand?" or "Do you have any questions?" Instead ask open-ended questions to verify a patient's understanding.

- "I've given you a lot of information (e.g., about your insulin) to remember. Please explain it (e.g., how it affects your blood sugar) to me so that I can be sure that I gave you the information you want and need to take good care of yourself."
- "What will you tell your wife (or husband/partner/child) about the changes we made to your medications today?"
- "We've gone over a lot of information today about how you might change your diet, and I want to make sure I

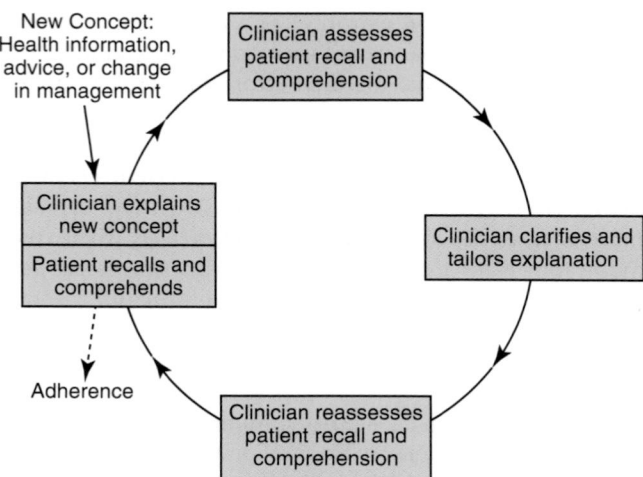

New Concept: Health information, advice, or change in management

Clinician assesses patient recall and comprehension

Clinician explains new concept

Patient recalls and comprehends

Clinician clarifies and tailors explanation

Adherence

Clinician reassesses patient recall and comprehension

FIG 21.4 Using teach-back technique to close the loop. (From the U.S. Health Resources and Services Administration.)

explained everything clearly. In your own words, please review what we talked about. How will you make it work at home?"

Teach-back is not intended to test a patient but rather to confirm the clarity of your communication (AHRQ, 2015). Many patients are embarrassed by their inability to sort out health information or instructions. By regarding teach-back as a test of your communication skills, you take responsibility for the success or failure of the interaction and create a shame-free environment for your patients. Following are helpful hints to consider when trying the teach-back method (AHRQ, 2015).

- Plan your approach. Think about how you will ask your patient to teach back in a shame-free way. Keep in mind that some situations are not appropriate for teach-back.
- Use handouts, pictures, and models to reinforce your teaching.
- "Chunk and check." Do not wait until the end of the visit to initiate teach-back. Chunk out information into small segments, and have the patient or family caregiver teach it back. Repeat several times during a visit.
- Clarify and check again. If teach-back uncovers a misunderstanding, explain things again using a different approach. Ask patients to teach-back again until they are able to correctly describe the information in their own words. If they parrot your words back to you, they may not have understood.
- Start slowly and use teach-back consistently. Practice. It will take a little time, but once it is part of your routine, teach-back can be done without awkwardness.
- Use the show-me method. When prescribing new medicines or changing a dose, research shows that even when patients correctly say when and how much medicine they will take, many will make mistakes when asked to demonstrate the dose.
- Clarify. If a patient cannot remember or accurately repeat your instructions, clarify your information, and allow him or her to teach it back again (see Fig. 21.4).

BOX 21.6 PATIENT TEACHING

Medication and Nutritional Adherence

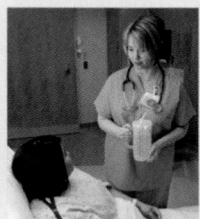

Marina knows it is important for Ms. Tatum to understand her health problems and prescribed treatments. Thus Marina plans to use teach-back to ensure Ms. Tatum understands how to effectively manage her diabetes.

OUTCOME

At the end of the teaching session, Ms. Tatum will be able to:
- Describe how she plans to make healthy food choices at the shelter and neighborhood store

TEACHING STRATEGIES
- Create a shame-free environment by demonstrating a general attitude of helpfulness.
- Use nonmedical language and define in plain language all medical terms.
- Sit instead of stand, and speak slowly.
- Use pictures, models, and written handouts to help Ms. Tatum better remember relevant information.
- Have Ms. Tatum prepare a meal plan.

EVALUATION
- Use the principles of teach-back to evaluate patient/family caregiver learning:
  - "What foods do you plan to include in a daily diet?"
  - "We've gone over a lot of information today about changes you plan to make to your diet. In your own words, please review what we talked about. How will you make it work for you?"

Although it takes time to get used to teach-back, studies show that it does not take longer to perform once it becomes a part of your routine (AHRQ, 2015). Box 21.6 provides an example of how Marina used some of these strategies to educate Ms. Tatum on how to take oral insulin and manage her diet.

Working With Interpreters

The National CLAS Standards (OMH, n.d.) ensure that qualified interpreters be provided to patients with limited English proficiency. The CLAS standards require you to notify patients both verbally and in writing of their rights to receive language assistance. If a health care setting does not have timely access to an interpreter, a more feasible option is the use of a telephone service, which provides an on-call trained interpreter connected by phone (Juckett and Unger, 2014). Ensure that interpreters are competent in medical terminology and understand issues of confidentiality and impartiality. Do not use a patient's family members to interpret for you or other health care providers. When you begin a patient interview with an interpreter present, you should speak in the first person ("I" statements), not the third person (e.g., "tell her," "he said"), and speak directly to the patient, as the interpreter functions as an inconspicuous translator for the conversation (Juckett and Unger, 2014). Have the interpreter sit next to or slightly behind the patient. Look at the patient instead of looking at the interpreter and speak in short sentences, then wait for the interpreter to convey them (Juckett and Unger, 2014). Avoid using jargon, acronyms, and jokes; attempts at humor are often lost in interpretation. Ask the patient for feedback and clarification at regular intervals. Be observant of the patient's nonverbal and verbal behaviors. At the end of a conversation thank both the patient and the interpreter.

CULTURAL ENCOUNTER

In every health care setting you will directly interact with patients from culturally diverse backgrounds. This interaction is a cultural encounter, which has two goals (Campinha-Bacote, 2011). One goal is to communicate in a way that generates a wide variety of responses and to send and receive both verbal and nonverbal communication accurately and appropriately in each culturally different context. The second goal is to continuously interact with patients from culturally diverse backgrounds to validate, refine, or modify existing values, beliefs, and practices about a cultural group.

CULTURAL DESIRE

Engaging with people we perceive as "different" from us can be threatening and difficult. It generally takes more effort and patience than engaging with patients who are more similar to us. Cultural desire refers to having the motivation to engage patients so that you can understand them from a cultural perspective. It is the pivotal and key construct of cultural competence, for it is a nurse's desire that evokes the entire process of cultural competence (Campinha-Bacote, 2003). Cultural desire involves the concept of caring (see Chapter 20). Establishing a caring relationship with a patient requires you to enter into the patient's world view. Cultural desire includes a genuine passion to be open and flexible with others, to accept differences and build on similarities, and to be willing to learn from others as cultural informants (Campinha-Bacote, 2003).

You will care for patients who display behaviors that may be in direct moral conflict with your values (e.g., abortion, substance abuse, spouse abuse). For example, you are asked to care for a young male gang member whose beliefs about violence and respect for life are in direct contrast to yours. Yet you care for this patient nonjudgmentally and with respect. Acquiring the willingness to practice cultural desire requires a respect and acceptance of all human beings. The LEARN Model (Campinha-Bacote, 2003) can assist with this process. The mnemonic *LEARN* represents the process of listening, explaining, acknowledging, recommending, and negotiating:

- *Listen* to the patient's perception of the problem. Be nonjudgmental and use encouraging comments such as, "Tell me more" or "I understand what you are saying."
- *Explain* your perception of the problem.
- *Acknowledge* not only the differences between the two perceptions of the problem but also the similarities. Recognize the differences, but build on the similarities.

- *Recommendations* must involve the patient.
- *Negotiate* a treatment plan, considering that it is beneficial to incorporate selected aspects of the patient's culture into the plan.

Applying the LEARN mnemonic will help you to reflect at each patient encounter. You recognize that each patient is unique, but you are responsible for understanding what "unique" truly means so that you can engage patients in a patient-centered approach to care.

KEY POINTS

- Cultural competence is necessary for a nurse to provide patient-centered care.
- A health disparity that involves differences in the burden of disease, injury, violence, or opportunities to achieve optimal health experienced by socially disadvantaged groups is preventable.
- Health care systems and providers contribute to the problem of health disparities as a result of inadequate resources, poor patient-provider communication, a lack of culturally competent care, system fragmentation, and inadequate access to language services.
- Oppression occurs on many levels—individual, cultural, and institutional. It has a profound effect on the individual and group experiences of people living in oppression.
- Cultural awareness self-examines the dynamics of your own race, ethnicity, and culture and is necessary so that you can gain knowledge about and appreciate the diversity of patients from different cultures.
- Cultural desire is the pivotal and key construct of cultural competence. It is your desire to engage with patients who have cultural differences that evokes the entire process of cultural competence.
- People who are marginalized are more likely to have poor health outcomes and to die at an early age because of a complex interaction between individual behaviors, public and health policy, cultural factors, and quality of health care.
- Teach-back is an ongoing process of asking patients for feedback through explanation or demonstration and of presenting information in a new way until you feel confident that you communicated clearly.
- A person's culture and life experiences shape his or her world view about health, illness, and health care.

REFLECTIVE LEARNING

Before your next clinical assignment when you are assigned to a patient with a different cultural background from your own, spend some time with self-examination. Ask yourself these questions:

- How do you perceive this patient?
- Are you aware of your biases?
- What do you know about the patient's culture, and how different is it from your own?

REVIEW QUESTIONS

1. Which of the following is an example of a health disparity? (Select all that apply.)
   1. A patient who has a homosexual sexual preference
   2. A patient unable to access primary care services
   3. Patients living with a chronic disease
   4. A family who relies on public transportation
   5. A patient who has had a history of smoking for 10 years

2. A 35-year-old woman has Medicaid coverage for herself and 2 young children. She missed an appointment at the local health clinic to get an annual mammogram because she has no transportation. She gets the annual screening because her mother had breast cancer. Which of the following are social determinants of this woman's health? (Select all that apply.)
   1. Medicaid insurance
   2. Annual screening
   3. Mother's history of breast cancer
   4. Lack of transportation
   5. Woman's age

3. During a nursing assessment a patient displayed several behaviors. Which behavior suggests the patient may have a health literacy problem?
   1. Patient has difficulty completing a registration form at a medical office
   2. Patient asks for written information about a health topic
   3. Patient speaks Spanish as primary language
   4. Patient states unfamiliarity with a newly ordered medicine

4. Health care organizations must provide which of the following based on Federal civil rights laws? (Select all that apply.)
   1. Provide language assistance services at all points of contact free of charge
   2. Provide auxiliary aids and services, such as interpreters, note takers, and computer-aided transcription services
   3. Use patients' family members to interpret difficult topics
   4. Ensure that interpreters are competent in medical terminology
   5. Provide language assistance to all patients who speak limited English or are deaf

5. Match the cultural concepts on the left with the correct definitions on the right.
   1. _____ Etic world view
   2. _____ World view
   3. _____ Cultural desire
   4. _____ Intersectionality
   5. _____ Emic world view

   a. Factor that shapes how people perceive others and how they relate to reality
   b. Insider's perspective in an intercultural encounter
   c. A policy model that describes factors and power structures that shape and influence life
   d. An outsider's perspective in an intercultural encounter
   e. The motivation of a health care professional to "want to" engage in cultural competency

evolve

Additional Review Questions, as well as rationales for all Review Questions, can be found on the Evolve website.

1, 2, 3, 5; 2, 1, 4, 5; 3, 1; 4, 1, 2, 4, 5; 5, 1d, 2a, 3e, 4c, 5b.

REFERENCES

Adams M, et al: *Teaching for diversity and social justice*, ed 2, New York, 2007, Routledge.

Agency for Healthcare Research and Quality (AHRQ): *What is cultural and linguistic competence*, 2013, http://www.ahrq.gov/professionals/systems/primary-care/cultural-competence-mco/cultcompdef.html.

Agency for Healthcare Research and Quality (AHRQ): *Health literacy universal precautions toolkit*; 2015. ed 2, http://www.ahrq.gov/professionals/quality-patient-safety/quality-resources/tools/literacy-toolkit/index.html.

Agency for Healthcare Research and Quality (AHRQ): *Health literacy measurement tools (revised)*, 2016a. http://www.ahrq

.gov/professionals/quality-patient-safety/quality-resources/tools/literacy/index.html.

Agency for Healthcare Research and Quality (AHRQ): *2015 National Healthcare Quality and Disparities Report and 5th Anniversary Update on the National Quality Strategy*; 2016b. http://www.ahrq.gov/research/

findings/nhqrdr/nhqdr15/index
.html.

American Medical Association (AMA):
*Health literacy and patient safety: help
patients understand*, 2007. Chicago,
American Medical Association
Foundation.

Arozullah AM, et al: Development and
validation of a short-form, rapid
estimate of adult literacy in medicine,
Med Care 45:1026, 2007.

Ball JW, et al: *Seidel's guide to physical
examination*, ed 8, St Louis, 2015,
Elsevier.

Campinha-Bacote J: Many faces: addressing
diversity in health care, *Online J Issues
Nurs* 8(1):2003. www.nursingworld.org/
MainMenuCategories/ANAMarketplace/
ANAPeriodicals/OJIN/TableofContents/
Volume82003/No1Jan2003/
AddressingDiversityinHealthCare.aspx.

Campinha-Bacote J: Delivering patient-
centered care in the midst of a cultural
conflict: the role of cultural competence,
Online J Issues Nurs 16(2):5, 2011.

Centers for Disease Control and Prevention
(CDC): CDC health disparities and
inequalities report—United States, 2013,
MMWR Morb Mortal Wkly Rep 62(Suppl
3):1, 2013. http://www.cdc.gov/mmwr/
pdf/other/su6203.pdf.

Centers for Disease Control and Prevention
(CDC): *Health literacy*; 2015. http://
www.cdc.gov/healthliteracy/learn/
understandingliteracy.html.

Centers for Medicare and Medicaid (CMS):
Core measures; 2016. https://www.cms.gov/
Medicare/Quality-Initiatives-Patient
-Assessment-Instruments/QualityMeasures/
Core-Measures.html.

Chavez AF, Guido-DiBrito F: *Racial and
ethnic identity, new directions for adult
and continuing education*, no. 84, Winter
1999, Jossey-Bass Publishers.

Colby SL, Ortman JM: *Projections of the size
and composition of the U.S. population:
2014 to 2060*, US Census Bureau, March
2015, https://www.census.gov/content/
dam/Census/library/publications/2015/
demo/p25-1143.pdf.

Conrad P, Barker K: The social construction
of illness, *J Health Soc Behav* 51(1):S67,
2010.

Edelstein S: *Food, cuisine and cultural
competency for culinary, hospitality and
healthcare professionals*, Sudbury, MA,
2011, Jones & Bartlett.

Gucciardi E, et al: Designing and delivering
facilitated storytelling interventions for
chronic disease self-management: a

scoping review, *BMC Health Serv Res*
16:249, 2016.

Helms JE: Black and white racial identity:
theory, research, and practice. In
*Contributions in Afro-American and
African studies*, New York, NY, 1990,
Greenwood Press. No. 129.

Houston TK, et al: Culturally appropriate
storytelling to improve blood pressure:
a randomized trial, *Ann Intern Med*
154(2):77, 2011.

Institute for Intersectionality Research and
Policy: *Intersectionality*, 2016, https://
www.sfu.aaca/iirp/aboutus.html.

Institute of Medicine (IOM): *Crossing the
quality chasm: a new health system for
the 21st century*, Washington DC, 2001,
National Academy of Sciences, National
Academies Press.

Juckett G, Unger K: Appropriate use of
medical interpreters, *Am Fam Physician*
90(7):476, 2014.

Lee SD, et al: Short assessment of health
literacy—Spanish and English: a
comparable test of health literacy for
Spanish and English speakers, *Health
Serv Res* 45(4):1105, 2010.

Lie D, et al: What do health literacy and
cultural competence have in common?
Calling for a collaborative health
professional pedagogy, *J Health
Commun* 17:13, 2012.

Moskowitz GB, et al: Implicit stereotyping
and medical decisions: unconscious
stereotype activation in practitioners'
thoughts about African Americans,
Am J Public Health 102(5):996,
2012.

Mutha S, et al: *Bringing equity into quality
improvement: an overview and
opportunities ahead*; 2012. San Francisco,
Healthforce Center at UCSF.

National Center for Education Statistics
(NCES): *The health literacy of America's
adults: results from the 2003 National
Assessment of Adult Literacy*, Washington,
DC, 2006, US Department of Education,
http://nces.ed.gov/pubsearch/
pubsinfo.asp?pubid=2006483.

National Institutes of Health (NIH): *Plain
language at NIH*; n.d.. https://www
.nih.gov/institutes-nih/nih-office
-director/office-communications
-public-liaison/clear-communication/
plain-language.

National Quality Forum (NQF): *Disparities*;
2016. http://www.qualityforum.org/
Topics/Disparities.aspx.

Office of Disease Prevention and Health
Promotion (ODPHP): *Disparities*; 2016.

https://www.healthypeople.gov/2020/
about/foundation-health-measures/
Disparities.

Office of Minority Health (OMH), US
Department of Health and Human
Services (USDHHS): *Think cultural
health: CLAS and continuing education*;
n.d.. https://www.thinkculturalhealth
.hhs.gov/index.asp.

Pew Research Center: *5 key takeaways about
views of race and inequality in America*;
2016. http://www.pewresearch.org/fact
-tank/2016/01/18/5-facts-about
-race-in-america/.

Purnell LD: *Transcultural health care: a
culturally competent approach*, ed 4,
Philadelphia, 2013, FA Davis.

Substance Abuse and Mental Health
Services Administration (SAMHSA):
Improving cultural competence;
2014. Treatment Improvement
Protocol (TIP) Series No. 59. HHS
Publication No. (SMA) 14-4849.
Rockville, MD, Substance Abuse
and Mental Health Services
Administration.

Terkildsen MD, Wittrup I: Negotiating
experience in patient involvement—
challenges of practicing storytelling in
health care conversations, *Tidsskrift for
Forskning i Sygdom og Samfund, nr*
22:45–65, 2015.

The Joint Commission (TJC): *Core measure
sets*, Chicago, 2016, TJC. http://www
.jointcommission.org/core_measure
_sets.aspx.

Transcultural C.A.R.E. Associates: *The
process of cultural competence in the
delivery of healthcare services*; 2015.
http://transculturalcare.net/the-process
-of-cultural-competence-in-the
-delivery-of-healthcare-services/.

United Health Foundation: *America's annual
report health rankings*; 2015. http://
assets.americashealthrankings.org/app/
uploads/2015ahr_annual-v1.pdf.

Walker RL, et al: Ethnic group differences
in reasons for living and the moderating
role of cultural worldview, *Cultur Divers
Ethnic Minor Psychol* 16(3):372,
2010.

Wilson DK, et al: *Exploring the role of digital
storytelling in pediatric oncology patients'
perspectives regarding diagnosis*; February
17, 2015. *Sage Open*, http://sgo.sagepub
.com/content/5/1/2158244015572099.

World Health Organization: *Social
determinants of health*; 2016. http://
www.who.int/social_determinants/
sdh_definition/en/index.html.

CHAPTER

22

Spiritual Health

evolve MEDIA RESOURCES

http://evolve.elsevier.com/Potter/essentials

- Audio Glossary
- QSEN Activity and Review Questions Answers and Rationales

OBJECTIVES

- Describe the relationship among faith, hope, and spiritual well-being.
- Compare and contrast the concepts of religion and spirituality.
- Discuss the relationship of spirituality to an individual's total being.
- Assess a patient's spirituality and spiritual health.
- Discuss nursing interventions designed to promote spiritual health.
- Establish presence with patients.
- Evaluate how patients attain spiritual health.

KEY TERMS

agnostic, p. 580
atheist, p. 580
connectedness, p. 586
faith, p. 580

holistic, p. 578
hope, p. 581
self-transcendence, p. 579
spiritual distress, p. 581

spiritual well-being, p. 580
spirituality, p. 578
transcendence, p. 579

The word *spirituality* comes from the Latin word *spiritus,* which refers to breath or wind. The spirit gives life to a person. It signifies whatever is at the center of all aspects of a person's life. **Spirituality** is an awareness of one's inner self and a sense of connection to a Supreme Being, nature, or some purpose greater than oneself. It includes personal beliefs that help a person maintain hope and get through difficult situations (March and Caple, 2016). A person's health depends on a balance of physical, psychological, sociological, cultural, emotional, developmental, and spiritual variables. This **holistic** view of health is the focus and heart of nursing practice. Spiritual care is often an overlooked part of nursing; however, the spiritual dimension does not exist in isolation from our physical and psychological being (Collins-McNeil et al., 2015). Spirituality is an important factor that helps people achieve the balance needed to maintain health

and well-being and to cope with illness. Current evidence shows that spirituality positively affects health, quality of life, health promotion behaviors, and disease prevention activities (Conway-Phillips and Janusek, 2014; Jones et al., 2015).

Nurses and other health care providers often fail to recognize the spiritual dimension of human nature. In addition, some health care providers do not believe in God or a Supreme Being or believe that they do not have time to address spiritual needs. Frequently people think of the concepts of spirituality and religion interchangeably, but spirituality is a much broader and more unifying concept than religion (Dahlkemper, 2016; Carson, 2017). Florence Nightingale believed that spirituality is a force that provides energy needed in a healthy hospital environment. She also believed that caring for a person's spiritual needs is just as important as caring for his or her physical needs (O'Brien, 2014).

CASE STUDY *Victoria Timms*

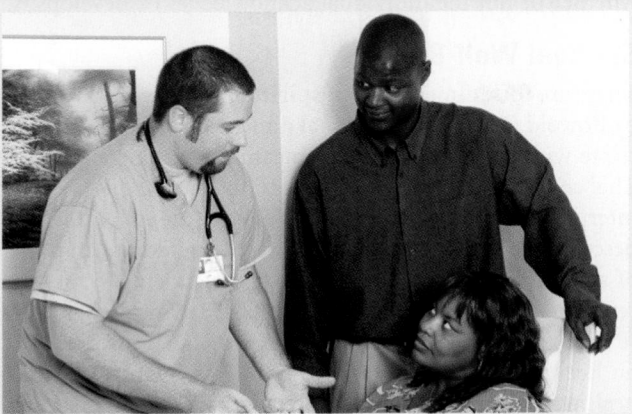

Victoria Timms is a 44-year-old nurse manager who was diagnosed 3 months ago with breast cancer. She is married to Joe, an accountant, and is the mother of two children: Davis, who is 17 years old, and Pamela, who is 15. Victoria describes her family as being very close and supportive. Surgeons removed Victoria's cancerous tumor and two involved lymph nodes. Because of the lymphatic involvement, Victoria is at increased risk for the cancer to spread. Victoria has completed a course of radiation and now visits the local cancer clinic with her husband three times a week for chemotherapy treatments. Both Victoria and Joe discuss their concern for their children. Davis and Pamela attend young adult education and prayer meetings weekly. Davis, a senior in high school, is beginning to look at colleges for next year. Davis and Pamela shared with Victoria that they are very worried about her cancer diagnosis and health.

Jeff is a 38-year-old student nurse assigned to the oncology clinic. Jeff's preceptor, a nursing case manager, assigns Jeff to follow Victoria during her clinic visits. Jeff is in his last semester at school and hopes to get a position in the clinic after graduation. Victoria's experience is significant for Jeff because he has children who are the same age as Victoria's and he wonders how his children would react if he or his spouse became ill.

During one of their clinic visits Victoria and Joe appear very calm and relaxed when discussing cancer therapy. Joe explains, "We both have a lot of faith in God." Victoria responds, "Even though I know I have cancer, I hope to be able to continue to go to church with my family and my children. My family is very supportive, and together I know that we'll make it through this experience. But I'm worried about my children. With God's help, I can help them cope with my illness better."

The human spirit is powerful, and spirituality has different meanings for different people. Your personal spiritual health is important to your values and beliefs and can influence your attitudes toward spiritual care, professional commitment, and caring (Chiang et al., 2016). Therefore you need to understand your own spirituality to integrate spirituality into your patients' care. Nursing care involves helping patients use their spiritual resources as they identify and explore what is meaningful in their lives and find ways to cope with illness and stressors of life (Ramezani et al., 2014).

SCIENTIFIC KNOWLEDGE BASE

The relationship between spirituality and health is not fully understood. However, people often are healthier when they believe in a higher power. Current evidence shows a link connecting the mind, body, and spirit. The biopsychosocial-spiritual model shows the interconnectedness between the body, mind, and spirit. The model provides a holistic approach to caring for patients and includes spirituality as an important factor impacting health and illness (Mark and Lyons, 2014). An individual's beliefs and expectations often have effects on his or her physical and psychological well-being. Many individuals use spiritual and religious practices as a way to cope with illness (Trevino and McConnell, 2015). For example, engagement in prayer, reading of scripture, and meditation increased a sense of empowerment leading to improved mental health (Hipolito et al., 2014). Laughter has a positive effect on life satisfaction, anxiety, mood, and pain reduction (Gilbert, 2014). A person's inner beliefs and convictions are powerful resources for healing. Positive emotions such as joy, interest, contentment, pride, and love help individuals flourish by building on their physical, psychological, and social resources and lead to resiliency and improved emotional well-being (Fredrickson, 2001). As a nurse, you will be more successful in helping patients achieve desirable health outcomes after learning to support patients and their families spiritually.

NURSING KNOWLEDGE BASE

Current research supports the link between spirituality and health. Thus it is important for you to understand spiritual health and the concepts of spirituality, spiritual well-being, faith, religion, and hope to provide supportive spiritual care.

Spirituality

Definitions of spirituality differ. However, experts agree that it is complex and diverse (Timmins et al., 2014; March and Caple, 2016). It is unique for each individual and exists in everyone, regardless of religious beliefs. Our culture, development, life experiences, beliefs, and ideas about life influence our definition of spirituality. Spirituality exists in all people, regardless of their religious beliefs; it gives people the *energy* needed to maintain health and cope with difficult situations. Current definitions of spirituality include five distinct but overlapping constructs (Fig. 22.1).

Self-transcendence refers to connecting to your inner self, which allows one to go beyond oneself to understand the meanings of experiences. For example, people with a high level of self-transcendence feel a connectedness to other living beings and the environment. In contrast, **transcendence** is the belief that there is a positive force outside of and greater than oneself that allows one to develop new perspectives that are beyond physical boundaries (Hatamipour et al.,

Spirituality

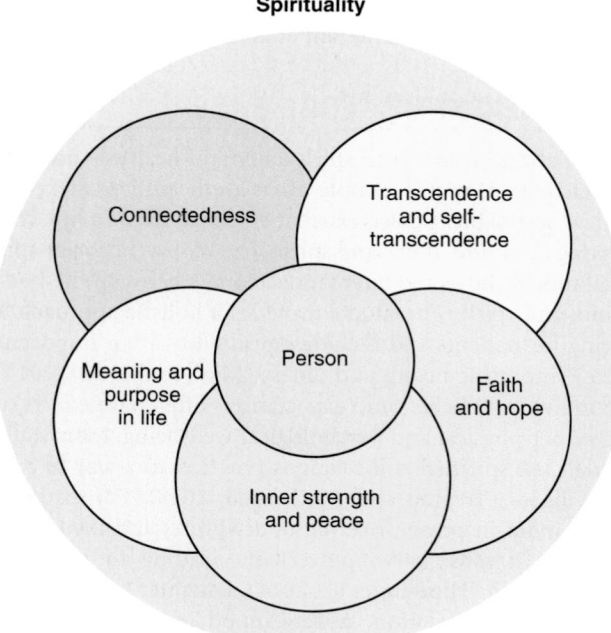

FIG 22.1 The concept of spirituality has five distinct but overlapping constructs.

2015). Examples of transcendent moments include the feeling of awe when holding a new baby or watching the sun rise over the mountains. Spirituality offers a sense of *connectedness* intrapersonally (connected with oneself), interpersonally (connected with others and the environment), and transpersonally (connected with God, the unseen, or a higher power). Through connectedness patients are able to move beyond the stressors of everyday life and find comfort, faith, hope, peace, and empowerment (Hakanson and Ohlen, 2016). *Inner strength* is an energy source that instills hope, provides motivation, and promotes a positive outlook on life even during difficult times. *Inner peace* fosters calm and positive feelings despite life experiences of chaos, fear, and uncertainty (Viglund et al., 2014). These feelings help people feel comforted and find peace even in times of great distress (Hatamipour et al., 2015). Finally, spirituality helps people find *meaning and purpose in life* in both negative and positive life events (Dobratz, 2016).

Spirituality is an important concept for individuals who either do not believe in the existence of God (**atheist**) or who believe that any ultimate reality is unknown or unknowable (**agnostic**). Atheists search for meaning in life through their work and relationships with others. It is important for agnostics to discover meaning in what they do or how they live because they find no ultimate meaning for the way things are. They believe that we, as people, bring meaning to what we do.

Spirituality is an integrating theme in life. A person's concept of spirituality begins in childhood and continues to grow throughout adulthood (Johnston Taylor et al., 2015). Spirituality represents the totality of one's being, serving as the overriding perspective that unifies the various aspects of an individual. It spreads throughout the physiological,

psychological, and sociocultural dimensions of a person's life, whether or not the individual acknowledges or develops it.

Spiritual Well-Being

There are four dimensions of **spiritual well-being** as defined by Rowold (2011). The personal dimension refers to how you relate with yourself in finding meaning and purpose in life. The communal dimension relates to the quality of your interpersonal relationships. The environmental dimension describes how you interact in the world, including your sense of awe with the environment. The transcendental dimension refers to the relationship between you and some higher power (e.g., God, Buddha). Spiritual well-being has a positive effect on health and leads to spiritual health. If you are spiritually healthy, you experience joy, forgive yourself and others, accept hardship and mortality, experience enhanced quality of life, and have a positive sense of physical and emotional well-being (Rowold, 2011; Cottrell, 2016).

Faith

In addition to being a part of the definition of spirituality, the concept of **faith** has other common definitions. Faith allows a person to have firm beliefs about something despite the lack of physical evidence. Although many associate faith with religious beliefs, faith can exist without them (O'Brien, 2014). Faith is a cultural or institutional religion such as Buddhism, Christianity, or Islam. It also is a relationship with a divinity, higher power, authority, or spirit that incorporates a reasoning faith (belief) and a trusting faith (action). Reasoning faith is a person's belief and confidence in something for which there is no proof. It is an acceptance of what our reasoning cannot explain. Sometimes it involves a belief in a higher power, spirit guide, God, or Allah. Faith also is how a person chooses to live life. In this sense it enables action. Patients who are ill frequently have a positive outlook on life and continue to participate in daily activities rather than resigning themselves to the symptoms of their disease. In these cases a patient's faith often becomes stronger because illness is viewed as an opportunity for personal growth (Granero-Molina et al., 2014). *For example, in the case study, Victoria is living with breast cancer. She has faith; thus she has a positive outlook on life and continues to complete daily activities rather than giving into the symptoms caused by her breast cancer. Her faith becomes stronger because she views her cancer as an opportunity for growth.*

Religion

Religion is associated with the "state of doing," or a specific system of practices associated with a particular denomination, sect, or form of worship. Religion refers to the system of organized beliefs and worship that a person practices to outwardly express spirituality. Many people practice a faith or belief in the doctrines of a specific religion or sect such as the Lutheran church within Christianity or Orthodox Judaism. People from different religions view spirituality differently. For example, a Buddhist believes in Four Noble Truths: life is suffering, suffering is caused by clinging, suffering can be eliminated by eliminating clinging, and to eliminate clinging and suffering one follows an eightfold path. The path includes the right understanding, intention, speech, action, livelihood, effort, mindfulness, and concentration. This path promotes wisdom, moral behavior, and meditation. A Buddhist turns inward, valuing self-control, whereas a Christian looks to the love of God to provide enlightenment and direction in life.

When providing spiritual care to patients, you need to know the differences between religion and spirituality. Although closely related, these terms are not synonymous. Religious care helps patients follow their belief systems and worship practices. Spiritual care helps people maintain personal relationships and a relationship with a Supreme Being or life force to identify meaning and purpose in life.

Hope

Spirituality and faith bring hope. When a person has the attitude of living for and looking forward to something, hope is present. Hope is multidimensional and gives comfort while a person endures hardship and personal challenges. It usually refers to a source of energy that helps a person plan and achieve goals (Griggs and Walker, 2016) and is used by patients to sustain themselves during illness (Dunn, 2016). It is closely associated with faith. It is energizing, giving individuals a motivation to achieve and the resources to use toward that achievement. People express hope in all aspects of their lives as a force that helps them deal with life stressors. It is a valuable personal resource and brings comfort when people face a loss (see Chapter 27) or a challenge that seems difficult to achieve (Griggs and Walker, 2016).

Spiritual Health

People gain spiritual health by finding a balance between their life values, goals, and belief systems and their relationships within themselves and with others. Throughout life a person sometimes grows more spiritual, becoming increasingly aware of the meaning, purpose, and values of life. In times of stress, illness, loss, or recovery, a person often turns to previous ways of responding or adjusting to a situation. Often these coping styles lie within the person's spiritual beliefs.

Spiritual beliefs change as people grow and develop (Table 22.1). Spirituality begins as children learn about themselves and their relationships with others. When you understand a child's spiritual beliefs, it is easier to care for and comfort the child (Darby et al., 2014; Johnston Taylor et al., 2015). As children mature into adulthood, they experience spiritual growth by entering into lifelong relationships. An ability to care meaningfully for others and self is evidence of a healthy spirituality. A majority of older adults describe themselves as spiritual and often turn to important relationships and give themselves to others (Touhy and Jett, 2018).

THE EFFECT OF ILLNESS ON SPIRITUALITY

When illness, loss, grief, or a major life change affects a person, spiritual resources help the person move to recovery.

Without spiritual resources, concerns and doubts develop within an individual. Spiritual distress is "a state of suffering related to the impaired ability to experience and integrate meaning and purpose in life through connectedness with self, others, art, music, literature, nature, and/or a power greater than oneself" (NANDA International, 2014). Spiritual distress causes doubt, a loss of faith, and a sense of feeling alone or abandoned. Individuals question their spiritual values, raising questions about their way of life and purpose for living. Spiritual distress also occurs when there is conflict between a person's beliefs and a prescribed health treatment plan or the inability to practice usual rituals.

Acute Illness

Sudden, unexpected illness that threatens a patient's life, health, and/or well-being creates significant spiritual distress. For example, an older man who has a heart attack and a young adult who is injured in a motor vehicle accident both face crises that threaten their spiritual health. The illness or injury creates an unanticipated scramble to integrate and cope with new realities (e.g., disability). People look for ways to remain faithful to their beliefs and value systems through use of spiritual resources. Often conflicts develop around a person's beliefs and the meaning of life. Anger is common; sometimes patients express it against God, their families, themselves, and their nurses or other health care providers. The strength of patients' spirituality influences their ability to cope with and recover from sudden illness. Having a better understanding of your patients' illnesses and conditions helps you spiritually support them (Sweat, 2015). You play a key role in helping patients resolve feelings of spiritual distress. You create a healing environment and maximize recovery by enhancing their spiritual well-being (Estores and Frye, 2015).

Chronic Illness

Patients with chronic illnesses often experience debilitating symptoms that permanently change their lifestyles. The uncertain and long-term nature of chronic illness and the potential for outcomes such as pain, changes in body image, and the need to confront death all lead to spiritual distress. Patients struggle with questions about the meaning and purpose of their lives because their independence is threatened, which often causes fear, anxiety, and powerlessness. The nursing diagnosis *Spiritual Distress* is appropriate to use for patients who experience these symptoms. A person's spirituality is a significant factor in how he or she adapts to the changes resulting from chronic illness. Successfully adapting to these changes strengthens a person spiritually, but it sometimes takes a long-term plan to help a patient with a chronic illness achieve spiritual well-being. As a nurse, you are in a unique position to help patients reevaluate their lives and achieve spiritual health (Box 22.1). Patients who have a sense of spiritual well-being are often better able to cope with their illnesses and experience enhanced quality of life (Carron, 2016). Exploring the meaning of pain and suffering with patients allows you to spiritually support them during their illnesses (Sweat, 2015).

TABLE 22.1   RELATIONSHIP BETWEEN DEVELOPMENTAL STAGE AND SPIRITUAL BELIEFS

ERICKSON'S DEVELOPMENTAL STAGE	SPIRITUAL BELIEFS
Trust vs. mistrust—birth to 18 months	Spiritual well-being provided by parents Trust provides basis for hope Love, affection, security, and a stimulating environment promote spirituality
Autonomy vs. shame and doubt—18 to 36 months	Fascination with magic and mystery Often believes that illness is related to bad behavior Begins to learn difference between right and wrong Imitates parents' spiritual or religious actions; recites prayers and sings simple religious songs, but does not understand their meanings Interprets meanings literally
Initiative vs. guilt—3 to 6 years	Feels guilty when not acting responsibly Influenced by spiritual and religious stories, examples, moods, and actions Models moral behaviors of parents Begins to ask about God or Supreme Being
Industry vs. inferiority—6 to 12 years	Wants to learn about spirituality Has a clear picture of God or Supreme Being, morality, and difference between right and wrong Sorts fantasy from fact Demands proof of reality and believes literal meanings of spiritual stories
Identity vs. identity confusion—adolescence (12-18 years of age)	Reflects on inconsistencies in stories Begins to question spiritual practices, forms own opinions, and occasionally discards parents' beliefs Abstract reasoning leads to exploration of moral issues Spirituality comes from connectedness with family, nature, and God or Supreme Being
Intimacy vs. isolation and loneliness—young adulthood (18-35 years of age)	Establishes self-identity and world view Forms independent beliefs, attitudes, and lifestyles Uses principles to solve problems when individual's and society's rules conflict
Generativity vs. stagnation—middle-age adulthood (35-65 years of age)	Develops appreciation of past spiritual experiences Embraces people from different faiths and religions Reviews value system during crisis Values others
Ego identity vs. despair and disgust—older adulthood (65 years of age and older)	Values love and interactions with others Focuses on overcoming oppression and violence Beliefs vary based on many factors such as gender, past experiences, religion, economic status, and ethnic background

Data from Edelman CL, Mandle CL: *Health promotion throughout the life span,* ed 8, St Louis, 2014, Elsevier; and Hockenberry MJ, Wilson D: *Wong's nursing care of infants and children,* ed 10, St Louis, 2015, Elsevier.

Terminal Illness

Terminal illness commonly causes fears of physical pain, isolation, the unknown, and dying. When patients feel uncertain about what death means, they are susceptible to spiritual distress. Spirituality helps patients and families find resolution and peace by helping them prepare for and accept death (Petersen, 2014). Individuals experiencing a terminal illness often find themselves reviewing their life and questioning its meaning. Common questions they ask may include, "Why is this happening to me?" or "What have I done?" Terminal illness affects family and friends just as much as the patient. It causes members of the family to ask important questions about the meaning of life and how the illness will affect their relationship with the patient (see Chapter 27).

When caring for dying patients, help them gain a greater sense of control over their illness, whether they are in a health care setting (e.g., the hospital) or at home. Dying is a holistic process encompassing the patient's physical, social, psychological, and spiritual health (Petersen, 2014; Finocchiaro, 2016).

Near-Death Experience

You may care for a patient or have a family member who has had a near-death experience (NDE). NDE is a psychological phenomenon in which people have either been close to clinical death or recovered after being declared dead. It is not associated with a mental disorder. Experts agree that NDE describes a powerfully close brush with physical, emotional, and spiritual death. For example, people who have an NDE after cardiopulmonary arrest often tell the same story of feeling themselves rising above their bodies and watching caregivers initiate lifesaving measures. Commonly patients

BOX 22.1 EVIDENCE-BASED PRACTICE

PICO Question: Does the use of spiritual care interventions improve patient outcomes?

SUMMARY OF EVIDENCE

Nursing care for patients needs to focus on mind, body, and spirit. It is important to include spiritual interventions in a patient's plan of care that will help to relieve spiritual distress and enhance spiritual well-being (Abuatiq, 2015). Providing spiritual care to patients helps a patient cope with illness and therapies (Trevino and McConnell, 2015). Researchers have found that spiritual interventions help decrease anxiety and reduce depression in patients with cancer (Pantuso, 2015). Spiritual interventions have also been found to contribute to spiritual well-being, improved psychological adaptation, and improved satisfaction for patients (Ramezani et al., 2014). Spiritual counseling, which includes praying with a patient, religious-specific rituals, and visits from pastoral care, had a positive effect on quality of life in patients with heart failure (Tadwalkar et al., 2014). Before providing spiritual care to patients it is important for nurses to assess for patients' cues to respect patient beliefs and autonomy (Johnston Taylor et al., 2014).

APPLICATION TO NURSING PRACTICE

- Use active listening and therapeutic communication to develop rapport with your patients (Ramezani et al., 2014).
- Offer to pray or read scripture with patients (Tadwalkar et al., 2014).
- Turn on the patient's favorite religious music station or television channel (Abuatiq, 2015).
- Conduct a spiritual assessment or history for each of your patients (Pantuso, 2015).
- Be nonjudgmental in your assessment and care of patients, showing respect for each patient's spiritual beliefs (Ramezani et al., 2014).
- Offer to contact pastoral care or the chaplain for the patient (Abuatiq, 2015).

BOX 22.2 SYNTHESIS IN PRACTICE

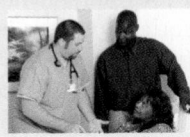

Jeff plans for Victoria and Joe's return to the oncology clinic. He spends time learning more about Victoria's disease and treatment plan so that he is able to explain what to expect as chemotherapy progresses. Jeff knows that Joe usually comes to the clinic, and Victoria describes him as a strong source of support. However, Jeff does not know enough about the couple's relationship and wants to explore this further. The role of family members in providing support, particularly regarding decision making, is important for Jeff to understand before he develops a plan of care. In reviewing information about loss and grieving, Jeff recognizes that Victoria shows acceptance of her disease because she is able to discuss cancer and the plan for treatment. Jeff knows that as patients begin to accept the diagnosis of a life-threatening disease, it is important to offer opportunities to share feelings and discuss future plans.

Jeff's previous experiences with patients who have cancer taught him that when patients express hope, they move forward and cope better with the challenges of their disease. During the last clinic visit Victoria stated that she hoped she would be able to continue to attend religious services at her church. Jeff reflected on that experience and thinks that Victoria and Joe have a strong sense of spiritual well-being that will help them cope with cancer. However, further assessment is necessary.

Jeff wants to completely assess Victoria and Joe's level of spiritual health. He is Lutheran and does not know very much about the Baptist faith, the couple's religion. However, he knows that the Baptist sense of community is very strong and that it is important to learn more about how members of the Timms' church play a role in offering support to the family. Jeff recognizes that spiritual well-being is more complex than religion. He spends time reflecting on his own value and belief systems so that he remains open and receptive to understanding Victoria and Joe's spiritual belief systems. By understanding his own beliefs, Jeff is also better able to help Victoria and Joe cope with Victoria's diagnosis of cancer.

---

who experience an NDE describe feeling totally at peace, having an out-of-body experience, being pulled into a dark tunnel, seeing bright light, and encountering people who preceded them in death. Instead of moving toward the light, they learn that it is not time for them to die, and they return to life (Johnson, 2015; Rawlings and Devery, 2015).

Patients who have an NDE are often reluctant to discuss it, thinking family or caregivers will not understand. Isolation and depression often occur. NDEs can be either positive or negative experiences (Johnson, 2015). However, individuals experiencing an NDE who discuss it openly with family or caregivers find acceptance and meaning from this powerful experience. They are often no longer afraid of death, and they have a decreased desire to achieve material wealth. They also report increased sensitivity to different chemicals such as alcohol and medications. After patients have survived an NDE, promote spiritual well-being by remaining open, giving patients a chance to explore what happened, and supporting them as they share the experience with significant others (Rawlings and Devery, 2015).

CRITICAL THINKING

Synthesis

Patient care requires you to apply what you know about a patient, your knowledge base, experience, and critical thinking attitudes and standards. Your synthesis of this information allows you to make sound decisions as you apply the nursing process. Critical thinking synthesis involves combining all available information to obtain a clear picture of the approach needed to provide patient-centered care.

You apply elements of critical thinking whenever you perform the nursing process with patients. Consider the scientific knowledge you have learned, your experience, critical thinking attitudes, and standards to ensure an individualized approach to patient care (Box 22.2).

Knowledge. The helping role is an important domain of nursing practice (Benner, 1984). Patients look to nurses for help that is different from the help they seek from other health care professionals. To effectively care for your patients' spiritual needs, you first need to be comfortable with your own spirituality (Delgado, 2015). By fostering your own personal, emotional, and spiritual health, you become a resource for your patient (Chiang et al., 2016). Use your awareness of your own spirituality as a tool when caring for yourself and your patients. Differentiate your personal spirituality from that of the patient. This becomes important during the delivery of care, when you need to be able to engage a patient spiritually rather than try to exercise personal spiritual convictions. Your role is not to solve the spiritual problems of patients but to provide an environment for them to express their spirituality (Johnston Taylor et al., 2014).

After becoming comfortable with your own spirituality, use your nursing expertise to anticipate your patients' personal issues and the resulting effect on spiritual well-being. Your knowledge about the concept of spirituality and a patient's faith and belief systems helps to provide appropriate spiritual care. Knowledge of a patient's values, beliefs, preferences, and needs provides additional insight into a person's spiritual practices. Application of therapeutic communication principles (see Chapter 11) and caring practices (see Chapter 20) helps you establish therapeutic trust with patients. An individual's spiritual beliefs are very personal. When you integrate patient preferences into spiritual care, you provide patient-centered care, respecting the diversity of your patient's experience (Box 22.3) (QSEN Institute, 2014).

When caring for patients who have a terminal illness or are experiencing some other type of loss, knowledge of loss and grief dynamics is important (see Chapter 27). Spirituality influences personal reactions to loss and response to grief. Also consider family dynamics while providing spiritual care (see Chapter 25). For many individuals their spiritual health is often integrated with their relationships among family members. Therefore consider the family's beliefs when planning spiritual care for your patient.

Finally a sound understanding of ethics and values (see Chapter 6) is essential when providing spiritual care. A person's values or beliefs about the worth of a given idea, attitude, or custom are linked to the individual's spiritual well-being. Application of ethical principles ensures respect for a patient's spiritual and religious convictions.

Experience. You often care for patients who are in spiritual distress. Use these experiences when helping others. Because spirituality is more than religion, you need to consider personal views and philosophies about life and reflect on whether your own spirituality is beneficial in helping patients. If you sense a personal faith and hope regarding life, it is likely that you will be better able to help patients. Previous personal and professional experiences with dying patients, patients with chronic disease, or patients who have experienced significant losses provide lessons in how to help patients face difficult challenges and how to offer support to family and friends.

BOX 22.3   PATIENT-CENTERED CARE

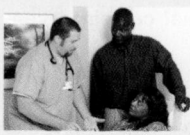 Jeff knows that patients' spiritual needs are often associated with their cultural, social, and ethnic background. Research shows that women generally express a deep relationship with God and strong moral and ethical values. Spirituality often provides a source of healing, coping, and peace. Furthermore, being connected with a caring community environment such as a neighborhood or church is particularly important for women who have breast cancer because caring communities provide great emotional and social support (Timmons, 2015). Jeff applies this information when he assesses Victoria's spiritual needs, validates that this perspective is shared by Victoria, and uses this understanding of breast cancer and spirituality to provide patient-centered care for Victoria and her family.

IMPLICATIONS FOR PRACTICE

- Jeff encourages Victoria and her family to strengthen their spiritual health as they continue to cope with Victoria's breast cancer diagnosis and cancer treatment.
- After asking Victoria if there are any communities with whom she feels connected, Jeff discovers that she is close to the members of her church and her work group.
- Jeff determines that Victoria's church has a parish nurse. With Victoria's permission he shares her health problems and concerns with the parish nurse who agrees to contact Victoria and arrange a time for them to meet.
- Jeff determines that Victoria and Joe have used prayer in the past to cope with different stressors. Thus Jeff prays with Victoria and Joe during their visits to the oncology clinic, encourages them to continue to read the Bible together at home, and encourages Joe to attend church even if Victoria is too ill to attend.
- Because breast cancer and its treatment often interfere with employment, Jeff explores ways that Victoria can remain connected with her peers at work to help her maintain this important source of support (Lewis et al., 2012).

Attitudes. Do not take a patient's reaction to illness or loss for granted. Humility becomes very important, particularly when caring for patients from diverse cultural and/or religious backgrounds. Recognize any limitations in your own knowledge about a patient's spiritual beliefs and religious practices and be willing to pursue the knowledge needed to provide appropriate, individualized care. Show genuine concern for patients as you ask them about their beliefs and how spirituality influences their health. Also exhibit integrity; realize the importance of refraining from expressing your opinions about religion or spirituality when they conflict with a patient's opinions. Finally show confidence in dealing with spiritual issues as you build a caring relationship with a patient. Confidence builds trust.

Standards. A nurse who thinks critically is thorough and ensures that information about a patient is significant and relevant when making decisions about his or her spiritual needs. The nature of a person's spirituality is complex and highly individualized. Therefore avoid making assumptions about a patient's religion and beliefs. Significance and relevance are standards of critical thinking that ensure that you explore the issues that are most meaningful to patients and most likely to affect their spiritual well-being. Apply ethical standards of care when providing spiritual care.

The Joint Commission (TJC) sets standards for quality health care. It requires health care organizations to acknowledge patients' rights to spiritual care and provide for patients' spiritual needs through pastoral care or others who are certified, ordained, or lay individuals. The standards also require that you assess your patients' religious preferences and provide for their beliefs and spiritual practices (TJC, 2016). The HealthCare Chaplaincy Network (2016) developed evidence-based indicators and metrics for quality spiritual care.

The American Nurses Association (ANA) Code of Ethics for Nurses (ANA, 2015) sets standards for quality nursing care. The Code of Ethics requires you to practice nursing with compassion by accepting the dignity and worth of all your patients regardless of their socioeconomic status, personal characteristics, or type of health problems. You promote an environment that respects your patients' values, customs, and spiritual beliefs.

NURSING PROCESS

Understanding a patient's spirituality and then appropriately identifying the level of support and resources needed require a broad perspective and an open mind. As a nurse, you make a commitment to care for and meet the spiritual needs of your patients. It is essential to respect each patient's personal beliefs. People experience the world and find meaning in life in different ways. Application of the nursing process from the perspective of a patient's spiritual needs is not simple. It goes beyond assessing his or her religious practices. Caring for your patients' spiritual needs requires you to be compassionate and remove any personal biases or misconceptions. Be willing to share and discover their meaning and purpose in life, illness, and health. Identify common values and respect unique commitments and values with your patients by having quiet conversations, listening effectively, and communicating using presence and therapeutic touch (Ramezani et al., 2014).

You need to recognize that not all patients have spiritual problems. Patients bring certain spiritual resources that help them live healthier lives, recover from illness, or face impending death. Supporting and recognizing the positive side of a patient's spirituality allows you to deliver safe, effective, patient-centered nursing care.

■■■ ASSESSMENT

Understanding your own spirituality is essential when you complete a spiritual assessment and provide spiritual care to your patients (Pullen et al., 2015). Remember that spirituality is very subjective and has different meanings for different people. You gather an accurate assessment of your patients' spirituality when you take time to build therapeutic relationships with them. Conduct an ongoing spiritual assessment the entire time you care for a patient. Talking about spirituality with a patient helps build a trusting relationship that often leads to conversations about spirituality and health outcomes (Carson, 2017). Focus your assessment on aspects of spirituality most likely to be influenced by life experiences, events, and questions in the case of illness and hospitalization (Table 22.2). Conducting an assessment is therapeutic for you and your patient because it conveys a level of caring and support.

One way to assess your patient's spiritual health is to ask the patient direct questions. This approach requires you to feel comfortable asking others about their spirituality. You start with a brief assessment and later follow with a more in-depth assessment (Hodge, 2015). Some health care agencies and researchers have created assessment tools to clarify values and assess spirituality. For example, the Spiritual Well-Being Scale (SWB) has 20 questions that assess a patient's relationship with God and his or her sense of life purpose and life satisfaction (Life Advance, 2009). The FICA assessment tool (Borneman et al., 2010) evaluates spirituality and is closely correlated to quality of life. *FICA* is an acronym stands for the following:

F—**Faith** or belief
I—**Importance** of spirituality
C—Individual's spiritual **Community**
A—Interventions to **Address** spiritual needs

Effective assessment tools such as the SWB and FICA help you remember important areas to assess. Patient responses to the assessment items on the tools indicate areas that you need to investigate further. *For example, Jeff used the FICA tool to assess Victoria's spirituality. Jeff's assessment shows that Victoria has*

TABLE 22.2	FOCUSED PATIENT ASSESSMENT		
FACTORS TO ASSESS	**QUESTIONS**	**PHYSICAL ASSESSMENT**	
Past experiences with loss	How would you describe the ways you cope spiritually when faced with difficult times?	Observe patient's facial expressions and mannerisms during the discussion.	
Fear of the unknown resulting from a terminal illness	Describe the people who mean the most to you. In what way do you look to them for support? Do you consider yourself a spiritual person? If so, what gives you comfort? If not, what provides you a sense of peace?	Fear is associated with anxiety. Be alert for changes in vital signs. Observe the patient's mood, willingness to initiate conversation, and interest in surroundings.	

a strong belief in God and prayer. Her church community is an important source of strength for both Victoria and Joe. They frequently pray together and attend church regularly. Remember, when using any spiritual assessment tool, do not impose your personal values on your patient. This is sometimes difficult, especially when a patient's values and beliefs are similar to yours, because it is very easy for you to make false assumptions. However, self-reflection without judgment is an important skill for you to develop. When you understand the overall approach to spiritual assessment, you can enter into thoughtful discussions with patients, gain a greater awareness of the personal resources they bring to a situation, and incorporate the resources into an effective plan of care.

Faith. Although individual definitions vary, faith helps people find meaning in their life experiences. When assessing a patient's faith, first determine his or her beliefs, especially beliefs that influence hope. For example, ask how a patient believes that a treatment will affect a newly diagnosed serious illness. Determine which of your patient's beliefs serve as a guide and help the patient find meaning in life events. Ask your patient if he or she is able to live according to his or her beliefs. Finally assess to what extent your patient interrelates with self, others, and a source of authority. Faith in an authority provides a sense of confidence that guides a person in exercising beliefs and experiencing growth. Assess a person's faith in an authority by asking, "To whom do you look to for guidance in life?" The patient's response to an open-ended question such as this will likely open the door for a meaningful discussion. Listen carefully and explore what is meaningful to the patient.

Determine if patients have a religious source of guidance that conflicts with their medical treatment plans. This seriously affects the treatment options that nurses and other health care providers are able to offer patients. For example, if a patient is a Jehovah's Witness, blood products are not an acceptable form of treatment. Christian Scientists often refuse any medical intervention, believing that their faith will heal them.

It is also important to understand a patient's philosophy of life. Asking a patient, "Describe for me what is most important in your life," or "Tell me what gives your life meaning or purpose," helps to assess the basis of his or her spiritual belief system. This information often reveals how illness, loss, or disability affects a person's life. A patient's religious practices, views about health, and response to illness influence how you will provide support.

Life and Self-Responsibility. Assessing spiritual well-being includes looking at your patient's life and self-responsibility. People who accept change, make decisions about their lives, and are able to forgive themselves and others in times of difficulty have a higher level of spiritual well-being. During illness patients often are unable to accept limitations or know what to do to regain a functional and meaningful life. Their sense of helplessness reflects spiritual distress. However, if a patient is able to adapt to changes and seek solutions for how to deal with any limitations, they are more responsible, and their spiritual well-being reflects an important coping

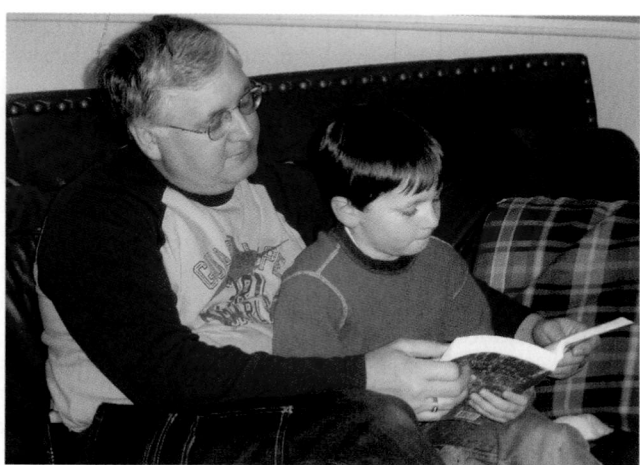

FIG 22.2 Praying or reading a religious text together enhances connectedness between parents and their children.

resource. Assess the extent to which a patient understands any limitations or threats posed by an illness and the way the patient chooses to adjust to them. Ask, "Tell me how you feel about the changes caused by your illness," and "How do these changes affect what you now need to do?"

Connectedness. Connectedness is a dimension of spirituality that is related to the human need of belonging. Patients who are connected to themselves, others, nature, God, or another Supreme Being usually report higher levels of physical and emotional health (Hakanson and Ohlen, 2016). Patients who pray use this form of personal communication to remain connected with God (Fig. 22.2). Praying provides a sense of hope, strength, and security and is woven into one's faith. Patients often use prayer when other treatments are ineffective (O'Brien, 2014). You help patients become or remain connected by respecting each patient's unique sense of spirituality. Assess whether a patient loses the ability to express a sense of relatedness to something greater than self. You assess a patient's connectedness by asking open-ended questions, "Is prayer something helpful to you? What feelings do you have after you pray?" or "Who do you believe is the most important person in your life?"

Life Satisfaction. Spiritual well-being is tied to a person's satisfaction with life and what the person has accomplished (Dobratz, 2016). When people are satisfied with life and how they are using their abilities, more energy is available to deal with new difficulties and resolve problems. You assess a patient's satisfaction with life by asking, "How happy or satisfied are you with your life?" or "Tell me to what extent you feel satisfied with what you have accomplished in life."

Fellowship and Community. Fellowship is one kind of relationship that an individual has with other people, including immediate family, close friends, associates at work or school, fellow members of a church, and neighbors. More specifically this includes the extent of the community of shared faith between people and their support networks. Many times social support from faith-based groups helps patients cope with illness and participate in health promotion behaviors (Plunkett et al., 2015). To assess a patient's supportive community, ask questions such as, "With whom do you bond or connect with?" "Who do you find to be the greatest source of support in times of difficulty?" or "When you've faced difficult times in the past, who has been your greatest resource?"

Explore the extent and nature of a person's support networks and their relationship with the patient. Do not assume that a given network offers the kind of support that a patient desires. For example, calling a patient's pastor to request a visit is inappropriate if the patient finds little fellowship with the pastor or the pastor's faith community. Does the patient have one significant fellowship or several? What level of support does the community give? Do they visit, say prayers, or support the patient's immediate family? Learn whether openness exists between a patient and the people with whom a fellowship has formed.

Ritual and Practice. The use of rituals and practice is easy to assess and helps you understand a patient's spirituality. Rituals include participation in a religious group or private worship, prayer, participating in sacraments such as baptism or communion, fasting, singing, meditating, scripture reading, making offerings or sacrifices, or enjoying nature. Different religions have different rituals for life events. For example, Buddhists practice baptism later in life and find burial or cremation acceptable at death. Muslims wash the body of a dead family member and wrap it in white cloth with the head turned toward the right shoulder. Orthodox and Conservative Jews have their newborn sons circumcised 8 days after birth. Determine whether illness or hospitalization has interrupted a patient's usual rituals or practices. A ritual provides a patient with structure and support during challenging times. If rituals are important to a patient, use them as part of your nursing intervention.

Vocation. Individuals express their spirituality daily in their work, play, and relationships. Spirituality is often a part of a person's identity and vocation in life. Determine if illness or hospitalization alters the ability to express some aspect of spirituality as it relates to a person's work or daily activities. Expression of spirituality is highly individual and includes showing an appreciation for life in the variety of things people do, living in the moment and not worrying about tomorrow, appreciating nature, expressing love toward others, and being productive. Assess how patients routinely express spirituality. Questions to ask include, "How has your illness affected the way you live your life spiritually at home or where you work?" or "How has your illness affected your ability to express what's important in life for you?"

Older Adult Considerations. Spirituality often plays a more pronounced and important role in the lives of older adults as they face an increased number of life transitions (Dahlkemper, 2016). Older adults often experience many losses, including the loss of a home, spouse, friends, and siblings. Although spirituality varies among older adults, it is strongly related to their ability to cope and manage stress (Edelman and Mandle, 2014). Supporting spirituality in older adults supports their dignity as people (Rykkje and Raholm, 2014). Older adults frequently participate in spiritual rituals and practices. They also often have a strong relationship with God or another Supreme Being, strive to find meaning and purpose in difficult situations, and need to connect with others (Rykkje and Rahom, 2014). Ask open-ended questions to assess spiritual needs of older adults (Abuatiq, 2015). Questions such as, "Which spiritual practices do you use most frequently?" and "What brings you hope?" help you identify spiritual needs and show that you care about and value the older adult.

Patient Expectations. Patients often need to make difficult health-related decisions, and many use spirituality to achieve a sense of well-being (Carson, 2017). Thus it is essential to take the time to establish a trusting and therapeutic relationship with your patients to accurately assess their expectations for health care and any spiritual implications. Active listening and maintaining presence leads to an accurate assessment of a patient's health care needs and how the patient's spirituality might affect achievement of those needs. To determine a patient's expectations, consider asking the following questions: "What are your goals for your care?" "How do you believe your faith or belief system will help you meet those goals?" "In what way can we support you? Would you like me to contact your minister, pastor, or rabbi to visit you?" Questions such as these indicate respect for your patient and allow you to include the patient's expectations in the plan of care.

■ ■ ■ NURSING DIAGNOSIS

When you review your patient's spiritual assessment, you know a great deal about the patient's spirituality. Exploring a patient's spirituality sometimes reveals responses to health problems that require nursing intervention, or it reveals a strong set of resources for the patient to use in coping. Use your critical thinking skills to analyze data and discover patterns of defining characteristics. Potential nursing diagnoses affected by spiritual health include the following:

- *Anxiety*
- *Ineffective Coping*
- *Fear*
- *Hopelessness*
- *Powerlessness*
- *Spiritual Distress*
- *Risk for Spiritual Distress*
- *Readiness for Enhanced Spiritual Well-Being*

As you identify nursing diagnoses for a patient, it is important to recognize the significance that spirituality has for all types of health problems. You may need to apply spiritual care principles if your patient has nursing diagnoses such as *Acute Pain, Chronic Pain, Fear, Anxiety,* and *Compromised Family Coping.*

Three nursing diagnoses accepted by NANDA International (2014) pertain specifically to spirituality. *Readiness for Enhanced Spiritual Well-Being* is based on defining characteristics that show a pattern of inner strength and interconnectedness that comes from inner faith and hope. Patients with this nursing diagnosis have a strong faith; are in harmony with self, others, and a higher power; and have a good sense of life purpose and meaning. A patient with enhanced spiritual well-being has resources on which to draw when faced with other nursing diagnoses. You help the patient explore how to use these resources when facing health problems.

The problem-focused nursing diagnoses of *Spiritual Distress* and the risk diagnosis of *Risk for Spiritual Distress* create different clinical pictures. Defining characteristics and risk factors from your assessment show patterns that reflect a person's actual or potential dispiritedness (e.g., expressing concern with the meaning of life and beliefs, anger toward God, and verbalizing conflicts about personal beliefs). Patients likely to be at risk for spiritual distress include patients who have poor relationships, have experienced a recent loss, or are experiencing some form of mental or physical illness.

Validate defining characteristics and clarify them with the patient before you make a diagnosis and develop a plan of care. With spiritual care the importance of your own spiritual well-being and perceptions cannot be overemphasized. Do not impose your personal beliefs. Be sure that any problem-focused diagnosis has an accurate related factor (e.g., a situational loss or relationship conflict) so your interventions are purposeful and goal directed.

■■■ PLANNING

During planning integrate the knowledge gathered from assessment and knowledge relating to resources and therapies available for spiritual care to develop an individualized plan of care (see Care Plan). Match a patient's diagnoses with evidence-based interventions that are supported and recommended in the clinical and research literature. Use a concept map (Fig. 22.3) to organize your patient's care and show how his or her medical diagnosis, assessment data, and nursing diagnoses are interrelated. Focus on building a caring relationship with the patient so that you enter into a healing relationship together.

◎ CARE PLAN

Readiness for Enhanced Spiritual Well-Being

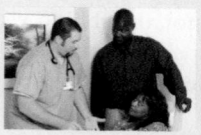

ASSESSMENT

Jeff learns that doctors told Victoria that her prognosis is promising, although she will need treatment to prevent spread of her disease. Joe has been helping Victoria more at home and has been trying to arrange work so that he is able to take her to the clinic. This means that he has less time in the evening to spend with the children. In the past Joe and Victoria have always had discussions with the children during mealtime, but recently this has been difficult. Jeff knows that current evidence shows many women use spirituality to cope with breast cancer; therefore he decides to assess Victoria's spirituality.

ASSESSMENT ACTIVITIES	FINDINGS[a]
Assess Victoria's connections with herself.	Victoria used to feel good about herself. However, since her cancer treatments, she is more tired and feels less positive at times. She states, **"I wish I had more hope about my prognosis."**
Assess Victoria's connections with her family and significant others.	Before Victoria's illness the **children were very close to their parents and shared their faith in God.** However, **now they are struggling with coping with Victoria's illness.** Victoria and Joe **attend their church regularly and hope to continue** doing so during the chemotherapy. **Members of their church have offered support** by taking Victoria to the clinic if Joe is unable.
Determine Victoria's connections with a power greater than herself.	Victoria **expresses a connectedness with her God,** "I don't feel alone; God is with me. I have a better appreciation of each day God gives me, and I believe God's strength will help me continue to be active in my church."

[a]**Defining characteristics/risk factors** are shown in **bold** type.

NURSING DIAGNOSIS: Readiness for Enhanced Spiritual Well-Being related to desire to be more connected with self, family, and God

---

PLANNING

GOAL

Victoria will restore connectedness with children within 2 months.

EXPECTED OUTCOMES (NOC)[b]

Spiritual Health

In 2 weeks Victoria, Joe, and children will discuss Victoria's beliefs about the future and her hope of having the cancer cured.

In 6 weeks Victoria will report son and daughter's ability to discuss fears with their mother.

◎ CARE PLAN—cont'd

Readiness for Enhanced Spiritual Well-Being

GOAL	EXPECTED OUTCOMES (NOC)[b]
Victoria will remain connected with herself, her husband, and God within 1 month.	By the end of this week, Victoria will make a formal time in her day to pray with family members. In 3 weeks Victoria will report that she and Joe are able to discuss their feelings and fears daily.

[b]Outcomes classification label from Moorhead S et al, editors: *Nursing outcomes classification (NOC)*, ed 5, St Louis, 2013, Mosby.

INTERVENTIONS (NIC)[c]	RATIONALE
Spiritual Support	
Use therapeutic communication (see Chapter 11) to establish presence and trust and demonstrate empathy with Victoria and Joe.	Establishing rapport, active listening, and trust is necessary to connect with patients who have spiritual needs (Pullen et al., 2015; March and Caple, 2016).
Pray with Victoria and her family.	When people pray, they often experience enhanced health outcomes and connectedness (O'Brien, 2014).
Encourage Victoria and her family to continue to attend church and participate in religious practices.	Active participation in faith communities and in religious activities helped support women's health and improved coping with illnesses (Plunkett et al., 2015; Dobratz, 2016).
Family Integrity Promotion	
Identify typical family coping mechanisms during a conference scheduled late in afternoon at the cancer clinic when the children are able to attend. Provide discussion of their mother's progress. Establish a presence and express a realistic hope of mother's prognosis.	Diagnosis of cancer causes the entire family to grieve. Providing spiritual care and spiritual support has a positive effect on coping and helps the family develop strategies for personal coping (Ramezani et al., 2014; Dobratz, 2016).
Encourage Joe to communicate frequently and openly with Victoria so that he can better understand her feelings and to create special times every day to talk about feelings and fears and connect with one another.	Maintaining a sense of connectedness helps improve psychological and mental health (Hakanson and Ohlen, 2016).

[c]Intervention classification labels from Bulechek GM et al, editors: *Nursing interventions classification (NIC)*, ed 6, St Louis, 2013, Mosby.

EVALUATION

NURSING ACTIONS	PATIENT RESPONSE/FINDING	ACHIEVEMENT OF OUTCOME
Ask Victoria about her daily routine. Determine if it includes time for prayer with the family.	Victoria reports that she spends at least 10 minutes every morning in prayer while sitting in her garden. Husband has joined her at times. She meditates for 10 to 15 minutes every day and reports that she is going to church regularly.	Victoria is attending to her spiritual health daily and is maintaining connections with herself and with God.
Ask Victoria and Joe about their relationship with themselves and their children.	Victoria and Joe set time aside every day to talk about what is happening that day, but they are having difficulty finding time to spend with their children because of their hectic school schedule.	Victoria is spending time with her husband regularly; she needs some help working out a schedule that will allow her to spend time with her children. Suggest that Victoria plan a family game night or some other fun family activity to allow time for enhanced interaction with children.

Goals and Outcomes. A spiritual plan of care includes realistic and patient-centered goals along with relevant outcomes. This requires you to work closely with each patient and engage together in setting goals and outcomes and ultimately choosing nursing interventions. In cases in which spiritual care requires helping patients adjust to loss or stressful situations, some goals are long-term (e.g., regaining spiritual comfort or affirming a purpose in life). Short-term goals such as renewing participation in religious practices are helpful to allow patients to move toward a more spiritually healthy situation. It is essential to include your patient when setting outcomes for spiritual care. For example, if you know

CONCEPT MAP

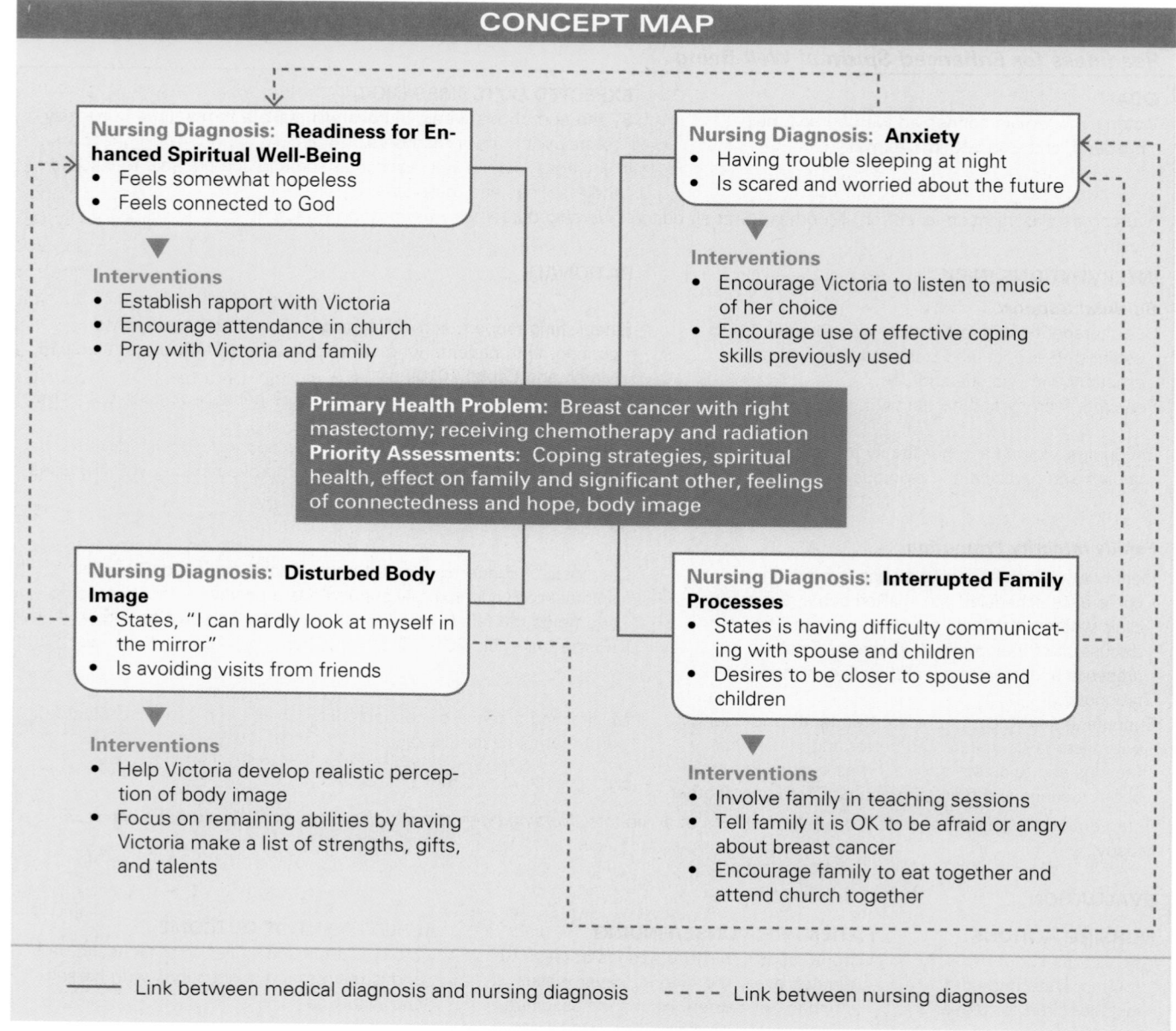

Nursing Diagnosis: Readiness for Enhanced Spiritual Well-Being
- Feels somewhat hopeless
- Feels connected to God

Interventions
- Establish rapport with Victoria
- Encourage attendance in church
- Pray with Victoria and family

Nursing Diagnosis: Anxiety
- Having trouble sleeping at night
- Is scared and worried about the future

Interventions
- Encourage Victoria to listen to music of her choice
- Encourage use of effective coping skills previously used

Primary Health Problem: Breast cancer with right mastectomy; receiving chemotherapy and radiation
Priority Assessments: Coping strategies, spiritual health, effect on family and significant other, feelings of connectedness and hope, body image

Nursing Diagnosis: Disturbed Body Image
- States, "I can hardly look at myself in the mirror"
- Is avoiding visits from friends

Interventions
- Help Victoria develop realistic perception of body image
- Focus on remaining abilities by having Victoria make a list of strengths, gifts, and talents

Nursing Diagnosis: Interrupted Family Processes
- States is having difficulty communicating with spouse and children
- Desires to be closer to spouse and children

Interventions
- Involve family in teaching sessions
- Tell family it is OK to be afraid or angry about breast cancer
- Encourage family to eat together and attend church together

——— Link between medical diagnosis and nursing diagnosis   - - - - Link between nursing diagnoses

FIG 22.3 Concept map.

that a patient wants to practice regular prayer and meditation, you state an outcome for the goal of regaining spiritual comfort as "Patient prays and meditates daily."

Setting Priorities. Spiritual care is very personalized. Your relationship with a patient allows you to understand your patient's priorities. If you have developed a mutually agreed-on plan with a patient, he or she is able to relate what is most important. Do not sacrifice spiritual priorities for physical care priorities. For example, if your patient is in acute distress, focus your care to help the patient gain a sense of control. As a person nears the end of life, spiritual care is possibly the most important intervention that you provide (Finocchiaro, 2016).

Collaborative Care. To ensure ongoing spiritual care, it sometimes becomes necessary to involve family, family caregivers, significant others, and clergy to lend support. This means that you learned from the assessment that individuals or groups have a fellowship with the patient. These individuals become involved in all levels of your care plan. The patient's support network help in sharing quiet moments of prayer and reading scripture to the patient as well as giving physical care. In a hospital setting the pastoral care department and chaplains are a valuable resource. Chaplains not only provide spiritual and/or pastoral care to patients and families but also help staff in crisis (Healthcare Chaplains Ministry Association [HCMA], 2013). Health care–based chaplains are typically available 24 hours a day to provide spiritual and pastoral support to patients and families (HCMA, 2013). These professionals provide insight about how and when to best support patients and families. When caring for patients with spiritual needs in the community setting, make a referral to a parish nurse if possible. Faith community nurses work in a variety of churches and other faith communities. They help bring people closer to God during times of illness and crisis (Balent and George, 2015). Practice of faith community nurses emphasizes health and healing within the faith community; they provide a variety of holistic nursing interventions to their patients, respecting their diverse needs (Dandridge, 2014).

■ ■ ■ IMPLEMENTATION

If a patient is in spiritual distress or has a health problem that requires the use of spiritual resources, a caring relationship between you and the patient is necessary (see Chapter 20). Both you and the patient must feel free to let go and discover together the meaning that illness or loss poses for the patient and the effect it has on the meaning and purpose of his or her life. When you achieve this level of understanding with a patient, it enables you to deliver care in a sensitive, creative, and appropriate manner.

Health Promotion. Spiritual care needs to be a central theme in promoting an individual's overall well-being because of its importance in health promotion (Vlasblom et al., 2015). Spirituality is one personal resource that influences the balance between health and illness. Churches often play an important role in health promotion, especially if there is minimal availability of other health promotion resources (Plunkett et al., 2015). You are able to use the interventions described here at any level of health care.

Establishing Presence. You contribute to a sense of well-being and provide hope for recovery when you spend quality time with your patients. Behaviors that establish your presence include giving attention, answering questions, listening, and having a positive and encouraging (but realistic) attitude. Presence is part of the art of nursing (Carson, 2017). Benner (1984) explains that presence involves "being with" a patient versus "doing for" a patient. Presence is being able to offer closeness with a patient physically, psychologically, and spiritually. It helps to prevent emotional and environmental isolation (see Chapter 20).

When health promotion is the focus of care, your presence becomes important in instilling confidence in patients' abilities to take the steps necessary to remain healthy. You convey a caring presence by listening to patients' concerns, willingly involving family in discussions about a patient's health, showing self-confidence when providing health instruction, and supporting your patients when they make decisions about their health.

Trust is fundamental to any relationship. The attitude you convey when first interacting with a patient sets the tone for all conversations (see Chapter 11). Actively listening to the meaning of what a patient says is most important. It involves paying attention to the person's words and tone of voice and

entering his or her frame of reference. By observing the patient's expressions and body language, you find cues to help him or her explore ways to achieve inner peace, take action, or manage pain. Your role as a nurse is not to solve patients' spiritual problems or impart your opinions but to provide an environment in which the patient can express spirituality.

Supporting a Healing Relationship. When giving spiritual care, look beyond isolated patient problems and recognize the broader picture of a patient's holistic needs. This is especially important when caring for older adults (Box 22.4). For example, do not look at a patient's back pain as just a problem to solve with quick remedies but rather look at how the pain influences his or her ability to function and achieve goals established in life. A holistic view enables you to assume a helping role so that you can establish a healing relationship (Benner, 1984). Three steps are evident when you establish healing relationships with your patients:

1. Mobilizing hope for you and for your patients
2. Finding an interpretation or understanding of the illness, pain, anxiety, or other stressful emotion that is acceptable to patients
3. Helping patients use social, emotional, or spiritual resources (Benner, 1984)

Mobilizing a patient's hope is central to a healing relationship. Hope helps people to face challenges in life (Broadhurst and

---

BOX 22.4 CARE OF THE OLDER ADULT
Supporting Older Adults' Spirituality

- There is an association between an older adult's spirituality and his or her ability to adjust or cope with illness and other life stressors (Manning, 2014).
- Older adults achieve spiritual resilience through frequent expressions of gratitude (e.g., via prayer, meditation, or discussions with friends) and finding ways to maintain purpose in life (e.g., helping family, volunteering) (Manning, 2014).
- Religious activities, attitudes, and spiritual experiences are very common among older adults. Older adults who experience spiritual well-being have better emotional health, experience a sense of peace that helps them accept life transitions, and experience to some extent improved physical health (Dahlkemper, 2016).
- Respecting privacy and dignity is an essential part of nursing care, especially when meeting spiritual needs of older adults (Rykkje and Raholm, 2014).
- Feelings of connectedness are important for older adults. Enhance connectedness by helping the older patient find meaning and purpose in life, listening actively to concerns, and being present (Dahlkemper, 2016).
- Beliefs in the afterlife increase as adults grow older. Make visits from clergy, social workers, lawyers, and even financial advisors available so that patients feel as though they have completed all unfinished business. Leaving a legacy to loved ones prepares the older adult to leave the world with a sense of meaning (Touhy and Jett, 2018). Legacies include oral histories, works of art, publications, photographs, or other objects of significance.

Harrington, 2015). You help patients find realistic things for which to hope. For example, a patient newly diagnosed with diabetes becomes hopeful when you help him learn how to manage the disease so as to continue a productive and satisfying way of life. Your focus on controlling the pain and other symptoms a terminally ill patient is experiencing raises hope that the patient will be able to attend her daughter's graduation and live each day to the fullest.

Hope has both short-term and long-term implications. From a long-term perspective, it gives individuals a determination to endure and carry on with life responsibilities. In the short-term, hope provides an incentive for constructive coping with obstacles and finding ways to realize the object of hope. Hope is future oriented and helps a patient work toward goals (Yarcheski and Mahon, 2016). You help patients achieve hope by working with them to find explanations for their situations that are mutually acceptable. Then help each patient realistically exercise hope. This includes supporting a patient's positive attitude toward life or a desire to be informed and make decisions.

To further support a healing relationship, know a patient's spiritual resources and needs. It is always important for patients to be able to express and exercise their beliefs and find spiritual comfort. When illness or treatment creates confusion or uncertainty for a patient, recognize the possible effect that this can have on the patient's well-being. How can spiritual resources be used and strengthened? Having a clear sense of what illness will be like helps a patient apply all resources toward recovery.

Acute Care. Within an acute care setting, support and enhancement of a patient's spiritual well-being are challenging when the focus of health care is on treatment and cure rather than care. Lack of time, lack of education or training, confusion over one's own spirituality, and patient privacy are other barriers to spiritual care in acute care settings (Rushton, 2014; Vlasblom et al., 2015). Patients often experience multiple stressors and feel like they are losing control. To overcome these challenges, display a soothing presence and supportive touch as you implement nursing interventions. Some patients are fearful of experiencing an illness that threatens their loss of control and they look for someone to offer competent direction. Your artful use of hands, encouraging words of support, promotion of connectedness, and calm and decisive approach establish a presence that builds trust. Work closely with patients to maximize resources that support their spirituality. For example, you build trust with your patients when you perform procedures competently. Promote connectedness and build trust by listening to a dying patient's concerns, providing reassurance and comfort, and helping a patient complete unfinished business.

Support Systems. Use of support systems is important in any health care setting. They serve as a human link connecting the patient, the nurse, and the patient's lifestyle before an illness. In today's society support comes from many areas, including family, friends, and support groups. Families often influence how patients perceive their illness. You enhance a

patient's support network when you include a patient's family and friends in planning care. A patient's support system often is a source of coping, faith, and hope.

When a patient depends on family, friends, spiritual advisors, and members of the clergy for support, encourage these individuals to visit the patient regularly. Make all the patient's visitors welcome on nursing units and ensure privacy during visits to provide spiritual comfort. If the patient desires, ask the pastoral care department or hospital chaplain to notify the patient's clergy of the patient's admission. Often illness and the hospital environment produce uncertainty that frightens family members and friends. Help the family feel welcome and use their support and presence to promote the patient's healing. For example, including family members in prayer is a thoughtful gesture if it is appropriate to the patient's religion and if family members are comfortable participating. Encouraging the family to bring meaningful religious symbols to the patient's bedside and facilitating the administration of sacraments, rites, and rituals offers significant spiritual support. Do not forget to support the family as well. When you support the family's spirituality and faith practices, you decrease their anxiety and feelings of uncertainty (Dobratz, 2016).

Diet Therapies. Food and nutrition are important aspects of nursing care. Food is also an significant component of some religious observances. For example, people in some Hindu and Islamic sects are vegetarian. Muslims are not allowed to eat pork, and they fast during the month of Ramadan. Orthodox Jewish patients observe kosher dietary restrictions. Native Americans have food practices influenced by individual tribal beliefs. Similar to many aspects of a particular culture or religion, food and the rituals surrounding the preparation and serving of food are important to a patient's spirituality. Integrate a patient's dietary preferences into daily care when possible, and consult with the dietitian in the health care institution. If a hospital or other health care agency cannot prepare food in the preferred way, ask the family to bring meals that are appropriate for dietary restrictions posed by the patient's condition.

Supporting Rituals. You become active in your patients' spiritual care by supporting their participation in spiritual rituals and activities. Plan care to allow time for religious readings, spiritual visitations, or attendance at religious services. Some churches and synagogues offer audiotapes of religious services. Allow family members to plan a prayer session or an organized reading when appropriate. Taped meditations, religious music, televised religious services, and some Internet sites provide other effective options. Be respectful of icons, medals, prayer rugs, or crosses that patients bring to a health care setting, and make sure that they are not lost or misplaced.

Restorative and Continuing Care

Prayer and Meditation. The act of prayer gives an individual the opportunity to renew personal faith and belief in a Supreme Being in a specific, focused way that is either highly ritualized and formal or spontaneous and informal.

Prayer is an effective coping resource for physical and psychological symptoms (O'Brien, 2014). Patients pray in private or pursue opportunities for group prayer with family, friends, or clergy. Some patients pray while listening to music. Be supportive of prayer by giving the patient privacy if desired, learning if the patient wishes to have you participate, and suggesting prayer when you know that it is a coping resource for the patient. Delgado (2015) found that nurses often pray for patients rather than with patients; sharing the fact that prayer has been offered gives patients support and comfort. If prayer is not suitable for a patient, alternatives include listening to calming music or reading a book, poetry, or inspirational texts selected by the patient.

QSEN ACTIVITY *Evidence-Based Practice*

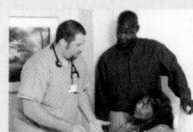

To provide evidence-based, patient-centered care to Victoria, Jeff wonders what effects prayer has on the severity of side effects of breast cancer treatment. He also wonders if the clinic nurses should routinely start praying with their patients. The manager of the clinic, who believes that Jeff's question may lead to an evidence-based practice change at the clinic, informs Jeff that the first step of the evidence-based practice process is to ask a clinical question.

- Using the PICO format, develop an appropriate and clinically relevant question that Jeff could use to guide his search of the current evidence (see Chapter 7).

evolve Answers to QSEN Activities can be found on the Evolve website.

BOX 22.5 PATIENT TEACHING

Meditation

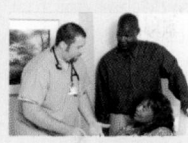

At one of her clinic visits, Victoria tells Jeff, "My friend told me yesterday that when she had cancer, she used meditation to help her cope with the side effects of her chemotherapy. I was thinking that I might try meditating to see if it would help me, but I don't know how to meditate. Can you help me?" Jeff develops the following teaching plan for Victoria:

OUTCOME
Victoria verbalizes feelings of relaxation and self-transcendence after meditation.

TEACHING STRATEGIES
- Provide a brief description of what will be taught.
- Give Victoria a patient-teaching sheet that describes how to meditate.
- Help Victoria identify at least one quiet place in her home that has minimal interruptions.
- Encourage her to use soft background noise such as a fan or soft music during meditation to block out distractions.
- Teach Victoria the steps of meditation—sit in a comfortable position with the back straight; breathe slowly; and focus on a sound, a prayer, or an image.
- Encourage Victoria to meditate for 10 to 20 minutes two times a day.
- Answer any questions.
- Reinforce information as needed.

EVALUATION
- Use the principles of teach-back to evaluate patient learning:
  - "What did you learn about yourself?"
  - "How did you feel after meditating?"

Meditation is effective in creating a relaxation response that reduces daily stress. Patients who meditate often state that they have an increased awareness of their spirituality and of the presence of God or a Supreme Being (Box 22.5). Meditation exercises give patients relief from pain, insomnia, anxiety, and depression and increase coping and the ability to relax (Starkweather, 2017). Meditation involves sitting quietly in a comfortable position with eyes closed and repeating a sound, phrase, or sacred word in rhythm with breathing while disregarding intrusive thoughts. Individuals who meditate regularly (twice a day for 10 or 20 minutes) experience decreased metabolism and heart rate, easier breathing, and slower brain waves. Chapter 34 addresses relaxation approaches.

■ ■ ■ EVALUATION

Patient Outcomes. Attainment of spiritual health is a lifelong goal. Patients experience the need to clarify values (see Chapter 6), reshape philosophies, and live the experiences that help to shape purpose in life. As you provide spiritual care, always evaluate whether the patient achieved planned outcomes and goals (Box 22.6). Compare the patient's level of spiritual health with the behaviors and perceptions noted in the nursing assessment. For example, if your assessment found a patient losing hope, the follow-up evaluation involves a discussion to determine if the patient has regained an attitude that life is worth living. Family and friends are a useful source of evaluative information. Successful outcomes reveal a patient developing an increased or restored sense of connectedness with family; maintaining, reviewing, or reforming a sense of purpose in life; and, for some, having a confidence and trust in a Supreme Being or higher power.

For patients with a serious or terminal illness, evaluation focuses on the goal of helping them retain faith and hope or express openly the uncertainties life poses. Evaluate how well a patient accepts an illness and whether hope has enabled the patient to recognize individual mortality and focus on living for each day. You cannot assume that all patients have faith in a higher power. However, your support helps patients find

BOX 22.6   EVALUATION

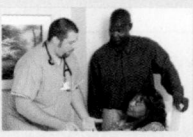

Victoria returns to the clinic 1 week after making a plan to enhance her spiritual health. A member of her church accompanies Victoria because Joe is out of town on a business trip. Jeff wants to evaluate whether Victoria continues to feel connected with herself, Joe, her children, and God. Jeff asks, "Tell me, Mrs. Timms, have you had a chance yet to try any of the approaches we talked about last week to give yourself, Joe, and the kids a chance to talk about their feelings? If so, what were the results?" Victoria reports, "Yes, I spend at least 10 minutes every morning in prayer while I sit in my garden, and I've been meditating for 10 to 15 minutes every day. Joe and I set aside at least 15 minutes a day to talk in private after the kids go to bed. If he's not in town, we talk on the phone. Joe and I planned a family dinner night last Saturday evening with the kids. We shared lots of funny family stories and began to talk with them about my cancer treatment. The kids really seemed to enjoy being together as a family. They asked many questions, and we talked about what they could do to help me. We also planned for the family to visit two colleges for Davis." Jeff also determines that Victoria has spoken with close friends from her church and they plan to visit her this week. Victoria states that she is going to see the physical therapist today.

In an effort to evaluate whether the clinic has met Victoria's expectations, Jeff asks, "Your faith is strong, and it is my hope you have felt comfortable in talking about your worries. Do you believe that we have helped you so far with your concerns about your family?" Victoria replies, "The best thing you've done is listen and recognize how important my family is to me. Your suggestions have helped so far; I am truly blessed to have met all of you nice people at the clinic."

DOCUMENTATION NOTE

"Visited the clinic for the third week of chemotherapy. Denies nausea but is complaining of some soreness in the mouth and a loss of hair. Asks questions readily and made an appointment with the physical therapist as recommended. States has enhanced her connectedness with herself and her family by taking time to pray and meditate, talking and listening with her family, and having fun with her children. Expresses hope that her children will feel less frightened over the diagnosis and states that they will be coming to the next clinic visit."

meaning in life and death, accept their destiny, and be at peace (Petersen, 2014).

Patient Expectations. You use critical thinking to evaluate whether your spiritual care met your patient's expectations and contributed to your patient's health. When you evaluate the effects of spiritual care, include your patient in the evaluation of outcomes. Ask the patient if you and the health care team met the patient's expectations and if there is anything you can do to enhance the patient's spiritual

well-being. Regarding the nurse-patient relationship, does your patient express trust and confidence in you? Taking time to ask a patient to reflect on the quality of the nurse-patient relationship is time well spent. Asking a patient, "Have you felt comfortable in saying what you feel is important to you spiritually?" determines whether you developed an effective healing relationship.

KEY POINTS

- Attending to a patient's spirituality ensures a holistic focus to nursing practice.
- Frequently the concepts of spirituality and religion are interchanged, but spirituality is a much broader and more unifying concept than religion.
- An individual's beliefs and spiritual well-being influence physical health status.
- Faith and hope are closely linked to a person's spiritual well-being, providing an inner strength for dealing with illness and disability.
- Research suggests that there is a link between a patient's spirituality and potential for healing.
- Acute and chronic illness, terminal illness, and NDEs pose spiritual problems for individuals.
- Providing appropriate spiritual care requires you to critically apply knowledge from principles related to caring, cultural care, loss and grief, and therapeutic communication.
- Avoid biases when assessing and planning spiritual care.
- Learning to practice caring and compassion helps you discover a patient's life values and meaning.
- Connectedness and fellowship with other people are a source of hope for a patient.
- Patients often have spiritual strengths that you use as resources to help them live healthier lives.
- Interruptions in or changes to customary religious practices affect the support that religion contributes to a person's well-being.
- Common religious rituals include private worship, prayer, singing, use of a rosary, and scripture reading.
- The personal nature of spirituality requires open communication and the establishment of trust between you and a patient.
- Establishing presence involves giving attention, answering questions, having an encouraging attitude, and conveying a sense of trust.
- Part of a patient's caregiving environment is the regular presence of family, friends, and spiritual advisors.

REFLECTIVE LEARNING

- Select a patient that you were assigned to care for this week and describe the spiritual needs of that patient.
- Discuss how you met the spiritual needs of one of your patients this week.
- Using the FICA assessment tool, complete a personal assessment of your own spirituality.

REVIEW QUESTIONS

1. The nurse is caring for a patient who had a stroke and has some right-side paralysis. The patient states, "I have been praying to God and I know that he will help me cope with my problems and give me the courage to face my challenges in rehabilitation." Which nursing diagnosis is this patient likely experiencing?
   1. *Spiritual Distress*
   2. *Ineffective Coping*
   3. *Risk for Spiritual Distress*
   4. *Readiness for Enhanced Spiritual Well-Being*

2. The nurse is assessing the spiritual beliefs of a 15-year-old patient. Based on the patient's developmental stage, what should the nurse expect to see?
   1. The patient questions why prayer is needed.
   2. The patient values the support of peers.
   3. The patient feels guilty for missing church.
   4. The patient requests to speak to the chaplain.

3. The nurse is caring for a woman who is recovering from a total hip replacement. During the assessment, the nurse learns that the patient is Roman Catholic. The patient tells the nurse is she very nervous about starting therapy. Based on this information, which of the following interventions does the nurse implement to enhance the patient's spiritual health? (Select all that apply.)
   1. Giving the patient an antianxiety medication
   2. Asking the patient if she would like to pray with the nurse
   3. Asking the patient if she would like pastoral care to visit
   4. Providing the patient privacy while she is praying the rosary
   5. Telling the patient that therapy will help her get home

4. A patient who is recovering after recently experiencing third-degree burns shows connectedness when she states:
   1. "My pain medicine helps me feel better."
   2. "I know I will get better if I just keep trying."
   3. "I see God's grace and become relaxed when I watch the sun set at night."
   4. "I feel so much closer to God after I read my Bible and pray."

5. The nurse is caring for a hospitalized patient who is of the Hindu faith. Which action by the nursing assistive personnel (NAP) required the nurse to intervene?
   1. The NAP gives the patient privacy during a prayer ritual.
   2. The NAP plans care around the patient's purity rituals.
   3. The NAP encourages the patient's family to visit with the patient.
   4. The NAP tells the patient that he or she must remove the amulet while in the hospital.

evolve

Additional Review Questions, as well as rationales for all Review Questions, can be found on the Evolve website.

1. 4; 2. 1; 3. 2, 3, 4, 4; 5. 4.

REFERENCES

Abuatiq A: Spiritual care for critical care patients, *Int J Nurs Clin Pract* 2:128, 2015.

American Nurses Association (ANA): *Code of ethics for nurses with interpretive statements*, Silver Spring, MD, 2015, ANA.

Balent KA, George NM: Faith community nursing scope of practice: extending access to healthcare, *J Christ Nurs* 32(1):34, 2015.

Benner P: *From novice to expert*, Menlo Park, CA, 1984, Addison-Wesley.

Borneman T, et al: Evaluation of the FICA tool for spiritual assessment, *J Pain Symptom Manage* 40(2):163, 2010.

Broadhurst K, Harrington A: A mixed method thematic review: the importance of hope to the dying patient, *J Adv Nurs* 72(1):18, 2015.

Carron R: Spirituality. In Larsen PD, editor: *Lubkin's chronic illness: impact and interventions*, ed 9, Burlington, MA, 2016, Jones & Bartlett.

Carson VB: Spirituality. In Giddens JF, editor: *Concepts for nursing practice*, ed 2, St Louis, 2017, Elsevier.

Chiang YC, et al: The impact of nurses' spiritual health on their attitudes toward spiritual care, professional commitment, and caring, *Nurs Outlook* 64(3):215, 2016.

Collins-McNeil J, et al: Spirituality: opportunities for advanced practice nursing and primary care, *J Christ Nurs* 32(2):75, 2015.

Conway-Phillips R, Janusek L: Influence of sense of coherence, spirituality, social support and health perception on breast cancer screening motivation and behavior in African American women, *ABNF J* 25(3):72, 2014.

Cottrell L: Joy and happiness: a simultaneous and evolutionary concept analysis, *J Adv Nurs* 72(7):1506, 2016.

Dahlkemper TR: *Anderson's caring for older adults holistically*, ed 6, Philadelphia, 2016, FA Davis.

Dandridge R: Faith community/parish nurse literature: exciting interventions, unclear outcomes, *J Christ Nurs* 31(2):100, 2014.

Darby K, et al: Understanding and responding to spiritual and religious needs of young people with cancer, *Cancer Nurs Pract* 13(2):32, 2014.

Delgado C: Nurses' spiritual care practices: becoming less, *J Christian Nurs* 32(2):116, 2015.

Dobratz MC: Building a middle-range theory of adaptive spirituality, *Nurs Science Quart* 29(2):146, 2016.

Dunn SL: Identifying and promoting hope in patients, *West J Nurs Res* 38(3):267, 2016.

Edelman CL, Mandle CL: *Health promotion throughout the life span*, ed 8, St Louis, 2014, Elsevier.

Estores IM, Frye J: Healing environments: integrative medicine and palliative care in acute care settings, *Crit Care Nurs Clin N Am* 27:369, 2015.

Finocchiaro DN: Supporting the patient's spiritual needs at the end of life, *Nursing* 46(5):57, 2016.

Fredrickson BL: The role of positive emotions in positive psychology, *Am Psychol* 56(3):218, 2001.

Gilbert R: Laughter therapy: promoting health and wellbeing, *Nurs Resident Care* 16(7):392, 2014.

Granero-Molina J, et al: Religious faith in coping with terminal cancer: what is the nursing experience?, *Eur J Cancer Care (Engl)* 23(3):300, 2014.

Griggs S, Walker RK: The role of hope for adolescents with a chronic illness: an integrative review, *J Pediatr Nurs* 31:404, 2016.

Hakanson C, Ohlen J: Connectedness at the end of life among people admitted to inpatient palliative care, *Am J Hosp Palliat Care* 33(1):47, 2016.

Hatamipour K, et al: Spiritual needs of cancer patients: a qualitative study, *Indian J Palliat Care* 21(1):61, 2015.

HealthCare Chaplaincy Network: *What is quality spiritual care in health care and how do you measure it?* 2016, https://www.healthcarechaplaincy.org/docs/research/quality_indicators_document_2_17_16.pdf.

Healthcare Chaplains Ministry Association (HCMA): *What is a chaplain?*, 2013, http://www.hcmachaplains.org/what-is-a-chaplain/.

Hipolito E, et al: Trauma-informed care: accounting for the interconnected role of spirituality and empowerment in mental health promotion, *J Spiritual Mental Health* 16:193, 2014.

Hodge DR: Administering a two-stage spiritual assessment in healthcare settings: a necessary component of ethical and effective care, *J Nurs Manage* 23:27, 2015.

Johnson S: Near-death experience in patients on hemodialysis, *Nephrol Nurs J* 42(4):331, 2015.

Johnston Taylor E, et al: Nurse religiosity and spiritual care, *J Adv Nurs* 70(11):2612, 2014.

Johnston Taylor E, et al: Spirituality and spiritual care of adolescents and young adults with cancer, *Semin Oncol Nurs* 31(3):227, 2015.

Jones A, et al: Relationships between negative spiritual beliefs and health outcomes for individuals with heterogeneous medical conditions, *J Spiritual Mental Health* 17:135, 2015.

Lewis PE, et al: Psychosocial concerns of young African American breast cancer survivors, *J Psychosoc Oncol* 30(2):168, 2012.

Life Advance: *The spiritual well-being scale*, 2009, http://www.lifeadvance.com/spiritual-well-being-scale.html.

Manning LK: Enduring as lived experience: exploring the essence of spiritual resilience for women in later life, *J Relig Health* 53(2):352, 2014.

March P, Caple C: *Spiritual needs of hospitalized patients*. In *CINAHL Nursing Guide*, April 29, 2016.

Mark G, Lyons A: Conceptualizing mind, body, spirit interconnections through, and beyond, spiritual healing practices, *Explore (NY)* 10(5):294, 2014.

NANDA International: *Nursing diagnoses: definitions and classification, 2015-2017*, ed 10, Oxford, 2014, Wiley-Blackwell.

O'Brien ME: *Spirituality in nursing: standing on Holy ground*, ed 5, Washington, DC, 2014, Jones & Bartlett.

Pantuso T: Spiritual interventions for patients with cancer, *Integr Med Alert* 18(7):79, 2015.

Petersen CL: Spiritual care of the child with cancer at the end of life: a concept analysis, *J Adv Nurs* 70(6):1243, 2014.

Plunkett R, et al: Healthy spaces in meaningful places: the rural church and women's health promotion, *J Holistic Nurs* 33(2):122, 2015.

Pullen L, et al: The relevance of spirituality to nursing practice and education, *Mental Health Pract* 18(5):14, 2015.

QSEN Institute: *Pre-licensure KSAs*, 2014, http://qsen.org/competencies/pre-licensure-ksas/.

Ramezani M, et al: Spiritual care in nursing: a concept analysis, *Int Nurs Rev* 61:211, 2014.

Rawlings D, Devery K: Near death experience and nursing practice: lessons from the palliative care literature, *Aust Nurs Midwifery J* 22(8):26, 2015.

Rowold J: Effects of spiritual well-being on subsequent happiness, psychological well-being, and stress, *J Relig Health* 50(4):950, 2011.

Rushton L: What are the barriers to spiritual care in a hospital setting?, *Br J Nurs* 23(7):379, 2014.

Rykkje L, Raholm MB: Understanding older people's experiences of dignity and its significance in caring—a hermeneutical study, *Int J Hum Caring* 18(1):17, 2014.

Starkweather A: Pain. In Giddens JF, editor: *Concepts for nursing practice*, ed 2, St Louis, 2017, Elsevier.

Sweat MT: How do I spiritually support those who are suffering and in pain?, *J Christian Nurs* 32(2):123, 2015.

Tadwalkar R, et al: The beneficial role of spiritual counseling in heart failure patients, *J Relig Health* 53:1575, 2014.

The Joint Commission (TJC): *Standard FAQ details: provision of care, treatment, and services (PC) (hospital and hospital clinics/hospital)*, 2016, https://www.jointcommission.org/standards_information/jcfaqdetails.aspx?StandardsFAQId=765&StandardsFAQChapterId=78&ProgramId=5&ChapterId=0&IsFeatured=False&IsNew=False&Keyword=spiritual.

Timmins F, et al: Spiritual dimensions of care: developing an educational package for hospital nurses in the Republic of Ireland, *Holist Nurs Pract* 28(2):106, 2014.

Timmons SM: Review and evaluation of faith-based weight management interventions that target African American women, *J Relig Health* 54:798, 2015.

Touhy TA, Jett KF: *Ebersole and Hess' gerontological nursing & healthy aging*, ed 5, St Louis, 2018, Elsevier.

Trevino KM, McConnell TR: Religiosity and spirituality during cardiac rehabilitation, *J Cardiopulm Rehabil Prev* 35:246, 2015.

Viglund K, et al: Inner strength as a mediator of the relationship between disease and self-rated health among old people, *J Adv Nurs* 70(1):44, 2014.

Vlasblom JP, et al: Effect of nurses' screening of spiritual needs of hospitalized patients on consultation and perceived nurses' support and patients' spiritual well-being, *Holist Nurs Pract* 29(6):346, 2015.

Yarcheski A, Mahon NE: Meta-analyses of predictors of hope in adolescents, *West J Nurs Res* 38(3):345, 2016.

Growth and Development

evolve EVOLVE MEDIA RESOURCES

http://evolve.elsevier.com/Potter/essentials
- Audio Glossary

- QSEN Activity and Review Questions Answers and Rationales

OBJECTIVES

- Compare the frameworks for growth and development as described by major developmental theorists.
- Identify the difference between growth and development.
- Describe the growth and development changes that occur from conception through old age.
- Identify factors that promote or interfere with normal growth and development at each stage of life.
- Specify the physical and psychosocial health concerns of infants, children, adolescents, and adults.

- Apply developmental theories when planning patient care across the life span.
- Identify specific nursing interventions for the health promotion of patients across the life span.
- Apply critical thinking skills to determine appropriate individualized teaching topics for patients across the life span.

KEY TERMS

As a nurse, you care for individuals of all ages. Human growth is an orderly, predictable process beginning with conception and continuing until death. Although development is less predictable, there are patterns of developmental tasks. Your knowledge of human development patterns will help you anticipate appropriate developmental tasks to help patients and families for whom you care.

SCIENTIFIC KNOWLEDGE BASE

Concept of Growth and Development

When the terms *growth* and *development* are used together, they refer to all of the many changes that take place throughout an individual's lifetime (Hockenberry et al., 2017). **Growth** is the measurable aspect of a person's increase in physical dimensions. Measurable growth indicators include changes in height, weight, teeth and bone, and sexual characteristics.

CASE STUDY *Crystal Taylor*

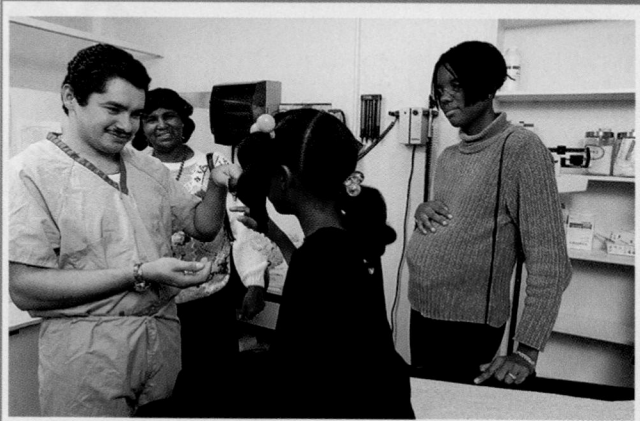

Crystal Taylor is a 25-year-old single parent of 2½-year-old Zachary and 6-year-old Monica, who has recently learned to ride a bicycle. Crystal smokes and is currently 6 months pregnant. She lives with her 44-year-old mother and 15-year-old brother. Crystal's 68-year-old maternal grandmother and aunt live next door and often help care for Zachary and Monica. Crystal has a strong family history for breast cancer. Her grandmother and aunt are both breast cancer survivors. Crystal mentioned that her mother has not had a mammogram or any other routine screenings. Crystal's family has used the health care center for years. She and Monica came to the clinic today for Monica's checkup before beginning school.

Louis Ruiz is a 28-year-old nursing student assigned to the clinic. He selected this family to follow throughout the semester. The clinic is Louis' first clinical experience as a nursing student, and he is eager to become involved in health promotion activities but is also anxious about his new role as a professional nurse.

Development is an interaction of biological, sociological, and psychological forces. Development occurs gradually and refers to changes in skill and capacity to function. These changes are qualitative in nature and difficult to measure in exact units. However, certain predictable characteristics are measurable such as development that proceeds from simple to complex. An example of this is learning to crawl before learning to walk.

Maturation is the biological plan for the predictable milestones for growth and development. Physical growth and motor development are a function of maturation. Examples of age-related behaviors that follow a specific sequence are sitting, walking, and running, which are a result of maturation.

A critical period of development refers to a specific phase or period when the presence of a function or reasoning has its greatest effect on a specific aspect of development. For example, if a child does not walk by 20 months, there is delayed gross-motor ability, which slows exploration and manipulation of the environment. The success or failure experienced within a phase affects a person's ability to complete the next phases.

Theories of Human Development

Developmental theories provide a framework for examining, describing, and appreciating human development. It is helpful to look at multiple theories to understand the person as a whole (Burns et al., 2017). Theories explain and predict behavior that is measurable and observable (Table 23.1). Some theories view development as a continuous process involving gradual, cumulative changes slowly over time. Others consider it as discontinuous, with distinct stages.

Sigmund Freud. Freud's psychoanalytic model of personality development is grounded in the belief that two internal biological forces drive the psychological change in a child: sexual (libido) and instinctive forces. The theory describes a series of five stages, each associated with a pleasurable zone serving as the focus of gratification. A child who successfully completes the stages develops a healthy personality. A fixation can result if a child does not progress through a stage. In the first stage, the oral stage, sucking and oral satisfaction are vital to life and very pleasurable. During the anal stage the focus of pleasure changes to anal zone. Children become increasingly aware of the pleasurable sensations of this body region. Through the toilet-training process the child learns how to control body functions. In stage 3, the phallic or Oedipal stage, the genital organs become the focus of pleasure. The child is learning the differences between genders. In stage 4, the latency stage, children repress sexual urges and channel them into productive activities that are socially acceptable. Stage 5, the genital stage, occurs during adolescence and is a turbulent time for the child and family. The child develops sexually and is interested in members of the opposite sex. Social activities begin to occur outside the family circle, and the child seeks more independence (Santrock, 2012).

Erikson's Eight Stages of Development. Erickson's theory describes eight stages of development (Erikson, 1963, 1997). Individuals need to accomplish particular tasks before successfully completing a stage (see Table 23.1). Each task is framed with opposing conflicts such as trust versus mistrust. Each stage builds on the successful attainment of the previous developmental conflict. In contrast to Freud, Erikson describes three additional stages: young adulthood, middle adulthood, and older adulthood. The task for stage 6, young adulthood, is intimacy versus isolation. This occurs as young adults develop a sense of identity and deepen their capacity to love others and care for them. Stage 7, generativity versus self-absorption and stagnation, presents the task for adults to accept themselves and be accepting of others. Middle-age adults achieve success by contributing to future generations through parenting and/or grandparenting, teaching, mentoring, or volunteering. The last stage, ego integrity versus despair, occurs through the aging process. Many older adults review their lives with a sense of satisfaction, whereas others may review their lives with a sense of failure. Older adults cope with losses such as the loss of loved ones, changes in

TABLE 23.1 COMPARISON OF MAJOR DEVELOPMENT THEORIES OF CHILDHOOD

DEVELOPMENTAL STAGE (APPROXIMATE AGE)	FREUD (PSYCHOSEXUAL DEVELOPMENT)	ERIKSON (PSYCHOSOCIAL DEVELOPMENT)	PIAGET (LOGICAL, COGNITIVE, AND MORAL DEVELOPMENT)	KOHLBERG (DEVELOPMENT OF MORAL REASONING)
Infancy (birth to 18 months)	Oral stage	Trust vs. mistrust Ability to trust others	Sensorimotor period Progress from reflex activity to simple repetitive actions	
Early childhood/toddler (18 months to 3 years)	Anal stage	Autonomy vs. shame and doubt Self-control and independence	Preoperational period—thinking using symbols; egocentric	Preconventional level Punishment-obedience orientation
Preschool (3–5 years)	Phallic stage	Initiative vs. guilt Highly imaginative	Use of symbols; egocentric	Preconventional level Premoral Instrumental orientation
Childhood (6–12 years)	Latent stage	Industry vs. inferiority Engaged in tasks and activities	Concrete operations period Logical thinking	Conventional level Good-boy, nice-girl orientation
Adolescence (12–19 years)	Genital stage	Identity vs. role confusion Sexual maturity, "Who am I?"	Formal operations period Abstract thinking	Postconventional level Social contract orientation
Young adulthood		Intimacy vs. isolation Affiliation and love		
Adulthood		Generativity vs. stagnation Production and care		
Maturity		Ego integrity vs. despair Renunciation and wisdom		

family, or losses in functional status. These changes challenge the person to adjust while continuing to live a full and rich life.

Piaget's Theory of Cognitive Development. Jean Piaget developed the theory of cognitive development, which describes children's intellectual organization and how they think, reason, and perceive the world. The theory includes four periods: sensorimotor, preoperational, concrete operations, and formal operations (see Table 23.1). As a child grows from infancy into adolescence, intellectual development progresses, starting with reflex and repetitive motion responses and progressing to the use of symbols and objects from the child's point of view, to logical thinking, and finally to abstract thinking (Burns et al., 2017).

Kohlberg's Moral Developmental Theory. According to Kohlberg's Moral Development Theory (1964), moral development is one component of psychosocial development. The theory describes how people justify their behaviors. Moral development continues throughout a person's lifetime. It depends on a child's ability to accept social responsibility

and integrate personal principles of justice and fairness. In addition, a child's knowledge of right and wrong and behavioral expression of this knowledge is founded on respect and regard for the integrity and rights of others (Burns et al., 2017). Cognitive development aids the progression of a person's morality from level to level.

Maslow's Theory of Human Needs. Abraham Maslow developed a theory of human needs from his study of healthy individuals without physical or mental illness (Fig. 23.1). He described an ordering (hierarchy) of needs that motivate human behavior. This ordering is often depicted as a pyramid composed of five levels (Maslow, 1970). When the most basic needs such as hunger and oxygen are met, a person strives to satisfy the needs for safety and security on the next highest level. Disturbances at lower levels interfere with the highest level, self-actualization, or the realization of one's potential. This theory has made a valuable contribution to understanding human development through its positive viewpoint and recognition of needs that motivate all humans. However, critics have noted that it does not differentiate according to age-groups.

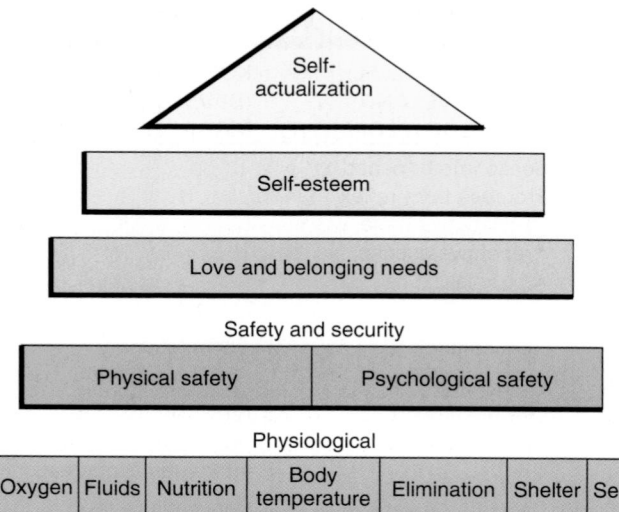

FIG 23.1 Maslow's hierarchy of needs. (From Maslow AH, et al: *Motivation and personality,* ed 3. Copyright ©1987. Reprinted by permission of Pearson Education, Inc., New York, New York.)

NURSING KNOWLEDGE BASE

A strong body of knowledge about growth and development gives you good insight regarding how individuals perceive an event or behave in response to a given situation at a particular age or stage of life. An overview of the stages of life and related health concerns follows.

Conception and Fetal Development

From the moment of conception, human development proceeds rapidly. The ovum and sperm each carry half the genetic material that guides biochemical processes essential to the developing organism. Intrauterine life generally lasts approximately 9 calendar or 10 lunar months, or 266 days, beginning with fertilization and ending with the birth of a baby. Pregnancy may be divided into three periods: germinal, embryonic, and fetal. The germinal period is about 2 weeks and occurs from the time of fertilization until implantation. The embryonic period extends from the second week until the eighth week after conception. During this time cells differentiate, and organs appear. The fetal period extends from 2 months after conception until birth.

Pregnancy is also divided into three trimesters. The first trimester is the first 3 calendar months. During this time, several organ systems are developing at the same time. The disruption of one system can affect the development of other systems.

The second trimester is from the third to the sixth prenatal months. Basic development of some organ systems continues during this time, and the functional capabilities of other systems are refined. By the end of the second trimester most organ systems are complete and able to function. The fetus weighs approximately 0.7 kg (1½ lb) and is approximately 30 cm (12 inches) long.

During the last 3 months of intrauterine life the fetus grows to approximately 50 cm (20 inches) in length. Weight increases to approximately 3.2 to 3.4 kg (7 to 7½ lb). The skin thickens, lanugo (soft, downy hair) begins to disappear, and the fetal body becomes rounder and fuller. A tremendous spurt in brain growth begins during this trimester and lasts well into the first few years of life. The central nervous system has established its total number of neurons and connections between neurons, and myelination of nerve fibers progresses rapidly. Damage to the central nervous system during the third trimester can potentially alter higher-level cognitive functions.

Health Promotion. Abnormalities in the genes or chromosomes alter health. Other health problems result from environmental factors (e.g., the mother's diet or tobacco use or alcohol use as in fetal alcohol syndrome). **Teratogens** are chemical or physiological agents capable of having adverse effects on a fetus. Exposure to potential teratogens can affect fetal development during any of the trimesters; however, vulnerability is increased during the first trimester when fetal cells are differentiating and organs are forming. Because the placenta is extremely porous, teratogens pass easily from mother to fetus. Some examples of teratogens are viruses, drugs (prescribed, over-the-counter, and street drugs), alcohol, and environmental pollutants such as cigarette smoke and lead.

The effect of these harmful agents on the fetus depends on the developmental stage in which exposure takes place. Some teratogens produce defects only if the fetus is exposed to the agent at a critical time when the vulnerable organ is developing.

Many drugs are teratogenic during the period of rapid organ growth in the first trimester. Barbiturates, alcohol, anticonvulsants, antibiotics, anticoagulants, and over-the-counter medications can cause fetal abnormalities. Health care providers weigh the benefits of prescribed medications against potentially harmful fetal effects. In addition, there is evidence that mothers who smoke deliver infants with lower birth weights than nonsmoking mothers.

Explore lifestyle changes that can help women abstain from tobacco, alcohol, and drugs not only during pregnancy but also while planning for pregnancy. Preconception counseling is a growing trend in health care. The goal is to secure the best outcome for mother, fetus, and significant others through good prenatal care.

Neonate

The neonatal period is the first 28 days of life. The newborn's physical functioning is primarily reflexive, and stabilization of major organ systems is the primary task of the body. The average full-term **neonate** weighs 3.4 kg (about 7½ lb), is 50 cm (20 inches) in length, and has a head circumference of 35 cm (14 inches). Neonates lose up to 10% of their birth weight in the first few days of life, primarily through fluid losses by respirations, urination, defecation, and low fluid intake. They usually regain the weight by the end of the second week of life.

Physically the neonate may have lanugo on the skin of the back, cyanosis of the hands and feet (acrocyanosis) especially during activity, and a soft protuberant abdomen. Behaviorally the newborn has periods of sucking, crying, sleeping, and activity. The newborn's movements are generally sporadic, but they are symmetrical and involve all extremities. Newborns respond to sensory stimuli, particularly the caregiver's face, voice, and touch.

Early cognitive development begins with innate behaviors, reflexes, and sensory functions. For example, the rooting reflex permits neonates to turn to the nipple instinctively when their cheek is stroked. Other automatic and involuntary reflexes help an infant respond to its environment. Newborns can focus on objects 20 to 25 cm (8 to 10 inches) from their faces and respond to auditory stimuli. Therefore you need to teach parents the importance of talking to their babies and providing appropriate visual stimulation.

Health Promotion. Parental concerns during the neonatal period most frequently center on the baby's crying, feeding, elimination, and sleeping behaviors (Box 23.1). New parents are not always aware of the newborn's immature immune system and need information about how to protect the baby from infection (e.g., avoiding exposure to crowds of people such as at church or the grocery store).

The American Academy of Pediatrics (AAP) recommends placing healthy neonates and infants on their backs while they sleep to decrease the risk for sudden infant death syndrome (SIDS) (AAP, 2015a). Side sleeping is not advised because it is not as safe as back sleeping. Help new parents by teaching the phrase "face up to wake up" as a reminder to always place babies on their backs. The AAP also recommends avoiding the use of thick bedding, sheepskins, waterbeds, or cushions. Research shows that these preventive measures are associated with a decreased incidence of SIDS (AAP, 2015b). Nurses help parents attain the knowledge and skills required to foster the newborn's physical, psychosocial, and cognitive well-being and development.

Infant

Growth and development are more rapid during the first 12 months of life than at any other time of life. The infant depends completely on caregivers to provide for basic needs of food, warmth, and comfort; love and security; and sensory stimulation.

Typically, infants double their birth weight by 5 to 6 months of age and triple it by 12 months of age. Their length increases about 1 inch per month during the first 6 months of life and then ½ inch per month to the end of the first year of life. Play is solitary, and it provides opportunities for the infant to develop many motor skills. Rattles, plastic stacking rings, and wooden blocks are a few examples of toys that promote fine-motor development of the hands and fingers (Fig. 23.2).

Health Promotion. Erikson (1963) described the task for the infant stage as trust. Basic trust is established by having caregivers meet their infant's needs in a timely manner. Infants who are neglected develop mistrust. Thus help parents understand the need to establish routines when caring for their infants' needs. Parents of newborns often need guidance

BOX 23.1 HEALTH PROMOTION GUIDELINES FOR PARENTS OF NEWBORNS

- Select a crib with slats less than approximately 6 cm (2⅜ inches) apart (Hockenberry et al., 2017) and with a mattress that fits snugly against the slats (AAP, 2015b).
- Do not put pillows or bumper pads in baby's crib (AAP, 2015b).
- Position infants on their backs in the crib, "face up to wake up" (AAP, 2015a).
- Know expected physiological newborn behaviors and variability of behavioral cycles (sleep-awake states).
- Understand principles and techniques for feeding method chosen; the AAP (2012) recommends breastfeeding, and breastfeeding mothers need support and interventions for minor problems such as sore nipples and temporary decline in milk production.
- Provide appropriate sensory stimulation techniques.
- Know feeding patterns and behaviors.
- Schedule well-baby visits and immunization schedule.
- Provide appropriate care measures including hygiene, dressing, comfort.
- Understand protective measures including asepsis, safety, cardiopulmonary resuscitation (CPR), thermoregulation.
- Cleanse the umbilical cord stump with alcohol until it falls off.
- Provide appropriate circumcision care.
- Identify signs and symptoms that require evaluation by health care professional.

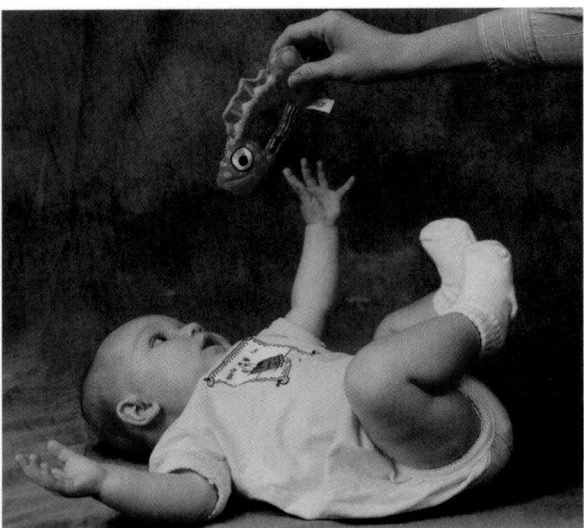

FIG 23.2 A 3-month-old infant focuses on a visual object and reaches toward it. (Courtesy Paul Vincent Kuntz, Texas Children's Hospital, Houston, TX. From Hockenberry ML, Wilson D: *Wong's nursing care of infants and children*, ed 10, St Louis, 2015, Mosby.)

in providing health promotion activities regarding feeding, crying, eliminating, and sleeping. Other health promotion activities for the 1- to 12-month-old infant are often related to dentition, immunizations, and safety.

The first tooth to erupt is usually one of the lower central incisors at the average age of 7 months. Most babies have six teeth by their first birthday (Hockenberry et al., 2017). The use of a chilled teething ring may soothe swollen, sore gums. Tooth decay is preventable by providing adequate fluoride through formula or otherwise cleaning inside the baby's mouth at least once a day with a wet washcloth as well as not allowing the baby to take the bottle to bed (Hockenberry et al., 2017).

Sleep varies from infant to infant. Most neonates sleep 10 to 20 hours a day. Sleep patterns vary as the infant grows; however, by 4 months of age most infants are sleeping at night with one to two naps during the day.

The quality and quantity of nutrition influence an infant's growth and development. Breastfeeding is recommended for infants (AAP, 2012). Breastfeeding is associated with a decreased frequency of gastroenteritis, otitis media, food allergies, diabetes, childhood leukemia, obesity, and pneumonia (Hockenberry et al., 2017). However, when a mother cannot or does not want to breastfeed, an acceptable alternative is iron-fortified commercially prepared formula. Infants should not have any type of cow's milk during the first year because the high protein content may increase the chance of food allergies (Hockenberry et al., 2017).

Immunizations have dramatically reduced infectious diseases over the past 50 years. Some parents choose not to vaccinate their children, citing fears regarding side effects of the vaccines. Although there are small risks from the vaccines, the risks of not receiving the vaccines are far more serious (AAP, 2017a; Centers for Disease Control and Prevention [CDC], 2017b). Nurses play a major role in helping community organizations promote immunizations and eliminate preventable childhood disease.

Infants' quickly developing motor skills increase their mobility and their ability to place all types of objects in their mouths. They need constant supervision when not sleeping. Help parents raise their level of awareness regarding potential hazards in their homes. Common accidents during infancy include automobile accidents, aspiration, burns, drowning, falls, poisoning, and suffocation (Box 23.2). The AAP recommends that infants should not sleep with a blanket until they are 1 year old. Some day care facilities recommend blanket sleepers and do not allow blankets in cribs (AAP, 2015a).

Acute Care. When an infant becomes ill, it is important that you maintain the infant's routine daily care. When this is impossible, limit the number of caregivers who have contact with the infant, and follow the parents' directions for care. If hospitalization is necessary, infants sometimes have difficulty establishing physical boundaries because of repeated bodily intrusions and painful sensations. Limiting these negative experiences and providing pleasurable sensations support early psychosocial development.

BOX 23.2 HEALTH PROMOTION GUIDELINES FOR PARENTS OF INFANTS

- Keep crib away from radiators, blast of air ducts, and cords from drapes or blinds.
- Understand expected growth and developmental norms.
- Provide play activities to stimulate gross-motor and fine-motor development.
- Encourage development of language.
- Identify readiness for weaning from breast or bottle to cup.
- Add solid foods (usually at 6 months) and other fluids by introducing only one new food at a time to assess for food allergies.
- Understand need for immunizations and immunization schedule.
- Implement safety measures related to use of approved car seats, falls, drowning, and use of mouth to explore everything in environment.
- Avoid exposure to secondhand smoke.
- Expect the baby to develop attachment, stranger awareness, and separation anxiety.
- Use voice, eyes, and facial gestures appropriately as disciplinary measures.
- Identify signs of illness, measures for assessment (temperature taking), and appropriate action.
- Use appropriate criteria to choose day care.

Toddler

The toddler period ranges from 12 to 36 months of age. The rapid development of fine-motor and gross-motor skills allows a child to participate in feeding, dressing, and toileting. Toddlers walk in an upright position with a broad-stance gait, bowed legs, protuberant abdomen, and arms flung out to the sides for balance. Soon the child begins to navigate stairs, run, jump, stand on one foot for several seconds, and kick a ball.

Because moral development is closely associated with cognitive ability, the moral development of toddlers is just beginning. Toddlers are also egocentric. They do not fully understand concepts of right and wrong. However, they do grasp that some behaviors bring pleasant results and others bring unpleasant results.

Toddlers are generally able to speak in short sentences. Common questions they ask are, "Who's that?" and "What's that?" By 3 years of age toddlers have a beginning mastery of speech; they are possessive of their toys and are often heard to say, "Mine!" They begin to learn that sharing is a desirable behavior when they offer parents toys to hold and the parents express pleasure. Play is frequently solitary in nature. However, toddlers often participate in parallel play, playing beside another child with a similar toy or object but not actively interacting through their play. Gradually the toddler's play begins to include the exchanging or sharing of objects when playing beside another toddler engaged in a similar activity.

Health Promotion. Slower growth rates often occur with a decrease in caloric needs and a smaller food intake. Confirming a child's pattern of growth with standard growth charts is reassuring to parents concerned about their child's decreased, fussy appetite, known as physiological anorexia. Encourage parents to offer a variety of nutritious foods, in reasonable servings, for mealtime and snacks (AAP, 2017b). Finger foods allow the toddler to be independent.

Toilet training is a major task of toddlerhood. The success of toilet training is based on three primary factors: physical ability to control anal and urethral sphincters (after the child learns to walk), the child's ability to recognize urge and communicate it to the parent, and the desire to please the parent by holding on and letting go at appropriate times. The average age for achieving control is 2 years for daytime and 3 years for nighttime control. Girls usually toilet train earlier than boys (Hockenberry et al., 2017).

Toddlers are developing autonomy and want to do things for themselves (Erikson, 1963). The natural curiosity and mobility of toddlers without good reasoning abilities make them an accident waiting to happen. Toddlers want to put everything into their mouths (e.g., bugs, bleach, electrical cords) or place their hands, feet, or entire bodies into dangerous places (e.g., electrical outlets, clothes dryers, tubs with very hot water). They need constant supervision unless they are in a totally childproofed area such as their crib or playpen. Toddlers have little awareness of physical safety, and accidents are the leading cause of death and injury. The most common accidents are burns, drowning, falls, motor vehicle accidents, and poisoning (National Center for Health Statistics, 2016). You can help parents anticipate the safety needs of their toddlers and make appropriate suggestions (Box 23.3).

Acute Care. When a toddler is ill, it is important to provide care consistent with the child's developmental needs. Use the responses of the child and parents to determine specific care for the child. For a young child, being separated from one's family in an unfamiliar environment during an illness is a stressful experience. Parents are more likely to remain with their young child when health care team members create a comfortable environment for them. Whenever possible encourage the family to bring in the child's favorite toy, blanket, or familiar object. If a significant caregiver cannot remain with the toddler, it is especially important that one nurse assume responsibility for providing the toddler with consistent and appropriate care. Limiting the number of strange caregivers helps establish trust and reduces separation anxiety for the toddler. During times of stress or illness children often regress to behaviors of an earlier time to provide comfort and security. This regression of behavior is often disturbing to parents, and they need reassurance that the behavior is normal and the child will return to more mature behavior patterns when the stressful situation is resolved.

Toddlers cannot clearly identify where they feel pain and often find anything that causes pressure intrusive or extremely painful. Reduce physical discomfort by keeping periods of

> **BOX 23.3   HEALTH PROMOTION GUIDELINES FOR PARENTS OF TODDLERS**
>
> - Stimulate gross-motor and fine-motor development through play (e.g., push/pull, nesting toys).
> - Read to child.
> - Establish good nutritional habits and teach how to feed self.
> - Give whole milk and limit to two to three glasses per day (AAP, 2017b).
> - Cut all food into bite-sized pieces and watch for choking with grapes, hot dogs, and marshmallows (AAP, 2017b).
> - Offer two to three healthy snacks per day (AAP, 2017b).
> - Encourage development of language.
> - Identify readiness and implement appropriate methods for toilet training.
> - Set limits on behavior while recognizing toddler's need for independence.
> - Set limits and provide firm, gentle discipline to resolve negativism and temper tantrums.
> - Expect continued separation anxiety and development of ritualism.
> - Implement safety measures including childproofing the home environment (e.g., storage of cleaning products and medication, use of car seats, selection of appropriate safe toys, pool and water precautions, outdoor play, placing plants out of reach and getting rid of poisonous ones).
>   - Keep electrical cords out of reach and cover unused electrical outlets.
>   - Block stairways and balconies and do not leave child unsupervised near water.
>   - Reduce risk for injuries (e.g., do not leave iron on ironing board, turn handles of saucepans and frying pans to inside of stove when cooking).
> - Understand continued need for immunizations (AAP, 2017a) and developmental assessments.

restraint or immobility to a minimum. A soft voice, physical contact, and a security item also comfort a child.

Preschool Child

Early childhood is the period between the ages of 3 and 5 years when children refine the mastery of their bodies and eagerly await the beginning of formal education. Many parents find this age-group more enjoyable than toddlerhood because children are more cooperative, share thoughts with greater accuracy, and interact and communicate more effectively. Physical development continues at a slow pace, whereas cognitive and psychosocial development accelerates. According to Erikson, this is the time when children develop a sense of moral responsibility (Erikson, 1963).

A 3-year-old can recognize people, objects, and events by their outward appearance. For example, 3-year-olds prefer having two nickels over a dime because it appears to be more. The continued egocentricity of early thinking makes it difficult to suggest acceptable alternatives to preschoolers. When they are hungry, they expect others also to be hungry, and they think they must eat now!

In addition, preschoolers are increasingly able to solve problems intuitively on the basis of one aspect of a situation. For example, they can classify objects according to either size or color but not both. They ask many questions. Erikson described the task for this stage as initiative versus guilt. Initiative is described as the point in which children see themselves as separate individuals. They also have a great sense of imagination. Adults often misinterpret preschoolers' "tall tales" as lying; however, they are actually presenting their own reality. Their imagination also contributes to the development of fears, the greatest of which in this age-group is the fear of bodily harm (Hockenberry et al., 2017). For example, preschool children are sometimes afraid of various animals, the dark, or procedures such as having their blood pressure measured.

Health Promotion. Ingestion of large amounts of carbohydrates and fats from junk foods results in unhealthy weight gain and undernourishment. Encourage parents to be role models for good eating habits and to offer their children a varied diet that prevents deficiencies and excesses. Children enjoy helping prepare healthy snacks such as fruit slices, carrot sticks, celery stuffed with peanut butter, and popcorn. Family meals also help improve the quality of food eaten.

Preschoolers require role models and instruction to develop good hygiene measures such as brushing their teeth after meals and sugary snacks, covering their mouths and noses when coughing or sneezing, keeping their fingers out of their noses and eyes, and washing their hands before eating and after using the toilet.

Accidents, specifically motor vehicle accidents (usually as a pedestrian), are the major cause of mortality for this age-group. Parents need education to help meet the health promotion needs of their child (Box 23.4). This is a good time to teach children what to do in case of fire, safety regulations for crossing the street, the need to ride in the back seat of the car buckled in an approved car seat, and how to get help when someone is hurt.

Acute Care. When preschoolers become ill, their beginning abilities to reason and understand make illness less stressful. Although they have developed object permanence and recognize that their parents still exist when out of sight, most tolerate only short absences without becoming distressed. Encourage parents to tell the child when they are leaving and when they will return in terms the child can understand (e.g., "I am leaving and will be back after lunch."). Be present when parents leave to provide distraction and support for the child. Reduce children's fear by allowing the child to sit up for assessments and procedures when possible and demonstrating procedures on another person or doll. Also allow the child to see and handle equipment and help with a procedure as appropriate. Encouraging parents to be present during procedures and leaving the room door open at night if the child requests it reduce fear as well. Simple and

---

BOX 23.4 HEALTH PROMOTION GUIDELINES FOR PARENTS OF PRESCHOOL CHILDREN

- Encourage parents to support their child's sense of initiative and recognizing that the child will be unable to complete all activities begun.
- Understand nutritional requirements for optimal growth.
- Stimulate continued progress in development of motor skills, language, cognitive skills, and social skills, (e.g., reading to the child, using play groups, encouraging the child to do small chores and activities for the family).
- Recognize signs of common childhood communicable diseases and implement measures to reduce their risk and spread.
- Begin instruction for personal safety (e.g., do not talk to strangers, tell an adult about inappropriate touching, strangers in the area).
- Use criteria to evaluate preschool education programs.
- Help preschoolers learn about health, including nutrition, exercise, and rest.
- Implement safety measures related to motor vehicles, tricycles, and fire.
- Be prepared for child's increased sexual curiosity and use correct anatomical terminology.
- Identify signs of child abuse, know how to protect children, and be aware of community agencies available for assistance.

---

factual information is especially important to this age-group because of their great sense of imagination (Hockenberry et al., 2017).

School-Age Child

The foundation for adult roles in work, recreation, and social interaction occurs during the "middle years" of childhood (6 to 12 years of age). Great developmental strides are made in physical, cognitive, and psychosocial skills. Children become "better" at things. For example, they run faster and farther as proficiency and endurance develop.

Educational experience in school expands a child's world and transitions him or her from a life of relatively free play to one of structured play, learning, and work. The school and home influence growth and development. For optimal development to occur, a child has to learn to cope with the rules and expectations of school and peers. School-age children have some reasoning and logical thoughts, and they adopt their parents' moral standards to seek their approval.

School-age children become more graceful as they gain increasing control over their bodies (Fig. 23.3). Strength doubles, and large-muscle coordination improves. Participation in the basic gross-motor skills of running, jumping, balancing, throwing, and catching refines neuromuscular function and skills. Holding a pencil and printing letters and words are evidence of fine-motor coordination improvement in 6-year-olds. By 12 years of age, a child makes detailed drawings and writes sentences. Teachers often ask

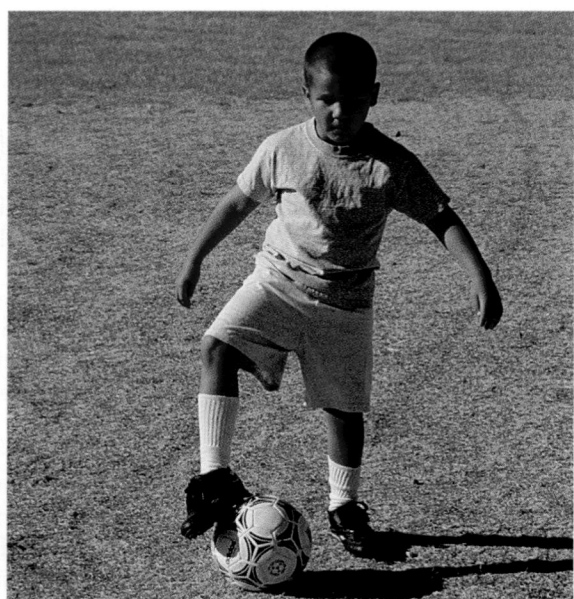

FIG 23.3 Coordination improves in school-age children as they gain control over their bodies.

BOX 23.5	HEALTH PROMOTION GUIDELINES FOR SCHOOL-AGE CHILDREN AND THEIR PARENTS

- Understand expected growth parameters and developmental tasks including middle childhood growth spurt and puberty.
- Enhance adjustment to school and reduce school-related stressors.
- Recognize the influence and importance of peers as they learn to follow rules and be competitive.
- Prepare for development and expression of sexuality including sex play (e.g., masturbation).
- Model safety practices.
- Teach children about personal safety (e.g., do not talk to strangers, tell an adult about inappropriate touching, strangers in the area, bullying).
- Monitor and limit recreational screen time (computer, video games, television) to 1 to 2 hours a day.
- Read violence and sexual language ratings on video and computer games and media.
- Reinforce Internet safety (e.g., placing the computer in an interactive family area rather than in the child's room, blocking inappropriate e-mail messages and pop-up messages, emphasizing the need to tell an adult when there is "something funny" on the screen or in the e-mail).
- Enforce recreational safety including helmets for sports, bicycling, and skateboarding.
- Substance abuse (tobacco, alcohol, drugs) including dangers, signs of use, and available community agency support.
- Discuss health promotion activities including nutrition, exercise, and safety.

school nurses to conduct fine-motor assessment of children if they observe a lack of these motor skills.

Children often lose all their primary teeth during the middle childhood years. The secondary teeth are much larger in proportion. Regular dental visits are essential and confirm that children are brushing their teeth with regularity and proper technique.

As children progress through school, there are many opportunities for them to gain a sense of competence as they learn reading, writing, and other academic skills. They also have the ability to follow the rules of a new authority person and to compete and cooperate with peers in play and work. Recognizing a child's achievements at home improves the child's developing self-esteem and often encourages self-motivation. Children's success in work and play leads to an increasing sense of independence and a need to participate in decisions that involve them. As children move through the middle years of childhood, they confront a number of stressors in school, in their home, and from peers.

The school-age child prefers same-sex peers to opposite-sex peers. In general, girls and boys view the opposite sex negatively. Peer influence becomes diverse during this stage.

Health Promotion. Accidents and injuries are major health problems and are the causative factor in a large number of deaths in this age-group. Motor vehicle accidents are the most frequent fatal accidents, followed by accidents involving drowning, fires, burns, and firearms. Other major causes of accidents involve recreational activity involving bicycles, swings, skateboards, and contact sports. Encourage parents of school-age children to have their children assume some responsibility for their own safety by establishing rules and acting as good role models (Box 23.5).

Blood pressure elevation in childhood is the single best predictor of adult hypertension. This recognition emphasizes the significance of making blood pressure measurement a part of every annual assessment of a school-age child (National Institutes of Health [NIH], 2015; Hockenberry et al., 2017). Measure a child's blood pressure on at least three separate occasions with the appropriate-size cuff and in a relaxed situation before concluding that the child's blood pressure is elevated and needs further medical attention.

Childhood obesity is a prominent health problem, which increases a child's risk for hypertension, diabetes, coronary artery disease, and other chronic health problems. In addition, overweight children are frequently the targets of teasing and bullying, and these children are less likely to be chosen for team or peer activities. Daily exercise and maintaining normal body weight are important as both interventions and prevention (Kovalskys et al., 2016; Hockenberry et al., 2017).

Acute Care. During illness school-age children usually tolerate the absence of their parents better than younger children because of their reasoning abilities. Although they understand that their parents often need to be elsewhere, they want and expect daily visits and phone calls and texts. The items that school-age children often bring from home such as their own pillows and favorite books give them a sense of security and independence. During times of illness and hospitalization, honesty, factual information, and interest in their concerns are helpful in establishing a trusting relationship with school-age children.

School-age children are usually able to pinpoint their pain, describe it with moderate assistance, and sometimes attempt to explain its cause. They often use play to cope with their pain or withdraw in an attempt to deal with their discomfort. They are usually aware that they receive medication for pain but sometimes do not ask for it until the pain is intense. They are quick to learn to use a scale to assess their discomfort. Most school-age children are eager learners who enjoy learning to find their pulse, read a thermometer, or operate the blood pressure machine during hospitalization. Many are able to help check their urine for sugar or protein or learn to do their own fingersticks for blood samples. School-age children who become ill are often threatened by a loss of their recently developed independence by needing to use a bedpan, having help with bathing, having to be on bed rest, or having someone else select their food choices.

Preadolescent

At present children experience more emotional and social pressures than they did 30 years ago. As a result, children 10 to 12 years of age are now having experiences that were once unique to 14- and 15-year-old youths. This transitional period between childhood and adolescence is preadolescence. Others refer to this period as *late childhood, early adolescence, pubescence,* and *transescence.* Physically it refers to the beginning of the second skeletal growth spurt, when the physical changes such as the development of pubic hair and female breasts begin. Children also become more social, and their behavioral patterns become much less predictable.

Puberty. A wide variation exists between the sexes and within the same sex as to when the physical changes of puberty begin. Use the ranges of normal growth to assess the progress of growth for an adolescent patient. As with increases in height and weight, the pattern of sexual changes is more significant than their time of onset. Large deviations from normal time frames require attention. Visible and invisible changes take place during puberty as a result of hormonal changes.

The physical changes of puberty enhance achievement of sexual identity. These changes encourage the development of masculine and feminine behaviors. If these physical changes involve deviations, the person has more difficulty developing a comfortable sexual identity.

Girls attain 90% to 95% of their adult height by **menarche,** the onset of menstruation, and reach their full height by 1 to 2 years after menarche. Boys continue to grow taller until 18 to 20 years of age. Adolescents are sensitive about physical changes that make them different from peers. Thus they are generally interested in the normal pattern of growth and their personal growth curves.

Adolescent

Adolescence is the transition from childhood to adulthood, usually between 13 and 18 years of age but sometimes extending until graduation from college. The term *adolescence* refers to the psychological maturation of an individual, whereas puberty refers to the point when reproduction is possible. A steady progression of physical, social, cognitive, psychological, and moral changes characterizes this period. This is a period when adolescents search for a sense of identity (Erikson, 1963). The adaptations required by these changes push adolescents to develop individualized coping mechanisms and styles of behaviors, which they will continue to use or adapt throughout life.

Physical Development. Although timing varies greatly, physical changes occur rapidly during adolescence. Sexual maturation follows the development of primary and secondary sexual characteristics. Primary characteristics are the physical and hormonal changes necessary for reproduction. Secondary characteristics differentiate males from females externally.

Adolescents depend on the development of secondary sex characteristics to define their maleness or femaleness. In addition, this helps them feel secure and like their peers. Cultural attitudes, expectations of sex role behavior, and available role models also influence sexual identity. The masculine and feminine behaviors that teenagers see and the expectations they perceive for behaving as a man or woman affect how they express sexuality. Adolescents master age-appropriate sexuality when they feel comfortable with sexual behaviors, choices, and relationships.

Language development is complete by adolescence, although vocabulary continues to expand. The primary focus becomes developing diverse communication skills to use effectively in many situations, which the person will refine later in life. Adolescents need to communicate thoughts, feelings, and facts to peers, parents, teachers, and other people of authority.

Developing moral judgment depends on cognitive and communication skills and peer interaction. Moral development, begun in early childhood, matures. Adolescents learn to understand that rules are cooperative agreements that can be changed to fit the situation rather than absolutes. They learn to apply rules by using their own judgment rather than simply to avoid punishment as in the earlier years. They judge themselves by internalized ideals, which often lead to conflict between personal and group values.

Adolescents are more likely to engage in risk-taking behaviors that often jeopardize their safety. The prefrontal area of the brain, which is responsible for impulse control, is not fully developed until 25 years of age. Adolescents have a sense of invulnerability, which also increases risk-taking behavior (CDC, 2017c). The incidence of motor vehicle accidents, sexually transmitted infections (STIs), and substance experimentation and addiction increases during adolescence.

The search for personal identity is the major task of adolescent psychosocial development. Teenagers establish close

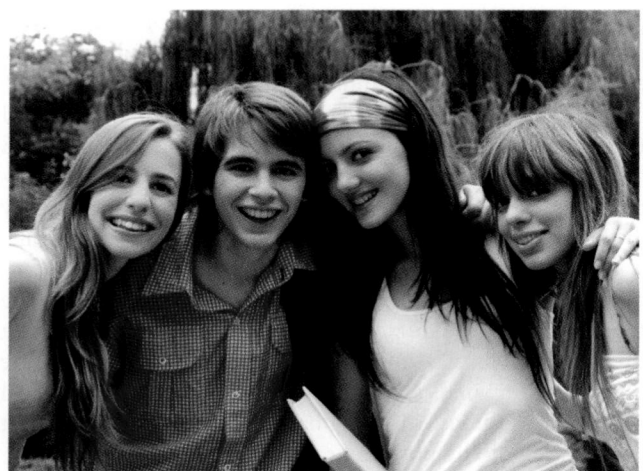

FIG 23.4 Peer interactions help increase self-esteem during puberty.

peer relationships or remain socially isolated (Fig. 23.4). Erikson (1963) sees identity (or role) confusion as the prime task of this stage. Teenagers need to become emotionally independent from their parents and yet retain family ties. They also need to develop their own ethical systems based on personal values.

Health Promotion. A component of personal identity is perception of health. Healthy adolescents evaluate their own health according to feelings of well-being, ability to function normally, and absence of symptoms. Health problems causing severe or long-term alteration of these factors permanently alter self-identity. Along with parents, you help adolescents take responsibility for their own health status and practices (Box 23.6).

The major causes of mortality in adolescents are injuries, homicide, and suicide (CDC, 2014; Hockenberry et al., 2017). Motor and other vehicular accidents, pregnancy, STIs, and substance abuse are major causes of morbidity. Mental disorders, chronic illness, and eating disorders are other causes.

Health services for adolescents need to be readily available, affordable, and approachable for teens to use them. Adolescents tend to use school-based programs. Health care providers need skills in interviewing adolescents and identifying individuals more at risk. Successful health promotion activities actively involve teenagers at all times. Involving teens in organizations that promote responsible behaviors such as Students Against Destructive Decisions (SADD) is a key element. Through your efforts in the school and community you can make many contributions to help meet the *Healthy People 2020* objectives (Office of Disease Prevention and Health Promotion [ODPHP], 2017). Wearing seat belts when in a motor vehicle and refraining from texting while driving are important topics to emphasize with adolescents.

Social media is a very important part of a teenager's life. Social networking can help teenagers stay connected with family and friends, but it can also present issues such as cyberbullying and leave them vulnerable to dangerous

---

BOX 23.6 HEALTH PROMOTION GUIDELINES FOR ADOLESCENTS AND THEIR PARENTS

- Set clear, reasonable limits for acceptable behavior and consequences for breaking the rules.
- Enforce automobile safety including driver's education course; use of seat belts; risks to self and others associated with drinking, drugs, and driving; use of helmets by bicyclists and motorcyclists (CDC, 2017a).
- Develop a mutual plan so that the adolescent never gets into a car when the driver has been drinking or the adolescent never drives if he or she has been drinking; plan to include who to call to pick up the adolescent.
- Become aware of warning signs of depression and suicide, alternatives to suicide, and methods to deal with a suicidal peer.
- Understand the potential of social isolation and excessive use of computer for recreational activities (e.g., searching the Internet, solitary computer games).
- Discuss threats to safety from the Internet and social media (e.g., identity theft, sexual predators, cyberbullying).
- Deal with peer pressure, school-related stressors, anger, and violent feelings through decision-making skills, conflict resolution, and positive coping strategies.
- Prevent unintentional injuries (e.g., classes on use of firearms, danger of swimming alone or under the influence of alcohol or drugs).
- Discuss sexual experimentation and measures to prevent STIs and pregnancy including abstinence, transmission of infection, symptoms of disease, prophylactic measures, and community organizations that provide assistance.
- Support development of sexual identity (i.e., heterosexual, homosexual, bisexual).
- Complete routine HIV testing and encourage vaccination for HPV for at-risk adolescents.
- Teach breast awareness and testicular self-examination.

HIV, Human immunodeficiency virus; *STIs,* sexually transmitted infections.

---

situations. It is important for adolescents to know to be wary of strangers, not share personal information, keep passwords private, and notify their parents if they have an uncomfortable online experience (Nemours Foundation, 2014).

Substance abuse is a major concern with teenagers. Adolescents are at risk for experimental or recreational substance use. When you assess a risk, educate to prevent accidents related to substance abuse, and counsel adolescents in rehabilitation.

Suicide is the second leading cause of death in people between 15 and 34 years of age (CDC, 2015). Depression and social isolation commonly precede a suicide attempt, but suicide most likely results from a combination of several factors. Be alert to the following warning signs, which often occur for at least 1 month before a suicide attempt (Hockenberry et al., 2017):

1. Decrease in school performance
2. Withdrawal

3. Loss of initiative
4. Loneliness, sadness, or crying
5. Appetite and sleep disturbances
6. Verbalization of suicidal thoughts

Make immediate referrals to mental health professionals when your assessment suggests that an adolescent is considering suicide. Guidance helps the adolescent focus on the positive aspects of life and strengthens coping abilities.

Sexual experimentation is common among adolescents. Peer pressure, physiological and emotional changes, and societal expectations contribute to heterosexual and homosexual relations. In a recent CDC survey of high school students (2017d), 41% admitted to having sexual intercourse. Of those who had sexual intercourse within the previous three months, 43% did not use a condom the last time they had sex, and 21% used alcohol or drugs previous to having intercourse. The risk-taking behaviors of adolescent sexual activity and drug use make adolescents vulnerable to the threat of human immunodeficiency virus (HIV) infection, human papilloma virus (HPV), and acquired immunodeficiency syndrome (AIDS).

The United States has one of the highest rates of teenage pregnancy in the world (CDC, 2017e). Adolescent pregnancy occurs across socioeconomic classes, in public and private schools, among all ethnic and religious backgrounds, and in all parts of the country (Hockenberry et al., 2017).

Acute Care. Hospitalization imposes rules and separates adolescents from their usual support system, restricts their independence, and threatens their personal identity. Adolescents who are forced into dependency or have their need for privacy ignored respond with frustration, anger, or self-assertion. Most hospitals allow peers to visit. Many adolescents welcome peer visitors, and hospitals often allow patients to go to a lounge or cafeteria with them. However, some adolescents isolate themselves until they are able to compete on an equal basis with peers. A mobile device is often the lifeline between adolescents and their friends and helps them maintain their place in their social group.

Adolescents who are more independent from their parents usually do well with intermittent visiting but expect some type of daily contact. Some adolescents request that their parent remain with them throughout the hospitalization, demonstrating that they also experience regression with the stress of illness. It is important that you address the patient rather than the parents during the assessment process.

Adolescents usually describe and locate their pain with minimal assistance. They are usually aware of the medication they receive for pain and like to be in control of when you give it to them. Many of them are able to use distraction and relaxation techniques to decrease their discomfort.

Young Adult

Adult developmental changes are based on earlier characteristics that help shape subsequent behaviors. Each person's development is a unique process. Young adulthood is defined as the ages between 20 and 30 (Leifer, 2013). During this phase the individual moves away from the family and marries or remains single. Young adults are active and adapt to new experiences and newly acquired independence.

Young adults have reached physical maturity, have achieved the highest level of cognitive ability according to Piaget, and are expected to exhibit a high degree of psychosocial maturity. Many young adults recognize that they are continuously in the process of becoming more mature in their behavior.

Physical Development. Young adults usually complete their physical growth by the age of 20. They are usually at their peak of health and less commonly experience severe illnesses compared with other adults. Although physical changes associated with aging have begun, the effects are not great enough to be noticed or require attention.

Cognitive Development. Rational thinking habits and flexibility of thought increase steadily through the adult years. Formal and informal educational experiences, general life experiences, and occupational opportunities dramatically increase conceptual, problem-solving, and motor skills. A rich, stimulating environment for the growing and maturing adult encourages the development of full creative potential. An understanding of how adults learn helps you develop teaching plans for them (see Chapter 12).

Psychosocial Development. The emotional health of young adults is related to their ability to effectively address personal and social tasks. According to developmental theorists, certain patterns or trends are relatively predictable. Once young adults begin to work in their chosen area, they have more time and energy to select a mate (if they have not already done so) and develop a greater sense of intimacy. Many choose to marry, but an increasing number of young adults are choosing to remain single.

Identifying a preferred occupational area is a major task. When individuals know their skills, talents, and personality characteristics, occupational choices are easier, and they are generally more satisfied with their choices. In the young and middle adult years, job satisfaction is a major factor in achievement and responsibility.

The developmental tasks of young adults are potentially filled with stressful situations. Most young adults have the physical and emotional resources and support systems to meet the many challenges, tasks, and responsibilities they face. You often help them develop time-management skills or mobilize their resources and support systems, especially when one of their immediate family members is ill or hospitalized.

Health Promotion. Health teaching and counseling are directed at helping young adults improve their health habits. Understanding the dynamics of behavior and habits helps you design interventions that help young adults develop or reinforce health-promoting behaviors. You become a teacher and facilitator. Remember that although you do not always change young adults' habits, you are able to raise their level of knowledge regarding the potential impact of behavior on health. Young adults have control of and are responsible for their own behaviors. Explain psychological principles of changing habits, offer information about health risks, and provide positive reinforcement of health-directed behaviors and decisions. Minimize barriers to change such as lack of knowledge or motivation to bring about change.

Young adults are generally active and have no major health problems. However, their fast-paced lifestyles put them at risk for illnesses or disabilities during their middle or older adult years. Motor vehicle accidents and violence are the greatest cause of mortality and morbidity among young adults. Poor adherence to routine screening schedules puts young adults at risk for severe illnesses because of failed early detection. Encourage your young adult patients to follow cancer screening guidelines for breast awareness, testicular self-examination (TSE), and genital self-examination (see Chapter 16).

Family stressors occur at any time. Family life has peaks, when everyone in the family works together, and valleys, when everyone appears to pull apart (see Chapter 25). Situational stressors occur during events such as births, deaths, illnesses, marriages, divorces, and job losses. A psychosocial assessment allows you to identify areas of particular stress for the young adult (see Chapter 26). After identifying these stressors, work with the patient to modify the stress response.

Acute Care. Many young adults do not experience hospitalization, but when they do it is often threatening because it interferes with their employment and fulfillment of family responsibilities. Scheduled hospitalizations allow adults to effectively plan to meet the needs of their families and expectations of their employment. Unanticipated hospitalizations often cause chaos for adults and all the people directly involved in their lives. If young adults do not have a strong support system, they usually welcome your help to establish priorities and mobilize their resources. Adults are often impatient with the time and energy requirements that a chronic health problem requires for good management. Support groups often help patients deal with these challenges.

Middle-Age Adult

Middle adulthood usually refers to the years between 40 and 65. For many it is a period when one has both grown children and older adult parents. Most have experienced personal and career achievements and socioeconomic stability. Using leisure time in satisfying and creative ways is a challenge that, if met satisfactorily, enables middle-age adults to prepare for retirement.

Physical Changes. Accepting and adjusting to the physiological changes of middle age is one of the major developmental tasks of this age period. Because middle adulthood spans 25 years, many of the physical changes described usually do not occur until later in the developmental period. Middle-age adults use much energy to adapt self-concept and body image to physiological realities and changes in physical appearance. Table 23.2 summarizes these expected physical assessment findings.

Climacteric. Climacteric is the decline of reproductive capacity and accompanying changes brought about by the decrease in sexual hormones. It affects men and women differently. Men begin to experience decreased fertility, but they are able to continue to father children. Menopause, when a woman stops ovulating and menstruating, occurs when 12 months have passed since the last menstrual flow.

Cognitive Development. Changes in the cognitive function of middle-age adults are few except during illness or trauma. Performance on intelligence tests indicates increases in some areas, particularly verbal abilities and tasks involving stored knowledge. Although middle-age adults sometimes perform more slowly and are not as adept at solving new or unusual problems, the ability to solve practical problems based on experience peaks at midlife because of the ability for integrative thinking.

Psychosocial Development. According to Erikson (1963), the primary developmental task of the middle-age adult years is to achieve generativity, which is the willingness to establish and guide the next generation and care for others. Many find particular joy in helping their children and other young people become productive and responsible adults.

Expected changes in the middle-age adult involve expected events such as children moving away from home (the empty-nest syndrome) or unexpected events such as a marital separation or the death of a spouse or parent. Another increasingly common situation is that many middle age adults find themselves caring for both their own children still living at home and an elderly parent. For this reason, middle age adults are frequently referred to as the "sandwich generation." These changes result in stress that affects the middle-age adult's overall level of health.

Career changes occur by choice or as a result of changes in the workplace or society as a whole. In recent decades, middle-age adults more often change occupations because they find themselves less satisfied with their present employment. In some cases, technological advances or changes in the direction of industry force them to change work situations. Such changes, especially when unanticipated, result in stress that affects family relationships, self-concept, and financial security for the later years.

Marital changes that occur during middle age include death of a spouse, separation, divorce, and the choice of remarrying or remaining single. An adult goes through a period of loss and grief during which it is necessary to adapt to the change in marital status.

The increasing life span in the United States and Canada has led to increased numbers of older adults in the population. Therefore, greater numbers of middle-age adults address the personal and social issues confronting their aging parents. Adult children frequently assume partial or total caregiving responsibilities for their older parents. This means that adult children help with personal care, decision making, housekeeping, financial matters, transportation, and medical care management tasks. The burden placed on adult

TABLE 23.2 PHYSICAL ASSESSMENT FINDINGS IN THE MIDDLE-AGE ADULT

BODY SYSTEM	NORMAL OR EXPECTED FINDINGS
Integument	Intact Appropriate distribution of pigmentation Slow, progressive decrease in skin turgor Graying and loss of hair
Head and neck	Symmetry of scalp, skull, and face
Eyes	Visual acuity by Snellen chart less than 20/50 Loss of accommodation of lens to focus light on near objects Pupillary reaction to light and accommodation Normal visual fields and extraocular movements Normal retinal structures
Ears	Normal auditory structures; acuity of high-pitched sounds declines
Nose, sinuses, and throat	Patent nares and intact sinuses, mouth, and pharynx Location of trachea at midline Nonpalpable lateral thyroid lobes
Thorax and lungs	Increased anteroposterior diameter Respiratory rate 10–20 breaths/min and regular Normal tactile fremitus, resonance, and breath sounds
Heart and vascular system	Normal heart sounds Systole: S_1 less than S_2 at base Diastole: S_1 less than S_2 at apex Point of maximal impulse: at fifth intercostal space in midclavicular line and 2 cm or less in diameter Vital signs 　Temperature: 36.0°–37.6° C (96.8°–99.6° F) 　Pulse: 60–100 beats/min (conditioned athlete, 50 beats/min) 　Blood pressure: less than 120 mm Hg systolic; less than 80 mm Hg diastolic All pulses palpable
Breasts	Decreased size resulting from decreased muscle mass Normal nipples and areola
Abdomen	No tenderness or organomegaly Decreased strength of abdominal muscles
Female reproductive system	Change in menstrual cycle and duration and quality of menstrual flow "Hot flashes" Change in cervical mucosa
Male reproductive system	Normal penis and scrotum Prostatic enlargement in some men
Musculoskeletal system	Decreased muscle mass Decreased range of joint motion
Neurological system	Appropriate affect, appearance, and behavior Lucidity and appropriate level of cognitive ability Intact cranial nerves Adequate motor responses Responsive sensory system

family caregivers increases if they are also employed and continuing to raise children. Most caregivers are women, and women spend 50% more time in caregiving roles than men. The average caregiver is 50 years of age and is married and employed (Family Caregiver Alliance, 2015). The middle-age adult and the older adult parent often have conflicting relationship priorities. The older adult often desires to remain independent, whereas the adult child strives to protect the parent. Negotiations and compromises are useful in defining and resolving such problems.

Health Promotion. Because middle-age adults experience physiological changes and face certain health realities, their perceptions of health and health behaviors are often important factors in maintaining health. Middle-age adults are more prone to stress-related illnesses such as heart attacks,

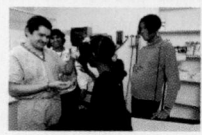

BOX 23.7 PATIENT-CENTERED CARE

As Louis prepared to help develop health promotion activities for Crystal and her family, he read about the impact of a patient's culture on health care practices. Louis knows that it is important to respect his patient's cultural beliefs and practices, but he also understands the value of routine health screenings (Kidd et al., 2015). Because there is a strong family history for breast cancer, Louis wants to help Crystal and her mother develop breast health practices. He knows that breast cancer survival rates are increasing, but he also recognizes that cultural beliefs and practices influence adherence to breast cancer screening. Although the 5-year survival rate for breast cancer is steadily improving, the survival rate for African American women remains lower than that of women of other races. African American women are not as diligent as Caucasian women in having routine clinical breast examinations (CBEs) or mammograms (Kidd et al., 2015). Louis learns that Crystal's mother, at age 44, has not yet had a mammogram. Her risk for cancer makes her a candidate for screening. More African American women delay breast cancer screening and at the time of diagnosis often have late-stage breast cancer (Kidd et al., 2015). Louis wants to learn if Crystal's mother has talked with her physician about screening.

IMPLICATIONS FOR PRACTICE
- Assess Crystal and her mother to determine their family's beliefs and practices about breast awareness, CBE, and mammography.
- Ask Crystal about the role of their family's spirituality and spiritual practices in coping with illness, symptoms, and other life stressors.
- Contact the breast health center at the city clinic. Determine if Crystal and her mother desire to be introduced to culturally specific breast health practices from a female health care provider.

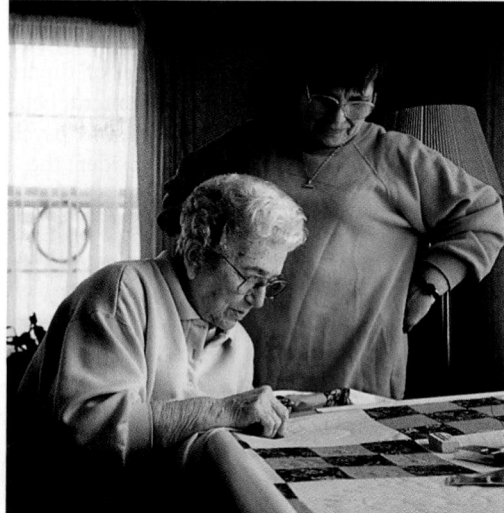

FIG 23.5 Quilting keeps this older adult active.

hypertension, migraine headaches, backache, arthritis, cancer, and autoimmune diseases.

The leading causes of death in people between 45 and 64 years of age are heart disease, cancer (primarily lung, breast, and colorectal), stroke, accidental injuries, and chronic obstructive pulmonary diseases. Middle-age adults need to continue the same recommended health practices outlined in the discussion on the young adult. It is important that you understand cultural implications when providing health screening to your patients (Box 23.7). Encourage middle-age patients to follow cancer screening guidelines (see Chapter 16).

When middle-age adults seek health care, you need to develop goals for positive health behaviors. For example, women need to increase the calcium in their diets to decrease the risk for osteoporosis. In addition, organizations such as exercise and fitness clubs give men and women the opportunity to participate in many physical activities. These activities help improve balance, coordination, and activity tolerance.

Acute Care. Middle-age adults have the same family and occupational concerns regarding hospitalization as young adults. There is sometimes less stress because of the security of employment or because the children who are still at home are usually old enough to care for themselves. However, underinsured middle-age adults face serious financial threats. Middle-age adults are at risk for a decline in their physical health. Chronic health problems such as sickle cell anemia, arthritis, asthma, diabetes, cancer, and lung disease require ongoing medical care and often brief hospitalizations. The middle-age adult is usually interested in his or her health and wants to be informed.

Older Adult

Most older adults are physically active, intelligent, and socially engaged (Fig. 23.5). Extended life spans allow many older adults to enjoy their retirement by pursuing interests for which they previously had little time. The number of older adults in the United States continues to grow. In addition, statistics project that the diversity of this population will increase. By 2050, it is expected that the older adults from minority groups (e.g., African American, American Indians, Asian/Pacific Islanders, Hispanics, and Islamic) will account for 33% of adults older than 65 years of age (Vincent and Velkoff, 2010).

Older adulthood traditionally begins after retirement, but the time when people retire varies greatly. It is not unusual for people who write about older adults to divide them into the "young old," who are vital, vigorous, and active, and the "old old," who are frail and infirm. The fastest growing subset is people older than 90 years of age, whose growth rate tripled between 1980 and 2010 and is expected to quadruple between 2010 and 2050 (Ortman et al., 2014). **Geriatrics** is the branch of health care dealing with the physiology and psychology of aging and with the diagnosis and treatment of diseases affecting older adults. Gerontology is the study of all aspects of the aging process and its consequences.

Nursing care of older adults poses special challenges because of diversity in patients' physical, cognitive, and psychosocial health. Older adults vary in level of function and productivity. Before making a health assessment, be aware of the normal expected findings on physical and psychosocial assessment for an older adult and consider the normal changes of aging.

Physical Development. An older adult must adjust to the physical changes of aging. These changes are not associated with a disease state but are the normal changes anticipated with aging. Table 23.3 describes the common types of physiological changes. They occur in all people but take place at different rates and depend on accompanying circumstances in an individual's life.

TABLE 23.3	COMMON PHYSICAL CHANGES OF AGING
SYSTEM	**NORMAL OR EXPECTED FINDINGS**
Integument	
Skin color	Brown age spots and spotty pigmentation in areas exposed to sun; pallor even in absence of anemia
Moisture	Dry, scaly
Temperature	Extremities cooler; perspiration decreased
Texture	Decreased elasticity; wrinkles; folding, sagging
Fat distribution	Decreased on extremities; increased on abdomen
Hair	Thinning and graying on scalp; axillary and pubic hair and hair on extremities sometimes decreased; facial hair in men decreased; chin and upper lip hair present in women
Nails	Decreased growth rate
Head and Neck	
Head	Nasal and facial bones sharp and angular; loss of eyebrow hair in women; men's eyebrows become bushier
Eyes	Decreased visual acuity; decreased accommodation; reduced adaptation to darkness; sensitivity to glare; diminished light reflex
Ears	Decreased pitch discrimination; diminished hearing acuity
Nose and sinuses	Increased nasal hair; decreased sense of smell
Mouth and pharynx	Use of bridges or dentures; decreased sense of taste; atrophy of papillae of lateral edges of tongue; occasionally change in voice pitch
Neck	Thyroid gland nodular; slight tracheal deviation resulting from muscle atrophy
Thorax and Lungs	Increased anteroposterior diameter; increased chest rigidity; increased respiratory rate with decreased lung expansion
Heart and Vascular System	BP remains within normal limits, less than 120/80 mm Hg (NIH, 2015); BP between 120/80 and 139/89 mm Hg is considered prehypertension; elevations in BP are not a normal aspect of aging, and older adults need minor elevations monitored (NIH, 2015); peripheral pulses easily palpated; pedal pulses weaker, and lower extremities colder, especially at night; orthostatic hypertension common
Breasts	Diminished breast tissue; pendulous
Gastrointestinal System	Decreased salivary secretions, which makes swallowing more difficult; decreased peristalsis; decreased production of digestive enzymes, hydrochloric acid, pepsin, and pancreatic enzymes, leading to indigestion and constipation
Reproductive System	
Female	Decreased estrogen; decreased uterine size; decreased secretions; atrophy of epithelial lining of vagina; vaginal dryness
Male	Decreased testosterone; decreased sperm count; erections less firm and slower to develop; decreased testicular size
Urinary System	Decreased renal filtration and renal efficiency; subsequent loss of protein from kidney; nocturia
Female	Urgency and stress incontinence from decrease in perineal muscle tone
Male	Frequent urination resulting from prostatic enlargement
Musculoskeletal System	Decreased muscle mass and strength; bone demineralization (more pronounced in women); shortening of trunk from intervertebral space narrowing; decreased joint mobility; decreased range of joint motion; kyphosis (usually in women); slowed reaction time
Neurological System	Decreased rate of voluntary or automatic reflexes; decreased ability to respond to multiple stimuli; insomnia; shorter sleeping periods

BP, Blood pressure.
Modified from Ebersole P, et al: *Toward healthy aging: human needs and nursing response,* ed 9, St Louis, 2016, Mosby.

Cognitive Development.

Older adults often remain alert and highly perceptive until the time of their death. Nevertheless, the misconception that older adults always have cognitive impairments and suffer from memory loss and confusion persists. Because cognitive impairment occurs in this age-group, be aware of the nature and type of these impairments.

Certain aspects of short-term memory (e.g., numbers) decrease with age; however, visual memory, which allows a person to remember how to read, remains strong. Long-term memory for newly learned information decreases significantly with age, but recall for distant experiences and procedural experiences (e.g., driving) do not seem to be affected in the later years of life. Both intelligence and memory vary greatly among individuals. Most older people who want and need to learn new skills and information do so when the skills and information are presented more slowly over a long period. Continuing mental activity is essential to keeping older adults alert (Leifer, 2013).

Three common conditions affecting cognition in older adults are delirium, dementia, and depression (Box 23.8). It is important that you learn how to distinguish among these three conditions to select appropriate interventions for your patients. Use a valid assessment tool such as the Mini-Mental State Examination (MMSE) to accurately assess for patients' cognitive changes. Take the time to learn how to correctly use these cognitive assessment tools (Saczynski et al., 2015).

Delirium is an acute confusional state and requires prompt assessment. It is a potentially reversible cognitive impairment that often has physiological causes such as electrolyte imbalance, hypoglycemia, infection, and medications. In addition, very slight body temperature alterations cause delirium in older adults. This condition often accompanies infections such as pneumonia. The characteristics of delirium usually include fluctuations in cognition that develop over a short time such as a reduced ability to focus, sustain, or shift attention; there are also acute changes in mood, arousal, and self-awareness. Other signs are hallucinations, transient incoherent speech, disturbed sleep pattern, and disorientation.

Dementia is a broad category of disorders that refers to a generalized impairment of intellectual functioning that interferes with social and occupational functioning. Dementia differs from delirium in that it is a gradual, progressive, irreversible dysfunction. The many causes of dementia include neurological disorders, vascular disorders, inherited disorders, and infections (NIH, 2017). Thus early recognition is important, requiring you to make thorough observations of patient behavior, neurological function (see Chapter 16), and laboratory diagnostic studies. Family and friends are valuable resources in detecting behavioral changes, as this disorder may go unnoticed by people who see the patient infrequently.

Alzheimer disease is the most common form of dementia. It is a progressive loss of memory (amnesia), loss of ability to recognize objects (agnosia), loss of the ability to perform familiar tasks (apraxia), and loss of language skills (aphasia). As the disease progresses some patients also experience changes in personality and behavior such as anxiety,

---

BOX 23.8 EVIDENCE-BASED PRACTICE

PICO Question: What interventions best help reduce anxiety for adult children caring for parents with dementia?

SUMMARY OF EVIDENCE

Older adults in the United States who require assistance because of chronic illnesses or disabilities frequently receive help from their family to live independently. According to the Pew Research Center, 39% of American adults reported that they were unpaid caregivers in 2013, an increase from 30% in 2010 (Desilver, 2013). Most caregivers are women, and nearly half of them report providing complex nursing tasks (Reinhard et al., 2014). Research indicates that informal caregivers are more likely to experience anxiety than the general population. Nurses can assess risk factors for anxiety in caregivers to enhance positive caregiving outcomes. Helping caregivers to identify and develop healthy coping skills such as problem solving, positive reappraisal, assertiveness, and control of negative thoughts reduces anxiety (del-Pino-Casado et al., 2014).

APPLICATION TO NURSING PRACTICE

- Encourage adult children to discuss caregiving plans with their parents to give them a sense of control in assuming the caregiving role (Day et al., 2014).
- Encourage adult children who are going to be assuming a caregiving role to discuss resources with their siblings (Day et al., 2014).
- Help caregivers locate community support groups and respite resources.
- Encourage caregivers to reconcile their work schedules, when possible, with family caregiving responsibilities.
- Assess caregivers for work flexibility to identify high-risk groups.
- Assess caregivers for compassion fatigue (Day et al., 2014).
- Encourage caregivers to identify and develop healthy coping skills (del-Pino-Casado et al., 2014).

---

suspiciousness, agitation, and delusions or hallucinations (Alzheimer's Association, 2017).

Ischemic vascular dementia (IVD) is the second most common form of dementia. It can be characterized by either an abrupt loss of function, usually from a stroke, or general slowing of cognitive abilities. The person may have difficulty with cognitive tasks such as planning. For some people the condition develops slowly with a gradual loss of function and/or thinking (Ebersole et al., 2016).

Depression among older adults is increasing. This diagnosis was once overlooked and assumed to be a normal response to aging, physical losses, or other life events. Depression is treatable and often reversible. Health care workers must look at the possible underlying or contributing factors in an attempt to find the proper treatment methods (NIH, 2017).

Psychosocial Development.

The older adult must adapt to many psychosocial changes. Among the more common transitions with aging are retirement, volunteerism, and loss of spousal roles (Ebersole et al., 2016). Despite these changes, the older adult has the potential for developing new and fulfilling life patterns.

Most older adults want to work as long as they are physically able (Ebersole et al., 2016). The time a person chooses to retire is often based on type of work, status achieved, and length of time employed. When a patient describes retirement, it is important to know whether the individual is fully retired, partially retired, or retired from one position to assume another.

Retirement represents a developmental stage that may occupy 30 years of one's life. It also represents a highly productive and fulfilling period of life. Retirement affects more individuals than the retired person; it affects spouses, adult children, and grandchildren. In addition, the retired person may be spending more time alone for the first time in his or her life.

Reminiscence, or life review, is a technique that facilitates an individual's preparation for the end of life. It is an adaptive function of older adults that allows them to recall the past to assign new meaning to past experiences. Reminiscence is the natural way that older adults revive their past in an attempt to establish order and meaning. There is evidence that life review in older adults enhances psychological well-being and positively impacts their quality of life (O'Shea et al., 2014).

Death. Most older adults experience death of spouses, friends, and sometimes children. These losses require individuals to go through a process of grieving (see Chapter 27). Some experience loss when they lose a partner after many years in a satisfying relationship (Ebersole et al., 2016). For many older adults, the grief associated with loss of a spouse lasts for many years; thus they require support from family, nurses, and other health professionals. Show warmth and caring to help patients feel they are not alone.

A common misconception is that the death of an older adult is always a blessing and the culmination of a full and rich life. Many dying older adults still have life goals and are not emotionally prepared to die.

Aloneness and Loneliness. With advancing age, more people live alone. This is particularly common for older Caucasian women. However, living alone is not equivalent to the feeling of loneliness. A person can be surrounded by others yet still feel lonely. Ebersole et al. (2016) define loneliness as an affective state of longing and emptiness, whereas being alone is to be solitary, apart from others, and undisturbed. Many patients choose to be alone or isolated simply because of the desire for privacy or an opportunity for self-reflection and creativity. Loneliness is sometimes a passive and painful emotion, influenced by psychological, economic, sociological, and physiological factors.

Housing and Environment. Changes in social roles, family responsibilities, and health status influence an older patient's choice of living arrangements. An older adult sometimes needs to change living arrangements because of the death of a spouse or a change in health status. A change in an older patient's living arrangements requires an extended period of adjustment during which assistance and support

will be needed from family and friends and health care professionals.

Health Promotion. The possibility of an individual being reasonably healthy and fit in later life depends on his or her lifestyle. Older adults need to continue the same recommended health practices introduced in the section on young adults. Some need encouragement to maintain a pattern of physical exercise and activity. It is not too late for an older person to begin an exercise program; however, older adults need to have a complete physical examination, which usually includes a stress cardiogram or stress test. Assessment of activity tolerance helps you and the patient plan a program that meets physical needs while allowing for physical impairments (Box 23.9).

Most older adults are in good health; however, chronic medical conditions increase dramatically with age. The effect of a chronic health problem on mobility and independence depends greatly on the individual. Most older adults can take charge of their lives and assume responsibility for preventing disability.

Sensory impairments are common in older adults (see Chapter 39). These changes are frequently the result of the normal aging process. Help the older adult identify resources

---

BOX 23.9 CARE OF THE OLDER ADULT
Health Promotion and Independence

- Provide information from the American Association of Retired Persons (http://www.aarp.org) regarding supplemental health insurance, group discounts for older adults, and medical and legal information.
- Discuss housing alternatives to aid in decisions regarding the sale of the home, relocation to another area of the country, or retirement communities.
- Instruct about health maintenance programs such as exercise activities that are designed to increase exercise tolerance, flexibility, and socialization (Nishiguchi et al., 2015).
- Encourage having annual influenza and routine pneumonia vaccines, especially when chronic illness is present (CDC, 2017b).
- Teach about safe and appropriate administration of prescribed drugs including purpose; effect; possible other prescription, over-the-counter, or dietary interactions; and reportable side effects.
- Encourage use of one pharmacy for prescription and over-the-counter preparations (Kaufman, 2017).
- Explain the importance of being sure to tell health care providers about all prescription drugs, over-the-counter preparations, and supplements that the individual takes (Maher et al., 2014).
- Discuss environmental safety issues (e.g., home lighting, floor coverings, stairs, shoes, electrical cords) to reduce the risk for falling.
- Educate about nutritional aspects related to disease (e.g., low-fat diet with hypertension, need for a balanced diet with reduced total calories because of aging changes and lower energy expenditures).

to help correct visual and auditory problems. The sense of touch usually remains strong. Older adults who become victims of social isolation are often deprived of touching and holding, which convey affection and friendliness. The touch of nurses and all caregivers who work with older adults serves to provide sensory stimulation; reduce anxiety; relieve physiological and emotional pain; orient older adults to reality; and provide comfort, particularly during the dying process.

Adults older than 65 years of age are the greatest users of prescription drugs. Many drugs interact with one another, potentiating or negating the effect of another drug. Some drugs cause confusion; affect balance; cause dizziness, nausea, or vomiting; or promote constipation or urinary frequency. Polypharmacy, the use of multiple prescription medications, administration of more medications than are indicated clinically, or excessive use of over-the-counter (OTC) medications, is a common problem. Older adults are vulnerable to the effects of polypharmacy because of the physiological changes of aging and comorbidities, which with the combined effects of multiple medications have the potential to cause new health problems (Maher et al., 2014; Kaufman, 2017).

Acute Care. Hospitalization is often disturbing to older adults because they are not accustomed to the environment and routines. Even older adults who live independently with some assistance from their families become temporarily disoriented by the strange surroundings of a hospital. Monitor patients for confusion and encourage frequent visitation by family members. Use reality orientation to reorient the older adult who has been disoriented by a change in environment, surgery, illness, or emotional stress.

Reality orientation is a communication modality used for making a patient aware of time, place, and person (Ebersole et al., 2016). The major purposes of reality orientation include the following:

- Restoring patients' sense of reality
- Improving their level of awareness
- Promoting socialization
- Elevating patients to a maximal level of independent functioning
- Minimizing confusion, disorientation, and physical regression

Environmental changes within a hospital such as the bright lights and lack of windows in intensive care and the noise from nearby roommates often lead to disorientation and confusion. A patient's environment and the nursing personnel are constantly changing in the hospital, and the immediate environment is unstable, making coping and adaptation difficult. Anticipate some disorientation and/or confusion when older adults are hospitalized, and incorporate reality orientation interventions into their care.

When an older adult is hospitalized or has an acute or chronic illness, the related physical dependence makes it difficult for the person to maintain a positive body image. Take the time to help the older adult maintain a pleasant appearance and present a socially acceptable image.

CRITICAL THINKING

Synthesis

Patient care requires you to apply what you know about a patient, your knowledge base, experience, and critical thinking attitudes and standards. Your synthesis of this information allows you to make sound decisions as you apply the nursing process. Critical thinking synthesis involves combining all available information to obtain a clear picture of the approach needed to provide patient-centered care.

Consider the scientific knowledge you have learned when individualizing patient care. In addition to your knowledge, you and your patients bring unique backgrounds and personal experiences to each care setting. Although you do not always discuss these individual perspectives openly, they influence your care. Both you and your patients have preexisting ideas as to how to best meet their developmental needs.

Knowledge. Before you initiate assessment, review the developmental theories that relate to your patient. In addition, as you work with your patients in attaining an optimal level of health, it is essential that you know the expected physical developmental milestones, psychosocial developmental crises, cognitive development, and health concerns for each age-group.

Another important area of knowledge to consider when caring for a patient's developmental needs is that of cultural awareness (see Chapter 21). Together with the patient, explore the cultural variations in family roles and relationships as they influence an individual's development to have a clear understanding of patient needs.

Experience. Use your experiences caring for or teaching patients from infancy to older adulthood to help you understand how thought processes change as people grow and develop. Your experiences help you determine different approaches to engage patients of various ages in their care. Your family, social, and educational experiences with individuals of various ages make it easier for you to determine age-specific appropriate or inappropriate behaviors and health concerns.

Attitudes. Humility is an important attitude for you to apply when collecting data about a patient's developmental history. It is easy to form opinions about patients' developmental needs based on a developmental theory and related psychosocial principles. However, as is the case in any nursing situation, do not assume that you know what a patient's needs are without assessing the developmental stage and needs of the patient. Often information about a patient's health practices reflects his or her cultural background, which is sometimes very different from yours. Creativity is a valuable critical thinking attitude when you assess an infant or child. Often you incorporate play or other activities into the assessment to better visualize a child's physical developmental capacities.

Standards. Use critical thinking standards to ensure that you are making the right decisions. When developing a plan of care that incorporates growth and development principles and approaches, strive to apply the intellectual standards of relevance and completeness. It is important that you use a developmental approach that fits with a patient's level of maturation. *For example, in the case study, asking Zachary to attempt a motor skill such as coloring a detailed picture or successfully using eating utensils is not within his ability, is irrelevant, and is inappropriate for promoting developmental enrichment.* When selecting a plan of care, you need to be sure that the plan uses psychosocial, cognitive, and physical approaches that complement and strengthen a patient's developmental abilities.

Use professional standards, such as the CDC (2017b) or AAP (2017a) standards for immunization (Box 23.10), when providing care to patients of various age-groups. Similarly, the American Cancer Society lists a variety of health screening standards for adults. Refer to these standards when providing patient education.

NURSING PROCESS

▪▪▪ ASSESSMENT

Nursing assessment of individuals across the life span requires you to be familiar with the physiological, cognitive, and psychosocial changes that occur during each stage of development and the health concerns for each age-group. Table 23.4 is an example of a focused assessment for a school-age child such as Crystal's daughter Monica. Several assessment tools facilitate concise but comprehensive data collection for individuals of various ages. Observe the interactions between the patient and any family member present during the health history, physical assessment, and developmental assessment. The data gathered provide information regarding the patient's lifestyle, level of functioning and coping skills, family relationships, lifestyle habits, health concerns, and health promotion activities.

Throughout life, illness and hospitalization are stressful experiences. Many factors affect the ability of individuals to cope such as their developmental level, their coping skills, their previous experiences with illness and hospitalization, and the seriousness of the diagnosis. The degree to which an illness interferes with activities of daily living and lifestyle and the availability of a support system also have an impact on how individuals cope. Be sure your assessment demonstrates an awareness of specific patient concerns at various stages of life.

Older Adult Considerations. Older adults have certain assessment parameters that must be observed or measured to help them maintain a safe and optimum level of health. You need to assess for your patient's ability to read and understand printed health information. Seventy percent of adults over 60 years of age have difficulty using printed materials; this difficulty ranges from actually being able to see the print

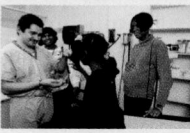

BOX 23.10 SYNTHESIS IN PRACTICE

Louis selected Crystal Taylor and her family to follow throughout this semester of his nursing program. As he prepares to begin an assessment, he focuses on 6-year-old Monica, whom Crystal has brought to the clinic for a checkup before beginning school. Louis recalls the physical, psychosocial, and cognitive developmental characteristics that are typical of the older preschool child and prepares to use this information as a basis for his observations. He plans to engage Monica in play activities with dolls to ensure that observations of her physical abilities are relevant and complete. He is also interested in any concerns that Crystal has regarding Monica's health. In preparation for doing anticipatory guidance with Monica and her mother, he reviews types of accidents common among her age-group and appropriate health promotion activities. He is also interested in observing the quality of the interaction between Monica and her mother and assessing how Crystal copes with being a single parent.

As the parent of a 4-year-old, Louis knows the importance of immunizations in keeping children free of many contagious diseases with serious consequences, and he is aware that children are not admitted to school without the completion of certain immunizations. His own child has made him very conscious of the great fear that young children have for bodily harm and the fact that Monica may have difficulty cooperating with an injection. He recalls the approach he has used to help his own son cooperate with and recover from the discomfort of an injection. Louis refers to the standards for immunizations that the American Academy of Pediatrics, the American Academy of Family Physicians, and the Centers for Disease Control and Prevention to determine Monica's immunization needs. Louis knows that the key to having a positive effect on the practice of health promotion activities by Crystal and her family members is the development of trust through positive interactions.

Louis' nursing instructors have informed him that he is responsible for encouraging health promotion activities among his patients. He recognizes that *Healthy People 2020: National Objectives for Improving Health* is a guide for choosing health promotion activities for Crystal's family (see Chapter 2). He knows he cannot be judgmental toward Crystal as a single parent and that he needs to assess the resources she has to support health promotion in her family. Understanding that Crystal probably has some definite ideas about parenting and health promotion ensures that Louis is complete in assessing patient needs and offering appropriate suggestions to support Crystal and her family.

to interpreting the printed health care information. Be aware of any cognitive, visual, or auditory challenges your patient might have and, if these are present, provide adequate time for your patient to respond to assessment questions or examination (CDC, 2016).

Ask questions related to patient safety. For example, if the patient is ambulatory, ask if there have been any recent falls. In addition, ask if the patient feels steady when walking or climbing stairs. Assess activity tolerance and exercise patterns.

TABLE 23.4 FOCUSED PATIENT ASSESSMENT

FACTORS TO ASSESS	QUESTIONS	PHYSICAL ASSESSMENT
Home safety	Where do you keep household cleaners, medications?	Observe patient's home environment.
	Has your child had any accidents at home during the last year? If so, please tell me about them.	Observe child's play area.
	Does your family have a home evacuation plan and a meeting place?	Along with parent, play out a situation when the home needs to be evacuated (e.g., fire) and observe evacuation drill and congregation of family at meeting place.
	Where do you keep your computer? Does your child have unsupervised use of the Internet? Do you have any parental controls that block unsafe sites?	If able, observe child's use of home computer if home visit is made.
Health promotion activities	Does your child have all immunizations? How current are your immunizations? Where do you keep this information?	Conduct an immunization history. Measure height and weight and compare with standards.
	Tell me about your child's usual food intake.	
Sibling interaction	How do your children get along? Do they play together?	Observe child playing and interacting with sibling.
	Are there any changes in your child's behavior, independence?	

If the patient lives alone, is he or she able to safely administer medication or other therapies, such has oxygen? Also determine the patient's support system. Are there family caregivers? Are friends assisting as caregivers?

Patient Expectations. During assessment, determine what patients and/or their families expect from caregivers. Remember that patients' expectations and preferences vary based on their developmental stage and culture as well as on their ethnic and social backgrounds. In the hospital setting, determine if family members want to participate in the care of a patient. You begin each day with a brief assessment to determine any changes in your patient's condition. Ask your patient, "What is your goal for today? And how can I help you meet your goal?" In the outpatient setting, assess the patient's and/or family's needs and preferences during the visit. At the beginning of a home visit ask, "What do you think is most important for us to accomplish today?" When preparing to leave ask, "Have I met your expectations for this visit?"

■ ■ ■ NURSING DIAGNOSIS

Your nursing assessment of a patient and, when appropriate, the family reveals clusters of data from the nursing history, physical examination, and developmental assessment. These data include defining characteristics and risk factors, which you analyze through critical thinking to select the nursing diagnoses that apply. Accuracy is important because the defining characteristics differentiate the problem-focused or health promotion nursing diagnoses that apply to the clinical situation. For example, *Parental Role Conflict* and *Impaired Parenting* are two distinctly different problem-focused nursing diagnoses. Carefully review all information before selecting the nursing diagnosis that applies to the needs of the patient and family. Defining characteristics for a problem-focused nursing diagnosis of *Ineffective Sexuality Pattern* include factors such as difficulties or limitations in sexual functioning, expressions of concern about sexuality, and inappropriate verbal and nonverbal sexual behavior. Following are more examples of nursing diagnoses for patients with developmental problems throughout the life span:

- *Risk for Delayed Development*
- *Caregiver Role Strain*
- *Compromised Family Coping*
- *Readiness for Enhanced Health Management*
- *Risk for Injury*
- *Impaired Social Interaction*

In the second part of a problem-focused or health promotion nursing diagnostic statement, related factors of a patient's response to the health problem are stated. The related factors revealed in the assessment data allow you to target specific interventions toward the patient's diagnosis. For example, the nursing diagnosis of *Ineffective Sexuality Pattern* might be related to the stress of an impaired relationship with a significant other, fear of pregnancy, or lack of a significant other. The related factors are different, and each requires different nursing strategies.

■ ■ ■ PLANNING

Goals and Outcomes. The plan addresses each identified nursing diagnosis and appropriate goals, patient outcomes, and interventions for the alleviation or resolution of the diagnosis. The goal for each nursing diagnosis identifies a specific and measurable patient outcome that is realistic and reflects the patient's highest level of wellness and independence in function. An example of a goal is "Patient will acquire healthy physical and mental health behaviors within 3 months." An example of an outcome is "Patient participates in scheduled exercise activities within 6 weeks." See the Care Plan for detailed examples of goals and outcomes.

◎ CARE PLAN

Ineffective Health Maintenance

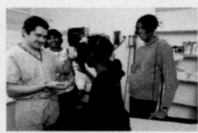

ASSESSMENT

Louis knows that this family has multiple health promotion needs. He wants to ensure that the children are on target with their growth and development and developmental tasks, especially Monica, who is entering school. In addition, he wants to determine any of Crystal's concerns as she enters the last trimester of her pregnancy.

ASSESSMENT ACTIVITIES	FINDINGS[a]
Complete height and weight examination on Monica.	Monica is in the 60th percentile for weight and the 75th percentile for height of a 6-year-old.
Using the Denver II (Denver Developmental Screening Test), observe Monica as she completes developmental tasks.	Monica balances on each foot for 6 seconds. Monica defines words such as "house" and "banana." Monica can copy a square. Crystal says that Monica independently brushes her teeth and dresses, prepares her own cereal, and plays board games. Monica enjoyed showing and telling Louis about the pictures she is coloring and often giggles.
Ask Crystal about how the children interact with one another.	Crystal explains that **Monica is very protective of and bossy with her brother,** and she always **wants to sit on Crystal's lap when Crystal is holding Zachary.**
Ask about immunizations and safety concerns.	Crystal is **unsure of the status of the children's immunizations and states, "I'm not sure they help."** Crystal states that all medications and cleaning agents are locked in a cabinet in the garage and she has the only key. Crystal states that she is **concerned about Monica riding her bike without the training wheels.** Monica **tries to play with a cigarette lighter.**
Ask Crystal about preparation for the new baby.	Crystal states that she has **done nothing.** Monica **asks how the baby will get out.** Crystal **asks about suggestions to prepare her children for the arrival of the new baby.**
Ask Crystal about her tobacco use.	Crystal states that she **smokes half a pack of cigarettes daily and would like to quit.**

[a]**Defining characteristics/risk factors** are shown in **bold** type.

NURSING DIAGNOSIS: Ineffective Health Maintenance related to a lack of knowledge regarding age-related health promotion activities

---

PLANNING

GOALS	EXPECTED OUTCOMES (NOC)[b]
	Knowledge: Health Promotion
Crystal will become more knowledgeable about health concerns related to her children's ages within the next 3 months.	Crystal will begin to discuss the safety needs of her children with all other family members who participate in their care before her next clinic visit. Crystal will talk to other family caregivers and Monica about protecting Monica from the danger of playing with fire before the next clinic visit. Crystal will talk to other family members about the importance of making sure that Monica always wears a safety helmet when riding her bicycle. Crystal will begin to prepare Monica and Zachary for the birth of a sibling within the next month by letting them feel the baby move, help pack the bag for the hospital, and reading age-appropriate books on childbirth.

Ineffective Health Maintenance

GOALS

Crystal will become more knowledgeable about smoking cessation strategies within the next month.

EXPECTED OUTCOMES (NOC)[b]

Crystal will implement smoking cessation activities within the next month.
Crystal will begin to remove/clean smoke residue from residence.

Health-Promoting Behavior

Crystal will keep her children's appointments for well-baby or well-child checkups and have the children receive appropriate immunizations during the next clinic visit.
Crystal will insist that Monica always wear her bicycle helmet when riding her bicycle.
Crystal will stop smoking within 1 month.

[b]Outcome classification labels from Moorhead S, et al, editors: *Nursing outcomes classification (NOC)*, ed 5, St Louis, 2013, Mosby.

INTERVENTIONS (NIC)[c]

Health Education

Provide Crystal with literacy-appropriate handouts that describe safety measures according to age of child.

Discuss with Crystal measures to decrease Monica's risk for playing with fire.

Provide Crystal with a list of books about preparing children for a new sibling.

Help Crystal develop a smoking cessation plan.

Discuss the importance of removing secondhand smoke residue from the residence.

Decision-Making Support

Provide Crystal with a pocket schedule for required childhood immunizations.

Provide a copy of her children's actual immunization records.

RATIONALE

Written information both provides initial information and allows for a quick review of information whenever needed (Guzys et al., 2015).

Adults need to keep potentially hazardous items out of reach of children; a lighter or a match is an adult tool (Hockenberry et al., 2017).

The list helps Crystal find these books in a bookstore or at the local library.

Research shows that assessing readiness to quit smoking is essential for a successful outcome and opens up communication between the patient and the nurse (McGrath et al., 2014).

Secondhand smoke residue contains toxins that build up on surfaces where smoking has occurred. Children coming into contact with carpeting and furniture are exposed to highly toxic particles.

Immunization education that includes immunization schedules, appointment reminder methods, and the importance of routine immunizations is essential.

[c]Intervention classification labels from Bulechek GM, et al, editors: *Nursing interventions classification (NIC)*, ed 6, St Louis, 2013, Mosby.

EVALUATION

NURSING ACTIONS	PATIENT RESPONSE/FINDING	ACHIEVEMENT OF OUTCOME
Ask Crystal to describe safety measures she has implemented in her home.	Crystal continues to lock up medicines, cleaning agents, lighters, and matches in her home. Crystal was able to get her grandmother to move medicines and cleaning agents to a locked cabinet. Crystal requested that all family members insist that Monica wear a helmet when riding her bicycle.	Crystal's home is improved for safety. Crystal is modifying her grandmother's home for safety risks. Crystal is making sure that there is consistency among caregivers in providing safe care.
Ask Crystal to describe what she plans to do to keep her children current on their immunizations.	Crystal states she is not sure when their next appointment is, but she has it written down on her calendar. Crystal provided child's school with an up-to-date record of immunizations.	This is ongoing. Reinforce when the next scheduled immunizations are to be administered.
Ask Crystal if she received list of books and tapes to prepare children for arrival of new sibling.	Children were able to talk about the "almost new baby." "Baby is coming for Halloween."	Preparation for new sibling is progressing but remains ongoing.
Ask Crystal how she is doing in regard to her smoking cessation plan.	Crystal quit smoking 2 weeks after her last clinic visit, although at times she still has strong cravings for a cigarette.	Crystal continues to follow her smoking cessation plan by using resources to help her cope with tobacco cravings.
Ask Crystal about her progress in removing smoke residue from her home.	Crystal has had window treatments, carpets, and upholstery cleaned.	Home environment is remediated from smoke residue.

Collaboration with patients and their families is essential when determining goals and outcomes. Patients' degree of participation in planning depends on their developmental status and physiological and psychological condition. For example, because young children are often unable to articulate feelings and needs, their parents need to become involved in establishing goals. The participation of patients and their families in this process increases their motivation for achievement of identified goals and outcomes.

Setting Priorities. During the planning phase of the nursing process, formulate a plan of care directed toward the identified nursing diagnoses. Patients and their families often have multiple nursing diagnoses, and these diagnoses often interact with one another. Address the nursing diagnoses in order of priority, giving the most pressing problems immediate attention. Base your priorities of nursing diagnoses on factors such as the nature of the problem (e.g., whether it is life threatening, interferes with activities of daily living, or affects level of comfort) and the degree of importance attributed to it by the patient or family. Maslow's theory of human needs is helpful as a guide when prioritizing nursing diagnoses. A high-priority nursing diagnosis is not always a physiological problem. *For example, Louis has concerns over the fact that Crystal is unsure about the children's immunization schedule; thus he views knowledge deficit as a priority for care in the initial clinic visit, especially when immunizations are necessary.*

Collaborative Care. Collaboration and consultation with other members of the health care team provide valuable resources for patient care. Such collaboration identifies community resources to help parents of a child with developmental disabilities or help a family find adult day care activities for an older adult. These resources often help to provide continuity in discharge planning.

Begin discharge planning at the time of admission to the hospital because the length of stay is usually very brief. Effective planning involves the health care team, the patient, and the patient's support system. Make sure that you individualize nursing interventions for the patient, and modify them accordingly for home-based or hospital-based nursing care. Make needed referrals to community agencies to coincide with the patient's arrival home.

■■■ IMPLEMENTATION

Provide developmental interventions in collaboration with the patient and the family or significant others. It is important that you keep patients and their families as active as possible in this process. Appropriate interventions for both the patient's developmental level and his or her unique needs will support and promote normal developmental processes.

Many of the interventions related to your patients' developmental stage include a component of patient education (see Chapter 12). Patient education is an effective tool to teach your patients about health promotion practices, desired

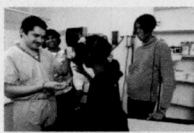

QSEN QSEN ACTIVITY *Teamwork and Collaboration*

As indicated in the case study, Crystal needs help from a variety of health care team members. It is important that Louis collaborate and communicate effectively with other members of the health care team to achieve the best possible outcome for Crystal and her family.

• How can Louis best communicate, collaborate, and integrate the skills of the other health care team members to help Crystal and her family achieve her health goals?

evolve Answers to QSEN Activities can be found on the Evolve website.

behavioral changes, and the need for age-appropriate screening practices. However, patients from different cultures or countries have different languages and beliefs that affect their ability to understand or talk to a health care provider (Mogobe et al., 2016). Effective patient education considers your patient's health literacy, and it is planned according to the patient's needs (Box 23.11).

Earlier in this chapter nursing strategies for health promotion and acute care were discussed for each age-group. Restorative care measures for older adults were also outlined. Refer to each of the developmental age-groups for specific interventions regarding age-related health concerns. It is important to remember to incorporate a patient's developmental needs into any plan of care, regardless of the nature of the patient's health problem. Whether the patient has serious physiological alterations or merely is seeking health promotion information, developmental care considerations ensure a more individualized and thorough nursing approach.

■■■ EVALUATION

Patient Outcomes. During evaluation measure the patient's progress and the degree to which the planned interventions were effective in meeting the expected outcomes and goals of care (see Case Study). Evaluate a patient's behavioral response to the interventions, and determine the success or failure of the nursing action. For example, have the patient describe positive health promotion activities or how poor habits changed. Visit the home to observe if recommendations for making the home safer are followed.

Collaborate with your patient and/or family caregiver to determine how the expected outcomes were achieved or why the outcomes were not met. This review helps you and the patient determine if the outcomes were realistic and appropriate or if there is a need to modify an approach. Ongoing evaluation is necessary to ensure that progress toward defined goals is achieved (Box 23.12).

Patient Expectations. Nurse-patient relationships are often long-term when you start a developmental plan of care.

BOX 23.11   PATIENT TEACHING

Immunizations

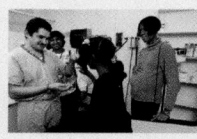

Louis knows that he is developing a therapeutic nurse-patient relationship with Crystal. Crystal told Louis that she wants to provide good health care for her children, but she does not understand the suggested immunization schedule for them.

OUTCOME

At the end of the teaching session, Crystal is able to state the routine immunization schedule for her children.

TEACHING STRATEGIES

- Provide Crystal with the American Academy of Pediatrics schedule for routine immunizations (AAP, 2017a).
- Using Crystal's personal calendar, highlight the dates when the immunizations are due.

- Provide Crystal with the phone contact for the appropriate clinic for immunizations.
- Show Crystal how to safely keep a permanent record of the immunizations.
- Tell Crystal to provide only copies of the immunization records to the children's school.

EVALUATION

- Use the principles of teach-back to evaluate patient/family caregiver learning:
  - "Tell me when your children's next immunizations are due."
  - "Let's look at your personal calendar to schedule an appointment for immunizations."
  - "Tell me where would be a safe place to keep the children's immunization records."

BOX 23.12   EVALUATION

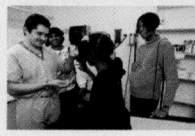

Louis sees Crystal 1 month later when she returns to the clinic for a scheduled prenatal visit. She left the children at home with their grandmother. While Crystal waits to see her primary caregiver, Louis takes the opportunity to evaluate the progress she has made in meeting expected outcomes. Crystal proudly shares with Louis that she has not had a cigarette in over 2 weeks. Louis asks Crystal if she has been able to find any of the books on the list he had given her about preparing young children for the birth of a sibling. Crystal reports that the librarian helped her locate two books, one appropriate for her toddler and the other one for Monica. She adds that the children loved the books and want her to read them every night at bedtime. Louis asks her if she thinks the content of the books was the kind of information she wanted to share with her children, and she replies that they explained childbirth so simply that it really made it easy for her to talk about the new baby with both children.

During the previous clinic visit, Louis gave Crystal pamphlets that described important safety measures for infants and young children. He asks her if she has discussed any of this information with any family members. Crystal tells him that her mother and grandmother have looked at the pamphlets and told her that it is a big responsibility to watch grandchildren and it is very hard to keep up with them. She also reports that they have all talked to Monica about not playing with candles, matches, or lighters, and Crystal locks up these items as well. She tells Louis about the evening news on television, which told a story about a child who hid in her bedroom playing with

a lighter and caught herself and the mattress on fire and almost died. The story scared Monica, and they talked about what young children should do if anything caught fire around them. She says Monica often talks about the situation and asks what happened to the little girl on television. Crystal also discussed with her family members the importance of Monica wearing a safety helmet every time she rides her bicycle.

Crystal asks Louis if he will be there for her next prenatal appointment, and he tells her that he plans to be. He asks if there is anything in particular that she would like to talk about next time. Crystal replies, "Just tell me how I can manage a new baby and my other two at the same time!" Before leaving, Crystal tells Louis she likes having him be with her at each clinic visit and that he has given her helpful information. Louis is satisfied that they are developing a therapeutic relationship and that he has helped her develop her knowledge base for managing health promotion activities for her children.

DOCUMENTATION NOTE

After the primary caregiver documented Crystal's prenatal visit, Louis adds the following documentation in Crystal's clinic chart:

"While waiting for primary caregiver, reports she has not smoked in over 2 weeks and has begun to prepare her two children for the birth of a new sibling through reading books and talking about the event. States she has shared safety measures for children, particularly in regard to fire and bicycle safety, with family caregivers. Has requested additional information pertaining to childrearing; will assess further during next visit."

Always remember to determine if a patient's expectations of care are continuing to be met, because a patient's expectations will change over time. To add to the complexity of evaluation, expectations sometimes vary when family members are involved. Basic to understanding the expectations of the patient and family members is trust. When you and a patient have established trust, it becomes easier to evaluate on a frequent basis how your relationship with the patient is proceeding and whether the patient senses that his or her health care needs are being adequately and professionally addressed.

KEY POINTS

- Growth and development are orderly, predictable, interdependent processes that continue throughout the life span.
- Growth is most rapid during the prenatal and infancy stages and then slows until the second skeletal growth spurt announces that puberty is approaching.
- People progress through similar stages of growth and development but at an individual pace and with individual behaviors.
- Theories of growth and development provide nurses with a framework for understanding individual behaviors.
- Know normal physiological, cognitive, and psychosocial developmental changes across the life span to determine potential problems and promote normal development.
- Patients need specific immunizations throughout life, not just in childhood.
- Young adults have few health problems but need to develop positive health habits and behaviors to avoid problems in middle and late adulthood.
- Common health concerns of middle-age adults involve normal hormonal changes, stress-related illnesses, situational stressors, screening for health problems, and adoption of positive health habits.
- The health concerns of older adults are often related to chronic illnesses, lifestyle changes, functional ability changes, accidents, and infectious diseases.

REFLECTIVE LEARNING

- Think about a patient you cared for recently and identify Piaget's stage of growth and development you would expect this patient to be in. Do you think this patient has completed the tasks associated with this stage of growth and development? Why or why not?
- Hospitalized children frequently revert back to previous stages of growth and development. Give an example of behaviors you expect to see in a 3-year-old hospitalized child.
- How might you approach patient teaching with a teenager who has begun experimenting with tobacco differently than with an adult smoker?

REVIEW QUESTIONS

1. Following a recent hospitalization, a mother indicates that she is concerned because her 3-year-old daughter suddenly started sucking her thumb again. Which of the following is the best nursing response?
   1. "Toddlers often suck their thumbs."
   2. "Your child may have seen another patient suck her thumb and is imitating the behavior."
   3. "It is not unusual for children to seek out prior comfort behaviors during or following an illness or trauma."
   4. "Your child probably is teething."

2. Sequence the skills in the expected order of gross-motor development beginning with the earliest skill:
   1. Move from prone to sitting unassisted
   2. Sit down from standing position
   3. Sit upright without support
   4. Roll from abdomen to back
   5. Turn from side to back

3. A newly diagnosed 36-year-old patient with type 1 diabetes shares with you that he is frustrated with the time it takes to prepare meals, monitor his exercise and blood sugar, and worry about his insulin coverage. Which of the following actions would be most appropriate? (Select all that apply.)
   1. Provide additional patient education materials that are easy to read
   2. Refer this patient to a diabetes support group
   3. Suggest that the patient make an appointment with a registered dietitian
   4. Suggest ways to modify his schedule
   5. Refer the patient to his endocrinologist

4. The mother of your 14-year-old patient is concerned because she believes her daughter spends too much time worrying about what her friends think. You can help this mother by explaining that this is normal behavior and that her daughter is in which stage of psychosocial development?
   1. Autonomy versus shame and doubt
   2. Initiative versus guilt
   3. Industry versus inferiority
   4. Identity versus role confusion

5. Chronic illness (e.g., diabetes mellitus, hypertension, rheumatoid arthritis) may affect a person's roles and responsibilities during middle adulthood. When assessing the health-related knowledge base of both the middle-age patient with a chronic illness and his or her family, the assessment should include which of the following? (Select all that apply.)
   1. Medical course of the illness
   2. Prognosis for the patient
   3. Socioeconomic status
   4. Coping mechanisms of the patient and family
   5. Need for community and social services

evolve

Additional Review Questions, as well as rationales for all Review Questions, can be found on the Evolve website.

1. 3; 2. 5, 4, 3, 1, 2; 3. 1, 2, 3, 4, 4; 5. 1, 2, 4, 5.

REFERENCES

Alzheimer's Association: *Know the ten signs and symptoms of Alzheimer's*, 2017, The Alzheimer's Association, http://www.alz.org/10-signs-symptoms-alzheimers-dementia.asp.

American Academy of Pediatrics (AAP): Policy statement: breastfeeding and the use of human milk, *Pediatrics* 129(3):e827, 2012.

American Academy of Pediatrics (AAP): *Where we stand: back to sleep*, 2015a. https://www.healthychildren.org/English/ages-stages/baby/sleep/Pages/Where-We-Stand-Back-To-Sleep.aspx.

American Academy of Pediatrics (AAP). *New crib standards: what parents need to know*, 2015b. http://www.healthychildren.org/English/ages-stages/baby/sleep/Pages/New-Crib-Standards-What-Parents-Need-to-Know.aspx.

American Academy of Pediatrics (AAP): *Immunization schedule*, 2017a. https://www.aap.org/en-us/advocacy-and-policy/aap-health-initiatives/immunization/Pages/Immunization-Schedule.aspx.

American Academy of Pediatrics (AAP): *Toddler—food and feeding*, 2017b. https://www.aap.org/en-us/advocacy-and-policy/aap-health-initiatives/HALF-Implementation-Guide/Age-Specific-Content/Pages/Toddler-Food-and-Feeding.aspx.

Burns CE, et al: *Pediatric primary care*, ed 6, St Louis, 2017, Elsevier.

Centers for Disease Control and Prevention (CDC): *National Center for Injury Prevention and Control: 10 leading causes of death by age group, United States*, 2015. https://www.cdc.gov/injury/images/lc-charts/leading_causes_of_death_age_group_2015_1050w740h.gif.

Centers for Disease Control and Prevention: *Older adults: are you communicating effectively*, 2016. https://www.cdc.gov/healthliteracy/developmaterials/audiences/olderadults/index.html.

Centers for Disease Control and Prevention (CDC): *Motor vehicle safety: teen drivers: get the facts*, 2017a. https://www.cdc.gov/motorvehiclesafety/teen_drivers/teendrivers_factsheet.html.

Centers for Disease Control and Prevention (CDC): *Vaccine Information Statements (VIS)*, 2017b, http://www.cdc.gov/vaccines/hcp/vis/index.html.

Centers for Disease Control and Prevention (CDC): *National Center for Health Statistics: adolescent health*, 2017c. https://www.cdc.gov/nchs/fastats/adolescent-health.htm.

Centers for Disease Control and Prevention (CDC): *Sexual risk behaviors: HIV, STD, teen pregnancy prevention*, 2017d. https://www.cdc.gov/healthyyouth/sexualbehaviors/.

Centers for Disease Control and Prevention (CDC): *About teen pregnancy*, 2017e. https://www.cdc.gov/teenpregnancy/about/index.htm.

Day JR, et al: Compassion fatigue in adult daughter caregivers of a parent with dementia, *Issues Ment Health Nurs* 35:796, 2014.

del-Pino-Casado R, et al: Coping, subjective burden and anxiety among family caregivers of older dependents, *J Clin Nurs* 23(23/24):3335, 2014.

Desilver D: *As population ages, more Americans becoming caregivers*, 2013. http://www.pewresearch.org/fact-tank/2013/07/18/as-population-ages-more-americans-becoming-caregivers/.

Ebersole P, et al: *Toward healthy aging: human needs and nursing response*, ed 9, St Louis, 2016, Mosby.

Erikson E: *Childhood and society*, New York, 1963, WW Norton.

Erikson E: *The lifecycle completed*, New York, 1997, WW Norton.

Family Caregiver Alliance: *Women and caregiving: facts and figures*, 2015. https://www.caregiver.org/women-and-caregiving-facts-and-figures.

Guzys D, et al: A critical review of population health literacy assessment, *BMC Public Health* 15(1):1, 2015.

Hockenberry M, et al: *Wong's essentials of pediatric nursing*, ed 10, St Louis, 2017, Mosby.

Kaufman G: Polypharmacy and older people, *Nurse Prescribing* 15(3):140, 2017.

Kidd A, et al: Mammography: review of the controversy, health disparities, and impact on young African American women, *Clin J Oncol Nurs* 19(3):52, 2015.

Kohlberg L: Development of moral character and moral ideology. In Hoffman ML, Hoffman LNW, editors: *Review of child development research*, vol 1, New York, 1964, Russell Sage Foundation.

Kovalskys I, et al: Childhood obesity and bullying in schools of Argentina: analysis of this behavior in a context of high prevalence, *J Child Obes* 1(3):10, 2016.

Leifer G: *Growth and development across the lifespan*, ed 2, St Louis, 2013, Saunders.

Maher RL, et al: Clinical consequences of polypharmacy in elderly, *Expert Opin Drug Saf* 13(1):57, 2014.

Maslow AH: *Motivation and personality*, ed 3, Upper Saddle River, NJ, 1970, Prentice Hall.

McGrath CA, et al: Smoking cessation in primary care: implementation of a proactive telephone intervention, *J Am Assoc Nurse Pract* 26:248, 2014.

Mogobe KD, et al: Language and culture in health literacy for people living with HIV: perspectives of health care providers and professional care team members, *AIDS Res Treat* 2016, Article ID 50515707, 2016.

National Center for Health Statistics: *Health, United States, 2015: in brief, Hyattsville, MD*, 2016. http://www.cdc.gov/nchs/data/hus/hus15_inbrief.pdf.

National Institutes of Health (NIH): *Description of high blood pressure*, 2015. http://www.nhlbi.nih.gov/health/health-topics/topics/hbp.

National Institutes of Health (NIH): *Senior health: depression*, 2017. http://nihseniorhealth.gov/depression/aboutdepression/01.html.

Nemours Foundation: *KidsHealth: Teaching kids to be smart about social media*, 2014. http://kidshealth.org/en/parents/social-media-smarts.html?WT.ac=ctg#catfamily.

Nishiguchi S, et al: A 12-week physical and cognitive exercise program can improve cognitive function and neural efficiency in community-dwelling older adults: a randomized controlled trial, *J Am Geriatr Soc* 63(7):1355, 2015.

Office of Disease Prevention and Health Promotion (ODPHP): *Healthy People 2020*, 2017. https://www.healthypeople.gov/2020/topics-objectives.

Ortman JM, et al: *An aging nation: the older population in the United States*, 2014. https://www.census.gov/prod/2014pubs/p25-1140.pdf.

O'Shea E, et al: The impact of reminiscence on the quality of life of residents with dementia in long-stay care, *Int J Geriatr Psychiatry* 29:1062, 2014.

Reinhard S, et al: *Family caregivers providing complex chronic care to their spouses*, 2014. http://www.aarp.org/home-family/caregiving/info-04-2014/family-caregivers-providing-complex-chronic-care-to-spouses-AARP-ppi-health.html.

Saczynski JS, et al: The Montreal Cognitive Assessment: creating a crosswalk with the Mini-Mental State Examination, *J Am Geriatr Soc* 63(11):2370, 2015.

Santrock JW: *Life span development*, ed 13, New York, 2012, McGraw-Hill.

Vincent GK, Velkoff VA: *The next four decades: the older population in the United States: 2010 to 2050*, U.S. Census Bureau, Current Population Reports, 2010. https://www.census.gov/prod/2010pubs/p25-1138.pdf.

evolve MEDIA RESOURCES

http://evolve.elsevier.com/Potter/essentials
- Audio Glossary

- QSEN Activity and Review Questions Answers and Rationales

OBJECTIVES

- Discuss factors that influence the following components of self-concept: identity, body image, and role performance.
- Identify stressors that affect self-concept, self-esteem, and sexuality.
- Describe the components of self-concept as each relates to Erikson's developmental stages.

- Reflect on ways in which your self-concept and nursing actions affect your patient's self-concept and self-esteem.
- Discuss your role in maintaining or enhancing a patient's sexual health.
- Apply the nursing process to promote a patient's self-concept and sexual health.

KEY TERMS

body image, p. 626
gender identity, p. 626
identity, p. 626
role performance, p. 627

self-concept, p. 624
self-esteem, p. 627
sexual dysfunction, p. 629
sexual identity, p. 626

sexual orientation, p. 626
sexuality, p. 625
sexually transmitted infections (STIs), p. 630

Self-concept and sexuality include a complex mixture of unconscious and conscious thoughts, beliefs, opinions, and attitudes. As a nurse, you care for patients who face a variety of health problems that threaten their self-esteem and sexuality. For example, patients who experience a loss of body function or a change in their physical appearance are at risk for experiencing a change in self-concept and sexual health needs. Help your patients adjust to alterations in self-concept and sexuality to promote successful adjustment and positive health outcomes.

SCIENTIFIC KNOWLEDGE BASE

Self-concept is your subjective view of who you are. Self-concept, or how you *think* about yourself, directly affects self-esteem, or how you *feel* about or value yourself. Classic research conducted by Franken (1994) noted that self-concept is, perhaps, the basis for all motivated behavior. One's self-concept gives rise to possible selves, and it is possible selves that create the motivation for behavior. Because self-concept is related to self-esteem, Franken (1994) further notes that people who have strong self-esteem have a clearly differentiated self-concept. When people know themselves, they can maximize outcomes because they know what they can and cannot do.

What you think and how you feel about yourself affect the way in which you care for yourself physically and emotionally. Self-concept influences the way in which you care for others. You need to have knowledge of factors that affect self-concept and self-esteem. Be aware of differences in self-concept and

CASE STUDY *Paul Taylor*

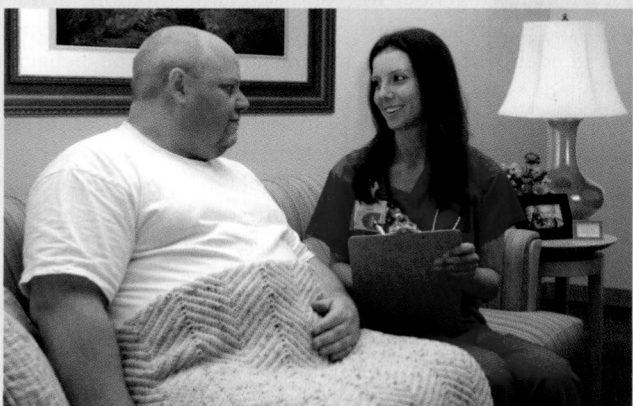

Paul Taylor, a 53-year-old man, had a stroke while working at his job as a construction manager. He did not know that he had hypertension because he had not been getting annual checkups. Mr. Taylor woke up in the hospital bed to find that he could not move his right hand and arm, and he also had weakness of the right leg. He was unable to care for himself or to turn himself for days after the stroke. With daily rehabilitation activities, he is finally able to transfer from his bed into a chair. His body image has dramatically changed from that of a strong man to that of a helpless individual. Mr. Taylor worries about being a burden to his family, and both he and his wife, Meredith, are terrified about what lies ahead. Although Mrs. Taylor works, their savings are minimal. The family is concerned they will not have enough money for their children's college education without both incomes. Mr. Taylor's role as primary breadwinner for the family will be drastically changed if his condition does not improve.

Mr. Taylor's self-esteem lessens as his recovery and rehabilitation move slowly. His self-concept has changed from that of a strong laborer, one who did his own plumbing and car repairs, to a man who must rely on others. Although he is now at home in the rehabilitation process, Mr. Taylor is not able to perform tasks for the family and waits until his wife and son get home to help him with things that require strength. Moreover, because of the sexual side effects of the antihypertensive medication he is taking, there is a lack of intimacy with his wife, and this is affecting their relationship. Mr. Taylor's adaptation capabilities are stretched, and he is reevaluating his identity. He has no clear role within the family, his body image has drastically altered, his sexual health has suffered, and his self-esteem has never been lower.

Maria Kendal is a 25-year-old nursing student assigned to care for Mr. Taylor. She recognizes that changes in health status often result in stressors that affect a person's self-concept and sexuality. Such stressors influence a person's ability to interact with others and function effectively. Maria's knowledge of self-concept and sexuality helps to identify stressors that affect Mr. Taylor and promote effective planning to support his growth and adaptation to change.

self-esteem across age, gender, ethnicity, socioeconomic status, and other cultural variables to individualize your approach to patient care (see Chapter 21).

Sexuality is a broad term that refers to all aspects of being sexual including how you choose to identity yourself sexually and with whom you choose to be intimate. It is a part of who you are as a person and is important for overall health. Sex is considered a basic physiological need, and sexual intimacy throughout the life span is equally important for sexual health. Healthy sexuality enables people to develop and maintain their fullest potential. Sexuality includes a person's thoughts and feelings about the body, a sense of femaleness and maleness, romantic and erotic attachments to others, and attitudes toward sexual functioning. Our sexual health is based on our ability to form healthy relationships with others.

NURSING KNOWLEDGE BASE

To provide evidence-based care to patients, incorporate professional nursing knowledge from the humanities and sciences, nursing research, and clinical practice. A broad knowledge base allows you to have a holistic view of patients, promoting quality patient care that best meets the self-concept and sexual health needs of each patient and family.

Development of Self-Concept

The development of self-concept is a complex process that involves many factors. It begins at birth and continues throughout life. Erikson's psychosocial theory of development describes key tasks that individuals face at various stages of development (Erikson, 1963). Each stage builds on the tasks of the previous stage. Completing each developmental stage successfully leads to a solid sense of self.

Use Erikson's theory to identify the stage of psychosocial development of a patient based first on the patient's biological age and then adjusted based on any significant life events. You apply this knowledge when you assess a patient's psychosocial development stage by determining how the patient is handling the developmental tasks of that stage. Adolescence is a particularly critical developmental period when many variables including school, family, and friends affect self-concept and self-esteem (Mantilla et al., 2014). Awareness of lifelong developmental tasks (Box 24.1) will allow you to select individualized nursing actions tailored to your patient's needs.

Components and Interrelated Terms of Self-Concept and Sexuality

A positive self-concept gives a sense of meaning and wholeness to a person. Nurses care for patients who experience threats to the various components of self-concept including identity, body image, role performance, and self-esteem. Sexuality also influences self-concept. Likewise, identity, body image, role performance, and self-esteem affect sexual health. Although overlap exists among concepts, this chapter presents each one separately.

BOX 24.1 ERIKSON'S DEVELOPMENTAL TASKS AND IMPACT ON SELF-CONCEPT AND SEXUALITY

TRUST VS. MISTRUST (BIRTH TO 18 MONTHS)
- Develops trust from consistency in caregiving and nurturing interactions with caregivers
- Distinguishes self from environment

AUTONOMY VS. SHAME AND DOUBT (18 MONTHS TO 3 YEARS)
- Begins to communicate likes and dislikes
- Increasingly independent in thoughts and actions
- Appreciates body appearance and function (including dressing, feeding, talking, and walking)

INITIATIVE VS. GUILT (3 TO 5 YEARS)
- Takes initiative
- Identifies with a gender
- Enhances self-awareness
- Increases language skills including identification of feelings

INDUSTRY VS. INFERIORITY (6 TO 12 YEARS)
- Incorporates feedback from peers and teachers
- Increases self-esteem with new skill mastery (e.g., reading, math, sports, music)
- Sexual identity strengthens
- Aware of strengths and limitations

IDENTITY VS. ROLE CONFUSION (12 TO 18 YEARS)
- Accepts body changes and maturation
- Examines attitudes, values, and beliefs; establishes goals for the future
- Feels positive about expanded sense of self

INTIMACY VS. ISOLATION (18 TO 35 YEARS)
- Has intimate relationships with family and significant others
- Has stable, positive feelings about self
- Experiences successful role transitions and increased responsibilities

GENERATIVITY VS. SELF-ABSORPTION (35 TO 55 OR 65 YEARS)
- Able to accept changes in appearance and physical endurance
- Reassesses life goals
- Shows contentment with aging

EGO INTEGRITY VS. DESPAIR (55 OR 65 YEARS TO DEATH)
- Feels positive about one's life and its meaning
- Interested in providing a legacy for the next generation

Identity involves the sense of individuality and being distinct and separate from others. Being "oneself" or living a life that is genuine and authentic is the basis of true identity. The achievement of identity is necessary for intimate relationships because identity is expressed in relationships with others. Sexuality is a part of identity. **Sexual identity** is how

a person thinks about himself or herself sexually, and includes gender identity, gender role, and sexual orientation. **Gender identity** is a person's private view of maleness and femaleness, and gender role is the feminine and masculine behavior exhibited. Assessing one's gender identity and **sexual orientation,** defined as a person's sexual identity in relation to the gender to which they are attracted, requires you to be accepting of responses that fall within the LGBTQ+ (Lesbian, Gay, Bisexual, Transgender, Queer, Questioning, Asexual, and others) continuum (Strong and Folse, 2015). Racial or cultural identity develops from identifying and socializing within an established group and through incorporating the responses of individuals who do not belong to that group into one's self-concept. The opinion or approval of others affects self-esteem differently among racial and cultural groups.

As a person grows and develops, so does his or her self-concept and sexuality. Each stage of development brings changes in sexual functioning, sexual focus, and sexual relationships. Your knowledge of sexual development and changes throughout the life span is essential to provide individualized and complete nursing care. An adult has achieved physical maturation but is continuing to explore and define emotional maturation in relationships. Even into adulthood people struggle with questions about who they are, how they want to present themselves, and what type of partners they find most attractive. It helps to have a clear sense of your own sexual identity because it influences your ability to form open relationships, which is needed to support your patients' sexual health. You will provide care to individuals whose sexual orientation and sexual identity is heterosexual (attracted to different-sex partners), lesbian or gay (same-sex partners), bisexual (both male and female partners), transgender (gender identity or expression is different from sex at birth), queer (an umbrella term representing all individuals who fall out of the gender and sexuality binary "norms"), questioning (exploring one's sexual orientation or identity), asexual or aromantic (does not experience sexual or romantic attraction), fluid (fluctuating mix of options), pansexual (sexual attraction to members of all gender identities and expressions), and cisgender (gender identity, gender expression, and biological sex all align) as well as uniquely defined by your patient (VandenBos, 2015). You will also care for patients who are involved in intimate relationships with several partners and for patients whose sexual relationships occur outside of marriage or a committed relationship. You may not learn a great deal about a patient's sexual preferences even if you ask direct questions. What you do learn will depend on the time you spend and your ability to establish therapeutic relationships with your patients. As a caregiver, you must learn to accept a person's sexual orientation and sexual identity and help the individual understand the implications that his or her health condition has on maintaining healthy sexual relationships and on achieving positive health outcomes.

Body image involves attitudes related to the perception of the body including physical appearance, femininity and masculinity, youthfulness, health, and strength. These views are not always the same, as the person's actual physical structure or appearance is ever changing. *When a change in health status occurs, as in the case of Mr. Taylor, an individual sometimes has exaggerated disturbances in body image.* The way others view a person's body and the feedback offered are also influential. For example, a husband who is controlling and violent tells his wife that she is fat and ugly and that no one else would want her. Over the years of marriage, she incorporates this criticism into her self-concept.

Cultural and societal attitudes and values influence body image and sexuality. Some cultures are more accepting of individuals who are slightly overweight because this body type represents being healthy and prosperous. Racial and ethnic background play an integral role in body satisfaction and the differences among groups. Race, gender, and the social environment (family, peers, media) also affect a person's body image, particularly in adolescence. For example, identification and pride in ethnic background can act as a partial buffer against advertisements, magazines, television, and movies depicting the thin-ideal white image and help vulnerable teenage girls feel more comfortable with themselves and their appearance (Schooler and Daniels, 2014). Furthermore body image is more favorable in cultures in which people describe more reasonable views about physical appearance, report less social pressure for thinness, and have less tendency to base self-esteem on body image. Body art such as tattoos and piercings is increasingly common among all ages of individuals and has become a popular way to express individuality, which is part of one's body image.

Body image depends only partly on the reality of the body. When physical changes occur, individuals may or may not incorporate these changes into their body image. For example, a patient who experiences significant weight loss may not perceive herself as thin and tells you that there is still a "fat person" inside. Body image issues are often associated with negative self-concept and self-esteem. Most men and women experience some degree of body dissatisfaction, which often affects body image and overall self-concept.

Normal developmental changes such as puberty and aging have a more obvious effect on body image than on other aspects of self-concept. Hormonal changes during puberty and menopause in later adulthood influence body image. The development of secondary sex characteristics and changes in body fat distribution have a tremendous impact on the self-concept of an adolescent. Changes associated with aging (e.g., wrinkles; graying hair; decrease in visual acuity, hearing, and mobility) affect body image in older adults.

Role performance is the way in which a person views his or her ability to carry out significant roles. Common roles include mother or father, wife or husband, daughter or son, sister or brother, employee or employer, and nurse or patient. For example, stating, "I am a good father" or "I am a caring and competent nurse" reflects a positive self-concept and self-esteem. Each role involves meeting certain expectations. *In the case of Mr. Taylor, his roles as a husband, father, and employee require him to earn a salary as a construction manager and to support his wife and children. Fulfillment of these expectations leads to an enhanced sense of self. Difficulty or failure to meet role expectations leads to decreased self-esteem or altered self-concept.*

Self-esteem is an individual's overall sense of personal worth or value. It is positive when one feels capable, worthwhile, and competent. Once established, basic feelings about the self tend to be constant, even though sometimes fluctuation exists. A situational crisis such as a hospitalization often temporarily affects one's self-esteem.

Self-evaluation is an ongoing mental process. A positive sense of self-worth, or self-esteem, is important for determining how an individual functions in the world. A person's ability to contribute in a meaningful way to society often affects self-concept and self-esteem. Some individuals who are chronically ill feel a sense of worthlessness. Your acceptance of a patient as an individual with worth and dignity helps to maintain and improve the patient's self-esteem.

Stressors Affecting Self-Concept and Sexuality

A self-concept stressor is any real or perceived change that threatens identity, body image, or role performance (Fig. 24.1). An individual's perception of the stressor is the most important factor in determining his or her response. *For example, Mr. Taylor's stroke caused a deficit that makes him believe he will no longer be able to be the active construction site manager he has been. This perception of what the stroke will mean to his lifestyle can lead to depression or anxiety. However, another man may view his stroke as a message to slow down and enjoy his life.*

Any change in health is a stressor that potentially affects self-concept. A physical change in the body leads to an altered body image, affecting identity and self-esteem. Chronic illnesses often alter role performance, which frequently impacts a person's identity and self-esteem. Living with a chronic illness requires a person to cope with a lost sense of self while a new self emerges. After adjustment to the loss, the person has to develop a new self-concept. For example, the loss of a partner sometimes leads to a loss of identity and a lower self-esteem.

A crisis occurs when a person cannot cope with stressors with usual methods of problem solving and adaptation. Any crisis potentially challenges self-concept and self-esteem. *Some crises, such as Paul Taylor's stroke, directly affect all components of self-concept.* If people are unable to adapt to such stressors, their health is at risk, and illness often results.

Identity Stressors. Stressors throughout life affect an individual's identity; identity is particularly vulnerable during adolescence, which is a time of great change. Adolescents are trying to adjust to the physical, emotional, and mental changes of increasing maturity, which can result in insecurity and anxiety. For example, an adolescent who wants to be identified as part of the popular crowd at school develops a poor self-concept if not included in that group. Although social media and social networking sites (e.g., Facebook, Instagram, Snapchat, Twitter, YouTube) provide opportunities to connect with others and to feel included in groups,

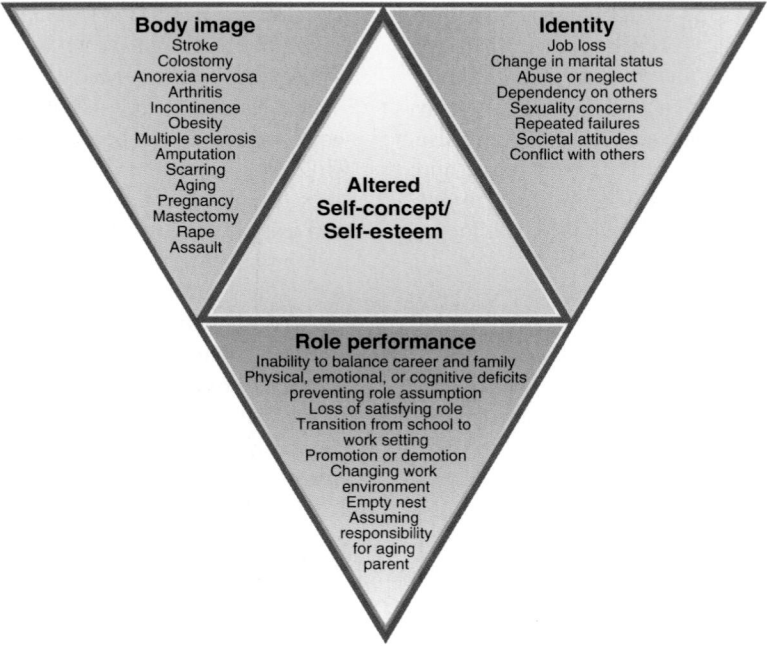

FIG 24.1 Common stressors that influence self-concept.

individuals who are ignored (e.g., messages unread or un-opened) or are the recipient of mean posts are at risk for negative self-concept responses. A decline in self-concept occurs in people who are bullied and cyberbullied on social media (Box 24.2). Low self-esteem is associated with individuals who commit peer aggression including cyberbullying (Toledano et al., 2015). Family and cultural factors can influence self-concept resulting in negative health practices such as cigarette smoking, at-risk drinking or drug use, and unsafe sexual practices. Promoting a change in a patient's self-concept demands an evidence-based approach supported by the entire health care team.

An adult generally has a stable identity and thus a more developed self-concept than an adolescent. Once a person has established his or her identity, the mature adult is better able to handle stressors such as marriage, divorce, meno-pause, aging, and retirement. Job satisfaction and overall performance in adulthood are also linked to self-esteem. Self-enhancing opportunities such as exploring new ideas, solving problems in creative ways, and learning new skills predict job satisfaction and commitment as well as promote self-concept clarity and self-esteem (McIntyre et al., 2014). Sometimes when individuals lose a job, their sense of self diminishes, they lose motivation to be socially active, and they may even become depressed. If a person's identity is tied to a job, retirement can alter the person's self-perceptions and self-care practices. Some people at retirement begin to reevaluate their identities and accomplishments. Many older people are working past the traditional retirement age or change careers after retirement. Some do so because of a financial need, whereas others have a desire to remain involved and produc-tive. Sometimes loss of a significant other leads a person to reexamine aspects of his or her identity.

Body Image Stressors. Changes in the appearance or function of a body part require a body image adjustment. An individual's perception of the change and the relative impor-tance placed on body image in the individual's self-concept affect the significance of the loss or change. For example, if a woman considers her breasts key to her femininity, a mastec-tomy negatively affects her body image. Changes in the appearance of the body such as an amputation, facial disfig-urement, or burns are obvious stressors affecting body image. Surgical procedures, potentially undetected by others, have a significant impact on an individual. Elective changes such as breast augmentation or reduction also affect body image. Chronic illnesses such as heart and lung disease involve a change in function (less tolerant of exercise) in which the body no longer performs at an optimal level. Physical changes associated with aging or treatment for medical conditions can negatively affect body image as well. In addition, the effects of pregnancy, significant weight gain or loss, medication management of an illness, and radiation therapy all change body image. Negative body image sometimes leads to adverse health outcomes.

Many people associate success with a specific body part or function. For example, some athletes consider their bodies and physical activities to be the focus of personal success. Their adaptation and rehabilitation is often affected if an injury prevents future participation in athletics. Body image changes require reevaluation of long-accepted self-perceptions and alterations in lifestyle.

Role Performance Stressors. Throughout life, a person undergoes many role changes. Normal changes associated with maturation result in changes in role performance. For example, when a couple has a child, both the man and the

BOX 24.2. EVIDENCE-BASED PRACTICE

PICO Question: Does cyber aggression reduce self-concept and increase depression and anxiety in adolescents?

SUMMARY OF EVIDENCE

Bullying, including cyberbullying, is one type of youth violence that threatens an adolescent's self-concept and well-being. Nationwide, electronic bullying is increasing with 15.5% of students reporting being cyberbullied during the past 12 months through e-mail, chat rooms, instant messaging, websites, or texting (Kann et al., 2016). The prevalence of electronic bullying was higher among female than male students and highest among white female students followed by black and Hispanic female students. White male students were cyberbullied more than black or Hispanic male students. Individuals who experience cyber aggression report lower self-esteem and self-concept, whereas individuals who engage in peer aggression do not report higher levels of popularity or freedom from anxiety (Toledano et al., 2015). Adolescents who are being bullied or who are bullying others are at increased risk for depression and anxiety as well as suicide, especially when they experience additional threats to safety such as being threatened or injured at school (Pham & Adesman, 2017).

APPLICATION TO NURSING PRACTICE

- Conduct a thorough assessment for depression and anxiety as well as risk for suicide in individuals who engage in or who report bullying (Pham & Adesman, 2017; Toledano et al., 2015).
- When completing a social history, a priority nursing action is assessment of child and adolescent coping strategies, conflict resolution, and stress management as related to the use of social media and texting (Kann et al., 2016).
- Educate adolescents about what to do if they observe cyberbullying or are victims of cyberbullying and provide school and community resources (Toledano et al., 2015).

woman need to adjust to new parenting roles and changes in their personal relationship. When a middle-age woman with young children assumes responsibility for the care of her older parents, she adapts to the increased demands of this new role. Acute and chronic illnesses alter a person's ability to carry out various roles, which affects self-esteem and identity.

All people must adapt to changes that occur with aging. Role performance changes associated with retirement differ for men and women. Many women have adjusted to several different roles throughout their lifetime and are more likely than men to have developed friendships that are not work related. Adjusting to changes in role performance has an impact on the marital relationship. Changes in role performance after the loss of a spouse or partner also affect self-concept. A widow who has never paid bills or who needs to learn to cook needs help to change roles.

Self-Esteem Stressors. Individuals with high self-esteem are generally better able to cope with demands and stressors than individuals with low self-esteem. Low self-worth contributes to feeling unfulfilled and misunderstood and results in depression and anxiety. Illness, surgery, or injuries that change lifestyle patterns also influence feelings of self-worth. Chronic illnesses such as diabetes, arthritis, and heart disease that interfere with the ability to engage in activities contributing to feelings of worth or success affect self-esteem. Self-esteem and health behaviors are intertwined. Self-concept guides health behaviors and influences health-related actions (Thomas and Moring, 2014).

Self-esteem stressors vary with developmental stages and differ across the life span. A child's self-worth lessens if the child feels unable to meet his parents' expectations or if his parents harshly criticize or inconsistently discipline him. The self-esteem of an adolescent is also vulnerable because he or she expends so much energy worrying about appearance, searching for identity, and being overly concerned about what others think. At-risk behaviors and stressors such as smoking, hazardous alcohol consumption, and unprotected sexual activities often signal self-esteem disturbances in adolescents. Stressors affecting the self-esteem of an adult include failures at work and in relationships, and stressors in older adults include retirement and the death of friends. Box 24.3 discusses ways to promote self-concept, self-esteem, and healthy sexuality in older adults.

Sexuality Stressors. You will work with patients who are making decisions or dealing with issues related to sexuality on a regular basis, including issues related to contraception, infertility, sexual dysfunction, and sexual satisfaction. Understanding some of the decisions and issues that patients face increases your effectiveness in helping them reach their maximum level of sexual health.

LGBTQ+ individuals have unique stressors related to their sexual identity and sexual orientation, which is the emotional, romantic, or sexual attraction to others. Peer, family, and social support is often lacking. It is important to increase efforts to ensure a culturally competent and knowledgeable nursing workforce while eliminating health disparities and improving patient outcomes in vulnerable populations including the LGBTQ+ community. Nurses are in a unique position to support a patient and provide education and resources based on his or her individual needs. LGBTQ+ patients experience barriers to health care that include fear of discrimination, insensitivity, and lack of knowledge about their specific health needs. This places LGBTQ+ individuals at high risk for health issues such as sexually transmitted infections (STIs), human immunodeficiency virus (HIV), depression, and victimization (Strong and Folse, 2015). Health care providers need to tell patients that it is important to disclose sexual preferences and behaviors, as many patients do not make the connection between sexuality and physical health (Fuzzell et al., 2016).

Alterations in sexual health occur as a result of a variety of situations such as illness, infertility, trauma, and abuse. Sexual dysfunction involves problems with desire, arousal, or orgasm. Erectile dysfunction is a common problem among older men. It is generally related to chronic diseases such as

BOX 24.3   CARE OF THE OLDER ADULT

Promoting Self-Concept, Self-Esteem, and Sexuality

It is important to understand how self-concept and self-esteem change across the life span. Although self-concept is sometimes negatively affected in older adults as a result of a number of life changes, sexuality remains important to the older adult's well-being (Haesler et al., 2016). However, in some individuals, aging promotes improved coping strategies that protect against the declining feelings of self-esteem despite the physical and emotional changes associated with aging (Touhy and Jett, 2016). Nursing interventions aimed at enhancing self-concept and self-esteem in older adults are essential, particularly during experiences of illness, injury, or disability. Improving sexual health knowledge and changing negative attitudes of health care providers toward older adults are essential to ensure positive patient outcomes (Haesler et al., 2016):

- Clarify what the life changes mean and the impact on self-concept and sexuality for the older adult (Touhy and Jett, 2016).
- Be alert to preoccupation with physical complaints. Assess complaints thoroughly; if no physical explanation exists, encourage the older adult to verbalize needs (e.g., fear, insecurity, loneliness) in a nonphysical way (Touhy and Jett, 2016).
- Identify positive coping mechanisms.
- Reinforce positive coping strategies and support and teach new strategies (Stuart, 2013).
- Provide opportunities for the patient and partner to discuss changes in sexuality and possible solutions (Haesler et al., 2016).
- Encourage reminiscence (see Chapter 23) through the review of old photographs and use of storytelling (Chan et al., 2014).
- Communicate that the older adult is worthwhile by actively listening to and accepting the older adult's feelings, being respectful, and praising healthy behaviors (Touhy and Jett, 2016).
- Reinforce the older adult's self-care and efforts at independence, and provide additional time to complete self-care tasks (Touhy and Jett, 2016).

diabetes, kidney disease, alcohol dependence, depression, neurological disorders, vascular insufficiency, and diseases of the prostate (Touhy and Jett, 2016). Side effects of medications or medical conditions also contribute to sexual dysfunction. Examples of common medications that can cause sexual dysfunction include statins, antihypertensives, antidepressants, antipsychotics, and benzodiazepines. Causes of sexual dysfunction are both physiological and psychological. Sometimes the cause of sexual dysfunction cannot be identified or is a result of a combination of several factors.

Because sexual dysfunction sometimes results from the use of medications, it is important to include a discussion of sexual side effects in patient teaching. Your patient is more likely to adhere to a treatment plan if you discuss side effects of medications that alter sexual function with both partners

and the patient can make an informed decision. A person's current state of health greatly influences sexual response (from desire to arousal to orgasm). The availability of sexual performance–enhancing medications such as sildenafil (Viagra) and tadalafil (Cialis) has changed the lives of many couples. However, these medications to treat erectile dysfunction are not without risk and are contraindicated in men with coronary artery disease and men taking common cardiac drugs.

Changes in physical appearance and concerns about physical attractiveness affect sexual functioning. The loss of sexual activity and the absence of a self-concept that includes being a sexual person are not inevitable aspects of aging. Some older people face health concerns and societal attitudes that make it difficult for them to continue sexual activity. Although declining physical abilities sometimes make sex as they knew it painful or impossible, with intervention older adults can experiment with and learn alternative ways of sexual expression.

Hormonally stimulated changes brought on by developmental maturation are also stressors that affect sexuality across the life span. Menarche, the onset of menstrual cycle in girls, is occurring at an earlier age in the United States, and some adolescent girls are unaware that it is normal to grow pubic, underarm, and body hair and deposit more fat on their hips and breasts, all of which also affect body image. Early maturation in girls is linked to negative health outcomes throughout the life span such as obesity and cardiovascular disease. As boys approach puberty, physical changes include nocturnal emissions and ejaculation, increasing sexual desire, and increased hygiene needs.

Patient teaching needs to include instruction on breast and testicular self-examinations (see Chapter 16) and prevention of sexually transmitted infections (STIs), which are spread through oral, anal, or vaginal sexual contact. Mutually monogamous relationships, delayed sexual debut, and consistent use of latex condoms reduce the risk of STIs as well as unplanned pregnancies (Kerpelman et al., 2016). Risky sexual behavior is reduced in adolescents with solid self-esteem; you can support an adolescent's sexual and psychological health by providing health information and reinforcing deliberate sexual decision making (Kerpelman et al., 2016).

Human papillomavirus (HPV) is the most common STI in the United States. Approximately 79 million people in the United States are infected with HPV including roughly 14 million new infections each year with most of these infections occurring in adolescents and young adults (Centers for Disease Control and Prevention [CDC], 2016). The Gardasil 9 vaccine is recommended for boys and girls in early adolescence (11 or 12 years of age) to decrease the risk for cancers of the cervix, vagina, vulva, penis, anus, and throat as well as genital warts associated with HPV (CDC, 2016). The greatest benefit occurs when individuals receive the vaccines before sexual activity or exposure to the virus. Two doses of the 9-valent HPV vaccine are recommended for preteens, and three doses are recommended for older adolescents and young adults.

BOX 24.4	SIGNS AND SYMPTOMS THAT MAY INDICATE CURRENT SEXUAL ABUSE OR A HISTORY OF SEXUAL ABUSE

- Unexplained bruises, lacerations, or abrasions, especially around breasts, genital, or anal areas
- Unexplained vaginal or anal soreness or bleeding
- Unexplained genital or sexually transmitted infection
- Frequent visits to health care providers
- Headaches
- Gastrointestinal problems
- Abdominal pain
- Dysmenorrhea
- Premenstrual syndrome
- Sleep pattern disturbances
- Nightmares

- Repetitive dreams
- Depression
- Social withdrawal
- Anxiety
- Eating disorders
- Substance abuse
- Decreased self-esteem
- Difficulty developing trust
- Difficulties with intimate relationships
- Impaired school or work performance
- Reports of being sexually assaulted or raped

Note: No physical symptoms may be present.

Modified from Stuart GW: *Principles and practice of psychiatric nursing*, ed 10, St Louis, 2013, Mosby.

Older women experiencing menopause, which is the cessation of menstrual periods, experience changes in vaginal lubrication and sexual interest. Most menopausal woman recognize the importance of maintaining an active sex life; however, many report reduced sex drive, decreased sexual interest, and mood changes that may require intervention by a health care provider (Touhy and Jett, 2016). High levels of self-esteem and sexual quality of life are associated with successful aging in postmenopausal women (White and Taliaferro, 2016).

Sexual abuse, assault, and rape are also stressors that affect self-concept. Be alert to clues that suggest abuse (Box 24.4). In addition, observe the interaction between the patient and partner for additional clues. Controlling behaviors such as speaking for the person or refusing to leave him or her alone with a caregiver are suggestive of emotional and perhaps physical or sexual abuse. If you suspect abuse, interview the patient privately, as a patient will probably not admit to problems of abuse with the abuser present. The following questions are useful: "Are you in a relationship in which someone is hurting you?" "Have you ever been forced to have sex when you didn't want to?" When you recognize or report abuse, mobilize treatment immediately for the person experiencing the abuse and for the family. The most important factor to consider is the safety of the person who has experienced sexual violence. Often all family members require therapy to promote healthy interactions and relationships.

The Nurse's Influence on the Patient's Self-Concept and Sexuality

You have the ability to positively influence a patient's self-concept. Your acceptance of a patient with an altered self-concept helps promote positive change. Your words and actions convey sincere interest and acceptance and have a profound effect on patients. When a patient's physical appearance has changed, both the patient and the family watch your verbal and nonverbal responses and reactions to the changed appearance. A positive and matter-of-fact approach to care provides a model for the patient and family to follow. It is important that health care providers understand the

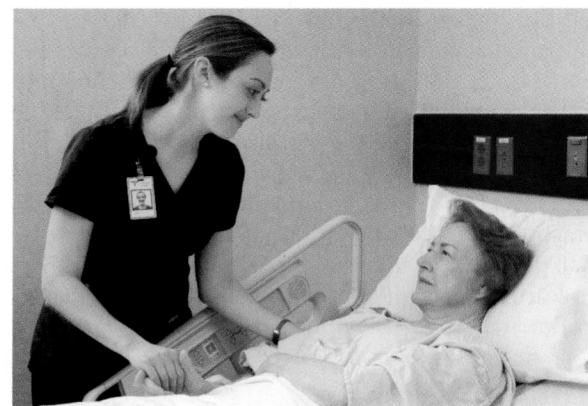

FIG 24.2 Nurses use touch and eye contact to enhance a patient's self-esteem.

degree to which self-esteem and sexuality affect patient outcomes.

How you respond to patients who have experienced changes in body appearance sets the stage for how they come to see themselves. The patient with a change in body functioning or appearance is often extremely sensitive to your verbal and nonverbal responses (Fig. 24.2). Building a trusting nurse-patient relationship and appropriately including a patient in decision making will support most patients' self-concepts (see Chapter 11). Sometimes individualized approaches including supporting the use of alternative healing techniques or methods of spiritual expression help a patient adapt to changes in self-concept.

Your actions, expressions, and what you say affect your patient's body image. For example, you have a positive influence on the body image of a patient who has had disfiguring surgery by showing acceptance of the surgical scar. A shocked or disgusted facial expression causes a patient to develop a negative body image. It is very important to monitor your responses toward each patient. Matter-of-fact statements such as "This wound is healing nicely" or "This looks healthy" enhance the body image of a patient.

Inadvertent nonverbal communication, such as frowning or grimacing when performing procedures, can have a profound effect on patients. Your nonverbal behavior conveys the level of caring that exists for your patient and affects his or her self-esteem. For example, when a patient who is incontinent perceives that you find the situation unpleasant, it threatens the patient's self-concept. Anticipate your own reactions, acknowledge them, and focus on the patient instead of the unpleasant task or situation. Put yourself in the patient's position to lessen his or her embarrassment, frustration, and anger.

When you consider the sexuality of patients, think about your own knowledge regarding sexual development, sexual orientation, sexual response, STIs, contraception, and alterations in sexual health. Your own sexuality, sexual experiences, and communication style are valuable when trying to understand your patient's experiences. Be sure not to convey your feelings to patients. Attempts at self-exploration teach us about our bodies and the potential for providing pleasure. Your attitude about masturbation may have stemmed from personal experience or from values or beliefs communicated by other people. Games such as "doctor" and "nurse" may have provided early sex play and exploration. In addition, your own sexual experiences add to understanding the complexities of a first sexual encounter or the challenges of sexual interactions when you or an intimate partner is ill. In addition to personal experiences related to sexuality, use what you have learned through working with other patients as you assess and develop trust with current patients.

CRITICAL THINKING

Synthesis

Patient care requires you to apply what you know about a patient, your knowledge base, experience, and critical thinking attitudes and standards. Your synthesis of this information allows you to make sound decisions as you apply the nursing process. Critical thinking synthesis involves combining all available information to obtain a clear picture of the approach needed to provide patient-centered care. Your nursing expertise allows you to anticipate and respond to stressors that affect your patient's self-concept and sexual health. Consider changes in your patient's identity, body image, role performance, and self-esteem as important aspects of care (Box 24.5).

Knowledge. Use knowledge about how various medications, certain medical conditions, and chronic symptoms such as dyspnea, pain or fatigue influence your patient's ability to perform self-care and function at an optimal level, affect your patient's mood, and impact sexuality. When you care for patients who have alterations in self-concept, be particularly alert to the patient who is experiencing chronic pain or fatigue. Chronic pain often causes decreased sexual function, irritability, and decreased sleep. Patients with chronic fatigue often feel exhausted and lack the energy for sexual interaction. These types of changes negatively affect self-

---

BOX 24.5	SYNTHESIS IN PRACTICE

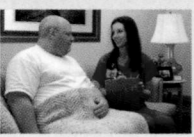

As Maria prepares to care for Mr. Taylor, she thinks about what she knows about self-concept, body image, and sexuality. She realizes that Mr. Taylor's stroke and resulting neurological deficits along with the sexual side effects of his antihypertensive medications are significant stressors. Mr. Taylor's independence is threatened because he is in the hospital and dependent on the nurses for most of his care. He may never be able to go back to work again, and he does not consider himself a strong man anymore. His role as provider for his family is also threatened. Maria recognizes the significance of these changes and their potential influence on his self-concept, body image, and sexuality.

Maria's father had a stroke 2 years ago. Although his neurological symptoms eventually improved enough to allow him to go back to work, Maria remembers the struggle her father went through as he coped with the physical and emotional changes that the stroke created. Maria's experience as a single mother also provides insight into what it is like to assume a new role within a family. She uses these two different experiences to guide her assessment of Mr. Taylor's concerns.

Maria needs to learn as much as she can about Mr. Taylor's thoughts and feelings about his self-concept, body image, and sexuality. To do this she realizes that she must first establish a trusting relationship with him and his wife, Meredith. Because Maria feels uncomfortable discussing sexuality with her patients, she reviews the PLISSIT assessment of sexuality (see Box 24.7) the night before she cares for Mr. Taylor and writes out some questions that she wants to ask him. Maria also plans to talk with Mr. and Mrs. Taylor about their relationship before his stroke.

---

concept. Also, gather knowledge about your patient's cultural background. Culture influences the importance that people place on such things as appearance, role performance, and acceptance by others (see Chapter 21).

Experience. Throughout life all individuals, including nurses, experience self-concept issues. Personal memories of changes in appearance or times when you were unable to carry out usual roles because of a temporary illness help you to be empathetic with patients who are experiencing stressors to their self-concept or sexuality. Past experiences with patients who have experienced changes in self-concept or self-concept stressors provide useful insight into how to work effectively with a current patient.

Attitudes. Use critical thinking attitudes such as humility, fairness, and responsibility and accountability when caring for a patient with threats to self-concept and sexuality. Always admit what you do not know about a patient's own values and beliefs about their sexuality or self-concept, and obtain the knowledge needed to develop a relevant plan of care. Be fair, and do not allow bias or prejudice affect how you care for patients with sexual preferences different from your own. Show professional behaviors, including acceptance, respect, and compassion and being accountable for an individualized plan of care.

Standards. There are several codes of professional conduct for nurses; each reflects an ethical commitment to the principle of respect for patient autonomy. Autonomy means that individuals have the freedom to choose their own life plan. Support your patients' autonomy to make choices and live in an authentic way consistent with personal values and beliefs to help them develop and maintain a strong and positive self-concept.

NURSING PROCESS

▪▪▪ ASSESSMENT

When assessing self-concept and self-esteem, focus on all components (identity, body image, and role performance) and on behaviors suggestive of altered self-concept, self-esteem, or sexuality (Box 24.6). Also, assess for actual and potential self-concept stressors (see Fig. 24.1). Determining a patient's current and past coping patterns is also important. If a patient shows mood changes such as depression, a mental status examination may also be helpful (see Chapter 16). In addition to direct questioning, you effectively gather much of the data regarding self-concept by observing a patient's nonverbal behavior and paying attention to what he or she says. Take note of the way patients talk about the people in their lives because this provides clues to both stressful and supportive relationships. It also suggests key patient roles and obligations.

Apply your knowledge of developmental stages (see Box 24.1) to determine what aspects of self-concept are likely to be important to the patient, and inquire about these aspects of the person's life. For example, ask a 67-year-old male patient about his life now that retirement is approaching and what is now most important to him. Spend time asking a school-age patient how he or she has adjusted to transferring to a new school and whether he or she has been able to make friends. Conversations with individual patients will likely provide data relating to role performance, identity, self-esteem, stressors, and coping patterns. At appropriate times, specific questions are useful (Table 24.1).

Bullying is very common in schools and any other locations in which children gather and interact. In the case of school-age children and adolescents, assess for signs of bullying (Youth Connection, 2005; Johns Hopkins, n.d.):

- Damaged or missing clothing and belongings
- Unexplained cuts, bruises, or torn clothes
- Lack of friends
- Frequent claims of having lost pocket money, possessions, packed lunches, or snacks
- Fear of school or of leaving the house
- Avoidance of places, friends, family members, or activities adolescents once enjoyed
- Unusual routes to and from school or the bus stop
- Poor appetite, headaches, stomachaches
- Mood swings
- Trouble sleeping
- Lack of interest in schoolwork
- Talk about suicide
- Uncharacteristic aggression toward younger siblings or family members

Depending on the environment, some young people—such as LGBTQ+ youth, youth with disabilities, and socially isolated youth—may be at an increased risk of being bullied (American Society for the Positive Care of Children, 2017). Ask parents (when appropriate) if they have noticed any of the behaviors that may indicate bullying.

A complete nursing history also needs to include a few questions related to a person's sexual health. Start with a general statement such as "Sex is an important part of life and can be affected by health status" and follow with open-ended questions such as "Tell me how you would describe your sexual health" or "Share with me any questions or concerns you have about how your health or medications will affect your sex life." Once you approach the topic, a patient is able to talk about concerns and explore possible ways to resolve the problem. When you address sexuality in a sensitive, relaxed, matter-of-fact manner, patients feel safe to bring up areas of concern. Use gender-neutral terms and questions when completing a sexual history. For example, say "partner" versus "husband" or "wife" and "chest" versus "breast." The intimacy of a nurse-patient relationship, whether it is involved in providing physical care or discussing the impact of a recent diagnosis, provides a unique opportunity for discussing a person's sexual concerns. The acronym *PLISSIT* is a helpful format for discussing sexuality with patients (Box 24.7). PLISSIT describes a step-wise model that is still relevant for intervening with sexual concerns with progressively more intensive intervention steps (Petersen, 2017).

Assessment of sexuality involves physical, psychological, social, and cultural variables. It is sometimes unnerving to inquire about another person's sexual functioning. You may worry that a patient does not appreciate being asked about sexuality and sexual practices. However, patients want to know how medications, treatments, and surgical procedures influence their ability to perform sexually and the impact on

---

BOX 24.6	**BEHAVIORS SUGGESTIVE OF ALTERED SELF-CONCEPT AND SEXUALITY**

- Avoidance of eye contact
- Slumped posture
- Unkempt appearance
- Overly apologetic
- Hesitant speech and/or withdrawn
- Overly critical or angry
- Frequent or inappropriate crying

- Negative self-evaluation
- Excessively dependent
- Hesitant to express views or opinions
- Lack of interest in what is happening
- Passive attitude
- Difficulty making decisions

TABLE 24.1 FOCUSED PATIENT ASSESSMENT

FACTORS TO ASSESS	QUESTIONS	PHYSICAL ASSESSMENT
Identity	How would you describe yourself?	Note verbal and nonverbal responses. Watch for hesitant speech, poor eye contact, and slumped posture. Derogatory answers (e.g., "I don't know; there's not too much worth mentioning") raise concern and need further assessment.
Body image	Which aspects of your appearance do you like? Describe any aspects of your appearance that you would like to change.	Determine patient's ability to identify something positive about appearance or body functions (e.g., "People have always told me I have nice eyes" or "I'm strong"). People who do not identify positive characteristics often have negative body image and poor self-esteem.
Self-esteem	Tell me about the things you do that make you feel good about yourself. How do you feel about yourself? If you were to describe yourself to someone else, which characteristics would you use?	Observe verbal and nonverbal responses. With prompting, most patients can identify something favorable. Statements about not having any strengths or not being able to do anything well raise concern and require additional assessment.
Role performance	Tell me about your primary roles (e.g., partner, parent, friend, sister, professional role, volunteer). How effective are you at carrying out each of these roles? Do you have any barriers to fulfilling your roles?	Listen for the number of primary roles identified. Many primary roles will put the patient at risk for role conflicts and role overload. Patients who do not think that these roles are met adequately may be experiencing alterations in self-concept.
Sexuality	How has your illness, medication, or surgery affected your sex life? Are your needs for intimacy being met? Do you have any concerns about your sexual functioning?	Identify concerns about sexual functioning (e.g., erectile dysfunction in men, changes in vaginal lubrication in women) or overall change in sex drive. Determine if patient is hesitant to bring up issues of sexuality.

BOX 24.7 PLISSIT MODEL FOR ASSESSING AND APPROACHING SEXUALITY

Permission—Permission for health care provider to discuss sexuality issues and for patient to continue to do what he or she is already doing. Allieviates unnecessary guilt, anxiety, and concerns about normality.

Limited **I**nformation—Health care provider assesses and clarifies misinformation, dispels and explores myths, and provides accurate factual sexual information.

Specific **S**uggestions—Health care provider offers practical ideas and exercises directly related to the patient's particular problem (only when the nurse is clear about the problem).

Intensive **T**herapy—Long-term therapy. Provides individualized therapy by referring to a professional with advanced training if necessary.

Modified from Annon J: The PLISSIT model: a proposed conceptual scheme for the behavioral treatment of sexual problems, *J Sex Educ Ther* 2(2):1, 1976; Petersen Z: *The Wiley-Blackwell handbook of sex therapy*, 2017, Wiley-Blackwell.

sexual relationships. With experience, you come to recognize that many patients welcome the opportunity to talk about their sexuality, especially when they are having trouble in sexual functioning.

It is important to first understand the reasons for changes in a patient's perceived sexual health. How a person responds to any physical or functional change in sexuality and intimacy following an illness depends on the person's self-concept, support of sexual partner, and attitudes regarding sexuality. Many health professionals fail to address the sexual needs of their patients. To promote sexual health, assess the effect of a diagnosis and its treatment and medications on your patient's perception of sexuality or sexual performance as you develop a treatment plan. For example, when caring for a man who has had a heart attack, you might say, "Following a heart attack, men have questions about sexuality such as when they are able to resume sexual intercourse" and then ask "Do you have questions like this that I can answer?" In the case of a patient with spinal cord injury resulting in paralysis, say, "It is natural for you to have concerns about being able to perform sexually. Would you like to discuss any concerns that you have?" Various physical factors positively or negatively influence sexual desire and function. Sexual intercourse sometimes results in pain or discomfort from arthritis, angina, endometriosis, or lack of vaginal lubrication. Anticipation that sex may hurt such as during the postpartum period or after surgery lessens sexual desire. Learn to what extent these physical factors affect a patient's sexual performance.

QSEN QSEN ACTIVITY *Quality Improvement*

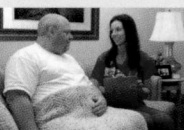

Discharge instructions given to patients following a myocardial infarction do not always include counseling regarding resumption of sexual activity. You realize that some patients may be hesitant to bring up this subject but know that sexually active adults report higher quality of life than adults who are not sexually active. You ask a group of nurses on a cardiac care unit to find out more about their discharge teaching and discover that some nurses say they do not feel knowledgeable about this topic.

- What strategies could help improve the discharge teaching on this topic?
- How should the nurses measure if any changes in their approach have beneficial effects?

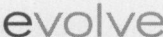 Answers to QSEN Activities can be found on the Evolve website.

Body image can also be affected by adherence to medical and treatment regimens. For example, many chemotherapy agents used in the treatment of cancer often result in infertility. Invite a patient to discuss sexual concerns by saying, "Tell me if you have any concerns about whether your chemo medicine will affect your ability to have children." Such risks seriously lessen the likelihood of patients adhering to their medications. Some medications affect sexual desire or cause physical changes that affect performance. Drinking alcohol or using drugs clouds judgment and results in sexual intercourse or other activities that lead to STIs or pregnancy. Gather a complete history of any medications or illicit drugs that the patient is taking or has taken in the past. You also need to obtain the same information for the patient's partner.

Another important area to assess is sexual decision making including patients' use of contraception and safe sex practices. Adolescents respond best to a question such as "Many people your age have questions about sexually transmitted infections or whether their bodies are developing at the right rate. What questions about sex can I answer?"

Older Adult Considerations. Reviewing sexuality changes associated with aging is also important. Many older women experience some type of sexual problem such as low desire or vaginal dryness. In men, the penis does not become firm as quickly and is not as firm as it is at a younger age. Ejaculation takes longer to achieve and is shorter in duration, and the erection often diminishes more quickly. When assessing sexual changes, you need to ask about a patient's past sexual experiences, perceptions, and difficulties. Start the

conversation by first asking permission to discuss intimate issues. It is important to have adequate knowledge about sexuality across the life span and to be aware of your own attitudes and beliefs while promoting sexual health in elderly patients (Atallah, 2016).

Your nursing assessment includes consideration of previous coping behaviors; the nature, number, and intensity of stressors; and a patient's internal and external resources. Knowing how a patient has dealt with self-concept stressors in the past provides insight into his or her style of coping. Not all patients address issues in the same way, but often a person uses a familiar coping pattern for newly encountered stressors. As you identify previous coping patterns, it is useful to determine whether these patterns contributed to healthy functioning or created more problems. For example, the use of drugs or alcohol during times of stress often creates additional stressors (see Chapter 26).

Exploring resources and strengths such as availability of significant others or prior use of community resources is important when formulating a realistic and effective plan. Women in midlife who are recently single because of separation, divorce, or widowhood may be unaware that they are at risk for unintended pregnancies and STIs. In addition, the physiological changes associated with aging such as changes in vaginal mucosa can place middle-age and older women at higher risk for genital infections. All mature adults need education about safe sex and STI screenings because they may be unaware of the health risks of unprotected sex. People 50 years of age and older are at risk for HIV, but they may be less aware of HIV risk factors than younger people and may take fewer precautions. Health care providers may not always test older people for HIV infection, and older people may not consider themselves to be at risk for HIV infection or may mistake HIV symptoms for symptoms of normal aging and not consider HIV as a cause (CDC, 2017).

Valuable assessment data often evolve from conversations with family and significant others. Sometimes significant others have insights into a person's way of dealing with stressors and knowledge about what is important to the person's self-concept. The way in which a loved one talks about a patient including his or her nonverbal behaviors provides information about what kind of support is available for the patient. Ask patients if they feel comfortable when they are relating to their partner and whether there is openness in the interaction.

Patient Expectations. The patient's expectations are also important to assess. Illnesses, trauma, and surgeries all have the potential to create bodily and psychological changes that affect a patient's perception of self-concept, body image, and sexuality. Asking a patient how he or she believes medical and nursing interventions will make a difference provides useful information regarding the patient's expectations. This also provides an opportunity to discuss the patient's goals. For example, when working with a patient who is experiencing anxiety related to an upcoming cancer surgery, ask the patient about his or her expectations and what changes to expect.

Also, verify what information the surgeon provided and the level of patient understanding. Determine if the patient is performing the relaxation exercises taught during the outpatient preoperative visit, and ask the patient about the effectiveness of these exercises. The patient's response provides valuable insight about his or her beliefs and attitudes regarding the effectiveness of the interventions and the potential need to modify the nursing approach. When nursing care involves consideration of a patient's self-concept, body image, and sexuality, you need to be sensitive and understanding and always maintain the patient's confidentiality.

■ ■ ■ NURSING DIAGNOSIS

Critically review and analyze assessment data to identify a patient's actual or potential problem areas. You rely on knowledge and experience, apply appropriate critical thinking attitudes and professional standards, and look for clusters of defining characteristics and risk factors that indicate nursing diagnoses. Possible nursing diagnoses related to self-concept and sexual functioning include the following:

- *Disturbed Body Image*
- *Disturbed Personal Identity*
- *Ineffective Role Performance*
- *Readiness for Enhanced Self-Concept*
- *Chronic Low Self-Esteem*
- *Situational Low Self-Esteem*
- *Sexual Dysfunction*
- *Ineffective Sexuality Pattern*

Forming nursing diagnoses about self-concept or sexuality is complex. For example, often isolated data are the defining characteristics for more than one problem-focused nursing diagnosis. If a person who has recently been laid off from work expresses a predominantly negative self-appraisal including inability to handle situations or events and difficulty making decisions, these characteristics suggest a nursing diagnosis of *Situational Low Self-Esteem related to inability to fulfill previous roles*. Assessing information regarding recent events in the patient's life and how the patient has viewed himself or herself in the past is important. Likewise, identifying a problem-focused nursing diagnosis regarding sexuality often requires you to clarify that defining characteristics exist and the patient perceives difficulty regarding sexuality. Clues to help you identify defining characteristics of a possible problem-focused nursing diagnosis include surgery of reproductive organs or changes in appearance, chronic fatigue or pain, past or current physical abuse, chronic illness, and developmental milestones such as puberty or menopause. Determining contributing factors is important. Interventions depend on selecting the correct related factors when you identify a problem-focused diagnosis. When you include all relevant contributing factors, you plan effectively. For example, the nursing diagnosis *Ineffective Sexuality Pattern related to difficulty with acceptance of recent loss and fear of pain* is appropriate for a woman who recently had a mastectomy. Further expanding the "related to" section to include more about how the mastectomy is affecting sexuality is

helpful. For example, altered sexuality is possibly related to postoperative pain or fear of pain, fear of diminished attractiveness, or difficulty in moving.

■ ■ ■ PLANNING

Goals and Outcomes. As you develop an individualized plan of care for your patient's nursing diagnoses, help the patient set realistic and meaningful expectations for care. Individualize goals, and set realistic and measurable outcomes. Collaborating with a patient in establishing realistic goals involves helping the patient identify alternative solutions and develop realistic goals based on them. This facilitates real change and encourages goal-setting behaviors. Always consult with the patient about whether the goals are perceived as realistic (see Care Plan). In addition, consult with significant others (when the patient consents) to develop a more comprehensive and workable plan. Once you formulate a goal, consider how the assessment data that illustrated the problem would change if the problem were diminished. Reflect these changes in the outcome criteria. As you develop your patient's plan of care, remember that patients have more than one interrelated problem (Fig. 24.3).

Setting Priorities. The care plan presents the goals, expected outcomes, and interventions for a patient with an alteration in self-concept or sexuality. Your interventions focus on helping the patient adapt to the stressors that led to the disturbance and supporting and reinforcing the development of coping methods. The patient often needs time to adapt to physical changes. Self-concept priorities include maximizing the patient's ability to address physical and psychological needs. Priorities for sexual health typically include resuming sexual activities the patient can successfully perform. Look for strengths in both the individual and the family, and provide resources and education to turn limitations into strengths. Patient teaching communicates the normalcy of certain situations (e.g., nature of a chronic disease, change in relationships, effect of a loss). It is important to determine your patients' needs and plan accordingly. For example, when caring for a patient whose sexual health is altered, include private time for your patient and partner to quietly sit in the room and have dinner and watch a movie without any interruptions.

Collaborative Care. The perceptions of significant others are important to incorporate into the care plan. Sometimes individuals who experienced deficits in self-concept before the current episode of treatment have established a system of support including mental health clinicians, clergy, and other community resources. Before involving the family, consider a patient's desires for significant others to be involved and cultural norms regarding who most frequently makes decisions in the family. Sexual conflict in marriage and intimacy issues stemming from past sexual assault or incest often require intensive treatment with mental health professionals. Resolving self-concept issues is a long-term goal and includes

◎ CARE PLAN

Situational Low Self-Esteem

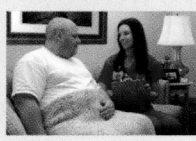

ASSESSMENT

After Maria completes Mr. Taylor's physical assessment and helps him with his self-care activities, she sits down with Mr. and Mrs. Taylor to discuss how the stroke has affected Mr. Taylor's self-concept and sexual health.

ASSESSMENT ACTIVITIES

Ask about identity concerns (e.g., sexuality, masculinity, and role of breadwinner). Ask how the stroke has affected Mr. Taylor's sense of self.

Observe Mr. Taylor's mood, affect, nonverbal communication, and interactions with others; interview family as appropriate.

[a]**Defining characteristics/risk factors** are shown in **bold** type.

FINDINGS[a]

Mr. Taylor **looks away, shakes his head,** and states, **"I feel less of a man."** Is not able to perform physical activities by self or fulfill role within family.

Mrs. Taylor reports that Mr. Taylor demonstrates **intermittent eye contact, frequent crying when alone, blank staring** at his flaccid hand, and **superficial conversations** with family members.

NURSING DIAGNOSIS: Situational Low Self-Esteem related to negative view of self as less than whole following stroke and uncertainty of future personal, family, and professional roles.

PLANNING

GOAL

Mr. Taylor will perceive fewer alterations in self-concept including low self-esteem, disturbed body image, and impaired sexuality by discharge.

EXPECTED OUTCOMES (NOC)[b]

Self-Esteem

Mr. Taylor will verbalize increased feelings of self-acceptance and self-worth within 4 days.

[b]Outcome classification labels from Moorhead S, et al, editors: *Nursing outcomes classification (NOC),* ed 5, St Louis, 2013, Mosby.

INTERVENTIONS (NIC)[c]

Self-Esteem Enhancement

Facilitate an environment and activities (e.g., writing in a journal, reflection, praying, talking with a nurse) that increase self-esteem.

Reinforce and encourage Mrs. Taylor to reinforce Mr. Taylor's statements of self-worth during care activities.

Sexual Counseling

Teach Mr. and Mrs. Taylor about the effects of his paralysis and medications on sexual function.

Discuss with the couple how they can try to make adaptations to have mutually satisfying sexual health.

RATIONALE

A therapeutic nurse-patient relationship promotes positive patient outcome including behavior change (Stuart, 2013).

Reinforcing positive self-esteem statements and activities improves quality of life and adaptive functioning (Mantilla et al., 2014).

When illness and/or treatments affect sexual performance, partners benefit from open discussion about the sexual performance side effects of medications and treatments (Santos-Iglesias et al., 2016).

Sexuality is a basic need and concern for both men and women. Many health care providers believe that patients do not expect their sexuality concerns to be addressed and treated in an acute care or rehabilitation setting (Haesler et al., 2016; Touhy and Jett, 2016).

[c]Intervention classification labels from Bulechek GM, et al, editors: *Nursing interventions classification (NIC),* ed 6, St Louis, 2013, Mosby.

EVALUATION

NURSING ACTIONS	PATIENT RESPONSE/FINDING	ACHIEVEMENT OF OUTCOME
Ask Mr. Taylor how effective he feels in his ability to identify and express feelings verbally and nonverbally.	Mr. Taylor reports, "I've been able to talk with my wife, even about my concerns that she won't find me attractive anymore."	Improved verbal and nonverbal communication noted.
Monitor changes in Mr. Taylor's statements about himself.	Mr. Taylor is making fewer negative comments and is evaluating body image more realistically but remains dissatisfied with appearance and strength of hand.	Small improvement in self-esteem; body image more realistic but remains negative. Discusses body image with wife and primary nurse.

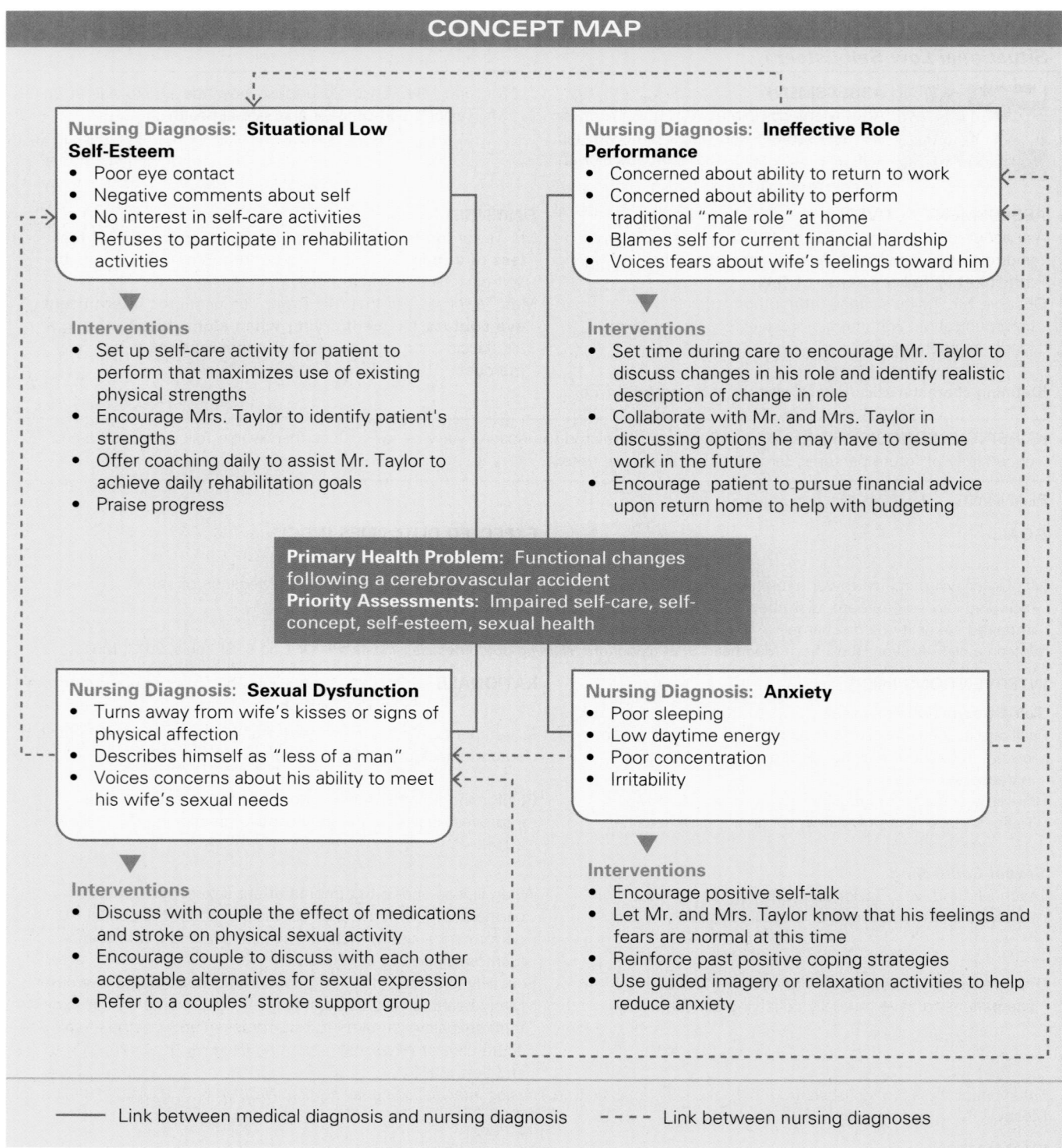

CONCEPT MAP

Nursing Diagnosis: Situational Low Self-Esteem
- Poor eye contact
- Negative comments about self
- No interest in self-care activities
- Refuses to participate in rehabilitation activities

Interventions
- Set up self-care activity for patient to perform that maximizes use of existing physical strengths
- Encourage Mrs. Taylor to identify patient's strengths
- Offer coaching daily to assist Mr. Taylor to achieve daily rehabilitation goals
- Praise progress

Nursing Diagnosis: Ineffective Role Performance
- Concerned about ability to return to work
- Concerned about ability to perform traditional "male role" at home
- Blames self for current financial hardship
- Voices fears about wife's feelings toward him

Interventions
- Set time during care to encourage Mr. Taylor to discuss changes in his role and identify realistic description of change in role
- Collaborate with Mr. and Mrs. Taylor in discussing options he may have to resume work in the future
- Encourage patient to pursue financial advice upon return home to help with budgeting

Primary Health Problem: Functional changes following a cerebrovascular accident
Priority Assessments: Impaired self-care, self-concept, self-esteem, sexual health

Nursing Diagnosis: Sexual Dysfunction
- Turns away from wife's kisses or signs of physical affection
- Describes himself as "less of a man"
- Voices concerns about his ability to meet his wife's sexual needs

Interventions
- Discuss with couple the effect of medications and stroke on physical sexual activity
- Encourage couple to discuss with each other acceptable alternatives for sexual expression
- Refer to a couples' stroke support group

Nursing Diagnosis: Anxiety
- Poor sleeping
- Low daytime energy
- Poor concentration
- Irritability

Interventions
- Encourage positive self-talk
- Let Mr. and Mrs. Taylor know that his feelings and fears are normal at this time
- Reinforce past positive coping strategies
- Use guided imagery or relaxation activities to help reduce anxiety

——— Link between medical diagnosis and nursing diagnosis   - - - - Link between nursing diagnoses

FIG 24.3 Concept map.

referrals to a clinical psychologist, advanced practice psychiatric nurse, social worker, or professional counselor.

■ ■ ■ IMPLEMENTATION

As with all the steps of the nursing process, a therapeutic nurse-patient relationship is central to implementing an effective plan for patients with self-concept or sexuality needs. Once you have developed goals and outcomes, consider nursing interventions that help move your patient toward his or her goals. Individualize any standard interventions to your patient. In the case of problem-focused nursing diagnoses, develop nursing interventions based on the "related to" component. Prioritizing interventions that affect the "related to" factors often decrease the problem reflected in the nursing diagnosis. *In the case of Mr. Taylor (see Care Plan), the "related to" component of the problem-focused nursing diagnoses focuses on the areas to explore when talking with the patient and family.*

Nursing interventions are designed to promote a patient's healthy self-concept and sexuality by helping patients regain or restore the elements that contribute to a strong and secure sense of self. The approaches that you choose vary according to the level of care required. Effective nursing care includes promoting sexual health in acute and restorative settings by helping patients understand their problems and exploring methods to deal with them effectively.

Health Promotion. Collaborate with patients and family caregivers to help develop healthy lifestyle behaviors that contribute to a positive self-concept. Interventions that support adaptation to stress such as proper nutrition (see Chapter 35), regular exercise within a patient's capabilities, adequate sleep and rest (see Chapter 33), stress-reducing practices (see Chapter 26), elimination of stressors, or risk reduction contribute to a healthy self-concept. A patient-centered approach to care is important to support patients who engage in high-risk behaviors and who have alterations in self-concept (Box 24.8). You are in a unique position to identify lifestyle practices that place a patient's self-concept at risk or are suggestive of altered self-concept. For example, a college student visits an outpatient clinic with complaints of being unable to sleep and anxiety attacks. In gathering the patient history, you learn of lifestyle practices such as too little rest, many life changes occurring simultaneously, irregular menstrual cycles, and excessive use of alcohol. These data suggest actual or potential self-concept disturbances. You then talk with the patient to determine how she views the various lifestyle elements, to facilitate her insight into behaviors, and to make appropriate referrals or provide needed health teaching.

Assessing a person's sexuality and providing useful sex education require good communication skills. Make sure that the environment and timing provide privacy, uninterrupted time, and patient comfort. For example, discuss contraception methods with a woman in an office rather than in the examination room when she is only partially clothed. Plan the discussion so that there are no interruptions, and sit down while showing your interest and readiness to support her needs.

Teaching topics on sexuality vary based on the age of the patient. Education offers explanations of normal developmental changes. For example, talk to a school-age child about the appearance of breast buds or pubic hair. When discussing sexual health with patients of childbearing age, always consider your patient's cultural and religious beliefs regarding contraception. The discussion includes the patient's desire for children, usual sexual practices, and acceptable methods of contraception. Review all methods of contraception to provide necessary information for an informed patient choice. Reinforce that the best method is the one the patient will use consistently. Teaching needs for an adult include

---

🌐 **BOX 24.8 PATIENT-CENTERED CARE**

Self-Concept and Impact on Adolescent Drinking Behaviors

Low self-concept may precede or perhaps even motivate adolescent drinking. Because many teens engage in behaviors that increase the potential for morbidity and mortality, helping youth develop a healthy self-concept may prevent health risk behaviors including teen drinking (Kann et al., 2016). The 2015 Centers for Disease Control and Prevention Youth Risk Behavior Survey found that among high school students, during the past 30 days 33% of underage teens drank some amount of alcohol, 18% binge drank, 8% drove after drinking alcohol, and 20% knowingly rode with a driver who had been drinking alcohol (Kann et al., 2016). Identifying risk and protective factors is important when creating drinking prevention programs. Enhancing opportunities to learn communication skills and engage in alternative behaviors may reduce drinking as an adolescent risk behavior.

IMPLICATIONS FOR PRACTICE
- Include stress management and self-esteem improvement in drinking prevention interventions.
- Assess for effective adolescent coping strategies such as effective communication, conflict resolution, and stress management.
- Family members, peers, teachers, and health care providers should instill adolescents' ethnic pride, which promotes self-concept and encourages protective factors against risk behaviors such as drinking.
- Address family, social, and behavioral factors during preadolescence and adolescence.
- Identify risk factors for early drug and alcohol use, including genetic predisposition, family environment, and ethnic identity.

---

details of physiological changes resulting from illness or treatment effects (Box 24.9).

Individuals need to learn more about safe sex practices when they have more than one sex partner or when their partner had other sexual experiences. Provide information on the signs and symptoms of STIs and interventions to decrease STI transmission such as the use of latex condoms and how to avoid high-risk sexual activities. Safe sex also means considering a patient's emotional risks within a relationship. Role play is a useful teaching tool to help a patient learn to say "no" or to negotiate with a partner to use a condom.

Acute Care. In the acute care setting you are likely to encounter patients who are experiencing potential threats to their self-concept because of the nature of the treatment and diagnostic procedures. Threats to a patient's self-concept result in anxiety and/or fear. You need to address numerous new stressors with your patient including a new diagnosis and the need to make changes in lifestyle after hospitalization. In the acute care setting, there is often more than one stressor, increasing the overall stress level for patients and their families.

BOX 24.9   PATIENT TEACHING

Promoting Sexual Function

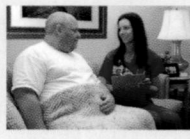 After talking with Mr. and Mrs. Taylor, Maria decides to develop a teaching plan that will help the couple adapt to the changes in sexuality that resulted from Mr. Taylor's stroke.

OUTCOME

Mr. and Mrs. Taylor will state at least three ways to attain a satisfactory level of sexual activity.

TEACHING STRATEGIES

- Provide information about normal sexual changes that occur with aging and changes following a stroke (Haesler et al., 2016). Be specific in explaining how Mr. Taylor's deficit will affect sexual performance.
- Encourage Mr. and Mrs. Taylor to discuss which types of intimate behavior provide the most sexual stimulation and satisfaction.
- Discuss side effects of medications that Mr. Taylor is taking that commonly alter sexual function and response. Describe the types of changes that may occur (Meiner, 2015).
- Encourage selection of a time of day when Mr. Taylor feels most rested and a comfortable and nonthreatening setting.
- Encourage alternative positions for intercourse (e.g., side-lying, lying on a bed with legs over the side) that decrease discomfort during intercourse (Touhy and Jett, 2016).

EVALUATION STRATEGIES

- Use the principles of teach-back to evaluate patient/family caregiver learning:
  - "Explain for me the plan you have put together to improve your sexual health."
  - "What specific medications are you taking that may change how you can perform sexually and have good sexual health?"

You also care for patients who are faced with the need to adapt to an altered body image because of surgery or other physical change. Often a visit by someone who has experienced similar changes and adapted to them is helpful. The timing of such a visit is important. Because it is often difficult to address these needs while in an acute care setting, appropriate follow-up and referrals including home care and information about support groups are essential. Be sensitive to a patient's level of acceptance of the change. Forcing confrontation with the change before a patient is ready delays the patient's acceptance. Signs that a patient is receptive to such a visit include the patient's asking questions related to how to manage an aspect of what has happened or looking at the changed area. As the patient expresses readiness to integrate the body change into his or her self-concept, you either let him or her know about groups that are available or ask if he or she wants you to make the initial contact. In addition, respond to the change with acceptance to model acceptance for both the patient and the family.

Both physical and psychological aspects of illness have the potential to affect sexuality. Never assume that sexual functioning is not a concern merely because of an individual's age or severity of prognosis. After identifying concerns, address them in the context of the patient's value system. When a patient experiences physical limitations to sexual performance, provide the following suggestions: planning sexual activity when the patient is rested, experimenting with positions that are more comfortable, encouraging partners to give one another more time, and encouraging the use of foreplay to achieve arousal.

Restorative and Continuing Care. Home care or restorative care environments provide opportunities to work with a patient to attain a more positive self-concept. Interventions designed to help a patient reach the goal of adapting to changes in self-concept or attaining a positive self-concept are based on the premise that a patient first develops insight and self-awareness concerning problems and stressors and then acts to solve the problems and cope with the stressors. You incorporate this approach into patient teaching for alterations in self-concept including situational low-self-esteem, which is sometimes present in the home care setting. Increase a patient's self-awareness by establishing a trusting relationship that allows the patient to openly explore thoughts and feelings. A priority nursing intervention is the expert use of communication skills to clarify the expectations of the patient and family as interventions are implemented. Open exploration makes the situation less threatening for the patient and encourages behaviors that expand self-awareness. Encourage the patient's self-exploration by accepting his or her thoughts and feelings, helping him or her to clarify interactions with others, and being empathetic. Also facilitate self-expression, and stress the patient's self-responsibility.

Promoting a patient's self-evaluation involves helping the patient define problems clearly and identify positive and negative coping mechanisms. Work closely with each patient to help analyze adaptive and maladaptive responses, consider alternatives, and discuss outcomes. Design opportunities that result in success, reinforce the patient's skills and strengths, and help the patient obtain needed assistance.

Teach patients to move away from ineffective coping mechanisms and develop successful coping strategies. Offering support when patients attempt to adopt health-promoting behaviors motivates patients to continue efforts at promoting health. Promoting adaptive, flexible coping is essential to intervening in self-concept alterations. Patients who are experiencing threats to or alterations in self-concept often benefit from collaboration with mental health and community resources to promote increased awareness. Knowledge of available community resources allows you to make appropriate referrals.

Use a nonjudgmental, respectful approach to encourage honest and open discussions about sexual health. Management of sexuality concerns is important as you promote sexual intimacy and provide closeness and closure between partners at the end of life. Give priority to patients in middle and older adulthood when you address sexuality concerns resulting from illness, medications, or physical changes. Provide information on how the specific illness will limit sexual activity and ideas for adapting or facilitating sexual activity. Interventions range from giving permission for a partner to lie in bed and hold a patient to coordinating nursing care and medications in a way that provides opportunity for privacy and intimacy. In the home environment, it is important to help patients create an environment comfortable for sexual activity. For example, this sometimes involves making recommendations for ways to rearrange a patient's bedroom to accommodate any limitations. Patients and partners need to know how to accommodate barriers such as Foley catheters or drainage tubes that make sexual positioning difficult.

Middle-age and older adults who are sexually active have greater independence, better overall health, and longer life expectancy. Older adults who report being highly satisfied with their sex lives report moderate to high sexual self-esteem (Santos-Iglesias et al., 2016). In the event of an extended hospital stay or admission to a rehabilitation or long-term care setting, facilities need to make proper arrangements for privacy during a patient's sexual experience. Staff at such facilities need to be educated about the importance of sexuality and ways to support intimacy and sexual expression among consenting adults. In addition, do not assume that all older patients are heterosexuals.

Establishing a therapeutic relationship is critical to successfully intervening with patients who have alterations in self-concept, whether care is focused on health promotion, dealing with an acute process, or addressing restorative care. To support the development of a positive self-concept in a patient, convey genuine caring for the patient. Then and only then do you establish a partnership with the patient to address underlying problems.

■■■ EVALUATION

Patient Outcomes. Expected outcomes for a patient with a self-concept disturbance include nonverbal behaviors indicating a positive self-concept, statements of self-acceptance, and acceptance of change in appearance or physical function (Box 24.10). For example, a patient who has difficulty making eye contact demonstrates a more positive self-concept by making more frequent eye contact and smiling during conversation. Adequate self-care practices and acceptance of the use of prosthetic devices are also outcomes that indicate progress. A positive attitude toward rehabilitation and increased movement toward independence facilitate a return to preexisting roles at work or at home. Patterns of interacting often reflect changes in self-concept. A patient who was hesitant to express his or her views more readily offers opinions and ideas as self-esteem increases.

Sometimes initial goals are unrealistic or require modification as the patient's condition changes. You and the patient need to revise the plan in these cases. Patient adaptation to

---

BOX 24.10   EVALUATION

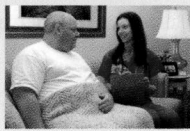

Because Mr. Taylor was in the hospital for 2 weeks, Maria could care for him and watch him adapt to the changes he experienced as a result of his stroke. On the last day that Maria cared for Mr. Taylor, he reported that he was going to a rehabilitation center that specializes in helping people who have had strokes. Mr. Taylor is able to complete most of his bath independently. Although his gait is a little unsteady, he can walk short distances with a walker. During his bath, he jokes, "I think my new haircut makes me look a lot younger!" This improvement in function and acceptance of self has helped Mr. Taylor become more satisfied with himself and his progress in therapy. Toward the end of his hospitalization, Mr. Taylor began to address concerns about changes in role performance. He is hopeful that he will be able to return to work after he leaves the rehabilitation center. Mr. and Mrs. Taylor have worked with a therapist who specializes in helping couples adapt to changes in sexuality following illness or surgery. Mr. Taylor states that the therapy sessions have helped him grow closer to his wife and have strengthened their relationship. Several of his bowling friends visited him last night. Mr. Taylor states, "I can't wait to get better. I have a lot of things to do and a lot to live for."

DOCUMENTATION NOTE

"Ability to perform ADLs improving. Only needs help to wash back during bath. Improvements in function have led to reports of enhanced self-esteem and acceptance of body image. Interacts affectionately with spouse and is maintaining relationships with friends. States, "I feel motivated to get better and return to work soon. I plan to continue to work on improving the weaknesses I still have while I am at the stroke rehabilitation center.""

---

major changes sometimes takes a year or longer, but the fact that this period is long does not suggest problems with adaptation. Look for signs that the patient has reduced some stressors and that some behaviors have become more adaptive. This requires follow-up discussions with the patient to determine if the level of satisfaction with sexual performance or sexual function has improved. Sometimes the patient achieved the goal and outcome criteria, but sexual functioning is still not ideal. Consider which other steps are appropriate. Changes in self-concept and sexuality take time. Although change is slow, care of the patient with a self-concept disturbance is rewarding.

Patient Expectations. Determine if patient's expectations are met regarding measures taken to improve self-concept and sexual health. After determining the achievement of targeted outcomes, ask if the patient thinks that nursing care was effective and supportive. Remain aware of any personal limitations in your ability to counsel the patient. In some cases, referrals to other health care providers are still necessary.

KEY POINTS

- Self-concept is an integrated set of conscious and unconscious attitudes and perceptions about the self.
- Components of self-concept are identity, body image, and role performance. Self-esteem and sexuality are closely related components.
- Each developmental stage involves factors that are important to the development of a healthy, positive self-concept.
- Identity is particularly vulnerable during adolescence.
- Body image is the mental picture of one's body and is not necessarily consistent with a person's actual body structure or appearance.
- Body image stressors include changes in physical appearance, structure, or functioning caused by normal developmental changes or illness.
- Self-esteem is the emotional appraisal of self-concept and reflects the overall sense of being capable, worthwhile, and competent.
- Self-esteem stressors include developmental and relationship changes, illness (particularly chronic illness involving changes in what were normal activities), surgery, accidents, and the responses of other individuals to changes resulting from these events.
- The nurse's self-concept and nursing actions often influence a patient's self-concept.
- Planning and implementing nursing interventions for self-concept disturbance involve expanding the patient's self-awareness, encouraging self-exploration, aiding in self-evaluation, helping formulate goals regarding adaptation, and helping the patient achieve these goals.
- Sexuality is related to all dimensions of health. Therefore address sexual concerns or problems as a routine part of nursing care.
- Sexual health involves physical and psychosocial aspects and contributes to an individual's sense of self-worth and positive interpersonal relationships.
- Development and life changes, ethical decisional issues, fertility, personal and emotional conflicts, illness, and hospitalization all affect a patient's sexuality.

REFLECTIVE LEARNING

- Describe a situation during a recent clinical experience in which your own self-concept or self-esteem influenced the care you provided.
- Consider a patient who was younger than 18 years of age or older than 50 years of age who would have benefited from a discussion of sexual health concerns and what factors interfered with your ability to provide the best care possible.
- Reflect on a statement a patient made during a recent clinical experience about identity, body image, role performance, self-esteem, or sexuality and how you could have improved your response.

REVIEW QUESTIONS

1. A 47-year-old divorced woman tells the nurse that she has just started dating again. Based on this information, the nurse realizes that the patient needs information about which of the following topics? (Select all that apply.)
   1. Breast self-examination and mammograms
   2. The HPV vaccine
   3. Safe sex practices and screenings for STIs
   4. Birth-control options
   5. Risks of sildenafil and tadalafil
2. A 64-year-old patient says that she has not been intimate with her partner since her mastectomy 2 months ago. The nurse realizes that the woman is having difficulty adjusting to changes in which of the following aspects of self-concept? (Select all that apply.)
   1. Self-esteem
   2. Sexuality
   3. Gender identity
   4. Body image
   5. Role identity
3. The nurse is educating a group of adolescents about HPV vaccines. The nurse knows that further instruction is needed when several of the youths state:
   1. "The vaccines will reduce my chances of getting genital warts."
   2. "The vaccines can only be given to females."
   3. "The vaccines protect me from cancers of the anus."
   4. "The vaccines work best when given before I get exposed to the virus."
4. A nurse is taking a sexual history during the admission process and wants to establish a relaxed and matter-of-fact approach to help the patient feel safe. Which of the following questions is the best example of this practice?
   1. Have you ever had a homosexual experience?
   2. Are you a heterosexual?
   3. Tell me how you would describe your sexual health.
   4. Tell me about your last 3 sexual partners.
5. A 70-year-old patient reports she is currently sexually active. Which of the following is most important for the nurse to ask?
   1. "Please tell me more about your sexual experiences."
   2. "Are you using water-based lubricants during intercourse?"
   3. "Are any of your medications causing vaginal dryness?"
   4. "What adjustments have you made in your sexual positions?"

evolve

Additional Review Questions, as well as rationales for all Review Questions, can be found on the Evolve website.

1, 3, 4; 2, 1, 2, 4; 3, 2, 4; 4, 3; 5, 1.

REFERENCES

American Society for the Positive Care of Children: *Bullying statistics and information*, 2017. http://americanspcc.org/bullying/statistics-and-information/?gclid=EAIaIQobChMIw8aDpKLF1QIVhlYNCh0JfgbEAAYAiAAEgKb8fD_BwE.

Atallah S: Cultural aspects in sexual function and dysfunction in the geriatric population: a review of the current literature and clinical overview of clinical interventions with efficacy, *Top Geriatr Rehabil* 32(3):156, 2016.

Centers for Disease Control and Prevention (CDC): *CDC recommends only two HPV shots for younger adolescents*, 2016. https://www.cdc.gov/media/releases/2016/p1020-hpv-shots.html.

Centers for Disease Control and Prevention (CDC): *HIV among people aged 50 and over*, 2017. https://www.cdc.gov/hiv/group/age/olderamericans/.

Chan M, et al: Reducing depression among community-dwelling older adults using life-story review: a pilot study, *Geriatr Nurs* 35(2):105, 2014.

Erikson E: *Childhood and society*, ed 2, New York, 1963, WW Norton.

Franken R: *Human motivation*, ed 3, Pacific Grove, CA, 1994, Brooks/Cole Publishing.

Fuzzell L, et al: I just think doctors need to ask more questions: sexual minority and majority adolescents' experiences talking about sexuality with healthcare providers, *Patient Educ Couns* 99:1467, 2016.

Haesler E, et al: Sexuality, sexual health, and older people: a systematic review of research on the knowledge and attitudes of health professionals, *Nurse Educ Today* 40:57, 2016.

Johns Hopkins Bloomberg School of Public Health: *The teen years explained: bullying*, n.d. http://www.jhsph.edu/research/centers-and-institutes/center-for-adolescent-health/_includes/_pre-redesign/Bullying_HQP.pdf.

Kann L, et al: Youth risk behavior surveillance—United States, 2015, *MMWR Surveill Summ* 65(SS-6):1, 2016.

Kerpelman JL, et al: Engagement in risky sexual behavior: adolescents' perceptions of self and the parent-child relationship matter, *Youth Soc* 48(1):101, 2016.

Mantilla EF, et al: Self-image and eating disorder symptoms in normal and clinical adolescents, *Eat Behav* 15:125, 2014.

McIntyre K, et al: Workplace self-expansion: implications for job satisfaction, commitment, self-concept clarity, and self-esteem among employed and unemployed, *Basic Appl Soc Psych* 36:59, 2014.

Meiner SE: Gerontologic assessment. In Meiner SE, editor: *Gerontologic nursing*, ed 5, St Louis, 2015, Mosby.

Petersen Z: *The Wiley-Blackwell handbook of sex therapy*, 2017, Wiley-Blackwell.

Pham TB, Adesman A: Increased risk of sadness and suicidality among victims of bullying experiencing additional threats to physical safety, *Int J Adolesc Med Health* Nov 23, 2017. doi:10.1515/ijamh-2017-0109.

Santos-Iglesias P, et al: Sexual well-being of older men and women, *Can J Hum Sex* 25(2):86, 2016.

Schooler D, Daniels EA: "I am not a skinny toothpick and proud of it." Latina adolescents' ethnic identity and responses to mainstream media images, *Body Image* 11:11, 2014.

Strong K, Folse VN: Assessing undergraduate nursing students' knowledge, attitudes and cultural competence in caring for lesbian, gay, bisexual, and transgender patients, *J Nurs Educ* 54(1):45, 2015.

Stuart GW: *Principles and practice of psychiatric nursing*, ed 10, St Louis, 2013, Mosby.

Thomas JJ, Moring JC: Development of a revised generalized health-related self-concept inventory, *Am J Health Behav* 38(4):614, 2014.

Toledano S, et al: Domain-specific self-concept in relation to traditional and cyber peer aggression, *J Sch Violence* 14:405, 2015.

Touhy TA, Jett K: *Ebersole and Hess' toward healthy aging: human needs and nursing response*, ed 9, St Louis, 2016, Elsevier.

Youth Connection: *Institute for youth development*, 2005. www.youthdevelopment.org.

VandenBos GR: *APA dictionary of psychology*, Washington, DC, 2015, American Psychological Association.

White AJ, Taliaferro D: Relationship between postmenopausal women's successful aging, global self-esteem, and sexual quality of life, *Int J Hum Caring* 20(2):102, 2016.

evolve MEDIA RESOURCES

http://evolve.elsevier.com/Potter/essentials
• Audio Glossary

• QSEN Activity and Review Questions Answers and Rationales

OBJECTIVES

• Examine current trends in the American family.
• Discuss how the term *family* reflects family diversity.
• Discuss common family forms and associated health implications.
• Explain how the relationship between family structure and patterns of functioning affects the health of individuals within a family and the family as a whole.

• Discuss the role of families and family members as caregivers.
• Compare and contrast nursing care that views family as context, family as patient, and family as system, and explain how these different perspectives influence nursing practice.
• Use the nursing process to provide for the health care needs of a family.

KEY TERMS

family, p. 645
family as context, p. 648
family as patient, p. 648

family as system, p. 648
family forms, p. 646

hardiness, p. 649
resiliency, p. 649

Y ou will care for many families as a nurse. Family nursing recognizes that health and illness are family events that affect all its members. Additionally, families affect how health care is accessed and delivered as well as the outcomes of health care. All families differ in structure, function, and process, and they change over time. Families face many challenges including the effects of health and illness, changing economics, childbearing and childrearing, changes in family dynamics, and caring for older parents. Family characteristics or attributes such as durability, resiliency, and diversity help families adapt to these challenges.

Family durability is a system of support and structure within a family that extends beyond the walls of the household. New members sometimes join a family (e.g., through divorce, remarriage, cohabitation). Extended families often include grandparents, aunts, uncles, cousins, and former spouses or partners. *For example, in the case study, Patrick and Michelle are part of an extended family because of their relationship with Lois. Michelle keeps her husband connected with her grandmother.* The people who make up a family may change. For example, parents may remarry, and children may leave home as adults, but the "family" transcends long periods and inevitable lifestyle changes.

Family resiliency is the ability of a family to cope with expected and unexpected stressors. *One stressor on the O'Connell family is Patrick's potential job loss. Not only does Patrick's job provide income and insurance benefits, but it also defines part of Patrick's role in his family. Patrick's and Michelle's resiliency will affect how they adjust to this stressor. For example, if Michelle needs to take a full-time job with benefits, will*

CASE STUDY *The O'Connell Family*

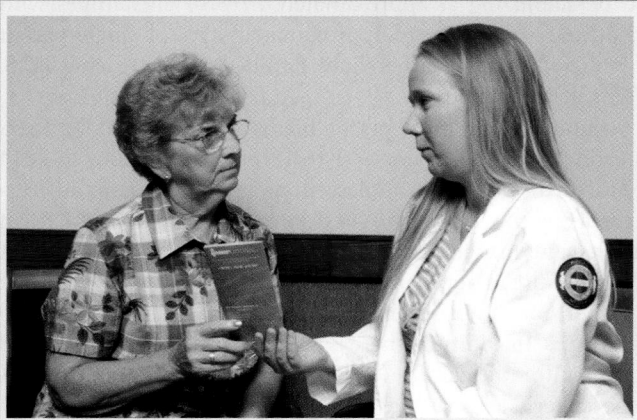

Patrick and Michelle O'Connell have been married for 10 years. Patrick is 44 years old and recently found out he may be laid off from his job. He has borderline hypertension and ranks his stress level as an 8 on a scale of 0 to 10. He enjoys playing computer games and playing with his 2 dogs and 2 cats. The family has health insurance through Patrick's job. Michelle is 42 years old, has a part-time job, and attends nursing school. They do not have children. Michelle was diagnosed with cervical cancer 3 months after their wedding and had a hysterectomy. Michelle is worried about their financial problems and the health problems of her 80-year-old grandmother, Lois. Michelle describes herself as spiritual and attends church occasionally.

Michelle is the oldest daughter in her family and the only one of the siblings to keep in regular contact with her grandmother. Her parents and sisters live out-of-state and are unable to visit often. Lois is more forgetful and does not tolerate physical activity well because she has severe heart failure. Lois' need for help at home will increase over time. Michelle worries that her grandmother will need to move in with her and her husband. If so, Michelle would need to get rid of her pets because of Lois' allergies, and her home would require major renovations.

Bethany, a nursing student, is in her community health rotation and is assigned to care for Lois. Lois lives alone in a clean mobile home. Although Lois receives Social Security and has Medicare, she cannot afford supplemental insurance.

Patrick be able and willing to take over household tasks and care for Lois? The family's ability to adapt to role changes, developmental milestones, and crises shows resilience (see Chapter 26). A family's goal is to survive, thrive, and grow as a result of challenges and new experiences.

Family diversity is the uniqueness of each family unit. As a nurse, you work with many different kinds of families. Some families experience marriage for the first time and have children in later life, whereas others of the same age are grandparents. You work with families that are headed by a single parent as well as two-parent families. Every person within a family unit has specific needs, strengths, and important developmental considerations.

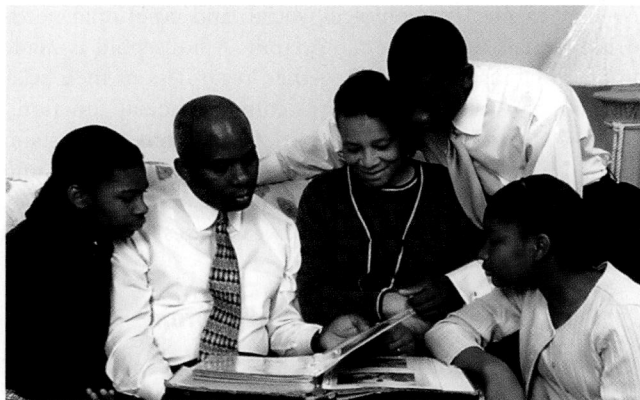

FIG 25.1 Family members have beliefs, values, and a set of relationships.

When you care for patients and their families you are responsible for first understanding the makeup (configuration), structure, function, and coping capacity of the family and then building on the family's relative strengths and resources (Duhamel et al., 2015). The goal of family-centered nursing care is to care for the family as a unit, advocating for, promoting, and providing for the well-being of the patient, family, and individual family members (Svavarsdottir et al., 2015; Wilson, 2016).

SCIENTIFIC KNOWLEDGE BASE

Concept of Family

For some, the term *family* creates a visual image of adults and children living together in a satisfying, harmonious manner. For others, this term has the exact opposite image. Families are more than a set of individuals, and a family is more than a sum of its individual members (Kaakinen et al., 2015). Families are as diverse as the individuals who are within them. Patients have deeply ingrained beliefs and values about their families that you need to respect. It is important that you understand how your patient defines a family. In other words, think of a **family** as a set of relationships that a patient identifies as family or as a network of individuals who influence one another's lives, whether there are actual biological or legal ties (Fig. 25.1).

Definition: What Is Family?

Defining family seems simple at first. However, there is no universally accepted definition. Different definitions cause debates among sociologists, psychologists, and legislators. The definition of family is significant and affects who is included on health insurance policies, who has access to children's school records, who files joint tax returns, and who has eligibility for sick-leave benefits or public assistance programs. A family is what an individual believes the family to be. It includes a set of interacting individuals who are related through biology or enduring commitments who usually socialize with each other (Kaakinen et al., 2015). Sometimes they divide household and economic responsibilities. Members in a family work together to meet the physical, social, and emotional needs of individuals within the family unit. A household is made up of individuals who live together, regardless of their relationship or whether they fulfill common social functions. When you provide individualized family care, understand that families take many forms and have diverse cultural and ethnic orientations. In addition, no two families are alike. Each family has its own strengths, weaknesses, resources, and challenges.

Current Trends and New Family Forms

Family forms are patterns of people who are identified as family members. Family living arrangements are more diverse and change more frequently when compared with the family forms several decades ago (Box 25.1). Although all families have some things in common, each family form has unique strengths and challenges. Maintain an open mind about who makes up a family to establish a therapeutic relationship with families and to ensure you are aware of a family's potential resources and concerns.

Families are constantly changing. People may marry later or delay childbirth; couples may choose to have fewer children or none at all. Approximately 53% of people 15 years of age and older are married (U.S. Census Bureau, 2016). However, the number of people living alone is expanding and accounts for approximately 14.5% of adults 18 years of age and older (U.S. Census Bureau, 2016). The measurement of divorce rates in the United States is complicated and inaccurate. However, most scholars agree that approximately 40% to 50% of marriages will end in divorce (Stanley, 2015;

Stanton, 2015). The number of single-parent families appears to be stabilizing at approximately 27% of all families with children. Mothers head approximately 85% of single-parent families; however, father-only families are increasing (U.S. Census Bureau, 2016).

Although the numbers of births to adolescent mothers steadily decreased from 1991 (61.8 births per 1000) to 2014 (24.2 births per 1000), adolescent pregnancy remains an ever-increasing concern (Office of Adolescent Health, 2016). Most adolescent mothers continue to live with their families. A teenage pregnancy has long-term consequences for the mother and often severely stresses family relationships and resources. In addition, there is an increased risk for continued poverty for the family (Romero et al., 2016). Teenage boys also experience stressors when their partner becomes pregnant (Hunt et al., 2015). They have poorer support systems and fewer resources to teach them how to parent (Kirven, 2014). As a result, both adolescent parents often struggle with the normal tasks of development and identity and need to accept a responsibility for which they are not ready physically, emotionally, socially, or financially.

In 2015 the U.S. Supreme Court ruled that state bans on same-sex marriage are unconstitutional. This ruling now allows gay and lesbian couples to be married in all 50 states (Pew Research Center, 2015). Approximately 40% of same-sex couples are married (Gates and Newport, 2015). Individuals in same-sex relationships have become more open about their sexual preferences and more vocal about their legal rights.

Factors Influencing Family Forms

Families face many challenges, including changing structures and roles related to the changing economic status of society. There are family challenges related to divorce and the aging of older members. Changing economic status, homelessness, and domestic violence also create challenges for families.

Economic Factors. Making ends meet is a daily concern for many people because of the declining economic status of families. Economics particularly affect families at the lower end of the income scale. Single-parent families are especially vulnerable. As a result, many families still have inadequate or no health insurance, and they have difficulty accessing health care. Of the nearly 72 million children younger than 18 years of age in the United States, 44%, or 31.4 million, live in low-income families, and another 21%, or 15.4 million, live in poor families (Jiang et al., 2016). Approximately 8% of children in low-income families and 7% in poor families do not have health insurance (Jiang et al., 2016). Ongoing legislation is working to make health insurance for families more affordable, but challenges in accessing health care in the United States persist (U.S. Department of Health and Human Services [USDHHS], 2017). *As you read in the case study, the O'Connell family is faced with a potential loss of income. Not only will this loss affect the family finances, but there is a potential loss of health insurance if Patrick loses his job.*

BOX 25.1   FAMILY FORMS

NUCLEAR FAMILY
A nuclear family consists of two adults (and sometimes one or more children).

EXTENDED FAMILY
An extended family includes relatives (grandparents, aunts, uncles, and cousins) in addition to the nuclear family.

SINGLE-PARENT FAMILY
A single-parent family is formed when one parent leaves the nuclear family because of death, divorce, or desertion or when a single person decides to have or adopt a child.

BLENDED FAMILY
A blended family is formed when parents bring unrelated children from prior or foster parenting relationships into a new, joint living situation.

ALTERNATIVE PATTERNS OF RELATIONSHIPS
These relationships include multiadult households, "skip-generation" families (e.g., grandparents caring for grandchildren, which commonly results from legal interventions such as when the parent is absent and there is no other parent available), communal groups with children, "nonfamilies" (adults living alone), and cohabitating partners.

Homelessness. Another factor influencing families is homelessness. The fastest growing segment of the homeless population is families with children. This includes complete nuclear families and single-parent families. More than 1.36 million children enrolled in public school are homeless (U.S. Department of Education, 2015).

Homelessness greatly affects the functioning, health, and well-being of the family and its members. Children of homeless families are often in fair or poor health and have higher rates of asthma, ear infections, stomach problems, mental illness, poor dental health, and poor immunization documentation. Usually the emergency department is the only access to health care.

Children who are homeless face barriers such as meeting residency requirements for public schools and inability to obtain previous enrollment records when enrolling and attending school. They frequently lack adult supervision to help them with homework and other school-related projects and issues. As a result, they are more likely to drop out of school, develop risky behaviors, and become unemployable. Homelessness greatly increases the risk for developing long-term health, psychological, and socioeconomic problems in families and children, posing a major challenge for our entire society (U.S. Interagency Council on Homelessness, 2016).

Adults who are homeless face health risks as well. They are more likely to have mental health issues and chronic health problems (U.S. Interagency Council on Homelessness, 2017). They are exposed to the elements and have poor nutrition and limited access to health care. When a shelter is present, it is usually an evening/night shelter only. Because adults who are homeless usually live "on the street," they are vulnerable to physical and emotional violence, injury, and trauma.

Domestic Violence. Domestic violence includes not only intimate partner relationships of spouses, live-in partners, and dating couples but also familial, elder, and child abuse. Abuse generally falls into one or more of the following categories: physical battering, sexual assault, and emotional or psychological abuse. It generally escalates over a period of time.

The cause of family violence is complex and multidimensional. Stress, poverty, social isolation, psychopathology, and learned family behaviors all are factors associated with violence. In addition, other factors such as alcohol and drug abuse, pregnancy, sexual orientation, and mental illness increase the incidence of abuse within a family. Although abuse sometimes ends when a person leaves a specific family environment, there are often negative long-term physical and emotional consequences (Futures Without Violence, 2017). One of these consequences includes moving from one abusive situation to another. For example, a child sees marriage as a way to leave an abusive home and in turn marries a person who continues the abuse within the marriage.

Structure

Family structure is based on which people make up the family, their relationships and interactions, and their interactions with other social systems (Kaakinen et al., 2015). The pattern of relationships is often numerous and complex. Each family has a unique structure and way of functioning. *For example, in the case study, Michelle has relationships with her husband, grandmother, employer, and colleagues in school. Each of these relationships has different demands, roles, and expectations.* Multiple relationships and their expectations are often sources for personal and family stress (see Chapter 26).

Family structure either enhances or detracts from a family's ability to respond to expected and unexpected stressors of daily life. Structures that are too rigid or flexible often threaten family functioning. Rigid structures specifically dictate who accomplishes different tasks and limit the number of people outside the immediate family allowed to assume these tasks. For example, in a rigid family the mother is often the only person who provides emotional support for the children and/or performs all the household chores. The husband is the only acceptable person to provide financial support, maintain the vehicles, do the yard work, and do all the home repairs. A change in the health status of the person responsible for a task places a burden on a rigid family because no other person is available, willing, or considered acceptable to assume that task. An extremely flexible structure also presents problems for the family. An absence of stability often impairs the ability to take action during a crisis or rapid change.

Function

Family functioning refers to the processes used by a family to achieve its goals. Specific functional aspects include how a family reproduces, interacts to socialize its young, cooperates to meet economic needs, and relates to the community or larger society. Family function includes communication among family members, goal setting, conflict resolution, nurturing, and use of internal and external resources. Although many families pursue these goals at various times during their development, providing psychological support remains an important goal throughout the life span.

Developmental Stages

Families, similar to individuals, change and grow over time. Although all families are unique, they have a basic pattern and similarity in experiences resulting in predictable stages. Each developmental stage has its own challenges, needs, and resources and includes tasks that need to be completed before a family is able to successfully move on to the next stage (Table 25.1).

NURSING KNOWLEDGE BASE

To care for families, you need a scientific knowledge base in family theory and family nursing. The two concepts interact to affect the care that you deliver to a family. All practice settings and health care environments emphasize family nursing.

Family Nursing: Family as Context, as Patient, and as System

In caring for a family, your goal is to help a family and its individual members reach and maintain maximum health in

TABLE 25.1 STAGES OF THE FAMILY LIFE CYCLE

FAMILY LIFE CYCLE STAGE	EMOTIONAL PROCESS OF TRANSITION: KEY PRINCIPLES	CHANGES IN FAMILY STATUS REQUIRED TO PROCEED DEVELOPMENTALLY
Unattached young adults	Accepting parent-offspring separation	Differentiating self in relation to family of origin Developing intimate peer relationships Establishing self in work/profession
Joining of families through marriage: newly married couple	Committing to new family system	Forming marital system Realigning relationships with extended families and friends to include spouse
Family with young children	Accepting new generation of members into system	Adjusting marital system to make space for children Taking on parenting roles Realigning relationships with extended family to include parenting and grandparenting roles
Family with adolescents	Increasing flexibility of family boundaries to include children's independence	Shifting parent-child relationships to permit adolescents to move into and out of system Refocusing on midlife marital and career issues Beginning shift toward concerns for older generation
Family with young adults	Accepting multitude of exits from and entries into family system	Renegotiating marital system as a couple Developing adult-to-adult relationships between grown children and parents Realigning relationships to include in-laws and grandchildren Dealing with disabilities and death of parents (grandparents)
Family without children		Refocusing on new career opportunities Refocusing on marital and career issues Renegotiating recreational activities
Family in later life	Accepting shifting of generational roles	Maintaining own or couple functioning and interests in face of physiological decline; exploring new familial and social role options Supporting more central role for middle generation Making room in system for wisdom and experience of older adults; supporting older generation without overfunctioning for them Retiring; change in role Dealing with loss of spouse, siblings, and other peers and preparing for own death; reviewing life and integrating

Data from Duvall EM, Miller BC: *Marriage and family development,* ed 6, Boston, 2005, Allyn & Bacon.

any given situation throughout and beyond an illness experience. Family nursing is based on the assumption that all people, regardless of age, are a member of some type of family form (see Box 25.1). *In the case study, Bethany meets with Michelle every 2 weeks and offers Michelle strategies that allow her to help Lois adapt to the physical limits of her heart disease. In addition, Bethany offers Patrick and Michelle strategies to prepare for the impending changes in their family life resulting from Lois' illness and changes in the family's finances.*

This chapter presents three different approaches for family nursing practice: (1) family as context, (2) family as patient, and (3) family as system. Family as system is a newer model and includes both relational and transactional concepts. All approaches recognize that a nursing intervention for one member influences all members and affects family functioning. Families are continually changing. As a result, the need for family support changes over time. Remember that a

family is more complex than simply a combination of individual members.

Family as Context. When you view the family as context, your primary focus is on the health and development of an individual member existing within a specific family environment. Although you focus the nursing process on an individual, you also assess the extent to which a family helps the individual meet basic needs. These needs vary, depending on an individual's developmental level and situation. Because families provide more than what is necessary or essential, you need to consider a family caregiver's ability to help a patient meet psychological needs as well.

Family as Patient. When you view the family as patient, the family processes and relationships (e.g., parenting or family caregiving) are your primary focus of care. Focus your nursing assessment on family processes instead of individual member characteristics. Concentrate on processes that are consistent with reaching and maintaining family and individual health. *In the case study, Bethany focuses on the O'Connell family as the patient.* Care is planned to meet not only a patient's needs but also the changing needs of the family. Use an interprofessional approach, especially when a family's needs are complex. Know the limits of nursing practice and make referrals when appropriate.

Family as System. Although you make theoretical and practical distinctions between the family as context and the family as patient, they are not necessarily mutually exclusive. When you care for the family as a system, you are caring for each family member (family as context) and the family unit (family as patient), using all community, social, and psychosocial resources. For example, when caring for a family who has a member living with dementia, you use the family as system approach by arranging to have all family caregivers meet with you to discuss challenges and concerns about the patient's health. After identifying the family's top concerns, you create a plan of care that includes the entire family and community resources such as the local agency on aging and a support group for families affected by dementia. You maintain close contact with the family, modifying the plan as new needs arise and priorities change.

Family and Health

Multiple factors influence the health of a family (e.g., its social resources, economic resources, geographical location, and genetic factors). The family is the primary social context in which health promotion and disease prevention take place. A family's beliefs, values, and culture strongly influence a family's structure and function. They also affect a family's communication patterns, roles, and health-promoting practices. Providing culturally appropriate family-centered interventions and teaching can improve family functioning and self-care (Deek et al., 2015).

Good health is not always highly valued; in fact, harmful practices are acceptable in some families. For example, some families have poor dietary habits such as eating high-caloric, high-fat diets. A long-term illness in one of the family members affects the well-being and health of the entire family. In addition, long-term habits such as smoking also affect the health of members in the family unit. Although illness strains relationships, research indicates that family members can be a primary force for coping (Gibbons et al., 2014).

Hardiness and resiliency moderate a family's stress and thus affect its health. Family hardiness is the internal strengths and durability of the family unit. A sense of control over the outcome of life, a view of change as beneficial and growth producing, and an active rather than passive orientation in adapting to stressful events characterize family hardiness (Resilience, Adaptation, and Well-Being, 2016). Resiliency helps individuals and families achieve healthy responses when experiencing stressful events. Resources and techniques that a family or individuals within the family use to maintain a balance or level of health enhance a family's resiliency. *Hardiness and resiliency are important for the O'Connell family. The strong marital bond between Patrick and Michelle helps them balance the new demands as Lois' health declines.*

Genetic factors reflect a family's heredity or genetic susceptibility to a disease that may or may not result in actual development of the disease (National Institutes of Health [NIH], 2017). Sometimes genetic factors and genetic counseling information help family members decide whether or not to test for the presence of a disease and/or have children. Some families choose not to have children; other families choose not to know genetic risks and have children; and other families choose to know the risk and then determine whether or not to have children. Some of these diseases such as heart or kidney disease are manageable. With genetic risks for certain cancers, a family member may choose to have prophylactic treatment to reduce the risk for developing the disease (e.g., a woman with risk for breast cancer has a double mastectomy). Families with genetic neurological diseases such as Huntington disease may choose not to have children. When families know of these risks, they have the opportunity to make informed decisions about their lifestyle and health behaviors, be more vigilant about changes in their health, and seek medical intervention earlier.

Acute or Chronic Illness

Any acute or chronic illness influences a family economically, socially, and functionally and affects a family's decision-making and coping resources. Hospitalization of a family member is stressful for the whole family. Hospital environments are scary, physicians and nurses are strangers, the medical language is difficult to understand, and family members are separated from one another.

During an acute illness such as a trauma, myocardial infarction, or surgery, family members are often left in waiting rooms anticipating information about their loved one. Communication and support among family members is often misunderstood because of fear and worry. Previous family conflicts sometimes rise to the surface, causing tension. In other families, illness brings families together (Mattila et al., 2014). In addition, a shortened length of stay often leads to fragmented care, which increases family and patient anxiety and often leads to readmissions (Yoo and Huber, 2014). When implementing a patient-centered or family-centered care model, include the family, allowing patients' family members, family caregivers, and surrogate decision makers to become active partners in decision making, care, advocacy, and quality-of-life issues (Price, 2016). A family-centered care approach will help your patients achieve the desired outcomes of care.

Chronic illnesses are a global health problem. The incidence of chronic illnesses is increasing, and adapting to them is challenging for families (Sav et al., 2015). Often a family needs to reorganize family patterns, interactions, social activities, work and household schedules, economic resources, and other family needs and functions to adapt to the chronic illness or disability. Families must also learn how to manage many aspects of their loved one's illness or disability (Gibbons et al., 2014). Astute nursing care helps a family prevent and/or manage medical crises, control symptoms, learn how to provide specific therapies, adjust to changes over the course of an illness, avoid isolation, obtain community resources, and resolve conflict. Partnering with families and the health care team helps you identify available health care and community resources for disease management (Garcia-Fernandez et al., 2014; Kennedy and Nordrum, 2015). As with all serious illnesses, caring for a family member whose chronic illness worsens is socially, emotionally, and financially devastating, and it affects the entire family.

Trauma. Trauma is a sudden unplanned event. Family members need to cope with the challenges of a severe, life-threatening event, which can include the stressors associated with an intensive care environment, anxiety and depression, and economic burden, not to mention the impact on a family's functioning and decision making (Ford et al., 2014). When caring for family members, answer their questions honestly. When you do not know the answer, find someone who does. Provide realistic assurance; giving false hope breaks the nurse-patient trust and affects how the family adjusts to "bad news." Take time to be sure that a family is comfortable. For example, bring them something to eat or drink, give them a blanket, or encourage them to get a meal. Sometimes telling a family that you will stay with their loved one while they are gone is all they need to feel comfortable in leaving.

End-of-Life Care. Although people frequently equate terminal illness with cancer, there are other terminal diseases (e.g., heart failure, neuromuscular diseases). When a family member becomes terminally ill, even if family members are prepared for their loved one's death, they still need information, support, assurance, and presence. The more you know about a family's cultural background and how family members interact with one another, their strengths, and their weaknesses, the better (see Chapter 21). Each family approaches and copes with end-of-life decisions differently. Give a family information about the dying process. Help set up home care and obtain hospice and other appropriate resources including grief support. Be sure that the family knows what to do at the time of death. If you are present at the time of death, be sensitive to a family's needs (e.g., provide for privacy and allow sufficient time for saying good-byes).

CRITICAL THINKING

Critical thinking is crucial in the care of patients and their families. As a nurse, you synthesize all aspects of critical thinking to give individualized, compassionate family care. The care of a family is an ongoing mutually acceptable relationship. As you provide family-centered care, you continually assess, analyze, and reflect on the changing needs and health care goals of your patients and their families.

Synthesis

Patient care requires you to apply what you know about a patient, your knowledge base, experience, and critical thinking attitudes and standards. Your synthesis of this information allows you to make sound decisions as you apply the nursing process. Critical thinking synthesis involves combining all available information to obtain a clear picture of the approach needed to provide patient-centered care (Box 25.2).

Knowledge. The health and functioning of each family member usually depend on the health of the family system as a whole. Family nursing care requires knowledge about growth and development, psychology, stress and coping, cultural competency, communication, family theories, sociology, and the family life cycle. When a family is in a transitional phase of the life cycle perspective (e.g., birth of a first child) or there is an additional stressor to the family unit (e.g., chronic illness), it creates considerable anxiety and stress within the family system.

BOX 25.2 SYNTHESIS IN PRACTICE

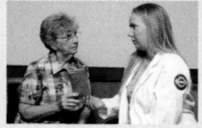

Bethany assesses Lois' health care needs. She analyzes the role strain on Michelle and its effect on her relationship with Patrick. Bethany also is aware of the effect of stress on Patrick's health status and management of his hypertension. She knows that Lois wants to stay in her home and Michelle wants to help that happen. Bethany asks if Michelle has any extended-family members. Michelle says that she has two sisters who live 4 and 6 hours away. They are willing to alternate visits every month to help.

If Bethany views the family as the context, she focuses on each member of the family. Lois' changes in health affect the family greatly, and Bethany's care helps Lois improve her ability to tolerate exercise and maximize her independence. In addition, Bethany helps Michelle reduce stress by teaching her relaxation and meditation techniques, helping her to plan "down time," and giving her some time-management techniques. Bethany assesses Patrick's knowledge of ways to manage his blood pressure (e.g., reducing the number of high-sodium foods and using stress-reduction techniques) and helps him plan "down time" as well.

When she views the family as a patient, Bethany assesses the family's goals for Lois' care and independence. She assesses their caregiving strengths, needs, and weaknesses as well as the resources available to the family as they assume the role of caregiver. She observes the impact that caregiving has on Michelle and Patrick and asks about Michelle's siblings who are helping with the care.

As Bethany views the family as a system, she needs to work with the entire family to help Lois transition from her own home. One possible solution to this problem is to help the family select an assisted-living community located halfway between the O'Connell home and the homes of Michelle's two sisters.

Experience. Your life experiences and nursing knowledge help you recognize and solve problems. Experiences in your own family help you design family-centered care. Carefully reflect on your past experiences and information you gained through these experiences. Remember that no two families are alike.

It is possible for illness to bring family members closer together. Conversely, illnesses, especially critical or life-threatening illnesses, have the potential to pull families apart. *In the case study, as Lois' health declines, Patrick and Michelle look for ways to help her. As the case study progresses, you see that Michelle reaches out to her siblings for help.*

Attitudes. Apply critical thinking attitudes such as creativity, perseverance, and risk taking, and keep an open mind to identify a patient's and family's needs. As you gain experience in caring for families, you will become more confident in how you communicate and provide family-centered care. As you assess a family's current situation, use fairness when you look at each family member's situation and perspective, and use this information to plan care.

Standards. As a nurse, you apply nursing standards (e.g., critical care, obstetrical) that pertain to a patient and family. *In the case study, Bethany applies gerontological nursing standards when offering guidelines for Lois care.* In addition, it is important to apply ethical principles when supporting family decisions such as helping family members accept the advance directives of their loved ones. You need to keep all information about a family confidential in all health care settings. In family-centered care there may be many health care providers; therefore follow documentation standards when recording pertinent information accurately and consistently (see Chapter 10).

NURSING PROCESS

The nursing process is the same whether your focus is family as patient, context, or system. It incorporates the needs of the family and the needs of the patient.

■■■ ASSESSMENT

Family assessment is a priority for providing family care and support. You have an essential role in helping families adjust to acute and chronic illnesses; however, you must first understand the family unit, what a patient's illness means to family members and family functioning, and the support the family needs (Kaakinen et al., 2015). Assess a patient and family thoroughly (Table 25.2). The family as a whole differs from individual members. The measure of family health is more than a summation of the health of all members. You need to include the form, structure, and function of the family; its developmental stage; and its progress toward or accomplishment of developmental tasks in your assessment. Begin assessment by considering the views of a patient toward the family. To determine the family form and membership, ask a patient to tell you about the family, by asking questions: "Who do you consider your family?" "Who do you talk with to share your concerns?" If a patient is unable to express a

TABLE 25.2 FOCUSED PATIENT AND FAMILY ASSESSMENT		
FACTORS TO ASSESS	**QUESTIONS**	**PHYSICAL ASSESSMENT**
Family resources	Do you have relatives and friends who do not live with you in your home?	Observe family member interaction.
	How does your family cope? What are your family's coping strengths/coping challenges or needs?	Observe for physical signs of stress or coping difficulties (e.g., rapid speech, difficulty focusing, weight gain/loss, increased blood pressure, heart rate) (see Chapter 26).
	How does your family obtain health services?	Review family's past medical experiences.
Family patterns	Which family members work outside the home? Describe what they do. How many hours do they usually work?	Observe communication patterns with individual family members.
	How does your family divide the work of the family such as household chores (e.g., housekeeping, shopping, and repairs), caring for children, and care of older parents?	Observe family members as they make decisions (e.g., regarding health care, discharge planning) to help obtain this information.
	How does your family make decisions (e.g., day-to-day decisions, financial decisions, and health care decisions)?	
Family function	Does your family have any short-term and long-term goals (e.g., for childrearing, retirement, health care)?	Observe communication and interaction patterns within the family.
	Have these goals changed because of your family member's illness?	

concept of family, ask with whom the patient lives, spends time, and shares confidences. Then ask the patient to confirm that people mentioned are part of the family: "Do you consider this person to be family or like family?"

Structure and Function. It is important to assess family structure and function and determine the effects of illness and the support the family requires (Kondrat et al., 2014). Family structure provides information about the composition of a family (e.g., whether it is a nuclear or extended family). To assess family structure, you ask questions such as the following: "Who are the members of your family?" "Who is the head of your household?" "Who is the wage earner?" "Who maintains your house?" To assess family functioning, ask questions to determine the power structure and patterning of roles and tasks: "How do you and your partner make financial decisions?" "How do you make decisions as a family?" "How are the tasks divided in your family (e.g., who does the laundry)?"

Family-Focused Care. Use a family-focused approach to enhance your nursing care and establish a relationship with a family. It is important to conduct a thorough assessment to identify potential and external resources. Successful assessment requires being family focused and building a relationship based on mutual respect and trust. The family needs to feel in control as much as possible, even as you ask assessment questions.

You may participate in conflict resolution between family members so that each member is able to confront and resolve problems in a healthy way. Ask questions that help a family identify external and internal resources as necessary. Ultimately your aim is to help a family reach a point of optimal function, given the family's resources, capacities, and desire to become healthier.

Assessment of family function includes determining the ability to cope with the current health problem or situation, need for social and emotional support for members, appropriateness of their routine goal setting, and progress toward achievement of developmental tasks (see Table 25.1). Because families' goals vary, make sure that your assessment of family health is flexible. During assessment determine whether a family has sufficient economic resources and if a family's social network is extensive enough to provide support.

Cultural Aspects. All families are different. Conduct a comprehensive, culturally sensitive family assessment to form an understanding of family life, values and beliefs, current changes in family life, and overall goals and expectations. It is important to assess a family's cultural background (see Chapter 21). Education, race, ethnicity, and the geographical location of the home affect structure, function, health beliefs, values, and the way a family perceives events. The United States is increasingly more diverse. A large number of immigrants enter the country daily, adding to both the number and the variety of ethnic groups that make up the population. U.S. health care institutions tend to operate from a white, middle-class perspective. Culturally diverse and immigrant

populations often have difficulty understanding and "fitting into" the health care system. If a patient speaks a language other than English, obtain a professional interpreter to help with your assessment (see Chapter 21).

Forming conclusions about families' needs based on cultural backgrounds requires critical thinking. Always remember that broad generalizations and biases about people and populations are often misleading (e.g., Asian Americans consume low-fat diets, people who live in poverty are unmotivated). Your personal biases do not help you understand the needs of a culturally diverse family. All families vary in meaningful and significant ways. You need to reflect on your own cultural values and beliefs and then carefully assess each family's differences and similarities to avoid arriving at inaccurate assumptions and stereotyping.

Knowing about a family's culture and how it affects a family's structure, functioning, health practices, and family celebrations helps you design family-centered care (Box 25.3). To determine the influence of culture on a family, ask patients about their cultural background. Then ask questions concerning cultural practices such as the following: "Tell me about the usual foods you eat at home." "Who cares for sick family members?" "Tell me about your past experiences with a family member being hospitalized. Tell me what that was like; were family members able to remain at the hospital?" "Describe for me health practices from your culture that you use regularly (e.g., acupuncture or meditation)." "What role do grandparents play in raising children?"

Community Assessment. Assess a family's home environment and community. When assessing a patient's home, determine the size of the home, provision for privacy, and safety factors such as presence of smoke detectors, safe bathrooms and stairwells (see Chapter 30). When assessing a community, determine the presence of health care resources, access to stores (e.g., grocery and drug stores), proximity of emergency services, and municipal services (see Chapter 4). Also assess if the patient and family's immediate community is considered safe. If there is a strong extended family, how far away does the extended family live from the patient? Do they live together, in the same neighborhood, or the same city? If the family lives together, how large is their living space?

Patient Expectations. Families, like individual patients, have certain expectations for care. Some families expect to be consulted as a whole unit when discussing care of their loved one. Others have a designated family caregiver and decision maker. Families sometimes expect the health care system to meet all their needs, not only those related to health issues. When assessing a family's expectations, be clear whether the family or the family member is the patient and receiver of care. Determining these expectations early in the assessment helps to avoid problems resulting from misunderstandings in the future.

Older Adult Considerations. Family structures and functions are changing rapidly in the United States; this is

BOX 25.3 FAMILY-CENTERED CARE

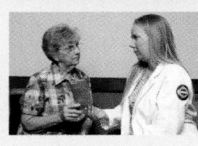

Bethany knows that families have unique perspectives and characteristics. They have different values, beliefs, and philosophies. The cultural heritage of a family often affects religious, childrearing, and nutritional practices; recreational activities; and health promotion behaviors. As she studies and reviews the literature, Bethany learns that nurses need to have cultural competence and sensitivity when caring for families. Incorporating cultural preferences helps provide family-centered and patient-centered care, which increases a patient's adherence to therapy, helps the family transition from hospital to home, and provides a unique aspect for care.

IMPLICATIONS FOR PRACTICE

- Focus on the needs of the family and understand the family's beliefs, values, customs, and roles when designing care (Ehrlich et al., 2015). Perceptions of events vary across cultural groups and affect families differently. For example, the care of a grandmother has great significance to an extended family.
- Family caregiving values, practices, and roles vary across cultures (Kung, 2016). Bethany knows that in some cultures it is disrespectful to place your elders in nursing homes. She knows that Lois' family wants to help her live as independently as possible.
- Intergenerational support and patterns of living arrangements are related to cultural background (Giger, 2017). For example, older adults from traditional Chinese, African American, Japanese, and Hispanic cultures are more likely to live in extended family households than white older adults.
- Health beliefs differ among various family forms and cultures. These beliefs affect a family's health care decisions about when and where to seek help. Trust in the health care system is a cross-cultural influence. When family members and caregivers have a sense of trust in the health care system, they are more likely to use the system as a resource for decision making (Stevens and Throud, 2015/2016).

partially due to the increase in the older adult population. When caring for a family with older adults, assess the role older adult members play in the family. For example, some grandparents are raising their grandchildren. As mentioned earlier, the incidence of chronic illness is increasing; however, many older adults live independently and are in good health despite having one or more illnesses. Determine the effects of illnesses on an older adult, and ask if there is anyone in the family who provides caregiving support for older family members. Also assess older adults for signs and symptoms of abuse and neglect. Most people who abuse older adults are family members, such as spouses and adult children (Kaakinen et al., 2015). Report any suspected abuse immediately. Be sensitive when assessing an older adult and his or her family. Be aware of underlying tensions within a family, and provide nonjudgmental support. Family dynamics are

based on a lifetime of relationships among family members and their actions (Evans et al., 2017; Kaakinen et al., 2015).

NURSING DIAGNOSIS

Use critical thinking when selecting nursing diagnoses. Diagnostic reasoning allows you to cluster relevant data and see patterns that support a patient's nursing diagnoses. The nursing diagnoses you select often include a patient's and family's health needs, current and potential health problems, and level of wellness. Examples of nursing diagnoses for family-focused care include the following:

- *Caregiver Role Strain*
- *Compromised Family Coping*
- *Disabled Family Coping*
- *Interrupted Family Processes*
- *Impaired Parenting*
- *Ineffective Role Performance*
- *Risk for Other-Directed Violence*

A nursing diagnosis that relates to family often focuses on a family's ability to cope with its current situation, whether it is an acute illness, an anticipated developmental transition, or negative behaviors that threaten short-term or long-term health. Appropriate use of internal and external resources helps a family cope with unexpected events that threaten health and stability. A nursing diagnosis often focuses on changes in family processes or roles of its members. For example, when an older adult experiences the worsening of a chronic condition, a family becomes extremely distressed and focuses only on the older adult, neglecting the needs of the other family members. Consider the diagnosis of *Caregiver Role Strain* a possibility when extended care of a family member is necessary.

The diagnostic statement indicates related factors contributing to the health problem. For example, a possible related factor is *unrealistic expectations. In the case study, Michelle initially wanted to assume responsibility for Lois. However, after making repeated trips to Lois' home and trying to support Patrick, Michelle becomes more stressed when trying to handle all the demands of care. In this case, the nursing diagnosis* Caregiver Role Strain *is appropriate. Another potential nursing diagnosis,* Interrupted Family Processes related to caregiving demands, *is the result of a change in the relationship between Michelle and Patrick. Because of caregiving demands, Michelle and Patrick are not able to relax and spend time together as a couple.*

PLANNING

Goals and Outcomes. After you develop nursing diagnoses, you prioritize the nursing diagnoses and plan care with the family. Goal setting is mutual. Collaborate with your patients and their families to develop a plan that is understandable, achievable, and acceptable to all members of the family. Establish concrete and realistic goals with a patient and family, and ensure the goals are compatible with the family's developmental stage. The plan of care for the O'Connell family is represented in a concept map (Fig. 25.2) and Care Plan.

CONCEPT MAP

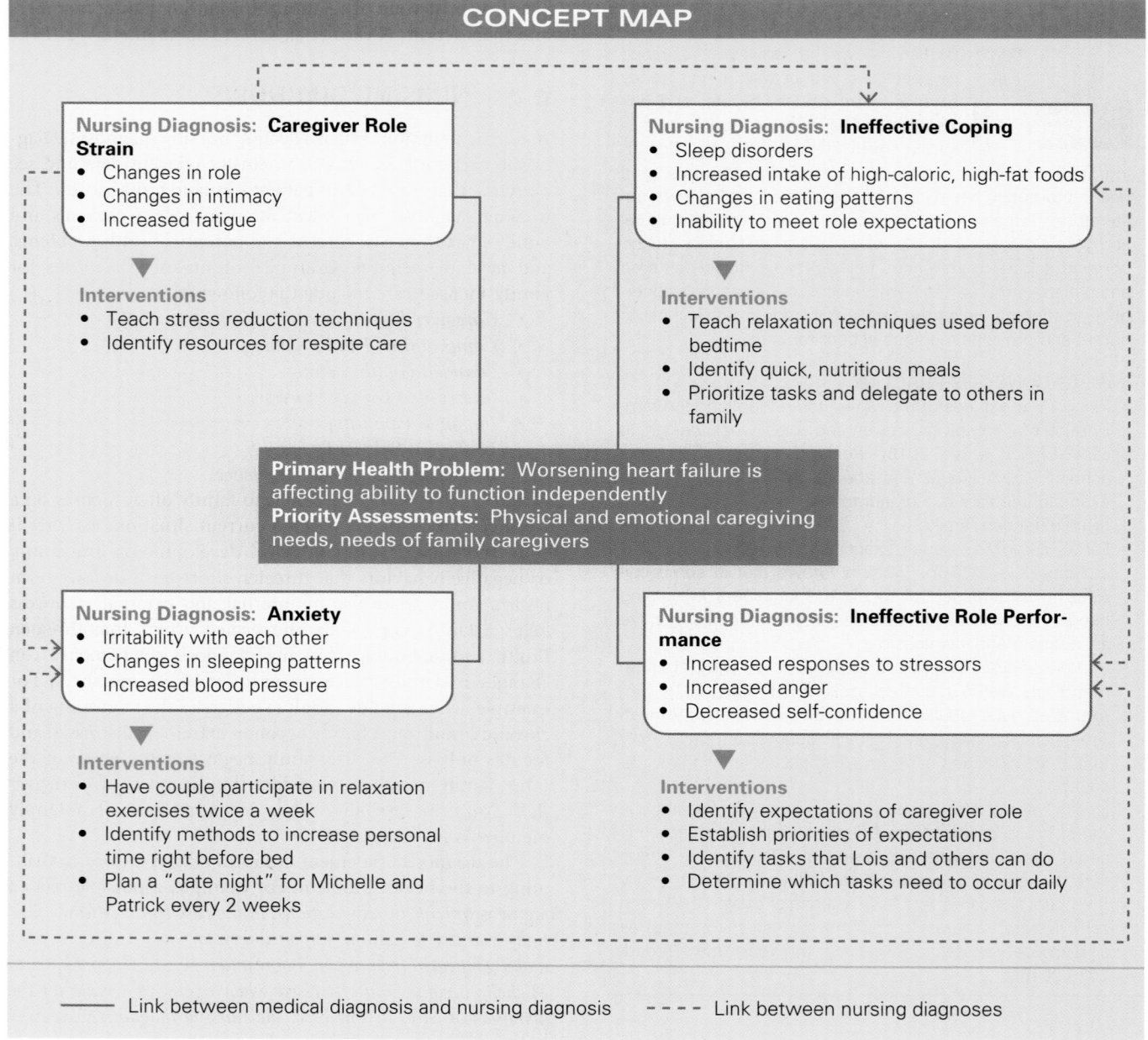

Nursing Diagnosis: Caregiver Role Strain
- Changes in role
- Changes in intimacy
- Increased fatigue

Interventions
- Teach stress reduction techniques
- Identify resources for respite care

Nursing Diagnosis: Ineffective Coping
- Sleep disorders
- Increased intake of high-caloric, high-fat foods
- Changes in eating patterns
- Inability to meet role expectations

Interventions
- Teach relaxation techniques used before bedtime
- Identify quick, nutritious meals
- Prioritize tasks and delegate to others in family

Primary Health Problem: Worsening heart failure is affecting ability to function independently
Priority Assessments: Physical and emotional caregiving needs, needs of family caregivers

Nursing Diagnosis: Anxiety
- Irritability with each other
- Changes in sleeping patterns
- Increased blood pressure

Interventions
- Have couple participate in relaxation exercises twice a week
- Identify methods to increase personal time right before bed
- Plan a "date night" for Michelle and Patrick every 2 weeks

Nursing Diagnosis: Ineffective Role Performance
- Increased responses to stressors
- Increased anger
- Decreased self-confidence

Interventions
- Identify expectations of caregiver role
- Establish priorities of expectations
- Identify tasks that Lois and others can do
- Determine which tasks need to occur daily

—— Link between medical diagnosis and nursing diagnosis   - - - - Link between nursing diagnoses

FIG 25.2 Concept map.

A family-focused approach enhances nursing practice. Family-centered goals view the family as context, patient, system, or a combination of the three. A patient's situation and availability of family members define the types of goals that are feasible, thus helping family members to confront and resolve conflict in a healthy way. An example of a goal is "The family will gain improved understanding of family caregiving," with the expected outcome being "Communication clearly describes the role and expectation for each caregiver."

Setting Priorities. You focus on a patient, a patient/family unit, or an entire family when setting priorities. Ensure a family and patient clearly understand and agree on the plan of care and priorities. The priorities for a patient and family are sometimes different. For example, your patient needs physiological or emotional stability, self-care, or to move to a rehabilitation facility. However, the family priorities include obtaining temporary housing so that they are near their ill family member, spiritual support, assistance with decision making, and understanding the complexities of the health care delivery system. The priorities of the family and patient often are different but require simultaneous interventions.

Collaborative Care. In today's health care environment, more family members are becoming caregivers, and the transition from hospital to home is often overwhelming. Including family caregivers in a patient's care helps prepare a family and patient for discharge (Dellenmark-Blom and Wigert, 2014).

◎ CARE PLAN

Caregiver Role Strain

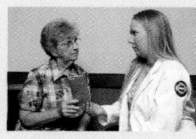

ASSESSMENT

Patrick and Michelle are caregivers to Michelle's grandmother, Lois, who has heart disease and is still living in her own home. Lois suffers fatigue and forgetfulness and has numerous caregiving demands. Michelle and Patrick argue frequently over how to best help Lois. They both recognize that although they are committed to caring for Lois, their caregiving responsibilities take time away from their marital, social, and professional relationships.

ASSESSMENT ACTIVITIES	**FINDINGS**[a]
Ask Michelle if she notices any changes in her sleeping or eating.	Michelle has **difficulty falling asleep** and remaining asleep. Michelle notes that she does not eat regularly, and when she eats it is frequently a high-fat, high-carbohydrate fast-food meal.
Ask Patrick to describe changes in lifestyle since Michelle increased her caregiving activities.	Time spent together is decreased. They have **increased arguments.** He complains about the time Michelle spends with her grandmother. He admits to doing less around the home to help Michelle.
Ask Patrick about changes in his health status.	Patrick's health care provider said that his **blood pressure is higher.**
Use a scale of 0 to 10 to ask Patrick and Michelle to rate their stress level.	Patrick rates his stress as an 8. Michelle rates her stress as a 7.
Ask Michelle to describe how she feels about taking care of her grandmother.	She describes being fearful of "not doing things well for her grandmother." She **feels anxious** when actually helping with tasks and when at home with Patrick.

[a]**Defining characteristics/risk factors** are shown in **bold** type.

NURSING DIAGNOSIS: Caregiver Role Strain related to Lois' increasing health care needs and unrealistic expectations

---

PLANNING

GOAL	**EXPECTED OUTCOMES (NOC)**[b]
	Caregiver Well-Being
Michelle and Patrick will gain improved understanding of stress and stress management techniques within 1 month.	Michelle and Patrick are able to identify four caregiving activities within 1 week. Michelle and Patrick meditate together 4 nights a week within 4 weeks.
Patrick and Michelle will use community-based resources within 1 month.	Michelle and Patrick contact the local council on aging within 3 weeks.

[b]Outcomes classification labels from Moorhead S, et al, editors: *Nursing outcomes classification (NOC)*, ed 5, St Louis, 2013, Mosby.

INTERVENTIONS (NIC)[c]	**RATIONALE**
Caregiver Support	
Discuss with Patrick and Michelle the effects of stress on themselves and the family.	For stress-reduction techniques to be effective, caregivers need guidance to identify specific stressors and their potential effects (Bazzano et al., 2015).
Listen to their individual concerns. Teach relaxation exercises and meditation techniques to reduce their stress response.	Teaching specific problem-solving and coping skills improves family caregiver's abilities to adjust to expectations and changes as patient's disease worsens (Leach et al., 2014; Bazzano et al., 2015).
Provide a list of support services such as community resources, assisted-living facilities, volunteers from faith-based groups, and the local council on aging to provide support and respite care for Patrick and Michelle.	Interprofessional care services such as physical therapy (PT), occupational therapy (OT), speech therapy, and Meals on Wheels support caregivers and reduce their caregiving burden (Greenwood et al., 2015). Promoting health maintenance and/or restoration assistance is complex and often requires community-based groups to help families reduce strain on caregivers (Niemelä et al., 2016).
Call Patrick and Michelle weekly to coach them in use of the caregiving and stress-reduction activities.	Helps satisfy caregivers' needs for hope, confidence, reinforcement, and safety (Steffen and Gant, 2016).

[c]Intervention classification labels from Bulechek GM, et al, editors: *Nursing interventions classification (NIC)*, ed 6, St Louis, 2013, Mosby.

Continued

⊙ **CARE PLAN—cont'd**

Caregiver Role Strain

EVALUATION

NURSING ACTIONS	PATIENT RESPONSE/FINDING	ACHIEVEMENT OF OUTCOME
Ask Patrick and Michelle how often they meditate each week and how they feel after they meditate.	Patrick and Michelle state that they meditate 3 times per week together. Michelle states, "It is difficult to find the time to meditate, but we are much more relaxed after we do it."	Meditation is effective. Need to work with couple to reinforce need to schedule meditation 4 times per week.
Ask Patrick, Michelle, and Lois to identify resources found through the local agency on aging.	Patrick and Michelle state they were able to locate resources through their church. The ladies from church come once a week to stay with Lois. Lois is happy with Meals on Wheels.	Michelle and Patrick have located community resources to help meet caregiving demands.

Collaborate with all appropriate family members when planning care, and always respect their needs, values, and beliefs. Collaboration with family members, whether the family is the patient or the context of care, is essential when determining family health goals. By offering alternative actions and asking family members for their own ideas and suggestions, you reduce a family's feelings of powerlessness. For example, offering options for how to rearrange a kitchen and plan meals to accommodate a family member's disability gives a family an opportunity to express their preferences, make choices, and ultimately feel as though they have contributed.

Collaborating with other disciplines such as physical therapy and social services increases the likelihood of a comprehensive approach to a family's health care needs, and it ensures better continuity of care. Making referrals to other disciplines is particularly important when discharge planning from a health care agency to home or an extended care facility or from home to an extended care facility (McCurry and Hunter Revell, 2015).

■■■ **IMPLEMENTATION**

Family nursing is used in a variety of health care settings, whether you are providing health promotion, acute care, or restorative and continuing care. Regardless of the setting, you apply some general facts about family nursing across all health care settings. Knowing about challenges for family nursing and principles for implementing family-centered nursing is important to help you develop individualized care for your patients and their families.

Health Promotion. Although people often learn health behaviors from their family, the primary focus on health promotion has traditionally been on individuals. When implementing family nursing, design health promotion interventions such as low-fat, low-carbohydrate meals or a family exercise program to improve or maintain the physical, social, emotional, and spiritual well-being of the family unit and its members (Duhamel et al., 2015). Link health promotion behaviors to the developmental stage of a family. For example, a childbearing family needs effective prenatal care, and a childrearing family needs encouragement to follow immunization schedules. Encourage patients and families to reach their optimum level of wellness. Strong families that adapt to transitions, crises, and change tend to have clear communication, problem-solving skills, a commitment to one another and to the family unit, and a sense of coherence and spirituality (Ngai and Ngu, 2014; Wen, 2014).

Whether you provide care for the family as context, patient, or system, nursing interventions increase family members' abilities to function and perform, remove health care barriers, and perform tasks that the family is not currently able to do. For example, you provide accurate health information about diagnosis and prognosis that helps a family caregiver understand and anticipate needs and concerns of a care recipient. Caregivers are not born knowing how to be caregivers, and patients are not born knowing how to accept dependency. A moderately flexible family structure is generally most beneficial and allows you to assist family members in making adjustments. Therefore your nursing interventions help a family move away from extremely rigid or extremely flexible structures (e.g., schedule for when to perform daily hygiene in the home, schedule for grocery shopping) if either extreme causes problems related to the health of an individual or the family as a whole.

Families do not always recognize their own strengths. Help family members recognize and use their unique strengths to improve their health and meet their goals. Family strengths often include clear communication, adaptability, healthy childrearing practices, support and nurturing among family members, and the use of crisis for growth. *In the case study, Michelle and Patrick developed a clear plan together to divide up household tasks. Bethany points out to Patrick and Michelle that their 10-year marriage probably endured a variety of crises and transitions. As a result, they are likely to have the capabilities to adapt to this latest challenge.* Prevention programs aimed at enhancing or developing these attributes are available for families and children in many communities. Be aware of family-oriented programs in your community to refer patients as needed.

Acute Care. The family is becoming more of the focus within the context of health care delivery in a managed care environment. Acute care settings discharge patients very quickly. Thus the complexities of today's acute health care settings require you to be astute in assessing, understanding, and supporting family and patient needs. The Synergy Model is useful in providing patient-centered and family-centered care. According to this model, nursing care reflects an integration of knowledge, skills, experiences, and attitudes needed to meet the needs of patients and their families (Swickard et al., 2014). The needs and characteristics of a patient and family drive nursing interventions. When there is synergy between a patient and family and a nurse, optimal patient outcomes result.

Include family caregivers in a patient's care during admission to better prepare them for their role and reduce stress following discharge to home (Dellenmark-Blom and Wigert, 2014). Provide education and encourage families to take an active role in their family member's care on admission. For example, if you are caring for a patient who will need to go home on insulin, you provide education about insulin administration and blood sugar management to the patient and family caregiver throughout the hospitalization. With shortened lengths of hospital stays and more complex family needs at the time of discharge, planning for discharge needs to begin before or on admission.

One expanding area in acute care for family caregivers is end-of-life care (Dosser and Kennedy, 2014). You help family members in their caregiving role by showing them how to perform specific aspects of physical care (e.g., dressing changes), helping them find home care equipment (e.g., oxygen therapy), and helping them identify community resources. Preparing members of a family for care activities and responsibilities helps caregiving become a meaningful experience for both caregiver and patient across health care settings.

Discharge Planning. Discharge planning with a family is important during the acute care phase of an illness. An open relationship between you and a patient and family leads to a family-centered plan of care at discharge, including coordination of resources in the community and the patient's home (Wrobleski et al., 2014). For example, when a patient is discharged with an open healing wound after surgery, the family caregiver needs to know how to take care of the wound and recognize complications and when to contact a health care professional. In some cases, a family also has home care services, which provide short-term assistance. Be sure the family caregiver is prepared for discharge (e.g., ensuring the caregiver knows where to obtain necessary supplies and when to contact the health care provider).

Communication. Clear communication is essential. Engage with family members to maintain open lines of communication with you and the health care team. This allows you to anticipate the needs of your patient, family members, and family caregivers and provide optimal care based on these unique needs (Weiss et al., 2014). For example, when a family member is ill, use caring practices to help immediate family members inform extended family about a patient's progress or setbacks. Identify who makes decisions for the family and consistently go to the decision maker. In some situations, the decision maker also needs help to develop a method to clearly communicate decisions made. Some families use blogs on the Internet to provide consistent information. Help a family determine if this is the best approach for their family needs and structure.

Likewise, it is important that the health care team uses communication techniques that are supportive, easy to understand, and advocate for a family's needs (Dosser and Kennedy, 2014). In addition, clear communication from the health care team makes medical terminology understandable and allows the family to understand their health care issues, types of decisions to be made, and possible health care outcomes (Box 25.4). Use clear plain language when you communicate, and provide professional interpreters if the patient or family does not speak English.

Restorative and Continuing Care. Family nursing emphasizes maintenance of a patient's functional abilities. This means working closely with a patient and family to provide well-timed and individually targeted information, practical guidance, and instructions to help a family caregiver understand the specific care a patient will require in the home (Lees et al., 2014). For example, when family caregivers help with medication administration, it is important for them to understand the importance and aspects of safe medication practices (Box 25.5).

When there are changes in a person's functional abilities, make sure that the home environment will accommodate a patient's strengths and limitations. Referral to home care nursing is essential. The patient may require occupational therapy or physical therapy as well. Clear, concise, and accurate communication with a home care nurse helps to provide continuity of care and facilitates the transition from hospital to home. Educate family members about providing ongoing care and making changes in the home so that the patient can become self-sufficient whenever possible.

Family Caregiving. Family caregiving is a social issue that is becoming more and more prevalent because of the aging population and the increase in chronic illnesses (Family Caregiver Alliance [FCA], 2016). Family caregivers are crucial to health care; they provide the majority of physical and emotional care to patients wishing to remain in their home (FCA, 2016). The fastest growing age-group is 65 years and older. This "graying" of America affects the family life cycle and is perhaps most significant for the middle generation who are part of the "sandwich generation" (Box 25.6). Caregivers in this generation need to balance their own needs with the needs of their offspring and their aging parents. This balance often occurs at the expense of caregivers' well-being and resources (O'Sullivan, 2015). It is also common for people in their 60s and 70s to be the major caregivers for one another; as a result, there are major caregiver concerns for this age-group (Box 25.7). Many caregivers report that support from professional health professionals is lacking (FCA, 2016).

The Family Caregiver Alliance (2016) reports that an average family caregiver spends 24.4 hours every week providing care to their family member; one in four are involved

BOX 25.4 EVIDENCE-BASED PRACTICE

PICO Question: Does the implementation of family-centered rounds improve patient outcomes and satisfaction with communication with the health care team?

SUMMARY OF EVIDENCE

Family-centered care focuses on the family as context. Although there is support for the principles of family-centered care, its implementation varies in clinical practice (Subramony et al., 2014). One way to support family-centered care is to implement family-centered rounding (Hastings et al., 2016). During family-centered rounds, the interprofessional health care team partners with the patient and family to engage them in the treatment plan (LaVela et al., 2016). Although the process of conducting family-centered rounds varies among health care agencies, the ultimate goal is to develop a therapeutic relationship with a patient and family, provide support, and develop a plan for discharge. Evidence shows that family-centered rounds enhance communication among the health care team and the family (LeGrow et al., 2014). Families and patients are satisfied with the level of communication and prefer being actively involved in their plan of care (Wrobleski et al., 2014).

APPLICATION TO NURSING PRACTICE

- Ensure that all members of the health care team take time to actively listen to family caregivers. Encourage team members to sit at the same level as the patient and family during rounds. A professional and compassionate approach by all health care team members involved in the rounds is valued by family members and enhances satisfaction with communication and care (LeGrow et al., 2014; Wrobleski et al., 2014; LaVela et al., 2016).
- Sharing information about a patient's health status, treatment, and discharge plans during family-centered rounds improves patient and family satisfaction with care and decreases use of health care resources after discharge (Wrobleski et al., 2014; LaVela et al., 2016).
- Conducting family-centered rounds often improves efficiency of nurse workflow because of improved communication between the health care team and family (Wrobleski et al., 2014; Hastings et al., 2016).
- Allow patients and families the opportunity to speak first during rounds to share their concerns before others speak to show respect to the family and develop a therapeutic relationship with the family (Subramony et al., 2014).
- Assess the needs of family caregivers in addition to the patient's needs during family-centered rounds. Family caregivers require support to maximize their caregiving role (LaVela et al., 2016).
- When implementing family-centered rounds, it is important that all health care team members buy into the idea and understand the process (Hastings et al., 2016).

BOX 25.5 PATIENT TEACHING

Medication Administration

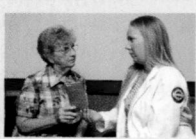

Michelle tells Bethany that Lois' medications were changed. Michelle needs to hold the digoxin if Lois' pulse is less than 60 beats/min. Michelle states she is afraid of giving her grandmother the wrong medication or giving the medication incorrectly.

OUTCOME

At the end of the teaching session, Michelle and Patrick will be able to prepare all of Lois' medications correctly and will be able to decide correctly if Lois needs to have her digoxin.

TEACHING STRATEGIES

- Provide Michelle and Patrick with a laminated card that lists all medications including action, side effects, precautions, and premedication assessments (e.g., need for pulse measurement before taking digoxin).
- Demonstrate to both Michelle and Patrick how to fill the weekly medication dispenser.
- Demonstrate how to take a pulse and explain rationale for pulse rate target.
- Provide Michelle and Patrick different real-life scenarios to give them opportunities to problem solve medication preparation and administration (e.g., "what would you do if Lois woke up with nausea and vomiting one morning?").

EVALUATION

- Use the principles of teach-back to evaluate patient/family caregiver learning:
  - "Tell me which medications require you to take Lois' pulse before administration."
  - "What would you do if you took Lois' pulse and it was 58 beats/min?"
  - "Describe what you would do with the medications if Lois were sick."

care services, coordinating health care provider visits, managing financial issues) (FCA, 2016).

Family caregiving occurs within the context of a family and is more than simply a series of tasks. Family caregivers provide ongoing emotional support for their loved ones, making decisions, becoming a patient advocate, and maintaining the integrity of the family unit (Dosser and Kennedy, 2014; Ehrlich et al., 2015). Whether it is a wife caring for a husband or a daughter caring for a mother, caregiving is an interactional process. The interpersonal dynamics among family members influence the ultimate quality of caregiving. Thus you have a key role in helping family members develop better communication and problem-solving skills to build the relationships needed for caregiving to be successful.

You will often need to teach family caregivers how to provide complex physical care for a patient (e.g., wound care, enteral nutrition, intravenous therapy). Recognize that family caregivers also have their own physical and emotional health care needs. Teach them how to meet their needs and set up respite times as appropriate to allow them time to care for themselves.

in caregiving tasks 41 hours or more each week. They provide basic tasks (e.g., shopping, cleaning, laundry, giving medications) an average of 13 days every month and help with activities of daily living (e.g., dressing, bathing, walking, helping with toileting) about 6 days a month. They spend 13 hours per month in other activities (e.g., researching diseases or

unrelieved. When stress reaches chronic and harmful levels, negative consequences follow. Selye's initial theory has evolved as scientists have learned more about the physiological responses to stress.

Neuroendocrine Stress Response

When there is a stressor within our environment, our sensory system is the first to play a role in the stress response. When someone confronts an oncoming car or hears an alarm, the eyes or ears (or both) send the information to the amygdala, an area of the brain that processes emotions (Harvard Medical School, 2016). The amygdala interprets the sensory images and sounds and, when it perceives danger, instantly sends a distress signal to the hypothalamus, which is the command center for responding to stress. When stress is perceived, the hypothalamus activates one of two systems: (1) the hypothalamic-pituitary-adrenal (HPA) axis, and (2) the sympathetic nervous system (SNS) (Miller & O'Callaghan, 2002; Smith & Vale, 2006). This results in a series of neural and endocrine adaptations known as the neuroendocrine stress response. A cascade of events allows the two systems to make the necessary physiological and metabolic changes required to maintain homeostasis. The effects of stress are both immediate and long-term (Fig. 26.1), with each response resulting in different physiological reactions from the two systems (Table 26.1).

Fight or Flight—Alarm

In the alarm stage described by Selye (1993), the hypothalamus communicates with the rest of the body through the

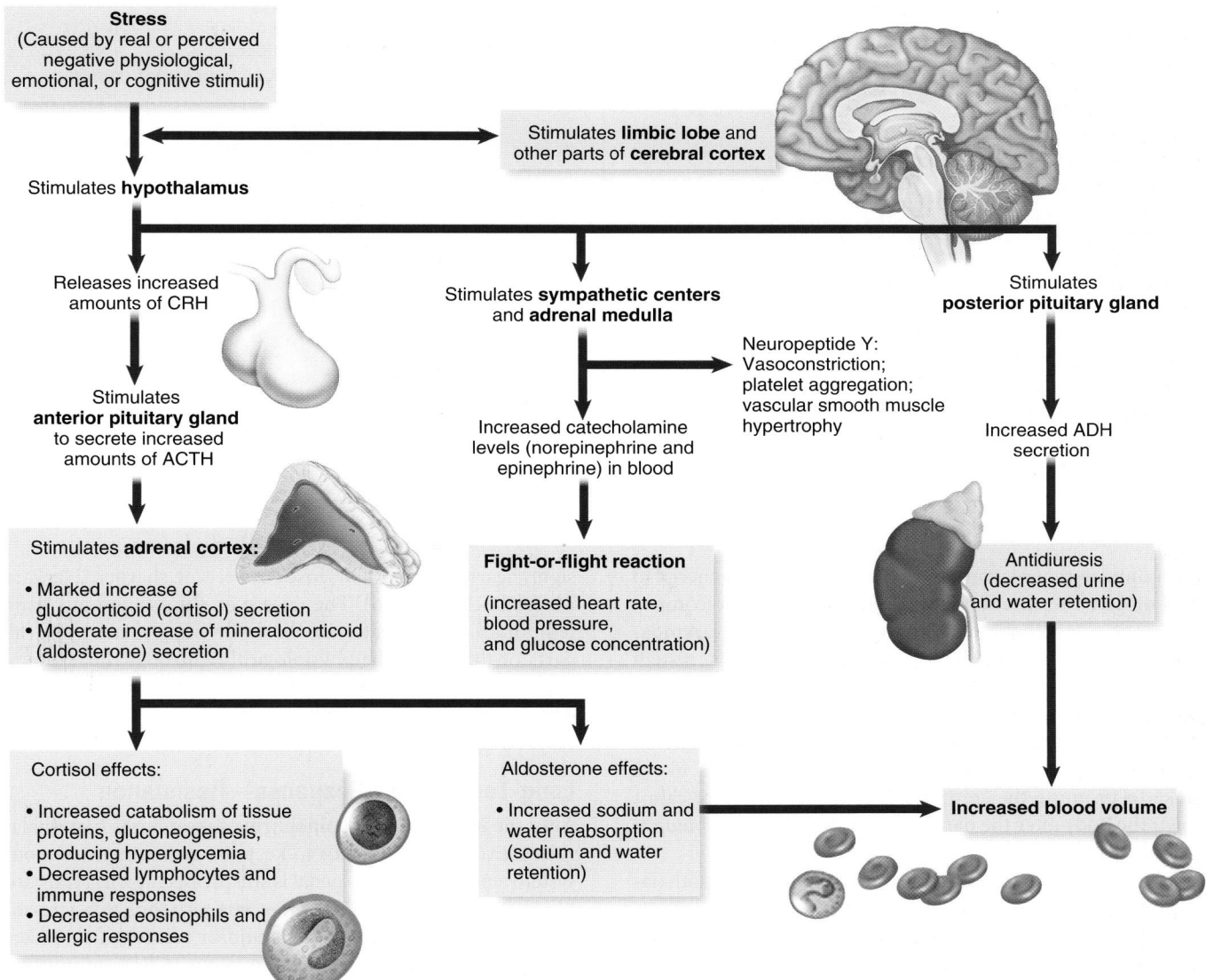

FIG 26.1 Short-term and long-term stress response. Some effects are immediate, such as the sympathetic fight-or-flight reaction, and some effects are longer-term, such as the hormonal effects. *ACTH,* Adrenocorticotropic hormone; *ADH,* antidiuretic hormone; *CRH,* corticotropin-releasing hormone. (From Patton KT: *Anatomy & physiology,* ed 10, St Louis, 2019, Elsevier.)

TABLE 26.1 INDICATORS OF STRESS

SYSTEM	ASSESSMENT FINDINGS	SYSTEM	ASSESSMENT FINDINGS
Physical		**Psychological**	
Cardiovascular	Tightness of chest Increased heart rate Elevated blood pressure	Cognitive	Forgetfulness/preoccupation Denial Poor concentration Inattention to detail Orientation to past instead of present Decreased creativity Slower thinking, problem solving, reactions Learning difficulties Apathy Confusion Decreased attention span Calculation difficulties Memory problems
Respiratory	Breathing shallow Tachypnea		
Neuroendocrine	Headaches, migraines Fatigue, exhaustion Insomnia, sleep disturbances Feeling uncoordinated Restlessness, hyperactivity Tremors (lips, hands) Profuse sweating (palms) Dry mouth Cold hands and feet		
Gastrointestinal/ genitourinary	Urinary frequency Nausea, diarrhea, vomiting Weight gain or loss of more than 10 lb Change in appetite Gastrointestinal bleeding	Emotional	Disruption of logical thinking Blaming others Lack of motivation to get up in the morning Crying tendencies Lack of interest Irritability Isolation Diminished initiative
Diagnostic	Blood in stools/vomitus Elevated blood glucose level Elevated cortisol levels		
Musculoskeletal	Backaches, muscle aches Bruxism (clenched jaw) Slumped posture	Behavior/lifestyle	Worrying Decreased involvement with others Withdrawal Change in interactions with others Increased or decreased food intake Increased smoking or alcohol intake Overvigilance to environment Excessive humor or silence No exercise
Reproductive	Amenorrhea Failure to ovulate Impotency in men Loss of libido		
Immunological	Frequent or prolonged colds/flu		

autonomic nervous system so that a person has the energy to fight or flee. The autonomic nervous system has two components: the sympathetic nervous system and the parasympathetic nervous system. The sympathetic nervous system functions like a gas pedal in a car for triggering the fight-or-flight response (Harvard Medical School, 2016), giving the body a burst of energy so that it can respond to perceived dangers. The parasympathetic nervous system acts like a brake to promote the "rest and digest" response that calms down the body after the danger has passed (Harvard Medical School, 2016).

When there is an initial perceived stressor, the hypothalamus activates the sympathetic nervous system for a short-term response by stimulating the release of epinephrine and norepinephrine from the adrenal gland. The response prepares a person for action by increasing heart and respiratory rates, dilating the bronchioles, diverting blood from the intestines to the brain and striated muscles, and increasing blood pressure and blood glucose levels. As a result, extra oxygen is sent to the brain, increasing a person's alertness and causing sight, hearing, and other senses to become sharper (Harvard Medical School, 2016). The release of glucose and fats from temporary storage sites in the body supply energy to all parts of the body. The physiological fight-or-flight response happens so quickly that people aren't aware of it. This is why a person can jump out of the way of an incoming car before even thinking about what he or she is doing.

Long-Term Stress Response—Resistance

After the initial surge of epinephrine subsides, the hypothalamus activates the HPA axis to keep the sympathetic nervous system activated (the gas pedal is still pressed down) (Harvard Medical School, 2016). The HPA axis responds to a stressor primarily through the synthesis and/or release of three key hormones: corticotropin-releasing factor (CRF), adrenocorticotropic hormone (ACTH), and the glucocorticoid hormone cortisol (COR) (Miller & O'Callaghan, 2002) (see Fig. 26.1). If the brain continues to perceive something as a threat, the hypothalamus releases CRF, which travels to the pituitary gland and triggers the release of ACTH. ACTH then travels to the adrenal glands, prompting the release of cortisol and vasopressin. Cortisol increases blood glucose, enhances the use of glucose by the brain, and increases the availability of substances for tissue repair. Vasopressin increases resorption of water by the kidneys and causes vasoconstriction, raising blood pressure. Thus the body stays revved up and on high alert. Cortisol will be released for several hours after encountering a stressor.

Once a certain blood concentration of cortisol is reached, the "protection" against stress is met and the cortisol exerts negative feedback to the hypothalamic release of CRF and the pituitary release of ACTH. At this point, systemic homeostasis returns (Alschuler, 2016). Homeostasis is a state of physiological balance in which the body has a chance to recover from the physiological activation experienced during stress. As cortisol levels fall, the parasympathetic nervous system acts as a "brake" to dampen the stress response (Harvard Medical School, 2016). Over time the body may experience an excessive state of activation that cannot be inhibited by the parasympathetic system. Alternatively, the ability of the parasympathetic system to respond to stress may be reduced. This pattern of response reflects the stages of resistance.

Exhaustion From Continued Stress

The release of cortisol during the normal stress response curbs bodily functions that are nonessential in or detrimental to a fight-or-flight situation. For example, immune system responses are altered and digestive system, reproductive system and growth processes are suppressed (Mayo Clinic, 2016). The body's stress-response system is usually self-limiting. Once a perceived threat has passed, hormone levels return to normal and the body adapts physiologically. However, when stressors are always present and a person constantly feels threatened or under attack, the fight-or-flight reaction stays turned on, exhaustion develops, and serious health consequences occur (Mayo Clinic, 2016). Individuals can become more vulnerable to infection and develop anxiety, depression, heart disease, weight gain, memory and concentration impairment, and sleep problems.

Immune Response

The immune system is integrated with other physiological processes and is sensitive to changes in central nervous system and endocrine functioning that occur during the stress response. The stress response directly influences the immune system (Huether and McCance, 2017). One effect of long-term stress is the influence of cortisol on T-lymphocyte cells, which are an essential component of cell-mediated immunity. T-cells respond to molecules called interleukins by way of a signaling pathway. Cortisol blocks T-cells from proliferating by preventing some T-cells from recognizing the interleukin signals. It also reduces inflammation due to inhibition of histamine secretion. Continued exposure to stress thus causes prolonged changes in the immune system, which can result in increased risk for infection, as well as high blood pressure, diabetes, and cancer (Janowski et al., 2014; Moreira et al., 2014).

Reaction to Psychological Stress

When a person encounters a stressor, there is an immediate process of primary appraisal or rating of the event. If primary appraisal results in the person identifying the event or circumstance as a harm, loss, threat, or challenge, the person experiences stress. At the same time, the person is also considering possible coping strategies or resources available to help deal with the event; this process is referred to as secondary appraisal. If demands placed on the person exceed the ability to cope, stress continues.

No single coping strategy works for everyone or for every stressor. Coping is important to physical and psychological health because stress is associated with a range of psychological and health outcomes (Doron et al., 2014). Effective coping strategies use a person's cognitive and behavioral traits to manage a stressor (Nielson and Knardahl, 2014). A person also copes differently at different times.

In stressful situations most people use a combination of physiological, problem-focused, and emotion-focused coping strategies. In other words, when under stress a person learns to relax physically (physiological), obtain information, take action to change the situation (problem-focused), and regulate emotions tied to the stress (emotion-focused). In some cases people avoid thinking about the situation or change the way they think about it without changing the actual situation itself.

Techniques used for stress management, to cope with generalized stress and arousal, aim to relax and soothe the body and mind. Physical relaxation aims to switch the body from sympathetic to parasympathetic dominance to restore homeostasis to the HPA axis. Other coping resources include problem-solving skills, financial status, social skills, supportive family and friends, physical attractiveness, health and energy, and personal stress management techniques such as optimism and mindfulness (O'Driscoll, 2013; van den Hurk et al., 2015). For example, physical exercise, relaxation strategies, and letting go of excess anger reduce physical and psychological tension. Exercise improves circulation and triggers the release of endorphins. The relaxation response, elicited by meditation or progressive muscle relaxation, restores parasympathetic function to lower blood pressure, pulse rate, and respiratory rate.

Psychological adaptive behaviors, or ego-defense mechanisms, regulate emotional distress and protect a person from anxiety and stress (Box 26.2). When you recognize that a patient is using an ego-defense mechanism such as denial or displacement, do not point this out to the patient or suggest that the defense mechanism is unhealthy. Denial often helps a patient reduce stress to a manageable level until he or she can cope with it. Displacement means transferring emotions from a stressful situation to a less anxiety-producing substitute. For example, this can happen if a patient acts angrily toward a nurse when the patient is worried about his or her illness, pain, or trauma. Accept the patient's response, listen, and try to learn the specific source of his or her emotions.

BOX 26.2 EXAMPLES OF EGO-DEFENSE MECHANISMS

COMPENSATION
Making up for a deficiency in one aspect of self-image by strongly emphasizing a feature considered an asset. (*Example:* A person who is a poor communicator relies on organizational skills.)

CONVERSION
Unconsciously repressing an anxiety-producing emotional conflict and transforming it into nonorganic symptoms (e.g., difficulty sleeping, loss of appetite).

DENIAL
Avoiding emotional conflicts by refusing to consciously acknowledge anything that causes intolerable emotional pain. (*Example:* A person refuses to discuss or acknowledge a personal loss.)

DISPLACEMENT
Transferring emotions, ideas, or wishes from a stressful situation to a less anxiety-producing substitute. (*Example:* A person transfers anger over a job conflict to a malfunctioning computer.)

IDENTIFICATION
Patterning behavior after that of another person and assuming that person's qualities, characteristics, and actions.

DISSOCIATION
Experiencing a subjective sense of numbing and a reduced awareness of one's surroundings.

REGRESSION
Coping with a stressor through actions and behaviors associated with an earlier developmental period.

Types of Stress

Stress arises from work, social, and family stressors that can be either chronic or acute. Examples include daily hassles, dysfunctional relationships, emotional trauma, and crisis. One person looks at a stimulus and sees it as a challenge, leading to mastery and growth. Another sees the same stimulus as a threat, leading to stress and a potential sense of loss. An individual with family responsibilities and a full-time job outside the home and who experiences a job loss or a chronic illness can experience chronic stress. Chronic stress occurs in stable conditions and from stressful roles. Living with a long-term illness produces chronic stress. Conversely, time-limited events that threaten a person for a relatively brief period (e.g., death of a family member or friend) provoke acute stress.

Posttraumatic stress disorder (PTSD) is a mental health problem that some people develop after experiencing or witnessing a life-threatening event, such as military combat, physical assault, or a natural disaster (U.S. Department of Veterans Affairs, 2016). The person responds with a sense of intense fear or helplessness. There are four types of PTSD symptoms: (1) reliving the event (bad memories, nightmares), (2) avoiding situations that remind the person of the event, (3) having more negative beliefs and feelings about oneself or the world, and (4) hyperarousal (anxiety, irritability, trouble sleeping) (U.S. Department of Veterans Affairs, 2016). Some people with PTSD experience flashbacks, or recurrent and intrusive recollections of the event. Depression and PTSD commonly occur together, and both are associated with self-destructive behaviors such as suicide attempts and substance abuse (Stevens et al., 2013).

A crisis implies that a person is facing a turning point in life. This means that previous ways of coping are not effective. There are three types of crises: (1) maturational or developmental crises, (2) situational crises, and (3) adventitious crises (Varcarolis, 2017). A new developmental stage such as marriage, birth of a child, or retirement requires new coping styles. Developmental crises occur as a person moves through the stages of life. External sources such as a job change, a motor vehicle crash, a death, or a severe illness provoke situational crises. An adventitious or social crisis is a rare and unexpected tragedy that may affect an entire community or population, such as a major natural disaster, man-made disaster, or violent crime.

Patient-centered care provides an important context for any crisis intervention (Gillespie and Gates, 2013). The vital questions for a person in crisis are: "What does this mean to you?" "How does it affect your life?" What causes extreme stress for one person is not always stressful to another. The perception of the event, situational supports, and coping mechanisms all influence return of equilibrium. A person either grows or regresses as a result of a crisis, depending on how he or she manages the situation (Gillespie and Gates, 2013; Varcarolis, 2017).

NURSING KNOWLEDGE BASE

Nursing Theory and the Role of Stress

Many nursing theories explain and describe stress. One of these models is the Neuman Systems Model. This model uses a systems approach to help you understand your patients' individual responses to stressors as well as responses of families and communities. A systems approach explains that a stressor at one place in a system affects other parts of the system; a system is a person, family, or community. Events are multidimensional and not caused or affected by only one thing. Every person develops a set of responses to stress that constitute the "normal line of defense" (Neuman and Fawcett, 2010; Turner and Kaylor, 2015). This line of defense helps to maintain health and wellness. Physiological, psychological, sociocultural, developmental, and spiritual influences buffer stress. When a patient cannot buffer stress, the normal line of defense is broken, resulting in disease. The Neuman Systems Model of nursing views a patient, family, or community as constantly changing in response to the environment and stressors.

Pender's Health Promotion Model focuses on promoting health and managing stress. Interventions associated with this model teach people to live in ways that enable them to be as healthy as possible and capable of assessing their own abilities and assets (see Chapter 2) (Pender and Murdaugh, 2015). This model supports increasing physical activity, improving diet and nutrition, and using stress-management strategies to become healthy and remain healthy (Sousa et al., 2015; Valek et al., 2015).

Situational, Maturational, and Sociocultural Factors

Potential stressors and coping mechanisms vary across the life span. For example, adolescence, adulthood, and old age bring different stressors related to separating from family, establishing oneself as an adult, and making a contribution to society. Likewise, coping strategies fluctuate from an emphasis on primarily emotional coping to problem solving as our minds grow and thinking develops.

Situational Factors. Stressors in the workplace that affect nurses and other health care professionals include high-acuity patient load, job environment, constant distractions, responsibility, conflicting priorities, and intensity of care (e.g., trauma, emergency, or critical care areas) (Najimi et al., 2012; Ianello and Balzarotti, 2014; Mealer et al., 2014). In addition, changing shifts increases fatigue and work-related stress. Coping strategies vary with the individual and the situation.

Some nurses often ease coping with shift work by knowing their own circadian rhythms. People who function best in the morning have the greatest difficulty with night work and changing shifts. As people age they tend to become more morning oriented. Morning people need to be counseled about the potentially negative effects of night work for them. In general, people doing shift work need to maintain as consistent a sleep and mealtime schedule as possible (Sabo, 2011; Lin et al., 2014).

Adjusting to chronic illness is a situational stress. The physical limitations posed by a disease state and the uncertainty associated with treatment and illness trigger stress in patients of all ages. Sometimes illness changes how people manage their stress. For example, Parelkar et al. (2015) found that cancer survivors who made active efforts to control stress changed their physical, psychosocial, and preventive health behaviors during and after cancer treatment. Having difficulty paying for treatment and limited access to health care providers also create stress. Although being a family caregiver for someone with a chronic illness such as Alzheimer disease is stressful, the actions of competent health care providers often help minimize the stress for family caregivers.

Maturational Factors. Stressors vary with life stage. Children identify stressors related to physical appearance, family dynamics, friendships, and school. Preadolescents experience stress related to self-esteem issues, hospitalizations, or changing family structure as a result of divorce or death of a parent. Adolescents experience stress as they search for identity with peer groups and separate from their families. In addition, they face stressful questions about using mind-

---

BOX 26.3 CARE OF THE OLDER ADULT

Coping Strategies

Some older adults report better mental health than younger adults because older adults appraise and cope with stress differently. Coping strategies to assist in healthy aging include the following:
- Organizing objects in the environment such as canes, walkers, handrails, hearing aids, amplifiers on telephones, and magnifying glasses to enhance daily functioning.
- Using life experiences and stress management techniques to cope with family, health, or residential stressors (Rayens and Reed, 2014).
- De-emphasizing health problems by using positive comparisons with peers and finding others who are more disabled with whom they can compare themselves.
- Using dyadic coping (two people), or joint coping, to compensate for memory problems and other physical deficits. The spouse or partner anticipates the other's needs and helps as needed. Anticipatory guidance can reduce the stress on both partners (Rayens and Reed, 2014).

---

altering substances, sex, jobs, school, and career choices. Stress for adults centers around major changes in life circumstances. These include the many milestones of beginning a family and a career, losing parents, seeing children leave home, and accepting physical aging. In old age, stressors include the loss of autonomy and mastery resulting from general frailty or health problems that limit stamina, strength, and cognition (Box 26.3).

Sociocultural Factors. Environmental and social stressors can lead to developmental problems. Potential stressors affect any age-group, but they are especially stressful for young people. These include prolonged poverty, physical handicap, and chronic illness. The vulnerability of children escalates when they lose relationships with parents and caregivers through divorce, abandonment, imprisonment, or death or when parents have mental illness or substance-abuse disorders. Furthermore, living under conditions of continuing violence, disintegrated neighborhoods, or homelessness affects people of any age, but these factors are especially stressful to young people (Pender and Murdaugh, 2015).

Cultural variations produce stress, particularly if a person's values differ from the dominant culture in aspects of gender roles, family relationships, and religious beliefs (Giger, 2016). Other aspects of cultural variations begin with language difference, geographical location, family relationships, time orientation, access to health care programs, and disparities in health care (Box 26.4). Uncertainty about immigration status and citizenship can contribute to increased stress.

Compassion Fatigue

Compassion fatigue is a term used to describe a state of burnout and secondary traumatic stress (Potter et al., 2013). Secondary traumatic stress is the stress that health care providers experience when witnessing and caring for others who

BOX 26.4   PATIENT-CENTERED CARE

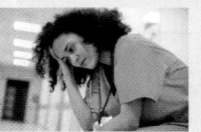

Copyright ©
gpointstudio/iStock/
Thinkstock.

Stress and anxiety sometimes lead to insomnia, as in Rachael's case. Cultural factors influence a person's health behaviors and also influence the quality of a person's sleep (Garcia, 2016). There are significant differences in sleeping habits and routines as well as rates of insomnia among ethnic groups (Giger, 2016).

IMPLICATIONS FOR PRACTICE

- Ask patients what their family members, especially their parents, do when they cannot sleep to learn about their cultural values associated with insomnia.
- Help patients connect their insomnia with the stress that they are experiencing by asking them what they think about while they are lying in bed awake.
- Ask patients with insomnia which coping strategies they have tried. Determine if their coping measures include culturally specific remedies.
- If folk or culturally specific remedies are used to improve sleeping, verify that these remedies do not interact with the patient's prescribed medication.

BOX 26.5   SYNTHESIS IN PRACTICE

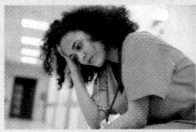

Copyright ©
gpointstudio/iStock/
Thinkstock.

When Becky talks with Rachael, she learns that Rachael worries about losing her job because of the declining quality of patient care on her unit. Rachael provides sole support for her family at this time. Becky also learns about her husband's recent illness and the effect it has on Rachael's overall well-being. Becky has also talked with Rachael's supervisor and knows that Rachael has been having headaches and difficulty concentrating when making decisions.

Becky takes time to reflect on other employees that she sees in the employee health office. Many of the RNs have had physical complaints of stress, including headaches, sleep problems, changes in eating habits, and flare-ups of existing medical problems. Becky wants to be thorough in assessing the responses and symptoms that Rachael is experiencing. Previous experience with other employees has taught Becky the importance of learning about the employee's family, the type of support they offer, and the person's appraisal of the situation.

are suffering. Examples include an oncology nurse who cares for patients undergoing surgery and chemotherapy over the long term for their cancer or a spouse who witnesses his wife deteriorating over the years from Alzheimer disease. Burnout occurs when perceived demands outweigh perceived resources (Potter et al., 2013). It is a state of physical and mental fatigue and exhaustion that often affects health care providers because of the nature of their work environment. Perceived inadequate staffing, long work shifts, demands of patient acuity, and dysfunctional relationships (patients and other care providers) serve as triggers for ongoing stress. Over time, giving of oneself in often intense caring environments can result in emotional exhaustion, leaving a nurse feeling irritable, restless, and unable to focus and engage with patients. This condition may be viewed as a failure of coping because it often occurs in situations in which there is a lack of social support, organizational pressures influencing staffing, and the inability of a nurse to practice self-care.

Compassion fatigue is a condition that can overwhelm health care providers and cause physical, mental, and emotional health issues (Hunsaker et al., 2015). The feelings of hopelessness and anxiety from compassion fatigue usually result in feelings of inadequacy and lower self-esteem. These factors can lead to the health care provider lashing out in an attempt to cope with these feelings and stress. This often manifests itself as *lateral violence,* which refers to a deliberate and harmful behavior demonstrated in the workplace by one employee to another. This includes health care providers engaging in bullying and potentially assaultive behaviors toward co-workers (Embree and White, 2010; Christie and Jones, 2013).

Early recognition of the risk for compassion fatigue is essential. A supportive work environment helps guide a nursing unit in designing communication techniques to identify, prevent, and adapt to potential compassion fatigue situations (Hunsaker et al., 2015).

CRITICAL THINKING

Synthesis

Patient care requires you to apply what you know about a patient, your knowledge base, experience, and critical thinking attitudes and standards. Your synthesis of this information allows you to make sound decisions as you apply the nursing process. Critical thinking synthesis involves combining all available information to obtain a clear picture of the approach needed to provide patient-centered care.

This approach helps you identify patients' specific health care needs and design individualized interventions (Box 26.5).

Knowledge. Physiological changes occur in a patient experiencing stress. Apply knowledge of the neuroendocrine stress response. Your knowledge of communication principles helps you assess the patient's behaviors. Consider your patient's perception of the stress. Determine his or her ability to cope with it. If the patient does not succeed with his or her usual coping skills, you need to refer him or her to crisis intervention counseling.

Experience. Your experience helps you better understand a patient's unique perception of stressors and responses to stress. View every person as an individual, recognizing that no two people are exactly alike. Experience with patients also helps you recognize responses to stress. In addition, your own personal experiences with stress and coping increase your ability to empathize with a patient temporarily immobilized by stress. Understanding a patient's position enables you to intervene more effectively.

Attitudes. Use confidence and believe that you and a patient are able to manage stress effectively. Patients respect your realistic advice and counsel and gain confidence from your belief in their ability to move past stressful events or illnesses. Patients experiencing a crisis often lack the ability, at least initially, to act on their own behalf. They require either direct intervention or guidance. You need to have an attitude of integrity through which you respect a patient's perception of or perspective about a stressor and his or her cultural beliefs. Make the effort to have patients explain their unique viewpoints and situations.

Standards. Accurately assess a patient's stress, coping mechanisms, and support system before intervening. Clearly and precisely understand a patient's perception of the stress and focus on factors significant to his or her well-being. In addition, select interventions that respect the individuality of the patient. Be especially aware of your ethical responsibility in caring for someone who has less independence because of being in a crisis state.

NURSING PROCESS

◼ ▦ ▢ ASSESSMENT

Assessment of a patient's stress level and coping resources requires that you first establish a trusting nurse-patient relationship. You ask the patient and family to share personal and sensitive information (see Chapter 11). Learn from the patient by asking questions and making observations of nonverbal behavior, interactions with the family, and the patient's environment. Synthesize the information you obtain and adopt a critical thinking attitude while observing and analyzing patient behaviors. Often a patient has difficulty describing the most bothersome aspects of a situation until someone else has time to listen and encourage the patient to explore it.

Subjective Findings. When you assess a patient's stress level and coping resources, sit with the patient in comfortable chairs in a private setting facing one another. Assume a listening posture, establish eye contact, and allow time for the patient to talk (Varcarolis, 2017). Gather information about the health status of the patient from his or her perspective: Is the patient experiencing physical signs of stress (see Table 26.1)? Begin the process of developing a trusting relationship.

Use the interview to determine a patient's view of the situation that provoked stress; assess the patient's perceptions of safety issues, coping resources, any possible maladaptive coping, and adherence to prescribed medical recommendations such as medication or diet (Table 26.2) (Varcarolis, 2017). Ask the patient to describe any prior stressful situations and how he or she adapted. Learn whether the patient

relies on the use of tobacco, alcohol, or drugs to cope with difficult issues. If the patient uses denial as a coping mechanism, be alert to whether the person overlooks necessary information you provide. Listen for any recurrent themes in the patient's conversation such as anger, powerlessness, or anxiety. As in all interactions with a patient, respect the confidentiality and sensitivity of the information shared.

If your patient is experiencing a crisis, assess safety concerns such as potential for self-harm or suicide and harm to others including homicide and the patient's ability to perform activities of daily living. Assessment includes determining the patient's emotions, behaviors, cognitive state, and precrisis level of functioning. In addition, assess for prior trauma, symptoms of mental illness, and use of legal and illegal drugs. Assess whether this crisis is a one-time situation or part of a pattern of a crisis-oriented life history. Finally assess alternatives, coping mechanisms, and support systems (Janowski et al., 2014).

Objective Findings. Obtain objective findings related to stress and coping by observing a patient's appearance and nonverbal behavior. Observe grooming and hygiene, gait, characteristics of the patient's handshake, actions of the patient while sitting, quality of speech, facial expression and eye contact, and the attitude of the patient toward you during the interview (see Chapter 16). During this part of the interview you need to keep in mind cultural norms that may influence a patient's responses. Before the interview begins or at the end of the interview, depending on the anxiety level of the patient, take basic vital signs to assess for physiological signs of stress such as elevated blood pressure, heart rate, or respiratory rate.

Older Adult Considerations. Assessment of an older adult should include a review of the patient's level of resiliency, which is defined by the American Psychological Association (APA) as "the process of adapting well in the face of adversity, trauma, tragedy, threats, or significant sources of stress," or "bouncing back" from difficult experiences. Many older adults experience high levels of well-being and quality of life, low stress, and recovery from adversities and consider themselves to be aging successfully despite the onset of chronic conditions (MacLeod et al., 2016). Tools have been designed to assess for resilience based on the APA definition of the concept. A review of the literature has shown that key characteristics of high resilience among adults 65 years of age and older include mental, social, and physical factors such as the following:

- **Mental:** Gratitude, happiness, lack of cognitive failure, optimism, adaptive coping
- **Social:** Community involvement, active with family and friends, sense of purpose, social support seeking
- **Physical:** ADL independence, high mobility, physical health

Ask patients to describe how well they believe they are aging. Consider questions such as: How would you describe your retirement? Tell me how you would describe your quality of life? How would you describe your ability to deal with

TABLE 26.2 FOCUSED PATIENT ASSESSMENT

FACTORS TO ASSESS	QUESTIONS	PHYSICAL ASSESSMENT
Patient safety	Describe for me any thoughts you might have of harming yourself. How are you sleeping? Describe for me any problems you have going to sleep or awakening during the night. How has your appetite changed? Tell me how stress affects your work. Describe any problems you are having concentrating. Have you had accidents at home, in the car, or on the job?	Observe for indicators of anxiety, anger, or tension. For example, you may observe such nonverbal behaviors as irritability, crying, and inappropriate laughing.
Perception of stressor	What do you believe is stressing you? What do you think about when you can't sleep? What does this situation or stressor mean in your opinion?	Observe for nonverbal indicators of stress such as rapid talking, crying, changes in posture (e.g., folding arms over chest). Listen for recurrent themes.
Available coping resources	Are you keeping in touch with your friends? How often do you see your family members? What have you done before to cope with similar problems or stress? What do you do for fun? How do you spend your leisure time?	Observe whether the person is alone or with others. Observe the person's communication skills. Observe if the person is able to ask for help. Observe developmental level. Assess sociocultural circumstances (Giger, 2016).
Maladaptive coping used	How much do you smoke? How much do you drink? If you use any over-the-counter or herbal medications for your stress, tell me what they are. How much coffee or soda do you drink in a day?	Observe for effects of smoking, alcohol, drugs, and caffeine (e.g., difficulty sleeping, nervousness, or difficulty concentrating).
Adherence to healthy practices	How long has it been since you saw a health care provider? How often do you go for regular check-ups? What type of a diet do you follow? Describe for me what you would call a regular meal at home. What type of exercise do you get?	Obtain vital signs and palpate for any tender areas. Obtain weight.

Copyright © gpointstudio/iStock/Thinkstock.

adversity or loss? Your assessment will reveal if patients have resources for coping with stressors and allow you to use those resources when helping patients face any health crises.

Three stressors common in the older adult population include loss of independence, relocation, and loss of a spouse or partner. Various factors can limit an older adult's independence; one common factor is changes in mobility. Changes in a person's musculoskeletal system (e.g., joint stiffness and pain associated with arthritis), effects of multiple medications on balance, or physical disability from previous injuries reduce mobility and increase the risk for falls (see Chapter 30). A person may report having stiffness in the back or legs and a lack of balance, which can increase the risk for falls. However, changes in mobility do not account for all losses of independence in an older adult. Cognitive decline resulting from dementia prevents patients from being able to problem solve and make the decisions necessary to maintain self-care. Visual changes associated with cataracts, glaucoma, or macular degeneration not only impact independence but also affect a person's safety and how that person views the environment. Changes in hearing acuity impact both the person and the spouse or partner. Often there is a decrease in communication and socialization.

Relocation stress occurs when an older adult must leave his or her familiar residence and relocate to the home of an adult child, a long-term care facility, or a memory care unit. Assessment findings that may reveal relocation stress include anxiety, depression, altered problem solving and insecurity, and physical symptoms related to a person's health status (Touhy and Jett, 2014). Relocation stress should not be confused with downsizing or with cognitive changes. Although there are stressors associated with any move, downsizing is usually planned, and the older adult chooses to live in a smaller home, sometimes to be near children and grandchildren.

The loss of a spouse or partner is another stressor for older adults. Spousal bereavement is a major source of life stress that often leaves people vulnerable to later problems such as chronic stress and depression. An older adult dealing with the death of a spouse or partner is often more likely to engage in risky health behavior, including smoking, abusing drugs or alcohol, failing to care for themselves, or generally becoming more inactive (Vitelli, 2015). Examples of assessment findings associated with this loss include loneliness, social isolation, grief, sorrow, anxiety, depression, use of alcohol or recreational drugs, and lack of interest in hobbies, family, and community.

Patient Expectations. Determine the importance of the meaning of the stressor to the patient and the ways in which the patient expects you and other health care providers to help him or her manage the stress. Ask the patient about the situation and allow time for the patient to discuss the situation and describe some priorities for coping with stress. For example, you are caring for a woman who has just found out about a breast mass identified on a routine mammogram. It is important for you to know what the patient wants and needs most from you. Ask her what she wants to know about the next steps (e.g., surgical or diagnostic procedure). Although some women in this situation identify their need for information about biopsy or mastectomy as their personal priority, other women need guidance and support in discussing how to share the news with family members.

Remember that in some cases nothing will change or improve the situation. Allowing a patient to use denial as a coping mechanism is helpful. Gaining an understanding of patient expectations does not mean that you exclude certain types of care that are important simply because a patient does not identify them as needs. However, when you ask a patient to describe personal expectations and priorities, you have a better awareness of his or her needs, and you are better able to ensure that these needs are addressed.

QSEN QSEN ACTIVITY *Safety*

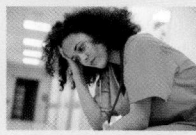
Copyright © gpointstudio/iStock/Thinkstock.

During her assessment of Rachael, Becky collects a great deal of information regarding the stressors that Rachael is experiencing. Through a process of systematic assessment Becky also identifies the coping strategies and mechanisms that Rachael uses most frequently. Becky now needs to identify ineffective coping patterns and the potential for adverse consequences of stress.

- How could the use of systematic assessment measures help Becky identify Rachael's coping patterns and the consequences of stress? What are some objective signs of ineffective coping that may threaten Rachael's safety? What are some possible subjective statements from Rachael that would also support ineffective coping?

evolve Answers to QSEN Activities can be found on the Evolve website.

■■■ NURSING DIAGNOSIS

Review your assessment findings to identify nursing diagnoses appropriate to a patient. When selecting a problem-focused nursing diagnosis, be sure there are defining characteristics applicable to the diagnosis. For example, major defining characteristics of *Ineffective Coping* include verbalization of an inability to cope and an inability to ask for help. You identify defining characteristics during the assessment (e.g., by asking the patient to identify his or her greatest concerns at the time of the interview or to relate experiences with stressors)

and, importantly, allow the patient sufficient time to answer (see Table 26.2). Your assessment should reveal risk factors if you identify a risk diagnosis. Observe for physiological and psychological indicators of stress. After selecting a problem-focused diagnosis, identify the related factor so that you can select appropriate interventions that are relevant and likely to resolve the diagnosis once they are implemented.

The nursing diagnoses that are most applicable to stress and coping focus on ineffective coping responses and the consequences of stress. Other appropriate diagnoses target a patient or family member who is ready for additional education regarding coping strategies. Examples of stress-related nursing diagnoses include the following:

- *Anxiety*
- *Compromised Family Coping*
- *Ineffective Coping*
- *Fear*
- *Moral Distress*
- *Relocation Stress Syndrome*
- *Stress Overload*
- *Post-Trauma Syndrome*

■■□ PLANNING

Goals and Outcomes. Desirable goals for people experiencing stress are (1) coping with the stressor, (2) family coping, and (3) psychosocial adjustment: life change. Expected outcomes are behavioral markers that show progress toward goal achievement. For example, if a patient is to cope with stress, outcomes may include increasing interaction with others and improved sleep. After setting goals and outcomes, select interventions for managing the specific stressor and improving coping (Varcarolis, 2017).

Plan care using nursing interventions designed within the framework of primary, secondary, and tertiary prevention. At the primary level of prevention, nursing interventions include preparing patients for turning points in life such as the birth of a baby or the death of a parent. Nursing interventions at the secondary level include actions directed at symptoms such as protecting the patient from self-harm. Tertiary-level interventions help a patient readapt and often include relaxation and time-management training.

Patients' perceptions of stress and coping depend on recognition of the problem and use of coping resources. Similarly, selecting appropriate interventions requires a partnership with a patient and support system, usually the family caregiver. In the case of a family or community stressor and impaired family or community coping, your view of the situation and resources would be broader (see Care Plan).

Setting Priorities. People experiencing stress often have multiple nursing diagnoses that interrelate to one another. Prioritizing their diagnoses is important in planning care (Fig. 26.2). One way to prioritize is to first ask questions: "What has happened that caused you to come for help today?" "What happened in your life that is *different*?" This requires some focusing by the patient. Next refer to your assessment

◎ CARE PLAN

Stress and Individual Coping

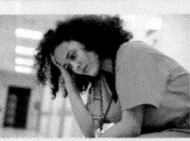
Copyright © gpointstudio/iStock/Thinkstock.

ASSESSMENT

During her initial contact with Rachael, Becky detects a great deal of anxiety but also some anger. Becky knows that it is important to build trust with Rachael as quickly as possible. She knows that Rachael's anger is not directed at her but reflects Rachael's frustration. As a single parent, Becky identifies with Rachael's crisis of being the sole financial support for the family. Yet Becky decides not to tell her life history to Rachael because she recognizes that no two persons have exactly the same experience or use the same coping strategies to get through difficult times. Becky wants to be able to work closely with Rachael and establish priorities that are realistic for her to achieve.

ASSESSMENT ACTIVITIES	FINDINGS[a]
Observe for signs of stress.	She observes Rachael frequently licking her lips, picking at her fingernails, and being easily startled. Rachael has **poor eye contact** and then bursts into tears and expresses feelings of being overwhelmed.
Measure vital signs.	Rachael's **vital signs show changes during interview:** pulse, 120 beats/min; respirations, 24 breaths/min; blood pressure, 168/84 mm Hg.
Ask about recent weight loss.	Rachael appears thin and pale and reports that she has lost 20 lb in the last 3 months.
Ask about changes in sleep.	Rachael **reports difficulty in falling and remaining asleep at night.**
Assess Rachael's perception of the stress.	Rachael expresses fear of losing her job and being **unable to support her family.** She also expresses feelings of shame and embarrassment. She thinks of herself as a **failure for not coping better.**
Ask about current coping methods.	Rachael admits to having **one to two glasses of wine** at night to help herself "unwind." Rachael acknowledges that this is something new for her to do each night.

[a]**Defining characteristics/risk factors** are shown in **bold** type.

NURSING DIAGNOSIS: Ineffective Coping related to increased pressure at work and multiple family stresses and responsibilities

---

PLANNING

GOAL	EXPECTED OUTCOMES (NOC)[b]
	Coping
Rachael will begin to manage stressors that have been taxing her individual resources within 3 weeks.	Rachael identifies her effective and ineffective coping patterns.
	Rachael verbalizes a decrease in stress.
	Rachael adds improved nutritional intake and regular exercise to her lifestyle.
	Rachael uses her personal support system.
	Rachael verbalizes need for assistance.

[b]Outcomes classification labels from Moorhead S, et al, editors: *Nursing outcomes classification (NOC)*, ed 5, St Louis, 2013, Mosby.

INTERVENTIONS (NIC)[c]	RATIONALE
Coping Enhancement	
Encourage Rachael to identify a realistic description of her changing roles.	A cognitive reappraisal helps Rachael reframe the poor patient satisfaction scores so that she does not take all the responsibility for them. How she defines the reality and the personal meaning it has for her directly affect her stress level (Varcarolis, 2017).
Help Rachael develop an objective appraisal of her situation.	Rachael's recognition of the stressor and her appraisal of her coping strategies help define the stressful situation and begin the process of establishing realistic expectations (Valek et al., 2015).
Explore Rachael's previous achievements.	Emphasizing the positive helps a person feel more optimistic, which leads to positive actions and results (Varcarolis, 2017).
Encourage Rachael to identify own strengths and abilities.	To manage stress and cope with change, people need to know their strengths and abilities and what is important to them (Nguyen-Rodriguez, et al., 2015).
Help Rachael break down complex goals into small, manageable steps.	Changing her cognitive view of her situation reduces Rachael's stress. Small successes accumulate for her and reduce the magnitude of her stress (Varcarolis, 2017).
Teach Rachael to explore some mindfulness training sessions.	Mindfulness courses and training programs reduce stress and promote well-being among health care workers (Raab, 2014).

⊚ CARE PLAN—cont'd

Stress and Individual Coping

INTERVENTIONS (NIC)ᶜ	RATIONALE
Teach Rachael meditation strategies to increase her resistance to stress.	Increasing resistance to stress is one of the primary modes for intervention for stress management (Pender and Murdaugh, 2015; Pender, 2016).

ᶜIntervention classification labels from Bulechek GM, et al, editors: *Nursing interventions classification (NIC),* ed 6, St Louis, 2013, Mosby.

EVALUATION

NURSING ACTIONS	PATIENT RESPONSE/FINDING	ACHIEVEMENT OF OUTCOME
Ask Rachael about her perception of stress in her life and changes she has made.	Rachael demonstrates less licking of her lips, picking at her fingernails, and being easily startled. She exercises by walking with her husband three times a week. Her blood pressure is 140/82 mm Hg, and pulse is 88 beats/min during the next session. She has a 3-lb weight gain and is eating healthy foods. She resports not drinking wine to reduce her stress. During the past week she began sleeping through the night.	Rachael is decreasing the effect of stress and is practicing healthy lifestyle habits.
Ask Rachael about the use of new and former support systems.	Rachael resumed a friendship with a neighbor. She now asks her husband for help at home and her co-workers for help at work. She has begun mindfulness training.	Rachael is increasing her use of personal support systems at home and work. Consider helping Rachael identify ways to incorporate mindfulness training as a support system for her staff.

data, where you learned about the patient's perception of the event, available situational supports, and what the patient usually does about a problem that he or she is not able to solve. Be aware that some personality traits are associated with passive coping strategies and cause high stress levels (Afshar et al., 2015). As in all areas of nursing, your priority is to ensure the safety of the patient and others in the patient's environment. For example, if a patient is potentially suicidal, determine if he or she is at risk for harming himself or herself. Examples of questions to ask include: How are you coping with what's been happening in your life? Do you ever feel like just giving up? Are you thinking about dying? Are you thinking about hurting yourself? (Mayo Clinic, 2015).

Offering a patient the opportunity to talk about feelings may reduce the risk of acting on suicidal feelings. If you suspect suicidal intention, ask for more information, such as whether the person has attempted suicide previously, has a plan for committing suicide, and has the means to carry out the specific plan. These questions are sometimes difficult to ask, but a patient who is highly stressed and has thought about suicide at some point is usually relieved when someone else brings up the subject.

Prioritize diagnoses by determining the degree of disruption in a person's life with regard to work, school, home, and family. When you thoroughly assess a patient, you are able to prioritize problems, ensure the patient's safety, and begin the problem-solving process (Varcarolis, 2017).

Collaborative Care. An effective plan requires you to collaborate appropriately with health care providers. There are times when nursing practice alone does not meet all of a patient's needs. Patients experiencing stress from medical conditions or psychiatric disorders present needs that make it necessary for you to consult with advanced practice mental health nurses, psychiatrists, psychologists, pastoral care professionals, or psychiatric social workers. Such a multidisciplinary approach to care addresses the holistic needs of your patients. Have the patient and family caregivers partner in care when appropriate. Recognize the need for collaboration and consultation; inform the patient about potential resources; and make arrangements for consultations, group sessions, or therapy as needed.

■ ■ ■ ■ IMPLEMENTATION

Health Promotion. Intervention for relieving stress has a three-pronged approach: (1) decrease stress-producing situations, (2) increase resistance to stress, and (3) learn skills that reduce physiological response to stress (Pender and Murdaugh, 2015; Pender, 2016). First help patients reduce the frequency of stress-inducing situations by using strategies such as instituting positive workplace habits, avoiding excessive change, and effectively managing one's personal time (Hunsaker et al., 2015). Next increase a patient's resistance to stress by building resiliency and recommending physical and psychological conditioning, which includes enhancing self-esteem, increasing assertiveness, setting realistic goals, and building coping resources. Finally use relaxation strategies to reduce physiological arousal (Pender and Murdaugh, 2015). As a nurse, you educate patients

CONCEPT MAP

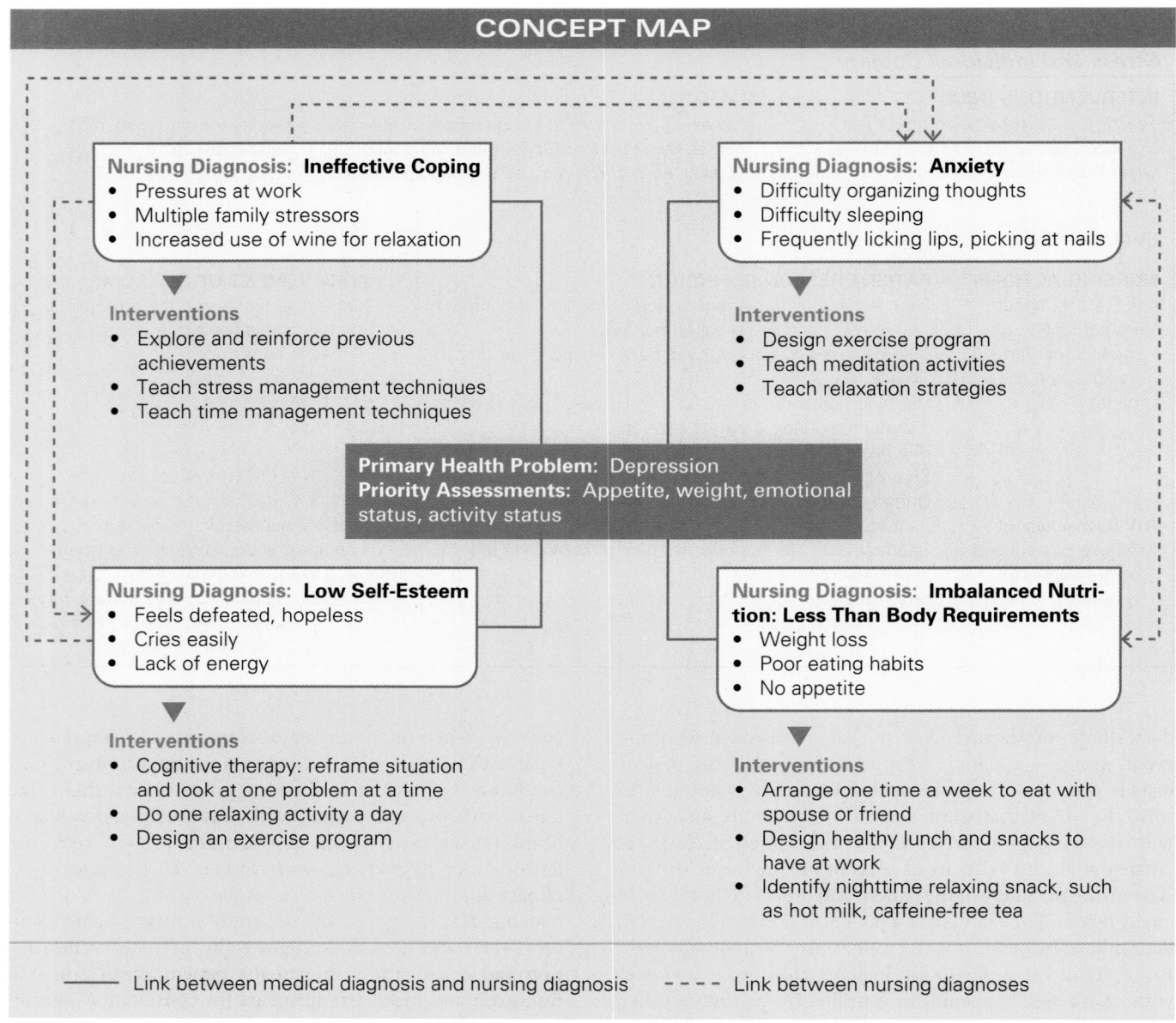

Nursing Diagnosis: Ineffective Coping
- Pressures at work
- Multiple family stressors
- Increased use of wine for relaxation

Interventions
- Explore and reinforce previous achievements
- Teach stress management techniques
- Teach time management techniques

Nursing Diagnosis: Anxiety
- Difficulty organizing thoughts
- Difficulty sleeping
- Frequently licking lips, picking at nails

Interventions
- Design exercise program
- Teach meditation activities
- Teach relaxation strategies

Primary Health Problem: Depression
Priority Assessments: Appetite, weight, emotional status, activity status

Nursing Diagnosis: Low Self-Esteem
- Feels defeated, hopeless
- Cries easily
- Lack of energy

Interventions
- Cognitive therapy: reframe situation and look at one problem at a time
- Do one relaxing activity a day
- Design an exercise program

Nursing Diagnosis: Imbalanced Nutrition: Less Than Body Requirements
- Weight loss
- Poor eating habits
- No appetite

Interventions
- Arrange one time a week to eat with spouse or friend
- Design healthy lunch and snacks to have at work
- Identify nighttime relaxing snack, such as hot milk, caffeine-free tea

——— Link between medical diagnosis and nursing diagnosis   - - - - Link between nursing diagnoses

FIG 26.2 Concept map.

and families about the importance of stress reduction (Box 26.6).

Building Resiliency. Most programs aimed at improving a person's resilience recommend approaches that take a public health approach by suggesting general ways to prepare for challenges before they occur (MacLeod et al, 2016). One example is the APA's campaign to increase awareness of and provide resources for building resilience (APA, 2015). A Resilience Tool Kit recommends approaches to building resilience, including maintaining strong relationships and social support, becoming active in the community, thinking positively, and maintaining hopefulness.

Regular Exercise and Rest. A regular exercise program improves muscle tone and posture, controls weight, reduces tension, improves circulation, triggers the release of endorphins, and promotes relaxation. It is important for patients

to engage in exercise activities that promote stretching, improve balance, and increase conditioning. In addition, exercise reduces the risk for cardiovascular disease and improves cardiopulmonary functioning.

Regular rest and sleep help manage stress and stress-related fatigue. Encourage patients and their families to adopt regular sleep routines (see Chapter 33). People who are well rested are often able to manage stress, problem solve, and maintain control over some situations (Akerstedt et al., 2014).

Progressive Muscle Relaxation. Muscles tense during stressful thoughts and events. Physiological tension diminishes through a systematic approach to releasing tension in major muscle groups. In addition, this aids the parasympathetic nervous system to become dominant and achieve better balance. When helping a patient achieve a relaxed state, have

BOX 26.6 PATIENT TEACHING

Stress Reduction

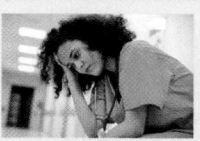

Copyright © gpointstudio/iStock/ Thinkstock.

Becky recognizes that Rachael wants to learn how to increase her resistance to stress. Becky develops the following teaching plan for Rachael.

OUTCOME

At the end of the teaching session, Rachael verbally identifies two methods to reduce her stress.

TEACHING STRATEGIES

- Meet with Rachael in a quiet and private setting at a time when Rachael has about 1 hour to talk without interruptions.
- Schedule a follow-up hour about a week after the first session.
- Encourage Rachael to focus on two stress-management strategies: regular exercise and mindfulness training.
- Ask Rachael to maintain a daily record of her physical exercise and mindfulness strategies.
- Explore with Rachael her support system, possibilities for continuing education, financial status, and her personal appearance, depending on her identified needs (Pender and Murdaugh, 2015).
- For developing insight about maintaining appropriate boundaries between work and personal space, explore with Rachael ways that she will increase awareness of her feelings of anger, pain, hurt, sadness, and joy. Discuss with her how she will recognize the limits of her responsibilities.
- Ask Rachael to keep a personal journal of her feelings for the next week.

EVALUATION

- Use the principles of teach-back to evaluate patient/family caregiver learning:
  - Review with Rachael her record of exercise and mindfulness activities during the week.
  - Ask Rachael to evaluate her progress toward her goal of increased resistance to stress.

the patient breathe deeply. Then direct the patient to relax muscles in areas that feel stiffened. Other controlled relaxation exercises such as yoga are effective in regulating stress responses and reducing blood pressure (Doron et al., 2014).

Support Systems. Patients experiencing stress benefit from a support system of family and friends who listen, offer advice, share recreation time, and provide emotional support (Doron et al., 2014). People with strong networks of friends, neighbors, and family tend to be healthier than people without support systems. Many organizations such as the American Heart Association, the American Cancer Society, local hospitals and churches, and mental health organizations offer support group services to individuals. Acceptable support systems vary by cultural group. For example, one cultural group might rely heavily on church

members for support. Another cultural group values individual privacy and prefers to avoid a self-help group with "strangers."

Mindfulness-Based Stress Reduction (MBSR). Mindfulness is a moment-to-moment present awareness with an attitude of nonjudgment, acceptance, and openness (Lengacher et al., 2014). MBSR meditative practice is effective in reducing stressful psychological and physical symptoms or perceptions. It is an intervention that emphasizes optimism and positive emotions to enhance happiness, improve resilience, and boost well-being more effectively than reducing negative behaviors (MacLeod et al., 2016).

MBSR is effective in stress management and symptom control with certain chronic conditions including some cancers (Lengacher et al., 2015). Mindfulness training helps people learn to self-regulate awareness, identify their feelings, and implement effective changes. People use cognitive exercises and subjective experiences to process images or feelings (van den Hurk et al., 2015). These feelings are then evaluated as pleasant or unpleasant. A patient learns strategies to enhance the pleasant experiences and replace the unpleasant experiences. MBSR can be used in a variety of settings. For example, MBSR can help people control their stress response to illnesses and treatments, allow employees to manage job-related stress, and help students manage classroom stress and test anxiety.

Assertiveness Training. Assertiveness training teaches individuals to communicate effectively regarding their needs and desires. The ability to resolve conflict with others through assertiveness training reduces stress. Teaching assertiveness in a group setting increases the benefits of the experience because the participants can see the how people in the group interact with one another.

Stress Management in the Workplace. Dealing with stress in the workplace as a health care provider requires a different approach for stress management. Rapid changes in health care systems and technology, organizational restructuring, ability to retain qualified staff, and changing regulatory demands place stress on nurses. Additional causes of job stress include patient acuity levels, particular job assignments, difficult schedules, shift work, fear of failure, and inadequate support services. Compassion fatigue occurs as a result of chronic stress and is associated with the human service professions (Hunsaker et al., 2015; Potter et al., 2013).

It is important that nurses participate in self-care practices (Box 26.7). Some settings such as oncology put nurses at a higher risk for experiencing compassion fatigue because nurses see patients frequently return for care as their clinical conditions deteriorate. Recently researchers found that in other high-stress clinical settings such as critical care, trauma, and emergency departments, resilience training and clinical debriefing improved nurses' abilities to manage stress, thus reducing burnout and nursing staff turnover (Hunsaker et al., 2015; Ianello and Balzarotti, 2014; Mealer et al., 2014). Shift work and changes in schedule also contribute to work-related stress. Allowing nurses to self-schedule has been shown to

BOX 26.7 **EVIDENCE-BASED PRACTICE**

PICO Question: Does resilience training for managing workplace stress improve nurse job satisfaction?

SUMMARY OF EVIDENCE

Nurses in all health care settings need to cope with high patient acuity rates and short staffing. These factors are work-related stressors (Kennedy et al., 2014). Other factors such as control of work assignment, lateral violence, leadership structure, and empowerment also create work-related stress. The presence of resiliency, or stress resistance, was found to be the strongest predictor of likelihood of staying in a nursing position. Stress resiliency often contributes to a sense of empowerment and job satisfaction (Mealer et al., 2014).

Traumatic work stress occurs in high-acuity settings such as emergency departments and critical care units and areas where nurses and patients develop long-term relationships such as oncology units (de Boer et al., 2013; Perez et al., 2015). Compared with nurses experiencing adverse levels of stress, nurses who are highly resistant to stress typically have good social networks, are more optimistic, and have good role models (Mealer et al., 2014). Nurses are more resistant to workplace stress and are more likely to continue working as nurses when they have friends and loved ones with whom they can talk, have a sense of spiritual connection, and are more optimistic (Perez et al., 2015).

APPLICATION TO NURSING PRACTICE

- Learn stress reduction techniques that are appropriate for the health care environment and ones that can be used during working hours (Perez et al., 2015).
- Assess support systems, coping mechanisms, and strategies to identify ways to help deal with stress positively.
- Consider joining a support group of other nurses to help discuss strategies for dealing with workplace stress (Perez et al., 2015).
- Work with staff and administration to provide resiliency and mindfulness training to help improve work-related stressors (Mealer et al., 2014; Raab, 2014).
- Have a confidant with whom you can talk and share your difficult patient care experiences.

provide some autonomy and choice in scheduling, which often reduces job-related stress, improves sleep quality, and improves collaboration and teamwork (Nguyen-Rodriguez et al., 2015).

If you recognize feelings of compassion fatigue, learn how to identify perceived threats that are sources of stress (e.g., angry co-worker, added patient assignment, sense of not getting work done) and practice relaxation when you perceive them (Edward et al., 2014). Being able to relax at a time of perceived threat helps to switch off sympathetic dominance and allows you to think more clearly with purpose. In addition, identify the limits and scope of your responsibilities at work. Recognize what you can and cannot control and try to separate your work from your home life. Engage in activity that is creative and active so that the stress of work will not intrude your thinking. Strengthening friendships outside of the workplace, socially finding ways for personal "recharging" of emotional energy, and spending off-duty hours in interesting activities all help reduce burnout.

Acute Care

Crisis Intervention. When stress overwhelms a person's usual coping mechanisms and demands mobilization of all available resources, the stress becomes a crisis. **Crisis intervention** is different from counseling. It requires excellent nurse-patient communication skills (see Chapter 11). Crisis intervention provides more direction than brief psychotherapy or counseling. It focuses on how intensely a patient views his or her problems as intolerable or how emotionally unstable a patient is. Knowledgeable members of the interdisciplinary health care team are able to initiate crisis intervention (Varcarolis, 2017).

Crisis intervention begins with defining the problem, ensuring patient safety, and providing support. First determine that a patient is safe and not at risk for injury to self or others. Then help the patient examine alternatives, make plans, and obtain a commitment to positive action. Ideally these last three steps are completed collaboratively with a patient, but a patient in crisis may be unable to participate actively and may need a very directive approach or a crisis interventionist.

When using crisis intervention, help a person become aware of present feelings such as anger, grief, guilt, or tension. Using open-ended questions elicits feelings and responses with deeper meaning. Closed-ended questions provide important information early in the crisis intervention process. Focus on the specific problem and help a patient avoid all-encompassing, catastrophic interpretations. You may need to provide guidance and direction for obtaining resources and assistance. Provide an atmosphere of calm acceptance, yet be aware of situations that require a direct approach to ensure the safety of the patient. Capitalize on a patient's strengths when helping patients identify coping strategies, such as previous hobbies, an interest in music or sports, or religious faith (Krageloph et al., 2015).

Restorative and Continuing Care. A person under stress recovers when the stress disappears or coping strategies succeed. However, a person who experienced a crisis has changed, and the effects sometimes last for years or for the rest of the person's life. In the final stage of adapting to a crisis, a patient acknowledges the long-term implications of the crisis. If a person successfully copes with a crisis and its consequences, he or she becomes more mature and healthy. When a person has recovered from a stressful situation, teach him or her stress-management skills to reduce the number and intensity of the stress responses in future situations.

■ ■ ■ EVALUATION

Patient Outcomes. Evaluation of the goals and expected outcomes of care is important in determining the effectiveness of your nursing interventions and if the patient is coping well

BOX 26.8   EVALUATION

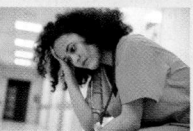

Copyright © gpointstudio/iStock/ Thinkstock.

Three weeks after their initial discussion, Rachael makes her routine appointment at the employee health office to see Becky. Becky is relieved to see that Rachael is less anxious and looking better. Her previously assessed nervous behaviors are no longer present. Feeling less drained, Rachael is making progress on developing professional and personal boundaries. Her neighbors and friends know about her situation and provide casseroles for the family to eat. Rachael accepts this help by reminding herself that it is only temporary. She is encouraged by the insight she gets from individual and group counseling sessions. Although the Bennett family has not yet found full resolution for their stress, they are making progress toward achievable, short-term goals.

DOCUMENTATION NOTE

"Reports that she feels 'more hopeful.' Blood pressure is 140/82 mm Hg, and pulse is 88 beats/min. Weight increased by 3 lb since her last visit, and this week began sleeping through the night. States is going with husband to a family support group meeting held every week at the rehabilitation facility."

with the identified stress. Assess a patient's perception of the effectiveness of the plan. Review the behaviorally stated, measurable goals, and evaluate whether or not the patient has met the criteria for success as stated in the outcomes. To evaluate a patient experiencing stress, observe patient behaviors, and talk with the patient and family, if appropriate (Box 26.8).

Remember that coping with stress takes time. If the nursing interventions have not been effective in helping the patient achieve targeted goals, reevaluate the strategies implemented and revise the plan of care in consideration of the patient's current health status. Include the patient during any revision. Refer your patient to appropriate resources if you are in a setting in which your contact with a patient ends before achieving goals or resolution so as not to delay or interrupt progress.

Patient Expectations. Maintain ongoing communication with patients regarding the plan of care. Patients under severe stress often experience feelings of powerlessness, vulnerability, and loss of control. Actively involve patients and families in problem identification (assessment), prioritizing, goal setting, problem solving, and evaluation. Involving patients in these processes gives them an opportunity to direct their energy in a positive way and moves them toward taking greater responsibility for health maintenance and promotion.

Engage your patient as a partner in his or her health care to set the stage for open communication. This gives the patient a sense of control and begins to promote independence, which are both crucial to the patient's successful resolution of the situation. A patient-centered environment gives the patient the opportunity to give important feedback to you

about interventions that are successful and data to support the achievement of outcomes. Patient feedback also helps you better understand why some interventions fail to meet the established goals.

KEY POINTS

- The general adaptation syndrome (GAS), an immediate physiological response to stress, involves the autonomic nervous system and the endocrine system.
- When stress is perceived by the sensory system, impulses to the hypothalamus activate one of two systems: the hypothalamic-pituitary-adrenal (HPA) axis and the sympathetic nervous system (SNS).
- Physiological responses to stress also include immunological changes.
- Stress makes people ill as a result of both increased levels of powerful hormones such as cortisol that change bodily processes and coping choices that are unhealthy such as not getting enough rest or a proper diet or use of tobacco, alcohol, or caffeine.
- Posttraumatic stress disorder begins when a person experiences, witnesses, or is confronted with a traumatic event and responds with intense fear or helplessness. There are four types of symptoms of PTSD: reliving the event, avoiding situations that remind the person of the event, having more negative beliefs and feelings about oneself or the world, and hyperarousal.
- Compassion fatigue is a state of burnout and secondary traumatic stress that can overwhelm health care providers and result in feelings of hopelessness, inadequacy, and anxiety.
- A person experiences psychological stress only if he or she evaluates the event or circumstance as a personal threat; this is called *primary appraisal.*
- Stress includes work stress, family stress, chronic stress, acute stress, daily hassles, trauma, and crisis.
- Potential stressors and coping mechanisms vary across the life span, from childhood through adolescence, adulthood, and old age and from one culture to another.
- Coping, a process that constantly changes to manage demands on a person's resources, means making an effort to manage psychological stress.
- Resiliency is an important coping resource that you can promote in patients by suggesting general ways for them to prepare for challenges before they occur.
- Unmanaged workplace stress affects nurses' job satisfaction and patient satisfaction.

REFLECTIVE LEARNING

- Consider a recent new clinical experience and list the personal stressors you faced.
- Think about caring for a patient from a different culture. What information did you need to have about yourself and your patient's culture to fully understand how the patient would perceive a stressor?

- Nursing is a rigorous academic program that is often very stressful. Identify three long-term strategies that you can use to deal with academic stress.

REVIEW QUESTIONS

1. Your co-worker tells you that she "no longer cares about her patients." You conclude that she is experiencing compassion fatigue. Which other signs and symptoms do you expect to find? (Select all that apply.)
   1. Hopelessness
   2. Flashbacks
   3. Anxiety
   4. Fatigue
   5. Loss of pleasure in activities
   6. Depression
2. Which signs and symptoms do you expect to assess in a patient who is in the alarm stage of the neuroendocrine stress response? (Select all that apply.)
   1. Increased heart rate
   2. Return of vital signs toward baseline
   3. Dilated pupils
   4. Decreased hormone levels
   5. Increased respirations
   6. An irregular pulse and atrial fibrillation
3. A young father is in the primary care clinic for a routine appointment for management of his type 2 diabetes. During the assessment he tells you that his wife suddenly left him. They have two children. His wife left without the children, so he is now a single parent to two school-aged children 8 and 10 years of age. You suspect that this man is experiencing a developmental crisis. Which of the following questions are appropriate for providing information about the impact of this crisis? (Select all that apply.)
   1. Who can you talk to on a routine basis?
   2. What do you do when you feel lonely?
   3. Is there any change in your diabetes?
   4. I know this must be hard for you. Let me tell you what might help.
   5. Tell me about any changes you have experienced in lifestyle habits, such as sleeping, eating, smoking, and drinking.

4. After a health care provider has informed a patient that he has colon cancer, a nurse enters the room and finds the patient gazing out the window in thought. Which of the following are appropriate responses or nursing actions at this time? (Select all that apply.)
   1. "I know another patient whose colon cancer was cured by surgery."
   2. Straighten the patient's bed and room
   3. "Have you thought about how you are going to tell your family?"
   4. "Would you like for me to sit down with you for a few minutes so you can talk about this?"
   5. Sit quietly with the patient
   6. Leave the patient alone to allow him time to think
5. A nurse experiencing work-related stress should take which of the following actions first?
   1. Determine the particular cause of the workplace stress for him or her
   2. Begin a walking-based exercise program
   3. Use relaxation strategies
   4. Increase assertiveness and set realistic goals

evolve

Additional Review Questions, as well as rationales for all Review Questions, can be found on the Evolve website.

1. 1, 3, 4, 5; 2. 1, 3, 5; 3. 1, 2, 5; 4. 4, 5; 5. 3.

REFERENCES

Afshar H, et al: The association of personality traits and coping styles according to stress levels, *J Res Med Sci* 20:353, 2015.

Akerstedt T, et al: Do sleep, stress, and illness explain daily variations in fatigue? A prospective study, *J Psychosom Res* 76:280, 2014.

Alschuler L: The HPA axis, *Integrative Therapeutics*, 2016. http://www .integrativepro.com/Resources/ Integrative-Blog/2016/The-HPA-Axis.

American Psychological Association (APA): *The road to resilience*, 2015. http://www.apa.org/helpcenter/ road-resilience.aspx.

Christie W, Jones S: Lateral violence in nursing and the theory of the nurse as wounded healer, *Online J Issues Nurs* 19(1):2013.

de Boer J, et al: Critical incidents among intensive care unit nurses and their need for support: explorative interviews, *Brit Assoc Crit Care Unit* 19(4):166, 2013.

Doron J, et al: Coping profiles, perceived stress and health-related behaviors: a cluster analysis approach, *Health Promot Int* 30:88, 2014.

Edward K, et al: Nursing and aggression in the work place: a systematic review, *Br J Nurs* 23(12):653, 2014.

Embree JL, White AH: Concept analysis nurse-to-nurse lateral violence, *Nurs Forum* 45(3):1266, 2010.

Garcia DS: Evaluation of three behavioral theories for application in health promotion strategies for women, *Adv Nurs Sci* 34(2):165, 2016.

Giger J: *Transcultural nursing*, ed 7, St Louis, 2016, Mosby.

Gillespie GL, Gates DM: Using proactive coping to manage the stress of trauma patient care, *J Trauma Nurs* 20:44, 2013.

Harvard Medical School: Understanding the stress response, *Harvard Health Publications*, 2016. http://www.health.harvard.edu/staying-healthy/understanding-the-stress-response.

Huether SE, McCance KL: *Understanding pathophysiology*, ed 6, St Louis, 2017, Mosby.

Hunsaker S, et al: Factors that influence the development of compassion fatigue, burnout, and compassion satisfaction in emergency department nurses, *J Nurs Scholarsh* 47(2):186, 2015.

Ianello P, Balzarotti S: Stress and coping strategies in the emergency room, *Emerg Care J* 10:72, 2014.

Janowski K, et al: Emotional control, styles of coping with stress and acceptance of illness among patients suffering from chronic somatic disease, *Stress Health* 30:34, 2014.

Kennedy F, et al: Work stress and cancer researchers: an exploration of challenges, experiences, and training needs of UK cancer researchers, *Eur J Cancer Care (Engl)* 23:462, 2014.

Krageloph CU, et al: Spirituality quality of life and spiritual coping: evidence for a two-factor structure of the WHOQOl spirituality, religiousness, and personal belief module, *Health Qual Life Outcomes* 13:26, 2015.

Lengacher CA, et al: Mindfulness based stress reduction (MBSR (BC)) in breast cancer: evaluating fear of recurrence (FOR) as a mediator of psychological and physical symptoms in a randomized control trial (RCT), *J Behav Med* 37:185, 2014.

Lengacher CA, et al: The effects of mindfulness-based stress reduction on objective and subjective parameters in women with breast cancer: a randomized controlled study, *Psychooncology* 24:424, 2015.

Lin SH, et al: The impact of shift work on nurses' job stress, sleep quality and self-perceived health status, *J Nurs Manag* 22:604, 2014.

MacLeod S, et al: The impact of resilience among older adults, *Geriatric Nurs* 37(4):266, 2016.

Mayo Clinic: *Suicide and suicidal thoughts. Suicide: What to do when someone is suicidal*, 2015. http://www.mayoclinic.org/diseases-conditions/suicide/in-depth/suicide/art-20044707.

Mayo Clinic: *Chronic stress puts your health at risk*, 2016. http://www.mayoclinic.org/healthy-lifestyle/stress-management/in-depth/stress/art-20046037.

Mealer M, et al: A qualitative study of resilience and posttraumatic stress disorder in United States ICU nurses, *Intensive Care Med* 38:1445, 2014.

Miller DB, O'Callaghan JP: Neuroendocrine aspects of the response to stress, *Metabolism* 51(6 Suppl 1):5, 2002.

Moreira S, et al: Combined exercise circuit session acutely attenuates stress-induced blood pressure reactivity in health adults, *Braz J Phys Ther* 18:38, 2014.

Najimi A, et al: Causes of job stress in nurses: a cross-sectional study, *Iran J Nurs Midwifery Res* 17(4):301, 2012.

Neuman B, Fawcett J: *The Neuman systems model*, ed 5, Upper Saddle River, NJ, 2010, Pearson.

Nguyen-Rodriguez ST, et al: Coping mediates the effects of depressive symptoms on sleep problems, *Am J Health Behav* 39(2):183, 2015.

Nielson MB, Knardahl S: Coping strategies: a prospective study of patterns, stability, and relationships with physiological distress, *Scand J Psychol* 55:142, 2014.

O'Driscoll MP: Coping with stress: a challenge for theory, research, and practice, *Stress Health* 29:89, 2013.

Parelkar P, et al: Stress coping and changes in health behavior among cancer survivors: a report from the American Cancer Society's study of cancer survivors II (SCS-II), *J Psychosoc Oncol* 31:136, 2015.

Pender N: *Health promotion model*, 2016. http://www.nursing-theory.org/theories-and-models/pender-health-promotion-model.php.

Pender N, Murdaugh CL: *Health promotion in nursing practice*, ed 7, Upper Saddle River, NJ, 2015, Pearson.

Perez GK, et al: Promoting resiliency among palliative care clinicians: stressors, coping strategies, and training needs, *J Palliat Med* 18(4):332, 2015.

Potter P, et al: Evaluation of a compassion fatigue resiliency program for oncology nurses, *Oncol Nurs Forum* 40(2):180, 2013.

Raab K: Mindfulness, self-compassion, and empathy among health care professionals: a review of the literature, *J Health Care Chaplain* 20:95, 2014.

Rayens MK, Reed DB: Predictors of depressive symptoms in older rural couples: the impact of work, stress, and health, *J Rural Health* 30:59, 2014.

Sabo B: Reflecting on the concept of compassion fatigue, *Online J Issues Nurs* 16(1):1, 2011.

Selye H: History of the stress concept. In Goldberger L, Breznitz S, editors: *Handbook of stress: theoretical and clinical aspects*, ed 2, New York, 1993, Free Press.

Smith SM, Vale WW: The role of the hypothalamic-pituitary-adrenal axis in neuroendocrine response to stress, *Dialogues Clin Neurosci* 8(4):383, 2006.

Sousa P, et al: Measuring heal promoting behaviors: cross cultural validation of the Health-Promotion Lifestyle Profile-II, *Int J Nurs Knowl* 26(2): 54, 2015.

Stevens D, et al: Posttraumatic stress disorder increases risk for suicide attempt in adults with recurrent major depression, *Depress Anxiety* 30:940, 2013.

Touhy TH, Jett KF: *Ebersole and Hess' gerontological nursing & healthy aging*, ed 4, St Louis, 2014, Mosby.

Turner SB, Kaylor SD: Neuman systems model as a conceptual framework for nurse resilience, *Nurs Sci Q* 28(3):213, 2015.

U.S. Department of Veterans Affairs, National Center for PTSD: *What is PTSD?* 2016. https://www.ptsd.va.gov/public/ptsd-overview/basics/what-is-ptsd.asp.

Valek RM, et al: Psychological factors associated with weight loss maintenance. Theory-driven practice for nurse practitioners, *Nurs Sci Q* 28(2):129, 2015.

van den Hurk DG, et al: Mindfulness-based stress reduction for lung cancer patients and their partners: results of a mixed methods pilot study, *Palliat Med* 29:652, 2015.

Varcarolis EM: *Essentials of psychiatric mental health nursing*, ed 3, St Louis, 2017, Elsevier.

Vitelli R: Grief, loneliness and losing a spouse, *Psychology Today*, March 16, 2015. https://www.psychologytoday.com/blog/media-spotlight/201503/grief-loneliness-and-losing-spouse.

Waude A: General adaptation syndrome, *Psychologist World*, 2016. https://www.psychologistworld.com/stress/general-adaptation-syndrome.

evolve MEDIA RESOURCES

http://evolve.elsevier.com/Potter/essentials
- Audio Glossary
- QSEN Activity and Review Questions Answers and Rationales

OBJECTIVES

- Discuss five categories of loss.
- Review grief and loss theories.
- Compare and contrast types of grief.
- Discuss variables that influence a person's response to grief.
- Identify assessment parameters in a patient experiencing loss and grief.
- Identify nursing interventions for helping patients cope with loss, death, and grief.
- Develop a care plan for a patient, family caregivers, and family members experiencing loss and grief.
- Discuss principles of palliative and hospice care.
- Identify ways to educate and involve family caregivers in providing palliative care.
- List the steps in caring for a body after death.
- Discuss the role of the nurse when caring for patients at the end of life.

KEY TERMS

acceptance, p. 684
actual loss, p. 683
anger, p. 684
anticipatory grief, p. 685
autopsy, p. 698
bargaining, p. 684
bereavement, p. 684
complicated grief, p. 685
denial, p. 684
depression, p. 684

disenfranchised grief, p. 685
disorganization and despair, p. 684
grief, p. 684
hope, p. 694
hospice care, p. 693
maturational losses, p. 683
mourning, p. 684
necessary losses, p. 683
normal or uncomplicated grief, p. 685
numbing, p. 684

palliative care, p. 691
perceived loss, p. 683
postmortem care, p. 698
reorganization, p. 684
reminiscence, p. 685
resilience, p. 685
situational loss, p. 683
yearning and searching, p. 684

Grief and loss affect a person's health physically, psychologically, socially, and spiritually. Patients at the end of life need knowledge, compassion, and expert nursing care as they live with illnesses that cannot be cured and come to the end of their lives. As a result, care at the end of life is enhanced when nurses provide holistic, patient-centered and family-centered care (Dobrina et al., 2016).

Situations that involve loss and grief can also bring out stress, fear, and uncertainty in caregivers (Coelho et al., 2015). Fortunately nursing knowledge regarding the care of people who are grieving and dying has expanded in the last decade for patients and family caregivers (Barrere and Durkin, 2014; American Association of Colleges of Nursing [AACN], 2016).

CASE STUDY *The Kelly Family*

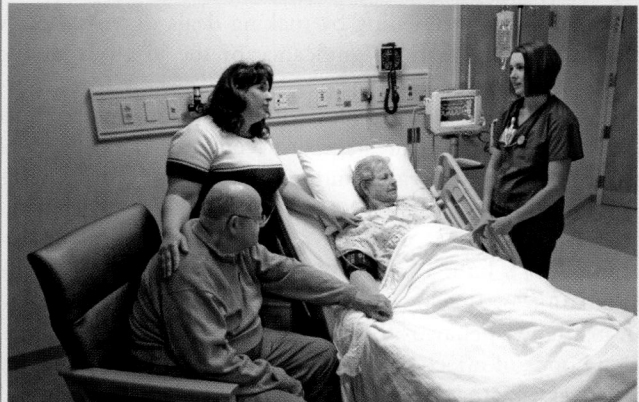

Mrs. Kelly is a 79-year-old woman who has end-stage heart disease secondary to diabetes mellitus. Her quality of life has declined greatly because of shortness of breath, anorexia, fatigue, lack of sleep, decreased strength, and poor oxygenation. She takes pain medication for severe back pain and frequently has constipation. She was admitted to the hospital 4 times in the past year for heart failure or for care of venous stasis ulcers. She is now in the intensive care unit for chest pain and heart failure. Tests indicate that her heart function is worsening. Mrs. Kelly no longer wants to be hospitalized every time her medical condition deteriorates, and she wants to go home to die. Mrs. Kelly is being evaluated for home hospice care and will temporarily receive home care.

Mrs. Kelly lives with her husband of 54 years. Her daughter, Lilly, visits her parents every day. Lilly does not agree with the plan to begin hospice care. She believes that her mother is "giving up" too soon. Mr. Kelly does not understand hospice and is not sure if he will be a good caregiver.

Nursing student Jennifer Brown will be caring for the Kelly family as she learns how to give care in the home. She has never taken care of a person at the end of life in a home setting and feels anxious about her abilities to care for Mrs. Kelly. She will be taking care of Mrs. Kelly's symptoms and physical needs and the family's grief issues.

SCIENTIFIC KNOWLEDGE BASE

Loss

Throughout our lives from birth to death we form attachments and suffer losses. We become independent from our parents, leave home to attend school, begin careers, and form new lifelong relationships. Growing up is natural and positive, yet throughout life we experience **necessary losses.** Often losses are replaced by something different or better. For example, a person leaves behind family members to begin college but makes new friends and begins a meaningful career. Other necessary losses, such as death of a loved one, challenge a person's sense of security and coping skills.

How we perceive loss depends on what we value. Our family, friends, society, culture, and faith traditions shape our priorities and help us determine what matters most in life. A person experiences loss when a meaningful object, person,

TABLE 27.1 TYPES OF LOSS

DEFINITION	IMPLICATIONS OF LOSS
Loss of external objects (e.g., misplacement, theft, destruction by nature)	Extent of grieving depends on object's value, sentiment attached to it, and its usefulness.
Loss of a known environment (e.g., moving from a neighborhood, hospitalization, a new job, moving to a long-term care facility)	Loss occurs through maturational or situational events and with injury or illness. Loneliness in an unfamiliar setting threatens self-esteem and makes grieving difficult.
Loss of a significant other (e.g., divorce; loss of a family member, friend, trusted nurse, or pet; family rifts)	Significant others meet a person's need for psychological safety, love and belonging, and self-esteem.
Loss of an aspect of self (e.g., body part, psychological or physiological function, job; financial uncertainty)	Illness, injury, or developmental changes result in a loss that causes changes in body image, self-concept, and level of independence.
Loss of life (e.g., death of family member, friend, or acquaintance; own death)	Loss of a life creates grief for those left behind. Persons facing death often fear pain and loss of control or independence.

body part or function, emotion, or idea is no longer present. There are several types of loss (Table 27.1). People experience an **actual loss** when they can no longer touch, hear, see, or have near them valued people or objects. Examples include the loss of a body part, pet, friend, life partner, or job. People feel grief when a valued object becomes worn out, lost, stolen, or destroyed by disaster. A child often grieves after losing a favorite toy. A **perceived loss** is uniquely experienced by a grieving person and is often less obvious to others. A perceived loss is very real to the person who has had the loss. For example, a person perceives that she is less loved by her parents and experiences a loss of self-esteem. Other people often misunderstand perceived losses.

People experience **maturational losses** as they go through a lifetime of normal developmental processes. For example, when a child goes to school for the first time he or she spends less time with his or her parents, leading to a change in the parent-child relationship. Grieving maturational losses help a person cope with the change. **Situational loss** occurs as a result of an unpredictable life event. A situational loss often involves multiple losses. For example, a divorce begins with the loss of a life companion but often leads to financial strain, changes in living arrangements, less contact with one's children, and loss of friends who were part of the couple's married life.

How an individual interprets the meaning of any loss and the type of loss influences how that person grieves. People respond to loss differently. For some people the loss of a possession or pet causes the same level of grief as the loss of a person. The value that people place on an absent object or changed social status influences their emotional response to the loss.

People experience multiple losses when they become ill or need to be hospitalized. They often lose their privacy, modesty, sense of safety, and control over body functions and daily routines. Chronic, debilitating illness often adds financial concerns, requires job changes, threatens independence, forces changes in lifestyle, and challenges family relationships.

Death is the ultimate loss. Although death is a part of life, its mysterious, uncertain character often produces anxiety and fear (Momtaz et al., 2015). Death ends relationships with family and friends and separates people from the physical presence of those important to them. Persons at the end of life and their caregivers often experience sorrow; uncertainty; fear; or physical and spiritual challenges throughout the dying process. Death can also lead to personal growth and a meaningful reprioritization of life. Close friends and caregivers of a dying person are reminded of their own mortality. Most people do not want to become dependent on others at the end of life, yet they do not want to die alone.

Facing death often brings out emotions such as guilt, anger, sadness, and fear. Some family members and family caregivers, fearful of the intensity of the experience, withdraw at a time when the dying person most needs their love and support. A person's basic beliefs and values, culture, and spirituality and the quality of emotional support influence the way a person and family approach dying. They need individually designed, compassionate end-of-life care.

Grief

Grief is the emotional response to a loss. People grieve in different ways, based on their experiences, cultural expectations, and spiritual beliefs (Schonfeld et al., 2015; Wienclaw, 2016) (see Chapters 21 and 22). Grief involves mourning, the conscious and unconscious behaviors associated with loss. Bereavement includes grief and mourning, the inner feelings and outward behaviors of a survivor. Many theorists describe the grief process that occurs with any loss. The following classic grief theories describe general psychological and behavioral characteristics and patterns (Harris and Winokuer, 2016). Theories provide a framework for nurses to plan nursing care for individuals experiencing grief. Grieving is an individual experience, and an individual may not go through all the steps or patterns described in grief theories (Wienclaw, 2016).

Kübler-Ross' Five Stages of Grief. Kübler-Ross' classic theory (1969) identifies five responses to loss: denial, anger, bargaining, depression, and acceptance. Individuals in the denial stage act as though nothing has changed. They cannot believe or understand that a loss has occurred. In the anger stage a person resists the loss, is angry about the situation, and sometimes becomes angry with God. During bargaining the individual postpones awareness of the loss and tries to prevent it from happening by making deals or promises. A person realizes the full significance of the loss during the depression stage. When depressed, the person feels overwhelmingly lonely or sad and withdraws from interactions with others. During the stage of acceptance the individual begins to accept the reality and inevitability of loss and looks to the future.

Bowlby's Four Phases of Mourning. Attachment, the foundation of Bowlby's four phases of mourning (1980), is an instinctive behavior that leads to the development of lifelong bonds of affection between children and their primary caregivers. In the numbing phase a person has periods of extremely intense emotion and reports feeling "stunned" or "unreal." The yearning and searching phase evokes emotional outbursts, tearful sobbing, and acute distress. To move forward people need to experience this painful phase of grief. Common physical symptoms include tightness in the chest and throat, shortness of breath, a feeling of weakness and lethargy, insomnia, and loss of appetite. During the phase of disorganization and despair an individual spends much time thinking about how and why the loss occurred. The person often expresses anger at anyone he or she believes to be responsible. Gradually this phase gives way to an acceptance that the loss is permanent. During the final phase of reorganization, the person accepts unaccustomed roles, acquires new skills, and builds new relationships.

Worden's Four Tasks of Mourning. The four tasks of mourning theory (Worden, 1982) describe how individuals help themselves through mourning and ask others for help. Although the time needed varies from person to person, moving through Worden's tasks typically takes at least 1 year.

- *Task I: Accept the reality of the loss.* People experience a period of disbelief and surprise that a loss has happened, even when a death is expected. In this phase people realize that a person or object is gone and will not return.
- *Task II: Work through the pain of grief.* It is impossible to experience a loss without some degree of emotional pain. Individuals who deny or suppress the pain often prolong their grief.
- *Task III: Adjust to the environment in which the deceased is missing.* A person does not realize the full impact of a loss for at least 3 months. After the first few weeks after a death, visitors and friends become less attentive, and a person experiences the full impact of the loss. Adjustment happens as a person takes on roles formerly filled by the deceased and participates in new activities.
- *Task IV: Emotionally relocate the deceased and move on with life.* People who move on with life do not forget the deceased or devalue the relationship but begin the difficult task of giving the deceased a less central place in their emotional life. Eventually a person is able to love other people without loving the deceased person less.

Rando's R Process Model. Rando's model of mourning (1993) is specific to western society. Mourning is an action-oriented process involving recognizing the loss, reacting to the pain of separation, reminiscence, relinquishing old attachments, and readjusting to life after loss. Reminiscence is an important activity in grief and mourning. In **reminiscence** a person recollects and reexperiences the deceased and the relationship by mentally or verbally reliving and remembering the person and past experiences.

Postmodern Grief Theories. The phase and task theories described in the previous paragraphs often have limited empirical evidence and may not consider cultural differences (Harris and Winokuer, 2016). Recent studies about grief focus on the multiple ways that people react to loss based on their personal, cultural, and social circumstances. Research suggests that people do not grieve in predictable, linear stages, and they do not necessarily complete the grieving tasks (Hall, 2014). Instead they move back and forth between stages, experience phases in an overlapping manner, or do not exhibit typical emotions (e.g., depression or anger) or grief behaviors. People rarely "get over" a significant loss but instead learn to live with loss. They can experience distress associated with the loss for a lifetime. People who demonstrate **resilience** accept their loss over time and return to their preloss level of functioning. Because people experience grief differently, you need to listen as people tell their stories and engage them as their story unfolds (Harris and Winokuer, 2016).

Theories of loss, death, grief, or mourning help you understand common shared feelings and behaviors. Use these theories to develop individualized interventions based on a patient's experiences.

Types of Grief

Normal Grief. **Normal or uncomplicated grief** consists of commonly expected emotional and behavioral reactions to a loss (e.g., resentment, sorrow, anger, crying, loneliness, temporary withdrawal from activities). When persons feel supported and valued as they grieve, they often come to view the experience later as growth producing and positive.

Anticipatory Grief. The process of "letting go" before an actual loss or death has occurred is called **anticipatory grief.** For example, after a person and family members accept the reality of a terminal diagnosis, they begin saying good-bye and complete life affairs before death occurs. After a prolonged dying process a patient's family members often do not respond with shock and disbelief at the time of death, and feelings of sadness mingle with some relief that the suffering is over. There are risks associated with anticipatory grieving. On one hand, some family members begin withdrawing emotionally from the patient as a self-protective mechanism, leaving the patient with less support as death approaches. On the other hand, if a person thought to be near death survives longer than anticipated, others can have difficulty reconnecting or feel resentful that the stressors associated with anticipating a death continue.

Complicated Grief. **Complicated grief** happens when a person has difficulty progressing through the loss experience. The person does not accept the reality of the loss, and the intense feelings associated with acute grief do not go away (Sierra Hernandez et al., 2016). A person experiencing complicated grief feels strain in relationships and finds it hard to go forward in life. Characteristics of complicated grief include intense yearning for the loss; intrusive thoughts of the death; and disturbing emotions of anger, avoidance, or disbelief (Guldin, 2014; Waller et al., 2016).

Disenfranchised Grief. Individuals experience disenfranchised grief when they cannot openly acknowledge a loss or receive full social support from others. This type of grieving is difficult for others to understand. **Disenfranchised grief** occurs in situations in which others view a person's loss as insignificant or invalid. For example, a grieving woman does not experience support from her parents when experiencing the loss of her ex-husband. People often experience disenfranchised grief when a loss is deeply private or secretly experienced (e.g., early miscarriage or death of a family member as a result of alcoholism).

NURSING KNOWLEDGE BASE

Nurses care for people who have experienced all types of losses and who express their grief in different ways. You use interventions supported by research and evidence-based practice to help patients during difficult life transitions. Nurses need knowledge of the multiple factors that influence a person's response to loss and grief.

Factors Influencing Loss and Grief

Human Development. A person's age and stage of development affect the ability to understand loss (see Chapter 23). Expressions of grief evolve as individuals mature. For example, toddlers cannot understand the permanence of death but feel anxiety over loss of objects and separation from parents. Although school-age children are able to understand the significance of loss more completely, they see their loss as a challenge to their emerging identity or self-concept. Adolescents do understand the significance of loss. For some adolescents, coping with the loss of a parent or sibling is often difficult. Some adolescents have problems with school, withdraw from family and/or friends, or increase risk-taking behaviors. Young adults, who are just beginning their independent lives, find the loss of a parent or sibling life-changing. Young adulthood is a time when adult relationships with parents or siblings begin, and they grieve for the loss of the past and new relationship. Middle-age adults often use grief experiences to reexamine or reprioritize their lives. Older adults anticipate grief as they encounter declining physical function or life opportunities, give up employment or social status, or lose loved ones.

Psychological Perspectives of Grief and Loss. Individuals respond to loss by using their usual coping strategies. Sometimes when people experience multiple losses or lose something of great significance, their usual coping strategies are inadequate. At the end of life people often find new coping mechanisms and new resources to maintain control and stability (Rodrigo, 2014; Bell Meisenhelder et al., 2016) (see Chapter 26).

Socioeconomic Status.
Socioeconomic status influences access to resources and support for coping with loss. Generally people feel greater burden from a loss when they lack financial, educational, or occupational resources. For example, a person with limited financial resources is unable to replace a home lost in a fire or afford the medical care needed to manage a newly diagnosed disease.

Nature of Personal Relationships.
If you gain information about the quality and meaning of a relationship that a person had with the deceased, you will better understand a person's grief. If the two people were close and well-connected, the surviving person often finds it very difficult to cope with the loss. If there was conflict or abuse in the relationship, the survivor often feels guilt, remorse, regret, or relief.

Nature of the Loss.
The visibility of a loss influences the amount of support a person receives. For example, a family who loses a home in a tornado gets strong support from the community, whereas a family in the same community who loses an early-term pregnancy experiences less support. Many people empathize with the first very public loss. In the case of a private loss, fewer people know about it or appreciate its significance. People respond differently to sudden, unexpected, or stigmatized deaths (e.g., suicide) than to anticipated or seemingly inevitable losses. Individuals who lose a family member from suicide often express guilt and self-blame for not intervening before the death (Honeycutt and Praetorius, 2016).

Culture and Ethnicity.
Patient-centered, culturally competent care focuses on respecting individual differences including cultural and religious responses to grief and loss (Box 27.1). Cultural belief systems provide the structures and interpretations that people need to cope with change, loss, illness, or death. For example, in western societies many people grieve privately and restrain their emotions. In other cultures, it is acceptable to have public demonstrations of grief that communicate the significance of their loss to others. Although members of a cultural or religious group often share similar beliefs, each person still responds in his or her own unique way. Gain knowledge and appreciation of values and beliefs as they apply to each individual's culture (Schonfeld et al., 2015).

⊕ BOX 27.1 PATIENT-CENTERED CARE

Cultural awareness is essential to patient-centered care. Awareness includes a recognition of patient and family cultural preferences and practices along with self-awareness of one's own culture. An awareness of biases and prejudices inherent in your own culture enhances your ability as a nurse to be more responsive to others (Lonneman, 2015). People across the world rely on culturally specific rituals and mourning practices to achieve a sense of acceptance and inner peace and participate in socially accepted expressions of grief. One's culture greatly influences behaviors and rituals expected at the time of loss and death. However, all individuals in a culture will not react the same to loss and grief (Wienclaw, 2016). Institutional guidelines and end-of-life care procedures should provide standards based on compassion, maintaining privacy and dignity, and respect for all patients', family caregivers', and family members' cultural beliefs and practices. Expert end-of-life care allows time for patients and their families to make private and public preparations and complete unfinished communication. Understanding the uniqueness of cultural expectations at the end of life helps you know what questions to ask.

The National Consensus Project for Quality Palliative Care Clinical Practice Guidelines for Quality Palliative Care (Dahlin, 2013) recommends culturally sensitive care to include:

- Respect of the patient's and family's cultural preferences and practices that influence the reaction to loss, grief, and death.
- Implementation of a culturally relevant plan of care that identifies the needs and strengths of the individual's cultural preferences and practices.

- Communication in a language that is understood by the patient, family caregiver, and family members. If the patient or family does not understand the language used by the health care providers, professional interpreter services are recommended.
- Referrals to community services that are responsive to cultural needs such as dietary restrictions or prayer services.

The availability of multilingual clinical staff, written material in the patient's and family's preferred language, and accessibility of professional interpreter services demonstrate a commitment to culturally sensitive care (Mixer et al., 2015).

IMPLICATIONS FOR PRACTICE
- Self-reflection about one's cultural preferences, practices, biases, and prejudices can enhance the nurse's cultural awareness (Lonneman, 2015).
- Assess patient and family cultural preferences and practices for care at the end of life.
- Implement a culturally sensitive plan of care that supports end-of-life and postmortem care.
- Access professional interpreter services to communicate in the patient's and family's preferred language.
- Ensure that end-of-life and postmortem care is culturally sensitive by communicating the patient's and family's preferences to the health care team.
- Assure patient and family that their postmortem care will be consistent with their cultural practices as communicated to the health care team.

Spiritual Beliefs. People use their faith in a higher power, a community of friends, their sources of hope and meaning in life, and religious rituals and practices to cope with life challenges and grief (Finocchiaro, 2016; Van Hook, 2016) (see Chapter 22). Regardless of their beliefs, all people have a need for love, meaning, and purpose. A loss often provokes questions related to spiritual values and the meaning of life. Spirituality may help patients buffer the stress of chronic illness and other life challenges (Rafferty et al., 2015; Van Hook, 2016).

CRITICAL THINKING

Synthesis

Patient care requires you to apply what you know about a patient, your knowledge base, experience, and critical thinking attitudes and standards. Your synthesis of this information allows you to make sound decisions as you apply the nursing process. Critical thinking synthesis involves combining all available information to obtain a clear picture of the approach needed to provide patient-centered care. You apply elements of critical thinking whenever you perform the nursing process with patients. Each patient for whom you care has different developmental, spiritual, and cultural backgrounds. Consider all these dimensions when you apply critical thinking in developing a comprehensive and holistic plan of care (Box 27.2).

Knowledge. Knowledge of loss and grief theories helps you understand a patient's unique responses to grief, loss, and death. Applying knowledge of therapeutic communication principles (see Chapter 11) allows you to have helpful discussions with patients and family caregivers to better understand their experience and perspectives. When loss is related to a particular disease or illness, knowledge about the disease process helps you design educational interventions and offer a realistic description of what to expect. Understanding cultural and religious diversity allows you to individualize your approach. Finally, principles of caring (see Chapter 20) and family dynamics (see Chapter 25) enable you to provide inclusive, compassionate care.

Experience. Most of us have experienced some type of loss. Personal experience with loss prepares you to understand and empathize with others going through difficult times. You need to reflect on your own mortality as well. Each time you care for a patient or family member who is coping with grief, loss, or death, you gain valuable life wisdom and experience. Reflect on these experiences and apply what you have learned when caring for other patients.

Attitudes. Critical thinking attitudes of risk taking, self-confidence, and humility help you make accurate assessments and decisions about your patients (see Chapter 8). Many nurses become anxious when caring for dying patients or people coping with grief and loss. Confidence helps you understand that, even if there is nothing you can do or say to change the situation, patients need your compassionate presence and a personal connection. Confidence helps you accept the responsibility to remain present even in difficult situations. By silently sharing a moment of sadness with a patient or family caregiver, you communicate caring and send the message that you respect and accept their feelings in the moment. You cannot know everything there is to know about a patient's loss. Humility helps you put aside personal assumptions about how the patient interprets loss to better hear his or her concerns and remain present with the patient in his or her grief or loss (Harris and Winokuer, 2016).

Standards. The use of appropriate standards guides you during the assessment phase of the nursing process so that you gather the data most pertinent to the patient's situation. Professional standards including bioethical principles (see Chapter 6), the *Dying Person's Bill of Rights* (Box 27.3) (Barbus, 1975), the End-of-Life Nursing Consortium basic and advanced curricula for end-of-life care (American

---

BOX 27.2 SYNTHESIS IN PRACTICE

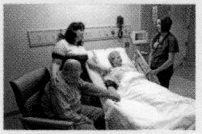

Before Jennifer meets the Kelly family for the first time, she reviews the information needed to complete a thorough assessment. She identifies the key symptoms to look for in a patient with end-stage heart disease with chronic pain and will be sensitive to any embarrassment that Mrs. Kelly feels about her constipation and decreased functional abilities. Jennifer understands that people experience grief differently, and she understands that not all members of the Kelly family agree on the plan of care.

Jennifer worries that she will be asked questions for which she has no answer. She feels more comfortable talking about heart disease than about end-of-life decisions and care. She knows that attitudes of humility and willingness to take risks will help her form helping, trusting relationships. If the family members ask her difficult questions about death or to predict what will happen, Jennifer plans to use open-ended questions to explore their concerns. She knows that she cannot "fix things" for the Kelly family, but she can assure them that they will have help. If family members share intense emotions, Jennifer will listen carefully and validate their feelings.

Jennifer will ensure that Mrs. Kelly's pain is well managed before asking about her other priorities for care. She knows that Mr. Kelly and Lilly have never given end-of-life care; therefore she plans to provide teaching for their priority concerns. She anticipates that they will want to learn how to help Mrs. Kelly conserve her energy, give medications, help with ambulation, and position her for comfort. Jennifer knows that above all she will honor patient and family preferences, culture, and religious traditions during this meaningful event in the Kelly family.

Association of Colleges of Nursing [AACN], 2016), the Hospice and Palliative Nurses Association [HPNA] standards of practice for clinical education (HPNA, 2015), and American Nurses Association [ANA] and Hospice and Palliative Nurses Association [HPNA] *Palliative Nursing: Scope and Standards of Practice* (2014) are available. The National Institute on Aging (NIA, 2015) offers guidelines for the care of older adults at the end of life.

BOX 27.3 THE DYING PERSON'S BILL OF RIGHTS

- I have the right to be treated as a living human until I die.
- I have the right to maintain a sense of hopefulness, however changing its focus may be.
- I have the right to be cared for by those who can maintain a sense of hopefulness, however changing this might be.
- I have the right to express my feelings and emotions about my approaching death in my own way.
- I have the right to participate in decisions concerning my care.
- I have the right to expect continuing medical and nursing attention even though "cure" goals must be changed to "comfort" goals.
- I have the right not to die alone.
- I have the right to be free from pain.
- I have the right to have my questions answered honestly.
- I have the right to retain my individuality and not be judged for my decisions that may be contrary to beliefs of others.
- I have the right to expect that the sanctity of the human body will be respected after death.
- I have the right to be cared for by caring, sensitive, knowledgeable people who will attempt to understand my needs and be able to gain some satisfaction in helping me face my death.

From Ferrell BR, Coyle N: An overview of palliative nursing care, *Am J Nurs* 102(5): 32, 2002. Copyright © Wolters Kluwer Health, Inc.

NURSING PROCESS

■■■ ASSESSMENT

Begin with an open heart and mind and an accepting, humble attitude as you assess a patient or family experiencing a loss (Dosser and Kennedy, 2014). The assessment process continues with all patient interactions. Be aware that any assumptions you make can interfere with the accuracy of your assessment. Do not assume that other people react to loss or grief as you do or that a particular behavior necessarily indicates grief. For example, crying expresses different feelings—grief, relief, sorrow, happiness, or gratitude. Encouraging patients to tell stories about their loved one gives them an opportunity to provide information in a natural, unstructured, and meaningful way. Remain aware of verbal and nonverbal communication as you ask questions and gather information about the way patients, family caregivers, and other family members experience their grief (Table 27.2).

Provide opportunities in a therapeutically safe environment for patients and family members to talk about their feelings with others. To maintain confidentiality and encourage conversation, talk to patients and family members separately unless they want to speak together. Listen carefully while observing responses and behaviors. Assume a neutral but interested perspective and remain alert for nonverbal cues such as facial expressions, voice tones, and avoidance of certain topics. Collaborate with other members of the health care team to complete your assessment.

Type and Stages of Grief. Most people exhibit some signs and symptoms of grief in situations of serious illness, loss, or impending death (Box 27.4). Your assessment becomes more specific as you begin to observe behaviors, listen to patients' conversations, and identify their type and/or stage of grief. Understanding grief theories helps you assess a situation accurately. For example, a patient who complains of loneliness and difficulty falling asleep may be in a yearning

---

TABLE 27.2 FOCUSED PATIENT ASSESSMENT

FACTORS TO ASSESS	QUESTIONS	PHYSICAL ASSESSMENT
Phase of grief	Tell me how you are feeling now. Validate patient's feelings: • You seem (angry/sad); tell me more about that.	Observe patient's behaviors: • Frequent sighing or crying • Withdrawn behaviors (e.g., decreased communication, silence, does not want visits) • Poor eye contact • Unwilling to talk about feelings and disagreements
Family member's response to loss	It can be very difficult to deal with these kinds of decisions. What do you think your wife is going through right now? What are *you* feeling right now? You feel guilt/sadness/regret because ...? Do you believe you could have changed what is happening?	Observe nonverbal behaviors as members of family interact: • Tone of conversation • Frequency of interaction • Detachment behaviors (e.g., changing topic, walking away) • Seeking physical closeness

BOX 27.4 SYMPTOMS OF NORMAL GRIEF

FEELINGS
- Sadness
- Anger
- Guilt or self-reproach
- Anxiety
- Loneliness
- Fatigue
- Helplessness
- Shock/numbness (lack of feeling)
- Yearning
- Relief

COGNITION (THOUGHT PATTERNS)
- Disbelief
- Confusion
- Preoccupation about the deceased
- Sense of the presence of the deceased
- Guilty thoughts
- Sense of despair

PHYSICAL SENSATIONS
- Hollowness in the stomach
- Tightness in the chest
- Tightness in the throat
- Oversensitivity to noise
- Sense of depersonalization ("Nothing seems real.")
- Feeling short of breath
- Muscle weakness
- Lack of energy
- Dry mouth

BEHAVIORS
- Sleep disturbances
- Appetite disturbances
- Dreams of the deceased
- Sighing
- Crying
- Carrying objects that belonged to the deceased

or searching phase. To gather more data, ask questions such as, "When did the loss occur?" or "How long have you been feeling this way?" Ask patients to describe their losses, how their lives have changed, and how they are adapting. Focus assessment questions on sleeping patterns, eating habits, and socializing behaviors. You understand the patient's grief better by assessing in detail the factors that influence grieving (Table 27.3).

Coping Resources. Determine which coping patterns and resources a patient typically uses to get through difficult challenges. Use open-ended questions when you want to learn more about coping patterns: "Tell me how you usually adjust to change or loss." Use direct questioning to find out if certain activities (e.g., relaxation exercises, massage, meditation, reading, or exercise) help a patient cope with stress (see Chapter 26). Include interventions patients use in your care plan. Also assess family caregivers' coping patterns and methods. If they are coping well, their care for the patient is enriched.

End-of-Life Decisions. Patients who have the capacity to make their own decisions should be encouraged to express their wishes for end-of-life care. Look for information about a patient's advance directives or medical durable power of attorney (a person who will make decisions for a patient if the patient cannot make health care decisions) in the patient's medical record (see Chapter 5). If there is no information in the record, ask if a patient has either of these legal documents and place a copy in the chart. If a person does not have an advance directive, ask the patient and/or family about their

preferences including their wishes for the use of life-sustaining measures, where the patient prefers to die, and their expectations about pain control and symptom management (Institute of Medicine [IOM], 2015; Price, 2016). If you feel uncomfortable assessing a patient's wishes, find a health care team member (e.g., social worker or spiritual care provider) who has experience with discussing sensitive, complex issues.

Older Adult Considerations. Thoroughly assess older adults who are experiencing grief and loss. Ask questions about recent relationships that they have lost, significant life events, and other stressful events that are happening at this time. Many times older adults experience several stressful events all at once. The risk for impaired grieving increases with the number of stressors being experienced simultaneously. Explore ways that an older adult has coped with loss previously, and assess the social and economic effect of the loss to help you develop appropriate, patient-centered nursing interventions that support healthy coping (Dockendorff, 2014).

Patient Expectations. A patient's perceptions, preferences, and expectations for care influence how you prioritize nursing diagnoses. Use current evidence to guide your assessment of a patient's and family members' expectations about the end of life (Box 27.5). Attend to acute, distressing symptoms before attempting to discuss a patient's care expectations. If a patient is in severe pain, he or she is less able to identify other needs. Assess patient or family caregiver expectations by asking questions such as, "What is the most important thing I could do to help you at this time?" Ask the family if they understand health care team members' roles and offer clarification if necessary. Early communication about expectations and goals provides clarity and helps prevent misunderstandings.

■ ■ ■ NURSING DIAGNOSIS

You review and interpret a patient's assessment data to cluster defining characteristics and risk factors to identify relevant nursing diagnoses. Several nursing diagnoses apply to patients who experience loss, grief, or death. In addition to diagnoses specific to grieving, you likely diagnose problems related to a patient's physical or mental states. Clustering data concerning patient or family behaviors, actual or potential losses, observed coping mechanisms, and information about the nature and meaning of loss leads to individualized nursing diagnoses. Examples of nursing diagnoses frequently identified in situations of grief, loss, and end of life include the following:

- *Death Anxiety*
- *Ineffective Denial*
- *Fear*
- *Grieving*
- *Complicated Grieving*
- *Hopelessness*
- *Social Isolation*
- *Spiritual Distress*

TABLE 27.3 ASSESSMENT OF FACTORS INFLUENCING GRIEVING

FACTORS	AREAS/SUGGESTED QUESTIONS TO EXPLORE
Hope	Explore goals, worth, adaptations to future changes. *Examples:* Tell me what you think about your treatment plan. What do you expect will happen to you? What do you most want to accomplish?
Nature of relationships	Explore functions of family, community, society. *Examples:* How have you and your husband coped during other hospitalizations? Tell me about your relationship with _____. Will it change? I see that you have lots of cards from church friends. Tell me about your church activities.
Social support system	Explore availability of family caregivers, friends, timing, family needs. *Examples:* How do other people best give you help? Tell me about the family/friends who are available to help you. Tell me about the people you talk to about your _____.
Nature of loss	Explore actual versus perceived losses; death issues; impact on roles. *Examples:* How is the loss affecting your daily life? What past experiences have you had with loss? Tell me how you usually cope with disappointment or loss.
Cultural and spiritual beliefs	Values, practices, beliefs, and attitudes are shaped by culture and spiritual beliefs. *Examples:* How would you describe your beliefs regarding death? Who makes health care decisions in your family/culture? Tell me about your family's/culture's funeral practices.
Personal life goals	Actual or perceived losses affect future decisions and options. *Examples:* What type of life changes may occur as a result of your diagnosis/loss? How does this loss change your personal goals? Tell me what you know about advance directives.

BOX 27.5 EVIDENCE-BASED PRACTICE

PICO Question: How can nurses improve their knowledge, skills, and attitude toward culturally sensitive nursing care at the end of life?

SUMMARY OF EVIDENCE
Patients and families require special care at the end of life. Assessing the patient's and family members' cultural expectations about death and dying is important to patient-centered care (Bhat et al., 2015). Identifying the spiritual, religious, life habits, and ethnic beliefs of patients and families is the cornerstone of a quality cultural assessment (Bhat et al., 2015). Nurses can ask specific questions (e.g., "Are there cultural traditions that you wish to share with us?") to gain insight into their patients' needs. It is also important to ask questions about where patients wish to die and help patients and family caregivers make appropriate plans for the end of life. Assessment tools can reduce cultural bias. For example, the Hope tool minimizes cultural biases about spirituality by asking the patient and family members about their "source of hope, strength, comfort and peace" (Blaber et al., 2015). End-of-life care improves when nurses participate in specialized nursing education about patients' and family members' cultural needs. Nurses and nursing assistants who participated in an educational program about end-of-life care reported improved awareness and sensitivity toward their patient's and family's culture (Mager and Lange, 2016). Web-based education is used to strengthen nursing care of dying patients and their families. Nurses self-reported improved cultural competency after participating in three Internet learning modules about best practices in end-of-life care (Bhat et al., 2015). Nurses facilitate interdisciplinary interventions by identifying patients who have cultural-based misconceptions about end-of-life care (Perrin and Kazanowski, 2015). Patients and family members feel supported when nurses and other health care providers communicate a consistent message to manage their symptoms (Perrin and Kazanowski, 2015).

APPLICATION TO NURSING PRACTICE
- Use a culturally sensitive tool when gathering data from the patient and family members about end-of-life care.
- Assess patient and family members' cultural expectations and goals about death and dying.
- Collaborate with other health care providers such as social workers to address misconceptions about end-of-life care.
- Engage in open conversations to help patients, family caregivers, and health care providers make death plans consistent with patient preferences.

Some patients have several nursing diagnoses. For example, if you are caring for a patient who cries often, displays anger, and reports nightmares, you have identified defining characteristics that are common with *Ineffective Coping* and *Spiritual Distress*. Look for other behaviors and symptoms to validate your selection of an accurate nursing diagnosis. Also identify the appropriate related factor for each problem-focused or health promotion diagnosis. For example, *Complicated Grieving related to loss of the ability to walk due to lower limb paralysis* requires different interventions than *Complicated Grieving related to the loss of a pregnancy*. Clarification of the related factor helps you select appropriate interventions.

■■■ PLANNING

Plan your nursing care to meet a patient's and family caregivers' holistic needs, and select interventions to alleviate symptoms as much as possible. Patient input, preferences, and priorities are of primary importance in planning end-of-life care (see Care Plan).

Goals and Outcomes. Establish realistic goals and expected outcomes. Consider the patient's available resources such as supportive family caregivers, methods for coping, spiritual beliefs, and physical energy when establishing goals of care. For example, if a patient who is terminally ill has the diagnosis of *Powerlessness related to cancer diagnosis and treatment,* a goal of "Patient will discuss expected course of disease" is realistic if the patient has accepted his diagnosis enough that he can talk about the disease without excessive anxiety. An expected outcome of "Patient participates in series of short planned teaching discussions about disease" takes into account a patient's need for short, nonthreatening sessions to reduce uncertainty and anxiety.

Goals of care for a patient dealing with loss can be long-term or short-term, depending on the nature of the loss, the patient's grief, and how long the patient has to live. Because a patient often moves back and forth between phases of grief, be prepared to revise goals and outcomes with patient input. Some nursing care goals include accommodating grief, accepting the reality of a loss, and renewing relationships.

Setting Priorities. When a patient has multiple nursing diagnoses, it is not possible to address all of them at the same time. Address the patient's most urgent physical or psychological needs first and then gather information about his or her expectations and preferences for prioritizing care. If the patient meets a high-priority goal, address other unmet needs. *For example, in the case study, Mrs. Kelly (see Care Plan) has been visited by a physical therapist and is beginning to feel more secure using a walker, but she continues to have problems with constipation. Jennifer, the nursing student, needs to reassess Mrs. Kelly's bowel pattern and frequency and recommend dietary or medication changes. Jennifer bases goal setting and prioritization on the patient's expectations and preferences. If*

Mrs. Kelly wants comfort interventions and spiritual support more than help with her constipation, Jennifer needs to address Mrs. Kelly's spiritual needs first.

Collaborative Care. End-of-life care draws on the resources of an interdisciplinary team. Social workers, spiritual care providers, and psychologists have skills to help patients, family caregivers, and family members deal with grief, anger, or depression. A pain-management specialist offers an individualized plan to address chronic pain. A coordinated team approach ensures that a patient's plan of care will be managed well and thoroughly addressed. When patients choose to go home for end-of-life care, home care and hospice nurses collaborate closely with the family and other health care providers to ensure continuity of care.

■■■ IMPLEMENTATION

Health Promotion. A person experiencing grief needs support as he or she learns how to live with loss and move toward grief recovery (Lloyd Jones, 2015). People facing significant disability, loss of body function, or even death want to achieve optimal physical and emotional well-being. Patients and family members feel sadness or emotional turmoil along the way but still want to cope with their life stressors. Nurses help patients learn how to deal with their loss; make effective decisions about their health care; and adjust to the disappointment, frustration, and anxiety created by their loss. Many times patients at the end of life wish to maintain as much self-care and independence as possible (Tipseankhum et al., 2016). With effective care and support, patients at the end of life often experience high levels of wellness.

Grief and Loss Support in Acute, Restorative, and Continuing Care Settings

Palliative Care. Interventions for patients with serious chronic illnesses or patients near the end of life are based on a philosophy of total care called *palliative care*. **Palliative care** is practiced in any setting and focuses on the prevention, reduction, or relief of physical, emotional, social, and spiritual symptoms of disease or treatment at the end of life when cure is no longer possible. People of any age or diagnosis receive palliative care at any time and in any setting. Expert palliative care involves an interdisciplinary team composed of health care professionals (i.e., nurses, social workers, spiritual care professionals, nutritionists, physicians, psychologists, and pharmacists). Therapists who use complementary healing interventions (e.g., massage, music, healing touch, or aromatherapy) also work with palliative care teams (Nyatanga, 2015). The World Health Organization (WHO, 2016) summarizes palliative care philosophy and practice as follows:

- Affirms life and regards dying as a normal process
- Neither hastens nor postpones death
- Provides relief from pain and other distressing symptoms

◎ CARE PLAN

Loss and Grief

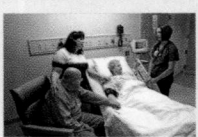

ASSESSMENT

Jennifer makes her first home visit 1 week after Mrs. Kelly's discharge from the hospital. Jennifer sees that Mrs. Kelly has a worried look on her face and she seems distressed. Mrs. Kelly cannot independently perform many activities of daily living because of shortness of breath. She is able to eat only small amounts of food and reports that she feels dizzy, weak, and "wobbly" when walking to the commode. Mrs. Kelly shares her feelings with Jennifer and asks many questions. While talking about her family, Mrs. Kelly states, "My daughter Lilly doesn't know what to do to help me."

ASSESSMENT ACTIVITIES

Arrange time to talk to Mrs. Kelly alone and observe her emotions.

Ask Mrs. Kelly about how she thinks her family is doing.

Ask Mr. Kelly about his feelings and needs.

FINDINGS[a]

Mrs. Kelly cries when she talks about her family and worries that she is a "burden" on them. She states, **"I know this is very hard for my husband to accept, but I feel alone when people don't seem to understand what I am going through."**

She confides that **her husband avoids talking about "what is really happening,"** and she says that he keeps talking about the trips they will take in the future. Lilly is tired and has not been sleeping well.

He talks about plans for a summer vacation, still 9 months away.

He appears sad and anxious.

He talks about **his fear of not knowing what to do when her symptoms worsen.**

He states, "I still can't believe that she wants to die instead of staying here with Lilly and me."

[a]**Defining characteristics/risk factors** are shown in **bold** type.

NURSING DIAGNOSIS: Compromised Family Coping related to stress of impending death of wife/mother

---

PLANNING

GOAL

Family understands the symptoms of end-stage heart condition within 2 weeks.

Family caregivers are able to provide palliative care interventions within 3 weeks.

The family develops affirming relationships within 3 weeks.

EXPECTED OUTCOMES (NOC)[b]

Caregiver Performance: Direct Care

Mr. Kelly describes end-stage heart disease in 1 week.

Mr. Kelly identifies the symptoms his wife may experience within 2 weeks.

Mr. Kelly and Lilly describe the palliative care that Mrs. Kelly will need in the next 2 weeks.

Mr. Kelly and Lilly provide hygiene and comfort needs within 3 weeks.

Caregiver-Patient Relationship

Mrs. Kelly shares feelings about her life and relationship with husband and daughter within 2 weeks.

Mr. Kelly and Lilly verbalize their understanding of Mrs. Kelly's need for their support within 1 month.

[b]Outcomes classification labels from Moorhead S, et al, editors: *Nursing outcomes classification (NOC)*, ed 5, St Louis, 2013, Mosby.

INTERVENTIONS (NIC)[c]

Coping Enhancement

Ask Mrs. Kelly to reminisce by sharing stories with her family.

Discuss with Mr. Kelly and Lilly the value of reminiscence as part of looking back and evaluating life and its meaning.

Caregiver Support

Involve the Kelly family in a discussion about symptom recognition and management.

RATIONALE

Encouraging patients to tell stories about events and people allows them to sense that life was meaningful and worth living (Keall et al., 2015).

Engaging in this process helps to move the family along the process of anticipatory grieving (Keall et al., 2015).

Even with a poor prognosis, social support and prompt symptom relief help maintain a higher quality of life for the patient and family.

◎ **CARE PLAN—cont'd**

Loss and Grief

INTERVENTIONS (NIC)ᶜ	RATIONALE
Offer the Kelly family a chance to ask questions about end-stage heart disease, the projected course of the condition, and Mrs. Kelly's wishes regarding the use of medications.	Clarifying expectations better prepares individuals to face changes that will happen as the disease progresses (Kim et al., 2016).
Explain that setting easily achievable goals helps give hope. Enlist family help to establish goals for the next week.	Restructuring goals to be short-term and achievable is a means of supporting and sustaining hope in terminally ill patients (Kim et al., 2016).

ᶜInterventions classification label from Bulechek GM, et al, editors: *Nursing interventions classification (NIC)*, ed 6, St Louis, 2013, Mosby.

EVALUATION

NURSING ACTIONS	PATIENT RESPONSE/FINDING	ACHIEVEMENT OF OUTCOME
Ask Mr. Kelly and Lilly about any changes they see in Mrs. Kelly.	Both note that Mrs. Kelly has less activity tolerance, but that she is able to rest with oxygen in place. They ask Mrs. Kelly if she is having pain more frequently instead of waiting until Mrs. Kelly states that she is in pain.	Mr. Kelly and Lilly are more skillful in recognizing subtle symptoms in Mrs. Kelly's status, and they are more proactive in controlling her symptoms.
Observe family caregiving activities and their level of comfort and involvement in care.	After 1 week Mr. Kelly and Lilly note that they are more at ease with their care activities.	Family continues to increase their knowledge of and ability to provide palliative care.
Ask Mrs. Kelly to describe her feelings after sharing stories and life review with family.	After 2 weeks the Kelly family notices that they look forward to sharing these stories and are becoming at ease with Mrs. Kelly's decision and their role in palliative care.	Developing and strengthening the relationship between Mrs. Kelly and her family remain ongoing.

- Integrates psychological and spiritual aspects of patient care
- Offers a support system to help patients live as actively as possible until death
- Offers a support system to help families cope during the patient's illness and their own bereavement
- Enhances the quality of life
- Uses a team approach to meet the needs of patients and families

Above all, palliative care ensures that patients with advanced chronic illness or patients near death receive care that is as free of avoidable pain and suffering as possible; is consistent with patient and family wishes; and is consistent with clinical, cultural, and ethical standards.

Hospice Care. **Hospice care** provides services for patients who are at the end of life. Many people do not know about this option for care and depend on you to explain hospice services and care philosophy to them. Patients who meet the criteria for hospice care no longer receive treatment to cure their disease and are terminally ill (Harrison and Connor, 2016). Hospice teams provide physical, emotional, and spiritual care for patients, family caregivers, and family members in many settings (i.e., home, hospital, or extended care facilities). Hospice care focuses exclusively on palliative care interventions to relieve the symptoms and burdens of illness or treatment and help patients live as fully as possible until

death. Nurses base hospice care on a patient's goals and support patient and family preferences for maintaining comfort and a high quality of life. Hospice programs are built on the following core beliefs and services:

- Patient and family as the unit of care
- Coordinated home care with access to inpatient and nursing home beds when needed
- Symptom management
- Provision of an interdisciplinary care team
- Medical and nursing services available at all times
- Bereavement follow-up after a patient's death
- Use of trained volunteers for visitation and respite support

For a patient to receive home hospice care, a family caregiver must be living in the home. The family caregiver receives support from professional and volunteer hospice team members who are available 24 hours a day. If a patient receiving home hospice care goes to the hospital for the management of acute symptoms, a nurse can use a hospice-to-hospital hand-off tool to communicate a patient's status and care goals to promote patient safety (Darrah and O'Connor, 2016). Fig. 27.1 illustrates the relationship between palliative care and hospice.

Communicate Therapeutically. A trusting nurse-patient relationship enables you to support patients in grief and to provide palliative care. Trust develops as you relate to patients

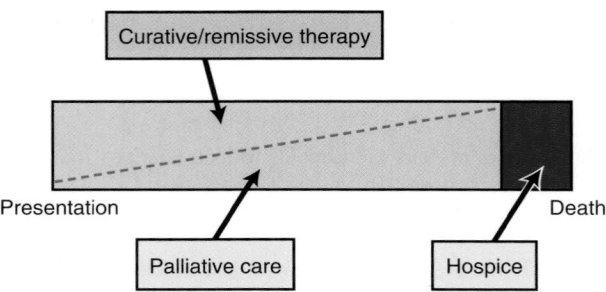

FIG 27.1 Continuum of palliative and hospice care. (From Emanuel L, et al: *Education in palliative and end of life care (EPEC) curriculum: the EPEC Project,* Chicago, 2003, Northwestern University Press.)

and family members with an open, nonassuming communication style (Harris and Winokuer, 2016). Open-ended questions invite patients to expand on their thoughts and tell their stories. Closed-ended questions usually lead patients to give short answers (yes or no).

Use active listening, learn to be comfortable with silence, and use prompts (e.g., "go on" or "tell me more") to encourage continued conversation. Verbally empathize with the patient's grief and build a trusting relationship by offering your caring presence using intentional, meaningful touch (Bezemer and Kress, 2014; Harris and Winokuer, 2016).

Some people do not want to talk about their feelings of loss or grief with others. Do not take a person's inability or lack of desire to communicate with you personally. Some people cope with stress and loss by talking things out, whereas others need to process their loss privately before they can talk to others. Cultural or gender expectations also influence the degree to which people talk about their loss. If patients do not want to share feelings or concerns, convey a willingness to be available if they want to talk later. When you are respectful of patients' personal or cultural values and their need for dignity, respect, and privacy, a therapeutic relationship will develop.

Grief brings out intense feelings such as anger, denial, depression, or guilt. People often become demanding and accusing and take out their anger on family or caregivers. Recall that denial, anger, and depression are normal reactions to loss. Reflect on how you react to people who exhibit intense feelings or negative behaviors. If you show fear or disappointment when people express intense emotions, they do not find it easy to confide in you. Offer support by saying, "I can see this is very upsetting to you. I just want you to know I am available to talk if you want." Avoid creating barriers to communication such as denying a patient's grief, offering false reassurance, or offering unsolicited advice (see Chapter 11).

Do not avoid a topic that a patient who is dying wishes to discuss. When you sense that patients want to talk, find the time to listen. In a busy acute care setting you need to reprioritize your responsibilities so that you can talk to your patients when they are ready. Respond to questions openly and honestly. Provide information to help patients understand their condition, consider the benefits and burdens of treatment choices, and clarify their personal values and goals.

Promote Hope and Spiritual Well-Being. Hope, a concept relevant to the human spirit, is the anticipation of a continued good or an improvement or lessening of something unpleasant. Hope energizes and comforts people and enhances their coping skills as they face personal challenges. To help patients feel more hopeful, remind them of their strengths and reinforce their expressions of courage, positive thinking, and realistic goal setting. Patients feel more hopeful when they have a sense of control. In a recent qualitative study, patients diagnosed with terminal cancer identified the importance of their family involvement and sense of hope for the future. The study results suggest that nurses can ease a patient's suffering by respecting the patient's sense of hope and encouraging family involvement in care (Nilmanat et al., 2015). Offer information to patients about their illness, correct misinformation, and clarify patient's perceptions. Patients can behave in hopeful ways also. Help them practice healthy behaviors (e.g., enjoying meals, talking with friends, and getting rest) and suggest that they develop a workable schedule for each day. People give hope to one another. Encourage patients to nurture important relationships. When people have strong relationships and a sense of emotional connectedness to others, they know that help is available. Nurses connect with patients to foster hope (Nilmanat et al., 2015).

Facilitate Mourning. Nursing interventions often help people acknowledge the reality of their loss. Discuss how and when the loss or illness occurred, under what circumstances, and other similar topics to help make the event more real and place it in perspective. Support efforts to live in the face of disability or in cases when the family must face being without the deceased person. Ask the people involved to identify and prioritize concerns and then facilitate the development of a plan to address their concerns. Encourage them to rely on their support network of family members, friends, professionals, and community resources. Suggest that they begin by reaching out to others in welcoming groups (e.g., religious communities or volunteer activities).

- Reinforce the understanding that people grieve differently and that feelings change or resolve over time. Some people have "anniversary reactions" (heightened or renewed feelings of loss or grief) months or years after a loss. They worry that they are losing ground when signs of grief reappear after a period of relative calm. Offer reassurance that anniversary reactions are common and encourage pleasant reminiscence.
- Provide continuing support. Patients and their families need to talk about their loved one and need support long after their loss. If you see the patient or family caregiver after an extended time, it is appropriate to ask them how they are doing after the loss. This gives them the opportunity to talk and lets them know that their loved one is remembered.

Manage Symptoms. Expert palliative care focuses primarily on managing the distress caused by unwanted symptoms of disease or side effects of treatments. Worry or fear concerning symptoms heightens a patient's perception of distress. Assess the character of a patient's symptoms carefully and individualize therapies. See Chapter 34 for a detailed discussion of both pharmacological and nonpharmacological pain management strategies, which are essential to achieve high-level palliative care. Patients at the end of life commonly experience other physical symptoms (e.g., dyspnea, fatigue, urinary incontinence, or nausea), psychological symptoms (e.g., anxiety, fear, or depression), social symptoms (e.g., loneliness, isolation, or loss of community), and spiritual symptoms (e.g., hopelessness, despair, or loss of meaning). A comprehensive care plan addresses symptoms identified by a patient as most distressing (Matzo and Sherman, 2015). See Table 27.4 for a summary of nursing implications of commonly experienced symptoms.

Maintain Dignity and Self-Esteem. You enhance patients' self-esteem by helping them maintain a pleasing physical appearance. Cleanliness, absence of body odors, attractive clothing, and personal grooming often elevate a patient's mood. Demonstrate respect, patience, and willingness when helping patients with toileting and bathing, especially as they become increasingly dependent on caregivers. Patients experience added grief and embarrassment when they can no longer tend to their basic needs. Include patients in making care decisions (e.g., how to perform personal hygiene, diet preferences, and timing of activities). Inform patients in advance about activities and their anticipated effects. Provide privacy while giving care and give patients and family members quiet, uninterrupted time together.

Prevent Feelings of Abandonment and Isolation. Many people fear dying alone. In hospitals or extended care facilities, answer patients' nurse call system promptly and assure them that caregivers are available throughout the day and night. Be readily available to answer questions or interpret changes in a patient's condition. Offer your comforting presence and use gentle touch when providing care (Fig. 27.2). Unless family members need privacy or are remaining with the patient around the clock, avoid placing patients in a private room. Patients who are actively dying often feel a sense of involvement and companionship when sharing a room and have more opportunities to interact with staff and visitors.

Family members who are having difficulty accepting a patient's impending death sometimes avoid visits. When family members visit, reassure them that their presence is important, encourage interaction, and offer information about what the patient was talking about or has recently experienced. Encourage family members to discuss normal family activities, reminisce about enjoyable times, and ask about the patient's concerns. Suggest simple and appropriate tasks for family members to perform (e.g., offering help with meals, simple hygiene or comfort activities, or filling out a menu).

Some people feel lonely or fearful at night and want a family member to stay with them. In acute care settings or extended care facilities, allow visitors to remain with a patient who is dying and relax other visiting restrictions (e.g., visits from children and number of visitors) to accommodate the patient's circumstances. Know how to contact family members so that they can be notified at any time if a patient wants to see them or if the patient's condition changes. Older adults often have a smaller support group and age-related needs at the end of life (Box 27.6).

Provide a Comfortable and Peaceful Environment. Promote patient comfort by repositioning, keeping bed linens dry, and controlling environmental temperature and noise. Keep the patient's immediate surroundings pleasant and clean. Open curtains so that patients can experience the natural changes from day to night. Remove sources of unpleasant odors (e.g., stale food and used bedpans or emesis basins) promptly. Pictures, cherished objects, cards from friends and family, or plants create a comforting and familiar

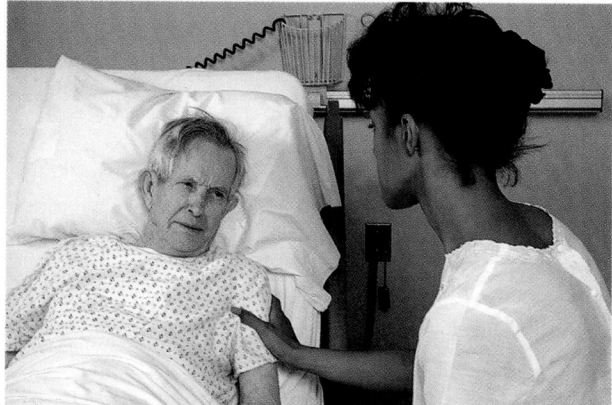

FIG 27.2 Offer your calm, comforting presence, and use gentle touch when providing care.

BOX 27.6 CARE OF THE OLDER ADULT

Family Caregiver Concerns

- Older adults exhibit resilience. Others around them can learn from their courage and ability to respond to life challenges graciously, accepting life with integrity and wholeness (Boman et al., 2015).
- Older adults are at risk for complicated grieving secondary to multiple losses, potential for cognitive impairment, or decreased physical abilities. Other risks include depression, loneliness, and accompanying functional decline.
- Pain is often underreported and undertreated in older adults, particularly in patients with dementia or cognitive impairments.
- Side effects of pain medications are often more pronounced in older adults (Paladini et al., 2015).
- Older adults benefit from the same therapeutic techniques as persons in other age-groups and have opportunities for growth and development through their loss experiences (Boman et al., 2015).
- Older adults are likely to be cared for across multiple health care settings, increasing the risk of fragmentation of care from one setting to another (Brown and Bub, 2016).

TABLE 27.4 MANAGING SYMPTOMS IN TERMINALLY ILL PATIENTS

SYMPTOMS	CHARACTERISTICS OR CAUSES	NURSING IMPLICATIONS
Pain	Pain can be related to the disease process, medical interventions, chronic conditions, prolonged bed rest, or pressure injuries.	Address pain reports promptly; provide medication as ordered and multiple nonpharmacological measures such as massage, repositioning, relaxation, guided imagery, or reiki (Kisvetrová et al., 2016) (see Chapter 34).
Discomfort	Discomfort can result from any source of physical irritation (e.g., dehydration, immobility) that causes pressure injuries and pain. As patients approach death, they breathe through the mouth, the tongue becomes dry, and lips become dry and cracked.	Provide thorough skin care including daily baths; lubrication of skin; and dry, clean bed linens to reduce irritants (see Chapter 31). Provide oral care at least every 2 to 4 hours. Use soft toothbrushes or foam swabs dipped in water for frequent mouth care. Apply a light film of petroleum jelly to lips and tongue (see Chapter 31).
	Blinking reflexes diminish near death; eyes often remain open, causing drying of cornea.	Gently remove crusts from eyelid margins. Use artificial tears to reduce corneal drying (see Chapter 31).
Fatigue	Increased metabolic demands, disease progression, pain, and declining heart function cause weakness and fatigue. Exhaustion phase of general adaptation syndrome causes energy depletion.	Help patient to identify valued or desired tasks; conserve energy for only those tasks. Help with activities of daily living. Plan frequent rest periods in a quiet environment and pace nursing care activities.
Nausea	Occurs as a side effect of medications, disease progression, or a result of severe pain.	Give antiemetic: provide oral care at least every 2 to 4 hours; offer clear liquids and ice chips; avoid liquids that cause stomach acidity such as coffee, milk, and citrus juice (Moradian and Howell, 2015).
Constipation	Opioid medications and immobility slow peristalsis. Lack of bulk in diet or reduced fluid intake occurs as appetite decreases.	Increase fluid and fiber intake if possible. Administer prophylactic stool softeners (Huang et al., 2015).
Diarrhea	Diarrhea results from some disease processes and side effects of medications.	Assess for fecal impaction. Confer with health care provider to change medication if possible. Provide low-residue diet.
Urinary incontinence	Incontinence results from disease progression, decreased level of consciousness.	Protect skin from irritation or breakdown (see Chapter 38). Change linens frequently. Use indwelling urinary catheter or condom catheters if indicated (Farrington et al., 2014).
Decreased appetite	Decreased blood flow to intestines at the end of life causes anorexia. Nausea and vomiting decrease appetite.	Give patients whatever food or fluids they enjoy. Offer frequent small meals, small portions, and/or snacks rather than large meals. Do not force people to eat. Offer small portions of desired foods or home-cooked meals if patient prefers (Ní Bhuachalla et al., 2016).
Dyspnea or shortness of breath	Disease progression involves lung tissue (e.g., pneumonia, pulmonary edema). Anemia reduces oxygen-carrying capacity. Anxiety increases oxygen demands. Fever increases oxygen demands.	Provide ordered treatments for underlying cause. Maximize lung expansion and ease of breathing (e.g., position patient upright, provide supplemental oxygen if ordered; decrease anxiety or fever). Give medications (e.g., bronchodilators, anxiolytics, inhaled steroids, opioids) to suppress cough and ease breathing (Maeda and Hayakawa, 2016). Provide antipyretics as ordered.
Anxiety	Anxiety has physical causes such as shortness of breath, pain, fear of death, spiritual concerns, and relationship concerns.	Give anxiolytics as ordered (Thekdi et al., 2015). Offer self as healing presence and provide information to decrease uncertainty (Hawthorn, 2015). Discuss spiritual or relational issues causing anxiety or fear (Finocchiaro, 2016). Collaborate with spiritual care professionals. Discuss feelings/reasons associated with the anxiety.

environment for patients and family members (Regan et al., 2014). Offer the patient frequent body massage if desired and provide opportunities for patients to hear their favorite music (Nyatanga, 2015; Pische, 2015; Clements-Cortes, 2016). A comfortable environment often helps patients relax, promotes sleep, and minimizes severity of symptoms.

Support Family Members. When a patient chooses to be at home at the end of life, family members become primary caregivers. Caring for a person dying at home is often rewarding yet physically exhausting and emotionally and spiritually stressful (Jaffray et al., 2016). Family caregivers benefit from education regarding the physical, emotional, and spiritual issues that often arise through each phase of the dying process (Box 27.7). They also need information about home care services, hospice, and community service resources. Hospice

programs offer respite care for family caregivers to temporarily relieve them of their duties so that they can get needed rest and rejuvenation. In some cases families need assistance and support in making the difficult decision about nursing home placement.

Provide family members with a description of common symptoms the patient will likely experience, the signs and symptoms of impending death, and the implications for care (Box 27.8). Encourage family members to talk openly with their loved one to give everyone a chance to discuss lingering concerns or requests. Family members often appreciate the opportunity to share their concerns with you in private. As death approaches encourage the use of silent vigil at the patient's bedside, touch, and verbal reassurances that the person is loved and not alone. After death help family caregivers notify the funeral home, other family members, and friends who were not present at the bedside; arrange for safe transportation of the body; and gather the patient's belongings.

Provide Care After Death. Provide a private area for the family to discuss organ donation if this is an option. Professionals educated in organ procurement and transplant procedures (e.g., transplant coordinators, social workers, or spiritual care providers) make the first contact with family members regarding requests for donation of organs or tissues. They consider the family's personal, religious, and cultural needs and discuss which tissues or organs are suitable for transplant; offer a description of the process, costs, and impact of donation on funeral plans; and answer family members' questions. For example, many people do not understand "brain death." For their loved one to donate major organs (e.g., heart, lungs, and liver), the body must be kept in good functional condition so the organs do not become damaged before donation. The patient remains on a ventilator until his or her organs are removed. Family members often believe that the person is still alive because his or her heart is still beating. Be available to reinforce explanations of the organ-retrieval process during this most stressful, tragic time. Nonvital tissues such as corneas, skin, long bones, and middle ear bones can be removed at the time of death

---

BOX 27.7 PATIENT TEACHING

Preparing the Dying Patient's Family

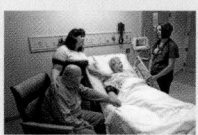 Jennifer establishes a teaching plan for Mr. Kelly and Lilly to help them learn how to perform palliative care interventions.

OUTCOME

At the end of the teaching session Mr. Kelly and Lilly demonstrate ways to help Mrs. Kelly with activities of daily living, pain management, and mobility safety.

TEACHING STRATEGIES

- Describe and demonstrate techniques for helping a person experiencing fatigue to eat safely and select easily chewed and swallowed foods.
- Demonstrate bathing, mouth care, and other hygiene measures and allow family to perform a return demonstration.
- Show video on simple transfer techniques and use of walker to prevent injury to themselves and the patient. Observe family members practice the techniques.
- Describe ways the family can promote patient's comfort (e.g., frequent rest periods, giving massage, repositioning).
- Discuss medication purposes and side effects.
- Discuss ways to assess fatigue, bowel and bladder symptoms, and shortness of breath.
- Demonstrate how to assess pain, record pain intensity, and give medications.
- Teach family to recognize signs and symptoms of impending death and who to call in an emergency and when death occurs.
- Invite questions from family and provide information as needed.

EVALUATION

- Use the principles of teach-back to evaluate patient/family caregiver learning:
  - "Mr. Kelly and Lilly, tell me what we discussed about the purpose and dosage of pain medications and how frequently you can administer them to Mrs. Kelly."
  - "Mr. Kelly and Lilly, tell me how you can use hospice services and who you will call when Mrs. Kelly dies."

BOX 27.8 SIGNS OF IMPENDING DEATH

- Minimal intake of food or water
- Increased sleeping and decreased consciousness
- Disorientation and restlessness
- Decreased urinary output and/or incontinence
- Cool hands and feet
- Noisy breathing
- Irregular breathing patterns with long pauses
- At the time of death, you will note:
  - Absence of breathing and heartbeat
  - Bowel and bladder release
  - Unresponsiveness
  - Eyes fixed on a certain spot
  - Dilated pupils

without maintaining vital functions. If the patient left no communication regarding his or her preferences for organ donation, family members make that decision with support and conversation. Review your state laws regarding organ retrieval and the formal consent process.

A nurse assumes responsibility for **postmortem care** (i.e., care of the body after death) (Box 27.9). Give postmortem care with dignity and sensitivity and in a manner consistent with a patient's religious or cultural beliefs. Because a body undergoes many physical changes after death, provide postmortem care as soon as possible to prevent tissue damage or disfigurement of body parts. For example, immediately after death, elevate the head of the bed to 30 degrees or place the patient's head on pillows to prevent pooling of blood, which can discolor the face.

Be aware that federal and state laws require that health care agencies formulate policies and procedures based on current laws to validate death, identify potential organ or tissue donors, request autopsy, and provide postmortem care. Following some deaths family members are asked to consent to an **autopsy,** the surgical dissection of a body after death to determine cause of death or how the person died or to contribute to knowledge of the disease. State legislation determines when an autopsy must be obtained, usually when death may have resulted from accident, homicide, or suicide. You alter your approach to care of the body after death if an autopsy is planned.

Nurses coordinate all aspects of care surrounding a patient's death. If a hospitalized patient dies while in a semiprivate room, transfer the other patient temporarily to another room to provide privacy for the deceased patient and family and avoid exposing the roommate to the stressors related to postmortem care. Use postmortem care guidelines to make the body appear as natural and comfortable as possible.

After a patient's death shift your care to surviving family members. Make all appropriate resources available to them.

BOX 27.9 CARE OF THE BODY AFTER DEATH

HEALTH CARE PROVIDER RESPONSIBILITIES
1. Confirm the time of death and take appropriate actions.
2. Determine the need for autopsy and order autopsy if indicated.
3. A staff member educated in making requests for organ and tissue donation discusses with family the donation options.

NURSE RESPONSIBILITIES
1. Perform hand hygiene and apply clean gloves.
2. Provide care with dignity and sensitivity to the patient and family members. Place the patient in a supine position and elevate the head of the bed 30 degrees or elevate with pillows to prevent discoloration of the face as you prepare for and complete postmortem care.
3. Check orders for any specimens to be collected or special postmortem instructions such as autopsy or retrieval of donated tissues.
4. Ask family members if and how they would like to help care for the body. Make arrangements for a member of the professional staff (e.g., spiritual care provider) to stay with family members if they do not wish to participate in body care. Ask family members if they have any special requests for body preparation (e.g., shaving, a special gown, Bible or rosary with the body).
5. Ask family about shaving male facial hair. Some cultures or religions prohibit shaving facial hair or cutting hair.
6. Remove all catheters, tubes, or indwelling devices from the patient's body except in the case of autopsy. In that case, leave medical devices in place. Remove medical equipment, supplies, and dirty linens from the room to create a clean, natural environment.
7. Bathe the body thoroughly, keeping the head of the bed elevated; apply clean sheets.
8. Brush and comb patient's hair. Apply patient's hairpiece, if possible, for natural appearance.
9. Position according to protocol. Close eyes gently by holding eyelids down briefly. Some cultural groups prefer that the eyes remain open. Dentures remain in the mouth to maintain facial alignment.
10. Cover the body with a clean sheet up to the chin with arms outside covers if possible.
11. Lower the lighting and reduce unpleasant odors as able.
12. Dispose of supplies, remove gloves, and perform hand hygiene.
13. Give family members an opportunity to view the body and accompany them to the bedside. Some will not want to view their dead loved one; assure them that either choice is acceptable.
14. Encourage the family to say good-bye with words and touch.
15. Do not rush the process of family visitation and body viewing. Once the family is more comfortable, *ask* if they would like to be left alone. Tell them how to find you easily.
16. Ask which personal belongings remain with or on the body. Give remaining personal items to a family member and document a description of the item and the date and time you transferred the belongings to the family's possession.
17. Do not throw away any personal belongings left behind by the family. Call a family member to describe the items and arrange for someone to retrieve the items they want to keep.
18. Apply name tags to the body according to agency protocol, usually on the right big toe and/or outside a shroud before transporting the body. Clearly mark the outside of the shroud if the body presents an isolation or contamination risk.
19. Document all care and any observations of injury to the skin in the nursing notes.
20. Remain sensitive to other hospitalized patients or visitors when transporting the body. Cover the body with a clean sheet and avoid moving it past groups of visitors when transporting it to the morgue or funeral home.
21. Follow all agency protocols and policies and comply with national or state laws regarding end-of-life issues.

They may want their family priest, minister, or rabbi to be with them; or they may appreciate the presence of the spiritual care staff at the health care agency. Social workers and counselors also offer valuable support. Remember that this is a very stressful but important event in the family's history. Do all you can to calmly and smoothly facilitate family members' requests, attend to their needs, and ask them about their preferences. Some family members prefer to be left alone and are unable to talk about the event until they have processed it privately.

Document all the activities surrounding a death carefully to provide an accurate record of the final events of a patient's life. Sometimes your summary of activities is used for risk management or legal investigations. Include in your documentation the time and date of death, the name of the health care provider who pronounces the death, organ or tissue donation status (e.g., request made and donation decision), preparation of the body, medical devices left in or on the body, valuables or belongings left with the patient (e.g., dentures, glasses, or wedding ring) or given to the family (e.g., clothing, mail, or photographs), time of discharge, and destination of the body (e.g., morgue at the agency or funeral home). Become familiar with the policies and procedures for postmortem care used in your agency and be sure that your care and documentation reflect those guidelines.

QSEN QSEN ACTIVITY *Teamwork and Collaboration*

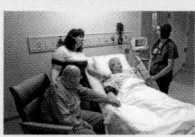

The nurse needs to consider the multiple concerns that Mrs. Kelly and her family have about providing care at home. Although Mr. Kelly is at home with his wife, he is not able to provide for all of her needs, and he will need respite care. Mrs. Kelly has lost strength as a result of decreased activity, shortness of breath, and back pain. She has a decreased appetite and no longer wants to help prepare meals. She feels anxious about the changes in her life and impending death and worries about how her family is coping.

- How can the hospice nurse ensure collaboration among the health care team?
- How will teamwork and interprofessional collaboration help Mrs. Kelly achieve her goal of staying in her home for end-of-life care?

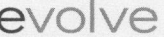 Answers to QSEN Activities can be found on the Evolve website.

■■■ EVALUATION

Patient Outcomes. Nurses care for patients and families at various times during a grief experience. Use your observations of behaviors and symptoms to evaluate how a patient or family is coping with loss and progressing through the grief process. Critical thinking ensures that the evaluation process is thorough and relevant to a patient's situation.

BOX 27.10 EVALUATION

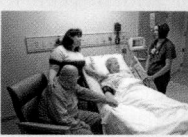

Two weeks after discussing her plan of care with the Kelly family, Jennifer observes Mr. Kelly helping his wife with her bath. He explains that Lilly is "taking a break to catch up on her school work." Mr. Kelly has obtained a walker, and Mrs. Kelly states that she feels less afraid of walking. Walking relieves the back pain that has become worse with bed rest. Mrs. Kelly explains that she and Lilly have enjoyed looking through old photo albums together, and yesterday Mr. Kelly "wanted to join in the fun, too." Mr. Kelly tells Jennifer that his wife still reports some problems with constipation. He carefully records her pain medication schedule and frequency of bowel movements. He also tells Jennifer that he and his daughter received information about a support group for family caregivers sponsored by the hospital palliative care service.

DOCUMENTATION NOTE

"Uses walker to ambulate in the home. States she feels more secure. Husband involved in bathing. Husband and daughter working together in care activities. Bath in progress at time of visit. Skin has no redness, tenderness, or evidence of tissue breakdown. Continues to have problems with constipation. Assessed current bowel medication regimen and bowel movement frequency. States has some constant back pain, but current pain medication keeps in control. Sleeps well at night, waking once a night for pain medication. Family contacted palliative care team regarding support group."

Refer to the goals and expected outcomes in your care plan and compare actual behaviors with expected outcomes to determine the patient's progress and make revisions to the care plan as needed. For example, if the goal is to have a patient share her feelings about death through reminiscing, you evaluate her verbal and nonverbal communication for cues that reflect normal grieving and healthy coping. Patient responses determine if the problem is resolving, if the patient needs new interventions, or if you need to revise existing strategies. Include patients and family members as active participants in the evaluation process (Box 27.10).

Patient Expectations. Maintain open lines of communication with patients so that they feel free to evaluate their nursing care honestly. Patients who have a good relationship with you comfortably discuss their perceptions of care. Consider it a sign of a trusting relationship when a patient or family caregiver offers feedback or suggestions to improve their care. When providing end-of-life care, ask often about patient and family satisfaction. Revise the care plan to include changing patient needs or requests for a different approach. Similarly, be encouraged when patients or family caregivers tell you that the care plan is helping them achieve their established goals.

Nurses' Self-Evaluation. Nurses who care for patients at the end of life and their family members often find their work to be very fulfilling and rewarding (Stodart, 2014). However, experiencing repeated deaths of patients can feel overwhelming at times. Nurses grieve too. If you work in an area in which you experience multiple losses and fail to acknowledge your own feelings of loss, you may begin to feel overwhelmed by intense emotions (e.g., frustration, anger, guilt, sadness, or dissatisfaction with life) and become vulnerable to compassion fatigue (Boyle, 2015).

Frequently evaluate your own emotional well-being. We all have feelings and memories about previous illnesses and death. Use self-reflection or journaling to determine if your personal sadness is related to a patient or to a past unresolved personal experience. Knowing more about your own grief and past experiences helps you care for others more insightfully. Being a professional caregiver involves knowing when to get away from a stressful situation and how best to take care of one's self. Many nurses, especially nurses who routinely provide hospice care, attend a viewing at the mortuary or the funeral to show support for the family, honor the deceased's memory, and cope with their own grief. As a caregiver you were an important part of the patient's story at a very meaningful time of life. Develop your own support systems, take restful time away from your work, and find a person with whom you can safely share your feelings and concerns. Physical and spiritual well-being help to restore your energy and enjoyment in your work (Hylton Rushton et al., 2015).

KEY POINTS

- The type and meaning of a loss influence how a person experiences and expresses grief.
- Individuals move back and forth through the phases or tasks of grieving, experience them simultaneously over a period of time, or do not experience them at all.
- A person's age, developmental stage, beliefs, roles, culture, relationships, and socioeconomic status influence reactions to loss and expressions of grief.
- When assessing patients experiencing grief or loss, do not make assumptions about how you think they feel. Ask them to share their experience in their own words and tell their stories.
- Therapeutic communication fosters the development of trust and provides an opportunity for patients and family members to talk about their concerns.
- Nursing care of a patient who is grieving or at the end of life focuses on enhancing a patient's sense of identity, dignity, and self-esteem and maintaining the highest possible quality of life.
- Patients of any age or diagnosis benefit from palliative care at any time in the course of their illness.
- Palliative and hospice care principles include involving patients and family caregivers in developing the plan of care; helping patients make informed choices; providing relief for physical, emotional, or spiritual symptoms; and offering support from an interdisciplinary team.
- Provide education and opportunities for family caregivers who want to be involved in end-of-life care.

- Provide care of a body after death and care for surviving family members with respect and sensitivity for their preferences and culture and/or religion and based on evidence-based protocols and standards.
- Nurses benefit from acknowledging and attending to their own grief when caring for patients at the end of life and their family members.

REFLECTIVE LEARNING

- Consider patient or family encounters you have had in the clinical setting, and discuss potential or real losses that the patient or family experienced.
- Culture influences how patients and families cope with losses. Discuss your personal expectations about loss and the grieving process. How are your expectations similar or different from other cultural expectations?
- Nurses encounter many patients or families who are grieving. Recognizing that nurses also grieve, what can you do to care for yourself?

REVIEW QUESTIONS

1. Which of the following statements made by a patient with a new diagnosis of end-stage heart failure best illustrates the numbing phase of loss?
   1. "I am in shock; how can this be really happening?"
   2. "I have always eaten healthy food and exercised. Why me?"
   3. "This must have happened because I smoked as a teenager and didn't care."
   4. "I think my disease will actually kill me."
2. A patient's family members ask the nurse what bodily changes they should expect when their relative's death is imminent. Which points does the nurse include in the teaching? (Select all that apply.)
   1. Warm hands and feet
   2. Noisy breathing
   3. Limited intake of food
   4. Consistent shallow breaths
   5. Reduction of urine output
   6. Orientation to person, place, and time
3. A patient's husband asks the nurse to explain what grief is. Which points does the nurse include in the teaching? (Select all that apply.)
   1. Individuals grieve with all the steps or patterns described in grief theories.
   2. Complicated grief occurs when a person has difficulty progressing through the loss experience.
   3. Grief is the emotional response to a loss.
   4. People grieve based on their experiences, cultural expectations, and spiritual values.
   5. Disenfranchised grief occurs when people discuss their losses with strangers.
   6. Anticipatory grief begins when family hear the diagnosis of a terminal illness.

4. A patient diagnosed with a progressive neurological disease believes she will live independently until her death. Which of the following statements is appropriate to begin your assessment of the patient's care decisions?
    1. "Tell me what you already know about your disease."
    2. "Many people are afraid of what hospice care means."
    3. "Palliative care is different than hospice care."
    4. "I think you do not understand what will happen as this disease progresses."

5. A patient diagnosed with end-stage lung disease asks about palliative care. Which of the following statements about palliative care are accurate? (Select all that apply.)
    1. A patient with end-stage lung disease can receive palliative care.
    2. When a patient chooses palliative care, the patient stops all acute treatments.
    3. People must be considered as having less than 6 months to live to be eligible for palliative care.
    4. Palliative care must be started when the patient is in the hospital.
    5. Palliative care interventions focus on providing symptom relief and maintaining a high quality of life.

evolve

Additional Review Questions, as well as rationales for all Review Questions, can be found on the Evolve website.

1. 1; 2, 3, 5; 3. 3, 4; 4. 1; 5. 1, 5.

REFERENCES

American Association of Colleges of Nursing [AACN]: *ELNEC fact sheet*, 2016, http://www.aacn.nche.edu/elnec/about/fact-sheet.

American Nurses Association [ANA] and Hospice and Palliative Nurses Association [HPNA]: *Palliative nursing: Scope and standards of practice*, Silver Spring MD, 2014, Author.

Barbus A: The dying person's bill of rights, *Am J Nurs* 75:99, 1975.

Barrere C, Durkin A: Finding the right words: the experience of new nurses after ELNEC education integration into a BSN curriculum, *Medsurg Nurs* 23(1): 35, 2014.

Bell Meisenhelder J, et al: Spiritual coping at the end of life, *J Hosp Palliat Nurs* 18(1): 66, 2016.

Bezemer J, Kress G: Touch: a resource for making meaning, *Aust J Lang Literacy* 37(2):78, 2014.

Bhat AM, et al: Advancing cultural assessments in palliative care using web-based education, *J Hosp Palliat Nurs* 17(4):351, 2015.

Blaber M, et al: Spiritual care: which is the best assessment tool for palliative settings? *Int J Palliat Nurs* 21(9):434, 2015.

Boman E, et al: Inner strength as identified in narratives of elderly women, *ANS Adv Nurs Sci* 38(1):10, 2015.

Boucher N: Direct engagement with communities and interprofessional learning to factor culture into end-of-life health care delivery, *Am J Public Health* 106(6):996, 2016.

Bowlby J: *Attachment and loss, vol 3, Loss, sadness, and depression*, New York, 1980, Basic Books.

Boyle D: Compassion fatigue: the cost of caring, *Nursing* 45(7):50, 2015.

Brown H, Bub L: Care transitions across the continuum: improving geriatric competence, *Geriatr Nurs* 37(1):69, 2016.

Clements-Cortes A: Development and efficacy of music therapy techniques within palliative care, *Complement Ther Clin Pract* 23:125, 2016.

Coelho A, et al: Prolonged grief in palliative family caregivers: a pilot study in a Portuguese sample, *Omega (Westport)* 72(2):151, 2015.

Dahlin C: *The national consensus project for quality palliative care clinical practice guidelines for quality palliative care*, ed 3, 2013, https://www.hpna.org/multimedia/NCP_Clinical_Practice_Guidelines_3rd_Edition.pdf.

Darrah N, O'Connor N: Toward safer transitions: a curriculum to teach and assess hospital-to-hospice handoffs, *J Pain Symptom Manage* 51(6):961, 2016.

Dobrina R, et al: Mutual needs and wishes of cancer patients and their family caregivers during the last week of life: a descriptive phenomenological study, *J Holist Nurs* 34(1):32, 2016.

Dockendorff DT: Healthy ways of coping with losses related to the aging process, *Educ Gerontol* 40(5):363, 2014.

Dosser I, Kennedy C: Improving family carers' experiences of support at the end of life by enhancing communication: an action research study, *Int J Palliat Nurs* 20(12):611, 2014.

Farrington N, et al: Indwelling urinary catheter use at the end of life: a retrospective audit, *Br J Nurs* 23(9): S10, 2014.

Finocchiaro D: Supporting the patient's spiritual needs at the end of life, *Nursing* 46(5):58, 2016.

Guldin M: Complicated grief—a challenge in bereavement support in palliative care: an update of the field, *Prog Palliat Care* 22(3):138, 2014.

Hall C: Bereavement theory: recent developments in our understanding of grief and bereavement, *Bereave Care* 33(1):9, 2014.

Harris DL, Winokuer HR: *Principles and practices of grief counseling*, ed 3, New York, 2016, Springer.

Harrison K, Connor S: First Medicare demonstration of concurrent provision of curative and hospice services for end-of-life care, *Am J Public Health* 106(8):1405, 2016.

Hawthorn M: The importance of communication in sustaining hope at the end of life, *Br J Nurs* 24(13):702, 2015.

Honeycutt A, Praetorius R: Survivors of suicide, *Illn Crises Loss* 24(2):104, 2016.

Hospice and Palliative Nurses Association (HPNA): *HPNA standards for clinical education of hospice and palliative nurses*, 2015, http://hpna.advancingexpertcare.org/wp-content/uploads/2015/08/HPNA-Clinical-Education-Standards.pdf.

Huang T, et al: Effectiveness of individualized intervention on older residents with constipation in nursing home: a randomized controlled trill, *J Clin Nurs* 24:3449, 2015.

Hylton Rushton C, et al: Burnout and resilience among nurses practicing in high-intensity settings, *Am J Crit Care* 24(5):418, 2015.

Institute of Medicine (IOM): *Dying in America: improving quality and honoring individual preferences near the end of life*, 2015, http://www.nationalacademies.org/hmd/~/media/Files/Report%20Files/2014/EOL/Report%20Brief.pdf.

Jaffray L, et al: Evaluating the effects of mindfulness-based interventions for informal palliative caregivers: a systematic literature review, *Palliat Med* 30(2):118, 2016.

Keall R, et al: Therapeutic life review in palliative care: a systematic review of quantitative evaluations, *J Pain Symptom Manag* 49(4):759, 2015.

Kim B, et al: The effects of dying well education program on Korean women with breast cancer, *Appl Nurs Res* 30:64, 2016.

Kisvetrová H, et al: Dying care interventions in the intensive care unit, *J Nurs Scholarsh* 48(2):142, 2016.

Kübler-Ross E: *On death and dying*, New York, 1969, Macmillan.

Lloyd Jones S: The psychological miscarriage: an exploration of women's experience of miscarriage in the light of Winnicott's "primary maternal preoccupation," the process of grief according to Bowlby and Parkes, and Klein's theory of mourning, *Br J Psychother* 31(4):437, 2015.

Lonneman W: Teaching strategies to increase cultural awareness in nursing students, *Nurse Educ* 40(6):285, 2015.

Maeda T, Hayakawa T: Combined effect of opioids and corticosteroids for alleviating dyspnea in terminal cancer patients: a retrospective review, *J Pain Palliat Care Pharmacother* 30(2):106, 2016.

Mager D, Lange J: The ELDER project, *J Hosp Palliat Nurs* 18(1):26, 2016.

Matzo M, Sherman D: *The interprofessional practice of palliative care nursing. Palliative care nursing: quality care to the end of life*, ed 4, New York, 2015, Springer.

Mixer S, et al: The relationship between the nursing environment and delivering culturally sensitive perinatal hospice care, *Int J Palliat Nurs* 21(9):424, 2015.

Momtaz Y, et al: Spousal death anxiety in old age, *Omega (Westport)* 72(1):69, 2015.

Moradian S, Howell D: Prevention and management of chemotherapy-induced nausea and vomiting, *Int J Palliat Nurs* 21:216, 2015.

National Institute on Aging (NIA): *End of life: helping with comfort and care*, 2015, https://www.nia.nih.gov/health/publication/end-life-helping-comfort-and-care/introduction.

Ní Bhuachalla É, et al: Good nutrition for cancer recovery—a nutritional resource for the treatment of cancer-induced weight loss, *Nutr Bull* 41(2):151, 2016.

Nilmanat K, et al: Moving beyond suffering: the experiences of Thai persons with advanced cancer, *Cancer Nurs* 38(3):224, 2015.

Nyatanga B: Using complementary therapies in palliative care, *Br J Community Nurs* 20(4):203, 2015.

Paladini A, et al: Chronic pain in the elderly: the case for new therapeutic strategies, *Pain Physician* 18(5):E864, 2015.

Perrin OK, Kazanowski M: End-of-life care. Overcoming barriers to palliative care consultation, *Crit Care Nurse* 35(5):46, 2015.

Pische K: Integrative and holistic oncology nursing, *Beginnings* 35(3):19, 2015.

Price J: Informed shared decision-making in planning for the end of life, *Br J Nurs* 25(7):381, 2016.

Rafferty K, et al: Spirituality, religion, and health: the role of communication, appraisals, and coping for individuals living with chronic illness, *J Relig Health* 54(5):1880, 2015.

Rando T: *Treatment of complicated mourning*, Champaign, IL, 1993, Research Press.

Regan A, et al: Improving end of life care for people with dementia, *Nurs Stand* 28(48):39, 2014.

Rodrigo L: A rare kind of light at the end of a rare kind of tunnel: trauma of a life-altering, chronic, degenerative disease and its redemption, *J Loss Trauma* 19(6):584, 2014.

Schonfeld D, et al: Grief across cultures, *NASN Sch Nurse* 30(6):350, 2015.

Sierra Hernandez C, et al: Use of referential language in short-term group psychotherapy for complicated grief, *Group Dyn* 20(1):10, 2016.

Stodart K: Self-care vital for palliative nursing team, *Nurs N Z* 20(4):24, 2014.

Thekdi SM, et al: Psychopharmacology in cancer, *Curr Psychiatry Rep* 20(15):522, 2015.

Tipseankhum N, et al: Experiences of people with advanced cancer in home-based palliative care, *Pac Rim Int J Nurs Res Thail* 20(3):238, 2016.

Van Hook MY: Spirituality as a potential resource for coping with trauma, *SWC* 43(1):13, 2016.

van Wijngaarden E, et al: Ready to give up on life: the lived experience of elderly people who feel life is completed and no longer worth living, *Soc Sci Med* 138:261, 2015.

Waller A, et al: Assisting the bereaved: a systematic review of the evidence for grief counselling, *Palliat Med* 30(2):133, 2016.

Wienclaw R: Grief and bereavement, *Grief & Bereavement Research Starters Sociology* 3:1, 2016.

Worden JW: *Grief counseling and grief therapy*, New York, 1982, Springer.

World Health Organization (WHO): *Palliative care*, 2016, http://www.who.int/ncds/management/palliative-care/introduction/en/.

evolve MEDIA RESOURCES

http://evolve.elsevier.com/Potter/essentials
- Audio Glossary
- Case Study Continuation

- QSEN Activity and Review Questions Answers and Rationales
- Video Clip

OBJECTIVES

- Describe the role of the musculoskeletal and nervous systems in the regulation of activity and exercise.
- Discuss physiological and pathological influences on body alignment and joint mobility.
- Describe how to assess patient body alignment and levels of activity and exercise.
- Formulate nursing diagnoses for patients experiencing alterations with activity and exercise.

- Develop an individualized nursing care plan for a patient with impaired physical mobility.
- Discuss the national patient initiatives and regulations in relation to patient handling and movement.
- Evaluate the nursing care plan for maintaining patient activity and exercise.

KEY TERMS

active range-of-motion (ROM) exercises, p. 719
activities of daily living (ADLs), p. 704
antagonistic muscles, p. 706
antigravity muscles, p. 706
cartilage, p. 706
center of gravity, p. 704
crutch gait, p. 722
ergonomics, p. 708

extension, p. 706
footboards, p. 705
friction, p. 705
gait, p. 712
hemiplegia, p. 707
isometric contraction, p. 705
isotonic contraction, p. 705
joint, p. 705
ligaments, p. 706
mechanical lift, p. 718

muscle tone, p. 704
orthostatic hypotension, p. 718
posture, p. 704
proprioception, p. 706
range of motion (ROM), p. 712
side rail, p. 725
supine, p. 710
tendons, p. 706

Patients require regular activity and exercise with the levels depending on their health conditions. Nurses assist patients in maintaining or improving their level of activity and exercise. Walking, turning, lifting, or carrying all are common actions used to provide nursing care. Such activities require muscle exertion. As a nurse, you need to practice proper body mechanics and remain knowledgeable about current research, standards, and guidelines concerning safe transfer and positioning techniques to reduce the risk for injury (Box 28.1). This includes knowledge of the actions of muscle groups; understanding of the factors involved in the coordination of body movement; and familiarity with the integrated functioning of the skeletal, muscular, and nervous systems.

CASE STUDY *Mr. Indelicato*

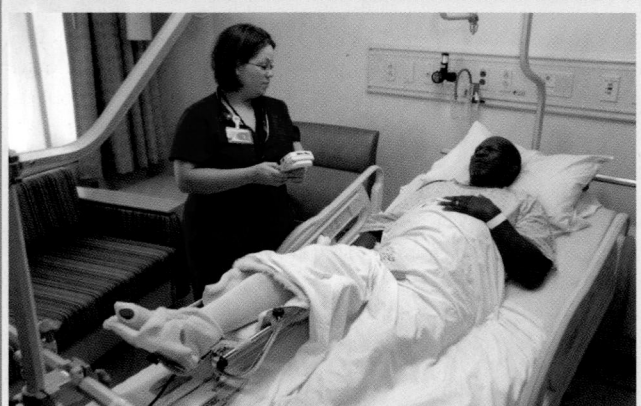

Mr. Indelicato is a 72-year-old man who has been hospitalized for surgery on his right knee. His general level of health is good. He does not have underlying chronic illnesses and relates the problem with his knee to previous sports injuries. He reports, "I twisted my knee" at least 6 times over the last 30 years while playing racquetball. He first sought medical advice and treatment approximately 6 years ago. His last injury to his knee was approximately "5 or 6 years ago, and it hasn't worked the same since." He tried various treatments including physical therapy, rest, and pain medication. His only preoperative medication is ibuprofen 600 mg every 6 to 8 hours. He has not taken his ibuprofen for the past few days because of the impending surgery. He wants the surgery so he can get back to being active. He and his wife enjoy golf, tennis, and bike riding. Mr. Indelicato's wife is also very healthy.

Marilyn Sweeney is a 30-year-old nursing student. She just finished a clinical rotation on a general surgical unit and is spending the remaining 6 weeks in the orthopedic/rehabilitation division of the agency. Her assignment is to follow Mr. Indelicato through his surgery and rehabilitation.

SCIENTIFIC KNOWLEDGE BASE

Regular physical activity and exercise contribute to both physical and emotional well-being (Edelman et al., 2014; Covan, 2015). Knowing the physiology and regulation of body mechanics, exercise, and activity helps you to provide individualized patient care.

Overview of Exercise and Activity

The coordinated efforts of the musculoskeletal and nervous systems provide the foundation for body mechanics to maintain balance, posture, and body alignment during lifting, bending, moving, and performing activities of daily living (ADLs). Performing these activities correctly decreases the risk for musculoskeletal system injury, preventing muscle strain and excessive use of muscle energy.

Body Alignment. Body alignment refers to the relationship of one body part to another along a horizontal or vertical line. Correct alignment reduces strain on musculoskeletal

BOX 28.1 EVIDENCE-BASED PRACTICE

PICO Question: Does the use of lift devices compared with good body mechanics for positioning adult patients reduce injuries to nurses?

SUMMARY OF EVIDENCE

Musculoskeletal disorders are the most prevalent and debilitating occupational health hazard among nurses. There has been some improvement in the incidence of musculoskeletal injuries in health care workers. The total recordable injury incidence rate for hospitals is 6.0 per 100 full-time employees (Bureau of Labor Statistics, 2016). Back injuries among health care workers are estimated to cost $10,689 per case, creating an economic burden and a major health concern (VISN8, 2014; NIOSH, 2016). NIOSH recommends standards for manual lifting of patients be minimized in all cases and eliminated when feasible (VISN8, 2014; NIOSH, 2016). In addition, many facilities have limited-lift policies (LLPs) that minimize patient handling by nurses and instead use lift devices to reduce on-the-job injuries (Stevenson, 2014). There is strong evidence for the use of ergonomic solutions being effective in reducing musculoskeletal pain and injuries in care providers (Nelson and Baptiste, 2004). These solutions are divided into three categories: engineering, administrative, and behavioral controls.

APPLICATION TO NURSING PRACTICE

- Consider the risk associated with a patient handling task. Assess factors such as a patient's weight; transfer distance; confined workspace; unpredictable patient behavior; and awkward positions such as stooping, bending, and reaching.
- Use engineering controls: Patient handling technology includes lateral lift aids, sliding boards, and specialized hospital beds that rotate (Nelson and Baptiste, 2004). Lift devices reduce on-the-job injuries (Anderson et al., 2014).
- Behavioral practice controls: As a nurse, be sure you are trained in mobility and handling techniques such as manual patient lifting, training in proper use of lifting equipment and devices, and the use of unit-based peer leaders or "lift teams" (Nelson and Baptiste, 2004).
- The American Nurses Association (ANA, 2015, 2016) has standards for use of safe, efficient lifting techniques including assistive equipment and devices to promote safe patient transfer and prevent injury to patients and health care workers.
- Administrative controls: Follow work practices and policies that reduce or prevent exposure to ergonomic risks. Minimize manual lifting of patients in all cases and eliminate lifting when possible (VISN8, 2014; NIOSH, 2016). Some agencies have "no lift" policies.

structures, maintains adequate muscle tone, and contributes to balance.

Body Balance. You achieve body balance when you balance a relatively low center of gravity over a wide, stable base of support. A vertical line falls from the center of gravity through the base of support. The base of support is the foundation. When the vertical line from the center of gravity does not fall through the base of support, the body loses balance.

Posture also enhances body balance. The term *posture* means maintaining optimal body position. It means a position that most favors function; requires the least muscular work to maintain; and places the least strain on muscles, ligaments, and bones (Huether and McCance, 2017).

Maintain proper body alignment and posture. First, widen your base of support by separating your feet to a comfortable distance. Second, bring the center of gravity closer to your base of support to increase balance. Bend your knees and flex the hips until squatting, and maintain proper back alignment by keeping your trunk erect.

Coordinated Body Movement. Weight is the force exerted on a body by gravity. When you lift an object, you must overcome the weight of the object and be aware of its center of gravity. In symmetrical objects the center of gravity is located at the exact center of the object. The force of weight is always directed downward. An object that is unbalanced has its center of gravity away from the midline and falls without support. Similar to unbalanced objects, patients who fail to maintain balance with their center of gravity are unsteady, placing them at risk for falling. Promptly intervene with patients with an unbalanced center of gravity.

Friction. Friction is the effect of rubbing or the force between two objects rubbing against each other. As you turn, transfer, or move a patient up in bed, you need to overcome friction. Remember, the greater the surface area of the object you move, the greater the friction generated.

A patient who is acutely ill or immobilized produces greater friction during movement. Thus when possible use some of a patient's strength and mobility when lifting, transferring, or moving a patient up in bed. You do this by explaining the procedure and telling the patient when to move. For instance, you decrease friction when patients are able to bend their knees and lift their hips while being moved up in bed. You also reduce friction by safe lifting techniques rather than pushing a patient. Lifting has an upward component and decreases the pressure between a patient and the bed or chair. The use of a lift sheet or transfer board reduces friction because you are able to move the patient more easily along the surface of the bed.

Exercise and Activity. Exercise is physical activity used to condition the body, improve health, and maintain fitness. Sometimes exercise is also a therapeutic measure. A patient's individualized exercise program depends on the patient's activity tolerance or the type and amount of exercise or activity that the patient is able to perform. Physiological, emotional, and developmental factors influence a patient's activity tolerance.

An active lifestyle is important for maintaining and promoting health and psychological well-being (Edelman et al., 2014; Covan, 2015). The best program of physical activity includes one that is a combination of exercises that produce different physiological and psychological benefits. Three categories of exercise are isotonic, isometric, and resistive isometric. Isotonic exercises (e.g., walking, swimming, jogging, bicycling) cause muscle contraction and change in muscle length (isotonic contraction). Isotonic exercises enhance circulatory and respiratory functioning; increase muscle mass, tone, and strength; and promote osteoblastic activity that combats osteoporosis.

Isometric exercises (e.g., quadriceps set exercises, contraction of the gluteal muscles) involve tightening or tensing muscles without moving body parts (isometric contraction). This form of exercise is ideal for patients who do not tolerate increased activity. A patient who is immobilized in bed can perform isometric exercises. The benefits are increased muscle mass, tone, and strength, thus decreasing the potential for muscle wasting; increased circulation to the involved body part; and increased osteoblastic activity.

Resistive isometric exercises are exercises in which an individual contracts the muscle while pushing against a stationary object or resisting the movement of an object (Kim et al., 2015). A gradual increase in the amount of resistance and length of time that the muscle contraction is held increases muscle strength and endurance. Examples of resistive isometric exercises are push-ups and hip lifting, in which a patient in a sitting position pushes with the hands against a surface such as a chair seat and raises the hips. In some health care settings, footboards are placed on the end of beds; patients push against them to move up in bed. Resistive isometric exercises help promote muscle strength and provide sufficient stress against bone to promote osteoblastic activity.

Physical activity not only benefits a patient's overall health but also is reported to reduce psychological and physical stress (Childs and deWit, 2014). Consider a patient's knowledge of exercise and activity, their values and beliefs about exercise in relation to health, barriers to a program of exercise and physical activity, and current exercise habits. Readiness to developing an exercise program plays an important role in the development of an exercise program.

Regulation of Movement

Coordinated body movement involves the integrated functioning of the skeletal, muscular, and nervous systems. Because these three systems cooperate so closely in mechanical support of the body, they are often considered as a single functional unit.

Skeletal System. Bones perform five functions in the body: support, protection, movement, mineral storage, and hematopoiesis (blood cell formation). To provide support, bones serve as the framework and contribute to the shape, alignment, and positioning of body parts. Bones provide movement, using their joints as levers for muscle attachment (Huether and McCance, 2017).

Joints. An articulation, or joint, is the connection between bones. Each joint is classified according to its structure and degree of mobility. Joints are classified as fibrous, cartilaginous, or synovial connective structures (Huether and

McCance, 2017). Fibrous joints have a ligament or membrane that unites two bony surfaces such as the paired bones of the tibia and fibula. They are flexible and permit limited movement. The cartilaginous joint has little movement but is elastic. This type of joint allows for bone growth while providing stability such as the joint between the sternum and second rib. The synovial, or true, joint is a freely movable joint. Bony surfaces are covered by cartilage and connected by ligaments lined with a synovial membrane. An example is the hip joint.

Ligaments, Tendons, and Cartilage. Ligaments are white, shiny, flexible bands of fibrous tissue that bind joints and connect bones and cartilages. They are elastic and aid joint flexibility and support. In some areas of the body, they also have a protective function. Tendons are white, glistening, fibrous bands of tissue that connect muscle to bone. Tendons are strong, flexible, and inelastic and occur in various lengths and thicknesses. Cartilage is nonvascular, supporting connective tissue with the flexibility of a firm, plastic material. The gristle-like nature of cartilage permits it to sustain weight and serve as a shock-absorber pad between articulating bones (Huether and McCance, 2017).

Skeletal Muscles.
In addition to facilitating movement, muscles determine body form and contour. Skeletal muscles span at least one joint and attach to both articulating bones. When contraction occurs, one bone is fixed, while the other moves. The origin is the point of attachment that remains still; the insertion is the point that moves when the muscle contracts (Huether and McCance, 2017).

Muscles Concerned With Movement. The muscles of movement are near the skeletal region, where a lever system causes movement (Huether and McCance, 2017). The lever system makes the work of moving a weight or load easier. Movement occurs when specific bones such as the humerus, ulna, and radius and the associated joints such as the elbow act as levers. Thus the force applied to one end of a bone to lift a weight at another point tends to rotate the bone in the opposite direction of the applied force. Muscles that attach to bones of leverage provide the necessary strength to move an object.

Muscles Concerned With Posture. Gravity pulls on parts of the body all the time; muscles exert pull on bones in the opposite direction to keep the body in position. Muscles accomplish this counterforce by maintaining a low level of sustained contraction. Poor posture places more work on muscles to counteract the force of gravity. This leads to fatigue and eventually interferes with bodily functions and causes deformities.

Muscle Groups. The nervous system coordinates the antagonistic, synergistic, and antigravity muscle groups that maintain posture and initiate movement. Antagonistic muscles bring about movement at the joint. During movement the active mover muscle contracts, while its antagonist relaxes. For example, during extension of the arm, the active mover, the triceps brachii, contracts, and the antagonist, the biceps brachii, relaxes.

Synergistic muscles contract to accomplish the same movement. For example, when you flex your arm, you increase the strength of the contraction of the biceps brachii by contracting the synergistic muscle, the brachialis.

Antigravity muscles stabilize joints. These muscles continuously oppose the effect of gravity on the body and permit a person to maintain an upright or sitting posture. In an adult, the antigravity muscles are the extensors of the leg, the gluteus maximus, the quadriceps femoris, the soleus muscles, and the muscles of the back.

Skeletal muscles support posture and carry out voluntary movement. The muscles are attached to the skeleton by tendons, which provide strength and permit motion.

Nervous System.
The nervous system regulates movement and posture. The motor strip, the major voluntary motor area, is located in the cerebral cortex (precentral gyrus) of the brain. Most motor fibers descend from the motor strip and cross at the level of the medulla. The motor fibers from the right motor strip initiate voluntary movement for the left side of the body, and motor fibers from the left motor strip initiate voluntary movement for the right side of the body. Transmission of the impulse from the nervous system to the musculoskeletal system is an electrochemical event that requires a neurotransmitter (i.e., a chemical that transfers the electrical impulse from the nerve to the muscle).

Proprioception. The nervous system also regulates posture. Posture requires coordination of proprioception and balance. Proprioception is the awareness of the position of the body and its parts and depends on impulses from the inner ear and receptors in joints and ligaments (Huether and McCance, 2017). Proprioceptors located on nerve endings in muscles, tendons, and joints monitor proprioception. While a person carries out ADLs, proprioceptors monitor muscle activity and body position. When a person walks, the proprioceptors on the bottom of the feet monitor pressure changes. Thus when the bottom of the moving foot comes in contact with the walking surface, the individual automatically moves the stationary foot forward.

Balance. The cerebellum and the inner ear control balance through the nervous system. The major function of the cerebellum is to coordinate all voluntary movement. Within the inner ear are the fluid-filled semicircular canals. When you rotate your head suddenly in one direction, the fluid remains stationary for a moment while the canal turns with the head. This allows a person to change position suddenly without losing balance. Conditions affecting the cerebellum or inner ear impair balance and increase patients' risk for falling.

Principles of Transfer and Positioning Techniques

Using principles of safe patient transfer and positioning during routine activities decreases work effort and places less strain on musculoskeletal structures (Box 28.2). In addition to following these principles in your own practice it is important to teach these principles to patients and family

BOX 28.2 PRINCIPLES OF SAFE PATIENT TRANSFER AND POSITIONING

- Mechanical lifts and lift teams are essential when a patient is unable to assist.
- When a patient is able to assist, remember the following principles:
  - The wider the base of support, the greater the stability of the nurse.
  - The lower the center of gravity, the greater the stability of the nurse.
  - The equilibrium of an object is maintained as long as the line of gravity passes through its base of support.
  - Facing the direction of movement prevents abnormal twisting of the spine.
  - Dividing balanced activity between arms and legs reduces the risk of back injury.
  - Leverage, rolling, turning, or pivoting requires less work than lifting.
  - When friction is reduced between the object to be moved and the surface on which it is moved, less force is required to move it.

2015). Bones are porous, short, bowed, and deformed; as a result, children experience curvature of the spine and shortness of stature. Scoliosis is a structural curvature of the spine associated with vertebral rotation. Muscles, ligaments, and other soft tissues become shortened. This affects balance and mobility in proportion to the severity of abnormal spinal curvatures (Huether and McCance, 2017).

Disorders of Bones, Joints, and Muscles. Osteoporosis is a common disorder of aging in which bone mass or density is reduced. The bone remains biochemically normal but has difficulty maintaining integrity and support. Many factors cause this, varying from hormonal imbalances to insufficient intake of nutrients (foods that contain calcium and vitamin D) (Huether and McCance, 2017).

Inflammatory and noninflammatory joint diseases and articular disruption all alter joint mobility. Some characteristics of inflammatory joint disease (e.g., arthritis) are inflammation or destruction of the synovial membrane and articular cartilage and systemic signs of inflammation. Noninflammatory diseases such as those resulting from a traumatic injury have none of these characteristics, and the synovial fluid is normal (Huether and McCance, 2017).

Central Nervous System Damage. Damage to any component of the central nervous system that regulates voluntary movement results in impaired body alignment and mobility. For example, you are caring for a patient who experienced head trauma with damage to the motor strip in the cerebrum. As a result the patient could experience symptoms of limited or complete loss of movement based on where the damage occurred. The amount of voluntary motor impairment is directly related to the amount of destruction of the motor strip. A patient with a right-sided cerebral hemorrhage and damage to the right motor strip usually has left-sided hemiplegia or paralysis.

Musculoskeletal Trauma. Trauma to the musculoskeletal system sometimes results in bruises, contusions, sprains, and fractures. A fracture is a disruption of bone tissue continuity. Fractures most commonly result from direct external trauma. They also occur because of some deformity of the bone, as with pathological fractures of osteoporosis.

NURSING KNOWLEDGE BASE

Application of nursing knowledge from scientific evidence allows you to think critically about the holistic needs of patients. Nursing knowledge as it pertains to activity and exercise helps you assess, identify, and intervene when patients have decreased activity tolerance or physical limitations that affect their ability to exercise (see Chapter 29).

Safe Patient Handling

Nurses are exposed to overexertion from the hazards related to lifting and transferring patients in many settings such as inpatient nursing units, long-term care facilities, and the

caregivers. Teaching family caregivers how to properly transfer or position a family member who is hospitalized increases and reinforces the family's knowledge about proper transfer and position techniques once the patient returns home.

The U.S. National Institute of Occupational Safety and Health (NIOSH) released federal ergonomic guidelines to prevent musculoskeletal injuries in the workplace (VISN8 Patient Safety Center [VISN8], 2014; NIOSH, 2016). Half of all back pain in the workplace is associated with manual lifting tasks. The most common back injury is strain on the lumbar muscle group, which includes the muscles around the lumbar vertebrae. Injury to these areas affects the ability to bend forward, backward, and from side to side and decreases the ability to rotate the hips and lower back (Stevenson, 2014).

Manual lifting is the last resort. Do *not* use manual lifting when you need to lift most or all of a patient's weight. Before lifting assess the weight to be lifted, the assistance needed, and the resources available. Use safe patient–handling equipment and refer to algorithms for safe handling and movement in conjunction with agency lift teams to reduce the risk of injury to a patient and health care team members (Table 28.1).

Pathological Influences on Body Alignment, Mobility, and Activity

Many pathological conditions affect body alignment and mobility, including congenital defects; disorders of bones, joints, and muscles; central nervous system damage; and musculoskeletal trauma.

Congenital Defects. Congenital abnormalities can affect the musculoskeletal system by altering alignment, balance, and appearance. Osteogenesis imperfecta is an inherited disorder that affects bone. Some characteristics of this disorder are fractures and bone deformity (Hockenberry and Wilson,

TABLE 28.1 PREVENTING LIFT INJURIES IN HEALTH CARE WORKERS

ACTION	RATIONALE
When planning to move a patient, arrange for adequate help. If your institution has a lift team, use it as a resource.	A lift team is properly trained in techniques to prevent musculoskeletal injuries.
Use patient-handling equipment and devices such as height-adjustable beds, ceiling-mounted lifts, friction-reducing slide sheets, and air-assisted devices (Stevenson, 2014).	These devices reduce caregiver muscular strain during patient handling.
Encourage patient to help as much as possible during repositioning or transfer.	Promotes patient's independence and strength while minimizing workload.
Keep back, neck, pelvis, and feet aligned. Avoid twisting.	Reduces risk of injury to lumbar vertebrae and muscle groups. Twisting increases risk of injury.
Flex knees; keep feet wide apart and aligned with shoulders.	A broad base of support increases stability.
Position yourself close to patient (or object being lifted).	Reduces horizontal reach and stress on caregiver's back.
Use arms and legs (not back).	Leg muscles are stronger, larger muscles capable of greater work without injury.
Slide patient toward yourself with a slide board or pull sheet. When transferring a patient onto a stretcher or bed, a slide board is more appropriate.	Sliding requires less effort than lifting. Pull sheet minimizes shearing forces, which can damage patient's skin.
Person with the heaviest load coordinates efforts of team involved by counting to three.	Simultaneous lifting minimizes the load for any one lifter.
Perform manual lifting as last resort and only if it does not involve lifting most or all of a patient's weight (Stevenson, 2014).	Lifting is a high-risk activity that causes significant biochemical and postural stressors.

operating room (Anderson et al., 2014). Manually lifting and transferring patients contributes to the high incidence of work-related musculoskeletal problems and back injuries in nurses and other health care staff. Evidence-based research has shown that safe patient handling interventions significantly reduce overexertion injuries by replacing manual patient handling with safer methods guided by ergonomic principles (NIOSH, 2016). **Ergonomics** refers to the design of work tasks to best suit the capabilities of workers. In the case of patient handling, it involves the use of mechanical equipment and safety procedures to lift and move patients. Many states have laws that mandate safe patient handling in health care agencies. Health care agencies are implementing comprehensive safe patient–handling programs in all parts of the United States. Comprehensive safe patient–handling programs include the following elements (VISN8, 2014):

- An ergonomics assessment protocol for health care environments
- Patient assessment criteria and algorithms for safe patient handling and movement (e.g., the Banner Mobility Assessment Tool [BMAT] [Boynton et al., 2014)
- Special equipment kept in convenient locations to help transfer patients
- Back injury resource nurses
- An "after-action review" that allows the health care team to apply knowledge about moving patients safely in different settings
- A no-lift policy

Transfer Techniques. Nurses provide care for immobilized patients whose positions must be changed, who must be moved up in bed, or who must be transferred from a bed to a chair or from a bed to a stretcher. Although nurses use many transfer techniques, knowledge of ergonomics and safe patient handling is crucial in maintaining caregiver and patient safety. Assess every situation that involves patient handling and movement to minimize risk of injury. Use the patient's strength when lifting, transferring, or moving when possible. Involving the patient also increases participation in self-care, thus promoting a sense of accomplishment. In addition to handling patients safely, nurses need to assume an active role in their workplaces to ensure that a culture of safety exists and that appropriate patient-handling equipment is readily available (Anderson et al., 2014).

Factors Influencing Activity and Exercise

Factors influencing activity and exercise include growth and development changes, behavioral aspects, and a patient's cultural background. Consider these areas of knowledge and incorporate into the plan of care.

Growth and Development. Throughout the life span the appearance and functioning of the body undergo change. Knowledge of growth and development (see Chapter 23) helps you anticipate types of activities that patients are able to perform. A newborn infant's spine is normally flexed and lacks the anteroposterior curves of an adult. As growth and stability increase, the thoracic spine straightens, and the lumbar spinal curve appears, which allows sitting and standing. As an infant grows, musculoskeletal development permits support of weight for standing and walking. A toddler's posture is awkward because of the slight swayback and protruding abdomen (Hockenberry and Wilson, 2015). From the third year through the beginning of adolescence, the musculoskeletal system continues to grow and develop. Greater coordination enables a child to perform tasks that require fine-motor skills.

A middle-age adult should normally have full musculoskeletal function; however, for people 45 to 64 years of age, the percentage of adults with two or more common chronic conditions has increased (Lee and Ory, 2013). The lack of physical activity is recognized as a risk factor for chronic diseases (Partnership to Fight Chronic Disease, 2012). Adults frequently fail to meet national physical activity guidelines (e.g., being active for at least 30 minutes of moderate intensive activity for most days of the week) (Lee and Ory, 2013). Physical activity is important for health promotion and disease prevention across an individual's life span with older adults having less engagement in physical activity than younger age groups. The percentages of adults participating in physical activity that meet the national physical activity guidelines were 19.2% among people 45 to 54 years of age, 15.9% among people 55 to 64 years of age, and 13.6% among people 65 to 74 years of age (Lee and Ory, 2013). With aging, changes in musculoskeletal function further limit patient activity.

Behavioral Aspects

Take into consideration a patient's knowledge of exercise and activity, barriers to a program of exercise and physical activity, and current exercise behavior or habits. One barrier to exercise is whether a patient has a chronic disease. Symptoms of one chronic condition (e.g., difficulty breathing related to asthma) interferes with another condition (diabetes), preventing the patient from engaging in needed regular exercise (Lee and Ory, 2013). Patients are more open to developing an exercise program if they are at the stage of readiness to change their behavior (Tsang et al., 2015). Patients' decisions to change behavior and include a daily exercise routine in their lives often occur gradually with repeated information individualized to their needs and lifestyle.

Cultural Background

Exercise and physical fitness are beneficial to all people. However, there are cultural differences regarding the extent to which people exercise. A study has shown that leisure physical activity comprises only 10% of total nonwork physical activity among adults (Saffer et al., 2013). The study showed that nonwork physical activity is significantly lower among African Americans, Hispanics, and other racial/ethnic groups as well as among men as a result of educational disadvantages, socioeconomic status, time constraints, and residential location. Individuals with a low level of education and minority racial/ethnic groups tend to have higher levels of physical

---

🌐 BOX 28.3 PATIENT-CENTERED CARE

Lack of physical activity is one of the risk factors associated with type 2 diabetes. In the United States, type 2 diabetes is more prevalent in African Americans and Native Americans. Physical activity is identified as having an important role in the prevention and treatment of type 2 diabetes, yet a disproportionate number of African Americans and Native Americans are disadvantaged and lack access to the health care system and regular exercise (Hernandez et al., 2014; Scarton et al., 2014).

IMPLICATIONS FOR PRACTICE

- Physical inactivity is a modifiable risk factor for the development of type 2 diabetes. Prevention and treatment programs need to focus heavily on exercise and be tailored to the activity tolerance of the individual patient.
- Support promotion of physical activity through formal programs in schools, churches, and government agencies within communities.
- Incorporate motivational factors into exercise programs such as providing a healthy snack or meal for participants and furnishing each patient with a log to monitor weight loss and blood glucose levels.
- Development of an exercise/prevention program needs to remove potential barriers such as transportation and cost to facilitate commitment to the program.

---

activity at work but lower levels of nonwork physical activity. The difference may limit the positive effects of physical activity on an individual's health because nonwork physical activity has a stronger positive association with health relative to work physical activity (Saffer et al., 2013). When developing a physical fitness program for diverse populations, consider their education regarding the value of exercise and learn about what motivates individuals to exercise and which activities are appropriate and enjoyable (Box 28.3).

CRITICAL THINKING

Synthesis

Patient care requires you to apply what you know about a patient, your knowledge base, experience, and critical thinking attitudes and standards. Your synthesis of this information allows you to make sound decisions as you apply the nursing process. Critical thinking synthesis involves combining all available information to obtain a clear picture of the approach needed to provide patient-centered care (Box 28.4).

Knowledge. When you begin the process of problem solving for patient care, consider a variety of concepts and synthesize them together to provide the best outcome for your patient. Knowledge of the musculoskeletal system, exercise physiology, and health alterations that create problems for a patient in the area of exercise and activity provides the foundation for decision making and planning care.

BOX 28.4   SYNTHESIS IN PRACTICE

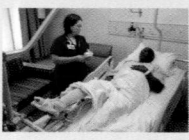

As Marilyn prepares to assess Mr. Indelicato, she reviews musculoskeletal anatomy and physiology and exercise physiology. She gathers information about the expected surgery, anticipated recovery, and physical therapy. During her previous rotation she cared for postoperative patients and knows relevant postoperative care measures to promote patient comfort and the implications of inactivity on postoperative recovery.

Marilyn knows that it is important to assist Mr. Indelicato in a prompt, immediate postoperative recovery and engage him in a steady, progressive physical therapy program. Although she has cared for patients who have required physical therapy, Marilyn has never cared for a patient requiring continuous passive motion (CPM) equipment. She found and read literature about this equipment, and she consulted with the physical therapist who will be assigned to Mr. Indelicato. The use of CPM has been found to improve bending of the knee slightly and the person's quality of life in select cases but may have no effects on pain or function (Harvey et al., 2014). Nonetheless Marilyn learns how to apply the device correctly to guarantee Mr. Indelicato's safety. Marilyn approaches this clinical experience with energy and creativity. She plans to collaborate and implement individualized care to promote Mr. Indelicato's activity and improve his range of motion.

Experience. Past experiences with exercise or caring for patients with problems related to activity and exercise help you anticipate patients' needs such as pain control, positioning, transferring, and support of ADLs. Visits to a physical or occupational therapy unit in a hospital or community setting increase your experiential base.

Attitudes. Attitudes of creativity and perseverance are essential because problems with activity and exercise are often prolonged. The more creative your approach for improving activity tolerance and mobility skills, the greater the chance for a patient's success. This is especially important with children. For example, creating a game that incorporates the goal of improving activity tolerance and provides feedback through colorful stickers elicits better cooperation and participation from a child (Hockenberry and Wilson, 2015).

Standards. Professional standards and guidelines such as those from the American Nurses Association (ANA, 2015, 2016), U.S. Department of Health and Human Services (USDHHS, 2010), NIOSH (VISN8, 2014; NIOSH, 2016), and the American College of Sports Medicine (Garber, 2011) concerning the use of assistive equipment and devices to safely transfer and position patients provide valuable safety guidelines for you and your patients. In addition, these standards help you promote a patient's independence while safely adhering to the prescribed rehabilitation plan.

NURSING PROCESS

Apply the nursing process and use a critical thinking approach in your care of patients. The nursing process provides a clinical decision-making approach for you to develop and implement an individualized plan of care.

■■■ ASSESSMENT

An assessment includes a patient's regular activity level and tolerance and information about preillness functioning. Assess body alignment and posture with a patient standing, sitting, or lying down. Table 28.2 presents examples of factors to assess, related questions, and physical assessment techniques for assessing activity tolerance.

Through assessment you are able to determine patients' normal physiological changes in growth and development; deviations related to poor posture, trauma, muscle damage, or nerve dysfunction; and any learning needs. In addition, assessment provides opportunities for you to observe patients' posture and obtain important information about other factors that contribute to poor alignment such as fatigue, malnutrition, and psychological problems.

Body Alignment. The first step in assessing body alignment is to help a patient feel at ease so that the patient does not assume unnatural or rigid positions. Begin by having the patient stand if he or she is able, then have the patient sit. Place the patient in the supine position by removing pillows and positioning supports from the bed (if not contraindicated) to assess alignment in the recumbent position.

Standing. Assessment of the patient's alignment normally reveals the following:
- The head is erect and midline.
- Body parts are symmetrical.
- The spine is straight with normal curvatures (cervical concave, thoracic convex, and lumbar concave).
- The abdomen is comfortably tucked in.
- The knees are in a straight line between the hips and ankles and slightly flexed.
- The feet are flat on the floor and pointed directly forward and slightly apart to maintain a wide base of support.
- The arms hang comfortably at the sides (Fig. 28.1).

A patient's center of gravity is in the midline, and the line of gravity is from the middle of the forehead to a midpoint between the feet. Laterally the line of gravity runs vertically from the middle of the skull to the posterior third of the foot (Ball et al., 2015; Patton and Thibodeau, 2016).

Sitting. Assess your patient for the following: The head is erect, and the neck and vertebral column are in straight alignment; the body weight is distributed on the buttocks and thighs; the thighs are parallel and in a horizontal plane (be careful to avoid pressure on the popliteal nerve and blood supply); the feet are supported on the floor; and the forearms are supported on the armrest, in the lap, or on a table in front of the chair.

TABLE 28.2 FOCUSED PATIENT ASSESSMENT

FACTORS TO ASSESS	QUESTIONS	PHYSICAL ASSESSMENT
Range of motion (ROM)	To what extent you have limited movement in your joints? Do you have a history of connective tissue disorders, fractures, or damage to ligaments or tendons?	Observe patient's gait and ability to carry out ADLs. Inspect joints for deformity. Measure ROM of affected joints.
Pain	Do you experience pain or discomfort on movement? Do you need pain medication before ambulating (with assistance) or other exercise? Please rate your pain on a scale of 0 to 10 with 10 representing the worst pain.	Inspect joints for redness or swelling indicating potential inflammatory process. Observe for objective signs of pain such as grimacing, moaning, increasing respiratory rate, pulse, and blood pressure. (**Note:** These objective signs are not always present, and it is best to ask patient if pain is present.)
Activity tolerance	Do you feel fatigued? Tell me in what way muscle weakness affects your ability to perform daily activities. Do you feel short of breath, palpitations, light-headed, or dizzy?	Observe for signs of fatigue. Observe patient's performance of ADLs. Observe patient for paleness, obtain vital signs, and compare with baseline measures.

ADLs, Activities of daily living; *ROM,* range of motion.

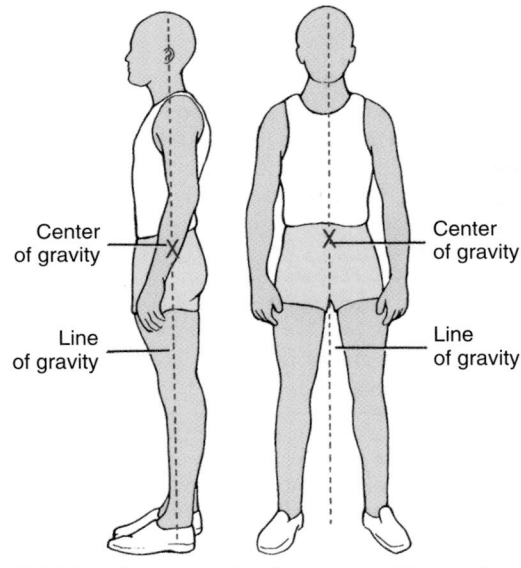

FIG 28.1 Correct body alignment with standing.

Assessment of alignment in the sitting position is particularly important for patients with neuromuscular disorders, muscle weakness, muscle paralysis, or nerve damage. A patient with these alterations has diminished sensation in affected areas and is unable to perceive pressure or decreased circulation. Proper sitting alignment reduces the risk for musculoskeletal system damage.

Recumbent. Position your patient in the lateral side-lying position with all but one pillow and all positioning supports removed from the bed. Make sure that the vertebrae are in straight alignment without observable curves. This assessment provides baseline data concerning a patient's body alignment while in bed. Conditions that create a risk for damage to the musculoskeletal system when lying down include impaired mobility (e.g., spinal curvature), use of immobilization devices (e.g., traction), decreased sensation (e.g., hemiparesis from a stroke), impaired circulation (e.g., diabetes), and lack of voluntary muscle control (e.g., spinal cord injuries).

When a patient is unable to change position voluntarily, assess the position of body parts while the patient is lying down. Make sure that the vertebrae are in straight alignment without any observable curves. Normally the extremities are in alignment and do not cross over one another. The head and neck are aligned without excessive flexion or extension.

Mobility. The adequacy of a patient's mobility affects his or her coordination and balance while sitting, standing, and walking; the ability to carry out ADLs; and the ability to participate in an exercise program. The assessment of mobility has five components: sitting, standing, range of motion (ROM), gait, and exercise.

Sitting. Your observation includes noting if a patient can sit on the side of the bed or in a chair upright. A patient's ability to do so affects his or her ability to perform self-care activities such as feeding self and performing hygiene activities. When assessing the ability of patients to sit, allow them to use a side rail (when present). Skill 28.2 describes the Banner Mobility Assessment Tool (BMAT), a validated tool that includes a component for assessment of a patient's mobility while sitting (Boynton et al., 2014). Success with the sitting maneuver indicates good sitting mobility.

Standing. Do not rely on a patient's self-report that he or she is able to stand independently without support. This commonly occurs when nurses rush to admit or transfer patients to their care units. When you assess a patient's ability to stand, it is appropriate to have them use an assistive device for support. The BMAT (Boynton et al., 2014) includes a measure for assessing a patient while standing. A patient should be able to raise the buttocks off the bed and hold for a count of five (Boynton, et al., 2014). The ability to achieve this maneuver indicates good mobility and balance (see Skill 28.2).

Range of Motion. Observing range of motion (ROM) is one of the first assessment techniques used to determine the degree of limitation or injury to a joint. Assess ROM to clarify the extent of joint stiffness, swelling, pain, limited movement, and unequal movement. Chapter 29 presents a thorough ROM assessment. Limited ROM indicates inflammation such as arthritis, fluid in the joint, altered nerve supply, or contractures. Increased mobility (beyond normal) of a joint indicates connective tissue disorders, ligament tears, and possible joint fractures.

Gait. Gait is the manner or style of walking including rhythm, cadence, length of stride, and speed. Assessing gait allows for conclusions about balance, posture, and the ability to walk without assistance (see Chapter 16). While a patient walks, look for conformity, a regular smooth rhythm and symmetry in the length of leg swing; smooth swaying related to the gait phase; and a smooth symmetrical arm swing (Ball et al., 2015). An abnormal gait is a common risk factor for patient falls.

Exercise. Exercise is physical activity. It can be used for body conditioning, improving health, maintaining fitness, providing therapy for correcting a deformity, or restoring the body to a maximal state of health. During assessment, determine a patient's level and frequency of exercise (Box 28.5). Determine whether a patient participates in sufficient physical activity by comparing your findings with the Centers for Disease Control and Prevention (CDC, 2015) recommendations, as follows: Adults need at least 2 hours and 30 minutes (150 minutes) of *moderate-intensity aerobic activity* (i.e., brisk walking) every week and *muscle-strengthening activities* on 2 or more days a week that work all major muscle groups (legs, hips, back, abdomen, chest, shoulders, and arms). The activity can be spread across a week. Your assessment of the patient's activity provides baseline information for both exercise and activity tolerance. In addition, baseline information is beneficial when establishing a patient's exercise and rehabilitation plan after an illness or injury. When a person exercises, physiological changes occur in body systems (Box 28.6).

Exercise improves muscle tone, size, and strength and cardiopulmonary conditioning. As a result an individual is able to exercise longer with each strengthening of the muscles. Exercise also enhances joint mobility because the exercise itself requires movement of body parts.

Activity Tolerance. Activity tolerance is the type and amount of exercise or work that a person is able to perform without undue exertion or injury (Box 28.7). Observe patients after ambulation, self-bathing, or sitting in a chair for several hours, and assess their verbal report of fatigue and weakness. Do they exhibit difficulty breathing or report being short of

---

BOX 28.5 GENERAL GUIDELINES FOR INITIATING AN EXERCISE PROGRAM

STEP 1: ASSESS FITNESS LEVEL
- Seek approval from a health care provider to begin. Are there any limitations to consider before determining the exercises in the fitness program?
- Record baseline fitness scores such as pulse rate, how long it takes to walk 1 mile, waist circumference, and body mass index.

STEP 2: DESIGN THE FITNESS PROGRAM
- Consider fitness goals. Make goals attainable.
- Plan a logical progression of activities (e.g., walk 1 mile and gradually increase the pace).
- Build the program into a daily routine.
- Plan the fitness program with creativity and different activities.

STEP 3: ASSEMBLE EQUIPMENT
- Choose athletic shoes designed for the chosen exercise.
- Try equipment at a fitness center before purchasing to make sure that it fits into the fitness program.
- Buy used fitness equipment.
- Try homemade equipment (e.g., half-gallon milk jugs filled with sand for weights).

STEP 4: GET STARTED
- Start slowly, including a warm-up and cool-down period.
- Divide exercise time throughout the day if time or fatigue is a barrier. Ten minutes of exercise 3 times a day instead of a single 30-minute workout may be better for some patients' schedules and medical conditions.

STEP 5: MONITOR PROGRESS
- Repeat fitness assessment at 6 weeks and then every 3 to 6 months.
- If losing motivation: set new goals, exercise with a friend, or try new activities.

Modified from the American Academy of Orthopaedic Surgeons: *Rehabilitation exercise and conditioning handouts,* 2012, http://orthoinfo.org/topic.cfm?topic=A00672; and Mayo Clinic Tools for Healthier Lives: *Fitness programs: 5 steps to getting started,* 2014, http://www.mayoclinic.org/healthy-lifestyle/fitness/in-depth/fitness/art-20048269?pg=1.

---

breath after exercise? Assess heart rate and blood pressure response to activity by comparing with baseline rates at rest. Both heart rate and blood pressure should increase. When you care for a patient who is relatively healthy and able to exercise regularly, assess what the patient sets as his or her target heart rate during exercise. Use this finding to determine if the patient has set an adequate target rate for exercise training (American Heart Association [AHA], 2015).

Older Adult Considerations. Older adults who experience a disease or debilitating illness often experience a decline in physical activity and changes in joints that predispose to problems with mobility and limit joint flexibility.

BOX 28.6   EFFECTS OF EXERCISE

CARDIOVASCULAR SYSTEM
- Increased cardiac output
- Improved myocardial contraction, thereby strengthening cardiac muscle
- Decreased resting heart rate
- Improved venous return

PULMONARY SYSTEM
- Increased respiratory rate and depth followed by a quicker return to resting state
- Improved alveolar ventilation
- Decreased work of breathing
- Improved diaphragmatic excursion

METABOLIC SYSTEM
- Increased basal metabolic rate
- Increased use of glucose and fatty acids
- Increased triglyceride breakdown

- Increased gastric motility
- Increased production of body heat

MUSCULOSKELETAL SYSTEM
- Improved muscle tone
- Increased joint mobility
- Improved muscle tolerance to physical exercise
- Possible increase in muscle mass
- Reduced bone loss

ACTIVITY TOLERANCE
- Improved tolerance
- Decreased fatigue

PSYCHOSOCIAL FACTORS
- Improved tolerance to stress
- Reports of "feeling better"
- Reports of decrease in illness (e.g., colds, influenza)

Data from Huether SE, McCance KL: *Understanding pathophysiology*, ed 6, St Louis, 2017, Mosby.

BOX 28.7   FACTORS INFLUENCING ACTIVITY TOLERANCE

PHYSIOLOGICAL FACTORS
- Skeletal abnormalities
- Muscular impairments
- Endocrine or metabolic illnesses (e.g., diabetes mellitus, thyroid disease)
- Hypoxemia
- Decreased cardiopulmonary function
- Decreased endurance
- Impaired physical stability
- Pain
- Sleep pattern disturbance
- Prior exercise patterns
- Infectious processes and fever

EMOTIONAL FACTORS
- Anxiety
- Depression
- Chemical addictions
- Motivation

DEVELOPMENTAL FACTORS
- Age
- Sex
- Pregnancy
- Physical growth and development of muscle and skeletal support

In addition, chronic conditions increase in older adults, and certain medications (e.g., cardiovascular medication or diuretics, or changes in dosages of these medications) affect a person's activity and exercise tolerance. It is important for older adults to exercise and remain active. A program of exercise promotes health and improves illness, trauma, and rehabilitation outcomes (CDC, 2015). As people age they lose lifelong partners and friends, and opportunities for exercise and activities lessen.

Patient Expectations. In assessing a patient's expectations concerning body alignment, joint mobility, or activity, determine your patient's perception of what is normal or acceptable in regard to mobility. For example, if exercising is painful or tiresome to patients, they may lack adherence and commitment to desired interventions. Some patients are content with their present ROM or mobility and do not perceive a need for improvement. Often they are unaware of the implications of inactivity.

■■■ NURSING DIAGNOSIS

Data from your nursing assessment including a patient's knowledge of or motivation to be active and alterations in body alignment, joint mobility, and neurological function are the defining characteristics or risk factors to support a nursing diagnosis. In the case of activity and exercise alterations, nursing diagnoses will focus on a patient's ability or desire to move. A nursing diagnostic label must be accurate to appropriately direct nursing interventions. For example, the diagnoses *Impaired Physical Mobility* and *Fatigue* are different with respect to the type of nursing interventions such as positioning techniques or exercise measures.

A patient's assessment provides related clusters of risk factors or defining characteristics that lead to the identification of nursing diagnoses including the following examples:
- *Activity Intolerance*
- *Chronic Pain*
- *Fatigue*
- *Risk for Injury*
- *Impaired Physical Mobility*
- *Impaired Sitting*
- *Impaired Walking*
- *Sedentary Lifestyle*

If you select a problem-focused nursing diagnosis such as *Impaired Physical Mobility*, select a related factor that is relevant and will further aid you in intervention selection. For example, *Impaired Physical Mobility related to pain* will require different interventions than *Impaired Physical Mobility related to activity intolerance*.

■■■ PLANNING

Use data gathered during assessment and critical thinking to develop an individualized plan of care based on the nursing diagnoses for your patients. Once you identify the relevant nursing diagnoses, collaborate with the patient and family, integrate the needs associated with the diagnoses with the goals and outcomes of care, and select care priorities. The plan of care will include appropriate interventions that will allow you to maintain or optimize the patient's exercise and activity levels (Fig. 28.2).

Goals and Outcomes. Once you define appropriate nursing diagnoses, collaborate with the patient to set goals and expected outcomes that are relevant, appropriate, and

timely. Each outcome provides a measure for later evaluating the success of your nursing interventions. For example, the goal of achieving optimum ROM in the right knee has the outcome of achieving 90-degree flexion in the right knee by discharge. While you care for the patient, you will conduct reassessments to evaluate if right knee flexion improves. Other common goals that you might select for a patient with activity and exercise alterations include adoption of a regular exercise program, remaining injury-free, or ambulation without

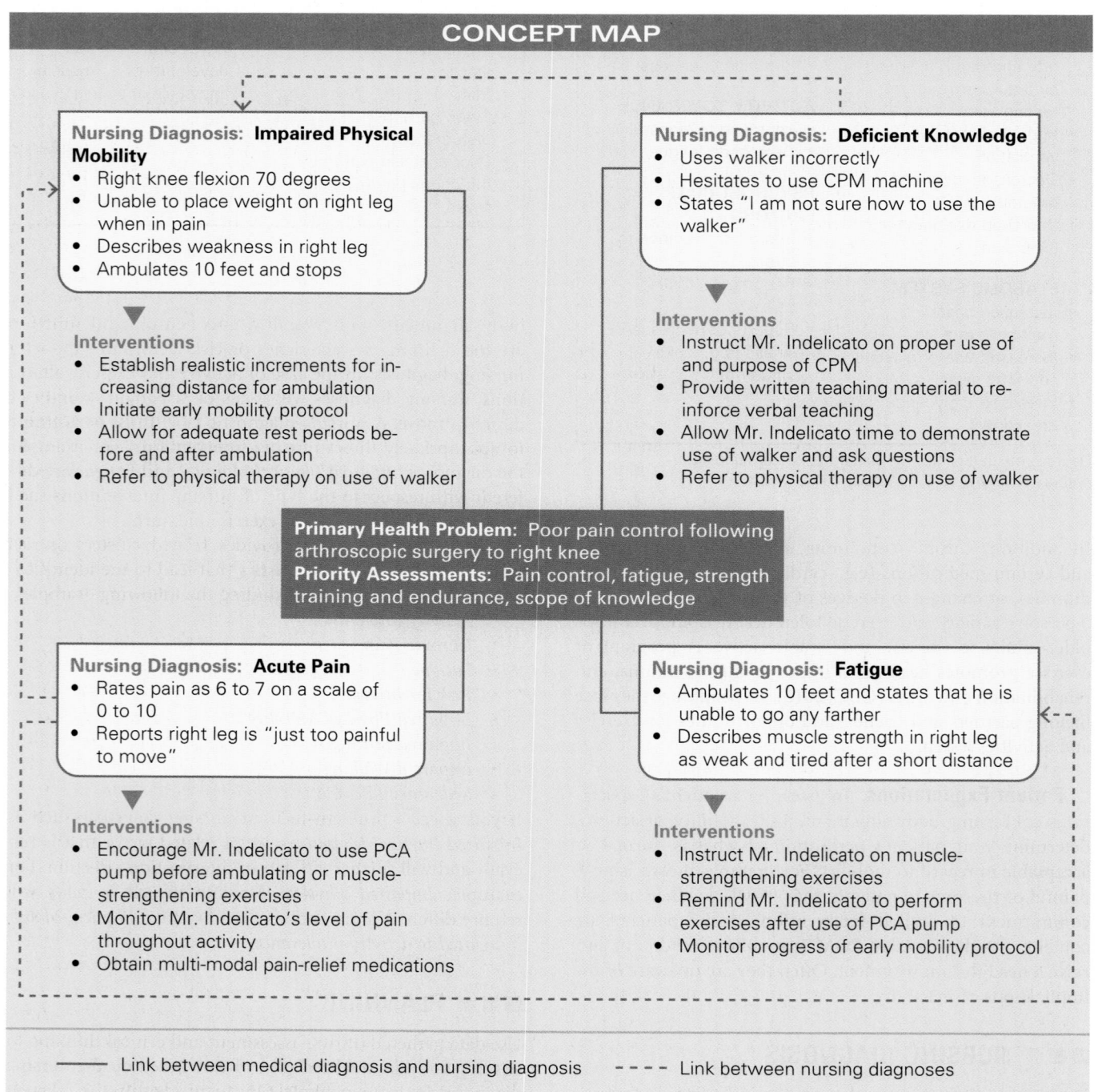

CONCEPT MAP

Nursing Diagnosis: Impaired Physical Mobility
- Right knee flexion 70 degrees
- Unable to place weight on right leg when in pain
- Describes weakness in right leg
- Ambulates 10 feet and stops

Interventions
- Establish realistic increments for increasing distance for ambulation
- Initiate early mobility protocol
- Allow for adequate rest periods before and after ambulation
- Refer to physical therapy on use of walker

Nursing Diagnosis: Deficient Knowledge
- Uses walker incorrectly
- Hesitates to use CPM machine
- States "I am not sure how to use the walker"

Interventions
- Instruct Mr. Indelicato on proper use of and purpose of CPM
- Provide written teaching material to reinforce verbal teaching
- Allow Mr. Indelicato time to demonstrate use of walker and ask questions
- Refer to physical therapy on use of walker

Primary Health Problem: Poor pain control following arthroscopic surgery to right knee
Priority Assessments: Pain control, fatigue, strength training and endurance, scope of knowledge

Nursing Diagnosis: Acute Pain
- Rates pain as 6 to 7 on a scale of 0 to 10
- Reports right leg is "just too painful to move"

Interventions
- Encourage Mr. Indelicato to use PCA pump before ambulating or muscle-strengthening exercises
- Monitor Mr. Indelicato's level of pain throughout activity
- Obtain multi-modal pain-relief medications

Nursing Diagnosis: Fatigue
- Ambulates 10 feet and states that he is unable to go any farther
- Describes muscle strength in right leg as weak and tired after a short distance

Interventions
- Instruct Mr. Indelicato on muscle-strengthening exercises
- Remind Mr. Indelicato to perform exercises after use of PCA pump
- Monitor progress of early mobility protocol

——— Link between medical diagnosis and nursing diagnosis   - - - - Link between nursing diagnoses

FIG 28.2 Concept map. *CPM,* Continuous passive motion; *PCA,* patient-controlled analgesia.

assistance. Corresponding outcomes would include patient participates in 20 minutes of walking daily, patient does not incur a fall before discharge, or patient participates in gait training daily. The plan of care considers risks for injury and preexisting health concerns. It is especially important to have knowledge of your patient's previous functional status and home environment.

Setting Priorities. Consider the patient's most immediate needs when selecting priorities of care. Determine the immediacy of any problem (e.g., pain, lack of knowledge about exercise, reduced ROM) by the effect the problem has on a patient's mental and physical health. For example, if a patient is in acute pain, relieving pain is a priority before you begin exercise therapy. Safety becomes a priority whenever you are assisting with the many skills associated with the care of patients with activity intolerance, improper body mechanics, or impaired mobility. For example, you must use caution to avoid a patient fall during transfer. Your priorities change from short-term to long-term when you plan for a patient's return to their home. For patients who remain disabled or limited in mobility, be sure that family caregivers are prepared to help with positioning and transfer techniques. When you perform skills that promote a patient's activity in the acute care setting, always be vigilant in monitoring your patients and supervising nursing assistive personnel in carrying out activities to prevent complications and potential injury.

Collaborative Care. Planning also involves an understanding of the resources necessary to maintain a patient's motor function and independence. Collaboration with other members of the health care team, such as physical or occupational therapists, is important in the provision of appropriate exercises and adaptive approaches to self-care. Long-term rehabilitation is sometimes necessary, and you begin discharge planning when a patient enters the health care system. In addition, always individualize a plan of care (see Care Plan).

■ ■ ■ IMPLEMENTATION

Health Promotion. A goal of the Healthy People 2020 (HealthyPeople.gov, 2015) initiative is to improve health, fitness, and quality of life through daily physical activity. This goal is based on guidelines that suggest that regular physical activity can improve the health and quality of life of Americans of all ages, regardless of the presence of a chronic disease or disability (USDHHS, 2008a, 2008b). As a nurse, you may work in outpatient settings with the opportunity to plan health promotion activities. It is crucial to educate patients and family caregivers about the importance of regular physical activity and exercise and how these activities can be incorporated into daily routines (see Box 28.5 and Skill 28.1).

With the increase in exercise awareness more community centers, shopping malls, and exercise facilities have indoor walking areas. Thus people are able to plan for walking as an exercise in climate-controlled and safe environments. Family and community gardens offer another method of exercise and help a person maintain and improve balance. Community centers, local adult education classes, and exercise facilities have exercise classes geared to a variety of age-groups and families. In addition, some facilities have exercise classes geared to individuals with chronic illnesses such as cardiac or pulmonary disease. All of these resources focus on improving exercise and activity.

Encourage patients to exercise daily; moderate 15- to 30-minute exercise is beneficial to maintain fitness, weight levels, and glycemic (blood sugar) control. The CDC (2015) recommends adults need at least 2 hours and 30 minutes (150 minutes) of moderate-intensity aerobic activity each week. If a patient is actively exercising, be sure the patient is setting an adequate target heart rate for vigorous exercise. The AHA (2015) recommends that a person's target heart rate should be between 50% and 85% of his or her maximum heart rate. Maximum heart rate is approximately 220 minus age.

Always encourage older adults or patients with underlying medical conditions to consult with their health care provider before beginning a vigorous exercise program. Direct patient-centered health promotion activities toward maintaining and/or improving exercise and activity that help return a patient to independence and a maximal state of health after trauma or illness. Although some patients require formal rehabilitation, many of these activities are implemented in a patient's home or neighborhood. Recommend approaches that help older adults increase exercise and activity, use proper body mechanics, and prevent injury (Box 28.8).

Acute Care

Early Mobility. Recently concerted efforts have been made in hospitals to increase inpatients' activity and mobility levels as soon as possible to prevent deconditioning and other complications of immobilization (see Skill 28.1). The AACN (2013) now recommends an early progressive mobility protocol for critical care patients (refer to agency policy for protocols). When patients are transferred out to general nursing units, early mobility protocols should continue. This is often a challenge because staff nurses on general units often have difficulty routinely ambulating patients because of overall patient care demands, access to equipment, or unfamiliarity with transfer skills (see Skill 28.2). However, early mobilization has been found to be a nursing intervention that provides positive outcomes for critical care, cardiovascular, neurological (stroke), and orthopedic patient populations (Pashikanti and Von Ah, 2012). Early mobility protocols typically involve a progressive series of specific mobility interventions (e.g., ROM, sitting on side of bed, ambulating to chair, ambulating) to help patients attain and/or maintain their baseline mobility status. Some hospitals have designated special mobility teams or mobility assistants to engage patients in early ambulation and activity.

Walking. Walking increases exercise tolerance, circulation, and joint mobility. In the normal walking posture, the

⊚ CARE PLAN

Impaired Physical Mobility

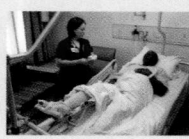

ASSESSMENT

Mr. Indelicato is a 72-year-old man hospitalized for surgery on his right knee. Over the past 5 years he has experienced pain and decreased mobility. He is now experiencing his first postoperative day following total right knee replacement using fast-track protocol. His incision is healing, and there is no edema or redness.

ASSESSMENT ACTIVITIES	FINDINGS[a]
Assess Mr. Indelicato's pain level.	Mr. Indelicato is **hesitant to ambulate** or participate in active exercises on his first postoperative day using the early mobility protocol. He rates his **pain as 6 to 7 on a scale of 0 to 10** and is using a patient-controlled analgesia (PCA) pump. He states, **"I can't put all my weight on my right leg. It's just too painful."**
Assess Mr. Indelicato's baseline mobility and endurance.	His degree of knee flexion is now 70 degrees. He is able to ambulate 10 feet with a walker but states, "I can't go any farther." In addition, he further describes his right leg as feeling weak and tired after walking a short distance.
Assess Mr. Indelicato's knowledge about proper use of his walker.	The nurse observes Mr. Indelicato using the walker incorrectly.

[a]**Defining characteristics/risk factors** are shown in **bold** type.

NURSING DIAGNOSIS: Impaired Physical Mobility related to pain, muscle weakness, and limited joint motion.

PLANNING

GOALS

Mr. Indelicato will obtain a tolerable level of pain during self-care activities.

Mr. Indelicato will gain optimal functioning of the right knee with independent, purposeful movement on discharge.

Mr. Indelicato will use walker properly while ambulating.

EXPECTED OUTCOMES (NOC)[b]

Self-Care: Activities of Daily Living

Mr. Indelicato's pain is below 3 at rest and below 5 with activity on a scale of 0 to 10 with oral pain relief medication by discharge.

Mr. Indelicato is able to climb stairs, dress independently, and go to the toilet independently by discharge.

Mobility

Mr. Indelicato ambulates 4 times with aid of walker, each time increasing distance, without reports of increasing fatigue by discharge.

Ambulation

Mr. Indelicato performs a return demonstration of proper use of walker.

[b]Outcome classification labels from Moorhead S, et al, editors: *Nursing outcomes classification (NOC)*, ed 5, St Louis, 2013, Mosby.

INTERVENTIONS (NIC)[c]

Exercise Therapy: Ambulation

Encourage Mr. Indelicato to use patient-controlled analgesia (PCA) pump at least 20 minutes before ambulation.

Advance patient to multimodal analgesia for pain control by day 2 postoperatively. Practices will vary, but multimodal analgesics usually include oral acetaminophen, celecoxib, and oxycodone (OxyContin) at prescribed intervals.

Initiate early mobility protocol by having Mr. Indelicato sit in bed or on side of bed (dangle) before standing to ambulate.

RATIONALE

Peak actions of analgesic occur as patient begins activity (Schofield, 2014).

There is mounting evidence that multimodal analgesia provides superior pain relief, while speeding up functional recovery, minimizing the adverse effects of traditional opioid-based analgesia, increasing patient satisfaction, and reducing length of hospital stay (Halawi et al., 2015).

Allowing patient to dangle before changing positions helps reduce or prevents orthostatic hypotension, maintains safety, and prevents injury to patient.

CARE PLAN—cont'd

Impaired Physical Mobility

INTERVENTIONS (NIC)[c]	RATIONALE
Have Mr. Indelicato ambulate (marching in place, walking in halls), increasing time and distance each day of hospitalization.	Gradually increasing physical activity and setting realistic goals for ambulation encourage activity in older adults (Doherty-King et al., 2014).
Collaborate with physical therapist in instructing Mr. Indelicato and family caregiver on proper use of walker and how to climb stairs. Provide written material that reinforces verbal instructions. Have patient return demonstrate stair walking.	Providing instructions in a quiet environment and giving written instructions in large, easy-to-read print enhances learning for older adults (Touhy et al., 2014). Return demonstration ensures patient safety.

Self-Care Assistance

Consult with occupational therapist to prepare patient to learn how to dress self and use the toilet with minimal assistance.	Preserves patient's sense of independence.

[c]Intervention classification labels from Bulecheck GM, et al, editors: *Nursing interventions classification (NIC)*, ed 6, St Louis, 2013, Mosby.

EVALUATION

NURSING ACTIONS	PATIENT RESPONSE/FINDING	ACHIEVEMENT OF OUTCOME
Ask Mr. Indelicato to rate the level of pain on a scale of 0 to 10.	Mr. Indelicato rates his pain at a 3 and states, "I am able to walk now that my knee doesn't hurt so badly anymore."	Mr. Indelicato's pain is under control, and he is able to ambulate with minimal discomfort.
Observe Mr. Indelicato's range of motion (ROM).	Able to perform ROM.	Outcome met. Mr. Indelicato expresses understanding of need for ROM.
Observe Mr. Indelicato use toilet and dress self.	Patient is a bit hesitant to rotate correctly before sitting on toilet seat. Needs assistance with applying pants.	Continue therapy sessions.
Monitor distance Mr. Indelicato ambulates.	Mr. Indelicato ambulates within 12 hr postoperatively 60 feet, then ambulates twice postoperative day 2 for a total of 140 feet using walling.	Ambulation is progressing. Continue ambulation sessions up to discharge. Demonstrates correct use of walker.

head is erect; the cervical, thoracic, and lumbar vertebrae are aligned; the hips and knees have appropriate flexion; and the arms swing freely in alternation with the legs. Illness or trauma reduces activity tolerance, sometimes requiring you to assist the patient with walking or having the patient use assistive devices such as crutches, canes, or walkers.

Helping a patient walk requires preparation. Your initial assessment should have included a patient's activity tolerance, strength, coordination, and balance to determine the type of assistance needed. Also reassess a patient's orientation and determine if there are any signs of distress before you assist the patient with ambulation.

Also assess the environment for safety before ambulation. Remove obstacles and be sure that the floor is clean and dry. Establish rest points in case the patient's activity tolerance decreases or the patient becomes dizzy. Also make sure that the patient wears supportive, nonslip shoes.

When preparing a patient who is in bed for ambulation, dangling is an important technique. You help the patient to a sitting position with the legs dangling off the side of the bed and have him or her rest for 1 to 2 minutes before standing (see Skill 28.1). The longer the period of immobility, the

greater are the physiological changes. This is especially true with changes in circulation. When a patient has been flat for extended periods, blood pressure drops when the patient stands. Dangling helps to prevent this. After standing, have the patient remain stationary for 1 or 2 minutes before moving. If the patient becomes dizzy, the bed is still nearby, and you are able to quickly ease him or her back to bed.

There are several methods to help a patient with ambulation. Always apply a gait belt to support a patient and maintain a midline center of gravity. Make sure that he or she does not lean to one side while walking because this causes the center of gravity to no longer be at midline, which distorts balance and increases risk for falling.

Return a patient who appears unsteady or complains of dizziness to the closest bed or a chair. If the patient has a syncopal episode or begins to fall, assume a wide base of support with one foot in front of the other, thus supporting the patient's body weight. Gently lower the patient to the floor, protecting his or her head. Although lowering a patient to the floor is not difficult, practice this technique with a friend or classmate before attempting it in a clinical setting (Fig. 28.3). Assess the patient for injuries at this time and

BOX 28.8 CARE OF THE OLDER ADULT

General Guidelines for Initiating an Exercise Program With the Older Adult

- Encourage older adults to avoid prolonged sitting and to get up and stretch. Frequent stretching decreases joint contractures. Supervised resistance and aerobic exercise training in older adults both significantly improved physical function (Parreira et al., 2014; Chmelo et al., 2015).
- Maintain proper body alignment when sitting. Proper alignment minimizes joint and muscle stress.
- Teach older adults how to use stronger joints or larger muscle groups to manipulate items such as spray cans and container lids. Efficient distribution of workload decreases joint stress and pain.
- Provide resources for planned exercise programs. Proper exercise activities slow further bone loss and prevent fractures in older adults with osteoporosis (Wallace et al., 2014).
- It is never too late to begin an exercise program (Edelman et al., 2014). Be sure that older adults consult a health care provider before beginning an exercise program, particularly if they have heart, lung, or other illnesses.

notify the patient's health care provider. Even if the patient is stable, obtain the assistance of a lift team to help you get the patient off the floor and back in bed or a chair.

Lifting Techniques. In the clinical setting, patient care activities place health care providers at risk for injury during patient handling (see Chapter 29). Recently the rate of injuries in occupational settings has increased dramatically. The most common back injury is strain on the lumbar muscle group, which includes the muscles around the lumbar vertebrae. Injury to these areas affects the ability to bend forward, backward, and side to side and to rotate the hips and lower back.

Lifting activities are necessary in acute care and restorative care settings. For example, you may care for an individual who is wheelchair dependent and healthy but needs assistance moving from bed to chair or chair to commode, or you may care for an individual who is unable to assist with any transfer and needs to be lifted from bed to chair or bed to stretcher. In any setting, you need to know and use proper lifting techniques. Before lifting, assess the weight that you will lift and what assistance, if any, you need. If you need help, assess if a second person is adequate or if you need to use a mechanical lift. Once you determine the amount of assistance you need, follow these steps:

1. Keep the weight you are lifting as close to your body as possible; this action places the object in the same plane as the lifter and close to the center of gravity for balance.
2. Bend at the knees; this maintains the center of gravity and uses the stronger leg muscles to do the lifting (Fig. 28.4). Avoid twisting. Twisting overloads the spine and leads to serious injury.

3. Tighten abdominal muscles and tuck the pelvis; this provides balance and helps protect the back.
4. Keep your trunk erect and knees bent so that multiple muscle groups work together in a coordinated manner.

Remember that injuries are not only related to lifting. You spend time in many activities involving bending and twisting that also cause injury (e.g., lifting and carrying supplies and equipment and pushing and pulling equipment (Anderson et al., 2014).

Moving and Transferring Patients. Patients require various levels of assistance to move up in bed, move to the side-lying position, or sit up at the side of the bed. For example, a young, healthy woman needs only a little support as she sits at the side of the bed for the first time after childbirth, whereas an older man needs help from two or more nurses to do the same task 1 day after abdominal surgery. When moving or transferring a patient always ask the patient to help to the fullest extent possible. To determine what the patient is able to do alone and how many people are needed to help move the patient in bed, assess whether the patient's illness contradicts exertion (e.g., cardiovascular disease). As a rule of thumb, *get help* to transfer a patient. If you or any other caregiver needs to lift more than 15.9 kg (35 lb) (Anderson et al., 2014; NIOSH, 2016), use assistive devices for the transfer (Fig. 28.5). Through the use of assessment tools and patient movement algorithms, you determine the safest method by which to move the patient. Explain the assistive device and procedure and determine the patient's understanding before the transfer. For example, a patient recently medicated for postoperative pain is too lethargic to understand instruction; thus to ensure safety, two nurses are necessary to move him or her. Then determine the patient's level of comfort. It is also important to evaluate your personal strength and knowledge of the procedure.

A safe transfer (e.g., moving from chair to bed, from bed to wheelchair) is the first priority. Proper use of body mechanics enables you to move, lift, or transfer patients safely and protects you from injury to your musculoskeletal system (see Skill 28.2). Prevent self-injury by using correct posture, minimal muscle strength, and effective body mechanics and lifting techniques Transferring is a skill that helps patients regain optimal independence as quickly as possible. Physical activity maintains and improves joint motion, increases strength, promotes circulation, relieves pressure on skin, and improves urinary and respiratory functions. It also benefits the patient psychologically by increasing social activity and mental stimulation and providing a change in environment. Thus mobilization plays a crucial role in a patient's rehabilitation.

When preparing to transfer patients, consider the type of problems that can develop. A patient who has been immobile for several days or longer is often weak or dizzy or sometimes develops initial orthostatic hypotension (a drop in blood pressure of 40 mm Hg or more systolic or 20 mm Hg or more diastolic when rising from a sitting position within 15 seconds of standing) when transferred (Frith et al., 2014; Lewis et al., 2014; Mills et al., 2014). A patient with

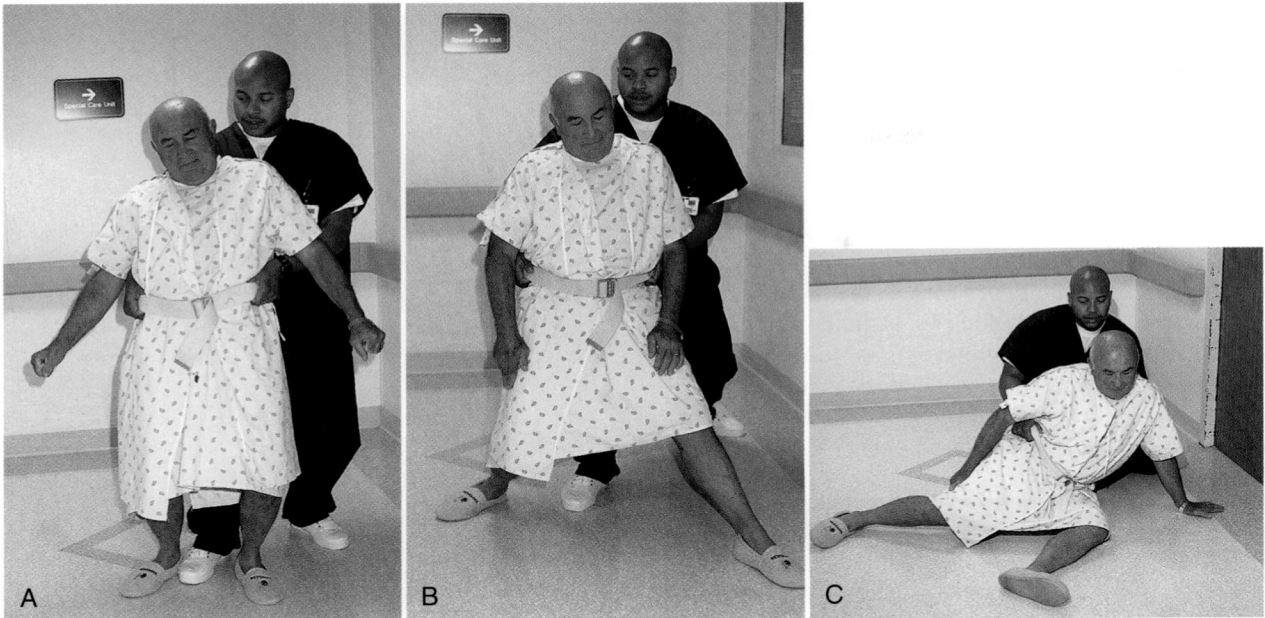

FIG 28.3 **A,** Stand with feet apart to provide broad base of support. **B,** Extend one leg and let patient slide against it to floor. **C,** Bend knees to lower body as patient slides to floor.

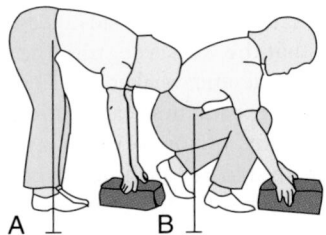

FIG 28.4 Incorrect **(A)** and correct **(B)** body position for lifting.

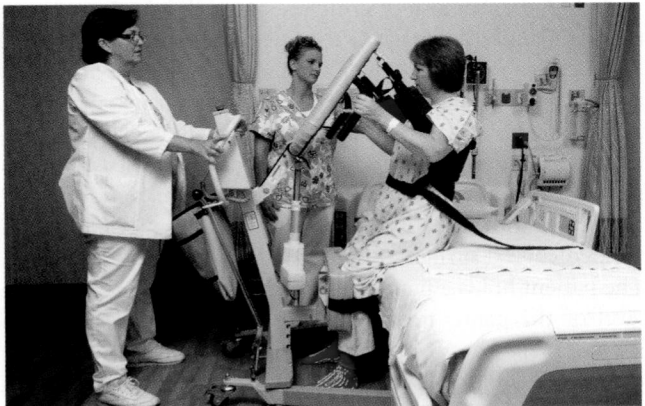

FIG 28.5 Patient grasps handles as nurse enables motorized lift.

neurological deficits sometimes has paresis (muscle weakness) or paralysis unilaterally or bilaterally, which complicates safe transfer. A flaccid arm sustains injury during transfer if unsupported. As a general rule use a gait belt and obtain assistance for mobilization of patients with neurological deficits.

Range-of-Motion Exercises. The easiest intervention to maintain or improve joint mobility for patients—and one that you are able to coordinate with other activities—is the use of ROM exercises. In **active range-of-motion (ROM) exercises** a patient is able to move his or her joints. In contrast, you move the patient's joints in passive ROM exercises. The use of these exercises enables you to evaluate a patient's response to improve the patient's joint mobility (see Chapter 29). Unless contraindicated, the nursing care plan includes exercising each joint through as nearly a full ROM as possible. Initiate passive ROM exercises as soon as a patient loses the ability to move the extremity or joint (see Chapter 29).

Joints that are not moved periodically develop contractures, a permanent shortening of a muscle followed by the eventual shortening of associated ligaments and tendons. Over time the joint becomes fixed in one position, and a patient loses normal use of it. For a patient who does not have voluntary motor control, passive ROM exercises are the exercises of choice.

Older adults experiencing a decline in physical activity and changes in joints often have limited mobility and joint flexibility. Use a variety of recommended approaches to help older adults maximize movement and prevent injury.

At times, mechanical devices are available to move joints through continuous passive motion (CPM). A physician orders this machine to be set at certain degrees of joint mobility with increasing flexion and extension as the goal. Patients who have historically used the CPM machine have had total joint replacement surgery. However, use of the CPM has decreased in practice over the last 10 years with implementation of fast-track rehabilitation following total knee arthroplasty.

Restorative and Continuing Care. Restorative and continuing care for activity and exercise involves implementing strategies to promote further exercise progression and to assist a patient in ADLs after a patient no longer needs acute care. In collaboration with other health care professionals such as physical and occupational therapists, you promote activity and exercise by reinforcing patients to continue and sustain an exercise plan. Patients requiring assistive devices for ambulation need instruction on how to use canes, walkers, or crutches appropriately, depending on the patient's condition. Restorative and continuing care includes activities and exercises that restore and improve optimal functioning in a patient with chronic musculoskeletal illnesses such as arthritis, trauma, and other chronic illnesses such as coronary artery disease (CAD).

QSEN QSEN ACTIVITY *Informatics*

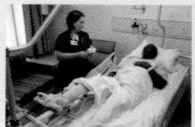

Marilyn meets with Mr. Indelicato at the outpatient rehabilitation setting 5 weeks after surgery on his right knee. He states, "I don't feel like I'm making progress or improvement; this is so frustrating. I can't keep track of when or if I did my exercises for the day." Marilyn notices that over the past several weeks Mr. Indelicato has entered his appointment times into his smartphone. She tells him that she will program his smartphone to help record his exercises each day.

- What is the appropriate response to Mr. Indelicato's statements? Should Marilyn recommend the use of smartphone technology to address his concerns? Explain your answer.

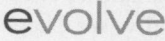 *evolve*   Answers to QSEN Activities can be found on the Evolve website.

Assistive Devices for Walking

Walkers. Walkers are extremely light, movable devices, approximately waist high and made of metal tubing (Fig. 28.6). They have four widely placed, sturdy legs. A walker is fitted correctly by having the patient step inside the walker. The person's elbow should bend comfortably, approximately 15 to 30 degrees, while holding onto the handgrips. When the person relaxes the arms at the side of the body, the top of the walker should line up with the crease on the inside of the wrist (Pierson and Fairchild, 2013; American Academy of Orthopaedic Surgeons, 2015). Box 28.9 describes steps for instructing a patient on use of a walker.

Canes. Canes are lightweight, easily movable devices, held approximately waist high, made of wood or metal. Two common types of canes are the single straight-legged cane and the quad cane. The single straight-legged cane is used to support and balance a patient with decreased leg strength. Make sure that a patient keeps the cane on the stronger side of the body (Pierson and Fairchild, 2013). Stand on the patient's weak side to provide support (Pierson and Fairchild, 2013). For maximum support when walking, the patient places the cane forward 15 to 25 cm (6 to 10 inches), keeping

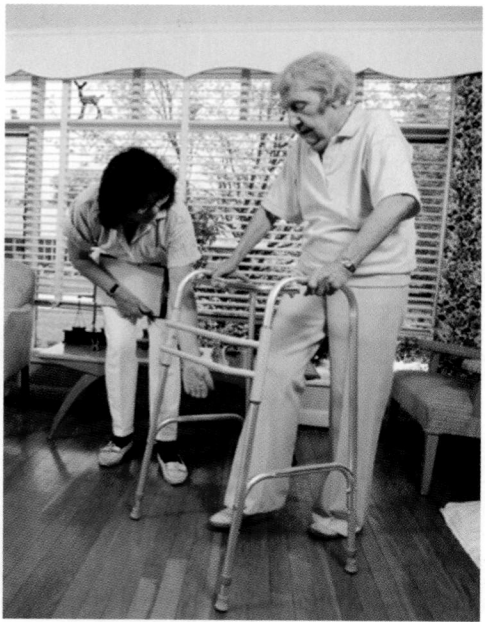

FIG 28.6 Patient using walker.

body weight on both legs. The patient moves the weaker leg to the cane, which divides body weight between the cane and the stronger leg. The patient then advances the stronger leg past the cane so that the weaker leg and the body weight are supported by the cane and weaker leg. During walking the patient continually repeats these same three steps. Teach the patient that two points of support such as both feet or one foot and the cane need to be touching the ground at all times.

The quad cane provides the most support and is used when there is partial or complete leg paralysis or some hemiplegia (Fig. 28.7). You teach the patient the same three steps used with the straight-legged cane.

Crutches. The use of crutches is usually temporary such as after ligament damage to the knee or a fracture to the leg. A crutch is a wooden or metal staff. The two types of crutches are the double adjustable Lofstrand or forearm crutch (Fig. 28.8) and the axillary wooden or metal crutch. The forearm crutch has a handgrip and a metal band that fits around a patient's forearm. The metal band and the handgrip are adjustable to fit a patient's height. The axillary crutch has a padded curved surface at the top, which fits under the axilla. The patient holds a handgrip in the form of a crossbar at the level of the palms to support the body. It is important to measure crutches for the appropriate length and teach patients to use their crutches safely. This includes teaching a patient to achieve a stable gait, ascend and descend stairs, and rise from a sitting position. You, or a physical therapist, teach the patient safety measures and guidelines associated with the use of crutches including maintenance of the crutches themselves as follows:

- Make sure that the rubber tips are attached securely to the crutches. Worn tips should be replaced immediately, as they increase surface friction and prevent crutches from slipping.

BOX 28.9 PATIENT TEACHING

Walker Safety

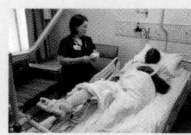 The physical therapist (PT) told Marilyn that Mr. Indelicato will need a walker for a short time because of limited weight bearing on the affected knee. It is important that Mr. Indelicato begins to use the walker before discharge. Marilyn and the PT work together to develop the following teaching plan.

OUTCOME

Patient states the steps needed for safe walker use.

TEACHING STRATEGIES

- Ensure patient's elbow bends at approximately 30 degrees while holding onto walker grips.
- Ensure the top of the walker aligns with the crease on the inside of the wrist when patient relaxes the arms at the side of the body (Pierson and Fairchild, 2013).
- Instruct patient to not lean over the walker or walk behind it so as to not lose balance and fall.
- Patient should walk upright and place one leg, or the injured leg, into the middle area of the walker. Caution patient to not step close to the front bar. Have the patient keep the walker still as walking into it.
- Have patient push straight down on the grips of the walker as he or she brings the other leg forward. Have the patient repeat the process by moving the walker forward and stepping into it one leg at a time.
- Patient or family caregiver should inspect walker regularly for worn tips or missing screws in the metal frame.

EVALUATION

- Use the principles of teach-back to evaluate patient/family caregiver learning:
  - "Tell me what we discussed about the proper placement of your wrist and arms when using the walker."
  - "Tell me what we discussed about the correct way to walk when using the walker."
  - "Tell me what we discussed about ways to maintain walker safety."

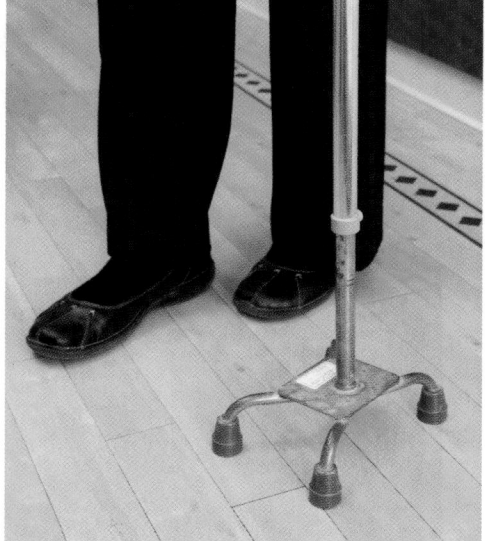

FIG 28.7 Base of quad cane.

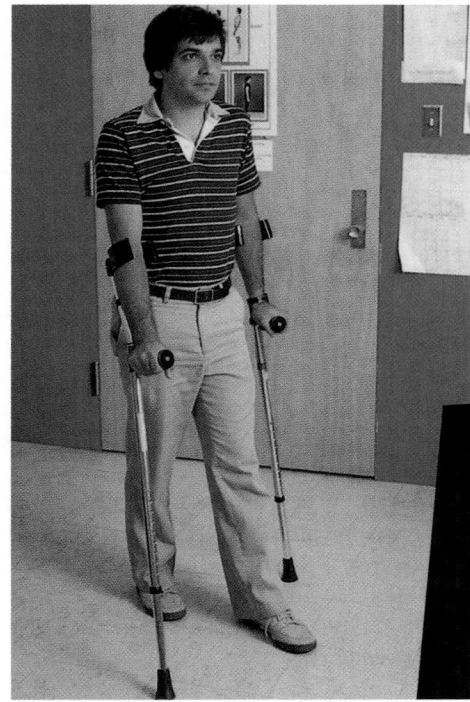

FIG 28.8 Double adjustable Lofstrand or forearm crutch.

- Inform the patient about the importance of keeping the crutch tips dry. Water decreases surface friction and increases the risk of crutches slipping.
- Show the patient how to inspect the structure of wooden crutches for cracks that decrease the ability of the crutch to support weight. Bends in aluminum crutches alter body alignment, increasing the risk for further damage to the musculoskeletal system.
- Give the patient a list of medical suppliers in the community to obtain repairs, new rubber tips, handgrips, and crutch pads as need arises.
- Suggest that the patient investigate the possibility of having a set of spare crutches and tips.

Measuring for Crutches. The axillary crutch is the more common crutch used. Measurement of a patient for a crutch includes the patient's height, the angle of elbow flexion, and the distance between the crutch pad and the axilla. When fitting a crutch, ensure that the length of the crutch is two to three finger widths from the axilla, and position the tips approximately 2 inches lateral and 4 to 6 inches anterior to the front of the patient's shoes (Fig. 28.9) (Pierson and Fairchild, 2013).

Position the handgrips so that the axillae are not supporting the patient's body weight. Pressure on the axillae increases risk to underlying nerves, which sometimes results in partial paralysis of the arm. Determine correct position of the

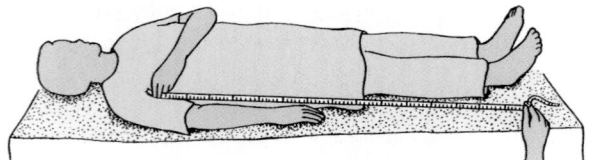

FIG 28.9 Measuring for crutch length.

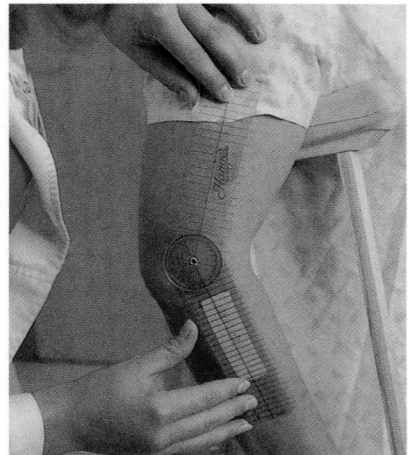

FIG 28.10 Using goniometer to verify correct degree of elbow flexion for crutch use.

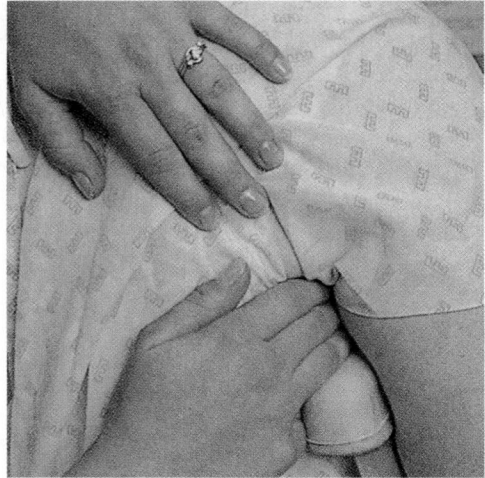

FIG 28.11 Verifying correct distance between crutch pad and axilla.

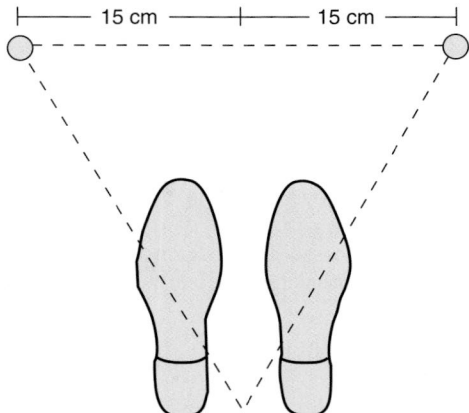

FIG 28.12 Tripod position, basic crutch stance.

handgrips with the patient upright, supporting weight by the handgrips with the elbows slightly flexed at 20 to 25 degrees (Pierson and Fairchild, 2013). Elbow flexion may be verified with a goniometer by a physical therapist (Fig. 28.10). When you determine the height and placement of the handgrips, verify that the distance between the crutch pad and the patient's axilla is approximately 2 inches (two to three finger widths) (Fig. 28.11).

Crutch Gait. A patient assumes a crutch gait by alternately bearing weight on one or both legs and then on the crutches. The physical therapist determines the appropriate gait by assessing a patient's functional abilities, strength and weight-bearing ability, and the disease or injury that resulted in the need for crutches.

This section summarizes the basic crutch stance and the three standard gaits: four-point alternating gait, three-point alternating gait, and two-point gait. The basic crutch stance is the tripod position, formed when the crutches are placed 15 cm (6 inches) in front of and 15 cm to the side of each foot (Fig. 28.12). This position improves the patient's balance by providing a wider base of support. The body alignment of the patient in the tripod position includes erect head and neck, straight vertebrae, and extended hips and knees. No weight should be borne by the axillae. The tripod position is used before crutch walking.

The four-point alternating or four-point gait gives stability to a patient but requires weight bearing on both legs. Each leg is moved alternately with each opposing crutch so

that three points of support are on the floor at all times (Fig. 28.13A).

Three-point alternating or three-point gait requires a patient to bear all of the weight on one foot. In a three-point gait a patient puts weight on both crutches and then on the uninvolved leg and repeats the sequence (Fig. 28.13B). The affected leg does not touch the ground during the early phase of the three-point gait. Gradually the patient progresses to touchdown and full weight bearing on the affected leg.

The two-point gait requires at least partial weight bearing on each foot (Fig. 28.13C). The patient moves a crutch at the same time as the opposite leg so the crutch movements are similar to arm motion during normal walking.

People with paraplegia who wear weight-supporting braces on their legs frequently use the swing-through gait. With weight placed on the supported legs, the patient places the crutches one stride in front and then swings to or through the crutches while they support his or her weight.

Crutch Walking on Stairs. Walking up or down stairs with a single crutch and using the support of a handrail poses a risk for patients to fall. Perform this skill carefully. Apply a gait belt securely around the patient's waist. Be sure there are no obstacles on the stairs, such as stacks of magazines or other items. To walk up the stairs, have the patient hold the handrail with one hand (strong leg next to railing) (Fig. 28.14). You carry the crutch positioned next to the handrail in your nondominant hand as the patient holds the other crutch. Stay behind the patient holding the gait belt with your dominant hand. Then have the patient support his or her weight evenly between the handrail and crutch. The patient next places some weight on the crutch and then steps up on the first step with the weight-bearing foot. Have the patient get his or her balance. Next, instruct the patient to straighten the uninvolved knee and lift his or her body weight, bringing the crutch and affected leg up the stair. The patient repeats the sequence of steps until patient reaches the top of the stairs. Observe patient's balance and level of fatigue.

Walking down steps basically involves the same steps with the patient holding the handrail with the involved leg next to the railing. You again carry the other crutch in your hand that is not grasping gait belt. Have the patient bend his or her strong knee while moving the crutch and involved leg down a step (Fig. 28.15, Step 1). The patient then supports his or her weight evenly between the handrail and crutch. Hold onto the patient's gait belt at all times. Be sure that the patient has good balance. Have the patient slowly bring the uninvolved or stronger leg down a step and caution the patient not to hop (Fig. 28.15, Step 2). Continue sequence (Fig. 28.15, Step 3).

The American College of Foot and Ankle Surgeons (ACFAS, 2016) recommends a safer method for patients to move up and down steps with crutches. Basically, the patient sits on the stairs and uses both arms and the weight-bearing foot and leg to lift himself or herself up or down, one step at a time. A family caregiver or nurse places the crutches at the top or bottom of the stairs before the patient begins.

Sitting in a Chair With Crutches. Sitting in a chair with crutches also involves phases and requires a patient to transfer weight (Fig. 28.16). First the patient gets positioned at the center front of the chair with the posterior aspect of the legs touching the chair. Then the patient holds both

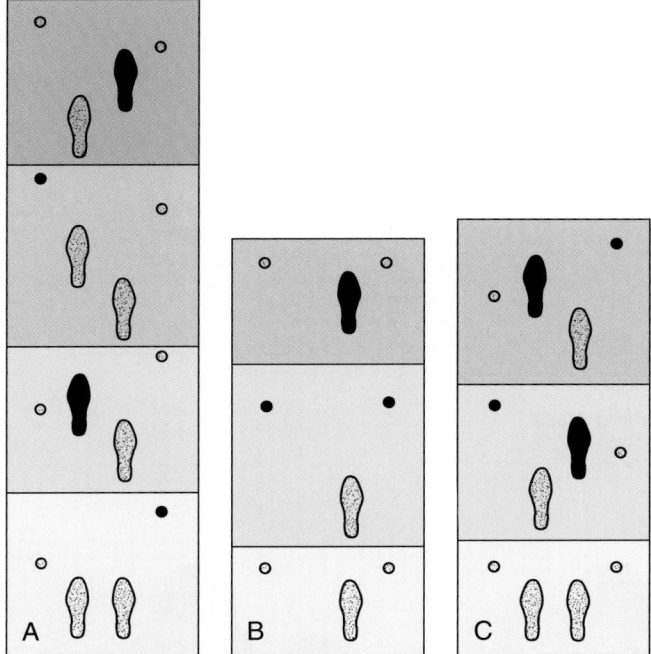

FIG 28.13 **A,** Four-point alternating gait. Solid feet and crutch tips show foot and crutch tip moved in each of the four phases. (Read from bottom to top.) **B,** Three-point gait with weight borne on unaffected leg. Solid foot and crutch tips show weight bearing in each phase. **C,** Two-point gait with weight borne partially on each foot and each crutch advancing with opposing leg. Solid areas indicate leg and crutch tips bearing weight.

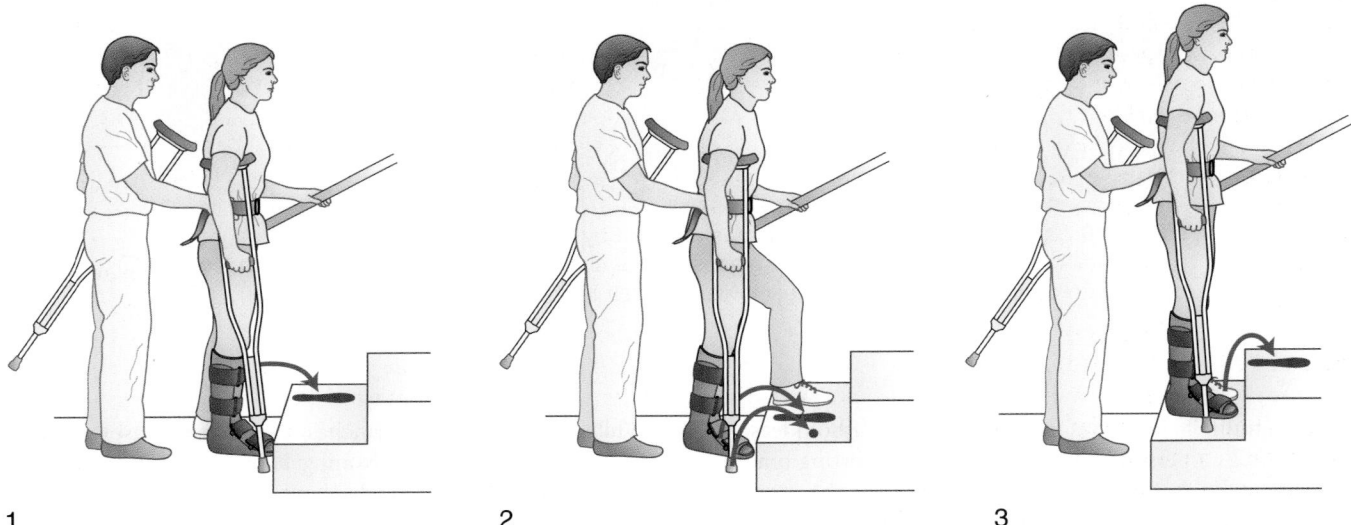

1   2   3

FIG 28.14 Patient position to begin ascending stairs.

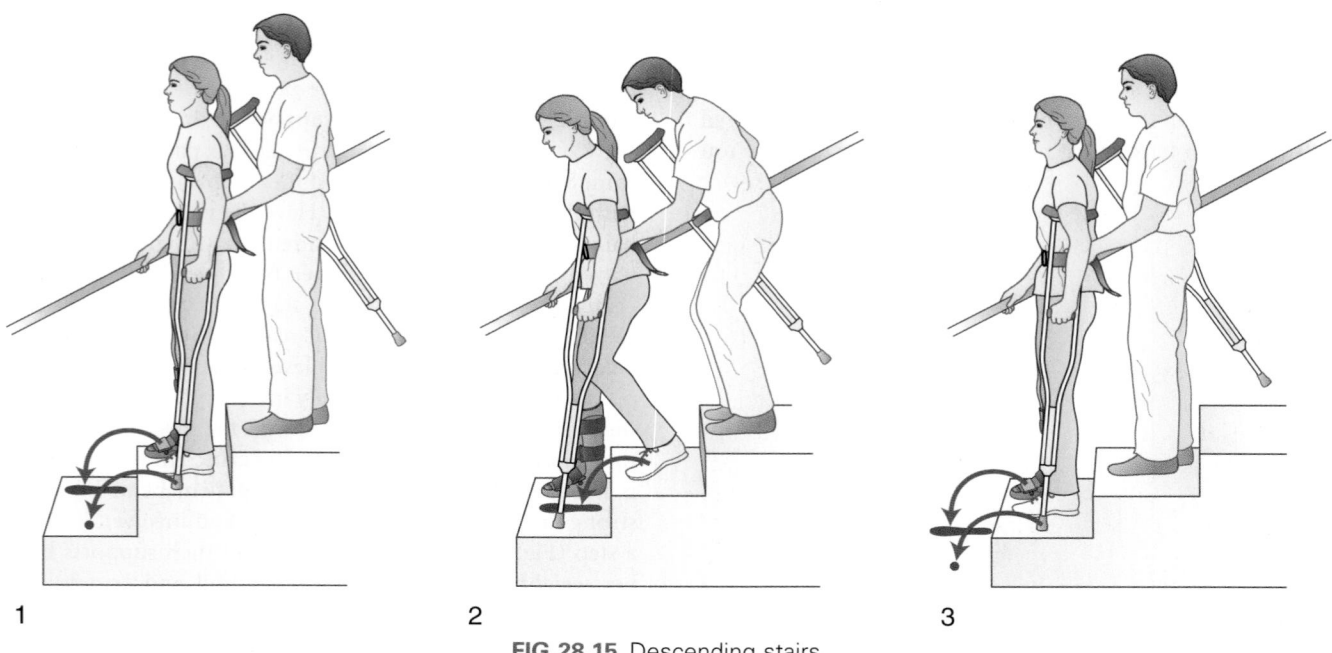

FIG 28.15 Descending stairs.

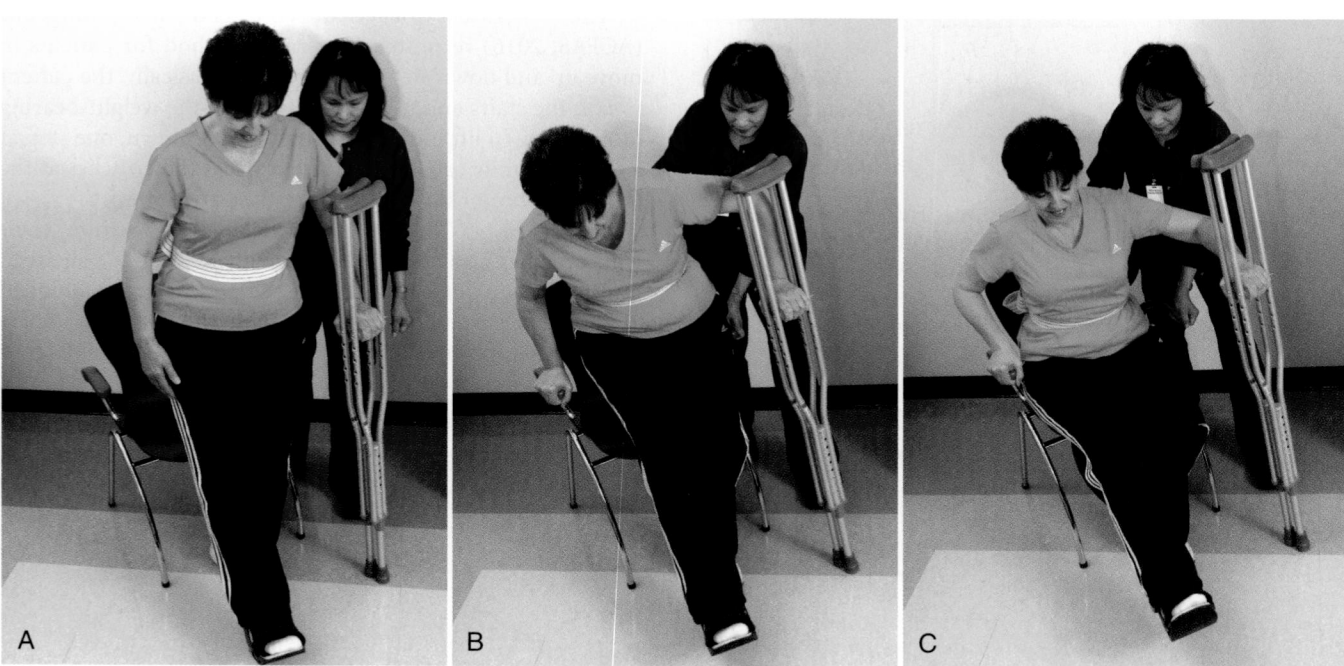

FIG 28.16 Sitting on chair. **A,** Both crutches are held by one hand. Patient transfers weight to crutches and unaffected leg. **B,** Patient grasps arm of chair with free hand and begins to lower herself into chair. **C,** Patient completely lowers herself into chair.

crutches in the hand opposite the affected leg. If both legs are affected (e.g., a person who wears weight-supporting braces), the patient holds the crutches in the hand on the stronger side. With both crutches in one hand, the patient supports his or her body weight on the unaffected leg and crutches.

While still holding the crutches, the patient grasps the arm of the chair with the remaining hand and lowers the body into the chair. To stand, the patient reverses the procedure and, when fully erect, assumes the tripod position before beginning to walk.

■■■ EVALUATION

Patient Outcomes. You evaluate a patient's response to all nursing interventions by comparing a patient's actual response with the expected outcomes for each goal. You evaluate specific outcomes designed to demonstrate improved activity and exercise tolerance. You revise the plan if the patient does not achieve the expected outcomes. For example, a patient may achieve improved joint ROM as determined by measuring the ROM, but if exercise tolerance is still poor (accelerated heart rate, shortness of breath), there may be a need to increase duration of exercise. The success in meeting each outcome is based on the use of evaluative measures such as ROM, ability to ambulate, distance of ambulation, and activity/exercise tolerance (Box 28.10). In many cases, evaluation will occur in the long-term (e.g., weeks or months) before patients regain full function.

Patient Expectations. To evaluate a patient's perception of whether expectations were met, ask the patient the extent to which the patient perceives he or she reached desired activity levels. Also evaluate if the patient perceives whether he or she is able to follow any activity restrictions and how to use any assistive devices at home, when applicable. What is acceptable or anticipated on your part is sometimes vastly different from what a patient and family members anticipate or accept. Ask patients to describe their satisfaction with the plan of care.

BOX 28.10 EVALUATION

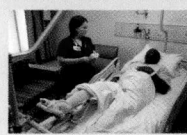

Marilyn began to care for Mr. Indelicato 5 weeks ago, and she has followed him in the outpatient physical therapy setting over the past 4 weeks. He progressed steadily, increasing both weight bearing and range of joint motion of his affected knee. Mr. Indelicato's pain was difficult to manage. He expected pain to be completely resolved on hospital discharge and did not expect it to follow his physical therapy. Marilyn and the physical therapist worked with Mr. Indelicato and his orthopedic surgeon to identify pain-control measures following physical therapy. Currently Mr. Indelicato takes 650 mg of acetaminophen 45 minutes before physical therapy and every 8 to 12 hours thereafter. He reports that his pain is now almost totally gone. He is working on increasing strength so that he is able to return to golf and bike riding. He says he will probably give up racquetball and tennis.

DOCUMENTATION NOTE

"Weight bearing and range of motion continue to improve. States that he takes 650 mg acetaminophen 45 minutes before coming to therapy and every 8 to 12 hours as needed for pain. Rates pain a 1 when exercising. States "Would like to begin riding bike and playing golf again in next 1 to 2 months.""

SAFETY GUIDELINES FOR NURSING SKILLS

Ensuring patient safety is an essential role of the professional nurse. To ensure patient safety, communicate clearly with members of the health care team, assess and incorporate the patient's priorities of care and preferences, and use the best evidence when making decisions about your patient's care. When performing the skills in this chapter, remember the following points to ensure safe, individualized patient care:

- Clear the immediate environment where a patient will walk of any obstacles or clutter.
- Monitor a patient's activity tolerance throughout any extended ambulation.
- Mentally review the steps of a transfer before beginning to ensure safety of both the patient and you.
- Assess the patient's mobility and strength to determine the assistance that the patient is able to offer during transfer. Stand on patient's weak side when assisting (Pierson and Fairchild, 2013).

- Determine the amount and type of assistance required for transfer including type of transfer equipment and the number of personnel it will take to safely transfer and prevent harm to the patient and health care providers.
- Raise the **side rail** on the side of the bed opposite of where you are standing to prevent the patient from falling out of bed on that side.
- Make sure all personnel understand how lift and transfer equipment functions before it is used.
- Educate patients about how equipment functions to reduce their anxiety and enlist their cooperation.
- Arrange equipment (e.g., intravenous [IV] lines, feeding tube, Foley catheter) so that it will not interfere with the transfer process.
- Evaluate patient for correct body alignment and pressure risks after a transfer.

SKILL 28.1   PROMOTING EARLY ACTIVITY AND EXERCISE

DELEGATION CONSIDERATIONS

The skill of promoting early activity and exercise for inpatients can be delegated to nursing assistive personnel (NAP) trained in transfer and assisted ambulation skills. In the outpatient setting education regarding activity and exercise cannot be delegated. Within inpatient settings the nurse directs the NAP by:

- Explaining the level of progressive mobility a patient has achieved
- Explaining any restrictions in range-of-motion (ROM) exercises to perform
- Explaining if there are any weight-bearing precautions or if patient needs to use assistive device
- Explaining criteria to use to stop assisted ambulation or sitting if patient cannot tolerate activity

EQUIPMENT

- Inpatient
  - Pulse oximeter
  - Gait belt
  - Appropriate assistive devices (e.g., cane, walker)
- Outpatient
  - Appropriate devices, depending on type of exercise recommended (e.g., 2.2-kg [5-lb] weights, resistance bands)

STEP	RATIONALE
ASSESSMENT	
1. Identify patient using at least two identifiers (e.g., name and birthday or name and medical record number) according to agency policy.	Ensures correct patient. Complies with The Joint Commission standards and improves patient safety (TJC, 2018).
2. Perform hand hygiene. Gather baseline assessment of vital signs and oxygen saturation (if available).	Reduces transmission of microorganisms. Allows you to evaluate patient's response to activity/exercise.
3. Assess patient's pain level; ask patient to rate pain on scale of 0 to 10.	Determines if there is need for an analgesic before mobilizing or ambulating inpatient. In outpatient settings data will allow you to counsel patient as to best time to try more strenuous exercise.
4. Assess patient's beliefs, values, and perceptions regarding current health status and confidence in being capable of performing exercise.	Perceived self-efficacy is a judgment of capability. The outcomes that people anticipate depend largely on their judgments of how well they will be able to perform in given situations.
5. Review patient's medical history for conditions that could influence or contraindicate mobility/exercise (e.g., dysrhythmias, recent myocardial infarction, stroke, paralyzed extremity, neuromuscular disease, peripheral neuropathy, current pregnancy). Review health care provider's order for early mobility or exercise program. Obtain physician clearance for outpatient exercise.	Examples of conditions that may contraindicate or require adjustments to activity. Patients should have medical clearance to begin activity/exercise program.
6. Implement Inpatient Early Mobility Protocol Screening— this example describes screening for a protocol to begin in intensive care unit (ICU) (AACN, 2013).	Protocol established for ICU patients; however, different screening criteria can be used based on the patient population (e.g., surgical ICU versus medical ICU). Also different criteria are likely used when patients have been transferred out of an ICU.

> **Clinical Decision Point.** Similar protocols to the one developed by AACN are being adopted on acute care inpatient units as well.

STEP	RATIONALE
7. Perform safety screening (MOVE) (AACN, 2013). **M:** Assess patient's myocardial stability.	
• No evidence of active myocardial ischemia has occurred over last 24 hours.	Ensures cardiac stability. Exercise can initiate ischemic attack or worsen dysrhythmias.
• No dysrhythmia requiring new antidysrhythmic drug has occurred over last 24 hours.	
O: Assess oxygenation status; must be adequate on:	Medical stability involves having sufficient perfusion to maintain normal organ function. Activity assessment criteria allow for early ambulation.
• FiO_2 0.6 or less.	
• Positive end expiratory pressure (on ventilator) less than 10 cm H_2O.	
• *Option:* Heart rate less than 120 beats/min at rest, mean arterial blood pressure 60 to 110 mm Hg, respiratory rate less than 28 breaths/min.	

STEP	RATIONALE
V: Minimal vasopressors: • No increase of any vasopressor has occurred for last 2 hours.	Change in vasopressor dose could lead to side effects such as tachycardia, dysrhythmias, and blood pressure changes such as orthostatic hypotension (Burchum and Rosenthal, 2016).
E: Patient engages to voice of caregiver. • Patient responds appropriately to verbal stimulation/commands.	Patient must be alert and responsive, able to follow directions.
8. Outpatient assessment a. Identify patient's activity/exercise history: • Which type of regular daily exercise do you perform at home? • Do you exercise or play a sport at least 3 times a week? • On a scale of 0 to 5 with 0 being no daily exercise and 5 being strenuous regular exercise daily, how would you rate yourself? • How long have you been exercising regularly?	Provides information on patient's motivation or willingness to exercise regularly. Allows you to plan exercise that complements and advances patient's activity level.
b. Ask patient to what extent he or she enjoys exercising and what his or her beliefs are about ability to exercise.	Factors positively associated with adult physical activity (HealthyPeople.gov, 2015).
c. Determine if patient has social support from peers, family, or spouse.	Factors positively associated with adult physical activity (HealthyPeople.gov, 2015).
d. Determine if patient has access to facility or area to exercise. Is neighborhood considered safe?	Absence of facility or sense of safety discourages activity/exercise.
e. Consider these factors in your assessment: patient's age, income level, time available to exercise, rural resident, overweight, being disabled.	Factors negatively associated with adult participation in activity (HealthyPeople.gov, 2015).
f. Have patient rate level of quality of life based on current activity level.	Serves as baseline to measure long-term benefits of exercise.

PLANNING

STEP	RATIONALE
1. Inpatient: Consult with physical therapist (PT) regarding role in protocol to provide planned active resistance exercise for patients. If PT is available in home health, consult on types of exercises suited for outpatient's mobility restrictions.	Progressive resistance exercise (PRE) is method of increasing ability of muscles to generate force.
2. All patients: Explain benefits and reasons for activity/exercise. Do so in a way that matches patient's beliefs and values regarding recovery or maintaining health.	Exercise self-efficacy is an important predictor of the adoption and maintenance of exercise behaviors. Self-efficacy is the belief and conviction that one can perform a given activity successfully (Fletcher and Banasik, 2001; Shieh et al., 2015).
3. Inpatients: Explain precautions that will be taken to prevent falls during ambulation (gait belt, assisted walking, monitoring for dizziness).	Patients may have a fear of falling. Explanation may relieve anxiety.
4. Inpatients: As patient progresses to ambulating, try to schedule ambulation around patient's other activities.	Avoids overexertion of patient. Organizes nursing care activities.
5. Perform hand hygiene. Prepare equipment and supplies.	Reduces transmission of microorganisms. Ensures organized procedure.

IMPLEMENTATION

1. Inpatient Early Progressive Mobility Protocol (AACN, 2013)
   Each patient starts at a different level, depending on his or her medical status and ability to participate in mobility.

SKILL 28.1 PROMOTING EARLY ACTIVITY AND EXERCISE—cont'd

STEP	RATIONALE
Level 1 • Initiate passive ROM exercises 3 times daily (see Table 29.3 in Chapter 29). Turn patient every 2 hours. • Help patient to sitting position in bed (e.g., stretcher chair or elevating head of bed to 45 degrees) and maintain for 20 minutes 3 times daily. • Obtain a PT consultation if patient is alert to determine if strengthening exercises are indicated.	This level is designed for patients who are medically unstable to tolerate activity and/or have bed rest orders because of a medical condition.
Level 2 • Continue passive ROM exercises 3 times daily. • Turn patient every 2 hours. • Help patient to sitting position in bed and maintain for 20 minutes 3 times daily. • Initiate sitting patient on edge of bed or lift patient to chair (using safe mobility techniques). • Obtain PT consultation for mobility/strengthening program (e.g., active resistance exercise).	Patient begins to progress, he or she is starting to be able to sit independently on edge of bed or tolerate sitting up in a chair. Principles of active resistance exercise: (1) to perform small number of repetitions until fatigue, (2) to allow sufficient rest between exercises for recovery, and (3) to increase resistance as ability to generate force increases. There is some evidence that PRE improves endurance and ability to generate muscle force, which can carry over into an improved ability to do everyday tasks (Taylor et al., 2005).
Level 3 • Continue passive ROM exercises 3 times daily. • Turn every 2 hours. • Help patient to sitting position in bed and maintain for 20 minutes 3 times daily; sitting on edge of bed unsupported (but supervised). • Active transfer to chair with the patient sitting up in chair 20 minutes 3 times daily. • PT to continue with strengthening program as ordered.	Patient progresses to transfer training, prewalking activities.
Level 4 • Continue passive ROM 3 times daily. • Turn every 2 hours. • Active transfer to chair with patient sitting up in chair 20 minutes 3 times daily sitting on edge of bed unsupported (but supervised). • PT to continue with strengthening program. • Initiate ambulation. Apply gait belt securely around patient's waist. Have patient ambulate (marching in place, walking in halls). **Note:** Ambulation time/distance should increase daily during hospitalization.	Patients can still be in ICU during this phase or out on general nursing unit. Progression of mobility (amount of help required and distance walked) should occur until hospital discharge.

2. Outpatient Exercise and Activity Promotion
  a. Initiate an exercise program that contains any of the following components:
  • Warm-up (5 to 10 minutes)
  • Strengthening exercises
  • Endurance exercises
  • Balance exercises
  • Flexibility exercises
  Consider consulting PT to help develop complete exercise program that would fit needs of your patient. A good overview of exercise programs can be found at http://health.gov/paguidelines/guidelines.
	Warm-up directs needed blood flow to muscles and prepares body for exercise. Warming up is important for preventing injury. Flexibility exercises help prevent tightness of muscles and improve joint ROM. Loss of ROM or muscle tightness can impede a person's function.
	Cool downs help body recover from exercises.

b. Recommend strength training for adults in collaboration with PT.	Strength training has been shown to improve strength and bone density and can be beneficial for older adults.
c. AHA (2015) recommends aerobic exercise at least 150 minutes per week of moderate exercise or 75 minutes per week of vigorous exercise (or combination of moderate and vigorous activity). This includes activities (e.g., climbing stairs; playing sports; or aerobic activities such as walking, jogging, swimming, or biking).	Designed to improve overall cardiovascular health.

STEP	RATIONALE
d. Recommend balance exercises for older adults to decrease risk of falls. Have patient be sure to have something sturdy nearby to hold onto (wall or chair) if he or she becomes unsteady.	Helps to improve person's balance while standing or sitting and may decrease risk of falls.
• Perform exercises: standing on one foot, walking heel to toe, balance walking, back leg raises, side leg raises. Have patient do strength exercises while holding back of chair (back leg raises, side leg raises) 2 or more days per week but not on any 2 days in a row (National Institute on Aging [NIA], 2016).	
e. Recommend patient perform cool down (5 to 10 minutes) after exercising: quadriceps stretch, hamstring/calf stretch, chest and arm stretch, neck, upper back, and shoulder stretch.	Exercises help muscles relax and become more flexible.

EVALUATION

1. Measure vital signs and oxygen saturation during activity/exercise and compare findings with baseline.	Determines patient's exercise tolerance.

Clinical Decision Point. Terminate physical activity when (Adler and Malone, 2012):
- **Heart rate is greater than a 20% decrease in resting value or less than 40 beats/min or greater than 130 beats/min.**
- **Oxygen saturation shows greater than 4% drop from baseline or less than 88% to 90%.**
- **Blood pressure: Systolic pressure is greater than 180 mm Hg or greater than 20% decrease in systolic/diastolic or orthostatic hypotension.**
- **Respirations: Less than 5 breaths/min or greater than 40 breaths/min.**
- **Terminate exercise if dizziness lasts 60 seconds or fainting or diaphoresis occurs; change in breathing pattern occurs with increase in accessory muscle use, extreme fatigue, or severe dyspnea with respiratory rate greater than baseline by more than 20 breaths/min (Myszenski, 2014).**

2. Evaluate patient's pain severity using 0-to-10 pain scale.	Exercises can increase muscle discomfort.
3. After patient has reached level 4 of inpatient mobility protocol or after outpatient has been exercising more than 2 to 3 months, evaluate level of confidence in performing exercises.	Determines self-efficacy and likelihood of continued participation in exercise.
4. **Use Teach-Back:** "We've talked about doing a warm-up and cool down as part of your exercise plan. Tell me why each is important." Revise your instruction now or develop plan for revised patient/family caregiver teaching if patient/family caregiver is not able to teach back correctly.	Determines patient's/family caregiver's level of understanding of instructional topic.

RECORDING AND REPORTING

- Record in the inpatient medical record or clinic record results of patient screening, type of exercise implemented, pre-exercise and postexercise assessments, and patient's tolerance in nurses' notes in electronic health record (EHR) or chart.
- Document your evaluation of patient learning.
- Report to health care provider any signs or symptoms indicative of exercise intolerance.

UNEXPECTED OUTCOMES AND RELATED INTERVENTIONS

- Patient has abnormal vital sign response or decrease in oxygen saturation requiring termination of exercise. (In home setting be sure that patient or family caregiver knows patient's normal pulse range and when to terminate exercise.)
  - Return patient to chair or bed immediately using safe patient-handling principles.
  - Notify health care provider.
  - Continue to monitor vital signs until patient's condition stabilizes.
- Patient develops chest pain and/or discomfort during exercise.
  - Return patient to chair or bed immediately using safe patient-handling principles.
  - Notify health care provider.
  - Prepare for possible electrocardiogram.
  - Continue to monitor vital signs until patient's condition stabilizes.
  - In home setting, have caregiver call 911.

SKILL 28.2   USING SAFE AND EFFECTIVE TRANSFER TECHNIQUES

View Video!

DELEGATION CONSIDERATIONS

The skill of effective transfer techniques can be delegated to trained nursing assistive personnel (NAP). The nurse is responsible to initially assess patient's readiness and ability to transfer. The nurse directs the NAP by:

- Assisting and supervising when moving patients who are transferred for the first time after prolonged bed rest, extensive surgery, critical illness, or spinal cord trauma.
- Explaining the patient's mobility restrictions, changes in blood pressure to look for, or sensory alterations that may affect safe transfer (e.g., medicated or confused).
- Explaining what to observe and report back to the nurse, such as dizziness or the patient's ability to assist.

EQUIPMENT

- Gait belt, sling, or lapboard (as needed)
- Nonskid shoes, bath blankets, and pillows
- Wheelchair (position chair at 45- to 60-degree angle to bed, lock brakes, remove footrests, and lock bed brakes)
- Stretcher (position next to bed, lock brakes on stretcher, lock brakes on bed)
- Mechanical/hydraulic lift (use frame, canvas strips or chains, and hammock or canvas strips)
- Stand-assist lift device

STEP	RATIONALE

ASSESSMENT

1. Identify patient using at least two identifiers (e.g., name and birthday or name and medical record number) according to agency policy

Ensures correct patient. Complies with The Joint Commission standards and improves patient safety (TJC, 2018).

2. Refer to medical record for most recent recorded weight and height for patient.

A factor used to determine if mechanical transfer device or friction-reducing device is needed for transfer.

3. Review history and assess patient's specific risk for falling or being injured during transfer (e.g., neuromuscular deficit, visual loss, motor weakness or incoordination, fear of falling, bone loss).

Causes risk for tripping or losing balance.

4. Assess previous mode of transferring to bed or chair (if applicable).

Determines mode of transfer and assistance required to provide continuity.

5. Assess patient's specific risk of falling or being injured when transferred (e.g., neuromuscular deficits, motor weakness, calcium loss from bone, cognitive and visual dysfunction, altered balance).

Certain conditions increase risk of falling or potential injury.

6. Perform hand hygiene.

Reduces transmission of microorganisms.

7. Assess patient's mobility: including ability to sit up on side of bed or chair, and ability to stand. *Option:* administer the Banner Mobility Assessment Tool (BMAT) (Boynton et al., 2014).

The BMAT is an assessment tool to guide a patient through a 4-step functional task list to identify the level of mobility a patient can achieve. This assessment aids in determining the patient's level of mobility (e.g., Mobility Level 1) and recommends the equipment and tools needed to safely lift, transfer, and mobilize the patient.

   a. **Sit and Shake:** From a semireclined position, ask patient to sit upright and rotate to a seated position at the side of the bed; patient may use bedrail. Note patient's ability to maintain bedside position. Ask patient to reach out and grab your hand and shake, making sure patient reaches across his or her midline.

If patient fails to Sit and Shake: Use total lift with sling and/or positioning sheet and/or straps, and/or use lateral transfer devices such as rollboard, friction-reducing device (slide sheets/tube), or air-assisted device.

   b. **Stretch and Point:** With patient in seated position at the side of the bed, have patient place both feet on the floor (or stool) with knees no higher than hips. Ask patient to stretch one leg and straighten the knee, then bend/flex the ankle and point the toes. If appropriate, repeat with the other leg.

If patient fails Stretch and Point: Use total lift for patient unable to bear weight on at least one leg; use sit-to-stand lift for patient who can bear weight on at least one leg.

   c. **Stand:** Ask patient to elevate off the bed or chair (seated to standing) using an assistive device (cane, bedrail). Patient should be able to raise buttocks off bed and hold for a count of five. May repeat once.

If patient fails Stand: Use nonpowered raising/stand aid (default to powered sit-to-stand lift if no stand aid available), use total lift with ambulation accessories, or use assistive device (cane, walker, crutches).

   d. **Walk** (march in place and advance step): Ask patient to march in place at bedside, then ask patient to advance step and return each foot. Patient should display stability while performing tasks. Assess for stability and safety awareness.

If patient cannot Walk: Use nonpowered raising/stand aid (default to powered sit-to-stand lift if no stand aid available), use total lift with ambulation accessories, or use assistive device (cane, walker, crutches).

STEP	RATIONALE
8. Assess for weakness, dizziness, or risk for orthostatic (postural) hypotension (e.g., previously on bed rest, first time arising from supine position after surgical procedure, history of dizziness when arising).	Determines risk of fainting or falling during transfer. Immobilized patients have decreased ability of autonomic nervous system to equalize blood supply, resulting in initial drop of 40 mm Hg systolic or more in blood pressure when rising from sitting position (Frith et al., 2014; Lewis et al., 2014; Mills et al., 2014).
9. Assess activity tolerance, noting for fatigue during sitting and standing.	Determines ability of patient to help with transfer.
10. Assess proprioceptive function (awareness of posture and changes in equilibrium) including ability to maintain balance while sitting in bed or on side of bed and tendency to sway toward one side.	Determines stability of patient's balance for transfer and risk for falls.
11. Assess sensory status including central and peripheral vision, adequacy of hearing, and presence of peripheral sensation loss.	Determines influence of sensory loss on ability to make transfer. Visual field loss decreases patient's ability to see in direction of transfer. Peripheral sensation loss decreases proprioception. Patients with visual and hearing losses need transfer techniques adapted to deficits.

Clinical Decision Point. Patients with hemiplegia may "neglect" one side of the body (inattention to or unawareness of one side of body or environment), which distorts perception of the visual field. If patient experiences neglect of one side, instruct him or her to scan all visual fields when transferring.

STEP	RATIONALE
12. Assess level of comfort (e.g., joint discomfort, muscle spasm) and measure level of pain using scale of 0 to 10. Offer prescribed analgesic 30 minutes before transfer. (**Note:** Patient will require assistance when analgesic has been given.)	Pain reduces patient's motivation and ability to be mobile. Pain relief before transfer enhances patient's ability to participate (Schofield, 2014).
13. Assess vital signs.	Vital sign changes, such as increased pulse and respiration and drop in blood pressure, indicate activity intolerance (see Chapter 15).
14. Assess patient's cognitive status including ability to follow verbal instructions, short-term memory, and recognition of physical deficits and limitations to movement.	Determines patient's ability to follow directions and learn transfer techniques.

Clinical Decision Point. Patients with head trauma or cerebrospinal fluid loss may have perceptual cognitive defects that create safety risks. If the patient has difficulty comprehending, simplify instructions by providing one step at a time and maintain consistency.

STEP	RATIONALE
15. Assess patient's level of motivation such as eagerness versus unwillingness to be mobile and perception of value of exercise.	Altered physiological and psychological conditions reduce a patient's desire to engage in activity.
16. Assess special transfer equipment needed for home setting and previous mode of transfer (if applicable).	Prior teaching of family caregivers and support people, assessing home for safety risks and functionality, and providing applicable aids greatly enhance transfer ability at home.

PLANNING

1. Perform hand hygiene. Gather appropriate equipment.	Reduces transmission of microorganisms. Ensures safe and organized procedure.
2. Determine number of people needed to assist with transfer by referring to proper algorithm. Do not start procedure until all caregivers are available.	Ensures safe patient transfer. Algorithms for safe patient handling and movement are available at https://cseany.org/wp-content/uploads/2014/02/SPHMALGORITHMS.PDF.
3. Verify that bed brakes are locked.	Provides for patient and caregiver safety, preventing inadvertent movement of bed.
4. Explain procedure to patient and family.	Increases patient participation and family caregiver knowledge of continued care of patient on discharge (Wrobleski et al., 2014).

SKILL 28.2 USING SAFE AND EFFECTIVE TRANSFER TECHNIQUES—cont'd

View Video!

STEP	RATIONALE

IMPLEMENTATION

1. Perform hand hygiene.

2. Assist patient from supine position to sitting position on edge of bed with bed positioned so that top of mattress is even with your elbows.

3. Allow patient to sit on the side of the bed for a few minutes. Have patient alternately flex and extend feet, and move lower legs up and down. Ask if patient feels dizzy; if so, check blood pressure. Have patient relax and take a few deep breaths until dizziness subsides and balance is gained. If dizziness lasts more than 60 seconds, return patient to bed (Frith et al., 2014; Mills et al., 2014). Recheck blood pressure.

Reduces transmission of microorganisms.
Reduces strain on your back.

Allows patient's circulation to equilibrate to reduce chance of orthostatic hypotension.

Clinical Decision Point. Remain in front of patient until patient regains balance, and continue to provide physical support to weak or cognitively impaired patient.

---

4. Transfer patient from bed to chair:

   a. Have a chair in position at 45-degree angle with one side against bed, facing foot of bed.

   Positions chair with easy access for transfer.

   b. Place bed in low position or to point where patient's feet are comfortably on the floor.

   Provides patient stability when transferring.

   c. *If patient has partial weight bearing with upper body strength or caregiver must lift more than 15.9 kg (35 lb), use mechanical lift or transfer aid with minimum of two or three caregivers (see Fig. 28.5): Follow guidelines of lift manufacturer to apply.*

   The use of mechanical lift devices is strongly recommended to transfer a patient to reduce risk for musculoskeletal injury (Degelau et al., 2012; Occupational Safety and Health Administration [OSHA], 2014, n.d.).

Clinical Decision Point. If patient demonstrates weakness or paralysis of one side of the body, place chair on patient's strong side.

---

   d. *If patient has partial weight bearing, is cooperative and able to stand, and has upper body strength, use stand-and-pivot technique with one caregiver (VISN8, 2014):*

   (1) Apply gait belt. Be sure that it completely circles the waist. Place the belt low and be sure that it is snug. Avoid placing the belt over any IV lines, incisions, or drainage tubes.

   Gait belt allows you to maintain stability of patient during transfer and reduces risk for falling (Degelau et al., 2012; OSHA, 2014).

   (2) If not already in place, help patient apply stable, nonskid shoes or socks. Place patient's weight-bearing or strong leg forward on floor, with weak foot back.

   Nonskid soles decrease risk for slipping during transfer. Always have patient wear nonskid shoes or socks during transfer; bare feet increase risk for falls. Patient will stand on stronger or weight-bearing leg.

   (3) Spread your feet apart. Then flex hips and knees, aligning knees with patient's knees.

   Ensures balance with wide base of support.
   Flexing knees and hips lowers your center of gravity to object to be raised; aligning your knees with patient's knees allows for stabilization of knees when patient stands.

   (4) Grasp gait belt, keeping your palms up, along patient's sides (see illustration).

   Gait belt allows you to move patient at center of gravity. Patients should never be lifted by or under their arms.

   (5) Rock patient up to standing position on count of three while straightening hips and legs and keeping knees slightly flexed (see illustration). While rocking patient in back-and-forth motion, make sure that your body weight is moving in the same direction as patient's weight to ensure that you and patient are moving in same direction simultaneously. Unless contraindicated, patient may be instructed to use hands to push up if applicable.

   Rocking motion gives patient's body momentum and requires less muscular effort to lift him or her.

STEP	RATIONALE
(6) Maintain stability of patient's weakened leg with your knee.	Ability to stand can often be maintained in weak limb with support of knee to stabilize.
(7) Pivot on foot farthest from chair.	Maintains support of patient while allowing adequate space for patient to move.
(8) Instruct patient to use armrests on chair for support and ease into chair (see illustration).	Increases patient stability.
(9) Flex hips and knees while lowering patient into chair.	Prevents injury from poor body mechanics.
(10) Assess patient for proper alignment in sitting position. Provide support for weakened extremity. You can use a sling or lap board to support an injured or flaccid arm. Stabilize leg with bath blanket or pillow.	Prevents injury to patient from poor body alignment.
(11) Proper alignment for sitting position: Head is erect, and vertebrae are in straight alignment. Body weight is evenly distributed on buttocks and thighs. Thighs are parallel and in horizontal plane. Both feet are supported on floor, and ankles are comfortably flexed. A 2.5- to 5-cm (1- to 2-inch) space is maintained between edge of seat and popliteal space on posterior surface of knee.	Prevents stress on intravertebral joints. Prevents increased pressure over bony prominences and reduces damage to underlying musculoskeletal system.
e. *If patient is not able to cooperate (regardless of ability to bear weight) or has no upper body strength:* Use ceiling or floor hydraulic lift to transfer patient from bed to chair (VISN8, 2014).	Research supports use of mechanical lifts to prevent musculoskeletal injuries (ANA, 2013a, 2013b). Use of ceiling-mounted lifts is a popular choice because of availability of lift in each patient's room (see illustration).
(1) Bring mechanical floor lift to bedside or lower ceiling lift and position properly.	Ensures safe elevation of patient off bed.
(2) Position chair near bed and allow adequate space to maneuver lift.	Prepares environment for safe use of lift and subsequent transfer.
(3) Raise bed to high position with mattress flat. Lower side rail on side near chair.	Allows you to use proper body mechanics.
(4) Have a second nurse positioned at opposite side of bed.	Maintains patient safety, preventing fall from bed.

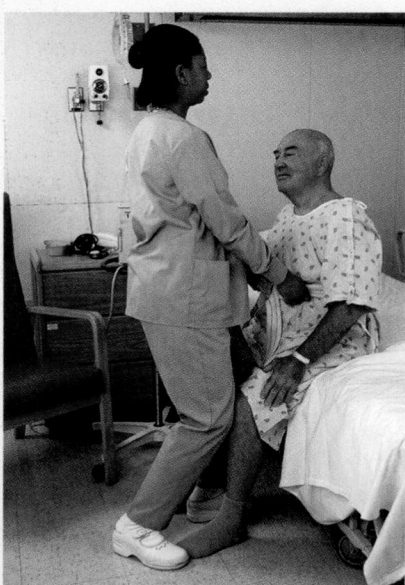

STEP 4d(4) Nurse flexes hips and knees, aligns knees with patient's knee, and grasps gait belt palms up.

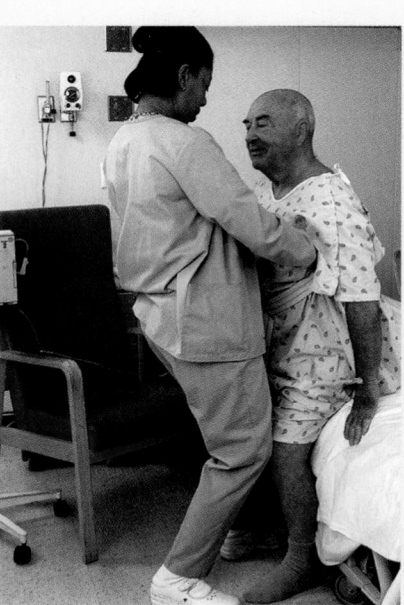

STEP 4d(5) Nurse rocks patient (who is able to assist) to standing position.

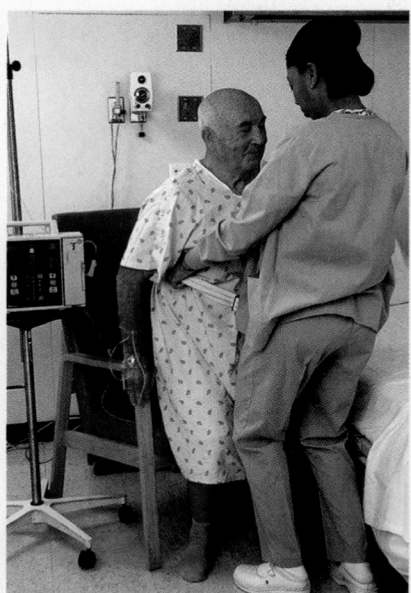

STEP 4d(8) Patient uses armrests and is guided to sit in chair.

SKILL 28.2 USING SAFE AND EFFECTIVE TRANSFER TECHNIQUES—cont'd

View Video!

STEP	RATIONALE
(5) Roll patient on side away from you.	Positions patient for placement of lift sling.
(6) Place hammock or canvas strips under patient to form sling. With two canvas pieces, lower edge fits under patient's knees (wide piece), and upper edge fits under patient's shoulders (narrow piece).	Two types of seats are supplied with mechanical/hydraulic lift: hammock style is better for patients who are flaccid, weak, and need support; canvas strips can be used for patients with normal muscle tone. Hooks should face away from patient's skin. Place sling under patient's center of gravity and greatest portion of body weight.
(7) Roll patient back toward you as second nurse pulls hammock (straps) through.	Ensures sling is in proper position before lift.
(8) Return patient to supine position. Be sure hammock or straps are smooth over bed surface. Sling should extend from shoulders to knees (hammock) to support patient's body weight equally.	Completes positioning of patient on mechanical/hydraulic sling.
(9) Remove patient's glasses if appropriate.	Swivel bar is close to patient's head and could break eyeglasses.
(10) Place horseshoe base of a floor lift under the patient's bed (on side with chair).	Positions lift efficiently and promotes smooth transfer.
(11) Lower horizontal bar to sling level by following manufacturer directions. Lock valve if required.	Positions hydraulic lift close to patient. Locking valve prevents injury to patient.
(12) Attach hooks on strap (chain) to holes in sling. Short chains or straps hook to top holes of sling; longer chains hook to bottom of sling (see manufacturer's directions).	Secures hydraulic lift to sling.
(13) Elevate head of bed to Fowler's position.	Positions patient in sitting position.
(14) Have patient fold arms over chest.	Prevents injury to patient's arms during transfer.
(15) Either use power cord to turn on lift or pump hydraulic handle using long, slow, even strokes until patient is raised off bed (see illustration). For ceiling lift turn on control device to move lift.	Ensures safe support of patient during elevation.
(16) Use lift to raise patient off bed and use steering handle to pull lift from bed as you and other nurse maneuver patient to chair. Have second nurse alongside patient.	Lifts patient off bed safely, nurse's position reduces any risk of patient falling from sling.
(17) Roll base of lift around chair. Release check valve slowly and lower patient into chair (see manufacturer directions and see illustration).	Positions lift in front of chair in which patient is to be transferred. Safely guides patient into back of chair as seat descends.

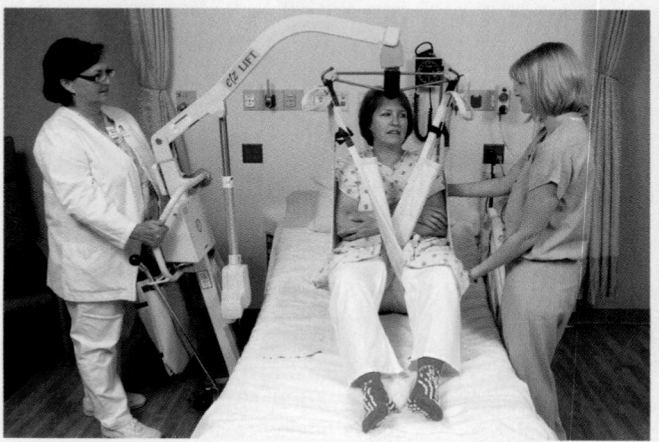

STEP 4e(15) Patient lifted in hydraulic lift above bed.

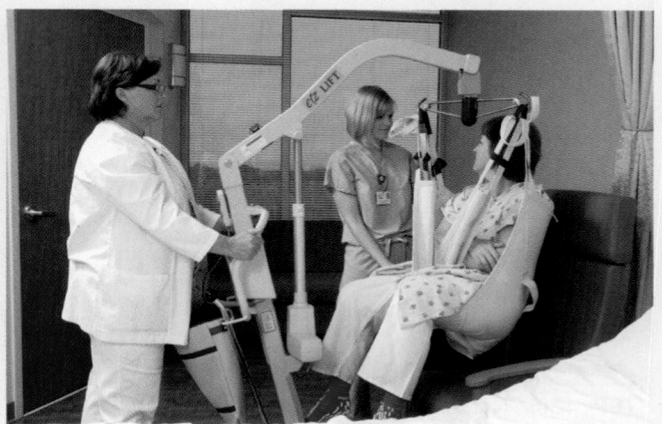

STEP 4e(17) Use of hydraulic lift lowers patient into chair.

STEP	RATIONALE
(18) Close check valve as soon as patient is down in chair and straps can be released.	If valve is left open, boom may continue to lower and injure patient.
(19) Remove straps and roll mechanical/hydraulic lift out of patient's path.	Prevents damage to skin and underlying tissues. Provides patient.
(20) Check patient's sitting alignment and correct if necessary.	Prevents injury from poor posture.
5. Perform lateral transfer from bed to stretcher:	The three-person lift (using lift sheet) for horizontal transfer from bed to stretcher is no longer recommended and is discouraged (Anderson et al., 2014; OSHA, 2014). Physical stress can be decreased significantly by using slide board or friction-reducing board positioned under lift sheet beneath patient. In addition, patient is more comfortable using this method.
a. Can patient assist?	Patient's level of strength and weight determine level of assistance required for safe transfer. During any patient transferring task, if any caregiver is required to lift more than 15.9 kg (35 lb) of a patient's weight, the patient is considered fully dependent, and an assistive device is used (OSHA, 2014, n.d.).
(1) If patient can assist, caregiver needed only to stand by for safety, with stretcher and bed locked as patient moves to stretcher (VISN8, 2014).	
(2) If patient is partially able or not at all and weighs less than 90.7 kg (200 lb), use friction-reducing device or lateral transfer board (VISN8, 2014).	
(3) If patient is partially able or not at all and weighs more than 90.7 kg (200 lb), use a ceiling lift with supine sling or a mechanical lateral transfer device with three caregivers (VISN8, 2014).	
b. Lateral transfer with friction-reducing device—slide board (see illustration) or air-assisted device:	Maintains alignment of spinal column. Ensures that bed does not move inadvertently.
(1) Lower head of bed as much as patient can tolerate. Be sure to lock bed brakes.	
(2) Cross patient's arms on chest.	Prevents injury to arms during transfer.
(3) Lower side rails. To place slide board under patient, position two nurses on side of bed toward which patient will be turned. Position third nurse on other side of bed.	Distributes weight equally between nurses.
(4) Fanfold lift sheet on both sides.	Provides strong handles to grip lift sheet without slipping.
(5) On count of three, logroll patient onto side toward the two nurses. Turn patient as one unit with a smooth, continuous motion.	Maintains body in alignment, preventing stress on any part.

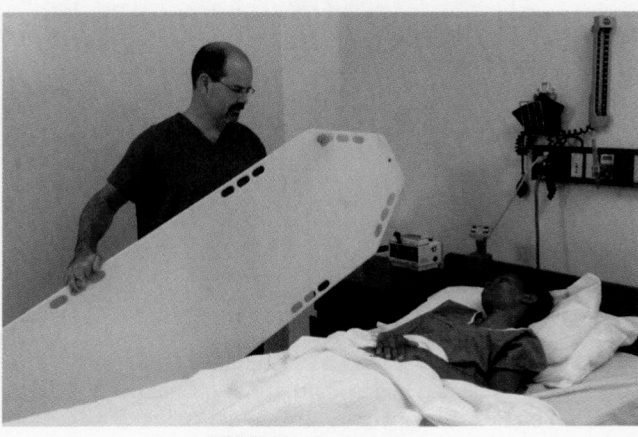

STEP 5b Slide board.

SKILL 28.2   USING SAFE AND EFFECTIVE TRANSFER TECHNIQUES—cont'd

View Video!

STEP	RATIONALE
(6) Place slide board under lift sheet (see illustrations). Option: Apply air-assisted device.	Prevents friction from contact of skin with board.
(7) Gently roll patient back onto slide board.	
(8) Line up stretcher so that surface is ½ inch lower than bed (VISN8, 2014). Lock brakes on stretcher. Instruct patient not to move.	Ensures that stretcher does not move inadvertently during transfer.
(9) Two nurses position themselves on side of stretcher while the third nurse positions self on side of bed without stretcher. All three nurses place feet widely apart with one foot slightly in front of the other and grasp friction-reducing device.	

Clinical Decision Point. A nurse may also be positioned at the head of patient's bed to protect and support his or her head and neck if patient is weak or unable to assist.

(10) Holding fan folded lift sheet and one nurse counting to three, the two nurses pull lift sheet across slide board positioning patient onto stretcher. The third nurse holds slide board in place (see illustrations). Option: Inflate air-assisted device and slide patient across bed onto stretcher.	Slide board remains stationary and provides slippery surface to reduce friction and allows patient to transfer easily to stretcher.

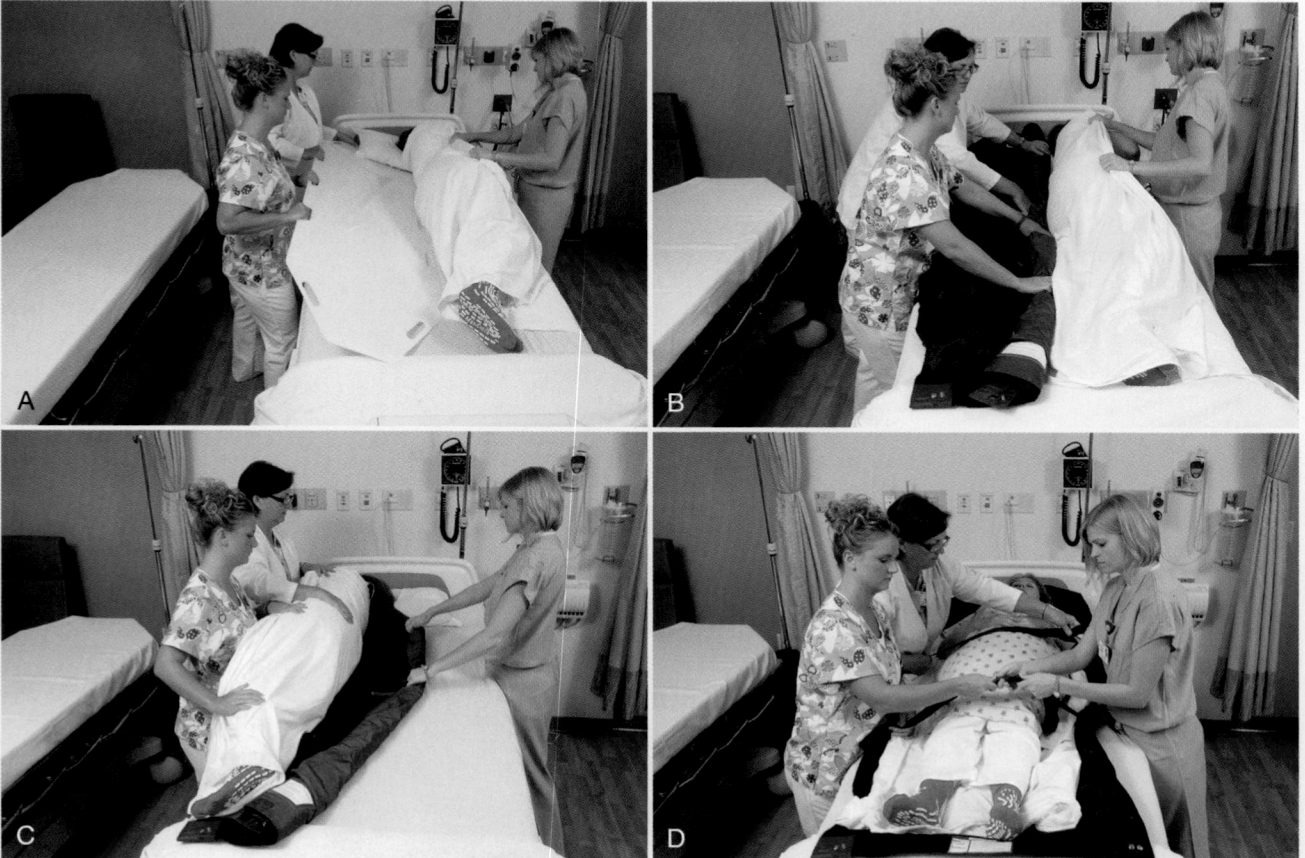

STEP 5b(6) A, Two caregivers placing slide board under lift sheet. **B,** Two caregivers place air-assisted device under patient. **C,** Patient rolls to opposite side, while other caregiver unrolls air-assisted device. **D,** Secure safety straps.

STEP	RATIONALE
(11) Position patient in center of stretcher. Raise head of stretcher if not contraindicated. Raise stretcher side rails. Cover patient with blanket.	Provides for patient comfort.
6. Perform hand hygiene.	Reduces transmission of microorganisms.

EVALUATION

1. Evaluate vital signs. Ask if patient feels tired or dizzy.	Evaluates patient's response to postural changes and activity.
2. Observe for correct body alignment and presence of pressure points on skin.	Minimizes risk for immobility complications.
3. Ask if patient experienced pain during transfer; measure current pain level.	Determines need for additional pain control or alteration of technique of transferring.
4. **Use Teach-Back:** "We have discussed how to transfer from the bed to the chair. Tell me the steps you take to move safely from the bed to a chair." Revise your instruction now or develop a plan for revised patient/family caregiver teaching if patient/family caregiver is not able to teach back correctly.	Determines patient's/family caregiver's level of understanding of instructional topic.

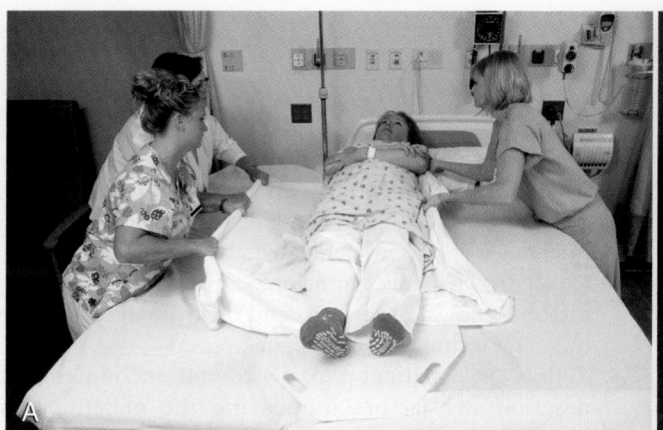
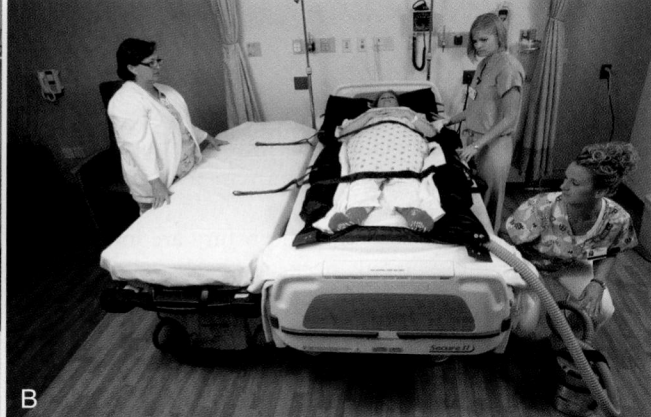
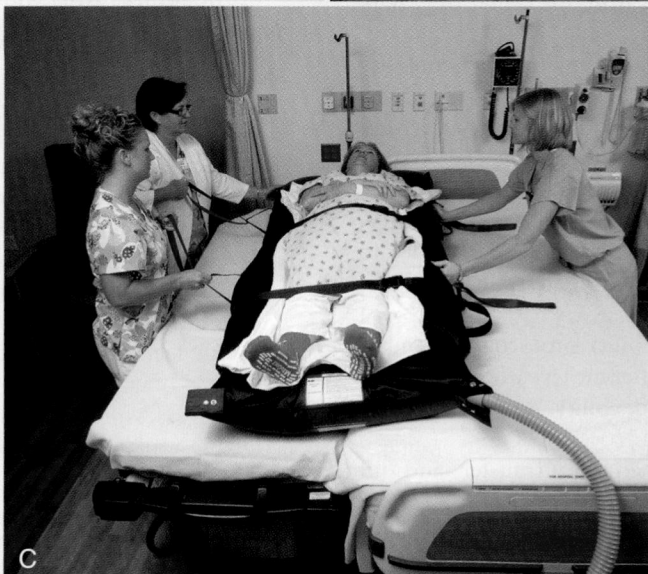

STEP 5b(10) A, Transfer of patient to stretcher using slide board. **B,** Inflating air-assisted transfer device. **C,** Transfer of patient using air-assisted device.

RECORDING AND REPORTING

- Record procedure including pertinent observations— weakness, ability to follow directions, weight-bearing ability, balance, ability to pivot, number of personnel needed to assist, assistive device used, amount of assistance (muscle strength) required, and patient's response— in nurses' notes in electronic health record (EHR) or chart.

- Document your evaluation of patient learning.
- Report transfer ability and assistance needed to next shift or other caregivers. Report progress or remission to rehabilitation staff (physical therapist, occupational therapist).

UNEXPECTED OUTCOMES AND RELATED INTERVENTIONS

- Patient unable to comprehend and follow directions for transfer.
  - Reassess continuity and simplicity of instructions.
- Patient sustains injury on transfer.
  - Evaluate incident that caused injury (e.g., inadequate assessment, change in patient status, improper use of equipment).
  - Complete occurrence report according to agency policy.

- Patient is unable to stand for time required to transfer to chair.
  - Provide for adequate assistance during transfer.
  - Assess for orthostatic changes in blood pressure when transferring patient.

■ KEY POINTS

- Muscles primarily associated with movement are located near the skeletal region, where movement results from leverage.
- Muscles primarily associated with posture are located in the lower extremities, trunk, neck, and back.
- Body alignment is the positioning of joints, tendons, ligaments, and muscles in various body positions.
- Body balance is achieved when there is a wide base of support, the center of gravity falls within the base of support, and a vertical line falls from the center of gravity through the base of support.
- Conditions that affect body alignment and mobility include postural abnormalities, altered bone formation or joint mobility, impaired muscle development, central nervous system damage, and musculoskeletal system trauma.
- Assessment of a patient's mobility enables you to determine the patient's coordination, balance, and ability to complete ADLs and makes it possible to evaluate or plan an exercise program.
- When implementing early mobility protocols remember that each patient starts at a different level, depending on his or her medical status and ability to participate in mobility.
- Apply proper algorithms when you transfer and lift patients.
- Assistive devices such as canes, crutches, and walkers require specific techniques to walk safely.

■ REFLECTIVE LEARNING

- Reflect on a patient experience you had today where a patient needed to perform an activity but was unable to because of voiced complaints of pain and describe what interventions you implemented.
- Recall any challenges in helping a patient transfer during a recent clinical experience and describe the safe patient handling techniques you applied.
- Reflect on a patient experience you encountered and describe any factors influencing the patient's activity tolerance. How did you intervene for this patient problem?

■ REVIEW QUESTIONS

1. Which of the following indicates that additional assistance is needed to transfer a patient from the bed to the stretcher?
   1. The patient is 5 feet 6 inches and weighs 120 lb (54.4 kg).
   2. The patient speaks and understands English.
   3. The patient received an injection of morphine 30 minutes ago for pain.
   4. You feel comfortable handling a patient of this size and level of cooperation.
2. Which assessment data does the nurse gather before transferring a patient from the bed to a stretcher? (Select all that apply.)
   1. Patient's weight
   2. Patient's level of cooperation
   3. Patient's ability to assist
   4. Presence of medical equipment
   5. 24-hour calorie intake

3. Which of the following are necessary safety precautions when ambulating a patient? (Select all that apply.)
   1. Placing a gait belt around patient's waist
   2. Clear the immediate environment of safety hazards
   3. Having patient wear well-fitting rubber-soled shoes or slippers
   4. Having at least three people present to assist patient
   5. Being sure that no pain medication was given for at least 3 hours before ambulation
4. Place the first five steps of Assessment for the performance of the Skill of Safe and Effective Transfer Techniques in the correct order.
   1. Perform hand hygiene.
   2. Directly assess physical capacity of a patient to transfer.
   3. Assess for weakness, dizziness, or risk for orthostatic (postural) hypotension.
   4. Identify the patient using at least two identifiers.
   5. Refer to medical record for most recent recorded weight and height for patient.

5. The nurse recognizes that a decline in physical activity and joint changes that decrease flexibility experienced by the older adult will most likely:
   1. Increase the patient's risk for falls and injuries
   2. Result in less stress on the patient's joints
   3. Decrease the amount of work of the patient to move
   4. Allow for mobility despite the aging effects on the patient's joints

evolve

Additional Review Questions, as well as rationales for all Review Questions, can be found on the Evolve website.

1. 3; 2. 1, 2, 3, 4; 3. 1, 2, 3; 4. 4, 1, 2, 3, 5; 5. 1.

REFERENCES

Adler J, Malone D: Early mobilization in the intensive care unit: a systematic review, *Cardiopulm Phys Ther J* 23(1):5, 2012.

American Academy of Orthopaedic Surgeons: *How to use crutches, canes, and walkers*, 2015. http://orthoinfo.aaos.org/topic.cfm?topic=A00181.

American Association of Critical-Care Nurses (AACN): *Early progressive mobility protocol*, 2013. https://www.aacn.org/docs/EventPlanning/WB0007/Mobility-Protocol-szh4mr5a.pdf.

American College of Foot and Ankle Surgeons (ACFAS): *Instructions for using crutches*, 2016. http://www.acfas.org/footankleinfo/crutches.htm.

American Heart Association (AHA): *Target heart rates*, 2015. http://www.heart.org/HEARTORG/HealthyLiving/PhysicalActivity/FitnessBasics/Target-Heart-Rates_UCM_434341_Article.jsp#.

American Nurses Association (ANA): *Safe patient handling and mobility interprofessional standards*, Silver Spring, MD, 2013a, The American Nurses Association.

American Nurses Association (ANA): *ANA leads initiative to develop national safe patient handling standards*, Silver Springs, MD, 2013b, The American Nurses Association.

American Nurses Association (ANA): *Nursing: scope and standards of practice*, ed 3, Silver Spring, MD, 2015, The American Nurses Association.

American Nurses Association (ANA): *Handle with care fact sheet*, 2016. http://www.nursingworld.org/MainMenuCategories/ANAMarketplace/Factsheets-and-Toolkits/FactSheet.html.

Anderson MP, et al: Safe moving and handling of patients: an interprofessional approach, *Nurs Stand* 28(46):37, 2014.

Ball J, et al: *Seidel's guide to physical examination*, ed 8, St Louis, 2015, Mosby.

Boynton T, et al: Banner Mobility Assessment Tool for nurses: instrument validation, *Am J SPHM* 4(3):86–92, 2014.

Burchum JR, Rosenthal LD: *Lehne's pharmacology for nursing care*, ed 9, St Louis, 2016, Elsevier.

Bureau of Labor Statistics (BLS): *Employer reported workplace industries and illnesses—2015*, 2016. http://www.bls.gov/news.release/pdf/osh.pdf.

Centers for Disease Control and Prevention (CDC): *How much physical activity do adults need?*, 2015. https://www.cdc.gov/physicalactivity/basics/adults/.

Childs E, deWit H: Regular exercise is associated with emotional resilience to acute stress in healthy adults, *Front Physiol* 5:1, 2014.

Chmelo EA, et al: Heterogeneity of physical function response to exercises training in older adults, *J Am Geriatr Soc* 63(3):462, 2015.

Covan EK: Benefits of exercise for body, mind, and spirit, *Health Care Women Int* 36(3):255, 2015.

Degelau J, et al: *Institute for Clinical Systems Improvement (ICSI). Prevention of falls (acute care). Health care protocol*, Bloomington, MN, 2012, Institute for Clinical Systems Improvement (ICSI). https://pdfs.semanticscholar.org/59cb/ea99bce55e2928e58311a5ff8451508c2488.pdf.

Doherty-King B, et al: Frequency and duration of nursing care related to older patient mobility, *J Nurs Scholarsh* 46(1):20, 2014.

Edelman CL, et al: *Health promotion throughout the life span*, ed 8, St Louis, 2014, Mosby.

Fletcher JS, Banasik JL: Exercise self-efficacy, *Clin Excell Nurse Pract* 5(3):134, 2001.

Frith J, et al: Measuring and defining orthostatic hypotension in the older person, *Age Aging* 43(2):168, 2014.

Garber CE, et al: Position stand: the recommended quantity and quality of exercise for developing and maintaining cardiorespiratory, musculoskeletal, and neuromotor fitness in apparently healthy adults: guidance for prescribing exercise, *Med Sci Sports Exerc* 43(7):1334, 2011.

Halawi MJ, et al: Multimodal analgesia for total joint arthroplasty, *Orthopedics* 38(7):e616, 2015.

Harvey LA, et al: Continuous passive motion following total knee arthroplasty in people with arthritis, *Cochrane Database Syst Rev* (2):CD004260, 2014.

HealthyPeople.gov: *Physical activity*, 2015. http://www.healthypeople.gov/2020/topics-objectives/topic/physical-activity.

Hernandez R, et al: Correlates of self-care in low-income African American and

Latino patients with diabetes, *Health Psychol* 33(7):597, 2014.

Hockenberry MJ, Wilson D: *Wong's nursing care of infants and children*, ed 10, St Louis, 2015, Mosby.

Huether SE, McCance KL: *Understanding pathophysiology*, ed 6, St Louis, 2017, Mosby.

Kim MK, et al: Effects of different types of exercise on muscle activity and balance control, *J Phys Ther Sci* 27(6):1875, 2015.

Lee W, Ory MG: The engagement in physical activity for middle-aged and older adults with multiple chronic conditions: findings from a community health assessment, *J Aging Res* 2013:152868, 2013.

Lewis S, et al: *Medical-surgical nursing: assessment and management of clinical problems*, ed 9, St Louis, 2014, Mosby.

Mills P, et al: Five things to know about orthostatic hypotension in the older adult, *J Am Geriatr Soc* 62(9):1822, 2014.

Myszenski A: *The essential role of lab values and vital signs in clinical decision making and patient safety for the acutely ill patient*, 2014. http://www.occupationaltherapy.com/ot-ceus/course/essential-role-lab-values-and-2029.

National Institute of Occupational Health and Safety (NIOSH): *Safe patient handling and movement (SPHM)*, 2016. http://www.cdc.gov/niosh/topics/safepatient/.

National Institute on Aging (NIA): *Exercise and physical activity*, 2016. https://go4life.nia.nih.gov/sites/default/files/nia_exercise_and_physical_activity.pdf.

Nelson A, Baptiste A: Evidence-based practices for safe patient handling and movement, *Online J Issues Nurs* 9(3):Manuscript 3, 2004. www.nursingworld.org/MainMenuCategories/ANAMarketplace/ANAPeriodicals/OJIN/TableofContents/Volume92004/No3Sept04/EvidenceBasedPractices.aspx.

Occupational Safety and Health Administration (OSHA): *Safe patient handling: preventing musculoskeletal disorders in nursing homes*, 2014. https://www.osha.gov/Publications/OSHA3708.pdf.

Occupational Safety and Health Administration (OSHA): *Worker safety in hospitals*, n.d., https://www.osha.gov/dsg/hospitals/.

Parreira RB, et al: Older adults present better back endurance than young adults during a dynamic trunk extension exercise, *J Back Musculoskelet Rehabil* 27(2):153, 2014.

Partnership to Fight Chronic Disease: *Needs great, evidence lacking for people with multiple chronic conditions*, 2012. http://www.fightchronicdisease.org/sites/fightchronicdisease.org/files/docs/MCC%20White%20paper%20October%202012%20-%20final%20draft.pdf.

Pashikanti L, Von Ah D: Impact of early mobilization protocol on the medical-surgical inpatient population: an integrated review of literature, *Clin Nurse Spec* 26(2):87, 2012.

Patton KT, Thibodeau GA: *Anatomy and physiology*, ed 9, St Louis, 2016, Mosby.

Pierson F, Fairchild S: *Principles and techniques of patient care*, ed 5, St Louis, 2013, Saunders.

Saffer H, et al: Racial, ethnic, and gender differences in physical activity, *J Hum Cap* 7(4):378, 2013.

Scarton LJ, et al: Needs and concerns of family caregivers of American Indians, African Americans, and Caucasians with type 2 diabetes, *Clin Res* 25(2):597, 2014.

Schofield PA: The assessment and management of peri-operative pain in older adults, *Anaesthesia* 6(1):54, 2014.

Shieh C, et al: Association of self-efficacy and self-regulation with nutrition and exercise behaviors in a community sample of adults, *J Community Health Nurs* 32(4):199, 2015.

Stevenson JM: Looking forward by looking back: helping to reduce work-related musculoskeletal disorders, *Work* 47(1):137, 2014.

Taylor NF, et al: Progressive resistance exercise in physical therapy: a summary of systematic reviews, *Phys Ther* 85(11):1208, 2005.

The Joint Commission (TJC): *2018 National Patient Safety Goals*, Oakbrook Terrace, IL, 2018, The Commission. http://www.jointcommission.org/standards_information/npsgs.aspx.

Touhy T, et al: *Ebersole and Hess' gerontological nursing and healthy aging*, ed 4, St Louis, 2014, Mosby.

Tsang M, et al: Examination of the readiness to learn and the best teaching method regarding health education and promotion within the Chinese elderly population, *Nurs Res* 64(2):2015.

U.S. Department of Health and Human Services (USDHHS): *Physical activity guidelines for Americans*, Washington, 2008a, HHS.

U.S. Department of Health and Human Services (USDHHS): *Physical activity guidelines advisory committee report*, Washington, 2008b, HHS.

U.S. Department of Health and Human Services (USDHHS): *Safe patient handling & lifting standards for a safer American workforce*, 2010. http://www.help.senate.gov/imo/media/doc/Collins4.pdf.

VISN8 Patient Safety Center (VISN8): *Safe patient handling and movement algorithms*. https://cseany.org/wp-content/uploads/2014/02/SPHMALGORITHMS.PDF.

Wallace R, et al: Effects of a 12-week community programme on older people, *Art and Science* 26(1):20, 2014.

Wrobleski DM, et al: Discharge planning rounds to the bedside: a patent- and family-centered approach, *Medsurg Nurs* 23(2):111, 2014.

evolve MEDIA RESOURCES

http://evolve.elsevier.com/Potter/essentials

- Audio Glossary
- Case Study Continuation

- QSEN Activity and Review Questions Answers and Rationales
- Video Clip

OBJECTIVES

- Describe the concepts of mobility and immobility.
- Discuss the physiological and psychosocial changes associated with immobility, and identify the impact changes have on nursing interventions.
- Describe complications associated with the physiological changes of immobility.
- Explain the techniques for assessing body alignment and impaired mobility.
- Identify appropriate nursing diagnoses for patients with impaired mobility.
- Discuss the importance of no-lift policies for patients and health care providers.

- Discuss the appropriate decision-making process when choosing equipment needed for safe patient handling and movement.
- Develop an individualized nursing care plan for patients with impaired mobility.
- Compare and contrast active and passive range-of-motion exercises.
- Discuss risks for development of deep vein thrombosis and appropriate interventions to use for prevention.
- Describe the techniques for repositioning patients in bed.
- Evaluate patient outcomes of nursing care for improving or maintaining mobility.

KEY TERMS

abduction, p. 751

activity tolerance, p. 748

adduction, p. 751

anthropometric measurements, p. 752

atelectasis, p. 745

bed rest, p. 744

body alignment, p. 743

body mechanics, p. 768

cerebellum, p. 743

deep vein thrombosis (DVT), p. 744

disuse osteoporosis, p. 746

diuresis, p. 745

dorsiflexion, p. 745

exercise, p. 742

foot boot, p. 767

footdrop, p. 745

friction, p. 766

hand-wrist splints, p. 768

hospital-associated deconditioning (HAD), p. 742

hyperextension, p. 767

hypostatic pneumonia, p. 745

immobilization, p. 742

instrumental activities of daily living (IADLs), p. 769

ischemia, p. 743

joint contracture, p. 745

mobility, p. 742

negative nitrogen balance, p. 745

orthostatic hypotension, p. 744

osteoporosis, p. 744

pathological fractures, p. 744

plantar flexion, p. 760

pressure injury, p. 746

prone, p. 767

pulmonary embolus, p. 752

range of motion (ROM), p. 748

recumbence, p. 744

thromboprophylaxis, p. 760

thrombus, p. 744

trapeze bar, p. 768

trochanter rolls, p. 767

venous thromboembolism (VTE), p. 752

CASE STUDY *Mr. Paul Rogers*

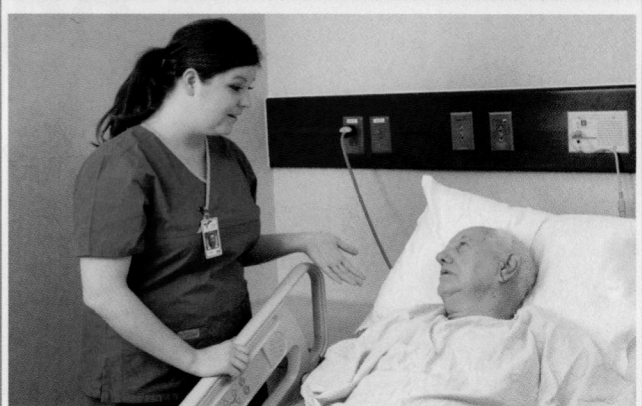

Mr. Paul Rogers, an 81-year-old widower, is hospitalized as a result of an ischemic stroke that occurred 24 hours ago. He has left-sided paralysis with decreased sensation. He currently is on bed rest. He has had type 2 diabetes mellitus for the past 15 years. There is no history of smoking or use of alcohol. He lives by himself since the death of his wife 4 years ago but has a son and daughter who live within a 25-minute drive. Both are married and visit him several times during the week. His son and daughter are now concerned as to whether he will be able to live alone in the future. He weighs 185 lb and is 6 feet 1 inch tall. Before his stroke, Mr. Rogers cooked for himself. He followed his prescribed diet "OK" but did admit that he likes cake, ice cream, and sweets. His daughter tries to monitor his blood sugar and brings diabetic diet meals on the weekends.

Abby Goodman, a 20-year-old nursing student, is assigned to Mr. Rogers for the week. Abby has reviewed the care for a patient who has had a stroke, including **mobility** impairment and prevention of complications. She has also reviewed possible nursing diagnoses for patients who have had a stroke that are appropriate for Mr. Rogers because of his age, impaired mobility, and medications.

The capacity to move around freely in the environment is a critical element for health as discussed in Chapter 28. It serves many purposes and requires the functioning of the nervous, cardiopulmonary, and musculoskeletal systems. When patients experience conditions that seriously threaten their ability to remain mobile, nurses take actions to reduce or prevent the effects of **immobilization**. Understanding the effects immobilization has on the function of all body systems and implementing evidence-based practices and safe patient handling are essential to protecting the safety of both patients and nurses. Immobilization is the physical restriction of movement to a body part. Nurses care for patients who become immobilized as a result of serious illness, traumatic injuries, or medical treatments. Examples of patients likely to become immobilized are patients with chronic illness; elderly patients; disabled patients; patients paralyzed by stroke or spinal cord injury; surgical patients who have postoperative

complications; and patients with multiple trauma, coronary artery disease, and obstetrical complications (preeclampsia). The longer a patient is immobilized, the greater risk for **hospital-associated deconditioning (HAD)**. HAD is the loss of muscle mass, functional reserve, and decreased activity tolerance and the functional decline in activities of daily living (ADLs) and mobility regardless of a specific neurological or orthopedic insult. The deconditioning from inactivity during hospitalization can negatively affect a patient's recovery resulting in longer length of stay (LOS) and development of medical complications such as pressure injuries, deep vein thrombosis (DVT), and falls and create the need for postdischarge rehabilitation. Studies have shown that hospitalized older adults are 61 times more likely to develop disability in ADLs than older adults who are not hospitalized (Falvey et al., 2015). Thus it is a priority among health care providers to limit the duration of immobility for any patient. It is a nurse's responsibility to know the effects of immobility, recognize the contributing factors that place each patient at risk for being immobile, and implement preventive strategies.

SCIENTIFIC KNOWLEDGE BASE

Depending on the degree of immobility and deconditioning a patient is experiencing, the effects can be far reaching. Apply the knowledge you acquired from Chapter 28 to keep patients active and to safely assist them when they are able to transfer out of bed. As a nurse, it is important that you understand the types of pathological conditions that can cause patients to become immobile and the effects immobility and deconditioning have on physiological function.

Pathological Influences on Mobility

Chapter 28 described the regulation of movement and the importance of activity and **exercise** for a patient's well-being. A brief discussion of four pathological influences that can affect a patient's mobility follows.

Postural Abnormalities. Acquired or congenital abnormalities interfere with the functioning of the musculoskeletal system. Changes to bones, muscles, and supporting structures alter functioning and may result in pain, impaired alignment, and impaired mobility. Knowledge about the characteristics, causes, and treatment of common postural abnormalities is necessary when you lift, transfer, and position patients (Table 29.1). In addition, chronic postural abnormalities are associated with diminished functional ability and frequent falls.

Muscle Abnormalities. Chapter 28 describes the role muscles play in the regulation of movement. Injuries and disease can lead to numerous alterations in musculoskeletal function. One example of this would be patients with muscular dystrophy who experience progressive, symmetrical weakness and wasting of skeletal muscle groups with increasing disability and deformity (Huether and McCance, 2017).

TABLE 29.1 POSTURAL ABNORMALITIES

ABNORMALITY	DESCRIPTION	CAUSE	POSSIBLE TREATMENTS[a]
Torticollis	Inclining of head to affected side, in which sternocleidomastoid muscle is contracted	Congenital or acquired condition	Surgery, heat, support, or immobilization, depending on cause and severity; gentle ROM
Lordosis	Exaggeration of anterior convex curve of lumbar spine	Congenital condition Temporary condition (e.g., pregnancy)	Spine-stretching exercises (based on cause)
Kyphosis	Increased convexity in curvature of thoracic spine	Congenital condition Rickets, osteoporosis Tuberculosis of spine	Spine-stretching exercises, sleeping without pillows, using bed board, bracing, spinal fusion (based on cause and severity)
Scoliosis	Lateral S- or C-shaped spinal column with vertebral rotation; unequal heights of hips and shoulders	Sometimes a consequence of numerous congenital, connective tissue, and neuromuscular disorders	Approximately half of children with scoliosis require surgery Nonsurgical treatment with braces and exercises
Congenital hip dysplasia	Hip instability with limited abduction of hips and occasionally adduction contractures (head of femur does not articulate with acetabulum because of abnormal shallowness of acetabulum)	Congenital condition (more common with breech deliveries)	Maintenance of continuous abduction of thigh so that head of femur presses into center of acetabulum Abduction splints, casting, surgery
Knock-knee (genu valgum)	Legs curved inward so that knees come together as person walks	Congenital condition Rickets	Knee brace; surgery if not corrected by growth
Bowlegs (genu varum)	One or both legs bent outward at knee, which is normal until 2–3 years of age	Congenital condition Rickets	Slowing rate of curving if not corrected by growth With rickets, increase of vitamin D, calcium, and phosphorus intake to normal ranges
Clubfoot	95%: Medial deviation and plantar flexion of foot (equinovarus) 5%: Lateral deviation and dorsiflexion (calcaneovalgus)	Congenital condition	Casts, splints such as Denis Browne splint, and surgery (based on degree and rigidity of deformity)
Footdrop	Inability to dorsiflex and invert foot because of peroneal nerve damage	Congenital condition Trauma Improper position of immobilized patient	None (cannot be corrected) Prevention through physical therapy Bracing with AFO
Pigeon toes	Internal rotation of forefoot or entire foot; common in infants	Congenital condition Habit	Growth; wearing reversed shoes

AFO, Ankle-foot orthotic; *ROM,* range of motion.
[a]Severity of condition and cause dictate treatment, which is individualized to patient's needs.
Data from Huether SE, McCance K: *Understanding pathophysiology,* ed 6, St Louis, 2017, Mosby.

Damage and Disorders Affecting the Central Nervous System. The influence of the central nervous system on movement, balance, and posture is discussed in Chapter 28. Damage to portions of the central nervous system that regulate voluntary movement results in impaired movement, body alignment, balance, and coordination. Trauma from a head injury, ischemia from a stroke (cerebrovascular accident [CVA]), or bacterial infection such as meningitis can damage the cerebellum or the motor strip in the cerebral cortex. The cerebellum coordinates voluntary movements such as posture, balance, coordination, and speech resulting in smooth and balanced muscular activity. Damage to the cerebellum will alter any one of these functions. Motor impairment, the ability to initiate voluntary movement, is directly related to the amount of destruction of the motor strip. Damage to the left motor strip causes paralysis or impaired function on the right side of the body, whereas damage to the right motor strip causes alterations on the left side of the body.

Neuromuscular diseases such as amyotrophic lateral sclerosis, Parkinson disease, multiple sclerosis, and myasthenia gravis affect the nerves that control the voluntary muscles. These diseases affect the function of neurons, which transmit signals that control these muscles. When the neurons become unhealthy or die, communication between the nervous system and muscles breaks down, causing muscle weakness and wasting.

Direct Trauma to the Musculoskeletal System. Fractures most commonly result from direct external trauma, but they also occur as a consequence of some deformity of the bone (e.g., pathological fractures of osteoporosis or osteogenesis imperfecta). Young children are usually able to form new bone more easily than adults and as a result have fewer complications after a fracture. Treatment often includes positioning the fractured bone in proper alignment and immobilizing it to promote healing and restore function. Even this temporary immobilization results in some muscle atrophy, loss of muscle tone, and joint stiffness. Adults 65 years of age and older have both an increased rate of trauma and an increased predisposition to fractures from even minimal force as a result of reduced bone density (Southerland and Barrie, 2014). This makes older adults a high-risk population for traumatic fracture.

Immobility

In addition to the effects of trauma and disease, a patient's mobility can be restricted for therapeutic reasons such as when bed rest is ordered. Therapeutic reasons for bed rest include decreasing the oxygen needs of the body, reducing cardiac workload and pain, and allowing the debilitated or ill patient to rest. The duration of bed rest depends on the type and nature of an illness or injury and the patient's prior state of health. For example, a patient returning from major surgery might be ordered to remain on bed rest for only a few hours. A patient with a serious systemic infection and cardiac complications might require bed rest for several days. Whatever the cause of a patient's immobility, the extent of the immobilization depends on the length and severity of illness, presence of pain, cognitive and emotional status such as depression, and overall physical condition. It is essential to remember that the hazardous effects of immobility are imposed on each of the systems of a patient's body (Box 29.1) (Huether and McCance, 2017). The greater the extent and longer the duration of immobility, the more pronounced the effects.

Cardiovascular Changes. Immobility initially results in an increased heart rate (resting tachycardia) with the heart rate rising slightly each day. The heart rate increase becomes exaggerated even with mild exertion. The patient has decreased stroke volume (approximately 15% in 2 weeks), but the cardiac output is relatively unchanged. The cardiac muscle mass may decrease depending on the duration of immobility. The effects on circulation include pooling of blood in the legs. Blood vessels may lose their ability to constrict in response to postural change; as a result venous return, stroke volume, and blood pressure are decreased. When a patient rises from a sitting position, orthostatic hypotension, a decrease in blood pressure of 40 mm Hg or more systolic or 20 mm Hg or more diastolic, may occur within 15 seconds of standing

---

| BOX 29.1 | **PATHOPHYSIOLOGY OF IMMOBILITY** |

PHYSIOLOGICAL OUTCOMES
- ↓ Basal metabolic rate
- ↓ Gastrointestinal motility
- ↓ Nutrients/fluids
- ↓ Appetite
- Shift in electrolyte balance
- ↓ O_2 availability/ischemia
  - ↓ O_2/CO_2 exchange
  - ↑ Respiratory muscle weakness
  - ↓ Lung expansion
  - ↑ Atelectasis/hypostatic pneumonia
- ↓ Cardiac output
  - ↑ Cardiac workload
  - ↑ Oxygen demand
  - ↑ Dependent edema
  - ↑ Clot formation (deep vein thrombosis)
- ↑ Muscle atrophy
  - ↓ Strength/flexibility/endurance
  - ↑ Joint contractures
- ↑ Disuse osteoporosis
- ↑ Bone resorption

PSYCHOLOGICAL OUTCOMES
- ↑ Stressors
- ↑ Depression
  - ↓ Self-identity
  - ↓ Self-esteem
- ↑ Behavioral changes
- ↑ Changes in sleep-wake cycles
- ↓ Coping successes
- ↑ Isolation
- ↑ Passive behaviors
- ↑ Sensory deprivation/overload

DEVELOPMENTAL OUTCOMES
- ↑ Dependence
- ↑ Regression in development

(Frith et al., 2014; Lewis et al., 2014; Mills et al., 2014). Prolonged bed rest also increases the workload of the heart producing a need for more oxygen.

Prolonged recumbence (a position of lying down at rest) leads to circulatory fluid volume loss with a fluid shift to the thoracic area. The patient begins to diurese (excrete more urine) because of protein loss. With a decrease in plasma volume the hematocrit will increase but then fall as the red blood cell mass later decreases. Immobilized patients are at risk for a deep vein thrombosis (DVT). A thrombus is an accumulation of platelets, fibrin, clotting factors, and cellular elements of the blood attached to the interior wall of a vein or artery, sometimes occluding the lumen of the vessel. Three factors, known as Virchow's triad, contribute to venous thrombus formation: (1) blood stasis resulting from decreased blood flow and increased viscosity, (2) hypercoagulability resulting from a change in clotting factors or increased platelet activity, and (3) vessel trauma (Huether and McCance,

2017). The first two factors are physiological responses to immobility. A DVT places a patient at risk for pulmonary emboli, which is a life-threatening complication.

Respiratory Changes.

There is a potential decrease in lung volumes secondary to muscle weakness and restricted ventilation from the positioning that is associated with bed rest. A patient is unable to easily deep breathe and expand the lungs. The patient will have a reduction in vital capacity, residual volume, functional residual capacity, and expiratory reserve. Clinically an easy sign to detect is the increase in respiratory rate. There is also dependent stasis of secretions within the airways. These conditions often contribute to the development of atelectasis (collapse of alveoli) and hypostatic pneumonia (inflammation of the lung from stasis or pooling of secretions). General muscle weakness reduces a patient's ability to cough. Mucus accumulates, particularly when the patient lies supine, providing an excellent medium for bacterial growth. Thus hypostatic pneumonia may result.

Metabolic Changes.

Immobility disrupts normal metabolic functioning, decreasing the metabolic rate and altering the metabolism of carbohydrates, proteins, and fats. There is impaired glucose tolerance and hyperinsulinemia with the muscles developing insulin resistance. A patient's basal metabolic rate (BMR) decreases in response to reduced cellular energy because of the decreased ability of the body to use insulin. Because glucose cannot enter the cells, the body begins to break down its protein stores for energy resulting in a negative nitrogen balance and increased oxygen demands. However, in the presence of an infection, immobilized patients have an increased BMR. Fever and wound repair add to cellular oxygen requirements (see Chapter 35).

Fluid and Electrolyte Balances.

Major shifts in blood volume occur in immobile patients. Diuresis (increased urine excretion) occurs as a result of the increased blood flow to the kidneys. Diuresis causes the body to lose electrolytes such as potassium and sodium and reduces serum calcium levels. Immobility increases calcium resorption (loss) from the bones causing hypercalcemia, a release of excess calcium into the circulation. The loss of calcium may result in pathological bone fractures if the patient's kidneys cannot respond appropriately to treatment.

Gastrointestinal Changes.

An immobile patient has decreased fluid intake and appetite. There is also a decrease in the transit time in the esophagus and stomach. These changes along with reduced small bowel motility result in constipation. With an increase in inactivity, there is the development of hypercalcemia, which depresses peristalsis. Constipation is sometimes so severe that fecal impaction develops, and if left untreated, a partial or complete bowel obstruction can occur (see Chapter 37).

Musculoskeletal Changes.

The effects of immobility are devastating to the muscular system. There is a decrease in muscle mass and tension, characterized by a decrease in muscle fiber diameter and muscle atrophy. This is ongoing as long as immobility continues. The body composition also changes with decreases in lean body mass and increased body fat. The body loses muscle strength when muscles atrophy from inactivity. The rate of muscle decline varies with the degree of immobility, but it is rapid while mobility and weight bearing are restricted. These effects are especially devastating to patients who are marginally functional with their ADLs. As immobility progresses and muscles are not exercised, muscle mass continues to decrease, and the size of the muscles decreases. Immobility affects the leg muscles the most, which explains the difficulty that older patients have in getting up from a chair after periods of bed rest.

Skeletal changes cause a decreased passive range of motion (ROM) of joints secondary to connective tissue or muscle shortening. A joint contracture is a preventable, abnormal, and possibly permanent condition characterized by limited movement or fixation of the joint. When a contracture occurs, the joint cannot maintain full ROM (Fig. 29.1), leaving the joint in a nonfunctional position. Factors that contribute to contractures include positioning patients out of alignment, failure to reposition frequently, pain and edema that limit joint movement, and the muscle imbalance that occurs in patients with paralysis or spastic muscles.

One common and debilitating deformity that can result from bed rest is footdrop (Fig. 29.2), which is a gait abnormality involving a significant weakness of ankle and toe dorsiflexion (Pritchett et al., 2016). A footdrop involves the dropping of the forefoot that happens secondary to weakness, irritation or damage to the sciatic or peroneal nerve, or paralysis of the muscles in the anterior portion of the lower leg. A patient has a steppage gait because the patient tends to walk with an exaggerated flexion of the hip and knee to prevent the toes from catching on the ground during the swing phase of walking (Pritchett et al., 2016). Peroneal neuropathy with an overt footdrop is a known risk factor for falling (Poppler et al., 2016). A footdrop can be temporary or permanent. When a patient becomes immobilized, it is critical to provide regular ROM and proper positioning to prevent footdrop.

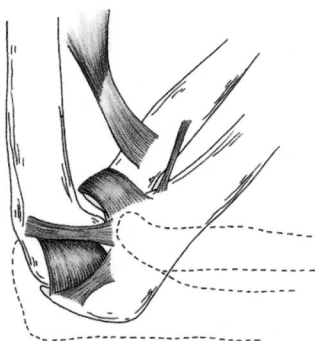

FIG 29.1 Flexion contracture of elbow resulting in permanent flexion of joint. Normally the elbow is able to extend to 90-degree angle *(dotted line)* and 180-degree angle *(not shown)*.

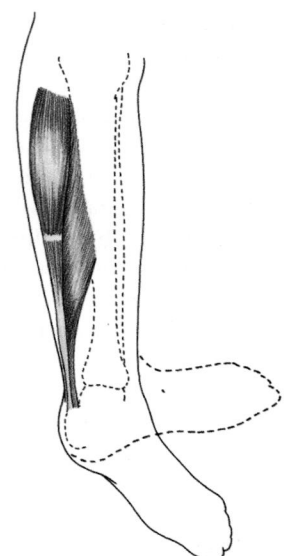

FIG 29.2 Footdrop. Ankle is fixed in plantar flexion.

Disuse osteoporosis is a disorder characterized by increased bone resorption from immobilization. Osteoporosis peaks at 4 to 6 weeks with bone density decreasing 40% after 12 weeks (in the case of patients with spinal cord injury). There is a decreased rate of bone formation, and weight-bearing bones are the first to lose bone mass. Osteoporosis can lead to pathological fractures even with minor trauma such as coughing violently. If patients have osteoporosis at the time of admission, nurses must recognize that they are at high risk for accelerated bone loss if immobilized. Patients with identified risk of osteoporosis need encouragement to eat the current recommended dietary allowances for calcium and foods such as milk fortified with vitamin D, leafy green vegetables, yogurt, and cheese.

Integument Changes. The direct effect of pressure on the skin by immobility is compounded by metabolic changes. Older adult patients and patients with paralysis have a greater risk for developing pressure injuries (see Chapter 38). A **pressure injury** has been defined by the National Pressure Ulcer Advisory Panel (NPUAP, 2016) as:

> Localized damage to the skin and/or underlying soft tissue usually over a bony prominence or related to a medical or other device. The injury can present as intact skin or an open ulcer and may be painful. The injury occurs as a result of intense and/or prolonged pressure or pressure in combination with shear.

When a patient lies in bed or sits in a chair, the weight of the body is on bony prominences. The longer the pressure is applied, the longer the period of ischemia (i.e., temporary decrease of blood flow to tissue) and the greater the risk for skin breakdown. Because of the change of circulation, any break in the integrity of the skin is difficult to heal in the immobilized patient. Impaired perfusion increases the risk of pressure injuries, and cognitive disturbances can make

prophylactic measures more difficult (Anders et al., 2010). Chapter 38 describes pressure injuries in detail.

Urinary Elimination Changes. Patients who remain recumbent have difficulty voiding because of positioning restrictions. This becomes complicated when physiological changes shift blood flow to the kidneys causing diuresis and an increased need to void. In the upright position urine normally flows from the renal pelvis into the ureter to the bladder because of gravity. When a patient is in bed, the kidneys and ureters move toward a more level plane, and urine tries to move from the kidney to the bladder against gravity. Because the peristaltic contractions of the ureters are not strong enough to overcome gravity, the renal pelvis fills before urine enters the ureters. This condition, called *urinary stasis*, increases a patient's risk for urinary tract infection (UTI) and renal calculi or calcium stones. The stones lodge in the renal pelvis and pass through the ureters. Immobilized patients are also at risk for calculi because of altered calcium metabolism and resulting hypercalcemia (see Chapter 36).

NURSING KNOWLEDGE BASE

The science of nursing has contributed significantly to better understanding how to manage complications of immobility including pressure injuries (Chapter 38) and elimination problems (Chapters 36 and 37). In addition, nurse researchers have contributed to the knowledge necessary for nurses to understand the nature of movement and immobility in the clinical setting so that they can determine the safest way to move patients. Because nursing has a holistic focus, nursing knowledge has contributed to understanding the effects of immobility on the physiological and psychosocial aspects of patient care as well.

Safe Patient Handling

Nurses are exposed to the hazards related to the lifting and transferring of patients. This is especially true in settings such as hospitals and long-term care facilities. Patient-handling tasks most frequently associated with low back pain are lifting and forceful movements (American Nurses Association [ANA], 2016). Manually lifting and transferring patients contributes to the high incidence of work-related musculoskeletal problems and back injuries in nurses and other health care staff (Anderson et al., 2014; Stevenson, 2014). Current evidence shows that many nurses frequently transfer to different positions in a work setting or leave the profession because of work-related injuries (ANA, 2016). Implementing evidence-based interventions and programs (e.g., proper use of lift devices and lift teams) reduces injuries to patients and reduces the number of work-related injuries experienced by health care providers, which improves the health of the nurse and reduces indirect costs to the health care agency (e.g., workers' compensation and replacing injured workers). The American Nurses Association (ANA) has been advocating for safe patient handling since initiating the policy in 1992 and establishing standards in 2012 (ANA, 2012). The

Association of Safe Patient Handling Professionals (ASPHP, www.asphp.org/certification/) offers certifications for health care professionals and hospitals. The focus should be on safe handling and transfer to avoid injury to patients and nurses.

Several states have laws that mandate safe patient handling in health care agencies or are in the process of passing legislation. Health care agencies are implementing comprehensive safe patient-handling programs in all parts of the United States. These programs include the following elements: an ergonomics assessment protocol for health care environments, patient assessment criteria, algorithms for patient handling and movement, special equipment kept in convenient locations to help transfer patients, back-injury resource nurses, "after-action reviews" or safety huddles that allow the health care team to apply knowledge about safe patient moving in different settings, and a no-lift policy (Department of Health and Human Services [DHHS], 2010; VISN 8 Patient Safety Center [VISN8], 2014).

Psychosocial Effects

Immobilization reduces a patient's independence and creates a sense of loss. As a result, there are emotional, intellectual, sensory, and sociocultural responses. The most common emotional changes are depression, social isolation, sleep-wake disturbances, and impaired coping.

Some immobilized patients become depressed because of changes in self-concept (see Chapter 24). Depression is an affective disorder characterized by exaggerated feelings of sadness, melancholy, dejection, worthlessness, emptiness, helplessness, and hopelessness (Parker, 2012). It results from worrying about present and future levels of health, finances, and family needs. Because immobilization removes patients from their daily routines, they have more time to worry about disability. Worrying quickly increases patients' depression, causing withdrawal. Withdrawn patients often do not want to participate in their own care and are unwilling to take part in other activities.

Immobilized patients require vigilant nursing care such as repositioning at least every 2 hours or more often to avoid physical complications. Because of the need for frequent repositioning, it is important to organize care activities together including nursing and medical interventions to ensure that a patient gets sufficient sleep (see Chapter 33). Disruption of normal sleeping patterns causes further behavioral changes and affects coping patterns.

Long-term immobility or bed rest affects usual coping patterns. Some immobilized patients withdraw and become passive. The passive patient demonstrates little interest in achieving independence or participating in care. Assess a patient's normal coping mechanisms and develop a nursing care plan that is based on patient strengths and encourages patient input as much as possible.

Developmental Effects

Developmental effects of immobility more commonly affect very young and older adult patients. The immobilized young or middle-age adult experiences few, if any, changes.

When an infant, toddler, or preschooler is immobilized, it is usually because of trauma or the need to correct a congenital skeletal abnormality. Prolonged immobilization delays a child's motor skill and intellectual development (Hockenberry and Wilson, 2015).

Prolonged immobilization alters adolescent growth patterns as well. In addition, adolescents who experience immobility often are behind peers in gaining independence and accomplishing certain skills such as obtaining a driver's license, a major milestone for many teenagers. Social isolation is another concern for this age-group when immobilization occurs, although computers and smartphones reduce this concern considerably.

A healthy adult patient who is briefly immobile may not experience the hazards of immobility; however, if the immobilization is prolonged or the patient has one or more chronic conditions, all physiological systems are at risk. In addition, the role of the adult often changes with regard to the family or social structure. Some adults lose their jobs, which affects their self-concept.

Immobilization in older adult patients increases their physical dependence on others and accelerates functional losses in physiological systems (Touhy and Jett, 2014). Immobilization in this patient group usually results from a degenerative disease, neurological trauma, or chronic illness. For some patients immobilization occurs gradually and progressively; whereas for others, especially patients who have had a CVA, loss of mobility is sudden. Develop nursing care plans that encourage patient independence.

CRITICAL THINKING

Synthesis

Patient care requires you to apply what you know about a patient, your knowledge base, experience, and critical thinking attitudes and standards. Your synthesis of this information allows you to make sound decisions as you apply the nursing process. Critical thinking synthesis involves combining all available information to obtain a clear picture of the approach needed to provide patient-centered care. Gather information from a variety of sources when caring for patients. Integrating knowledge and experience makes it possible to determine physical, psychosocial, and developmental needs of immobilized patients. The needs of immobile patients are multiple and complex.

Knowledge. Knowledge of anatomy, physiology, and pathophysiology helps you anticipate how patients are affected by limitations in mobility. Applying such knowledge helps you to understand the bodily structures affected and the impact on patients. Your assessment of any patient's limitations should focus on the pathophysiological changes that exist compared with the changes you expect so that you can develop an appropriate plan of care that is comprehensive and will prevent complications.

Understand the importance of a patient's culture and traditions regarding activity and what it means to be immobile

---

🌐 **BOX 29.2   PATIENT-CENTERED CARE**

Cultural factors influence many aspects of patients' lives including time orientation, health care practices, and nutrition. Not as much attention has been given to the impact of cultural factors on mobility and exercise. You know that being immobile even for a short period of time can result in a number of hazards for a patient. Therefore knowing a patient's cultural practices helps you plan care. Unhealthy lifestyles are associated with socioeconomic factors such as social class, education, geographic location, and income. This is the case with physical activity and obesity. In addition, not having social support and certain ethnic customs may cause people to be inactive.

IMPLICATIONS FOR PRACTICE

- Help patients plan physical activities that are culturally appropriate (Owiti et al., 2014; Purnell, 2014).
- Make exercise programs that are flexible, affordable, and accommodate family and community culture yet keep patients safe from negative patient outcomes (Owiti et al., 2014; Purnell, 2014).
- Incorporate cultural beliefs and desired patient outcomes when designing the plan of care (Owiti et al., 2014; Purnell, 2014).

(Box 29.2). Also apply knowledge of patients' developmental stages to assess their current functional and mobility status and health care needs. Application of knowledge gained from the study of human growth and development is essential for accurately selecting appropriate interventions for mobility alterations. Concepts for patient teaching are based on developmental stages and are vital in preparing patients for rehabilitation following immobilization.

Abby knows that she needs to respect Mr. Rogers' need to be independent and desire to participate in his care as much as possible. She realizes their difference in age and understands that Mr. Rogers probably has his "own way of doing things." She approaches this clinical experience with patience and creativity and plans to implement individualized care to increase Mr. Rogers' activity level, keep him as independent as possible, prevent hazards of immobility, and help him progress through the acute phase of his care by addressing his anticipated needs associated with that of a patient who has had a stroke.

Experience. Taking care of patients who had mobility restrictions in the past allows you to anticipate patients' needs for comfort, pain control, positioning, and support of ADLs. Your experience with a variety of exercise strategies helps develop health promotion activities or rehabilitation plans for assigned patients.

Attitudes. Attitudes for critical thinking allow you to make reasoned judgments and solve patient problems. Design creative solutions to improve a patient's mobility status such as collaborating with occupational therapy to select self-care activities that require a patient to use weakened muscle groups. The attitude of perseverance is essential

for coordinating patient care and working with patients experiencing psychological and developmental changes resulting from immobilization. Use discipline and be thorough in your assessment and approach to planning care, considering patients' needs once they return home and how family caregivers can become involved.

Standards. Promote a patient's independence while adhering to the prescribed rehabilitation plan and maintaining safety. Professional standards such as those for safe patient handling are important when developing a plan of care because they establish scientifically proven guidelines for selecting effective nursing interventions. Since 2003 in the *Position Statement on Elimination of Manual Patient Handling to Prevent Work-Related Musculoskeletal Disorders,* the ANA has prompted the use of evidence-based research to develop policies for safe patient handling (ANA, 2015, 2016). The leadership of the ANA (2015) set standards for safe patient handling and continues to review and revise these policies to help nurses develop policies and procedures for the safe use of transfer and positioning equipment within their facilities. Such policies result in decreased injuries to nurses and patients.

When discharging patients from a health care agency, instructions must be clear and explicit. Use the ethical standard of autonomy in supporting patients in making decisions about their discharge needs. Evaluate discharge teaching by having patients demonstrate required actions to ensure that they understand them completely and can perform them correctly, thereby validating the quality of the teaching sessions.

Synthesis of knowledge, experience, attitudes, and standards is important in developing an individualized care plan with the immobilized patient. This plan of care prevents complications, promotes rehabilitation, and expedites discharge.

NURSING PROCESS

■■■ ASSESSMENT

Mobility assessment focuses on patients' past and present mobility and the potential effects of being immobile. The greater the extent and the longer the duration of immobility, the more pronounced the consequences. A patient with complete mobility restrictions is continually at risk for the hazards of immobility. You must thoroughly assess each body system for these risks. Table 29.2 presents an example of a focused patient assessment that includes a review of a patient's mobility, pain associated with movement, and **activity tolerance**.

Mobility. When a patient is immobile, assessment focuses on the status of the musculoskeletal system and includes ROM, muscle strength, activity tolerance, and posture and alignment. Assessment of **range of motion (ROM)** is important as a baseline measurement to compare and evaluate whether loss in joint mobility is developing or has occurred. Refer to Table 29.3 for normal joint ROM to compare with findings when you assess a patient's ROM. Be sure to assess all joints in the body. Ask questions about and physically

TABLE 29.2 FOCUSED PATIENT ASSESSMENT

FACTORS TO ASSESS	QUESTIONS	PHYSICAL ASSESSMENT
Mobility	Describe for me how difficult it is for you to walk or get around. Do you have problems with steps? Describe for me how your ability to get around affects your ability to care for yourself.	Observe patient's gait as he or she walks. Observe patient sit and rise from chair. Observe patient while performing self-care activities.
Pain	Do you have any pain or discomfort on movement? Ask patient to rate pain on a 0-to-10 pain scale. Please tell me about your pain. When did it start? How long does it last? Can you get relief? Would you like your pain medication before I help you walk?	Observe for objective signs of pain such as grimacing; moaning; increasing respiratory rate, pulse, and blood pressure. Inspect joints for redness or swelling, indicating potential inflammatory process. Watch if patient favors one leg or knee when walking, sitting, or changing position. Use appropriate pain scale for patients who cannot verbalize their pain.
Endurance and activity	Are you feeling tired now? In what way does feeling weak or tired affect your ability to bathe or wash yourself, get to the bathroom, or dress yourself? Are you having shortness of breath, either when resting or moving; palpitations; light-headedness or dizziness?	Observe for signs of fatigue. Observe patient's performance of ADLs. Observe patient for pallor; obtain baseline vital signs. Monitor oxygen saturation before and after activity.

ADLs, Activities of daily living.

TABLE 29.3 RANGE-OF-MOTION EXERCISES

BODY PART	TYPE OF JOINT	TYPE OF MOVEMENT	RANGE (DEGREES)	PRIMARY MUSCLES
Neck, cervical spine	Pivotal	Flexion: Bring chin to rest on chest.	45	Sternocleidomastoid
		Extension: Return head to erect position.	45	Trapezius
		Hyperextension: Bend head back as far as possible.	10	Trapezius
		Lateral flexion: Tilt head as far as possible toward each shoulder.	40–45	Scalenes
		Rotation: Turn head as far as possible in circular movement.	180	Sternocleidomastoid, upper trapezius
Shoulder	Ball and socket	Flexion: Raise arm from side position forward to position above head.	45–180	Coracobrachialis, deltoid, pectoralis major
		Extension: Return arm to position at side of body.	180	Latissimus dorsi, teres major, triceps brachii
		Shoulder extension: Move arm behind body, keeping elbow straight.	0–60	Latissimus dorsi, teres major, deltoid
		Internal rotation: With elbow flexed and shoulder abducted, rotate shoulder by moving arm until thumb is turned inward and toward back.	70–90	Pectoralis major, latissimus dorsi, subscapularis
		External rotation: With elbow flexed and shoulder abducted, move arm until thumb is upward and lateral to head.	90	Infraspinatus, teres minor
		Circumduction: Move arm in full circle (circumduction is combination of all movements of ball-and-socket joint).	360	Deltoid, coracobrachialis, latissimus dorsi, teres major

Continued

TABLE 29.3 RANGE-OF-MOTION EXERCISES—cont'd

BODY PART	TYPE OF JOINT	TYPE OF MOVEMENT	RANGE (DEGREES)	PRIMARY MUSCLES
Elbow	Hinge	Flexion: Bend elbow so that lower arm moves toward its shoulder joint and hand is level with shoulder.	150	Biceps brachii, brachialis, brachioradialis
		Extension: Straighten elbow by lowering hand.	150	Triceps brachii
Forearm	Pivotal	Supination: Turn lower arm and hand so that palm is up.	70–90	Supinator, biceps brachii
		Pronation: Turn lower arm so that palm is down.	70–90	Pronator teres, pronator quadratus
Wrist	Condyloid	Flexion, move palm toward inner aspect of forearm.	80–90	Flexor carpi ulnaris, flexor carpi radialis
		Extension: Move fingers and hand posterior to midline, bring dorsal surface of hand back as far as possible.	70–80	Extensor carpi radialis brevis, extensor carpi radialis longus, extensor carpi ulnaris
		Radial deviation: Bend wrist medially toward thumb.	Up to 30	Flexor carpi radialis brevis, extensor carpi radialis brevis, extensor carpi radialis longus
		Ulnar deviation: Bend wrist laterally toward fifth finger.	30	Flexor carpi ulnaris, extensor carpi ulnaris
Fingers	Condyloid hinge	Flexion: Make fist.	90	Lumbricales, interosseus volaris, interosseus dorsalis
		Extension: Straighten fingers.	90	Extensor digiti quinti proprius, extensor digitorum communis, extensor indicis proprius
		Hyperextension: Bend fingers back as far as possible.	30–60	Extensor digitorum
		Abduction: Spread fingers apart.	30	Interosseus dorsalis
		Adduction: Bring fingers together.	30	Interosseus volaris
Thumb	Saddle	Flexion: Move thumb across palmar surface of hand.	90	Flexor pollicis brevis
		Extension: Move thumb straight away from hand.	90	Extensor pollicis longus, extensor pollicis brevis
		Abduction: Extend thumb laterally (usually done when placing fingers in abduction and adduction).	30	Abductor pollicis brevis and longus
		Adduction: Move thumb back toward hand.	30	Adductor pollicis obliquus, adductor pollicis transversus
		Opposition: Touch thumb to each finger of same hand.		Opponens pollicis, opponens digiti minimi
Hip	Ball and socket	Flexion: Move leg forward and up.	110–120	Psoas major, iliacus, sartorius
		Extension: Move leg back beside other leg.	90–120	Gluteus maximus, semitendinosus, semimembranosus
		Hyperextension: Move leg behind body as far as possible.	30–50	Gluteus maximus, semitendinosus, semimembranosus
		Abduction: Move leg laterally away from body.	30–50	Gluteus medius, gluteus minimus
		Adduction: Move leg back toward midline position and beyond if possible.	20–30	Adductor longus, adductor brevis, adductor magnus
		Internal rotation: Turn foot and leg toward other leg.	45	Gluteus medius, gluteus minimus, tensor fasciae latae
		External rotation: Turn foot and leg away from other leg.	45	Obturatorius internus, obturatorius externus, quadratus femoris, piriformis, gemellus superior and inferior, gluteus maximus
		Circumduction: Move leg in circle.	120–130	Psoas major, gluteus maximus, gluteus medius, adductor magnus

TABLE 29.3 RANGE-OF-MOTION EXERCISES—cont'd

BODY PART	TYPE OF JOINT	TYPE OF MOVEMENT	RANGE (DEGREES)	PRIMARY MUSCLES
Knee	Hinge	Flexion: Bring heel back toward back of thigh.	120–130	Biceps femoris, semitendinosus, semimembranosus, sartorius
		Extension: Return leg to floor.	120–130	Rectus femoris, vastus lateralis, vastus medialis, vastus intermedius
Ankle	Hinge	Dorsal flexion: Move foot so that toes are pointed upward.	20–30	Tibialis anterior
		Plantar flexion: Move foot so that toes are pointed downward.	45–50	Gastrocnemius, soleus
Foot	Gliding	Inversion: Turn sole of foot medially.	35 or less	Tibialis anterior, tibialis posterior
		Eversion: Turn sole of foot laterally.	10 or less	Peroneus longus, peroneus brevis
Toes	Condyloid	Flexion: Curl toes downward.	30–60	Flexor digitorum, lumbricalis pedis, flexor hallucis brevis
		Extension: Straighten toes.	30–60	Extensor digitorum longus, extensor digitorum brevis, extensor hallucis longus
		Abduction: Spread toes apart.	15 or less	Abductor hallucis, interosseus dorsalis
		Adduction: Bring toes together.	15 or less	Adductor hallucis, interosseus plantaris

examine a patient for stiffness, swelling, pain, and limited movement, and compare sides for unequal movement (see Chapter 16). If a patient has restricted ROM, your information will help you collaborate with a physical therapist (PT) to select the type of ROM exercise a patient is able to perform so that you can reduce risk of complications. ROM exercises are active (the patient moves all joints through their ROM unassisted), passive (the patient is unable to move independently, and the nurse moves each joint through its ROM), or somewhere in between. For example, provide support for a weak patient while the patient performs most of the movement. Some patients are able to move some joints actively, whereas the nurse passively moves others. Ligaments, muscles, and the nature of the joint limit patients' mobility, and some joint movements are specific to their location in the body. Abduction and adduction of the arms and legs are an example of this specific type of movement. Abduction is the movement of an extremity away from the midline of the body, and adduction is the movement of an extremity toward the midline of the body.

The major musculoskeletal changes expected during assessment of an immobilized patient include decreased muscle strength, loss of muscle tone and mass, and contractures. Patients with musculoskeletal injuries or chronic conditions require careful palpation of joints and extremities to minimize discomfort. Because immobilized patients are weakened, determine if difficulty in moving joints is the result of fatigue or decreased ROM. Remember that the patient's total musculoskeletal system must be evaluated from the head and neck down to the toes. Any limitation not identified early can result in the patient developing a permanent complication that will impact mobility in the future.

Activity tolerance is the type and amount of exercise or work that a person is able to perform without undue exertion or injury. Many of the patients who have become immobilized may be very limited in their ability to walk. When they are, their heart rate and blood pressure should increase. Assessment of activity tolerance is necessary when planning activities such as ADLs or assisted walking. This assessment includes data from physiological, emotional, and developmental domains (see Chapter 28). This assessment is applicable in all clinical settings.

Observing a patient's posture and alignment while sitting and lying in bed helps to determine the type of assistance the patient requires for safe repositioning (i.e., notice which method the patient uses to push up in bed or if the patient grabs onto objects to steady himself or herself). Aligning patients properly within their own restrictions helps to reduce discomfort and placement of stress on weakened or injured extremities.

As activity is incorporated into the plan of care, monitor patients' tolerance and assess for dyspnea, shortness of breath, fatigue, chest pain, or a change in heart rate or blood pressure. The weak or acutely ill patient is unable to sustain even slight changes in activity because of the increased demand for energy. Seemingly simple tasks such as eating and moving in bed often result in extreme fatigue. When a patient experiences decreased activity tolerance, carefully assess how much time he or she needs to recover. Decreasing recovery time indicates improving activity tolerance.

Patients who are depressed, worried, or anxious are frequently unable to tolerate exercise. Depressed patients tend to withdraw rather than participate. Patients who worry or are frequently anxious expend a tremendous amount of mental energy and often report feeling fatigued. Because of this they also experience physical and emotional exhaustion.

Respiratory System. Perform a respiratory assessment at least every 2 hours for acutely ill patients with restricted activity. Monitor the patient's respiratory rate and oxygen saturation.

Inspect chest wall movements for symmetry, and auscultate the lungs to identify regions of diminished breath sounds (see Chapter 16). Focus auscultation for adventitious lung sounds on the dependent lung fields because pulmonary secretions tend to accumulate in the lower lobes. If a patient has an atelectatic area (an area of collapsed alveoli), breath sounds are asymmetrical. A complete respiratory assessment identifies the presence of secretions and is used to determine appropriate nursing interventions for optimal respiratory function.

Metabolic System. When assessing a patient's metabolic functioning, measure intake and output and review laboratory data to evaluate fluid and electrolyte status (see Chapter 18). Assess the patient's nutritional status to determine the risk for nitrogen imbalance (see Chapter 35). A patient whose mobility is restricted often has a reduced appetite, altered gastrointestinal function, and a reduced capacity to self-feed.

Anorexia commonly occurs in immobilized patients. Assess food intake and the environment for unpleasant odors or noises that interfere with appetite. You can avoid nutritional imbalances if you learn the patient's previous dietary patterns and food preferences early in the immobilization period (see Chapter 35).

In addition to height and weight, anthropometric measurements include mid upper-arm circumference and triceps skinfold measurements. These measures are more commonly assessed by a registered dietitian and used to determine if there is a loss of muscle mass. A decrease in mid upper-arm circumference measured in centimeters or triceps skinfold measured in millimeters indicates a decline in muscle mass. After the initial assessment take this measurement every 2 to 4 weeks, depending on the patient's age, previous physical condition, and amount of immobility.

If an immobilized patient has a wound, the speed of healing indicates how well the body delivers nutrients to the tissues for use (see Chapter 35). The normal progression of wound healing indicates that the metabolic needs of the injured tissues are being met.

Cardiovascular System. Cardiovascular assessment of the immobilized patient includes monitoring blood pressure and heart rate and assessing the arteriovenous system. Because of the risk for orthostatic hypotension, measure blood pressure when a patient moves from lying to a sitting or standing position. These measurements document the patient's tolerance to postural changes and are vital to know when transferring the patient from one position or location to another.

Assess heart rate including the apical pulse. Lying down increases cardiac workload and results in an increased pulse rate. In some patients, particularly older adults, the heart does not tolerate the added workload, and a form of cardiac failure develops. A third heart sound, heard at the apex, is an early indication of congestive heart failure.

Monitoring peripheral pulses allows you to evaluate the ability of the heart to pump blood and the condition of the arterial system. Immediately document and report the absence of a peripheral pulse in the lower extremities to the patient's health care provider, especially if the pulse was present previously. Checking for capillary refill (see Chapter 16) assesses tissue perfusion and arterial function. Also note the color of extremities, as changes in venous and arterial function will alter skin color.

Edema sometimes develops in the extremities of patients who have had a tissue injury or whose heart is unable to handle the increased workload of bed rest. Because edema moves to dependent body regions as a result of gravity, assessment of the immobilized patient includes checking for dependent edema in the sacrum, legs, and feet (see Chapter 16). If the heart is unable to tolerate the increased workload, peripheral body regions such as the hands, feet, nose, and earlobes are colder than central body regions.

Venous thromboembolism (VTE) is a blood clot in the vein. It is related to two life-threatening conditions: DVT is a clot in a deep vein, usually in the leg, and a pulmonary embolus is a deep vein clot that breaks free from a vein wall, travels to the lungs, and blocks some or all of the blood supply (American Heart Association [AHA], 2015). VTE is a hazard of immobility as well as other medical conditions. Venous emboli that travel to the lungs are sometimes life threatening. More than 90% of all pulmonary emboli begin in the deep veins of the lower extremities (Huether and McCance, 2017). To assess the venous system for the presence of a DVT, determine if the patient is experiencing leg pain by gently palpating under the thighs and along the calves. Note any tenderness, and look for redness. Gently palpate for presence of edema. Carefully compare findings in both legs; unilateral redness, tenderness, and edema indicate possible DVT. Also consider the patient's risk factors for a DVT (Box 29.3). The Wells score is an objective and widely used measure for determining a patient's risk for a DVT (Box 29.4) (Wells et al., 1998; Modi et al., 2016). When you identify clinical indicators of a possible DVT, report to a health care provider immediately and include the Wells score as appropriate. If a patient has antiembolic stockings or a sequential compression device (SCD) or mobile compression device (MCD) remove the stockings or device once every 8 hours or according to agency policy and reassess the calves and thighs.

Measure bilateral calf circumference and record it daily as an alternative assessment for DVT. To do this, mark a point on each calf 10 cm down from the midpatella. Measure the circumference each day using this mark for placement of the tape measure. Unilateral increases in calf circumference are an early indication of thrombosis (Lewis et al., 2014). If the patient has a history of DVT, measurement of the thighs should also be conducted daily because the upper thigh is a common site for clot formation. Many hospitals now order Doppler ultrasound scans to assess blood flow in arteries and veins to detect presence of clots. There is a high prevalence of asymptomatic DVTs especially among elderly patients.

Skin Integrity. Continually assess the skin for signs of pressure injury formation especially over bony prominences.

BOX 29.3 RISK FACTORS FOR DEVELOPING DEEP VEIN THROMBOSIS

- Surgery
- Trauma
- Long periods of not moving (bed rest, sitting, long car or airplane trips)
- Cancer and cancer therapy
- Past history of deep vein thrombosis
- Increasing age
- Pregnancy and postpartum period 4–6 weeks after giving birth
- Use of birth control methods that contain estrogen or hormone therapy for menopause symptoms
- Certain illnesses including heart failure, inflammatory bowel disease, and some kidney disorders
- Hypertension
- Hyperlipidemia
- Nephrotic syndrome
- Autoimmune disease including systemic lupus erythematosus
- Obesity
- Smoking
- Varicose veins
- Having a tube in a main vein (sometimes needed to give medications over a period of time)
- Having thrombophilia, one of several diseases in which the blood does not clot correctly

From Geerts WH, et al: Prevention of venous thromboembolism: The Seventh ACCP Conference on Antithrombotic and Thrombolytic Therapy, *Chest* 126(suppl):338S, 2004.

BOX 29.4 WELLS SCORE

PARAMETER	SCORE
Active cancer (patient receiving treatment for cancer within previous 6 months or currently receiving palliative treatment)	1
Paralysis, paresis, or recent plaster immobilization of lower extremities	1
Recently bedridden for 3 days or more or major surgery within previous 12 weeks requiring general or regional anesthesia	1
Localized tenderness along distribution of deep vein system	1
Entire leg swollen	1
Calf swelling at least 3 cm more compared with asymptomatic leg	1
Pitting edema localized to symptomatic leg	1
Collateral superficial veins	1
Previously documented deep vein thrombosis (DVT)	1
Alternative diagnosis as likely or greater than that of DVT	2
Wells scoring system for DVT: −2 to 0, low probability; 1 to 2 points, moderate probability; 3 to 8 points, high probability.	

From Modi S, et al: Wells criteria for DVT is a reliable clinical tool to assess the risk of deep venous thrombosis in trauma patients, *World J Emerg Surg* 11:24, 2016.

Inspect for redness, tenderness, edema, and actual skin breakdown. If you find an area of redness, check for blanching (see Chapter 38). Nonblanchable redness (hyperemia) is an early indicator of impaired skin integrity, but damage to underlying tissue is sometimes more progressive. *All* immobilized patients are at high risk for developing pressure injuries, regardless of age. Use of valid, objective scales such as the Braden Scale or the Gosnell Scale determines a patient's risk for pressure injury formation. The type of risks then directs the interventions most appropriate to prevent or treat ulcers and an objective measure for increasing risk.

Elimination Systems. Assess a patient's elimination status each shift and the total intake and output every 24 hours (see Chapter 18). Inadequate intake and output or fluid and electrolyte imbalances increase the risk for renal system impairment, ranging from recurrent infections to kidney failure. Dehydration also increases the risk for skin breakdown, thrombus formation, respiratory infections, and constipation.

Assessment of elimination also includes auscultation for bowel sounds, the frequency and consistency of bowel movements, and the patient's typical urine and bowel elimination patterns (see Chapter 37). Accurate assessment and identification of patient problems enable you to intervene before constipation leads to fecal impaction and urinary incontinence develops.

Pain. Pain is a common factor in many conditions that cause immobility such as trauma, postoperative restrictions, and musculoskeletal conditions. Carefully assess the character of a patient's pain (see Chapter 34). Use a pain scale that is appropriate to a patient's developmental level to assess pain severity. When you notice a change in a patient's activity level, a more thorough assessment of pain may be necessary. You compare a patient's baseline level of pain with the level of pain following interventions such as repositioning to determine your success in minimizing patient discomfort.

Psychosocial Condition. Changes in psychosocial status usually occur slowly. Observe for changes in emotional status (e.g., depression) and behavioral changes. Common reactions to immobilization when a patient is on bed rest include boredom and feelings of isolation, depression, and anger. Listen carefully to family if they report emotional changes. Examples of change that indicate psychosocial concerns are a cooperative patient who becomes less cooperative or an independent patient who asks for more help than is necessary. Continual communication with family members is vital because they can identify and report changes in a patient's personality.

Assess patients' readiness to improve their level of independence. Be prepared to adapt teaching and motivational strategies to meet their expectations and needs.

Identify and correct any changes in a patient's sleep-wake cycle such as difficulty falling asleep or frequent awakenings (see Chapter 33). Many sleep disruptions are preventable with an assessment of prior sleep habits and early intervention when you suspect problems. Consider instituting a "quiet-time" rule to promote rest. Nurses can prevent or minimize most stimuli that interrupt the sleep-wake cycle (e.g., nursing activities, a noisy environment, or discomfort). Some medications such as analgesics, sleeping pills, or cardiovascular drugs also cause sleep disturbances.

Observe for changes in the use of normal coping mechanisms to adapt to immobilization. Decreasing coping ability causes patients to become disoriented, confused, or depressed. Identifying how a patient usually copes with loss is vital (see Chapter 27). Change in a person's mobility status, whether permanent or temporary, produces a grief reaction.

Development. Include developmental considerations in an assessment. Assess a young child's developmental stage before immobilization and then after immobilization to determine whether the child has been meeting developmental tasks and is progressing normally. The parents will often need to provide this information. Developmental delays or regression occur with prolonged bed rest. Reassure parents that these developmental changes are usually temporary.

Immobilization of a family member changes the family's functioning. The family's response to this change often leads to role changes, stress, and anxieties. Children seeing parents who are immobile sometimes have difficulty understanding what is happening and have difficulty coping. A decline in developmental functioning of a patient of any age needs prompt investigation to determine why the change occurred and interventions that can return the patient to an optimal level of functioning as soon as possible (see Chapter 23).

Fall Risks. Patients of all ages are at risk for falling. In the acute care setting, patients recovering after periods of immobilization have a high risk for falling especially their first time out of bed. Complete any fall risk assessment tool by using a valid instrument provided by your health care agency (e.g., Hendrich II Fall Risk Model) not only at the time of admission but also when you believe the patient's risk has changed (see agency policy) (Touhy and Jett, 2014). Know what the level of a patient's mobility was before immobilization and consider whether the reason for immobility likely affects the patient's gait, posture, strength, or balance. A patient who becomes unable to perform a timed get up and go test is a fall risk (see Chapter 30). Assessment for fall risks also includes a patient's home and community to identify factors that are risks to the patient's mobility and safety regardless of the individual's age.

Older Adult Considerations. Immobility significantly affects an older adult's level of health, independence, and functional status (Box 29.5). Your assessment enables you to determine his or her ability to meet needs independently and adapt to developmental changes such as declining physical functioning and altered family and peer relationships. As a person grows older, activity tolerance changes. Muscle mass is reduced, and posture and the composition of bones change.

BOX 29.5   CARE OF THE OLDER ADULT

Improving Overall Well-Being for Older Adults via Exercise and Physical Activity

Research has indicated that physical activity and exercise have many benefits when started early in life. However, it has been shown that when older adults including older adults with chronic conditions participate in aerobic and resistance exercise training, they benefit as well. Therefore include such activities in your plan of care, and encourage older adults to continue them after discharge (Parreira et al., 2014; Chmelo et al., 2015). Chapter 28 provides additional guidelines.

- Older adults including older adults with chronic health conditions and sedentary lifestyles can benefit from aerobic and resistance exercise training (Parreira et al., 2014; Chmelo et al., 2015).
- Guidelines for exercises that can be continued after discharge are available to share with older adults so they can begin an exercise program regardless of their physical limitations.
- Including aerobic and resistance exercise training in the older adult's daily routine helps to reduce the occurrence of depression and improve and/or maintain cognitive functioning.

There are often changes in the cardiorespiratory system such as decreased maximum heart rate and decreased lung compliance that affect the intensity of exercise. As age progresses some older individuals still exercise but do so at a reduced intensity. The more inactive a patient is, the more pronounced are these activity changes.

Abrupt changes in an older adult's personality often have a physiological cause such as surgery, a medication reaction, a pulmonary embolus, or an acute infection. For example, compromised older patients have confusion as their primary symptom with an acute UTI or fever. Identifying confusion is an important component of your assessment. Acute confusion in older adults is not normal, and a thorough nursing assessment is the priority.

Patient Expectations. In assessing a patient's expectations concerning how long immobility might last and the care he or she is to receive, you determine your patient's perception of what is normal or acceptable in regard to mobility. For example, if movement is more painful or tiresome than anticipated, a patient may be less willing to adhere and commit to desired interventions. If the patient has pain associated with the condition causing immobility, determine what level of pain (on a scale of 0 to 10) he or she is willing to tolerate (Box 29.6). Patients expect their pain to be managed and only they can tell you if expectations are met.

Some patients are content with their present mobility and do not perceive a need for improvement. In contrast, a patient who is active normally may expect to be able to engage in exercise or activity that is not yet realistic for his or her condition. Unless there is a real threat to health maintenance,

BOX 29.6 EVIDENCE-BASED PRACTICE

PICO Question: Does the reliability of assessment of older adults' pain improve with use of pain scales compared with relying solely on self-reported pain for hospitalized older patients?

SUMMARY OF EVIDENCE

Studies have shown that pain is a common occurrence with older adults and that it is commonly undertreated. The reasons for this include the belief that pain is just a normal part of aging, misconceptions about addiction to pain medications, and a lack of routine pain assessment of older adults (Guo et al., 2015). Persistent pain has been associated with functional impairments, falls, slow rehabilitation, depression, anxiety, decreased socialization, and increased health costs. Thus management of pain in older adults must be achieved (Stewart, 2014). Three tools have been found to be highly effective when used to assess pain in older adult patients: the Numeric Rating Scale, the Verbal Descriptor Scale, and the Faces Pain Scale–Revised. All three were used in community and acute and long-term care settings and could be used with cognitively impaired older adults (Pasero and McCaffery, 2011; Whittemore and Sauda, 2015). By using these scales consistently, pain in hospitalized older adults can be assessed properly and managed effectively (Guo et al., 2015). Once pain is effectively managed, a patient's ability and willingness to become mobile and active often increases, and the risk for falling is reduced.

APPLICATION TO NURSING PRACTICE

- Assess for pain as frequently as you assess the other vital signs.
- Evaluate the management of the pain control; if inadequate, advocate for another intervention (e.g., another medication or dose) (Stewart, 2014).
- Evaluate the pain-management regimen in relation to patient activities such as physical therapy and ambulation, and modify pain interventions to increase patient comfort during activity.
- Use one of the three pain scales to assess your patient's level of pain, even if the patient also has cognitive impairments (Pasero and McCaffery, 2011; Whittemore and Sauda, 2015).
- Use the same scale consistently for the most effective management of the patient's pain (Guo et al., 2015).

Mobility and *Risk for Disuse Syndrome.* The diagnosis of *Impaired Physical Mobility* applies to the patient who has limitation in independent, purposeful physical movement of the body or of one or more extremities (Herdman and Kamitsuru, 2014) but is not completely immobile. The diagnosis of *Risk for Disuse Syndrome* applies to the patient who is immobile and at risk for multisystem problems because of prescribed or unavoidable musculoskeletal inactivity (Herdman and Kamitsuru, 2014). Beyond these diagnoses, the list of potential diagnoses is extensive because immobility affects multiple body systems. For example, an immobilized or partially immobilized patient can have one or more of the following nursing diagnoses:

- *Ineffective Airway Clearance*
- *Risk for Constipation*
- *Risk for Disuse Syndrome*
- *Risk for Falls*
- *Impaired Bed Mobility*
- *Impaired Physical Mobility*
- *Impaired Sitting*
- *Risk for Impaired Skin Integrity*

The list of potential nursing diagnoses related to immobility is more extensive when alterations in physical, psychosocial, or developmental functioning occur. Often these problems are interrelated, and it is imperative that nursing care focus on all dimensions.

Most often the physiological dimension is the major focus of nursing care for patients with impaired mobility, and the psychosocial and developmental dimensions are neglected. Yet all dimensions are important to health. During immobilization some patients experience decreased social interaction and stimuli. These patients frequently use the call bell to request minor physical attention when their real need is greater socialization. Nursing diagnoses for health needs in developmental areas reflect changes from the patient's normal activities. Immobility may lead to a developmental crisis if the patient is unable to resolve problems.

Selecting appropriate related factors for each problem-focused nursing diagnosis allows you to select the most appropriate interventions. For example, *Impaired Physical Mobility* related to lower extremity weakness versus general fatigue requires different nursing approaches. Individualize nursing diagnoses for selecting patient-centered goals, outcomes, and interventions (Box 29.7).

■■■ PLANNING

Consider each nursing diagnosis to plan for the appropriate therapeutic interventions. Recognize how a patient's multiple nursing diagnoses interact with and affect one another (Fig. 29.3). Often an intervention that you plan will be appropriate for more than one nursing diagnosis. As you plan care synthesize information using critical thinking. Apply appropriate standards. For example, apply skin-care guidelines from the Agency for Healthcare Research and Quality (AHRQ, 2014) and the Wound, Ostomy and Continence Nurses Society (WOCN, 2013) to select interventions

forcing patients to accept perspectives not in accordance with their own beliefs is a breach of standards of care.

■■■ NURSING DIAGNOSIS

Assessment reveals clusters of data that indicate if a patient is at risk or if a mobility problem exists. The clusters of data include pertinent defining characteristics or risk factors that support the nursing diagnoses.

A patient who is experiencing an alteration in mobility often has one or more nursing diagnoses. Two diagnoses directly related to immobilization are *Impaired Physical*

BOX 29.7   SYNTHESIS IN PRACTICE

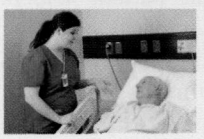

As Abby prepares to assess Mr. Rogers, she reviews the pathophysiology of stroke and the associated hazards of immobility. She gathers knowledge about the effect a stroke can have on physical movement and the expected physical therapy and rehabilitative measures Mr. Rogers will likely undergo. During a previous clinical experience Abby cared for a patient who received a cardiac valve and was given anticoagulant therapy. She knows that a medication that Mr. Rogers is receiving is also an anticoagulant and Mr. Rogers' bleeding times must be monitored very closely. The therapeutic range must be maintained to prevent clots in the deep veins, but he must also be monitored for any overt or covert episodes of bleeding. Movement is important in the prevention of complications anticipated in a patient who has had an ischemic stroke as well as for general well-being. He will also wear antiembolic stockings to prevent venous stasis.

for the prevention of pressure injuries. Because of the effect immobilization has on a patient's deconditioning, adopt protocols for fall prevention (Staggs et al., 2015). Critical thinking ensures that the patient's plan of care integrates all that you know about the individual and key critical thinking elements.

A care plan for an immobilized patient should focus on prevention of physical, psychosocial, and developmental complications. For example, providing for ROM exercises and patient repositioning is a first step in preventing serious complications such as pneumonia or contractures. In addition, routine provision of diversional activities stimulates a patient and may help to reduce depression or a sense of powerlessness. Individualize a plan in which the patient is able to participate as much as possible.

Goals and Outcomes. Patients at risk for hazards of immobility require nursing care plans directed at meeting their actual and potential needs (see Care Plan). It is important to develop patient-centered goals and outcomes aimed at preventing or reducing the complications of immobility, restoring function, and reducing risks associated with immobility such as DVT or constipation. Incorporate goals into the plan that consider the patient's own preferences and level of mobility expected as much as possible. For example, a goal of "patient will achieve normal joint function of right elbow in three weeks" will have accompanying outcomes such as "joint ROM extension of right elbow increases 5 degrees each week" and "patient achieves desired pain control to initiate exercise." Set realistic expectations for care and include the patient's family caregiver when possible. Set goals that are individualized, realistic, and measurable.

A family caregiver who does too much or too little in an attempt to help the patient seriously impedes the patient's progress. Watching a family member walk slowly and with

effort seems cruel, and some family caregivers excessively perform tasks that patients need to learn to do for themselves. Patients often experience immobility for a long time. Develop goals and expected outcomes to help the patient achieve his or her highest level of mobility and ensure progressive improvement over time.

Setting Priorities. The effect that immobilization problems have on a patient's mental and physical health determines the urgency of any problem. Set priorities when planning care to ensure that immediate needs are met first. This is particularly important when patients have multiple diagnoses. For example, relieve a patient's pain first before implementing exercises and mobility activities. Because you can delegate many of the skills associated with care of the immobile patient such as turning, positioning, and applying antiembolic stockings, it is easy to overlook *potential* complications until they occur. It is especially important in priority setting that you do not overlook potential complications such as pressure injuries or disuse syndrome and that you address these complications as part of the care plan. Reinforce prevention strategies in the plan of care. Plan on delegating clearly to nursing assistive personnel the need to carry out activities aimed at preventing complications of immobility.

Collaborative Care. A collaborative approach is especially important when providing care with and for a patient with impaired mobility. PTs are a resource for developing a plan involving treatment techniques that promote the ability to move, reduce pain, restore function, and prevent disability (American Physical Therapy Association [APTA], 2016). They collaborate with nurses to determine the type of ROM or strengthening exercises necessary. An occupational therapist (OT) helps patients improve or maintain skills for day-to-day activities (e.g., dressing, grooming, getting into a car) and well-being (American Occupational Therapy Association [AOTA], 2017). Both a PT and OT can assist home health nurses in assessing the condition of a patient's home to determine how to adapt therapies to help the patient return to a safe environment.

Wound care specialists and respiratory therapists are experts at preventing pressure injuries and respiratory complications, respectively, as they relate to immobility. Proper nutrition is essential for wound healing and prevention of skin breakdown; therefore a registered dietitian contributes significantly to the plan of care, especially if the patient is older or experiencing nutritional difficulties. You may also need to refer the patient to a mental health advanced practice nurse, licensed social worker, or psychologist to assist with coping or psychosocial issues.

Discharge planning begins when a patient first enters the health care system. In anticipation of the patient's discharge from an agency, make appropriate referrals to a case manager or a discharge planner to ensure the patient's needs are met at home. Consider the patient's home environment when planning therapies to maintain or improve mobility and reduce

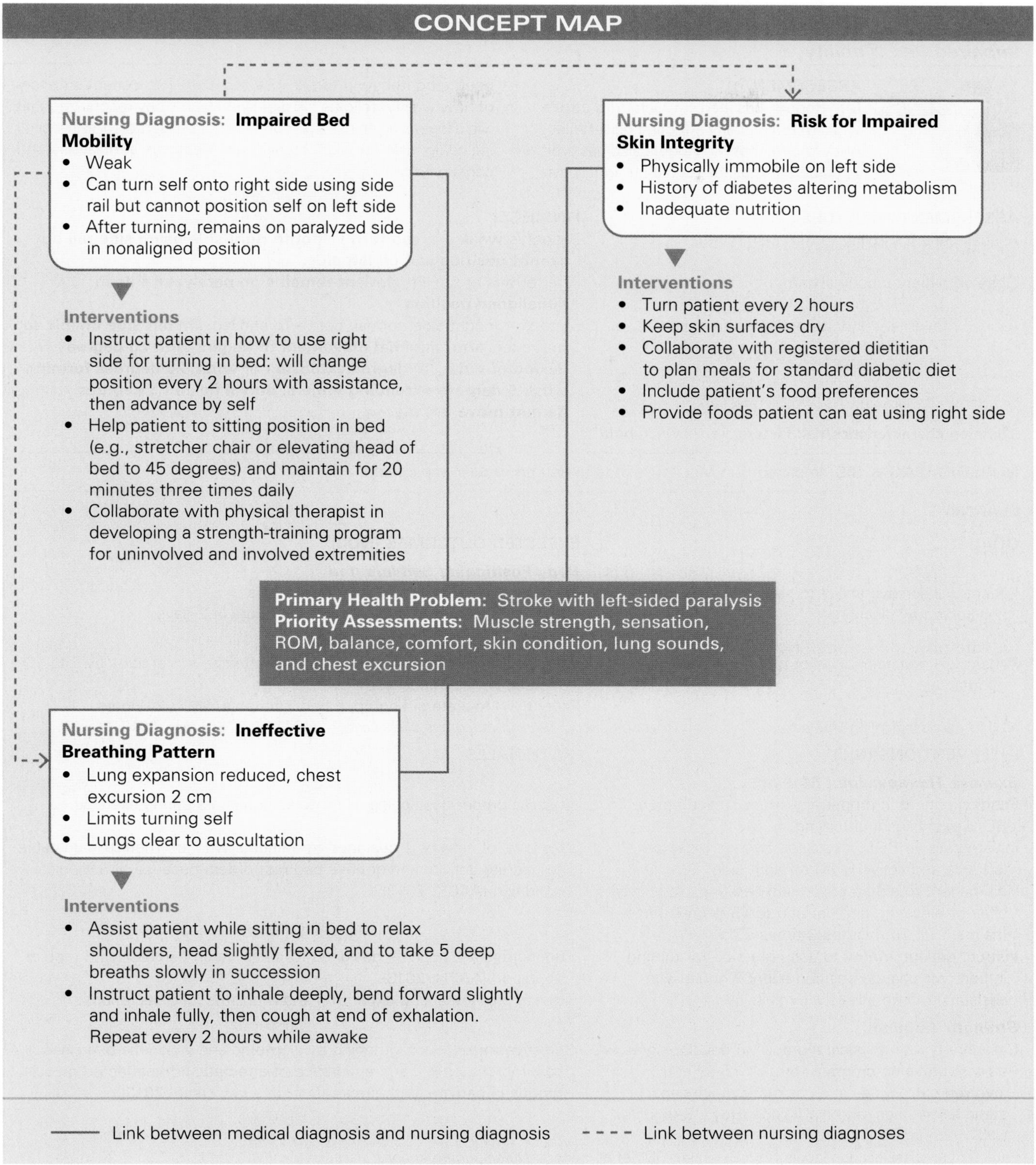

CONCEPT MAP

Nursing Diagnosis: Impaired Bed Mobility
- Weak
- Can turn self onto right side using side rail but cannot position self on left side
- After turning, remains on paralyzed side in nonaligned position

▼

Interventions
- Instruct patient in how to use right side for turning in bed: will change position every 2 hours with assistance, then advance by self
- Help patient to sitting position in bed (e.g., stretcher chair or elevating head of bed to 45 degrees) and maintain for 20 minutes three times daily
- Collaborate with physical therapist in developing a strength-training program for uninvolved and involved extremities

Nursing Diagnosis: Risk for Impaired Skin Integrity
- Physically immobile on left side
- History of diabetes altering metabolism
- Inadequate nutrition

▼

Interventions
- Turn patient every 2 hours
- Keep skin surfaces dry
- Collaborate with registered dietitian to plan meals for standard diabetic diet
- Include patient's food preferences
- Provide foods patient can eat using right side

Primary Health Problem: Stroke with left-sided paralysis
Priority Assessments: Muscle strength, sensation, ROM, balance, comfort, skin condition, lung sounds, and chest excursion

Nursing Diagnosis: Ineffective Breathing Pattern
- Lung expansion reduced, chest excursion 2 cm
- Limits turning self
- Lungs clear to auscultation

▼

Interventions
- Assist patient while sitting in bed to relax shoulders, head slightly flexed, and to take 5 deep breaths slowly in succession
- Instruct patient to inhale deeply, bend forward slightly and inhale fully, then cough at end of exhalation. Repeat every 2 hours while awake

———— Link between medical diagnosis and nursing diagnosis   - - - - Link between nursing diagnoses

FIG 29.3 Concept map.

the risk of falls. Referrals to home care or outpatient therapy are often needed. This should include assessing the patient's mobility within the community (e.g., how the patient with limited mobility will get to and return from the required health care appointments).

■ ■ ■ IMPLEMENTATION

Nursing interventions for the completely or partially immobilized patient focus on health promotion and prevention of complications. Many patients with limited mobility function

◎ CARE PLAN

Impaired Bed Mobility

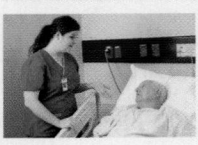

ASSESSMENT

Mr. Rogers has had an ischemic stroke with limited mobility affecting his left side. Abby knows that Mr. Rogers also has type 2 diabetes mellitus, which might have been a contributing factor to the stroke. The patient's history of how well he follows his diet is unclear. Abby recognizes that Mr. Rogers is at risk for complications related to immobility including risk for skin breakdown, reduced ventilation, and constipation.

ASSESSMENT ACTIVITIES	FINDINGS[a]
Assess patient's ability to turn self in bed.	Patient is **weak** and **can turn self onto right side using side rail but cannot position self on left side.**
Observe patient's body alignment.	After efforts at turning, **patient remains on paralyzed side in nonaligned position.**
Assess movement and strength in extremities.	Strength on right side normal, both arm and leg. On **left side unable to move left arm, minimal movement in fingers with 20-degree flexion of wrist, 10-degree extension of wrist, 20 degrees forming a fist, 5 degrees extending fingers, dorsal flexion 5 degrees. Cannot move left leg.**

[a]**Defining characteristics/risk factors** are shown in **bold** type.

NURSING DIAGNOSIS: Impaired Bed Mobility related to neuromuscular impairment

---

PLANNING

GOAL	EXPECTED OUTCOMES (NOC)[b]
	Body Positioning Self-Initiated
Patient will achieve ability to self-initiate positioning by discharge.	Patient will learn how to turn self in 2 days.
	Patient will initiate turning every 2 to 3 hours in 2 days.
	Endurance and Joint Movement
Patient will maintain range of motion (ROM) and endurance.	Patient will maintain or improve ROM in affected extremities by 5 to 10 degrees (wrist, hands, feet) by discharge.
	Patient will tolerate sitting up in bed 3 times a day in 24 hours.

[b]Outcome classification labels from Moorhead S, et al, editors: *Nursing outcomes classification (NOC)*, ed 5, St Louis, 2013, Mosby.

INTERVENTIONS (NIC)[c]	RATIONALES
Exercise Therapy: Joint Mobility	
Position patient in proper alignment supine before ROM exercises and turning.	Ensures proper positioning of muscles and joints during exercise.
Initiate passive ROM exercises 3 times a day on left side and active ROM on right side.	This level of activity is designed for patients who are medically unstable to tolerate activity and/or have bed rest orders because of a medical condition (AACN, 2013).
Help patient to sitting position in bed (e.g., stretcher chair or elevating head of bed to 45 degrees) and maintain for 20 minutes 3 times a day.	
Instruct patient in how to use right side for turning in bed; will change position every 2 hours with assistance, then advance by self.	Turning every 2 hours is designed for patients on bed rest with medical condition (AACN, 2013).
	Turning promotes lung expansion and mobilizes lung secretions.
Strength Training	
Collaborate with physical therapist in developing a strength training program for uninvolved and involved extremities such as static quadriceps, static hamstrings, and hip flexion (Royal Berkshire NHS Foundation Trust, 2016).	Selective muscle strengthening by isometric and isokinetic exercises can improve power and endurance of affected and unaffected muscle groups in patients with stroke (Dobkin and Dorsch, 2013).

[c]Intervention classification labels from Bulechek GM, et al, editors: *Nursing interventions classification (NIC)*, ed 6, St Louis, 2013, Mosby.

CARE PLAN—cont'd

Impaired Bed Mobility

EVALUATION

NURSING ACTIONS	PATIENT RESPONSE/FINDING	ACHIEVEMENT OF OUTCOME
Measure Mr. Rogers' ROM of extremities on left side.	ROM of extremities on right side remain within normal limits. Left side flexion and extension of wrists improved by 10 degrees. Able to close fist to 45 degrees. Dorsiflexion improved by 5 degrees.	ROM is maintained on unaffected side and improving on left side.
Observe patient's ability to self-initiate turning.	Patient able to use side rail to pull and turn toward left side; requires assistance with alignment. Has been able to move hips to turn toward right side and raise right shoulder. Needs assistance.	Improving self-initiated turning from supine to side lying, but requires assistance.

QSEN ACTIVITY Teamwork and Collaboration

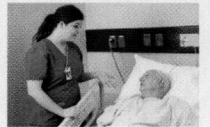

Abby is meeting with the physical therapist to discuss Mr. Rogers' case so that the therapist can provide the appropriate level of quality care.

• What information has Abby learned in caring for Mr. Rogers that would be valuable to communicate to the therapist in planning appropriate therapies?

evolve — Answers to QSEN Activities can be found on the Evolve website.

BOX 29.8 PATIENT TEACHING

Fall Prevention

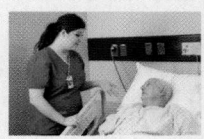

Mr. Rogers lives alone with family living nearby. The daughter plans to have her father stay with her family until he is able to regain the strength needed to walk more safely in the home. Abby examined the evidence-based research on risks of falls in older adults in a community setting (Goodwin et al., 2014; Touhy and Jett, 2014). Therefore she decided to teach Mr. Rogers and his family how to prepare the daughter's and patient's home to prevent risks of falls.

OUTCOME

At the end of the teaching session, Mr. Rogers and his daughter will list three fall preventive measures to take in preparation for discharge to home.

TEACHING STRATEGIES

• Plan a teaching session at a time when the patient is rested, there is reduced noise in the environment, and his family is in attendance.
• Recommend use of a fall safety checklist in the home focusing on rooms the patient will primarily use (e.g., bedroom, bathroom, and family room).
• Reinforce with the patient and family exercises recommended by the physical therapist.
• Develop a continence management program with fluids and adequate fruits and vegetables.
• Instruct the daughter on what steps to take if her father falls in the home (see Chapter 30).

EVALUATION

• Plan home visit to observe patient performing exercises.
• Use the principles of teach-back to evaluate patient/family caregiver learning:
  • "Tell me three ways you can make the home safer when you will be walking."
  • "Tell me what would be the plan of action if your father should fall."

---

are in home or assisted-living settings; thus they require active intervention to prevent complications that might necessitate hospitalization. Specific interventions in the acute care setting focus on reducing severity of complications that have developed (e.g., by positioning and transferring patients correctly). Direct restorative and continuing care interventions to regain and maximize functional mobility and independence.

Health Promotion. When patients have some level of mobility, health promotion activities aim to keep individuals mobile as much as possible and to prevent falls (see Chapter 30). For patients who have mobility alterations and require assistance with activity, researchers have established a series of algorithms to be used to lift and transfer patients safely, preventing injury to the health care provider and the patient (see Chapter 28) (VISN8, 2014).

Fall prevention measures are implemented in the home and health care setting when a patient is identified to be at risk for falls (Box 29.8). Multiple variables have been investigated to assist in determining how to decrease the risk for falls in acute care settings through implementation of evidence-based fall prevention activities (Titler et al., 2016). Implementation of the Targeted Risk Factor Fall Prevention Bundle including scheduled rounding, keeping essential items within reach, and familiarizing a patient with his or her surroundings resulted in a reduction of falls that was statistically insignificant; however, the severity of the injuries from the falls was decreased from major and moderate to minor (Titler et al., 2016).

Structured exercise programs for immobile patients improve their endurance, strength, overall health, and feelings of well-being. Chapter 28 presents in greater detail the importance of exercise and activity for general well-being. Older patients need special consideration. Deconditioning and disuse along with disease conditions account for much of the functional decline in older adults. However, this is not a developmental norm of aging. By incorporating exercise into an older patient's care plan and collaborating with a PT, it is possible to prevent disuse syndrome for these patients.

Respiratory System.   Interventions aim to promote expansion of the chest and lungs and prevent stasis of pulmonary secretions. Regular exercise and activities such as changing the position of patients at least every 2 hours allow the dependent lung regions to reexpand, maintain the elastic recoil property of the lungs, and clear the dependent lung regions of pulmonary secretions (see Chapter 32). Your assessment findings determine areas of the lungs affected and if patients need more frequent exercising and position changes. Stagnant secretions accumulating in the bronchi and lungs of the immobilized patient lead to the growth of bacteria and subsequent development of pneumonia. Changing the patient's position reduces stagnation of secretions, rotates the dependent lung, and mobilizes secretions.

Make sure that the immobile patient has a fluid intake of at least 2000 mL per day, if not contraindicated, to help keep mucociliary clearance intact. In patients free from infection and with adequate hydration, pulmonary secretions appear thin, watery, and clear. It is easy for the patient to remove these secretions with coughing. Without adequate hydration secretions become thick, tenacious, and difficult to remove. One method for removing pulmonary secretions is chest physiotherapy (CPT). The use of this technique drains secretions from specific segments of the bronchi and lungs into the trachea and helps the patient expel the secretions by coughing (see Chapter 32). Combine coughing with deep-breathing exercises and have the patient do these on a regular schedule.

Metabolic System. Adequate nutrition is essential to prevent tissue breakdown for patients of any age who are immobile. Therefore the plan of care must be designed to incorporate enough carbohydrates, proteins, and fats to combat the effects of immobility. Carbohydrates meet energy requirements; proteins are necessary for tissue repair and to counter negative nitrogen balance. Fats prevent further breakdown of nutritional stores. Determine the patient's specific caloric and diet prescription from the nutritional assessment. Collaborate with the registered dietitian for any dietary restrictions related to other medical conditions or for patients not consuming the necessary nutrients. The nutritional deficit results in complications such as pressure injuries, which could be fatal for the older patient (see Chapter 35).

Cardiovascular System. Interventions designed to promote a healthy cardiovascular system involve approaches for minimizing and preventing venous thrombus formation. Patients with preexisting cardiovascular conditions and patients who have undergone certain types of surgery will require **thromboprophylaxis**, the prevention of thromboembolic disease, in the home setting. Adherence to prescribed anticoagulants, proper positioning, and safe use of anti-embolic stockings help reduce thrombus formation. Every patient and family caregiver must understand the patient's specific risk for development of VTE (Skinner and Moran, 2007). Because DVTs can be clinically silent and present no symptoms at all, home health nurses must conduct ongoing assessments of the vascular system of patients. Because there are DVTs that present classic symptoms of the disease, it is important for patients and family caregivers to know the signs and symptoms.

When patients take anticoagulants at home, provide appropriate patient education. Patients must understand their risk for bleeding. If patients take anticoagulants such as enoxaparin, which is administered subcutaneously, the continuing care plan may include services offered by an outpatient anticoagulation clinic; coordination of care facilitated by the attending physician's office; or the administration of therapy in the home by a home health nurse, the patient, or the patient's support system (Skinner and Moran, 2007).

Patients at risk for DVT should maintain adequate hydration by drinking water or juice and avoiding alcoholic beverages. Patients benefit from long-term lifestyle modifications including smoking cessation, achieving a body mass index that is 25 kg/m^2, maintaining a normal blood pressure, achieving glycemic control, and managing lipid levels (Skinner and Moran, 2007). When patients who take anticoagulants plan to travel long distances, review the following recommended guidelines: avoid flights of more than 6 hours' duration, avoid wearing constrictive clothing around the lower extremities or waist, avoid dehydration, and perform frequent calf muscle stretching. Patients who travel should also be instructed to carry their medications with them (do not store in baggage) and never double doses because of a missed dose (AHA, 2016).

It is also important to teach patients to avoid crossing the legs, sitting for prolonged periods of time, wearing tight clothing that constricts the legs or waist, putting pillows under the knees, and massaging the legs. All of these factors can reduce circulation to the extremities. ROM exercises reduce the risk for contractures and help to prevent thrombi (see Table 29.3). Activity contracts the skeletal muscles, which exerts pressure on the veins to promote venous return and thus reduce venous stasis. Specific exercises that help prevent thrombophlebitis are ankle pumps, foot circles, hip rotation, and knee flexion. Ankle pumps, sometimes called *calf pumps,* include alternating **plantar flexion** and dorsiflexion. Foot circles require the patient to rotate the ankle. While the patient is supine (lying on back) or sitting, he or she rotates the hip joint by rotating the entire leg and pointing the toes inward and outward. Knee flexion involves alternately extending and flexing the knee. These exercises are usually done each hour while awake and are aimed at preventing thrombi; they are sometimes called *antiembolic exercises.*

Musculoskeletal System. The immobilized or partially immobilized patient needs exercise to prevent excessive muscle atrophy, decreased endurance, and joint contractures. The amount of activity required to prevent physical disuse syndromes is 2 hours in a 24-hour period; therefore schedule exercise regularly throughout the day based on individual patient needs and tolerance.

If a patient is unable to move any part or all of the body, teach family caregivers how to perform passive ROM exercises for all immobilized joints at least 3 or 4 times a day unless contraindicated. If one extremity is paralyzed, teach the patient to perform passive ROM on the paralyzed limb and encourage him or her to engage in active ROM with all other extremities (see Table 29.3). Encourage patients to use mobile extremities during ADLs (e.g., dressing) as much as possible. The bath is an excellent time to perform ROM.

The best nursing intervention is establishing an individualized progressive exercise program. A progressive exercise program gradually increases the patient's physical activity to reverse the deconditioning associated with immobility (see Chapter 28). Depending on the setting and resources available, collaborate with physical therapy for the exercise program.

Skin Integrity. The major risk to the skin from restricted mobility is the formation of pressure injuries. Early identification of high-risk patients (e.g., wheelchair-bound patients, patients with stroke) helps to prevent them. Interventions aimed at prevention are positioning, skin care, and use of pressure-relief devices (see Chapter 38). Family caregivers and patients must know the importance of changing position routinely if a patient is confined to a bed or wheelchair. The patient's ability and need to reposition will depend on his or her activity level, perceptual ability, status of peripheral circulation, and daily routines. For example, a person in a wheelchair learns to move the buttocks and hips up and off of the wheelchair seat every 15 to 20 minutes. Although turning patients confined to bed is essential, it is sometimes necessary to use pressure relief devices for relieving pressure (see Chapter 38). Normally the time that a mobile patient sits uninterrupted in a chair is 1 hour or less, but this time interval must be individualized. Uninterrupted pressure causes skin breakdown. Teach chair-bound patients who are able to move to shift their weight every 15 to 20 minutes, and provide a pressure-reducing device for the chair (AHRQ, 2014).

Elimination System. Health promotion interventions for maintaining optimal urinary functioning are to keep the patient well hydrated without causing bladder distention and the reflux of urine into the ureters and renal pelvis. This helps to prevent renal calculi and UTIs. Timely toileting prevents bladder distention. Educate patients and family caregivers about making sure that the patient's urine is light yellow and comparable in amount to the fluid intake by monitoring total fluid intake and output each day in the home.

A patient who continually dribbles urine and whose bladder is distended likely has reflex incontinence. If the immobilized patient does not have voluntary control of bladder elimination, bladder retraining is necessary. Teaching patients how to perform Kegel exercises is effective (see Chapter 36). Patients with stroke and with paralysis may require insertion of a straight or indwelling Foley catheter

(see Chapter 36) if the patient experiences ongoing bladder distention. Educate patients and family caregivers on how to perform these procedures and take measures to reduce UTIs.

Have patients and family caregivers keep a record of the frequency and consistency of bowel movements. A diet rich in fruits and vegetables helps to facilitate normal peristalsis. Insoluble fiber is necessary to facilitate both the passage of stool and adequate water intake. Patients should drink at least 6 to 8 glasses of water daily, unless contraindicated, to help promote bowel elimination. If a patient is unable to maintain normal bowel patterns, initiate a bowel-training program (e.g., stool softeners, cathartics, or enemas) (see Chapter 37).

Psychosocial Problems. Health promotion for the immobilized patient requires anticipation of changes in psychosocial status and intervention with preventive measures. Encourage patients to participate in routine and informal socialization. Encourage visits to the home by friends. Help family caregivers learn the importance of keeping patients involved in decisions about their care and engaging them in conversation and self-help activities. Plan activities to give patients in health care settings the opportunity to interact with the staff. If possible, place these patients in a room with other mobile patients. If the patient remains in a private room, ask staff members to visit periodically throughout waking hours. Provide stimuli to maintain orientation and entertain the patient.

Encourage patients to wear their glasses or dentures and to shave or apply makeup. These are normal activities to enhance body image. Encourage patients to perform as much self-care as possible. Make sure that hygiene and grooming articles are within easy reach.

Developmental Changes. Plan care to stimulate a patient, especially a young child, mentally and physically. Incorporate play activities within a patient's mobility restrictions into the nursing care plan. For example, puzzles help patients develop fine-motor skills. Health promotion for older adults requires matching mobility needs with the patient's developmental limitations. Older adults benefit when exercise routines are mildly progressive. Walking, aquatic exercise, swimming, and gardening are good ways to promote ROM and endurance.

Acute Care. Patients in acute care settings demonstrate more rapid and pronounced complications of immobility because of the presence of multisystem involvement. In these patients design nursing interventions to reduce the impact of immobility on body systems and prepare the patient for restorative and continuing care. Use interventions combined with those outlined in the health promotion section to return the patient to an optimal level of function.

Respiratory System. A patient with more serious mobility limitations requires aggressive pulmonary hygiene (see Chapter 32). Encourage patients to sit up in bed routinely and to cough and deep breathe every 1 to 2 hours while awake to expand all lobes of the lungs and prevent atelectasis. Coughing reduces the stasis of pulmonary secretions. Some immobile patients, particularly after surgery, need to use an incentive spirometer to aid in deep breathing.

Postoperative patients who have undergone general anesthesia especially need to cough and deep breathe to prevent atelectasis and stasis of secretions. Timely pain management for incision discomfort is essential. Patients cough more effectively when their pain is under control. If a patient becomes drowsy from medication, actively reinforce coughing and deep breathing. Encouraging early ambulation (see Chapter 28) helps prevent multiple pulmonary complications.

Immobilized patients and patients on bed rest are generally weakened. The cough reflex gradually becomes inefficient as the weakness progresses. If a critically ill patient is too weak or unable to cough up secretions, maintain the patient's airway by using suctioning techniques (see Chapter 32). This usually involves oral or nasotracheal suctioning and suctioning of artificial airways. Suspect hypostatic bronchopneumonia if the patient develops a productive cough with greenish yellow sputum, fever, and pain on breathing.

Cardiovascular System. After prolonged bed rest (or long period of not moving), patients become deconditioned and usually have an increased heart rate, a decrease in pulse pressure, and a drop in blood pressure with an increase in fainting when rising to a sitting or standing position (Lewis et al., 2014). Attempt to have patients move as soon as their physical condition allows, even if this involves only sitting up in bed, dangling feet at the bedside, or moving to a chair (see Chapter 28). This activity maintains muscle tone and increases venous return. Isometric exercises (i.e., activities that involve muscle tension without muscle shortening) do not have any beneficial effect on preventing orthostatic hypotension, but they improve activity tolerance (see Chapter 28).

Chapter 28 provides details on the techniques for transferring patients from bed to chair. When transferring a patient from a supine position into a chair, move the patient gradually. First obtain a baseline blood pressure and pulse with the patient in the supine position. Then raise the patient to a high-Fowler's position and measure blood pressure and pulse again to detect decreases in blood pressure or elevations in pulse. Leave the patient in this position for 2 minutes to allow the body to adapt. Monitor the patient for dizziness or light-headedness. The patient is now ready to sit at the side of the bed with the feet on the floor. If there is no dizziness, help the patient to a chair. When transferring an immobile patient for the first time, make sure to use the appropriate safe patient handling and movement algorithm (Fig. 29.4) (VISN8, 2014).

It is also important to direct nursing interventions at reducing cardiac workload. When a patient moves up in bed or strains on defecation, a Valsalva maneuver occurs. During a Valsalva maneuver a patient holds his or her breath and strains, increasing intrathoracic pressure, which decreases venous return and cardiac output. When the strain is released, venous return and cardiac output immediately increase, and systolic blood pressure and pulse pressure rise. These pressure changes produce a reflex bradycardia that can be associated with sudden cardiac death, particularly in patients with heart disease. Teach the patient to breathe out while moving or being lifted up in bed to avoid straining.

Because a DVT is a hazard of immobility, interventions that reduce the risk for thrombus formation in the immobilized patient such as leg exercises, encouraging fluids, wearing compression devices, and position changes must be incorporated into the plan of care. Instruct preoperative patients in leg exercises before their surgery (see Chapter 40). Interventions such as antiembolic elastic stockings and SCDs/MCDs require a health care provider's order and are often found as part of routine postoperative protocols.

Elastic stockings help to maintain pressure on the muscles of the lower extremities and therefore promote venous return. Make sure to measure the patient's lower extremities correctly to ensure proper fit and apply the stockings properly (Box 29.9). Remove and reapply stockings at least every 8 hours or according to agency policy. Improper application of stockings can reduce circulation in the lower extremities. Always observe the status of circulation to the extremities (see Chapter 16), and be sure stockings do not roll down the leg. Patients are usually discharged home with these stockings. Be sure that patients learn how to apply them correctly and how to observe the status of circulation to the extremities. Instruct patients on the signs of allergic reactions, thrombophlebitis, or skin irritation so they can report changes to their health care provider.

SCDs consist of inflatable plastic sleeves wrapped around the legs and secured with Velcro. The tubing that inflates the sleeves extends from the sleeve at the patient's ankles. The sleeves are connected to an air pump that alternately inflates and deflates, providing rhythmic, external extremity compression (see Box 29.9). The pump is mounted on the end of a patient's bed. Use of SCDs on the legs decreases venous stasis by increasing venous return. Studies have shown that the use of compression devices along with pharmacotherapy helps prevent thromboembolic disease (Colwell et al., 2010; Colwell, 2011; Nam et al., 2015). Postoperative patients are encouraged to ambulate even when SCD therapy is in use. However, you must remove SCDs for ambulation, as they often are associated with patient falls when left on.

MCDs act physiologically in much the same manner as SCDs. In addition MCDs such as the ActiveCare+S.F.T. have a synchronized flow technology that uses an internal sensor to apply pressure around the legs in sync with respiratory-related changes in venous phasic flow to optimize peak venous velocity at lower applied pressures (United Health Care [UHC], 2012). The disposable, inflatable compression sleeves wrap around the lower legs and fasten with Velcro (Topfer, 2016). The sleeves connect to a lightweight pump. MCDs have an advantage over SCDs that have cords extending from the patient's ankles and cannot be worn during ambulation. An MCD cord extends from the lower leg upward and connects to a controller unit that can be worn on a shoulder strap during ambulation (Topfer, 2016). Patients are able to wear the device safely during ambulation. MCDs are designed to increase inpatient compliance with ambulation during hospitalization (UHC, 2012). MCDs have been shown to be more comfortable and easier to wear than SCDs. Certain models of MCDs can detect if the sleeves are being worn and records the number of hours of utilization. Patients often remove

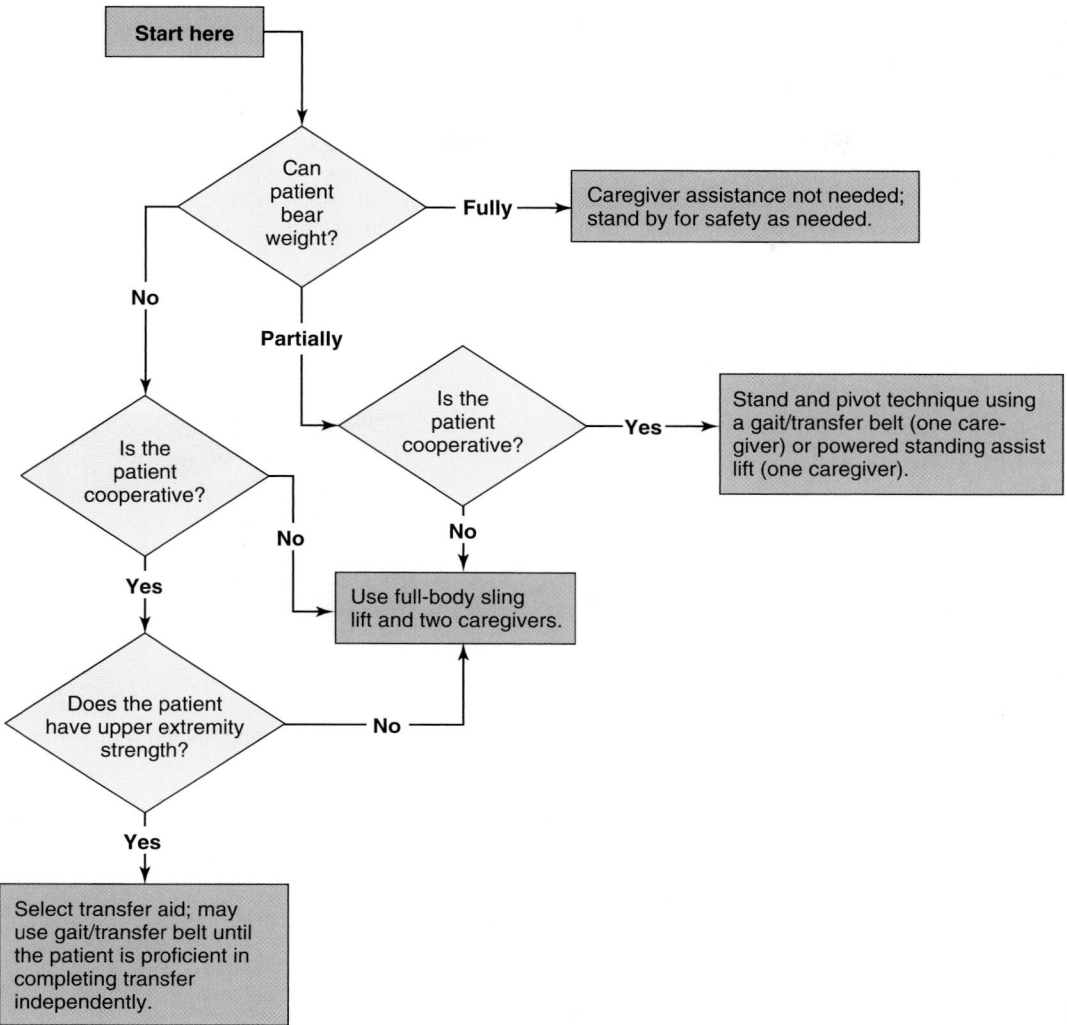

FIG 29.4 Algorithm used to transfer patient to and from bed to chair, chair to toilet, chair to chair, or car to chair. (From VISN8 Patient Safety Center [VISN8]: *Safe patient handling and movement algorithms,* 2014. https://cseany.org/wp-content/uploads/2014/02/SPHMALGORITHMS.PDF.)

SCDs or MCDs because of discomfort, warmth around the legs, local rash, or noise from the inflation machine (Colwell et al., 2010); it is important to encourage patient adherence when compression devices are in place.

Immobilized patients are frequently on thromboprophylactic (preventive) low-dose heparin therapy to minimize the risk for VTE. Heparin is an anticoagulant that suppresses clot formation. This therapy requires a health care provider's order. Low-molecular-weight (LMW) heparins such as ardeparin and enoxaparin are prescribed in place of older forms of unfractionated heparin. LMW heparins have a more predictable anticoagulant effect. The drugs are given subcutaneously, usually every 12 hours until the risk for DVT declines. LMW heparin compared with unfractionated heparin reduces the occurrence of major hemorrhage as a side effect (Lewis et al., 2014). Local irritation such as erythema, hematoma, and urticaria at injection sites is common. However, it is still wise to monitor the patient for signs of bleeding (e.g., increased bruising, guaiac-positive stools, bleeding gums). Report any occurrence of hemorrhage immediately.

BOX 29.9 PROCEDURAL GUIDELINES

View Video!

Applying Antiembolic Compression Stockings and Compression Devices

DELEGATION CONSIDERATIONS

The skill of applying and maintaining graduated compression stockings and intermittent sequential compression devices (SCDs) and mobile compression devices (MCDs) can be delegated to nursing assistive personnel (NAP). The nurse initially determines the size of elastic stockings and assesses the patient's lower extremities for any signs and symptoms of a deep vein thrombosis (DVT) or impaired circulation. The nurse directs the NAP to:

- Remove SCD sleeves before allowing a patient to get out of bed.
- Report to the nurse if a patient's calf or thigh appears larger than the other or is red, tender, hot, or swollen or if the patient complains of calf pain.
- Report to the nurse if there are signs of allergic reactions to elastic (redness, itching, or irritation).
- Report to the nurse if the patient is routinely removing the compression device from the legs.

EQUIPMENT

Tape measure, powder or cornstarch *(optional)*, graduated compression stockings or Velcro compression device sleeves, SCD/MCD insufflator with air hoses attached, compression device pump, hygiene supplies, *option:* cotton stockinette with MCD

STEPS

1. Review medical record for order for SCD or graduated compression stockings.
2. Identify patient using at least two patient identifiers (e.g., name and birthday or name and account number) according to agency policy (TJC, 2018).
3. Review medical record to assess patient for risk factors for developing DVT (see Box 29.3).
4. Assess for contraindications for use of elastic stockings or compression devices:
   a. Dermatitis or open skin lesions on area to be covered by stockings/sleeves
   b. Recent skin graft to lower leg
   c. Decreased arterial circulation in lower extremities as evidenced by cyanotic, cool extremities and/or gangrenous conditions affecting the lower limbs
   d. If signs/symptoms of a DVT are present do not manipulate the leg to place stockings on the legs.
5. Perform hand hygiene. Assess condition of patient's skin (area to be covered by stockings/sleeves) and circulation to the legs. Palpate pedal pulses; note any palpable veins; and inspect skin over lower extremities for edema, skin discoloration, warmth, and presence of lesions.
6. Assess patient's or family caregiver's knowledge of previous use of elastic compression stockings or compression devices.
7. Explain procedure and reason for applying elastic stockings or SCD/MCD.
8. Position patient in supine position.
9. Perform hand hygiene. Bathe patient's legs as needed. Dry thoroughly. Perform hand hygiene.
10. Apply graduated compression hose.

a. Use tape measure to measure patient's leg to determine proper elastic stocking size (follow package directions).
b. *Option:* Apply a small amount of powder or cornstarch to legs provided that patient does not have sensitivity.
c. Turn elastic stocking inside out: Place one hand into stocking, holding heel of stocking. Take other hand and pull stocking inside out until reaching the heel (see illustration).

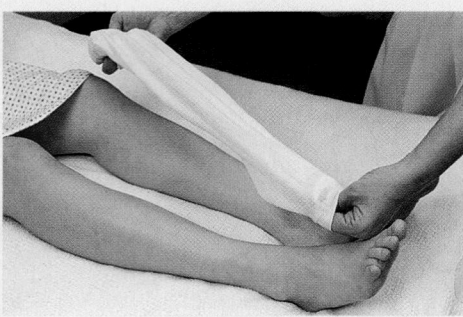

STEP 10c Turn stocking inside out; hold heel and pull through.

d. Place patient's toes into foot of elastic stocking up to the heel, making sure that stocking is smooth (see illustration).

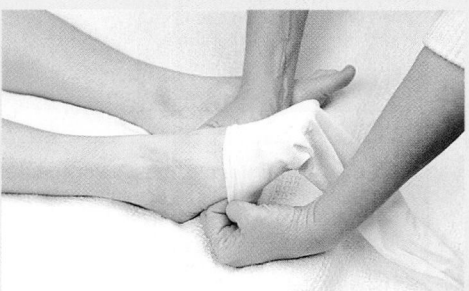

STEP 10d Place toes into foot of stocking.

e. Slide remaining portion of stocking over patient's foot, making sure that toes are covered. Make sure that foot fits into toe and heel position of stocking. Stocking will now be right side out (see illustration).

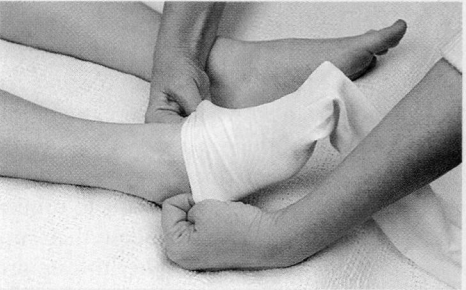

STEP 10e Slide remaining portion of stocking over foot.

BOX 29.9 PROCEDURAL GUIDELINES—cont'd

Applying Antiembolic Compression Stockings and Compression Devices

f. Slide stocking up over patient's calf until sock is completely extended. Be sure that stocking is smooth and that no ridges or wrinkles are present (see illustration).

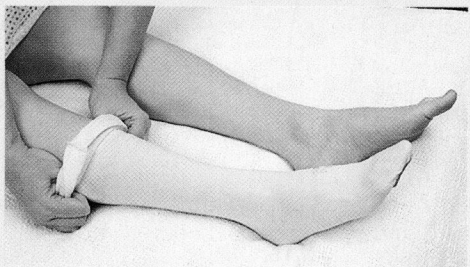

STEP 10f Slide sock up leg until completely extended.

g. Instruct patient not to roll stockings partially down, to avoid wrinkles, to avoid crossing legs, and to elevate legs while sitting.

11. Apply SCD sleeves.
 a. Remove SCD sleeves from plastic cover; unfold and flatten onto bed.
 b. Arrange SCD sleeve under patient's leg according to leg position indicated on inner lining of sleeve.
 c. Place patient's leg on SCD sleeve. Back of ankle should line up with ankle marking on inner lining of sleeve.
 d. Position back of knee with popliteal opening on inner sleeve (see illustration).

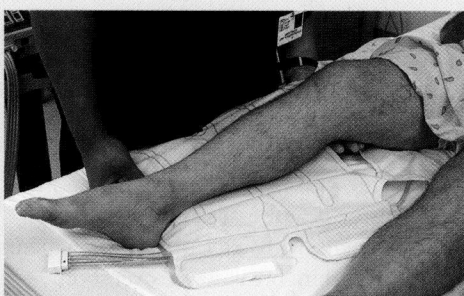

STEP 11d Position back of patient's knee with popliteal opening.

 e. Wrap SCD sleeve securely around patient's leg. Check fit of SCD sleeve by placing two fingers between patient's leg and sleeve (see illustration).

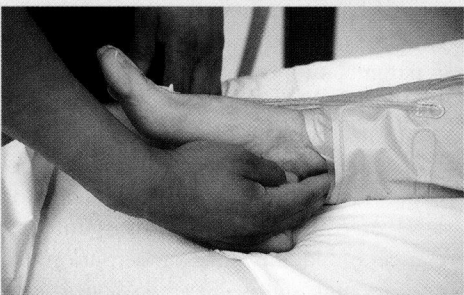

STEP 11e Check fit of the SCD sleeve.

f. Attach SCD sleeve connector to plug on mechanical unit. Arrows on connector line up with arrows on plug from mechanical unit (see illustration).

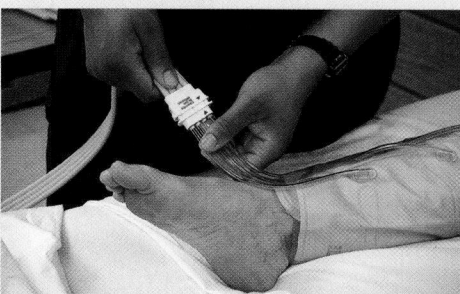

STEP 11f Align arrows when connecting plug to mechanical unit.

g. Turn mechanical unit on. Green light indicates that unit is functioning. Monitor functioning SCD through one full cycle of inflation and deflation.

12. Apply MCD sleeve (example used: Calf Sleeve ActiveCare+S.F.T. Application).
 a. A cotton stockinette is provided along with the calf sleeves. Apply over patient's calves.
 b. Wrap sleeve smoothly around patient's calf and fasten it beginning at the top, moving toward the bottom (see illustration).
 c. Place two fingers between patient's calf and sleeve to be sure it is snug but not too tight.
 d. The device has two identical extension tubes. Use either end of the extension tube to connect to the sleeve or device pump (see illustration).
  (1) Connect one end of the extension tube to the sleeve connector. The white arrows should be pointed toward each other.
  (2) Connect the other end of the extension tube to the device pump. The white arrow should be facing upward.
 e. Press the power switch located at the back of the device to "ON" position. After turning the device on, the Configuration Setup Screen is shown on the LCD screen, and the sleeves should immediately start to inflate from the bottom to the top.
 f. Wait 60 seconds for the automatic operation of the device. The device automatically identifies which sleeves are connected and selects the suitable treatment mode, which will be displayed on the main LCD screen.

13. Position patient comfortably, then perform hand hygiene.

Clinical Decision Point. Caution patient to not exit bed and walk with SCD in place. Have patient call for assistance. The patient may walk with MCD in place.

---

14. Remove compression stockings or SCD/MCD sleeves at least once per shift (e.g., long enough to inspect skin for irritation or breakdown and to determine patient's comfort level).

BOX 29.9 PROCEDURAL GUIDELINES—cont'd

Applying Antiembolic Compression Stockings and Compression Devices

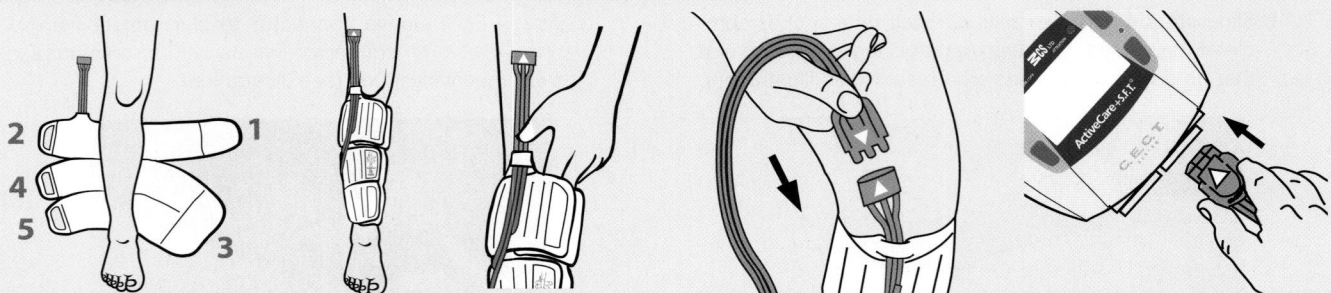

STEP 12b Application of ActiveCare MCD to calves. (Courtesy Zimmer Biomet.)

STEP 12d Application of ActiveCare MCD connector hose to pump. (Courtesy Zimmer Biomet.)

15. Evaluate skin integrity and circulation to patient's lower extremities as ordered (see agency policy).
16. Educate patient/family caregiver about how to care for stockings (keep two pair and wash one daily) and precautions to take to prevent DVT at home (Centers for Disease Control and Prevention [CDC], 2015):
    • Stay active and move around as much as possible.
    • When sitting for long periods of time such as when traveling for more than 4 hours, get up and walk around every 2 to 3 hours, drink plenty of water, and exercise your legs while you're sitting by raising and lowering your heels while keeping your toes on the floor, raising and lowering your toes while keeping your heels on the floor, and tightening and releasing your leg muscles.
    • Wear loose-fitting clothes.
17. Use the principles of teach-back to evaluate patient/family caregiver learning:
    • To a family caregiver: "Show me how you will put the elastic compression stockings on your mother."
    • To a patient: "Tell me what you could do to prevent a DVT from forming if you were traveling."
18. Document condition of lower extremities, application of stockings/SCD, patient education, and patient response in medical record.

When you suspect DVT, do not massage the area; report assessment findings to the health care provider immediately; and elevate the leg, with no pressure on the area of the leg with the suspected thrombus. If the patient complains of shortness of breath or severe chest pain, suspect a pulmonary embolus, which is a deep vein clot that breaks free from a vein wall and travels to the lungs and blocks some or all of the blood supply. Immediately place the patient in high-Fowler's position, check the patient's oxygen saturation, and apply oxygen. This complication is life threatening and requires prompt medical attention and activation of the Rapid Response Team if required by agency policy.

Musculoskeletal System. The immobilized patient needs exercise to prevent excessive muscle atrophy and joint contractures. For patients on bed rest, incorporate sitting up in bed and active ROM exercises into their daily schedules. Patients with impaired nervous, skeletal, or muscular system functioning and significant weakness often require help positioning to attain and maintain body alignment.

Positioning Techniques. Patients with impaired nervous or musculoskeletal system functioning, patients with increased weakness, and patients restricted to bed rest benefit from therapeutic positioning. During patient positioning determine areas of bony prominences where pressure, friction, and shear cause the most wear and tear. Through the use of proper positioning and pressure-relief methods, you are able to protect these areas (see Chapter 38).

In general, you reposition patients as needed and at least every 2 hours if they are in bed and every 15 to 20 minutes if they are sitting in a chair or wheelchair (AHRQ, 2014; Swafford et al., 2016). Improper positioning increases patients' risk for developing pressure injuries or contractions, especially patients who have underlying conditions such as diabetes mellitus or peripheral vascular diseases.

Reposition patients with contractures or patients who are at greater risk for skin breakdown over bony prominences more often than every 2 hours. New sensor devices are now being used in hospital settings. The devices are applied over bed mattresses and provide a visual image of the interface pressure between a patient's body and support surface or mattress (Wong et al., 2015). The images inform clinicians about areas of the skin under pressure and the need for repositioning strategies. Use of the pressure sensor devices has shown promise in the reduction of hospital-acquired pressure injuries (Behrendt et al., 2014).

Placing patients in positions that compromise peripheral blood flow also damages nerves. Every time you reposition a patient, make certain to check total body alignment, placement of extremities, skin condition, and joint ROM. The following also influence the frequency of position changes: level of comfort, amount of spontaneous movement, presence of edema, loss of sensation, and overall physical and mental status. Several devices are available to maintain a patient's body alignment after positioning.

Select the therapeutic position that maximizes your patient's comfort, safety, and ability to still use remaining function (see Skill 29.1).

Fowler's and Semi-Fowler's Positions. Elevate the head of the patient's bed to the desired level, and slightly elevate the patient's knees, avoiding pressure on the popliteal vessels. The head rests against the mattress or a small pillow for support. Use pillows to maintain natural alignment of the hands, wrists, and forearms. In semi-Fowler's position, the head of the bed is at a 30- to 45-degree angle; you use this position for patients who cannot tolerate a supine position such as patients with cardiac and respiratory problems. In Fowler's or high-Fowler's position, the head of the bed is 60 to 90 degrees. Patients with severe respiratory distress breathe more easily in a high-Fowler's position. A patient who remains in place in Fowler's or semi-Fowler's position for more than 2 hours (sometimes less) can develop common problems including the following:

- Increased cervical flexion because the pillow at the head is too thick and head thrusts forward
- Extension of the knees, allowing a patient to slide to the foot of the bed causing shear against the skin.
- Pressure on the posterior aspect of the knees, decreasing circulation to the feet
- External rotation of the hips
- Arms hanging unsupported at a patient's sides
- Unsupported feet or pressure on the heels
- Unprotected pressure points at the sacrum and heels
- Increased shearing force on the back and heels when you raise the head of the bed greater than 60 degrees

Supine Position. Position a patient supine by placing him or her flat on the back. A small, flat pillow supports the head, neck, and upper shoulders (Perry et al., 2017). When a patient is immobile, use pillows, **trochanter rolls**, heel boots, hand rolls, or arm splints to increase comfort and reduce injury to the skin or musculoskeletal system. The risk for aspiration into the tracheobronchial tree (see Chapter 35) is greater with this position; avoid the supine position when the patient is confused, agitated, experiencing a decreased level of consciousness, or at risk for aspiration. Make sure that the mattress is firm enough to support the cervical, thoracic, and lumbar vertebrae. Avoid pressure on the back of the legs and heels. Use a **foot boot** to prevent footdrop (Fig. 29.5), maintain proper alignment, and provide freedom of movement for the feet. Patients who remain in the supine position for too long can develop the following problems:

- Cervical flexion from a too thick pillow being placed under the head
- Pressure over the occiput from the head staying flat on the mattress
- Shoulders unsupported and internally rotated
- Elbows extended
- Thumb not in opposition to the fingers
- Hips externally rotated
- Feet unsupported
- Unprotected pressure points at the vertebrae, coccyx, elbows, heels, and occipital region of the head

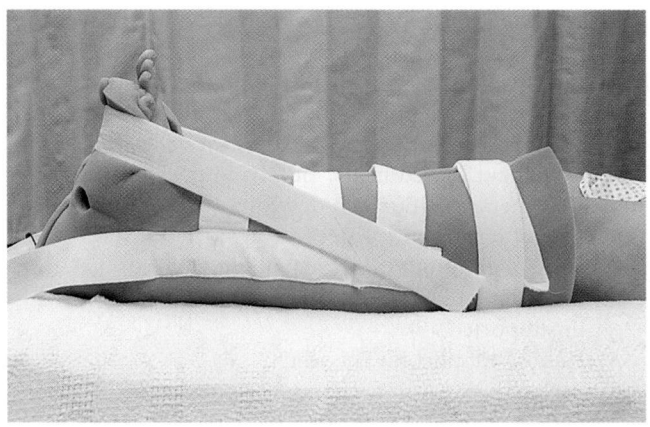

FIG 29.5 Foot boot with lower leg extension.

Prone Position. When **prone,** a patient is in the face-down position. Although it is not a position commonly used for patients, it is used for critically ill patients on mechanical ventilation and who have acute respiratory distress syndrome (ARDS). Use of prone position ventilation has been shown to improve oxygenation in selected patients with ARDS (Henderson et al., 2014). Before placing a patient in the prone position, assess his or her medical record for any possible complications such as increasing intracranial pressure or cardiopulmonary disease. Also assess current vital signs.

Help the patient lie on the abdomen. Have the patient turn the head to the side; this facilitates respiration and drainage of oral secretions. Place a pillow under the head for comfort and relief from pressure. As an alternative place a wedge under the patient's chest or arms flexed over the head if it is more comfortable. Place a pillow under the lower leg; this promotes relaxation. If a pillow is unavailable, make sure that a patient's ankles are in dorsiflexion over the end of the mattress. Body alignment is poor when the ankles are continuously in plantar flexion and the lumbar spine remains in **hyperextension**. Sometimes lung expansion is compromised in this position, especially in patients who are obese. Monitor your patient for signs of respiratory distress. You assess for and correct any of the following potential trouble points:

- Neck hyperextension
- Hyperextension of the lumbar spine
- Plantar flexion of the ankles
- Unprotected pressure points at the chin, elbows, hips, knees, and toes

Thirty-Degree Lateral Position. In the 30-degree lateral position, a patient is supported on the right or left side with the opposite arm, thigh, and knee flexed and resting on the bed. Place a pillow under the patient's head to keep the head, neck, and spine in alignment. Both arms are placed in slightly flexed positions with the upper arm supported with a pillow. The dependent hip is brought forward so that the angle from hip to mattress is approximately 30 degrees. Less pressure is placed directly on the bony prominence compared with just a side-lying position. The upper leg is flexed at the hip and knee and positioned on a small pillow (Perry et al., 2017). The 30-degree lateral position is recommended as a position to avoid development of pressure injuries (Swafford et al., 2016). A patient placed in the side-lying position instead of 30-degree lateral position can develop:

- Lateral flexion of the neck
- Spinal curves out of normal alignment
- Shoulder and hip joints internally rotated, adducted, or unsupported
- Lack of support for the feet
- Lack of protection for pressure points at the ear, shoulder, anterior iliac spine, trochanter, and ankles
- Excessive lateral flexion of the spine if the patient has large hips and a pillow is not placed superior to the hips at the waist

Sims' Position. In Sims' position, a patient is semiprone on the right or left side with the opposite arm, thigh, and knee flexed and resting on the bed. Sims' position differs from the side-lying position in the distribution of the patient's weight. In this position you place the patient's weight on the anterior ilium, humerus, and clavicle. Trouble points common in Sims' position include the following:

- Lateral flexion of the neck
- Internal rotation, adduction, or lack of support to the shoulders and hips
- Lack of support for the feet
- Lack of protection for pressure points at the ilium, humerus, clavicle, knees, and ankles

Several devices are available for maintaining proper patient positioning (see Table 29.4). Pillows are commonly used to support body alignment. Before using a pillow, determine whether it is the proper size and consistency. A thick pillow under a patient's head causes excessive cervical flexion. A thin pillow under bony prominences is inadequate to protect skin and tissue from damage. When additional pillows are unavailable, use folded sheets, blankets, or towels as positioning aids. Elevate a patient's calves on pillows or use a heel protector to avoid pressure on the heels. A trochanter roll prevents external rotation of the hips when the patient is in a supine position (Fig. 29.6). Hand rolls maintain the hand, thumb, and fingers in a functional position (Fig. 29.7). **Hand-wrist splints** are individually molded for a patient to maintain proper alignment of the thumb. A **trapeze bar** is a triangular device that hangs from a securely fastened overhead bar that is attached to the patient's bedframe (Fig. 29.8). It is a useful device for helping to increase patient independence when moving in bed, maintain upper body strength, and reduce friction from movement in bed.

Safe Patient Handling and Movement. Before attempting any movement or transfer always explain the process and equipment being used to the patient in terms that are appropriate for his or her developmental stage. Patients unable to move themselves safely from one location to another must depend on the nursing staff to choose the appropriate piece of equipment with which to facilitate that transfer.

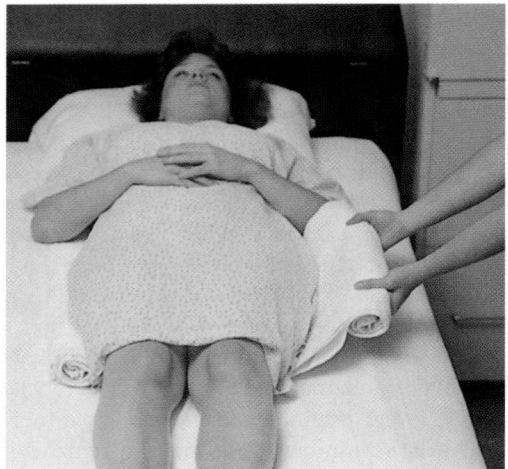

FIG 29.6 Trochanter roll.

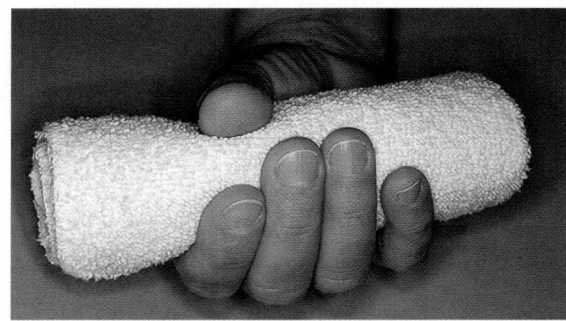

FIG 29.7 Hand roll.

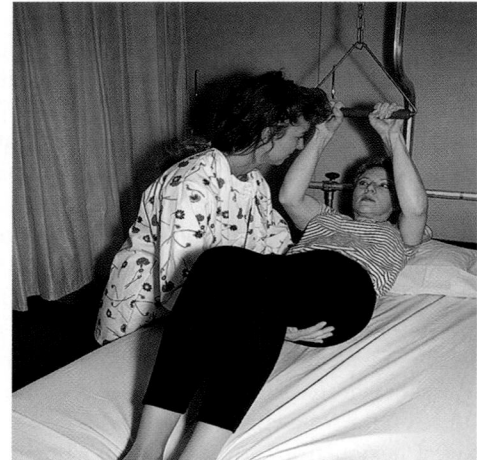

FIG 29.8 Patient using a trapeze bar.

Algorithms (VISN8, 2014) were designed just for this purpose (see Fig. 29.4).

Transfer Techniques. Nurses often provide care for immobilized patients whose positions must be changed, who must be moved up in bed, or who must be transferred from a bed to a chair or from a bed to a stretcher. As noted earlier, **body mechanics** alone do not protect a nurse from injury to

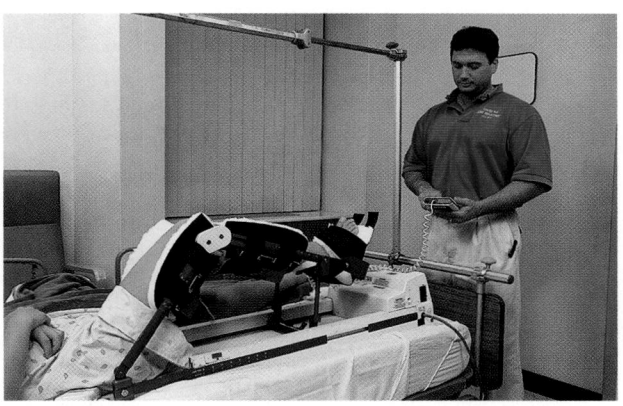

FIG 29.9 Continuous passive range-of-motion machine.

the musculoskeletal system when moving, lifting, or transferring patients. Although nurses use many transfer techniques, knowledge of ergonomics and safe patient handling is crucial in maintaining caregiver and patient safety. See Chapter 28 for safe transfer techniques.

Assess every situation that involves patient handling and movement to minimize risk of injury. After completing the assessment, use an algorithm to guide decisions about safe patient handling. Use the patient's strength when lifting, transferring, or moving when possible. Involving the patient has the added bonus of increasing participation in self-care, promoting a sense of accomplishment. In addition to handling patients safely, nurses need to assume an active role in their workplaces to ensure that a culture of safety exists and that appropriate patient-handling equipment is readily available (ANA, 2015).

Range of Motion. Some orthopedic and neurological conditions require ROM exercises more frequently or for longer duration to restore an injured joint or extremity to maximal function. Patients with such conditions may use automatic equipment for passive ROM exercises. The continuous passive motion (CPM) machine moves an extremity within a prescribed range for a specific period (Fig. 29.9). This method is beneficial when a patient gradually increases ROM of a particular joint. For example, it is used for patients who have had total knee replacement surgery. Research has shown that CPM probably improves the ability to bend the knee slightly but may not lessen pain or improve overall function (Harvey et al., 2014). The device is applied immediately after surgery and is removed only when a patient is receiving physical therapy. Over time the patient progresses to flexing and extending the joint without the aid of the CPM.

Active ROM exercises also maintain function of the musculoskeletal system. Have patients participate in active ROM and collaborate with a PT if needed to establish an individualized progressive exercise program when possible. A progressive exercise program gradually increases a patient's physical activity to reverse the deconditioning associated with immobility. Progressive exercise programs are successful in patients with musculoskeletal, neurological, cardiopulmonary, renal, and other chronic diseases.

Integumentary System. The major risk to skin integrity from restricted mobility is the formation of pressure injuries. Continuous use of tools such as the Braden Scale to monitor high-risk patients helps prevent pressure injuries (see Chapter 38). Interventions aimed at preventing prolonged pressure should prevent or delay the development of the ulcers until the patient is able to move more freely or be out of bed. Change the immobilized patient's position according to the patient's activity level, perceptual ability, treatment protocols, and daily routines.

Psychosocial Problems. Establish a balance between rest, the physiological effects of bed rest, and a patient's psychosocial needs. Promote a patient's comfort and keep interventions to a minimum in a stable patient who is able to turn in bed unassisted. Having to stay in bed causes restlessness, anxiety, and general discomfort. Keep hygiene and grooming articles within easy reach. Encourage patients to wear their glasses or dentures and to shave or apply makeup. These activities help maintain body image, thus improving the patient's outlook.

Nurses provide stimuli to maintain a patient's orientation. If possible place the patient in a room with others who are mobile and interactive. If a private room is required, ask staff members to visit throughout the shift to provide meaningful interaction. Access to daily news helps patients keep track of events and time. Bedside conversations at appropriate moments familiarize the patient with nursing activities, meals, and visiting hours. Books help occupy the patient when he or she is alone. The patient can participate in craft activities; also, radio, television, or computers provide stimulation and help pass the time.

Actively engage patients in their plan of care whenever possible. For example, have a patient discuss concerns related to immobility, plans for discharge to a nonacute setting, and how the family can be involved. If the plan of care is not improving the patient's coping patterns, collaborate with a mental health and advanced practice nurse, counselor, social worker, spiritual adviser, or other health care professional and incorporate their recommendations into the plan of care.

Developmental Changes. Immobilization or restricted mobility of an older adult requires complex care and innovative approaches because older adults are at risk for cognitive changes and depression as a result of immobilization, chronic illnesses, and medications. It is important to focus on activities to promote cognitive awareness of the patient's surroundings (see Chapter 23). Give explanations before starting care and involve the patient in decision making. Plan nursing care to allow the older adult patient to perform as many ADLs as possible by allowing extra time for routine activities. Not only are older adults more susceptible to the hazards of immobility, but also the consequences of immobility appear more quickly and become severe more rapidly.

Restorative and Continuing Care. The goal of restorative and continuing care for the immobilized patient is to maximize independence, increase endurance, and prevent injury. Restorative interventions focus on finding ways for patients with mobility limitations to perform instrumental activities of daily living (IADLs) such as shopping, preparing meals, banking, taking medications, and ADLs. Often patients with mobility issues are transferred to rehabilitation centers to work on improving IADLs. Provide the rehabilitation center with a complete report to ensure patient safety and continuity of care (The Joint Commission [TJC], 2018). This is a routine part of a patient hand-off.

Use many of the same interventions for mobility as described in the health promotion and acute care sections, but the emphasis in restorative care is working collaboratively to help patients adjust in the home or in an extended-care facility. Often occupational or physical therapy is ordered. Work collaboratively with OTs and PTs, and reinforce exercises and teaching. Patients often must learn how to use and care for assist devices. Common items used to help the patient adapt to mobility limitations include walkers; canes; wheelchairs; and devices such as toilet seat extenders, reaching sticks, special eating utensils, and clothing with Velcro closures.

■■■■ EVALUATION

Patient Outcomes. Evaluate the efficacy of interventions for reducing the risks of immobility by comparing the patient's actual responses to the expected outcomes for each goal. If expected outcomes are not achieved, revise the plan of care. Base the success in meeting each outcome on the use of evaluative measures such as ROM status, exercise tolerance, skin integrity, and fluid intake.

Evaluate outcomes designed to demonstrate normal function of specific systems and prevent complications (Box 29.10). For example, are the lungs clear; are any areas of skin showing signs of skin breakdown; is the patient's joint ROM improving? Evaluation provides evidence of whether you are meeting the outcomes set with the patient during the planning phase of care. If the answers to the questions indicate that outcomes are being met, the plan is working; if not, you need to reassess and revise the plan with input from the patient.

Patient Expectations. People often take movement for granted. Patients who are immobile and dependent on others for some or all of their needs sometimes become overly dependent or try to do too much themselves too early. Finding the balance between independence and dependence is a difficult task. Patients want control over their mobility

---

BOX 29.10 EVALUATION

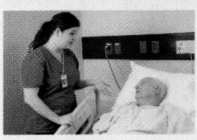

It has been 5 days since Mr. Rogers' stroke. He has increased his strength and has been able to begin walking with the use of a walker. He will be discharged to a rehabilitation facility before going home. During his stay in the hospital Abby taught Mr. Rogers the importance of following the American Diabetes Association (ADA) diet. In addition, she worked with Mr. Rogers and his physical therapist in deciding which exercises he can perform on his own in the rehabilitation facility as well as when he returns home. Abby also made sure that Mr. Rogers' children understood his medications and exercises so they could work with him as well. Mr. Rogers must concentrate on increasing his strength and mobility, reducing his weight by following an ADA diet as prescribed by his primary health care provider, and keeping up with his physical activities and exercises.

DOCUMENTATION NOTE
"Mr. Rogers discharged to rehabilitation facility in a.m. He has been able to demonstrate safe transfer techniques as taught and is able to use a walker with assist of one. His children verbalized understanding of his medications and exercises so they could work with him as well when discharged to home from the rehabilitation facility. Mr. Rogers verbalized the importance of reducing his weight by following an ADA diet as prescribed by his primary health care provider and keeping up with his physical activities and exercises."

---

that is personally satisfactory. For patients who are completely dependent on others for care, control over how and when things are done is very important. Do caregivers treat them as adults? Patients who are dependent on others for care sometimes see their demands as the only control they have over their lives.

For most patients with mobility problems, lack of control is often a major issue. Do they think that staff are considerate, and do staff protect their privacy? Are patients' preferences taken into consideration when planning care? Do caregivers talk to them or ignore them? It is important to recognize that immobility possibly leads to fear, anger, grief, withdrawal, or hostility. If you are sensitive to these reactions and help the patient work through them instead of responding negatively, you can make a big difference in the patient's outcomes.

SAFETY GUIDELINES FOR NURSING SKILLS

Ensuring patient safety is an essential role of the professional nurse. To ensure patient safety, communicate clearly with members of the health care team, assess and incorporate the patient's priorities of care and preferences, and use the best evidence when making decisions about your patient's care. When performing the skills in this chapter, remember the following points to ensure safe, individualized patient care:

- Know your patients' risks for complications of immobility.
- Inspect the skin routinely for development of early signs of pressure injuries.
- The use of elastic stockings can impair circulation if stockings are not correctly applied.
- Follow safe patient-handling guidelines when positioning patients

SKILL 29.1 MOVING AND POSITIONING PATIENTS IN BED

View Video!

DELEGATION CONSIDERATIONS

The skills of moving and positioning patients in bed and maintaining correct body alignment can be delegated to nursing assistive personnel (NAP). The nurse directs the NAP by:

- Explaining about any moving and positioning restrictions (e.g., avoid prone position unless clinically indicated, patient has one-sided weakness) and type of safe patient-handling devices needed.
- Designating specific times throughout the shift that NAP must reposition the patient.
- Providing information regarding patient's individual needs for body alignment (i.e., patient with spinal cord injury), ability to assist, and number of other caregivers needed to assist.

EQUIPMENT

- Pillows, lift sheet
- *Options:* friction-reducing device, ceiling lift or mechanical floor lift
- Therapeutic boots/splints *(optional)*
- Trochanter roll
- Sandbag
- Hand rolls
- Clean gloves

STEP	RATIONALE

ASSESSMENT

1. Identify patient using at least two identifiers (e.g., name and birthday or name and medical record number) according to agency policy.

   Ensures correct patient. Complies with The Joint Commission standards and improves patient safety (TJC, 2018).

2. Perform hand hygiene.

   Prevents transmission of microorganisms.

3. Assess patient's range of motion (ROM), current body alignment, and level of pain while patient is lying down.

   Provides baseline data for later comparisons. Determines ways to improve position and alignment.

4. Assess for risk factors that contribute to complications of immobility.

   Increased risk factors require patient to be repositioned more frequently.

   a. Reduced sensation: cerebrovascular accident (CVA), spinal cord injury, or neuropathy.

   With reduced sensation, patient has difficulty moving and poor awareness of involved body part. Patient is unable to position body part and protect it from pressure.

   b. Impaired mobility: Traction, arthritis, CVA, spinal cord injury, hip fracture, joint surgery, or other contributing disease processes.

   Traction, bone fractures, surgery, or arthritic changes of affected extremity result in decreased ROM. Loss of function as a result of CVA or spinal injury can lead to contractures.

   c. Impaired circulation: Arterial insufficiency.

   Decreased circulation predisposes patient to pressure injuries.

   d. Age: Very young and older adult patients.

   Premature and young infants require frequent turning because their skin is fragile. Normal physiological changes associated with aging predispose older adults to greater risks for developing complications of immobility.

5. Assess patient's level of consciousness.

   Determines need for special aids or devices. Patients with altered levels of consciousness may not understand instructions and may be unable to assist with positioning.

6. Assess patient for presence of pain; rate on scale of 0 to 10 (with 0 being no pain and 10 being worst ever).

   Pain reduces patient's motivation and ability to be mobile. Pain relief before transfer enhances patient participation (Schofield, 2014).

7. Assess condition of patient's skin (apply gloves if needed), especially over bony prominences. (Dispose of gloves and perform hand hygiene.)

   Provides baseline to determine effects of positioning. Reduces transmission of microorganisms.

8. Perform observations to assess patient's physical ability to help with moving and positioning, which may be affected by age, level of consciousness, disease process, strength, ROM, and coordination.

   Enables you to use patient's mobility, strength, and coordination during positioning. Determines need for additional help. Ensures patient and nurse safety.

9. Assess for sensory loss (vision and hearing) (see Chapter 16).

   Deficits affect patient's ability to cooperate during repositioning procedures.

10. Apply clean gloves (as needed) to assess for presence of incisions, drainage tubes, and equipment (e.g., traction). Empty drainage bags before positioning. Remove and dispose of gloves. Perform hand hygiene.

    Alters positioning procedure and type of position in which to place patient. Eliminates barriers to moving patient. Reduces transmission of microorganisms.

SKILL 29.1   MOVING AND POSITIONING PATIENTS IN BED—cont'd

View Video!

STEP	RATIONALE
11. Assess motivation of patient and ability of family caregivers to participate in moving and positioning if patient to be discharged home.	Indicates whether instruction is necessary before discharge.
12. Refer to medical record for most recent recorded weight and height for patient.	Information needed to determine if mechanical lift, mechanical transfer device, or friction-reducing device is needed for moving patient up in bed.
13. Check health care provider's orders before positioning patient.	Some positions may be contraindicated in certain situations (e.g., spinal cord injury; hip fracture; respiratory difficulties; certain neurological conditions; presence of incisions, drains, or tubing).

PLANNING

1. Gather appropriate equipment.	Ensures an organized procedure.
2. Determine number of people needed to assist with transfer by referring to proper algorithm. Do not start procedure until all caregivers are available.	Ensures safe patient transfer. Algorithms for safe patient handling and movement are provided at http://www.washingtonsafepatienthandling.org/images/VA_Algorithms_for_Safe_Patient_Handling_Movement.pdf.
3. If patient perceives level of pain to be enough to avoid movement, offer an analgesic 30 minutes (if ordered) before repositioning.	Will lessen discomfort when positioning extremities. **Note:** An analgesic may not be available as frequently as a patient will require turning.
4. Perform hand hygiene. Verify that bed brakes are locked.	Reduces transmission of microorganisms. Provides patient and caregiver safety.
5. Remove all pillows and devices used in previous position.	Reduces interference from bedding during positioning procedure.
6. Explain procedure to patient and/or family using plain language.	Increases patient participation and/or family knowledge of continued care of patient on discharge (Wrobleski et al., 2014).

IMPLEMENTATION

1. Perform hand hygiene.	Reduces transmission of microorganisms.
2. Close door to room or bedside curtains.	Provides for patient privacy.
3. Raise level of bed to comfortable working height, level with your elbows.	Raises level of work toward nurse's center of gravity and reduces risk for back injuries.
4. Help patient move up in bed.	This is not a one-person task unless patient can fully assist (VISN8, 2014). Pulling patients who have migrated in bed carries an extremely high risk of caregiver injury (VISN8, 2014)
a. Can the patient assist?	Determines degree of risk in repositioning patient and technique required to safely assist patient.
(1) Fully able to assist.	Promotes patient independence.
(a) Stand at bedside to assist with positioning of tubing and equipment as patient moves.	
(b) Have patient place feet flat on mattress, grasp either side rails or overhead trapeze, and on a count of three lift hips up and push legs so that body moves up in bed.	
(2) Partially able to assist.	
(a) Encourage patient to assist using a repositioning device (slide board) (VISN8, 2014).	Repositioning device reduces friction as patient is moved up in bed.
(b) Patient weighs less than 200 lb (90.7 kg): Use a friction-reducing sheet or slide board and two or three caregivers (VISN8, 2014).	

STEP	RATIONALE

(c) Patient weighs more than 200 lb (90.7 kg): Use a friction-reducing device and at least three caregivers (VISN8, 2014).

(i) Using a friction-reducing device (three nurses), position patient supine with head of bed flat. A nurse stands on each side of bed.

Prevents friction from contact of skin with board.

(ii) Remove pillow from under head and shoulders and place it at head of bed.

(iii) Turn patient side to side to place friction-reducing device under lift sheet on the bed, with device extending from shoulders to thighs or ankles (see Skill 28.2).

(iv) Return patient to supine position.

(v) Have two nurses grasp lift sheet (one on each side of bed) firmly, and have third nurse hold onto end of friction-reducing device.

Slide board remains stationary, provides a slippery surface to reduce friction, and allows patient to move up in bed easily.

(vi) Nurses place their feet apart with forward-backward stance. Flex knees and hips. On count of three, shift weight from front to back leg and move patient and lift sheet to desired position up in bed.

Clinical Decision Point. If patient has a stage III or IV pressure injury, take care to avoid shear (VISN8, 2014).

---

(3) Patient unable to assist.

(a) Use appropriate number of caregivers and appropriate safe handling devices (e.g., supine sling with ceiling lift, floor-based lift and two or more caregivers) (VISN8, 2014).

Repositioning patients manually is associated with a high risk of musculoskeletal injury (VISN8, 2014).

Clinical Decision Point. Protect patient's heels from shearing force by having another caregiver lift heels while moving patient up in bed.

---

5. Position patient in bed in one of the following positions. Ensure correct body alignment. Protect pressure areas.

Prevents injury to musculoskeletal system and integument. Even positioning patient side to side requires use of safe handling algorithm (VISN8, 2014).

a. Can the patient assist? Follow appropriate guidelines described in Steps 4a(1)–(3).

b. Begin with patient lying supine and move up in bed following Step 4.

Positioning patient initially near head of bed allows for repositioning using entire bed surface.

c. **Position patient in supported semi-Fowler's (see illustration) or Fowler's position.**

(1) With patient lying supine, elevate head of bed 45 to 60 degrees if not contraindicated.

Increases comfort, improves ventilation, and increases patient's opportunity to socialize or relax.

(2) Rest head against mattress or on small pillow.

Prevents flexion contractures of cervical vertebrae.

(3) Use pillows to support arms and hands if patient does not have voluntary control or use of hands and arms.

Prevents shoulder dislocation from effect of downward pull of unsupported arms, promotes circulation by preventing venous pooling, and prevents flexion contractures of arms and wrists.

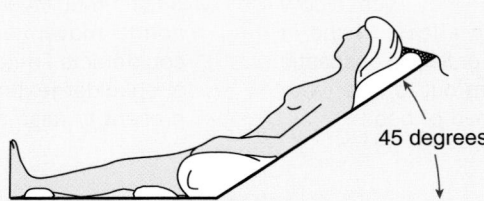

45 degrees

STEP 5c Supported semi-Fowler's position.

SKILL 29.1   MOVING AND POSITIONING PATIENTS IN BED—cont'd

View Video!

STEP	RATIONALE
(4) Position small pillow at lower back.	Supports lumbar vertebrae and decreases flexion of vertebrae.
(5) Place small pillow or roll under thigh.	Prevents hyperextension of knee and occlusion of popliteal artery from pressure from body weight.
(6) Support calves with pillows.	Heels should not be in contact with bed to prevent prolonged pressure of mattress on heels. This is sometimes referred to as *floating* heels.

d. Position hemiplegic patient in supported semi-Fowler's or Fowler's position.

(1) Elevate head of bed 45 to 60 degrees.	Increases comfort, improves ventilation, and increases patient's opportunity to relax. Adjust head of bed according to patient's condition. For example, patients with increased risk for pressure injuries remain at 30-degree angle.
(2) Position patient in Fowler's position as straight as possible.	Counteracts tendency to slump toward affected side. Improves ventilation and cardiac output; decreases intracranial pressure. Improves patient's ability to swallow and helps prevent aspiration of food, liquids, and gastric secretions.
(3) Position head on small pillow with chin slightly forward. If patient is totally unable to control head movement, avoid hyperextension of neck.	Prevents hyperextension of neck. Too many pillows under head may cause or worsen neck flexion contracture.
(4) Provide support for involved arm and hand by placing arm away from patient's side and supporting elbow with pillow.	Paralyzed muscles do not automatically resist pull of gravity as normal muscles do. As a result, shoulder subluxation, pain, and edema may occur.
(5) Place rolled blanket (trochanter roll) firmly alongside patient's legs.	Ensures proper alignment. Prevents external rotation of hips, which contributes to contractures.
(6) Support feet in dorsiflexion with therapeutic boots or splints.	Prevents plantar flexion contractures or footdrop by positioning patient's ankle in neutral dorsiflexion. Position foot so that heel is aligned in opening of splint to prevent pressure. Other therapeutic boots or splints are manufactured with thick padding to cushion heel and prevent pressure injuries.

e. Position patient in supported supine position.

(1) Place patient supine with head of bed flat.	Necessary for properly aligning patient.
(2) Place small rolled towel under lumbar area of back.	Provides support for lumbar spine.
(3) Place pillow under upper shoulders, neck, and head.	Maintains correct alignment and prevents flexion contractures of cervical vertebrae.
(4) Place trochanter rolls or sandbags parallel to lateral surface of patient's thighs.	Reduces external rotation of hip.
(5) Place patient's feet in therapeutic boots or splints.	Maintains feet in dorsiflexion. Prevents plantar flexion contractures or footdrop.
(6) Place pillows under pronated forearms, keeping upper arms parallel to patient's body (see illustration).	Reduces internal rotation of shoulder and prevents extension of elbows. Maintains correct body alignment.
(7) Place hand rolls in patient's hands. Consider physical therapy referral for use of hand splints.	Reduces extension of fingers and abduction of thumb. Maintains thumb slightly adducted and in opposition to fingers.

f. Position hemiplegic patient in supine position.

(1) Place head of bed flat.	Necessary for positioning in supine position.
(2) Place folded towel or small pillow under shoulder or affected side.	Decreases possibility of pain, joint contracture, and subluxation. Maintains mobility in muscles around shoulder to permit normal movement patterns.
(3) Keep affected arm away from body with elbow extended and palm up. Position affected hand in one of recommended positions for flaccid or spastic hand. (Alternative is to place arm out to side, with elbow bent and hand toward head of bed.)	Maintains mobility in arm, joints, and shoulder to permit normal movement patterns. (Alternative position counteracts limitation of ability of arm to rotate outward at shoulder [external rotation]. External rotation must be present to raise arm overhead without pain.)

STEP	RATIONALE
(4) Place folded towel under hip of involved side.	Diminishes effect of spasticity in entire leg by controlling hip position.
(5) Flex affected knee 30 degrees by supporting it on pillow or folded blanket.	Slight flexion breaks up abnormal extension pattern of leg. Extensor spasticity is most severe when patient is supine.
(6) Support feet with soft pillows at right angle to leg.	Maintains foot in dorsiflexion and prevents footdrop. Pillows prevent stimulation to ball of foot by hard surface, which has tendency to increase muscle tone in patient with extensor spasticity of lower extremity.
g. Position patient in 30-degree lateral (side-lying) position (one nurse).	This position is recommended to prevent development of pressure injuries by reducing direct contact of trochanter with support surface (see Chapter 38).
(1) Lower head of bed completely or as low as patient can tolerate.	Provides position of comfort for patient and removes pressure from bony prominences on back.
(2) Lower side rail and position patient on side of bed opposite direction toward which patient is to be turned. Move upper trunk, supporting shoulders first; then move lower trunk, supporting hips (*Option:* use sliding board to move to side of bed).	Provides room for patient to turn to side.
(3) Raise side rail and go to opposite side of bed.	
(4) Flex patient's knee that will not be next to mattress. Keep foot on mattress. Place one hand on patient's upper bent leg near hip, and place other hand on patient's shoulder.	Use of leverage makes turning to side easy.
(5) Roll patient onto side toward you.	Rolling decreases trauma to tissues. In addition, patient is positioned so that leverage on hip makes turning easy.
(6) Place pillow under patient's head and neck.	Maintains alignment. Reduces lateral neck flexion. Decreases strain on sternocleidomastoid muscle.
(7) Place hands under patient's dependent shoulder and bring shoulder blade forward.	Prevents patient's weight from resting directly on shoulder joint.
(8) Position both arms in slightly flexed position. Support upper arm with pillow level with shoulder; other arm on mattress.	Decreases internal rotation and adduction of shoulder. Supporting both arms in slightly flexed position protects joint. Ventilation improves because chest is able to expand more easily.
(9) Place hands under dependent hip and bring hip slightly forward so that angle from hip to mattress is approximately 30 degrees.	The 30-degree lateral position reduces pressure on trochanter; designed to prevent pressure injury.
(10) Place small tuck-back pillow behind patient's back. (Make by folding pillow lengthwise. Smooth area is slightly tucked under patient's back.)	Provides support to maintain patient on side.

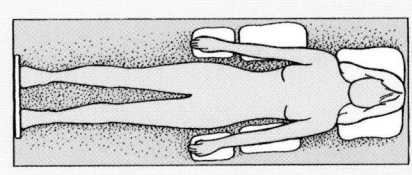
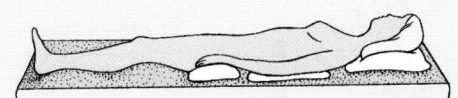
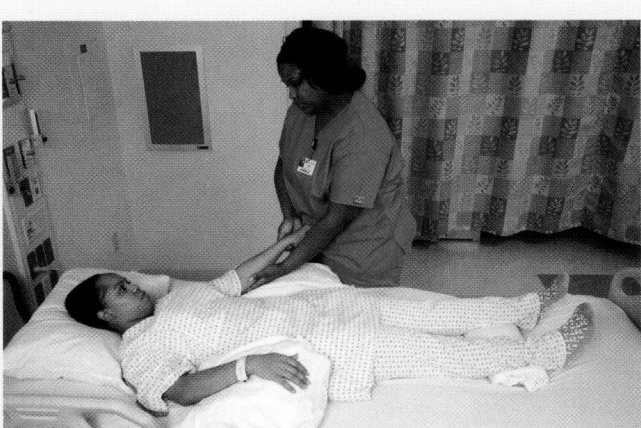

STEP 5e(6) Supported supine position with pillows in place.

View Video!

SKILL 29.1 MOVING AND POSITIONING PATIENTS IN BED—cont'd

STEP	RATIONALE
(11) Place pillow under semiflexed upper leg level at hip from groin to foot (see illustration).	Flexion prevents hyperextension of leg. Maintains leg in correct alignment. Prevents pressure on bony prominences.
(12) Place sandbags parallel to plantar surface of dependent foot. May use ankle-foot orthotic on feet if available.	Maintains dorsiflexion of foot.
h. Position patient in Sims' (semiprone) position.	
(1) Lower head of bed completely.	Provides for proper body alignment while patient is lying down.
(2) Place patient supine on side of bed opposite direction toward which he or she is to be turned. Move upper trunk, supporting shoulders, first, followed by lower trunk, supporting hips.	Prepares patient for position.
(3) Move to other side of bed and turn patient on side. Position in lateral position, lying partially on abdomen, with dependent shoulder lifted out and arm placed at patient's side	
(4) Place small pillow under patient's head.	Maintains proper alignment and prevents lateral neck flexion.
(5) Place pillow under flexed upper arm, supporting arm level with shoulder.	Prevents internal rotation of shoulder. Maintains alignment.
(6) Place pillow under flexed upper legs, supporting leg level with hip.	Prevents internal rotation of hip and adduction of leg. Flexion prevents hyperextension of leg. Reduces mattress pressure on knees and ankles.
(7) Place sandbags parallel to plantar surface of foot or apply foot boots (see illustration).	Maintains foot in dorsiflexion. Prevents plantar flexion contractures or footdrop.
i. Position patient in prone position using two nurses.	In certain patients with pulmonary conditions such as acute respiratory distress syndrome use prone position to improve oxygenation.
(1) With head of bed flat and one nurse standing on each side of bed, roll patient to one side while placing arm on side to be turned alongside of body. For patients with hemiplegia, move toward unaffected side.	Prepares patient for positioning.
(2) Roll patient over arm positioned close to body, with elbow straight and hand under hip. Position on abdomen in center of bed.	Positions patient correctly so that alignment can be maintained.
(3) Turn patient's head to one side and support with small pillow.	Reduces flexion or hyperextension of cervical vertebrae.

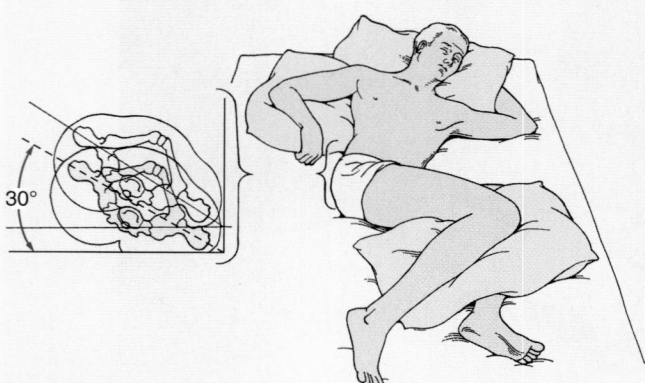

STEP 5g(11) The 30-degree lateral position with pillows in place.

30°

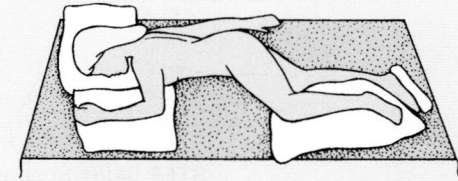

STEP 5h(7) Sandbag supporting right foot in dorsiflexion.

STEP	RATIONALE
(4) Place small pillow under patient's abdomen below level of diaphragm.	Reduces pressure on breasts of female patients and decreases hyperextension of lumbar vertebrae and strain on lower back. Improves breathing by reducing mattress pressure on diaphragm.
(5) Support arms in flexed position level at shoulders.	Maintains proper body alignment. Reduces risk for joint dislocation.
(6) Support lower legs with pillow to elevate feet (see illustration).	Prevents footdrop.
6. Logroll patient (three nurses).	

Clinical Decision Point. A nurse supervises and assists the **NAP** when there is a health care provider's order to logroll a patient. Patients with a spinal cord injury or who are recovering from neck, back, or spinal surgery often need to keep the spinal column in straight alignment to prevent further injury.

STEP	RATIONALE
a. Place small pillow between patient's knees.	Prevents tension on spinal column and adduction of hip.
b. Cross patient's arms on chest.	Prevents injury to arms.
c. Position two nurses on side toward which patient is to be turned and one nurse on side where pillows are to be placed (see illustration).	Distributes weight equally between nurses during turning.
d. Fanfold lift sheet alongside of patient that will be turning.	Provides strong handles to grip lift sheet without slipping.
e. With one nurse grasping lift sheet at lower hips and thighs and the other nurse grasping lift sheet at patient's shoulders and lower back, on count of three roll patient as one unit in a smooth, continuous motion (see illustration).	Maintains proper alignment by moving all body parts at the same time, preventing tension or twisting of spinal column.
f. Nurse on opposite side of bed places pillows along length of patient for support (see illustration).	Maintains patient in side-lying position.

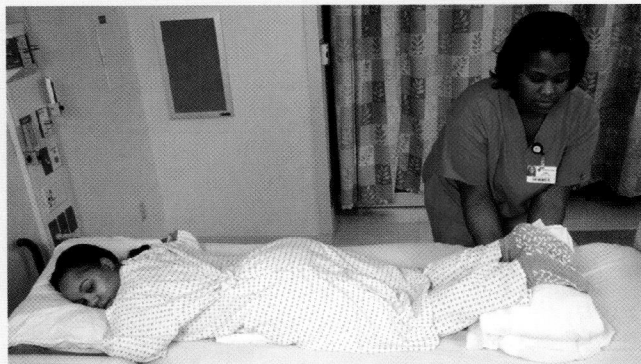

STEP 5i(6) Prone position with pillows supporting lower legs.

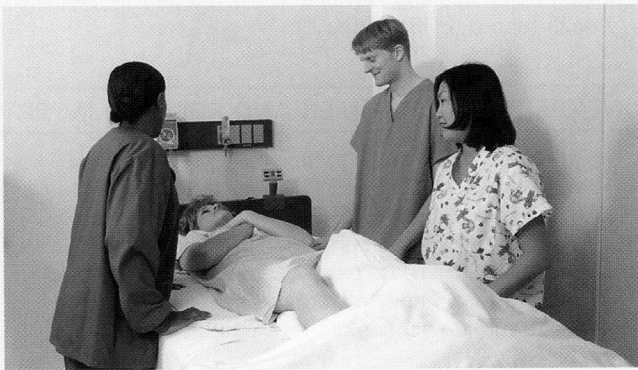

STEP 6c Preparing patient for logrolling.

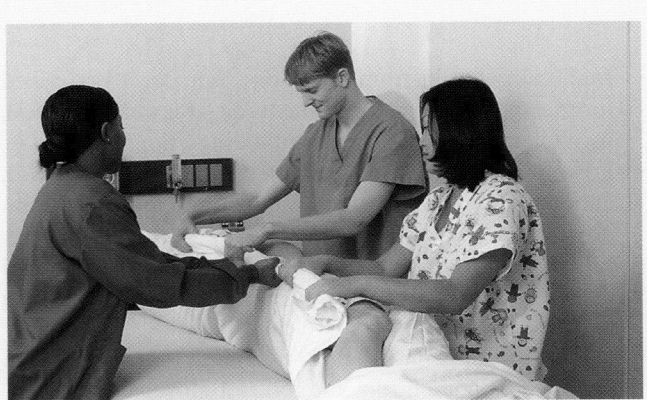

STEP 6e Logrolling patient onto side.

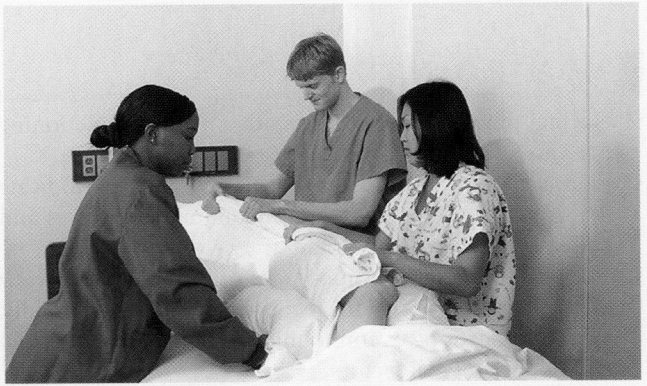

STEP 6f Placing pillows along patient's back for support.

SKILL 29.1 MOVING AND POSITIONING PATIENTS IN BED—cont'd

View Video!

STEP	RATIONALE
g. Gently lean patient as a unit back toward pillows for support.	Ensures continued straight alignment of spinal column, preventing injury.
7. Once patient is repositioned be sure nurse call system is in an accessible location within patient's reach. Perform hand hygiene.	Ensures patient safety. Reduces transmission of microorganisms.

EVALUATION

1. Assess patient's body alignment, position, and level of comfort. Patient's body should be supported by adequate mattress, and vertebral column should be without observable curves.	Determines effectiveness of positioning. Additional supports (e.g., pillows, bath blankets) may be added or removed to promote comfort and correct body alignment.
2. Measure ROM of affected joints.	Determines if joint contracture is developing.
3. Observe for areas of erythema or breakdown involving skin.	Provides ongoing observation regarding patient's skin and musculoskeletal system. Indicates complications of immobility or improper positioning of body part.
4. **Use Teach-Back:**"I want to be sure I explained the steps we are going to use to move and position you in bed. Can you repeat the steps you can follow to move up in bed?" Revise your instruction now or develop a plan for revised patient/family caregiver teaching if patient/family caregiver is not able to teach back correctly.	Determines patient's/family caregiver's level of understanding of instructional topic.

RECORDING AND REPORTING

- Record time and position change of patient throughout shift, observations (e.g., condition of skin, joint movement, patient's ability to assist with positioning), and whether positioning devices were needed in electronic health record (EHR) or chart.

- Record your evaluation of patient/caregiver learning.
- Report observations at change of shift and document in nurses' notes in EHR or chart.

UNEXPECTED OUTCOMES AND RELATED INTERVENTIONS

- Joint contractures develop or worsen.
  - Increase frequency of ROM exercises to affected and immobilized areas.
  - Consider PT consultation for different positioning.
- Skin shows localized areas of erythema and breakdown.
  - Increase frequency of repositioning.
  - Place turning schedule above patient's bed.

- Patient avoids moving.
  - Medicate with analgesia as ordered by health care provider to ensure patient's comfort before moving.
  - Allow pain medication to take effect before repositioning.

▮ KEY POINTS

- Normal physical mobility depends on intact functioning nervous and musculoskeletal systems.
- Findings from evidence-based nursing research indicate that safe patient handling prevents injuries to nurses and patients when moving patients.
- The assessment of an immobilized patient includes review of body systems likely affected; the patient's risks for falls; and complications of immobility, pain, and psychosocial and developmental factors.

- Immobility results from illness or trauma or is prescribed for therapeutic reasons; it presents hazards in the physical, psychological, and developmental dimensions.
- Pressure injuries and deep vein thrombosis (DVT), although often preventable, are two of the most common physical hazards of immobility.
- Effects of immobility include depression, behavioral changes, changes in the sleep-wake cycle, decreased coping abilities, and developmental delays.
- Patient-handling tasks most frequently associated with low back pain are lifting and forceful movements.

- Patients with impaired body alignment require nursing interventions to maintain them in the supported Fowler's, supine, prone, 30-degree side-lying, and Sims' positions.
- The clinical signs of a DVT may be silent, but when symptoms are present a DVT is characterized by unilateral redness, tenderness, and edema over a calf or thigh.
- Adequate hydration reduces immobility-related complications in the respiratory and elimination systems.
- Elastic antiembolic stockings, sequential compression devices, and mobile compression devices improve venous return and help prevent the potentially life-threatening complication of DVT.
- The primary evaluation criterion for nursing care in the developmental dimension for immobilized patients is the prevention of any measurable decline in functioning or delay in development.

REFLECTIVE LEARNING

- Reflect on a recent clinical experience where a patient needed to ambulate but was not able because of voiced complaints of pain and describe what interventions you implemented.
- Recall any challenges in patient repositioning experienced during a clinical day and describe any safe patient-handling techniques you applied.
- Reflect on a patient experience you encountered today and describe the risks the patient had because of reduced mobility.

REVIEW QUESTIONS

1. An older adult has limited mobility as a result of a total knee replacement. During assessment you note that the patient has difficulty breathing while lying flat. Which of the following assessment data support a possible pulmonary problem related to impaired mobility? (Select all that apply.)
   1. Blood pressure 128/84 mm Hg
   2. Respirations 26 per minute on room air
   3. Heart rate 114 beats/min
   4. Crackles heard on auscultation
   5. Pain reported as 3 on scale of 0 to 10 after medication

2. A patient is receiving 5000 units of heparin subcutaneously every 12 hours to prevent venous thromboembolism while on prolonged bed rest. Because bleeding is a potential side effect of this medication, the nurse should continually assess the patient for which findings? (Select all that apply.)
   1. Increased bruising
   2. Pale yellow urine
   3. Bleeding gums
   4. Guaiac-positive stools
   5. Skin turgor

3. The nurse observes the NAP apply and monitor a patient's sequential compression device (SCD) appropriately when the following is observed.
   1. Initial patient measurement is made around the calves.
   2. NAP verifies fit of SCD by placing two fingers between patient's leg and SCD sleeve.
   3. Sleeves are wrapped directly over the leg from ankle to knee.
   4. NAP removes SCD sleeves every 2 hours during placement.

4. The effects of immobility on the cardiac system include which findings? (Select all that apply.)
   1. Thrombus formation
   2. Increased cardiac workload
   3. Weak peripheral pulses
   4. Orthostatic hypotension
   5. Increased stroke volume

5. Identify the order in which elastic stockings should be applied.
   1. Evaluate skin integrity and circulation.
   2. Identify patient using at least two identifiers.
   3. Pull the remainder of the stocking over the patient's heel and on up the leg.
   4. Turn the stocking inside out holding heel.
   5. Slide stocking over patient's foot, making sure that toes are covered.
   6. Assess condition of patient's skin.
   7. Use tape measure to measure patient's legs to determine proper stocking size.

evolve

Additional Review Questions, as well as rationales for all Review Questions, can be found on the Evolve website.

1, 2, 3, 4; 2, 1, 3, 4; 3, 2; 4, 1, 2, 4; 5, 2, 6, 7, 4, 5, 3, 1.

REFERENCES

Agency for Healthcare Research and Quality (AHRQ): *Pressure injury prevention and treatment*, 2014. http://www.ahrq.gov/professionals/systems/hospital/pressureulcertoolkit/index.html.

American Association of Critical-Care Nurses (AACN): *Early progressive mobility protocol*, 2013. https://www.aacn.org/docs/EventPlanning/WB0007/Mobility-Protocol-szh4mr5a.pdf.

American Heart Association (AHA): *What is venous thromboembolism (VTE)?* 2015. http://www.heart.org/HEARTORG/Conditions/More/What-is-Venous-Thromboembolism-VTE_UCM_479052_Article.jsp#.WHjsvEszWpo.

American Heart Association (AHA): *A patient's guide to taking warfarin*, 2016. http://www.heart.org/HEARTORG/Conditions/Arrhythmia/PreventionTreatmentofArrhythmia/A-Patients-Guide-to-Taking-Warfarin_UCM_444996_Article.jsp#.WHj0X0szWpo.

American Nurses Association (ANA): *ANA leads initiative to develop national safe patient handling standards*, 2012. http://www.nursingworld.org/FunctionalMenuCategories/MediaResources/PressReleases/2012-PR/ANA-Leads-National-Safe-Patient-Handling-Standards.pdf.

American Nurses Association (ANA): *Nursing: scope and standards of practice*, ed 3, ANA, 2015, Silver Spring, MD.

American Nurses Association (ANA): *Handle with care fact sheet*, 2016. http://www.nursingworld.org/MainMenuCategories/ANAMarketplace/Factsheets-and-Toolkits/FactSheet.html.

American Occupational Therapy Association (AOTA): *Occupational therapy: improving function while controlling costs*, 2017. http://www.aota.org/About-Occupational-Therapy/Professionals.aspx.

American Physical Therapy Association (APTA): *Role of a physical therapist*, 2016. http://www.apta.org/PTCareers/RoleofaPT/.

Anders J, et al: Decubitus ulcers: pathophysiology and primary prevention, *Dtsch Arztebl Int* 107(21):371, 2010.

Anderson MP, et al: Safe moving and handling of patients: an interprofessional approach, *Nurs Stand* 28(46):37, 2014.

Behrendt R, et al: Continuous bedside pressure mapping and rates of hospital-associated pressure ulcers in a medical intensive care unit, *Am J Crit Care* 23(2):127, 2014.

Bulechek GM, et al, editors: *Nursing interventions classification (NIC)*, ed 6, St Louis, 2013, Mosby.

Centers for Disease Control and Prevention (CDC): *Venous thromboembolism (blood clots)*, 2015. http://www.cdc.gov/ncbddd/dvt/facts.html.

Chmelo EA, et al: Heterogeneity of physical function response to exercises training in older adults, *J Am Geriatr Soc* 63(3):462, 2015.

Colwell CW Jr, et al: Thrombosis prevention after total hip arthroplasty, *J Bone Joint Surg Am* 92(3):527, 2010.

Colwell CW Jr: What is the state of the art in orthopaedic thromboprophylaxis in lower extremity reconstruction? *Instr Course Lect* 60:283, 2011.

Department of Health and Human Services (DHHS): *Safe patient handling & lifting standards for a safer American workforce*, 2010. http://www.help.senate.gov/imo/media/doc/Collins4.pdf.

Dobkin BH, Dorsch A: New evidence for therapies in stroke rehabilitation, *Curr Atheroscler Rep* 15(6):331, 2013.

Falvey JR, et al: Rethinking hospital-associated deconditioning: proposed paradigm shift, *Phys Ther* 95(9):1307, 2015.

Frith J, et al: Measuring and defining orthostatic hypotension in the older person, *Age Ageing* 43(2):168, 2014.

Goodwin VA, et al: Multiple component interventions for preventing falls and fall-related injuries among older people: systematic review and meta-analysis, *BMC Geriatr* 14:15, 2014.

Guo LL, et al: Evaluation of two observational pain assessment scales during the anesthesia recovery period in Chinese surgical older adults, *J Clin Nurs* 24(1/2):212, 2015.

Harvey LA, et al: Continuous passive motion after knee replacement surgery, *Cochrane Database Syst Rev* (2):CD004260, 2014. http://www.cochrane.org/CD004260/MUSKEL_continuous-passive-motion-after-knee-replacement-surgery.

Henderson WR, et al: Does prone positioning improve oxygenation and reduce mortality in patients with acute respiratory distress syndrome?, *Can Respir J* 21(4):213, 2014.

Herdman TH, Kamitsuru S, editors: *NANDA International nursing diagnoses: definitions & classification 2015-2017*, Oxford, 2014, Wiley Blackwell.

Hockenberry M, Wilson D: *Wong's nursing care of infants and children*, ed 10, St Louis, 2015, Mosby.

Huether S, McCance K: *Understanding pathophysiology*, ed 6, St Louis, 2017, Mosby.

Lewis L, et al: *Medical-surgical nursing: assessment and management of clinical problems*, ed 9, St Louis, 2014, Elsevier.

Mills P, et al: Five things to know about orthostatic hypotension and aging, *J Am Geriatr Soc* 62(9):1822, 2014.

Modi S, et al: Wells criteria for DVT is a reliable clinical tool to assess the risk of deep venous thrombosis in trauma patients, *World J Emerg Surg* 11:24, 2016.

Nam D, et al: Mobile compression devices and aspirin for VTE prophylaxis following simultaneous bilateral total knee arthroplasty, *J Arthroplasty* 30:447, 2015.

National Pressure Ulcer Advisory Panel (NPUAP): *National Pressure Ulcer Advisory Panel (NPUAP) announces a change in terminology from pressure ulcer to pressure injury and updates the stages of pressure injury*, 2016. https://www.npuap.org/national-pressure-ulcer-advisory-panel-npuap-announces-a-change-in-terminology-from-pressure-ulcer-to-pressure-injury-and-updates-the-stages-of-pressure-injury/.

Owiti JA, et al: Cultural consultation as a model for training multidisciplinary mental healthcare professionals in cultural competence skills: preliminary results, *J Psychiatr Ment Health Nurs* 21(9):814, 2014.

Parker K: Psychosocial effects of living with a leg ulcer, *Nurs Stand* 26(45):52, 2012.

Parreira RB, et al: Older adults present better back endurance than young adults during a dynamic trunk extension exercise, *J Back Musculoskelet Rehabil* 27(2):153, 2014.

Pasero C, McCaffery M: *Pain assessment and pharmacologic management*, St Louis, 2011, Elsevier.

Perry AG, et al: *Clinical nursing skills and techniques*, ed 9, St Louis, 2017, Elsevier.

Poppler L, et al: Subclinical peroneal neuropathy: a common, unrecognized, and preventable finding associated with a recent history of falling in hospitalized patients, *Ann Fam Med* 14(6):526, 2016.

Pritchett JW, et al: *Foot drop*, Medscape 2016, http://emedicine.medscape.com/article/1234607-overview.

Purnell L: *Guide to culturally competent health care*, ed 3, Philadelphia, 2014, FA Davis.

Royal Berkshire NHS Foundation Trust: *Exercises during bedrest*, 2016. http://www.royalberkshire.nhs.uk/patient-information-leaflets/Therapies/bed-rest-exercises—physiotherapy-march-2014.htm.

Schofield PA: The assessment and management of peri-operative pain in older adults, *Anaesthesia* 6(1):54, 2014.

Skinner N, Moran P: *CMAG: deep vein thrombosis*, Case Management Society of America, 2007. http://www.cmsa.org/portals/0/pdf/CMAG_DVT.pdf.

Southerland LT, Barrie M: *Fractures in older adults*, Trauma Reports, 2014. https://www.ahcmedia.com/articles/118940-fractures-in-older-adults.

Staggs VS, et al: Challenges in defining and categorizing falls on diverse unit types, *J Nurs Care Qual* 30(2):106, 2015.

Stevenson JM: Looking forward by looking back: helping to reduce work-related musculoskeletal disorders, *Work* 47(1):137, 2014.

Stewart C: What do we mean by "older adults' persistent pain self-management":

a concept analysis, *Pain Med* 15(2):214, 2014.

Swafford K, et al: Use of a comprehensive program to reduce the incidence of hospital-acquired pressure ulcers in an intensive care unit, *Am J Crit Care* 25(2):152, 2016.

The Joint Commission (TJC): *2018 National Patient Safety Goals*, Oakbrook Terrace, IL, 2018, The Commission, http://www.jointcommission.org/standards_information/npsgs.aspx.

Titler MG, et al: The effect of a translating research into practice intervention to promote use of evidence-based fall prevention interventions in hospitalized adults: a prospective pre-post implementation study in the U.S., *Appl Nurs Res* 31:52–59, 2016.

Topfer L: Portable compression to prevent venous thromboembolism after hip and knee surgery: the ActiveCare System. In *CADTH issues in emerging health technologies*, 2016. https://www.ncbi.nlm.nih.gov/books/NBK378970/.

Touhy T, Jett K: *Ebersole and Hess' gerontological nursing and healthy aging*, ed 4, St Louis, 2014, Mosby.

United Health Care (UHC): *TechFlash: ActiveCare+SFT® portable compression device for venous thromboembolism prevention after joint arthroplasty*, 2012. http://www.njha.com/media/41054/vte_1_techflash.pdf.

VISN8 Patient Safety Center (VISN8): *Safe patient handling and movement algorithms*, 2014. https://cseany.org/wp-content/uploads/2014/02/SPHMALGORITHMS.PDF.

Wells PS, et al: Use of a clinical model for safe management of patients with suspected pulmonary embolism, *Ann Intern Med* 129(12):997, 1998.

Whittemore D, Sauda V: *Pain management in older adults*, 2015. http://www.une.edu/sites/default/files/Pain%20Management%20PracticesDeb%20W%20and%20Val%20.pdf.

Wong H, et al: Efficacy of a pressure-sensing mattress cover system for reducing interface pressure: study protocol for a randomized controlled trial, *Trials* 16:434, 2015.

Wound Ostomy and Continence Nurses Society (WOCN): *Pressure ulcer reduction case study*, 2013. http://c.ymcdn.com/sites/www.wocn.org/resource/resmgr/Publications/WOC_Nurse_Utilizes_Skin_Care.pdf.

Wrobleski DM, et al: Discharge planning rounds to the bedside: a patent- and family-centered approach, *Medsurg Nurs* 23(2):111, 2014.

evolve MEDIA RESOURCES

http://evolve.elsevier.com/Potter/essentials
- Audio Glossary
- QSEN Activity and Review Questions Answers and Rationales
- Video Clips

OBJECTIVES

- Describe environmental hazards that pose risks to patient safety.
- Discuss the importance of national patient safety resources and standards for promoting patient safety.
- Describe factors that create a culture of safety.
- Describe the nurse's role in prevention of serious reportable events.
- Assess risks to patients' safety within health care settings and the home.
- Identify relevant nursing diagnoses associated with risks to safety.

- Explain approaches for establishing a restraint-free environment.
- Identify factors to consider in the use of restraints.
- Develop a nursing care plan for patients whose safety is threatened.
- Describe developmentally appropriate nursing interventions for reducing risks for falls, fires, poisonings, and electrical hazards.
- Describe methods to evaluate interventions designed to maintain or promote patient safety.
- Describe approaches to reducing violence in the health care workplace.

KEY TERMS

carbon monoxide, p. 785
chemical restraints, p. 799
heat exhaustion, p. 786
hypothermia, p. 786

immunization, p. 787
pathogen, p. 787
restraint, p. 799

serious reportable events (SREs),
  p. 783
workplace violence, p. 790

Patient safety is the most pressing issue facing health care today. The Institute of Medicine (IOM) report (2000), *To Err Is Human: Building a Safer Health System,* was a pivotal publication that brought patient safety to the forefront of health care in the United States. The report indicated that 44,000 to 98,000 people die each year as a result of preventable medical errors. Shortly thereafter, the IOM published a second book, *Crossing the Quality Chasm: A New Healthcare System for the 21st Century* (IOM, 2001).

The second report recommended fundamental changes in the organization and delivery of health care in the United States. The report also identified the need to focus on introducing processes and approaches for improving the quality of care delivered to patients. This included forming new rules to redesign and improve health care, building organizational supports for change, applying evidence to health care delivery, and using information technology.

CASE STUDY *Mr. Gonzales*

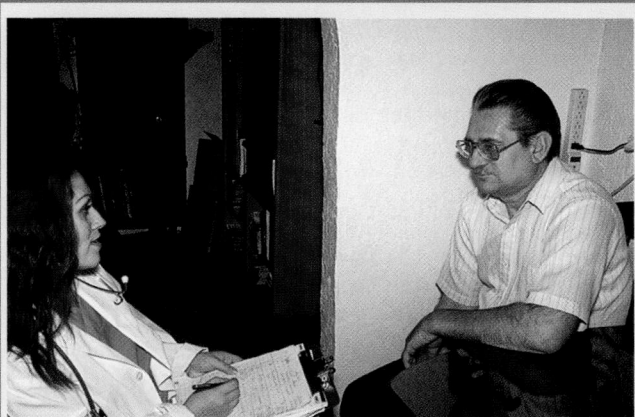

Mr. Gonzales is a 73-year-old man who has lived alone in a senior apartment building since his wife died 6 months ago. He and his wife were born in Mexico but came to live in the United States shortly after they were married. He is retired from a produce warehouse where he worked for 42 years. He and his wife raised three sons. Carlos, the son who lives the closest, is 30 minutes away by car. Carlos visits Mr. Gonzales every week to socialize and take him shopping. Mr. Gonzales is generally healthy but takes medication for high blood pressure. He also has decreased visual acuity, hearing loss from the noisy warehouse job, and some "arthritis" in his knees. He expects to live at least as long as his father, who lived to be 92 years old. Since his wife's death, Mr. Gonzales has attended Catholic mass every day at his parish church, where his wife had attended daily.

Joani Green, a 25-year-old married mother of two, is currently a nursing student at the local college. As part of the clinical requirements, she and her study partner are conducting health screenings and providing health promotion education for the residents of the apartment building where Mr. Gonzales lives. Part of her screening will include safety screenings and risk assessment of Mr. Gonzales' home environment.

BOX 30.1 THE JOINT COMMISSION 2018 HOSPITAL NATIONAL PATIENT SAFETY GOALS

- **Identify patients correctly.**
  - Use at least two ways to identify patients.
  - Make sure that the correct patient gets the correct blood.
- **Improve staff communication.**
  - Get important test results to the right staff person on time.
- **Use medicines safely.**
  - Before a procedure, label medicines that are not labeled.
  - Take extra care with patients who take medicines to thin their blood.
  - Record and pass along correct information about a patient's medicines.
- **Use alarms safely.**
  - Make improvements to ensure that alarms on medical equipment are heard and responded to on time.
- **Prevent infection.**
  - Use hand cleansing guidelines from the Centers for Disease Control and Prevention or the World Health Organization.
  - Use proven guidelines to prevent infections that are difficult to treat.
  - Use proven guidelines to prevent infection of the blood from central lines.
  - Use proven guidelines to prevent infection after surgery.
  - Use proven guidelines to prevent infections of the urinary tract that are caused by catheters.
- **Identify patient safety risks.**
  - Find out which patients are most likely to try to commit suicide.
- **Prevent mistakes in surgery.**
  - Make sure that the correct surgery is done on the correct patient and at the correct place on the patient's body.
  - Mark the correct place on the patient's body where the surgery is to be done. Pause before the surgery to make sure that a mistake is not being made.

From The Joint Commission (TJC): *2018 National Patient Safety Goals,* Oakbrook Terrace, IL, 2018, The Commission. https://www.jointcommission.org/assets/1/6/2018_HAP_NPSG_goals_final.pdf.

Much of the force behind the changes for improving safety in health care settings comes from regulatory and accreditation agencies. The Joint Commission (TJC) and the Centers for Medicare and Medicaid Services (CMS) stress the importance of error prevention and patient safety. The Speak Up campaign encourages patients to take a role in preventing health care errors by becoming active, involved, and informed participants in their health care (TJC, 2017b). For example, patients are encouraged to ask health care workers if they have washed their hands before providing care. The 2017 TJC National Patient Safety Goals (Box 30.1) are specifically directed at reducing the risk of medical errors.

The National Quality Forum (NQF, 2017a) has the mission of improving the quality of health care in the United States. The NQF focuses on building consensus on national priorities and goals for performance improvement in health care. The organization also endorses national consensus standards for measuring and publicly reporting the performances of

health care institutions. The *National Voluntary Consensus Standards for Public Reporting of Patient Safety Events* (NQF, 2011) is a report that offers a framework for publicly reporting patient safety events, indicators, and measures about health care organizations to consumers. The NQF patient safety measures (e.g., falls with injury, incidence of pressure injuries, and central line–associated bloodstream infections) are standards for judging health care quality. These measures are also used by organizations such as TJC and CMS. The NQF also endorses an updated list of 29 serious reportable events (SREs) (Box 30.2) that are a major focus for patient safety initiatives (NQF, 2017b). CMS now denies payment to hospitals for any hospital-acquired conditions resulting from or complicated by the occurrence of certain SREs that were

BOX 30.2 NATIONAL QUALITY FORUM LIST OF SERIOUS REPORTABLE EVENTS

SURGICAL OR INVASIVE PROCEDURE EVENTS
- Surgery or other invasive procedure performed on wrong site
- Surgery or other invasive procedure performed on wrong patient
- Wrong surgical or other invasive procedure performed on patient
- Unintended retention of foreign object in patient after surgery or other invasive procedure
- Intraoperative or immediately postoperative/postprocedure death in ASA class 1 patient

PRODUCT OR DEVICE EVENTS
- Patient death or serious injury associated with use of contaminated drugs, devices, or biologicals provided by health care setting
- Patient death or serious injury associated with use or function of a device in patient care in which device is used for functions other than intended
- Patient death or serious injury associated with intravascular air embolism that occurs while being cared for in health care setting

PATIENT PROTECTION EVENTS
- Discharge or release of patient/resident of any age who is unable to make decisions to other than authorized person
- Patient death or serious injury associated with patient elopement (disappearance)
- Patient suicide, attempted suicide, or self-harm that results in serious injury while being cared for in health care setting

CARE MANAGEMENT EVENTS
- Patient death or serious injury associated with medication error (e.g., errors involving wrong drug, wrong dose, wrong patient, wrong time, wrong rate, wrong preparation, or wrong route of administration)
- Patient death or serious injury associated with unsafe administration of blood products
- Maternal death or serious injury associated with labor or delivery in low-risk pregnancy while being cared for in health care setting
- Death or serious injury of neonate associated with labor or delivery in low-risk pregnancy

- Patient death or serious injury associated with a fall while being cared for in health care setting
- Any stage 3, stage 4, and unstageable pressure injuries acquired after admission/presentation to health care setting
- Artificial insemination with wrong donor sperm or wrong egg
- Patient death or serious injury resulting from irretrievable loss of irreplaceable biological specimen
- Patient death or serious injury resulting from failure to follow up or communicate laboratory, pathology, or radiology test results

ENVIRONMENTAL EVENTS
- Patient or staff death or serious injury associated with electric shock in the course of patient care process in health care setting
- Any incident in which system that is designated for oxygen or other gas to be delivered to patient contains no gas or wrong gas or is contaminated by toxic substances
- Patient or staff death or serious injury associated with a burn incurred from any source in the course of patient care process in health care setting
- Patient death or serious injury associated with use of physical restraints or bedrails while being cared for in health care setting

RADIOLOGIC EVENTS
- Death or serious injury of patient or staff associated with introduction of metallic object into magnetic resonance imaging (MRI) area

POTENTIAL CRIMINAL EVENTS
- Any instance of care ordered or provided by someone impersonating physician, nurse, pharmacist, or other licensed health care provider
- Abduction of patient/resident of any age
- Sexual abuse/assault on patient or staff member within or on grounds of health care setting
- Death or serious injury of patient or staff member resulting from physical assault (i.e., battery) that occurs within or on grounds of health care setting

Copyright © 2018 National Quality Forum.

not present on admission (Box 30.3). Some hospital-acquired conditions are nurse-sensitive indicators, meaning that nursing interventions directly affect their development.

Health care organizations strive to create a culture of safety, where adverse events are consistently minimized despite carrying out complex and hazardous work (AHRQ, 2016). A culture of safety requires a commitment that acknowledges the high-risk nature of the activities of an organization, the decision to focus on achieving consistently safe operations, a just culture in which individuals can report errors without fear or reprimand, and an organizational commitment of resources. These organizations foster a patient-centered just culture by continually focusing on performance improvement efforts, empowering employees

to actively participate in the safety activities of the organization, risk-management findings, and safety reports to design a safe work environment (see Chapter 7) (Boysen, 2013). A safer work environment requires all staff to receive continuing education and have access to appropriate resources (Box 30.4).

As part of the health care team, you have the professional responsibility to engage in activities that support a patient-centered safety culture. Quality and Safety Education for Nurses (QSEN) was developed to meet the challenge of preparing future nurses to have the knowledge, skills, and attitudes needed to continuously improve the quality and safety of the health care systems where they work (QSEN Institute, 2017). The QSEN safety competency requires you

BOX 30.3 **2016 CENTERS FOR MEDICARE AND MEDICAID SERVICES HOSPITAL-ACQUIRED CONDITIONS AND PRESENT-ON-ADMISSION INDICATORS**

- Foreign object retained after surgery
- Air embolism
- Blood incompatibility
- Stage 3 and stage 4 pressure ulcers
- Falls and trauma: fracture, dislocation, intracranial injury, crushing injury, burn, other injuries
- Manifestations of poor glycemic control: diabetic keto-acidosis, nonketotic hyperosmolar coma, hypoglycemic coma, secondary diabetes with ketoacidosis, and secondary diabetes with hyperosmolarity
- Catheter-associated urinary tract infections
- Vascular catheter-associated infections
- Surgical site infection, mediastinitis, following coronary artery bypass graft (CABG)
- Surgical site infection following bariatric surgery for obesity: laparoscopic gastric bypass, gastroenterostomy, laparoscopic gastric restrictive surgery
- Surgical site infection following certain orthopedic procedures: spine, neck, shoulder, elbow
- Surgical site infection following cardiac implantable electronic device (CIED)
- Deep vein thrombosis and pulmonary embolism following certain orthopedic procedures: total knee replacement or hip replacement
- Iatrogenic pneumothorax with venous catheterization

From Centers for Medicare and Medicaid Services (CMS): *Hospital-acquired conditions,* 2012, http://www.cms.gov/Medicare/Medicare-Fee-for-Service-Payment/HospitalAcqCond/Hospital-Acquired_Conditions.html.

to "minimize risk of harm to patients and providers through both system effectiveness and individual performance." Use of critical thinking skills (see Chapter 8) coupled with application of the nursing process (see Chapter 9) enables you to become a provider of safe patient care and an active participant in health promotion.

SCIENTIFIC KNOWLEDGE BASE

Safety (i.e., freedom from psychological and physical injury) is a basic human need. Health care provided in a safe manner and within a safe community environment is essential for well-being of patients. Vulnerable groups that require help in achieving a safe environment include infants, children, older adults, ill or injured people, people with physical and mental disabilities, people who are illiterate, and people who live in poverty. To be effective, you need to understand factors that contribute to a safe environment in the home or health care agency and be able to thoroughly assess the environment for threats to safety. Understanding how alterations in mobility, sensory function, and cognition affect patients' safety is also important (see Chapters 29 and 39). A safe environment

BOX 30.4 **RESOURCES RELATED TO SAFETY AND SAFETY INITIATIVES**

- The Joint Commission: http://www.jointcommission.org/topics/patient_safety.aspx
- Agency for Healthcare Research and Quality: http://www.psnet.ahrq.gov
- Institute for Healthcare Improvement: http://www.ihi.org/ihi
- U.S. Department of Veterans Affairs: http://www.patientsafety.va.gov/
- Centers for Medicare and Medicaid Services: http://www.cms.gov
- Quality Improvement Organization Support Center: http://www.qualitynet.org
- National Quality Forum: http://www.qualityforum.org/Home.aspx
- ECRI Institute: http://www.ecri.org

includes meeting basic human needs, reducing physical hazards, and reducing transmission of pathogens.

Basic Human Needs

The physiological needs of adequate oxygen, nutrition, and favorable temperature and humidity are basic human needs often at risk from various environmental hazards. People need to meet these basic needs before physical and psychological safety and security can be addressed.

Oxygen. Patients who require supplemental oxygen in health care settings can be at risk because oxygen is highly flammable. Fire can occur when oxygen therapy is combined with smoking or exposure to a heat source, which can cause severe burns or death. Strict codes regulate the use and storage of medical oxygen in health care agencies. This is not the case in the home environment. In the home, smoking combined with home oxygen use is by far the leading cause of burns, reported fires, deaths, and injuries. Be sure to administer oxygen safely and provide patients and family caregivers the information needed to manage oxygen in the home (see Chapter 32).

Know factors in a patient's environment that decrease the amount of available oxygen. For example, an improperly functioning heating system is a hazard in the home. A furnace, stove, or fireplace that is not properly vented introduces carbon monoxide into the environment. Carbon monoxide affects a person's oxygenation by binding strongly with hemoglobin, preventing the formation of oxyhemoglobin, and reducing the supply of oxygen delivered to the tissues (see Chapter 32). Low concentrations of oxygen cause nausea, dizziness, headache, and fatigue. Higher concentrations are often fatal. Unintentional, non–fire-related (UNFR) carbon monoxide poisoning is one of the most common causes of poisoning in the United States and results in approximately 15,000 emergency department visits annually (Centers for Disease Control and Prevention [CDC], 2011).

Nutrition. Meeting nutritional needs requires knowledge about healthy food and food safety. Chapter 35 details the principles of balanced nutrition and therapeutic diets. Health care agencies are required to meet State Board of Health regulations for storage, preparation, and provision of food. In the home some patients do not know how to properly refrigerate, store, and prepare food. A patient needs a refrigerator with a freezer compartment to keep perishable foods fresh. An adequate, clean water supply is necessary for drinking and to wash fresh produce and dishes. Regular garbage collection is necessary to maintain sanitary conditions. Foods need to be adequately cooked to kill any residing organisms. If a patient does not prepare or store foods properly, it increases the risk for infections and food poisoning from bacteria such as *Escherichia coli, Salmonella,* or *Listeria.* Groups at highest risk for food poisoning are children, pregnant women, older adults, and people with compromised immune systems.

Temperature. A person's comfort zone is usually between 18.3°C and 23.8°C (65° F and 75° F). Temperature extremes, which often occur during the winter and summer, affect comfort, productivity, and safety. Exposure to severe cold for prolonged periods may cause frostbite and accidental **hypothermia** (see Chapter 15). Older adults, infants, young children, patients with cardiovascular conditions, patients who have ingested drugs or excess alcohol, and people who are homeless are at high risk for hypothermia. Prolonged exposure to extreme heat changes body electrolyte balance and raises the core body temperature, resulting in heatstroke or **heat exhaustion.** People of any age can be at risk for heat exhaustion when the weather is extremely hot, regardless of humidity.

Physical Hazards

More than 31.7 million nonfatal injuries take place each year, with most occurring inside or outside of the home (CDC, 2017c). Physical hazards in the environment threaten a person's safety and often result in physical or psychological injury or death. Unintentional injuries are the fourth leading cause of death for Americans of all ages (Kochanek et al., 2016). Motor vehicle accidents are the leading cause, followed by poisonings and falls. Additional environmental hazards include fire and disasters. Your role as a nurse is to educate patients about common safety hazards and how to prevent injury, while placing emphasis on hazards to which patients are more vulnerable.

Motor Vehicle Accidents. Vehicle design and equipment such as seat belts, air bags, and laminated windshields that remain in one piece when impacted have improved vehicular safety. State laws relating to licensing of young drivers, safety belt use, child restraint use, and motorcycle helmets exist for protection of drivers. It is important that children ride in child safety seats and booster seats appropriate for their age and weight and the type of car. The American Academy of Pediatrics (AAP, 2017) recommends the following:

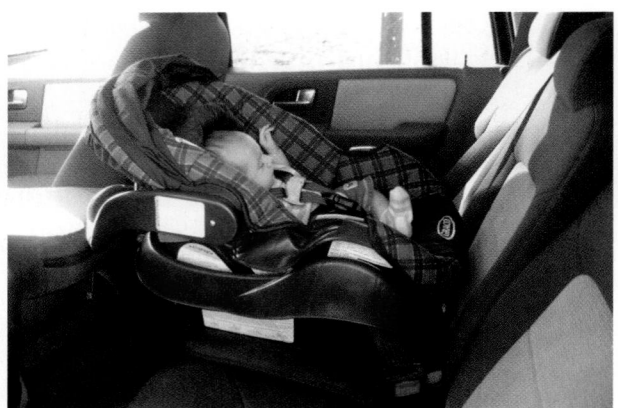

FIG 30.1 Rear-facing infant car seat. (Courtesy Brian and Mayannyn Sallee, Las Vegas, NV.)

1. All infants and toddlers should ride in a rear-facing car safety seat (CSS) until they are 2 years of age or until they reach the highest weight or height allowed by the manufacturer of their CSS.
2. Children who have outgrown the rear-facing weight or height limit for their CSS should use a forward-facing CSS with a harness for as long as possible, up to the highest weight or height allowed by the manufacturer of their CSS.
3. All children whose weight or height exceeds the forward-facing limit for their CSS should use a belt-positioning booster seat until the vehicle seat belt fits properly, typically when they have reached 4 feet 9 inches in height and are between 8 and 12 years of age. All children younger than 13 years of age should ride in the back seat.
4. When children are old enough and large enough for the vehicle seat belt to fit them correctly, they should always use lap-and-shoulder seat belts for the best protection.

Nearly all cars and trucks made after September 2002 are equipped with a LATCH (Lower Anchors and Tethers for Children) system for installing child safety seats (Fig. 30.1). There are lower anchors in the back seat where the seat cushions meet and tether anchors located behind the seat either on the panel behind the seat or seat back, ceiling or floor. All lower anchors are rated for a maximum weight of 65 lb (total weight includes car seat and child) (AAP, 2017).

According to the CDC, the risk of motor vehicle accidents is higher among 16- to 19-year-old drivers than any other age-group (CDC, 2017b). Teens tend to underestimate dangerous situations or are unable to recognize hazardous situations (e.g., texting while driving). In addition, they tend to speed and allow shorter headways, ride with intoxicated drivers, and drive after using alcohol and drugs. Teens have the lowest rate of seat belt use. Elderly drivers are keeping their licenses longer and driving more miles than in the past. Age-related decline in vision and cognitive functioning (ability to reason and remember) and physical changes affect driving abilities of some older adults (CDC, 2017d). On the positive side, older adults have a higher incidence of seat belt usage, they tend to drive when road conditions are the safest, and they are less likely to drink under the influence of alcohol.

Poison. A poison is any substance that impairs health or destroys life when ingested, inhaled, or absorbed by the body. Almost any substance is potentially poisonous if too much is taken. Poisons impair the function of every major organ system. Health care providers are at risk from chemicals such as chemotherapy drugs and toxic cleaning agents. Sources of poison in people's homes include medicines, other solid and liquid substances, gases, and vapors. Toddlers, preschoolers, and young school-age children have a greater risk for accidental poisoning in the home because they often ingest household cleaning solutions, medications, or personal hygiene products. Emergency treatment is needed when a person ingests a poisonous substance or comes in contact with a chemical that is absorbed through the skin. A poison control center is the best resource for patients and parents needing information about the treatment of an accidental poisoning. The American Association of Poison Control Centers supports the 55 poison centers in the United States to prevent and treat poison exposures. Poison centers offer free, confidential medical advice 24 hours a day, 7 days a week through the Poison Help line at 1-800-222-1222.

Fire. Home fires are a major cause of death and injury. In 2014 U.S. fire departments responded to 367,500 home structure fires, which caused 11,825 civilian injuries and 2745 civilian deaths (Ahrens, 2015). Smoking materials such as cigarettes, cigars, and pipes are a primary source of home fires. Many fatal fires result from individuals falling asleep while smoking in bed or a failure to keep fresh batteries in home smoke detectors. The improper use of cooking equipment and appliances, particularly stoves, is another source for in-home fires. Smoke detectors and carbon monoxide detectors need to be placed strategically throughout a home. Multipurpose fire extinguishers need to be near the kitchen and any workshop areas.

Falls. Among adults 65 years of age and older, falls in the home are the leading cause of unintentional death (CDC, 2017a). Common physical hazards that lead to falls in the home include inadequate lighting, barriers along normal walking paths and stairs, and a lack of safety devices (e.g., walkers or handrails). Falls often involve accidental contact with objects on stairs or floors and low-standing furniture. Falls can result in serious injury such as fractures or internal bleeding depending on the height of the fall, body position on impact, and impact surface.

Disasters. Serious injury or death may result when a natural disaster such as a flood, hurricane, tornado, or wildfire strikes. These types of disasters can also leave many people homeless. Bombings, another type of disaster, are a likely form of a terrorist attack to occur (Terrorism Research, n.d.). National preparedness for all disasters has progressed during the last decade. Hospitals have plans and drills for internal and external disasters (Veenema et al., 2016). Medical and public health professionals have joined the disaster preparedness community, the U.S. federal government has increased investment in preparedness, and community partners and participants are involved in disaster preparedness (Inglesby, 2011).

Pathogen Transmission. Pathogens and parasites pose a threat to patient safety. A pathogen is any microorganism capable of producing an illness. The most common means of transmission of pathogens is by the hands. The most effective way to limit the transmission of pathogens is the medical aseptic practice of hand hygiene. Pathogens are also transmitted through human blood and body fluids and by insects (e.g., mosquitoes carrying malaria) and rodents (see Chapter 14).

Health care agencies need to properly process biohazardous wastes (e.g., needles, surgical dressings, sharps and syringes) to prevent the risk for pathogen exposure to the general population and employees. You also need to clean or dispose of bed linens and patient gowns contaminated by body fluids in proper containers to reduce potential exposure to pathogens.

Immunization. Immunization is the process by which resistance to an infectious disease is produced or increased. The body acquires active immunity after a small amount of weakened or dead organisms and modified toxins from the organism (toxoids) is injected into the body. Passive immunity occurs when antibodies produced by other people or animals are introduced into a person's bloodstream for protection against a pathogen. Nurses must know immunization guidelines and inform members of the public about the importance of immunization in maintaining the health of their children and themselves.

Pollution. A healthy environment is free of pollutants (i.e., harmful chemical or waste materials discharged into the water, soil, or air). Air pollution is the contamination of the atmosphere with a harmful chemical. Prolonged exposure to air pollution increases the risk of pulmonary disease. In urban areas industrial waste and vehicle exhaust commonly contribute to air pollution. Cigarette smoke is another primary air pollutant. Improper disposal of radioactive and bioactive waste products can cause land pollution. Water pollution is the contamination of lakes, rivers, and streams, usually by industrial pollutants. If the public water supply becomes contaminated, the public must use bottled or boiled water for drinking and cooking. Flooding often damages water treatment stations and thus requires use of bottled or boiled water. Excessive noise is another form of pollution that presents significant health risks.

NURSING KNOWLEDGE BASE

Factors Influencing Patient Safety

A person's developmental level, lifestyle habits, mobility status, sensory and cognitive function, and safety awareness all influence threats to safety. As a nurse, be familiar with each patient's risks and the risks that are present within a health care setting.

Developmental Level

Infant, Toddler, and Preschooler. Injuries are a major cause of death during infancy, especially for children 6 to 12 months old (Hockenberry and Wilson, 2015). The leading causes of injury to infants are falls, ingestion injuries (poison, foreign body ingestion, and medication), and burns. Aspiration often occurs from the ingestion of foreign material such as small toys and food items. The nature of an injury is closely related to an infant's normal growth and development. Children at these early stages are curious; they explore their environment and because of an increase in oral activity put objects in their mouths. Accidents involving young children are largely preventable. Accident prevention requires targeted health education for parents and the removal of dangers whenever possible.

School-Age Child. When children enter school, their environment expands to include the school itself, transportation to and from school, and after-school activities. Although school-age children learn how to perform more complicated motor activities, they are often uncoordinated. Instruct parents and teachers about safe practices to follow at school and during play. Teach school-age children who are involved in team and contact sports how to use protective safety equipment. Head injuries resulting from falls, motor vehicle injuries, and bicycle injuries are a major cause of pediatric deaths (Hockenberry and Wilson, 2015). Playground safety is especially important during the summer months.

Adolescent. As children enter adolescence, they develop greater independence and a sense of identity. The adolescent begins to separate emotionally from the family, and the peer group begins to have a stronger influence. Adolescents typically have wide variations that swing from childlike to mature behavior (Hockenberry and Wilson, 2015). Adolescents often engage in risk-taking behaviors such as smoking, drinking alcohol, and using drugs. Environmental clues of substance abuse include the presence of drug-oriented magazines, beer and liquor bottles, drug paraphernalia, blood spots on clothing, and wearing long-sleeved shirts in hot weather and dark glasses indoors. Psychosocial clues include failing grades, change in dress, increased absenteeism from school, isolation, increased aggressiveness, and changes in interpersonal relationships. Substance abuse increases the risk for accidents such as drowning and motor vehicle accidents. According to the Insurance Institute for Highway Safety (IIHS, 2016), the fatal crash rate per mile driven for 16- to 19-year-olds in the United States is nearly 3 times the rate for drivers 20 years of age and older. Teens are at higher risk for fatal crashes because of their immaturity and driving inexperience.

Adult. Threats to an adult's safety are often related to lifestyle habits. For example, a patient who uses alcohol or drugs excessively is at greater risk for motor vehicle accidents. Adults experiencing high levels of stress are at a greater risk for accidents and stress-related illnesses such as headaches, depression, gastrointestinal disorders, and infections.

Older Adult. The physiological changes associated with aging, effects of multiple medications, psychological factors, and acute or chronic disease increase an older adult's risk for falls and other types of accidents. More than one-fourth of adults 65 years of age and older falls each year, but less than half tell their health care providers (CDC, 2017a). Falls are the major cause of injury leading to death among adults 65 years of age and older. They are also the most common cause of nonfatal injuries and hospital admissions for trauma.

Most falls occur within or around the home, specifically in the bedroom, bathroom, and kitchen. Environmental factors such as broken stairs, icy sidewalks, inadequate lighting, throw rugs, and exposed electrical cords cause many accidents. Older adults typically fall while transferring from beds, chairs, and toilets; getting into or out of bathtubs; tripping over carpet edges or doorway thresholds; slipping on wet surfaces; or descending stairs. Fear of falling is common among older adults both with and without a history of falling (Chang et al., 2016). As a result of their fear, many older adults avoid activities or change the way in which they walk and position themselves, making them more at risk for falling. It is important to ask what specific conditions increase an individual's fear of falling so hazards in the home can be removed.

Other Risk Factors

Lifestyle. Lifestyle choices increase safety risks. People who drive or operate machinery while under the influence of chemical substances or work at jobs that are dangerous are at greater risk for injury. People who are preoccupied by stress or anxiety are more accident-prone because they fail to recognize the source of potential accidents such as a cluttered stair or stop sign.

Impaired Mobility. A patient with impaired mobility has many kinds of safety risks. Immobilization predisposes a patient to physiological and emotional hazards, which further restrict mobility and independence (see Chapter 29). Patients with disabilities are at greater risk for injury when entering motor vehicles and buildings that are not accessible.

Sensory Impairments. Patients with visual, hearing, tactile, or communication impairments such as aphasia or language barrier are at greater risk for injury. Such patients are not always able to perceive a potential danger or express need for assistance (see Chapter 39).

Cognitive Impairments. Cognitive impairments associated with delirium, dementia, and depression place patients at greater risk for injury. These conditions contribute to altered concentration and attention span, impaired memory, and orientation changes. Patients with these alterations become easily confused about their surroundings and are more likely to experience falls and burns.

Safety Awareness. Some patients are unaware of safety precautions such as keeping medicine, poisonous plants, or other poisons away from children or reading the expiration date on food products. This may be the result of their educational background, low health literacy, health beliefs, or access to informational resources.

Risks in the Health Care Agency

Environmental safety pertains not only to a patient's home and community but also to a health care agency. There are risks in health care agencies that you need to address.

Chemical Exposure. Various forms of chemicals used in patient care can be an environmental risk. Chemicals found in some medications such as chemotherapy agents, anesthetic gases, cleaning solutions, and disinfectants are potentially toxic if ingested or inhaled. Safety data sheets (SDSs) are resources available in any health care agency. These sheets provide information on the chemical composition of a material, first aid measures for exposure, proper disposal methods, and technical information such as the physical and chemical properties of the material (Occupational Safety and Health Administration [OSHA], n.d.a).

Falls. Falls often occur in health care settings. Up to 50% of patients are at risk for falls while hospitalized, and 30% to 35% of patients who fall sustain an injury (The Joint Commission Center for Transforming Healthcare [TJCCTH], 2017). Falls contribute to a patient's functional decline and increased health care use. A fall can cause lasting pain and suffering and may limit physical, psychological, and social function, placing additional burdens on families and society. According to TJC (2014), approximately 11,000 fatal falls occur in the hospital annually. Inpatient falls add about 6.3 days to a patient's stay and cost about $14,000 (TJCCTH, 2017). Every health care institution has initiatives in place to reduce falls including use of special fall risk assessment tools, fall prevention protocols, fall alert signs, and identification bands. Causes of falls are multifactorial. Common risk factors for falls in hospital settings are broken down into two categories: intrinsic and extrinsic.

- *Intrinsic factors* are patient related and include physiological conditions such as vision disturbances, urinary/stool frequency or incontinence, mental impairment, gait and balance disorders, polypharmacy, and older age.
- *Extrinsic factors* are environmentally related and include room clutter, loose electrical cords, and liquid spills.

Effectively preventing falls requires an interdisciplinary, evidence-based approach (ECRI Institute, 2016) (Box 30.5).

Patient-Inherent Accidents. Patient-inherent accidents are accidents (other than falls) in which a patient is the primary reason for the event. Examples are self-inflicted cuts, injuries, and burns; ingestion or injection of foreign substances; self-mutilation or setting fires; and pinching fingers in drawers or doors. Diagnosis of a seizure disorder places a patient at risk for a patient-inherent accident. Place patients with seizure disorders on seizure precautions, which include protecting a patient from harm during a seizure, assisting with airway management if indicated, and administering antiseizure medications as ordered.

BOX 30.5 EVIDENCE-BASED PRACTICE

PICO Question: Does a multifactorial fall-intervention program compared with single interventions reduce incidence of falls among hospitalized patients?

SUMMARY OF EVIDENCE

Research shows that fall prevention is successful with an interdisciplinary approach; using only one intervention is not successful (TJC, 2015). Hospitals need to use multiple evidence-based fall prevention interventions aimed at a patient's specific risk factors to reduce falls and falls with injuries. Interventions include fall-risk assessments, door/bed/patient fall-risk alerts (e.g., bed alarms, signs, identification bands), environmental and equipment modifications, staff and patient safety education, improved medication management (evaluating polypharmacy), and additional assistance with transfer and activities of daily living (showering, toileting, and dressing). Current research shows that an interdisciplinary approach and hourly rounds, or rounding tailored to patient-specific needs, aid in fall reduction with successful implementation over time (Stanford Health Care, 2017; AHRQ, 2013; TJCCTH, 2017; ECRI Institute, 2016; CDC, 2017a).

APPLICATION TO NURSING PRACTICE

- Educate patient and family members about safe mobility practices (e.g., how to move safely with IV pole or indwelling urinary catheter).
- Provide patient and family with information on fall risk indicators and safety tips to prevent falls related to risk indicators (ECRI Institute, 2016).
- Use bed or chair alarms when appropriate with rapid response.
- Keep beds in lowest position with wheels locked (TJCCTH, 2017).
- Communicate mobility needs with other care members of the team (e.g., "provide assistive device" or "assist to bathroom") (ECRI Institute, 2016).
- Round on patients at least hourly or more tailored if needed (ECRI Institute, 2016; TJCCTH, 2017).
- Implement fall prevention bundle (fall risk armband, skid-proof socks, gait belt use) (TJCCTH, 2017).

Procedure-Related Accidents. Health care providers cause procedure-related accidents. These accidents include medication and fluid administration errors, incorrect placement of external devices, and improper performance of procedures such as dressing changes. Always follow the policies and procedures of an organization and standards of nursing practice to prevent procedure-related accidents. For example, correct use of body mechanics and transfer techniques reduces the risk for injuries when moving and lifting patients (see Chapter 28). All staff need to be aware that distractions and interruptions contribute to procedure-related accidents and need to be limited.

Equipment-Related Accidents. Equipment-related accidents result from an electrical hazard or malfunction, disrepair, or misuse of equipment. To avoid rapid infusion of

IV fluids, all general-use and patient-controlled analgesic pumps need to have free-flow protection devices. To avoid accidents, do not operate medical equipment without adequate instruction. If you discover a faulty piece of equipment, replace it with the proper working equipment, place a tag on the faulty one, take it out of service, and promptly report any malfunctions. Assess potential electrical hazards to reduce the risk of electrical fires, electrocution, or injury from faulty equipment. In health care settings the clinical engineering staff make regular safety checks of equipment. Facilities must report all suspected medical device–related deaths to both the Food and Drug Administration (FDA, 2016) and the product manufacturer.

Workplace Safety

Violence is becoming a familiar occurrence in hospitals, nursing homes, and other health care settings. The sources of violence include patients, visitors, intruders, and co-workers. The National Institute for Occupational Safety and Health (NIOSH, 2017) defines workplace violence as the act or threat of violence, ranging from verbal abuse to physical assault, directed toward persons at work or on duty. The impact of workplace violence ranges from psychological issues (e.g., posttraumatic stress disorder [PTSD], compassion fatigue) to physical injury or death. In a study involving 6300 RNs and licensed practical nurses (LPNs), nursing staff most often reported workplace violence–induced anger, frustration, fear, stress, and irritability, with 13% of staff reporting long-term difficulty with these symptoms following an event (Gerberich et al., 2004).

From 2002 to 2013, incidents of serious workplace violence (incidents requiring victims to take days off to recuperate) were 4 times more common in health care than in private industry (OSHA, n.d.c). However, workplace violence occurs on a continuum. Bullying, verbal threats, and name calling are common. Patients are most commonly the source of violence in health care settings resulting from hitting, kicking, beating, and shoving (OSHA, n.d.c). Risk factors for workplace violence caused by patients include overcrowded waiting areas in health care agencies, working in isolation from co-workers, working in high-crime areas, having a mobile workplace, transporting patients, poor environmental design, access to firearms, and working with volatile patients (McPhaul et al., 2008). Many incidents of violence are not reported (OSHA, n.d.c). Patients who exhibit violent behavior are often repeat offenders. Although situations can escalate quickly, they can often be minimized or prevented before they can get out of control (Crisis Prevention Institute [CPI], 2016).

CRITICAL THINKING

Synthesis

Patient care requires you to apply what you know about a patient, your knowledge base, experience, and critical thinking attitudes and standards. Your synthesis of this information allows you to make sound decisions as you apply the nursing process. Critical thinking synthesis involves combining all

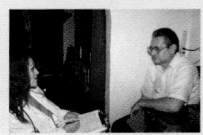

BOX 30.6   SYNTHESIS IN PRACTICE

Joani completed a health screening on Mr. Gonzales. She knows that she needs to incorporate knowledge about fall and environmental risks as they relate to Mr. Gonzales' age, level of independence, health status, and expectations. Mr. Gonzales is the third patient Joani has cared for in the home; thus she is also able to draw on her past experiences. As Joani integrates knowledge with her previous experience, she remembers that Mr. Gonzales values his independence. Therefore she considers ways to develop a plan of care to meet Mr. Gonzales' safety needs while helping him maintain his independence. She discovers that the lighting in his home is poor and that several throw rugs are near the chairs and bedside. The health screening revealed that Mr. Gonzales has decreased visual acuity and has not had a new pair of glasses for 3 years. He fell in his apartment about a month ago but did not have any injuries; he did not tell his son about his fall.

available information to obtain a clear picture of the approach needed to provide patient-centered care (Box 30.6).

Knowledge. When caring for a patient's safety needs, begin by reflecting on the knowledge you have about common safety risks and a patient's developmental level. You need a complete picture of a patient's physical, cultural, physiological, psychosocial, and environmental information to protect a patient from injury. Consider information from pharmacology (e.g., medications being taken and possible interactions) and information about environmental hazards. Apply your assessment findings regarding a patient's environment and where most activities of daily living occur. Because all patients are different, prioritize factors that are threats to their safety and concentrate on probable threats. After you consider a patient's specific strengths, weaknesses, developmental level, and environment, work with the patient and family to determine a patient-centered approach.

Experience. Use clinical and personal experience to recall safety incidents that occurred with other patients or your own family and the specific circumstances that led to a situation. For example, if your grandmother fell because she tripped on a throw rug, use the experience of your grandmother's fall and apply the knowledge gained when you assess a patient's home for safety hazards during a home visit.

Attitudes. Using a professional attitude and critical thinking ensures that your plan of care for a patient's safety is comprehensive. For example, show perseverance in identifying all potential safety risks and threats. Be responsible for collecting unbiased, accurate data that are relevant to a patient's safety. It is important to show discipline to thoroughly assess a patient's home environment. View all situations as opportunities to protect a patient. Once they occur, injuries cause pain, immobility, loss of income, or even death.

TABLE 30.1 FOCUSED PATIENT ASSESSMENT

FACTORS TO ASSESS	QUESTIONS	PHYSICAL ASSESSMENT
Environment	Describe times you have fallen in the past. Where do the falls commonly happen? Have you ever burned yourself?	Inspect the home environment both inside and outside for potential hazards; focus on the kitchen and bathroom.
Sensory	When do you wear your glasses? When was the last time you had your eyes checked? Can you easily hear during phone conversations?	Observe patient's ability to read printed material accurately and ability to move about within the home. Assess ability to hear normal spoken word.
Physical mobility	How does your (arthritis, surgery, impaired gait) affect the way you walk and move around? Do you exercise? Describe how you exercise each day. Are you able to move around safely at home?	Observe patient's posture, gait, and balance during activities of daily living.

Standards. The American Nurses Association (ANA) *Nursing: Scope and Standards of Practice, Third Edition* (ANA, 2015a) includes the concept of safety, stating that nurses will implement nursing interventions competently in a safe and appropriate manner. The ANA *Code of Ethics for Nurses* (ANA, 2015b) includes safety issues, describing a nurse's responsibility to promote, advocate for, and strive to protect the health, safety, and rights of patients. Regulatory agencies such as TJC (2017a) and OSHA (n.d.b) define standards and guidelines related to safety in health care settings.

NURSING PROCESS

■■■ ASSESSMENT

To conduct a thorough patient assessment, consider possible threats to a patient's safety including the patient's immediate environment and any individual risk factors (Table 30.1). When you care for patients in the home, perform a home safety assessment to look for factors that are hazards within the home (Box 30.7). A thorough safety assessment covers topics such as adequacy of lighting, presence of safety devices, conditions (e.g., flooring, steps) that pose risks for falls, and safety of the kitchen and bathrooms. To assess a home, walk through the rooms with the patient and discuss how the patient normally conducts daily activities and whether the environment poses problems. For example, when assessing adequacy of lighting, inspect areas where a patient moves and works, particularly outside walkways, steps, interior halls, and doorways. Getting a sense of a patient's routines helps you recognize safety hazards.

Assessment of patients' risk factors for falling is a priority in health care settings. Many different fall assessment instruments are available such as the Morse Fall Scale (Morse, 2009); use the one chosen by your health care agency. Assess both intrinsic and extrinsic factors that increase a patient's risk. Intrinsic factors include a previous history of falling, age 65 years or older, reduced vision, orthostatic hypotension,

BOX 30.7 HOME SAFETY ASSESSMENT

Look for the following factors when assessing the safety of a home:
- Proper lighting inside and outside
- Storage areas within easy reach
- Appliances in good working order
- Extension cords placed along walls
- Presence of smoke detectors and a fire extinguisher
- Presence of carbon monoxide detector
- Flammable objects away from stove or heaters
- Gas pilot lights lit
- Hot water thermostat set to 120° F or less
- Handrails or grip bars installed
- Nonskid surfaces in bathroom and tub or shower
- Floor coverings secured and floors free of clutter
- Furniture and assistive devices to promote ease of mobility
- Medications stored properly and not outdated
- Telephone accessible with readily available emergency phone numbers

gait instability, lower limb weakness, balance problems, urinary incontinence, frequency or need for assisted toileting, use of walking aids, agitation or confusion, and effects of medications (e.g., sedatives, hypnotics, anticonvulsants, certain analgesics) (Plaksin, 2014). Extrinsic factors include factors within the hospital environment. Does the placement of equipment pose barriers when a patient attempts to ambulate? Does positioning of a patient's bed allow the patient to safely reach items on a bedside table? Does a patient need assistance with ambulation? Are self-care items at the bedside, and is the nurse call system arranged for accessibility? Another area of risk includes wheelchair-related falls involving older adults and people with disabilities. Patients are at risk for falls during transfer tasks and reaching while seated in a wheelchair. Finally be sure that equipment is safe to use. Collaborate with the hospital clinical engineering staff if you have any questions about equipment functions.

BOX 30.8 CARE OF THE OLDER ADULT

Physical Assessment Findings in Older Adults That Increase the Risk for Accidents

MUSCULOSKELETAL CHANGES
- Muscle strength decreased
- Joints becoming less mobile
- Brittle bones caused by osteoporosis
- Posture changes; some kyphosis common
- Limited range of motion (ROM)
- Change in walking gait

NERVOUS SYSTEM CHANGES
- Slower voluntary or autonomic reflexes
- Decreased ability to respond to multiple stimuli
- Decreased sensitivity of touch

SENSORY CHANGES
- Decreased peripheral vision and lens accommodation
- Decreased night vision and ability to adjust to changes in light
- Development of opacity (cataracts) in lens
- Increased stimuli threshold for light touch and pain
- Impaired hearing because high-frequency tones are less perceptible

GENITOURINARY CHANGES
- Increased nocturia
- Increased occurrence of incontinence

Modified from Touhy TA, Jett K: *Ebersole and Hess' toward healthy aging,* ed 9, St Louis, 2016, Mosby.

Your nursing history includes data about a patient's level of wellness to determine if any underlying conditions pose a further threat to safety. Patients with conditions such as osteoporosis and bleeding disorders are more at risk for injury from falls. When you believe that a patient is a fall risk, assess for a fear of falling. Signs that a person is fearful of falling include concern or worry during walking, sweating or shaking while walking, clutching people or objects while walking, and reluctance to change position or walk. Other fall risk factors to assess include a patient's activity tolerance, level of cognition, presence of painful conditions, muscle strength in extremities, balance, and vision (see Chapter 16). Consider a patient's developmental level when you analyze your data. Review the type and number of medications that a patient is taking and if the patient is undergoing any procedures that pose risks.

Older Adult Considerations. When you assess older adults, recognize the types of physical changes that increase their risk for injury (Box 30.8). Research shows that even slight changes in walking speed and stride length can be a strong predictor for a patient fall (Mignardot et al., 2014). An assessment approach used within health care agencies is the timed "get up and go" test (Mathias et al., 1986). Have the older adult wear regular footwear, sit back in a comfortable chair with an armrest, and use his or her normal assist device (if needed). Have a watch with a second hand or a digital

second display ready. On the word "go," time the person as he or she performs the following:

1. Stands up from the arm chair
2. Stands still momentarily
3. Walks 10 feet (3 m) (in a line)
4. Turns around
5. Walks back to chair
6. Turns around
7. Sits down

Time the effort and observe the patient for postural stability, steppage, stride length, and sway.

Normally a person completes the task in less than 10 seconds; an abnormal response is more than 20 seconds.

Patient Expectations. Patients expect to be safe in health care settings and in their homes. However, there are times when their view of what is safe does not agree with that of health care providers and standards of care. For this reason conduct a patient-centered assessment that includes a patient's own perceptions of his or her risk factors, knowledge of how to adapt to such risks, and previous experience with accidents. Ask what a patient expects from your care. For example, ask, "How can I provide care that will make you feel safe?" or "After we walk through your home, tell me what we need to do to help you feel safe." Patients usually do not purposefully put themselves in danger; however, when they are uninformed or inexperienced, threats to their safety can occur. Always ask patients or family members about their ideas for ways to reduce hazards in their environment.

■ ■ ■ NURSING DIAGNOSIS

Gather data from your nursing assessment and analyze clusters of defining characteristics to identify relevant nursing diagnoses. Be thorough in analyzing risk factors and defining characteristics. For example, the two nursing diagnoses of *Risk for Injury* and *Risk for Falls* have similar risk factors. In the case of *Risk for Falls* the risk factors are specific to conditions that increase fall risk, whereas risk factors for *Risk for Injury* are broader and cover areas such as infection and malnutrition risks. Nursing diagnoses for patients with safety risks include the following:

- *Risk for Falls*
- *Impaired Home Maintenance*
- *Risk for Injury*
- *Deficient Knowledge related to safety risks*
- *Risk for Poisoning*
- *Risk for Suffocation*
- *Risk for Trauma*

Include specific related or contributing factors so that the diagnosis allows you to individualize your nursing care. For example, the nursing diagnosis *Impaired Home Maintenance* could be related to injury or sensory alteration (e.g., visual). An injury that affects a person's mobility leads you to select such nursing interventions as placing handrails near toilets, showers, and bathtubs or teaching the proper use of safety devices such as side rails, canes, or crutches. Visual impairment (as the related factor) leads you to select different interventions such as keeping the area well lit or keeping eyeglasses clean, handy, and well protected. When you do not identify the correct related factor, the use of inappropriate interventions increases a patient's risk for injury.

■■■ PLANNING

Patients who have safety risks require a nursing care plan with interventions that prevent and minimize the intrinsic and extrinsic threats to safety. Design interventions to create a safe environment and help a patient feel safe to interact freely within that environment. The total plan of care addresses all aspects of patient needs and uses resources of the health care team and the community when appropriate.

Goals and Outcomes. Collaborate with the patient, family members, and other members of the health care team when you plan and set goals of care. Remember to keep goals realistic, within the resources available to a patient. When you involve a patient and family in planning, they become more alert to safety risks and potential hazards. *For example, in the case study, Joani identifies the goal for Mr. Gonzales of "Patient will not fall." Expected outcomes include "Patient removes barriers to reaching the bathroom" and "Patient improves mobility in using lower extremities." Joani discusses the goal with Mr. Gonzales and his son, suggesting that they discuss ways the patient's bedroom and bath can be made safer and consider if there is a way to get Mr. Gonzales involved in an exercise program (see Care Plan).*

Setting Priorities. Prioritize a patient's nursing diagnoses and interventions that are most important in terms of risk to safety and health promotion. In some situations you need to select more than one nursing diagnosis that best represents a patient's particular needs. *For example, in the case study*

Joani identifies the nursing diagnoses Risk for Falls, Impaired Physical Mobility, and Fear (Fig. 30.2). She establishes risk for falls as the first priority. After completing a comprehensive home safety assessment with Mr. Gonzales and his son, Joani focuses nursing interventions on modifying the home. They discuss together the factors within the home that pose risk for injuries and falls. Once both Mr. Gonzales and his son understand Mr. Gonzales' health risks, Joani can focus on specific interventions for reducing Mr. Gonzales' fear of falling and improving mobility to prevent falls and injuries.

Collaborative Care. It is important to collaborate with patients and health care workers from other disciplines such as social work and occupational and physical therapy in planning a patient's care. Having appropriate resources within the home, being able to perform activities of daily living safely, and being able to move about with minimal risk are key factors in helping patients return to safe environments in their homes. Hospitalized patients also need to learn how to identify and select resources that are available within their community after they return home. For example, an older adult may need to go to an adult day care center during weekdays when family members are working and unable to provide regular assistance.

■■■ IMPLEMENTATION

QSEN (2017) outlines recommended skills to ensure nurse competency in patient safety. These include skills involving safe nursing practice during direct care, as follows:

- Demonstrate effective use of technology and standardized practices that support safety and quality.
- Demonstrate effective use of strategies to reduce risk of harm to self or others.
- Use appropriate strategies to reduce reliance on memory (e.g., forcing functions, checklists).

◎ CARE PLAN

Risk for Falls

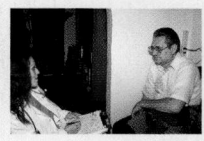

ASSESSMENT

Joani knows that people with impaired vision and mobility are at increased risk for injury. She knows that she also needs to assess Mr. Gonzales' fall risks more thoroughly. When Joani meets with Mr. Gonzales, she learns that he fell in his home about 3 months ago. He expresses concern about his safety, "I'm afraid I might fall again. My knees make it harder to go upstairs." He wants to remain independent and live to a "ripe old age" but admits that his fear of falling causes him to participate in fewer social activities. His son has talked with him about getting a cane to help him walk, but so far Mr. Gonzales has declined.

ASSESSMENT ACTIVITIES	FINDINGS[a]
Inspect Mr. Gonzales' home environment for safety hazards.	Joani discovers **throw rugs on the floors** near the chairs and at the bedside and **poor lighting** in the bedroom and bathroom.
Conduct a physical assessment to determine Mr. Gonzales' risk factors for falling.	Mr. Gonzales is unable to read the labels on his medication bottles. His last visual examination was 3 years ago. Gait assessment reveals that Mr. Gonzales does not pick his feet up very high off the floor. He has reduced strength in his right leg. His movements are stiff and slow, especially when standing up from a chair. Joani also learns that Mr. Gonzales exercises infrequently.

Continued

◎ CARE PLAN—cont'd

Risk for Falls

ASSESSMENT ACTIVITIES	FINDINGS[a]
Joani asks Mr. Gonzales what he knows about fall risks and ways to prevent them.	Mr. Gonzales has **limited knowledge** about fall risks except that he knows to use caution with stairs. He says that his doctor talked about things to be aware of after his fall, but **he can't recall the information.**

[a]**Defining characteristics/risk factors** are shown in **bold** type.

NURSING DIAGNOSIS: Risk for Falls

PLANNING

GOAL	EXPECTED OUTCOMES (NOC)[b]
	Safe Home Environment
Mr. Gonzales' fall risk will be reduced within 2 months.	Mr. Gonzales lists hazards in his apartment within 1 week.
	Mr. Gonzales reduces modifiable hazards in his apartment by 100% within 1 month.
	Personal Safety Behavior
Mr. Gonzales improves balance and mobility in using lower extremities.	Mr. Gonzales will participate in a prescribed exercise program.
	Mr. Gonzales will use assist device correctly.

[b]Outcome classification labels from Moorhead S, et al, editors: *Nursing outcomes classification (NOC)*, ed 5, St Louis, 2013, Mosby.

INTERVENTIONS (NIC)[c]	RATIONALE
Environmental Management: Safety	
Review and discuss with Mr. Gonzales and his son the risks for accidents and falls. After completing a home safety checklist, recommend the following:	Identifying fall hazards in the home helps to prevent falls (CDC, 2015). Home modification includes multiple interventions that can reduce fear of falling and incidence of falls (Keall et al., 2014).
• Removing throw rugs	
• Increasing lighting	
• Installing nonslip surface in shower, decks, and porches	
• Clearing pathways from bedroom to bathroom	
Arrange for Mr. Gonzales to visit an optometrist and get a new prescription for eyeglasses.	Routine eye examinations are recommended as part of a comprehensive program to reduce falls in older adults. Early detection of visual disturbances can provide early interventions to prevent falls in the home (Hong et al., 2014).
Exercise Promotion	
Consult with Mr. Gonzales' health care provider about a physical therapy evaluation to recommend an exercise regimen for Mr. Gonzales and determine if an assist device is needed.	Organized exercise targeted on fall prevention can reduce the rate of falls and falls with injury. Balance training, gait and functional training, strengthening, flexibility, and endurance also contribute to reduction of falls and injury severity (El-Khoury et al., 2013).

[c]Intervention classification labels from Bulechek GM, et al, editors: *Nursing interventions classification (NIC)*, ed 6, St Louis, 2013, Mosby.

EVALUATION

NURSING ACTIONS	PATIENT RESPONSE/FINDING	ACHIEVEMENT OF OUTCOME
Visit and observe Mr. Gonzales' apartment for elimination of threats to safety.	Throw rugs are removed or replaced with rubber-backed rugs.	Mr. Gonzales has reduced home hazards. Knowledge about barriers and risk factors within the apartment has improved but may need reinforcement.
	Lighting is increased to 75 watts except in bedroom.	
	Mr. Gonzales identifies most factors in home that increase his risk for falling.	
Reassess motor, sensory, and cognitive status.	Mr. Gonzales has new glasses and is able to read medication bottle labels.	Improved visual acuity.
	Mr. Gonzales will start an exercise program established by physical therapist (PT) in 1 week.	Still has reduced strength in right leg and problem with gait. Will reevaluate in 2 weeks after exercise program begins.
	Mr. Gonzales is not in need of assist device as determined by PT.	Discontinue recommendation for assist device at this time.

CONCEPT MAP

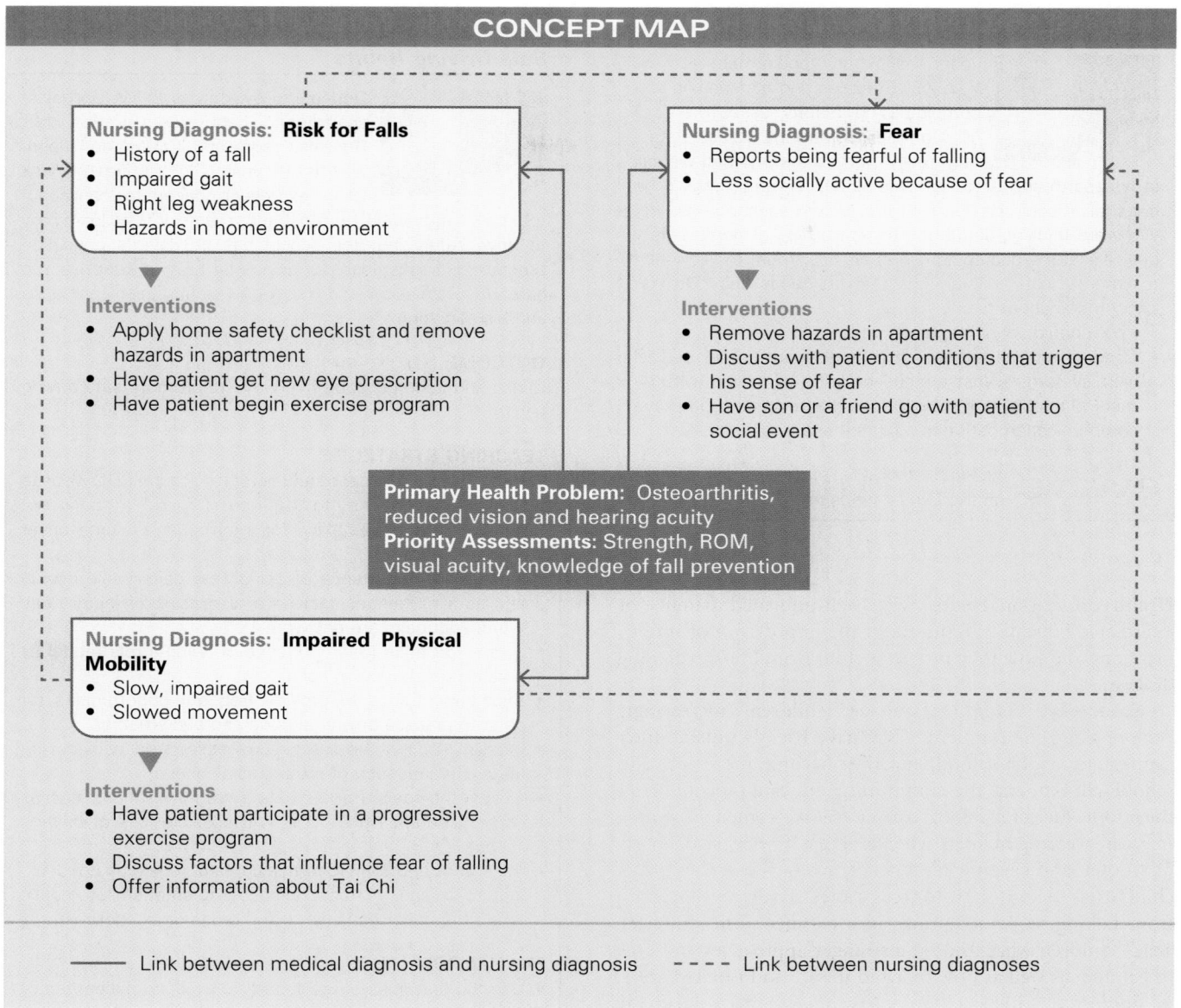

Nursing Diagnosis: Risk for Falls
- History of a fall
- Impaired gait
- Right leg weakness
- Hazards in home environment

Interventions
- Apply home safety checklist and remove hazards in apartment
- Have patient get new eye prescription
- Have patient begin exercise program

Nursing Diagnosis: Fear
- Reports being fearful of falling
- Less socially active because of fear

Interventions
- Remove hazards in apartment
- Discuss with patient conditions that trigger his sense of fear
- Have son or a friend go with patient to social event

Primary Health Problem: Osteoarthritis, reduced vision and hearing acuity
Priority Assessments: Strength, ROM, visual acuity, knowledge of fall prevention

Nursing Diagnosis: Impaired Physical Mobility
- Slow, impaired gait
- Slowed movement

Interventions
- Have patient participate in a progressive exercise program
- Discuss factors that influence fear of falling
- Offer information about Tai Chi

——— Link between medical diagnosis and nursing diagnosis   - - - - Link between nursing diagnoses

FIG 30.2 Concept map.

Direct nursing interventions toward maintaining a patient's safety in all settings. Always be safety conscious when you intervene to promote health, implement illness prevention measures, and prevent patient harm and injury.

Health Promotion. Health promotion requires a person to be in a safe environment and practice a lifestyle that minimizes risk of injury. There are both passive and active strategies aimed at health promotion. Passive strategies include public health measures and government legislative interventions (e.g., sanitation and clean water laws). Active strategies require an individual to be actively involved through changes in lifestyle (e.g., wearing seat belts or installing outdoor lighting along walking paths) and participation in wellness programs. As a nurse, you can participate in health promotion activities by supporting legislation; acting as a positive role model; and recommending safety measures in the home, school, neighborhood, and workplace.

Developmental Interventions

Infant, Toddler, and Preschooler. Growing, curious children need adults to protect them from injury. Educate parents or guardians about reducing risks of injuries to children, and teach ways to promote safety in the home. Some examples are preventing access to poisonous substances; creating a safe sleeping environment; using car seats correctly; using safe, age-appropriate toys; and teaching young children safety rules (e.g., proper use of scissors, how to walk in parking lots with parents) (see Chapter 23). Children typically trust their environment and never perceive that they are in danger.

QSEN **QSEN ACTIVITY** *Informatics*

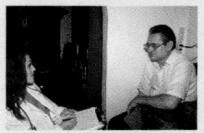

Joani makes an appointment to visit with Mr. Gonzales and his son. As she completes her safety assessment of Mr. Gonzales' apartment, his son states, "I'm really worried that my dad will fall in his apartment. Since he lives alone, I'm afraid that, if he does fall, it could be hours or days before anyone finds him. We were thinking about getting some type of home safety device that my dad could use in his apartment to allow him to communicate to someone that he needs help. Do you know much about them?"

- How should Joani respond?
- Conduct an Internet search to investigate home medical alert systems. What are the benefits of having a home medical alert system? How does this technology improve communication between a patient and a responder?

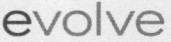

Answers to QSEN Activities can be found on the Evolve website.

Health promotion begins with well-informed parents or guardians. Educate parents about the importance of immunizations and how they protect a child from life-threatening diseases.

School-Age Child. School-age children increasingly explore their environment. They have friends outside their immediate neighborhood, and they become more active in school, church, and the community. Educate parents about the importance of children wearing seat belts whenever riding in a car; wearing helmets when riding a bicycle, skateboard, or scooter; and keeping adults informed of where they are. A child needs to know how to cross a street safely and to refrain from talking to or accepting rides or gifts from strangers. Teach children what to do if a stranger approaches and how to get help as well as how to avoid unsafe and isolated areas.

Adolescent. Risks to an adolescent's safety involve many factors outside the home because adolescents spend much of their time away from home and with their peer group. Adults serve as role models for adolescents, and they can help teens minimize safety risks by setting expectations and providing examples and education. Because adolescence is a time when sexual physical characteristics develop, adolescents often begin to have physical relationships with others. They need prompt, accurate instructions about abstinence and safe sexual practices. It is also important to educate them and their families about signs of school violence including bullying, fighting, weapon use, gang violence, and electronic aggression (CDC, 2017e). Adolescents may benefit from developing better social skills and social problem solving with peers. Although most schools have drivers' education programs, when teens learn to drive, they need education about complying with rules and regulations regarding safe driving and the use of a car (Box 30.9).

Adult. Risks to young and middle-age adults frequently result from lifestyle factors such as childrearing, high-stress

BOX 30.9 PATIENT TEACHING

Safe Driving Habits

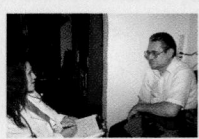

During a follow-up visit to Mr. Gonzales' apartment, Joani meets Carlos, Mr. Gonzales' son, and Carlos' son John, who is 16 years old. During the visit Carlos expresses concern to Joani about his son's safety while driving. Carlos wants John to learn how to drive safely, but the school has no driver's education program. He asks Joani for advice on how to keep his son safe. Joani develops the following teaching plan for Carlos and his son John.

OUTCOME
Carlos and John describe five ways to promote safe driving habits.

TEACHING STRATEGIES
- Recommend that Carlos and his son go to the CDC website "Parents Are the Key to Safe Teen Drivers" (http://www.cdc.gov/parentsarethekey) for information on teen driver safety.
- Explain the importance of using seat belts while driving and as a passenger. Include a discussion of injury rates when seat belts are not worn.
- Stress to Carlos the importance of being a role model by practicing safe driving habits.
- Encourage Carlos to provide frequent opportunities for John to practice driving in good and bad weather.
- Explain to John the safety risks associated with driving under the influence of drugs and alcohol.
- Explain the costs associated with traffic violations such as higher insurance premiums and possible loss of driver's license.
- Ask Carlos and John to form a contract regarding not drinking and driving. Instruct John never to enter an automobile when the driver has been using drugs or alcohol.

EVALUATION
- Use the principles of teach-back to evaluate patient/family caregiver learning:
  - "Carlos, tell me how you will provide opportunities for John to practice driving."
  - "Carlos, describe for me how you will demonstrate safe driving habits to John."
  - "John, tell me what you would do if you were drinking at a party and needed to get home."
  - "John, identify for me the risks of driving without a seat belt."

states, inadequate nutrition, use of firearms, and abuse of drugs or alcohol. In this fast-paced society there also appears to be more expression of anger. This anger can quickly precipitate motor vehicle collisions resulting from "road rage." Help adults understand their safety risks and guide them in making lifestyle modifications by referring them to resources such as classes to help quit smoking and for stress management or employee assistance programs. Encourage them to exercise regularly, maintain a healthy diet, practice relaxation techniques, and get adequate sleep (see Chapters 28 and 32 to 34).

Older Adult. Elimination of threats to the safety of the older adult focuses primarily on accident prevention. Advancing age and concurrent physiological changes predispose older adults to falls. Table 30.2 lists nursing interventions designed to prevent falls and compensate for the physiological changes of aging. Certain disease states common to older adults such as arthritis or strokes increase the chance of injury (Box 30.10). The effects of many medications such as sedatives, diuretics, and anticoagulants also increase the chance of injury.

Provide information about neighborhood resources to help an older adult maintain an independent lifestyle. Older adults frequently relocate to new neighborhoods and must get acquainted with new resources such as modes of transportation, church schedules, and food resources (e.g., Meals on Wheels). Information about assistance resources such as daily "hello" programs, emergency services, and elder-abuse hot lines is also helpful.

Environmental Interventions. Nursing interventions directed at eliminating environmental threats include interventions associated with a person's basic needs as well as general preventive measures.

Basic Needs. Nurses contribute to a safer environment by helping patients meet their basic needs. When administering oxygen, follow the principles of medication administration and use precautions to prevent accidental fires. Contact with heat or a spark is needed to trigger combustion. When oxygen is in use, post "No Smoking" and "Oxygen in Use" signs in patients' hospital rooms and in their homes. Do not use oxygen around electrical equipment or flammable products. Store oxygen tanks upright in carts or stands to prevent tipping or falling over. Chapter 32 outlines guidelines for proper oxygen administration. A home medical provider and home health nurse educate patients who require oxygen in the home about safe oxygen use.

Food safety requires a patient and family to understand the following principles of food preparation:
- Proper refrigeration, storage, and preparation of food decrease risk of foodborne illnesses. Store perishable foods in refrigerators to maintain freshness.
- Thaw frozen foods in the refrigerator.
- Wash hands for at least 15 seconds before preparing food.

TABLE 30.2   MEASURES TO PREVENT FALLS IN OLDER ADULTS

MEASURE	RATIONALE
Home or Health Care Agency	
Stairs	
Install treads with uniform depth of 25.4–28 cm (10–11 inches) and 19–19.7 cm (7½–7¾ inches) risers (vertical face of steps).	When stairs are of uniform size, older adults do not have to continually look at the stairs and adjust their gait.
Install uniform-textured or plain-colored surfaces on each tread, and mark edge of tread with contrasting color.	Uniform textures or color help to decrease vertigo. Marking edge of tread provides obvious visual clue to end of stair.
Ensure proper lighting of each tread. Block sun or light bulb glare with translucent shades or screen or use lower-wattage bulbs.	Older adults' vision is unable to adjust quickly to changes in lighting.
Ensure adequate head room so that user does not have to duck to avoid hitting his or her head while going up or down the stairs.	Sudden changes in head position often result in dizziness, which increases risk for falling.
Remove protruding objects from staircase walls.	Decreased peripheral vision prevents older adults from seeing objects at their sides. Moving to avoid protruding objects disrupts balance.
Maintain outdoor walkways and stairs in good condition and free of holes, cracks, and splinters.	Decreased visual acuity prevents patient from seeing any structural defect. If older adults shuffle their feet when walking, it is easy to trip on uneven surfaces.
Handrails	
The space between the handrail and wall should be 40–50 mm for smooth walls and 60 mm for rough texture walls and 0.85–0.95 m (33½–37½ inches) from the floor (United Nations Enable [UNE], 2004).	Ample distance needed to allow older adults to grasp handrail firmly for support.
Secure handrail firmly to support user's weight, especially at bottom and top of stairway.	Older adults have greatest risk for falling at top and bottom of stairs because they shift their center of gravity, making balance unstable.
Install grab bars in bathroom near toilet and tub (ADABathroom.com, 2017).	Enables patient to have support while rising from sitting to standing position.

Continued

TABLE 30.2 MEASURES TO PREVENT FALLS IN OLDER ADULTS—cont'd

MEASURE	RATIONALE
Floors	
Ensure that patients wear properly fitting shoes or slippers with nonskid surface.	Reduces chances of slipping.
Secure all carpeting, mats, and tile; place nonskid backing under small rugs.	Sudden slip causes dizziness and inability to regain balance.
Place bath mats or nonskid strips on bathtub or shower stall floors.	Wet surfaces increase the risk for falling.
Secure electrical cords against baseboards.	Prevents tripping.
Health Care Agency	
Orientation	
Admit disoriented patients to a room near nurses' station.	Provides for more frequent observation by nursing staff.
Maintain close supervision of confused patients.	Confused patients often attempt to wander out of bed or room.
Show patient how to use nurse call system at bedside and in bathroom and place in an accessible location within patient's reach. Instruct patient to call for assistance with movement as needed.	Convenient location and use of the nurse call system are essential to patient safety.
Place bedside tables and over-bed tables close to patient. Place articles within easy reach.	Prevents patients from searching or overreaching for items.
Keep bed in low position. Have patient rise from bed or chair slowly.	Prevents dizziness resulting from postural hypotension.
Leave one side rail up and one down on side where oriented and ambulatory patient gets out of bed.	Patients are able to use side rail for support when getting in and out of bed and to position self once in bed.
Transport	
Lock bed and wheelchair when transferring patient from bed to wheelchair or back to bed.	Provides stability and support during transfer.
Place side rails in up position and secure safety straps around patient on stretcher.	Prevents patients from rolling off stretchers.

BOX 30.10 CARE OF THE OLDER ADULT

Safety Education

- Because of visual impairments in older adults, teach older adults to keep living areas well lighted and free of clutter, keep eyeglasses in good condition, and avoid night driving.
- Older adults have musculoskeletal changes that make movement difficult and increase the risk for falling. Teach older adults to keep assistive devices (canes, handrails in tub and bathroom, and elevated seats) in proper working order and to use nonskid strips in bathtubs (Touhy and Jett, 2018).
- Advise older adults to avoid smoking in bed, lower thermostats on water heaters, avoid overloading electrical outlets, and install and maintain smoke and carbon monoxide detectors in the house (Touhy and Jett, 2018).
- Driving helps older adults stay mobile and independent, yet they are more likely to have automobile accidents as a result of decreased hearing and visual acuity, altered depth perception, slowed reaction time, and poor peripheral vision. Advise

older adults to drive only short distances and in the daylight; avoid driving in inclement weather; use side and rearview mirrors carefully; look behind them toward their blind spot before changing lanes; and keep a window rolled down to hear sirens and horns.
- Teach older adults about the proper handling and storage of medications and safe methods of scheduling and taking them (Touhy and Jett, 2018).
- Older adults have physiological changes that often result in slower metabolism of drugs. Teach patients about drug interactions and signs and symptoms of drug toxicity to report to their health care provider (Burcham and Rosenthal, 2016).
- Some older adults have irreversible dementia. Help family caregivers understand the nature of dementia. Teach family caregivers to match expectations with the patient's capabilities; to incorporate earlier life skills and interests; and to provide a calm, caring, and structured environment.

- Rinse fruits and vegetables thoroughly.
- Avoid cross-contamination of one food with another during preparation, especially with poultry.
- Use separate cutting boards for vegetables, meat, and poultry.
- Cook foods adequately to kill any residual organisms.
- Refrigerate foods at 4°C (40°F) within 2 hours of cooking; label leftovers with the date.

General Preventive Measures. Adequate lighting and security measures in and around a home including the use of night-lights, exterior lighting, and locks on doors and windows reduce a person's risk for injury from falls or crime. Local police departments and community organizations often hold safety classes on how not to become a victim of crime.

Help parents reduce the risk of accidental poisoning by teaching them to keep hazardous substances out of children's reach. Older adults are also at risk for poisoning because diminished eyesight may cause an accidental ingestion of toxic substances. When older adults have impaired memory, accidental overdose of prescription medications may occur. Educate patients or family caregivers about keeping medications in original containers that are labeled in large print. Recommend the use of medication organizers that are filled once a week. Have patients keep poisonous substances out of the bathroom and properly discard old and unused medications.

To control pathogen transmission, teach patients how and when to wash hands (e.g., following toileting, before and after food preparation, before eating, before wound care). Nurses use Standard Precautions when caring for all patients to protect themselves from contact with blood and body fluids (see Chapter 14). Patients also need to know how to dispose of infected material such as wound dressings and used needles in the home. The Environmental Protection Agency (EPA) encourages disposal of used needles by way of community drop-off programs, household hazardous waste facilities, or sharps mail-back programs or by using home needle destruction devices (Illinois EPA, 2015). Encourage patients to contact their local community governments for guidelines on waste disposal methods.

Acute Care. Nurses implement specific interventions to ensure patient safety in acute care settings. You are responsible for making a patient's hospital room safe. Explain and demonstrate to patients how to use a nurse call or intercom system. Always place a call device close to a patient at the conclusion of any care activity. Respond quickly to nurse call systems and bed/chair alarms so that patients do not attempt to get up on their own. Many falls occur as patients try to get out of bed unassisted. Keep the environment around the bedside free from clutter. Also be prepared to conduct hourly rounds, a practice that many health care agencies have adopted. During rounding, address toileting, turning, pain control, and hydration.

Falls. Patient-centered care is important. Nurses need to partner with their patients in recognizing fall risks and taking preventive action. Target fall prevention strategies to specific patient risks. For example, if a patient has postural hypotension, you choose a low bed and have the patient dangle the legs for 5 minutes on the side of the bed before trying to ambulate. You give a patient with a history of urinary incontinence a bedside commode to use. Remember, patient situations change. Prevention of falls and fall-related injuries requires diligent ongoing nursing assessment and engagement of the entire health care team in the implementation of patient-specific interventions (Degelau et al., 2014). TJC Speak Up campaign was created for patients to follow in the home and hospital (TJC, 2017b). It offers tips and actions to help people reduce their risk of falling, whether at home or in a health care agency.

Health care settings use color-coded wristbands to help communicate a patient's safety risk. In 2008 the American Hospital Association (AHA) issued a recommendation that hospitals standardize wristband colors: red for patient allergies, yellow for fall risk, and purple for do-not-resuscitate preferences. This recommendation came after a near-miss incident in which a nurse, working in two different hospitals, placed a wrong-colored band on a patient. Many state hospital associations and communities are now standardizing colors to reduce confusion both within and across health care organizations (AHA, 2008).

Modifying a patient's environment reduces fall risks. For example, a patient who is morbidly obese needs a bed, wheelchair, or commode specifically designed to support the additional weight. A patient with impaired mobility benefits from organizing the home so that it is unnecessary to walk up or down stairs. In a health care agency, use a gait belt for patients needing assistance to transfer or ambulate. Remove excess furniture and equipment and make sure that patients wear rubber-soled shoes/slippers to walk or during transfer. Use additional safety equipment and safe patient-handling techniques when moving and positioning patients (see Chapter 29). Also provide a clear path to the bathroom and keep rooms well lit to promote safe ambulation. Inspect canes, walkers, and crutches to be sure that rubber tips are intact and connections are tight and that the assistive devices are at the appropriate height for the patient. Additional devices to use at a patient's bedside include a low bed, bedside commode, nonskid floor mat, and overhead trapeze (Fig. 30.3).

Restraints. Patients who are confused or disoriented or who repeatedly try to remove medical devices (e.g., IV lines or dressings) may temporarily need restraints to keep them safe. Restraints are not a solution to a patient problem but rather a temporary means to maintain patient safety. You must exhaust all alternatives before placing patients in restraints. Federal and state laws prohibit Medicare- and Medicaid-certified nursing homes from using restraints unless they are medically needed. **Chemical restraints** are medications such as anxiolytics and sedatives used to manage a patient's behavior and are not a standard treatment for a patient's condition. A physical **restraint** is any manual method, physical or mechanical device, material, or equipment that immobilizes or reduces the ability of a patient to

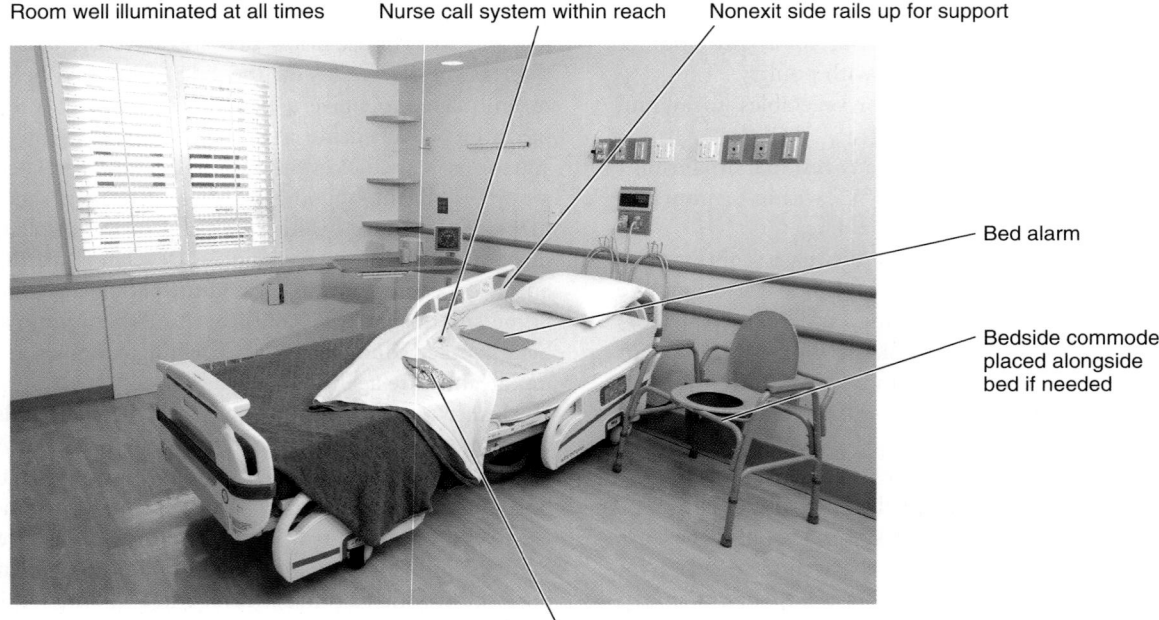

Room well illuminated at all times   Nurse call system within reach   Nonexit side rails up for support

Bed alarm

Bedside commode placed alongside bed if needed

Nonskid footwear available

FIG 30.3 Safe patient room environment.

move arms, legs, body, or head freely. A restraint does not include devices such as orthopedically prescribed devices, protective helmets, or methods that involve physically holding a patient to conduct an examination or test, protecting a patient from falling out of bed, or permitting a patient to participate in activities without the risk of physical harm (TJC, 2017a).

The use of restraints is associated with serious complications resulting from immobilization such as pressure injuries, pneumonia, constipation, and incontinence. Loss of self-esteem, humiliation, and agitation are also serious concerns. Because of these risks, legislation emphasizes reducing the use of restraints. Regulatory agencies such as TJC and CMS enforce standards for the safe use of restraint devices. A restraint-free environment (neither physical nor chemical restraints) is your first goal for all patients. Always try alternatives before using restraints (Box 30.11).

For patients who continue to try to ambulate without assistance, use low beds and electronic bed/chair alarm devices. Specially designed low beds reduce the distance from the edge of a mattress to the floor, making a potential fall out of bed safer because the bed is closer to the floor. Use a low bed with an adjacent mat on the floor. Alarm devices warn nursing staff that a patient is attempting to leave a bed or chair unassisted. There are a variety of types including a device with a knee band that sounds an alarm when the patient reaches a near-vertical position. An infrared type of alarm is affixed to a headboard or bedframe, allowing a patient to move freely within a bed. If a patient tries to leave the bed, the infrared beam detects motion and sends out an alarm tone. Other safety devices include pressure-sensitive strips placed beneath a patient under the buttocks or a tether alarm that is clipped to a patient's gown. Alarm devices help

---

BOX 30.11   ALTERNATIVES TO RESTRAINTS

- Orient patients and family members to the environment; explain all procedures and treatments.
- Provide companionship and supervision; use trained sitters; adjust staffing and involve family.
- Offer diversionary activities such as music, puzzles, crocheting, activity aprons, and folding towels. Enlist ideas and support from family.
- Assign confused or disoriented patients to rooms near nurses' stations and observe them frequently.
- Use calm, simple statements and physical cues as needed.
- Use de-escalation, time-out, and other verbal intervention techniques when managing aggressive behaviors.
- Provide appropriate visual and auditory stimuli (e.g., family pictures, clock, calendar).
- Remove cues that promote leaving the room (e.g., close doors to block view of stairs, do not wear street clothes).
- Promote relaxation techniques and normal sleep patterns.
- Institute exercise and ambulation schedules as allowed by patient's condition; consult physical therapist for mobility and exercise program.
- Attend frequently to needs for toileting, food and liquid, and pain management.
- Camouflage IV lines with clothing, stockinette, or Kling dressing.
- Evaluate all medications and ensure timely and effective pain management.
- Eliminate bothersome treatments as soon as possible. For example, discontinue tube feedings and begin oral feedings as quickly as patient's condition allows.
- Use protective devices such as hip pads, helmet, skid-proof slippers, and nonskid strips near bed.

avoid physical restraints and, when responded to immediately, can prevent patient falls.

When restraints are required to protect a patient or others, involve the patient and family in the decision to use them. Help them adapt to this change by explaining the purpose of the restraint, expected care while the patient is in restraints, and that the restraint is temporary and protective. It is a requirement for nursing homes to obtain informed consent from family members before using restraints.

For legal purposes, know agency-specific policies and procedures for appropriate use and monitoring of restraints. The use of a restraint must be clinically justified and part of a patient's prescribed medical treatment and plan of care. A physician's order based on a face-to-face assessment of a patient is required. The order must be current, stating the type and location of the restraint, and specify the duration and circumstances under which it will be used. The orders need to be renewed within a specific time frame according to agency policy. In hospitals each original restraint order and renewal is limited to 4 hours for adults (18 years of age and older), 2 hours for children 9 through 17 years of age, and 1 hour for children younger than 9 years of age (CMS, 2015; TJC, 2017a). Orders may be renewed to the time limits for a maximum of 24 consecutive hours. Restraints are not to be ordered prn. Always make ongoing assessments of patients who are restrained. Properly document the behaviors that led to application of restraints, the procedure used in restraining, the condition of the body part restrained (e.g., color and pulse of extremity), and the evaluation of the patient response. Always remove a restraint periodically and assess if it continues to be necessary. Follow specific guidelines when using physical restraints (see Skill 30.1). The use of restraints must meet one of the following objectives:

1. Reduce the risk for patient injury from falls
2. Prevent interruption of therapy such as traction, IV infusions, nasogastric tube feeding, or Foley catheter
3. Prevent the confused or combative patient from removing life-support equipment
4. Reduce the risk for injury to self or others

Collaborate with other members of the health care team to design fall prevention programs and a restraint-free environment for patients. The goal is to discontinue the use of restraints as soon as possible.

Side Rails. When used correctly, side rails help to increase a patient's mobility and/or stability when in bed or moving from a bed to chair. Although they are the most commonly used physical restraint, side rails increase the occurrence of falls when patients attempt to get out of bed and crawl over a rail. There are a variety of beds with different side-rail designs. A patient needs to have a route to exit a bed safely and maneuver freely within the bed; in this case side rails are not considered a restraint. For example, raising only the two side rails at the top of the bed so that the lower part of the bed is open gives a patient room to exit a bed safely. Side rails used to prevent a patient such as one who is sedated from falling out of bed are not considered a restraint. Always know agency policy about the use of side rails. Be sure that a bed is in the lowest position possible when side rails are raised. Always assess the risk of using side rails compared with not using them. Check their condition; bars between the bedrails need to be spaced close together to prevent entrapment. A potential exists for trapping a person's head and body in gaps and openings between the bedframe and mattress.

The use of side rails alone for a patient who is disoriented often causes more confusion and further injury. Frequently a patient who is confused or determined to get out of bed because of pain, toileting needs, or anxiety tries to climb over a side rail or out at the foot of the bed. Either attempt often results in a fall. To reduce a patient's confusion, focus your interventions first on the cause, such as a response to a new medication, dehydration, or pain. Frequently nurses mistake a patient's attempt to explore his or her environment or to self-toilet as confusion. Use of a low bed reduces the distance between the bed and floor, facilitating a roll rather than a fall from the bed. If all efforts to reduce confusion or restlessness fail and the patient is at risk for serious injury to self or others, a restraint is sometimes necessary. A less restrictive restraint for the cognitively impaired patient is the Posey Bed Canopy. The canopy is a bed enclosure that allows a patient freedom of movement within a protected environment. However, remember that the goal is to remove the restraint at the earliest possible time.

Fires. Although smoking is usually not allowed in health care settings, smoking-related fires continue to pose a significant risk because of unauthorized smoking in beds or bathrooms. Institutional fires typically result from an electrical or anesthetic-related fire. The best intervention is to prevent fires. Nursing measures include complying with the smoking policies of an agency and keeping combustible materials away from heat sources. Box 30.12 highlights fire intervention guidelines in health care agencies. Regardless of where a fire occurs, always have an evacuation plan in place. Know where fire extinguishers and gas shut-off valves are located and how to activate a fire alarm.

BOX 30.12   FIRE INTERVENTION GUIDELINES IN HEALTH CARE AGENCIES

- Keep phone number for reporting fires visible on the telephone at all times.
- Know fire drill and evaluation plan of an agency.
- Know location of all fire alarms, exits, extinguishers, and oxygen shut-off.
- Use the mnemonic **RACE** to set priorities in case of fire:
  - **R**—Rescue and remove all patients in immediate danger.
  - **A**—Activate the alarm. Always do this before trying to extinguish even a minor fire.
  - **C**—Confine a fire by closing doors and windows and turning off oxygen and electrical equipment.
  - **E**—Extinguish a fire with an appropriate extinguisher.

Some health care agencies have fire doors that are held open by magnets and close automatically when a fire alarm sounds. It is important to keep equipment from blocking these doors. All personnel evacuate patients when appropriate. Patients who are close to the fire, regardless of its size, are at risk of injury and need to be moved to another area. If a patient requires oxygen but not life support, discontinue the oxygen, which is combustible and will fuel an existing fire. If the patient is on life support, maintain the patient's respiratory status manually with a bag-valve mask (e.g., Ambu bag) (see Chapter 32) until you move the patient away from the fire. Direct patients who can walk by themselves to move to a safe area or have them help move patients in wheelchairs. Move patients who are bedridden from the scene by a stretcher, their bed, or a wheelchair or have one or two rescuers carry them. If you have to carry a patient, do so correctly (e.g., two-man carry). Another two-rescuer technique is the chair carry, in which the patient is seated in a chair and both rescuers carry the chair. If you must carry a patient, be careful not to overextend your physical limits for lifting because an injury to you can result in further injury to the patient. If fire department personnel are on the scene, they help to evacuate patients.

After a fire has been reported and patients are out of danger, you and other personnel need to take measures to contain or put out the fire such as closing doors and windows, turning off oxygen and electrical equipment, and using a fire extinguisher. There are three types of extinguishers based on causes of fires: type A for paper and rubbish, type B for grease and anesthetic gas, and type C for electrical. There is also a multipurpose extinguisher (ABC) to use for all types of fires. To use an extinguisher correctly, remember the word **PASS** and follow these steps:

- **P**ull the pin. Hold the extinguisher with the nozzle pointing away from you and release the locking mechanism.
- **A**im low. Point the extinguisher at the base of the fire.
- **S**queeze the lever slowly and evenly.
- **S**weep the nozzle from side to side.

Electrical Accidents. Electrical equipment used in health care settings is regularly inspected and maintained. The clinical engineering departments of hospitals inspect biomedical equipment such as beds, IV infusion pumps, and ventilators. You know that a piece of equipment is safe to use when you see a safety inspection sticker with an expiration date. Decrease the risk for electrical injury and fire by using properly grounded and functional equipment. The ground prong in an electrical outlet carries any stray electrical current back to the ground. Remove equipment that is not in proper working order or that sparks when plugged in or is out of service, and notify appropriate hospital staff.

Radiation. Radiation is a health hazard in health care settings where radiation and radioactive materials are used in the diagnosis and treatment of patients. Hospitals have strict guidelines concerning the care of patients who are receiving radiation and radioactive materials. Know your agency-established protocols. To reduce your exposure to radiation, limit the time spent near the source, make the distance from the source as great as possible, and use shielding devices such as lead aprons. Staff who work near radiation must wear devices that track the cumulative exposure to radiation.

Disasters. As a nurse, be prepared to respond to and care for a sudden influx of patients during a disaster. TJC (2017a) requires hospitals to have an emergency-management plan that addresses identifying possible emergency situations and their probable impact, maintaining an adequate amount of supplies, and having a formal response plan. The plan must include actions to be taken by staff and steps to restore essential services and resume normal operations after an emergency. Infection control practices are critical in the event of a biological attack. You must manage all patients with suspected or confirmed bioterrorism-related illnesses with Standard Precautions (see Chapter 14). Additional precautions including airborne or contact isolation precautions are needed for diseases such as smallpox and pneumonic plague. Most infections associated with biological agents are not transmissible from patient to patient. However, limit the transport and movement of patients only to movement that is essential for treatment.

Workplace Violence Prevention. Being able to work in a safe environment is central to job satisfaction. As a nurse, it is important to be aware of your risks of being exposed to violence in the setting where you work. Nurses do not always know what acts constitute violence (Stene et al., 2015). A study involving nurses in emergency departments found that nurses often underreport violence, and as a direct result resources are not recognized or provided (Stene et al., 2015). It is important to recognize the patients who are most likely to enact violence. Research has shown that the five most common predictors of patient violence are confusion/cognitive impairment, anxiety, agitation, shouting/demanding, and a history of physical aggression (Kim et al., 2012).

An assessment tool is available for nurses to use to predict patients who are likely to act violently. The Aggressive Behavior Risk Assessment Tool (ABRAT) is a simple, easy-to-use assessment tool with acceptable interrater reliability, sensitivity, and specificity that may identify patients likely to commit an act of violence while on a medical-surgical unit and in long-term care (Kim et al., 2012; Berry et al., 2017). Behaviors in patients who may become violent include staring, eye contact, threatening tone and volume of voice, anxiety, mumbling, and pacing. If you face a violent situation, use the following tips for reducing violence (CPI, 2016):

1. Be nonjudgmental and empathic of patient's feelings.
   - Whatever the patient's problem is, it can be highly important to him or her.
2. Respect personal space.
   - Stand 1.5 to 3 feet away from a patient who is escalating. Allowing personal space helps reduce a patient's anxiety and can help you prevent acting-out behavior.
   - If you must enter personal space to administer care, first explain what you are doing and why.

3. Use nonthreatening nonverbal communication.
   - As a patient loses control, he or she does not listen to what you have to say. Instead, the patient reacts to your nonverbal communication (see Chapter 11).
   - Keep your voice tone, facial expressions, and movements neutral.
4. Do not overreact.
   - Stay calm, rational, and professional. Use positive thoughts such as, "I can manage this," and "I know what to do."
5. Focus on feelings.
   - Some people have trouble identifying how they really feel in a situation. Watch and listen carefully for the patient's real message.
6. Redirect or refocus any challenging questions, such as "Why does it always take so long for the doctor to see me?" or "Who's going to make me go to that test?"
   - Restate your request or directive; do not ignore the patient.
   - Bring the discussion back to how you can work together.
7. Set limits.
   - If patients become belligerent, defensive, or disruptive, give them *clear, simple, and enforceable limits.*
   - Speak clearly and offer a positive choice first.
8. Choose wisely what you insist on.
   - Be thoughtful in deciding *which rules are negotiable and which are not.* For example, if a patient is unwilling to walk at a given time, can you allow the patient to choose a time best for them?
   - When patients have options and flexibility, you may be able to avoid an altercation.
9. Allow silence for reflection.
   - Silence gives a person a chance to reflect on what is happening and how to proceed.
10. Allow time for the patient to make a decision.
    - Give patients a few moments to *think through what you have said.* A person's stress increases when they feel rushed.

If you find that you work in a setting where violence occurs, be sure to take care of yourself. Dealing with potentially violent patients is very stressful and sometimes dangerous. Find positive ways to care for yourself away from work. Use stress-management strategies (see Chapter 26).

■■■ EVALUATION

Patient Outcomes. Evaluate the outcomes of your care by comparing a patient's response with the expected outcomes for each goal of care. This requires you to reassess a patient's condition to measure actual responses. When the expected outcomes are not achieved, revise your interventions. It is also

---

BOX 30.13 EVALUATION

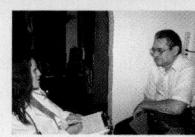

It has been 2 weeks since Joani implemented Mr. Gonzales' plan of care. She recommended modifications after conducting the home safety checklist. Mr. Gonzales' son helped to remove throw rugs in his father's home and adjust lighting. He plans to install a nonslip surface in the shower next week. With a new pair of glasses and after attending two sessions of a recommended exercise program, Mr. Gonzales is beginning to sense that his walking is improving. He tells Joani, "I feel a bit more relaxed moving around. I'm not as hesitant."

DOCUMENTATION NOTE

"Mr. Gonzales' home has improved lighting and fewer obstacles along walking path. He verbalizes benefit from his exercise program and is exercising on his own by walking twice a day. He states that he is less 'hesitant' to move about. No report of injury."

---

possible that new nursing diagnoses have developed. Apply evaluative measures (reassessments) to determine a patient's progress toward outcomes and goals. An example of a goal is "Family caregiver will modify the environment based on the patient's motor and sensory developmental needs." A possible outcome for this goal is "Family caregiver modifies all hazards in the home within 2 weeks." Evaluative measures include "Observe environment for elimination of threats to safety," and "Reassess motor and sensory status for appropriate environmental modifications." Evaluate outcomes by comparing what you planned with what resulted, and evaluate how well you implemented the plan (Box 30.13). Examine the planned interventions for appropriateness and effectiveness in each situation. By accomplishing goals and outcomes you validate effective care.

Patient Expectations. Patient-centered care requires a thorough evaluation of a patient's perspective related to safety and whether the patient's expectations have been met. Expectations as a result of care include restoration of health, reduction in fall risks, a safer home environment, and improved recognition of safety risks. Patients are often unaware of the dangers in their homes and workplaces. Many patients make adjustments to keep themselves and loved ones safe and free of injury once you identify the dangers. Ask a patient questions such as the following: "Are you satisfied with the changes made to your home?" "Do you feel safer as a result of changes we made?" "Are you still afraid of falling?" Involve family members in the evaluation, especially if they live with the patient and provide assistance in the home.

SAFETY GUIDELINES FOR NURSING SKILLS

Ensuring patient safety is an essential role of the professional nurse. To ensure patient safety, communicate clearly with members of the health care team, assess the patient's risks, incorporate priorities of care and preferences, and use the best evidence when making decisions about your patient's care. When performing the skills in this chapter, remember the following points to ensure safe, individualized patient care.

- Always attempt restraint alternatives (see Box 30.11) before using a restraint.
- If a restraint is needed, always use the least restrictive device.
- Because restraints limit a patient's ability to move freely, make clinical judgments appropriate to the patient's condition and agency policy.

SKILL 30.1 APPLYING PHYSICAL RESTRAINTS

View Video!

DELEGATION CONSIDERATIONS

The skills of assessing a patient's behavior and level of orientation, the need for restraints, the appropriate restraint type, and the ongoing assessments required while a restraint is in place cannot be delegated to nursing assistive personnel (NAP). However, applying and routinely checking a restraint can be delegated to NAP. The nurse directs the NAP by:

- Reviewing correct placement of the restraint and how to routinely check the patient's circulation, skin condition, and breathing.

- Reviewing when and how to change a patient's position and provide range-of-motion (ROM) exercises, toileting, and skin care.
- Instructing the NAP to notify the nurse immediately if there is a change in level of patient agitation, skin integrity, circulation of extremities, or patient's breathing.

EQUIPMENT

- Proper restraint (e.g., belt, wrist, mitten)
- Padding (if needed)

STEP	RATIONALE

ASSESSMENT

1. Identify patient using at least two identifiers (e.g., name and birthday or name and medical record number) according to agency policy.
2. Perform hand hygiene.
3. Assess for underlying causes of agitation and cognitive impairment leading to patient-initiated medical device removal.
   a. Assess for life-threatening physiological impairments.

   b. Assess for respiratory impairments, neurological impairments, fever and sepsis, hypoglycemia and hyperglycemia, alcohol or substance withdrawal, and fluid and electrolyte imbalance.
   c. Notify physician of change in mental status and compromised physiological status.
   d. Obtain baseline or premorbid cognitive function from family caregivers.
   e. Establish whether the patient has history of dementia or depression.
   f. Review medications that cause risk for falling to identify drug-drug interactions, adverse effects.
   g. Review current laboratory values.
4. Assess patient's current behavior (e.g., confusion; disorientation; agitation; restlessness; combativeness; inability to follow directions; repeated removal of tubing, dressing, or other therapeutic devices). Does patient create a risk to other patients?

Ensures correct patient. Complies with The Joint Commission standards and improves patient safety (TJC, 2018).
Prevents the spread of microorganisms.

Conditions might lead to patient-initiated medical device removal. Identification of life-threatening impairments might lead to more appropriate medical or pharmacological treatment, eliminating need for restraints.

Family caregivers provide excellent source of information for patient's behavior patterns and past history.

If patient's behavior continues despite treatment or restraint alternatives, use of restraint is indicated. You use the least restrictive type of restraint.

STEP	RATIONALE
5. If restraint alternatives failed earlier, confer with health care provider. Review agency policies and state laws regarding restraints. Obtain a current health care provider's order. Order must include purpose, type, location, and time or duration of restraint. Determine if signed consent for use of restraint is necessary (long-term care). Orders for nonviolent or non–self-destructive patients are written and renewed according to agency policy. Orders for self-destructive or violent patients are limited to select time limits and renewed only for a maximum of 24 consecutive hours (TJC, 2017a).	A health care provider's order for the least restrictive type of restraint is required.

Clinical Decision Point. A licensed independent health care provider responsible for the care of the patient evaluates the patient in person within 1 hour of initiation of restraint used for management of violent or self-destructive behavior that jeopardizes the physical safety of the patient, staff, or others. An RN or a physician assistant may conduct the in-person evaluation if trained in accordance with the requirements and consults with the aforementioned health care provider after the evaluation as determined by hospital policy (TJC, 2017a). *Always use the least restrictive restraint possible (e.g., mitts, elbow extenders)* (TJC, 2017a).

STEP	RATIONALE
6. Review manufacturer's instructions for restraint application before entering patient's room. Determine most appropriate size restraint.	You need to be familiar with all devices used for patient care and protection. Incorrect application of restraint device results in patient injury or death.
7. Assess the patient's or family caregiver's knowledge of restraints and the reasons for use.	Encourages cooperation; minimizes risks and anxiety. Identifies teaching needs.

PLANNING

1. Provide privacy.	Reduces patient anxiety and promotes cooperation.
2. Prepare and gather restraint equipment.	Ensures an organized approach for application of restraints.
3. Instruct patient and family about the use of restraints and associated nursing care.	Promotes patient and family cooperation and increases understanding of need for restraints.

IMPLEMENTATION

1. Perform hand hygiene. Adjust bed to proper height and lower side rail on side of patient contact. Be sure patient is comfortable and in proper body alignment.	Allows you to use proper body mechanics and prevents injury during restraint application. Positioning prevents contractures and neurovascular injury while restraint is in place.
2. Inspect area where restraint is to be placed. Note if there is any nearby tubing or device. Assess condition of skin, sensation, adequacy of circulation, and range of joint motion.	Restraints sometimes compress and interfere with functioning of devices or tubes. Assessment provides baseline to monitor patient's response to restraint.
3. Pad skin and bony prominences (as necessary) that will be under restraint.	Reduces friction and pressure from restraint to skin and underlying tissue.
4. Apply proper-size restraint. **Note:** Refer to manufacturer's directions.	
a. *Mitten restraint:* Thumbless mitten device restrains patient's hands. Place hand in mitten, being sure Velcro strap is around wrist and not forearm (see illustration).	Prevents patient from dislodging or removing medical device, removing dressings, or scratching but allows greater movement than a wrist restraint. It is considered a restraint alternative if untethered and patient is physically and cognitively able to remove it.
b. *Elbow restraint (freedom splint):* Restraint consists of rigidly padded fabric that wraps around the arm and is closed with Velcro. The upper end has a clamp that hooks to the sleeve of a patient's gown or shirt (see illustration). Insert arm so that elbow joint rests against padded area, keeping joint extended.	Commonly used with infants and children to prevent elbow flexion (e.g., with IV line placed in antecubital fossa). Restraint keeps elbow extended, making it difficult to remove or disrupt a medical device.

SKILL 30.1 APPLYING PHYSICAL RESTRAINTS—cont'd

View Video!

STEP	RATIONALE
c. *Belt or body restraint:* Have patient in sitting position in bed. Apply belt over clothes, gown, or pajamas. Be sure to place restraint at waist, not chest or abdomen. The slot in belt may be positioned in the front for limited movement or rear for increased movement. Remove wrinkles or creases in clothing. Bring ties through slots in belt. Help patient lie down in bed. Have patient roll to side and avoid applying belt too tightly. Ensure that straps secured to bedframe are snug so that belt does not slide to sides of bed (see illustrations). *Option:* Apply restraint net if an intent is to limit patient turning.	Restrains center of gravity and prevents patient from rolling off stretcher or sitting up while on stretcher or from falling out of bed. Tight application interferes with ventilation if belt moves up over abdomen or chest.

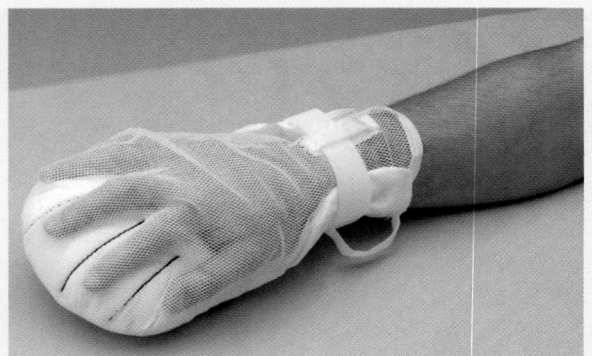

STEP 4a Mitten restraint. (Courtesy Posey Company, Arcadia, CA.)

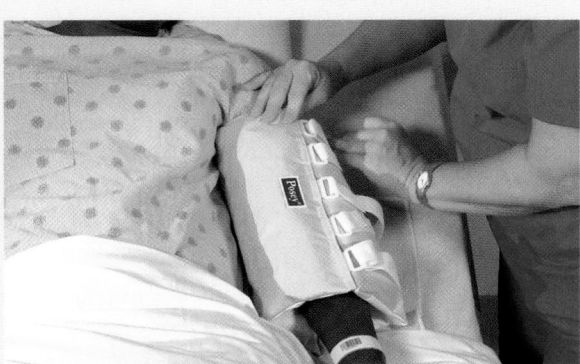

STEP 4b Freedom elbow restraint.

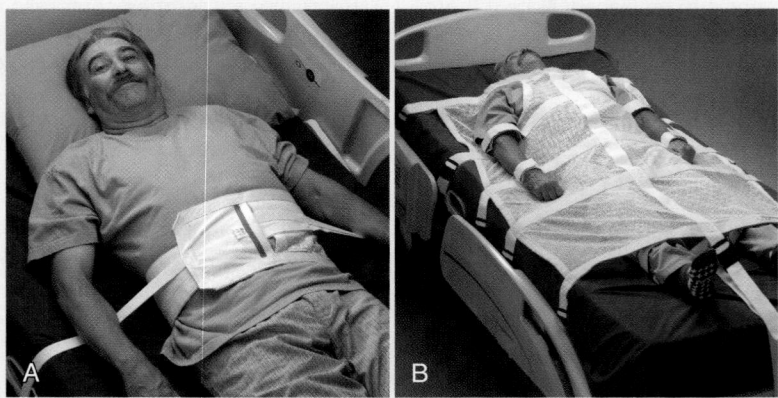

STEP 4c A, Properly applied belt restraint allows patient to turn in bed. **B,** *Option:* Restraint with net limits patient's ability to turn.

STEP	RATIONALE
d. *Extremity (ankle or wrist) restraint:* Restraint made of soft quilted material or sheepskin with foam padding. Wrap limb restraint around wrist or ankle with soft part toward skin and secure snugly (not tightly) in place by Velcro strap (see illustration). Insert two fingers under secured restraint (see illustration).	Restraint designed to immobilize one or all extremities. Maintain immobilization of extremity to protect patient from fall or accidental removal of therapeutic device (e.g., IV tube, Foley catheter). Tight application interferes with circulation and potentially causes neurovascular injury.

Clinical Decision Point. Patient with wrist and ankle restraints is at risk for aspiration if positioned supine. Place patient in lateral position or with head of bed elevated rather than supine.

STEP	RATIONALE
5. Attach restraint straps to portion of bedframe that moves when raising or lowering head of bed. Be sure straps are secure. *Do not attach to side rails.* Attach restraint to chair frame for patient in chair or wheelchair, being sure buckle is out of patient's reach.	Properly positioned strap does not tighten and restrict circulation when bed is raised or lowered.
6. Secure restraints on bedframe with quick-release buckle (see illustration). *Do not tie strap in a knot.* Be sure that buckle is out of patient's reach.	Allows for quick release in an emergency.
7. Double check and insert two fingers under secured restraint one more time. Assess proper placement of restraint including skin integrity, pulses, skin temperature and color, and sensation of restrained body part.	Provides baseline to later evaluate if injury develops from restraint.
8. Reposition patient, provide comfort and toileting measures, provide nutrition and fluids, and evaluate patient condition. If patient is violent or noncompliant, remove one restraint at a time and/or have staff assistance while removing restraints.	Provides an opportunity to attend to patient's basic needs and determine need for continuation.

Clinical Decision Point. Do not leave a patient who is violent or aggressive unattended while restraints are off.

STEP	RATIONALE
9. Secure nurse call or intercom system within patient's reach.	Allows patient, family, or caregiver to obtain assistance quickly.
10. Leave bed or chair with wheels locked. Keep bed in lowest position.	Prevents bed or chair from moving if patient tries to get out. If patient falls with bed in lowest position, this reduces chance of injury.
11. Perform hand hygiene.	Reduces transmission of microorganisms.

EVALUATION

1. After application, evaluate patient for signs of injury every 15 minutes (e.g., circulation, vital signs, ROM, physical and psychological status, and readiness for discontinuation). Perform visual checks if patient is too agitated to approach.	Frequent evaluation prevents injury to patient and ensures removal of restraint at earliest possible time. Frequency of monitoring guides staff in determining appropriate intervals for evaluation based on patient's needs and condition, type of restraint used, risk associated with use of chosen intervention, and other relevant factors.

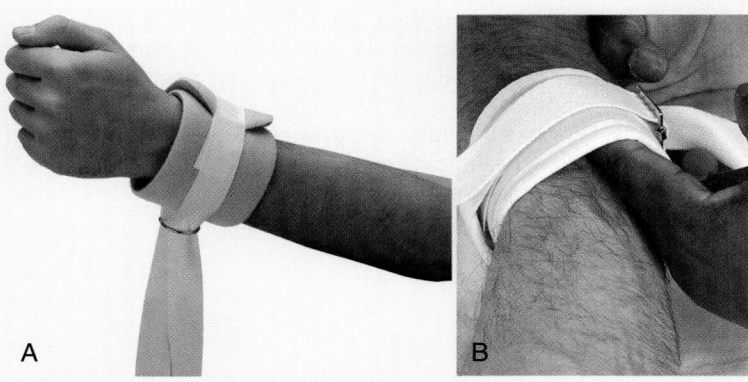

STEP 4d A, Extremity restraint. **B,** Check restraint for constriction by inserting two fingers under restraint.

STEP 6 Quick-release buckle makes it easier to disconnect and evacuate patients in an emergency.

SKILL 30.1   APPLYING PHYSICAL RESTRAINTS—cont'd

View Video!

STEP	RATIONALE
2. Evaluate patient's need for toileting, nutrition and fluids, hygiene, and elimination/release of restraints at least every 2 hours.	Prevents injury to patient and attends to basic needs.
3. Evaluate patient for any complications of immobility.	Early detection of skin irritation, restricted breathing, or reduction in mobility prevents serious adverse events.
4. Licensed health care provider or RN trained according to CMS requirements needs to evaluate patient within either 1 hour or 4 hours after initiation of restraints, depending on Medicare status of hospital (see agency policy).	Determines patient's immediate situation, reaction to restraints, medical and behavioral condition, and need to continue or terminate restraints (CMS, 2015).
5. After 24 hours, before writing a new order, the health care provider who is responsible for the patient's care must see and reassess patient.	Ensures that restraint application continues to be medically appropriate.
6. Observe IV catheters, urinary catheters, and drainage tubes to determine that they are positioned correctly and that therapy remains uninterrupted.	Reinsertion is uncomfortable and increases risk for infection or interrupts therapy.
7. Observe patient's behavior and reaction to presence of restraint.	Restraints can increase restlessness and agitation, resulting in harm.
8. **Use Teach Back:** "We have talked about the reason we are using restraints on your father. Can you tell me that reason? I want to be sure you understand." Revise your instruction now or develop a plan for revised patient/family caregiver teaching if patient/family caregiver is not able to teach back correctly.	Determines patient's/family caregiver's level of understanding of instructional topic.

RECORDING AND REPORTING

- Record nursing interventions and restraint alternatives tried on restraint flow sheet or in nurses' notes in electronic health record (EHR) or chart.
- Record patient's behavior before restraints were applied, level of orientation, and patient's/ family caregiver's understanding of explanation of purpose of restraint and consent (when required).
- Record the purpose for restraint, type and location, time applied, time ending the restraints, and routine observations made every 15 minutes (e.g., skin color, pulses, sensation, vital signs, behavior) in the flow sheets or nurses' notes.
- Record patient's level of orientation and behavior after restraint application. Record times patient was evaluated, attempts to use alternatives, and patient's response when restraint was removed.

UNEXPECTED OUTCOMES AND RELATED INTERVENTIONS

- Patient experiences impaired skin integrity.
  - Evaluate need for continued use of restraint and if alternatives can be used.
  - If restraint still needed, be sure it is applied correctly and provide adequate padding.
  - Check skin under restraint for abrasions and remove restraints more often. Provide appropriate skin care, and change wet or soiled restraints.
- Patient becomes more confused or agitated.
  - Determine cause of the behavior and eliminate if possible; consult with health care provider.
  - Determine need for more or less sensory stimulation and make any stimulation meaningful.
  - Reorient as needed, and try restraint-free options.
- Patient has neurovascular injury (e.g., cyanosis, pallor, and coldness of skin or complains of tingling, pain, or numbness).
  - Remove restraint immediately, stay with patient, and notify health care provider.
  - Protect extremity from further injury.

KEY POINTS

- A culture of safety requires a commitment that acknowledges the high-risk nature of the activities of an organization, the determination to achieve consistently safe operations, a blame-free environment, and an organizational commitment to resources.
- Vulnerable groups that require help in achieving a safe environment include infants, children, older adults, people who are ill or injured, people with physical and mental disabilities, people with poor literacy skills, and people who live in poverty.
- Your role as a nurse is to educate patients about common safety hazards and how to prevent injury while placing emphasis on hazards to which patients are more vulnerable.
- In the community a safe environment means that basic needs are achievable, physical hazards are reduced, transmission of pathogens and parasites is reduced, pollution is controlled, and sanitation is maintained.
- Caring for patients requires assessment of safety risks based on their developmental stage.
- Threats to an adult's safety are frequently associated with lifestyle habits.
- In older adults, the physiological changes associated with aging, effects of multiple medications, psychological factors, and acute or chronic disease increase risk for falls and other types of accidents.
- Risks to patient safety within a health care agency include falls and patient-inherent, procedure-related, and equipment-related accidents.
- Common risk factors for falls in hospital settings are broken down into two categories: intrinsic (patient related) and extrinsic (environmentally related).
- Nurses are responsible for making patients' hospital rooms safe.
- Restraints are not a solution to a patient problem. Exhaust all alternatives before placing patients in restraints.
- A medical order for a restraint must be current, stating the type and location of restraint, and specify the duration and circumstances under which it will be used.
- Side rails are the most commonly used physical restraint and increase the occurrence of falls when patients attempt to get out of bed by crawling over a rail.
- Continually evaluate the nursing care plan to promote safety to identify new or continued risks to a patient.

REFLECTIVE LEARNING

- Consider the patients you interacted with today and describe their age-specific safety risks.
- Thinking back over your past week of interacting with patients, identify factors that created a culture of safety as well as opportunities you saw for creating or improving a culture of safety.
- Consider the patients you interacted with today and their safety risks. What types of interventions would you include in your nursing care plan to help prevent and minimize the intrinsic and extrinsic threats to their safety?

REVIEW QUESTIONS

1. A nurse discovers an electrical fire in a patient's room. Which action should the nurse take first?
   1. Turn off the oxygen to the wall unit
   2. Evacuate any patients/visitors in immediate danger
   3. Close all doors and windows
   4. Use water from the sink in the patient room to extinguish fire
2. Which of the following activities reflect a culture of safety within a health care agency? (Select all that apply.)
   1. A hospital purchases a new bar-code system to check patient identification during medication administration.
   2. A hospital requires nurse managers to submit an annual safety plan for high-risk patients.
   3. A nurse commits an error while administering a high-risk medication and is released from her position.
   4. A hospital enforces routine monthly checks of electrical equipment.
   5. A nurse is treated unfairly after reporting a medication error.
3. The nurse finds a 68-year-old woman wandering in the hallway and exhibiting confused behavior. The patient says that she is looking for the bathroom. Which interventions are appropriate to ensure the safety of the patient? (Select all that apply.)
   1. Ask the physician or health care provider to order a restraint.
   2. Insert a urinary catheter.
   3. Provide scheduled toileting rounds every 2 to 3 hours.
   4. Consult with the health care provider about ordering an antianxiety medication.
   5. Keep the bed in low position with the side rails down.
   6. Keep the pathway from the bed to the bathroom clear.
4. Place the following steps for applying a wrist restraint in the correct order.
   1. Pad the skin overlying the wrist.
   2. Insert two fingers under secured restraint to be sure that it is not too tight.
   3. Be sure that patient is comfortable and in correct anatomical alignment.
   4. Secure restraint straps to bedframe with quick-release buckle.
   5. Wrap limb restraint around wrist or ankle with soft part toward skin and secure snugly.

5. Which of the following patients are at risk for falls because of intrinsic factors? (Select all that apply.)
    1. A patient with a tendency to have postural hypotension
    2. A patient whose hospital room has a bedside commode and suction machine blocking the path to the bathroom
    3. A patient who has bathroom floor mats that are thin and frayed
    4. A patient who has dementia and has cataracts
    5. A patient whose bed is placed in the highest position

evolve

Additional Review Questions, as well as rationales for all Review Questions, can be found on the Evolve website.

1, 2; 2, 1, 2, 4; 3, 3, 5, 6; 4, 3, 1, 5, 2, 4; 5, 1, 4.

REFERENCES

Agency for Healthcare Research and Quality (AHRQ): *Preventing falls in hospitals*, 2013. https://www.ahrq.gov/professionals/systems/hospital/fallpxtoolkit/index.html.

Agency for Healthcare Research and Quality (AHRQ): *Culture of safety*, 2016. http://psnet.ahrq.gov/primer.aspx?primerID=5.

Ahrens M: *Home structure fires*, National Fire Protection Association, 2015. http://www.nfpa.org/news-and-research/fire-statistics-and-reports/fire-statistics/fires-by-property-type/residential/home-structure-fires.

American Academy of Pediatrics (AAP): *Car seats: information for families*, 2017. http://www.healthychildren.org/English/safety-prevention/on-the-go/pages/Car-Safety-Seats-Information-for-Families.aspx.

American Hospital Association (AHA): *Quality advisory: implementing standardized colors for patient alert wristbands*, 2008. http://www.aha.org/advocacy-issues/tools-resources/advisory/2008/080904-quality-adv.pdf.

American Nurses Association (ANA): *Nursing: scope and standards of practice*, ed 3, Silver Spring, MD, 2015a, ANA.

American Nurses Association (ANA): *Code of ethics for nurses with interpretive statements*, Silver Spring, MD, 2015b, ANA.

ADABathroom.com: *Your source for ADA compliance in the bathroom*, 2017. http://www.adabathroom.com.

Berry B, et al: Utility of the Aggressive Behavior Risk Assessment Tool in long-term care homes, *Geriatr Nurs* 2017. http://www.gnjournal.com/article/S0197-4572(17)30041-1/abstract.

Burcham JR, Rosenthal LD: *Lehne's pharmacology for nursing care*, ed 9, St Louis, 2016, Elsevier.

Boysen P: Just culture: a foundation for balanced accountability and patient safety, *Ochsner J* 13(3):400, 2013. https://www.ncbi.nlm.nih.gov/pmc/articles/PMC3776518/.

Centers for Disease Control and Prevention (CDC): *Carbon monoxide exposures—United States, 2000-2009*, Atlanta, GA, 2011. https://www.cdc.gov/mmwr/preview/mmwrhtml/mm6030a2.htm.

Centers for Disease Control and Prevention (CDC): *Check for safety: a home fall prevention checklist for older adults*, 2015. https://www.cdc.gov/steadi/pdf/check_for_safety_brochure-a.pdf.

Centers for Disease Control and Prevention (CDC): *Important facts about falls*, 2017a. https://www.cdc.gov/homeandrecreationalsafety/falls/adultfalls.html.

Centers for Disease Control and Prevention (CDC): *Teen drivers: get the facts (motor vehicle safety)*, 2017b. https://www.cdc.gov/motorvehiclesafety/teen_drivers/teendrivers_factsheet.html.

Centers for Disease Control and Prevention (CDC): *Nonfatal injury reports*, 2017c. https://webappa.cdc.gov/sasweb/ncipc/nfirates.html.

Centers for Disease Control and Prevention (CDC): *Older adult drivers*, 2017d. http://www.cdc.gov/motorvehiclesafety/older_adult_drivers/.

Centers for Disease Control and Prevention (CDC): *About school violence*, 2017e. http://www.cdc.gov/ViolencePrevention/youthviolence/schoolviolence/index.html.

Centers for Medicare and Medicaid Services (CMS): *State operations manual. Appendix A: survey protocol, regulations, and interpretive guidelines for hospitals*, 2015. https://www.cms.gov/Regulations-and-Guidance/Guidance/Manuals/Downloads/som107ap_a_hospitals.pdf.

Chang HT, et al: Factors associated with fear of falling among community-dwelling older adults in the Shih-Pai study in Taiwan, *PLoS ONE* 11(3):e0150612, 2016.

Crisis Prevention Institute (CPI): *CPI's top 10 de-escalation tips*, 2016. https://www.crisisprevention.com/CPI/media/Media/download/PDF_DT.pdf.

Degelau J, et al: *Prevention of falls (acute care). Health care protocol*, Bloomington, MN, 2014, Institute for Clinical Systems Improvement.

ECRI Institute: *Falls*, 2016. https://www.ecri.org/components/HRC/Pages/SafSec2.aspx?tab=1.

El-Khoury F, et al: The effect of fall prevention exercise programmes on fall induced injuries in community dwelling older adults: systematic review and meta-analysis of randomised controlled trials, *BMJ* 347(7934):1, 2013.

Food and Drug Administration (FDA): *Report a problem to the FDA*, 2016. http://www.fda.gov/safety/reportaproblem/.

Gerberich SG, et al: An epidemiological study of the magnitude and consequences of work related violence: the Minnesota Nurses' Study, *Occup Environ Med* 61(6):495, 2004.

Hockenberry M, Wilson D: *Wong's nursing care of infants and children*, ed 10, St Louis, 2015, Mosby.

Hong T, et al: Visual impairment and the incidence of falls and fractures among older people: longitudinal findings from the Blue Mountains eye study, *Invest Ophthalmol Vis Sci* 55:7589, 2014.

Illinois Environmental Protection Agency (EPA): *Safe options for home needle disposal*, 2015. http://www.epa.illinois.gov/Assets/iepa/waste-management/medication-disposal/sharps-fact-sheet.pdf.

Inglesby TV: Progress in disaster planning and preparedness since, *JAMA* 306(12):1372, 2011.

Institute of Medicine (IOM) Committee on Quality of Health Care in America: *To err is human: building a safer health system*, Washington, DC, 2000, National Academies Press.

Institute of Medicine (IOM) Committee on Quality of Health Care in America: *Crossing the quality chasm: a new health system for the 21st century*, Washington, DC, 2001, National Academies Press.

Insurance Institute for Highway Safety (IIHS): *Fatality facts: teenagers 2015*, Arlington, VA, 2016, The Institute. http://www.iihs.org/iihs/topics/t/teenagers/fatalityfacts/teenagers.

Keall M, et al: Home modifications to reduce injuries from falls in the home injury prevention intervention (HIPI) study: a cluster-randomised controlled trial, *Lancet* 385(9964):1, 2014.

Kim S, et al: Usefulness of Aggressive Behaviour Risk Assessment Tool for prospectively identifying violent patients in medical and surgical units, *J Adv Nurs* 68(2):349, 2012.

Kochanek KD, et al: Deaths: final data for 2014. *National Vital Statistics Reports*, 2016. https://www.cdc.gov/nchs/data/nvsr/nvsr65/nvsr65_04.pdf.

Mathias S, et al: The get up and go test, *Arch Phys Med Rehabil* 67:387, 1986.

McPhaul KM, et al: Environmental evaluation for workplace violence in healthcare and social services, *J Safety Res* 39:237, 2008.

Mignardot J, et al: Gait disturbances as specific predictive markers of the first fall onset in elderly people: a two-year prospective observational study, *Front Aging Neurosci* 6:22, 2014.

Morse JM: *Preventing patient falls: establishing a fall intervention program*, ed 2, New York, 2009, Springer Publishing.

National Institute for Occupational Safety and Health (NIOSH): *Occupational violence*, 2017. https://www.cdc.gov/niosh/topics/violence/default.html.

National Quality Forum (NQF): *National voluntary consensus standards for public reporting of patient safety events*, Washington DC, 2011, NQF. http://www.qualityforum.org/Publications/2011/02/National_Voluntary_Consensus_Standards_for_Public_Reporting_of_Patient_Safety_Event_Information.aspx.

National Quality Forum (NQF): *Mission and vision*, Washington DC, 2017a. http://www.qualityforum.org/About_NQF/Mission_and_Vision.aspx.

National Quality Forum (NQF): *List of SREs*, 2017b. http://www.qualityforum.org/Topics/SREs/List_of_SREs.aspx#sre1.

Occupational Safety and Health Administration (OSHA): *Hazard communication standard: safety data sheets*, n.d.a. https://www.osha.gov/Publications/HazComm_QuickCard_SafetyData.html.

Occupational Safety and Health Administration (OSHA): *What is healthcare?* n.d.b. https://www.osha.gov/SLTC/healthcarefacilities/index.html.

Occupational Safety and Health Administration (OSHA): *Workplace violence in healthcare*, n.d.c. https://www.osha.gov/Publications/OSHA3826.pdf.

Plaksin J: Falls in older adults—risk factors and strategies for prevention, *Clinical Correlations: The NYU Langone Online Journal of Medicine*, 2014. http://www.clinicalcorrelations.org/?p=8114.

QSEN Institute: *QSEN Institute*, 2017. http://qsen.org/.

Stanford Health Care: *Nursing: patient centered care and education*, 2017. https://stanfordhealthcare.org/health-care-professionals/nursing/patient-care/fall-prevention.html.

Stene J, et al: Workplace violence in the emergency department: giving staff the tools and support to report, *Perm J* 19(2):e113, 2015.

Terrorism Research: *Types of terrorist incidents*, n.d. http://www.terrorism-research.com/incidents/.

The Joint Commission (TJC): Center for Transforming Healthcare aims to prevent inpatient falls with injury, *Joint Commission Online*, 2014. http://www.jointcommission.org/assets/1/23/jconline_April_30_14.pdf.

The Joint Commission (TJC): *Preventing falls and fall-related injuries in health care facilities*, 2015. http://www.jointcommission.org/assets/1/18/SEA_55.pdf.

The Joint Commission (TJC): *Comprehensive accreditation manual for hospitals*, Chicago, 2017a, TJC.

The Joint Commission (TJC): *Speak up initiatives*, 2017b. http://www.jointcommission.org/speakup.aspx.

The Joint Commission (TJC): *2018 National Patient Safety Goals*, Oakbrook Terrace, IL, 2018, The Commission. https://www.jointcommission.org/standards_information/npsgs.aspx.

The Joint Commission Center for Transforming Healthcare (TJCCTH): *Targeted solutions tool for preventing falls*, 2017. http://www.centerfortransforminghealthcare.org/tst_pfi.aspx.

Touhy T, Jett K: *Ebersole and Hess' gerontological nursing & healthy aging*, ed 5, St Louis, 2018, Elsevier.

United Nations Enable (UNE): *Accessibility for the disabled—a design manual for a barrier free environment*, 2004. http://www.un.org/esa/socdev/enable/designm/AD2-05.htm.

Veenema TG, et al: Nurses as leaders in disaster preparedness and response—a call to action, *J Nurs Scholarsh* 48(2):187, 2016.

evolve MEDIA RESOURCES

http://evolve.elsevier.com/Potter/essentials
- Audio Glossary
- QSEN Activity and Review Questions Answers and Rationales
- Video Clips

OBJECTIVES

- Describe factors that influence personal hygiene practices.
- Perform a comprehensive assessment of a patient's hygiene needs.
- Discuss factors that affect the condition of the skin, mouth, hair, scalp, nails, and feet.
- Identify common problems involving the skin, feet, nails, hair, and scalp.
- Discuss appropriate interventions for hygiene problems.
- Correctly perform hygiene procedures for care of a patient's skin, perineum, feet, nails, mouth, eyes, ears, and nose.

- Explain the importance of foot care for a patient with diabetes.
- Discuss conditions that place patients at risk for impaired oral mucous membranes.
- Describe how hygiene for older adults differs from hygiene for younger patients.
- Make an occupied and unoccupied hospital bed.
- Identify ways to foster patient-centered care when providing hygiene care.
- Incorporate safety measures into hygiene care activities.

KEY TERMS

alopecia, p. 822
dental caries, p. 814
denture stomatitis, p. 829
edentulous, p. 820
effleurage, p. 837

gingivitis, p. 814
maceration, p. 830
mucositis, p. 826
pediculosis capitis, p. 822
perineal care, p. 832

skin tears, p. 824
stomatitis, p. 824
xerosis, p. 824

Personal hygiene influences your patients' comfort, safety, and well-being. Hygiene includes cleaning and grooming activities that maintain personal body cleanliness and appearance. A variety of personal, social, and cultural factors influence hygiene practices.

Because hygiene care requires close contact with your patients, use communication skills (e.g., listening, reflecting, focusing) to promote caring therapeutic relationships (see Chapter 11). When providing hygiene, you can integrate other nursing activities including patient assessment and interventions such as range-of-motion (ROM) exercises, application of dressings, or inspection and care of IV sites. Assess each patient's ability to perform hygiene care; ensure privacy; convey respect; and foster a patient's independence, safety, and comfort.

CASE STUDY *Mrs. Winkler*

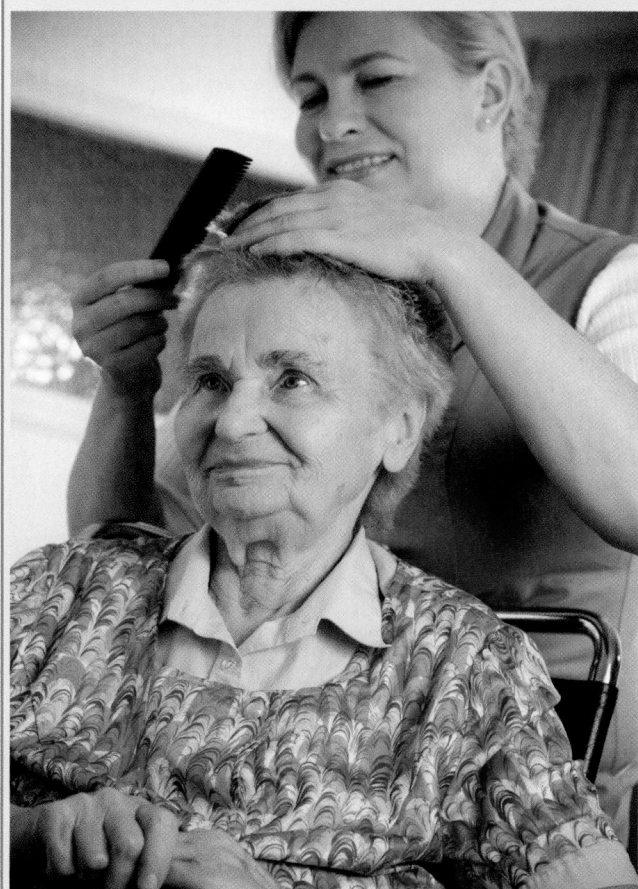

Copyright © AlexRaths/iStock/Thinkstock.

Mrs. Winkler is a 78-year-old woman with a medical history of rheumatoid arthritis and diabetes mellitus. She is a newly admitted resident of an extended care facility. The arthritis has resulted in chronic pain and deformity in her hands and knees. The pain and joint deformity have caused Mrs. Winkler to have limited ability to use her hands and thus a decreased ability to perform hygiene independently. Jamie Johnson is a nursing student assigned to care for Mrs. Winkler today, which includes helping Mrs. Winkler with her hygiene care.

Jamie needs to provide patient-centered personal hygiene while giving attention to Mrs. Winkler's comfort level. When hygiene needs are not fulfilled, patients may experience complications including skin or oral mucosa breakdown and infections.

One of Jamie's nursing priorities is to review the effect of dependency on Mrs. Winkler's self-esteem and implement care that helps Mrs. Winkler meet self-care needs. Even at an optimal level of functioning with assistance, Mrs. Winkler is at risk for self-care deficits, impaired skin integrity, impaired oral mucosa, and risk for infection.

During hygiene care, Jamie assesses Mrs. Winkler's readiness to learn health promotion practices. Jamie wants to preserve as much of Mrs. Winkler's independence as possible, ensure privacy, and foster physical well-being.

SCIENTIFIC KNOWLEDGE BASE

Providing hygiene for patients requires an understanding of the anatomy and physiology of the skin, nails, oral cavity, eyes, ears, and nose. Whether patients perform their own hygiene or you help them, effective hygiene techniques promote the normal structure and function of body tissues.

Skin

The skin serves several functions including protection, secretion, excretion, body temperature regulation, and cutaneous sensation (Table 31.1). The layers of the skin include the epidermis, the dermis, and the subcutaneous tissue (also known as the *hypodermis*), which shares some of the protective functions of the skin.

The epidermis (outer layer) shields underlying tissues against water loss and injury, prevents entry of disease-producing microorganisms, and generates new cells to replace the dead cells that are continuously shed from the outer surface of the skin. Bacteria (normal flora) commonly reside on the outer epidermis. Normal flora inhibits disease-producing microorganisms.

The dermis supports the epidermis and contains nerve fibers, blood vessels, sebaceous and sweat glands, and hair follicles. Sebaceous glands secret sebum, an oily fluid that softens and lubricates the skin, slows water loss from the skin, and exerts bactericidal action.

The subcutaneous tissue functions as a heat insulator, supports upper skin layers in withstanding stresses and pressure, and anchors the skin loosely to underlying structures such as muscle. The subcutaneous tissue layer contains blood vessels, nerves, lymph tissue, and loose connective tissue filled with fat cells.

Bacteria reside on the outer surface of the skin. The resident bacteria are normal flora. These normal flora do not cause illness; rather, they inhibit disease-producing microorganisms from reproducing. Because a part of the skin is usually exposed to environmental irritants, and the skin is an active organ sensitive to physiological changes within the body, some skin problems are common. The skin often reflects a change in a person's physical condition by alterations in color, thickness, texture, turgor, temperature, and moisture (see Chapter 16).

Hygiene practices often affect skin status, with both beneficial and negative effects on the skin and its functions. For example, long baths and use of hot water can lead to dry, flaky skin and loss of protective oils.

Oral Cavity and Teeth

The oral cavity consists of the lips, the cheeks, the tongue and its muscles, and the hard and soft palates. Mucous membranes continuous with the skin line the oral cavity. Normal oral mucosa glistens and is pink, soft, moist, smooth, and without lesions. Healthy gums fit tightly around each tooth and are pink, moist, and smooth.

Several glands secrete saliva into the oral cavity. Saliva cleanses the mouth, dissolves food chemicals to promote

TABLE 31.1 FUNCTIONS OF THE SKIN AND IMPLICATIONS FOR CARE	
FUNCTION/DESCRIPTION	**IMPLICATIONS FOR CARE**
Protection Epidermis is a relatively impermeable skin layer that prevents entrance of microorganisms. Although microorganisms reside on skin surfaces and in hair follicles, relative dryness of the surface inhibits bacterial growth. Sebum removes bacteria from hair follicles. Acidic pH of skin further slows bacterial growth.	Weakening of epidermis occurs by scraping or stripping its surface during use of dry razors, tape removal, or improper turning or positioning techniques. Excessive dryness causes cracks and breaks in skin and mucosa that allow bacteria to enter. Emollients soften and prevent moisture loss, soaking improves moisture retention, and hydration of mucosa prevents dryness. Constant exposure to moisture causes maceration or softening, which interrupts dermal integrity and promotes ulcers and bacterial growth. Keep bed linen and clothing dry. Misuse of soap, detergents, cosmetics, deodorant, and depilatories causes chemical irritation. Alkaline soaps neutralize the protective acid condition of the skin. Cleansing removes excess oil, sweat, dead skin cells, and dirt, which promote bacterial growth. Minimize friction to avoid loss of stratum corneum, which increases risk for pressure injuries.
Sensation The skin contains sensory organs for touch, pain, heat, cold, and pressure.	Smooth out linen to remove sources of mechanical irritation. Make sure that bath water is not too hot or too cold.
Temperature Regulation Radiation, evaporation, conduction, and convection control body temperature.	Factors that interfere with heat loss can alter temperature control. Wet bed linen or gowns increase heat loss. Excess blankets or bed coverings conserve heat and interfere with heat loss through radiation and conduction. Coverings conserve heat.
Excretion and Secretion Sweat promotes heat loss by evaporation. Sebum lubricates skin and hair.	Perspiration and oil sometimes harbor microorganism growth. Bathing removes excess body secretions, but excessive bathing causes dry skin.

taste, moistens food to enable bolus formation, and contains enzymes that start the breakdown of starchy foods. Medications, exposure to radiation, dehydration, and mouth breathing may impair salivary secretion in the mouth.

A normal tooth consists of the crown, neck, and root. Healthy teeth appear in a variety of shades of white, smooth, shiny, and aligned. The condition of the oral cavity reflects overall health and indicates oral hygiene needs (see Chapter 16).

Difficulty in chewing develops when the gums surrounding the teeth become inflamed or infected or when teeth are lost or become loosened. Regular oral hygiene helps to prevent gingivitis (inflammation of the gums), plaque, and dental caries (tooth decay produced by interaction of food with bacteria that forms plaque).

Eyes, Ears, and Nose

Chapters 16 and 39 describe the structure and function of the eyes, ears, and nose. Specialized glands in the auditory canal secrete cerumen, which traps foreign bodies and repels insects. In some people cerumen builds up and becomes impacted. The eyes contain sensitive nerve endings and secrete tears, which contain substances to cleanse and lubricate the eye and protect it from bacteria. Patients with alterations in one or more of the senses often need help to meet their hygiene needs.

Feet, Hands, and Nails

The feet, hands, and nails require special attention to prevent infection, odor, and injury. The condition of a patient's hands and feet affects the patient's ability to perform hygiene care. Discomfort and reduced ability to bear weight, ambulate, or manipulate the hands places a patient at risk for losing self-care ability.

The nails are epithelial tissues that grow from the root of the nail bed, located in the skin at the nail groove hidden by a fold of skin called the *cuticle*. A normal healthy nail appears transparent, smooth, and convex, with a pink nail bed and translucent white tip. The appearance of the nails reflects level of self-care. Inadequate nutrition and disease cause changes in the shape, thickness, and curvature of the nail (see Chapter 16).

Hair

Special hair-care practices focus on care of the scalp, axilla, and pubic areas. Hair growth, distribution, and pattern are indicators of a person's health status (see Chapter 16). Hormonal changes, emotional and physical stress, aging, intake of toxins (e.g., arsenic, cocaine), gender, race, nutrition, infection, and certain diseases affect hair characteristics. A person's appearance and sense of well-being often depend on the way the hair looks and feels. Illness or disability sometimes prevents patients from maintaining daily hair care.

NURSING KNOWLEDGE BASE

Individualized patient-centered hygiene care considers a patient's hygiene preferences, ability to perform care, and level of assistance needed to ensure safe hygiene. Because no two individuals perform hygiene care the same way, you must individualize patient care by assessing a patient's unique hygiene practices and preferences. Hygiene care requires you to know your patient and use therapeutic communication skills to promote a trusting therapeutic relationship. The time you spend with patients during hygiene care allows you to convey caring and more thoroughly assess patients' needs. Personal hygiene activities promote comfort, foster a positive self-image, and help prevent infection and disease.

Physical and Mental Status

Patients with limitations or disabilities resulting from disease and/or injury often lack the physical energy and dexterity to perform hygiene self-care safely. Limited mobility caused by a variety of factors (e.g., physical injury, weakness, surgery, pain, prolonged inactivity, medication effects, and presence of an indwelling catheter or IV line) affects a patient's ability to handle and manipulate hygiene supplies, use a washcloth, or walk to the bathroom.

Safety is a priority for a patient with a sensory deficit. Sensory deficits not only impair a patient's ability to perform care but also place him or her at risk for injury. For example, the inability to feel that bath water is too hot can lead to burn injury.

Chronic illnesses (e.g., cardiac disease, chronic lung disease, cancer, or neurological disorders) often exhaust or incapacitate a patient. Patients who become fatigued need assistance with hygiene and periods of rest during care to allow them to participate.

Pain that accompanies illness and/or injury often limits a patient's ability to tolerate hygiene and grooming activities or perform self-care. Pain may limit ROM, resulting in impaired use of the arms or hands or limited ability to move about in the environment. Sedation and drowsiness associated with analgesics used for pain management also limit a patient's ability to participate in care and could result in injury from a fall, such as when walking to the bathroom.

Acute and chronic cognitive impairments such as stroke, brain injury, psychoses, and dementia often leave a patient unable to perform self-care independently. Patients with cognitive impairments may be unaware of their hygiene and grooming needs. Because of impaired ability to interpret stimuli, some patients with dementia become fearful and agitated during hygiene care, resulting in aggressive behavior (Zimmerman et al., 2014). To provide safe, effective patient care, you need to consider the effects of cognitive impairment on your patient and modify hygiene care appropriately.

Socioeconomic Status

A person's economic resources influence the type and extent of hygiene practices used in the home. Be sensitive in considering that patients' economic status affects their ability to maintain hygiene. A patient with limited funds may be unable to afford basic supplies such as deodorant or shampoo or may be unable to make needed modifications to ensure safety in the home, such as adding nonskid surfaces and grab bars in the bathroom.

Developmental Stage

Apply your knowledge of physical and psychosocial developmental changes as you assess your patients and plan, implement, and evaluate hygiene care (see Chapter 23). A patient's developmental stage affects not only the normal condition of body tissues and structures but also his or her ability to perform proper hygiene care. Family customs affect hygiene practices during childhood and adolescence, such as the frequency or time of bathing and whether teeth brushing is performed.

According to Erikson (1963), children in the early-childhood stage strive to develop a sense of autonomy and independence. Caregivers can foster this development by supervising toddlers during hygiene care while allowing them to attempt the care.

During the preschool stage of "initiative versus guilt," a child exerts control over the environment and becomes more independent. During this stage, caregivers need to encourage children to explore hygiene care while helping them make appropriate care choices.

When children enter school, they must cope with the social demands of that environment including the influence of peers. Caregivers must recognize that personal hygiene habits may change during this stage as the child struggles to fit in with his or her peer group (e.g., a young boy might rebel against a daily bath during this stage).

During adolescence, a teen tries to develop a sense of self and personal identity. He or she may experiment with a variety of hygiene and grooming choices; it is important for teens to be able to express their personal style as they develop their individual identities.

Middle and older adults have specific routines for hygiene practices. They prefer to perform their own hygiene when possible and must be allowed to make decisions in how hygiene is administered.

Skin. A neonate's skin is relatively immature and thin, with the epidermis and dermis being loosely bound together. Friction against the skin layers may easily cause damage.

Handle neonates carefully during bathing. Any break in the skin may result in an infection.

A toddler's skin layers become more tightly bound together, resulting in greater resistance to skin injury and infection. However, because a toddler is more active and does not have established independent hygiene habits, caregivers must provide thorough hygiene and teach good hygiene habits.

During the school-age years, children are active and are exposed to skin injuries from falling, playing sports, or just play. When the skin is no longer intact the child is at risk for infection. School-age children need teaching and reinforcement about effective skin hygiene practices to promote healing of minor injuries and prevent skin infections.

During adolescence, the skin grows and matures. Sebaceous glands become more active, predisposing adolescents to acne. Sweat glands become fully functional during puberty. More frequent bathing and shampooing and the use of deodorants become necessary to reduce body odors and reduce oils on skin and hair.

The condition of an adult's skin condition depends on hygiene practices and exposure to environmental irritants. The skin is normally elastic, well hydrated, firm, and smooth. With aging, the rate of epidermal cell replacement slows, and elastic collagen fibers shrink. The skin thins and loses resiliency, becoming fragile and subject to bruising and breaking. As the production of lubricating substances from skin glands decreases, the skin becomes dry and itchy (Meiner, 2015). These changes often lead to dry, cracked skin. Although excessive bathing with hot water and/or harsh soap causes the skin to become increasingly dry, a 5- to 10-minute bath or shower adds moisture to the skin (American Academy of Dermatology [AAD], 2016).

Mouth. At approximately 6 to 10 months of age, infants begin teething, with the first permanent teeth erupting at about 6 years of age (Hockenberry and Wilson, 2015). By age 13 years, most children have 28 of their permanent teeth. The last of the permanent teeth to erupt are the third molars or "wisdom teeth," which usually begin to erupt between ages 17 and 21 years.

From adolescence through middle adulthood, the teeth and gums remain healthy if the person follows healthy eating patterns and oral care practices. As a person ages, many factors may contribute to poor oral health including age-related changes of the mouth, chronic diseases such as diabetes mellitus, physical disabilities involving hand grasp or strength, lack of attention to oral care, and medications (e.g., chemotherapy) that have side effects on the oral cavity. With aging, gums lose vascularity and tissue elasticity, which results in poor fitting dentures for patients who no longer have their own teeth.

Eyes, Ears, and Nose. Chapter 39 describes changes in hearing, vision, and olfaction across the life span. Alterations in sensory function often require modifications in hygiene care. Use your knowledge of developmental changes when planning hygiene care.

Feet and Nails. With aging, chronic foot problems are more likely to develop because of poor foot care, improper fit of footwear, or systemic disease. Older adults sometimes do not have the strength, flexibility, visual acuity, or manual dexterity to care for their feet and nails. Common problems of the feet affecting older adults include corns, calluses, bunions, hammertoe, and fungal infections. Painful feet result from a variety of deformities, weak structure, injuries, and diseases such as diabetes and rheumatoid arthritis (Meiner, 2015).

Hair. Throughout life, changes in the growth, distribution, and condition of the hair affect hair hygiene and grooming. As boys reach adolescence, shaving becomes a part of routine grooming. As girls reach puberty, they often begin to shave their legs and axillae. With aging, scalp hair becomes thinner and drier, and shampooing is needed less often.

Personal Preferences

Patients have individual preferences regarding the timing of bathing, shaving, and performing hair and oral care. Some patients prefer to shower, whereas others prefer to bathe at a sink or in bed. Patients may prefer specific hygiene products. Knowing these desires and preferences helps you take a patient-centered approach to hygiene. Learn a patient's preferences, allowing the patient to make personal choices whenever possible and promoting patient involvement and independence (Burman et al., 2013).

Cultural Variables

A patient's cultural beliefs and practices influence hygiene care. People from diverse cultural backgrounds follow different self-care practices. Some ethnic or social groups may not place the same importance on maintaining cleanliness as other groups (Giger, 2013).

Some patients take a bath or shower daily and use deodorant. People from other cultures, however, may not be sensitive to body odor, may prefer to bathe less often, and may not use deodorant. Avoid expressing disapproval when caring for a patient whose hygiene practices differ from yours. Do not force changes in hygiene practices unless the practices affect a patient's health or treatments. First identify a patient's beliefs and hygiene practices. Be tactful when speaking with the patient or family member, provide information, and allow the patient choices. Know the possible impact of a patient's cultural beliefs on the type and timing of hygiene care. In some situations, you may need to schedule the bath after mealtime or discard bath water that is too hot.

Religious beliefs also may guide hygiene practices. Some women practice modesty in dress when in the presence of men and avoid touching or having proximity to men (Giger, 2013). Clothing can include head covering, long sleeves, and long slacks or skirts covering the legs. Ensure that these patients receive care that follows their cultural hygiene practices and protects their privacy. This includes privacy during bathing and toileting activities, appropriate bed clothing, and same-gender caregivers for hygiene care.

CRITICAL THINKING

Synthesis

Patient care requires you to apply what you know about a patient, your knowledge base, experience, and critical thinking attitudes and standards. Your synthesis of this information allows you to make sound decisions as you apply the nursing process. Critical thinking synthesis involves combining all available information to obtain a clear picture of the approach needed to provide patient-centered care (Box 31.1).

Knowledge. Knowledge of the anatomy and physiology of the skin, oral cavity, nails, and sensory organs helps you understand the implications of proper hygiene for a patient's total health status. As you develop more knowledge about pathological conditions, you will understand factors that increase the risk for hygiene problems. Apply this knowledge to guide the questions you ask patients about their hygiene practices as you assess their needs and their self-care status. For example, knowing the pathophysiology of diabetes and its potential effects on circulation and sensation is the scientific knowledge base you need to determine a patient's practices and implement safe and effective foot care.

Also apply your knowledge of physical assessment skills (see Chapter 16) when providing hygiene. Examine the skin, oral and nasal cavities, eyes and ears, peripheral circulation, sensorimotor function, and degree of ROM while you meet hygiene needs to use time efficiently. This technique also will produce a database for identifying hygiene problems and monitoring a patient's progress over time.

Use your knowledge of comfort and safety measures when planning and implementing hygiene care. For example, give analgesic medications in a timely manner to reduce pain before performing hygiene care. Ensure a patient's safety by using aids to limit slipping or falling and by checking water temperature to prevent burns.

Experience. Draw on your own experiences when providing for your patients' hygiene needs. You may have helped family members with their hygiene. An early clinical experience often includes patient hygiene. As your experience increases, your comfort and expertise in meeting the specific hygiene needs of your patients increase as well.

Attitudes. Multiple critical thinking attitudes apply when providing hygiene. Display curiosity; be thorough in your assessment of the patient's skin, nails, sensory organs, and oral cavity. Strive to learn the patient's personal and cultural preferences. Use creativity to collaborate with patients and determine the best way to meet individual hygiene needs. Be creative and supportive to help patients develop new hygiene practices or adapt existing ones when illness or loss of function impairs self-care abilities. For example, your patient may need to adapt to showering instead of a tub bathing because of physical limitations.

Because of variations in patients' physical strength and hygiene practices, be flexible in your approach to care. Encourage a patient to participate in determining how and when care is provided. For example, you may need to include rest periods to prevent exhaustion during hygiene care. Demonstrate responsibility and accountability when designing a plan of care that promotes your patient's comfort and well-being.

Standards. Critical thinking standards ensure that assessment of hygiene needs is relevant, consistent, and accurate. Apply professional standards of care in your practice. For example, when caring for patients with diabetes, apply standards of the American Diabetes Association (2014) to ensure that you provide proper foot care. Recommendations from the American Dental Association (2017) are the guidelines for teaching oral care.

Apply standards of professional responsibility to advocate for your patient. For example, apply the ethical standard of autonomy by letting your patient choose the timing and type of bath when possible. Adhere to the principle of beneficence by using evidence-based, patient-centered bathing measures with a patient who is cognitively impaired and becomes agitated or aggressive when bathed (Zimmerman et al., 2014). Promote your patients' independence as much as possible while still protecting their safety.

NURSING PROCESS

■■■ ASSESSMENT

Assessment of a patient's hygiene status and self-care abilities requires you to complete a nursing history and physical assessment. You do not routinely assess all body regions before providing hygiene; much of your assessment will occur as you perform hygiene the first time. However, you must

---

BOX 31.1 SYNTHESIS IN PRACTICE

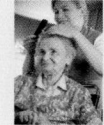

Copyright © AlexRaths/ iStock/ Thinkstock.

Before entering Mrs. Winkler's room, Jamie reviews and synthesizes knowledge about the effect of chronic illness in general and Mrs. Winkler's chronic illness on functional independence, reviews principles of therapeutic communication, and reviews the pathophysiological effects of rheumatoid arthritis and diabetes mellitus.

From previous clinical experience, Jamie has learned that patients want and need to provide input about their nursing care. By applying the ethical standard of autonomy, Jamie encourages Mrs. Winkler to make decisions about how to proceed with her hygiene care by engaging her in a therapeutic conversation.

Jamie learns that Mrs. Winkler wants to clean her face and hands and care for her dentures before breakfast. But then she tells Jamie that she cannot do these things by herself and that she does not want to be "any trouble." Jamie uses this information to determine that reassuring Mrs. Winkler and helping her with hygiene before breakfast are priorities.

conduct a brief history to identify priority areas and plan patient-centered hygiene care (Table 31.2).

While helping a patient with personal hygiene, carefully assess the skin, nails, oral cavity, hair and scalp, and sensory organs (see Chapter 16). Visually inspect and palpate tissue, noting injury to skin integrity. Pay attention to characteristics such as cleanliness of skin and hydration of oral mucosa, which are most affected by hygiene practices. Assessment data help you identify hygiene-related issues and plan the type and extent of hygiene care required.

Observe the patient as you give care to detect problems associated with inadequate hygiene practices. Also, assess a patient's ability to tolerate hygiene procedures that are often exhausting. During hygiene care, assess for a variety of health issues and thus better set health care priorities.

Self-Care Ability. Assess the patient's ability to independently perform hygiene care safely or ability to help with hygiene care. You need to assist when a patient is unable to bathe or perform skin care. To determine whether a patient requires a bed bath rather than a tub bath or shower, assess the patient's balance, activity tolerance, muscle strength and coordination, and the availability of treatment-related tubs or equipment. Your hygiene options are limited when bed rest is ordered or the patient is able to sit in a chair for only a short period of time.

Be alert for activity intolerance during hygiene care. Observe respirations, noting changes in rate and depth and/ or any shortness of breath. Observe for changes in skin color. Palpate the pulse to detect changes in rate and regularity and question the patient about dizziness, weakness, or fatigue. If a patient shows signs of intolerance and is up in a chair, return the patient to bed to reduce the cardiovascular and respiratory demand and help prevent injury from a fall. To foster safety with bathing, assess a patient's ability to detect thermal and tactile stimuli.

The degree of assistance a patient needs during bathing also depends on his or her vision, ability to sit without support and perform hand grasps, and degree of active ROM of extremities. Observe your patient's physical ability to perform eye, ear, and nose care. Assess your patient's ability to care for any sensory aids. Patients who have limited upper-extremity mobility, have reduced vision, are seriously fatigued, or are unable to grasp small objects such as a hearing aid battery or contact lenses require assistance. Evidence shows that changes in manual dexterity or cognitive function play a key role in hygiene and oral health practices (Pandey et al., 2014).

When patients have self-care limitations, family caregivers often help with home care. In the hospital setting, nurses begin discharge planning early in each hospitalization. The nurse is responsible for assessing whether a patient needs hygiene care assistance and ensuring that appropriate plans are made for care after discharge. When you determine that a patient has specific postdischarge hygiene care needs, the discharge plan should include arrangements for a home assessment and evaluation to guide an individualized plan of care.

TABLE 31.2   FOCUSED PATIENT ASSESSMENT

FACTORS TO ASSESS	QUESTIONS	PHYSICAL ASSESSMENT
Skin care	Which skin care products do you use? Tell me about any skin problems bothering you.	Inspect condition of skin and bony prominences. Observe skin surfaces and skinfolds for presence of irritation, dirt, odor, or debris.
Mouth care	Are you having any mouth pain, or have you noticed any sores in your mouth? Do you wear dentures or a partial plate?	Inspect condition of teeth, gums, and mouth. Observe patient performing mouth care or eating to determine presence of oral pain or discomfort that impairs hygiene practices. Observe fit of dentures.
Assistance with hygiene	Do you use any aids to help you with your bath such as grab bars in your tub or shower? Which parts of personal hygiene can you do for yourself? For which parts of hygiene care do you need help? How can I make helping you with your hygiene easier and more pleasant?	Observe patient's use of assistive devices, noting proper, safe use. Complete an environmental assessment to detect presence of safety devices or hazards related to hygiene care. Observe patient during hygiene activities, noting activities that are difficult for patient to perform.
Tolerance of hygiene	Does bathing/showering and mouth care cause any symptoms such as shortness of breath, pain, or fatigue? What do you do to minimize these symptoms? What can I do to help you complete hygiene care most comfortably?	Observe patient before, during, and after hygiene. Palpate pulse, noting rate and rhythm changes. Observe breathing pattern, noting rate and ease of breathing. Observe patient for pallor and diaphoresis. Notice facial expressions that indicate pain.

Copyright © AlexRaths/iStock/ Thinkstock.

In addition, you must assess your patient's cognitive status. A patient with impaired cognitive function may be unaware of hygiene care needs or less able to follow instructions and help with care. In the home setting, patients with dementia may begin to lose their ability to perform hygiene self-care activities.

An early warning sign of dementia is poor judgment. Patients may pay less attention to grooming or keeping themselves clean (Alzheimer's Association, 2017). In the hospital setting, you may need to consult with therapists or specialists for patients with cognitive deficits. Such consultation usually requires an order from a health care provider.

Assessment of the Skin. Assess the skin, noting color, texture, thickness, turgor, temperature, and hydration (see Chapter 16). Pay special attention to characteristics of any lesions. Note dryness of the skin indicated by flaking, redness, scaling, and cracking.

Discovering common skin problems influences how you administer hygiene care (Table 31.3). When caring for patients with dark skin pigmentation, know the assessment techniques and skin characteristics unique to highly pigmented skin (see Chapters 16 and 38). Determine the degree of cleanliness by observing the appearance of the skin and detecting body odors that indicate previous inadequate cleansing or excessive perspiration caused by fever or pain.

Inspect less obvious or difficult-to-reach skin surfaces such as under the breasts or scrotum, around a female patient's perineum, or in the groin for redness, excessive moisture, and soiling or debris. Separate skinfolds carefully for inspection and palpation. Assess the condition and cleanliness of the perineal and anal areas during hygiene and with each toileting when patients require hygiene assistance. Most people consider these areas to be private. Be sensitive in your approach.

Assess for characteristics of skin problems that can be caused by hygiene care. Is the skin dry from excessive bathing or from the use of hot water or irritating soap? Does the patient have a rash caused by an allergic reaction to a skincare product?

Some conditions place patients at increased risk for impaired skin integrity (see Chapter 38). For example, be particularly alert when assessing patients with reduced sensation, vascular insufficiency, altered cognition, incontinence, nutrition or hydration alterations, body secretions, and decreased mobility. Carefully assess the skin in dark-skinned patients at risk for pressure injury (see Chapter 38). Patients may be unaware of skin problems because they cannot feel pain or pressure or see their skin in some places (e.g., the back or the feet). Carefully assess the skin under orthopedic devices (braces, splints, casts), under medical devices the patient may lie over (e.g. drainage tube), and under items such as tape.

Assessment of the Feet and Nails. A variety of common foot and nail problems can be caused by inadequate hygiene and are often detected during hygiene care (Table 31.4).

TABLE 31.3 COMMON SKIN PROBLEMS

PROBLEM	CHARACTERISTICS	IMPLICATIONS	INTERVENTIONS
Dry skin	Flaky, rough texture caused by lack of moisture in outer stratum corneum, resulting in less pliable epidermis; most common on anterior surfaces of lower legs, knees, elbows, and backs of hands	Skin may crack, bleed, and become inflamed. As a result, redness, pruritus, and discomfort may develop. Skin may become infected if epidermal layer cracks.	Effective treatment of dry skin does not include limiting frequency of bathing but lies in bathing with warm, not hot, water and using moisturizers (nonpetroleum). Use super-fatted soap (e.g., Dove) for cleansing. Rinse body of all soap well because residue left can cause irritation and breakdown. Add moisture to air through use of humidifier. Increase fluid intake when skin is dry. Use moisturizing lotion to aid healing process; lotion forms protective barrier and helps maintain fluid within skin.
Hirsutism	Excessive growth of body and facial hair, especially in women	Hair may cause negative body image by giving a woman a male appearance.	Shaving is safest method to remove hair. Electrolysis and laser permanently remove hair. Tweezing and bleaching are temporary.
Skin rashes	Skin eruption that may result from overexposure to sun or moisture or from allergic reaction; appears flat or raised, localized or systemic, pruritic or nonpruritic	If patient scratches skin, inflammation and infection occur. Rashes also cause discomfort.	Wash area thoroughly and apply antiseptic spray or lotion to prevent further itching and aid healing process. Warm or cold soaks may relieve inflammation and promote comfort.

Continued

TABLE 31.3   COMMON SKIN PROBLEMS—cont'd

PROBLEM	CHARACTERISTICS	IMPLICATIONS	INTERVENTIONS
Contact dermatitis (From Morison MJ: *Nursing management of chronic wounds,* Edinburgh, 2001, Mosby.)	Inflammation of skin characterized by abrupt onset with erythema, pruritus, pain, and appearance of scaly, oozing lesions; seen on face, neck, hands, forearms, trunk, and genitalia	Dermatitis is often difficult to eliminate because person is usually in continual contact with substance causing skin reaction. Substance is sometimes hard to identify.	Identify and avoid contributing agents (e.g., cleansers, cosmetics, latex, poison ivy or oak). Treatment consists of removing contributing agent and applying over-the-counter topical steroids or calamine lotion. In some cases prescription steroids may be ordered. Patients may find that tepid baths provide comfort.
Abrasion (From Lanzi GL: Facial injuries in sports, soft tissue injuries [abrasions, contusions, lacerations], *Clin Sports Med* 36[2]:287, 2017.)	Scraping or rubbing away of epidermis; results in localized bleeding and later weeping of serous fluid	Infection occurs easily as result of loss of protective skin layer.	Wash abrasions with mild soap and water. Dressing or bandage could increase risk for infection because of retained moisture.

Problems sometimes result from abuse or poor care of the feet and hands such as nail biting, improperly trimming nails, exposure to harsh chemicals, and wearing poorly fitting shoes. Ask patients the type of footwear they wear and their usual foot and nail care practices.

Assess patients with diseases that affect peripheral circulation and sensation for adequate circulation and sensation of the feet. Palpate the dorsalis pedis and posterior tibial pulses and assess for intact sensation to light touch, pinprick, and temperature (see Chapter 16). Observe the patient's gait. A variety of common foot problems cause pain and changes in gait.

Inspect the fingernails and toenails for lesions, dryness, inflammation, or cracking, which are often associated with a variety of common nail problems (see Table 31.4) or with nail-care practices. The cuticle that surrounds the nail can grow over the nail and become inflamed if the patient does not perform periodic nail care.

Ask patients whether they often polish their nails and use polish remover because chemicals in these products can cause excessive nail dryness. Some diseases change the condition, shape, and curvature of the nails (see Chapter 16). Inflammatory lesions and fungus of the nail bed cause thickened, horny nails that can separate from the nail bed.

Examine all skin surfaces of the feet including areas between the toes and over the entire sole of the foot. Poorly fitting shoes may irritate the heels, soles, and sides of the feet. Inspect the feet for lesions, noting areas of dryness, inflammation, or cracking.

Observe your patient's gait. Painful foot disorders and decreased sensation cause limping or an unnatural gait. Ask whether the patient has foot discomfort and identify factors that aggravate the pain. Foot problems sometimes result from bone or muscle changes or poorly fitting footwear.

Assessment of the Oral Cavity.   Inspect all areas of the mouth carefully for color, hydration, texture, and lesions (see Chapter 16). Patients may develop oral problems as a result of inadequate oral care or disease (e.g., oral malignancy) or as a side effect of medications, radiation, and chemotherapy. Localized pain or tenderness and infection accompany many common oral problems (Box 31.2).

Apply clean gloves and palpate any tender areas or lesions. If an older adult is edentulous (without teeth) and wears complete or partial dentures, assess underlying gums and palate. Observe for cleanliness and use olfaction to detect halitosis. If you identify an oral problem, notify the patient's health care provider. Early identification of poor oral hygiene

TABLE 31.4 COMMON FOOT AND NAIL PROBLEMS

PROBLEM	CHARACTERISTICS	IMPLICATIONS	INTERVENTIONS
Callus	Thickened portion of epidermis consisting of mass of horny, keratotic cells; usually flat and painless; found on undersurface of foot or on palm of hand; caused by local friction or pressure	Foot calluses often cause discomfort when wearing tight-fitting shoes.	Refer patient to podiatrist; do not self-treat. Use of orthotic devices cushions and redistributes weight and pressure off calluses.
Corns	Keratosis caused by friction and pressure from shoes; mainly on toes, over bony prominence; usually cone shaped, round, and raised; calluses with painful core	Conical shape compresses underlying dermis, making it thin and tender. Tight shoes aggravate pain. Tissue attaches to bone if allowed to grow. Patient may have alteration in gait because of pain.	Refer patient to podiatrist. Avoid use of oval corn pads, which increase pressure on toes. Use wider, softer shoes.
Plantar warts	Fungating lesion that appears on sole of foot; caused by papillomavirus	Warts are sometimes contagious, are painful, and make walking difficult.	Refer patient to podiatrist.
Athlete's foot (tinea pedis)	Fungal infection of foot; scaliness and cracking of skin between toes and on soles of feet; small blisters containing fluid appear, apparently induced by constricting footwear (e.g., sneakers)	Athlete's foot can spread to other body parts, especially hands. It is contagious and often recurs.	Feet should be well ventilated. Drying feet well after bathing and applying powder help prevent infection. Wearing clean socks or stockings reduces incidence. Health care provider orders application of griseofulvin, miconazole nitrate, or tolnaftate.
Ingrown nails	Toenail or fingernail growing inward into soft tissue around nail; results from improper nail trimming, poor shoe fit, or heredity	Ingrown nails cause localized pain in presence of pressure; some become infected.	Treatment is frequent warm soaks (exception: patient with diabetes or other vascular diseases such as Berger disease) in antiseptic solution and removal of part of nail that has grown into skin. Teach patient proper nail-trimming techniques. Refer to podiatrist.
Paronychia	Inflammation of tissue surrounding nail after hangnail or other injury; occurs in people who frequently have their hands in water; common in patients with diabetes	Area sometimes becomes infected.	Treatment is warm compresses or soaks (exception: patient with diabetes) and local application of antibiotic ointments. Paronychia can be prevented by careful manicuring.
Foot odors	Result of excess perspiration promoting microorganism growth; faulty foot hygiene or improper footwear causes foot odor	Odor frequently embarrasses patient.	Frequent washing, use of foot deodorants and powders, and clean footwear prevent or reduce this problem.

BOX 31.2 COMMON ORAL PROBLEMS

DENTAL CARIES (CAVITIES)
- Most common among young people
- Buildup of plaque causes acid destruction of tooth enamel; initially appears as chalky, white discoloration of the tooth

PERIODONTAL DISEASE (PYORRHEA)
- Most common after age 35
- Involves destruction of gingiva (gums) and other supporting structures with bleeding gums, inflammation, and receding gum lines, which may lead to tooth loss

OTHER PROBLEMS
- Oral mucositis (oral erythema, ulceration, and pain)
- Glossitis (inflammation of the tongue)
- Gingivitis (inflammation of the gums)
- Halitosis (bad breath)
- Cheilitis (cracked lips)
- Oral malignancy (mouth lumps or ulcers)

BOX 31.3 ASSESSMENT OF HAIR

PHYSICAL CHANGES
- Assess condition of hair and scalp (see Chapter 16).
  - Consider age-appropriate changes.
  - Consider racial or ethnic differences.
- Determine reasons for change in distribution or loss of hair.
- Check oiliness and texture of hair.
- Inspect scalp for lesions, inflammation, infection, or parasites.

SELF-CARE ABILITY
- Assess patient's ability to grasp comb or brush and raise arm for brushing or combing.
- Determine patient's ability to physically care for hair.
- Does patient become easily fatigued?

HAIR-CARE PRACTICES
- Assess patient's preferences in hair styling.
- Identify patient's preferences for hair care and shaving products.
- Assess adequacy of patient's hygiene practices.
- Determine patient's perceptions of own appearance.
- Assess patient's socioeconomic background.

practices and common oral problems reduces the risk for gum disease and dental caries or cavities.

Include specific questions and observations for a patient with dentures or a dental appliance. Observe oral tissue under dentures and appliances for evidence of pressure areas or irritation. Note size and location of any lesions. Question patients about any problems associated with dental devices including tender areas and poor fit.

Assessment of the Hair and Hair Care. Routine assessment of the condition of the hair and scalp (Box 31.3) reveals problems and determines the frequency and type of care needed (Table 31.5). Observe your patient's ability to perform hair care. A person's overall appearance and feeling of well-being often are related to the look and feel of the hair. Illness, disability, arthritis, fatigue, and physical barriers (e.g., cast or IV access) reduce a patient's ability to maintain daily hair care. Assess the hair of a patient who is immobilized for tangles, and check hair around and beneath dressings for sticky blood residue or antiseptic solutions.

Cultural and personal preferences influence the patient's choice of hairstyle and hair-care practices. Assess patient's usual practices and discuss any potential associated problems.

In community health and home care settings, it is important to inspect the hair and scalp for lice. If you suspect pediculosis capitis (head lice), protect yourself against infestation by handwashing and using gloves or tongue blades to inspect the hair and scalp (Centers for Disease Control and Prevention [CDC], 2016). Notify the patient's health care provider if you identify lice.

Alopecia (loss of hair) may result from chemotherapy medications, hormonal changes, damaging hair-care practices, genetic predisposition, or psychological impairment. If you note alopecia, be sure to question your patient about

specific hair-care practices, especially the types of products used and heat application during hair care.

Assessment of the Eyes, Ears, and Nose. Carefully inspect all external eye structures (see Chapter 16). Redness indicates possible allergic or infectious conjunctivitis. The crusty drainage associated with infectious conjunctivitis easily spreads from one eye to the other. Wear gloves to examine the eyes and perform hand hygiene before and after the examination.

Determine whether the patient wears contact lenses, especially if he or she enters the health care agency in an unresponsive or confused state. An undetected contact lens may cause corneal injury when left in place too long.

Assessment of the external ear structures includes inspection of the auricle and external ear canal (see Chapter 16). Observe for the presence of accumulated cerumen (earwax) or drainage in the ear canal. Note evidence of local inflammation. Ask patients about tenderness on palpation of the external ear or the presence of pain, and ask how they usually clean their ears.

Inspect the nares for signs of inflammation, discharge, lesions, edema, and deformity (see Chapter 16). If your patient has any type of tubing in the nares (e.g., oxygen, nasogastric), observe for tissue damage (pressure injury), localized tenderness, inflammation, drainage, and bleeding.

If your patient has eyeglasses, contact lenses, an artificial eye, or hearing aids, ask your patient how he or she cares for them. Watch your patient perform care when possible for additional assessment data.

TABLE 31.5 HAIR AND SCALP PROBLEMS

PROBLEM	CHARACTERISTICS	IMPLICATIONS	INTERVENTIONS
Dandruff	Scaling of the scalp accompanied by itching; in severe cases dandruff on eyebrows	Dandruff may cause embarrassment; if it enters the eyes, conjunctivitis often develops.	Shampoo regularly (preferably daily) with over-the-counter dandruff shampoo or medicated shampoo. Make an appointment with health care provider if symptoms do not respond to over-the-counter treatments.
Ticks	Small gray-brown parasites that burrow into skin and suck blood	Ticks sometimes transmit Rocky Mountain spotted fever, Lyme disease, and tularemia.	Removal of tick (CDC, 2015): Use fine-tipped tweezers to grasp tick as close to the skin's surface as possible. Pull upward with steady, even pressure. Do not twist or jerk tick; this can cause the mouth parts to break off and remain in the skin. If this happens, remove the mouth parts with tweezers. If you are unable to remove mouth parts easily with clean tweezers, leave them alone and let the skin heal. After removing the tick, thoroughly clean the bite areas and your hands with rubbing alcohol and iodine scrub or soap and water. Save tick in plastic bag and store in freezer if it is necessary to identify the type of tick. If you develop a rash or fever within several weeks of removing a tick, see your health care provider.
Pediculosis capitis (head lice)	Tiny grayish-white parasitic insects that attach to hair strands; eggs look like oval particles, resemble dandruff; bites or pustules may be found behind ears and at hairline	Head lice are difficult to remove and if not treated spread to furniture and other people. They do not carry disease, cannot jump or fly, and are carried by animals.	Wearing gloves, check entire scalp with tongue depressor or special lice comb. *Caution against use of products containing lindane because the ingredient is a neurotoxin known to cause adverse reactions* (CDC, 2016). Check hair for nits and comb with a nit comb for 2–3 days until all lice and nits have been removed. Vacuum infested areas of home and car upholstery.
Pediculosis corporis (body lice)	Tend to cling to clothing, making them difficult to see; body lice suck blood and lay eggs on clothing and furniture	Patient itches constantly; scratches on skin become infected; hemorrhagic spots appear on skin where lice are sucking blood.	Have patient bathe or shower thoroughly; after drying skin, apply lotion for eliminating lice; after 12–24 hours have patient take another bath or shower; bag infested clothing or linen until laundered.
Pediculosis pubis (crab lice)	Found in pubic hair; grayish-white with red legs	Lice spread through bed linen, clothing, furniture, or sexual contact.	Shave hair off affected areas; cleanse as for body lice; if lice were sexually transmitted, patient needs to notify partner.
Alopecia	Balding patches; hair becomes brittle and broken; caused by improper use of hair curlers and picks, tight braiding, hot styling tools, genetics, and certain diseases	Patches of uneven hair growth and loss alter patient's appearance.	Stop hair-care practices that damage hair (e.g., teasing hair, hair picks, tight braiding, excessive heat when blow-drying).

Patients at Risk for Hygiene Problems. Some patients present risks that require more attentive and rigorous hygiene care (Table 31.6). These risks result from side effects of medications or other medical therapy; lack of knowledge; immobilization; inability to perform hygiene; or a physical condition that potentially injures the skin, feet and nails, hair, or oral cavity structures.

Determine if a patient is at risk for any hygiene problems and follow through with a complete assessment. Identifying risks and initiating preventive care as soon as possible reduce injury to skin, feet, nails, and oral mucosa.

Older Adult Considerations. Changes associated with aging affect hygiene needs of older adults. Observe for xerosis (abnormal dryness of the skin), which is marked by cracking of the skin, especially on the extremities but also on the trunk and face (Touhy and Jett, 2014). Question older adults about itching, which accompanies xerosis. Observe for evidence of skin trauma caused by scratching. Assess the usual frequency and duration of bathing, temperature of the water, and type of products used for skin care. Long baths with hot water and harsh soaps can cause the skin of the older adult to become dry and easily damaged. Although dry skin may be a part of aging or the effect of environmental factors, overly dry skin often indicates more serious systemic disease or dehydration.

Assess an older adult's fluid and nutrient intake because inadequacies can contribute to drying of the older adult's skin. The dermis loses about 20% of its thickness with aging (Meiner, 2015). Therefore carefully examine older adults' skin for damage, especially when they have limited movement or impaired sensation. Skin tears (traumatic wounds in which the epidermis separates from the dermis) occur easily in thin skin because of minor trauma such as bumping of an extremity or removing of tape.

Reduced circulation with advancing age can lead to yellowing, thickening, and brittleness of fingernails and toenails. Remember that these changes may require more attention to nail care, which the patient may be unable to perform because of loss of close vision acuity or limited manual dexterity (Touhy and Jett, 2014).

Common foot problems of older adults include corns and calluses. Observe carefully for evidence of chemical burns or ulcerations that sometimes occur with over-the-counter preparations and for evidence of damage from the use of razor blades or scissors to trim the corns or calluses (Touhy and Jett, 2014).

Patient Expectations. Hygiene is very personal. Each of your patients has unique expectations about his or her own hygiene practices. Most patients expect to continue their routine grooming practices. When you give or help with

TABLE 31.6   RISK FACTORS FOR HYGIENE PROBLEMS

RISKS	HYGIENE IMPLICATIONS
Oral Problems	
Patients who are unable to use upper extremities because of paralysis, weakness, or restriction (e.g., cast or dressing)	Patient lacks upper-extremity strength or hand dexterity needed to brush teeth.
Dehydration, inability to take fluids or food by mouth (NPO)	Causes excess drying and fragility of mucosa; increases accumulation of secretions on tongue and gums.
Presence of nasogastric or oxygen tubes; mouth breathers	Causes drying of mucosa, which increases risk for breakdown and infection.
Chemotherapeutic drugs	Drugs kill rapidly multiplying cells including normal cells lining oral cavity. Ulcers and inflammation (stomatitis) develop with resulting discomfort.
Broad-spectrum antibiotics	Destroy normal oral flora, allowing overgrowth of opportunistic microbes.
Over-the-counter lozenges, cough drops, antacids, and chewable vitamins	Medications contain large amounts of sugar. Repeated use increases sugar or acid content in mouth, increasing risk for tooth and gum problems.
Altered blood clotting caused by medications or disease states	Predisposes to bleeding gums spontaneously or with oral care.
Endotracheal intubation with mechanical ventilation	Creates potential for VAP. Use of routine oral hygiene and 0.12% chlorhexidine gluconate rinse reduces risk of VAP (Munro, 2014; Nicolosi et al., 2014).
Radiation therapy to head and neck	Causes oral mucositis, which affects all mucosal folds within oral cavity, resulting in erythema, ulceration, and pain (NCI, 2016).
Oral surgery, trauma to mouth, placement of oral airway	Cause trauma to oral cavity with swelling, ulcerations, inflammation, and bleeding.
Immunosuppression; altered blood clotting	Predisposes to inflammation, infection, and bleeding gums.

TABLE 31.6 RISK FACTORS FOR HYGIENE PROBLEMS—cont'd

RISKS	HYGIENE IMPLICATIONS
Diabetes mellitus	Predisposes to dryness of mouth, gingivitis, periodontal disease, and loss of teeth.
Poorly fitting dentures	Food trapped under dentures causes mouth odor; increases risk for oral mucosa breakdown and stomatitis.
Inadequate brushing and flossing of teeth	Predisposes patients to periodontal disease.
Cardiovascular disease	Linked to periodontal disease.
Skin Problems	
Immobilization	Dependent body parts are exposed to pressure from underlying surfaces. The inability to turn or change position increases risk for pressure injury.
Reduced sensation caused by stroke, spinal cord injury, diabetes, local nerve damage	Patient does not receive normal transmission of nerve impulses when excessive heat or cold, pressure, friction, or chemical irritants are applied to skin.
Limited protein or caloric intake and reduced hydration (e.g., fever, burns, gastrointestinal alterations, poorly fitting dentures)	Limited caloric and protein intake predisposes to impaired tissue synthesis. Skin becomes thinner, less elastic, and smoother with loss of subcutaneous tissue. Poor wound healing results. Reduced hydration impairs skin turgor.
Excessive secretions or excretions on skin from perspiration, urine, watery fecal material, and wound drainage	Moisture is medium for bacterial growth and causes local skin irritation, softening of epidermal cells, and skin maceration.
Presence of external medical devices (e.g., cast, restraint, bandage, dressing)	Device exerts pressure or friction against surface of skin increasing risk for pressure injury (Makic, 2015).
Vascular insufficiency	Arterial blood supply to tissues is inadequate or venous return is impaired causing decreased circulation to extremities. Tissue ischemia and breakdown occur. Risk for infection is high.
Foot Problems	
Patient unable to bend over or has reduced visual acuity	Patient is unable to fully see entire surface of each foot, making it difficult to adequately assess condition of skin and nails.
Decreased sensation	Patient is unable to sense pressure, heat or cold, or pain. Patient requires education on importance of regular foot inspection; possible referral to podiatrist.
Eye Care Problems	
Reduced dexterity and hand coordination	Physical limitations create inability to safely insert, remove, or cleanse contact lenses.

VAP, ventilator-associated pneumonia.

hygiene care, ask your patient questions to determine preferred personal care items such as soap, lotion, toothpaste, and deodorant; the type of bath desired and preferred time to bathe; and grooming preferences such as hair styling, makeup, and shaving.

Each culture has unique personal hygiene practices. When you care for patients from other cultures, learn as much as possible about your patient's culture and respect the customs, beliefs, and practices associated with the culture.

Recognize that some patients are sensitive to invasion of personal space and to the gender of caregivers. When assessing patients, ask open-ended questions and give the patient a choice. For example, ask questions such as following: "How would you prefer that I bathe you?" "Are you comfortable

with someone helping you?" "Would you feel more comfortable having a nurse of the same gender bathe you?" "Would you prefer someone from your family to help you?"

■■■ NURSING DIAGNOSIS

Thorough assessment of a patient's hygiene status and self-care abilities identifies defining characteristics and risk factors that support nursing diagnoses. Identifying defining characteristics enables you to select the correct problem-focused or health promotion nursing diagnosis. The identification of risk factors allows you to identify a risk nursing diagnosis. For example, you observe a generally unkempt appearance in a patient coming to the clinic. You initially think the patient has either *Bathing Self-Care Deficit* or *Activity Intolerance*. On closer assessment, you observe swollen joints, weakness, and limited ROM in the dominant hand. Questioning of the patient indicates that he or she cannot turn on or turn off the basin or tub faucets. Your critical thinking skills and analysis of the defining characteristics help you accurately determine the problem-focused diagnosis of *Bathing Self-Care Deficit*.

If a patient has a risk nursing diagnosis (e.g., *Risk for Impaired Skin Integrity*), your plan will be focused on prevention. For example, a patient with redness over the sacral area, limited mobility, and stool incontinence will require measures different from those of a patient with an actual skin lesion. Frequent repositioning, management of incontinence, and use of specialty support surfaces will be chosen interventions. The patient with an actual lesion will require wound care.

The selection of a related factor allows you to correctly identify a problem-focused nursing diagnosis. You choose interventions aimed at eliminating the related factor so that the diagnosis can be resolved. A diagnosis of *Impaired Oral Mucous Membrane related to malnutrition* and a diagnosis of *Impaired Oral Mucous Membrane related to chemical trauma* require different interventions. When chemotherapy injures the oral mucosa, follow cancer nursing guidelines regarding oral care for mucositis (Eilers et al., 2014). When the diagnosis is related to nutritional problems, work with a dietitian to provide an appropriate therapeutic diet. Although many nursing diagnoses often apply to patients in need of hygienic care, the following list offers are examples of commonly associated nursing diagnoses:

- Activity Intolerance
- Bathing Self-Care Deficit
- Dressing Self-Care Deficit
- Impaired Oral Mucous Membrane
- Risk for Activity Intolerance
- Risk for Infection

■■■ PLANNING

During planning, use collected data and critical thinking to develop an individualized plan of care. Identify patient goals and outcomes, set priorities, and plan for continuity of care. Rely on knowledge, experience, and established standards of care, including evidence-based guidelines, when developing a patient-centered plan of care. Include the patient and collaborate with other health care providers (e.g., occupational or physical therapists) in developing a plan that will meet relevant outcomes.

Goals and Outcomes. Partner with the patient and family to identify goals and outcomes, and develop an individualized plan of care based on the patient's nursing diagnoses (see Care Plan). Establish goals that integrate a patient's self-care abilities, risks, preferences, and resources. Focus on improving both self-care abilities and the condition of the skin and oral cavity. State patient outcomes in measurable and achievable terms within a patient's limitations.

In addition, work with the patient to select individualized hygiene measures.

You will care for a variety of patients with varying self-care abilities and hygienic needs. For example, you and the patient who has right-sided paralysis establish the following goal: "Patient's skin will remain free of breakdown." Then you create a series of realistic individualized expected outcomes, such as the following:

- Patient's skin is clean, dry, and intact without signs of inflammation.
- Patient's skin remains elastic and well hydrated.
- Patient's skin is free of pressure areas.

Setting Priorities. A patient's condition influences your priorities for hygiene care. Set priorities based on the assistance required by the patient, the extent of hygiene problems, and the patient's nursing diagnoses. For example, patients who are seriously ill usually need a daily bath because of increasing body secretions, but they are often unable to bathe independently because of a variety of factors (e.g., fatigue, impaired physical mobility, decreased level of consciousness). Some patients at home require a visit from a home care aide to help with a tub bath or shower. Patients who are normally inactive during the day and have skin that tends to be dry may need to bathe only twice a week, whereas a patient with urinary and bowel incontinence needs perineal cleansing with each episode of soiling. A patient with acute pain requires a bath but needs pain medications before the bath. Plan to use assistive devices to ensure a patient's optimal level of independence and safety. For example, a patient with partial paralysis who has difficulty getting out of the tub needs a tub chair, handrails, or extra personnel for help.

Timing is also important in planning hygiene care. Being interrupted in the middle of the bath for an x-ray examination frustrates and embarrasses patients. If a patient is tired after extensive diagnostic tests, rest is an important patient priority. In these situations, delaying hygiene and allowing the patient to rest are best.

Collaborative Care. Plan for care throughout a patient's hospital stay. Anticipate the need for postdischarge hygiene assistance when a patient is admitted. Collaborate with other services and health care providers including a social worker, occupational therapist, physical therapist, and home care agencies. For example, physical therapists help patients with strengthening exercises needed for bathing, and occupational therapists fit patients with assistive devices that allow patients to pick toileting items. Collaborate with the social worker to help gain access to community resources for hygiene activities and equipment.

Ensure continuity of care when patients are discharged to a rehabilitation facility or home. When your patient needs help because of a self-care deficit, family caregivers must be included in the plan of care. Consider the equipment and procedures needed so that the patient and family caregiver know about the skills to provide and have access to the necessary equipment on discharge.

⊚ CARE PLAN

Bathing Self-Care Deficit

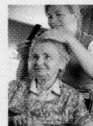

ASSESSMENT

As Jamie is talking with Mrs. Winkler about helping her with her bath before breakfast is served, Mrs. Winkler says, "It's just so hard for me to take care of myself. My arthritis makes my hands and knees hurt, and my fingers are so crippled I can hardly use them. I wish I could do more for myself."

Copyright © AlexRaths/
iStock/Thinkstock.

ASSESSMENT ACTIVITIES	FINDINGS[a]
Ask Mrs. Winkler what care is important to her this morning.	Mrs. Winkler says, "I want to clean my dentures and mouth and feel clean and look nice without it hurting too much. But I don't want to be any trouble."
Assess Mrs. Winkler's ability to bathe, perform oral hygiene care, and dress.	Mrs. Winkler admits, "I have trouble using my hands. My hands are so crippled and hurt so much that I **can't hold on to things like my hairbrush or toothbrush without pain. I can't even squeeze my own washcloth or turn the water faucets.** I sometimes can't even button or zip my clothes. I must let someone else dress me. Sometimes my knees hurt so much that **I can't walk to the bathroom by myself. I have to ask someone to help me."** Leaned heavily on nurse when transferring from bed to chair at bedside, did not bear full weight. Observed deformities of knee and hand (fingers and wrists) joints.
Ask Mrs. Winkler if she would like some rest periods during her morning hygiene.	Mrs. Winkler says that she would like to work in 30-minute sections with a short break and give her muscles a 10- to 15-minute rest period.

[a]**Defining characteristics/risk factors** are shown in **bold** type.

NURSING DIAGNOSIS: Bathing Self-Care Deficit related to musculoskeletal impairment and pain

PLANNING

GOALS

Mrs. Winkler will be involved in directing caregivers who give or assist with her personal hygiene care within the next 2 days.

Mrs. Winkler will use assistive devices for bathing within the next week.
Mrs. Winkler will accept help from caregiver as needed and be satisfied with the bathing experience within the next week.

EXPECTED OUTCOMES (NOC)[b]

Self-Direction of Care

Mrs. Winkler states two personal preferences for hygiene care today.
Mrs. Winkler selects the bathing assistive devices she wishes to use within 2 days.

Self-Care: Bathing

Mrs. Winkler helps with bathing by using padded shower chair, bath mitt, and large-grip shower spray mounted in shower within the next week.
Mrs. Winkler regulates water flow and temperature in shower using lever handles within the next week.
Mrs. Winkler states satisfaction with use of assistive devices and help from caregiver when needed within the next week.

[b]Outcome classification labels from Moorhead S, et al, editors: *Nursing outcomes classification (NOC)*, ed 5, St Louis, 2013, Mosby.

INTERVENTIONS (NIC)[c]

Self-Care Assistance: Bathing/Hygiene

Share results of Katz ADLs Index with Mrs. Winkler and include her when selecting assistive devices for bathing.
Coordinate with social services, occupational therapy, and home care services to obtain selected assistive devices for Mrs. Winkler.
Teach Mrs. Winkler how to safely use her assistive devices by going over printed material and demonstrating and supervising her use of the devices. Allow adequate time for instruction and practice, and encourage expression of concerns and questions.

RATIONALE

Determining patient's preferences and expressed needs and including these in the plan of care foster patient-centered care (Burman et al., 2013).
RN coordinates care delivery.

Teaching plan addresses the three domains of learning (cognitive, affective, and psychomotor) and multiple teaching methods (Meiner, 2015).

[c]Intervention classification labels from Bulechek GM, et al, editors: *Nursing interventions classification (NIC)*, ed 6, St Louis, 2013, Mosby.

Continued

◎ **CARE PLAN—cont'd**

Bathing Self-Care Deficit

EVALUATION

NURSING ACTIONS	PATIENT RESPONSE/FINDING	ACHIEVEMENT OF OUTCOME
Ask Mrs. Winkler to state two personal preferences for hygiene care.	Mrs. Winkler states that she prefers her care in the morning after breakfast and a shower instead of taking a bath.	Able to be involved in direction of care and express personal preferences for type and timing of hygiene care.
Ask Mrs. Winkler to state which bathing assistive devices she has selected.	Mrs. Winkler states that she would like to try the padded shower chair, the bath mitt, the lever shower controls, and the large-grip shower spray.	Able to be involved in direction of care and express personal preferences by selecting bathing assistive devices.
Ask Mrs. Winkler if her hygiene preferences were considered and if hygiene needs were satisfactorily met by the caregiver.	Mrs. Winkler states, "You were so kind and gentle. I appreciate that. You helped me but also let me do what I could. My joints feel better after the warm shower, and I feel clean. I am pleased with my care."	Verbally expresses satisfaction with hygiene care including level of fulfillment and caregiver consideration of preferences and personal needs.
Observe patient during shower to note use of assistive devices.	Observed Mrs. Winkler safely maneuver the handheld spray and use the padded shower chair and bath mitt. Mrs. Winkler was not able to adequately grasp the lever shower controls and needed help to regulate flow and temperature of the shower.	Able to safely use all assistive devices except for lever shower control. Need to search for another adaptation, perhaps increasing diameter of levers by using foam overlays.
Caregiver asks patient to state level of satisfaction with use of assistive devices and help from caregiver.	Mrs. Winkler stated, "I feel so much happier since I can do more of my shower now. I love the bath mitt and the handheld shower spray. The lever handles are better than the old knobs, but I still have some trouble grasping them in my hands."	Verbally expresses satisfaction with all assistive devices except for lever shower control.

■■■ **IMPLEMENTATION**

Basic patient care often includes hygiene interventions. Regardless of patient characteristics or variations in setting, all patients require attention to hygiene. Include family caregivers in all educational interventions when appropriate.

Health Promotion. To promote healthy hygiene and self-care practices, educate and counsel patients and their family caregivers on proper hygiene techniques. Always emphasize ways to avoid injury and reinforce infection control practices. Incorporate adaptations regarding patient's lifestyle, functional status, living arrangements, and preferences when teaching about hygiene care.

Skin Care. Teach patients ways to promote healthy skin. Demonstrate how to routinely inspect the skin for changes in color or texture, and instruct the patient to report changes or abnormalities to the health care provider. Instruct patients to handle the skin gently, avoiding excessive or rough rubbing.

Advise against use of hot water for bathing and excessively long bathing sessions to prevent loss of oils and excessive drying of skin. Also, encourage patients to drink adequate fluids and to eat a balanced diet including foods rich in antioxidants, vitamins, and minerals. Emphasize safety concerns in the home or environment. Examples include failure to adjust the water temperature when bathing or showering and slipping on wet surfaces in the bathroom. Instruct patients to use sunscreen, even in winter months, to protect the skin from sun exposure. Ensure that patients understand that healthy and intact skin protects them from infections.

Oral Care. Teach patients proper brushing and flossing techniques. The American Dental Association (ADA) (2017) guidelines for effective oral hygiene include brushing the teeth for 2 minutes at least twice a day with ADA-accepted fluoride toothpaste. A soft-bristled toothbrush with a straight handle and a brush small enough to reach all areas of the mouth cleans best. Older patients with reduced dexterity and grip may require a toothbrush with a larger handle.

Demonstrate how to brush all tooth surfaces thoroughly. Recommend that patients not share toothbrushes with family members or drink directly from a single bottle of mouthwash. Cross-contamination occurs easily. Instruct patients to rinse the toothbrush thoroughly after each use, store it upright between uses, and obtain a new toothbrush every 3 or 4 months (ADA, 2017). Avoid using toothbrush covers, which can create a moist, enclosed environment that promotes bacterial growth.

Daily dental flossing removes food particles, plaque, and tartar between teeth. To floss, the patient inserts waxed or unwaxed dental floss between all tooth surfaces, one at a time (ADA, 2017). A seesaw motion is needed to pull the floss between teeth, removing food and debris caught between teeth. Place a mirror in front of the patient to help you guide the patient in holding the floss and cleaning between the teeth. Applying toothpaste to the teeth before flossing puts fluoride in direct contact with tooth surfaces.

Teach the patient that diet influences plaque formation and the development of dental caries. Including acidic fruits in the patient's diet helps reduce plaque formation. A well-balanced diet contributes to the integrity of oral tissues. To prevent tooth decay, patients sometimes need to change eating habits (e.g., reduce intake of carbohydrates, especially sweet snacks, between meals). Encourage all patients to visit a dentist regularly for checkups.

Teaching about common gum and tooth disorders (see Box 31.2) and methods to prevent these problems may motivate patients to follow recommended oral hygiene practices. If a patient's finances limit options, look for a local dental hygiene clinic or dental school that offers low-cost dental care.

Patients with dentures require instruction in proper care of their dentures and prevention of associated complications, such as **denture stomatitis**, which is inflammation of the oral mucosa in contact with a denture surface (Box 31.4). Teach the patient to remove and rinse dentures after eating by running water over them. Placing a towel in the sink helps reduce the chance of breaking the dentures if dropped.

Instruct the patient to clean the mouth after removing dentures and use a soft-bristled toothbrush on any remaining natural teeth and on the tongue and palate. Dentures must be brushed at least once daily with denture cleanser and a denture brush to remove food, plaque, and other deposits. Instruct the patient to avoid damaging the dentures by avoiding stiff-bristled brushes, strong cleansers, and regular toothpaste. Toothpastes with whitening agents are particularly abrasive and should not be used on dentures.

Advise the patient to remove dentures, soak them overnight (perhaps in a denture cleansing solution), and rinse well before replacing in the morning. Emphasize that taking the dentures out at night helps prevent denture stomatitis (Tay et al., 2014). Emphasize that patients with dentures should schedule regular dental checkups. The patient should report any damage to dentures and any change in fit or development of tenderness or sore mouth.

Care of Eyes, Ears, and Nose. Teach patients how to safely clean the eyes, ears, and nose. Encourage patients to clean the eyes by washing with a clean washcloth moistened in water. Explain or demonstrate how to clean from the inner to the outer canthus. Use a different section of the washcloth for each eye to limit transmission of infection.

Explain that routine ear care includes cleaning the ear with the end of a moistened washcloth rotated gently into the ear canal. Gentle, downward retraction of the ear at the entrance of the ear canal usually causes visible cerumen to loosen and slip out. Instruct your patient to never use objects such as bobby pins, toothpicks, paper clips, or cotton-tipped applicators to remove earwax. These objects can injure the ear canal and rupture the tympanic membrane. In addition, they may cause earwax to become impacted within the ear canal.

Teach the patient to remove secretions from the nose by gently blowing into a soft tissue. Caution a patient against harsh blowing, which creates pressure capable of injuring the

---

BOX 31.4 PATIENT TEACHING

Preventing Denture Stomatitis

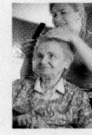

Copyright © AlexRaths/ iStock/ Thinkstock.

Mrs. Winkler wears full dentures. She does not usually remove her dentures at night. She finds it difficult to care for her dentures because of the deformity and pain in her hands. Usually she cleans her dentures only once a day, and she does not rinse her mouth after eating because she is reluctant to ask others for help. To help Mrs. Winkler prevent denture stomatitis, Jamie develops the following teaching plan for her.

OUTCOME

At the end of the teaching session, Mrs. Winkler will help perform preventive oral and denture care correctly.

TEACHING STRATEGIES

- Teach Mrs. Winkler the signs and symptoms of denture stomatitis (e.g., redness and swelling under dentures, especially on upper palate, and small red sores on roof of mouth).
- Remind Mrs. Winkler that although her mouth may not hurt or be sore, she may experience mouth discomfort when her dentures are in place or when inserting or removing dentures.
- Teach stomatitis prevention strategies:
  - Rinse mouth and dentures after eating.
  - Brush dentures when they are removed for the night (Tay et al., 2014).

- Visit a dentist twice a year to check denture fit and ensure that dentures are intact and smooth.
- Clean dentures weekly with effervescent denture cleaner.
- Instruct Mrs. Winkler to go to her dentist immediately if her dentures are damaged, or if she thinks they are damaged.
- Teach Mrs. Winkler that denture stomatitis often is caused by the following:
  - Poorly fitting dentures
  - Wearing dentures while sleeping
  - Inadequate cleansing and buildup of the yeast *Candida albicans*
- Give Mrs. Winkler printed material about denture stomatitis so that she can review the material after one-on-one instruction.

EVALUATION

- Use the principles of teach-back to evaluate patient/family caregiver learning.
  - "What are the signs and symptoms of denture stomatitis?"
  - "What will you do when symptoms of denture stomatitis occur?"
  - "State ways you can help prevent recurrence of denture stomatitis."
  - "Show me how you will care for your dentures."

eardrum, nasal mucosa, and even sensitive eye structures. Bleeding from the nares is a key sign of harsh blowing.

Nail and Foot Care. Routine nail care includes soaking to soften cuticles and layers of horny cells, thorough cleansing, drying, and proper nail trimming. The one exception is a patient who has diabetes. *Never recommend soaking the nails if a person has diabetes or other peripheral vascular or circulatory conditions, because soaking increases the risk for infection.*

Teach patients to avoid the use of harsh chemicals or long soaks in the tub. Prolonged soaking leads to softening or maceration of the tissue and can promote tissue injury. Demonstrate proper trimming and filing techniques. For ongoing home care, instruct patients or their family caregivers to use sharp manicure scissors or clippers to trim the nails straight across and then round the tips by filing in a gentle curve. Explain that trimming is easiest when the nails are soft, such as after the bath, but that the patient should be sure that nails have dried before filing to prevent splitting.

Prevent drying of nails and cuticles by rubbing hand lotion into the fingernails and cuticles. Instruct the patient to limit nail damage by not using fingernails as tools for prying things and not biting them or picking at the cuticles. The patient should carefully clip hangnails instead of pulling them off.

People with diabetes develop many types of foot complications associated with nerve damage and poor blood flow to the lower extremities. Foot injuries in the patient with diabetes can quickly turn into a serious problem with slow healing, infection, and the possibility of amputation. If a patient has diabetes or any other condition affecting peripheral circulation or sensation, recommend a podiatrist for regular examinations and trimming of nails (American Podiatric Medical Association [APMA], 2016). Instruct patients to report any of the following to their health care provider: changes in nail shape or color, bleeding around the nails, thinning or thickening of the nails, and redness, swelling, or pain around the nails.

When teaching patients who have diabetes about foot and nail care, advise them to use the following guidelines in a routine nail-care program (American Diabetes Association, 2014):

- Receive a thorough foot examination at least once a year.
- Inspect the feet daily including tops and soles of the feet, heels, and areas between the toes.
- Use a mirror to inspect all surfaces or ask a family caregiver to check daily.
- Wash feet daily with lukewarm water. Gently but thoroughly pat the feet dry, especially between the toes.
- Keep skin soft and smooth by rubbing a thin coat of lotion over toes and bottoms of feet but not between toes where the increased and prolonged moisture can lead to maceration.
- Wear shoes and clean, dry socks always; never go barefoot. Check inside shoes before wearing them for rough areas or objects that may rub against the foot.

- If you can see and reach your toenails, trim them straight across and square; file the edges smooth.
- Keep the blood flowing to your feet by putting them up when sitting, wiggling your toes, and moving your ankles up and down for 5 minutes 2 or 3 times a day. Do not cross your legs for long periods. Do not smoke.
- Protect the feet from hot and cold. Do not use heating pads or electric blankets, and always wear shoes at the beach or on hot pavement.

Hair Care. To best promote hair and scalp health, instruct the patient to keep hair clean, combed, and brushed regularly. Be sure to follow the practices of the patient's cultural preferences (Box 31.5). Frequent brushing helps to keep hair clean and distributes oil evenly along hair shafts. Combing prevents hair from tangling.

Patients also may need to know how to check for and remove parasites (see Table 31.5). Tell patients to notify their primary health care provider of changes in the texture and distribution of hair, which may indicate a systemic problem.

Acute Care. The variety and timing of hygiene care vary across health care settings and according to individual patient needs. In the acute care setting, factors such as frequent diagnostic and treatment plans and extensive hygiene care resulting from acute illness or injury affect scheduling of care.

Bathing and Skin Care. Consider a patient's normal grooming routines including preferred hygiene products and preferred time of day for hygiene care. The extent, type, and timing or frequency of bathing and the methods used depend on the patient's physical abilities, health problems, and degree of hygiene needed.

Use the tub bath or shower to give a more thorough bath than a bed bath (see Skill 31.1). Cleanse the skin at the time of any soiling and at routine intervals. Problems such as incontinence, wound drainage, or excessive diaphoresis require more frequent cleansing to promote comfort and prevent skin breakdown and infection.

A patient with overly dry skin is predisposed to skin impairment. Use soap and lotions that contain emollients to hydrate dry skin. Use the opportunity of a complete bath to reassess a patient's skin and help with joint ROM exercises. Regardless of the type of bath (Box 31.6), use the following guidelines when bathing a patient:

- *Provide privacy.* Close the door and/or pull room curtains around the bathing area. Expose only the areas being bathed by using proper draping.
- *Maintain safety.* Keep side rails up and the bed in low position when away from the bedside. **Note:** You need a health care provider's order (see agency-specific policy) for restraint use when side rails serve as a restraint (see Chapter 30). Be sure nurse call system is in an accessible location within patient's reach if leaving the bedside even temporarily. Protect patients from injury by assessing and controlling the bath water temperature. This is especially important for older adult patients and

BOX 31.5 PATIENT-CENTERED CARE

Some patients have hair that is dry, fragile, and prone to breakage and damage. In addition, the hair tends to be naturally dry. Some cultural ethnic hairstyles may excessively pull the hair (e.g., braids, cornrows, weaves). These styles are implicated in the development of traction alopecia, the most common form of permanent hair loss (American Academy of Dermatology, 2012).

When your patient has dry, fragile hair, carefully observe for evidence of hair damage and developing hair loss. Ask for details about hair-care practices and hairstyles that might pull the hair. Include teaching about the risk of traction alopecia and ways to prevent or reduce this risk and promote healthy hair. Recognize that the choice of hairstyle and hair-care practices belongs to each patient; your role is to provide information and support for an informed decision (American Academy of Dermatology, 2012).

IMPLICATIONS FOR PRACTICE

- Wash hair once a week or every other week; too-frequent washing dries the hair, but buildup of hair care products also dries.
- Use conditioner each time hair is washed, paying special attention to the ends.
- For individuals who work out regularly, rinse the hair to remove salty sweat buildup; apply conditioner after the water rinse.

- Use hair-care products with natural ingredients such as olive oil, Shea butter, aloe vera, or glycerin because these agents help hair retain moisture. Avoid lanolin-containing or greasy products; they may moisturize, but they also clog pores on the scalp.
- Avoid shampoos containing sulfates, which dry the hair.
- Hot oil treatments twice a month add moisture and elasticity to dry hair.
- Use heat protectant on hair after washing and before heat styling. Products with silicone provide heat shielding and hydration.
- Have hair relaxers applied only by a professional hair stylist to minimize hair damage.
- Avoid too-frequent use of relaxers including touch-ups; allow 8 to 12 weeks between applications.
- Avoid overuse of thermal straightening devices; limit heat use to no more than once a week. Ceramic combs or irons with a dial temperature are safest.
- Protect the hair by wrapping it in a satin scarf or bonnet before bedtime.
- Braids, cornrows, and weaves can damage hair if too tight or in place too long. If these styles hurt, they are potentially damaging.
- Report even slight thinning of the hair or change in hair texture to your health care provider because this can be the start of hair loss.

BOX 31.6 TYPES OF BATHS

- **Complete bed bath:** Bath administered to totally dependent patient in bed (see Skill 31.1).
- **Partial bed bath:** Bed bath that consists of bathing only body parts that would cause discomfort if left unbathed such as the hands, face, axillae, and perineal area. Partial bath also includes washing the back and providing a backrub. Give a partial bath to patients who are dependent and need partial hygiene or patients who are bedridden and cannot reach all body parts.
- **Sponge bath at the sink:** Involves bathing from a bath basin or sink with patient sitting in a chair. Patient can perform part of the bath independently. You help patient with hard-to-reach areas.
- **Tub bath:** Involves immersion in a tub of water that allows more thorough washing and rinsing than a bed bath. Patient may still require assistance. Some institutions have tubs equipped with lifting devices to help move patients in and out of the tub when necessary.
- **Shower:** Patient sits or stands under a continuous stream of water. The shower provides more thorough cleansing than a bed bath but can be fatiguing.
- **Bag bath/travel bath:** Contains several soft, nonwoven cotton cloths that are premoistened in a solution of no-rinse surfactant cleanser and emollient. The bag bath offers ease of use, reduced bathing time, and patient comfort.
- **Chlorhexidine gluconate (CHG) bath:** Antimicrobial agent used to reduce incidence of hospital-acquired infections on skin, invasive lines, and catheters (Cassir et al., 2015; Boonyasiri et al., 2016; Shah et al., 2016).

patients with reduced sensation such as patients with diabetes, peripheral neuropathy, or spinal cord injuries. Use assistive devices such as bath chairs when indicated. Place a chair in the shower for a patient with weakness or poor balance. Both tubs and showers must have grab bars for patients to hold during entry and exit and for maneuvering during the bath or shower.

- *Maintain warmth.* Keep the room warm to prevent chilling. Prevent drafts and keep windows closed. Cover your patient, exposing only the body part being washed. Moisture on the skin causes excessive heat loss through evaporation.
- *Promote independence.* Encourage your patient to participate with bathing as much as possible. Offer assistance as needed, but assess carefully for activity intolerance.
- *Anticipate needs.* Implement actions to address the patient's need to use the bedpan or urinal and to receive relief from pain or nausea before hygiene care. Bring all needed items including linen, hygiene products, and new gown before initiating bath.

A complete bed bath, tub bath, or shower (see Skill 31.1) may exhaust a patient. Be alert for the patient's activity intolerance during hygiene care. Observe respirations, noting changes in rate and depth or any shortness of breath. Observe for changes in skin color. Palpate the pulse to detect changes in rate and regularity and question the patient about dizziness, weakness, or fatigue. If the patient experiences activity intolerance (e.g., rapid, irregular heart rate) during care, seek assistance, return him or her to bed, and observe carefully for improvement with rest. Provide a partial bed bath to a patient who needs only partial hygiene, who is too debilitated or unable to tolerate a complete bed bath, or who can perform self-care but needs help with completing the bath.

The use of bath basins with soap and water became an issue after a recent study conducted in intensive care units. Researchers found that when baths were given with regular soap and water, bath basins become a reservoir for bacteria, which possibly leads to transmission of hospital-acquired infections. Research shows a link between waterborne pathogens and the development of biofilm (multiple colonies of microorganisms attached to a surface such as a bath basin). The formation of a biofilm combined with transmission of organisms through patient contact with a nurse's unwashed hands can create a reservoir of bacteria that can be transferred to and maintained in a patient's bath basin (Strouse, 2015).

In contrast, researchers found using chlorhexidine gluconate (CHG) 4% solution in place of standard soap and water in wash basins reduces bacterial growth in basins (Powers et al., 2012; Shah et al., 2016) and reduces critical care–acquired methicillin-resistant *Staphylococcus aureus* (MRSA) (Petlin et al., 2014). Be sure to air-dry bath basins completely, and do not use the basin to store supplies.

Another alternative to using CHG in bath basins is the use of CHG 2%–impregnated disposable washcloths. The CHG in the washcloth acts quickly, has broad-spectrum microorganism coverage, continues antimicrobial activity up to 24 hours after application, and is rinse free and disposable (Agency for Health Care Research and Quality [AHRQ], 2013). Research shows that compared with the use of antimicrobial washcloths, daily bathing with CHG 2%–impregnated cloths reduces a patient's risk of becoming infected with multidrug-resistant organisms (Climo et al., 2013; Cassir et al., 2015). Some reports show a risk of skin irritation after repeated use; thus bathing the patient with the cloths every other day may be an option. Another option is the bag bath. The bag bath contains a no-rinse surfactant, a humectant to trap moisture, and an emollient. The bag bath does not contain CHG. When using cloths or the bag bath, no bath basin is needed.

Health care–associated infections (HAIs) are one of the most common adverse events that occur during hospitalization. HAIs cause prolonged hospitalization and a high rate of fatalities resulting in a large financial burden. Several studies have tested the effect of interventions to reduce these central line infections (Box 31.7). Among the interventions tested is daily bathing with chlorhexidine-impregnated cloths or chlorhexidine liquid soap (e.g., Hibiclens). Findings consistently validate significant reductions in colonization and infection after use of chlorhexidine for bathing (Munoz-Price et al., 2012; Climo et al., 2013).

Patients with dementia require special considerations in bathing. Assess patients entering long-term care facilities for cognitive and functional status (Hall et al., 2013). Patients with cognitive impairments sometimes become more confused and combative as a result of pain, fatigue, weakness, anxiety from exposure during a bath, and discomfort from a

---

BOX 31.7   EVIDENCE-BASED PRACTICE

PICOT Question: Does daily bathing with chlorhexidine compared with traditional soap-and-water bathing reduce the rate of hospital-acquired infections in hospitalized adults?

SUMMARY OF EVIDENCE

Health care–associated infections (HAIs) are one of the most common adverse events during hospitalization, especially among critically ill patients (Cassir et al., 2015). Central line–associated bloodstream infections are one of the most frequent HAIs in the United States, with a mortality of up to 25% (Chen et al., 2013; Shah et al., 2016). Daily bathing with 2% chlorhexidine cloths substantially reduces bacterial colonization on patients' skin and bloodstream HAIs including methicillin-resistant *Staphylococcus aureus* (MRSA) and vancomycin-resistant *Enterococcus* (VRE) infections (Climo et al., 2013; Cassir et al., 2015; Shah et al., 2016). Studies conducted on general medicine units showed a substantial decrease in the risk of acquiring an infection from MRSA and VRE infections when using chlorhexidine gluconate (CHG) (Cassir et al., 2015; Shah et al., 2016).

APPLICATION TO NURSING PRACTICE

- The Joint Commission (TJC) recommends the use of evidence-based practices to prevent HAIs (Rubin et al., 2013).
- Develop a policy and procedure to adopt use of chlorhexidine for bathing patients at high risk of developing HAIs (i.e., specifically central line–associated bloodstream infections) (Rubin et al., 2013; Shah et al., 2016).
- Provide educational programs for nursing staff on the effectiveness of chlorhexidine for bathing in the reduction of HAIs.
- Adopt evidence-based care for central line hubs, including use of chlorhexidine to cleanse the hubs (Chen et al., 2013; Cassir et al., 2015) (see Chapter 18).

---

cold or drafty bathing area. Calmly speaking to the patient in a conversational but informative voice and using a calm, organized approach to bathing has been shown to be effective (Hall et al., 2013).

A thermal towel bath reduces agitation compared with tub baths. This is a person-centered, in-bed approach in which a nurse uses a large towel, one or two regular-size towels, washcloths, a bath blanket, and no-rinse soap and water (Hall et al., 2013).

Perineal Care. Cleansing patients' genital and anal areas is called perineal care. It is part of a complete bed bath but also is performed at other times as needed. Factors that create the need for more perineal care include urinary and bowel incontinence, presence of indwelling urinary catheters, menstruation, vaginal drainage or draining wounds, and obesity.

Prolonged contact of urine on the skin can alter the normal protective skin flora by raising the pH of the skin. Contact with moisture from incontinence weakens the skin, making it more prone to damage from friction (Voegeli, 2016). Stool remaining on the skin contains active fecal enzymes that damage the skin. Bacteria in the feces also can penetrate the skin and contribute to secondary infections. Incontinence-related dermatitis increases the risk for pressure injuries (Beeckman et al., 2014).

Encourage patients to perform their own perineal care if they are able. You may feel embarrassed about providing perineal care, particularly to a patient of the opposite gender. Similarly, a patient may feel embarrassed. Do not let these feelings cause you to overlook a patient's perineal hygiene needs. When staffing permits, use a gender-congruent caregiver. A professional, dignified, and sensitive approach reduces embarrassment and helps put the patient at ease.

If the patient performs perineal care without assistance, various issues such as vaginal or urethral discharge, perineal irritation, and unpleasant odors may go undetected. Emphasize the importance of perineal care in preventing skin breakdown and infection. Be alert for complaints of burning during urination or localized soreness, excoriation, or pain in the perineum. Inspect vaginal and perineal areas and the bed linen for evidence of discharge and use your sense of smell to detect abnormal odors.

Oral Care. When patients become ill, many factors influence their need for oral hygiene. Base the frequency of care on the condition of the oral cavity and a patient's level of comfort (Box 31.8). Some patients require oral hygiene every 1 to 2 hours.

Patients who are unconscious or have artificial airways (e.g., endotracheal or tracheal tubes) need special precautions with oral care because they often do not have a gag reflex (Box 31.9). These patients require meticulous and frequent oral hygiene. CHG mouth rinse further helps to reduce ventilator-associated pneumonia (VAP) in these patients (El-Rabbany et al., 2015).

While providing hygiene to an unconscious patient, you must protect the airway from aspiration. The safest practice is to have two nurses provide the care. You can delegate nursing assistive personnel (NAP) to participate. One nurse does the actual cleaning, and the NAP removes secretions using oral suction (see Chapter 32).

While cleansing the oral cavity, use a small oral airway or a padded tongue blade to hold the mouth open. Never use your fingers. A human bite is highly contaminated. Explain

---

BOX 31.8 PROCEDURAL GUIDELINES

Performing Oral Hygiene

DELEGATION CONSIDERATIONS

The skill of oral hygiene (including toothbrushing and rinsing) can be delegated to nursing assistive personnel (NAP). However, the nurse is responsible for assessing the patient's gag reflex to determine whether the patient is at risk for aspiration. The nurse instructs the NAP about:

- Types of changes in oral mucosa (e.g., presence of lesions or open sores) to report to the nurse.
- Positioning the patient to avoid aspiration.
  - Keeping head of bed (HOB) raised 30 to 45 degrees
  - Immediately reporting to the nurse excessive patient coughing or choking during or after oral hygiene.
- Reporting bleeding of oral mucosa or gums, patient report of pain, and any changes in oral mucosa (e.g., open areas or lesions).
- Not flossing when the patient has a bleeding tendency.

EQUIPMENT

Soft-bristle toothbrush; nonabrasive fluoride toothpaste; dental floss; chlorhexidine gluconate (CHG) 0.12% (optional; see agency policy); tongue depressor; glass with cool water, normal saline, or antiseptic mouth rinse (optional depending on patient preference); moisturizing lubricant for lips (optional); dental floss; emesis basin; face towel; paper towels; clean gloves; penlight; linen bag or hamper

STEPS

1. Identify patient using at least two identifiers (e.g., name and birthday or name and medical record number) according to agency policy.
2. Review medical record and identify presence of common oral cavity problems: dental caries, chalky white discoloration of tooth or presence of brown or black discoloration; gingivitis, inflammation of gums; periodontitis, receding gum lines, inflammation, gaps between teeth; halitosis, bad breath; cheilitis, cracked lips; dry, cracked, and coated tongue.
3. Determine patient's oral hygiene practices such as frequency of brushing and flossing, type of toothpaste and mouthwash used, last dental visit and frequency of dental visits.
4. Perform hand hygiene and apply clean gloves.
5. Using tongue depressor and penlight, inspect integrity of lips, teeth, buccal mucosa, gums, palate, and tongue; also, assess for gag reflex and ability to swallow (see Chapter 16).
6. Confirm presence of common oral problems.
7. Remove gloves and perform hand hygiene.
8. Explain procedure to patient, discussing patient's preferences and willingness to help with oral care.
9. Assess patient's ability to grasp and manipulate toothbrush.
10. Place paper towels on over-bed table and arrange other equipment within easy reach.
11. Provide privacy by closing room doors and drawing room divider curtain. Raise bed to comfortable working position. Raise head of bed (if allowed) and lower near side rail. Move patient or help him or her move closer to side. Place patient in side-lying position if needed (if aspiration risk). Place towel over patient's chest.
12. Apply clean gloves.
13. Apply enough toothpaste to brush to cover extent of bristles. Hold brush over emesis basin. Pour small amount of water over toothpaste.

Continued

BOX 31.8 PROCEDURAL GUIDELINES—cont'd

Performing Oral Hygiene

14. Patient may help with brushing. Hold toothbrush bristles at 45-degree angle to gum line (see illustration A). Be sure that tips of bristles rest against and penetrate under gum line. Brush inner and outer surfaces of upper and lower teeth by brushing from gum to crown of each tooth. Clean biting surfaces of teeth by holding top of bristles parallel with teeth and brushing gently back and forth (see illustration B). Brush sides of teeth by moving bristles back and forth (see illustration C).

15. Have patient hold brush at 45-degree angle and lightly brush over surface and sides of tongue (see illustration). Avoid initiating gag reflex.

16. Allow patient to rinse mouth thoroughly by taking several sips of cool water, swishing water across all tooth surfaces, and spitting into emesis basin. Use this time to observe patient's brushing technique and teach importance of regular hygiene.

17. Have patient rinse mouth with antiseptic rinse for 30 seconds. Then have patient spit rinse into emesis basin. Help wipe patient's mouth.

18. *Option:* Floss or allow patient to floss between all teeth (see illustration).

19. Allow patient to rinse mouth thoroughly with cool water and spit into emesis basin. Help wipe patient's mouth.

20. Inspect oral cavity to determine effectiveness of oral hygiene and rinsing. Ask patient if mouth feels clean or if there are any sore or tender areas. Remove towel and place in linen bag.

21. **Use Teach-Back:** "I want to be sure you know how often to brush your teeth and floss. Tell me how often you should floss your teeth." Revise your instruction now or develop a plan for revised patient/family caregiver teaching if patient/family caregiver is not able to teach back correctly.

22. Help patient to comfortable position, raise side rail, and lower bed to original position.

23. Clean and dry basin before returning basin and nondisposable supplies.

24. Remove gloves and perform hand hygiene.

25. Record relevant observations, condition of oral cavity, amount of care patient could perform, and whether additional instruction is needed.

26. Document your evaluation of patient/family caregiver learning.

27. Report bleeding, pain, or presence of lesions to nurse in charge or health care provider.

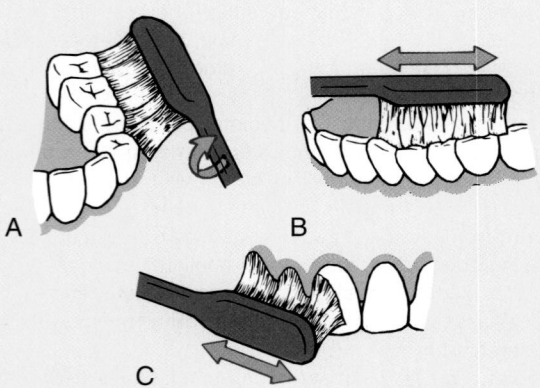

STEP 14 A to **C,** Directions of brush for toothbrushing.

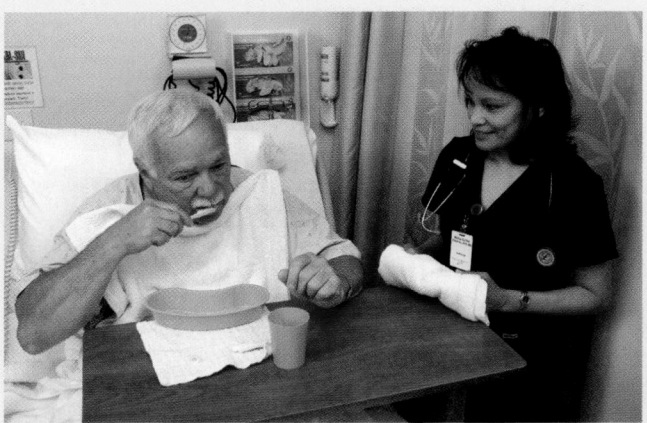

STEP 15 Nurse observes patient's toothbrushing technique including brushing of tongue.

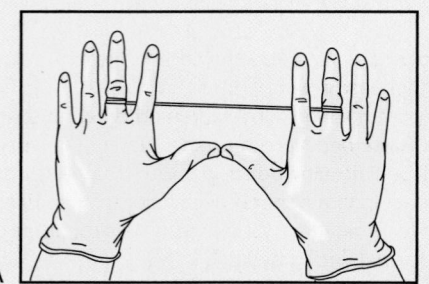
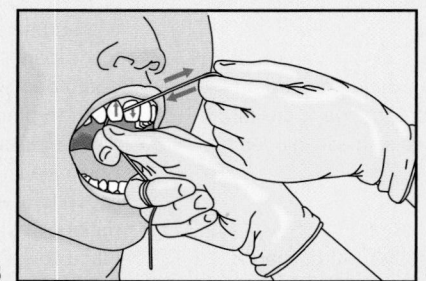
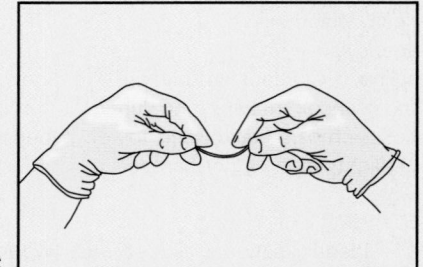

STEP 18 Flossing. **A,** Dental floss is held between middle fingers to floss upper teeth. **B,** Floss is moved in up-and-down motion between teeth. Floss is moved up and down from crown to gum line. **C,** Floss is held with index fingers to floss lower teeth.

the steps of mouth care and the sensations the patient will feel. Inform the patient when the procedure is completed.

Proper oral hygiene requires keeping the mucosa moist and removing secretions that can lead to infection. Researchers have found that foam stick applicators stimulate the mucosal tissues but are ineffective in removing debris from the teeth. Limit the use of foam swabs to situations in which gentle cleansing is required. Examples include patients who have bleeding tendencies or sustained trauma to the oral cavity (Kiyoshi-Teo and Blegen, 2015). A child-size toothbrush fits more easily around an endotracheal tube than an adult-size toothbrush.

Current evidence-based practice guidelines include guidelines for oral care in patients on mechanical ventilation. Microorganisms colonize in the oral pharynx of these patients. These microorganisms frequently move from the oral pharynx into the lungs, leading to VAP. Dental plaque also has been implicated as a reservoir for microorganisms, leading to VAP. Current evidence supports the use of antiseptic chlorhexidine rinse as part of oral hygiene because it

---

QSEN QSEN ACTIVITY *Evidence-Based Practice*

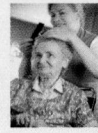
Copyright © AlexRaths/ iStock/ Thinkstock.

Today the student nurse Jamie changes clinical rotations. She is orienting to the medical intensive care unit and shadowing one of the nurses there. Jamie observes that many of the patients in the unit are on ventilators. Throughout the morning, she observes oral care being performed. She notices that different nurses perform the care in different ways. She recalls hearing in class about research regarding oral care, use of chlorhexidine, and ventilator-associated pneumonia. Jamie wants to be ready to provide evidence-based oral care in her next experience.

- To clarify her search for evidence-based information, what would be Jamie's PICO question?
- Where should Jamie look for the best evidence regarding her question?

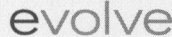 Answers to QSEN Activities can be found on the Evolve website.

BOX 31.9 PROCEDURAL GUIDELINES

Performing Oral Hygiene for a Patient Who Is Unconscious or a Debilitated Patient

DELEGATION CONSIDERATIONS

The skill of providing oral hygiene to an unconscious or debilitated patient can be delegated to nursing assistive personnel (NAP). The nurse is responsible for assessing the patient's gag reflex. The nurse instructs the NAP to:

- Have another NAP assist and properly position patient for mouth care.
- Be aware of aspiration precautions.
- Use an oral suction catheter for clearing oral secretions (see Chapter 32).
- Report signs of impaired integrity of oral mucosa to the nurse.
- Report any bleeding of mucosa or gums, excessive coughing, or choking to the nurse.

EQUIPMENT

Small pediatric, soft-bristled toothbrush; toothette sponges or suction toothbrushes for patients for whom brushing is contraindicated; antibacterial solution per agency protocol (e.g., chlorhexidine gluconate [CHG]); fluoride toothpaste; water-based mouth moisturizer; tongue blade; penlight; oral suction equipment; oral airway (uncooperative patient or patient who shows bite reflex); water-soluble lip lubricant; glass with cool water; face and bath towel; emesis basin; clean gloves

STEPS

1. Identify patient using at least two identifiers (e.g., name and birthday or name and medical record number) according to agency policy.
2. Review medical record for presence of oral cavity problems (see Box 31.8).
3. Perform hand hygiene and apply clean gloves.

4. Assess for presence of gag reflex by placing tongue blade on back half of tongue.

> **Clinical Decision Point. Patients with impaired gag reflex still require oral care but have a higher risk for aspiration. Keep suction equipment available when caring for patients who are at risk for aspiration.**

5. Inspect condition of oral cavity. Confirm presence of oral problems.
6. Remove gloves. Perform hand hygiene.
7. Explain procedure to patient, even if patient is unconscious.
8. Pull curtain around bed or close room door.
9. Place towel on over-bed table and arrange equipment. If needed, turn on suction machine and connect tubing to suction catheter.
10. Raise bed to appropriate working height. Unless contraindicated (e.g., head injury, neck trauma), position patient in Sims' or side-lying position. Turn patient's side of face toward mattress in dependent position with head of bed elevated at least 30 degrees.
11. Apply gloves.
12. Lower side rail. Place towel under patient's head and one across chest. Place emesis basin under patient's chin.
13. If patient is uncooperative or having difficulty keeping mouth open, insert an oral airway. Insert upside down and turn airway sideways and over tongue to keep teeth apart. Insert when patient is relaxed if possible. Do not use force.

> **Clinical Decision Point. Never place fingers into the mouth of a patient who is unconscious or debilitated. This could occlude the airway. In addition, the normal response is to bite down.**

Continued

BOX 31.9   PROCEDURAL GUIDELINES—cont'd

Performing Oral Hygiene for a Patient Who Is Unconscious or a Debilitated Patient

14. Clean mouth using brush moistened in water. Apply toothpaste or use antibacterial solution first to loosen crusts. Hold toothbrush bristles at 45-degree angle to gum line. Be sure that tips of bristles rest against and penetrate under gum line. Brush inner and outer surfaces of upper and lower teeth by brushing from gum to crown of each tooth, then clean biting surfaces of teeth by holding top of bristles parallel with teeth and brushing gently back and forth (see Box 31.8). Brush sides of teeth by moving bristles back and forth. Use a toothette sponge if patient has a bleeding tendency or use of toothbrush is contraindicated. Suction any accumulated secretions. Moisten brush with clear water or CHG solution to rinse. Use brush or toothette to clean roof of mouth, gums, and inside cheeks. Gently brush tongue, but avoid stimulating gag reflex (if present). Repeat rinsing several times, and use suction to remove secretions. Use towel to dry off lips (see illustration).

15. Apply thin layer of water-soluble moisturizer to lips (see illustration).

16. Inform patient that procedure is complete. Return patient to comfortable and safe position.

17. Raise side rails as appropriate and return bed to locked, low position. Be sure nurse call system is in an accessible location within patient's reach.

18. Clean equipment and return to its proper place. Place soiled linen in dirty laundry bag.

19. Remove and dispose of gloves in proper receptacle and perform hand hygiene.

20. To evaluate condition of oral cavity, apply clean gloves and use tongue blade and penlight to inspect oral cavity.

21. Ask debilitated patient if mouth feels clean.

22. **Use Teach-Back:** "I explained what is needed to reduce your husband's risk of choking on secretions in his throat. Tell me the ways you will prevent him from choking when you give mouth care at home." Revise your instruction now or develop a plan for revised patient/family caregiver teaching if patient/family caregiver is not able to teach back correctly.

23. Record relevant observations (objective and subjective), relevant details of procedure, and information about specific equipment uses and patient response as related to specific skill.

24. Document your evaluation of patient/family caregiver learning.

25. Report unexpected responses (e.g., ulceration, bleeding, choking) to nurse or health care provider.

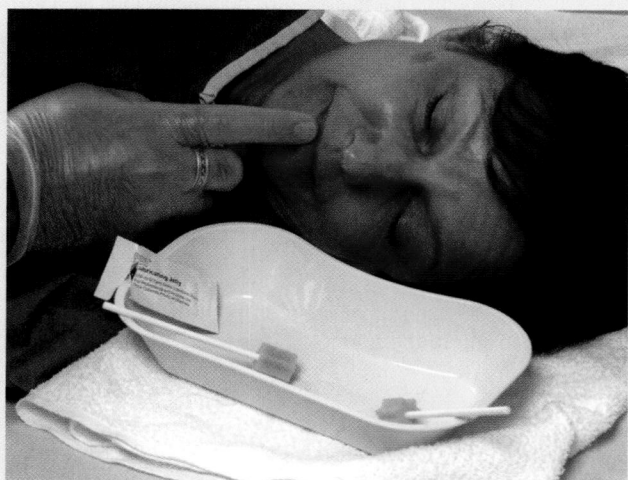

STEP 14 Cleaning lips and mucosa around oral airway with toothette.

STEP 15 Application of water-soluble moisturizer to lips.

reduces the risk for VAP in high-risk groups (Labeau et al., 2011; Munro, 2014; El-Rabbany et al., 2015).

Patients receiving cancer chemotherapy, immunosuppressive agents, head and neck radiation therapy, or nasogastric intubation or who have an infection of the mouth are susceptible to mucositis. Mucositis causes burning, pain, and a change in the patient's food and fluid tolerance. For these patients, brush with a soft toothbrush for at least 90 seconds twice a day, floss gently once a day, use sodium bicarbonate rinses, and include dental professionals in the plan of care (Eilers et al., 2014). Omit flossing if patients have excessive bleeding, use anticoagulants, or have thrombocytopenia. Normal saline rinses on awakening in the morning, after each meal, and at bedtime help clean the oral cavity. Patients can increase the rinses to every 2 hours if needed. Instruct patients with mucositis to avoid alcohol and commercial mouthwash that contains alcohol and to stop smoking. Consult with the health care provider to obtain topical or oral analgesics for pain control. Assess a patient's fluid and nutritional status regularly to detect inadequate food and fluid intake caused by oral discomfort (National Cancer Institute [NCI], 2016).

Denture Care. When patients become disabled, someone must assume responsibility for denture care (Box 31.10). Dentures are a patient's personal property and must be handled with care because they break easily. To prevent warping, keep them covered in water when they are not being worn, and always store them in an enclosed, labeled cup with the cup placed in a drawer in the patient's bedside stand. Discourage patients from removing their dentures and placing them on a napkin or tissue, on the bed, or in a chair because they could easily be thrown away.

Backrub. A backrub usually follows the bath. It promotes relaxation, relieves muscular tension, and reduces pain perception. Evidence shows that **effleurage** (long, light, gliding strokes used in a massage) may reduce anxiety, heart rate, and

---

BOX 31.10 PROCEDURAL GUIDELINES

View Video!

Cleaning Dentures

DELEGATION CONSIDERATIONS

The skill of cleaning dentures can be delegated to nursing assistive personnel (NAP). The nurse instructs the NAP to:
- Not use hot or excessively cold water when caring for dentures.
- Inform the nurse if there are cracks in dentures.
- Inform the nurse of any sores or irritation on patient's gums or in oral cavity.
- Inform the nurse if the patient has any oral discomfort.

EQUIPMENT

Soft-bristle toothbrush or denture toothbrush, denture-cleaning agent or toothpaste, denture adhesive *(optional)*, glass of water, emesis basin or sink, washcloth, gauze (4 × 4–inch), clean gloves, denture cup (for storage)

STEPS

1. Identify patient using at least two identifiers (e.g., name and birthday or name and medical record number) according to agency policy.
2. Assess environment for safety (e.g., check room for spills, make sure that equipment is working properly and that bed is in locked, low position).
3. Perform hand hygiene.
4. Ask patient if dentures fit and if there is any gum or mucous membrane tenderness or irritation. Ask patient about denture care and product preferences.
5. Determine if patient has necessary dexterity to clean dentures independently or requires assistance.
6. Position patient comfortably sitting up in bed or assist patient to walk from bed to a chair placed in front of sink.
7. Fill emesis basin with tepid water. (If using sink, place washcloth in bottom of sink and fill sink with approximately 2.5 cm [1 inch] of water.)
8. Apply clean gloves.
9. Ask patient to remove dentures. If patient is unable to do this independently, grasp upper plate at front with thumb and index finger wrapped in gauze and pull downward. Gently lift lower denture from jaw and rotate one side downward to remove from patient's mouth. Place dentures in emesis basin or sink lined with washcloth and filled with 2.5 cm (1 inch) of water.
10. Apply cleaning agent to brush and brush surfaces of dentures (see illustration). Hold dentures close to water. Hold brush horizontally and use back-and-forth motion to clean biting surfaces. Use short strokes from top of denture to

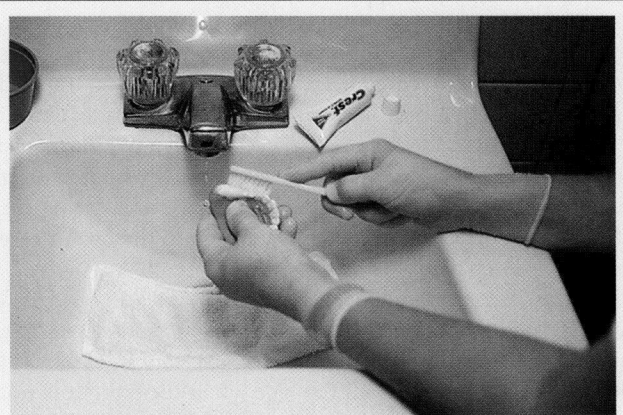

STEP 10 Brushing surface of dentures.

biting surfaces to clean outer teeth surfaces. Hold brush vertically and use short strokes to clean inner teeth surfaces. Hold brush horizontally and use back-and-forth motion to clean undersurface of dentures.
11. Rinse dentures thoroughly in tepid water. If water is too cold, dentures can crack. If water is too hot, dentures can become warped and no longer fit.
12. Some patients use an adhesive to seal dentures in place. Apply a thin layer to undersurface before inserting.
13. If patient needs help with inserting dentures, moisten upper denture and press firmly to seal it in place. Insert moistened lower denture (if applicable). Ask if dentures feel comfortable.
14. **Use Teach-Back:** "I explained the importance of regular cleansing of your dentures. Tell me why it is important to clean your dentures daily." Revise your instruction now or develop a plan for revised patient/family caregiver teaching if patient/family caregiver is not able to teach back correctly.
15. Some patients prefer to store their dentures to give gums a rest and reduce risk for infection. Store in tepid water in an enclosed, labeled denture cup. Keep denture cup in a secure place labeled with patient's name to prevent loss when not worn (e.g., at night, during surgery).
16. Dispose of supplies. Remove and discard gloves and perform hand hygiene.
17. Return patient to a comfortable position. Be sure nurse call system is in an accessible location within patient's reach.

respiratory rate (Zullino et al., 2005). Research shows that slow-stroke back massages of 3 minutes' duration and hand massages of 10 minutes' duration significantly improve both physiological and psychological indicators of relaxation in older adults (Harris and Richards, 2010).

Always ask whether a patient would like a backrub or whether he or she prefers gentle instead of deep massage because some patients dislike physical contact. In addition, review the patient's record for any contraindications to a massage such as spinal cord injury, rib fracture, and other painful conditions.

Care of Eyes, Ears, and Nose. Give special attention to cleansing the eyes, ears, and nose during a patient's bath. Focus care on preventing infection and maintaining normal organ function.

Basic Eye Care. A patient who is unconscious requires more frequent eye care. Secretions collect along the lid margins and inner canthus when the blink reflex is absent or when the eye does not close completely. When an eye remains open, you may need to apply an eye patch over the affected eye to prevent corneal drying and irritation. Administer lubricating eyedrops according to the health care provider's orders.

Eyeglasses. Although eyeglasses are made of hardened glass or plastic that is impact resistant to prevent shattering, you must use caution when handling or cleaning glasses. In addition, protect them from damage when the patient is not wearing them by placing them in a case and putting them in a drawer of the bedside table. Clean the lenses with cool water and use a soft cloth for drying to avoid scratching them. Avoid using paper towels for cleaning or drying glasses. Plastic lenses scratch easily; special cleansing solutions and drying tissues are available.

Contact Lenses. Contact lenses are relatively easy to apply and remove. If patients are able, have them remove daily-wear lenses nightly for cleaning and disinfection. A patient may wear extended-wear lenses overnight and remove them at least weekly for cleaning and disinfection.

Care of contact lenses includes proper cleaning, insertion and removal, and storage. When patients require help to clean their contact lenses, first perform hand hygiene and then clean and disinfect the lenses with the appropriate contact lens solution. Before reinsertion, rinse the lenses with an appropriate solution such as sterile saline. Instruct the patient to never use saliva or homemade solutions when cleaning contact lenses to avoid potential eye infections and to clean the contact lens case frequently with warm water and allow to air dry.

When patients are admitted to hospitals or health care agencies in unresponsive or confused states, you must determine if they wear contact lenses and whether the lenses are in place. If a seriously ill patient is wearing contact lenses and no one detects this, severe corneal injury results. If you determine that your patient has contact lenses in place and the patient cannot remove them, seek assistance in removing the lenses from the patient's eyes. After you have removed the lenses, be sure to document their removal, the condition of

the patient's eyes after removal, and whether you gave the lenses to a family member or placed them with the patient's valuables.

Ear Care. To properly clean the outer ear, insert one end of a cotton swab along the pinna or outer shell of the ear at the top. Then swipe clean by moving the cotton swab down, following the curve of the ear. Place the end of the cotton swab at the opening of the ear canal and gently wipe the entrance of the ear canal clean. Do not occlude the ear with the swab or try to clean the inside. This can damage the tympanic membrane and cause earwax to become impacted in the ear.

When earwax is impacted, you can usually remove it by irrigation, which requires a health care provider's order. Review the order for type of solution and ear to receive the irrigation. Before irrigation, ask if your patient has a history of perforated eardrum and inspect the tympanic membrane to be sure that it is intact. Your patient cannot have an ear irrigation if the tympanic membrane is perforated. Visually inspect the pinna and external meatus for redness, swelling, drainage, and presence of foreign objects. If an object (e.g., dried bean) is in the ear canal, do not perform irrigation. Use an otoscope to inspect deeper portions of the auditory canal (see Chapter 16). Determine the patient's ability to hear in the affected ear before irrigation.

To irrigate the ear, have a patient sit or lie on the side with the affected ear up. Place a curved emesis basin under the affected ear. For adults and children older than 3 years of age, gently pull the pinna up and back. In children 3 years of age or younger, the pinna should be pulled down and back. Using a bulb irrigating syringe, gently wash the ear canal with warm solution (37° C [98.6° F]), being careful not to occlude the canal, which results in pressure on the tympanic membrane. Direct the fluid slowly and gently toward the superior aspect of the ear canal, maintaining the flow in a steady stream. Periodically during the irrigation, ask if the patient is experiencing pain, nausea, or vertigo. These symptoms indicate that the solution is too hot or too cold or is being instilled with too much pressure. After the canal is clear, wipe off any moisture from the ear with cotton balls and inspect the canal for remaining earwax.

Nasal Care. If a patient cannot remove nasal secretions, help by using a wet washcloth or a cotton-tipped applicator moistened in water or saline. Never insert the applicator beyond the length of the cotton tip. You also can remove excessive nasal secretions through gentle nasal suctioning (see Chapter 32).

When patients have nasogastric, feeding, or endotracheal tubes inserted through the nares, change the tape anchoring the tube at least once a day. When the tape becomes moist from nasal secretions, the skin and mucosa can easily become macerated (softened by soaking). Friction from a tube causes tissue injury. Anchor tubing correctly with tape or fixative devices to minimize tension or friction on the nares (see Chapter 37).

Nail and Foot Care. Routine nail and foot care includes soaking to soften cuticles and layers of horny cells, thorough cleaning, drying, and proper nail trimming. In some settings or with some patients, such as a patient with diabetes mellitus or peripheral vascular disease, you need a health care provider's order to trim toenails. Sit patients in a chair if possible when providing foot and nail care. When patients are immobilized, you perform care while they are in bed (Box 31.11).

Recognize conditions that place a patient at increased risk for amputation such as uncontrolled diabetes, peripheral neuropathy, limited joint mobility, bony deformity, peripheral vascular disease, and a history of skin ulcers or previous amputation. Observe for changes that indicate peripheral neuropathy or vascular insufficiency (Box 31.12).

Hair Care. Patients appreciate the opportunity to have their hair brushed and combed before others visit them. Long hair easily becomes matted when a patient is confined to bed, even for a short period. Blood and topical medications also cause tangling when lacerations or incisions involve the scalp. Frequent brushing and combing keep long hair neatly groomed. Braiding helps to avoid repeated tangles. Ask permission before braiding a patient's hair.

To brush hair, part it into two sections and separate each into two more sections. It is easier to brush smaller sections of hair. Brushing from the tip of the hair ends and moving to the scalp minimizes pulling. Moistening the hair with water or an alcohol-free detangle product makes the hair easier to comb. Do not cut a patient's hair without consent.

The frequency of shampooing depends on a patient's preferences and the condition of the hair. Remind patients they may need more frequent shampooing if they are on constant bed rest or have excess perspiration or treatments that leave blood or solutions in their hair. A patient who can take a shower or bath usually shampoos the hair independently. Use a shower chair for a patient who is ambulatory but becomes tired or faint. Handheld shower nozzles allow patients to wash the hair during a tub bath or shower.

If a patient can sit in a chair, you usually shampoo the hair in front of a sink. If a patient sits at the bedside, shampoo the hair as the patient leans forward over a wash basin. If bending is limited or contraindicated (e.g., after eye surgery or neck injury), teach the patient and family caregivers the degree of bending allowed.

Transfer patients who cannot sit but can be moved to a stretcher for transportation to a sink or shower equipped with a handheld nozzle. Place a towel or small pillow under the patient's head and neck, allowing the head to hang slightly over the edge of the stretcher. Use caution when shampooing patients with neck injuries because hyperextension of the

---

BOX 31.11 PROCEDURAL GUIDELINES

Performing Nail and Foot Care

DELEGATION CONSIDERATIONS

The skill of nail and foot care of patients *without diabetes* or *circulatory compromise* can be delegated to nursing assistive personnel (NAP). The nurse instructs the NAP about:

- Not trimming patient's nails (unless permitted by agency or health care provider).
- Special positioning considerations.
- Reporting any breaks in skin, redness, numbness, swelling, or pain to the nurse.

EQUIPMENT

Washbasin, emesis basin, washcloth, towels, nail clippers (check agency policy), soft nail or cuticle brush, plastic applicator stick, emery board or nail file, lotion, disposable bath mat, paper towels, linen bag, clean gloves if drainage is present

STEPS

1. Identify patient using at least two identifiers (e.g., name and birthday or name and medical record number) according to agency policy.
2. Verify health care provider's order for cutting nails.
3. Determine patient's knowledge of nail and foot care.
4. Explain procedure to patient. Inform patient that proper soaking requires several minutes.
5. Pull curtain around bed or close room door to provide privacy.
6. Help patient who is ambulatory sit in chair and place disposable bath mat on floor under patient's feet. Help patient who must stay in bed to supine position with head of bed elevated 45 degrees and place waterproof pad on mattress (keep side rail up until ready to begin).
7. Perform hand hygiene and apply clean gloves. Inspect all surfaces of fingers, toes, feet, and nails. **Note:** You can do this inspection during the bath. Pay close attention to areas of dryness, inflammation, or cracking. Also, inspect areas between toes, heels, and soles of feet. Inspect socks for stains. Remove gloves.
8. Fill washbasin with warm water. Test water temperature. Place basin on floor or lower side rail and place basin on pad on mattress. Have patient immerse feet. If patient has diabetes mellitus, peripheral neuropathy, or peripheral vascular disease, go to Step 12 to begin foot care.
9. Fill emesis basin with warm water and place basin on towel on over-bed table. Test water temperature.
10. Have patient place fingers in emesis basin and arms in comfortable position.
11. Allow feet and fingernails to soak 5 to 10 minutes.

Clinical Decision Point. If patient has diabetes mellitus, peripheral neuropathy, or peripheral vascular disease, skip this step and go straight to Step 12.

---

12. Clean gently under fingernails with end of plastic applicator stick. Do this while fingers are immersed unless patient has diabetes (see illustration).

Continued

BOX 31.11 PROCEDURAL GUIDELINES—cont'd

Performing Nail and Foot Care

13. Trim nails straight across at level of finger or follow curve of finger, ensuring that you do not cut down into nail grooves (see illustration). Use disposable emery board and file nail to ensure that there are no sharp corners. (Verify agency policy on nail care regarding filing and trimming.)
14. Use a soft cuticle brush or nailbrush to clean around cuticles. Remove hands from basin and dry completely.
15. Move over-bed table away from patient. Begin foot care by scrubbing callused areas of feet with washcloth.
16. Scrub callused areas of feet and clean between toes with washcloth.
17. Dry feet thoroughly and trim or cut toenails (see Step 13).
18. Apply lotion to feet and hands. Rub in thoroughly. Do not leave excess lotion between toes.
19. Help patient back to bed and into comfortable, safe position. Be sure nurse call system is in an accessible location within patient's reach.

20. Sanitize equipment according to organizational policy and return equipment to proper place. Emery boards should be disposable. Dispose of soiled linen in dirty laundry bag. Remove and dispose of gloves. Perform hand hygiene.
21. During evaluation, inspect nails, areas between fingers and toes, and surrounding skin surfaces.
22. **Use Teach-Back:** "We discussed how to prevent infection in the skin around your nails. Tell me the tips you should follow to protect your feet from infection." Revise your instruction now or develop a plan for revised patient/family caregiver teaching if patient/family caregiver is not able to teach back correctly.
23. Record condition and appearance of nails and feet, condition of circulation, and care and instructions provided.
24. Document your evaluation of patient/family caregiver learning.
25. Report any breaks in the skin, reddened or tender areas, or any discomfort.

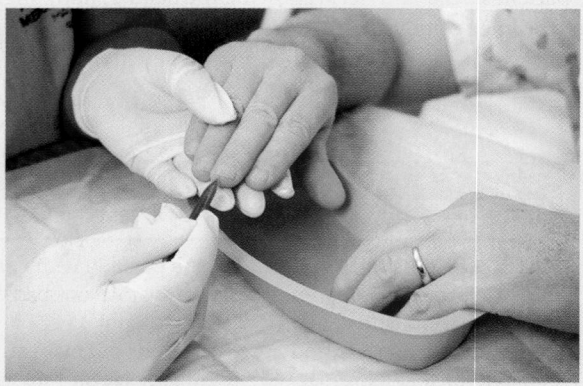

STEP 12 Clean under fingernails.

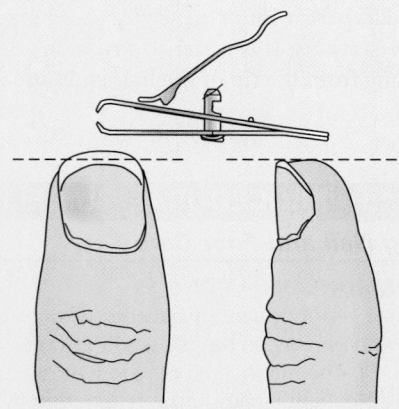

STEP 13 Trim nails straight across when using nail clipper.

BOX 31.12 SIGNS OF PERIPHERAL NEUROPATHY OR VASCULAR INSUFFICIENCY

PERIPHERAL NEUROPATHY	VASCULAR INSUFFICIENCY
• Muscle wasting of lower extremities	• Decreased hair growth on legs and feet
• Foot deformities	• Absent or decreased pulses
• Soft tissue infection of lower extremities	• Infection of the foot
• Abnormal gait	• Poor wound healing
• Decreased or absent vibratory, touch, temperature, or painful stimuli	• Thickened nails
	• Shiny appearance of the skin
	• Blanching of the skin on elevation

neck can cause further injury. You need a health care provider's order to shampoo the hair of patients with neck injuries. Another option is to wash the patient's hair in the bed (Box 31.13).

When patients are unable to move, sit in a chair, be transferred to a stretcher, or tolerate a wet hair-washing procedure, you can use various dry shampoo products. Read manufacturer guidelines carefully. In general, you massage these products into the patient's hair and scalp. Some products require you to apply a towel to remove excess oil and dirt, whereas others require you to brush the product through the patient's hair.

Shaving. Shave facial hair after a bath or shampoo. Some women prefer to shave their legs or axillae while bathing. Use caution when helping a patient shave to avoid cutting the patient with the razor blade. Patients prone to bleeding (e.g.,

BOX 31.13 PROCEDURAL GUIDELINES

Shampooing Hair of Bed-Bound Patient

View Video!

DELEGATION CONSIDERATIONS

The skill of shampooing the hair of bed-bound patients and the use of a disposable shampoo product can be delegated to nursing assistive personnel (NAP). The nurse instructs the NAP about:

- Proper way to position a patient with a head or neck mobility restriction.
- Knowledge of care for lice, stressing steps to take to prevent transmission to other patients.

EQUIPMENT

Bath towels, clean gloves, clean gown *(optional)* (if patient has known head lice), clean comb and brush
Regular shampoo: Washcloth, shampoo, hair conditioner *(optional)*, hydrogen peroxide *(optional)*, water pitcher with warm water, plastic shampoo board, wash basin, waterproof pad, saline *(optional)*
Disposable shampoo: Disposable shampoo cap product

STEPS

1. Identify patient using at least two identifiers (e.g., name and birthday or name and medical record number) according to agency policy.
2. Review medical record to determine that there are no contraindications to procedure. Check agency policy for health care provider order as needed. Certain medical conditions such as head and neck injuries and spinal cord injuries place patient at risk for injury because of positioning and manipulation of patient's head and neck.
3. Make sure that bed is in locked, low position (QSEN, 2014).
4. Perform hand hygiene and apply gloves. Inspect condition of hair and scalp. This determines if special shampoos or treatments are necessary (e.g., dandruff, lice, removal of blood). If draining head wounds are suspected, apply clean gloves. If lice are present, wear disposable gown and gloves. Remove gloves and perform hand hygiene.
5. Explain procedure to patient, using simple language.
6. Assemble equipment at bedside including pitcher with warm water.
7. Provide privacy by closing room door or curtain dividers. Raise bed to comfortable working height and lower side rail on side on which you will stand.

8. **Shampooing bed-bound patient with shampoo board:**
   a. Apply clean gloves. Place waterproof pad under patient's shoulders, neck, and head.
   b. Position patient supine with head and shoulders at top edge of bed. Place shampoo board under patient's head and washbasin under end of trough spout (see illustration). Be sure that trough spout extends beyond edge of mattress.
   c. Place rolled towel under patient's neck and bath towel over patient's shoulders.
   d. Brush and comb patient's hair.
   e. Ask patient to hold towel or washcloth over eyes.
   f. Test water temperature. Slowly pour water from pitcher over hair until it is completely wet (see illustration). If hair contains matted blood, apply hydrogen peroxide to dissolve clots and rinse with saline. Apply small amount of shampoo.
   g. Work up lather with both hands. Start at hairline and work toward back of neck. Lift head slightly with one hand to wash back of head. Shampoo sides of head. Massage scalp by applying pressure with fingertips.
   h. Rinse hair with water. Make sure that water drains into basin. Repeat rinsing until hair is free of soap. (If you need to refill pitcher, raise side rail when leaving bedside.)
   i. Apply conditioner or cream rinse if requested and rinse hair thoroughly.
   j. Wrap patient's head in bath towel. Dry face with cloth used to protect eyes. Dry off any moisture along neck or shoulders.
   k. Dry patient's hair and scalp. Use second towel if first one becomes saturated.
   l. Comb hair to remove tangles and dry with dryer if desired.
   m. Apply oil preparation or conditioning product to hair if desired by patient.
   n. Variation for patients with coarse, curly hair: Condition hair after washing. To untangle hair, use wide teeth of comb. Beginning at nape of neck, comb small subsections of hair, starting at hair ends. Continue to work through small sections until hair is free of tangles.

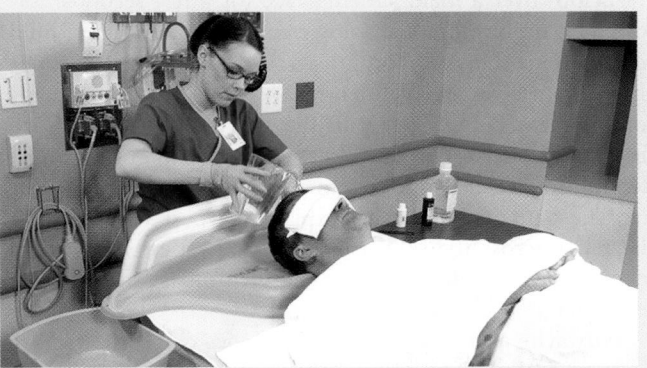

STEP 8b Patient positioned over shampoo board.

STEP 8f Nurse pouring water over patient's hair.

Continued

View Video!

BOX 31.13   PROCEDURAL GUIDELINES—cont'd

Shampooing Hair of Bed-Bound Patient

o. Help patient to comfortable position and complete styling of hair. Be sure nurse call system is in an accessible location within patient's reach.

p. Dispose of supplies. Store reusable supplies. Remove gloves and perform hand hygiene.

9. **Shampooing with disposable shampoo product:**

a. Patient can be sitting on chair or in bed. Apply clean gloves.

b. Comb hair to remove any tangles or debris.

c. Open package, apply cap, and secure all hair beneath cap (see illustration).

d. Massage head through cap. Check fitting around head to maintain correct fit.

e. Massage 2 to 4 minutes according to directions on package; additional time may be required for longer hair or hair matted with blood.

f. Discard cap in trash; do not dispose of in toilet because it may clog plumbing.

g. If patient desires, towel dry hair. Brush or comb patient's hair.

h. Remove gloves. Perform hand hygiene.

i. Help patient to comfortable position, and be sure nurse call system is in an accessible location within patient's reach.

10. Inspect condition of hair and scalp.

11. **Use Teach-Back:** "During the shampoo we discussed ways to reduce the risk of getting exposed to lice in your home. Tell me three ways to reduce the chance of exposing yourself and others to lice." Revise your instruction

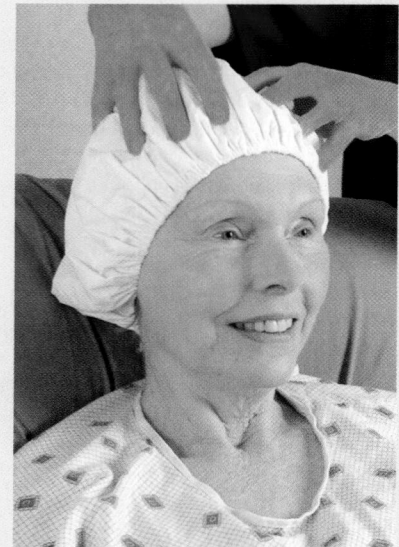

STEP 9c Patient wearing disposable shampoo cap.

now or develop a plan for revised patient/family caregiver teaching if patient/family caregiver is not able to teach back correctly.

12. Record relevant observations (objective and subjective), condition of scalp and skin, and patient comfort.

13. Document your evaluation of patient/family caregiver learning.

---

patients receiving anticoagulants or high doses of aspirin, patients with bleeding disorders such as thrombocytopenia and leukemia) must use an electric razor. Before you use an electric razor, check it for electrical hazards. Use an electric razor on only one patient to eliminate the risk of infection transmission.

When using a razor blade for shaving, you must soften the skin to prevent pulling, scraping, and cuts. Placing a warm washcloth over a male patient's face for a few seconds, followed by application of shaving cream or a lathering of mild soap, softens the skin. You must shave patients who cannot shave themselves independently. To avoid causing discomfort or razor cuts, gently pull the skin taut and use short, firm razor strokes in the direction the hair grows. Short downward strokes work best to remove hair over the upper lip. The patient usually can explain the best way to move the razor across the skin. Facial hair of African Americans tends to be curly and becomes ingrown unless shaved close to the skin.

Mustache and Beard Care. Mustaches or beards require daily grooming. Grooming keeps food particles and mucus from collecting in the hair. You must groom a patient's mustache and beard if the patient is unable to carry out self-care.

Comb out beards gently, and obtain a patient's permission before trimming or shaving off a mustache or beard.

Restorative and Continuing Care. Hygiene care may be scheduled less often in extended care facilities and nursing homes than in the acute care setting. Most patients in extended care facilities are older adults. Both the normal effects of aging and abnormal changes such as urinary and bowel incontinence and increased incidence of dementia create special challenges for nurses caring for patients in continuing and restorative care.

Bathing and Skin Care. Changes associated with aging include thinning, dryness, and roughness of the skin. These changes result in the need to adapt skin care for older adults (Box 31.14). The thinning of the skin and loss of elasticity associated with aging contribute to the increased frequency of skin tears, which often occur where an age-related purpura has already formed. Ayello and Fulmer (2012) recommend the following interventions to reduce the risk of skin tears: Use a standardized assessment tool to determine skin tear risk; use a no-rinse, one-step bath product instead of the traditional washcloth, soap, and water bathing method; implement measures to limit trauma, such as wearing long

BOX 31.14 CARE OF THE OLDER ADULT

Skin Changes With Aging

- Skin changes associated with aging include thinning, dryness, and roughness. Epithelial renewal may take 30% to 50% longer in older adults because keratinocytes become smaller and regeneration slows (Touhy and Jett, 2014).
- The dermis loses approximately 20% of its thickness with aging (Meiner, 2015).
- The American Academy of Dermatology (2016) recommendations for care of aging skin include:
  - Bathing daily using warm (not hot) water, limiting bath or shower time to 5 to 10 minutes.
  - Closing bathroom door to maximize humidity.
  - Using only mild cleansers; avoiding deodorant bars, perfumed soaps, and any products with alcohol.
  - Gently patting skin dry.
  - Applying moisturizer within 3 minutes of getting out of bath or shower; this maximizes trapping of moisture in skin.
  - Moisturizing more frequently throughout the day as needed.
  - Selecting correct type of moisturizer. Ointments and creams are better suited for dry skin than lotions.
  - Using moisturizers with hyaluronic acid, which helps skin hold water; dimethicone and glycerin can draw water to skin and keep it there. Mineral oil, lanolin, and petrolatum work well to trap moisture in skin.
  - Checking any antiaging products for presence of retinoids or an alpha hydroxy acid, which can irritate and dry skin.
  - Protecting hands by wearing gloves when out in cold, dry air; applying hand cream after each handwashing; and wearing waterproof gloves if hands are frequently in water.
  - Wearing sunscreen with a sun protection factor (SPF) of 30 or higher on all exposed skin daily, even in winter.
  - Using lip balm with an SPF of at least 30.
  - Seeing a dermatologist.

---

sleeves and pants, providing adequate light to reduce the chance of bumping into items, and making the environment safe for patients who wander; and educate all staff and family caregivers on the risk for skin tears and ways to prevent them.

Bathing often creates discomfort for patients with dementia. Confusion makes people feel vulnerable during bathing, resulting in screaming, crying, and even aggressively lashing out at caregivers. Research shows that using nontraditional bathing techniques and educating caregivers to provide person-centered care ease the conflict and reduce aggressive, negative behaviors associated with bathing activities (Hall et al., 2013). Use person-centered techniques such as covering the patient with towels as much as possible, avoiding rushing, using favorite soaps and no-rinse products, and padding the shower chair for comfort.

Oral Care. Implement measures to prevent denture stomatitis, also called *denture sore mouth*. Denture stomatitis is a disease of the mouth and gums caused by ill-fitting dentures and poor dental hygiene habits (Tay et al., 2014). Measures to prevent denture stomatitis include rinsing the dentures after meals, cleaning them carefully, soaking them overnight, brushing and flossing remaining teeth, and teaching patients and family caregivers how to prevent this complication.

Hearing Aid Care. Hearing aids amplify sound in a controlled manner; the hearing aid receives normal low-intensity sound inputs and delivers them to the patient's ear as louder outputs. Hearing aids come in a variety of types (see Chapter 39). Box 31.15 outlines care for a patient with a hearing aid including patient teaching.

Patient's Room Environment. A patient's room should be safe and large enough to allow patients and their visitors to move about freely. Control room temperature, ventilation, noise, and odors.

BOX 31.15 CARE AND USE OF HEARING AIDS

Follow these guidelines when caring for a patient's hearing aids and when teaching patients about care of hearing aids:
- Perform hand hygiene before handling the hearing aid.
- Check battery by holding hearing aid in your hand and turning up volume. If battery is working, you hear a "whistle." This is feedback noise.
- After inserting or applying the hearing aid, slowly turn up volume to one-third to one-half volume to obtain a comfortable hearing level for talking at 1 yard.
- A whistling sound while patient is wearing hearing aid indicates incorrect earmold insertion, improper fit of hearing aid, or buildup of earwax or fluid.
- Do not wear hearing aid under heat lamp or hair dryer or in very wet, cold weather.
- Do not store hearing aid in warm place such as a windowsill or in a car. Heat can change the shape of the earmold, causing hearing aid to not fit properly.
- Remove battery from hearing aid when aid is not being used for a day or longer.
- Avoid dropping hearing aid or twisting cord.
- Remove hearing aid before radiological examination or radiation therapy to avoid damage.
- Protect hearing aid from water, alcohol, aerosol sprays, perspiration, and cologne.
- Use manufacturer-recommended cleaning solution and soft, lint-free cotton cloth to clean earmold. Regularly remove earwax from hearing aid with a wax loop or device supplied with aid.

Data from National Institute on Deafness and Other Communication Disorders (NIDCD): *Hearing aids*, 2016, https://www.nidcd.nih.gov/health/hearing-aids.

Maintaining Comfort. Depending on a patient's age and physical condition, maintain the room temperature between 20° C and 23° C (68° F and 73.4° F). Infants, older adults, and acutely ill patients often need a warmer room. However, patients with certain illnesses benefit from cooler room temperatures to help reduce the body's metabolic demands. Protect acutely ill patients, infants, and older adults from drafts by ensuring that they are adequately dressed and covered with a lightweight blanket.

An effective ventilation system prevents stale air and odors from lingering in the room. Good ventilation reduces lingering odors caused by draining wounds, emesis, bowel movements, and used bedpans and urinals. Always empty and cleanse bedpans and urinals promptly. Room deodorizers help remove many unpleasant odors; however, be sure that your patient is not allergic or sensitive to the deodorizer itself.

Make every effort to limit the noise level, especially when patients are trying to sleep. Explain the source of unfamiliar noises such as an IV pump or a pulse oximeter alarm.

Proper lighting helps ensure safety and comfort. A brightly lit room usually stimulates the patient, whereas a darkened room promotes rest and sleep. Adjust room lighting by closing or opening drapes, regulating over-bed and floor lights, and closing or opening room doors. When entering a patient's room at night, avoid abruptly turning on the overhead light unless necessary.

Room Equipment.
Although rooms can vary across health care settings, the typical room contains a bed, over-bed table, bedside stand, and chairs (Fig. 31.1). An over-bed table rolls on wheels and adjusts to various heights over the bed or a chair. The over-bed table is an ideal working space for performing procedures. It also serves as a surface for meal trays, toiletry items, and objects that a patient often uses. Clean the top of the over-bed table with an antiseptic cleaner before using it for meals. Do not place a bedpan or urinal on the table. Use the bedside stand to store a patient's personal possessions and hygiene equipment. Patients often use bedside stands for their telephone, water pitcher, and drinking cup.

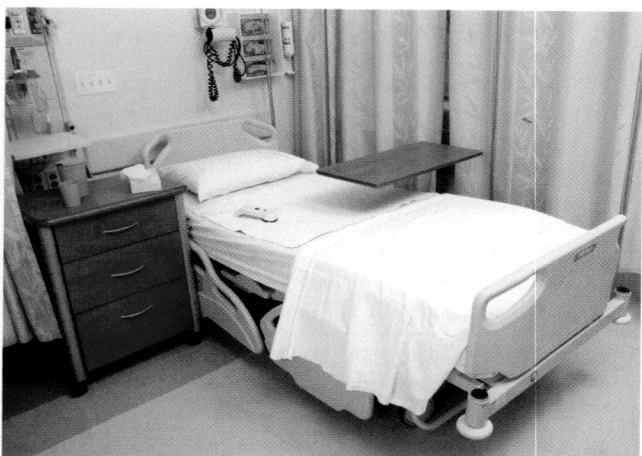

FIG 31.1 Room furniture.

Most patient rooms contain a straight-backed chair or an upholstered lounge chair with arms. Armless straight-backed chairs are convenient when temporarily transferring a patient from the bed such as during bed making. Upholstered lounge chairs or recliners tend to be more comfortable for patients who can sit for longer times.

Each room usually has an over-bed light and floor-level night lighting. Patients often have access to lighting controls via their nurse call system. Additional portable or built-in examination lighting provides extra light during bedside procedures.

Other equipment usually found in a patient's room includes a nurse call system, a television set, a wall-mounted blood pressure gauge, oxygen and vacuum wall outlets, and personal care items. Special equipment designed for promoting comfort or positioning patients includes footboards and foot boots, special mattresses, and bed boards.

Beds.
Patients who are seriously ill may remain in bed for a long time. The typical hospital bed has a firm mattress on a metal frame that you can raise and lower horizontally and that can be placed in various positions. You vary the bed positions to promote patient comfort, minimize symptoms, promote lung expansion, and improve access during procedures (Table 31.7). You change the position of an electric bed by using electrical controls usually incorporated into the nurse call system or in a panel on the side or foot of the bed. Become familiar with use of the bed controls. Instruct patients in the proper use of controls and caution them against raising the bed to a position that causes harm. Maintain the bed height at the lowest horizontal position when a patient is unattended.

Patients who are at risk for falling often are placed on low beds in the hospital (see Chapter 30). Special beds and mattress options (e.g., low-pressure mattresses, rotation beds) may be used with patients who are at risk for pressure injuries (see Chapter 38).

All beds contain safety features such as locks on the wheels or casters. Lock the wheels when a bed is stationary to prevent accidental movement. Side rails help patients to move more efficiently in bed and prevent accidents. Do not use side rails to restrict a patient from moving in bed. Using side rails as a restraint requires a health care provider's order (see Chapter 30). You can remove the headboard from most beds. This is important when the medical team needs easy access to the head such as during cardiopulmonary resuscitation.

Bed Making.
Keep a patient's bed clean and comfortable by regularly checking linen to ensure it is clean, dry, and free of wrinkles. When patients are diaphoretic, have draining wounds, or experience incontinence, check frequently for wet or soiled linen.

You usually make the bed in the morning after the patient's bath or while the patient is bathing, in a shower, sitting in a chair eating, or out of the room for procedures or tests. Throughout the day, straighten linen that becomes loose or wrinkled. In addition, check the bed linen for food particles after meals and for wetness or soiling. Change linen that becomes soiled or wet.

When changing bed linen, follow basic principles of medical asepsis by keeping soiled linen away from your uniform. Place soiled linen in linen bags before placing in the linen hamper. To avoid air currents that spread microorganisms, never shake linen. To avoid transmitting infection, do not place soiled linen or linen bags on the floor. Immediately place any clean linen that touches the floor or any unclean surface into a dirty linen container.

During bed making, use safe patient–handling procedures and proper body mechanics (see Chapter 25). Always raise the bed to the appropriate height before changing linen so that you do not have to bend or stretch over the mattress.

A patient's privacy, comfort, and safety are important when you make a bed. If the patient is confined to bed, organize bed-making activities to conserve time and energy. Use side rails, keep the nurse call system within a patient's reach, and maintain the proper bed position. After making a bed, return the bed to its lowest horizontal position and verify that the wheels are locked to prevent falls.

When you make an unoccupied bed, follow the same basic principles used for making an occupied bed (Box 31.16). When possible, make the bed while it is unoccupied (Box 31.17). The surgical, recovery, or postoperative bed is a modified version of the unoccupied bed. Fold the top

TABLE 31.7 COMMON BED POSITIONS

POSITION		DESCRIPTION	USES
Fowler's		Head of bed raised to angle of 45 degrees or more; semisitting position; foot of bed may also be raised at knee	Used during meals and oral medication administration, nasogastric tube insertion, and nasotracheal suction. Promotes lung expansion.
Semi-Fowler's		Head of bed raised approximately 30 degrees; incline less than Fowler's position; foot of bed may also be raised at knee	Promotes lung expansion. Used when patients receive gastric feedings to reduce regurgitation and risk for aspiration.
Trendelenburg's		Entire bed tilted with head of bed down	Used for postural drainage. Facilitates venous return in patients with poor peripheral venous perfusion.

Continued

TABLE 31.7   COMMON BED POSITIONS—cont'd

POSITION	DESCRIPTION	USES
Reverse Trendelenburg's 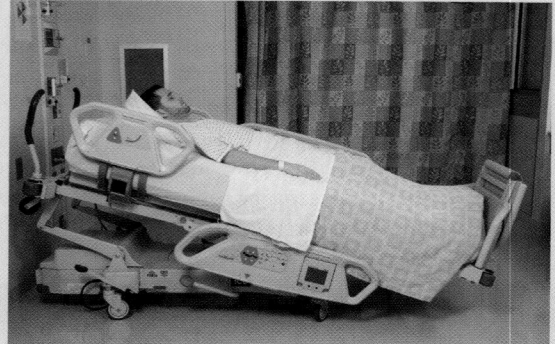	Entire bedframe tilted with foot of bed down	Used infrequently. Promotes gastric emptying. Prevents esophageal reflux.
Flat 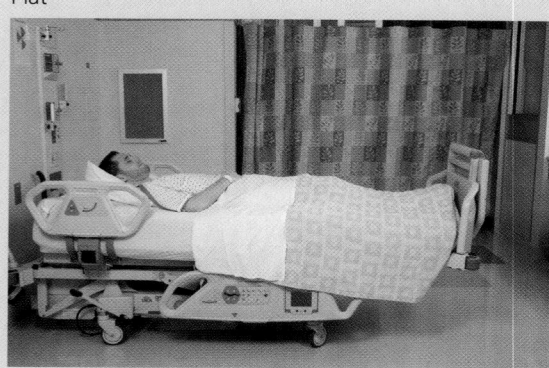	Entire bedframe horizontally parallel with floor	Used for patients with vertebral injuries and in cervical traction. Used for patients who are hypotensive. Generally preferred by patients for sleeping.

BOX 31.16   PROCEDURAL GUIDELINES

Making an Occupied Bed

DELEGATION CONSIDERATIONS

The skill of making an occupied bed can be delegated to nursing assistive personnel (NAP). The nurse reviews any precautions or activity restrictions. The nurse instructs the NAP about:

- Any activity or positioning restrictions for the patient including need to use equipment for lifting and positioning patient.
- Looking for wound drainage, dressing materials, drainage tubes, or IV tubing that becomes dislodged or is found in linens.
- Obtaining help from other caregivers for positioning a patient during linen change and the importance of using proper body mechanics and supporting patient alignment.
- Using special precautions (e.g., aspiration precautions or positioning for tube feeding infusion; see Chapter 35).

EQUIPMENT

Linen bags, mattress pad (*optional* depending on agency practice; needs to be changed only when soiled), bottom sheet (flat or fitted), drawsheet (*optional*), top sheet, blanket (*optional* depending on patient preference), bedspread, waterproof pads and/or bath blankets (*optional*), pillowcases, bedside chair or table, clean gloves (*optional*), paper towels or washcloth, disinfectant (Fig. 31.2).

STEPS

1. Review medical record and assess restrictions concerning patient mobility and/or positioning.
2. Perform hand hygiene and gather needed supplies, being sure not to let clean linen touch your uniform. Arrange equipment on bedside chair or over-bed table. Remove unnecessary equipment such as a dietary tray or items used for hygiene. Pull curtain and close door.
3. Make sure equipment is working properly and that bed is in locked position and appropriate number of side rails are raised).
4. Explain procedure to patient including that he or she will be asked to turn on side and roll over linen.
5. Perform hand hygiene. Apply clean gloves if patient was incontinent or if drainage is present on linen.
6. Adjust bed height to comfortable working position with bed flat if patient can tolerate. Lower raised side rail on side where you will be standing. Loosen all top linen. Remove bedspread and blanket separately, leaving patient covered with top sheet. Place soiled bedspread and/or blanket in linen bag and discard. If bedspread to be reused, fold and place and/or blanket over back of chair.

BOX 31.16 PROCEDURAL GUIDELINES—cont'd

Making an Occupied Bed

7. Cover patient with bath blanket in the following manner: unfold bath blanket over top sheet. Ask patient to hold top edge of bath blanket. If patient cannot help, tuck top of bath blanket under shoulders. Grasp top sheet under bath blanket at patient's shoulders and bring sheet down to foot of bed. Remove sheet and discard in linen bag.

8. Position patient on far side of bed, turned onto side and facing away from you. **Note:** This is when another caregiver can help by standing at bedside across from you. Be sure that side rail in front of patient is up. Encourage patient to use side rail to turn. Adjust pillow under patient's head.

9. Loosen bottom linens, moving from head to foot. With seam side down (facing the mattress), fanfold soiled drawsheet and bottom sheet toward patient. Tuck edges of linen just under buttocks, back, and shoulders. Do not fanfold mattress pad if it is to be reused (see illustration).

10. Wipe off any moisture on exposed mattress with paper towel. Clean and disinfect and dry mattress surface (check agency policy).

11. Apply clean linen to exposed half of bed:
    a. Place clean mattress pad (if used) on bed by folding it lengthwise with center crease in middle of bed. Fanfold top layer over mattress. (If pad is reused, simply smooth out any wrinkles.)
    b. If using flat sheet for bottom sheet, unfold sheet lengthwise so that center crease is situated lengthwise

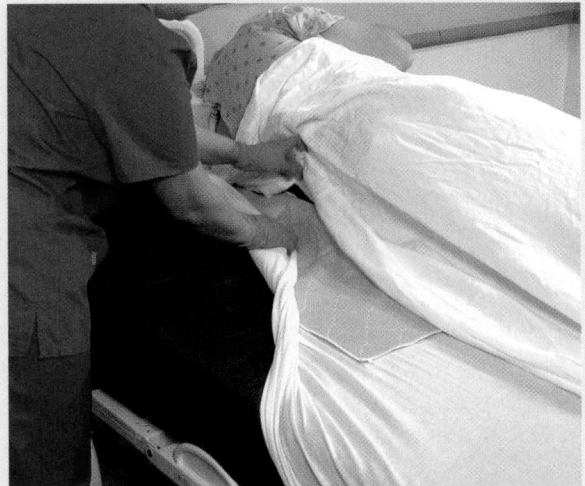

STEP 9 Tuck all soiled linen from one side of bed alongside patient's back.

along center of bed. Fanfold top layer of sheet toward center of bed alongside patient. Smooth bottom layer of sheet over mattress and bring edge over closest side of mattress. If using fitted sheet, pull sheet smoothly over mattress ends.
    c. Allow edge of flat unfitted sheet to hang about 25 cm (10 inches) over mattress edge. Make sure that lower hem of bottom flat sheet lies seam down and even with bottom edge of mattress.

12. If flat sheet is used for bottom sheet, miter bottom flat sheet at head of bed:
    a. Face head of bed diagonally. Place hand away from head of bed under top corner of mattress, near mattress edge, and lift.
    b. With other hand, tuck top edge of bottom sheet smoothly under mattress so that side edges of sheet above and below mattress meet when brought together.
    c. Face side of bed and pick up top edge of sheet at approximately 45 cm (18 inches) from top of mattress (see illustration).
    d. Lift sheet and lay it on top of mattress to form a neat triangular fold, with lower base of triangle even with mattress side edge (see illustration).
    e. Tuck lower edge of sheet, which is hanging free below the mattress, under mattress. Tuck with palms down without pulling triangular fold (see illustration).
    f. Hold part of sheet covering side of mattress in place with one hand. With the other hand, pick up top of triangular linen fold and bring it down over side of mattress. Tuck this part under mattress (see illustrations).
    g. Tuck remaining part of sheet under mattress, moving toward foot of bed. Keep linen smooth.

13. *Optional:* Open clean drawsheet so that it unfolds in half. Lay centerfold along middle of bed lengthwise and position sheet so that it is under patient's buttocks and torso. Fanfold top layer of drawsheet toward patient with edge along patient's back. Smooth bottom layer out over mattress and tuck excess edge under mattress (keep palms down).

14. Place single waterproof pad over drawsheet *(optional)* with centerfold against patient's side. Fanfold top layer toward patient.

15. Advise patient that rolling over thick layer of linens is necessary and that he or she will feel a lump. Have patient roll slowly toward you over the layers of linen, rolling like a log (see illustration). Have patient lie still and raise side rail on working side before going to other side of bed.

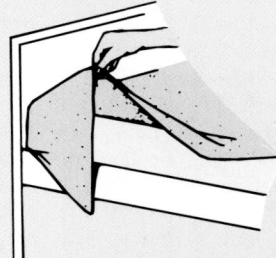

STEP 12c Top edge of sheet picked up.

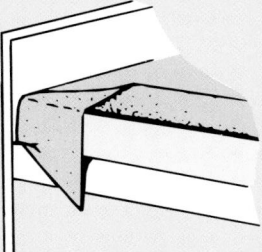

STEP 12d Sheet on top of mattress in a triangular fold.

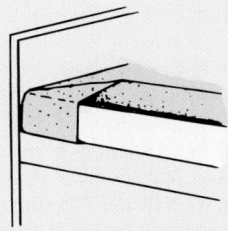

STEP 12e Lower edge of sheet tucked under mattress.

Continued

BOX 31.16 **PROCEDURAL GUIDELINES—cont'd**

Making an Occupied Bed

16. Lower side rail. Help patient to comfortable position on other side as needed. Loosen edges of soiled linen from under mattress.

17. Remove all soiled linen by folding it into a bundle or square with soiled side turned in. Discard in linen bag. If necessary, wipe mattress with antiseptic solution and dry mattress surface before unfolding and applying clean linen.

18. Pull clean, fanfolded linen smoothly over edge of mattress from head to foot of bed. Help patient roll back into supine position (if preferred). Reposition pillow.

19. If using a fitted sheet, pull it smoothly over mattress ends. If using a flat sheet, miter top corner of bottom sheet (see Steps 12a–g). When tucking corner, be sure that sheet is smooth and free of wrinkles.

20. Facing side of bed, grasp remaining edge of bottom flat sheet. Lean back, keep back straight, and pull while tucking excess linen under mattress. Proceed from head to foot of bed. (Avoid lifting mattress during tucking to ensure fit.)

21. Smooth fanfolded drawsheet out over bottom sheet. Grasp edge of sheet with palms down, lean back, and tuck sheet under mattress. Tuck from middle to top and then to bottom.

22. Place top sheet over patient with centerfold lengthwise down middle of bed. Open sheet from head to foot and unfold over patient. Ask patient to hold clean top sheet or tuck sheet around his or her shoulders. Remove bath blanket and discard in linen bag.

23. Place blanket on bed, unfolding it so that crease runs lengthwise along middle of bed. Unfold blanket to cover patient. Make sure that top edge is parallel with edge of top sheet and 15 to 20 cm (6 to 8 inches) from edge of top sheet.

24. Place spread over bed according to Step 22. Be sure that top edge of spread extends about 2.5 cm (1 inch) above edge of blanket. Tuck top edge of spread over and under top edge of blanket.

25. Make cuff by turning edge of top sheet down over top edge of blanket and spread.

26. Standing on one side at foot of bed, lift mattress corner slightly with one hand and tuck sheet and blanket together under mattress. Be sure that lines are loose enough to allow movement of patient's feet. Making a horizontal toe pleat is an option.

27. Make modified mitered corner with top sheet, blanket, and spread (follow Step 12a–e). After making the triangular fold, do not tuck tip of the triangle under the mattress (see illustration).

28. Raise side rail. Make other side of bed. Spread out sheet, blanket, and bedspread evenly. Fold top edge of spread over blanket and make cuff with top sheet (see Step 25); make modified mitered corner (see Step 27).

29. Change pillowcase:
    a. Have patient raise head. While supporting neck with one hand, remove pillow. Allow patient to lower head.
    b. Remove soiled case by grasping pillow open end with one hand and pulling case back over pillow with other hand. Discard case in linen bag.
    c. Grasp clean pillowcase at center of closed end. Gather case, turning it inside out over the hand holding it. With same hand pick up middle of one end of pillow. Pull pillowcase down over pillow with other hand.
    d. Be sure that pillow corners fit evenly into corners of pillowcase. Place pillow under patient's head.

30. Place nurse call system in an accessible location within patient's reach. Return bed to comfortable position and height. Open room curtains and rearrange furniture. Place personal items within easy reach on over-bed table or bedside stand.

31. Place dirty linen in hamper or chute. Remove gloves (if worn); dispose and perform hand hygiene.

32. Ask if patient feels comfortable.

33. Use this time to inspect skin for areas of irritation.

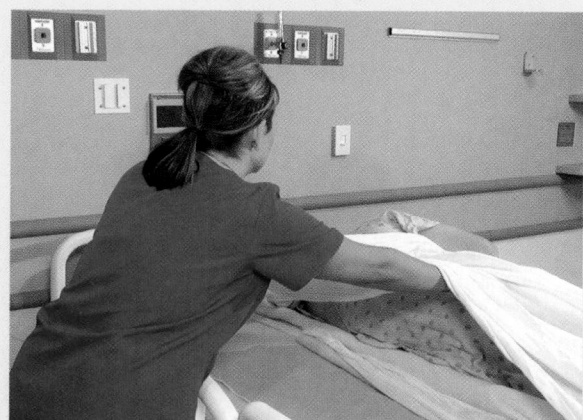

STEP 15 Patient begins rolling over layers of linen.

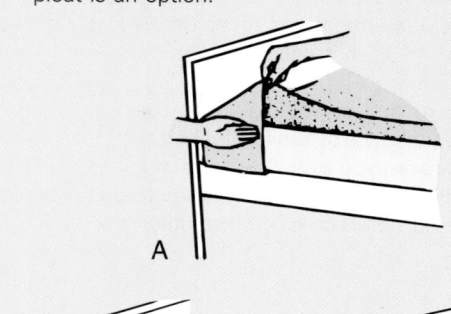

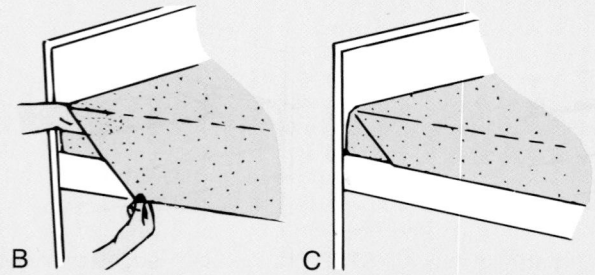

STEP 12f Triangular fold placed over side of mattress, sheet tucked under mattress.

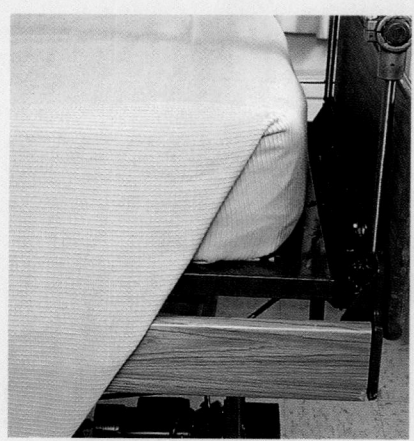

STEP 27 Modified mitered corner.

BOX 31.17 PROCEDURAL GUIDELINES

Making an Unoccupied Bed

DELEGATION CONSIDERATIONS

The skill of making an unoccupied bed can be delegated to nursing assistive personnel (NAP). The nurse instructs the NAP about:

- Position or activity restrictions that apply to patient's ability to get out of and back into bed.
- Any special linens to use if patient is on an airflow or other pressure reduction mattresses.

EQUIPMENT

Linen bag, mattress pad (change only when soiled), bottom sheet (flat or fitted), drawsheet *(optional)*, top sheet, blanket, bedspread, waterproof pads *(optional)*, special linens for support surface mattress *(optional)*, pillowcases, bedside chair or table, clean gloves (if linen is soiled), washcloth or paper towel, antiseptic cleanser

STEPS

1. Perform hand hygiene and arrange supplies at bedside.
2. Assess environment for safety (e.g., check room for spills, make sure equipment is working properly and that bed is in locked position).
3. Assess activity orders or restrictions in mobility to determine whether patient can get out of bed for procedure. Help patient to bedside chair or recliner.
4. If patient has been incontinent or if excess drainage is on linen, gloves are necessary.
5. Lower side rails on both sides of bed and raise bed to comfortable working position.
6. Remove soiled linen and place in laundry bag. Avoid shaking or fanning linen.
7. Reposition mattress and wipe off any moisture with a washcloth or paper towel moistened in antiseptic solution. Dry thoroughly.
8. Apply all bottom linens on one side of bed (before moving to opposite side):
   a. Be sure that fitted sheet is placed smoothly over mattress.
   b. To apply a flat unfitted sheet, allow about 25 cm (10 inches) to hang over sides of mattress edges. Make sure that lower hem of sheet lies seam down, even with bottom edge of mattress. Pull remaining top part of sheet over top edge of mattress.
9. While standing at head of bed, miter top corner of bottom sheet (see Box 31.16, Steps 12a–g).
10. Tuck remaining part of unfitted sheet under mattress from head to foot of bed.
11. *Optional:* Apply drawsheet, laying centerfold along middle of bed lengthwise. Smooth drawsheet over mattress and tuck excess edge under mattress, keeping palms down.
12. Move to opposite side of bed and spread bottom sheet smoothly over edge of mattress from head to foot of bed.
13. Apply fitted sheet smoothly over each mattress corner. For an unfitted sheet, miter top corner of bottom sheet (see Step 9), making sure that corner is taut.
14. Grasp remaining edge of unfitted bottom sheet and tuck tightly under mattress while moving from head to foot of bed.
15. Smooth folded drawsheet over bottom sheet and tuck under mattress, first at middle, then at top, and then at bottom.
16. If needed, apply single waterproof pad over bottom sheet or drawsheet.
17. Place top sheet over bed with vertical centerfold lengthwise down middle of bed. Open sheet out from head to foot, being sure that top edge of sheet is even with top edge of mattress.
18. Make horizontal toe pleat: stand at foot of bed and make fanfold in sheet 5 to 10 cm (2 to 4 inches) across bed. Pull sheet up from bottom to make fold approximately 15 cm (6 inches) from bottom edge of mattress.
19. Tuck in remaining part of sheet under foot of mattress. Place blanket over bed with top edge parallel to top edge of sheet and 15 to 20 cm (6 to 8 inches) down from edge of sheet. (*Optional:* Apply additional spread over bed.)
20. Make cuff by turning edge of top sheet down over top edge of blanket and spread.
21. Standing on one side at foot of bed, lift mattress corner slightly with one hand; with other hand tuck top sheet, blanket, and spread under mattress. Be sure that toe pleats have not been pulled out.
22. Make modified mitered corner with top sheet, blanket, and spread. Standing on one side at foot of bed, lift mattress corner slightly with one hand and tuck sheet and blanket together under mattress. Be sure that lines are loose enough to allow movement of patient's feet. Making a horizontal toe pleat is an option (see Box 31.16, Step 26).
23. Go to other side of bed. Spread out sheet and blanket evenly. Make cuff with top sheet and blanket. Make modified corner at foot of bed.
24. Apply clean pillowcase (see Box 31.16, Step 29).
25. Be sure nurse call system is in an accessible location within patient's reach on bedrail or pillow, and return bed to height allowing for patient transfer. Help patient to bed.
26. Arrange patient's room. Remove and discard supplies. Perform hand hygiene.

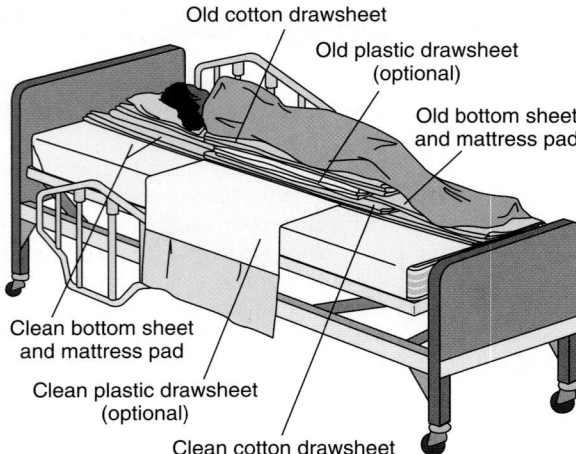

Old cotton drawsheet

Old plastic drawsheet (optional)

Old bottom sheet and mattress pad

Clean bottom sheet and mattress pad

Clean plastic drawsheet (optional)

Clean cotton drawsheet

FIG 31.2 Equipment for making an occupied bed.

BOX 31.18 EVALUATION

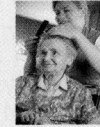

Copyright © AlexRaths/ iStock/ Thinkstock.

Jamie includes Mrs. Winkler in the plan to increase her self-care ability and feel more satisfied with her situation. She collaborates with occupational therapy and social services to obtain the assistive devices that Mrs. Winkler selects. After using the devices, Mrs. Winkler verbally expresses satisfaction with both her involvement in hygiene care planning and with the caregivers' consideration of her preferences and needs. She states that she is much happier with her care using the assistive devices except for the shower lever handles. Jamie observes Mrs. Winkler performing care with the assistive devices, noting that she can use the devices easily and safely except for the shower levers. Jamie alters the plan to include seeking a way to make the levers larger to allow Mrs. Winkler to move them without needing to grasp them with her arthritic hands.

DOCUMENTATION NOTE
Observed using assistive devices (bath mitt, padded shower chair, handheld shower spray, and shower levers); able to manipulate all devices without assistance except for shower levers. She states, "The levers are better than the old knobs, but I still have some trouble grasping them in my hands. I feel so much happier since I can do more of my shower now." Referral for occupational therapy for ideas to improve lever grasp.

covers of the surgical bed to one side or fanfold them to the bottom third of the bed so that you can easily transfer the patient into the bed after a procedure. When a patient is discharged, send all bed linen to the laundry. Housekeeping personnel usually clean and disinfect the mattress and bed and apply new bed linen after discharge. Many agencies have "nurse servers" either within or just outside the patient's room where a daily supply of linen is stored. To help control costs and prevent infection transmission, avoid bringing excess linen into the patient's room. Once you bring linen into a patient's room, even if the linen has not been used, it must be laundered before being used by another patient.

■■■ EVALUATION

Patient Outcomes. Evaluation of hygiene measures occurs while giving care and on completion of hygiene activities (Box 31.18). For example, while bathing a patient, inspect the skin carefully to determine whether soiling or drainage is effectively removed. Observe for any skin blistering or irritation. Evaluate the effectiveness of hygiene care by asking patients whether they feel more comfortable and relaxed. Observe a patient's behavior during and after hygiene care to detect discomfort that might be caused by movement and activities associated with hygiene care. Is the patient restless or relaxed? Does the patient's facial expression suggest a feeling of comfort? Is there any body odor?

Conduct ongoing evaluation because hygiene care often takes time to improve a patient's condition. For example, oral lesions and skin excoriation usually need repeated hygiene interventions. Use ongoing evaluative measures to determine whether the patient's condition and level of comfort improve over time. Throughout evaluation, consider the goals of care and evaluate whether expected outcomes have been achieved. Use the established expected outcomes as the standards for evaluation.

Patient Expectations. During assessment, you collect data about a patient's expectations for care. During and after care, learn from the patient whether care is provided in an acceptable manner. Determine the patient's satisfaction with your care by asking questions such as the following: "Do you think your bath helped you feel more comfortable?" "Are there ways that we can do a better job with your hygiene care?" Knowing and addressing a patient's expectations and any concerns fosters a caring therapeutic relationship.

SAFETY GUIDELINES FOR NURSING SKILLS

SAFETY CONSIDERATIONS

To ensure patient safety, communicate clearly with members of the health care team, assess and incorporate a patient's priorities of care and preferences, and use the best evidence when making decisions about your patient's care. When performing the skills in this chapter, remember the following points to ensure safe, individualized patient care:

- Patients who are totally dependent on a caregiver require help with personal hygiene measures. Always perform hygiene measures while moving from cleanest to less clean or dirty areas. This often requires you to change gloves and perform hand hygiene during care activities.
- Use clean gloves when you anticipate contact with nonintact skin or mucous membranes or when there is or may

likely be contact with drainage, secretions, excretions, or blood during hygiene care.

- When using water or solutions for hygiene care, be sure to test the temperature to prevent burn injury.
- Use principles of body mechanics and safe patient handling to avoid injury to patient or self when performing hygiene care (Quality and Safety Education for Nurses [QSEN], 2014).
- You are responsible and accountable for the care provided. Give proper direction to NAP when delegating hygiene measures.

SKILL 31.1 BATHING AND PERINEAL CARE

View Video!

DELEGATION CONSIDERATIONS

The skill of bathing and perineal care can be delegated to nursing assistive personnel (NAP). The nurse directs the NAP about:

- Not massaging reddened skin areas.
- Reporting early signs of impaired skin integrity including redness or pallor.
- Reporting perineal drainage, discomfort, or tenderness.
- Proper ways to position male and female patients with musculoskeletal limitations and indwelling catheters.
- Reporting patient fatigue or patient's report of pain during hygiene care.

EQUIPMENT

- Bar soap and soap dish or chlorhexidine 4% liquid soap (e.g., Hibiclens)

- *Option:* chlorhexidine gluconate (CHG) cloths or disposable bag bath cloths.
- 4 to 6 washcloths
- Bath towels
- Bath blanket
- Toiletry items (deodorant, powder)
- Body lotion (**Note:** if using CHG soap, use a lotion that is hospital approved such as Aloe Vesta)
- Toilet tissue or hygiene wipes
- Warm water
- Clean hospital gown or patient's own pajamas or gown
- Laundry bag
- Clean gloves (when risk for contacting body fluids)
- Wash basin (used for bath water only)

STEP	RATIONALE
ASSESSMENT	
1. Identify patient using at least two identifiers (e.g., name and birthday or name and medical record number) according to agency policy.	Ensures correct patient. Complies with The Joint Commission standards and improves patient safety (TJC, 2018).
2. Review medical record for orders for specific precautions concerning patient's movement or positioning and whether there is an order for a therapeutic bath. Note and confirm with patient any allergies or sensitivities to bath products.	Prevents accidental injury to patient during bathing activities. Determines level of assistance required by patient. Prevents allergic reactions to hygiene products during bathing.
3. Check for health care provider's therapeutic bath order; if there is an order, note type of solution, length of time for bath, and body part to be attended.	Therapeutic baths are ordered for specific physical effect, which usually includes promotion of healing or soothing effects.
4. Perform hand hygiene. Assess room environment for safety (e.g., check room for spills, make sure that equipment is working properly and that bed is in locked, low position).	Reduces transmission of microorganisms. Identifies safety hazards in patient environment that could cause or potentially lead to harm (QSEN, 2014).
5. Assess patient's fall risk status (if partial bathing out of bed or self-bath is to be performed).	Allows you to anticipate needed precautions such as having patient sit on chair in front of a basin.

SKILL 31.1   BATHING AND PERINEAL CARE—cont'd

View Video!

STEP	RATIONALE
6. Assess patient's tolerance for bathing: activity tolerance, comfort level during movement, cognitive ability, musculoskeletal function, and presence of shortness of breath.	Determines patient's ability to perform or tolerate bathing and level of assistance required (e.g., tub bath, partial bed bath).
7. Assess patient's cognitive (Mini-Mental State Examination) and functional status (e.g., Barthel Index of Activities of Daily Living [Hall et al., 2013] to measure self-care ability). For patients with suspected dementia, observe behavior especially after telling patient it is bath time; does patient become agitated?	Every person entering a long-term care setting needs to be formally assessed for cognitive and functional status (Hall et al., 2013). Functional status assesses a patient's capacity for self-bathing and the amount of supervision/assistance and/or needed to accomplish ADL tasks. Every attempt should be made to avoid bathing people against their will (Hall et al., 2013).

Clinical Decision Point. Patients with dementia may become agitated and aggressive during bathing. Consider using alternative bathing procedures such as bag wipes. Maintain a calm, nonthreatening, quiet environment using therapeutic communication.

STEP	RATIONALE
8. Assess patient's visual status, ability to sit without support, hand grasp, ROM of extremities.	Determines degree of assistance patient needs for bathing. ROM may be delegated to assistive personnel.
9. Assess for presence of equipment (e.g., IV line, oxygen tubing, indwelling urinary catheter).	Affects how you plan bathing activities and positioning. Helps determine how to set up supplies.
10. Assess for allergy or sensitivity to CHG.	If allergy exists, select another cleansing solution.
11. Assess patient's comfort on a 0- to 10-pain scale.	Bathing can soothe and comfort patient. Provides baseline measure.
12. Assess patient's bathing preferences: frequency and time of day preferred, type of hygiene products used, and other factors related to patient preferences.	Patient participates in plan of care. Promotes patient's comfort and willingness to cooperate. Includes cultural or personal hygiene preferences into care.
13. Ask if patient has noticed any problems related to condition of skin and genitalia: excess moisture, inflammation, drainage or excretions from lesions or body cavities, rashes or other skin lesions.	Provides you with information to direct physical assessment of skin and genitalia during bathing and influences selection of skin care products.
14. Before or during bath, assess condition of patient's skin. Note presence of dryness, indicated by flaking, redness, scaling, and cracking.	Provides a baseline for comparison over time in determining if bathing improves condition of skin.
15. Identify risks for skin impairment: older age, immobilization, reduced sensation, nutrition and hydration, excess skin moisture or drainage, shear or friction on skin, vascular insufficiencies, presence of external devices. *Option:* Use a pressure injury assessment tool (e.g., Braden Scale).	Prompt identification of risk factors reduces the likelihood of injury to the skin resulting from pressure, impaired tissue synthesis, softening of or friction on tissues, and impaired circulation (AHRQ, 2014).
16. Assess patient's knowledge of and perceptions of importance of skin hygiene, preventive measures to take, and common skin problems encountered (see Table 31.3).	Determines patient's willingness to learn and type of instruction required.
17. Assess patient's or family caregiver's knowledge of skin hygiene in terms of its importance, preventive measures to take, and common problems.	Determines patient's learning needs.

PLANNING

STEP	RATIONALE
1. Provide privacy and prepare bedside environment for patient safety.	Helps the student/nurse think about the steps needed need to remove clutter from over-bed or bedside table, removing barriers.
2. Prepare and organize equipment and supplies. If it is necessary to leave room, be sure nurse call system is in an accessible location within patient's reach.	Avoids interrupting procedure or leaving patient unattended to retrieve missing equipment.
3. Explain procedure and ask patient for suggestions on how to prepare supplies. If partial bath, ask how much of bath patient wishes to complete. If using CHG, explain benefit of reducing infection and that solution leaves a sticky feeling.	Promotes patient's cooperation and participation. Patients who prefer using their own bathing supplies may need to discuss benefits of CHG.

STEP	RATIONALE

IMPLEMENTATION

1. Perform hand hygiene and apply clean gloves. Offer patient bedpan or urinal. Provide toilet tissue and dispose of any excrement properly. Provide patient towel and moist washcloth.

   Patient will feel more comfortable after voiding. Prevents interruption of bath.

   a. Remove bedpan or urinal, dispose of contents, remove gloves and perform hand hygiene.

2. If patient has nonintact skin or skin is soiled with drainage, excretions, or body secretions, apply new pair of clean gloves before beginning bath.

   Reduces transmission of microorganisms.

3. Raise bed to comfortable working height. Verify that bed is in locked position.

   Reduces strain on back.
   Prevents bed from moving.

4. Lower side rail closest to you. Bring patient toward you and help patient assume a comfortable supine position, maintaining body alignment.

   Maintains patient's comfort throughout the bath. Safe patient handling minimizes strain on care provider's muscles. If patient is overweight or unable to assist with positioning, use another caregiver or lift device (see Chapter 29).

5. Complete or partial bed bath:

   a. Verify that patient is not allergic to latex.

      Prevents allergic reaction if latex gloves are used.

   b. Place bath blanket over patient and loosen and remove top covers without exposing patient. If possible, have patient hold top of bath blanket while you remove linen. Place soiled linen in laundry bag. Take care to not allow linen to touch your uniform. *Optional:* Use top sheet when bath blanket is not available or if patient prefers top sheet.

      Bath blanket provides warmth and privacy during bath.

   c. Remove patient's gown or pajamas.

      Provides full exposure of body parts during bathing.

      (1) If using gown with ties or snaps on sleeves for patient with IV line, upper-extremity injury, or limited ROM, unsnap or untie and remove gown.

      (2) If regular gown is used and patient has limited upper-extremity ROM or IV access, remove gown from *unaffected side first.*

         Undressing unaffected side first allows easier manipulation of gown over body part with reduced ROM.

      (3) Remove gown from arm with IV line (see illustrations A–C). Remove IV bag and tubing from pole, and slide IV container and tubing through arm of patient's gown. Rehang IV container and check flow rate (see illustration D). Regulate if necessary.

         Manipulation of IV tubing and container may disrupt flow rate. Do *not* delegate regulation of IV flow rate to NAP.

      (4) If IV pump is in use, turn pump off, clamp tubing, remove tubing from pump, and proceed as in Step (3). Reinsert tubing into pump, unclamp tubing, and turn pump on at correct rate. Observe flow rate and regulate if necessary. *Do not disconnect tubing.*

         Regulation is necessary to prevent improper infusion of fluids. Do *not* delegate regulation of IV pump to NAP.
         Disconnecting IV tubing places patient at risk of introduction of microorganisms into IV line.

   d. Raise side rail. Lower bed temporarily to lowest position and raise to comfortable working height on return. Place basin and supplies on over-bed table. Check water temperature and have patient place fingers in water to test temperature tolerance. Place plastic container of bath lotion in bath water to warm if desired.

      Maintains patient's safety while you leave bedside. Keeping bed at working height during bath prevents back strain. Warm water promotes comfort, relaxes muscles, and prevents unnecessary chilling. CHG is most effective at full strength. Testing temperature prevents accidental burns. Bath water warms lotion for application to patient's skin.

SKILL 31.1   BATHING AND PERINEAL CARE—cont'd

View Video!

STEP	RATIONALE
e. Lower side rail, remove pillow if tolerated, and raise head of bed 30 to 45 degrees if allowed. Place bath towel under patient's head. Place second bath towel over patient's chest.	Helps your access to patient. You do not have to reach across bed, minimizing strain on back muscles.
	Removal of pillow makes it easier to wash patient's ears and neck. Placing towels prevents bed linen and bath blanket from getting soiled or wet.
f. Wash face.	

Clinical Decision Point. If using CHG solution in bath water, do not use to wash face. Use clear water only or mild soap and water on the face.

(1) Ask if patient is wearing contact lenses.	Prevents accidental injury to eyes.
(2) Fold washcloth around fingers of your hand to form a mitt (see illustration). Immerse mitt in water and wring thoroughly.	Mitt retains water and heat better than loosely held washcloth; keeps cold edges from brushing against patient and prevents splashing.

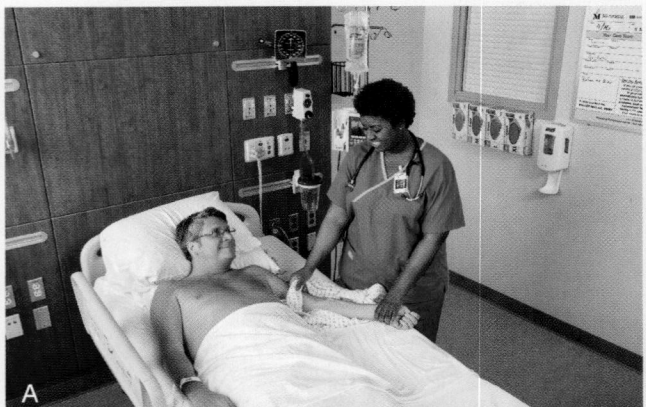
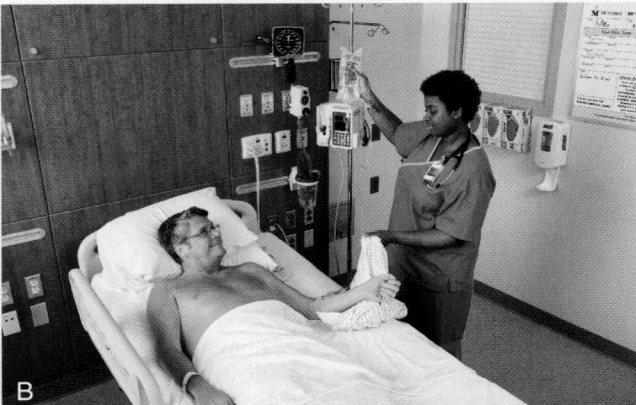
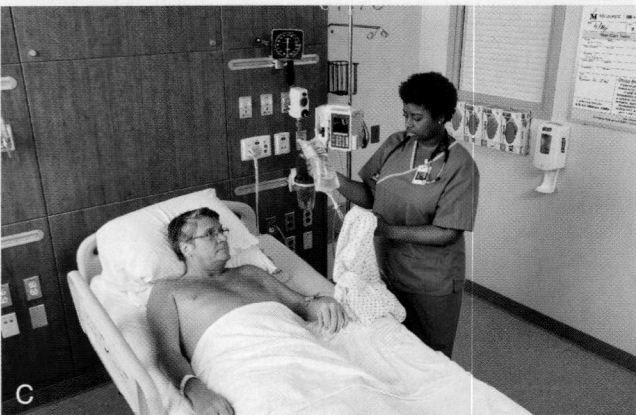
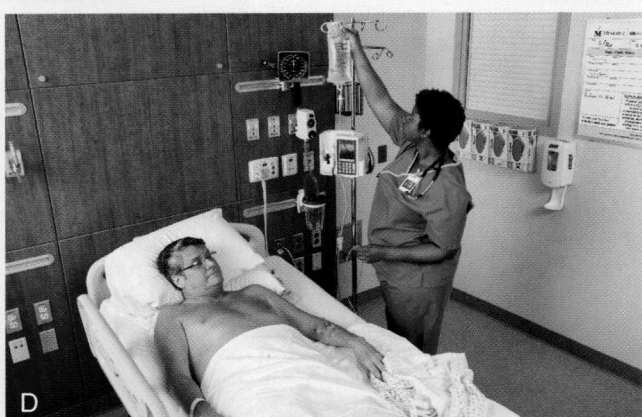

STEP 5c(3) A, Remove patient's gown. **B,** Remove IV bag from pole. **C,** Slide IV tubing and bag through arm of patient's gown. **D,** Rehang IV bag.

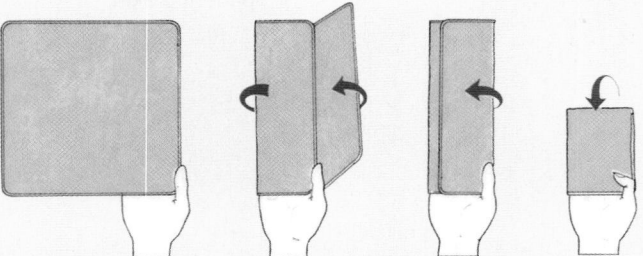

STEP 5f(2) Steps for folding washcloth to form a mitt.

STEP	RATIONALE
(3) Wash patient's eyes with plain warm water. Use different section of mitt for each eye. Move mitt from inner to outer canthus (see illustrations). Soak any crusts on eyelid for 2 to 3 minutes with damp cloth before attempting removal. Dry eyes thoroughly but gently.	Soap irritates eyes. Use of separate sections of mitt reduces infection transmission. Bathing eye from inner to outer canthus prevents secretions from entering nasolacrimal duct. Pressure can cause internal injury.
(4) When using soap and water, ask if patient prefers to use soap on face. Otherwise wash, rinse, and dry forehead, cheeks, nose, neck, and ears without using soap. (Men may wish to shave at this point or wait until after bath.)	Soap tends to dry face, which is exposed to air more than other body parts.
g. Wash trunk and upper extremities.	
(1) Remove bath blanket from patient's arm that is closest to you. Place bath towel lengthwise under arm. Bathe arm with soap and water using long, firm strokes from distal to proximal areas (fingers to axilla).	Towel prevents soiling of bed. Soap lowers surface tension and facilitates removal of debris and bacteria when friction is applied during washing. Long, firm strokes stimulate circulation; moving distal to proximal promotes venous return.
(2) Raise and support arm above head (if possible) to wash, rinse, and dry axilla thoroughly (see illustration). Apply deodorant or powder to underarms if desired or needed.	Movement of arm exposes axilla and exercises normal ROM of joint. Rinsing removes alkaline residue from soap. Drying prevents excess moisture, which can cause skin maceration or softening.

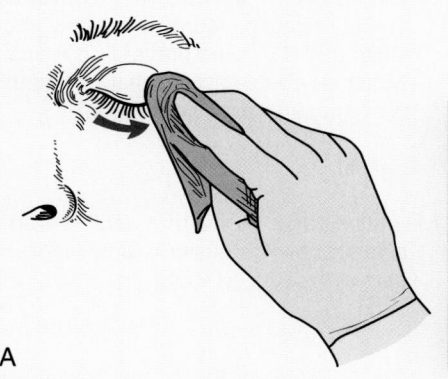 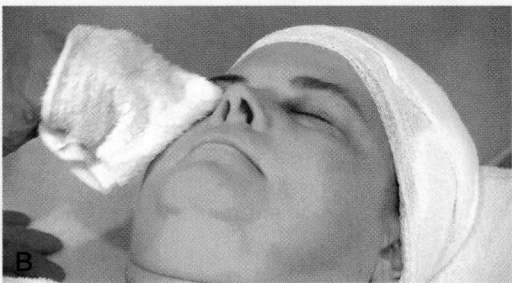

STEP 5f(3) Wash eye from inner to outer canthus. **A,** Direction for cleansing eye. **B,** Washing eye from inner to outer canthus.

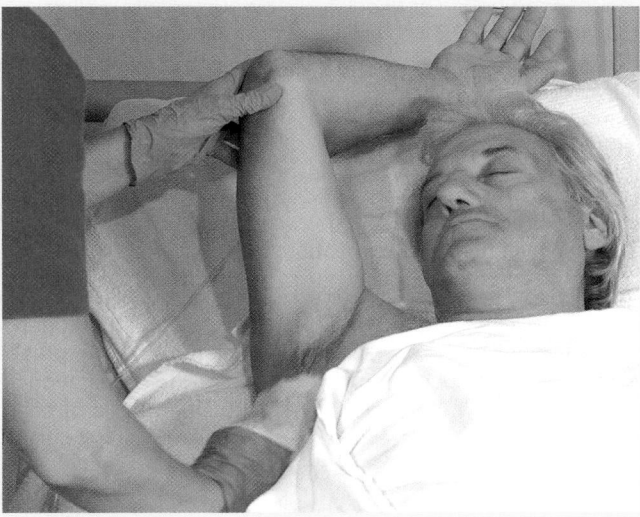

STEP 5g(2) Position of patient's arm for washing axilla.

SKILL 31.1 BATHING AND PERINEAL CARE—cont'd

View Video!

STEP	RATIONALE
(3) Move to other side of bed and repeat Steps (1) and (2) with other arm.	Provides for better access to patient and helps prevent back strain.
(4) Place bath towel across patient's chest so that it covers chest and arms, and fold bath blanket down to umbilicus. While lifting edge of towel away from chest with one hand, bathe chest with mitted washcloth on other hand using long, firm strokes. Take special care to wash skinfolds under the breasts of a female patient. It is often necessary to lift breast upward while bathing underneath it. Keep patient's chest covered between wash and rinse. Rinse and dry well.	Draping prevents unnecessary exposure of body parts. Towel maintains warmth and privacy. Secretions and dirt collect easily in areas of tight skinfolds. Skin under breasts is vulnerable to excoriation if not kept clean and dry.
h. Wash hands and nails (see Box 31.11).	
i. Check temperature of bath water and change water when cool or soapy. (See agency policy regarding changing water when using CHG solution.)	Warm water maintains patient's comfort. Alkaline soap residue is irritating to skin and can decrease normal protectiveness of acid pH.

Clinical Decision Point. If patient is at risk for falling, be sure that two side rails are up before obtaining fresh water. Lower bed when it is necessary to leave bedside. Note: Having all side rails raised is considered a restraint. Check agency policy.

j. Wash abdomen.	
(1) Place bath towel lengthwise over chest and abdomen. (Two towels may be needed.) Fold bath blanket down to just above pubic region. With one hand lift bath towel. With mitted hand bathe and rinse abdomen, giving special attention to umbilicus and skinfolds of abdomen and groin. Stroke from side to side. Keep abdomen covered between washing and rinsing. Rinse and dry well.	Draping prevents unnecessary exposure of body parts. Towel maintains warmth and privacy. Keeping skinfolds clean and dry helps prevent odor and skin irritation. Moisture and sediment that collect in skinfolds predispose skin to maceration.
(2) Apply clean gown or pajama top. If an extremity is injured or immobilized, dress affected side first. (This step may be omitted until completion of bath; gown should not become soiled during remainder of bath.)	Maintains patient's warmth and comfort. Dressing affected side first allows easier manipulation of gown over body part with reduced ROM.
k. Wash lower extremities.	
(1) Cover chest and abdomen with top of bath blanket. Cover legs with bottom of blanket. Expose near leg by folding blanket toward midline. Be sure to keep other leg and perineum draped.	Prevents unnecessary exposure.
(2) Place bath towel under leg, supporting leg at knee and ankle. If appropriate, place patient's foot in bath basin to soak while washing and rinsing. (Bend patient's leg at knee; while grasping patient's heel, elevate leg from mattress slightly and place bath basin on towel.) If patient is unable to support leg, you can wash feet thoroughly with washcloth.	Towel prevents soiling of bed linen. Support of joint and extremity during lifting prevents strain on musculoskeletal structures. Sudden movement by patient could spill bath water. Soaking softens calluses and rough skin.

Clinical Decision Point. If patient has diabetes or peripheral vascular disease with impaired circulation and/or sensation, do not soak feet. Maceration of skin may predispose to infection.

(3) Wash leg using long, firm strokes from ankle to knee and from knee to thigh (see illustration). Do not rub or massage back of calf. Rinse and dry well. Clean foot, making sure to bathe between toes. Rinse and dry toes and feet completely. Clean and clip nails as needed (see Box 31.11). Remove and discard towel.	Promotes circulation and venous return. Excess massage of calf could loosen deep vein thrombus. Secretions and moisture may be present between toes, predisposing patient to maceration and breakdown. Avoid cutting nails of patient with diabetes. See agency policy for podiatric care.

STEP	RATIONALE

(4) Raise side rail, move to opposite side of bed, lower side rail, and repeat Steps (2) and (3) for other leg and foot. If skin is dry, apply moisturizer. When finished, cover patient with bath blanket.

Clinical Decision Point. Do not use long, firm strokes to wash lower extremities of patients with history of deep vein thrombosis or blood-clotting disorders. Use short, light strokes instead.

---

l. Cover patient with bath blanket, raise side rail for patient's safety, remove soiled gloves, and perform hand hygiene. Change bath water.	Cooler bath water causes chilling. Clean water reduces microorganism transmission to perineal structures.
m. Provide perineal hygiene.	
(1) If patient is able to maneuver and handle washcloth, allow him or her to clean perineum on own.	Maintains patient's dignity and self-care ability.

Clinical Decision Point. CHG is safe to use on the perineum and external mucosa (AHRQ, 2013).

---

(2) Female patient	
(a) Apply pair of clean gloves. Lower side rail. Help patient into dorsal recumbent position. Note restrictions or limitations in patient's positioning. Place waterproof pad under patient's buttocks. Drape patient with bath blanket placed in shape of a diamond. Lift lower edge of bath blanket to expose perineum (see illustration).	Provides full exposure of female genitalia. If patient is totally dependent, provide assistance to support her in side-lying position and raise leg as perineum is bathed. If position causes patient discomfort, reduce degree of abduction in her hips.
(b) Fold lower corner of bath blanket up between patient's legs onto abdomen. Wash and dry patient's upper thighs.	Keeping patient draped until procedure begins minimizes anxiety. Buildup of perineal secretions soils surrounding skin surfaces.
(c) Wash labia majora. Use nondominant hand to gently retract labia from thigh; with dominant hand, wash carefully in skinfolds. Wipe in direction from perineum to rectum. Repeat on opposite side with separate section of washcloth. Rinse and dry area thoroughly.	Perineal care includes thorough cleaning of patient's external genitalia and surrounding skin. Skinfolds may contain body secretions that harbor microorganisms. Wiping front to back reduces chance of transmitting fecal organisms to urinary meatus.

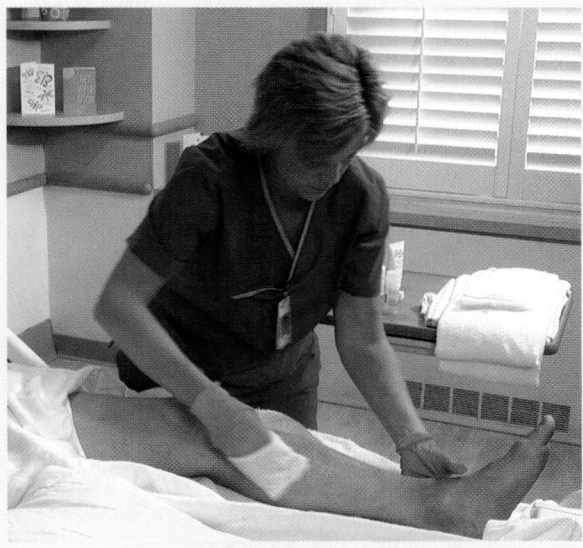

STEP 5k(3) Washing patient's leg.

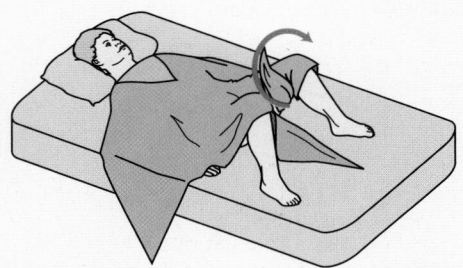

STEP 5m(2)(a) Drape patient for perineal care.

SKILL 31.1 BATHING AND PERINEAL CARE—cont'd

View Video!

STEP	RATIONALE
(d) Gently separate labia with nondominant hand to expose urethral meatus and vaginal orifice. With dominant hand, wash downward from pubic area toward rectum in one smooth stroke (see illustration). Wash middle and both sides of perineum. Use separate section of cloth for each stroke. Clean thoroughly around labia minora, clitoris, and vaginal orifice. Avoid placing tension on indwelling catheter if present, and clean area around it thoroughly.	Cleansing method reduces transfer of microorganisms to urinary meatus. (For menstruating women or patients with indwelling catheters, clean with cotton balls.)
(e) Provide catheter care using a CHG wipe or a clean washcloth to clean down along catheter from exit site (check agency policy) (see Chapter 36).	Reduces incidence of health care–associated urinary tract infection (Strouse, 2015).
(f) Rinse perineal area thoroughly. May use bedpan and pour warm water over perineal area. Dry thoroughly from front to back.	Rinsing removes soap and microorganisms more effectively than wiping. Retained moisture harbors microorganisms.
(g) Fold lower corner of bath blanket back between patient's legs and over perineum. Ask patient to lower legs and assume comfortable position.	
(3) Male patient	
(a) Apply pair of clean gloves. Lower side rail. Help patient to supine position. Note any restriction in mobility.	Provides full exposure of male genitalia. Position patients who are unable to lie supine on their side.
(b) Fold lower half of bath blanket up to expose upper thighs. Wash and dry thighs.	Buildup of perineal secretions soils surrounding skin surfaces.
(c) Cover thighs with bath towels. Raise bath blanket up to expose genitalia. Gently raise penis and place bath towel underneath. Gently grasp shaft of penis. If patient is uncircumcised, retract foreskin (see illustration). If patient has an erection, defer procedure until later.	Draping minimizes patient anxiety. Towel prevents moisture from collecting in inguinal area. Gentle but firm handling of penis reduces chance of an erection. Secretions capable of harboring microorganisms collect underneath foreskin.
(d) Wash tip of penis at urethral meatus first. Using circular motion, clean from meatus outward (see illustration). Discard washcloth and repeat with clean cloth until penis is clean. Rinse and dry gently.	Direction of cleaning moves from area of least contamination to area of most contamination to prevent microorganisms from entering urethra.
(e) Return foreskin to its natural position. This is extremely important in patients with decreased sensation in the lower extremities.	Tightening of foreskin around shaft of penis causes local edema and discomfort. Patients with reduced sensation do not feel tightening of foreskin.

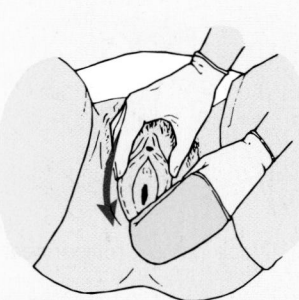

STEP 5m(2)(d) Clean from perineum to rectum (front to back).

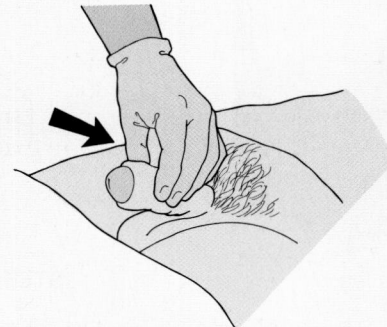

STEP 5m(3)(c) Retract foreskin.

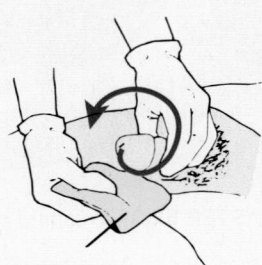

STEP 5m(3)(d) Use circular motion to clean tip of penis.

STEP	RATIONALE
(f) Gently clean shaft of penis and scrotum by having patient abduct legs. Pay special attention to underlying surface of penis. Lift scrotum carefully and wash underlying skinfolds. Rinse and dry thoroughly.	Vigorous massage of penis may cause an erection. Underlying surface of penis is an area where secretions accumulate. Abduction of legs provides easier access to scrotal tissues. Secretions collect easily between skinfolds.
(g) Provide catheter care as needed (see Step m(2)(e)). Avoid placing tension on indwelling catheter and clean area around it thoroughly. Provide catheter care (see Chapter 36).	Cleaning along catheter from exit site reduces incidence of nosocomial urinary tract infection.
n. Remove soiled gloves and discard in trash; raise side rail before leaving bedside to dispose of water and obtain fresh water.	Prevents transmission of infection. Protects patient from injury.
o. Wash back. (This follows both female and male perineal care.)	
(1) Perform hand hygiene and apply clean pair of gloves. Lower side rail. Help patient into prone or side-lying position (as applicable). Place towel lengthwise along patient's side and keep him or her covered with bath blanket.	Exposes back and buttocks for bathing while limiting exposure.
(2) Keep patient draped by sliding bath blanket over shoulders and thighs during bathing. Wash, rinse, and dry back from neck to buttocks using long, firm strokes.	Cleaning back before buttocks and anus prevents contamination of water.
(3) Move from back to buttocks and anus. Have patient remain in prone or side-lying position and keep covered to avoid chilling. Clean anus and buttocks area.	Exposes back and buttocks for bathing while limiting exposure.
(4) If fecal material is present, enclose in fold of underpad or toilet tissue and remove with disposable wipes.	Skinfolds near buttocks and anus may contain fecal secretions that harbor microorganisms.
(5) Clean buttocks and anus, washing front to back (see illustration). Clean, rinse, and dry area thoroughly. If needed, place a clean absorbent pad under patient's buttocks. Remove contaminated gloves. Raise side rail and perform hand hygiene.	Cleaning motion prevents contaminating perineal area with fecal material or microorganisms.
(6) Return to bed and lower side rail; give a back rub if appropriate or desired by patient.	Promotes patient relaxation. Back rubs are contraindicated in some cardiac patients.
p. Apply additional body lotion or oil to patient's skin as needed.	Moisturizing lotion prevents dry, chapped skin.
q. Remove soiled linen and place in dirty-linen bag. Clean and replace bathing equipment. Wash hands.	Reduces transmission of microorganisms.
r. Help patient dress. Comb patient's hair. Women may want to apply makeup. Help as needed.	Promotes patient's body image.
s. Make patient's bed (see Boxes 31.16 and 31.17).	Provides clean, comfortable environment.
t. Check function and position of external devices (e.g., indwelling urethral catheters, nasogastric tubes, IV lines).	Ensures that systems remain functional after bathing activities.
u. Place bed in lowest position.	Maintains patient's safety by decreasing height of bedframe from floor.
v. Place nurse call system and personal possessions in an accessible location. Leave room as clean and comfortable as possible.	Prevents transmission of infection. Clean environment promotes patient's comfort. Promotes patient's safety.
w. Perform hand hygiene.	Reduces transmission of microorganisms.
6. Commercial bag bath or CHG cleansing pack	
a. A cleansing pack contains six to eight premoistened towels for cleaning. Warm package contents in microwave following package directions. If you are bathing patient using warm commercial or CHG cloth, check temperature of cloth before use. Gloves diminish sense of heat.	Provides warm, soothing heat. CHG reduces bacteria for up to 24 hours and prevents infection (AHRQ, 2013). Prevents burn to skin.

SKILL 31.1 BATHING AND PERINEAL CARE—cont'd

View Video!

STEP	RATIONALE
b. Use all six CHG cloths in the following order (see illustration): • Cloth 1: Neck, shoulders, and chest • Cloth 2: Both arms, both hands, web spaces, and axilla • Cloth 3: Abdomen and groin/perineum • Cloth 4: Right leg, right foot, and web spaces • Cloth 5: Left leg, left foot, and web spaces • Cloth 6: Back of neck, back, and buttocks	Reduces transmission of microorganisms.
c. Firmly massage skin when using cloth. Allow skin to air dry for 30 seconds. Do not rinse. It is permissible to lightly cover patient with bath towel to prevent chilling.	Drying skin with towel removes emollient that is left behind after water/cleaner solution evaporates.
d. **Note:** If there is excessive soiling (e.g., in perineal region), use an extra cloth or conventional washcloths, soap, water, and towels.	
7. Tub bath or shower	
a. Consider patient's condition and review orders for precautions concerning movement or positioning of patient.	Prevents accidental injury to patient during bathing.
b. Schedule use of shower or tub.	Prevents unnecessary waiting, which causes fatigue.
c. Check tub or shower for cleanliness. Use cleaning techniques outlined in agency policy. Place rubber mat on tub or shower bottom. Place disposable bath mat or towel on floor in front of tub or shower.	Cleaning prevents transmission of microorganisms. Mats prevent slipping and falling.
d. Collect all hygienic aids, toiletry items, and linens requested by patient. Place within easy reach of tub or shower.	Placing items close at hand prevents possible falls when patient reaches for items.
e. Help patient move to bathroom if necessary. Have patient wear robe and nonskid slippers.	Assistance prevents accidental falls. Wearing robe and slippers prevents chilling.
f. Demonstrate how to use call signal for assistance.	Bathrooms are equipped with signaling devices in case patient feels faint or weak or needs immediate assistance. Patients prefer privacy during bath if safety is not jeopardized.
g. Place "occupied" sign on bathroom door.	Maintains patient's privacy.

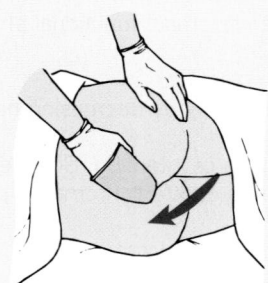

STEP 5o(5) Clean buttocks and anus, washing front to back.

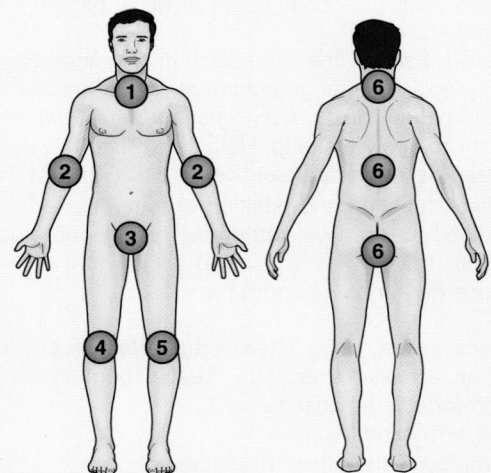

STEP 6b Using CHG bathing cloths. (From Agency for Healthcare Research and Quality [AHRQ]: *Appendix E. Training and educational materials: daily chlorhexidine bathing patient information,* 2013, Agency for Healthcare Research and Quality, Rockville, MD. http://www.ahrq.gov/professionals/systems/hospital/universal_icu_decolonization/universal-icu-ape.html.)

STEP	RATIONALE
h. Fill bath tub halfway with warm water. Check temperature of bath water, have patient test water, and adjust temperature if water is too warm. Explain which faucet controls hot water. If patient is taking shower, turn shower on and adjust water temperature before patient enters shower stall. Use shower seat or tub chair if needed (see illustration).	Adjusting water temperature prevents accidental burns. Older adults and patients with neurological alterations (e.g., diabetes, spinal cord injury) are at high risk for burn because of reduced sensation. Use of assistive devices facilitates bathing and minimizes physical exertion.
i. Instruct patient to use safety bars when getting in and out of tub or shower, and to pull cord to summon assistance (if available). Caution patient against use of bath oil in tub water.	Prevents slipping and falling. Oil causes tub surfaces to become slippery.
j. Instruct patient not to remain in tub longer than 10 or 15 minutes. Check on patient every 5 minutes.	Prolonged exposure to warm water causes vasodilation and pooling of blood in some patients, leading to light-headedness or dizziness.
k. Return to bathroom when patient signals and knock before entering.	Provides privacy.
l. For patient who is unsteady, drain tub of water before he or she tries to get out. Place bath towel over patient's shoulders. Help patient out of tub as needed and help with drying.	Prevents accidental falls. Patient may become chilled as water drains.

Clinical Decision Point. Weak or unstable patients need extra assistance in getting out of a tub. Planning for additional personnel is essential before attempting to help the patient. Lift equipment may be used for transfer in some cases. See agency policy.

m. Help patient as needed with getting dressed in clean gown or pajamas, slippers, and robe. (In home setting patient may put on regular clothing.)	Maintains warmth to prevent chilling.
n. Help patient to room and comfortable position in bed or chair.	Maintains relaxation gained from bathing.
o. Clean tub or shower according to agency policy. Remove soiled linen and place in dirty-linen bag. Discard disposable equipment in proper receptacle. Place "unoccupied" sign on bathroom door. Return supplies to storage area.	Prevents transmission of infection through soiled linen and moisture.
p. Perform hand hygiene.	Reduces transfer of microorganisms.

EVALUATION

1. Observe skin, paying particular attention to areas previously soiled, reddened, dry, or showing early signs of breakdown.	Techniques used during bathing leave skin clean and clear. Over time, dryness of skin diminishes. If patient shows areas of redness, use Braden Scale to measure risk for pressure injuries (see Chapter 38).
2. Observe ROM during bath.	Measures joint mobility.
3. Ask patient to rate level of comfort.	Determines patient's tolerance of bathing activities.
4. Ask patient to rate level of fatigue.	Determines patient's tolerance of bathing activities.

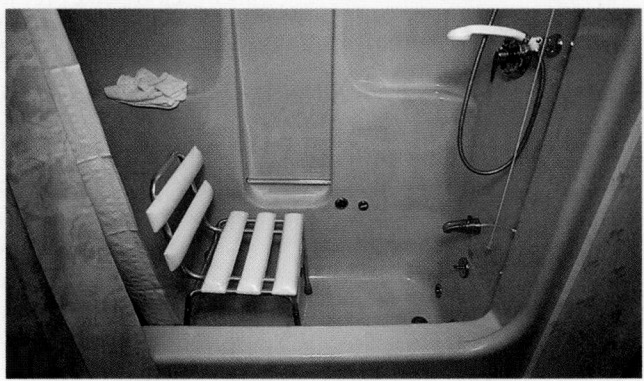

STEP 7h Shower seat for patient safety.

SKILL 31.1 BATHING AND PERINEAL CARE—cont'd

View Video!

STEP	RATIONALE
5. **Use Teach-Back:** "We talked about why it is important for you to have a daily bath while in the hospital. Please tell me why we are using bathing cloths for your bath. How will you be sure the area around your wound is bathed correctly once you get home?" Revise your instruction now or develop a plan for revised patient teaching if patient/family caregiver is not able to teach back correctly.	Determines patient's/family caregiver's level of understanding of instructional topic.

RECORDING AND REPORTING

- Record in nurses' notes in electronic health record (EHR), chart, or flow sheets amount of assistance provided, patient's participation in care, condition of skin, and any significant findings (e.g., reddened areas, breaks in skin, inflammation, ulcerations).

- Document your evaluation of patient/family caregiver learning.
- Report any skin irritations, breaks in skin, or ulcerations or patient's intolerance to activity to nurse in charge or health care provider.

UNEXPECTED OUTCOMES AND RELATED INTERVENTIONS

- Areas of excessive dryness, rashes, or pressure injuries appear on skin.
  - Complete pressure injury assessment (see Chapter 38).
  - Apply moisturizing lotions or topical skin applications per agency policy.
  - Limit frequency of complete baths. It may become necessary (if patient has a sensitivity to CHG) to switch to plain soap and water.
  - Obtain special bed surface.
- Patient becomes excessively tired or unable to cooperate or participate in bathing.
  - Reschedule bathing time when patient is more rested.
  - Provide pillow or elevate head of bed during bath for patient with breathing difficulties.

- Notify health care provider if this is a change in patient's fatigue level.
- Perform hygiene measures in stages between scheduled rest periods.
- The rectum, perineum, or genital area is inflamed or swollen or has foul-smelling odor.
  - Bathe perineal area frequently enough to keep clean and dry.
  - Obtain an order for a sitz bath.
  - Apply protective barrier ointment or antiinflammatory cream.
  - Report findings to health care provider.

KEY POINTS

- Various personal, social, cultural, and developmental factors influence patients' hygiene practices.
- Assess a patient's physical and cognitive ability to perform hygiene self-care and provide care according to the patient's needs and preferences.
- Incorporate knowledge of the factors influencing an individual patient's hygiene practices into hygiene care.
- Integrate physical assessment, wound care, teaching, and range-of-motion (ROM) exercises into hygiene care.
- Use communication skills and teaching to develop a caring relationship with the patient.
- Maintain privacy, comfort, and patient safety when providing hygiene care.

- Provide oral care for patients who are debilitated or unconscious; take precautions to reduce risk for ventilator-associated pneumonia (VAP) and aspiration.
- Patients who are immobilized and poorly nourished and who have reduced sensation or peripheral circulation are at risk for altered skin integrity; these patients require special nail, foot, and skin care.
- Patients with diabetes mellitus or other peripheral vascular diseases require special foot care practices.
- Maintain patient's environment clean and free of clutter.
- Base evaluation of hygiene care on the patient's sense of comfort, relaxation, well-being, and understanding of hygiene techniques.

REFLECTIVE LEARNING

- You are caring for a 30-year-old married man who has fractured both wrists. Think about the type of discharge patient education the patient and his wife will need. You want to educate the patient and his wife so that they can meet his hygiene needs of bathing, dressing, and toileting. How will you prepare this patient and his wife to work as a team?

- You need to give a complete bed bath to a patient from another culture. Reflect on the type of information about hygiene practices that you must include in your assessment of hygiene practices and personal preferences before you begin.

- You are providing home care assistance with foot care to a patient with diabetes. This is the first time you have cared for a patient with diabetes. Reflect on what you need to learn about diabetic foot care. Identify ways your instructor can be a resource as you prepare.

REVIEW QUESTIONS

1. The nurse is helping a new postoperative patient bathe at the sink. During the bath, the patient complains of feeling dizzy; the nurse observes that the patient is breathing rapidly and has a rapid pulse. What is the most appropriate response? (Select all that apply.)
   1. Finish the bath quickly
   2. Move the patient to a bed or chair
   3. Call for assistance
   4. Leave the patient alone to rest in the chair
   5. Instruct the patient to take deep breaths and try to relax

2. A nurse is caring for a patient who complains of sore feet but who also has decreased sensation in both feet. Which interventions should the nurse do? (Select all that apply.)
   1. Avoid cleaning the feet until an order from the health care provider is received
   2. Wash the feet with lukewarm water and then pat dry thoroughly
   3. Apply moisturizing lotion to the feet, especially between the toes
   4. File the toenails straight across
   5. Soak the feet in lukewarm water with Epsom salts for 20 minutes

3. While planning morning care, the nurse would assign the highest priority to which of these patients to receive a bath first?
   1. A patient who just returned to the nursing unit from surgery and is resting comfortably
   2. A patient who prefers a bath in the evening when his wife visits and can help him
   3. A patient who is febrile and whose skin is moist from perspiration
   4. A patient who has just returned from diagnostic testing and complains of being very fatigued

4. The nurse plans to talk with a female African American patient about hair care to prevent traction alopecia. Which points does the nurse include in the teaching? (Select all that apply.)
   1. Hairstyles do not contribute to traction alopecia.
   2. Hair should be washed daily.
   3. Avoid using excessive amounts of heat for styling hair.
   4. Select shampoos that contain sulfates.
   5. Avoid using relaxer treatments too frequently.

5. A clinical agency is starting to use chlorhexidine gluconate (CHG) 4% in a bath base basin for certain patients. Which points are important to remember? (Select all that apply.)
   1. Use one wash cloth, only once, for each body part.
   2. Patient's skin may feel sticky after bathing.
   3. Wipe off sticky residue from patient's skin.
   4. Wash patient's face with CHG 4%.
   5. One bottle of CHG solution is insufficient for a complete bath.

evolve

Additional Review Questions, as well as rationales for all Review Questions, can be found on the Evolve website.

1. 2, 3; 2. 2, 4; 3. 3; 4. 3, 5; 5. 1, 2.

REFERENCES

Agency for Healthcare Research and Quality (AHRQ): *Appendix E. Training and educational materials: daily chlorhexidine bathing patient information*, Rockville, MD., 2013, Agency for Healthcare Research and Quality. http://www.ahrq.gov/professionals/systems/hospital/universal_icu_decolonization/universal-icu-ape.html.

Agency for Health Care Research and Quality (AHRQ): *Preventing pressure ulcers in hospitals*, 2014, https://www.ahrq.gov/sites/default/files/publications/files/putoolkit.pdf.

Alzheimer's Association: *Ten early signs and symptoms of Alzheimer's disease*, 2017, http://www.alz.org/10-signs-symptoms-alzheimers-dementia.asp.

American Academy of Dermatology (AAD): *Handle with care: African-American hair needs special care to avoid damage*, 2012, http://www.aad.org/stories-and-news/news-releases/handle-with-care-african-american-hair-needs-special-care-to-avoid-damage.

American Academy of Dermatology (AAD): *Dermatologists' top tips for relieving dry skin*, 2016, https://www.aad.org/public/skin-hair-nails/skin-care/dry-skin.

American Dental Association: *Mouth healthy: brushing your teeth*, 2017, http://www.mouthhealthy.org/en/az-topics/b/brushing-your-teeth.aspx.

American Diabetes Association: *Foot care*, 2014, http://www.diabetes.org/living-with-diabetes/complications/foot-complications/foot-care.html.

American Diabetes Association: *Diabetes statistics*, 2016, http://www.diabetes.org/diabetes-basics/statistics/.

American Podiatric Medical Association (APMA): *Diabetes*, 2016, http://www.apma.org/learn/FootHealth.cfm?ItemNumber=980.

Ayello EA, Fulmer T: Preventing pressure ulcers and skin tears. In Boltz M, et al, editors: *Evidence-based geriatric protocols for best practice*, ed 4, New York, 2012, Springer, p 298.

Beeckman D, et al: A systemic review and meta-analysis of incontinence-associated dermatitis, incontinence, and moisture as risk factors for pressure ulcer development, *Res Nurs Health* 37:204, 2014.

Boonyasiri A, et al: Effectiveness of chlorhexidine wipes for the prevention of multidrug-resistant bacterial colonization and hospital-acquired infections in intensive care unit patients: a randomized trial in Thailand, *Infect Control Hosp Epidemiol* 36(3):245, 2016.

Burman M, et al: Linking evidenced based nursing practice and patient centered care through patient preferences, *Nurs Adm Q* 37(3):231, 2013.

Cassir N, et al: Chlorhexidine daily bathing: impact on health-care associated infections caused by gram-negative bacteria, *Am J Infect Control* 43:640, 2015.

Centers for Disease Control and Prevention (CDC): *Tick removal and test*, 2015, http://www.cdc.gov/lyme/removal/index.html.

Centers for Disease Control and Prevention (CDC): *Head lice: treatment*, 2016, https://www.cdc.gov/parasites/lice/head/treatment.html.

Chen W, et al: Effects of daily bathing with chlorhexidine and acquired infection of methicillin-resistant *Staphylococcus aureus* and vancomycin-resistant *Enterococcus*: a meta-analysis, *J Thorac Dis* 5(4):518, 2013.

Climo MW, et al: Effect of daily chlorhexidine bathing on hospital-acquired infection, *N Engl J Med* 368(6):533, 2013.

Eilers J, et al: Evidence-based interventions for cancer treatment–related mucositis, *Clin J Oncol Nurs* 18(Suppl 6):80, 2014.

El-Rabbany M, et al: Prophylactic oral health procedures to prevent hospital-acquired ventilator-associated pneumonia: a systematic review, *Int J Nurs Stud* 52(1):452, 2015.

Erikson E: *Childhood and society*, ed 2, New York, 1963, WW Norton.

Giger JN, editor: *Transcultural nursing: assessment and intervention*, ed 6, St Louis, 2013, Mosby.

Hall GR, et al: *Bathing persons with dementia*, Iowa City (IA), 2013, University of Iowa College of Nursing, John A. Hartford Foundation Center of Geriatric Nursing Excellence, p 58. http://www.guideline.gov/content.aspx?id=44984. National Guideline Clearing House.

Harris M, Richards KC: The physiological and psychological effects of slow-stroke back massage and hand massage on relaxation in older people, *J Clin Nurs* 19(7):917, 2010.

Hockenberry MJ, Wilson D: *Wong's nursing care of infants and children*, ed 10, St Louis, 2015, Mosby.

Kiyoshi-Teo H, Blegen M: Institutional guidelines on oral hygiene practices in intensive care units, *Am J Crit Care* 24(4):309, 2015.

Labeau SO, et al: Prevention of ventilator-associated pneumonia with oral antiseptics: a systematic review and meta-analysis, *Lancet Infect Dis* 11:845, 2011.

Makic MBF: Medical device–related pressure ulcers and intensive care patients, *J Perianesth Nurs* 30(3):36, 2015.

Meiner SE: *Gerontologic nursing*, ed 5, St Louis, 2015, Mosby.

Munoz-Price LS, et al: Effectiveness of stepwise interventions targeted to decrease central catheter-associated bloodstream infections, *Crit Care Med* 40(5):1464, 2012.

Munro CL: Oral health: something to smile about, *Am J Crit Care* 23(4):282, 2014.

National Cancer Institute (NCI): *Oral complications of chemotherapy and head/neck radiation (PDQr)—Health Professional Version*, 2016, http://www.cancer.gov/about-cancer/treatment/side-effects/mouth-throat/oral-complications-hp-pdq.

Nicolosi LN, et al: Effect of oral hygiene and 0.12% chlorhexidine gluconate oral rinse in preventing ventilator-associated pneumonia after cardiovascular surgery, *Respir Care* 59(4):504, 2014.

Pandey A, et al: Gerodontics: a boon for the oral health of geriatric patient, *Int Med J* 21(3):328, 2014.

Petlin A, et al: Chlorhexidine gluconate bathing to reduce methicillin resistant *Staphylococcus aureus*, *Crit Care Nurse* 34(5):17, 2014.

Powers J, et al: Chlorhexidine bathing and microbial contamination in patients' bath 186 basins, *Am J Crit Care* 21(5):338, 2012.

Quality and Safety Education for Nurses (QSEN): *Pre-licensure KSAs*, 2014, http://qsen.org/competencies/pre-licensure-ksas/.

Rubin C, et al: Chlorhexidine gluconate to bather or not to bathe?, *Crit Care Nurs Q* 36(2):233, 2013.

Shah H, et al: Bathing with 2% chlorhexidine gluconate, *Crit Care Nurs Q* 39:42, 2016.

Strouse AC: Appraising the literature on bathing practices and catheter-associated urinary tract infection preventions, *Urol Nurs* 35(1):11, 2015.

Tay LY, et al: Evaluation of different treatment methods against denture stomatitis: a randomized clinical study, *Oral Surg Oral Med Oral Pathol Oral Radiol Endod* 118:72, 2014.

The Joint Commission (TJC): *2018 National Patient Safety Goals*, Oakbrook Terrace, IL, 2018, The Commission. http://www.jointcomminssion.org/standards_information/npsgs.aspx.

Touhy TA, Jett K: *Ebersole and Hess' gerontological nursing and healthy aging*, ed 4, St Louis, 2014, Mosby.

Voegeli D: Incontinence-associated dermatitis: new insights into an old problem, *Br J Nurs* 25(5):256, 2016.

Zimmerman S, et al: Changing culture of mouth care: mouth care without a battle, *Gerontologist* 54(Suppl 1):25, 2014.

Zullino DF, et al: Local back massage with an automated massage chair: several muscle and psychophysiologic relaxing properties, *J Altern Complement Med* 11(6):1103, 2005.

evolve MEDIA RESOURCES

http://evolve.elsevier.com/Potter/essentials

- Audio Glossary
- Case Study Continuation

- QSEN Activity and Review Questions Answers and Rationales
- Video Clips

OBJECTIVES

- Describe the structure and function of the cardiopulmonary system.
- Identify the physiological processes of ventilation, perfusion, cardiac output, and respiratory gas exchange.
- Describe the interrelationship of cardiac output, preload, afterload, contractility, and heart rate.
- Describe the electrical conduction system of the heart.
- Describe the effects of a patient's health status, age, lifestyle, and environment on tissue oxygenation.

- Describe clinical outcomes as a result of disturbances in conduction, altered cardiac output, impaired valvular function, myocardial ischemia, and impaired tissue perfusion.
- Identify nursing interventions for promotion, maintenance, and restoration of cardiopulmonary function in all health care settings.
- Identify and describe clinical outcomes for hyperventilation, hypoventilation, and hypoxemia.

KEY TERMS

afterload, p. 869

atelectasis, p. 873

atrioventricular (AV) node, p. 870

cardiac index (CI), p. 869

cardiac output (CO), p. 869

cardiopulmonary rehabilitation, p. 896

cardiopulmonary resuscitation (CPR), p. 895

chest percussion, p. 891

chest physiotherapy (CPT), p. 890

chest tube, p. 893

compliance, p. 867

depolarization, p. 870

diaphragmatic breathing, p. 896

diastolic heart failure, p. 871

diffusion, p. 866

dyspnea, p. 878

dysrhythmia, p. 871

hemoptysis, p. 878

hemothorax, p. 893

high-frequency chest wall compression (HFCWC), p. 892

humidification, p. 889

hypercapnia, p. 868

hyperventilation, p. 868

hypoventilation, p. 868

hypoxemia, p. 868

hypoxia, p. 868

myocardial contractility, p. 869

myocardial infarction, p. 870

myocardial ischemia, p. 870

nebulization, p. 889

normal sinus rhythm (NSR), p. 870

orthopnea, p. 871

oxygen therapy, p. 885

perfusion, p. 866

pleural effusion, p. 893

pneumothorax, p. 893

postural drainage, p. 890

preload, p. 869

productive cough, p. 878

pursed-lip breathing, p. 896

repolarization, p. 870

respiration, p. 866

sinoatrial (SA) node, p. 870

stroke volume (SV), p. 869

surfactant, p. 867

systolic heart failure, p. 871

tension pneumothorax, p. 893

ventilation, p. 866

vibration, p. 892

wheezing, p. 878

CASE STUDY *Mr. King*

Mr. King is a 62-year-old man who is admitted to the hospital with a 6-day history of chest pain, shortness of breath, cough, and generalized malaise. Mr. King works as a salesman and lives with his wife. He has a history of chronic obstructive pulmonary disease (COPD) and alcohol abuse but is not drinking at present. Both Mr. and Mrs. King have smoked 2 packs per day for more than 40 years. Mr. King helped with the housework and states that he loves to tinker in the garden; however, lately he has been unable to do any of these activities. His wife states, "All he can do is sit in his chair and watch TV."

John Smith is the nurse assigned to Mr. King. After reviewing the medical record, John determines that Mr. King has health promotion needs such as smoking cessation and adding exercise to his daily routine. John determines that Mr. King is in respiratory distress while completing his morning assessment. It seems that every breath is a struggle. His respiratory rate is 26 breaths/minute, he is tachycardic with a heart rate of 110 beats/minute, his oxygen saturations are 86%, and he is extremely anxious. Everything that John had planned to do for Mr. King seems less important now. Mrs. King is at his side, watching John's every move and demanding something be done to make her husband breathe easier.

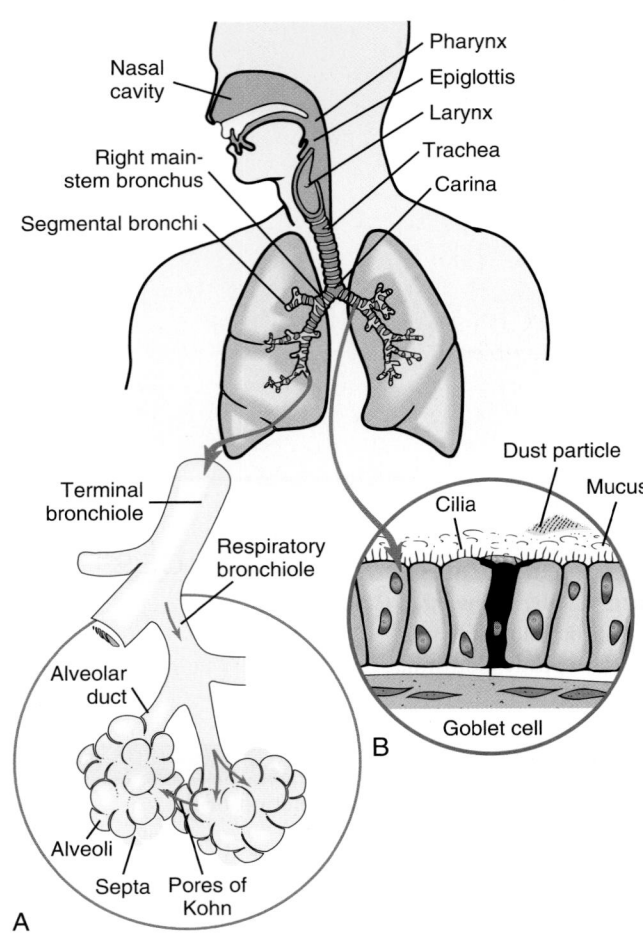

FIG 32.1 Structures of the respiratory tract. **A,** Pulmonary functional unit. **B,** Ciliated mucous membrane. (From Lewis SM, et al: Medical surgical nursing: assessment and management of clinical problems, ed 10, St Louis, 2017, Mosby.)

SCIENTIFIC KNOWLEDGE BASE

Oxygen is a basic human need. The heart and lungs supply the body with oxygen necessary for carrying out the respiratory and metabolic processes needed to sustain life. You will frequently care for patients who are unable to meet their oxygenation needs. This often results from ineffective gas exchange (lungs) or an ineffective pump (heart). Any condition that affects cardiopulmonary functioning directly affects the ability of the body to meet oxygen demands.

Cardiopulmonary Physiology

Respiration is the act of breathing with the exchange of oxygen and carbon dioxide (CO_2) during cellular metabolism. The airways of the lung transfer oxygen from the atmosphere to the alveoli, where the oxygen is exchanged for CO_2. Through the alveolar capillary membrane, oxygen transfers to the blood, and CO_2 transfers from the blood to the alveoli.

This occurs through the three steps of oxygenation: ventilation, diffusion, and perfusion. Ventilation is the movement of air in and out of the lungs, and diffusion is the movement of gases between the alveoli and the bloodstream. The heart supports perfusion, the transport of oxygenated blood to the cells and tissues (Giddens, 2017; Lewis et al., 2017).

Structure and Function of the Pulmonary System

The pulmonary system consists of two lungs, their numerous airways, the respiratory muscles and chest walls, pleural space, and the blood vessels that support them (Fig. 32.1). The right lung is composed of three lobes: the upper, middle, and lower lobes. The left lung has two lobes: the upper and lower lobes. The trachea enters the thorax and bifurcates, or branches out, into the right and left main-stem bronchus. The bronchi branch into smaller and smaller bronchioles, similar to a tree. The last branch of the airways ends at the alveoli, the exchanging unit of the lung. The blood flows through capillaries around the alveoli, allowing for diffusion of oxygen and CO_2 across the alveolar capillary membrane.

The alveoli are lined with a phospholipid, **surfactant**, which decreases the pressure needed to open the alveoli and prevents them from collapsing. Surfactant is essential for normal lung function. Without adequate amounts of surfactant, the alveoli would collapse on expiration, leading to impaired gas exchange.

Ventilation. Ventilation is the process of moving gases into and out of the lungs. It requires coordination of the muscular and elastic properties of the lungs and thorax. Gases move into and out of the lungs through pressure changes. Intrapleural pressure is negative, or less than atmospheric pressure (760 mm Hg at sea level). For air to flow into the lungs, intrapleural pressure becomes more negative, setting up a pressure gradient between the atmosphere and the alveoli. The diaphragm and external intercostal muscles contract to create a negative pleural pressure and increase the size of the thorax for inspiration. Relaxation of the diaphragm and contraction of the internal intercostal muscles allow air to escape from the lungs.

Successful ventilation depends on neuroreceptors and chemoreceptors in the lungs and central nervous system (CNS), muscles that support inspiration and exhalation, and **compliance**. Compliance is the ability of the lungs to distend or expand in response to increased intraalveolar pressure. It depends on the elasticity of the lungs and reflects how easily the lungs can expand. Appropriately controlled ventilation provides for adequate oxygen to meet a person's metabolic demands such as exercise, infection, or pregnancy. Ventilation promotes exhalation of metabolically produced CO_2, which is a determinant of acid-base status (see Chapter 18).

Neural and chemical regulators control ventilation The central nervous system (CNS) sends signals to maintain the rhythm and depth of ventilation, respiratory rate, and the balance between inspiration and expiration. Voluntary control of respiration delivers impulses to respiratory motor neurons by way of the spinal cord for control of respiration during speaking, eating, and swimming. Chemical regulation involves the activity of chemoreceptors located in the medulla, aortic bodies, and carotid bodies. Changes in blood concentration of oxygen (O_2), carbon dioxide (CO_2), and hydrogen ions (H^+) stimulate the chemoreceptors, which stimulate neural regulators to adjust the rate and depth of ventilation to maintain normal arterial blood gas levels. Chemical regulation occurs during physical exercise and emotional distress.

Lung volumes are determined by a person's age, gender, and height. Tidal volume is the amount of air exhaled after a normal inspiration. Residual volume is the amount of air left in the alveoli after a full expiration. Forced vital capacity is the maximum amount of air that can be removed from the lungs during forced expiration (McCance and Huether, 2014).

Oxygen Transport. The delivery of oxygen to the cells and tissues depends on the amount of oxygen entering the lungs (oxygenation) from the atmosphere, the person's ability to exchange gases in the alveoli, and the ability of the heart

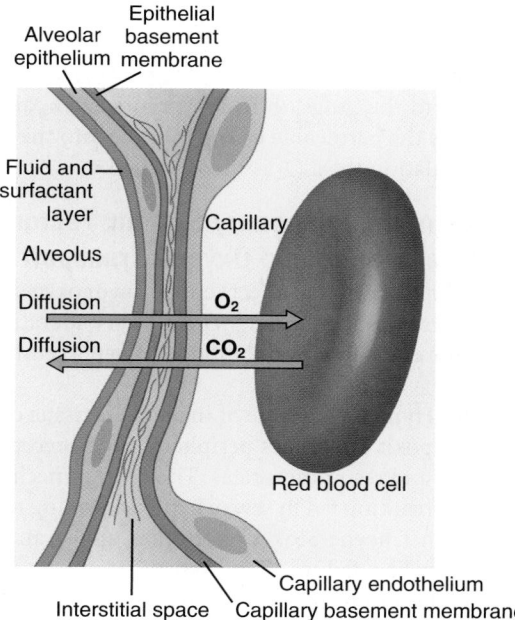

FIG 32.2 Diffusion: Gas-exchange membrane. (From Hall JE: *Guyton and Hall textbook of medical physiology,* ed 13, Philadelphia, 2016, Elsevier.)

to pump oxygenated blood to the cells and tissues (MacIntyre, 2014). Ventilation allows for movement of oxygen and CO_2 into and out of the lungs. Once oxygen has reached the alveoli, diffusion occurs. The thickness of the alveolar capillary membrane affects the rate of diffusion. Increased thickness of the membrane impedes diffusion because gas takes longer to transfer across the membrane. Patients with pulmonary edema or effusion have slow diffusion. Normally oxygen crosses the alveolar-capillary membrane and dissolves into the plasma (Fig. 32.2). It then moves into the red blood cells (RBCs) and binds with hemoglobin (Hgb) molecules. Hemoglobin transports most oxygen and serves as a carrier for both oxygen and CO_2. The Hgb molecule combines with oxygen to form oxyhemoglobin. The formation of oxyhemoglobin is easily reversible, allowing Hgb and oxygen to dissociate, which frees oxygen to enter tissues. The amount of dissolved oxygen in the plasma, the amount of Hgb, and the tendency of Hgb to bind with oxygen all influence the capacity of the blood to carry oxygen. Perfusion of oxygenated blood occurs in the capillary beds of the organs and tissues.

Carbon Dioxide Transport. Carbon dioxide is a product of cellular metabolism. The blood carries CO_2 in three ways: (1) dissolved in plasma, (2) as carbamino compounds, and (3) as bicarbonate. At the capillary level most CO_2 diffuses from the cells into the plasma, and the remaining CO_2 is dissolved in the plasma (PCO_2). The rest of the CO_2 rapidly moves into the RBCs and forms carbonic acid (H_2CO_3). The carbonic acid dissociates (separates) into hydrogen (H^+) and bicarbonate (HCO_3^-) ions. The H^+ ion binds to hemoglobin, which has released its oxygen, to form HHb and deoxyhemoglobin ($HbCO_2$); 23% of CO_2 is transported as $HbCO_2$. The

HCO_3^- ion moves out of the RBCs and back into the plasma (see Chapter 18). To help maintain acid-base balance, 70% of CO_2 is carried as HCO_3^-. Once the CO_2 is transported by the venous blood to the lungs, diffusion occurs again, and CO_2 quickly crosses the permeable gas membrane into the alveoli. Through ventilation the CO_2 is then exhaled.

Alterations of the Pulmonary System: Factors Affecting Ventilation and Oxygen Transport

Illnesses and conditions that affect ventilation or oxygen transport alter respiratory functioning. The primary alterations are hypoxia, hypoxemia, hypoventilation, and hyperventilation.

Hypoxia.   Hypoxia is a state of inadequate tissue oxygenation. Mild hypoxia stimulates peripheral chemoreceptors to increase heart and respiration rates. The central mechanisms that regulate breathing fail in severe hypoxia, leading to irregular respiration, Cheyne-Stokes respiration, apnea, and respiratory and cardiac failure. The tissues most sensitive to hypoxia are the brain, heart, and liver. Causes of hypoxia typically include the following:

- Hypoxemia, or low arterial concentrations of oxygen in the blood
- Inability of the tissues to extract oxygen from the blood, as in septic shock and cyanide poisoning
- Impaired delivery of oxygen to the tissues, which can be seen in cases of low cardiac output, sepsis, thyroid storm, or exercise (MacIntyre, 2014)
- Obstructive or restrictive pulmonary diseases
- Impaired ventilation from multiple rib fractures, spinal cord injury, neuromuscular diseases, or CNS depression resulting from medications or overdose

Signs and symptoms of hypoxia include tachycardia, tachypnea and dyspnea, peripheral vasoconstriction, dizziness, and mental confusion. Treatment aims to correct the cause and may include oxygen therapy, cardiac and respiratory stimulant drugs, and mechanical ventilation.

Hypoxemia.   Hypoxemia is an abnormal deficiency in the concentration of oxygen in arterial blood. Partial pressure of oxygen (PaO_2) less than 60 mm Hg is typically considered to be hypoxemic. Chronic hypoxemia stimulates RBC production by the bone marrow, leading to secondary polycythemia. Causes of hypoxemia include the following:

- Decreased diffusion of oxygen from the lung (alveoli) into the blood, as in pneumonia, asthma exacerbation, or atelectasis
- High altitudes
- Shunting of blood from the right side of the heart to the left side without exchange of gases in the lungs, as seen in some congenital heart defects

Symptoms of acute hypoxemia are similar to symptoms of hypoxia and include tachypnea, dyspnea, hypertension, hypotension, pallor, cyanosis, mental status changes (e.g., headache, anxiety, impaired judgment, confusion, euphoria, lethargy), and motor function changes (e.g., loss of coordination, weakness, tremors, restlessness, stupor, coma, death).

Hypoxemia may also cause dysrhythmias, diaphoresis, blurred or tunnel vision, and nausea and vomiting. Treatment for hypoxemia includes administration of oxygen and correction of the underlying cause.

Hypoventilation.   Hypoventilation occurs when ventilation is inadequate to meet the oxygen demands of the body or to have it eliminate CO_2. It can result from a decreased respiratory rate or a breathing pattern that is too shallow. This results in hypoxia or hypercapnia (arterial carbon dioxide [$PaCO_2$] level greater than 45 mm Hg) and respiratory acidosis. Causes of hypoventilation include the following:

- Impaired ventilation related to trauma, pain, infection, obstructive diseases (emphysema or sleep apnea), or fluid volume overload
- Alterations in neurological regulation of breathing, such as occurs with head or spinal cord injuries
- Alterations in chemical regulation of breathing

As ventilation decreases, $PaCO_2$ is elevated. Clinical signs and symptoms of hypoventilation include dizziness, occipital headache on awakening, lethargy, disorientation, decreased ability to follow instructions, dysrhythmias, hypertension, seizures, and possible coma or cardiac arrest.

When caring for patients with COPD and hypercapnia (high CO_2 levels), remember that administering excessive oxygen *may* result in hypoventilation and subsequent decrease in oxygenation. These patients have adapted to the higher CO_2 level, and the CO_2-sensitive chemoreceptors are no longer sensitive to increased CO_2 as a stimulus to breathe. Theoretically, their stimulus to breathe is a decreased PaO_2, or hypoxemia. Administering excessive oxygen to patients with COPD and hypercapnia satisfies the oxygen requirement of the body and *may* negate the stimulus to breathe. However, other factors are associated with the hypoxic drive to breathe, such as ventilation and perfusion. It should also be noted that not every patient with COPD retains CO_2 and has hypercapnia (Lewis et al., 2017).

Any patient with hypoventilation may retain CO_2, which leads to respiratory acidosis and ultimately respiratory arrest. If untreated, a patient's status rapidly declines, and death is possible. Treatment for hypoventilation involves treating the underlying cause, improving tissue oxygenation, restoring ventilation, and achieving acid-base balance.

Hyperventilation.   Hyperventilation is an increase in respiratory rate, resulting in excess amounts of CO_2 elimination. This causes a decrease in $PaCO_2$, or hypocapnia, and respiratory alkalosis. Causes of hyperventilation include severe anxiety, infection, head injury, medications (e.g., stimulants), and acid-base imbalance. Acute anxiety and the subsequent increased respiratory rate may cause loss of consciousness from excess CO_2 exhalation. An increase of 1° F in body temperature causes a 7% increase in metabolic rate, thereby increasing CO_2 production. The clinical response is increased rate and depth of respiration. Hypoxia associated with pulmonary embolus or shock also results in hyperventilation.

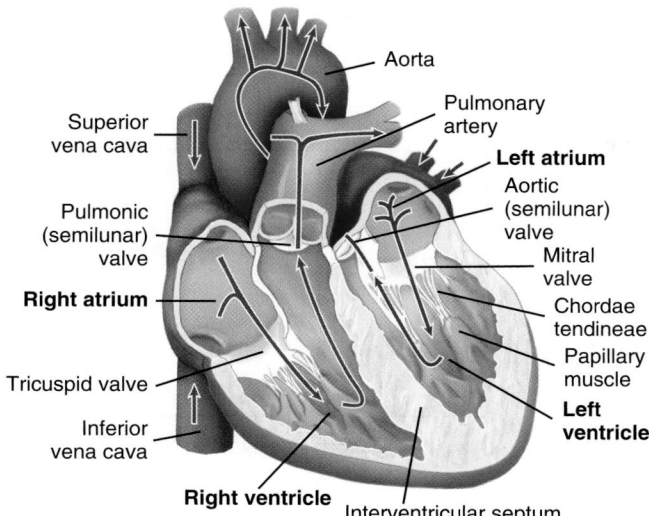

FIG 32.3 Schematic representation of blood flow through the heart. Arrows indicate direction of flow. (Modified from Lewis SM, et al: *Medical surgical nursing: assessment and management of clinical problems,* ed 10, St Louis, 2017, Mosby.)

TABLE 32.1	REGULATION OF BLOOD FLOW
REGULATOR	**DEFINITION**
Cardiac output (CO)	Amount of blood ejected from the ventricles per minute Normal range (adult): 4–8 L/min
Cardiac index (CI)	Measure of adequacy of cardiac output: cardiac index equals cardiac output divided by patient's body surface area Normal range (adult): 2.5–4 L/min/m³
Stroke volume	Amount of blood ejected from the ventricle with each contraction Normal range (adult): 50–75 mL per contraction
Preload	Amount of blood remaining in the ventricles at end of diastole, before the next contraction
Afterload	Resistance of the ejection of blood from the left ventricle
Myocardial contractility	Ability of the heart to contract and eject blood from the ventricles and prepare for the next contraction

Hyperventilation produces signs and symptoms of tachycardia, shortness of breath, chest pain, dizziness, lightheadedness, decreased concentration, paresthesia, circumoral and/or extremity numbness, tinnitus, blurred vision, and disorientation. Treatment involves treating the underlying cause, improving tissue oxygenation, restoring ventilation, reducing respiratory rate, and achieving acid-base balance.

Structure and Function of the Circulatory System

The circulatory system delivers oxygen, nutrients, and other substances to bodily tissues to support cellular life. During cellular metabolism, waste products accumulate. The system then removes waste products such as CO_2 and delivers them to the lungs and/or kidneys, where the wastes are eliminated. The pumping action of the heart supports the circulatory system. The four heart valves (tricuspid, pulmonic, mitral, and aortic) ensure the one-way flow of blood through the heart (Fig. 32.3).

Regulation of Blood Flow. There are multiple regulators of blood flow (Table 32.1). The heart muscle (myocardium) relaxes and contracts to support the regulation of blood flow. A cardiac cycle consists of two phases, contraction and relaxation. The contraction phase, also called systole, occurs when blood is ejected from the ventricles into the systemic circulation. The relaxation phase is called diastole, in which blood fills the ventricles.

The amount of blood ejected from the left ventricle each minute is termed **cardiac output (CO)**. A normal CO for a healthy adult is 4 to 8 L/minute. The CO is calculated as follows:

$$\text{Cardiac output (CO)} = \text{Stroke volume (SV)} \times \text{Heart rate (HR)}$$

Stroke volume (SV) is the amount of blood ejected from the ventricle with each contraction. The normal range for a healthy adult is 50 to 75 mL per contraction. Stroke volume is determined by preload, afterload, and myocardial contractility. **Preload** is the amount of blood at the end of ventricular diastole, before the next contraction. **Afterload** is the resistance to the ejection of blood from the left ventricle. The left ventricular pressure must be greater than the peripheral pressure to eject blood from the heart. **Myocardial contractility** is the ability of the heart to squeeze blood from the ventricles and prepare for the next contraction. Contractility is difficult to accurately measure because preload, afterload, and heart rate must remain constant. The heart rate, or beats per minute, is regulated by the sympathetic and parasympathetic systems. Normal limits for heart rate are between 60 and 100 beats/minute. **Cardiac index** is a measure of adequacy of the cardiac output. This calculation gives health care providers a more accurate calculation of cardiac function because it is more patient specific.

Conduction System. The heart's conduction system generates impulses that initiate the electrical/mechanical chain of events for a normal heartbeat. The rhythmic relaxation and contraction of the atria and ventricles depend on continuous, organized transmission of electrical impulses to the muscle. The conduction system generates, controls, and transmits these impulses (Fig. 32.4). The autonomic nervous system influences the rate of impulse generation, the transmission speed through the conductive pathway, and the strength of contractions through sympathetic and parasympathetic

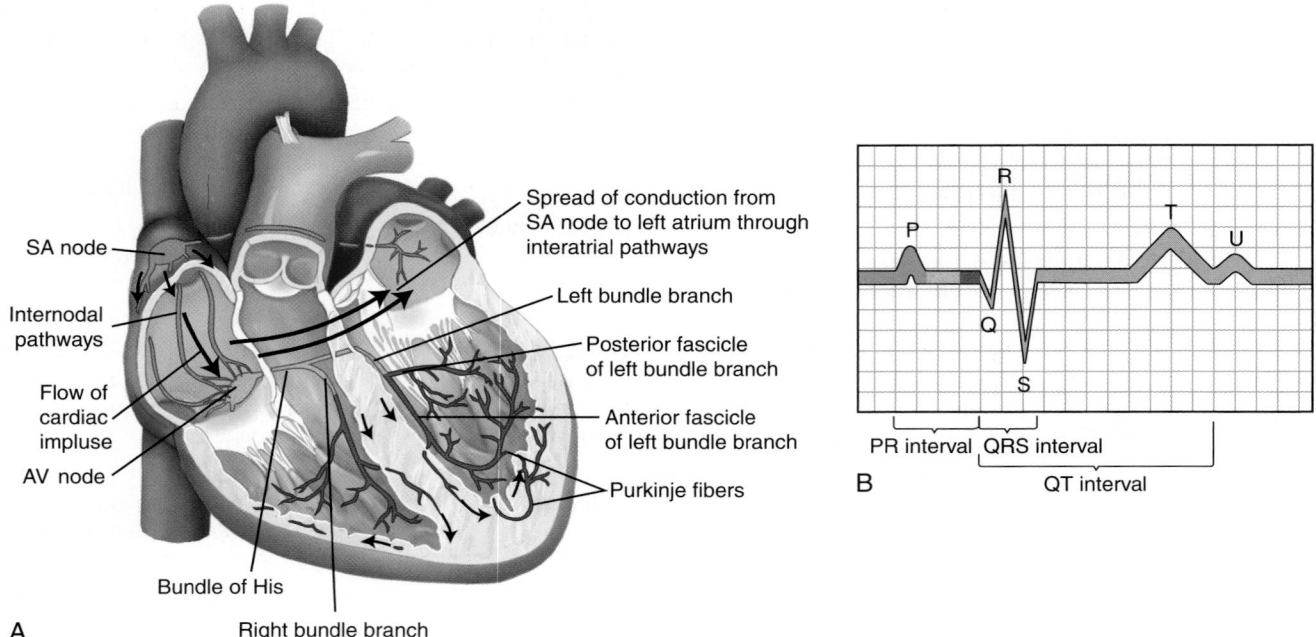

FIG 32.4 Conduction system of the heart. *AV*, Atrioventricular; *LA*, left atrium; *LV*, left ventricle; *RA*, right atrium; *RV*, right ventricle; *SA*, sinoatrial. (From Lewis SM, et al: *Medical surgical nursing: assessment and management of clinical problems*, ed 10, St Louis, 2017, Mosby.)

nerve fibers in the atria and ventricles. The vagus nerve (parasympathetic) also innervates sinoatrial and atrioventricular nodes and is able to reduce the rate of impulse generation.

The conduction system originates with the **sinoatrial (SA) node**, the "pacemaker" of the heart. The SA node is in the right atrium next to the entrance of the superior vena cava. Impulses begin at the SA node at an intrinsic rate of 60 to 100 beats/minute. Electrical impulses travel along interatrial and internodal pathways to the **atrioventricular (AV) node**. The AV node mediates impulse transmission between the atria and the ventricles. Delaying the impulse at the AV node before transmitting it through the bundle of His and ventricular Purkinje network assists atrial emptying.

An electrocardiogram (ECG) records the electrical activity of the conduction system as waves and complexes. An ECG monitors the rate, regularity, and path of the electrical impulse through the conduction system; however, it does not reflect the muscular work of the heart. The normal sequence of electrical impulses on the ECG is called **normal sinus rhythm (NSR)** (see Fig. 32.4). A normal ECG waveform consists of a P wave (atrial **depolarization**), QRS complex (ventricular depolarization), and T wave (ventricular **repolarization**). Depolarization is the electrical event occurring just before contraction of the cardiac chambers, whereas repolarization reflects the period of time when the heart is resting and the chambers are filling. Health care providers interpret the size, appearance, and sequence of waves to identify dysrhythmias and recognize the area of the heart affected.

Alterations of the Circulatory System

Conditions that affect cardiac rate, rhythm, strength of contraction, blood flow through the chambers, myocardial blood flow, and peripheral circulation alter cardiac functioning. Controllable risk factors for heart disease include smoking, hypertension, physical inactivity, obesity, diabetes, alcohol intake, high-fat/high-sodium diets, and high low-density lipoprotein (LDL or "bad cholesterol") levels and low high-density lipoprotein (HDL or "good cholesterol") levels. Uncontrollable risk factors include male gender, family history of heart disease, and ethnicity (Centers for Disease Control and Prevention [CDC], 2015a). Blacks, Caucasians, and Hispanics are at the greatest risk (Mozaffarian et al., 2015). Several genetic disorders lead to an increased risk of early heart attacks.

Decreased Cardiac Output. Failure of the myocardium to eject sufficient cardiac output to the systemic and pulmonary circulations results in heart failure. Failure of the myocardial pump results from primary coronary artery disease (CAD), valvular disorders, cardiomyopathic conditions, congenital heart defects, conduction disorders, and pulmonary disease.

Myocardial Ischemia. Myocardial ischemia occurs when the coronary artery does not supply sufficient blood to the heart muscle (myocardium). This condition results in chest pain, especially with activity. Angina pectoris is the result of decreased blood flow to the myocardium, often as a result of coronary artery spasms or other temporary constriction of the coronary arteries. When decreased myocardial blood perfusion is extensive or perfusion is completely blocked, the tissue becomes necrotic, and **myocardial infarction** occurs. Symptoms of myocardial infarction include severe or crushing chest pain, jaw pain, left arm pain, shortness of breath, and diaphoresis. Some people, particularly women, present with nonspecific symptoms of discomfort, weakness, and fatigue.

Impaired Valvular Function. Valvular heart disease is an acquired or congenital disorder of a cardiac valve characterized by stenosis, which obstructs blood flow, or valvular degeneration and regurgitation, which result in backflow of blood. When stenosis occurs in the aortic and pulmonic valves, the adjacent ventricles work harder to move the ventricular volume beyond the stenotic valve. When regurgitation occurs, there is a backflow of blood into an adjacent chamber, which causes either pulmonary or systemic congestion.

Left-Sided Heart Failure. Left-sided heart failure is characterized by impaired functioning of the left ventricle. It can be further classified as either systolic or diastolic failure. Systolic heart failure is an inability of the ventricle to adequately eject blood. Diastolic heart failure is the inability of the ventricle to relax and fill with blood during diastole. Left-sided heart failure is typically due to hypertension or CAD. In this type of heart failure, blood eventually backs up into the pulmonary veins, causing patients to present with pulmonary symptoms such as crackles on auscultation and complaints of fatigue, dyspnea, and orthopnea (difficulty breathing while lying down) (Lewis et al., 2017).

Right-Sided Heart Failure. Right-sided heart failure results from impaired functioning of the right ventricle, which is typically caused by pulmonary disease or pulmonary hypertension. An increase in pressure in the pulmonary system causes increased resistance in the right ventricle. The right ventricle fails as a result of this pressure. The patient then develops venous congestion in the systemic circulation, and on assessment you often identify distended jugular veins and peripheral edema. Right-sided heart failure may also result from untreated or end-stage left-sided heart failure.

Hypovolemia. Hypovolemia is a reduced circulating blood volume resulting from extracellular fluid losses that occurs in conditions such as shock and severe dehydration. If the fluid loss is significant, the body tries to adapt by increasing the heart rate and constricting peripheral vessels to increase the volume of blood returned to the heart and the cardiac output.

Disturbances in Conduction. A dysrhythmia is a disturbance in the formation or conduction of the heart's electrical impulse. Any rhythm not generated at the SA node is classified as a dysrhythmia. Dysrhythmias are primary conduction disturbances that occur as a response to ischemia, valvular abnormalities, anxiety, and drug toxicity (e.g., digoxin toxicity). Dysrhythmias also occur as a result of excess caffeine, alcohol, or tobacco use; following cardiothoracic surgery; or as a complication of acid-base or electrolyte imbalance, such as altered serum potassium levels (see Chapter 18).

Dysrhythmias are classified by their site of origin and cardiac response (Table 32.2). The cardiac response can be an increase in heart rate such as tachycardia (greater than 100 beats/minute), a decrease in heart rate such as bradycardia (less than 60 beats/minute), premature (early beat) atrial or ventricular beats, or blocked (delayed or absent beat) atrial or ventricular beats. Dysrhythmias often affect the pumping mechanism of the heart.

Factors Affecting Oxygenation

Alterations in oxygenation result from a decrease in oxygen-carrying capacity of blood, decreased inspired oxygen concentration, an increase in the metabolic demands of the body, and any alteration that affects a patient's chest wall movement.

Decreased Oxygen-Carrying Capacity. The Hgb molecule carries 97% of oxygen. Any process that decreases or alters Hgb, such as anemia or inhalation of toxic substances, decreases the oxygen-carrying capacity of blood. Anemia is the reduction in number of RBCs or a decrease in Hgb, the oxygen-carrying protein of RBCs. Acute blood loss or certain chronic diseases can result in anemia.

Carbon monoxide, a colorless and odorless gas, is a common toxic inhalant that decreases the oxygen-carrying capacity of blood. Carbon monoxide has a 230 to 300 times greater affinity for Hgb than oxygen, which can create a functional hypoxemia (Huether and McCance, 2017). Because of the strength of the bond, it is not easy for carbon monoxide to dissociate (break away) from Hgb, making it unavailable for oxygen transport.

Decreased Inspired Oxygen Concentration. When the concentration of inspired oxygen declines, the oxygen-carrying capacity of the blood decreases. An upper or lower airway obstruction limiting delivery of inspired oxygen to alveoli decreases the fraction of inspired oxygen concentration (FiO_2). Decreased environmental oxygen (the effect at high altitudes) or decreased delivery of inspired oxygen (e.g., incorrect oxygen concentration setting on respiratory therapy equipment) results in decreased FiO_2.

Increased Metabolic Rate. Increases in metabolism increase oxygen demand. Oxygen levels fall when the body is unable to meet an increased oxygen demand. An increased metabolism is a normal response of the body to pregnancy, infection, fever, wound healing, and exercise. Most people are able to meet increased oxygen demands and do not display signs of oxygen deprivation.

In patients with increased metabolic rates, CO_2 production also increases. If the condition, such as a fever, lasts for a period of time and the metabolic rate remains high, the body begins to break down protein stores resulting in muscle wasting and decreased muscle mass. Respiratory muscles such as the diaphragm and intercostals are also wasted. The body attempts to adapt to the increased CO_2 (hypercapnia) levels by increasing the rate and depth of respiration to eliminate the excess CO_2. The patient's work of breathing increases,

TABLE 32.2 COMMON BASIC CARDIAC DYSRHYTHMIAS

RHYTHM CHARACTERISTICS	ETIOLOGY	CLINICAL SIGNIFICANCE	MANAGEMENT
Sinus Tachycardia Regular rhythm, rate 100–180 beats/min (higher in infants), normal P wave, normal QRS complex	Rate increase is normal response to exercise; emotion; stressors such as pain, fever, heart failure, hypovolemia, or hyperthyroidism; and certain drugs (e.g., caffeine, nitrates, nicotine).	Patient may be unable to sustain increased workloads (increased myocardial oxygen consumption) brought on by persistent increases in heart rate; reduces myocardial perfusion.	Assess and support ABCs. Check vital signs. Consult health care provider. Correct underlying causative factors; remove offending drugs.
Sinus Bradycardia Regular rhythm, rate less than 60 beats/min, normal P wave, normal P–R interval, normal QRS complex	Rate decrease is normal response to sleep or a well-conditioned athlete; abnormal decreases in rate are caused by diminished blood flow to SA node, vagal stimulation, hypothyroidism, increased intracranial pressure, or certain drugs (e.g., digoxin, beta blockers, calcium channel blockers).	Depends on patient tolerance; has clinical significance when associated with signs of impaired cardiac output and symptoms of weakness, dizziness, hypotension, shortness of breath, syncope, or chest pain.	Assess and support ABCs. Check vital signs. Consult health care provider. Correct underlying causes; prepare for transcutaneous pacing; consider atropine; consider IV epinephrine or dopamine.
Atrial Fibrillation (A-FIB) Irregular atrial activity resulting in irregular ventricular response with resultant irregular cardiac rate and rhythm. No identifiable P wave. Rate determined by conduction of multiple atrial impulses across AV node	Usually due to heart disease (CAD, valvular disease, cardiomyopathy); also due to hypertension, excessive alcohol or caffeine intake, stress, cardiac surgery, or electrolyte imbalances (particularly potassium).	Loss of atrial kick (portion of cardiac output squeezed in the ventricles with a coordinated atrial contraction), pooling of blood in atria, and development of microemboli. Patients complain of fatigue, fluttering in the chest, and shortness of breath if ventricular response is rapid. Patients may have hypotension.	Assess and support ABCs. Check vital signs. Consult health care provider. Goal is to control ventricular rate and convert to normal sinus rhythm; may use pharmacological (amiodarone or ibutilide) or electrical cardioversion (shock delivered during the relative refractory period of cardiac cycle) if no thrombi are present. Prepare for rate control medication therapy such as calcium channel blockers or beta blockers. Treat underlying cause. Will also require blood thinners such as warfarin, dabigatran, apixaban, or rivaroxaban.
Ventricular Tachycardia Rhythm may be regular or irregular; rate 150–250 beats/minute; P wave is difficult to see on ECG, if present; QRS complex wide and bizarre and greater than 0.12 seconds in duration	Caused by irritable ventricular foci firing repetitively; caused by myocardial infarction, severe electrolyte imbalances, drug toxicity, and cardiomyopathy.	Often occurs before ventricular fibrillation; if condition persistent and rapid, causes decreased cardiac output because of decreased ventricular filling time. Patient may or may not have a pulse.	Assess and support ABCDs. Check vital signs. Consult health care provider. Prepare for IV amiodarone and epinephrine. Prepare for synchronized cardioversion (patient with a pulse). Prepare for CPR and unsynchronized cardioversion/defibrillation (patient without a pulse). Treat cause, if possible.

TABLE 32.2 COMMON BASIC CARDIAC DYSRHYTHMIAS—cont'd

RHYTHM CHARACTERISTICS	ETIOLOGY	CLINICAL SIGNIFICANCE	MANAGEMENT
Ventricular Fibrillation			
Irregular and chaotic rhythm with no discernible waves or rate	Usually due to acute MI or cardiomyopathy. Also can be seen in reperfusion after treatment for MI, hypoxemia, acidosis, altered potassium levels, and drug toxicity.	Ventricles are quivering, not pumping. Patient is unresponsive, pulseless, and apneic.	Immediate resuscitation is required. Begin ABCDs. In-hospital goals: Start CPR and defibrillate, preferably with biphasic defibrillator. Prepare to administer IV/IO epinephrine every 3–5 minutes.
Asystole			
Absence of electrical activity; no discernible rate or rhythm	Usually due to advanced cardiac disease.	Cardiac standstill. Patient is unresponsive, pulseless, and apneic.	Always assess rhythm in more than one ECG lead. Immediate resuscitation is required. Begin ABCDs. Initiate CPR. Prepare to administer IV/IO epinephrine every 3–5 minutes. Prepare for possible administration of vasopressin.

ABC, Airway, breathing, circulation; *ABCD*, airway, breathing, circulation, defibrillation; *AED*, automatic external defibrillator; *AV*, atrioventricular; *CAD*, coronary artery disease; *CPR*, cardiopulmonary resuscitation; *ECG*, electrocardiogram; *IO*, intraosseous; *IV*, intravenous; *MI*, myocardial infarction.
Data from Link MS, et al: Part 7: Adult advanced cardiovascular life support: 2015 American Heart Association guidelines update for cardiopulmonary resuscitation and emergency cardiovascular care, *Circulation* 132(suppl 2):s444, 2015; and Lewis S, et al: *Medical-surgical nursing: assessment and management of clinical problems*, ed 9, St Louis, 2017, Elsevier.

and the patient eventually displays signs and symptoms of hypoxemia, such as anxiety and restlessness.

As the hypoxemia worsens some patients develop cardiac dysrhythmias, develop cyanosis, and/or lose consciousness. Patients with pulmonary diseases are at greater risk for hypoxemia and hypercapnia (elevated $PaCO_2$ level). Patient assessments often show an increased rate and depth of respiration along with pursed-lip breathing and use of accessory muscles for respiration.

Conditions Affecting Chest Wall Movement.

Any condition that reduces chest wall movement decreases ventilation. If the diaphragm is unable to fully descend with breathing, the volume of inspired air decreases, delivering less oxygen to the alveoli and subsequently to tissues.

Musculoskeletal Abnormalities. Thoracic abnormalities such as abnormal structural shapes and muscle disease contribute to decreased oxygenation and ventilation. Structural abnormalities impairing oxygenation include conditions that affect the rib cage such as pectus excavatum and those that affect the spinal column such as kyphosis or scoliosis. The angle of curvature in kyphosis or scoliosis can progress with time, resulting in severe hypoventilation and eventual hypoxemia. Muscle diseases such as muscular dystrophy decrease diaphragmatic movement (i.e., the patient's ability to expand and contract the chest). This impairs ventilation

and often causes atelectasis (collapsed alveoli), hypercapnia, and hypoxemia.

Nervous System Diseases. Myasthenia gravis and Guillain-Barré syndrome are examples of nervous system diseases that result in hypoventilation. These diseases impair nervous and muscular control, causing reduced ventilation (hypoventilation).

Disease or trauma involving the brainstem and spinal cord can impair respiration. When the brainstem is affected, neural regulation of respiration is damaged, and abnormal breathing patterns develop. Damage to the spinal cord affects respiration in two ways. If the phrenic nerve is damaged, the diaphragm does not descend, reducing inspiratory lung volumes and causing hypoxemia. Cervical trauma at C3 to C5 levels can paralyze the phrenic nerve. Spinal cord trauma below the fifth cervical vertebra usually leaves the phrenic nerve intact but damages nerves that innervate the intercostal muscles, preventing anteroposterior chest expansion.

Trauma. Trauma to the chest wall also impairs inspiration. The patient with multiple rib fractures sometimes develops a flail chest, a life-threatening condition in which fractures cause instability in part of the chest wall. This causes paradoxical breathing in which the lung underlying the injured area contracts on inspiration and expands on expiration, making ventilation ineffective. Chest wall or upper abdominal incisions also decrease chest wall movement because incisional pain causes patients to inhale shallowly, which decreases chest wall movement.

NURSING KNOWLEDGE BASE

Your nursing knowledge prepares you to anticipate a patient's oxygenation needs. Knowledge of a patient's lifestyle patterns and developmental status allows you to anticipate cardiopulmonary problems.

Developmental Factors

The age and developmental level of a patient as well as the normal aging process can affect tissue oxygenation. Thus you need to identify developmental risk factors in your patients.

Premature Infants. Premature infants are at risk for respiratory distress syndrome, which is caused by surfactant deficiency and immature lung development. Surfactant is a chemical in the lung that maintains the integrity of the alveoli, preventing alveolar collapse. When surfactant is inadequate, infants are unable to keep their alveoli open, which impedes the exchange of respiratory gases. The surfactant-synthesizing ability of the lung develops at about 24 weeks of gestation, but surfactant-producing cells are not fully mature until 36 weeks of gestation. Premature infants are at risk for developing long-term lung issues such as chronic lung disease (bronchopulmonary dysplasia), particularly if they need mechanical ventilation or supplemental oxygen therapy. Premature infants and children younger than 1 year of age are at increased risk for contracting respiratory illnesses such as respiratory syncytial virus (Hockenberry et al., 2017).

Infants and Toddlers. Healthy full-term infants younger than 3 months of age are presumed to have a lower infection rate because of the protective function of maternal antibodies. The infection rate increases in infants from 3 to 6 months of age. Infants and toddlers are at risk for upper respiratory tract infections, especially when they are exposed to second hand smoke or other children. Upper respiratory tract infections are usually not dangerous, and infants and toddlers recover with little difficulty. Infants and toddlers are also at risk for airway obstruction because of their anatomically smaller airways and their tendency to place foreign objects in the mouth (Hockenberry et al., 2017).

School-Age Children and Adolescents. School-age children and adolescents are exposed to respiratory infections and respiratory risk factors such as secondhand smoke and are at risk to experiment with cigarette smoking and other recreational inhalants. A healthy child usually does not have adverse pulmonary effects from respiratory infections. However, a person who starts smoking in adolescence and continues to smoke into middle age has an increased risk for cardiopulmonary disease and lung cancer. School-age children and adolescents possess other cardiopulmonary disease risk factors such as obesity, inactive lifestyles, unhealthy diets, and excessive use of caffeinated or other energy drinks (Hockenberry et al., 2017).

Young and Middle-Age Adults. Young and middle-age adults are exposed to many cardiopulmonary risk factors including an unhealthy diet, lack of exercise, stress, excessive use of highly caffeinated energy drinks, and cigarette smoking. Reducing these modifiable factors sometimes decreases a patient's risk for cardiac or pulmonary diseases. Pregnancy causes changes in ventilation. As the fetus grows during pregnancy, the enlarged the uterus pushes abdominal contents up against the diaphragm. During the last trimester of pregnancy, the inspiratory capacity declines, resulting in dyspnea on exertion and increased fatigue.

Older Adults. The cardiac and pulmonary systems change throughout the aging process (Table 32.3). Normal changes of aging place an older adult at risk for complications in oxygenation, particularly when hospitalized. Older adults are at increased risk for the development of influenza and community-acquired pneumonia, which sometimes results in death. Because of these risks, this age-group should have the pneumonia vaccine and an annual flu vaccine (CDC, 2016b, 2016c).

Lifestyle Factors

Patients are exposed to numerous lifestyle factors that, either alone or in combination, affect cardiopulmonary function. Knowledge of these factors enables a nurse to consider the health promotion needs of patients.

Nutrition. Good nutrition affects cardiopulmonary function by supporting normal metabolic functions. A poor diet leads to risk factors affecting the heart and lungs such as obesity, hypertension, heart disease, and chronic lung disease. Inadequate nutrition occurs when nutritional intake does not meet nutritional needs of the body. Without essential nutrients, a patient may experience respiratory muscle wasting resulting in decreased muscle strength and respiratory excursion. Cough efficiency is reduced secondary to respiratory muscle weakness, putting a patient at risk for retention of pulmonary secretions. A patient with chronic lung disease usually requires a diet higher in calories because of the increased work of breathing. A diet with a moderate amount of carbohydrates is recommended to prevent an increase in CO_2 production.

Obesity affects the respiratory and the cardiovascular systems. Obesity leads to a decrease in lung expansion and an increase in oxygen demand to meet metabolic needs. Diets high in fat increase cholesterol and development of plaque in the coronary arteries, placing individuals at risk for CAD. Patients with nutritional alterations are at risk for anemia. There is a reduction in oxygen-carrying capacity if the diet has insufficient iron needed for Hgb and RBC synthesis.

Hydration. Fluid intake is essential for cellular health. Fluid intake depends on a patient's diet and disease processes

TABLE 32.3	CHANGES IN THE AGING CARDIOPULMONARY SYSTEM	
FUNCTION	**PATHOPHYSIOLOGICAL CHANGE**	**KEY CLINICAL FINDINGS**
Heart		
Muscle contraction	Ventricular wall thickened, collagen increased, and elastin decreased in heart muscle	Signs of decreased cardiac output (edema, shortness of breath, activity intolerance, inability to lie flat for extended time)
Blood flow	Heart valves, especially mitral and aortic valves, become thicker and stiffen	Systolic ejection murmur
Conduction system	SA node becomes fibrotic from calcification; decrease in number of pacemaker cells in SA node	Increased P–R, QRS, and Q–T intervals; decreased amplitude of the QRS complex; tachycardia more poorly tolerated
Arterial vessel compliance	Vessels become calcified; loss of arterial distensibility, decreased elastin in vessel walls, more tortuous vessels	Hypertension, with increase in systolic blood pressure
Lungs		
Breathing mechanics	Decreased chest wall compliance and loss of elastic recoil Decreased respiratory muscle mass and strength	Prolonged exhalation phase Decreased vital capacity and activity intolerance Decreased ability to clear secretions
Oxygenation	Decreased alveolar surface area, as alveoli are more fibrous and decreased CO_2 diffusion capacity	Decreased PaO_2 Slightly increased $PaCO_2$
Breathing control/ breathing pattern	Decreased responsiveness of central and peripheral chemoreceptors to hypoxemia and hypercapnia	Decreased tidal volume Increased respiratory rate
Lung defense mechanisms	Decreased number of cilia Decreased IgA production and humoral and cellular immunity Drier mucous membranes	Decreased airway clearance Increased risk for infection
Sleep and breathing	Decreased respiratory drive Decreased tone of upper airway muscles	Increased risk for aspiration and infection Snoring/obstructive sleep apnea

CO_2, Carbon dioxide; *IgA,* immunoglobulin A; *PaCO_2,* partial pressure of carbon dioxide; *PaO_2,* partial pressure of oxygen; *SA,* sinoatrial.
Data from Ball J, et al: *Seidel's guide to physical examination,* ed 9, St Louis, 2015, Elsevier; and Touhy T, Jett K: *Gerontological nursing and healthy aging,* ed 5, St Louis, 2018 Elsevier.

that require more or less water. Fluid volume overload or hypervolemia may lead to vascular congestion in patients with heart, kidney, or lung diseases. Dehydration or fluid volume deficit may result in dizziness, fainting, hypotension, a decrease in respiratory secretion production, or a thickening of respiratory secretions making it difficult for a patient to expectorate secretions.

Exercise. Exercise increases metabolic activity and oxygen demand of the body. The rate and depth of respiration increase, enabling a person to inhale more oxygen and exhale excess CO_2. A physical exercise program has many benefits (see Chapter 28). People who exercise daily for 30 to 60 minutes have a lower heart rate, lower blood pressure, decreased cholesterol, increased blood flow, and greater oxygen extraction by working muscles. The addition of weight training decreases the work of the heart by increasing the efficiency of the other muscles of the body.

Cigarette Smoking. Cigarette smoking is associated with heart disease, COPD, and lung cancer. Inhaled nicotine enables plaque to build up more quickly in the blood vessels, increases the risks for blood clot formation, and causes

vasoconstriction in the coronary and peripheral vessels. The risk for lung cancer is 15 to 30 times greater for a person who smokes than for a nonsmoker. Exposure to secondhand smoke increases the risk for lung cancer in a person who does not smoke and worsens other pulmonary problems such as asthma or COPD (CDC, 2016a).

Substance Abuse. Excessive use of alcohol and other drugs impairs tissue oxygenation. A patient who has chronic substance abuse usually has a poor nutritional intake that often causes a decreased intake of iron-rich foods leading to a decrease in Hgb production. Excessive use of alcohol and drugs such as barbiturates depresses the respiratory center, reducing the rate and depth of respiration and the amount of inhaled oxygen. Substances that are inhaled or smoked directly injure lung tissue, leading to permanent lung damage and impaired oxygenation. IV drug use places a person at risk for infections of the heart (endocarditis or myocarditis), blood clots, and transmitted diseases such as human immunodeficiency virus (HIV) and hepatitis.

Stress. Stress is a perceived threat that results in sympathetic stimulation (the fight-or-flight response). It often poses a demand that exceeds a patient's coping ability both physically and emotionally (see Chapter 26). Continuous stress adversely affects a patient's health and well-being. A continuous state of stress increases the metabolic rate and oxygen demand of the body. The body responds to stress by an increased rate and depth of respiration and increased cardiac output. Stressors also alter the normal response to illness and pain. Stress causes an increased release of cortisol, which affects the metabolism of fat and creates a risk for CAD and hypertension. Stressors are also often triggers for asthma attacks. Most people are able to adapt to physical or emotional stressors. Some patients, particularly patients with chronic illnesses or acute life-threatening illnesses, cannot tolerate the oxygen demands associated with stress.

Environmental Factors

The environment also influences oxygenation. The incidence of pulmonary disease is higher in smoggy, urban areas than in rural areas. In addition, a patient's workplace sometimes increases the risks for cardiopulmonary disease. Occupational pollutants include asbestos, talcum powder, dust, and airborne fibers. For example, tunnel workers exposed to dust from blasting, drilling, and rock transport have an increased risk for developing COPD. Construction workers may be at risk for asbestosis from asbestos exposure. This exposure leads to pulmonary fibrosis, a restrictive lung disease, and may lead to lung cancer.

CRITICAL THINKING

Synthesis

Patient care requires you to apply what you know about a patient, your knowledge base, experience, and critical thinking attitudes and standards. Your synthesis of this information allows you to make sound decisions as you apply the nursing process. Critical thinking synthesis involves combining all available information to obtain a clear picture of the approach needed to provide patient-centered care (Box 32.1).

Knowledge. When caring for patients with cardiopulmonary problems, you need to incorporate and apply knowledge and principles from physiology and pathophysiology; pharmacology; nutrition; and fluid, electrolyte, and acid-base balance. You will apply this knowledge in your interventions for health promotion and disease prevention. This knowledge prevents or helps to reduce at-risk behaviors and unhealthy lifestyles in your patients who are at risk for or have cardiopulmonary problems. This knowledge also allows you to anticipate clinical changes in patients in all situations. Also use knowledge from communication and patient education principles to deliver patient education.

Experience. In the acute care setting you care for patients with new or acute exacerbations of disease. When your patients require nursing management in the community or outpatient setting, they are usually stable, productive members of the community with little or no change in lifestyle. Use

---

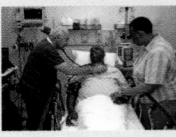

BOX 32.1 **SYNTHESIS IN PRACTICE**

John's knowledge of the physiology of pulmonary conditions helps him care for Mr. King. Mr. King's history reveals risk factors (alcohol abuse, sedentary lifestyle) and a 40-year history of smoking 2 packs per day; he still continues to smoke. John knows that the current increase in Mr. King's shortness of breath is due to his respiratory infection. The secretions are obstructing his alveolar capillary membrane, preventing oxygenation of blood in some parts of his lung. Because of John's experience working with patients who are addicted to inhaled nicotine, he recognizes the difficulty in quitting smoking. He knows that for some patients, the most effective time to encourage them to stop smoking is when they are in an acute care setting with an illness exacerbated by smoking. He knows that the education should also focus on Mrs. King, as she also smokes. John recognizes it is easier to quit smoking in a house in which no one else smokes. The acute phase is sometimes not the best time to educate patients and families about smoking cessation. John plans to assess both Mr. and Mrs. King about their readiness to receive smoking cessation education and desire to actually stop smoking.

John's attitude about his nursing care reflects his respect for the patient's autonomy and balances this with continually educating Mr. King about the risk factors of smoking. John knows the benefit of support systems in helping patients cope with chronic illnesses. He uses creativity and independent thinking to incorporate community and family resources into the plan of care. John will inquire about Mr. King's social supports and the availability of community programs to help him quit smoking. He reviews the standards set by the American Cancer Society to identify that tobacco use accounts for at least 32% of all cancer deaths and 83% of lung cancer deaths in men. He uses these facts and the resources at http://www.cancer.org to educate Mr. King and his wife about cancer statistics and methods to quit smoking.

---

your experience in caring for patients with cardiopulmonary diseases to recognize clinical changes and select effective interventions, especially lifestyle modifications that reduce cardiopulmonary risk factors.

Attitudes. You use critical thinking attitudes as you provide nursing care for patients with cardiopulmonary alterations. As a patient's advocate, determine if the patient is aware of his or her risk factors and then partner with the patient to find the best teaching approaches to reinforce learning or provide instruction. Do not be judgmental. Use discipline when providing health care information to your patients. For example, when deciding on the approach for a patient who has respiratory disease and still smokes, determine the patient's motivation to quit and preferred learning style.

Perseverance is also important in finding effective patient-centered solutions. For example, when a patient has severe cardiac disease and limited income, your solutions for promoting health and maintaining patient independence are complex. Sometimes you need to continue to provide the same information at each clinic visit. Often patients with chronic hypoxemia have a decreased short-term memory, and you need to reinforce information previously provided. Consider involving family caregivers as needed.

Standards. Nationally recognized organizations set forth best practices. The American Heart Association (AHA), American Lung Association (ALA), American Thoracic Society (ATS), American Cancer Society (ACS), American Association for Respiratory Care (AARC), Respiratory Nursing Society (RNS), and Agency for Healthcare Research and Quality (AHRQ) have specific guidelines for cardiopulmonary nursing care and disease management. The American Nurses Association (ANA) also has guidelines and standards for patient care. Each of these organizations reviews best practice standards and publishes its findings. Knowledge of the evidence that supports your practice enables you to provide safe and effective nursing care.

You use professional standards in the care of all patients. *In the care of Mr. King in the case study, these standards help to determine the appropriate medical and nursing interventions for a patient with pneumonia and COPD.*

NURSING PROCESS

■■■ ASSESSMENT

During assessment, thoroughly assess each patient and critically analyze findings to ensure that you make patient-centered clinical decisions for safe patient care.

Nursing History. The nursing history focuses on your patient's ability to meet oxygen needs and control symptoms. Ask questions that help a patient describe symptoms. Box 32.2 gives examples of assessment questions for you to ask your patient with cardiopulmonary conditions.

Risk Factors. Investigate familial, occupational, and environmental risk factors. Review the patient's family history of cardiovascular or lung disease. Document which blood relatives have cardiopulmonary disease, the type of condition, and their present level of health or age at time of death. Other family risk factors to assess include the presence of infectious diseases, particularly tuberculosis (TB). Determine who in the patient's household has the disease and the status of the treatment.

Exposure to certain inhaled environmental substances such as smog, cotton dust, silicon, mold, cockroaches, secondhand smoke, and asbestos is closely linked to respiratory disease. Investigate exposures in the patient's home and workplace. Ask the following questions:

- Are there environmental conditions that affect your breathing where you work?
- Have you recently traveled to countries or areas of the United States where you have been exposed to uncommon respiratory diseases?
- What is/was your occupation? Were you exposed to chemicals or inhalants?

| BOX 32.2 | **NURSING ASSESSMENT QUESTIONS** |

NATURE OF CARDIOPULMONARY PROBLEM
- Tell me the types of breathing problems you are having.
- Describe the problem you are having with your heart. Is there pain? Do you notice abnormal beats?
- Does this problem occur at a specific time during the day, after exercise, or all the time?

QUESTIONS TO ASK ASSOCIATED WITH BREATHING
- How has your breathing pattern changed?
- On a scale of 0 to 10, with 10 being the most severe, rate your shortness of breath.
- What helps your shortness of breath?
- Do you have a cough? Is the coughing increasing? Is it worse at a certain time of day?
- Describe your cough. Is it dry or moist?
- Are you having sputum or phlegm with coughing? What does it look like? Is this different? If so, when did you notice the change?

QUESTIONS TO ASK RELATED TO CHEST PAIN
- Are you having any chest pain? Show me where the pain is located. Does it occur with breathing in, breathing out, or both?
- What do you think causes the pain, and how long does it last? Is this a different type of pain? Does it occur with activity?
- On a scale of 0 to 10, with 0 being no pain and 10 the most severe pain, rate your chest pain at its worst. Is the severity of your pain different today?
- What do you do for this pain? Does it make the pain better?

QUESTIONS TO ASK REGARDING PREDISPOSING FACTORS
- Have you been around another person who had a cold, flu, or other respiratory illness?
- Tell me the medications you are taking. Are you taking any over-the-counter medications or any supplements? What are these?
- Do you smoke? If so, how much
- Have you been exposed to secondhand smoke?

QUESTIONS TO ASK REGARDING EFFECT OF SYMPTOMS ON PATIENT
- Tell me how these symptoms affect your daily activities. What effect do these symptoms have on your appetite, sleeping, and activity?

Assess for other risk factors such as exercise habits, presence and frequency of stress, tobacco use, and diet. Ask a patient to record what is eaten over 1 week to assess dietary habits and types of food eaten.

Fatigue. Fatigue is a subjective sensation reported as a loss of endurance. It is a common sign of prolonged exposure to stress and is often an early sign of worsening of an existing chronic cardiopulmonary disease. A visual analog scale is useful to objectively measure fatigue (see Chapter 34). Have patients rate their fatigue from 0 to 10, with 10 being the worst level of fatigue and 0 being no fatigue. Ask your patients the following questions about their perception of fatigue:

- When did you first notice the fatigue? What makes it get better or worse?
- Was the onset sudden or gradual? Is it related to any time of the day or is it constant throughout the day?
- In what way does the fatigue affect what you want to do?

Pain. Pain originating in the heart does not occur with respiratory variations. It is most often substernal and typically radiates to the left arm and jaw in men. Some women as well as some men have epigastric pain, complaints of indigestion, nausea or vomiting, or a choking feeling and dyspnea. Pericardial pain resulting from an inflammation of the pericardial sac is usually nonradiating and often occurs with inspiration or when lying supine. See Chapter 34 for pain assessment.

Pleuritic chest pain is peripheral and usually radiates to the scapular regions. Inspiratory maneuvers such as coughing, yawning, and sighing aggravate pleuritic chest pain. An inflammation or infection in the pleural space usually causes pleuritic chest pain. Patients often describe it as knifelike or sharp, and it increases in intensity with inspiration. Musculoskeletal pain is often present following exercise, rib trauma, and prolonged coughing episodes. Inspiratory movements aggravate the pain and are easily confused with pleuritic chest pain. When assessing pain in patients with cardiopulmonary disease, obtain information specific to cardiac or inspiratory pain (see Box 32.2)

Breathing Patterns. Dyspnea can be a subjective feeling of breathlessness as reported by the patient, or it can be observable labored breathing with shortness of breath (Ball et al., 2015). It is a clinical sign of hypoxia and/or hypoxemia. Dyspnea is associated with symptoms such as exaggerated respiratory effort, use of the accessory muscles of respiration, nasal flaring, and marked increases in the rate and depth of respirations. Collect data about your patient's breathing patterns. Use a visual analog scale to help patients objectively assess their perception of dyspnea (see Box 32.2). This will help to show change in a patient's breathlessness over time.

Dyspnea that occurs when a patient is sleeping is called paroxysmal nocturnal dyspnea (PND). The patient awakens in a panic, feels as if he or she is suffocating, and has a strong need to sit up to relieve the breathlessness. The cause of PND is probably resorption of fluid from dependent body areas when the patient is recumbent or reclining (Lewis et al., 2017).

Orthopnea is an abnormal condition in which a patient has difficulty breathing when lying down and has to use multiple pillows or to sit to breathe. The number of pillows required for sleep (e.g., two or three) quantifies the presence and severity of orthopnea.

Wheezing is not a breathing pattern but is a high-pitched musical sound caused by high-velocity movement of air through a narrowed airway. It is present in asthma, acute bronchitis, or pneumonia. It occurs on inspiration, expiration, or both. Determine any precipitating factors such as respiratory infection, allergens, exercise, or stress.

Cough. Cough is a sudden, audible expulsion of air from the lungs. Coughing is a protective reflex to clear the trachea, bronchi, and lungs of irritants and secretions. Some patients with chronic sinusitis cough only in the early morning, while trying to sleep, or immediately after rising from sleep. This clears the airway of sputum resulting from sinus drainage. Patients with chronic bronchitis generally produce sputum all day, although the body produces greater amounts after rising from a semi-recumbent or flat position. A productive cough produces sputum that is swallowed or expectorated. Collect data about the type, color, and quantity of sputum.

If a patient reports hemoptysis (bloody sputum), determine the source. Is it associated with coughing and bleeding from the upper respiratory tract, from sinus drainage, or from the gastrointestinal tract (hematemesis)? Describe the hemoptysis including amount, color, duration of bleeding, and presence of sputum. When hemoptysis develops, note if the patient is on anticoagulants.

Respiratory Infections. Determine if your patient has had a pneumococcal, pertussis, or flu vaccine in the past. Determine if the patient is on immunomodulators or immunosuppressant therapy or has a chronic lung disease because these patients are at higher risk of developing respiratory infections. Ask about any known exposure to TB and the results of the tuberculin skin test including type of test and date. Some patients with a history of IV drug use, blood transfusions, multiple unprotected sex partners, or a homosexual lifestyle are at a higher risk for developing HIV/acquired immunodeficiency syndrome (AIDS) infection. Patients with HIV/AIDS or in other immunocompromised states are at an increased risk of contracting a respiratory infection.

Medication Use. Assess your patient's knowledge and ability to correctly take medication (see Chapter 17). Include a family caregiver in your assessment if the caregiver assists with medication preparation or administration. Review what the patient understands about medication side effects and what or when to report to the health care provider.

Many herbals and over-the-counter (OTC) medications affect the heart rate and blood pressure and promote blood thinning. For example, the herb ma huang, a naturally occurring ephedrine, increases blood pressure and heart rate. Patients with cardiopulmonary disease should not use this herb. Patients with asthma should not use ephedrine-containing herbs because they can cause increased bronchospasm and respiratory arrest. Ginseng, garlic capsules, and *Ginkgo biloba* have properties similar to those of aspirin and decrease platelet aggregation, increasing the patient's risk for bleeding.

Illicit drugs often come diluted with talcum powder. This mixture causes pulmonary disorders resulting from the irritant effect of talcum powder on lung tissues.

Older Adult Considerations. The older adult has a wide range of normal heart rate, from the 40s to more than 100 beats/minute (Ball et al., 2015). When assessing older adults, additional assessment areas include functional and cognitive status, caregiver stress, patterns of health and health care, advanced directive and care planning, and the presence of geriatric syndromes (e.g., delirium, falls, dizziness, syncope, urinary incontinence). Other areas of assessment include sexual function, depression, alcoholism, hearing loss, and environmental safety (Touhy and Jett, 2018). Table 32.3 reviews factors that place older adults at increased risk for respiratory infections.

Patient Expectations. Knowing what a patient expects regarding his or her health and disease maintenance determines short-term and long-term needs and goals of care and the interventions needed to achieve the needs and goals. Knowing what a patient expects also helps you find appropriate educational tools and resources for the patient and family to use while at home. Determine what your patient expects from health care providers and other caregivers. Develop trust with patients and family caregivers and encourage them to be active participants in the development of a treatment plan.

Physical Examination. The physical examination includes a detailed, organized, and systematic evaluation of the entire cardiopulmonary system (Tables 32.4 to 32.6) (see Chapter 16). Be mindful of your patient's limitations such as breathlessness or fatigue. In some cases you have to complete your assessment in short sections to allow the patient to rest and recover. If your patient is breathless or fatigued, you may ask closed-ended questions with yes or no answers. Focus your initial assessment on your patient's immediate problems (Table 32.7).

Diagnostic Tests. Diagnostic tests determine adequacy of the cardiac conduction system, myocardial contraction, and blood flow. Tests measure the adequacy of ventilation and oxygenation and visualize structures of the respiratory and cardiac system. Some patients need an ECG, chest radiographic examination, pulse oximetry, laboratory tests (e.g., arterial blood gas levels, complete blood count, sputum analysis, cardiac enzyme levels), cardiac stress test, pulmonary function test, and cardiac catheterization.

TB skin testing is important to determine exposure to TB (CDC, 2016d). Patients from foreign countries often have received bacille Calmette-Guérin (BCG) vaccinations to prevent TB and will have a positive TB skin test. Testing in patients with altered immune function (e.g., older adults, HIV-positive patients, and patients undergoing chemotherapy) is less reliable. Health care providers will often use blood testing instead because it is more reliable in patients who have received BCG vaccinations. Chapter 17 describes the technique and what to evaluate for TB skin testing.

Many patients will have an initial chest radiographic examination if their TB skin test is positive. Repeat chest radiographs are recommended only if a patient develops symptoms such as hemoptysis, weight loss, fatigue, or night sweats. Definitive diagnosis depends on the presence of tubercle bacilli in the patient's sputum.

TABLE 32.4	INSPECTION OF CARDIOPULMONARY STATUS
ABNORMALITY	**CAUSE**
Eyes	
Xanthelasma (yellow lipid lesions in nasal portion of upper or lower eyelid)	Hyperlipidemia; abnormal lipid metabolism
Petechiae on conjunctivae	Bacterial endocarditis or bleeding disorder
Skin	
Peripheral cyanosis	Vasoconstriction and diminished blood flow; hypoxemia
Central cyanosis	Hypoxemia and/or hypoxia (late sign)
Decreased skin turgor	Dehydration (normal finding in older adults as a result of decreased skin elasticity)
Dependent edema	Heart failure
Fingertips and Nail Beds	
Cyanosis	Decreased cardiac output or hypoxia; sometimes the result of decreased circulation to affected limb or vasoconstriction secondary to cold
Splinter hemorrhages	Bacterial endocarditis
Clubbing of fingertips	Chronic hypoxemia
Mouth and Lips	
Cyanotic mucous membranes	Decreased oxygenation (hypoxia) **Note:** Lips may be more bluish in color in people with darker skin. This is a normal finding.
Pursed-lip breathing	Chronic lung disease; increased respiratory effort
Pallor	Anemia
Neck Veins	
Distention	Heart failure (typically right-sided); fluid overload
Nose	
Flaring nares	Respiratory distress; dyspnea; hypoxia
Nasal discharge	Color indicates allergy versus infection
Chest	
Barrel chest	COPD; may be a normal finding in older adults
Breathing pattern	Multiple (see Table 32.5)

COPD, Chronic obstructive pulmonary disease.
Data from Ball J, et al: *Seidel's guide to physical examination,* ed 9, St Louis, 2015, Elsevier; and Lewis S, et al: *Medical-surgical nursing: assessment and management of clinical problems,* ed 9, St Louis, 2017, Mosby.

TABLE 32.5 ASSESSMENT OF ABNORMAL CHEST WALL MOVEMENT

ABNORMALITY	CAUSE
Asymmetry: Unequal expansion of lungs	Chest wall injury; collapsed lung
Retraction: Visible sinking in soft tissues of chest that lie between and around firmer tissue (e.g., cartilage and bony ribs); retractions have specific beginning point and worsening, with need for increased inspiratory effort; possibly found at intercostal space, intraclavicular space, trachea, and substernally[a]	Any condition that causes increased inspiratory effort (e.g., airway obstruction, asthma, tracheobronchitis)
Paradoxical breathing: Asynchronous breathing; chest contraction during inspiration and expansion during expiration	Flail chest

[a]Infants can experience sternal and substernal retractions with only slight inspiratory effort because of chest pliability.

TABLE 32.6 RESPIRATORY PATTERNS

TYPE/PATTERN	RATE	CLINICAL SIGNIFICANCE
Eupnea	12–20 breaths/min	Normal rate in adult
Tachypnea	Greater than 20 breaths/min	Results from anxiety, pain, fever, respiratory infection, or other causes that lead to respiratory distress; can lead to respiratory alkalosis, paresthesia, tetany, and confusion
Bradypnea	Less than 10 breaths/min	Results from sleep, narcotic or sedative drug overdose, or CNS lesion; can lead to respiratory acidosis, disorientation, somnolence, and coma
Apnea	Periods of no respiration lasting greater than 20 seconds	Sometimes intermittent such as in sleep apnea or prolonged as in a respiratory arrest; sleep apnea can be treated with home CPAP; respiratory arrest needs emergency treatment
Kussmaul	Usually greater than 35 breaths/min	Breaths deep in nature; associated with metabolic acidosis states such as diabetic ketoacidosis
Cheyne-Stokes	Periods of increasing depths of breathing followed by period of apnea	Seen in seriously ill patients, typically with brain injury or drug-associated respiratory distress; may be seen in children and older adults during sleep
Ataxic or Biot	Irregular respirations of varying depths with irregular periods of apnea	Poor prognosis; associated with severe brain injury

CNS, Central nervous system; *CPAP,* continuous positive airway pressure.
Adapted from Ball J, et al: *Seidel's guide to physical examination,* ed 9, St Louis, 2015, Mosby.

TABLE 32.7 FOCUSED PATIENT ASSESSMENT

FACTORS TO ASSESS	QUESTIONS	PHYSICAL ASSESSMENT
Breathing pattern	When do you become short of breath? When lying down or after activities? Are you able to do your own personal hygiene without getting tired? How far can you walk without getting short of breath? How many pillows do you use to sleep at night?	Observe breathing pattern. Observe patient perform activities of daily living. Observe for use of pursed-lip breathing. Observe patient ambulating. Determine distance walked without shortness of breath. Observe patient's breathing patterns in different positions.
Airway patency	How often do you cough? Do you bring up any mucus when coughing? What does it look like? Is there anything that brings on your cough?	Monitor sputum for color, consistency, amount, and odor.
Chest pain	Do you have any chest pain? Is the pain only since you developed a fever? Is the pain worse when you breathe in?	Patient report of pain score on a visual analog scale of 0–10. Presence of splinting or grimacing, particularly with inspiration or deep breaths.

NURSING DIAGNOSIS

A patient with an altered level of oxygenation often has nursing diagnoses that are associated with conditions of cardiovascular or pulmonary origin. You base each problem-focused or health promotion nursing diagnosis on specific defining characteristics and include the related etiology. For risk diagnoses, base your diagnosis on risk factors (see Chapter 9).

During the assessment process you collect data that accurately reflects a patient's needs. For example, your objective findings in a patient who comes to the clinic with a diagnosis of pneumonia include nonproductive cough, breathlessness, crackles, tachypnea, shallow respirations, and pleuritic pain. These findings support the problem-focused diagnosis of *Ineffective Airway Clearance related to the presence of tracheobronchial secretions.*

Another example of a nursing diagnosis related to a patient with pneumonia is *Activity Intolerance related to imbalance between oxygen supply and demand.* The objective findings include crackles, nonproductive cough, restlessness, tachycardia, use of accessory muscles, and hypoxemia (PaO_2 less than 60 mm Hg). The subjective findings include the patient stating that he or she feels more short of breath with any sort of activity. Identifying the appropriate related factor, such as an imbalance between oxygen supply and demand, enables you to design nursing interventions (e.g., exercise strategies) to maximize the balance between a patient's oxygen supply and demand.

Possible nursing diagnoses for patients with oxygenation alterations include, but are not limited to, the following:

- *Activity Intolerance*
- *Ineffective Airway Clearance*
- *Ineffective Breathing Pattern*
- *Decreased Cardiac Output*
- *Fatigue*
- *Impaired Gas Exchange*
- *Risk for Infection*
- *Ineffective Peripheral Tissue Perfusion*

PLANNING

Goals and Outcomes. Patients with impaired oxygenation require patient-centered nursing care plans that are directed toward meeting their actual or potential oxygenation needs. Oxygenation goals for your patient often include having a patent airway, improving oxygenation, and increasing the level of independence and tolerance for activity (see Care Plan).

All goals must have measurable outcomes for you to determine whether they have been met. These include objective data such as oxygen saturation levels, laboratory and physical assessment findings, and vital signs. Quantify subjective findings such as the reported degree of breathlessness or pain on visual analog scales.

Patients have more than one nursing diagnosis, and often these diagnoses have an impact on one another (Fig. 32.5). It is important to include the patient and family caregiver in all care planning. Alterations in oxygenation are often chronic problems that affect the patient and family. The patient remains a member of the community despite the illness. Planning with the family and using community resources help patients adapt to activities of daily living.

Setting Priorities. A patient's clinical condition determines which nursing diagnosis takes priority while you care for the patient. For example, a patient who is short of breath and exhibiting signs and symptoms of *Impaired Gas Exchange* while sitting in a chair will not tolerate ambulating in the hallway, and this diagnosis takes priority over *Activity Intolerance*. A patient who reports a pleuritic chest pain score of 7 on a visual analog scale needs treatment of *Acute Pain* before you ask the patient to cough and clear the airways to address the problem of *Ineffective Airway Clearance*.

Collaborative Care. Impaired levels of oxygenation affect all aspects of your patient's life, not just the physical component. Planning care for a patient with a disturbance in oxygenation requires collaboration with other members of the health care team such as physical and occupational therapists and cardiac rehabilitation specialists. The respiratory therapist designs measures to improve breathing and cough control. Base your decision to delegate responsibility to nursing assistive personnel (NAP) on your assessment of the patient and the type of care he or she requires. Consider which tasks are safe to delegate and within the skill set of the NAP and how the patient will feel about the care that you have delegated. The priority is to maintain or improve the patient's oxygenation and meet the patient's needs. You are ultimately responsible for all total patient care.

When planning care for patients with impaired oxygenation, particularly as they transition to home, be sensitive to the needs of both the patient and the family. Chronic illness changes the dynamics of family relationships. Sometimes roles need to change, and the patient and family have difficulty coping. Provide an empathetic ear to both family members and the patient. Help them develop solutions that maintain the dignity of all parties and continue to support the family unit. Case managers or social service workers are often able to help patients and families identify and connect with community resources that offer support.

IMPLEMENTATION

Nursing interventions for patients with oxygenation alterations are diverse. Patients' cultural and religious beliefs may affect the selection of interventions (Box 32.3). Health promotion activities may result in healthier lifestyle habits. Symptom management aids in reducing the severity of cardiopulmonary problems. Interventions aimed at improving respiration and ventilation make it easier for patients to breathe.

◎ CARE PLAN

Oxygenation

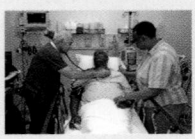

ASSESSMENT

John Smith begins his morning care for Mr. King, who is restless and anxious. He complains of difficulty breathing.

ASSESSMENT ACTIVITIES

Ask Mr. King how long he has had difficulty breathing.

Observe patient behaviors.
Auscultate Mr. King's lung fields.

Ask Mr. King to produce a sputum sample.

[a]**Defining characteristics/risk factors** are shown in **bold** type.

FINDINGS[a]

He replies, "My breathing has gotten worse over the past week." His vital signs are pulse rate 120 beats/min, temperature 102° F orally, **respiratory rate 36 breaths/min,** blood pressure 110/45 mm Hg, and **SpO$_2$ of 82%** on room air.
Patient is **restless** and **is short of breath when talking.**
On auscultation there are audible expiratory wheezes, crackles, and **diminished breath sounds** over right lower lobe.
Sputum is thick, **copious,** and discolored (yellow-green).

NURSING DIAGNOSIS: Ineffective Airway Clearance related to retained pulmonary secretions

---

PLANNING

GOAL

Pulmonary secretions will return to baseline levels within 24 to 36 hours.
Mr. King's oxygenation status will improve in 36 hours.

EXPECTED OUTCOMES (NOC)[b]

Respiratory Status: Gas Exchange

Mr. King's sputum will become less in amount, clear, white, and thinner in consistency within 36 hours.
Adventitious lung sounds will begin to clear within 24 hours.
Mr. King's respiratory rate will return to normal values.
Mr. King will clear airway secretions with coughing in 24 hours.
Mr. King's perceptions of dyspnea will improve within 24 hours.

[b]Outcome classification labels from Moorhead S, et al, editors: *Nursing outcomes classification (NOC),* ed 5, St Louis, 2013, Mosby.

INTERVENTIONS (NIC)[c]

Airway Management

Have Mr. King deep breathe and try to perform huff cough every 2 hours while awake. If patient is unable to cough, suction orally or nasopharyngeally.
Elevate the head of the bed 30 to 45 degrees. Encourage Mr. King to change positions frequently and to ambulate and sit in chair, according to early mobility protocol.

Encourage Mr. King to increase his fluid intake to at least 2000 mL/24 hours if his cardiac condition does not contraindicate it.
Avoid caffeinated beverages and alcohol; recommend water.

RATIONALE

Helps expectorate sputum; promotes gas exchange.

Elevating the head of the bed encourages better lung expansion, thereby promoting better gas exchange (Munro and Ruggiero, 2014). Mobilization facilitates expectoration of respiratory secretions (Lewis et al., 2017).
Fluids help hydrate patient and help reduce fever and dry mucous membranes and may help patient effectively expectorate secretions (Hong and Galvagno, 2013).
Caffeinated and alcoholic beverages promote diuresis and dehydration.

[c]Intervention classification labels from Bulechek GM, et al, editors: *Nursing interventions classification (NIC),* ed 6, St Louis, 2013, Mosby.

EVALUATION

NURSING ACTIONS	PATIENT RESPONSE/FINDING	ACHIEVEMENT OF OUTCOME
Auscultate chest.	Lung sounds are clear.	Outcome met.
Ask Mr. King how often he coughs and deep breathes.	Mr. King has completed a diary that shows he has been coughing and deep breathing every 2 hours while awake 85% of the time.	Mr. King is able to clear airways with coughing. Secretions are thin, and there is no evidence of infection. Outcome met.
Check flow sheet for recent vital signs.	Mr. King's last set of vital signs show heart rate 98 beats/minute, respiratory rate 20 breaths/minute, oral temperature 98.6° F, blood pressure 112/62 mm Hg, and SpO$_2$ 95% on room air.	Mr. King's vital signs are within normal limits. Outcome met.

CONCEPT MAP

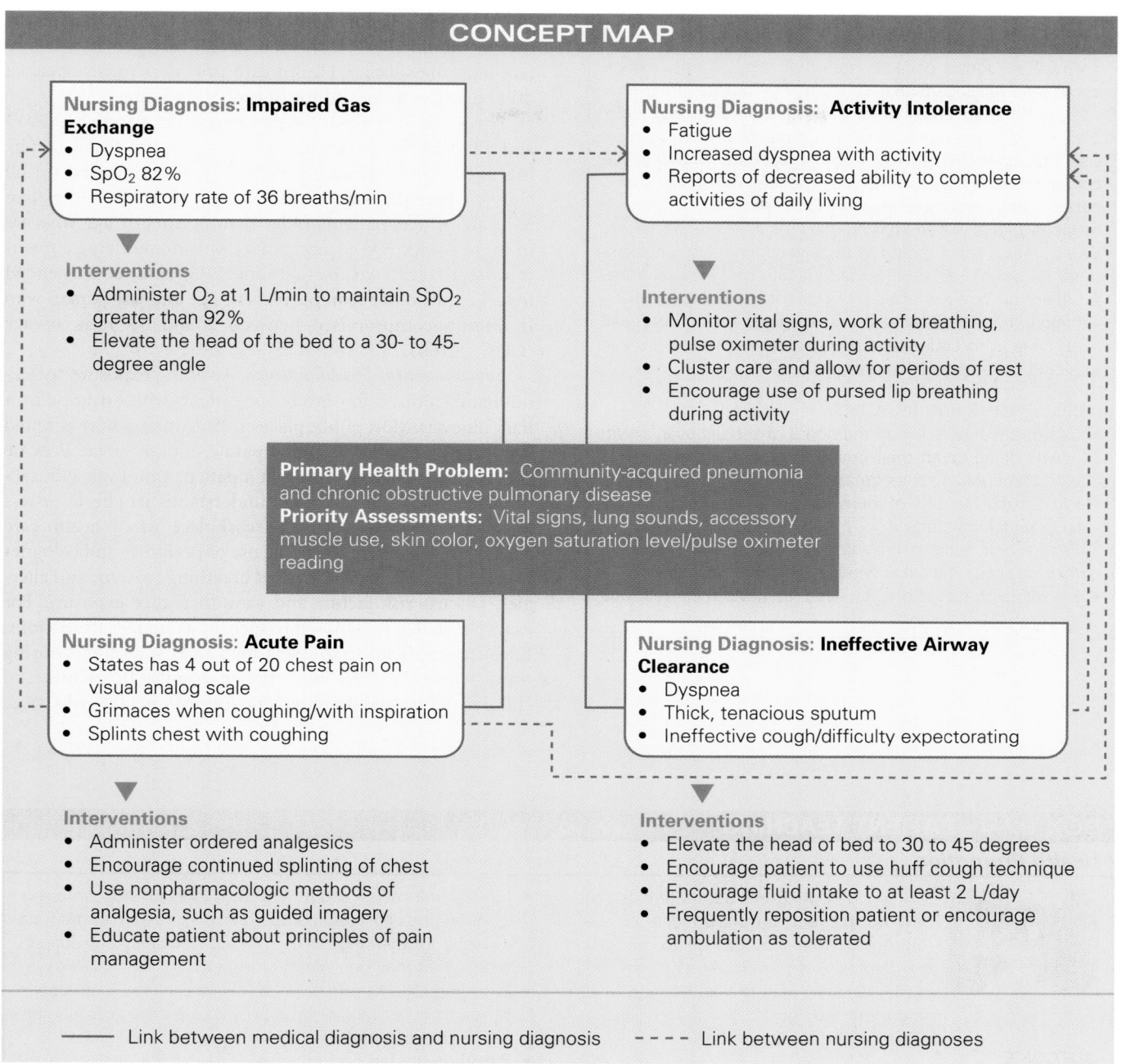

Nursing Diagnosis: Impaired Gas Exchange
- Dyspnea
- SpO$_2$ 82%
- Respiratory rate of 36 breaths/min

Interventions
- Administer O$_2$ at 1 L/min to maintain SpO$_2$ greater than 92%
- Elevate the head of the bed to a 30- to 45-degree angle

Nursing Diagnosis: Activity Intolerance
- Fatigue
- Increased dyspnea with activity
- Reports of decreased ability to complete activities of daily living

Interventions
- Monitor vital signs, work of breathing, pulse oximeter during activity
- Cluster care and allow for periods of rest
- Encourage use of pursed lip breathing during activity

Primary Health Problem: Community-acquired pneumonia and chronic obstructive pulmonary disease
Priority Assessments: Vital signs, lung sounds, accessory muscle use, skin color, oxygen saturation level/pulse oximeter reading

Nursing Diagnosis: Acute Pain
- States has 4 out of 20 chest pain on visual analog scale
- Grimaces when coughing/with inspiration
- Splints chest with coughing

Interventions
- Administer ordered analgesics
- Encourage continued splinting of chest
- Use nonpharmacologic methods of analgesia, such as guided imagery
- Educate patient about principles of pain management

Nursing Diagnosis: Ineffective Airway Clearance
- Dyspnea
- Thick, tenacious sputum
- Ineffective cough/difficulty expectorating

Interventions
- Elevate the head of bed to 30 to 45 degrees
- Encourage patient to use huff cough technique
- Encourage fluid intake to at least 2 L/day
- Frequently reposition patient or encourage ambulation as tolerated

——— Link between medical diagnosis and nursing diagnosis   - - - - Link between nursing diagnoses

FIG 32.5 Concept map.

Health Promotion. Maintaining a patient's optimal level of health reduces the number and severity of cardiopulmonary symptoms. Prevention of disease exacerbations and community-acquired infections is a goal of health promotion. Provide health education to help patients make choices for improving health practices (Box 32.4). Consider these patient education topics: regular blood pressure checkups and taking blood pressure medication as prescribed, following the DASH diet (NHLBI, 2015) and a proper caloric diet, getting an annual influenza vaccine and a pneumococcal vaccine, smoking cessation, and avoiding secondhand smoke exposure. Individualize patient teaching to meet the needs of each patient. Older adults have differing needs and respond differently than younger patients (Box 32.5).

Influenza and Pneumococcal Vaccine. Influenza is a viral infection that can cause serious complications in children, older adults, and patients with cardiopulmonary diseases. More than 970,000 patients were admitted to hospitals during the 2014–2015 season because of influenza (CDC, 2015b). The infection can lead to pneumonia and critical conditions requiring hospitalization. The CDC recommends annual influenza vaccines for all children 6 months of age and older

🌐 BOX 32.3   **PATIENT-CENTERED CARE**

You will encounter patients from different cultures, experiences, and religious faiths. Your patients' beliefs affect how you care for them and their families. Patients of various faiths may accept many routine health care practices such as exercise management. However, some patients who practice certain religions may avoid blood products, transfusions, and certain dietary recommendations. Other patients may consult religious elders when making their health care decisions. When caring for patients with cardiopulmonary illnesses, there is sometimes an urgency to health care interventions. A patient or family members may want to wait on an intervention until they speak with their religious leader. Your goal as a nurse is to understand and respect each patient's cultural and faith-based belief system.

IMPLICATIONS FOR PRACTICE

- Inform patients (such as members of the Jehovah's Witnesses faith) about their options including alternatives to blood products such as hetastarch and dextran.
- Provide the benefits of interventions in a respectful, nonjudgmental manner.
- Ensure that patients are informed about risks related to their choices, and acknowledge the possible outcomes.
- Be respectful of patients' need to have their religious leader present.

(CDC, 2016b). People with a history of Guillain-Barré syndrome should speak with their health care provider before receiving the vaccine. Health care providers must assess all other allergies before administering the vaccine.

There are two types of pneumococcal vaccine: PCV13 and PPSV23. Both vaccines protect patients from acquiring pneumococcal disease. PCV13 is recommended for all children younger than 5 years of age, all adults older than 65 years of age, patients older than 6 years of age who are immunocompromised, and adults who are receiving a pneumococcal vaccine for the first time. PPSV23 is recommended for all adults older than 65 years of age and any person who is immunocompromised between 2 and 64 years of age (CDC, 2016b).

Environmental Modifications. Avoiding exposure to secondhand smoke is important for patients with cardiopulmonary illnesses. Most public places and businesses have adopted a no-smoking policy or offer separate smoking areas. Provide counseling and support so that a patient who lives with secondhand smoke in the home understands its effects. Assess environmental hazards in the workplace. Many health care agency dress codes prohibit the use of perfumes and colognes because they often affect patient breathing patterns and allergies. Discuss risk factors and ways to reduce exposure. For example, pollen is a known trigger for asthma exacerbations. Encourage patients to shut windows and use air filters during times when there are high pollen counts. In infants and children secondhand smoke and environmental risks (e.g.,

BOX 32.4   **PATIENT TEACHING**

Health Promotion

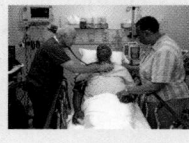 Mr. and Mrs. King are both interested in how to prevent hospitalizations in the future and what they can do to maintain their health. John Smith develops the following teaching plan to help Mr. and Mrs. King meet their goals.

OUTCOME

Mr. and Mrs. King will verbalize the steps they need to take to improve their health practices and reduce the risk for future hospitalizations.

TEACHING STRATEGIES

- Establish rapport with the Kings and maintain eye contact during the teaching session.
- Use words that the Kings understand; avoid medical jargon when possible.
- Set shared goals (in partnership with the Kings) that are realistic, meaningful, and achievable.
- With each topic, ask the Kings to repeat back the information you provide.
- Provide an overview of chronic obstructive pulmonary disease and pneumonia, signs and symptoms of exacerbation, medications, and follow-up appointments.

- Provide education about why they should stop smoking. Identify smoking cessation programs or resources that are available for the Kings to use. Assist in locating any support groups that may be available for them.
- Encourage Mr. King to balance activity and rest. Instruct him to report any changes in activity tolerance to his primary health care provider.
- Provide a written copy of material taught for reinforcement and reference.
- Allow time for questions and answer honestly, then summarize the material.

EVALUATION

- Use the principles of teach-back to evaluate patient/family caregiver learning.
  - "Tell me what you have learned about pneumonia and chronic obstructive pulmonary disease and signs and symptoms of it worsening."
  - "Tell me about some ways that you can quit smoking or the resources that are available to you to help you quit smoking."

BOX 32.5 CARE OF THE OLDER ADULT

Factors Affecting Cardiopulmonary Status

Older adults are at increased risk for developing a cardiopulmonary disorder (CDC, 2015a; Touhy and Jett, 2018). The cardiac and pulmonary systems are closely connected, and often a disturbance in one leads to a disturbance in the other. The following topics must be noted when caring for and educating an older adult:

- Older adults with hypertension have a higher risk of cardiovascular disease such as coronary heart disease, atrial fibrillation, and heart failure (Touhy and Jett, 2018).
- Risk-factor modification is important including smoking cessation, weight reduction, a low-cholesterol and low-salt diet, management of hypertension, and exercise.
- Healthy behavior changes sometimes slow or halt the progression of disease in an older adult. However, it is often difficult to get older adults to change long-term unhealthy habits.
- In older adults with underlying pulmonary diseases such as asthma and chronic obstructive pulmonary disease (COPD) mental status changes are often the first sign of worsening respiratory problems (Touhy and Jett, 2018).
- Ensure that educational materials are appropriate for the patient (e.g., large-print handouts for patients with vision disturbances, functioning hearing aids in place in patients with hearing loss).
- Interventions used when caring for older adults with chronic cardiopulmonary illness may need to focus on palliation and not cure.

pollution, cockroach infestation) increase risks for infection and asthma (Hockenberry et al., 2017).

Diet and Exercise. Advise patients to increase their activity levels with a minimum of 10 minutes at a time up to 2 hours and 30 minutes per week (National Heart, Lung, and Blood Institute [NHLBI], 2015). The goal is to achieve a target blood pressure of less than 120/80 mm Hg (Whelton et al., 2018). The risk factors for cardiac disease are lower when total cholesterol is less than 200 mg/dL, HDL is greater than 40 mg/dL in men and greater than 50 mg/dL in women, and LDL is less than 160 mg/dL (Lewis et al., 2017). A patient can reduce his or her blood pressure by 25 points by changing his or her lifestyle. Instruct patients on lifestyle modifications such as exercise and weight reduction by following the Dietary Approaches to Stop Hypertension (DASH) diet at http://dashdiet.org/default.asp.

Acute Care. Acute care interventions are directed toward halting the causative pathological processes that affect oxygenation. Nursing interventions also focus on shortening the duration and severity of an illness and preventing complications from illness or treatments such as hospital-acquired infection resulting from invasive procedures.

Dyspnea Management. Dyspnea is difficult to measure and treat, thus requiring individualized treatments for each patient. You will need to treat and stabilize the underlying processes that cause or worsen dyspnea, and then you will administer one or more of the four additional therapies:

1. Medications (e.g., bronchodilators, steroids, mucolytics, antianxiety drugs) to open the airways, decrease inflammation, thin secretions, or decrease anxiety
2. Oxygen therapy, as indicated and ordered, to treat hypoxia
3. Physical techniques (e.g., cardiopulmonary reconditioning, breathing techniques, cough control) to help mobilize secretions and strengthen the muscles used for breathing.
4. Psychosocial techniques (e.g., relaxation techniques, biofeedback, meditation) to lessen the sensation of dyspnea.

Oxygen Therapy. Some patients require oxygen therapy to keep a healthy level of tissue oxygenation. The goal of oxygen therapy is to prevent or relieve hypoxia. Any patient with impaired tissue oxygenation benefits from controlled oxygen administration. Oxygen is not a substitute for other treatments. It is a therapeutic gas that must be prescribed and adjusted only with a health care provider order. Oxygen is a drug with potentially dangerous side effects including the potential to cause hypoventilation in patients with COPD and hypercapnia. Continuously monitor the dosage or concentration. Routinely check the health care provider's orders to verify that the patient is receiving the prescribed oxygen concentration and flow rate. The six rights of medication administration also apply to oxygen administration (see Chapter 17).

Safety Precautions With Oxygen Therapy. Oxygen is a highly combustible gas and fuels fire readily. Although it does not spontaneously burn or cause an explosion, it can easily cause a fire to ignite if it contacts a spark from electrical equipment. With increasing use of outpatient oxygen therapy, patients and health care professionals need to be aware of the dangers of combustion. Chapter 30 describes steps to take in case of fire. Follow these oxygen safety precautions:

- Place an "Oxygen in Use" sign on the patient's room door or door of house.
- No smoking should be allowed on the premises.
- Keep oxygen delivery systems 10 feet from any open flames.
- Be sure electrical equipment in the room is functioning correctly and is grounded.
- Secure oxygen cylinders so that they do not fall over.

Patients discharged home on oxygen therapy need to have an environmental safety assessment (e.g., use of space/kerosene heaters or the presence of smokers who live or visit the home). Patients and family caregivers will also need special discharge instructions.

Oxygen Supply. Within health care settings, oxygen tanks or a permanent wall-piped system supplies oxygen to a patient's bedside. Oxygen tanks are transported on wide-based carriers that allow the tank to be upright at the patient's bedside. Regulators control the amount of oxygen delivered. One common type of oxygen tank has an upright flowmeter with a flow-adjustment valve at the top. A second type is a cylinder indicator with a flow-adjustment handle.

Methods of Oxygen Delivery. Nasal cannula, nasal catheter, face mask (Fig. 32.6), and a mechanical ventilator are ways to deliver oxygen to a patient (Table 32.8 and Box 32.6).

Home Oxygen. Home oxygen therapy is indicated in patients whose disease is stable with a PaO_2 of 55 mm Hg or less or an arterial oxygen saturation (SaO_2) of 88%. Patients with a PaO_2 of 55 to 59 mm Hg and signs of hypoxia qualify for long-term home oxygen therapy (McDonald, 2014). Home oxygen is usually administered by nasal cannula or face mask. If your patient has a permanent tracheostomy, a T tube or tracheostomy collar is necessary to provide humidified air to the airway. Patients requiring home oxygen need extensive teaching to be able to continue oxygen therapy at home efficiently and safely. This teaching includes oxygen safety, regulation of the amount of oxygen, obtaining and troubleshooting

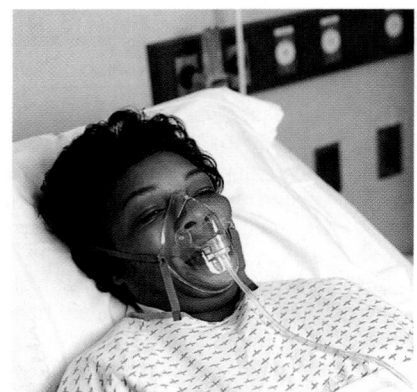

FIG 32.6 Simple face mask.

TABLE 32.8   OXYGEN DELIVERY SYSTEMS

DELIVERY SYSTEM	FLOW RATE; FiO₂ DELIVERED	ADVANTAGES	DISADVANTAGES
Low-Flow Delivery Devices			
Nasal cannula	1–6 L/min; 24%–44%	Safe and simple Easily tolerated Effective for low concentrations Does not impede eating or talking Inexpensive disposable	Unable to use with nasal obstructions Drying to mucous membranes Can dislodge easily May cause skin irritation breakdown over ears and in nares Patient's breathing pattern (mouth or nasal) affects exact FiO₂
Oxygen-conserving cannula (Oxymizer)	8 L/min; 30%–50%	Indicated for long-term O₂ use in the home Allows increased O₂ concentration and lower flow	Cannula cannot be cleaned More expensive than standard cannula
Simple face mask (see Fig. 32.6)	6–12 L/min; 35%–50%	Useful for short-term therapy such as patient transportation	Contraindicated for patients who retain CO₂ May make patient feel claustrophobic Therapy interrupted while eating or drinking Increased risk of aspiration
Partial nonrebreather mask[a]	10–15 L/min; 60%–90%	Short term delivery of increased FiO₂ Easily humidifies O₂ Does not dry mucous membranes	Hot and confining May irritate skin; tight seal is necessary Interferes with eating and talking Bag may twist or kink Should not totally deflate
High-Flow Delivery Devices			
Venturi mask	24%–50%	Provides specific amount of O₂ with humidity added Administers constant O₂	Mask and added humidity may irritate skin Therapy interrupted when patient eats Specific flow rate must be followed
High-flow nasal cannula	Adjustable FiO₂ (0.21–1.0) with modifiable low flow (up to 60 L/min)	Wide range of FiO₂ Can use on adults, children, and infants	FiO₂ dependent on patient respiratory pattern and input flow Risk for infection (Messika et al., 2015; Urden et al., 2016).

CO₂, Carbon dioxide; *FiO₂*, fraction of inspired oxygen concentration; *O₂*, oxygen.
[a]Reservoir bag should always remain partially inflated. Therefore flow rate must be high enough to prevent collapse of bag.

BOX 32.6 PROCEDURAL GUIDELINES

Applying a Nasal Cannula or Oxygen Mask

DELEGATION CONSIDERATIONS

The skill of applying (not adjusting oxygen flow) a nasal cannula or oxygen mask can be delegated to nursing assistive personnel (NAP) once the nurse confirms ordered therapy. The NAP cannot independently determine whether or not the oxygen delivery device can be applied. The nurse is responsible for assessing the patient's respiratory system and response to oxygen therapy and for setting up the device and liter flow, including the adjustment of oxygen flow rate. The nurse collaborates with the respiratory therapist when managing a patient receiving oxygen. The nurse directs the NAP by:

- Informing how to safely position and adjust the device (e.g., loosening the strap on mask).
- Instructing to inform the nurse immediately about any changes in vital signs; changes in pulse oximetry (SpO$_2$); changes in level of consciousness (LOC); skin irritation from the cannula, mask, or straps; or patient complaints of pain or breathlessness.
- Instructing personnel to provide extra skin care around patient's ears and nose.

EQUIPMENT

Oxygen nasal cannula or mask as ordered by health care provider, oxygen tubing (consider extension tubing), humidifier (if indicated), sterile water for humidifier, face shield as needed for risk of splash, clean gloves if secretions are present, oxygen source, oxygen flowmeter, appropriate "oxygen in use" signs, pulse oximeter, stethoscope. **Note:** When device is used in the home the medical equipment vendor will supply all the equipment.

STEPS

1. Identify patient using at least two identifiers (e.g., name and birthday or name and medical record number) according to agency policy. Compare identifiers with information on patient's MAR or medical record.
2. Review patient's medical record for medical order for oxygen, noting delivery method, flow rate, duration of oxygen therapy, and parameters for titration of oxygen settings.
3. Obtain patient's most recent SpO$_2$ value or most recent arterial blood gas (ABG) results if available.
4. Perform hand hygiene. Assess patient's respiratory status including symmetry of chest wall expansion, chest wall abnormalities (e.g., kyphosis), temporary conditions (e.g., pregnancy, trauma) affecting ventilation, respiratory rate and depth, sputum production, lung sounds, and signs and symptoms associated with hypoxia. **Note:** Apply face shield if risk of exposure to splashing mucus exists. Apply gloves if patient has oral or nasal secretions.

Clinical Decision Point. Excessive amounts of secretions, signs of respiratory distress (increased work of breathing, increased respiratory rate), presence of rhonchi on auscultation, excessive coughing, or decrease in SpO$_2$ can indicate a need for suctioning.

---

5. Observe for behavioral changes (e.g., apprehension, anxiety, confusion, decreased ability to concentrate, decreased LOC, fatigue, and dizziness).

Clinical Decision Point. Patients with sudden changes in their vital signs, LOC, or behavior may be experiencing profound hypoxia. Patients with subtle changes over time may have worsening of a chronic or existing condition or a new medical condition (Lewis et al., 2017).

---

6. Observe for patent airway and remove secretions by having patient cough and expectorate mucus or by suctioning. Remove and dispose of gloves and perform hand hygiene.
7. Explain procedure to patient and family.
8. Gather equipment/supplies.
9. Adjust bed to appropriate height and lower side rail on side nearest you. Check locks on bed wheel.
10. Apply new pair of gloves if patient has oral or nasal secretions.
11. Attach oxygen delivery device (e.g., cannula, mask) to oxygen tubing, and attach end of tubing to humidified oxygen source adjusted to prescribed flow rate.
    a. Place tips of the cannula into patient's nares. If tips are curved, they should point downward inside the nostrils. Then loop the cannula tubing up and over patient's ears. Adjust the lanyard so that the cannula fits snugly but not too tightly without pressure to patient's nares and ears.
    b. Apply a mask by placing it over patient's mouth and nose. Then bring the straps over patient's head and adjust to form a comfortable but tight seal.
12. Maintain sufficient slack on oxygen tubing and secure to patient's clothes.
13. Observe for proper function of oxygen delivery device:
    a. *Nasal cannula:* Cannula is positioned properly in nares; humidified oxygen flows through tips (see illustration).
    b. *Oxygen-conserving cannula (Oxymizer)* (see illustration): Fit as for nasal cannula. Reservoir is located under patient's nose or worn as a pendant.
    c. *Nonrebreathing mask* (see illustration): Apply as a regular mask. Contains one-way valves with a reservoir; exhaled air does not enter reservoir bag. Can be combined with a nasal cannula to provide higher FiO$_2$.
    d. *Simple face mask* (see Fig. 32.6): Select appropriate flow rate.
    e. *Venturi mask* (see illustration): Apply as regular mask. Select appropriate flow rate.

Continued

View Video!

BOX 32.6 PROCEDURAL GUIDELINES—cont'd
Applying a Nasal Cannula or Oxygen Mask

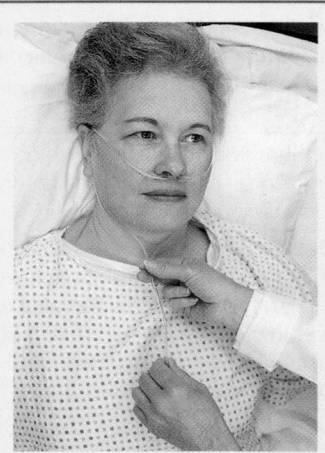

STEP 13a Nasal cannula adjusted for proper fit.

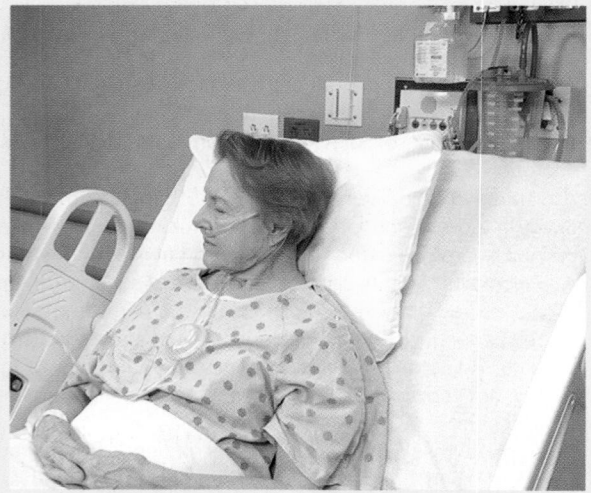

STEP 13b Reservoir nasal cannula/Oxymizer. (Copyright © Mosby's Clinical Skills: Essentials Collection.)

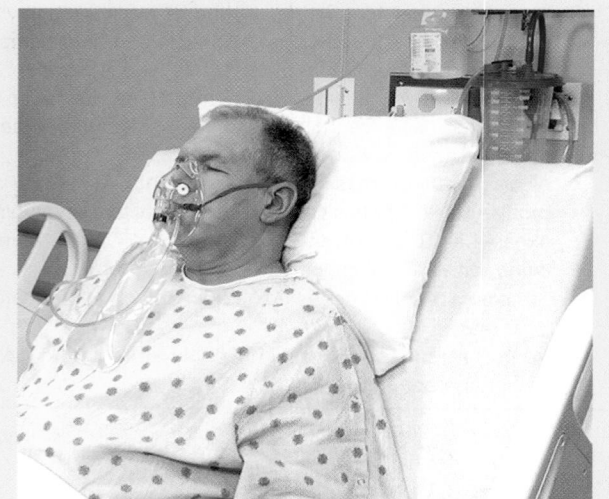

STEP 13c Nonrebreathing mask. (Copyright © Mosby's Clinical Skills: Essentials Collection.)

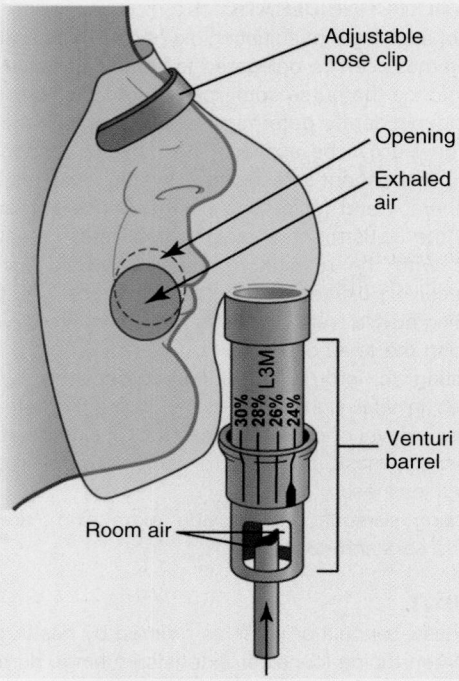

STEP 13e Venturi mask.

14. Verify setting on flowmeter and oxygen source for proper setup and prescribed flow rate.
15. Check cannula/mask every 8 hours or see agency policy. Keep humidifier filled at all times.
16. Post "Oxygen in use" signs on wall behind bed and at entrance to room.
17. Properly dispose of gloves (if used) and perform hand hygiene.
18. Monitor patient's response to changes in oxygen flow rate with SpO_2. (**Note:** Monitor arterial blood gases (ABGs) when ordered.
19. Auscultate lung sounds; observe chest excursion; inspect color of skin; and observe for decreased anxiety, improved LOC and cognitive abilities; decreased fatigue; and absence of dizziness. Measure vital signs.
20. Check adequacy of oxygen flow each shift or as agency policy dictates.
21. Observe patient's external ears, bridge of nose, nares, and nasal mucous membranes for evidence of skin breakdown.
22. **Use Teach-Back:** "I want to be sure I explained how oxygen will help you. Tell me one benefit of oxygen therapy." Revise your instruction now or develop a plan for revised patient/family caregiver teaching if patient/family caregiver is not able to teach back correctly.

equipment, how to use the prescribed home oxygen-delivery system, and when to contact local emergency medical services. A case coordinator or social worker usually assists with arranging for a home care nurse and oxygen vendor.

Mobilization of Pulmonary Secretions. The ability of a patient to mobilize pulmonary secretions out of lung airways is the difference between a short-term illness and a long recovery involving complications.

Hydration. Maintenance of adequate systemic hydration keeps mucociliary clearance normal for removing mucus and cellular debris from the respiratory tract. Excessive coughing to clear secretions is fatiguing and energy depleting. In patients with adequate hydration pulmonary secretions are thin, white, watery, and easily removable with minimal coughing. Unless contraindicated by a cardiac or renal condition, a fluid intake of 1500 to 2000 mL per day helps to keep pulmonary secretions thin and easy to expectorate (Lewis et al., 2017).

Humidification. Humidification (adding moisture to the inspired air) is necessary for patients receiving oxygen therapy at a high flow, typically greater than 4 L/minute. Oxygen humidification via a nasal cannula or face mask is achieved by bubbling oxygen through water. When using humidity, make sure to use sterile water. Also be sure to change the solution according to agency procedures. Humidification is a source for hospital-acquired infections because the moist environment supports the growth of pathogens.

Nebulization. Nebulization uses the aerosol principle to suspend a maximum number of water drops or particles of the desired size in inspired air. The moisture added to the respiratory system through nebulization improves mucus clearance and is used for administration of medications such as bronchodilators and mucolytic agents.

Maintenance of a Patent Airway. The airway is patent when the trachea, bronchi, and large airways are free from obstructions. You use three types of interventions to maintain a patent airway: coughing techniques, suctioning, and insertion of an artificial airway.

Coughing and Deep Breathing Techniques. Directed coughing is a deliberate maneuver that is effective when spontaneous coughing is inadequate. It allows a patient to remove secretions from the upper and lower airways. The normal series of events in a directed cough are deep inhalation, closure of the glottis, active contraction of the expiratory muscles, and glottis opening.

Cascade Cough. With a cascade cough, a patient takes a slow, deep breath and holds it for 2 seconds while contracting the expiratory muscles. Then the patient opens the mouth and performs a series of coughs throughout exhalation, thereby coughing at progressively lowered lung volumes. This technique promotes airway clearance and a patent airway to patients with large volumes of sputum.

Huff Cough. The huff cough is a more natural and gentler cough and is generally effective only for clearing the central airways. Have the patient sit or raise the head of the bed at least 45 degrees. The patient inhales slowly through the mouth while breathing through the diaphragm. The patient then forcefully exhales with his or her mouth open, creating a huff sound or saying the word "Huff." Have the patient repeat the huff process 2 to 3 times and then cough and expectorate the sputum. Reinforce to the patient that this type of coughing takes practice, and it can cause a sense of breathlessness when being performed (Lewis et al., 2017).

Quad Cough. The quad cough technique is for patients without abdominal muscle control such as patients with spinal cord injuries. While the patient breathes out with a maximal expiratory effort, the patient or you push inward and upward on the abdominal muscles toward the diaphragm, causing the cough. Evaluate cough effectiveness by the ability to expectorate sputum, a patient's report of swallowed sputum, and clearing of adventitious lung sounds.

Suctioning Techniques. When coughing does not effectively clear respiratory tract secretions, suctioning is indicated (see Skill 32.1). You need to use sterile technique for orotracheal, nasotracheal, and tracheal suctioning via an artificial airway because the tip of the catheter enters the sterile tracheal airway. The pharynx is considered clean; therefore oral and nasopharyngeal suctioning requires only clean technique. When suctioning both the oral pharynx and the trachea, always suction the nasotrachea and trachea (sterile) before oral pharyngeal (clean) secretions. Suctioning involves use of a round-tipped, flexible catheter with holes on the sides and end of catheter. When suctioning, you apply negative pressure (100 to 150 mm Hg for adults) during catheter withdrawal, never on insertion. It is indicated when rhonchi, gurgling breath sounds, and diminished breath sounds are audible on auscultation or when visible secretions are present after other methods have failed to remove secretions. There is no evidence to support suctioning on a scheduled basis (Myatt, 2015; Wiegand, 2017).

Oropharyngeal and Nasopharyngeal Suctioning. Use oropharyngeal or nasopharyngeal suctioning to help a patient who is able to cough effectively but is unable to clear secretions by expectorating or swallowing. Use a Yankauer or tonsillar tip suction catheter for oropharyngeal suctioning (Fig. 32.7). The catheter is made of rigid plastic with one large and several small eyelets through which mucus is removed. It is angled to facilitate removal of secretions from the mouth. Use

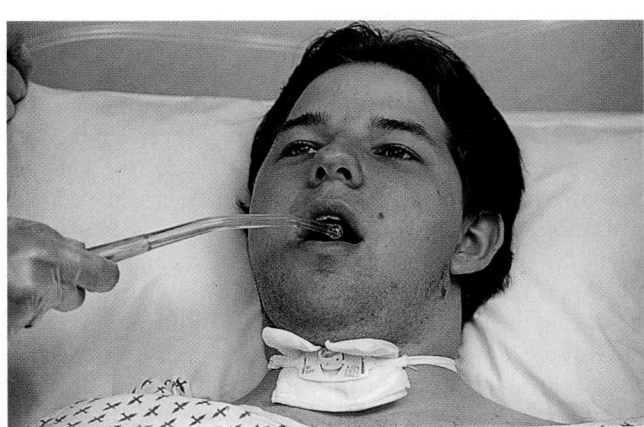

FIG 32.7 Oropharyngeal suctioning.

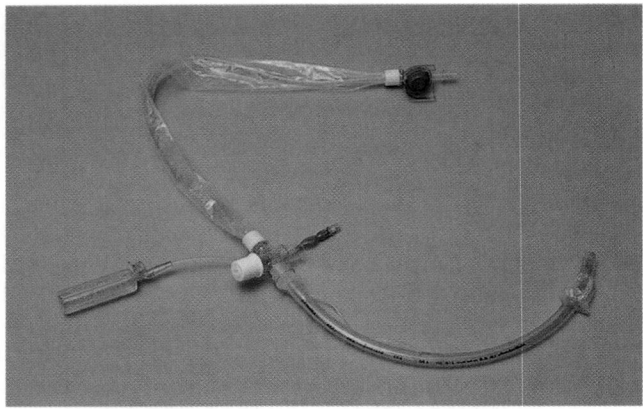

FIG 32.8 Ballard tracheal care closed suction.

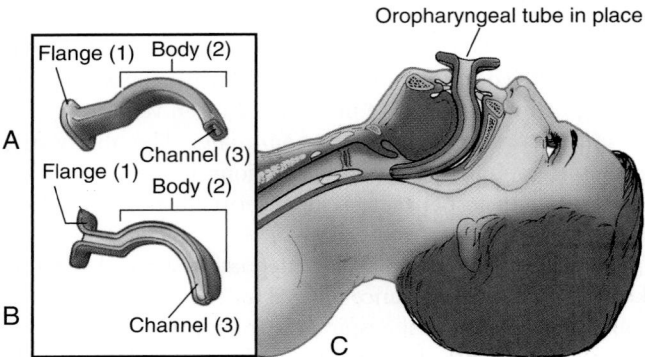

FIG 32.9 Artificial oral airways. (From Barnes TA: Emergency cardiovascular life support. In Kacmarek RM, et al, eds: *Egan's fundamentals of respiratory care,* ed 10, St Louis, 2013, Mosby.)

the Yankauer suction catheter when oral secretions are thick and plentiful. Do not use it in the nares because of its size.

Orotracheal and Nasotracheal Suctioning. Orotracheal or nasotracheal suctioning is necessary when a patient is unable to cough well enough to clear the airway but does not have an artificial airway in place. You pass a catheter through the mouth or nose and then into the trachea. The nose is the preferred route because stimulation of the gag reflex is minimal. The procedure is similar to nasopharyngeal suctioning, but the catheter tip enters the trachea.

Tracheal Suctioning. Perform tracheal suctioning through an artificial airway such as a tracheostomy tube or endotracheal tube. The catheter size should be as small as possible to prevent tissue injury. Two tracheal suctioning methods include use of a single catheter for one-time use and closed suctioning, which includes a multiple-use catheter. The suction catheter in closed suctioning is encased in a plastic sheath (Fig. 32.8). You use closed suctioning most often for patients who require mechanical ventilation because it decreases the patient's risk of having a hypoxic event during suctioning and helps to decrease the patient's risk of developing ventilator-associated pneumonia (VAP) (Box 32.7) (Branson et al., 2014). The practice of instilling normal saline into artificial airways to improve secretion removal could be harmful and is not recommended.

Artificial Airways. An artificial airway is for a patient with decreased level of consciousness, airway obstruction, or mechanical ventilation and who is unable to remove tracheo-bronchial secretions (see Skill 32.1). Patients with artificial airways who are on mechanical ventilation need specific oral hygiene care to prevent VAP (see Chapter 31) (see Box 32.7).

Oral Airway. The oral airway (Fig. 32.9), the simplest type of artificial airway, prevents obstruction of the trachea by displacing the tongue into the oropharynx. The oral airway extends from the teeth to the oropharynx, keeping the tongue in the normal position. Determine proper oral airway size by measuring the distance from the corner of the mouth to the angle of the jaw just below the ear. The length is equal to the distance from the flange of the airway to the tip. Use only the correct-size airway. If the airway is too small, the tongue will not stay in the anterior portion of the mouth; if too large,

it forces the tongue toward the epiglottis and obstructs the airway.

Insert the airway upside down, then turn the curve of the airway toward the cheek and place it over the tongue. When the airway is in the oropharynx, turn it so that the opening points downward. Correctly placed, the airway moves the tongue forward, away from the oropharynx and the flange. The flat portion of the airway rests against the patient's teeth. Incorrect insertion merely forces the tongue back into the oropharynx.

Tracheal Airway. An endotracheal or nasotracheal tube is a short-term artificial airway for administering mechanical ventilation. Tracheal tubes are for long-term use. These airways allow easy access to the trachea for deep tracheal suctioning. Because of the artificial airway, a patient no longer has normal humidification of the tracheal mucosa. Ensure that humidity is being supplied to the airway. Humidification is protective and helps reduce the risk for airway plugging. Most patients with tracheal airways cannot speak, and thus it is important to use written or nonverbal communication strategies.

Chest Physiotherapy. Chest physiotherapy (CPT) is external chest wall manipulation using postural drainage, percussion, vibration, high-frequency chest wall compression (HFCWC), or all of these for helping patients mobilize pulmonary secretions (Box 32.8). The AARC recommends that CPT be used in patients with cystic fibrosis and other diseases in which there is greater than 30 mL of sputum per day or in patients who have atelectasis on chest x-ray examination (Strickland et al., 2013). It has not been found to be effective in patients with uncomplicated pneumonia, patients with COPD for routine use, patients after surgery, or patients with respiratory muscle weakness (Strickland et al., 2013).

Postural Drainage. Postural drainage is the use of positioning techniques to drain secretions from specific segments of the lungs and bronchi into the trachea for expectoration (Table 32.9). Because some patients do not require postural drainage of all lung segments, adapt the procedure and position patients based on clinical assessment findings. For

BOX 32.7 EVIDENCE-BASED PRACTICE

PICO Question: In patients requiring mechanical ventilation, does the introduction of a ventilator care bundle compared with standard practices contribute to a reduction in ventilator-associated pneumonia (VAP)?

SUMMARY OF EVIDENCE

VAP develops in patients who receive mechanical ventilation for more than 48 hours (Institute for Healthcare Improvement [IHI], 2016). VAP is not easy to diagnose, as there is not a specific, sensitive test that can be used for diagnosis. Patients have increased fever, increased secretions, and pulmonary infiltrates (air spaces filled with fluid, exudate, or cells) seen on chest radiograph. Over time these infiltrates progressively increase, and the patient's lung functions decline. VAP increases the length of time the patient requires mechanical ventilation, which increases length of stay and health care costs. Mortality related to VAP approaches 50% (IHI, 2016).

Multiple VAP bundles are used by health care organizations to prevent VAP. Using these bundles reduces VAP incidence and mortality risk (Al-Thaqafy et al., 2014; Munro and Ruggiero, 2014; Kram et al., 2015; Lamb, 2015). The IHI Ventilator Bundle (IHI, 2012) and the multidisciplinary ABCDE Bundle are both series of interventions that, when implemented together, achieve significantly better outcomes than when implemented individually. The key components of these bundles are (IHI, 2012; Bounds et al., 2016):
- Elevation of the head of the bed to at least 30 degrees
- Daily "sedation vacations" and assessment of readiness to extubate
- Peptic ulcer disease prophylaxis
- Deep vein thrombosis prophylaxis
- Daily oral care with chlorhexidine
- Delirium prevention and management
- Early physical mobility

APPLICATION TO NURSING PRACTICE
- Unless contraindicated, maintain head of the bed elevation between 30 and 45 degrees to reduce aspiration of oropharyngeal and/or gastric fluids. Be aware of the increased risk of development of decubitus pressure injuries when patients are positioned with the head of the bed greater than 30 degrees (Munro and Ruggiero, 2014).
- Suction frequently to remove oropharyngeal and subglottic secretions to reduce the risk of early-onset VAP (Branson et al., 2014).
- Monitor ETT cuff pressure frequently to ensure there is an adequate seal to prevent aspiration of secretions (Branson et al., 2014).
- Provide daily oral care with chlorhexidine (IHI, 2012).
- Consult with health care providers to ensure that medications for deep vein thrombosis and peptic ulcer disease prophylaxis are ordered.
- Collaborate with other members of the health care team to ensure early mobilization of the patient.
- Always drain ventilator circuit condensation away from patient and into the appropriate receptacle (American Association of Respiratory Care [AARC], 2010; Wiegand, 2017).

BOX 32.8 CHEST PHYSIOTHERAPY CONSIDERATIONS

Nurses and respiratory therapists collaborate with health care providers to determine if chest physiotherapy (CPT) is best for a patient. Consultation also determines the position for the patient to assume during the procedure. Follow these guidelines:
- Know a patient's normal range of vital signs. CPT can be physically exhausting, and the activity can affect a patient's vital signs. The degree of change is related to the level of hypoxia, overall cardiopulmonary status, and tolerance of the procedure.
- Know a patient's current medications. Long-term steroid use increases the patient's risk for pathological rib fractures. Anticoagulants and nonsteroidal antiinflammatory drugs (NSAIDs) increase a patient's risk for bruising. Diuretics and antihypertensives cause fluid and hemodynamic changes.
- Know a patient's medical and surgical history. Conditions such as increased intracranial pressure, spinal cord injuries, abdominal aneurysm resection, severe osteoporosis, and thoracic trauma are contraindications for postural drainage and CPT.
- Know a patient's level of cognitive function. Participation in vibration and controlled cough CPT techniques is dependent on a patient's ability to understand and follow instructions. CPT may result in combative behavior in patients with confusion or delirium.
- Have suction machine equipment available to help clear the airway of secretions.
- Be aware of the patient's exercise tolerance. CPT maneuvers are fatiguing, and patients who are not used to physical activity may have little tolerance for this therapy.

example, some patients with left lower lobe bronchiectasis or pneumonia require postural drainage of only the affected region, whereas a patient with cystic fibrosis requires postural drainage of all segments.

Chest Percussion. **Chest percussion** is the manual external clapping of a patient's chest with cupped hands over the lung segments being drained. A mechanical device can also be used to loosen secretions from the bronchial walls. You perform chest percussion by alternating hand motion against the chest wall (Fig. 32.10). Perform percussion over a single layer of clothing, but not over buttons, snaps, or zippers. The single layer of clothing prevents directly slapping the patient's skin. Thicker or multiple layers of material dampen the percussions. When percussing the lung fields, be careful not to percuss the scapular area, or trauma will occur to the skin and underlying musculoskeletal structures. Percussion is contraindicated in patients with bleeding disorders, osteoporosis, or fractured ribs.

TABLE 32.9	POSITIONS FOR POSTURAL DRAINAGE
LUNG SEGMENT	**POSITION OF PATIENT**
Adult	
Left and right upper lobes	High-Fowler's
Apical Segments	
Right upper lobe—anterior segment	Supine with head elevated
Left upper lobe—anterior segment	Sitting on side of bed Supine with head elevated
Right upper lobe—posterior segment	Side-lying with right side of chest elevated on pillows
Left upper lobe—posterior segment	Side-lying with left side of chest elevated on pillows
Left and right middle lobes—anterior segment	Three-fourths supine position with dependent lung in Trendelenburg's position
Right middle lobe—posterior segment	Prone with thorax and abdomen elevated
Both lower lobes—anterior segments	Supine in Trendelenburg's position
Left lower lobe—lateral segment	Right side-lying in Trendelenburg's position
Right lower lobe—lateral segment	Left side-lying in Trendelenburg's position
Right lower lobe—posterior segment	Prone with right side of chest elevated in Trendelenburg's position
Both lower lobes—posterior segment	Prone in Trendelenburg's position
Child	
Sitting on nurse's lap, leaning slightly forward flexed over pillow	
Bilateral—middle anterior segments	Sitting on nurse's lap, leaning against nurse
Bilateral lobes—anterior segments	Lying supine on nurse's lap, back supported with pillow

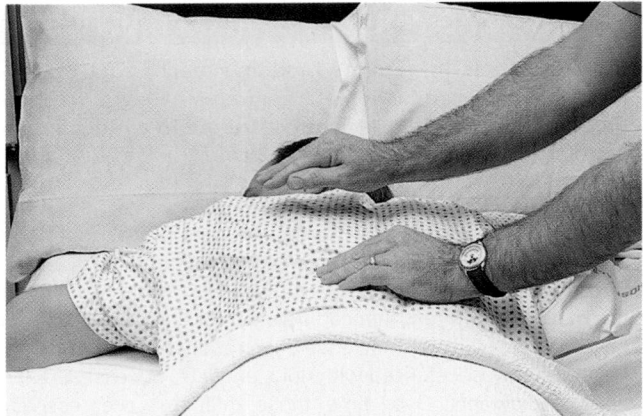

FIG 32.10 Chest wall percussion alternating hand motion against patient's chest wall.

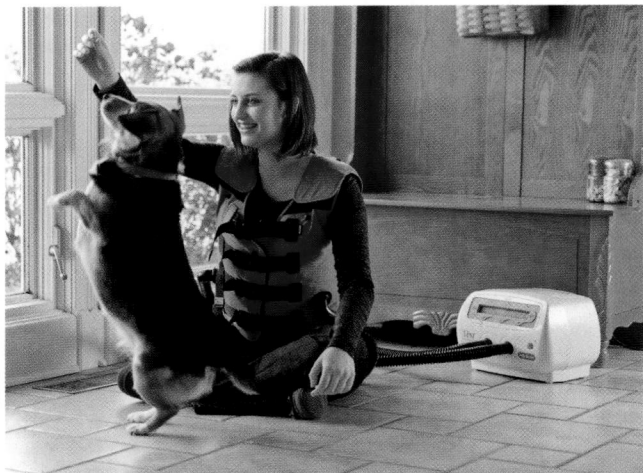

FIG 32.11 High-frequency chest wall oscillation vest for home use. (Copyright © 2012 Hill-Rom Services, Inc. Reprinted with permission. All rights reserved.)

Vibration. Vibration is a gentle shaking pressure applied to the chest wall only during exhalation to shake secretions into larger airways. This pressure can be applied either manually or with a commercially available device. Vibration may be tolerated better than percussion. You use vibration most often with patients with cystic fibrosis. It is not recommended for infants and young children.

High-Frequency Chest Wall Compression. High-frequency chest wall compression (HFCWC) consists of an inflatable vest that is attached to an air-pulse generator. The vest airway clearance system (Fig. 32.11) loosens and removes secretions from the airway by delivering high-frequency, small-volume expiratory pulses to a patient's external chest wall. This therapy benefits patients with neuromuscular disorders, cystic fibrosis, or ineffective cough and airway clear-

ance. HFCWC is also beneficial for patients who produce 25 to 30 mL of sputum per day, as it helps to decrease the viscosity of the mucus, making it easier for a patient to cough and clear the airway (Volsko, 2013).

Maintenance or Promotion of Lung Expansion. Nursing interventions to maintain or promote lung expansion include noninvasive techniques such as ambulation, positioning, incentive spirometry, and chest tube management.

Ambulation. Research shows that after 1 week of bed rest, muscle strength declines by as much as 20%, resulting in an increased oxygen demand, weakened respiratory muscles, and reduced functional status. Early ambulation increases a patient's general strength and lung expansion. Progressive mobilization from dangling the legs off a bed to standing and then walking is safe for all patients, including those who are intubated (Atkins and Kautz, 2014) (see Chapter 28). Support patients in being actively involved in ambulation as soon as possible.

Positioning. Healthy people maintain adequate ventilation and oxygenation by frequent position changes. When a person has restricted mobility, it increases his or her risk for respiratory impairment. Frequent position changes such as every 2 hours are a simple and cost-effective method for reducing a patient's risk for pooled airway secretions and decreased chest wall expansion.

The most effective position for patients with cardiopulmonary disease is the 45-degree semi-Fowler's position, using gravity to assist in lung expansion and reduce pressure from the abdomen on the diaphragm. Ensure that a patient does not slide down in bed, causing reduced lung expansion. When positioning a patient with unilateral lung disease such as a pneumothorax or atelectasis, position him or her with the healthy lung down. This position promotes better perfusion of the healthy lung and aeration of the diseased lung, improving oxygenation. In the presence of pulmonary abscess or hemorrhage, place the affected lung down to prevent drainage toward the healthy lung.

Incentive Spirometry. Incentive spirometry (IS) encourages voluntary deep breathing by providing visual feedback to patients about their inspiratory volume. It promotes deep inhalation to prevent atelectasis and other pulmonary postoperative complications (AARC, 2011; Cassidy et al., 2013). However, a recent review shows no evidence that IS prevents pulmonary complications following abdominal surgery (do Nascimento et al., 2014). It is effective in increasing lung expansion and thus is commonly used in postoperative care. The AARC (2011) recommends 5 to 10 breaths per session every hour while awake. Use incentive spirometry in combination with other pulmonary maneuvers such as deep breathing and coughing, early mobilization, and directed coughing (Restrepo et al., 2011; do Nascimento et al., 2014). Administer pain medications before incentive spirometry to help a patient breathe deeply.

There are two types of incentive spirometers. Flow-oriented incentive spirometers consist of one or more plastic chambers that contain freely moving colored balls. The patient inhales slowly with an even flow to elevate the balls and keep them floating as long as possible. This allows a maximally sustained inhalation. Volume-oriented incentive spirometry devices have a bellows that rises to a predetermined volume by an inhaled breath. An achievement light or counter is used to provide feedback. Some devices do not turn the light on unless the bellows is at a minimum desired volume for a specified period of time.

Chest Tubes. A chest tube is a catheter inserted through the rib cage into the pleural space to remove air, fluids, or blood; to prevent air or fluid from reentering the pleural space; or to reestablish normal intrapleural and intrapulmonic pressures. Chest tubes are typically 51 cm (20 inches) long and range in size from 12 F to 40 F. Large tubes drain blood, whereas smaller tubes drain air. Chest tubes are commonly used in patients after cardiac or thoracic surgery or in patients who have a chest trauma to promote lung reexpansion (see Skill 32.2). Once fluid or air is removed, a patient's oxygenation improves (Kane et al., 2013; Myatt, 2015).

A pneumothorax is a collapse of the lung caused by collection of air or other gas in the pleural space. The gas causes the lung to collapse because it changes the intrapleural pressure from negative to positive, exerting a counterpressure against the lung, making it unable to expand. A pneumothorax is commonly caused by chest trauma resulting in fractured ribs or secondary to chronic disease, or it can occur spontaneously. A patient with a pneumothorax feels sharp pain because atmospheric air irritates the parietal pleura. Dyspnea and tachycardia are common and worsen as the size of the pneumothorax increases.

A tension pneumothorax is a life-threatening situation that occurs from rupture in the pleura when air accumulates in the pleural space more rapidly than it is removed. Air is trapped in the pleural cavity between the chest wall and the lung. The volume of trapped air increases with each inspiration and is unable to escape with expiration, causing increased pressure on the lung, heart, and blood vessels of the thorax. If left untreated, the lung on the affected side collapses, and the mediastinum shifts to the opposite (unaffected) side leading to tracheal deviation, reduced venous return, and subsequent decrease in cardiac output. Tracheal deviation is a late sign and may be absent in some cases (Zarogoulidis et al., 2014). A large-bore cannula (needle decompression) or chest tube must be placed immediately to release the pressure (Bascom et al., 2016).

Hemothorax is an accumulation of blood in the pleural space, usually as the result of trauma. It produces a counterpressure and prevents the lung from full expansion. In addition to pain and dyspnea, signs and symptoms of shock develop if blood loss is severe. If it occurs with a pneumothorax, it is called a hemopneumothorax. Pleural effusions occur when fluid, in response to infection, inflammation, or cancer, enters the pleural space.

Disposable chest drainage systems such as the Thora-Seal (Covidien/Medtronic), Pleur-evac chest drainage system (Teleflex), or Atrium brand systems are one-piece molded plastic units that evacuate any volume of air or fluid with controlled suction (Fig. 32.12). The disposable units are cost-effective and safe. Each unit typically has three chambers: a water-seal chamber to prevent air from being drawn back into the pleural space, a chamber to collect fluid or blood, and a chamber for suction. The suction chamber facilitates removal of chest drainage and trapped air. Suction pressure is measured in centimeters of water and is usually set at −15 to −20 cm H_2O for adults. Children may require less pressure. Suction pressure is typically ordered by the health care

QSEN **QSEN ACTIVITY** *Teamwork and Collaboration*

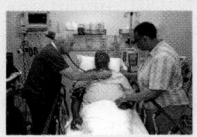

Mr. King continues to be hospitalized and you are collaborating with the nurse from the previous shift, who tells you Mr. King is being discharged in 2 days.
• What additional information do you need to receive from the nurse when assuming his care? Who will need to be consulted to help prepare the Kings for discharge and to manage Mr. King's illness at home?

evolve   Answers to QSEN Activities can be found on the Evolve website.

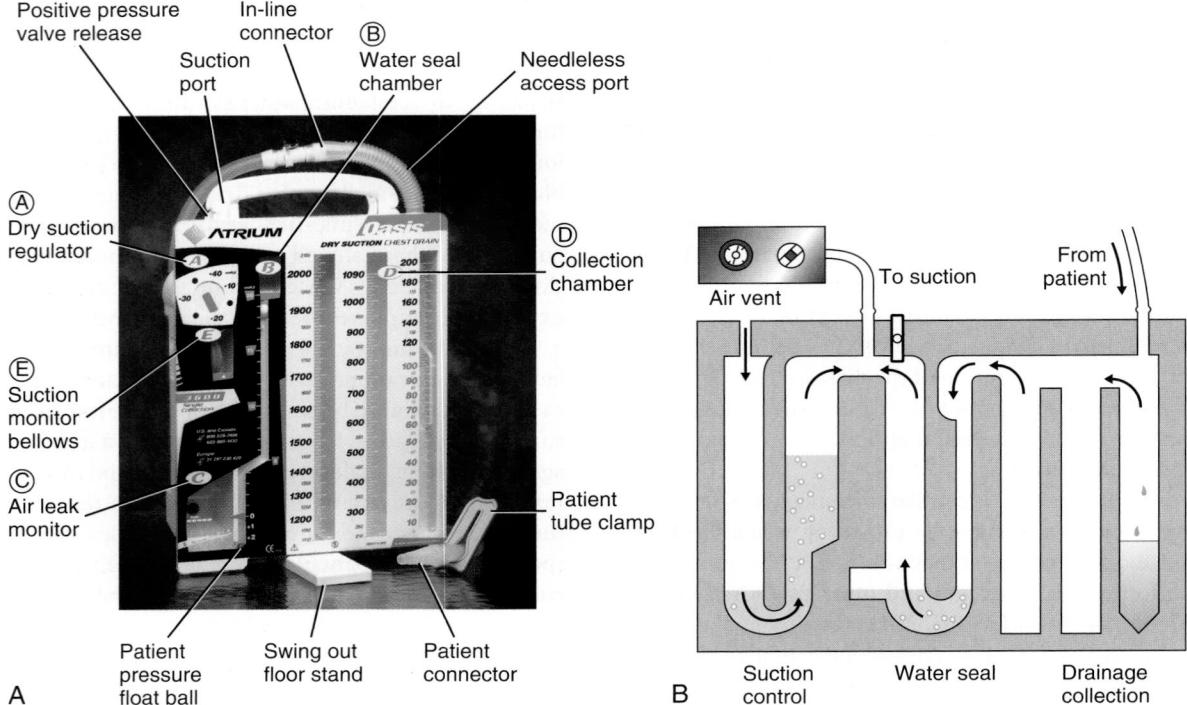

FIG 32.12 **A,** Dry suction chest drainage system. **B,** Schematic of drainage device. (**A** courtesy Atrium Medical Corp.)

provider. Your knowledge of the basics of chest tube management and troubleshooting maneuvers reduces a patient's risk for complications.

Special Considerations. Clamping chest tubes is contraindicated when a patient is ambulating or being transported, as it may cause a tension pneumothorax (Kane et al., 2013). The health care provider may choose to clamp a tube temporarily to determine if a patient has fluid or air accumulation. Clamping requires an order, and you must assess the patient frequently. Handle the chest drainage unit carefully and maintain the drainage device below the patient's chest. If the tubing accidentally disconnects from the collection unit, instruct the patient to exhale as much as possible and cough. This maneuver rids the pleural space of as much air as possible. Quickly cleanse the tip of the tubing and reconnect the tubing to the unit.

Chest Tube Removal. A physician, physician's assistant, or nurse practitioner usually removes a chest tube (verify agency policy). Prepare a patient by assessing the need for preremoval analgesia, obtaining the required medication orders, and instructing a patient about the process and what will be requested of him or her. There has been debate about the optimal timing of chest tube removal in relation to the respiratory cycle. Removal at full inspiration maximally expands the lungs and minimizes the potential space between the pleurae. Another recommendation is for chest tube removal at end expiration when the pressure difference between the chest cavity and the atmosphere is the least (Kwiatt et al., 2014). An occlusive dressing is applied immediately after tube removal to maintain a tight seal.

Noninvasive Ventilation. Noninvasive ventilation (NIV) maintains positive airway pressure and improves alveolar ventilation without the need for an artificial airway. This mechanical ventilator alternative reduces and reverses atelectasis, improves oxygenation, reduces pulmonary edema, and improves cardiac function. Positive airway pressure keeps the alveoli partially inflated, reducing the risk for atelectasis. If the patient has atelectasis, positive pressure assists in reinflation. Because the alveoli remain partially inflated, there is a continuous exchange of respiratory gas; as a result, the patient's oxygenation improves. NIV reduces pulmonary edema in patients with cardiac disease because the increased alveolar pressure forces interstitial fluid out of the lungs and back into the pulmonary circulation. In patients with obstructive sleep apnea, NIV helps to keep the airway open. Substantial reductions in mortality and the need for subsequent ventilation support are associated with NIV in patients with acute respiratory failure, especially in patients with COPD (Gale et al., 2015).

Continuous positive airway pressure (CPAP) maintains a steady stream of pressure throughout a patient's breathing cycle. It benefits patients with obstructive sleep apnea. In obstructive sleep apnea, the upper airway collapses during sleep and prevents normal airflow. When the airflow is interrupted, there is a drop in the patient's oxygen saturation, and frequent awakenings occur. CPAP uses continuous positive pressure to keep the airway open and prevent upper airway collapse. The patient breathes more normally, sleeps better, and has markedly reduced snoring. A CPAP setting of 5 cm H_2O provides 5 cm of pressure during inspiration

TABLE 32.10 PROBLEMS ASSOCIATED WITH CONTINUOUS POSITIVE AIRWAY PRESSURE

PROBLEM	CAUSE
Discomfort	Mask that fits over patient's nose is tight fitting. Oxygen flow rate causes dry mucous membranes.
Risks to skin integrity	Tight fit of mask causes pressure, diaphoresis, and increased risk for skin breakdown and pressure injuries.
Hypercapnia	Although CPAP improves alveolar function, which increases CO_2 clearance from the blood, it also causes air trapping. In some patients this causes increased CO_2 levels.
Gastric distention	CPAP forces more air into the stomach, which causes distention and discomfort in some patients. Severe gastric distention impedes diaphragmatic motion and reduces lung volumes.
Noise	Some patients find the machine very noisy and that it interferes with sleep.
Psychosocial	Relationship with sleep partner is difficult. There are possible sensations of claustrophobia.

CO_2, Carbon dioxide; *CPAP*, continuous positive airway pressure.
Data from Pooboni S: Noninvasive ventilation procedures, *Medscape,* 2013, http://emedicine.medscape.com/article/1417959 -overview.

and expiration. The usual CPAP setting is 5 to 20 cm H_2O. However, there are disadvantages to this device (Table 32.10).

Bi-level positive airway pressure (BiPAP) works by providing assistance during inspiration and preventing alveolar closure during expiration. It provides two levels of pressure: inspiratory positive airway pressure (IPAP) and lower expiratory positive airway pressure (EPAP). During inspiration, BiPAP generates a preset positive-pressure support, which increases a patient's tidal volume and ultimately alveolar ventilation. This pressure support is decreased when the patient begins exhaling, which allows for easier exhalation. As a result there is an increase in functional residual capacity (amount of air remaining in the lungs at the end of expiration), reduced airway closure, expansion of an atelectatic area, and improved oxygenation.

The goals of NIV include improved ventilation and sleep, enhanced quality of life, reduction of morbidity, improvement of physical and physiological function, and cost-effectiveness. You prepare family caregivers and patients who are candidates for noninvasive ventilation for discharge by collaborating with a multidisciplinary team.

Restoration of Cardiopulmonary Functioning. The AHA publishes guidelines for cardiopulmonary care and resuscitation every 5 years. The AHA outlines the standards for basic and advanced life support for children and adults (Link et al., 2015). A cardiac arrest is a sudden cessation of cardiac output and circulation. When this occurs, the tissues do not receive oxygen, CO_2 is not transported from tissues, tissue metabolism becomes anaerobic, and metabolic and respiratory acidosis occurs. Permanent heart, brain, and other tissue damage occurs within 4 to 6 minutes.

Cardiopulmonary Resuscitation. A patient with an absent pulse and respiration is in cardiac arrest and requires immediate cardiopulmonary resuscitation (CPR). CPR is a basic emergency procedure of artificial respiration and manual external cardiac massage. The sequence for CPR is C-A-B: chest compression, early defibrillation, establishing an airway, and rescue breathing (Link et al., 2015). Chest compressions are fast, deep applications of pressure on the lower half of a patient's sternum. While standing to the side of your patient, you place your hands on the lower half of the patient's sternum and push down at least 2 inches (5 cm) and allow the chest to come back up. In some institutions, mechanical chest compression devices are used. Rescue breathing is combined with compressions and consists of performing the head tilt–chin lift maneuver to open the patient's airway and then give the breaths. In acute care agencies the breaths are typically delivered using a bag-valve-mask device (Lewis et al., 2017).

Defibrillation delivers an electrical current to the myocardium that stops all electrical activity and allows the heart's normal pacemaker to resume its normal electrical activity (Wiegand, 2017). Defibrillation is recommended within 5 minutes for an out-of-hospital sudden cardiac arrest and within 3 minutes for a patient in the hospital. In addition to health care providers, specific lay individuals in public locations with high risk of a witnessed cardiac arrest (e.g., casinos and sporting events) should be trained in using an automated external defibrillator (AED) (AHA, 2015). An AED is a portable device that administers an electrical shock through the chest wall to the heart (Box 32.9).

For witnessed sudden collapse of a child or for any adult victim, the recommendation is to activate the emergency response system by using your own mobile phone or the closest available phone, get the AED, and then begin chest compressions. If a child victim is unconscious and no one witnessed the collapse, the rescuer is to deliver chest compressions for 2 minutes and then activate the emergency response system. The rate of compressions for both adults and children is 100 to 120 per minute. The rescuer must allow full recoil of the chest after each compression to allow adequate filling of the heart.

The rate of compression varies with age. In children (1 to 8 years of age) and infants (younger than 1 year of age but not newborns) the ratio of compressions to breaths is 30:2 for one rescuer and 15:2 for two rescuers. For adults and adolescents, regardless of the number of rescuers, the compressions are 100 to 120 per minute at the rate of 30 compressions to 2 breaths (30:2). Continue until an AED is available and ready to analyze rhythm (AHA, 2015).

When a person is choking and has an obstructed airway, perform abdominal thrusts until the person becomes

BOX 32.9 AUTOMATED EXTERNAL DEFIBRILLATOR

- If you see a person suddenly collapse and pass out, or if you find a person already unconscious, confirm that the person cannot respond and is not sleeping.
- Check the person's respirations and pulse. If breathing and pulse are absent or irregular, prepare to use the AED as soon as possible.
- If no one knows how long the person has been unconscious, or if an AED isn't readily available, do 2 minutes of CPR. Then use the AED.
- Be sure the person is lying in a dry area, and stay away from wetness when delivering shocks.
- Turn on the AED's power. The device will give step-by-step instructions through voice prompts and prompts on a screen.
- Expose the person's chest. If the person's chest is wet, dry it. Apply AED conduction pads to the person's chest (as pictured on instructions).
- Check for metal jewelry, body piercings, underwire bras, and whether patient has an implanted medical device (check for medical alert bracelet).
- The AED has a built-in computer that assesses the victim's heart rhythm and determines if defibrillation is needed.
- Stand clear and announce, "Everyone stand back." Then push the AED "shock button."
- The AED can be used by nonmedical personnel.

Adapted from National Heart, Lung and Blood Institute. *How to use an automated external defibrillator.* 2011, Available at https://www.nhlbi.nih.gov/health/health-topics/topics/aed/howtouse.

unconscious. Then you perform CPR. You may sweep the mouth and remove the foreign body if you can see it (AHA, 2015).

Restorative and Continuing Care. Restorative and continuing care emphasize cardiopulmonary reconditioning as a structured rehabilitation program. Cardiopulmonary rehabilitation involves helping a patient achieve and maintain an optimal level of health through controlled physical exercise, nutrition counseling, relaxation and stress management techniques, prescribed medications, and oxygen administration. As physical reconditioning occurs, the patient's physical symptoms, anxiety, depression, or somatic concerns decrease. The patient and the rehabilitation team define the goals of rehabilitation, and patient and family caregiver teaching is individualized according to patient needs (American Association of Cardiovascular and Pulmonary Rehabilitation [AACVPR], 2016).

Respiratory Muscle Training. Respiratory muscle training improves strength and endurance, resulting in improved activity tolerance. Respiratory muscle training can decrease the presence of debilitating symptoms and prevent respiratory failure in patients with COPD.

Breathing Exercises. Breathing exercises include techniques to improve ventilation and oxygenation. The two basic techniques are pursed-lip breathing and diaphragmatic breathing.

Pursed-lip breathing involves deep inspiration and prolonged expiration through pursed lips to prevent alveolar collapse. Instruct the patient to sit up and then take a deep breath and exhale slowly through pursed lips, as if he or she were whistling. Patients need to gain control of the exhalation phase so that exhalation is longer than inhalation. The patient is usually able to perfect this technique by counting inhalation time and gradually increasing the count during exhalation.

Diaphragmatic breathing, or abdominal breathing, is more difficult and requires a patient to use the diaphragm instead of the chest accessory muscles. The patient concentrates on expanding the diaphragm during controlled inspiration. Teach the patient to place one hand on the chest and one hand on the belly. As the patient inhales the diaphragm descends (belly moves out), and as the patient exhales the diaphragm ascends (belly sinks in). Coach a patient to gently push on the abdomen with the lower hand to gently push on the diaphragm and help the patient exhale air. The exercise is often used with the pursed-lip breathing technique (COPD Foundation, 2016).

■■■■ EVALUATION

Patient Outcomes. You evaluate nursing interventions and therapies by comparing a patient's progress with the goals and desired outcomes of the nursing care plan. For example, your expected outcomes are directed toward improving SaO_2 levels, lung expansion on auscultation, and improved airway clearance as evidenced by improved lung sounds, improved oximetry measurements, and better expectoration of mucus. When measures directed to improve oxygenation are unsuccessful, modify the care plan by revising existing interventions or introducing new ones. For example, in patients who do not clear their airway by deep breathing and coughing, you may need to perform nasotracheal or orotracheal suctioning. Do not hesitate to notify the health care provider about a patient's decline in oxygenation status. Early recognition of a change in cardiopulmonary status and prompt notification help to avoid an emergent situation or the need for CPR.

Patients with chronic cardiopulmonary disease present a nursing challenge, particularly when they present with an acute illness. These patients require interventions that manage both the chronic symptoms and the symptoms associated with acute exacerbations or illness. For example, they may require home oxygen therapy to manage their COPD, but if they have pneumonia, they may have an increased oxygen requirement. Patients with cystic fibrosis, who often require home airway clearance therapy, may need an increase in frequency of their prescribed airway clearance therapy or a change in the therapy that they use. They may need to switch from manual CPT to HFCWC therapy. With chronic diseases, do not think in terms of recovery but rather health maintenance. A measurable outcome for a patient experiencing an acute exacerbation of a chronic illness is a return to baseline functional and cognitive status before this most recent exacerbation. This return of functional status helps to improve the patient's quality of life.

Patient Expectations. Individualize a patient's goals and make sure they are realistic and incorporate his or her expectations. What you perceive a patient needs can be different from what he or she expects of you and other health care providers. Some patients may want to learn how to cope with chronic disease. Others may simply want to know their prognosis and what will be the course of their illness. Some patients want information about how to perform airway clearance techniques. You must determine in your initial assessment of what a patient perceives is necessary for recovery, such as emotional support, knowledge, or improved self-care abilities. Then during evaluation determine if his or her expectations were met. Ask patients to describe whether they believe their expectations were met. Then proceed to evaluate, for example, if they believe they have the knowledge to better manage their disease. Do they now know more about their condition and ways to promote their health? Measuring achievement of patient expectations offers important evaluation information.

In the case study, management of Mr. King, who has COPD, depends on achieving three major goals: reduction of airflow obstruction, prevention or management of complications, and improvement in Mr. King's quality of life (Box 32.10).

BOX 32.10 EVALUATION

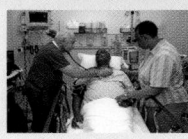

John cares for Mr. King throughout his hospital stay. On the day of his discharge, Mr. King is afebrile, his white blood cell counts are within normal limits, and his sputum cultures are negative. He does not require supplemental oxygen. He is able to teach back ways to prevent respiratory infections. Because he now practices pursed-lip breathing, his breathing is more controlled, relieving his subsequent anxiety. Mr. and Mrs. King both state they are going to try to quit smoking.

John observes Mr. King using the various breathing techniques that they have worked on together. Mr. King is able to perform activities of daily living. His wife appears less anxious: "I feel as though for the first time we have taken a small step to improve my husband's quality of life."

DOCUMENTATION NOTE

"Mr. King discharged to home. Able to teach back the purpose of breathing exercises and each medication, lists causes and symptoms of respiratory tract infection. Correctly demonstrated pursed-lip breathing. Has appointment in 1 week with community-based rehab program. Scheduled to see physician in 2 weeks."

SAFETY GUIDELINES FOR NURSING SKILLS

Ensuring patient safety is an essential role of the professional nurse. To ensure patient safety, communicate clearly with members of the health care team, assess and incorporate the patient's priorities of care and preferences, and use the best evidence when making decisions about your patient's care. When performing the skills in this chapter, remember the following points to ensure safe, individualized care:

- Know a patient's baseline range of vital signs. Patients with sudden changes in their vital signs, level of consciousness, or behavior are possibly experiencing profound hypoxia.
- Test all equipment before use. Have adequate supplies on hand. Verify that suction machine is generating adequate negative suction pressure.
- Perform tracheal suctioning before pharyngeal suctioning whenever possible. The mouth and pharynx contain more bacteria than the trachea. If oral secretions are abundantly present before beginning the procedure, suction the mouth with oral suction device.
- Use caution when suctioning patients with head injuries. Suctioning raises intracranial pressure (ICP). Reduce this risk by hyperventilating before suctioning, which produces hypocarbia that in turn induces vasoconstriction. Vasoconstriction reduces the potential increase in ICP.
- Limit the introduction of a catheter to 2 times with each suctioning procedure.

- Use caution when suctioning anyone with recent oral or head/neck surgery. Routine suctioning is avoided following tonsillectomy. Do not use or encourage agressive suctioning and excessive coughing in patients who have undergone throat surgery. These acts can aggravate the operative site, increasing the risk of infection or bleeding (Hockenberry et al., 2017).
- The routine use of normal saline instillation into the airway before endotracheal and tracheostomy suctioning is not recommended. Normal saline instillation in conjunction with endotracheal suction leads to the spread of microorganisms into the lower respiratory tract and decreases oxygenation saturation (Branson et al., 2014). Current evidence shows normal saline is not effective in thinning secretions or improving removal of secretions.
- Review your institutional policy before stripping or milking chest tubes. Most institutions have stopped this practice. Stripping causes a dangerous increase in intrathoracic pressure, which damages the lung tissue (Kane et al., 2013; American Association of Critical-Care Nurses [AACN], 2015). Chest drainage stripping or milking demonstrates no safety or efficacy benefits, slightly increases intrathoracic pressure, and risks tissue damage (AACN, 2015). Know policy and procedure if you are ordered to strip or milk a tube.

SKILL 32.1 SUCTIONING

View Video!

DELEGATION CONSIDERATIONS

The skill of nasotracheal suctioning and suctioning a new artificial airway cannot be delegated to nursing assistive personnel (NAP). When a patient has been assessed by the nurse to be stable, oropharyngeal and permanent tracheostomy tube suctioning can be delegated. The nurse directs the NAP about:

- Any modifications of the skill such as the need for supplemental oxygen.
- Appropriate suction limits and risks of applying excessive or inadequate suction pressure.
- Expected frequency of suctioning and color and volume of secretions.
- Risks of applying excessive or inadequate suctioning.
- How to avoid stimulating gag reflex with oropharyngeal suctioning.
- Immediately reporting any changes in patient's vital signs, pulse oximetry, level of consciousness, secretion color (bloody) and amount, unresolved coughing or gagging, difficulty breathing, or complaints of pain.

EQUIPMENT

- Stethoscope, pulse oximeter, end tidal CO_2 detector
- Portable or wall suction machine
- Connecting tubing

- Mask, goggles, gown or face shield if indicated (have available a manual self-inflating resuscitation bag-valve device/mask with appropriately sized mask and oxygen connecting tubing)

Oropharyngeal (Nonsterile) and Nasotracheal (Sterile) Suctioning

- Oropharyngeal—Clean suction catheter or Yankauer catheter, two clean gloves
- Nasotracheal—Sterile suction catheter (12 to 16 Fr) (smallest diameter preferred), two sterile gloves, sterile water-soluble lubricant
- Sterile basin with sterile water or normal saline (about 100 mL)
- Clean towel or paper drape

Endotracheal or Tracheostomy Suctioning

- 12 to 16-Fr catheter (no more than half of the internal diameter of artificial airway (Branson et al., 2014).
- Two sterile gloves or one sterile and one clean glove
- Sterile basin with normal saline (about 100 mL)
- Clean towel or sterile drape.

Closed System or In-Line Suctioning

- Closed-system or in-line suction catheter
- 5 to 10 mL normal saline in syringe or vials (to cleanse catheter)
- Two clean gloves

STEP	RATIONALE
ASSESSMENT	
1. Identify patient using at least two identifiers (e.g., name and birthday or name and medical record number) according to agency policy.	Ensures correct patient. Complies with The Joint Commission standards and improves patient safety (TJC, 2018).
2. Review laboratory data for sputum microbiology.	Certain bacteria are easier to transmit or require isolation because of virulence or antibiotic resistance.
3. Review patient's health care record for factors creating a risk for patient to be unable to clear airway: history of upper and lower airway obstruction, pulmonary disease, neuromuscular or neurological impairment, anatomical factors that influence upper or lower airway function, recent surgery, head or neck tumors, impaired mobility, decreased level of consciousness, nasal feeding tube, decreased cough or gag reflex, and decreased swallowing ability.	Factors can impair patient's ability to clear secretions from airway, accumulate secretions, and increase risk for retaining secretions, all requiring suctioning (Urden et al., 2016).
4. Review patient's health care record for factors that may affect volume and consistency of secretions.	Thickened or copious secretions increase risk for airway obstruction.
a. Fluid balance	Fluid overload increases amount of secretions. Dehydration promotes thicker secretions.
b. Lack of humidity	The environment influences secretion formation and gas exchange. Airway suctioning is needed when patient cannot clear secretions effectively.
c. Infection (e.g., pneumonia)	Patients are prone to increased secretions that are thicker and sometimes more difficult to expectorate.
5. Perform hand hygiene. Assess for signs and symptoms associated with hypoxia and hypercapnia: decreased SpO_2, increased and irregular pulse, increased respirations and blood pressure, apprehension, anxiety, irritability, lack of concentration, lethargy, decreased level of consciousness (especially sudden change), confusion, dizziness, fatigue, pallor, and cyanosis (very late sign of hypoxia).	Reduces transmission of microorganisms. Physical signs and symptoms resulting from decreased tissue oxygenation. Provides presuction baseline to measure effectiveness of suctioning.

STEP	RATIONALE
6. Assess for signs and symptoms of upper and lower airway obstruction: abnormal respiratory rate, adventitious lung sounds, nasal secretions, gurgling, drooling, restlessness, gastric secretions or vomitus in mouth, and coughing without clearing airway secretions and/or improving adventitious lung sounds.	Physical signs and symptoms result from secretions in upper and lower airways and decreased oxygen to tissues. Presuction assessment provides baseline data to identify need for suctioning and measure effectiveness of suction procedures (Branson et al., 2014).
7. Assess for excessive amounts of secretions or secretions visible in artificial airway, signs of respiratory distress (increased work of breathing, increased respiratory rate), presence of rhonchi on auscultation, excessive coughing, increased peak inspiratory pressures (if patient on mechanical ventilator), sawtooth pattern on ventilator monitor, changes in capnography waveform (if patient on mechanical ventilator), or decrease in patient's pulse oximeter (Branson et al., 2014).	Perform suctioning only as patient's condition indicates and not in a scheduled fashion (Lewis et al., 2017; Myatt, 2015).
8. Assess patency of ETT with capnography and/or end-tidal carbon dioxide (CO_2) detector.	ETT may become displaced or blocked by secretions. CO_2 detector is pH sensitive and can identify changes in CO_2 levels resulting from retained secretions (Walsh et al., 2011).
9. For endotracheal suctioning, assess patient's peak inspiratory pressure on volume-controlled ventilation or tidal volume on pressure-controlled ventilation.	Increased peak inspiratory pressure or decreased tidal volume may indicate airway obstruction (Urden et al., 2016).

Clinical Decision Point. Assess a patient's vital signs, pulse oximetry, end-tidal CO_2, and respiratory status before and continuously throughout suctioning procedure (Wiegand, 2017).

STEP	RATIONALE
10. Identify **contraindications to nasotracheal suctioning** (AARC, 2004): occluded nasal passages; nasal bleeding; epiglottitis or croup; acute head, facial, or neck injury or surgery; coagulopathy or bleeding disorder; irritable airway; laryngospasm or bronchospasm; gastric surgery with high anastomosis; myocardial infarction.	These conditions are contraindications because passage of a suction catheter through the nasal route traumatizes existing facial trauma and/or surgery, increases nasal bleeding, or causes severe bleeding. In the presence of epiglottitis or croup, laryngospasm, or irritable airway, passage of a suction catheter through the nose causes intractable coughing, hypoxemia, and severe bronchospasm necessitating emergency intubation or tracheostomy. Hypoxemia could worsen cardiac damage in myocardial infarction (AARC, 2004).
11. Assess patient's understanding of procedure and presence of any apprehension.	Reveals need for instruction or psychosocial support.

PLANNING

1. Provide privacy and place pulse oximeter on patient's finger, if not already in place. Take reading and leave oximeter in place. Prepare bedside environment for patient safety.	Provides continuous SpO_2 value to determine patient's response to suctioning. Providing privacy and preparing environment ensures a clean and distraction-free area for organizing necessary equipment.
2. Prepare and organize equipment. Place towel across patient's chest.	Ensures that you have the necessary equipment to implement all the interventions that need to be completed for patient.
3. Explain to patient how procedure will help clear airway and relieve breathing difficulty. Explain that temporary coughing, sneezing, gagging, or shortness of breath is normal during procedure.	Encourages cooperation and minimizes risks, anxiety, and pain of procedure.
4. Explain importance of and encourage coughing when catheter is introduced. Have patient practice coughing if able.	Facilitates secretion removal and reduces frequency and duration of suctioning.

IMPLEMENTATION

1. Perform hand hygiene and apply appropriate personal protective equipment (PPE) (mask with face shield or goggles; gown if splashing likely).	Reduces transmission of microorganisms.
2. Adjust bed to appropriate height (if not already done) and lower side rail on side nearest you. Check locks on bed wheel.	Minimizes caregiver muscle strain and prevents injury. Prevents the bed from moving.

SKILL 32.1 SUCTIONING—cont'd

View Video!

STEP	RATIONALE
3. Assist patient to comfortable position, typically semi-Fowler's or high Fowler's.	Reduces stimulation of gag reflex, promotes patient comfort and secretion drainage, and prevents aspiration.
4. Connect one end of connecting tubing to suction device and place other end in convenient location near patient. Turn suction device on and set suction pressure to as low a level as possible and yet able to effectively clear secretions. This value is typically between 100 and 120 mm Hg in adults (between 80 and 100 mm Hg in neonates) and should never be more than 180 mm Hg (Branson et al., 2014). Occlude end of suction tubing to check pressure.	Ensures equipment function. Excessive negative pressure damages tracheal mucosa and induces greater hypoxia (Wiegand, 2017).
5. If indicated, increase supplemental oxygen therapy to 100% as ordered by health care provider; encourage patient to deep breathe.	Hyperoxygenation provides some protection from suction-induced decline in oxygenation.
6. Prepare suction catheter for all types of suctioning.	
a. *One-time-use* catheter (open suction technique):	
(1) Using aseptic technique, open suction kit or catheter package. If sterile drape is available, place it across patient's chest or on bedside table. Do not allow suction catheter to touch any nonsterile surfaces.	Prepares catheter, maintains asepsis, and reduces transmission of microorganisms. Provides sterile surface on which to lay catheter between passes.
(2) Unwrap or open sterile basin and place on bedside table. Be careful not to touch inside of basin. Fill with about 100 mL sterile normal saline solution or water (see illustration).	Saline or water is used to clean tubing after each suction pass.
(3) If performing nasotracheal suctioning, open packet of water-soluble lubricant and apply a small amount onto sterile wrapper or kit without touching it. **Note:** Lubricant is not necessary for artificial airway suctioning.	Water-soluble lubricant helps avoid lipid aspiration pneumonia. Excessive amount of lubricant occludes catheter.
b. Closed (in-line) suction catheter:	
(1) Using aseptic technique, open suction catheter package and attach closed suction catheter to ventilation circuit by removing swivel adapter and placing closed suction catheter apparatus on ETT or TT. Connect Y on mechanical ventilator circuit to closed suction catheter with flex tubing.	Prepares catheter, maintains asepsis, and reduces transmission of microorganisms.

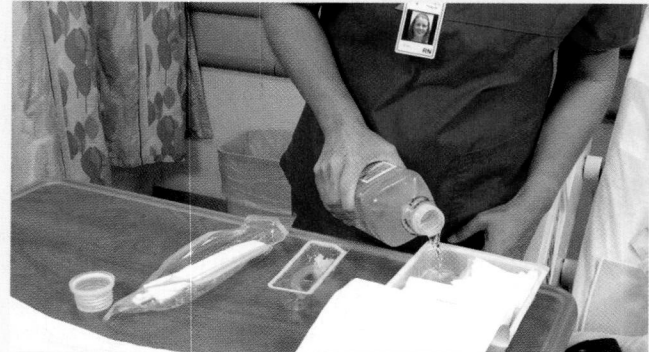

STEP 6a2 Pouring sterile saline into tray.

STEP	RATIONALE
(2) Connect one end of connecting tubing to suction machine; connect other end to end of closed system or in-line suction catheter. Check suction pressures.	Many closed system suction catheters require slightly higher suction pressures (consult manufacturer guidelines).
7. Apply gloves: a. Apply clean glove to each hand or dominant hand for oropharyngeal and closed suctioning. b. Apply sterile gloves to each hand or nonsterile glove to nondominant hand and sterile glove to dominant hand for nasopharyngeal, nasotracheal, and artificial airway suctioning.	Reduces transmission of microorganisms and maintains sterility of suction catheter.
8. Pick up suction catheter with dominant hand without touching nonsterile surfaces. Pick up connecting tubing with nondominant hand. Secure catheter to tubing (see illustration).	Maintains catheter sterility. Connects catheter to suction.
9. Place tip of catheter into sterile basin and suction a small amount of normal saline solution by occluding suction vent. **Note:** Skip this step with closed suctioning technique.	Ensures equipment function. Lubricates internal catheter and tubing.
10. Suction airway. a. **Oropharyngeal suctioning:** (1) Remove patient's oxygen mask if present. Nasal cannula may remain in place. Keep oxygen mask near patient's face.	Allows access to mouth. Reduces chance of hypoxia.

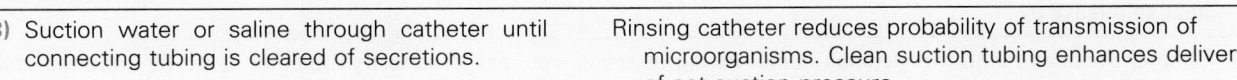

Clinical Decision Point. Be prepared to quickly reapply supplemental oxygen if SpO_2 value falls below 90% or respiratory distress develops during or at the end of oropharyngeal suctioning. Be prepared to use bag-valve-mask if patient has serious acute respiratory distress or decline in SpO_2.

STEP	RATIONALE
(2) Insert Yankauer catheter into mouth. Then apply suction and move catheter along gum line to pharynx. Suction until secretions have cleared. Encourage patient to cough. Repeat if needed. Replace oxygen mask if used.	Movement of catheter prevents suction tip from damaging oral mucosal surfaces and causing trauma. Coughing moves secretions from lower airway into mouth and upper airway.

Clinical Decision Point. Use caution when using a Yankauer tip suction catheter with a patient who had recent oral or head and neck surgery.

STEP	RATIONALE
(3) Suction water or saline through catheter until connecting tubing is cleared of secretions.	Rinsing catheter reduces probability of transmission of microorganisms. Clean suction tubing enhances delivery of set suction pressure.

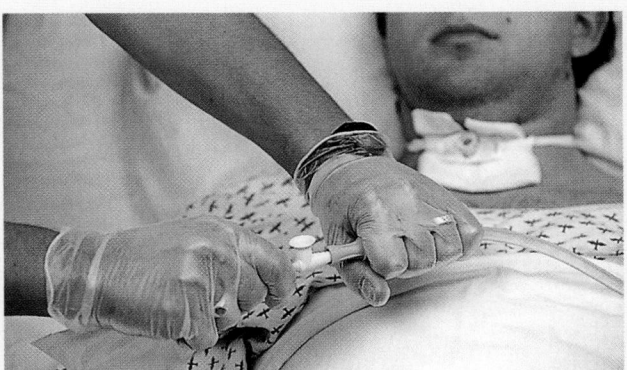

STEP 8 Attaching suction catheter to suction tubing.

SKILL 32.1   SUCTIONING—cont'd

View Video!

STEP	RATIONALE
(4) Turn off suction and place catheter in clean, dry area. If patient is able to suction self, place catheter within his or her reach and leave suction on.	Facilitates prompt removal of airway secretions for future suctioning.

b. **Nasopharyngeal and nasotracheal suctioning:**

STEP	RATIONALE
(1) Have patient take deep breaths, if able. Increase oxygen flow rate through cannula or mask if ordered.	Helps to decrease risks of hypoxemia.
(2) For nasotracheal suctioning, lightly coat distal 6 to 8 cm (2 to 3 inches) of catheter with water-soluble lubricant.	Lubricates catheter for easier insertion and reduces mucosal trauma.
(3) Remove oxygen delivery device, if applicable, with nondominant hand.	
(a) *Nasopharyngeal:* Without applying suction, have patient take a deep breath, and use dominant thumb and forefinger to insert catheter following natural course of naris; slightly slant catheter downward and advance to back of pharynx. Do not force through naris. In adults insert catheter approximately 20 cm (8 inches) into trachea until resistance is met or patient coughs, then pull back 1 to 2 cm (½ inch). In infants and children the suction catheter must not be passed any further than the suprasternal notch, which is the dip at the front base of the neck (Association of Paediatric Chartered Physiotherapists, 2015) (refer to agency policy).	Application of suction pressure while introducing catheter into nasopharynx increases risk for damage to mucosa and increases risk for hypoxia. Ensure that catheter tip reaches pharynx for suctioning.
Rule of thumb is to insert catheter distance from tip of nose (or mouth) to angle of mandible.	

Clinical Decision Point. Do not insert during swallowing or catheter will most likely enter esophagus. Never apply suction during insertion. Patient should cough; if patient gags or becomes nauseated, catheter is most likely in esophagus and you need to remove it.

Clinical Decision Point. If resistance is met during insertion, you may need to try the other naris. Do not force catheter through naris, as this will cause mucosal damage.

STEP	RATIONALE
(i) Apply intermittent suction for 2 seconds by placing and releasing nondominant thumb over catheter vent. Then slowly withdraw catheter while rotating it back and forth and applying intermittent suction. Total time should take about 10 to 15 seconds.	Intermittent suction for 10 to 15 seconds safely removes pharyngeal secretions. Suction time greater than 10 to 15 seconds increases risk for suction-induced hypoxemia (Branson et al., 2014).

STEP	RATIONALE
(b) *Nasotracheal* (without applying suction): Advance catheter using same procedure as nasopharyngeal through the naris. When just above entrance into larynx, have patient relax and then take a deep breath as you quickly advance catheter into trachea. Advance catheter in an adult approximately 20 cm (8 inches) into trachea (see illustration). Patient will begin to cough; pull back catheter 1 to 2 cm (½ inch) before applying suction. **Note:** In older children, insert 15 to 20 cm (6 to 8 inches); in infants and young children, insert 8 to 14 cm (3 to 5½ inches).	Inhalation opens glottis and facilitates entrance of catheter tip into trachea for suctioning.

Clinical Decision Point. Be sure to insert catheter during patient inhalation because epiglottis is open. When using the nasal approach, perform tracheal suctioning before pharyngeal suctioning whenever possible. The mouth and pharynx contain more bacteria than the trachea. If copious oral secretions are present before beginning procedure, first suction mouth with oral suction device such as a Yankauer.

Clinical Decision Point. When there is difficulty passing catheter, ask patient to cough or say "ahh" or try to advance catheter during inspiration. Both measures help to open the glottis to permit passage of catheter into the trachea.

STEP	RATIONALE
(i) Positioning option: In some instances, turning patient's head helps you insert catheter and suction more effectively. If you feel resistance after insertion of catheter, use caution, as it has probably hit the carina. Pull catheter back 1 to 2 cm (0.4 to 0.8 inches) before applying suction (AARC, 2004).	Turning patient's head to side elevates bronchial passage on opposite side. Turning head to right helps you suction left main-stem bronchus; turning head to left helps you suction right main-stem bronchus. Suctioning too deep may cause tracheal mucosa trauma.
(ii) Apply intermittent suction for no more than 10 to 15 seconds by placing and releasing nondominant thumb over catheter vent. Slowly withdraw catheter while rotating it back and forth between thumb and forefinger.	Suction time greater than 10 to 15 seconds increases risk for suction-induced hypoxemia (AARC, 2010; Branson et al., 2014). Intermittent suction and rotation of catheter prevent injury to tracheal mucosa. If catheter "grabs" mucosa, remove thumb to release suction.

Clinical Decision Point. Monitor patient's vital signs and oxygen saturation throughout suctioning process. Stop suctioning if there is a 20 beat/minute change (increase or decrease) in pulse or if SpO_2 falls below 90% or 5% from baseline.

STEP	RATIONALE
(4) Reapply oxygen delivery device and encourage patient to take some deep breaths, if able.	Helps to decrease risk of hypoxia. Increases patient comfort.
(5) Rinse catheter and connecting tubing with normal saline or water until cleared.	Secretions that remain in suction catheter or connecting tubing decrease suctioning efficiency.

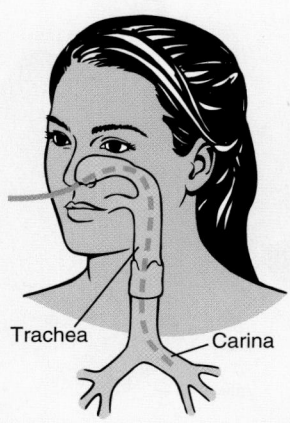

Trachea   Carina

STEP 10b(3)(b) Distance of insertion of nasotracheal catheter.

SKILL 32.1   SUCTIONING—cont'd

STEP	RATIONALE
(6) Assess for need to repeat suctioning. Do not perform more than two passes with catheter. Allow patient to rest at least 1 minute (Wiegand, 2017). Ask patient to deep breathe and cough.	Observe for alterations in cardiopulmonary status. Suctioning induces hypoxemia, irregular pulse, laryngospasm, and bronchospasm (Wiegand, 2017).
c. Artificial airway—one-time use catheter:	
(1) When patient has artificial airway (e.g., ETT or TT), hyperoxygenate patient with 100% oxygen for at least 30 to 60 seconds before suctioning by either pressing suction hyperoxygenation button on ventilator *or* increasing baseline FiO$_2$ level on mechanical ventilator. **Note:** Some mechanical ventilators have a button that when pushed delivers 100% oxygen for a few minutes and then resets to previous setting.	Preoxygenation decreases risk of decreased arterial oxygen levels while ventilation or oxygenation is interrupted and volume is lost during suctioning. Some models of resuscitation bags do not deliver 100% oxygen, so this is not the best way to oxygenate a patient (Wiegand, 2017). Consult with respiratory therapist if necessary.
(2) If patient is receiving mechanical ventilation, open swivel adapter or, if necessary, remove oxygen or humidity delivery device with nondominant hand.	Exposes artificial airway.

Clinical Decision Point. Suctioning can cause elevations in intracranial pressure (ICP) in patients with head injuries. Reduce this risk by presuction hyperoxygenation, which results in hypocarbia that in turn induces vasoconstriction. Vasoconstriction reduces the potential for increased ICP (Urden et al., 2016).

(3) Advise patient that you are about to begin suctioning. Without applying suction, gently but quickly insert catheter into artificial airway using dominant thumb and forefinger (try to time catheter insertion into artificial airway during inspiration) until you meet resistance or patient coughs; then pull back 1 cm (0.4 inch) (see illustration) (Wiegand, 2017).	Application of suction pressure while introducing catheter into trachea increases risk for damage to tracheal mucosa and increased hypoxia. Pulling back stimulates cough and removes catheter from mucosal wall so that catheter is not resting against tracheal mucosa during suctioning. Shallow suctioning is recommended to prevent tracheal mucosa trauma (AARC, 2010; Wiegand, 2017).

Clinical Decision Point. If unable to insert catheter past end of ET tube, the catheter is probably caught in the Murphy eye (i.e., side hole at distal end of ET tube that allows for collateral airflow in the event of tracheal main-stem intubation). If this happens, rotate catheter to reposition it away from Murphy eye or withdraw it slightly and reinsert with next inhalation. Usually the catheter meets resistance at the carina. One indication that the catheter is at the carina is acute onset of coughing because the carina contains many cough receptors. Pull the catheter back 1 cm (½ inch).

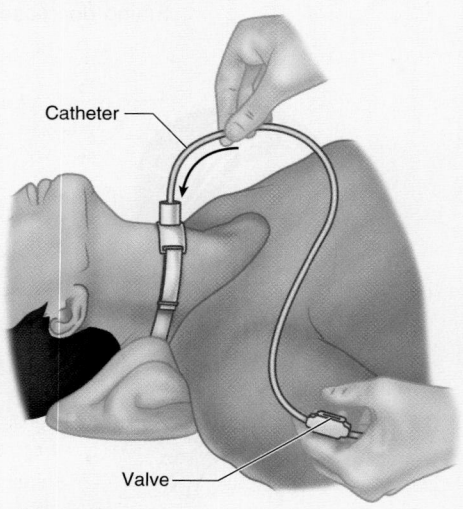

Catheter

Valve

STEP 10c(3) Suctioning tracheostomy.

STEP	RATIONALE
(4) Apply intermittent suction for 10 to 15 seconds (AARC, 2010; Branson et al., 2014). Apply intermittent suction by placing and releasing nondominant thumb over vent of catheter; slowly withdraw catheter while rotating it back and forth between dominant thumb and forefinger. Do not use suction for greater than 10 to 15 seconds. Encourage patient to cough. Watch for respiratory distress.	Suction time greater than 10 to 15 seconds increases risk for suction-induced hypoxemia (AARC, 2010; Branson et al., 2014). Intermittent suction and rotation of catheter prevents injury to tracheal mucosa. If catheter "grabs" mucosa, remove thumb to release suction.

Clinical Decision Point. If patient develops respiratory distress, immediately withdraw catheter and supply additional oxygen and breaths as needed. In an emergency, administer oxygen directly through catheter. Disconnect suction and attach oxygen at prescribed flow rate through catheter. If patient does not tolerate suctioning procedure, you may need to consider switching to closed (in-line) suctioning or allowing longer recovery times. Notify health care provider if patient develops significant cardiopulmonary compromise during suctioning (Urden et al., 2016; Wiegand, 2017).

STEP	RATIONALE
(5) If patient is receiving mechanical ventilation, close swivel adapter or replace oxygen delivery device. Hyperoxygenate patient for 30 to 60 seconds.	Reestablishes artificial airway. Helps to decrease risks of hypoxia.
d. Artificial airway suctioning—closed (in-line):	
(1) Hyperoxygenate patient (usually with 100% oxygen) by adjusting FiO_2 setting on ventilator or by using a temporary oxygen-enrichment program available on microprocessor ventilators, according to agency policy.	Preoxygenation decreases risk of decreased arterial oxygen levels while ventilation or oxygenation is interrupted and volume is lost during suctioning.
(2) Unlock suction control mechanism on suction catheter if required by manufacturer. Open saline port and attach saline syringe or vial.	Lock prevents catheter from accidentally migrating into airway when not in use. Unlocking catheter allows you to use it. The saline will be necessary to clean catheter between each suction pass.
(3) Pick up suction catheter enclosed in plastic sleeve with dominant hand. While patient inhales and without applying suction, insert catheter using a repeating maneuver of pushing catheter and sliding (or pulling) plastic sleeve back between thumb and forefinger until resistance is felt or patient coughs. Then pull back 1 cm (0.5 inch).	Application of suction pressure while introducing catheter into trachea increases risk for damage to tracheal mucosa and increased hypoxia. Pulling back stimulates cough and removes catheter from mucosal wall so that catheter is not resting against tracheal mucosa during suctioning.
(4) Encourage patient to cough and apply suction by continuously squeezing on suction control mechanism while withdrawing catheter over a period of no longer than 10 to 15 seconds.	It is difficult, if not impossible, to apply intermittent pulses of suction to a closed system catheter. Suctioning for longer periods of time increases risk of complications resulting from hypoxemia.
The following steps pertain to both open and closed tracheal suctioning:	
(5) Rinse catheter and connecting tubing with normal saline until clear. Use continuous suction.	Removes catheter secretions. Secretions left in tubing decrease suctioning efficiency and provide environment for microorganism growth.
(6) Assess patient's vital signs, cardiopulmonary status, and ventilator measures for secretion clearance. Repeat Steps (1) through (6) once or twice more to clear secretions. Allow adequate time (at least 1 full minute) between suction passes.	Suctioning can induce dysrhythmias, hypoxia, and bronchospasm and impair cerebral circulation or adversely affect hemodynamic stability (Wiegand, 2017).

Clinical Decision Point. Base the number of suction passes on patient assessment and presence of secretions. If secretions persist after two passes, allow patient more time to rest and recover from these procedures (Wiegand, 2017).

STEP	RATIONALE
(7) When pharynx and trachea are sufficiently cleared of secretions, perform oropharyngeal suctioning to clear mouth of secretions. Do not suction nose again after suctioning mouth.	Removes upper airway secretions. More microorganisms generally are present in mouth. Upper airway is considered "clean," and lower airway is considered "sterile." You can use same catheter to suction from sterile to clean areas (e.g., tracheal suctioning to oropharyngeal suctioning) but not from clean to sterile areas.

SKILL 32.1 SUCTIONING—cont'd

View Video!

STEP	RATIONALE
11. When suctioning is complete, disconnect the one-time use catheter from connecting tubing. Roll catheter around fingers of dominant hand. Pull glove off inside out so catheter remains coiled in glove. Pull off other glove over first glove in same way. Discard in appropriate receptacle. Turn off suction device. For closed suction catheter, ensure the catheter is pulled all the way back into sleeve, and if device has a locking mechanism, ensure that mechanism is locked.	Seals contaminants in gloves. Reduces transmission of microorganisms (Wiegand, 2017). Pulling closed suction catheter device back into sleeve ensures airway is not obstructed.
12. Remove towel or drape, place in laundry or appropriate receptacle, and reposition patient. (Apply clean gloves to continue personal care.)	Reduces transmission of microorganisms. Promotes comfort.
13. If indicated, readjust oxygen to original level because patient's blood oxygen level should have returned to baseline.	Prevents absorption atelectasis (i.e., tendency for airways to collapse if proximally obstructed by secretions). Prevents oxygen toxicity while allowing patient time to reoxygenate blood.
14. Discard remainder of normal saline into appropriate receptacle. If basin is disposable, discard into appropriate receptacle. If basin is reusable, rinse it out and place it in soiled utility room.	Reduces transmission of microorganisms.
15. Remove personal protective equipment and discard into appropriate receptacle. Perform hand hygiene.	Reduces transmission of microorganisms.
16. Place unopened suction kit on suction machine table or at head of bed.	Provides immediate access to suction catheter for next procedure.
17. Help patient to comfortable position and provide oral hygiene as needed. Wash face if secretions are present on patient's skin.	Prevents skin breakdown. Promotes comfort.

EVALUATION

1. Compare patient's vital signs, cardiopulmonary assessments, and end-tidal CO_2 ($EtCO_2$) and SpO_2 values before and after suctioning. If on ventilator, compare FiO_2 and tidal volumes and peak inspiratory pressures.	$PetCO_2$ is a noninvasive measurement of a patient's exhaled CO_2, and it can be used to help continuously monitor the amount of CO_2 in patients with artificial airways. Measures identify physiological effects of suction procedure (Wiegand, 2017).
2. Ask patient if breathing is easier and if congestion is decreased.	Provides subjective confirmation that suctioning procedure has relieved airway obstruction.
3. Auscultate lungs and compare patient's respiratory assessment before and after suctioning.	Provides objective information about any change in lung sounds.
4. Observe character of airway secretions.	Provides data to document presence or absence of respiratory tract infection or thickened secretions.
5. **Use Teach-Back:** "I need to suction your father and I want to be sure that I explained the suctioning procedure and when I need to do this procedure. Please, tell me why I'm having to suction your dad at this time." Revise your instruction now or develop a plan for revised patient/family caregiver teaching if patient/family caregiver is not able to teach back correctly.	Determines patient's/family caregiver's level of understanding of instructional topic.

RECORDING AND REPORTING

- Record in nurses' notes in electronic health record (EHR), chart, or flow sheets patient's presuctioning vital signs, cardiopulmonary status, and ventilation measures; need for and type of hyperoxygenation used; amount, consistency, color, and odor of secretions; size of catheter; route of suctioning.

- Record patient's response to suctioning and postsuctioning vital signs, cardiopulmonary status, and ventilation measures.
- Document your evaluation of patient/family caregiver learning.
- Report unexpected outcomes.

UNEXPECTED OUTCOMES AND RELATED INTERVENTIONS

- Patient has decrease in SpO_2, increased end-tidal CO_2, continued tachypnea, continued increased work of breathing, bronchospasm, and cardiac dysrhythmias.
  - Limit length of suctioning.
  - Determine need for more frequent suctioning, possibly of shorter duration.
  - Determine need for supplemental oxygen or increase in supplemental oxygen. Supply oxygen between suctioning passes as ordered.
  - Notify health care provider.
- Bloody secretions are returned after suctioning.
  - Determine amount of suction pressure used. May need to be decreased.
- Ensure that suction is completed correctly using intermittent suction and catheter rotation. Do not apply suction until after catheter has been pulled back 1 cm to prevent applying suction while catheter is touching the carina.
  - Evaluate suctioning frequency.
- Inability to obtain secretions during suction procedure.
  - Evaluate patient's fluid status and adequacy of humidification on oxygen delivery device.
  - Assess for signs of infection.
  - Determine need for chest physiotherapy.
  - Notify health care provider.

SKILL 32.2 CARE OF PATIENTS WITH CHEST TUBES

DELEGATION AND COLLABORATION

The skill of chest tube management cannot be delegated to nursing assistive personnel (NAP). The nurse directs the NAP about:

- Proper positioning of the patient with chest tubes to facilitate chest tube drainage and optimal functioning of the system.
- How to safely ambulate and transfer patient with chest drainage.
- Reporting changes in vital signs, pulse oximetry, complaints of chest pain or sudden shortness of breath, or excessive bubbling in water-seal chamber to the nurse immediately.
- Immediately notifying nurse if there is disconnection of drainage system, change in type and amount of drainage, sudden bleeding, or sudden cessation of bubbling.

EQUIPMENT

- Prescribed chest drainage system with suction source and setup (wall canister or portable)
  - *Water-seal system:* Add sterile water or normal saline (NS) solution to cover lower 2.5 cm (1 inch) of water-seal chamber. Pour sterile water or NS into suction control chamber if suction is to be used (see manufacturer directions).
  - *Waterless system:* Add vial of 30- to 45-mL sterile sodium chloride or water (for diagnostic air-leak indicator); 20-mL syringe, 21-gauge needle, and antiseptic swab (see manufacturer directions).
  - Dry suction system
- Suction tubing
- Clean gloves
- Sterile gauze sponges
- Local anesthetic with appropriate sized syringe and needle, if not an emergent procedure
- Chest tube tray (all items are sterile): knife handle (1), knife blade No. 10 or disposable safety scalpel No. 10, chest tube clamp, small sponge forceps, needle holder, size 3-0 silk sutures, tray liner (sterile field), curved 8-inch Kelly clamps (2), 4 × 4–inch sponges (10), suture scissors, hand towels (3), sterile gloves
- Dressings: petrolatum (Xeroform) gauze, split chest tube dressings, several 4 × 4–inch gauze dressings, large gauze dressings (2), and 2-inch or 4-inch tape (see agency procedure)
- Facemask, head cover, face shield, or goggles (as needed)
- Sterile gloves
- Two rubber-tipped hemostats (shodded) for each chest tube (for emergencies)
- 2.5-cm (1-inch) waterproof adhesive tape or plastic zip ties for securing connections
- Stethoscope, sphygmomanometer, and pulse oximeter

STEP	RATIONALE

ASSESSMENT

1. Identify patient using at least two identifiers (e.g., name and birthday or name and medical record number) according to agency policy.

2. Assess patient for known allergies. Ask patient if he or she has had a problem with medications, latex, or anything applied to skin.

3. Review patient's medication record for anticoagulant therapy or nonsteroidal antiinflammatory drugs (NSAIDs) including aspirin, warfarin, heparin, or platelet aggregation inhibitors.

Ensures correct patient. Complies with The Joint Commission standards and improves patient safety (TJC, 2018).

Antiseptic solutions are used to clean skin before tube insertion (Kane et al., 2013). Lidocaine is a local anesthetic administered to reduce pain. The chest tube will be held in place with tape and sutures.

Anticoagulants and NSAIDs can increase procedure-related blood loss.

SKILL 32.2 CARE OF PATIENTS WITH CHEST TUBES—cont'd

STEP	RATIONALE
4. Review patient's hemoglobin and hematocrit levels.	Parameters reflect if blood loss is occurring, which may affect oxygenation and other vital signs.
5. Perform hand hygiene. Perform a complete respiratory assessment, baseline vital signs, pulse oximetry, and level of cognition.	Reduces transmission of microorganisms. Determines level of respiratory distress. Cognitive changes indicate hypoxia.
a. Assess for signs and symptoms of increased respiratory distress and hypoxia (e.g., decreased breath sounds over affected lungs, cyanosis, asymmetrical chest movements, displaced trachea, shortness of breath, confusion).	Signs and symptoms associated with respiratory distress are related to type and size of pneumothorax, hemothorax, or preexisting illness. Signs of hypoxia are related to inadequate oxygen to tissues (Lewis et al., 2017).
b. Assess for sharp stabbing chest pain or chest pain on inspiration, hypotension, and tachycardia. If possible, ask patient to rate level of comfort on visual analog scale of 0 to 10.	Sharp stabbing chest pain, low blood pressure, and increased heart rate may indicate tension pneumothorax. Pneumothorax or hemothorax is painful, particularly with inspiration. In addition, discomfort is associated with presence of chest tube. As a result, patients tend to not cough or change position in an effort to minimize pain (Ball et al., 2015).
6. For patients who have chest tubes in place, observe:	
a. Chest tube dressing and site surrounding tube insertion.	Ensures that dressing is intact and occlusive seal remains without air or fluid leaks and that area surrounding insertion site is free of drainage or skin irritation. Leakage of air into tissue manifests as subcutaneous emphysema.
b. Tubing for kinks, dependent loops, or clots.	Maintains a patent, freely draining system, preventing fluid or air accumulation in chest cavity. When tubing is coiled, looped, or clotted, drainage is impeded (Mohammed, 2015).
c. Chest drainage system should be upright and below level of tube insertion.	Upright drainage system facilitates drainage and maintains water seal. If above site of insertion, fluid will drain back into patient (Mohammed, 2015; Lewis et al., 2017).
7. Determine patient's and family caregiver's knowledge of procedure and reason for tubes.	Encourages cooperation, minimizes risks and anxiety, and identifies teaching needs.

PLANNING

1. Provide privacy and prepare bedside environment by removing any items that are not needed for procedure.	Reduces interruptions and provides clean surface areas in the patient environment
2. Prepare and organize equipment and supplies. Place two rubber-tipped hemostats (for each chest tube) in an easily accessible position (e.g., taped to top of patient's headboard). These should remain with patient at all times, even during ambulation.	Ensures organized procedure. Chest tubes are double clamped under specific circumstances: (1) to assess for air leak, (2) to empty or quickly change disposable systems, (3) to assess if patient is ready to have tube removed.
3. Explain procedure and continued care of chest tube to patient and family caregiver.	Encourages cooperation and decreases anxiety.

IMPLEMENTATION

1. For tube insertion; check agency policy and determine whether informed consent is needed. Complete time-out procedure.	Invasive medical procedures typically require informed consent. Time-out is completed to determine right patient, procedure, and location of insertion or incision site (Kane et al., 2013).
2. Review health care provider's order for chest tube placement.	Insertion of a chest tube requires health care provider order.
3. Perform hand hygiene.	Prevents transmission of microorganisms.

STEP	RATIONALE
4. Administer premedication such as sedatives or analgesics as ordered 30 minutes before tube insertion.	Reduces patient anxiety and pain during procedure.
5. Set up water-seal system (or dry system with suction); see manufacturer guidelines.	
a. Remove sterile wrappers and prepare to set up a two- or three-chamber system.	Maintains sterility of system for use under sterile operating room conditions.
b. While maintaining sterility of drainage tubing, stand system upright and add sterile water or NS to appropriate compartments.	Reduces possibility of contamination.
(1) *Two-chamber system (without suction):* Add sterile solution to water-seal chamber, bringing fluid to required level as indicated.	Water-seal chamber acts as one-way valve so that air cannot enter pleural space (Kane et al., 2013).
(2) *Three-chamber system (with suction):* Add sterile solution to water-seal chamber. Add amount of sterile solution prescribed by health care provider to suction control chamber, usually 20 cm H_2O pressure. Connect tubing from suction control chamber to suction source. Tailor length of drainage tube to patient. **Note:** Suction control chamber vent must not be occluded when using suction (see Fig. 32.12).	Depth of fluid level dictates highest amount of negative pressure that can be present within system. For example, 20 cm of water is approximately 20 cm H_2O pressure. Any additional negative pressure applied to the system is vented into the atmosphere through suction control vent. This safety device prevents damage to pleural tissues from unexpected surge of negative pressure from suction source.
	After chest tube is inserted, turn up wall or portable suction device until water in suction control bottle exhibits continuous, gentle bubbling (Kane et al., 2013; Mohammed, 2015).

Clinical Decision Point. Remember when increasing suction that increased bubbling does not result in more suction to the chest cavity but serves only to evaporate the water more quickly.

STEP	RATIONALE
(3) *Dry suction system:* Fill water-seal chamber with sterile solution. Adjust suction control dial to prescribed level of suction; suction ranges from −10 to −40 cm H_2O pressure. Suction control chamber vent is never occluded when suction is used. **Note:** On a dry suction system, *do not* obstruct positive-pressure relief valve. This allows air to escape.	Automatic control valve on dry suction control device adjusts to changes in patient air leaks and fluctuation in suction source and vacuum to deliver prescribed amount of suction.
6. Set up waterless system (see manufacturer guidelines).	
a. Remove sterile wrappers and prepare to set up.	Maintains sterility of system for use under sterile operating room conditions.
b. For two-chamber system (without suction), nothing is added or needs to be done to system.	Waterless two-chamber system is ready for connecting to patient's chest tube after opening wrappers.
c. For three-chamber system (with suction), connect tubing from suction control chamber to suction source.	Suction source provides additional negative pressure to system.
d. Instill 15 mL of sterile water or NS into diagnostic indicator injection port located on top of system.	Allows observation of rise and fall in water in diagnostic air leak window. Constant left-to-right bubbling or rocking is abnormal and indicates air leak. This is not necessary for mediastinal drainage because there is no tidaling. In an emergency, system does not require water for set up.
7. Check system patency by:	Ensures functioning system.
a. Clamping drainage tubing that will connect to patient's chest tube.	
b. Connecting tubing from float ball chamber to suction source.	
c. Turning on suction to prescribed level.	

SKILL 32.2   CARE OF PATIENTS WITH CHEST TUBES—cont'd

STEP	RATIONALE
8. Turn off suction source and unclamp drainage tubing before connecting patient to system. Suction source is turned on again after patient is connected.	Having patient connected to suction when it is initiated could damage pleural tissues from sudden increase in negative pressure. Tubing that is coiled or looped may become clotted and cause tension pneumothorax (Kane et al., 2013).

Clinical Decision Point. Carefully monitor patient during procedure for changes in level of sedation. If patient is too sedated, patient will lose his or her respiratory drive and could potentially develop hypoxia.

STEP	RATIONALE
9. Provide psychological support to patient (Kane et al., 2013). Reinforce preprocedure explanation, and coach and support throughout insertion of tube(s).	Reduces patient anxiety and helps complete procedure efficiently.
10. Perform hand hygiene and apply clean gloves and any other PPE if you suspect exposure to fluid spray. Position patient for tube insertion so that side in which tube is to be inserted is accessible to health care provider.	Reduces transmission of microorganisms. For pneumothorax, place patient in lateral supine position. For hemothorax, place the patient in semi-Fowler's (Kane et al., 2013).
11. Assist health care provider with chest tube insertion by providing needed equipment and local anesthetic. Health care provider will anesthetize skin over insertion site, make small skin incision, insert clamped tube, suture it in place, and apply occlusive dressing.	Ensures smooth insertion.
12. Assist health care provider with attaching drainage tube to chest tube; remove clamp. Turn on suction to prescribed level.	Connects drainage system and suction (if ordered) to chest tube.
13. Tape or zip-tie all connections between chest tube and drainage tube. (**Note:** Chest tube is usually taped by health care provider at time of tube placement; check agency policy.)	Secures chest tube to drainage system and reduces risk for air leak that causes breaks in airtight system (Shlamovitz, 2014).
14. Check systems for proper functioning. Health care provider will order chest radiograph.	Verifies intrapleural placement of tube.
15. After tube placement, position patient in manner that promotes drainage of fluid or air.	Permits optimum drainage of fluid and/or air. Frequent repositioning promotes better drainage (Lewis et al., 2017).
a. Use semi-Fowler's or high-Fowler's position to evacuate air (pneumothorax) (Chotai, 2016).	
b. Use high-Fowler's position to drain fluid (hemothorax) (Chotai, 2016).	
16. Check patency of air vents in system	
a. Water-seal vent must have no occlusion.	Permits displaced air to pass into atmosphere.
b. Suction control chamber vent is not occluded when suction is used.	Provides safety factor of releasing excess negative pressure into atmosphere.
c. Waterless systems have relief valves without caps.	Provides safety factor of releasing excess negative pressure.
17. Position excess tubing horizontally on mattress next to patient. Secure with clamp provided so that it does not obstruct tubing.	Prevents excess tubing from hanging over edge of mattress in dependent loop. Drainage collected in loop can occlude drainage system, which predisposes patient to tension pneumothorax (Kane et al., 2013).
18. Adjust tubing to hang in straight line from chest tube to drainage chamber.	Promotes drainage and prevents fluid or blood from accumulating in pleural cavity (Mohammed, 2015).

Clinical Decision Point. Frequent gentle lifting of drain allows gravity to assist blood and other viscous material to move to drainage bottle. Patients with recent chest surgery or trauma need to have the chest drain lifted based on assessment of the amount of drainage; some patients might need chest tube drains lifted every 5 to 10 minutes until drainage volume decreases. However, when coiled or dependent looping of tubing is unavoidable, lift tubing every 15 minutes at a minimum to promote drainage (Kane et al., 2013).

STEP	RATIONALE
19. Be sure the two rubber-tipped hemostats are accessible to patient.	Chest tubes are double clamped when air leak is suspected, when there is a need to empty or change systems, or to assess if patient is ready for tube removal (Table 32.11).
20. Dispose of sharps in proper container, dispose of used supplies, and perform hand hygiene.	Reduces transmission of microorganisms.
21. Care of patient after chest tube insertion:	
a. Assess vital signs; oxygen saturation; chest wall movement; skin and mucous membrane color; breath sounds; rate, depth, and ease of respirations; and insertion site every 15 minutes for first 2 hours and then at least every shift (see agency policy).	Provides immediate information about procedure-related complications such as respiratory distress and leakage.
b. Monitor color, consistency, and amount of chest tube drainage every 15 minutes for first 2 hours and then hourly (see agency policy). Indicate level of drainage fluid, date, and time on write-on surface of chamber. Be aware of what is normal amount and color of drainage expected for patient condition.	Provides baseline for continuous assessment of type and quantity of drainage. Ensures early detection of complications. Pneumothorax typically has serous drainage with air. Hemothorax will initially have sanguineous drainage that transitions to serosanguineous and then serous. Drainage amounts can vary, but after surgery you can expect 100 to 300 mL/hr for the first few hours and then a decrease to less than 50 mL/hr (Kane et al., 2013).

TABLE 32.11 EMERGENCY CARE WITH CHEST TUBES

ASSESSMENT	INTERVENTION
1. Air leak: can occur at insertion site, at connection between tube and drainage, or within drainage device itself. Continuous bubbling occurs in water-seal chamber and water seal.	Locate leak by using rubber-tipped (shodded) hemostats to clamp tube at different intervals along tube, starting at patient's chest. If leak stops, the air is coming from patient—take dressing off, ensure tube is still in place, and notify health care provider. Do not leave chest tube clamped because this can cause collapse of lung, mediastinal shift, and eventual collapse of other lung from buildup of air pressure within pleural cavity. If bubbling continues, clamp tubing inch by inch to determine if there is a hole in tubing, loose connection, or problem with drainage device. If a leak is found in tubing or drainage device, change it. Use adhesive tape at all connections.
2. Break in chest drainage device	Place end of chest tube in bottle of sterile saline or water at 2-cm level. Notify health care provider immediately, and change drainage device according to manufacturer instructions.
3. Chest tube dislodgment	Apply dressing to chest tube site wound using petroleum gauze, dry gauze dressing, and adhesive tape. Notify health care provider immediately and obtain a STAT order for chest radiograph. Prepare for health care provider to insert another chest tube.
4. Tension pneumothorax: signs and symptoms include: • Severe respiratory distress • Low oxygen saturation • Chest pain • Absence of breath sounds on affected side • Tracheal shift to unaffected side • Tachycardia and hypotension	Assess chest tube for clamping or kinking of tubing. Notify health care provider immediately and obtain STAT order for chest x-ray film. Prepare for health care provider to insert another chest tube or perform needle decompression with large-bore needle. Have emergency equipment in patient's room to prepare for resuscitation if needed. **Note:** Leaving chest tube clamped can cause tension pneumothorax.
5. Drainage suddenly stops	Assess chest tube for clamping or kinking of tubing. Assess for presence of clots or fibrin within chest tube. Notify health care provider immediately, and obtain order to gently milk chest tube to reestablish chest drainage.
6. Excessive bleeding from chest tube.	Notify health care provider. Assess patient's vital signs and be prepared for resuscitation. Be prepared for surgical intervention.

SKILL 32.2 CARE OF PATIENTS WITH CHEST TUBES—cont'd

STEP	RATIONALE
(1) From mediastinal tube, expect less than 100 mL/hour immediately after surgery and no more than 500 mL in first 24 hours.	Sudden gush of drainage may result from coughing or changing patient's position, releasing pooled and/or collected blood rather than indicating active bleeding.
(2) From posterior chest tube, expect between 100 and 300 mL in first 3 hours after insertion, with 500 to 1000 mL expected in first 24 hours. Drainage is grossly bloody during first several hours after surgery and then changes to serous (Kane et al., 2013).	Acute bleeding indicates hemorrhage. Health care provider should be notified if there is more than 250 mL of bloody drainage in 1 hour (Kane et al., 2013).
(3) From anterior chest tube, expect little or no output from anterior chest tube that is inserted for pneumothorax (Kane et al., 2013).	
c. Observe chest tube dressing and skin around dressing for drainage. Dressing should be occlusive.	Drainage around tube may indicate blockage. Loose dressing increases risk of infection. Some patients may develop subcutaneous emphysema, which is a collection of air under the skin. You will palpate crepitus, or puffed out skin crackles (Mohammed, 2015).
d. Apply clean gloves. Palpate around tube for swelling and crepitus (subcutaneous emphysema) as noted by crackling.	Indicates presence of air trapping in subcutaneous tissues. Small amounts are commonly absorbed. Large amounts are potentially dangerous. Most occurrences of crepitus are minor (Mao et al., 2015).

Clinical Decision Point. Some patients may develop subcutaneous emphysema, which is a collection of air under the skin after chest tube placement that can occur if tubing is blocked or kinked. When this occurs a crepitus (a crackling sensation) is heard on auscultation.

STEP	RATIONALE
e. Check tubing to ensure it is free of kinks and dependent loops.	Promotes drainage.
f. Observe for fluctuation of drainage in tubing during inspiration and expiration (tidaling). Observe for clots or debris in tubing. Assess water-seal chamber for tidaling of water with patient's inspiration and expiration, and assess level of water.	If fluctuation or tidaling stops, it means that either the lung is fully expanded or the system is obstructed. In spontaneously breathing patient, fluid rises in water-seal or diagnostic indicator (waterless system) with inspiration and falls with expiration. The opposite occurs in patient who is mechanically ventilated. This indicates that system is functioning properly (Kane et al., 2013; AACN, 2015).
g. Keep drainage system upright and below level of patient's chest.	Promotes gravity drainage and prevents backflow of fluid and air into pleural space.
h. Check for air leaks by monitoring bubbling in water-seal chamber. Intermittent bubbling is normal during expiration when air is being evacuated from pleural cavity, but continuous bubbling during both inspiration and expiration indicates leak in system.	Absence of bubbling may indicate that lung is fully expanded in patient with pneumothorax. Check all connections and locate sources of air leak as described in Table 32.11.
22. Measure any drainage, and document time on surface of drainage system.	Provides assessment for type, quality, and quantity of drainage.
23. In patient with existing chest tube, apply sterile gloves (per agency policy) and change dressing if loose or saturated.	Check agency policy regarding whether or not dressing change is sterile or clean. Also know health care provider preference for need for petroleum gauze dressing around tube.
24. Remove and dispose of gloves and used supplies, if any, and perform hand hygiene.	Reduces transmission of microorganisms.
25. Assist patient to comfortable position: semi-Fowler's or Fowler's.	Ensures proper chest tube drainage and facilitates chest wall expansion.

STEP	RATIONALE

EVALUATION

1. Evaluate patient for decreased respiratory distress and chest pain. Auscultate patient's lungs and observe chest expansion.

Determines status of lung expansion.

2. Complete all assessment measures in Step 21 and Step 22. Compare with previous findings.

Provides data regarding respiratory status, level of oxygenation, and lung expansion.

> **Clinical Decision Point.** If no tidaling is present, drainage system could be blocked, the lungs could have reexpanded, or the system is attached to suction. Further investigation is warranted, and critical thinking on your part is needed. If bubbling is increased, an air leak may be present. See Table 32.11 for care of an air leak.

3. Evaluate patient's level of comfort on visual analog scale of 0 to 10, comparing level with comfort before chest tube insertion.

Indicates need for analgesia. Patients with chest tubes typically have pain, which makes it difficult to take deep breaths (Kane et al., 2013).

4. Evaluate patient's ability to use deep-breathing exercises while maintaining comfort.

Indicates patient's ability to promote lung expansion and prevent complications.

5. Assess suction control chamber.
   a. *Wet suction system:* Continuous gentle bubbling should be present.

Indicates chamber has appropriate suction and is functioning appropriately. No bubbling indicates that there is no suction, the suction is not high enough, or the air leak is so large that the suction is not high enough to evacuate the leak (Lewis et al., 2017).

   b. *Dry suction system (waterless system):* The float ball indicates the amount of suction the patient is receiving.

If the suction patient is receiving does not match amount ordered, adjust dial to reach prescribed setting.

> **Clinical Decision Point.** If chest tube drainage suddenly increases or if there is more than 100 mL/hour of bloody drainage (except for first 3 hours after surgery), inform health care provider immediately and remain with patient and assess vital signs, oxygen saturation by pulse oximetry, and cardiopulmonary status. This finding may indicate hemorrhage or perforation of the lung.

6. **Use Teach-Back:** "I want to be sure I explained why you need a chest tube. Tell me why you have it." Revise your instructions now or develop a plan for revised patient/family caregiver teaching if patient/family caregiver is not able to teach back correctly.

Determines patient's/family caregiver's level of understanding of instructional topic.

RECORDING AND REPORTING

- Record in nurses' notes in electronic health record (EHR), chart, or flow sheets relevant respiratory assessments, type of drainage device, amount of suction if used, amount and character of drainage in chamber, and presence or absence of an air leak. Document the integrity of dressing and color and type of drainage. If dressing change is performed, document dressing change with supplies used and wound assessment.

- Record level of patient comfort and pain and vital signs including oxygen saturation.
- Record your evaluation of patient/family caregiver learning.
- Report any unexpected outcomes immediately to nurse in charge and/or health care provider.

UNEXPECTED OUTCOMES AND RELATED INTERVENTIONS

- Patient develops respiratory distress, chest pain, decrease in breath sounds, marked cyanosis, asymmetrical chest movements, presence of subcutaneous emphysema around tube insertion site or neck, hypotension, tachycardia, or mediastinal shift.
  - Notify health care provider immediately.
  - Assess vital signs and pulse oximetry.
  - Prepare for chest x-ray.
  - Provide oxygen as ordered.

- Air leak is unrelated to patient's respirations.
  - Determine source of air leak (see Table 32.11).
  - Notify health care provider.
- Chest tube emergency occurs.
  - See Table 32.11.
  - Observe for mediastinal shift or respiratory distress (medical emergency).
  - Notify health care provider.

KEY POINTS

- The cardiopulmonary system consists of the heart, lungs, airways, and blood vessels, which function to provide oxygen to the tissues and to remove carbon dioxide (CO_2) and waste products from the body.
- Ventilation, diffusion, respiration, and perfusion are processes for providing adequate oxygenation from the alveoli to the blood.
- Cardiac output is determined by the patient's heart rate, strength of contraction, amount of blood in the ventricle, and amount of resistance the heart has to overcome to eject the blood.
- The process of inspiration and expiration is achieved with changes in lung pressures and volumes.
- Respiration is controlled by the central nervous system (CNS) and chemicals within the blood.
- Decreased hemoglobin levels, seen in patients with anemia or acute blood loss, alter a patient's ability to transport oxygen and can cause disturbances in oxygenation.
- Hypoventilation, seen in patients with musculoskeletal abnormalities or nervous system disease, causes CO_2 retention.
- A person's age, nutritional intake, hydration status, level of exercise, exposure to cigarette smoke (including secondhand smoke), substance abuse, environmental factors, and stress all affect the ability to exchange oxygen in the lungs and transport it to the tissues.
- Alterations in cardiac output caused by electrical or mechanical disturbances of the heart can negatively impact a person's ability to deliver oxygen to the tissues.
- Breathing exercises improve ventilation, oxygenation, and sensations of dyspnea.
- Chest physiotherapy, along with postural drainage, aids in mobilizing pulmonary secretions.
- Hydration, humidification, coughing, and suctioning techniques maintain a patent airway.
- Oxygen therapy improves levels of tissue oxygenation and can be delivered via nasal cannula, various types of oxygen masks, or mechanical ventilators via artificial airways.
- Positioning, incentive spirometry, chest tubes, and noninvasive ventilation help to promote lung expansion.
- Cardiopulmonary resuscitation (CPR) is necessary for cardiac arrest, an emergent complication of altered oxygenation and perfusion.

REFLECTIVE LEARNING

- You are assigned to care for a patient with a chest tube today. You perform an initial assessment and notice a large amount of bubbling in the water-seal chamber. What steps will you take? What is your priority assessment?
- You are walking in the patient hallway of your clinical agency. A visitor comes running out of a patient room and yells, "My husband is coughing and his oxygen alarm keeps beeping. Come help him!" What will you do? What are the priority assessments? What are possible interventions for this patient?
- You are providing education for a patient with chronic obstructive pulmonary disease who also smokes. The patient states that she does not want to quit smoking because she likes it too much, but that she hates feeling short of breath all the time. What will you say to your patient now? What are the important education points? What resources are available in your area for this patient?

REVIEW QUESTIONS

1. The nurse is caring for a patient with pneumonia. On entering the room, the nurse finds the patient lying supine in bed, coughing and short of breath, with a pulse oximeter reading of 95%. What should the nurse do first?
   1. Elevate the head of the bed to 45 degrees
   2. Apply oxygen via nasal cannula at 2 L/minute
   3. Encourage the patient to use the incentive spirometer
   4. Notify the health care provider
2. The nurse enters a patient's room to find the patient unresponsive and the cardiac monitor showing a rhythm of ventricular fibrillation. What is the priority intervention for the nurse to perform?
   1. Check a pulse
   2. Initiate CPR
   3. Administer epinephrine
   4. Defibrillate the patient
3. The nurse is performing discharge teaching for a patient with chronic obstructive pulmonary disease (COPD). What statement, made by the patient, indicates the need for more teaching?
   1. "Pursed-lip breathing is like exercise for my lungs and will help me strengthen my breathing muscles."
   2. "Huff coughing will help me get the mucus up out of my lungs."
   3. "I should make sure that I get the influenza vaccine every year."
   4. "I should limit my fluid intake to 1 liter per day because I don't want to produce excess sputum."
4. The nurse is caring for a patient with an endotracheal tube. What are reasons to suction this patient? (Select all that apply.)
   1. The airway has visible secretions.
   2. There is a written order to suction routinely every 4 hours.
   3. The patient exhibits excessive coughing.
   4. The patient shows a decrease in pulse oximeter reading.
   5. The patient has clear bilateral lung sounds.

5. The nurse is preparing to perform nasotracheal suctioning on a patient. Put the following steps in order of performance.
1. Assist patient to semi-Fowler's or high-Fowler's position, if able.
2. Perform hand hygiene.
3. Apply sterile gloves.
4. Lubricate catheter with water-soluble lubricant.
5. Apply suction.
6. Have patient take deep breaths.
7. Advance catheter through nares and into trachea.
8. Withdraw catheter.

evolve

Additional Review Questions, as well as rationales for all Review Questions, can be found on the Evolve website.

1. 1; 2, 4; 3, 4, 1, 3, 4; 5, 2, 1, 3, 6, 4, 7, 5, 8.

REFERENCES

Al-Thaqafy MS, et al: Association of compliance of ventilator bundle with incidence of ventilator-associated pneumonia and ventilator utilization among critical patients over 4 years, *Ann Thorac Med* 9(4):221, 2014.

American Association of Cardiovascular and Pulmonary Rehabilitation (AACVPR): *Cardiac rehab patient resources*, 2016, https://www.aacvpr.org/Resources/Resources-for-Patients/Cardiac-Rehab-Patient-Resources.

American Association of Critical-Care Nurses (AACN): *Evidence-based care of patients with chest tubes: 2015 AACN NTI ExpoEd*, Hudson, NH, 2015, Atrium. http://www.atriummed.com/EN/chest_drainage/Documents/NTI2015Evidence-BasedCareofPatientswithChestTubes.pdf.

American Association of Respiratory Care (AARC): AARC clinical practice guideline: nasotracheal suction—2004 revision and update, *Respir Care* 49:1080, 2004.

American Association of Respiratory Care (AARC): AARC clinical practice guideline: endotracheal suctioning of mechanical ventilation patients with artificial airways, *Respir Care* 55(6):758, 2010.

American Association of Respiratory Care (AARC): Clinical practice guideline: incentive spirometry, *Respir Care* 56(10):1600, 2011.

American Heart Association: *Highlights of the 2015 American Heart Association guidelines update for CPR and ECC*, 2015, https://eccguidelines.heart.org/wp-content/uploads/2015/10/2015-AHA-Guidelines-Highlights-English.pdf.

Association of Paediatric Chartered Physiotherapists: *Guidelines for nasopharyngeal suction of a child or young adult*, 2015, http://www.google.com/url?sa=t&rct=j&q=&esrc=s&source =web&cd=2&ved=0ahUKEwiD0YvclKrWAhUV52MKHfN_C-YQFggrMAE&url=http%3A%2F%2Fwww.csp.org.uk%2Fsites%2Ffiles%2Fcsp%2Fsecure%2Fguidelines_for_nasopharyngeal_suction_0_1.pdf&usg=AFQjCNG_DdEzSirI5FkYfkS96HZiCcS-aA.

Atkins JR, Kautz DD: Move to improve: progressive mobility in the intensive care unit, *Dimens Crit Care Nurs* 33(5):275, 2014.

Ball J, et al: *Seidel's guide to physical examination*, ed 9, St Louis, 2015, Elsevier.

Bascom R, et al: Restoring an air-free pleural space in pneumothorax, *Medscape*, 2016, available at http://emedicine.medscape.com/article/1959416-overview.

Bounds M, et al: Effect of ABCDE bundle implementation on prevalence of delirium in intensive care unit patients, *Am J Crit Care* 25(6):535, 2016.

Branson R, et al: Management of the artificial airway, *Respir Care* 59(6):974, 2014.

Cassidy MR, et al: I cough: reducing postoperative pulmonary complications with a multidisciplinary patient care program, *JAMA Surg* 148(8):740, 2013.

Centers for Disease Control and Prevention (CDC): *Heart disease risk factors*, 2015a, http://www.cdc.gov/heartdisease/risk_factors.htm.

Centers for Disease Control and Prevention (CDC): *Estimated influenza illnesses and hospitalizations averted by vaccination—United States, 2014-15 influenza season*, 2015b, http://www.cdc.gov/flu/about/disease/2014-15.htm.

Centers for Disease Control and Prevention (CDC): *What are the risk factors for lung cancer*, 2016a, https://www.cdc.gov/cancer/lung/basic_info/risk_factors.htm.

Centers for Disease Control and Prevention (CDC): *Get vaccinated*, 2016b, http://www.cdc.gov/flu/consumer/vaccinations.htm.

Centers for Disease Control and Prevention (CDC): *Pneumococcal vaccination*, 2016c, http://www.cdc.gov/vaccines/vpd-vac/pneumo/default.htm.

Centers for Disease Control and Prevention (CDC): *Tuberculin skin testing*, 2016d, http://www.cdc.gov/tb/publications/factsheets/testing/skintesting.htm.

Chotai P: Tube thoracostomy management, *Medscape*, 2016, http://emedicine.medscape.com/article/1503275-overview#a6.

COPD Foundation: *Breathing techniques*, 2016, http://www.copdfoundation.org/What-is-COPD/Living-with-COPD/Breathing-Techniques.aspx.

do Nascimento P, et al: Incentive spirometry for prevention of post-operative pulmonary complication in upper abdominal surgery, *Cochrane Database Syst Rev* (2):CD006058, 2014.

Gale N, et al: Adapting to domiciliary non-invasive ventilation in chronic obstructive pulmonary disease: a qualitative interview study, *Palliat Med* 29(3):268, 2015.

Giddens J: *Concepts for nursing practice*, ed 2, St Louis, 2017, Elsevier.

Hockenberry M, et al: *Essentials of pediatric nursing*, ed 10, St Louis, 2017, Elsevier.

Hong CM, Galvagno SM: Patients with chronic obstructive pulmonary disorder, *Med Clin North Am* 97(6):1095, 2013.

Huether S, McCance K: *Understanding pathophysiology*, ed 6, St Louis, 2017, Elsevier.

Institute for Healthcare Improvement (IHI): *How-to guide: prevent ventilator-associated pneumonia*, Cambridge, MA, 2012, Institute for Healthcare Improvement. http://www.ihi.org/resources/Pages/Tools/HowtoGuidePreventVAP.aspx.

Institute for Healthcare Improvement (IHI): *Ventilator-associated pneumonia: getting to zero … and staying there*, 2016, http://www.ihi.org/resources/pages/improvementstories/vapgettingtozeroandstayingthere.aspx.

Kane C, et al: Chest tubes in the critically ill patient, *Dimens Crit Care Nurs* 32(3): 111, 2013.

Kram S, et al: Implementation of the ABCDE bundle to improve patient outcomes in the intensive care unit in a rural community hospital, *Dimens Crit Care Nurs* 34(5):250, 2015.

Kwiatt M, et al: Thoracostomy tubes: a comprehensive review of complications and related topics, *Int J Crit Illn Inj Sci* 4(2):143, 2014.

Lamb KD: Year in review 2014: mechanical ventilation, *Respir Care* 60(4):606, 2015.

Lewis S, et al: *Medical-surgical nursing: assessment and management of clinical problems*, ed 9, St Louis, 2017, Elsevier.

Link M, et al: Part 7: Adult advanced cardiovascular life support: 2015 American Heart Association guidelines updates for cardiopulmonary resuscitation and emergency cardiovascular care, *Circulation* 132(Suppl 2):s444, 2015.

MacIntyre N: Tissue hypoxia: implications for the respiratory clinician, *Respir Care* 59(10):1590, 2014.

Mao M, et al: Complications of chest tubes: a focused clinical synopsis, *Curr Opin Pulm Med* 21:376, 2015.

McCance KL, Huether SE: *Pathophysiology: the biologic basis for disease in adults and children*, ed 7, St. Louis, 2014, Mosby Elsevier.

McDonald C: Oxygen therapy for COPD, *J Thorac Dis* 6(11):1632, 2014.

Messika J, et al: Use of high-flow nasal cannula oxygen therapy in subjects with ARDS: a 1-year observational study, *Respir Care* 60(2):162, 2015.

Mohammed H: Chest tube care in critically ill patient: a comprehensive review, *Egypt J Chest Dis Tuberc* 64:849, 2015.

Mozaffarian D, et al: *Heart disease and stroke statistics—2016 update. A report from the American Heart Association*, 2015, http://circ.ahajournals.org/content/early/2015/12/16/CIR.0000000000000350.

Munro N, Ruggiero M: Ventilator-associated pneumonia bundle reconstruction for best care, *AACN Adv Crit Care* 25(2):163, 2014.

Myatt R: Nursing care of patient with a temporary tracheotomy, *Nurs Stand* 29(26):42, 2015.

National Heart, Lung, and Blood Institute (NHLBI): *How is high blood pressure treated?*, 2015, https://www.nhlbi.nih.gov/health/health-topics/topics/hbp/treatment#.

Restrepo R, et al: Incentive spirometry: 2011, *Respir Care* 56(10):1600, 2011.

Shlamovitz GA: Tube thoracostomy, *Medscape*, 2014, http://emedicine.medscape.com/article/80678-overview#a1.

Strickland S, et al: AARC Clinical practice guideline: effectiveness of nonpharmacologic airway clearance therapies in hospitalized patients, *Respir Care* 58(12):2187, 2013.

The Joint Commission (TJC): *2018 National Patient Safety Goals*, Oakbrook Terrace, IL, 2018, The Commission. http://www.jointcommission.org/standards_information/npsgs.aspx.

Touhy T, Jett K: *Gerontological nursing and healthy aging*, ed 5, St Louis, 2018, Elsevier.

Urden L, et al: *Priorities in critical care nursing*, ed 7, St Louis, 2016, Elsevier.

Volsko TA: Airway clearance therapy: finding the evidence, *Respir Care* 58(10): 1669, 2013.

Walsh BK, et al: Capnography/capnometry during mechanical ventilation: 2011, *Respir Care* 56(4):503, 2011.

Whelton PK, et al: ACC/AHA/AAPA/ABC/ACPM/AGS/APhA/ASH/ASPC/NMA/PCNA guideline for the prevention, detection, evaluation, and management of high blood pressure in adults, *Hypertension* 71(1), 2017. doi:10.1161/HYP.0000000000000066.

Wiegand D: *AACN procedure manual for high acuity, progressive, and critical care*, ed 7, St Louis, 2017, Elsevier.

Zarogoulidis P, et al: Pneumothorax: from definition to diagnosis and treatment, *J Thorac Dis* 6(Suppl 4): S372, 2014.

evolve MEDIA RESOURCES

http://evolve.elsevier.com/Potter/essentials

- Audio Glossary
- Case Study Continuation

- QSEN Activity and Review Questions Answers and Rationales

OBJECTIVES

- Explain the effect the 24-hour sleep-wake cycle has on biological function.
- Discuss mechanisms that regulate sleep.
- Describe the normal stages of sleep.
- Explain the functions of sleep.
- Compare and contrast the characteristics of sleep for different age-groups.
- Identify factors that promote or disrupt sleep.
- Discuss characteristics of common sleep disorders.

- Summarize the elements of a sleep history and assessment.
- Describe interventions appropriate to promoting sleep for patients with various sleep disorders.
- Discuss differences in sleep interventions for patients of different age-groups.
- Describe ways to evaluate the effectiveness of sleep therapies.

KEY TERMS

biological clock, p. 918

cataplexy, p. 921

circadian rhythm, p. 917

excessive daytime sleepiness (EDS), p. 920

hypnotics, p. 934

insomnia, p. 920

melatonin, p. 934

narcolepsy, p. 920

nocturia, p. 922

nonrapid eye movement (NREM) sleep, p. 918

rapid eye movement (REM) sleep, p. 918

sedatives, p. 934

sleep, p. 921

sleep apnea, p. 920

sleep deprivation, p. 921

Physical and emotional health depend on adequate rest and sleep. Without proper amounts of rest and sleep, a person's ability to concentrate, make judgments, promote healing, and participate in daily activities decreases. To help patients gain needed rest and sleep, you need to understand the nature of sleep, the factors influencing it, and patients' sleep habits. Nurses care for patients who often have preexisting sleep disturbances and who develop sleep problems as a result of illness or being in the health care environment. Individulize your care based on patients' personal sleep habits and patterns of sleep to provide effective sleep therapies.

SCIENTIFIC KNOWLEDGE BASE

Physiology of Sleep

Sleep is a cyclical physiological process that alternates with longer periods of wakefulness. The sleep-wake cycle influences and regulates body functions and behavioral responses.

Circadian Rhythms. People experience cyclical rhythms as part of their everyday life. The most familiar rhythm is the 24-hour, day-night cycle known as the diurnal or circadian rhythm. The suprachiasmatic nucleus nerve cells in the

CASE STUDY *Walter Murphy*

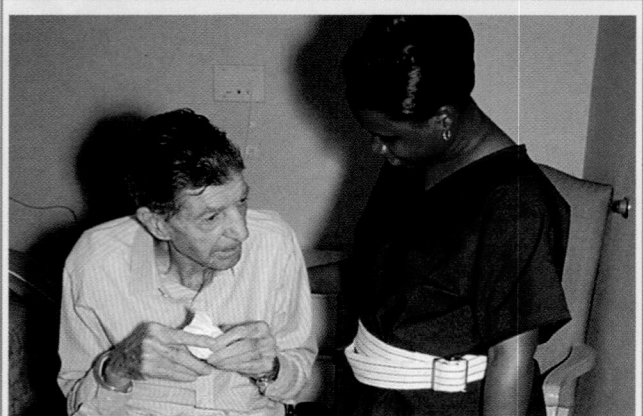

Walter Murphy is 82 years old and has resided in a skilled care facility for the last 3 months. His wife still lives at home but visits Mr. Murphy on a daily basis. Mr. Murphy is confined to a wheelchair as a result of osteoarthritis and weakness from a mild stroke he experienced 1 year ago. Although he has physical limitations, he is alert and oriented. Over the last several weeks, Mrs. Murphy found her husband to be very sleepy when visiting him just before lunchtime. Mr. Murphy tells his wife that he has trouble falling asleep at night, and once he does fall asleep, he reawakens frequently. Mrs. Murphy is concerned because her husband does not seem as alert or talkative during her visit.

Anna is a nursing student assigned to the skilled care facility as part of her clinical experience in caring for older adults. She worked as a nurse assistant during the last two summers in a skilled care facility, so she has experience in caring for patients in this setting. Anna's assignment is to care for Mr. Murphy over the next 4 weeks.

hypothalamus control the rhythm of the sleep-wake cycle and coordinate it with other circadian rhythms (Huether et al., 2017). Circadian rhythms influence the 24-hour pattern of major biological and behavioral functions such as predictable changes in body temperature, heart rate, blood pressure, hormone secretion, sensory acuity, and mood (Kryger et al., 2017).

Light and temperature affect all circadian rhythms including the sleep-wake cycle. External factors such as social activities and environmental stressors also affect circadian rhythms. Every person has a **biological clock** that is normally synchronized by exposure to light and activity. This explains why some people fall asleep at 8 p.m., whereas others go to bed at midnight or early in the morning. It also explains why people function best at different times of the day.

Hospitals or extended care facilities usually do not adapt care to an individual's sleep-wake cycle preferences. Typical hospital routines require nurses to interrupt patients' sleep to complete assessments or provide nursing care such as administering medications and changing dressings. Poor quality of sleep results when a person's sleep-wake cycle changes. Reversals in the sleep-wake cycle, such as when a person who is

normally awake during the day falls asleep during the day, sometimes indicate a serious illness.

When the sleep-wake cycle becomes disrupted (e.g., by working rotating shifts), other physiological functions change as well. For example, a new nurse who starts working the night shift experiences a decreased appetite and loses weight. Anxiety, restlessness, irritability, and impaired judgment are other common symptoms of sleep cycle disturbances. Failure to maintain a usual sleep-wake cycle negatively influences overall health.

Sleep Regulation. Sleep is a series of physiological states maintained by highly integrated central nervous system (CNS) activity that is associated with changes in the peripheral nervous, endocrine, cardiovascular, respiratory, and muscular systems (Huether et al., 2017). Specific sequential physiological responses and patterns of brain activity identify each sleep cycle. Instruments that measure physiological aspects of sleep include the electroencephalogram (EEG), which measures electrical activity in the cerebral cortex; the electromyogram (EMG), which measures muscle tone; and the electrooculogram (EOG), which measures eye movements.

The major sleep center is in the hypothalamus. Hypocretins (a form of peptide) secreted by the hypothalamus promote wakefulness and rapid eye movement (REM) sleep. Prostaglandin D_2, L-tryptophan, and growth factors also control sleep (Huether et al., 2017).

Researchers believe that several neuron groups within and next to the pontine and midbrain reticular formation work together to maintain alertness and wakefulness. Arousal, wakefulness, and maintenance of consciousness result from neurons in these areas releasing serotonin, norepinephrine, histamine, acetylcholine, and orexin (Kryger et al., 2017). Each of the neurotransmitters works on a distinct receptor to control sleep-wake patterns.

The homeostatic process (Process S), which primarily regulates the length and depth of sleep, and the circadian rhythms (Process C—"biological time clocks"), which influence the internal organization of sleep and timing and duration of sleep-wake cycles, operate simultaneously to regulate sleep and wakefulness (Kryger et al., 2017). Time of wake up is the intersection of Process S and Process C (Fig. 33.1).

Stages of Sleep. There are two sleep phases: **nonrapid eye movement (NREM) sleep** and **rapid eye movement (REM) sleep** (Box 33.1). In the classical definition of NREM sleep, an individual progresses through four stages during a typical 90-minute sleep cycle. The American Academy of Sleep Medicine defines three stages in NREM sleep, combining stages 3 and 4 (Kryger et al., 2017). The quality of sleep from stage 1 through stage 4 becomes increasingly deep. Lighter sleep is characteristic of stages 1 and 2, when a person is more easily arousable. Combined stages 3 and 4 involve a deeper sleep called *slow-wave sleep,* from which a person is more difficult to arouse (Kryger et al., 2017). REM sleep is the phase at the end of each 90-minute sleep cycle. During REM sleep there is increased brain activity associated with rapid eye movements and muscle atonia.

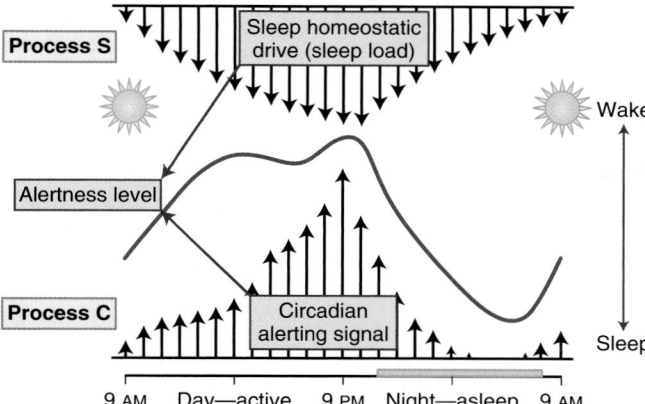

FIG 33.1 Two-process model of sleep regulation shows the time course of the homeostatic process *(Process S)* and the circadian process *(Process C)*. Process S rises during waking and declines during sleep. The intersection of Process S and Process C defines the time of wake-up. (From Daroff RB, et al: *Bradley's neurology in clinical practice,* ed 6, Philadelphia, 2012, Saunders.)

BOX 33.1 STAGES OF THE SLEEP CYCLE

NREM (75% OF NIGHT)

N1 (Formerly Stage 1)
- Stage of lightest level of sleep, lasting a few minutes.
- Decreased physiological activity begins with gradual fall in vital signs and metabolism.
- Sensory stimuli such as noise easily arouse sleeper.
- If awakened, person feels as though daydreaming has occurred.

N2 (Formerly Stage 2)
- Stage of sound sleep during which relaxation progresses.
- Arousal is still relatively easy.
- Brain and muscle activity continue to slow.

N3 (Formerly Stages 3 and 4)
- Called slow wave sleep.
- Deepest stage of sleep.
- Sleeper is difficult to arouse and rarely moves.
- Brain and muscle activity are significantly decreased.

REM SLEEP (25% OF NIGHT)
- Vivid, full-color dreaming occurs.
- Stage usually begins about 90 minutes after sleep has begun.
- Stage is typified by autonomic response of rapidly moving eyes, fluctuating heart and respiratory rates, and increased or fluctuating blood pressure.
- Loss of skeletal muscle tone occurs.
- Gastric secretions increase.
- It is very difficult to arouse sleeper.
- Duration of REM sleep increases with each cycle and averages 20 minutes.

Data from American Sleep Association: *What is sleep?,* 2017, https://sleepassociation.org/patients-general-public/what-is-sleep; Kryger M et al: *Principles and practice of sleep medicine,* ed 6, St Louis, 2017, Elsevier; National Sleep Foundation: *What happens when you sleep?,* 2017, https://sleepfoundation.org/how-sleep-works/what-happens-when-you-sleep.
NREM, Nonrapid eye movement; *REM,* rapid eye movement.

Sleep Cycle. Normally an adult's routine sleep pattern begins with a presleep period during which the person is aware only of a gradually developing sleepiness. This period normally lasts 10 to 30 minutes. Individuals experiencing difficulty falling asleep often remain in this stage for an hour or more. Once asleep, a person usually passes through four to six complete sleep cycles, each cycle consisting of four stages of NREM sleep and a period of REM sleep, for a total of 90 to 110 minutes (Huether et al., 2017).

With each successive cycle, stage 3 (combined stages 3 and 4) of NREM sleep shorten, and REM sleep lengthens. REM sleep lasts up to 60 minutes during the last sleep cycle. Not all people progress consistently through the usual stages of sleep. For example, a sleeper fluctuates back and forth for short intervals between NREM stages 2 and 3 before entering REM sleep. The amount of time spent in each stage varies. The number of sleep cycles depends on the total amount of time that the person spends sleeping.

Functions of Sleep

Sleep functions as a time of restoration, memory consolidation, and preparation for the next period of wakefulness (Huether et al., 2017). During NREM sleep biological functions slow. A healthy adult's heart rate decreases from a normal average of 70 to 80 beats/min to 60 beats/min or less during sleep, thus preserving cardiac function. Other biological functions that decrease during sleep are respirations, temperature, blood pressure, and muscle tone (Kryger et al., 2017).

Sleep restores biological processes. During NREM stage 3 sleep, the body releases human growth hormone for the repair and renewal of epithelial and specialized cells such as brain cells (Huether et al., 2017). Protein synthesis and cell division for the renewal of tissues also occur during rest and sleep. The basal metabolic rate lowers during sleep, which conserves the energy supply of the body (Huether et al., 2017).

REM sleep appears to be important for early brain development, cognition, and memory. Researchers associate REM sleep with changes in the brain including cerebral blood flow and increased cortical activity. In addition, there is increased oxygen consumption and epinephrine release. These changes are associated with memory storage and learning.

The benefits of sleep often go unnoticed until a person develops a problem resulting from sleep deprivation. Current estimates show that 50 to 70 million adults in the United States have some type of sleep-wake problem (Centers for Disease Control and Prevention [CDC], 2015). Sleep deprivation affects immune function, metabolism, nitrogen balance, and protein catabolism. A loss of REM sleep often leads to confusion and suspicion. Prolonged sleep loss alters various body functions (e.g., mood, motor performance, memory, equilibrium) (National Sleep Foundation, 2016b). Individuals with sleep problems are also more likely to have chronic diseases such as hypertension, diabetes, and obesity. They sometimes also experience poorer quality of life and productivity (Kohansieh and Makaryus, 2015). Millions of health care dollars are spent on indirect costs related to sleep deprivation such as motor vehicle and industrial accidents, litigation, property damage, hospitalization, medical errors, and death (Liu et al., 2016).

Dreams. Dreams during REM sleep are more vivid and elaborate than dreams during NREM sleep. Researchers believe REM dreams are functionally important to learning, memory processing, and adaptation to stress (Kryger et al., 2017). REM dreams progress throughout the night from dreams about current events to emotional dreams of childhood or the past. Personality influences the quality of dreams (e.g., a creative person may have very vivid, unusual dreams, whereas a depressed person may have dreams of helplessness). Dreams help people sort out immediate concerns or erase certain fantasies or nonsensical memories. Because most dreams are forgotten, many people have little dream recall and do not believe they dream at all. People who recall dreams vividly usually awaken just after a period of REM sleep.

Sleep Disorders

Sleep disorders are conditions that, if left untreated, cause disturbed nighttime sleep as well as potentially serious physiologic alterations. Many adults in the United States have significant sleep problems from inadequacies in either the quantity or the quality of their nighttime sleep and experience hypersomnolence on a daily basis (American Sleep Association [ASA], 2016). The American Academy of Sleep Medicine developed the International Classification of Sleep Disorders version 3 (ICSD-3), which classifies sleep disorders into eight major categories.

Insomnia. Insomnia is a symptom rather than the name of a disease and is experienced by patients who have chronic difficulty falling asleep, frequent awakenings from sleep, or nonrestorative sleep (Maness and Khan, 2015). It is commonly experienced by patients diagnosed with depression (Trauer et al., 2015). Insomnia leads to insufficient quantity and quality of sleep. It sometimes signals an underlying physical or psychological disorder and is more common in older adults and women.

Often people experience acute transient or temporary insomnia following situational stresses such as work or family problems, illness, or grief. Insomnia sometimes recurs, but between episodes a person is able to sleep well. However, a temporary case of insomnia caused by a stressful event can lead to chronic difficulty in getting enough sleep. Insomnia is often associated with poor sleep hygiene, which negates behaviors that promote sleep (Badin et al., 2016). If the condition continues, the fear of not being able to sleep is enough to cause wakefulness. During the day a person

with chronic insomnia feels sleepy, fatigued, depressed, and anxious.

Sleep Apnea. Sleep apnea is a disorder characterized by a lack of airflow through the nose and mouth for periods ranging from 10 seconds to 1 to 2 minutes during sleep. The person stops breathing during sleep. There are three types of sleep apnea: obstructive, central, and mixed, which has both an obstructive component and a central component.

The most common form of sleep apnea is obstructive sleep apnea (OSA), which is a cessation or stopping of airflow despite the effort to breathe. It occurs when muscles or soft structures of the oral cavity or throat relax during sleep. The upper airway becomes partially or completely blocked, and nasal airflow diminishes (hypopnea) or stops (apnea). The person tries to breathe because chest and abdominal movements continue, which often results in loud snoring sounds. When breathing is partially or completely diminished, the person becomes sufficiently hypoxic and must awaken to breathe. Structural abnormalities such as a deviated septum, nasal pharyngeal alterations, a narrow lower jaw, enlarged tonsils, or obesity predispose a patient to OSA. Smoking, increasing age (greater than 65 years of age), heart failure, alcohol use, large neck circumference, and menopause are increased risk factors (Qaseem et al., 2014; Schub, 2016). Serious OSA can lead to heart failure, hypertension, and coronary artery disease. About 10% to 17% of adults in the United States are affected by OSA (Qaseem et al., 2014). However, a large majority of people are undiagnosed and untreated (Kryger et al., 2017). Research shows that the risk for OSA is similar among African Americans, Asians, and Caucasians (Kryger et al., 2017).

Central sleep apnea (CSA) involves dysfunction in the respiratory control center of the brain. Pauses in breathing happen in the respiratory and pulmonary systems at the same time. The brain stops sending signals to muscles that control breathing. Conditions that are associated with CSA include stroke, degeneration of the cervical spine, obesity, and encephalitis. People with CSA tend to awaken during sleep and therefore complain of insomnia.

Excessive daytime sleepiness (EDS) is a common complaint in people experiencing OSA and CSA. Other common symptoms of OSA include fatigue, morning headaches, irritability, depression, difficulty concentrating, and decreased sex drive (Kryger et al., 2017). Lifestyle changes (including a weight-reduction program in people who are obese and improved sleep hygiene), bilevel positive airway pressure (BPAP or BiPAP), continuous positive airway pressure (CPAP), surgery, and oral repositioning devices for the jaw and tongue are treatment options (Rotenberg et al., 2016; Schub, 2016).

Narcolepsy. Narcolepsy is a rare CNS dysfunction of mechanisms that regulate sleep and wake states. EDS is the most common symptom. During the day a person suddenly feels an overwhelming wave of sleepiness and falls asleep, often at inappropriate times. This is commonly referred to as a sleep attack. Involuntary sleep episodes may be brief, lasting only a few seconds to minutes. It is possible for REM sleep to occur within 15 minutes of falling asleep. Unless recognized, others often mistake a person who suddenly and inappropriately falls asleep as being lazy, disinterested, or possibly drunk. Typically symptoms first occur in adolescence and are sometimes confused with EDS. Narcolepsy can occur with or without cataplexy. Cataplexy is a sudden muscle weakness during intense emotions such as anger or laughter that can occur at any time during the day. In a severe cataplectic attack, a patient loses voluntary muscle control and falls to the floor. Narcolepsy commonly includes frightening dreamlike experiences during the transition from a wake to a sleep state.

Narcolepsy is treated with stimulants or wakefulness-promoting drugs (e.g., sodium oxybate, modafinil) that only partially increase wakefulness and reduce sleep attacks. Prescribed antidepressants suppress cataplexy and other REM-related symptoms. Short daytime naps (no longer than 20 minutes) help reduce feelings of sleepiness. Exercising regularly, maintaining a regular nighttime sleep schedule, eating light meals high in protein, deep breathing, chewing gum, and taking vitamins are other management methods (Barateau et al., 2016; Kryger et al., 2017). People with narcolepsy need to avoid situations and activities that increase drowsiness (e.g., alcohol, heavy meals, exhausting activities, long-distance driving).

Sleep Deprivation. Sleep deprivation can be acute or chronic and results from insufficient or disrupted sleep. Causes include illness (e.g., fever, difficulty breathing, pain), emotional stress, medications, environmental disturbances (e.g., frequent interruptions in sleep during nursing care, noisy neighbors or pets), and variability in the timing of sleep as a result of shift work. Sleep disorders such as sleep apnea or insomnia can cause sleep deprivation. With sleep deprivation, there is a decrease in the quantity or quality of sleep and/or an inconsistency in the timing of sleep. Interrupted or fragmented sleep changes the normal sequencing of the sleep cycle. Cumulative sleep deprivation develops over time.

Individuals respond to sleep deprivation differently. Some patients experience a variety of physiological and psychological symptoms such as blurred vision, decreased reflexes, slow response time, headaches, memory problems, confusion, and irritability. The severity of symptoms is often related to the duration of sleep deprivation. The most effective treatment for sleep deprivation is elimination or correction of environmental factors and patient care activities that disrupt the sleep pattern. Nurses play an important role in identifying treatable sleep deprivation problems. Evidence suggests that chronic sleep deprivation is associated with obesity, type 2 diabetes, poor memory, depression, digestive problems, and development of cardiovascular disease (Kohansieh and Makaryus, 2015).

Parasomnias. Parasomnias are sleep disorders that can occur during arousal from REM sleep or partial arousal from NREM sleep. These disorders include sleepwalking, sleep eating, night terrors, nightmares, teeth grinding, and bed-wetting. Most parasomnias are more common in children, possibly because of brain immaturity, but they can also occur in adults. An individual often experiences more than one parasomnia. In all cases it is important to support patients experiencing a sleep disorder and maintain their safety.

NURSING KNOWLEDGE BASE

Sleep and Rest

When people are at rest, they usually feel mentally relaxed, free from anxiety, and physically calm. Rest does not imply inactivity, although everyone often thinks of it as settling down in a comfortable chair or taking a brief nap. Sleep is a recurrent, altered state of consciousness that occurs for sustained periods. When people get proper sleep, they feel that their energy has been restored. Adequate quality and quantity of sleep contribute to optimum health.

Sleep Requirements and Patterns Throughout the Life Span

Neonates. Sleep duration and quality vary among people of all age-groups. Neonates and infants up to 3 months of age average about 16 to 18 hours of sleep a day. Approximately 50% of this sleep is REM sleep, which stimulates higher brain centers (Hockenberry and Wilson, 2015).

Infants. Infants usually develop a nighttime pattern of sleep by 3 to 4 months of age. They sometimes take several naps during the day but usually sleep an average of 9 to 11 hours during the night. Infants spend about 30% of sleep time in the REM cycle. Infants commonly awake early in the morning, although they sometimes also awaken during the night.

Toddlers and Preschoolers. By 2 years of age, children usually sleep through the night and take daily naps. Total recommended sleep is 11 to 14 hours a day (Hirschkowitz et al., 2015). Some children stop taking naps altogether at age 3. Toddlers commonly awaken during the night, and the percentage of REM sleep continues to fall. Toddlers are often unwilling to go to bed at night. A preschooler sleeps an average of 12 hours a night (about 20% is REM). By 5 years of age preschoolers rarely take daytime naps (Hockenberry and Wilson, 2015) except in cultures in which a siesta is the custom. Preschoolers usually have difficulty relaxing or quieting down after long, active days and often have problems with bedtime fears, waking during the night, and nightmares.

School-Age Children. A school-age child usually does not require a nap. A 6-year-old averages 11 to 12 hours of sleep nightly, whereas an 11-year-old sleeps about 9 to 10 hours (Hockenberry and Wilson, 2015). Encouraging quiet activities usually persuades a 6- or 7-year-old child to go to bed. An older child often resists sleeping because of an unawareness of fatigue or a need to be independent.

Adolescents. Adolescents need 8 to 10 hours of sleep each night; however, the typical teenager gets less than $8\frac{1}{2}$ hours of sleep (National Sleep Foundation, 2016d). At a time when sleep needs actually increase, the typical adolescent is subject to a number of changes that often reduce the time spent sleeping (e.g., early start times for school; after-school social events, part-time jobs, worrying before sleep, and personal habits such as caffeine intake and viewing electronic devices (Wheaton et al., 2016). Adolescents typically stay up much later and may develop a circadian disorder called sleep phase delay. Adolescents with delayed sleep phase want to go to bed later, usually after midnight, and sleep later than what is typical, but this may not be possible with early school start times. The shortened sleep time in adolescents often results in EDS, which can impair waking, reduce performance in school, increase the risk of motor vehicle accidents and sports injuries, increase the use of alcohol, and lead to behavior and mood problems (Bartel et al., 2015).

Young Adults. Most young adults average 6 to $8\frac{1}{2}$ hours of sleep a night, but this varies. Young adults rarely take regular naps. They spend approximately 20% of sleep time in REM sleep, which remains consistent throughout the remainder of life. Healthy young adults require adequate sleep (7 to 9 hours per day) to participate in daily busy activities (Hirschkowitz et al., 2015). However, lifestyle demands and family relationships sometimes lead to insomnia. It is important that young adults learn to effectively cope with stressors and avoid unhealthy coping strategies. Pregnancy increases the need for rest and sleep. Common problems during the third trimester of pregnancy include restless legs syndrome (RLS), insomnia, periodic limb movements, and sleep-disordered breathing (Kryger et al., 2017).

Middle-Age Adults. During middle adulthood the total time spent sleeping at night declines. Health care providers often initially diagnose sleep disturbances among people in this age range even when the symptoms of a disorder have been present for several years. Because of stresses experienced in middle age, insomnia is a common occurrence. It is often experienced by menopausal women who may also develop restless leg syndrome (RLS) or periodic limb movements as a result of iron deficiency from menorrhagia.

Older Adults. Sleeping difficulties increase with age. Approximately 40% of older adults report problems with sleep (National Sleep Foundation, 2016a; Kryger et al., 2017). Older adults spend more time in stage 1 and less time in stages 3 and 4 (NREM sleep); some older adults have almost no NREM stage 4 sleep. Episodes of REM sleep tend to shorten. Older adults experience fewer episodes of deep sleep and more episodes of lighter sleep. They tend to awaken more often during the night, and it takes more time for them to fall asleep. Older adults increase the number of naps taken during the day to compensate. Older adults with insomnia often have

comorbid psychiatric illnesses or medical conditions, take medications that disrupt sleep patterns, or use drugs or alcohol (Touhy and Jett, 2018).

Factors Affecting Sleep

A number of factors (physical, psychological, and environmental) affect the quantity and quality of sleep. Often more than one factor combines to cause a sleep problem.

Physical Illness. Any illness or condition that causes pain, difficulty breathing, nausea, or mood problems such as anxiety or depression can result in sleep problems (Table 33.1). Individuals with such problems have trouble falling or staying asleep or may wake early. Illnesses or diseases also sometimes force patients to sleep in positions to which they are unaccustomed. For example, it is difficult for a patient with a leg immobilizer to rest comfortably.

Sleep-related breathing disorders are linked to increased incidence of nocturnal angina (chest pain), increased heart rate, electrocardiogram changes, high blood pressure, and risk of heart diseases and stroke (Huether et al., 2017).

Nighttime urination (**nocturia**) disrupts sleep and the sleep cycle. It is difficult to return to sleep after repeated awakenings, and a complete sleep cycle is prevented from occurring. Although this condition is most common in older people, it also affects a significant portion of younger people (Madhu et al., 2015). Nocturia also occurs in people with obstructive sleep apnea (OSA) because of release of atrial natriuretic peptide.

RLS is a neurological sensorimotor disorder that causes an irresistible urge to move the legs while they are at rest, sitting or lying. Symptoms are most severe in the evening and night and can severely disrupt a patient's sleep (National Sleep Foundation, 2016c).

Drugs and Substances. Numerous drugs cause sleepiness, insomnia, or fatigue as a side effect (Box 33.2). Medications prescribed for sleep often cause more problems than benefits. L-Tryptophan is a natural protein found in foods such as milk, cheese, and meats (e.g., turkey and chicken) and sometimes helps a person sleep. It is a precursor, or forerunner, to the neurotransmitter serotonin, which has a role in the sleep-wake cycle.

Lifestyle. A person's daily routine influences sleep patterns. For example, an individual who alternately works day and night shifts often has difficulty adjusting to an altered sleep schedule. Lifestyle changes that contribute to decreased quantity and quality of sleep include working an increased number of hours per day or week or at multiple jobs and spending more time on the Internet. Other alterations in routine that disrupt sleep patterns include performing unaccustomed heavy work or exercise, engaging in late-night social activities, and changing evening mealtime. Travel across time zones is a common factor associated with insomnia.

TABLE 33.1 ILLNESSES AND CONDITIONS THAT CAN ALTER SLEEP

ILLNESS/CONDITION	NATURE OF SLEEP ALTERATION
Respiratory disease (e.g., emphysema, asthma, bronchitis, allergic rhinitis, common cold)	Shortness of breath requires the use of two to three pillows to raise head and alters rhythm of breathing. Nasal congestion and sore throat impair breathing and ability to relax.
Coronary heart disease with episodes of chest pain and irregular heart rates	Heart disease causes frequent awakenings, sleep stage changes during sleep, and significant alterations in all stages of sleep.
Hypertension	Reduced length and depth of NREM sleep and a shortened REM latency period cause arousals and early morning awakening, resulting in fatigue.
Hypothyroidism	Decreases in slow-wave and REM sleep and increased movements during sleep contribute to daytime sleepiness.
Hyperthyroidism	Increase in metabolism causes insomnia resulting from increased time needed to fall asleep.
Nocturia (reduced bladder tone, heart failure, diabetes, urethritis, prostate disease)	Waking at night to urinate results in difficulty returning to sleep.
Gastric reflux	Burning pain in lower esophagus or nocturnal coughing increases when lying flat in bed.
Depression	Early morning awakenings with inability to return to sleep are worsened by anxiety or agitation.
Perimenopause	Waking at night is caused by hot flashes and sweating.
Pain	Delay in sleep onset, increased waking from sleep, and decreased slow-wave activity during sleep result in poor sleep quality. Pain is worsened by increased sympathetic activity, resulting in high cardiac heart rate.

NREM, Nonrapid eye movement; *REM,* rapid eye movement.

BOX 33.2 EFFECT OF MEDICATIONS AND OTHER SUBSTANCES ON SLEEP

HYPNOTICS
- Interfere with reaching deeper sleep stages
- Provide only temporary (1 week) increase in quantity of sleep
- Sometimes cause "hangover" feeling during day
- In some cases worsen sleep apnea in older adults

DIURETICS (ADMINISTERED LATE IN THE DAY)
- Cause nocturia, which leads to nighttime awakenings

ANTIDEPRESSANTS AND STIMULANTS
- Suppress REM sleep and decrease total sleep time

ALCOHOL
- Speeds onset of sleep and disrupts REM sleep
- Awakens person during night and causes difficulty returning to sleep

CAFFEINE
- Stimulant; prevents person from falling asleep
- Causes person to awaken during night

NICOTINE
- Causes decrease in sleep time
- Causes nighttime awakenings
- Causes difficulty staying asleep

BETA-ADRENERGIC BLOCKERS
- Cause nightmares and insomnia
- Cause awakening from sleep

BENZODIAZEPINES
- Increase sleep time
- Increase daytime sleepiness

OPIATES
- Suppress REM sleep
- Cause increased daytime drowsiness

ANTIHISTAMINES
- Cause drowsiness
- Cause insomnia when used in excess

ANTICONVULSANTS
- Decrease REM sleep
- Cause daytime drowsiness

REM, Rapid eye movement.

Usual Sleep Patterns and Excessive Daytime Sleepiness. Only 35% of adults report getting 8 hours of sleep a day regularly (University of Maryland Medical Center, 2016). The average American adult gets 7½ hours of sleep a night, but 35% of those report that their sleep quality is fair or poor (National Sleep Foundation, 2014; Liu et al., 2016). This leads to EDS during the day. A contributor to EDS is the use of technology close to bedtime, such as watching television, talking or texting on a cell phone, or reading information on electronic devices.

Sleepiness becomes pathological when it occurs at times when people need or want to be awake. People who temporarily experience sleep deprivation as a result of an active social evening or lengthened work schedule usually feel sleepy the next day. However, they are usually able to overcome these feelings even though they have difficulty performing tasks and remaining attentive. Chronic lack of sleep is much more serious than temporary sleep deprivation and causes serious alterations in the ability to perform daily activities. EDS is most difficult to overcome during sedentary tasks (e.g., driving).

Emotional Stress. Worry over personal problems or situations interferes with sleep. Emotional stress causes tension and often leads to frustration when sleep does not come. Stress also causes a person to try too hard to fall asleep, to awaken frequently during the sleep cycle, or to oversleep. Continued stress causes poor sleep habits in some cases.

Environment. The physical environment in which a person sleeps influences the ability to fall and remain asleep. Proper ventilation, a comfortable (usually cooler versus warmer) temperature, and a quiet, darkened or softly lit room are essential for restful sleep. A comfortable bed also affects sleep quality. Hospital beds are often harder than beds at home. If a person usually sleeps with another individual, sleeping alone during times of illness causes wakefulness. However, sleeping with a restless or snoring bed partner also disrupts sleep. It is best for older adults to avoid using beds for nonsleep activities such as watching television or reading.

Noise easily disturbs all patients, especially older adults because most of their sleep is in lighter sleep stages. This problem is greatest the first night a patient stays in a hospital or other agency, and often he or she experiences increased total wake time, increased awakening, and decreased REM sleep and total sleep time. Nursing activities are a source of increased sound levels. Noise from confused and ill patients and ringing of alarm systems and telephones are new and strange noises and make the hospital environment noisy and disruptive to sleep (Vincensi et al., 2016).

Hospitals across the United States are evaluated for their quality of care using the Hospital Consumer Assessment of Healthcare Providers and Systems (HCAHPS) survey (Centers for Medicare and Medicaid Services [CMS], 2014). The HCAHPS survey measures patients' perspectives on hospital care following discharge. The survey includes the topics of pain control and quietness of the hospital environment. Noise, pain management, and a hospital's general environment can negatively affect a patient's sleep and be a significant source of patient dissatisfaction, which affects survey scores and a hospital's reimbursement (see Chapter 3).

Exercise and Fatigue. Exercise and fatigue affect the ability to fall asleep and stay asleep. People who have a

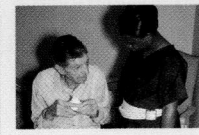

QSEN **QSEN ACTIVITY** *Quality Improvement*

While caring for Mr. Murphy, Anna overhears a number of other residents talking about the noise at night keeping them awake. Anna reports this to the charge nurse, who invites Anna to participate in a quality improvement project on noise reduction.

● How should Anna proceed with the project? Whom should she involve?

evolve   Answers to QSEN Activities can be found on the Evolve website.

relatively inactive lifestyle may not feel sleepy at bedtime, especially if they have spent extended periods in bed. A person who is moderately fatigued usually achieves restful sleep, especially if the fatigue results from enjoyable work or exercise. Exercising at least 2 or more hours before bedtime allows time for the body to cool and maintain a state of fatigue that promotes relaxation. However, excessive fatigue can make falling asleep difficult. This is common in adolescents who stay active with long hours involving school, extracurricular activities, and work.

Food and Caloric Intake. Following good eating habits is important for proper health including sleep. Eating a large, heavy, or spicy meal within 3 to 4 hours of bedtime sometimes results in indigestion. Alcohol consumed in the evening has insomnia-producing and diuretic effects. Coffee, tea, cola, and chocolate contain caffeine and xanthines that cause sleeplessness as a result of CNS stimulation.

Weight loss or weight gain influences sleep patterns. Weight gain contributes to OSA because of the increased size of the soft tissue structures in the upper airway (Kryger et al., 2017). Weight loss caused by semi-starvation diets sometimes causes sleep disorders such as reduced sleep and insomnia.

CRITICAL THINKING

You will apply elements of critical thinking whenever you perform the nursing process with patients.

Synthesis

Patient care requires you to apply what you know about a patient, your knowledge base, experience, and critical thinking attitudes and standards. Your synthesis of this information allows you to make sound decisions as you apply the nursing process. Critical thinking synthesis involves combining all available information to obtain a clear picture of the approach needed to provide patient-centered care. Many patients experience some type of sleep disorder, especially if sleeping in a new place. It is important not to overlook the problem or consider it as normal. Use of a

BOX 33.3   SYNTHESIS IN PRACTICE

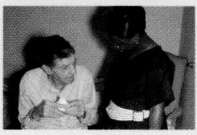

As Anna prepares to assess Mr. Murphy, she knows that it is important to consider sleep alterations in older adults. Because they typically have less deep sleep and more awakenings, it is important to consider which factors in the skilled care environment disrupt his sleep. She has learned that the pain from Mr. Murphy's osteoarthritis is a contributing factor to his sleep disturbances. His immobility resulting from the stroke adds discomfort. Anna also plans to assess Mr. Murphy's medications carefully to determine if any drugs are adding to a sleep alteration.

From Anna's experience in a skilled care facility, she knows that a resident's sleep is often fragmented. Furthermore, she read in a journal article that multiple factors affect sleep in patients residing in skilled nursing facilities, including physical illness, dementia, depression, sleep-disordered breathing, chronic bed rest, circadian rhythm disturbances, and the noise and lighting of the environment. She wants to be sure that her assessment considers all potential factors influencing Mr. Murphy's sleep pattern. She evaluates whether he has a roommate who stays up late or has multiple visitors, the presence of electrical equipment at his bedside, and the likelihood of noise coming from an outside hallway.

Anna will include Mr. Murphy's wife in the assessment to learn more about her perceptions of changes in his behavior. A complete assessment needs to be clear and precise; thus Anna plans to talk with Mr. Murphy more than one time to gather the necessary information and keep her patient from becoming fatigued.

critical thinking approach helps you correctly identify the nature of a sleep problem and initiate appropriate nursing care (Box 33.3).

Knowledge. To make decisions about the nature and cause of a patient's sleep problems, it is important to synthesize knowledge regarding the physiology and functions of sleep and factors that affect it. Knowledge of the pathophysiology of select disease processes further helps you understand the mechanisms for certain sleep problems. In addition, you need a thorough knowledge of pharmacological information because many medications that patients take contribute to sleeping difficulties. Another area of knowledge to synthesize is a patient's personal routine and cultural orientation. Infant care practices such as co-sleeping and the practice of regular siestas or naps are examples of cultural variations influencing sleep. Anticipate how such cultural factors ultimately influence an individual patient's ability to sleep.

Experience. You have experienced factors that have either disrupted or promoted your own ability to sleep. This personal experience is valuable when assessing patients'

sleep problems or in selecting therapies for sleep promotion. Previous clinical experience helps you to recognize the environmental and lifestyle variations that affect the quality and quantity of a patient's sleep.

Attitudes. It often takes a long time to find effective therapies for sleep alterations. For example, it is not easy to eliminate chronic insomnia in a short period. Perseverance and discipline are important critical thinking attitudes to use to develop a plan of care with effective solutions to manage a patient's sleep problems. The problems that result from sleep disruption also often require creative approaches. Sometimes an original idea is necessary to minimize or control environmental stressors in a patient's sleep environment.

Standards. When learning about a patient's sleep problem, you use numerous intellectual standards in conducting a nursing assessment. Always conduct a detailed sleep assessment to understand the nature of the sleep problem and potential causes and solutions. A clear, precise, specific, and accurate assessment is very important so that you establish an appropriate plan of care suited to a patient's specific sleep problem. Professional standards such as *Nursing: Scope and Standards of Practice* (American Nurses Association [ANA], 2015), *Management of Chronic Insomnia Disorder in Adults* (National Guideline Clearinghouse, 2016), and the *Perianesthesia Nursing Standards, Practice Recommendations and Interpretive Statements* (American Society of PeriAnesthesia Nurses [ASPAN], 2014) offer guidelines for care of patients with sleep disorders. Because patient satisfaction based on HCAHPS survey scores has become a priority in hospitals, many nursing units are developing unit-based standards to promote sleep for patients.

NURSING PROCESS

◼◼◻ ASSESSMENT

Assess a patient's sleep pattern to gather information about factors that usually influence sleep. Because sleep is a subjective experience, only the patient is able to report whether it is sufficient and restful. If a patient admits to or you suspect a sleep problem, gather a more detailed history. Aim your assessment at understanding the characteristics of any sleep problem and a patient's usual sleep habits so that you incorporate ways for promoting sleep into nursing care.

Sources for Sleep Assessment. Patients are your best resource for describing a sleep problem. Parents or bed partners offer information on patients' sleep patterns that reveal the nature of certain disorders. Obtain a child's sleep history from the parents. Older children often are able to relate the fears or worries that prevent them from falling asleep. Parents can describe typical behavior patterns that encourage or impair sleep. It is a good idea for parents of an infant to keep a 24-hour log of their infant's waking and sleeping behavior over a period of several days.

TABLE 33.2 FOCUSED PATIENT ASSESSMENT

FACTORS TO ASSESS	QUESTIONS	PHYSICAL ASSESSMENT
Bedtime routines	How do you prepare for bed? Tell me what time you typically go to bed each night.	Observe for dark circles under patient's eyes. Observe the number of times the patient yawns.
Bedtime environment	How much light is in your bedroom at night? What is the temperature of your room during the night? Do you listen to music to go to sleep?	Ask patient or sleeping partner about multiple patient position changes during sleep or frequent reawakenings.
Current life events	Tell me what hours do you normally work. Have you experienced any recent changes in your job or home responsibilities? Which activities do you do to relax outside of work? What hobbies do you have?	Observe patient's ability to concentrate on the conversation.

Sleep History. Obtain a brief sleep history from patients on admission to a health care agency. Determine usual bedtime, normal bedtime rituals, preferred environment for sleeping, and what time the patient usually rises. When you suspect a sleep problem, assess the quality and characteristics of sleep in greater depth (Table 33.2).

Sleep Pattern and Quality. Begin the sleep history with the patient's self-reported sleep pattern. Most patients give a reasonably accurate estimate of their sleep patterns, particularly if any changes have occurred. A visual analogue scale is an effective, subjective method for assessing sleep quality. Draw a straight horizontal line about 100 mm (4 inches) long. Add opposing statements such as "best night's sleep" and "worst night's sleep" at each end of the line. Ask the patient to place a mark along the horizontal line at the point that best matches his or her perception of the previous night's sleep. The distance of the mark along the line in millimeters offers a numerical value for satisfaction with sleep. Use the scale with the same patient repeatedly to show change in sleep over time. Do not use the scale to compare the quality of sleep for different patients.

The Epworth Sleepiness Scale (ASA, n.d.) is used to assess the degree of daytime sleepiness. A patient completes eight questions about the likeliness of being sleepy during certain activities (e.g., watching television, reading, and talking with someone) on a scale of 0 (would never doze or sleep) to 3 (high chance of dozing or sleeping). A score of 10 or more is considered sleepy. A score of 18 or more is very sleepy. The scale is available at http://epworthsleepinessscale.com/about-the-ess/.

Always have patients describe their usual sleep pattern in case there are significant changes created by a sleep disorder. Ask the following questions:

- What time do you usually get in bed?
- What time do you usually fall asleep? Do you do anything special to help you fall asleep?

- How many times do you wake up during sleep? Why do you think you awaken? What do you do about it?
- What time do you typically wake up? Do you use an alarm?
- What time do you get out of bed, and how long do you stay up once you have awakened?
- What is the average number of hours you sleep?
- Do you nap during the day? How many times? For how long? How do you feel when you wake?

Compare the assessment data with the pattern usually found for other patients of the same age and look for patterns that suggest problems. Sometimes patients with sleep problems show patterns very different from their usual one, and sometimes the change is relatively minor. Hospitalized patients usually need or want more sleep as a result of illness. However, some require less sleep because they are less active. Some patients who are ill think that it is important to try to sleep more than usual, eventually making sleeping difficult.

Description of Sleeping Problems. When a patient admits to or you suspect a sleep problem, ask open-ended questions to help the patient describe the problem fully. A general description of the problem followed by more focused questions usually reveals specific sleep characteristics. The STOP-BANG sleep assessment tool is a reliable evidence-based tool used to screen for OSA (Box 33.4) (Chung et al., 2016). You need to understand the nature of a sleep problem, its signs and symptoms, its onset and duration, its severity, predisposing factors or causes, and the overall effect on the patient. Examples of assessment questions include the following:

1. *Nature of the problem:* Tell me what type of problem you have with your sleep. Tell me why you think you are not getting enough sleep. Describe for me a recent typical night's sleep. How is this sleep different from your usual sleep?
2. *Signs and symptoms:* Have you been told that you snore loudly? Do you have headaches when awakening? (Ask

BOX 33.4 THE STOP-BANG QUESTIONNAIRE

Height _____ cm/inches   Weight _____ lb/kg
Age _____
Male/Female
BMI _____
Collar size of shirt: S, M, L, XL, or _____ cm/inches
Neck circumference* _____ cm

1. **S**noring
   Do you **s**nore loudly (louder than talking or loud enough to be heard through closed doors)?
   Yes   No
2. **T**ired
   Do you often feel **t**ired, fatigued, or sleepy during daytime?
   Yes   No
3. **O**bserved
   Has anyone **o**bserved you stop breathing during your sleep?
   Yes   No
4. Blood **P**ressure
   Do you have or are you being treated for high blood **p**ressure?
   Yes   No
5. **B**MI
   BMI more than 35 kg/m^2?
   Yes   No
6. **A**ge
   Age older 50 years old?
   Yes   No
7. **N**eck circumference (measure with approved measuring tape)*
   Neck circumference greater than 40 cm?
   Yes   No
8. **G**ender
   Gender male?
   Yes   No

Score of 4: High sensitivity of 88% for identifying severe OSA

Score of 5 or more: High risk of OSA; a score of 6 is more specific

Modified from Chung F, et al: Predictive performance of the STOP-BANG score for identifying obstructive sleep apnea in obese patients, *Obes Surg* 23(12):2050, 2013.
BMS, Body mass index; *OSA,* obstructive sleep apnea.
*Neck circumference is measured by staff.

bed partner or parents whether the patient has restful sleep or problems such as going to the bathroom frequently.)

3. *Onset and duration:* When did you notice the problem? How long has it lasted?
4. *Severity:* How long does it take you to fall asleep? How often during the week do you have trouble falling asleep or staying asleep?
5. *Predisposing factors:* Tell me what you do just before going to bed. Have you recently had any changes at work, school, or home? How would you describe your current mood, and have you noticed any recent changes?

Which medications or recreational drugs do you take regularly? Do you eat spicy or greasy foods or drink alcohol or caffeinated beverages? If so, how much do you eat or drink daily?

6. *Effect on patient:* How has the loss of sleep affected you? Tell me how it affects your day and ability to perform normal activities. (Ask a family member or friend about any changes in the patient's behavior since the sleep problem started.)

Sleep Diary. When a serious sleep problem exists, ask the patient and bed partner to keep a sleep-wake diary. Have them each complete the diary daily until they are scheduled to be seen for their next health care visit (at least 2 weeks is preferred); this will provide information on day-to-day variations in sleep-wake patterns over time. Entries in the diary often include 24-hour information on waking and sleeping activities such as exercise, work activities, mealtimes, and alcohol and caffeine intake. They should also include time and length of daytime naps, evening and bed routines, the time the patient tries to fall asleep, time and number of awakenings, and the time of morning awakening. The diary is most helpful if the patient is motivated to complete it thoroughly. Using a tape recorder is a helpful option for patients with visual impairment or who have difficulty writing. Do not use the diary for patients in the hospital.

Physical Illness. Assess for any physical or psychological problems that affect a patient's sleep. A review of known medical conditions reveals symptoms (e.g., pain, nausea, shortness of breath, acid reflux, fear) that interfere with the patient's normal sleep pattern. If a patient is scheduled for surgery, be sure to ask about a history of sleep apnea. Patients with sleep apnea who receive general anesthesia and pain medications after surgery have increased risk for developing airway obstruction during recovery (see Chapter 40). If the patient has recently had surgery, expect him or her to experience some disturbance in sleep.

Medications. Assess a patient's medication history including over-the-counter and prescribed drugs. If the patient takes medications for sleep, gather information about the type and amount used (see Box 33.2).

Current Life Events. Changes in lifestyle disrupt a patient's sleep. A patient's family situation or occupation offers clues to the nature of a sleep problem. Changes in job responsibilities, rotating shifts, and the recent birth of a child or loss of a family member can contribute to a sleep disturbance. Questions about social activities, recent travel, or mealtime schedules also help clarify the sleep assessment.

Emotional and Mental Status. If a patient is anxious, fearful, or angry, mental preoccupations seriously disrupt sleep. In this situation a patient experiences emotional stress related to illness or situational crises. Ask patients to explore feelings about relationships, work, or other situations.

Bedtime Routines. Ask how patients prepare for sleep. Assess for the habits that are beneficial compared with habits that disturb sleep. For example, does the patient perform strenuous exercise within 2 hours of going to sleep? Does he or she usually spend 1 to 2 hours cooling down or relaxing before sleep? Is the patient drinking fluids throughout the evening and night contributing to nocturia?

Bedtime Environment. Ask patients to describe their preferred bedroom conditions. For example, ask if the patient keeps the bedroom dark or softly lit and closes the door. Some patients listen to a radio or watch television or prefer a quiet environment if noise prevents them from falling asleep. Also ask about room temperature and ventilation. Some individuals need a fan to keep cool or for white noise. Assess the type of bed in which the patient sleeps. Does the patient sleep in the same bed every night? Is the mattress comfortable? Does the patient need several pillows or cushions in bed to sit up during sleep? Does the patient use a lounge chair/recliner to sleep? Information about the sleeping environment helps you design better sleeping conditions.

Behaviors of Sleep Deprivation. Some patients are unaware of how their sleep problems affect their behavior. Observe for irritability, disorientation (similar to a drunken state), and slurred speech. If sleep deprivation has lasted a long time, psychotic behavior such as delusions and paranoia develop. For example, a patient reports seeing strange objects or colors in the room, or the patient acts afraid when you or other health personnel enter the room suddenly or without warning.

Older Adult Considerations. Older adults have a harder time falling asleep and more trouble staying asleep compared with younger adults. Research suggests that much of sleep disturbance in older adults is attributed to physical and mental illnesses and medications used to treat the illnesses (Kryger et al., 2017). It is a common misconception that sleep needs decrease with aging. Older patients become sleepier in the early evening and wake earlier in the morning but still require 7 to 8 hours of sleep a day.

Older patients are more prone to RLS and should be assessed for the presence of this condition. Also assess older adults for the presence of chronic medical conditions associated with sleep disturbance such as heart failure or chronic obstructive pulmonary disease. Older adults frequently experience losses such as retirement and death of a loved one that may lead to emotional stress or depressive mood problems that reduce sleep efficacy (Meiner, 2015).

Patient Expectations. After assessing a patient's sleep history, determine the patient's expectations regarding nursing care. Use a caring and skilled approach to assess the patient's sleep needs and preferences. For example, ask, "Now that I understand more about your sleep habits and the recent problems you have had, what do you expect from us regarding your care?" or "To improve your sleep, what do you think is most important that we do for you?" The patient sometimes has a different view about the relationship of sleep and health from your own. Examining patient expectations and preferences helps to clarify any misconceptions. Ask the patient which interventions he or she prefers and how to implement them. In the hospital setting some patients are more concerned about being sure that you are checking

their condition routinely than about whether you disturb their sleep.

■■■■ NURSING DIAGNOSIS

Your assessment reveals clusters of data that include defining characteristics or risk factors for nursing diagnoses that are associated with sleep disturbances. If you identify a sleep pattern disturbance, it is helpful for you to specify the exact condition. By determining the nature of a sleep disturbance, you can design more effective interventions. Following is a list of potential nursing diagnoses that you may identify for a patient with a sleep problem:

- *Acute Confusion*
- *Ineffective Coping*
- *Fatigue*
- *Insomnia*
- *Disturbed Sleep Pattern*
- *Sleep Deprivation*
- *Ineffective Health Maintenance*
- *Readiness for Enhanced Sleep*

In the case of problem-focused diagnoses, your assessment needs to identify the probable cause or related factor for the sleep disturbance, such as a noisy environment or a high intake of caffeine. The cause becomes the focus of nursing interventions. For example, a hospitalized patient who experiences insomnia as a result of a noisy sleeping environment benefits from a reduction in hospital equipment noise or minimizing interruptions. If the insomnia is related to worry over a threatened marital separation, your interventions involve introducing coping strategies. If you define the probable cause or related factors incorrectly, the patient will not benefit from your care. There may be multiple factors for some patients. Validate your assessment with the patient or significant others.

■■■■ PLANNING

Goals and Outcomes. Develop a plan of care after identifying all relevant nursing diagnoses for a patient (Fig. 33.2) (see Care Plan). You develop an individualized care plan only after you understand how the nursing diagnoses relate to your patient's normal and current sleep pattern, his or her perception of the sleep problem, and the factors disrupting sleep. Together you and the patient develop realistic goals and outcomes. For example, the goal of "Patient will establish a healthy sleep pattern" includes outcomes such as "Patient falls asleep within a half hour of planned time" and "Patient has fewer than two awakenings during the night." This will be realistic if you know from your assessment that it now takes the patient 1 hour to fall asleep and that awakenings occur 3 or 4 times a night. The outcomes serve as measurable guidelines to determine goal achievement. An effective plan includes outcomes established over a realistic time frame that focus on improving the quality of sleep. This type of plan requires many weeks to accomplish.

CONCEPT MAP

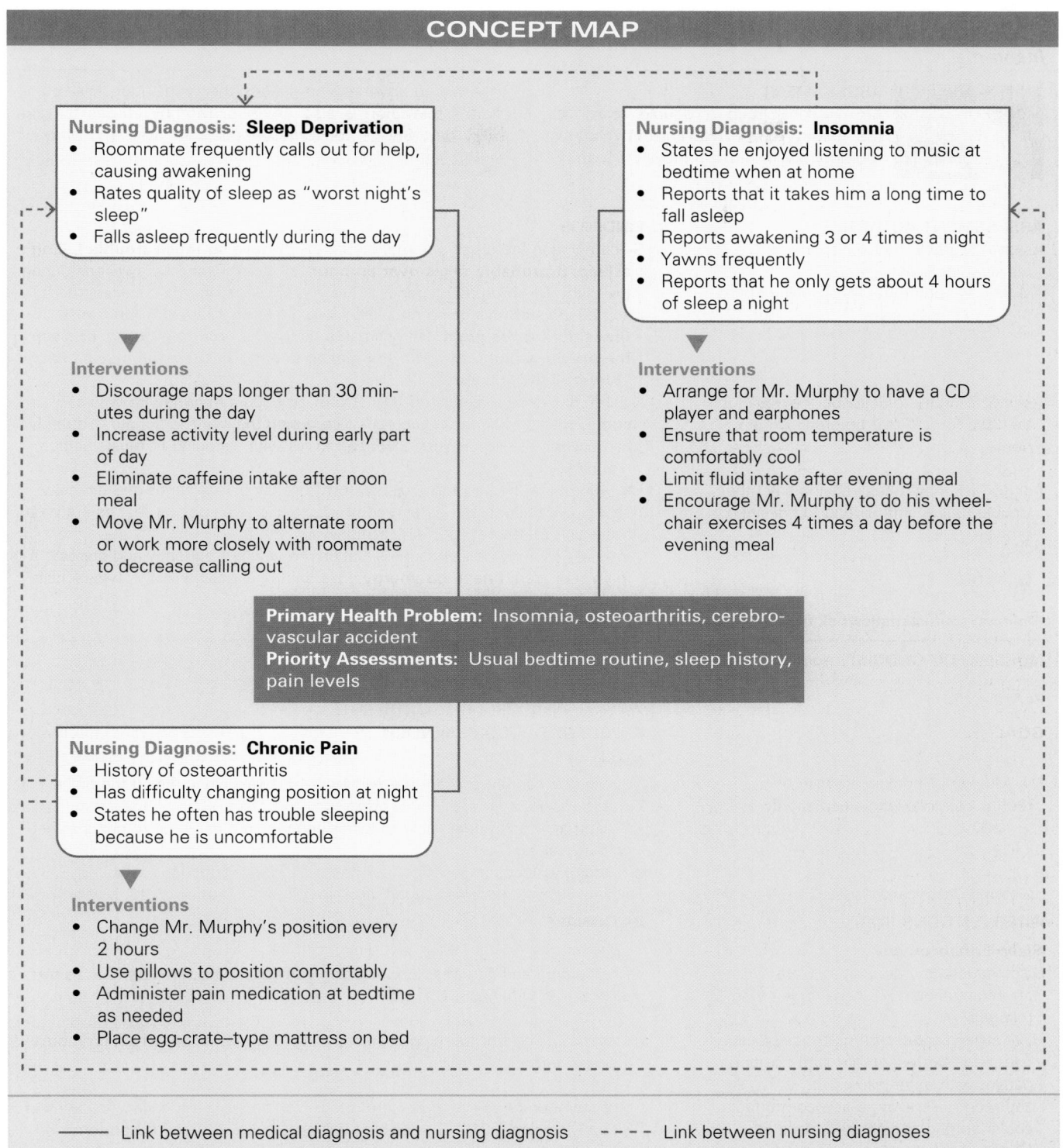

Nursing Diagnosis: Sleep Deprivation
- Roommate frequently calls out for help, causing awakening
- Rates quality of sleep as "worst night's sleep"
- Falls asleep frequently during the day

Interventions
- Discourage naps longer than 30 minutes during the day
- Increase activity level during early part of day
- Eliminate caffeine intake after noon meal
- Move Mr. Murphy to alternate room or work more closely with roommate to decrease calling out

Nursing Diagnosis: Insomnia
- States he enjoyed listening to music at bedtime when at home
- Reports that it takes him a long time to fall asleep
- Reports awakening 3 or 4 times a night
- Yawns frequently
- Reports that he only gets about 4 hours of sleep a night

Interventions
- Arrange for Mr. Murphy to have a CD player and earphones
- Ensure that room temperature is comfortably cool
- Limit fluid intake after evening meal
- Encourage Mr. Murphy to do his wheelchair exercises 4 times a day before the evening meal

Primary Health Problem: Insomnia, osteoarthritis, cerebrovascular accident
Priority Assessments: Usual bedtime routine, sleep history, pain levels

Nursing Diagnosis: Chronic Pain
- History of osteoarthritis
- Has difficulty changing position at night
- States he often has trouble sleeping because he is uncomfortable

Interventions
- Change Mr. Murphy's position every 2 hours
- Use pillows to position comfortably
- Administer pain medication at bedtime as needed
- Place egg-crate–type mattress on bed

——— Link between medical diagnosis and nursing diagnosis   - - - - Link between nursing diagnoses

FIG 33.2 Concept map.

Setting Priorities. Identify priority strategies and interventions to promote sleep using the data you gathered about the nature of the patient's problem. Together you and the patient identify and select the strategies and interventions that are most likely to be beneficial in the home or health care setting. The plan of care includes strategies that support positive sleep habits and patterns that fit the patient's living environment, cultural orientation, and lifestyle. For example, a patient decides that purchasing a new mattress to increase comfort is the first step toward improving sleep. In a health

◎ CARE PLAN

Insomnia

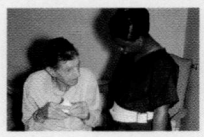

ASSESSMENT

Mr. Murphy is in a double room at the nursing home. He currently has a roommate who Anna notices frequently calls out to anyone who passes the room door. His roommate's television is also on. Mrs. Murphy comes to visit every day. She is concerned about how tired Mr. Murphy seems.

ASSESSMENT ACTIVITIES	FINDINGS[a]
Ask Mr. Murphy to describe the nature of his sleep problem.	Since being in the nursing home, he states, **"I have so much trouble falling asleep; it probably takes over an hour."** When asked if he awakens during the night, Mr. Murphy responds, "Are you kidding? No one can sleep here; something's always going on." Mr. Murphy admits to **waking up 3 or 4 times during the night.** He estimates that he had maybe **4 hours of sleep the previous night. Mr. Murphy places a mark on the analog scale near "worst night's sleep."**
Ask Mr. Murphy to rate the quality of previous night's sleep.	
Ask Mr. Murphy to describe the usual bedtime routine that he practiced at home.	Mr. Murphy usually slept from 10:30 p.m. to 6:00 a.m. when he was at home, usually waking up once or twice during the night to urinate. He rarely had difficulty falling asleep; according to his wife, listening to music helped him relax.
Ask Mr. Murphy if he is having any other trouble that is contributing to his sleep problem.	He reports that he has some discomfort from his osteoarthritis and difficulty changing positions and getting comfortable. He rates pain at rest as a 4 on a scale of 0 to 10.
Assess Mr. Murphy for signs of sleep problems.	While Mr. Murphy describes his situation, he yawns frequently and states, "I really feel tired. **I have no energy**." He shifts his position in his wheelchair multiple times.

[a]**Defining characteristics/risk factors** are shown in **bold** type.

NURSING DIAGNOSIS: Insomnia related to environmental barriers

---

PLANNING

GOAL	EXPECTED OUTCOMES (NOC)[b]
	Sleep
Mr. Murphy will obtain a sense of restfulness following sleep within 1 month.	Mr. Murphy has fewer than two self-reported awakenings during the night within 2 weeks.
	Mr. Murphy reports being able to fall asleep within a half hour of going to bed within 2 weeks.
	Mr. Murphy sleeps an average of 7 hours per night within 4 weeks.

[b]Outcome classification labels from Moorhead S, et al, editors: *Nursing outcomes classification (NOC)*, ed 5, St Louis, 2013, Mosby.

INTERVENTIONS (NIC)[c]	RATIONALE
Sleep Enhancement	
Discourage early morning and late afternoon napping or naps longer than 30 minutes.	Early morning and late afternoon napping interferes with sleeping (Centre for Clinical Interventions [CCI], n.d.).
Have an egg-crate–type mattress placed over bed mattress. Have staff position patient with extra pillows.	Increases comfort of sleeping position, enhancing relaxation, which promotes a sleep state.
Keep room temperature at a comfortable, cooler setting at night and make sure Mr. Murphy has a blanket as needed	Cooler temperatures are more comfortable for sleeping (American Academy of Sleep Medicine, 2016). The blanket will ensure Mr. Murphy is comfortable.
Encourage Mr. Murphy to decrease his fluids 2 to 4 hours before sleep.	Decreases number of times patient awakens to urinate (Meiner, 2015).
Relaxation Therapy	
Arrange for Mr. Murphy to have a personal music device with ear buds to play music of his choice when first going to bed.	Music therapy decreases situational anxiety and improves sleep efficiency (Meiner, 2015).
Arrange for Mr. Murphy to have some of his favorite reading material at his bedside.	Reading before bedtime is a rest-promoting activity.

CARE PLAN—cont'd

Insomnia

INTERVENTIONS (NIC)[c]	RATIONALE
Exercise Promotion	
Have Mr. Murphy get regular exercise (e.g., have him propel down hallways in wheelchair for 5 minutes 4 times a day before dinner).	Regular exercise improves sleep quality (Maness and Khan, 2015).

[c]Intervention classification labels from Bulechek GM, et al, editors: *Nursing interventions classification (NIC)*, ed 6, St Louis, 2013, Mosby.

EVALUATION

NURSING ACTIONS	PATIENT RESPONSE/FINDING	ACHIEVEMENT OF OUTCOME
Ask Mr. Murphy to use a visual analogue scale to rate the quality of his sleep at the end of each week.	At the end of the first week Mr. Murphy rates his quality of sleep as 6 out of 10. For the second week he rates his sleep at 8 out of 10.	Mr. Murphy is implementing sleep-hygiene measures. His sleep is improving because he rates his sleep as improving.
Ask Mrs. Murphy to evaluate her perceptions of Mr. Murphy's level of fatigue.	Mrs. Murphy states that her husband seems more awake, alert, and talkative when she visits. He does not nod off or nap in the early afternoon any more. She comments that he enjoys doing the wheelchair exercises.	The sleep-hygiene measures along with the exercises have contributed to improved sleep for Mr. Murphy, resulting in decreased daytime fatigue.
Ask Mr. Murphy at the end of 4 weeks to keep a record for a week of the length of time he estimates sleeping.	Mr. Murphy reports that he falls asleep within 30 minutes and generally wakes up 2 to 3 times a night. He reports that he is sleeping 6 hours a night.	Mr. Murphy's use of relaxation therapy and music has improved his sleep.

care setting you plan treatments or routines together to give the patient more time to rest. For example, you turn and reposition a patient at the same time you give him or her medication or perform a treatment such as suctioning to limit the number of nurse-patient contacts. All staff caring for the patient need to know the plan so that they cluster activities at times to reduce nocturnal awakenings. In a nursing home plan rest periods around the activities of other residents.

Collaborative Care. The nature of a sleep disturbance determines whether referrals to additional health care providers are necessary. For example, if a sleep problem is related to a situational crisis or emotional problem, refer the patient to a psychiatric clinical nurse specialist, pastoral care professional, or clinical psychologist for counseling. This ensures that you attend to the patient's problems not only in the health care setting but also in the home. Sharing information with a home care nurse on patient discharge is useful in planning interventions to ensure that the patient gets adequate sleep when home. When chronic insomnia is the problem, a medical referral or referral to a sleep center is beneficial.

IMPLEMENTATION

Your nursing interventions for improving the quality of a person's sleep largely focus on health promotion. In an acute care setting your focus becomes managing the environment to support a patient's normal sleep habits and keeping the patient safe. In long-term care or nursing home environments, give special considerations for promoting adequate sleep and rest.

Health Promotion. Helping patients to develop good sleep-hygiene practices is important. Educational interventions offer individuals in the community information for improving sleep hygiene practices (Box 33.5). Your specific interventions promote a person's normal sleep and rest pattern.

Environmental Controls. All patients require a sleeping environment with a comfortable room temperature and proper ventilation, minimal noise, a comfortable bed, and proper lighting. Infants sleep best when the room temperature is 18° C to 21° C (64° F to 70° F). Place healthy infants on their backs to sleep (Hockenberry and Wilson, 2015). The national "Safe to Sleep" campaign has been successful in teaching parents and infant caregivers to place infants on their backs for sleeping to reduce the incidence of sudden infant death syndrome (SIDS) (U.S. Department of Health and Human Services [USDHHS], n.d.). Children and adults vary more in regard to comfortable room temperature but usually sleep best in cooler environments. Some individuals prefer to sleep without covers. Older adults often require extra blankets, covers, or socks (Box 33.6).

BOX 33.5   EVIDENCE-BASED PRACTICE

PICO Question: Does the presentation of a sleep education program improve sleep-hygiene knowledge and behaviors in college students?

SUMMARY OF EVIDENCE

Good quality sleep is important for college students. Inadequate quantity and/or quality of sleep impacts learning abilities, leads to poor academic performance, affects both physical and mental health of students, and contributes to accidents (Gao et al., 2014; Dietrich et al., 2015). Nursing students demonstrated increased knowledge of good sleep-hygiene practices and of sleep disorders after a formal education program on sleep (Ye and Smith, 2015). A comprehensive sleep management program had a positive effect on sleep in college students (Gao et al., 2014). The students in the intervention group received education on sleep hygiene, music therapy, stimulus control, and relaxation therapy. The intervention group reported improved sleep quality, longer sleep duration, and less daytime dysfunction compared with the control group (Gao et al., 2014). Formal and comprehensive sleep education programs is an effective health promotion intervention that positively impacts sleep health in college students (Dietrich et al., 2015).

APPLICATION TO NURSING PRACTICE

- Sleep education programs in nursing curricula provide sleep education for future nurses (Ye and Smith, 2015).
- Sleep education programs using multiple strategies are effective in improving sleep (Gao et al., 2014).
- Teach patient muscle relaxation techniques and encourage them to perform within an hour before sleep (Gao et al., 2014).
- Listening to relaxing music for 30 minutes within 1 hour of sleep improves sleep quality (Gao et al., 2014).

BOX 33.6   CARE OF THE OLDER ADULT

Sleep Disturbances

SLEEP-WAKE PATTERN
- Maintain a regular rising time and bedtime.
- Eliminate early morning and late afternoon naps.
- If patient takes naps, limit to 20 to 30 minutes or less twice a day.
- Go to bed when sleepy.
- Use relaxation techniques and a regular bedtime routine to promote sleep.
- If unable to sleep in 15 to 30 minutes, get out of bed and do routine quiet activities.

ENVIRONMENT
- Expose to natural light or bright interior lights for 30 minutes to 2 hours daily, preferably soon after waking.
- Sleep where you sleep best.
- Keep noise to a minimum; use soft music to mask noise if necessary.
- Use night-light and keep path to bathroom free of obstacles.
- Set room temperature to preference.

MEDICATIONS
- Use sedatives and hypnotics as last resort; then use only for a short time if needed.
- Adjust medications being taken for other conditions and look for drug interactions that cause insomnia or EDS.

DIET
- Limit alcohol, caffeine, and nicotine in late afternoon and evening.
- Eat a light snack such as cereal and milk or cheese and crackers before bedtime.
- Decrease fluids 2 to 4 hours before sleep.

PHYSIOLOGICAL/ILLNESS FACTORS
- Elevate head of bed, and provide extra pillows as preferred.
- Use analgesics 30 minutes before bed to ease aches and pains.
- Use prescribed medications to control symptoms of chronic conditions.

EDS, Excessive daytime sleepiness.

Eliminate or reduce distracting noise so that the bedroom is as quiet as possible. In the home the television or the ringing of the telephone disrupts a patient's sleep. The television is too stimulating to watch before sleep and should not be watched in bed or immediately before going to bed (Brockmann et al., 2016). Family members become important participants in care when each has a different schedule for going to sleep. The cooperation of several people living with the patient is often required to reduce noise. Wearing ear plugs may help to reduce or eliminate distracting noises. Some patients sleep better with inside noises such as the hum of a ceiling fan.

Make sure that the bed and mattress provide support and comfortable firmness. Place a bed board under the mattress to add support. Sometimes extra pillows help a person position more comfortably in bed. The position of the bed in the room also makes a difference for some patients.

For a patient prone to confusion or falls, safety is critical. In the home a small night-light helps the patient become oriented to the room environment before arising to go to the bathroom. Beds set lower to the floor reduce the risk for falls when a patient stands. Remove clutter from the path a patient uses to walk from the bed to the bathroom. If a patient needs help in ambulating from the bed to the bathroom, have a small bell at the bedside to call family members or obtain a bedside commode.

Patients vary in regard to the amount of light that they prefer at night. Infants and older adults sleep best in softly lit rooms. Do not have light shining directly on their eyes. Small table lamps or night-lights prevent total darkness. For older adults this reduces the chance of confusion when arising from bed. If streetlights shine through windows or when patients nap during the day, a sleep mask or heavy shades, drapes, or slatted blinds are helpful.

BOX 33.7 PATIENT TEACHING

Improving Sleep

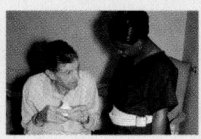 On one of her visits to the nursing home, Mrs. Murphy tells Anna that she is having trouble sleeping and does not feel rested. Anna asks Mrs. Murphy to describe her current sleep habits. Using what she knows about sleep-hygiene measures, Anna develops a teaching plan to help Mrs. Murphy improve her sleep.

OUTCOME

At the end of the teaching session, Mrs. Murphy develops a plan that includes effective sleep-hygiene practices.

TEACHING STRATEGIES

- Discuss with Mrs. Murphy the need to practice good sleep-hygiene habits regularly.
- Caution Mrs. Murphy against delaying bedtime or sleeping long hours during weekends or holidays to maintain her normal sleep-wake cycle.
- Explain to her not to use the bedroom and especially the bed for watching television, snacking, or other nonsleep activity.
- Encourage Mrs. Murphy to take a warm bath before bedtime.
- Encourage Mrs. Murphy to walk for 30 minutes every morning.
- Instruct Mrs. Murphy to play soft relaxing music at bedtime to help her fall asleep.
- Demonstrate and then practice relaxation techniques with Mrs. Murphy.
- Advise Mrs. Murphy that if she does not fall asleep within 20 minutes, she needs to get out of bed and do some quiet activity until feeling sleepy.
- Instruct Mrs. Murphy to avoid heavy meals for 3 hours before bedtime; a light snack including protein and carbohydrates helps.
- Answer questions that Mrs. Murphy has about sleep problems.

EVALUATION

- Use the principles of teach-back to evaluate patient/family caregiver learning:
  - Tell me three sleep-hygiene habits that we discussed to improve your sleep.
  - Demonstrate a relaxation technique you learned that promotes sleep.
  - Describe an appropriate bedtime snack that you would prepare for yourself.
  - Tell me the benefits of listening to soothing music at bedtime.

Promoting Bedtime Routines. Bedtime routines and sleep-hygiene measures relax patients in preparation for sleep. A person should go to sleep when he or she feels tired or sleepy. Patients and their bed partners need to learn techniques that promote sleep and conditions that interfere with it (Box 33.7). Encourage patients in the hospital to follow their at-home bedtime routine as much as possible.

Newborns and infants benefit from quiet activities such as holding them snugly in blankets, talking or singing softly, and gently rocking. A bedtime routine (e.g., same hour for bedtime or quiet activity) used consistently helps toddlers and preschool children avoid delaying sleep. Parents need to reinforce patterns of preparing for bedtime. Reading stories, allowing children to sit in a parent's lap while listening to music, and coloring are good sleep hygiene routines.

Adults need to avoid excessive mental stimulation just before bedtime. Reading a light novel, watching a relaxing television program, or listening to music helps a person relax. Progressive muscle relaxation exercises (see Chapter 34) and praying induce calm in patients.

Promoting Comfort. People fall asleep only after feeling comfortable and relaxed. You offer strategies that can reduce the minor irritants that keep people awake. Have family members change diapers before placing infants in bed. An extra blanket prevents chilling when trying to fall asleep. Encourage a patient to wear loose-fitting nightwear and to void before bedtime. Have family members give a relaxing back rub.

Patients with painful illnesses may benefit from the application of dry or moist heat, use of supportive dressings or splints, and proper positioning with the use of extra pillows for support. Patients with temporary acute pain (e.g., following surgery) may sleep better if the bed partner lets the patient sleep alone until the pain subsides. Also encourage the patient to take pain medications 30 to 60 minutes before going to bed.

You help patients with physical illness learn ways to control symptoms that disrupt sleep. For example, a patient with respiratory abnormalities needs to sleep with two pillows or in a semi-sitting position to ease the effort to breathe. The patient often benefits from taking prescribed bronchodilators before sleep to prevent airway obstruction.

Promoting Activity. Increasing daytime activity lessens problems with falling asleep. Always plan rigorous exercise at least 2 to 3 hours before bedtime. Research indicates that exercise is beneficial, particularly for older adults, to improve nighttime sleep. However, older adults with chronic diseases that influence their functional abilities are likely to have limited activity (Touhy and Jett, 2018). Recommend activities that are safe for older patients to perform, such as walking, swimming, wheelchair propulsion, and cycling on a stationary bike. Weight lifting using light weights (e.g., 2 to 5 lb) builds upper body strength and endurance. Activity and exercise often prove to be beneficial by improving activity endurance, mobility, and sense of well-being.

Stress Reduction. When patients feel emotionally upset, urge them to try not to force sleep. Otherwise insomnia often develops, and soon they will associate bedtime with the inability to relax. Encourage a patient who has difficulty falling asleep to get up and pursue a relaxing activity rather than staying in bed and thinking about sleep. When the emotional problem is ongoing and the patient finds little relief, encourage referral to an appropriate counselor.

Children often have problems going to bed and falling asleep. Have parents enter their children's rooms immediately after nightmares and talk to them briefly about their fears to provide a cooling-down period. Comforting children while they lie in their own bed is reassuring. Keeping a light on in the room also helps. Usually experts do not recommend that a child be allowed to sleep with parents; however, families approach sleep practices differently based on cultural traditions (Box 33.8).

Bedtime Snacks. Some people enjoy bedtime snacks, whereas others cannot sleep after eating. A bedtime snack containing protein and carbohydrates such as cereal and milk or cheese and crackers, which contain L-tryptophan, may help to promote sleep. A full meal before bedtime often causes gastrointestinal upset and interferes with the ability to fall asleep.

⊕ BOX 33.8 PATIENT-CENTERED CARE

Co-sleeping or bed sharing with children is often a culturally preferred habit or family tradition. Mothers younger than 20 years of age are more likely to practice co-sleeping (Keys and Rankin, 2015). Often mothers who are breastfeeding use this practice to have their babies close by (Cullen et al., 2016). Others believe co-sleeping is a way to keep infants safe because of the nearness. Parents may choose not to practice co-sleeping as they wish to promote self-sleep independence early in life (Matlock-Carr and Ward, 2015). Health care personnel in the United States discourage the practice of bed sharing because of safety issues. Bed sharing for newborns to 4-month-old infants is extremely risky and can result in death of the infant (Moon, 2017). As a nurse, be culturally sensitive when discussing co-sleeping practices with parents and developing sleeping plans for children.

IMPLICATIONS FOR PRACTICE

- Complete a thorough sleep assessment of the child and family.
- Discuss the risks of co-sleeping with parents. During the discussion remain culturally sensitive and respectful of the parents' views (Cullen et al., 2016).
- Co-sleeping has been linked to increased risk for SIDS under certain conditions such as parental smoking or alcohol or drug use.
- Instruct parents to avoid using alcohol or drugs that impair arousal. Decreased arousal prevents the parents from waking up if the child is having problems.
- Co-sleeping should only occur with parents and child and not another adult or child.
- Avoid soft bedding surfaces. Infants and children become entangled or have their heads covered if the bed contains loose coverings, pillows, or stuffed toys.
- Encourage parents to use light sleeping clothes, keep the room temperature comfortable, and not bundle the child tightly or in too many clothes.

SIDS, Sudden infant death syndrome.

Make sure that patients avoid drinking excess fluids or ingesting caffeine before bedtime. Coffee, tea, cola, and chocolate cause a person to stay awake or wake up throughout the night. Alcohol interrupts sleep cycles and reduces the amount of deep sleep. Caffeinated drinks and alcohol act as diuretics, which cause nocturia.

Pharmacological Approaches to Promoting Sleep. Melatonin is a neurohormone produced in the brain that helps control circadian rhythms. It is a popular nutritional supplement in the United States used to aid sleep. The recommended dose is 0.3 to 3 mg taken 2 hours before bedtime to improve sleep onset. Older adults with decreased levels of melatonin find it aids sleep (Emet et al., 2016). The short-term use of melatonin is considered safe with infrequent mild side effects of nausea, headache, and dizziness. Melatonin is a dietary supplement, not a drug, and is not regulated by the U.S. Food and Drug Administration (FDA).

Sedatives and hypnotics are groups of drugs that induce and/or maintain sleep. However, long-term use of these drugs disrupts sleep and leads to more serious problems. Benzodiazepines are a common classification of drug used to treat sleep problems when a change in sleep hygiene is not effective. Examples of benzodiazepines include temazepam, flurazepam, and triazolam. Benzodiazepines may cause psychological and physical dependence, and physical withdrawal symptoms may occur if the drug is not carefully tapered following long-term use (Burchum and Rosenthal, 2016). The use of benzodiazepines in older adults is potentially dangerous. Long-term use and high doses in older adults are associated with sedation and cognitive impairment leading to falls (Burchum and Rosenthal, 2016).

Trazodone is a serotonin antagonist and reuptake inhibitor (SARI) antidepressant often used in patients with depression or anxiety and insomnia. The most common side effects are daytime grogginess and orthostatic hypotension. Low-dose trazodone is often used as an alternative to benzodiazepines, especially in older patients.

Non-benzodiazepine receptor agonists appear to have better safety profiles and fewer adverse effects than benzodiazepines. They are also associated with a lower risk of abuse and dependence than benzodiazepines, although abuse and dependence do occur. Examples of medications in this class include zolpidem, zaleplon, and eszopiclone (Burchum and Rosenthal, 2016). A low dose of a short-acting medication such as zolpidem can be effective for short-term use (no longer than 2 to 3 weeks). Patients should avoid drinking alcohol while taking these drugs.

The use of nonprescription over-the-counter sleeping medications is not advisable. Over the long-term these drugs lead to further sleep disruption even when they initially seem effective. Help patients with optional sleep interventions that do not require the use of drugs.

Regular use of any sleep medication leads to tolerance, and withdrawal causes rebound insomnia. Make sure that all patients understand the possible side effects of sleep medications. In 2007, the FDA released a warning related to complex sleep-related behaviors such as sleep driving or sleep eating that have occurred with prescription sleep medications (FDA, 2016). Routine monitoring of patient response to sleeping medications is important.

Acute Care. The nursing interventions described for health promotion are applicable to a patient requiring acute care. The nature of the acute care setting requires you to be creative in finding ways to maintain the patient's normal sleep pattern.

Managing Environmental Stimuli. A challenge in the hospital is controlling noise. Implement ways to reduce noise such as conducting conversations and reports in a private area away from patient rooms and keeping necessary conversations to a minimum, especially at night (Flynn Makic et al., 2014). Provide patients with ear plugs or eye masks to decrease noise and light stimulation (Caple and March, 2016; Litton et al., 2016). Because many patients spend only a short time in hospitals, it is easy to forget the importance of establishing good sleep conditions. In a hospital setting plan nursing care activities to avoid waking patients. Try to schedule assessments, treatments, procedures, and routines for times when patients are awake. Perform nursing activities before the patient receives sleeping medication or begins to fall asleep. For example, you have a patient who had surgery. Before the patient gets ready for bed, change the surgical dressing, reposition the patient, administer pain medication, and check vital signs. Give medications and draw blood during waking hours when possible (Caple and March, 2016). Plan with other departments and services to schedule therapies at intervals that give patients time to rest. Whenever it becomes necessary to wake a patient, perform the activity as quickly as possible so the patient can fall back to sleep as soon as possible.

Safety. Safety precautions are important for patients who wake up during the night to use the bathroom and for patients with EDS. Set beds lower to the floor to lessen the chance of the patient falling when first standing. Remove clutter and move equipment from the path that a patient uses to walk from the bed to the bathroom. If a patient needs assistance in ambulating from the bed to the bathroom, make sure that the nurse call system is accessible within the patient's reach. Be sure that the patient knows how to turn the light on correctly.

If patients normally use a CPAP machine at home because of sleep apnea, it is important that they bring their home equipment with them to the hospital and use it every night. Check to make sure the mask is snug fitting and put on correctly so that the positive pressure is maintained (Schub, 2016) (see Chapter 32). In patients with sleep apnea who have surgery and receive general anesthesia, the anesthesia in combination with opioid medications used after surgery reduces the patient's defenses against airway obstruction. After surgery the patient achieves very deep levels of REM sleep that lead to muscle relaxation and airway obstruction. Use pain medication carefully in these patients. These patients need ventilator support in the postoperative period because OSA is linked to increased postoperative respiratory complications. Monitor the patient's breathing and oxygen saturation levels regularly (see Chapter 15). Notify the health care provider right away if the patient is difficult to arouse or is having trouble breathing.

Patients who experience EDS can fall asleep while sitting up in a chair or wheelchair. Position patients so that they do not fall out of the chair when sleeping. Elevating their feet on an ottoman or small bench may help to position them safely. A pillow placed in the patient's lap provides some support. If a patient enjoys leaning over an over-bed table while sitting in a chair, be sure that the table is locked and secure. Avoid using safety belts because they are considered restraints (see Chapter 30).

Comfort Measures. You make the patient more comfortable in an acute care setting by providing personal hygiene before bedtime. A warm bath or shower is very relaxing. Offer patients restricted to bed the opportunity to wash their face and hands. Toothbrushing and care of dentures also help to prepare the patient for sleep. Have patients void before going to bed so they are not kept awake by a full bladder. While a patient prepares for bed, help to position him or her off any potential pressure sites.

Removal of irritating stimuli also improves a patient's comfort for a restful sleep. Changing or removing moist dressings, repositioning drainage tubing, reapplying wrinkled compression hose, and changing tape on nasogastric tubes eliminate constant irritants to the patient's skin. When an IV site becomes irritated and painful, reinsertion of the IV line is usually recommended. Cleanse the perineal or anal area thoroughly for patients who are incontinent. Diaphoretic patients benefit from a cool bath and dry clothes or linens.

Restorative and Continuing Care. The quality of sleep in a long-term care or nursing home environment is often fragmented. Residents of a nursing home often have chronic disease, incontinence, and dementia and take multiple medications, all of which can disrupt sleep. Noise, light, and repositioning residents during linen changes are factors that cause patients to awaken. Besides care activities, residents in nursing homes themselves are sometimes very disruptive when they call out loudly to roommates or nursing staff.

In the long-term care environment many patients require rehabilitation or supportive care. The nature of their illnesses and treatment requirements disrupt sleep. For example, patients who are ventilator dependent likely get brief periods of sleep throughout the day rather than prolonged sleep because of ventilator alarm sounds and the need for occasional suctioning.

Maintaining Activity. In the restorative care setting try to limit the time residents spend in bed. In the nursing home serve meals in the resident dining area. Otherwise residents should be up in a chair for meals and for personal hygiene activities. It is also important to keep residents involved in social activities planned at the nursing home (e.g., card playing or arts and crafts). Regular exercise keeps people active and stimulated. It is also ideal to limit daytime napping to 30 minutes or less. Short naps taken in the midafternoon increase alertness and cognitive ability.

Residents with dementia often have disrupted sleep-wake cycles. They become easily fatigued and experience periods of insomnia (Meiner, 2015). In this situation activities and visits need to be shortened to allow the patient to maintain an adequate energy level. If a patient wakes up during the night, keeping the lights at a low level and using soothing techniques such as quiet music or a back rub promote returning to sleep.

Reducing Sleep Disruption. Use your knowledge about the many factors that disrupt sleep in restorative care settings to make the environment more conducive to sleep. Noise control is critical. Often staff within a nursing home speak louder because of hearing impairments of residents, even though raising one's voice does not improve hearing reception. Walking up close to a patient and talking in a normal but clear voice likely improves a patient's hearing and reduces the chance of waking a nearby roommate. Teach nursing assistive personnel (NAP) to be more sensitive to the sources of noise that disrupt patients' sleep.

■■■ EVALUATION

Patient Care. Individualize your evaluation of therapies designed to promote sleep and rest (Box 33.9). Patients in relatively good health often do not need as much sleep as patients whose physical condition is poor. If you have established realistic goals of care with your patient, the expected outcomes become guidelines for evaluating a patient's progress and response to interventions. Use evaluative measures shortly after trying a therapy. Use other evaluative measures after a patient awakens from sleep (e.g., asking a patient to describe the number of awakenings during the night). Together the patient and bed partner can usually provide accurate information. If the patient lives or sleeps alone, the evaluation may be unreliable. Families may be able to provide useful information when patients visit for brief weekend or holiday outings.

When a patient does not meet expected outcomes, revise the nursing measures based on the patient's needs or preferences. Document the patient's response to sleep therapies to maintain a continuum of care.

Patient Expectations. Review progress in the plan of care with your patient and determine if the patient's expectations were met. Does the patient believe that your interventions were helpful and useful? Did you incorporate the patient's typical sleep routine into the plan of care? For the hospitalized patient, did staff avoid unnecessary interruptions or excessive noise, giving the patient a chance to rest? The patient's perceptions are valuable sources of information regarding the overall success in improving the quality of the patient's sleep.

BOX 33.9   EVALUATION

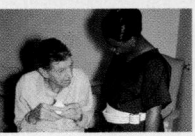

After 4 weeks at the skilled care facility, Anna advocated for Mr. Murphy and had him transferred to a new room. She has been monitoring his progress since he moved to his new room 2 weeks ago. Anna asks Mr. Murphy, "Tell me how our plan to improve your sleep has been working. Have the music and ear buds been helpful?" Mr. Murphy replies, "Well, it has helped to be down here at the end of the hall. It still is a bit noisy, especially if the nurses are working with people across the way. I've used the ear buds the last 2 weeks, and they've helped me relax and fall asleep in about 20 or 30 minutes." Anna questions Mr. Murphy further and learns that he is waking up 2 or 3 times during the night. However, during the last week he estimated getting about 6 hours of sleep, an improvement from a month ago. Mr. Murphy also reports that the staff has usually been good about reminding him to do his daily exercises with the wheelchair. He dislikes staying in his room and has exercised as much as possible.

Anna wants to know Mr. Murphy's level of satisfaction with her care. She asks, "Have I met your expectations so far? If not, tell me how I can better help you." Mr. Murphy replies, "You've been great. I know you can't make this place like home. There's so much to think about when you're here. I think about my wife a lot." Anna responds, "Tell me more. What do you mean, 'There's so much to think about'?" Anna recognizes that psychological and physical stressors alter sleep. She decides to reassess Mr. Murphy to determine if additional nursing interventions are appropriate.

DOCUMENTATION NOTE

"Reports some improvement in overall sleep quality. Able to fall asleep within 20 to 30 minutes using ear buds with music. Reports sleeping approximately 6 hours per night. Continues to experience awakenings, resulting from noise in outside hallway. Recommend closing room door at night to reduce noise further. Admits to thinking about his wife and other concerns. Will explore further with him."

▌ KEY POINTS

- The 24-hour sleep-wake cycle is a circadian rhythm that affects physiological function and behavior.
- During a typical night's sleep a person fluctuates between NREM stages 2, 3, and 4 before entering REM sleep. The amount of time in each stage varies.
- The number of hours of sleep needed by each person to feel rested varies.
- Long-term use of sleeping medications leads to difficulty in initiating and maintaining sleep.
- The hectic pace of a person's lifestyle, emotional and psychological stress, and drug and alcohol ingestion disrupt the sleep pattern.
- An environment with a darkened room, reduced noise, comfortable bed, appropriate temperature, and good ventilation promotes sleep.

- The most common type of sleep disorder is insomnia. Characteristics of insomnia include the inability to fall asleep, to remain asleep during the night, or to go back to sleep after waking up earlier than desired.
- Use your patient's self-report to determine if sleep is restful.
- When using environmental controls to promote sleep, consider the usual characteristics of the patient's home environment and normal lifestyle.
- Noise can disrupt sleep and enhance pain perception.
- The HCAHPS survey measures patients' perspectives on hospital care after discharge including quietness of the hospital environment.
- A bedtime routine of relaxing activities prepares a person physically and mentally for sleep.
- Important nursing interventions for promoting sleep in a hospital are establishing periods for uninterrupted sleep and decreasing noise.

▮ REFLECTIVE LEARNING

- Reflect on your own sleep-hygiene practices. What changes can you make to improve your sleep practices?
- Ask a patient about his or her sleep quality since being in the health care agency. How has your patient's sleep been affected?
- Working with two to three of your peers, develop a program on improving sleep for college-age students. Offer the program on your campus.

▮ REVIEW QUESTIONS

1. Which statements from a patient indicate an understanding of behaviors that often disrupt sleep? (Select all that apply.)
   1. "I will not watch television in bed."
   2. "I will not drink caffeine later in the day."
   3. "A short nap late in the evening will lead to a more restful night of sleep."
   4. "A glass of wine before bed will help me relax and sleep through the night."
   5. "I will try to develop a regular evening exercise program."

2. Mrs. Wilson is a 70-year-old patient who visits the medical clinic for a routine visit. Which nursing interventions would you recommend for this patient? (Select all that apply.)
   1. Limit fluids 2 to 4 hours before sleep
   2. Ensure that room is completely dark
   3. Ensure room temperature is comfortably cool
   4. Provide warm covers
   5. Encourage walking an hour before going to bed

3. Which statement made by the patient indicates an understanding of sleep-hygiene practices?
   1. "I drink a cup of warm milk in the evening about 30 minutes before bedtime."
   2. "If I exercise right before bedtime I will be tired and fall asleep faster."
   3. "I know that it is best for me to go to bed when I feel tired."
   4. "Long term use of hypnotics will cure my insomnia."

4. A nurse is completing a sleep history for a patient being assessed for obstructive sleep apnea (OSA). Which symptoms does the nurse expect the patient to report? (Select all that apply.)
   1. Nocturia
   2. Frightening dreamlike experiences
   3. Snoring
   4. Fatigue
   5. Increased sex drive

5. Which nursing interventions are appropriate to include in a plan of care to promote sleep for patients who are hospitalized? (Select all that apply.)
   1. Give patients a cup of coffee 1 hour before bedtime
   2. Plan vital signs to be taken before patients are asleep
   3. Turn television on 15 minutes before bedtime
   4. Have patients follow at-home bedtime schedule
   5. Close the door to patients' rooms at bedtime

evolve

Additional Review Questions, as well as rationales for all Review Questions, can be found on the Evolve website.

1. 1, 2, 5; 2. 1, 3, 4; 3. 1; 4. 1, 3, 4; 5. 2, 4, 5.

REFERENCES

American Academy of Sleep Medicine: *Healthy sleep habits*, 2016, http://www.sleepeducation.org/essentials-in-sleep/healthy-sleep-habits.

American Nurses Association (ANA): *Nursing: scope and standards of practice*, ed 3, Silver Springs, MD, 2015, ANA.

American Sleep Association (ASA): *Epworth Sleepiness Scale*, n.d., https://www.sleepassociation.org/epworth-sleep-scale/.

American Sleep Association (ASA): *What is insomnia?*, 2016, https://www.sleepassociation.org/patients-general-public/insomnia/insomnia.

American Society of PeriAnesthesia Nurses (ASPAN): *2015-2017 Perianesthesia Nursing Standards, Practice Recommendations and Interpretive Statements*, Cherry Hill, NJ, 2014, The Society.

Badin E, et al: Insomnia: the sleeping giant of pediatric public health, *Curr Psychiatry Rep* 18:47, 2016.

Barateau L, et al: Treatment options for narcolepsy, *CNS Drugs* 30:369, 2016.

Bartel KA, et al: Protective and risk factors for adolescent sleep: a meta-analytic review, *Sleep Med* 21:72, 2015.

Brockmann PE, et al: Impact of television on the quality of sleep in preschool children, *Sleep Med* 20:140, 2016.

Burchum JR, Rosenthal LD: *Lehne's pharmacology for nursing care*, ed 9, St Louis, 2016, Elsevier.

Caple C, March P: *Evidence-based care sheet: sleep and hospitalization*, 2016, Cinahl Information Systems.

Centers for Disease Control and Prevention (CDC): *Insufficient sleep is a public health problem*, 2015, http://www.cdc.gov/Features/dsSleep/index.html.

Centers for Medicare and Medicaid Services (CMS): *HCAHPS: patients' perspectives of care survey*, 2014, http://www.cms.gov/Medicare/Quality-Initiatives-Patient-Assessment-Instruments/HospitalQualityInits/HospitalHCAHPS.html.

Centre for Clinical Interventions (CCI): *Sleep hygiene*, n.d., http://www.cci.health.wa.gov.au/docs/Info-sleep%20hygiene.pdf.

Chung F, et al: STOP-Bang questionnaire: a practical approach to screen for obstructive sleep apnea, *Chest* 149(3):631, 2016.

Cullen D, et al: Infant co-bedding: practices and teaching strategies, *J Spec Pediatr Nurs* 21(2):54, 2016.

Dietrich SK, et al: The effectiveness of sleep education programs in improving sleep hygiene knowledge, sleep behavior practices and/or sleep quality of college students: a systematic review protocol, *JBI Database System Rev Implement Rep* 13(9):72, 2015.

Emet M, et al: A review of melatonin, its receptors and drugs, *Eurasian J Med* 48(2):135, 2016.

Flynn Makic MB, et al: Examining the evidence to guide practice: challenging practice habits, *Crit Care Nurse* 34(2):28, 2014.

Gao R, et al: Effects of comprehensive sleep management on sleep quality in university students in mainland China, *Sleep Biol Rhythms* 12:194, 2014.

Hirschkowitz M, et al: National Sleep Foundation sleep time duration recommendations: methodology and results summary, *Sleep Health* 1:40, 2015.

Hockenberry MJ, Wilson D: *Wong's nursing care of infants and children*, ed 10, St Louis, 2015, Mosby.

Huether SE, et al, editors: *Understanding pathophysiology*, ed 6, St Louis, 2017, Elsevier.

Keys EM, Rankin JA: Bed sharing, SIDS research, and the concept of confounding: a review for public health nurses, *Public Health Nurs* 32(6):731, 2015.

Kohansieh M, Makaryus AN: Sleep deficiency and deprivation leading to cardiovascular disease, *Int J Hypertens* 2015:615681, 2015.

Kryger MH, et al: *Principles and practice of sleep medicine*, ed 6, St Louis, 2017, Elsevier.

Litton E, et al: The efficacy of earplugs as a sleep hygiene strategy for reducing delirium in the ICU: a systematic review and meta-analysis, *Crit Care Med* 44(5):992, 2016.

Liu Y, et al: Prevalence of healthy sleep duration among adults: United States, 2014, *MMWR Morb Mortal Wkly Rep* 65(6):1, 2016.

Madhu C, et al: Nocturia: risk factors and associated comorbidities findings from the EpiLUTS study, *Int J Clin Pract* 69(12):1508, 2015.

Maness DL, Khan M: Nonpharmacologic management of chronic insomnia, *Am Fam Physician* 92(12):1058, 2015.

Matlock-Carr NL, Ward KS: Helping parents make informed decisions regarding bed-sharing, *Int J Childbirth Educ* 30(1):77, 2015.

Meiner SE: *Gerontologic nursing*, ed 5, St Louis, 2015, Elsevier.

Moon RY: *How to keep your sleeping baby safe, AAP policy explained*, 2017, https://www.healthychildren.org/English/ages-stages/baby/sleep/Pages/A-Parents-Guide-to-Safe-Sleep.aspx.

National Guideline Clearinghouse: *Management of chronic insomnia disorder in adults: a clinical practice guideline from the American College of Physicians*, 2016, https://www.guideline.gov/summaries/summary/50399/management-of-chronic-insomnia-disorder-in-adults-a-clinical-practice-guideline-from-the-american-college-of-physicians?q=insomnia.

National Sleep Foundation: *Lack of sleep is affecting Americans, finds the National Sleep Foundation*, 2014, https://sleepfoundation.org/media-center/press-release/lack-sleep-affecting-americans-finds-the-national-sleep-foundation.

National Sleep Foundation: *Aging and sleep*, 2016a, https://sleepfoundation.org/sleep-topics/aging-and-sleep.

National Sleep Foundation: *Depression and sleep*, 2016b, http://sleepfoundation.org/article/sleep-topics/depression-and-sleep.

National Sleep Foundation: *Restless legs syndrome (RLS) and sleep*, 2016c, http://www.sleepfoundation.org/article/sleep-related-problems/restless-legs-syndrome-rls-and-sleep. October 4, 2017.

National Sleep Foundation: *Teens and sleep*, 2016d, https://sleepfoundation.org/sleep-topics/teens-and-sleep.

Qaseem A, et al: Diagnosis of obstructive sleep apnea in adults: a clinical practice guideline from the American College of Physicians, *Ann Intern Med* 161(3):210, 2014.

Rotenberg BW, et al: Reconsidering first-line treatment for obstructive sleep apnea: a systematic review of the literature, *J Otolaryngol Head Neck Surg* 45:23, 2016.

Schub T: *Obstructive sleep apnea in adults*, 2016, Cinahl Information Systems.

Touhy T, Jett K: *Ebersole & Hess' gerontological nursing and healthy aging*, ed 5, St Louis, 2018, Elsevier.

Trauer JM, et al: Cognitive behavioral therapy for chronic insomnia, *Ann Intern Med* 163(3):191, 2015.

University of Maryland Medical Center: *Insomnia*, 2016, http://umm.edu/health/medical/altmed/condition/insomnia.

U.S. Department of Health and Human Services (USDHHS): *What does a safe sleep environment look like?*, n.d., https://www.nichd.nih.gov/sts/about/environment/Pages/look.aspx.

U.S. Food and Drug Administration (FDA): *Sleep problems*, 2016, https://www.fda.gov/forconsumers/byaudience/forwomen/ucm118563.htm.

Vincensi B, et al: Sleep in the hospitalized patient: nurse and patient perceptions, *Medsurg Nurs* 25(5):351, 2016.

Wheaton G, et al: Sleep duration and injury-related risk behaviors among high school students—United States, 2007-2013, *MMWR Morb Mortal Wkly Rep* 65(13):1, 2016.

Ye L, Smith A: Developing and testing a sleep education program for college nursing students, *J Nurs Educ* 54(9):532, 2015.

evolve MEDIA RESOURCES

http://evolve.elsevier.com/Potter/essentials

- Audio Glossary
- Case Study Continuation

- QSEN Activity and Review Questions Answers and Rationales
- Video Clip

OBJECTIVES

- Describe the physiology of pain.
- Identify components of the pain experience.
- Assess a patient experiencing pain.
- Develop appropriate nursing diagnoses for a patient experiencing pain.
- Describe guidelines for selecting and individualizing pain therapies.
- Describe nonpharmacological nursing interventions to manage pain.

- Discuss nursing implications for administering analgesics.
- Describe the sequence of interventions recommended in pain management
- Evaluate a patient's response to interventions that manage pain.

KEY TERMS

analgesics, p. 958
cutaneous stimulation, p. 956
endorphins, p. 941
epidural infusion, p. 961
guided imagery, p. 957

local anesthesia, p. 961
opioid, p. 958
patient-controlled analgesia (PCA), p. 959
prostaglandins, p. 940

relaxation, p. 957
transcutaneous electrical nerve stimulation (TENS), p. 956

You will encounter patients experiencing pain in all health care settings. Approximately 76 million people experience some degree or type of pain (The Joint Commission [TJC], 2017). Physiological, sociocultural, spiritual, psychological, and environmental factors influence the way patients interpret and experience pain. According to McCaffery's classic definition, "Pain is whatever the experiencing person says it is, existing whenever he says it does" (Pasero and McCaffery, 2011). Pain relief is not always achievable; however, nurses implement interventions to decrease pain, which can increase quality of life. Pain management involves more than administering analgesics. You need to understand how the pain experience affects a patient's ability to function and then use interventions that meet the unique needs of the patient (Pasero and McCaffery, 2011).

Pain is a leading public health problem in the United States. Many organizations have declared that pain management is a basic right of patients who are seriously ill. As a nurse, you are legally and ethically responsible for managing patients' pain. Effective pain management improves quality of life, promotes return to the previous level of activity, and decreases health care costs.

CASE STUDY *Mrs. Ellis*

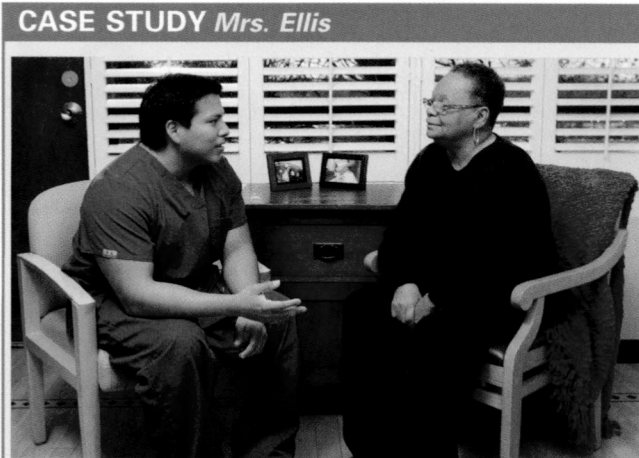

Mrs. Ellis is a 70-year-old woman with hypertension, diabetes, and rheumatoid arthritis. She is receiving care following a recent hospitalization to control her diabetes. Her current health priority is discomfort and disability associated with her rheumatoid arthritis. Arthritis has severely deformed her hands and feet. The pain in her feet is so severe that Mrs. Ellis can walk only short distances. The pain interferes with sleep and reduces her energy both physically and emotionally. Thus, she does not leave her home often. She has lived alone since her husband's death 6 years ago.

Jim is a nursing student assigned to make home visits with a home health nurse. Jim conducts assessments, performs procedures, and teaches health promotion under the direct supervision of the RN. This is Jim's first experience caring for a patient with severe chronic pain.

SCIENTIFIC KNOWLEDGE BASE

Nature of Pain

Pain is more than a single physiological sensation caused by a specific stimulus. It is subjective and highly individualized. The person experiencing pain is the only person who can confirm the existence of the pain and describe it. Pain is a physiological mechanism that protects an individual from a harmful stimulus. Pain warns of tissue damage and alerts the body to protect itself. Inability to express pain because of aphasia, airway intubation, or mental status changes does not mean that a patient is not experiencing pain. Carefully assess a patient's pain to identify the severity and effects of pain. Some patients such as patients with spinal cord injuries are unable to sense painful stimuli. You must take special precautions to protect these patients from additional injury (Pasero and McCaffery, 2011).

Physiology of Pain

There are four physiological processes of normal pain: transduction, transmission, perception, and modulation (Huether and McCance, 2017). Understanding each process helps you recognize factors that cause pain, symptoms that result, and the rationale for interventions for pain management.

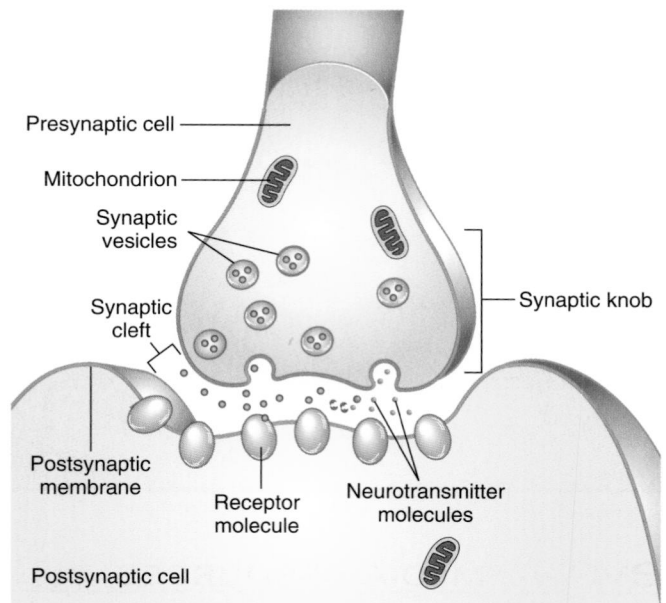

FIG 34.1 Chemical synapses involve transmitter chemicals (neurotransmitters) that signal postsynaptic cells. (From Patton KT, Thibodeau GA: *Anatomy & Physiology*, ed 7, St Louis, 2010, Mosby.)

Transduction. A thermal, mechanical, or chemical stimulus usually activates a pain event. Transduction converts energy produced by these noxious stimuli into electrical impulses. The process begins in the periphery when the pain-producing stimulus sends an impulse across a sensory peripheral pain nerve fiber, known as a nociceptor. Once transduction is complete, transmission of a pain impulse begins (Huether and McCance, 2017).

Transmission. Cellular damage from thermal, mechanical, or chemical injuries results in the release of excitatory neurotransmitters such as **prostaglandins,** histamine, bradykinin, and substance P (Fig. 34.1). These pain-sensitizing substances surround the pain fibers in the extracellular fluid, spreading the pain message and causing an inflammatory response. The pain stimulus enters the spinal cord via the dorsal horn and travels one of several routes until ending within the gray matter of the spinal cord. At the dorsal horn, substance P is released, causing a synaptic transmission from the afferent (sensory) nerve to spinothalamic tract nerves, which cross to the opposite side (Fig. 34.2) (Pasero and McCaffery, 2011).

Nerve impulses travel along afferent peripheral nerve fibers. Two types of peripheral nerve fibers conduct painful stimuli: the large, fast, myelinated A-delta fibers and the small, slow unmyelinated C fibers. The A fibers send sharp, localized, and distinct sensations that specify the source of the pain and detect its intensity. The C fibers relay slower impulses that are poorly localized, visceral, and persistent. For example, after stepping on a sharp object without shoes, a person initially feels a sharp localized pain, which is the

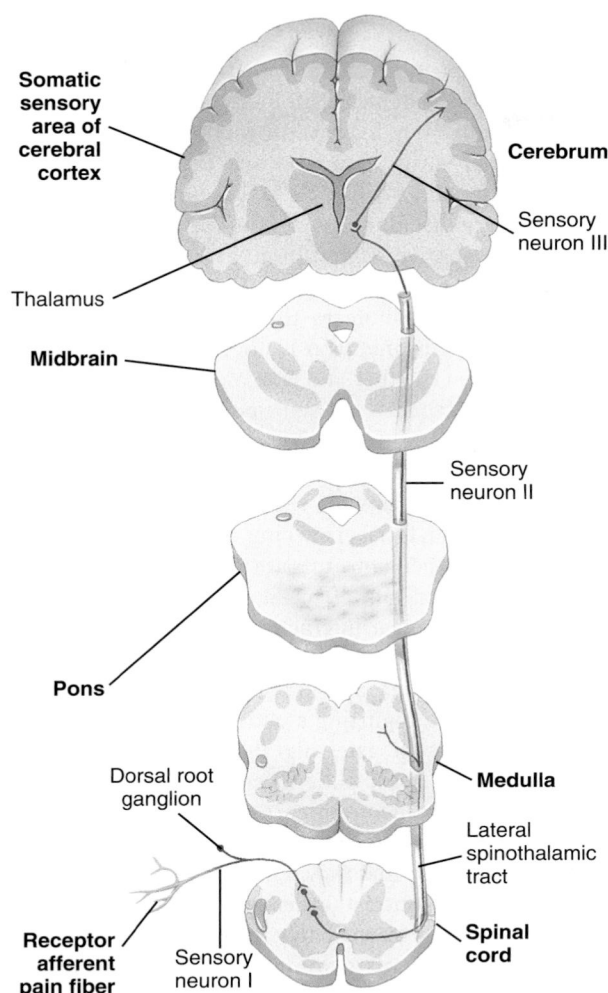

FIG 34.2 Spinothalamic pathway that conducts pain stimuli to the brain.

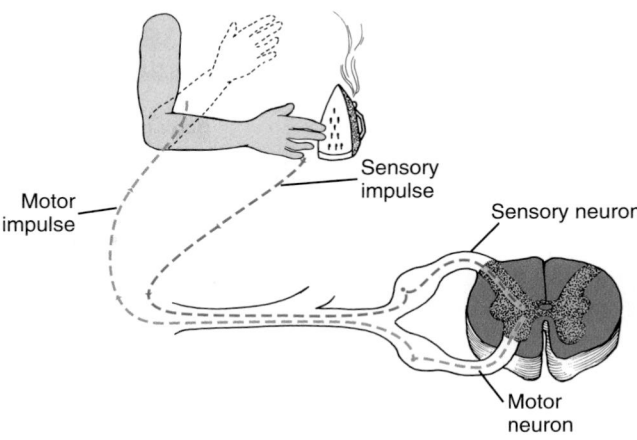

FIG 34.3 Protective pain reflex. Sensory impulse directly stimulates motor nerves, bypassing brain and causing withdrawal from pain stimulus.

result of A-fiber transmission, or first pain. Within a few minutes, the entire foot aches from C-fiber stimulation, or second pain.

Pain impulses travel up the spinal cord (see Fig. 34.2). When the impulse reaches the thalamus, the primary relay station of sensory impulses, it transmits information to higher centers in the brain where pain perception occurs.

Perception. As a pain impulse moves up the spinal cord toward the brain, the central nervous system extracts information such as location, duration, and quality of the pain impulse. Psychological and cognitive factors interact with neurophysiological factors. The thalamus is the first structure in the brain to process the impulse. It sends the impulse to many areas in the brain including the cerebral cortex, hypothalamus, and limbic system. Perception is that point in time when a patient becomes aware of the pain and attaches meaning to it. There is no one pain center in the brain that supports the complex nature of pain. Any factor that interrupts or influences normal pain perception, such as fatigue,

depression, or an analgesic, affects a person's awareness and response to pain.

Modulation. The fourth and final phase of the pain process is modulation. When a person perceives a harmful impulse, the brain releases inhibitory neurotransmitters such as endogenous opioids, serotonin, norepinephrine, and gamma-aminobutyric acid (GABA). The neurotransmitters hinder the transmission of pain to help produce an analgesic effect (Huether and McCance, 2017).

A protective reflex response also occurs with pain (Fig. 34.3). When a person is injured, a noxious stimulus from the skin travels along sensory neurons to the dorsal horn of the spinal cord where it synapses with spinal motor neurons. The impulse continues to travel along the spinal nerve to the skeletal muscle, creating a reflex arc and causing the person to withdraw from the source of the pain. For example, when you accidentally touch a hot iron, your hand reflexively withdraws from the hot surface. Pain processes require an intact peripheral nervous system and spinal cord.

Neurotransmitters. Neurotransmitters are substances that affect the sending of nerve stimuli (Box 34.1). They either excite or inhibit nerve transmission. Excitatory neurotransmitters such as substance P enhance transmission of the painful impulse. Inhibitory neurotransmitters such as endorphins decrease neuron activity through a synapse. Pain perception is influenced by balancing neurotransmitters and by the descending pain-control fibers originating from the cerebral cortex (Huether and McCance, 2017).

Gate Control Theory of Pain. The gate control theory suggests that gating mechanisms along the central nervous system can regulate and possibly block pain impulses (Mendell, 2014). The gating mechanism occurs within the spinal cord, thalamus, reticular formation, and limbic system. The brain determines whether the gate will be open or closed, either increasing or decreasing the intensity of the ascending pain impulse. The theory suggests that pain impulses pass through when the gate is open and not while it is closed.

BOX 34.1   NEUROPHYSIOLOGY OF PAIN: NEUROTRANSMITTERS

NEUROTRANSMITTERS (EXCITATORY)

Bradykinin
- Released from plasma that leaks from surrounding blood vessels at site of tissue injury
- Binds to receptors on peripheral nerves, increasing pain stimuli
- Binds to cells that cause chain reaction producing prostaglandins

Substance P
- Found in pain neurons of the dorsal horn (excitatory peptide)
- Needed to transmit pain impulses from periphery to higher brain centers
- Causes vasodilation and edema

Serotonin
- Released from brainstem and dorsal horn to inhibit pain transmission

Prostaglandins
- Generated through breakdown of phospholipids in cell membranes
- Increase sensitivity to pain

NEUROTRANSMITTERS (INHIBITORY)

Endorphins, Enkephalins, and Dynorphins
- Natural supply of morphine-like substances in the body
- Activated by stress and pain
- Located within brain, spinal cord, and gastrointestinal tract
- Cause analgesia when they attach to opiate receptors in the brain
- Present in high levels in people who have less pain than others with a similar injury

Closing the gate is the basis for nonpharmacological pain-relief interventions. The gate control theory suggests the importance of psychological variables (thoughts and feelings) and physiological sensations in the perception of pain. Using psychological, physiological, and pharmacological interventions to close the gate lowers pain intensity. For example, therapies such as exercise, heat, cold, massage, and transcutaneous electrical nerve stimulation (TENS) are thought to release endorphins, which close the gate and reduce perception of pain (Mendell, 2014).

Physiological Responses. When acute pain impulses travel up the spinal cord toward the brainstem and thalamus, the autonomic nervous system is stimulated as part of the stress response. Acute pain of low-to-moderate intensity and superficial pain cause the fight-or-flight response from the sympathetic branch of the autonomic nervous system and results in transient physiological responses (Table 34.1). If pain is unrelenting, severe, or deep, typically involving visceral organs, the parasympathetic nervous system is activated. Most patients adapt quickly, with physical signs such as vital signs returning to normal. As a result, your patient in pain does not always present with physical signs (Huether and McCance, 2017).

It is important to understand that patients with chronic pain do not have the same physiological responses as patients with acute pain. They may not demonstrate autonomic or sympathetic nervous system reactions. In addition, if you do not treat acute pain adequately, it can progress to chronic pain. It appears that unrelieved pain sensitizes and changes nerves (neuroplasticity), resulting in enhanced intensity, duration, and distribution of pain. These permanent neuroplastic changes contribute to the development of chronic pain syndromes. Chronic pain is not simply acute pain that lasts a long time (Huether and McCance, 2017).

Behavioral Responses. The response to pain is complex and variable, influenced by such factors as a person's culture, experiences with pain, meaning of pain, and ability to cope with stress. Be familiar with behavioral responses to pain. Clenching the teeth, facial grimacing, holding or guarding the painful part, and bent posture are common indications of acute pain. Chronic pain affects a patient's activity (eating, sleeping, hygiene, social interactions), thinking (confusion, forgetfulness, helplessness), or emotions (anger, depression, irritability, frustration) and quality of life (Huether and McCance, 2017). Recognizing a patient's unique response to pain is important in assessing the success of the pain-management plan. Some patients choose not to report pain if they believe that it inconveniences others or if it signals loss of self-control. Encourage your patients to accept pain-relieving measures so that they remain active and involved in daily activities. In contrast, other patients seek relief before pain occurs, having learned that prevention is easier than treatment. Help patients communicate their pain response effectively and do not question their report of pain (Pasero and McCaffery, 2011).

Types of Pain

The two types of pain that you most frequently observe in patients are acute (transient) and chronic (persistent). Millions of people experience pain every year. Pain results in increased health care costs and loss of income from being unable to work.

Acute/Transient Pain. Acute pain is protective, usually has an identifiable cause, is of short duration, and has limited tissue damage and emotional response. It is common after acute injury, disease, or surgery. Acute pain warns people of injury or disease; thus it is protective. It eventually resolves after the damaged tissue heals. Patients in acute pain are frightened, are anxious, and expect relief quickly. Acute pain is self-limiting; therefore the patient knows that an end is in sight. Because it usually has an identifiable cause and is usually of short duration, health care providers are willing to treat acute pain aggressively.

Acute pain often slows recovery because it interferes with a patient's ability to become active and involved in self-care. This decrease in self-care ability results in prolonged hospitalization and recovery from complications such as immobility,

TABLE 34.1 PHYSIOLOGICAL REACTIONS TO ACUTE PAIN

RESPONSE	CAUSE OR EFFECT
Sympathetic Stimulation[a]	
Dilation of bronchial tubes and increased respiratory rate	Provides increased oxygen intake
Increased heart rate	Provides increased oxygen transport
Peripheral vasoconstriction (pallor, elevation in blood pressure)	Elevates blood pressure with shift of blood supply from periphery and viscera to skeletal muscles and brain
Increased blood glucose level	Provides additional energy
Diaphoresis	Controls body temperature during stress
Increased muscle tension	Prepares muscles for action
Dilation of pupils	Affords better vision
Decreased gastrointestinal motility	Frees energy for more immediate activity
Parasympathetic Stimulation[b]	
Pallor	Causes blood supply to shift away from periphery
Muscle tension	Results from fatigue
Decreased heart rate and blood pressure	Results from vagal stimulation
Rapid, irregular breathing	Causes body defenses to fail under prolonged stress of pain
Nausea and vomiting	Causes return of gastrointestinal function
Weakness or exhaustion	Results from expenditure of physical energy

[a]Pain of low to moderate intensity and superficial pain.
[b]Severe or deep pain.

sleep deprivation, delayed wound healing, and pulmonary issues. Patients often focus all their energy on pain relief when acute pain persists. Efforts aimed at teaching and motivating a patient toward self-care are often hampered until pain is managed successfully. If not adequately controlled, acute pain can progress to chronic pain. When you relieve acute pain, a patient can direct full attention toward recovery.

Chronic/Persistent Pain. In contrast to acute pain, chronic pain is not protective. Chronic pain is prolonged, varies in intensity, and usually lasts longer than 3 to 6 months and beyond the expected or predicted healing time (Huether and McCance, 2017). It does not always have an identifiable cause and can greatly affect a person. Examples of chronic pain include arthritis, low back pain, myofascial pain, headache, and peripheral neuropathy. Chronic pain such as low back pain often results from nonprogressive or healed tissue injury. The pain is ongoing and often does not respond to treatment. Chronic pain is a major cause of psychological and physical disability, leading to problems such as job loss, sexual dysfunction, and social isolation. A person with chronic pain often does not show obvious symptoms and does not adapt to the pain. Associated symptoms include fatigue, insomnia, anorexia, weight loss, apathy, hopelessness, and anger. Sometimes patients with chronic pain consult with many health care providers to seek adequate pain relief. When this occurs, patients may inaccurately be judged as drug seekers. Nurses need to discourage patients from having multiple health care providers for treating pain and refer them to specialists. Pain centers use nonpharmacological and pharmacological strategies for a holistic approach to pain management (Pasero and McCaffery, 2011).

Chronic Episodic Pain. Pain that occurs sporadically over an extended period of time is episodic pain. Pain episodes last for hours, days, or weeks. Examples are migraine headaches and pain related to sickle cell crisis.

Cancer Pain. Not all patients with cancer have pain. For patients who do experience pain, 90% are able to have their pain managed with simple interventions (Burchum and Rosenthal, 2016). Some patients with cancer have acute and chronic pain. The pain is nociceptive or neuropathic. Nociceptive pain is more common and is the result of tissue injury. Neuropathic pain is related to peripheral nerve injury. Cancer pain is usually caused by tumor progression and related pathological processes, invasive procedures, treatment toxicities, infection, and physical limitations. A patient senses pain at the actual tumor site or distant to the site (called referred pain). Always assess reports of new pain by a patient with existing pain. Although the treatment of cancer pain has improved, undertreatment continues. Inadequate education of health care providers and fear of addiction lead to undertreatment of cancer pain (Burchum and Rosenthal, 2016).

Idiopathic Pain. Idiopathic pain is chronic pain in the absence of an identifiable physical or psychological cause or pain perceived as excessive for the extent of an organic pathological condition. An example of idiopathic pain is complex regional pain syndrome (CRPS). Research is needed to better identify the cause of idiopathic pain, thus leading to more effective treatment (Pasero and McCaffery, 2011).

NURSING KNOWLEDGE BASE

Knowledge, Attitudes, and Beliefs

Health care providers' knowledge affects pain management practices. Preconceptions about patients in pain often exist. Some health care providers do not believe a patient is experiencing pain unless the patient shows objective signs of pain. These assumptions about patients in pain influence your nursing assessment and seriously limit your ability to offer pain relief. Too often nurses allow misconceptions about pain to affect their willingness to provide pain relief (Box 34.2). Many nurses avoid acknowledging patients' pain because of fear of contributing to medication addiction. These fears and beliefs lead to mistrust, increased patient recovery time, complications, mortality, psychological problems, and increased cost (Pasero and McCaffery, 2011).

The failure of health care providers to assess pain accurately and consistently results in poor pain management and increased patient suffering. The Joint Commission has a pain standard that advises health care workers to assess and manage pain in all patients routinely (TJC, 2017). Many health care facilities implement this standard by recommending that pain be assessed as the "fifth vital sign."

Factors Influencing Pain

To accurately assess and then treat a patient's pain, be aware of the various factors that influence the pain experience.

Physiological Factors

Age. Developmental differences influence how patients of all ages react to pain. Infants demonstrate pain through crying, changes in vital signs, facial expression, and movement of extremities. Children have trouble understanding

pain and any treatments or procedures that cause pain. Children without full vocabularies have difficulty verbally describing and expressing pain to parents or caregivers. Toddlers and preschoolers are unable to recall explanations about pain, or they associate it with experiences that occur in various situations. A child's personality affects coping with pain.

Pain management for children is challenging and frequently results in undertreatment (Krauss et al., 2016). Children often describe treatments and procedures as the most difficult part of being sick or in a hospital. Analgesic doses are often ineffective because they are too small or given too infrequently. It is necessary for you to understand a child's response to pain. Self-reporting pain is the most accurate assessment, but if a child is too young or unable to speak, observe behavioral changes such as crying, whining, grimacing, muscle tension, unusual inactivity, and inconsolability as signs of pain (Burchum and Rosenthal, 2016). If a behavior such as crying changes after a child receives an analgesic, pain probably caused the behavior.

Pain in adolescents is usually related to an acute condition. Consider an adolescent's cognitive development, language skills, and growth and development needs when assessing pain and providing patient education.

Adults experience pain from acute and chronic conditions. Some health care providers are less accepting of reports of severe pain from younger adults than older adults. There may be an expectation of higher tolerance of pain in adults. Concern about drug-seeking behaviors and prescription drug abuse is also common among health care providers (Pasero and McCaffery, 2011).

Pain is not a natural part of aging. Likewise, pain perception does not decrease with age. However, older adults have a greater likelihood of developing pathological conditions, which are accompanied by pain. The older adult in pain, his or her family, and health care providers frequently take these conditions for granted or underestimate the pain. Serious impairment in functional status often accompanies pain in older adults. It reduces mobility, activities of daily living (ADLs), social activities, and activity tolerance in some older adults (Pasero and McCaffery, 2011).

Fatigue. Fatigue heightens pain perception. If it occurs along with sleeplessness, the perception of pain is even greater. Restful sleep often reduces pain perception.

Neurological Function. A patient's neurological function influences his or her pain experience. Any factor that interrupts or influences normal pain reception or perception (e.g., spinal cord injury, peripheral neuropathy) affects a patient's awareness of and response to pain.

Gender. Research on pain in men and women demonstrates differences in occurrence and response to pain related to gender. Chronic pain conditions occur more often in women than men. This is because some chronic pain conditions such as endometriosis occur only in women, and some such as chronic fatigue syndrome and fibromyalgia occur predominately in women. Reports of headache and joint pain are more common in women than men (Institute of Medicine [IOM], 2011).

BOX 34.2 COMMON BIASES AND MISCONCEPTIONS ABOUT PAIN

- Patients who are knowledgeable about opioids and make regular efforts to obtain them are drug seeking (addicted).
- There is no reason for patients to hurt when you cannot find a physical cause for pain.
- Administering analgesics regularly leads to patients' tolerance and physical drug dependence.
- The amount of tissue damage in an injury accurately indicates pain intensity.
- Health care providers are the best judge of the existence and severity of pain.
- Pain threshold and tolerance are the same for everyone.
- Pain is a natural outcome of growing old.
- Pain perception, or sensitivity, decreases with age.
- You use physical or behavioral signs of pain to verify the existence and severity of pain.
- Patients who fall asleep do not have pain.

Social Factors

Attention. The degree to which a patient focuses attention on pain influences pain perception. Increased attention frequently increases a person's pain, whereas distraction often decreases pain. By focusing a patient's attention and concentration on other stimuli such as having a patient listen to music or breathe rhythmically, you help turn his or her focus away from the pain. Usually increased tolerance for pain lasts only during the time of distraction.

Previous Experience. People learn from painful experiences. Previous experience includes pain that a patient has experienced personally and pain that a patient has heard about from someone else. Prior experience does not mean that a person accepts pain more easily in the future. Frequent episodes of pain without relief or bouts of severe pain produce anxiety or fear. In contrast, if a person repeatedly experiences the same type of pain that was successfully relieved in the past, it is easier for him or her to interpret the sensation. As a result, the person is better prepared to take steps to relieve the pain. A patient who has had no experience with a particular type of pain sometimes has an impaired ability to cope with it. You need to prepare your patient with a clear explanation of the type of pain to expect and methods to reduce it.

Family and Social Support. Patients often depend on the support and assistance of family members or friends when coping with pain. Family caregivers sometimes have misconceptions about pain and pain management. Some caregivers think patients should wait as long as possible before receiving pain medication and fear the possibility of addiction. It is your responsibility to educate the patient and family caregivers about the importance of early assessment and treatment of pain. The presence of a loved one usually minimizes anxiety and fear when a patient is experiencing pain. Absence of social support often makes the pain experience more stressful. The presence of parents is especially important for children in pain.

Spiritual Factors. Spirituality is an active searching for meaning to situations in which one finds oneself. Spiritual questions include, "Why has this happened to me?" and "Why am I suffering?" Often spiritual concerns include the loss of independence and becoming a burden to one's family. Be sensitive to a patient's spiritual needs and consider referral to a pastoral care professional (see Chapter 22).

Cultural Factors. Culture influences how people perceive the causes and meaning of pain as well as their reactions to and expressions of pain. Understanding cultural background and personal characteristics helps you more accurately assess pain and its meaning for patients (Box 34.3). People from some cultures appear to have a higher pain tolerance and avoid vocalizing to express their pain, whereas people from other cultures are more expressive with moaning and crying. The words used to describe pain may vary in different cultures. When patients do not speak the same language as you, you may find that their language does not have a word equivalent to "pain."

BOX 34.3 PATIENT-CENTERED CARE

Pain has both personal and cultural meanings. This influences the verbal expression of pain, individual reaction to pain, and pain treatment preferences. Disparities in pain perception, assessment, and treatment occur in all settings (Pasero and McCaffery, 2011).

IMPLICATIONS FOR PRACTICE

- Undertreatment of pain is often related to cultural differences.
- Ask a patient which word he or she prefers to use to describe pain. Many patients use *hurt* or *ache* to describe mild or moderate pain, reserving the word *pain* for severe discomfort.
- Use language-specific pain-intensity tools; these tools are available in many languages.
- Cultural responses to pain are often divided into two categories: stoic and emotive. One is not better than the other. Health care providers need to appreciate cultural variations of verbal and nonverbal responses to pain to accurately assess it.
- Recognize that communicating pain is not always acceptable within a culture.
- The meaning of pain differs among people of different cultures. Some people view pain as a punishment for the past, a part of life, or something to endure to enter heaven or progress to the next life.
- Biological variations of drug metabolism, dosing requirements, therapeutic response, and adverse effects are a function of race and ethnicity. It is important to assess the response to analgesics and not assume that an inadequate response is a nonadherence issue.
- Health care providers' beliefs about cultural groups and attitudes toward pain influence pain management. Self-awareness of potential cultural bias is essential to provide adequate pain management.

Psychological Factors

Meaning of Pain. The meaning that a patient attributes to pain affects the pain experience. Patients perceive pain differently if it suggests a threat, loss, punishment, or challenge. The degree and quality of pain perceived by a patient are related to its meaning.

Anxiety. High anxiety levels often increase pain perception, and pain usually causes anxiety. Autonomic arousal patterns are similar in pain and anxiety. Patients who worry about symptoms that are minor or nonexistent have health anxiety. The presence of health anxiety in patients who have pain negatively influences their response to pain and its associated treatments. Lowering a patient's health anxiety helps lower the patient's pain perception.

Depression. Patients with chronic pain are at a high risk of experiencing depression because they often experience many losses such as their ability to enjoy life, be in control, work, socialize, and be independent. Suicidal thoughts are relatively common; therefore you need to routinely assess for suicidal tendencies and reports of sleep disruption and deteriorating ability to function. As a nurse, be aware of the possibility of depression in patients with persistent pain and suggest a referral if symptoms of major depression emerge (Cheatle, 2014).

Coping Style. Pain sometimes causes feelings of loneliness. Frequently patients in pain feel a loss of control over their environment or the outcome of events, especially when their pain is difficult to manage. A patient's coping style influences the ability to cope with pain. Patients with internal loci of control perceive themselves as having personal control over their environments and the outcome of events. They ask questions, desire information, and like choices of treatment. In contrast, patients with external loci of control perceive other factors in their environments (e.g., nurses) as being responsible for the outcome of events. These patients tend to be less demanding, follow directions, and are more passive in managing their pain. They want specific instructions. Frequently patients with internal loci of control report less severe pain than patients with external loci.

CRITICAL THINKING

Synthesis

Patient care requires you to apply what you know about a patient, your knowledge base, experience, and critical thinking attitudes and standards. Your synthesis of this information allows you to make sound decisions as you apply the nursing process. Critical thinking synthesis involves combining all available information to obtain a clear picture of the approach needed to provide patient-centered care (Box 34.4).

Knowledge. It is important that you apply knowledge about the physiology of pain, along with the physiology of any underlying disease processes, to understand a patient's pain response, type of pain, and interventions needed for pain management. Knowledge and application of communication skills enhance the thoroughness of pain assessment. Once you have a clear picture of the physiological nature of a patient's condition, synthesis of knowledge regarding his or her psychological and sociocultural perspective becomes critical for an individualized approach to care. In addition, an understanding of pharmacological and nonpharmacological therapies helps you to work with a patient and health care providers in selecting pain therapies.

Experience. Caring for patients who have pain is an important part of a nurse's clinical experience. Because pain is so common, you will find that patients express pain in many ways. The degree of pain affects patients' behaviors and the actions they take to find relief. Such experience either positively or negatively affects your willingness to begin pain interventions. Furthermore, your own experience with pain emphasizes the importance of having someone who is supportive and understanding. Reflecting on the experiences of caring for patients in pain helps you search for better approaches for each new patient you meet.

BOX 34.4 SYNTHESIS IN PRACTICE

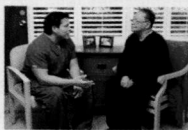

Jim is preparing for tomorrow's home visit with Mrs. Ellis. He reviews what he has learned about pain physiology and the pathophysiology of rheumatoid arthritis. This allows him to anticipate the need to carefully assess to what extent pain limits Mrs. Ellis' ability to walk and perform activities of daily living.

Jim plans to assess the location, duration, and aggravating and relieving factors influencing Mrs. Ellis' pain and any behavioral symptoms he observes. He plans to determine which pain scale Mrs. Ellis prefers to use to help him assess the severity of her pain. Because Mrs. Ellis is 70, Jim reviews gerontological principles and knows that he needs to take time to establish a trusting relationship to encourage a complete description of the pain experience. Jim recalls previous experiences with patients in chronic pain and interventions used to relieve pain. He remembers his own experiences with pain after sustaining a broken arm during a soccer game. These experiences make him sensitive to the personal and dynamic nature of each individual's pain experience.

Jim considers guidelines for the management of chronic pain. He wants to carefully clarify with Mrs. Ellis the extent to which the chronic arthritic pain and the acute exacerbations have affected her life. Jim needs to learn as much as he can about Mrs. Ellis' lifestyle and support systems to help her with pain relief and health promotion activities. Because Mrs. Ellis lives alone, Jim wants to assess if family or friends who live nearby can offer assistance.

Attitudes. Critical thinking attitudes ensure that you make decisions that are fair and responsible. When a patient is in pain, you need perseverance to find an approach that offers the patient some degree of relief. Quick solutions without follow-up aggravate a patient's discomfort. Learn as much as possible about a patient's pain, try various interventions, and continue different creative approaches until you discover an effective one. Accept a patient's report of pain and its severity, even if you question the severity of the pain reported (Pasero and McCaffery, 2011). When you are unable to help your patient achieve acceptable pain relief, you show humility when you ask for help from a peer or request consultation with a pain management specialist.

Standards. Professional standards, guidelines, and position statements are used to provide optimal evidence-based care for your patient having pain. Several professional organizations publish guidelines and standards of care for pain management. For example, the Oncology Nursing Society (ONS, 2017), the National Comprehensive Cancer Network (NCCN, 2017), and the National Cancer Institute (NCI, 2017) have published standards related to pain management for patients with cancer. The American Pain Society, the American Society of Regional Anesthesia and Pain Medicine, and the American Society of Anesthesiologists (Chou et al., 2016) have published joint guidelines for the management of postoperative pain.

The Centers for Disease Control and Prevention (CDC) published guidelines for health care providers who prescribe opioids for chronic pain (Dowell et al., 2016). Although you will not be the person prescribing medications for your patients, understanding these guidelines will help you be a patient advocate.

The Joint Commission (2017a) offers three standards for health care organizations to follow in pain management. The hospital:

- Educates all licensed independent practitioners on assessing and managing pain.
- Respects the patient's right to pain management.
- Assesses and manages the patient's pain.

NURSING PROCESS

◼◼◼◼ ASSESSMENT

A comprehensive assessment of pain gathers information about the cause of a person's pain and determines its effect on the person's ability to function. Accurate and factual pain assessment is necessary for determining a patient's responses, arriving at proper nursing diagnoses, and selecting appropriate therapies (Table 34.2). Pain assessment is one of the most frequent and difficult activities you perform. It is important to carefully interpret pain cues, and remember that psychological and physical components of pain influence a patient's reaction to it.

When assessing pain, be sensitive to a patient's level of discomfort and determine which level will allow your patient to function. For example, ask a patient in pain, "Which level of pain on a scale of 0 to 10 (with 0 being no pain and 10 being the worst pain you can imagine) allows you to walk down the hall?" If the patient answers that walking is possible when pain is at a level of 2, you then focus efforts on decreasing pain to that level. If pain is acutely severe, it is unlikely that the patient will provide detailed information. During an episode of acute pain, you primarily assess its location, severity, and quality. Collect a more detailed assessment when the patient is more comfortable, using the PQRSTU characteristics of pain (Table 34.3). A more comprehensive pain assessment takes time; you do this when the patient becomes more alert and attentive.

Pain always changes; it does not stay the same. Thus monitor pain on a regular basis along with vital signs. Many institutions now treat pain as the fifth vital sign. Pain

TABLE 34.2	**FOCUSED PATIENT ASSESSMENT**	
FACTORS TO ASSESS	**QUESTIONS**	**PHYSICAL ASSESSMENT**
Location of pain	Where is your pain located? Use your finger and point to where the pain is.	Depending on area of pain, use inspection to determine if body part is swollen, discolored, or warm to touch. Have patient use hand to locate area where pain originates and then spreads. Use light palpation over area identified by patient.
Aggravating factors	Describe your pain when you move. Do you do other things that make your pain worse? Tell me what makes the pain better.	When positioning body part aggravates pain, determine if range of motion is altered. Observe patient's facial expression and movement when patient attempts activity that typically aggravates pain.

TABLE 34.3	**IMPLICATIONS OF PAIN ASSESSMENT FOR NURSING INTERVENTIONS**
ASSESSMENT CRITERIA (PQRSTU)	**NURSING INTERVENTIONS**
Palliative or **P**rovocative factors—What makes your pain worse or better?	Avoid activities that cause or aggravate pain. Teach patient or family to avoid these activities.
Quality—How do you describe your pain?	Suggest changing pharmacological interventions if the quality of pain (neuropathic versus nociceptive) changes.
Relief measures—What do you do at home to gain pain relief?	Use measures that patient uses to relieve pain if they are safe and appropriate.
Region (location)—Show me where you hurt.	Position patient off affected area. Apply local treatments (e.g., elastic bandage, cold, heat, splinting) directly over painful site.
Severity—On a scale of 0 to 10, with 0 being no pain and 10 being the worst, how bad is your pain now?	Change or revise interventions, depending on success of one intervention in reducing severity.
Timing (onset, duration, and pattern)—Is your pain constant, intermittent, or both?	Administer analgesics so that peak action occurs when pain is most acute (e.g., during dressing change or exercise therapy).
U (effect of pain on patient)—What are you unable to do because of your pain?	Schedule activities that are important to patient during time of day when he or she feels least pain.

BOX 34.5   ROUTINE CLINICAL APPROACH TO PAIN ASSESSMENT AND MANAGEMENT (ABCDE)

A   **Ask** about pain regularly.

B   **Believe** patients and family caregivers in their report of pain and what relieves it.

C   **Choose** pain control options appropriate for patient, family, and setting.

D   **Deliver** interventions in timely, logical, and coordinated fashion.

E   **Empower** patients and their families.

From Maryniak K: Pain assessment and management, *RN.com,* 2013, https://lms.rn.com/courses/1773/presentation_html5.html.

assessment is *not* simply a number. Although pain assessment is a nursing function, nursing assistive personnel (NAP) also screen for pain and are responsible for informing a nurse immediately when a patient is having pain. This allows the nurse to confirm the assessment and provide appropriate therapy.

For patients with chronic pain, focus your assessment on the emotional impact and meaning of the experience and on its history and context. In addition, include level of function in your assessment because it is sometimes impossible to achieve complete pain relief. Teach family caregivers of patients with cancer how to assess pain so that they promote continuity of effective pain management (Box 34.5). In the home setting, involving family caregivers in pain assessment offers patients and families control over their experience. Be aware of possible errors in pain assessment. Bias (overestimating or underestimating level of pain), vague or unclear assessment questions, and use of unreliable or invalid pain assessment tools do not provide accurate data. Family caregivers' estimates of a patient's pain are not always accurate and should be used only when the patient is unable to verbalize or indicate pain intensity.

Older Adult Considerations. The ability of older adults to interpret pain is complicated. Older adults tend to use words such as *hurting* or *aching* instead of the word *pain* to describe their pain. In addition, older adults sometimes have more than one painful site. They often hesitate to discuss their pain because of concerns about bothering their health care providers. Frequently older adults believe they cannot change their pain and they simply must endure it. These barriers contribute to inadequate pain assessment and management (Lewis et al., 2014). Patients with a cognitive impairment or who are nonverbal (e.g., patients with aphasia or mental status changes) have trouble communicating pain and providing a detailed description. Thus you need to observe physical and behavioral cues when assessing pain (Huether and McCance, 2017).

Multiple diseases and vague symptoms affecting similar parts of the body further complicate the ability of older adults to interpret pain. When older patients have more than one source of pain, be sure to gather detailed assessments. Different diseases cause similar symptoms. For example, a patient who has a below-knee amputation continues to perceive pain from the foot that has been amputated (phantom pain) and has suture-line pain from the surgery. A patient who has a stroke sometimes has pain in the paralyzed arm and in areas of the body unaffected by the stroke.

Patient's Expression of Pain. A patient's self-report of pain is the most reliable indicator of the existence and intensity of pain (Burchum and Rosenthal, 2016). However, patients often fail to report or discuss pain. To complicate assessment, nurses frequently believe that patients will report pain if they have it, but patients often think that the health care providers know about their pain because that is their job. Do not assume that patients are pain free if they do not mention their pain intensity. Regularly *ask* patients about pain. Remember that pain varies from patient to patient, and pay attention to the nonverbal ways that patients communicate discomfort (Pasero and McCaffery, 2011). If patients sense that you doubt their pain exists, they share little information with you. Establish a caring relationship that allows for open communication. Refrain from using the phrase *complaining of pain* when discussing a patient's pain. It is better to use words such as *stating, telling,* or *reporting,* which is what the patient is doing.

Patients Unable to Self-Report Pain. Patients unable to communicate effectively often require special attention during assessment. Some examples are the following:

- Infants and children
- Patients who are critically ill, unconscious, or on life-support equipment
- Patients with dementia
- Patients who are aphasic
- Patients with an intellectual disability
- Patients at the end of life

These patients all require different assessment approaches. However, be alert for subtle behaviors that indicate pain (Box 34.6). Note a patient's vocal response (e.g., moaning, crying, gasping), facial movements (e.g., grimacing, clenched teeth, tightly closed eyes), and body movements (e.g., restlessness, pacing) or inactivity. Also assess social interaction. Does the patient avoid conversation or social contacts? Does the patient have a short attention span? Infants, children, and patients with cognitive impairments require simple assessment approaches involving close observation for changes in behavior. Monitor critically ill patients receiving medications that paralyze their muscles because these medications prevent them from being able to communicate their pain verbally or behaviorally. Often proxy pain ratings (e.g., the rating of pain by family caregivers) are useful. Do not assume that a patient is pain free if he or she is unable to report pain to you.

BOX 34.6   EVIDENCE-BASED PRACTICE

PICO Question: Does the use of individually tailored pain management plans help nurses better assess and manage pain in pediatric patients who cannot self-report their pain compared with using standard pain management interventions?

SUMMARY OF EVIDENCE

Recommendations related to pain assessment and management in pediatric patients who cannot self-report are found in current research and literature. Guidelines for the control of pain in children recommend validated tools for pain assessment as well as multimodal and multidisciplinary interventions (Ruest & Anderson, 2016). Many procedures done in the emergency department are painful and anxiety-producing for children, their parents, and their caregivers. Recommended tools for assessing pain in patients who are unable to use pain scales include vital signs, behaviors, and reporting by parents

(Krauss et al., 2016). Procedure-related pain can be decreased with simple age-specific nonpharmacological interventions. For example, oral sucrose and breast milk during procedures involving needles has been found to reduce crying in infants but not in older children (Ali et al., 2016; Krauss et al., 2016).

APPLICATION TO NURSING PRACTICE

- Develop an individualized patient-centric approach to managing pain in patients who cannot self-report.
- Use nonpharmacological interventions and nonopioid pain medications first to treat acute pain.
- Coordinate care with other health professionals (e.g., play therapists, child life specialists) and parents to encourage children to cooperate or to distract them from the procedure.
- Evaluate effectiveness and risk vs. benefit of nonpharmacological and pharmacological pain interventions.

After observing for behavioral clues, consider physiological parameters. Changes in heart rate, blood pressure, and respiratory rate and the presence of sweating may be associated with the presence of pain. However, physiological changes are the least reliable method for pain assessment because other factors such as dehydration or fever can affect them (Burchum and Rosenthal, 2016).

Characteristics of Pain. Only the patient can describe pain characteristics. Each characteristic presents implications for how you help to manage a patient's pain. The PQRSTU model is an effective tool for assessing pain in adults and determining interventions to relieve the pain (see Table 34.3).

Timing (Onset, Duration, and Pattern). Ask questions to determine the start, duration, and time sequence of pain. When did it begin? How long has it lasted? Does it occur at the same time each day? How often does it recur? It is sometimes easier to diagnose the nature of pain by identifying time factors. The onset of sudden and severe pain is easier to assess than gradual, mild discomfort. Knowing the time cycle of a patient's pain helps you intervene before the pain occurs or worsens.

Precipitating Factors. Determine the specific events or conditions that precipitate or aggravate pain. Ask a patient to describe activities that cause pain such as sitting, bending over, drinking coffee or alcohol, urination, swallowing, or stress. Ask the patient to demonstrate actions that cause painful responses such as coughing or turning in a certain manner. After identifying specific factors, it is easier to plan interventions to avoid worsening the pain.

Quality. There is no common pain vocabulary in general use. Patients describe pain in their own way. Patients often use *hurt* and *ache* to describe their pain, reserving the word *pain* for severe discomfort. Knowing the quality of pain helps to select appropriate therapies to treat it. When assessing the quality of pain, do not provide descriptive words for a patient. Assessment is more accurate if a patient describes the

sensation in his or her own words in response to open-ended questions. For example, say, "Tell me what your pain feels like." The only time you offer to list descriptive terms is when the patient is unable to describe pain.

There is some consistency in the way patients describe certain types of pain. People often describe the pain of a myocardial infarction (heart attack) as crushing or viselike. Some people describe the pain of a surgical incision as sharp and stabbing. Neuropathic pain is burning or electric-like. When a patient's description fits the pattern forming in your assessment, you are able to make a clearer analysis of the nature and type of pain. This leads to more appropriate pain management, as you treat different types of pain differently.

Relief Measures. Learn if a patient has an effective way of relieving pain such as changing position, pacing, rocking, eating, praying, or applying heat or cold to a painful site. A patient's methods are often ones that you can use for treatment. Determine if patients use relief measures safely in their home. Patients gain trust when they know you are willing to try their relief measures. They also gain a sense of control over the pain instead of the pain controlling them. Identify all health care providers. Patients with chronic pain are likely to try alternative health care methods.

Region/Location. To assess pain location, ask a patient to point to all areas of discomfort. To localize the pain more specifically, have the patient trace the area from the most severe point outward. This is difficult to do if pain is diffuse, involves several sites, or involves large parts of the body. Use a drawing showing the location of pain as the baseline if the pain changes. Use anatomical landmarks and descriptive terminology to record the pain location (e.g., "Pain is in the right upper quadrant of the abdomen"). Pain classified by location is also superficial or cutaneous, deep or visceral, localized or diffuse, referred or radiating.

Severity. One of the most subjective and therefore most useful characteristics for reporting pain is its severity or intensity. Nurses use a variety of pain scales to help patients communicate pain intensity. Many are available in foreign languages. Examples of pain intensity scales include the verbal descriptor scale (VDS), the numerical rating scale (NRS), and the visual analog scale (VAS) (Fig. 34.4). Use a scale to measure the current severity of a patient's pain. In addition, ask patients to rate their average pain and the worst pain they have had over the past 24 hours. This helps to determine an average pain intensity, allowing you to see trends.

An NRS requires patients to rate pain on a line scale of 0 to 10, with 0 representing no pain and 10 representing the worst pain the patient can imagine. These scales work best when assessing pain intensity before and after a therapy (e.g., ambulation or an analgesic). A VDS consists of a line with three- to six-word descriptors equally spaced along the line. Show the patient the scale and ask him or her to choose the descriptor that best represents the severity of pain. A VAS consists of a straight line without labeled subdivisions. The straight line shows a continuum of intensity and has labeled end points (no pain to pain as bad as it could possibly be). The patient indicates pain by marking the appropriate point on the line (Pasero and McCaffery, 2011).

An effective pain scale is easy to use, understandable, and not time consuming. If a patient can read and understand a scale easily, the description of pain is more accurate. If patients use a hearing aid or glasses, be sure that they are using them when answering pain-assessment questions or marking the pain scale. Descriptive scales are useful in assessing pain severity and evaluating changes in a patient's condition. Once you select a scale that works for a patient, be sure to use it consistently. Do not use pain-scale ratings to compare one patient with another but only to compare one patient's current pain level with what it was previously.

Several pain scales are available to assess pain in children. Wong and Baker (Wong-Baker FACES Foundation, 2016) developed the FACES pain rating scale to assess pain in children (Fig. 34.5). The scale shows drawings of six faces ranging from a very happy, smiling face for "no pain" to increasingly less happy faces to a final sad, tearful face for "worst pain." Children as young as 3 years of age can use the scale. The advantage is that patients do not have to interpret the meaning of numbers or adjectives. The faces clearly and quickly depict the concept of pain or discomfort (Wong-Baker FACES Foundation, 2016). Another tool designed to measure pain intensity in children is the Oucher pain scale (Beyer et al., 1992). The Oucher consists of two separate scales: the 0-to-10 scale on the left for older children and the six-picture photographic scale on the right for younger children (Fig. 34.6). There are Oucher scales for several common ethnic populations. Photographs of the face of a child in increasing levels of discomfort are designed to cue children into understanding what pain is and its severity. The child merely points to the selection, simplifying the task of describing the pain. There are additional pain rating tools for older children with verbal skills, neonates, and infants.

Effect of Pain on Patient. Pain alters a person's lifestyle and psychological well-being. For example, chronic/persistent pain often causes loss of control, loneliness, and an impaired quality of life. To understand a patient's pain experience, ask the patient what the pain prevents him or her from doing. Patients who live with daily pain or who have prolonged pain during a hospitalized illness are less able to participate in routine activities, which often leads to physical deconditioning. This deconditioning slows recovery of a patient who is

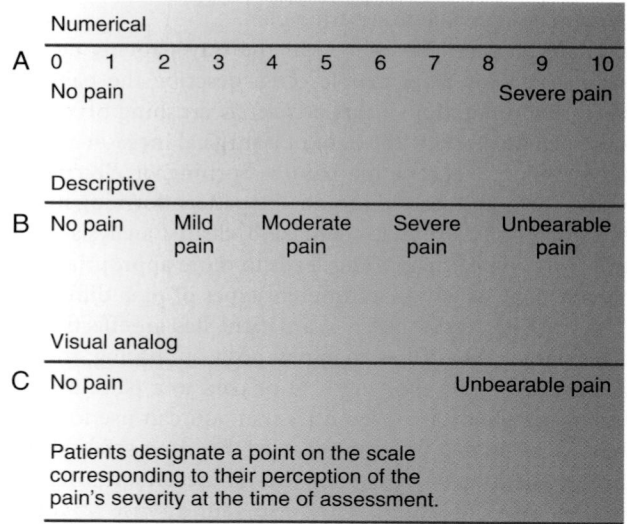

FIG 34.4 Sample pain scales. **A,** Numerical. **B,** Descriptive. **C,** Visual analog.

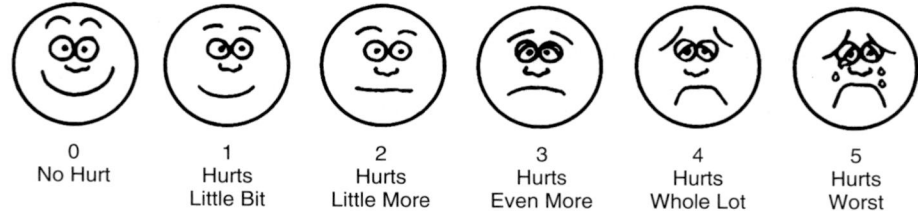

Brief word instructions: Point to each face using the words to describe the pain intensity. Ask the child to choose face that best describes own pain and record the appropriate number.

FIG 34.5 Wong-Baker FACES Pain Rating Scale. (Retrieved May 3, 2017, with permission from http://www.WongBakerFACES.org. Originally published in *Whaley & Wong's Nursing Care of Infants and Children.* © Elsevier Inc.)

Oucher®

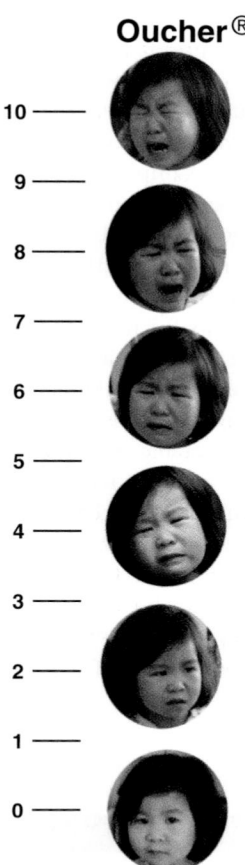

10 —
9 —
8 —
7 —
6 —
5 —
4 —
3 —
2 —
1 —
0 —

FIG 34.6 Asian girl version of Oucher pain scale. (The Asian versions of the Oucher scale [male and female] were developed and copyrighted in 2003 by CH Yeh [University of Pittsburgh] and CH Wang, Taiwan.)

BOX 34.7   ASSESSING THE INFLUENCE OF PAIN ON ACTIVITIES OF DAILY LIVING

SLEEP
- Does the patient have difficulty falling asleep?
- Does pain awaken the patient at night?
- Are sleeping pills or other aids needed?

HYGIENE
- Does pain hinder the patient's ability to bathe, dress, or perform other hygiene measures independently?
- Are family members or friends available or needed to help?

EATING
- Is the patient able to manipulate eating utensils?
- Can the patient chew and swallow without discomfort?

SEXUAL FUNCTIONING
- Do physical conditions such as arthritis or back pain prevent the patient from assuming usual positions during intercourse?
- Does pain or fatigue reduce the patient's desire for sex?
- Is the patient fearful that pain will increase with intercourse?

HOME MANAGEMENT AND WORK ACTIVITIES
- Is the patient able to perform usual housework chores?
- Does the patient's job require physical activity, and does pain limit activity now?
- If pain is related to emotional stress, does the patient's job involve tension-filled decision making?
- Does the patient need to stop activities momentarily to relieve pain?

SOCIAL ACTIVITIES
- Does the patient regularly socialize?
- To what extent has pain disrupted activities?

---

hospitalized. Assessment reveals the extent of the disability and the adjustments that will be necessary for participation in self-care (Box 34.7).

Concomitant Symptoms. Concomitant symptoms occur with pain and usually increase pain intensity. These include nausea, headache, dizziness, urge to urinate, constipation, depression, and restlessness. Certain types of pain have predictable symptoms. For example, severe rectal pain often causes constipation. These symptoms are as much a problem to a patient as the pain itself.

Patient Expectations. Patients rely on their caregivers to recognize and alleviate their physical discomfort. This may involve using a skilled and caring approach, trying a variety of comfort measures, and serving as an advocate for patients. You demonstrate caring when you provide patient-centered care tailored to an individual's needs. Always ask patients what they expect regarding their comfort needs. This includes asking not only which interventions they prefer but also how they think you should deliver them and how often. It is important to understand if patients expect full pain relief or if they simply hope to have their discomfort reduced. Full pain relief is often not possible. You must explain this to patients and clarify the level of comfort you can provide so that their expectations are realistic. When your patients ask for help because of pain, they expect you to respond promptly.

Documentation. Carefully assess and routinely document your patient's report of pain and the effectiveness of interventions. Use the assessment tool that is appropriate for your patient, and always use the same tool to reassess the patient's pain.

■ ■ ■ NURSING DIAGNOSIS

You make an accurate nursing diagnosis for your patient in pain only after reviewing all the assessment data and identifying patterns of risk factors or defining characteristics. Data collection and analysis reveal the presence of or potential for pain. Related factors focus on the nature of the pain and help identify interventions appropriate for problem-focused diagnoses. *Acute Pain related to physical trauma* and *Acute Pain related to natural childbirth processes* require very different nursing interventions.

In addition to *Acute Pain* and *Chronic Pain,* the following nursing diagnoses may be applicable to patients with pain (Herdman and Kamitsuru, 2014):

- *Ineffective Coping*
- *Fatigue*
- *Impaired Physical Mobility*
- *Dressing Self-Care Deficit*
- *Anxiety*
- *Social Isolation*
- *Risk for Delayed Surgical Recovery*

■■■ PLANNING

During the planning phase, you will identify priorities, appropriate patient-specific goals and outcomes, and interventions. The patient, family and interdisciplinary team collaborate to develop an appropriate plan.

Goals and Outcomes. Develop an individualized plan of care for each nursing diagnosis identified (see Care Plan).

Work with the patient and family to set realistic expectations for pain relief. Make sure that the patient understands that complete pain relief is not always possible, but it will be attempted. Individualize realistic goals for pain relief and levels of function with measurable outcomes (Pasero and McCaffery, 2011). For example, if a patient's baseline assessment reveals a pain severity consistently between 7 and 8 on the VAS, a realistic goal is for the patient to achieve the level of comfort that permits the patient to function. Although every patient is different, a pain severity outcome of 2 or 3 out of 10 usually allows for improved function or even full pain relief. Remember that no pain rating scale number offers an absolute guideline for a patient's perceived level of comfort. Thus it is essential that you always ask your patients what their current and acceptable pain levels are. However, pain ratings of 7 or higher on a 0-to-10 pain scale require urgent action by members of the health care team. For the goal "The patient will achieve a satisfactory level of pain relief within 24 hours," the following are possible outcomes:

- Reports pain at 3 or less
- Uses relaxation techniques before dressing change
- Able to dress self without a self-report of increased discomfort

---

◎ CARE PLAN

Chronic Pain

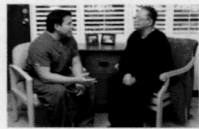

ASSESSMENT

When Jim enters Mrs. Ellis' four-room apartment, he finds the home to be in some disarray. Mrs. Ellis is sitting in the recliner in her living room, with clothing on the floor and soiled dishes on the nearby table. She reports that the pain she has been experiencing has made it very difficult to use her hands and walk between rooms. She is able to get to the bathroom, but it causes her to become fatigued. Her pain is constant and localized in the joints of her hands and knees.

ASSESSMENT ACTIVITIES

Ask Mrs. Ellis to select the pain scale that she prefers and rate her current pain intensity.

Ask Mrs. Ellis to rate her pain intensity when it is most severe.

Ask Mrs. Ellis what she does to control her pain.

Ask Mrs. Ellis if she has noticed any problems or side effects from taking the aspirin.

Observe Mrs. Ellis standing and walking to the kitchen. Measure the pain severity.

Ask Mrs. Ellis if she has friends or neighbors available to help her.

FINDINGS[a]

She rates the pain at the level of **3 on the FACES pain scale of 0 to 10.**

She rates the pain at 6 on the FACES pain scale of 0 to 10.

She currently takes aspirin for the pain; the pain **prevents her from being able to fall asleep;** when she does fall asleep, she **often reawakens at night.**

She reports "burning in the stomach" when she takes the aspirin.

She has **difficulty standing and an unsteady gait, with pain** at a level of 4.

She states, "I hate to be a bother, although my next-door neighbor has offered to help in the past."

[a]**Defining characteristics/risk factors** are shown in **bold** type.

NURSING DIAGNOSIS: Chronic Pain related to chronic joint inflammation

---

PLANNING

GOALS

Mrs. Ellis will report a sense of pain relief within 1 week.

EXPECTED OUTCOMES (NOC)[b]

Pain Level

Mrs. Ellis reports pain at 2 on the FACES pain scale of 0 to 10 following relaxation therapy and heat application.

CARE PLAN—cont'd

Chronic Pain

Mrs. Ellis will ambulate with less discomfort on self-report within 14 days.

Mrs. Ellis will be able to perform activities of daily living with less discomfort within 14 days.

Pain: Disruptive Effects

Mrs. Ellis demonstrates ability to rise to standing position without help within 1 week.

Mrs. Ellis demonstrates ability to walk from room to room with a walker with steady gait and at a pain severity of 3 or less in 2 weeks.

Mrs. Ellis is able to wash dishes and clean house at a pain severity of 3 or less in 2 weeks.

[b]Outcome classification labels from Moorhead S, et al, editors: *Nursing outcomes classification (NOC)*, ed 5, St Louis, 2013, Mosby.

INTERVENTIONS (NIC)[c]

Analgesic Administration

Discuss with Mrs. Ellis' primary health care provider the possibility of starting a disease-modifying antirheumatic drug (DMARD) (e.g., methotrexate), a biological response modifier (BRM) (e.g., infliximab [Remicade]), a nonsteroidal antiinflammatory drug (NSAID) (e.g., ibuprofen), or an analgesic (e.g., acetaminophen).

Consult with health care provider to allow Mrs. Ellis to take analgesics around the clock (e.g., every 4 hours) and plan activities such as ambulating, performing self-care activities, or going to sleep 30 minutes after a dose. Instruct her to take medication with a light snack or meal and a full glass of water. During instruction tell her that the drug relieves pain.

Cutaneous Stimulation

Have Mrs. Ellis place a sturdy stool in shower stall and run warm water continuously over joints of hands and feet.

Have Mrs. Ellis apply moist, warm compresses to joints of hands 3 times a day before dressing or other self-care activities.

Referral

Refer Mrs. Ellis to a physical therapist to determine possible need of a walker or other assistive devices.

RATIONALE

Different medications are used to control the pain and symptoms of rheumatoid arthritis. DMARDs cause immunosuppression; DMARDs, NSAIDs, and BRMs decrease inflammation; and DMARDs, NSAIDs, and analgesics relieve pain (Arthritis Foundation, n.d.).

Administer analgesics on a fixed schedule around the clock (Burchum and Rosenthal, 2016). Medication exerts peak effect when patient begins activities. Administration with meals and water reduces chance of gastrointestinal upset. An added positive effect occurs when the patient understands the action and purpose of the analgesic and believes that the medication will relieve pain.

Heat reduces pain associated with rheumatoid arthritis by improving blood flow and reducing stiffness of inflamed tissues.

Cutaneous stimulation inhibits transmission of pain.

Physical therapists teach effective exercise and ambulation techniques to reduce pain and conserve energy.

[c]Intervention classification labels from Bulechek GM, et al, editors: *Nursing interventions classification (NIC)*, ed 6, St Louis, 2013, Mosby.

EVALUATION

NURSING ACTIONS	PATIENT RESPONSE/FINDING	ACHIEVEMENT OF OUTCOME
Observe Mrs. Ellis' ability to stand and walk from living room to kitchen.	Mrs. Ellis is able to ambulate with walker from living room to kitchen; gait is slow but steady.	Mrs. Ellis is successfully ambulating with steady gait.
Ask Mrs. Ellis if she experiences discomfort during dressing and bathing.	Mrs. Ellis has less discomfort from bathing after using warm water over joints. Dressing is still causing some discomfort when manipulating buttons on clothing.	Cutaneous stimulation is providing some pain relief. Consider referring to occupational therapist to adapt clothes fasteners requiring less hand mobility.
Ask Mrs. Ellis to rate pain on FACES pain scale 30 minutes after analgesic is administered.	Mrs. Ellis rates pain at a level of 2 after receiving analgesic.	Mrs. Ellis continues to have discomfort, but it is less severe than before intervention.

An effective method for planning care is a concept map (Fig. 34.7). Patients who are in pain frequently have interrelated problems. As one problem worsens, other aspects of a patient's level of health also change. A concept map shows links or relationships among multiple nursing diagnoses, a patient's medical diagnosis, and associated interventions. This helps you learn how assessment findings and interventions can apply to more than one diagnosis so that you can form a comprehensive and holistic plan of care.

It is always important to remember that a successful plan of care requires development of a therapeutic relationship with a patient and family and a focus on education regarding pain. Helping patients learn how to manage their pain is an important goal of care. You help best by seeing each patient as a total person, listening carefully to concerns, attending promptly to the patient's needs, and respecting any response to pain. In the successful nurse-patient relationship, you recognize that a patient knows more about his or her own pain and is an important partner in identifying successful pain-relieving strategies.

Setting Priorities. When setting priorities in pain management, consider the type of pain that a patient is having and how it affects various body functions. Work with a patient to select interventions that are most appropriate for priority needs. For example, if a patient's acute pain is under control, focus attention on improving his or her appetite or ability to sleep. However, if the pain continues to be severe, preventing you from implementing other interventions, immediate pain relief becomes your priority. Priorities change as a patient's pain experience changes.

Collaborative Care. A comprehensive plan of care involves using the resources of a patient's family and friends.

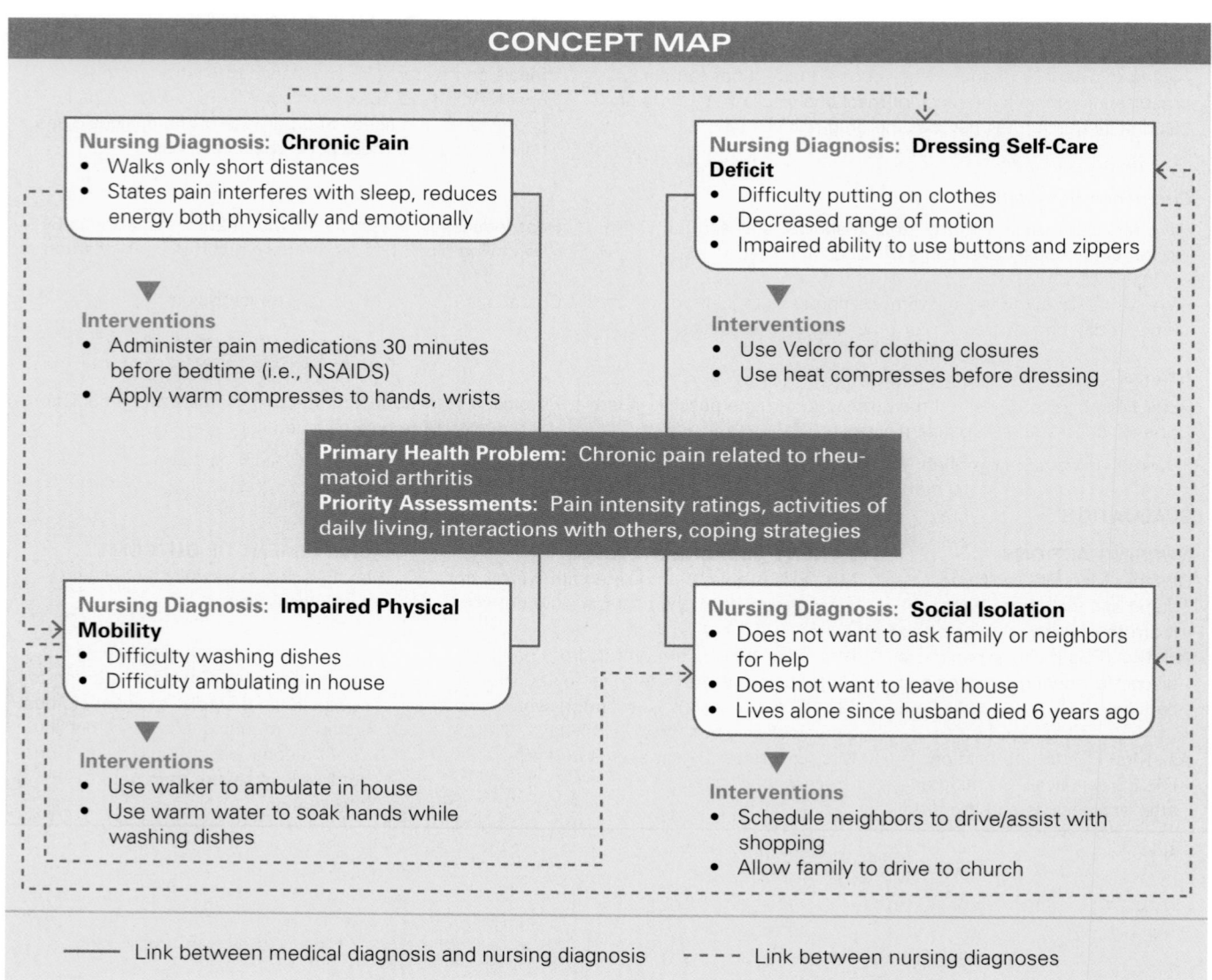

CONCEPT MAP

Nursing Diagnosis: Chronic Pain
- Walks only short distances
- States pain interferes with sleep, reduces energy both physically and emotionally

▼

Interventions
- Administer pain medications 30 minutes before bedtime (i.e., NSAIDS)
- Apply warm compresses to hands, wrists

Nursing Diagnosis: Dressing Self-Care Deficit
- Difficulty putting on clothes
- Decreased range of motion
- Impaired ability to use buttons and zippers

▼

Interventions
- Use Velcro for clothing closures
- Use heat compresses before dressing

Primary Health Problem: Chronic pain related to rheumatoid arthritis
Priority Assessments: Pain intensity ratings, activities of daily living, interactions with others, coping strategies

Nursing Diagnosis: Impaired Physical Mobility
- Difficulty washing dishes
- Difficulty ambulating in house

▼

Interventions
- Use walker to ambulate in house
- Use warm water to soak hands while washing dishes

Nursing Diagnosis: Social Isolation
- Does not want to ask family or neighbors for help
- Does not want to leave house
- Lives alone since husband died 6 years ago

▼

Interventions
- Schedule neighbors to drive/assist with shopping
- Allow family to drive to church

——— Link between medical diagnosis and nursing diagnosis   - - - - Link between nursing diagnoses

FIG 34.7 Concept map. *NSAIDs,* Nonsteroidal antiinflammatory drugs.

Family caregivers need to be prepared to assess a patient's pain and administer therapies safely at home. Discharge teaching in an acute care setting prepares a patient and family caregiver to understand the nature and extent of a patient's pain, the choice of therapies, and how to safely administer therapies. Family members or friends who show a disinterest or prejudice toward pain may slow a patient's recovery. Additional resources in planning care include nurse and physician specialists, Doctors of Pharmacology (PharmDs), physical therapists, occupational therapists, licensed massage therapists, social workers, and clergy. An oncology nurse specialist understands therapies for cancer pain. Physician pain specialists are experts on invasive therapies. PharmDs are knowledgeable about pharmacological treatments for pain. Physical therapists plan exercises that strengthen or relax muscle groups and lessen pain. Occupational therapists devise splints to support painful body parts. Licensed massage therapists offer massage that may relax muscles and block perceptions of pain. Clergy provide holistic support and offer strategies to relieve spiritual pain. If an agency does not have the resources to manage a patient's pain, refer the patient to a health care provider or agency that can provide the care needed.

Because patients are often transferred between departments of the same institution and sometimes between different institutions, documentation of the pain management plan is important for continuity of care. Record all discharge teaching and referrals implemented. A notation of who to call if pain consistently exceeds the pain-intensity goal is essential.

■■■ IMPLEMENTATION

Pain therapy requires an individualized approach, perhaps more so than any other health problem. The nature of pain and the extent to which it affects an individual's physical and psychosocial well-being determine the choice of pain-relief therapies. A nurse, patient, and frequently family caregiver are partners in pain management. You are responsible for administering and monitoring therapies ordered by health care providers for pain relief and independently providing pain-relief measures that complement the prescribed therapies. Implement any previously successful pain-relieving remedies used by a patient. Generally try the least invasive and safest therapy first. Do not delegate pain assessment and management to nursing assistive personnel (NAP). However, NAP may screen patients for the presence of pain by asking them if they are having pain. If a patient is in pain, the NAP reports this to the nurse for thorough assessment and evaluation.

Regardless of the type of therapies used, your ability to show compassionate care toward patients maximizes their pain control (see Chapter 20). You minimize pain through caring behaviors such as gentle handling and touch. Pain-relieving measures are more successful when you successfully convey compassion, maintain a patient's dignity, and consistently strive to minimize discomfort.

Health Promotion. When providing pain-relief measures, choose therapies suited to a patient's unique pain experience. Box 34.8 includes guidelines that are applicable for individualizing pain therapy (Pasero and McCaffery, 2011).

Maintaining Wellness. Patients who assume healthy behaviors are better able to manage the stress of living with painful conditions. Part of pain management is helping patients to actively participate in their own well-being whenever possible. Common holistic health approaches include wellness education, regular exercise, rest, attention to good nutrition and hygiene practices, and management of interpersonal relationships. Health promotion still involves the use of nonpharmacological and pharmacological therapies when a person develops more intense pain.

BOX 34.8 GUIDELINES FOR INDIVIDUALIZED PAIN THERAPY

- *Use different types of pain-relief measures.* This produces an additive effect in reducing pain and allows for changes in the character of pain.
- *Provide pain-relief measures before pain becomes severe.* It is easier to prevent severe pain than to try to relieve it after it occurs.
- *Use measures that a patient believes are effective.* A patient's beliefs make pain therapy successful; therefore, include these remedies unless they are harmful.
- *Some patients have ideas about pain-relief measures they are willing to use and times to use them.* Consider a patient's ability or willingness to participate in pain-relief measures.
- *Do not force participation.* Suggest measures that require little physical effort for patients unable to actively assist with pain therapy because of fatigue or altered levels of consciousness.
- *Choose pain-relief measures based on patient behavior that reflects the severity of pain.* Never administer a potent analgesic for mild pain. Only a patient can determine the potency of an effective therapy.
- *Depending on the therapy, ensure that you attempt a sufficient trial before abandoning it.* Pharmacological interventions particularly often need ATC administration for several days to attain and maintain therapeutic level and provide pain relief.
- *Keep an open mind about ways to relieve pain.* Rejecting nonconventional therapy leads to mistrust. Be sure that all therapies are safe.
- *Keep trying.* When efforts at pain relief fail, do not abandon the patient, but reassess the situation and consider alternative therapies.
- *Protect the patient.* Pain therapy does not cause more distress than the pain itself; you want to relieve pain without disabling the patient mentally, emotionally, or physically.
- *Educate the patient about pain.* Explain the cause of pain, times when you will give analgesics, and alternative therapies.

ATC, Around-the-clock.

There are interventions nurses can independently recommend. Measures that promote a sense of well-being by minimizing or avoiding discomfort include warm baths, massage, and a schedule of adequate rest. Chapter 33 discusses the effect that pain has on a patient's sleep pattern and ways to promote better sleep habits. Help patients find ways to plan rest periods before participating in exhausting activities. Patients with chronic pain need to rest before any social activities.

Some pain disables and immobilizes a person enough to impair the ability to perform self-care activities, which often results in feelings of social isolation, depression, and changes in self-concept. Change in function creates a significant loss to a patient. Help patients and family caregivers learn to discuss their feelings about the loss so that they can find ways to cope with pain and the lifestyle it imposes (see Chapter 27).

When pain limits a patient's mobility, you target health promotion at retaining function. For example, instruct patients and family caregivers in the safe and proper use of elastic bandages, braces, and splints that protect body parts. When a patient has chronic, disabling pain, instruct family caregivers in proper positioning techniques and ways to help the patient ambulate.

Refer patients who have difficulty eating, bathing, grooming, and dressing to an occupational therapist. Some agencies require a health care provider's order to begin occupational therapy. Devices designed to maintain function, even when finger movement or grasp is impaired, may help. The therapist attaches eating utensils, a comb, or a toothbrush to extension devices that have enlarged handles or splints for easy use. Velcro fasteners on clothing allow patients to remove or don clothing without assistance.

Some patients with pain avoid sexual activity. However, pain does not negate the need for sexual intimacy. Patients learn to express themselves sexually by assuming alternative positions during intercourse and learning about ways to make their partner feel sexually stimulated. Caution patients that some pain medications decrease libido and may cause impotency.

Nonpharmacological Pain-Relief Measures. There are many nonpharmacological or complementary therapies for pain relief that nurses use to promote health as well as manage acute and restorative care needs (see Chapter 19). Examples include massage, guided imagery, music, prayer, journaling, exercise, and relaxation techniques. Complementary therapies such as biofeedback and acupuncture require special training to perform. Use other therapies such as massage and relaxation to lessen the perception of pain, perhaps in combination with pharmacological measures (Burchum and Rosenthal, 2016). Combine pharmacological therapy with nonpharmacological therapies. Guidelines for chronic pain management from the CDC recommend using nonpharmacological therapy before opioids (Dowell et al., 2016). If opioids are needed, health care providers can add opioids, but only in combination with nonpharmacological approaches and nonopioid analgesics.

Reducing Pain Reception and Perception. One simple way to promote comfort is to remove or prevent painful stimuli. This is especially important for patients who are immobilized or have difficulty expressing themselves. For example, tighten and smooth wrinkled bed linen and be sure to position patients so that they are not lying on tubing and other equipment. Change wet dressings or bed linen immediately. Do not allow tubing from a Foley catheter to become kinked because bladder distention is uncomfortable. Remember to use safe patient-handling techniques when repositioning and lifting patients. Do not pull when positioning patients in correct anatomical alignment. Minimize exposure to skin irritants such as diarrhea stool or wound drainage. Many of these measures are easy for family caregivers to learn. Removing noxious stimuli is especially important for patients who are immobile. You can prevent pain by anticipating painful activities (e.g., ambulation or turning). Before performing a procedure, consider the patient's condition, aspects of the procedure that are painful, and ways to avoid causing pain. Consideration of the patient's comfort and a little extra time are needed to avoid pain-producing situations.

Anticipatory Guidance. Modifying anxiety directly associated with pain relieves the pain and adds to the beneficial effects of other pain-relief measures. Giving patients detailed descriptions of all medical procedures and expected postprocedural discomfort and giving instruction for decreasing treatment-related and mobility-related pain decrease pain and analgesic use. Provide patients with sufficient procedural and sensory information (e.g., prick of the needle during blood draw or burning during urinary catheter insertion) to satisfy their curiosity and enable them to prepare for and communicate pain.

Distraction. The reticular activating system inhibits painful stimuli if a person receives sufficient or excessive sensory input. With meaningful sensory stimuli, a patient can ignore or become unaware of pain. Pleasurable sensory stimuli reduce pain perception by the release of endorphins. Distraction directs a patient's attention to something else, thus reducing the awareness of pain. Distraction works best for short, intense pain lasting a few minutes such as during an invasive procedure or while waiting for an analgesic to become effective. Useful forms of distraction include singing, praying, describing photos out loud, telling jokes, and playing games. Music is helpful for managing acute and chronic discomfort, stress, anxiety, and depression by diverting a patient's attention and creating a relaxation response. Always let patients select the type of music they prefer. Patients may use earphones to enhance their concentration on the music. Evidence shows that music decreases the use of analgesics in some postoperative patients (Cole and LoBiondo-Wood, 2014).

Cutaneous Stimulation. Stimulation of the skin helps to relieve pain. A massage, warm bath, ice pack, and transcutaneous electrical nerve stimulation (TENS) are simple ways to reduce pain perception (Chou et al., 2016). How cutaneous stimulation works is unclear, but it may cause release of endorphins, thus blocking transmission of painful stimuli.

The gate control theory suggests that cutaneous stimulation activates larger, faster A-beta sensory nerve fibers that are sensitive to touch, pressure, and warmth. This decreases pain transmission through small-diameter A-delta and C fibers. Synaptic gates thus close to pain transmission.

Cutaneous stimulation gives patients and families some control over pain symptoms and treatment in the home. Using it properly helps to reduce muscle tension, resulting in less pain. When using cutaneous stimulation, eliminate environmental noise, help patients to assume comfortable positions, and explain the purpose of therapies. Do not use cutaneous stimulation directly on sensitive skin areas (e.g., burns, bruises, skin rashes, inflammation, underlying bone fractures).

Massage is effective for producing physical and mental relaxation, reducing pain, and enhancing the effectiveness of pain medication. Massaging the back, shoulders, hands, and/or feet relaxes muscles and promotes sleep. Massage conveys caring, and family caregivers can learn how to do this easily.

Cold and heat applications relieve pain and promote healing (Box 34.9) (see Chapter 38). The choice to use heat or cold is based on the origin of the pain and a patient's preferences and past experiences with pain relief using these methods. For example, moist heat often relieves the pain from a tension headache, and a cold pack reduces acute pain from inflammation. The use of heat or cold applications in the acute care setting requires a health care provider's order. When using any form of heat or cold application, instruct a patient to avoid injury to the skin by checking the temperature and not applying it directly to the skin. Older adults, confused patients, and patients with spinal cord or other neurological injuries and decreased sensation are at risk for burns from heating devices.

TENS stimulates the skin by passing mild electrical currents through external electrodes, blocking pain stimuli from reaching the brain. A patient places the electrodes directly over or near the site of pain and turns on a battery-powered transmitter to create a tingling electrical current when feeling pain. TENS is useful in reducing postoperative procedural pain (e.g., removing drains). The research evidence on the use of TENS for pain relief is often conflicting; however, TENS is safe, noninvasive, nonaddictive, inexpensive, and easy to use. It requires a health care provider's order (Chou et al., 2016).

Relaxation and Guided Imagery. Relaxation and guided imagery allow patients to alter affective motivational and cognitive pain perception. Relaxation is mental and physical freedom from tension or stress that provides individuals a sense of self-control. Potential physiological and behavioral changes associated with relaxation include decreased pulse, blood pressure, and respirations; heightened awareness; decreased oxygen consumption; a sense of peace; and decreased muscle tension and metabolic rate. Relaxation strategies include meditation, yoga, Zen, guided imagery, and progressive relaxation. Sometimes a combination is needed to achieve pain relief. The techniques require periodic reinforcement through encouragement and coaching.

For effective relaxation, a patient needs to be able to concentrate, participate, and cooperate. Teach relaxation techniques only when a patient is not anxious, in acute discomfort, or in severe pain. Explain the technique in detail. It sometimes takes several teaching sessions before patients effectively feel less pain. Patients can practice relaxation training indefinitely and usually with no side effects. Remove any noises or other irritating stimuli such as bright lights from the environment. Have a patient sit in a comfortable chair in proper alignment or lie in bed. A light sheet or blanket keeps the patient warm and comfortable. Describe common sensations that the patient will experience (e.g., decrease in temperature, feeling of heaviness, numbness of a body part). The patient uses these sensations as feedback. Acting as the coach, guide the patient slowly through the steps of the exercise.

In guided imagery, a patient creates an image in the mind, concentrates on that image, and gradually becomes less aware of pain. Initially ask the patient to think of a pleasant scene or experience that promotes using all senses. The patient describes the image, and you record it for later use. Use only

---

BOX 34.9 PATIENT TEACHING

Application of Moist Heat

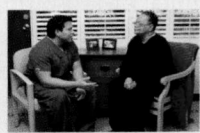 The application of moist heat for pain relief was recommended for Mrs. Ellis. Jim develops a teaching plan to help her learn how to implement this therapy.

OUTCOME
At the end of the teaching session, Mrs. Ellis will demonstrate proper application of moist heat to affected joints for pain relief.

TEACHING STRATEGIES
- Plan teaching session in quiet environment at time that is convenient for Mrs. Ellis.
- Avoid teaching during times of moderate-to-severe pain.
- Teach Mrs. Ellis about expected outcomes of use of moist heat to relieve chronic pain related to rheumatoid arthritis.
- Have Mrs. Ellis apply moist heat to painful areas while talking her through the procedure.
- To avoid burns, warn Mrs. Ellis against using water that is too hot or making the compress too hot.
- Summarize information taught and clarify questions or concerns.

EVALUATION
- Use the principles of teach-back to evaluate patient/family caregiver learning:
  - "Tell me what we discussed about how to apply moist heat to painful areas."
  - "Tell me why it is necessary to avoid using water or a compress that is too hot."

specific information given by the patient and make no changes in the image. The following is an example of a portion of a guided imagery exercise:

> Imagine yourself lying on a cool bed of grass with the sounds of water trickling over stones in a nearby stream. It's a warm day. You turn to see a patch of blue wildflowers in bloom, and you smell their fragrance.

Sit close enough so the patient can hear you but not so close that you are intrusive. A calm, soft voice helps the patient focus more completely on the suggested image. You speak continuously while the patient relaxes and focuses on the image. If the patient shows signs of agitation, restlessness, or discomfort, stop the exercise and begin again later when the patient is more at ease.

Progressive relaxation exercises involve the combination of controlled breathing exercises and a series of contractions and relaxation of muscle groups. A patient begins by breathing slowly from the diaphragm, allowing the abdomen to rise slowly. The chest remains still while fully expanding. Often a patient closes the eyes to focus on the exercise. When the patient establishes a regular breathing pattern, coach him or her to locate any area of muscular tension, think about how it feels, gently tense the muscles, and then completely relax them. This creates the sensation of removing all discomfort and stress. Gradually the patient relaxes the muscles without first tensing them. After achieving full relaxation, pain perception is lowered, and anxiety toward the pain experience lessens. If the patient becomes agitated or uncomfortable, stop the exercise. If the patient reports difficulty relaxing part of the body, slow the progression of the exercise and concentrate on the tensed body part. If the patient reports increased pain, focus on relaxing areas of muscle tension instead of consciously tensing the muscle. The patient may stop the exercise at any time. With practice the patient learns to perform relaxation exercises independently. Relaxation techniques are particularly effective for chronic pain, labor pains, and relief of procedure-related pain. The techniques are less effective for episodes of acute or severe pain.

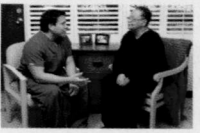

QSEN QSEN ACTIVITY *Patient-Centered Care*

As Jim continues to work with Mrs. Ellis, he becomes concerned about her safety related to living alone and having significant physical limitations. He suggests that she ask her niece or a friend to help her by coming to visit her routinely. Mrs. Ellis responds immediately that she does not want to be a burden to anyone. However, she does agree that her niece seems willing to help her.

- How can Jim include the niece in a patient-centered approach to Mrs. Ellis' pain management?

evolve   Answers to QSEN Activities can be found on the Evolve website.

Acute Care

Pharmacological Pain Therapy. All pharmacological agents require a health care provider's order. Your judgment in the use and management of analgesics with or without other pain therapies ensures the best pain relief possible. A systematic approach to pain assessment and appropriate treatment choices ensures a quick response for managing patient discomfort.

Analgesics. The most common treatment for pain relief is analgesics. However, health care providers still tend to undertreat patients because of incorrect drug information, concerns about addiction, anxiety over errors in using opioid analgesics, and administration of less medication than was ordered. Make sure that you understand the drugs available for pain relief and their pharmacological effects. Reassure patients that treatment of pain is necessary to aid recovery and that addiction is highly unlikely when analgesics are taken correctly.

There are three types of analgesics: (1) nonopioids including acetaminophen and nonsteroidal antiinflammatory drugs (NSAIDs); (2) opioids (traditionally called *narcotics*); and (3) adjuvants or coanalgesics, medications that enhance analgesics or analgesic properties (Burchum and Rosenthal, 2016).

Acetaminophen (Tylenol) is considered one of the most tolerated and safest analgesics available. It has no antiinflammatory effects, and its action is unknown. Its major adverse effect is toxicity to the liver. Acetaminophen is in a variety of over-the-counter (OTC) cold, flu, and allergy remedies. The maximum 24-hour dose is 4 g (the same limitation as aspirin). It is often combined with opioids (e.g., oxycodone [Percocet], hydrocodone [Vicodin], tramadol [Ultracet]) because it reduces the dose of opioid needed.

Nonselective NSAIDs such as aspirin and ibuprofen provide relief for mild-to-moderate acute intermittent pain such as pain from headache or muscle strain. Treatment for mild-to-moderate postoperative pain begins with an NSAID unless contraindicated (Burchum and Rosenthal, 2016). In contrast to opioids, NSAIDs do not depress the central nervous system, and they do not interfere with bowel and bladder function. However, chronic NSAID use is not recommended because it is associated with gastrointestinal bleeding, renal insufficiency, and bleeding tendencies. NSAIDs have antiinflammatory properties and work with opioids to relieve pain better than when given alone (Burchum and Rosenthal, 2016).

Opioid or opioid-like analgesics such as codeine, morphine, fentanyl, and hydromorphone are prescribed for moderate-to-severe pain. These analgesics act on higher centers of the brain and spinal cord by binding with opiate receptors to modify pain perception. Opioid-naïve patients have used opioids around-the-clock (ATC) less than approximately 1 week. A rare adverse effect of opioids in opioid-naïve patients is respiratory depression. Respiratory depression is clinically significant only if there is a decrease in the rate *and* depth of respirations from a patient's baseline assessment (Pasero and McCaffery, 2011). Patients who breathe deeply rarely have clinical respiratory depression. Sedation always occurs before respiratory depression. Closely monitor for sedation in opioid-naïve patients. If a patient develops respiratory depression, administer naloxone (Narcan) 0.4 mg diluted with 9 mL saline IV push at a rate of 0.5 mL every 2 minutes until the respiratory rate is greater than 8 breaths/minute with good depth. Evaluate patients who receive naloxone every 15 minutes for 2 hours because its duration is less than that of the opioid and respiratory depression can return. Additional adverse effects of opioids include nausea, vomiting, constipation, itching, urinary retention, and altered mental processes.

One way to maximize pain relief while potentially decreasing drug use is to administer analgesics on an ATC rather than as-needed (prn) basis (Burchum and Rosenthal, 2016). There are also a variety of extended-release or controlled-release oral opioid formulations with dosing intervals of 8, 10, 12, or 24 hours and transdermal patches with a dosing interval of 72 hours. These formulations maintain constant serum opioid concentration, minimizing toxic and subtherapeutic concentrations. They also lessen the severity of end-of-dose pain, allowing a patient to sleep through the night.

The current pharmacological approach to pain management is to provide multimodal analgesia. This approach combines drugs with at least two different mechanisms of action to optimize pain control. Medications are combined to target different sites in the peripheral or central pain pathways. Multimodal analgesia allows for lower-than-usual doses of each medication, thereby lowering the risk of side effects while providing good or better pain relief than giving each medication alone.

When a patient is converted from an IV to an oral form of opioid, know that the dose of the oral opioid is usually much higher than the IV dose because of the first-pass effect (Pasero and McCaffery, 2011). When a patient takes oral opioids, the opioids go to the liver first, where most of the medication is inactivated. Thus the body needs larger doses of oral opioids to achieve the same level of pain relief as the same opioid given intravenously. Know the comparative potencies of analgesics in oral and IV form. Also, know the route of administration that is most effective for a patient to achieve controlled, sustained pain relief. Equianalgesic charts show the conversion of one opioid to another and of parenteral forms of opioids to oral forms. These charts are available on nursing units, in the pharmacy, and in printed and online drug resources. Nurses on succeeding shifts need to know the route of administration that is most effective for a patient so that the patient has controlled, sustained pain relief.

Adjuvants or coanalgesics are drugs (e.g., steroids, anticonvulsants, antidepressants, muscle relaxants) originally developed to treat conditions other than pain that also have analgesic properties. For example, tricyclic antidepressants (e.g., nortriptyline), anticonvulsants (e.g., gabapentin), and infusional lidocaine successfully treat neuropathic pain. Corticosteroids relieve pain associated with inflammation and bone metastasis. Adjuvants have analgesic properties, enhance pain control, or relieve other symptoms associated with neuropathic pain such as anxiety, depression, and nausea. You give these alone or with analgesics (Burchum and Rosenthal, 2016). Sedatives, antianxiety agents, and muscle relaxants have no analgesic effect; however, they often cause drowsiness and impaired coordination, judgment, and mental alertness. Be aware of the risk for falls when a patient is taking these medications.

The proper use of analgesics requires careful assessment, application of pharmacological principles, and critical thinking (Box 34.10). Not all patients react the same way to analgesics. An orally administered analgesic usually brings the same relief as an injectable form.

Children require careful calculation of drug doses (see Chapter 17). Equianalgesia charts that convert recommended adult doses to children's doses are available. These charts consider age and body size. In addition, older adults require special dosing considerations (Box 34.11).

Patient-Controlled Analgesia. Patients benefit from having control over their pain therapy. Patient-controlled analgesia (PCA) is a safe method for a variety of painful conditions including but not limited to postoperative, traumatic, sickle cell crisis, cancer, and burn pain (Pasero and McCaffery, 2011). PCA is a drug-delivery system that allows patients to self-administer opioids with minimal risk of overdose, when they need medication, and without repeated parenteral injections (see Skill 34.1). The goal is to maintain a constant plasma level of analgesic to avoid the problems of intermittent dosing. Systemic PCA traditionally involves IV or subcutaneous administration.

PCA infusion pumps are portable and contain a cassette or chamber for a syringe. The PCA delivers a small preset dose of opioid. To receive a demand dose, a patient pushes a button attached to the PCA device. Systems are programmed to deliver a specified number of doses every 1 to 4 hours (depending on the pump settings) given every 5 to 15 minutes to avoid overdoses. On-demand doses typically add 1 mg of morphine every 10 minutes, with a limit set for every hour or every 4 hours. Most pumps have locked safety systems that prevent tampering by patients or family caregivers and are generally safe to be managed in the home. The typical PCA prescription relies on a series of "loading" doses (e.g., 3 to 5 mg of morphine repeated every 5 to 10 minutes until initial pain diminishes). A low-dose basal infusion (0.5 to 1 mg/hr) at night allows uninterrupted sleep; this option is commonly used for cancer pain. Use continuous basal infusions with caution in patients who are opioid naïve during the first 24 to 48 hours after surgery because of the possibility of respiratory depression from the combination of anesthetics with opioids (Pasero and McCaffery, 2011).

Benefits of PCA include better pain control, a need for less medication, and pain relief that does not depend on nurses' availability. Small PCA doses delivered at short intervals stabilize serum drug concentrations for sustained pain relief.

Patient preparation and teaching are critical to the safe and effective use of PCA. If PCA is ordered, patients having surgery receive teaching and demonstration of the PCA pump before surgery. Patients need to understand PCA and

BOX 34.10   NURSING PRINCIPLES FOR ADMINISTERING ANALGESICS

KNOW PATIENT'S PREVIOUS RESPONSE TO ANALGESICS

- Determine whether the patient obtained pain relief.
- Ask whether a nonopioid was as effective as an opioid.
- Identify previous doses and routes of administration to avoid undertreatment.
- Determine whether the patient has allergies.
- Know if the patient is at risk for using NSAIDs (e.g., history of gastrointestinal bleed or renal insufficiency) or opioids (e.g., history of obstructive sleep apnea).

SELECT PROPER MEDICATIONS WHEN MORE THAN ONE IS ORDERED

- Use nonopioid analgesics or opioid combination drugs (e.g., oxycodone with acetaminophen) for mild-to-moderate pain.
- Give opioids with nonopioids.
- In older adults avoid combinations of opioids.
- Fentanyl patches, morphine, or hydromorphone are opioids of choice for long-term severe pain.
- IV medications act more quickly and usually relieve severe, acute pain within 1 hour, whereas oral medications take up to 2 hours to relieve pain.
- Avoid intramuscular analgesics, especially in older adults.
- For chronic pain give oral extended-release formulations for longer, more sustained relief.

KNOW ACCURATE DOSAGE

- Remember that patients with severe pain generally need higher doses of analgesics.

- Adjust doses as appropriate for children and older patients.
- Large doses of opioids are acceptable in patients who are opioid tolerant but not in patients who are opioid naïve.
- When titrating opioids, it is important to titrate to effect or to uncontrollable side effects.
- Dosage typically requires adjustment over time.

ASSESS RIGHT TIME AND INTERVAL FOR ADMINISTRATION

- Administer analgesics as soon as pain occurs and before it increases in severity.
- An ATC administration schedule is best.
- Give analgesics *before* pain-producing procedures or activities.
- Know average peak and duration of action for drug so that you time drug administration to peak when pain is most intense.
- Give extended-release opioid formulations on an ATC basis and not prn.
- Avoid abruptly stopping opioids in patients who are opioid tolerant.

CHOOSE RIGHT ROUTE

- Oral route is generally preferred; IV route is preferred if patient is unable to swallow or has gastrointestinal problems.
- Avoid intramuscular and subcutaneous administration because these routes are painful and absorption is not reliable.

ATC, Around-the-clock; *NSAIDs,* nonsteroidal antiinflammatory drugs.
Modified from Pasero C, McCaffery M: *Pain assessment and pharmacological management,* St Louis, 2011, Mosby.

BOX 34.11   CARE OF THE OLDER ADULT

Principles of Pain Management in the Older Adult

- The presence of pain requires aggressive assessment and management.
- Older adults are at high risk for pain-inducing situations.
- Sometimes several pain-producing conditions coexist.
- Older adults are often fearful that pain will result in loss of independence, making them a burden to their family.
- Age-related changes in pain perception are most likely not clinically significant.
- Older patients experience faster onset, longer duration of action, and adverse effects from analgesics because of lower serum protein levels and reduced liver, renal, and cardiac function.
- Older adults may be more sensitive to analgesic and adverse effects of opioids. Thus, start with low doses of opioids and increase dose slowly as needed (Pasero and McCaffery, 2011).
- There is an increased risk for gastric and renal toxicity from NSAIDs among older adults.

NSAIDs, nonsteroidal antiinflammatory drugs.

be able to physically locate and press the button to deliver the dose (Pasero and McCaffery, 2011). PCA therapy is not appropriate for patients who are confused, have altered levels of consciousness, or are unable to understand how to use the equipment. Be sure to instruct family members not to "push the button" for patients. Use American Society for Pain Management Nursing (ASPMN) Authorized Agent Controlled Analgesia (AACA) guidelines to authorize a family member or nurse to administer the analgesic when appropriate (Cooney et al., 2013). In these cases, you select one family member or significant other to be the patient's primary pain manager. Check the patient's IV line or subcutaneous needle placement and PCA device regularly to ensure proper functioning. Most PCA devices track cumulative dosages and show the information when needed. Document drug doses carefully and record any wasted or unused opioid. Monitor the patient for adverse drug effects and pain management effectiveness. Use of PCA gives nurses and patients more flexibility in pain management.

Perineural Local Anesthetic Infusion. Perineural infusion pumps are an option for managing pain for a variety of adult and pediatric surgical procedures. An unsutured catheter from a surgical wound placed near a nerve or groups of nerves connects to a pump containing a local anesthetic. You set the pump on demand or continuous mode, and it is usually left in place for 48 hours. Patients learn how to discontinue the pump at home by pulling out the catheter and bringing it to their next health care provider visit.

Local Anesthetics. The loss of sensation to a localized body part is termed local anesthesia. Health care providers use local anesthetics including lidocaine, bupivacaine, and ropivacaine during brief surgical procedures such as suturing a wound. Local anesthetics are applied topically on skin and mucous membranes or are injected subcutaneously, perineurally, or intradermally to anesthetize a body part. The drugs produce temporary loss of sensation by inhibiting nerve conduction. Local anesthetics may also block motor and autonomic functions, depending on the amount used and the location and depth of an injection. Smaller sensory nerve fibers are more sensitive than large motor fibers. Thus a patient loses sensation before losing motor function; conversely motor function returns before sensation.

Local anesthetics cause side effects depending on their absorption into the circulation. Itching or burning of the skin or a localized rash is common after topical applications. Application to vascular membranes increases the chance of systemic effects such as a change in heart rate. Protect patients from injury until full sensory and motor function return because they can easily injure themselves without knowing it. You need to educate patients receiving local anesthesia by explaining insertion sites and warning them that they will temporarily lose sensory function. Injection is painful unless the health care provider first numbs the injection site. Prepare patients for such discomfort. Before a patient receives an anesthetic, assess for any medication allergies. Assess vital signs to monitor for systemic effects.

Epidural Analgesia. Epidural analgesia is a form of regional anesthesia and an effective therapy for the treatment of postoperative, labor and delivery, and chronic cancer pain. Epidural medications block transmission of pain stimuli in the spinal cord. Analgesia is short or long term, depending on a patient's condition and pain management needs. Short-term epidural analgesia is especially effective for pain after intrathoracic, abdominal, and orthopedic surgery. Long-term epidural therapy is effective for pain unresponsive to oral or parenteral medications. The advantages of epidural analgesia include the following:

- Production of excellent analgesia
- Occurrence of minimal sedation
- Long-lasting pain relief with fewer opioid doses
- Facilitation of early ambulation
- Avoidance of repeated injections
- No significant effect on sensation
- Little effect on blood pressure or heart rate
- Fewer pulmonary complications

Epidural analgesia is administered into the epidural space to block a group of sensory nerve fibers. It is administered through a catheter, which is usually placed in the operating room, postanesthesia care unit, or intensive care unit. The patient lies in the fetal position (lateral decubitus) to open the space between the vertebrae. The health care provider

administers a local anesthetic into the skin at the needle insertion site and then inserts a blunt-tip needle into the level of the vertebral interspace nearest to the area requiring analgesia (usually L4-L5). The health care provider advances a plastic catheter into the epidural space and then removes the needle (Fig. 34.8). The remainder of the catheter is secured with an occlusive dressing and taped up the back of the patient. A temporary catheter is sometimes connected to tubing positioned along the spine and over the patient's shoulder. You can place the end of the catheter on the patient's chest for easier access. Permanent catheters are tunneled through the skin and exit at the patient's side. Assessment of the insertion site and patency of the tubing are important nursing responsibilities (Pasero and McCaffery, 2011).

The epidural catheter is connected to a continuous epidural infusion pump, a port, or a reservoir, or it is capped for bolus injections. In many hospitals, only anesthesiologists or nurse anesthetists administer epidural anesthesia. Some institutions allow patients to deliver epidural analgesic doses (patient-controlled epidural analgesia [PCEA]) via a pump. To reduce the risk for accidental epidural injection of drugs intended for IV use, always place a brightly colored intermit-

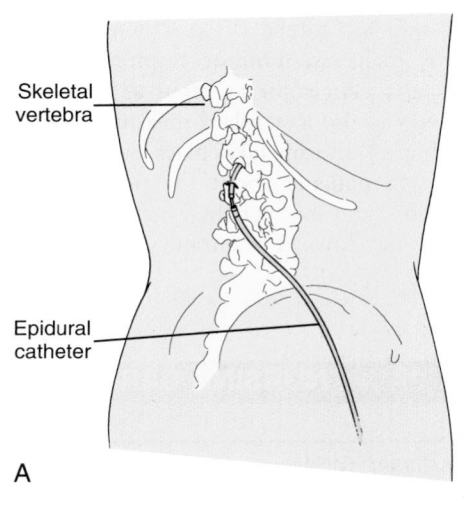

A

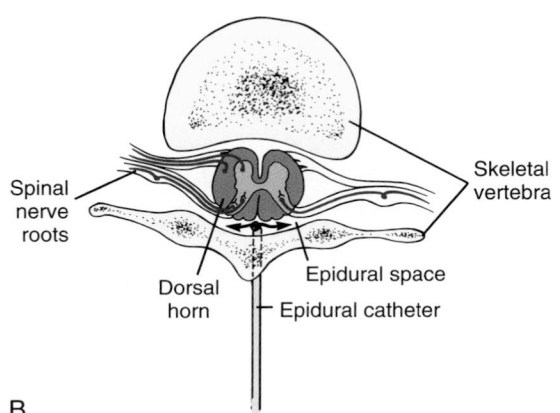

B

FIG 34.8 A, Epidural catheter inserted into L4-L5 space. **B,** Anatomical drawing of epidural space.

tent injection cap on the catheter tubing. You should label the catheter "epidural catheter" or use color-coded catheters and tubing to prevent accidental connections of IV tubing to the epidural catheter. Hospitals use tubing that has no access ports to minimize accidental introduction of IV medications. Administer continuous infusions through electronic infusion devices for proper control. Because of the catheter location, follow strict surgical aseptic technique when handling tubing to prevent a potentially fatal infection. Notify a health care provider immediately if any signs or symptoms of infection or pain at the insertion site develop (Pasero and McCaffery, 2011).

Medications used commonly for epidural analgesia include preservative-free solutions of morphine sulfate, hydromorphone, fentanyl, sufentanil citrate, bupivacaine, and clonidine. Sometimes your patient receives the combination of two of these solutions. *Do not administer supplemental doses of opioids or sedative/hypnotics because of possible additive central nervous system effects* (Pasero and McCaffery, 2011).

Table 34.4 summarizes nursing implications for managing epidural analgesia. Monitoring for drug effects differs, depending on whether infusions are intermittent or continuous. Some complications of epidural opioid use are respiratory depression (rare), nausea and vomiting, urinary retention, constipation, orthostatic hypotension, and pruritus (Pasero and McCaffery, 2011). When you start patients on epidural analgesia, monitor respiratory rate, respiratory effort, and skin color as often as every 15 minutes. Pulse oximetry is also a standard measurement. If a patient remains stable, monitoring takes place every hour (see agency policy). Inform patients about the potential for respiratory depression, and instruct them to notify you if breathing difficulty develops. If respiratory depression develops, turn off the infusion immediately and notify the health care provider.

Patients With Cancer Pain. Some cancer pain is intractable and difficult to treat. It becomes so debilitating that patients will try anything to gain relief. National Comprehensive Cancer Network (NCCN) guidelines promote treating cancer pain in a more comprehensive and aggressive manner, providing patients and family caregivers more options for pain relief. The best choice of treatment often changes when a patient's condition and the characteristics of pain change. Both nonpharmacological and pharmacological therapies are beneficial (NCCN, 2017).

Various medications and routes of administration provide relief for patients with cancer pain. Long-acting or controlled-release medications are very successful. These controlled-release medications (e.g., morphine [MS Contin, Roxanol SR], oxycodone [OxyContin]) relieve pain for 8 to 12 hours. A 72-hour fentanyl transdermal patch is also available. You can manage most cancer pain with oral or transdermal medications.

Administering analgesics to treat cancer-related pain requires applying principles different from the principles used to treat acute pain. The World Health Organization (WHO) recommends a three-step approach to managing cancer pain (Fig. 34.9) (Burchum and Rosenthal, 2016). Therapy begins with NSAIDs and/or adjuvants and progresses to strong opioids if pain persists. Side effects of opioids such as nausea and constipation are treated aggressively so that patients are able to continue using the opioids. Patients usually become tolerant to the side effects except for constipation. Health care providers should routinely order stimulant laxatives, not simple stool softeners, to prevent and treat constipation.

TABLE 34.4 NURSING CARE OF PATIENTS WITH EPIDURAL INFUSIONS	
GOAL	**ACTIONS**
Prevent catheter displacement	Secure catheter (if not connected to implanted reservoir) carefully to skin.
Maintain catheter function	Check external dressing around catheter site for dampness or discharge. (Leak of cerebrospinal fluid may develop.)
	Use transparent, adhesive dressing to aid inspection.
	Inspect catheter for breaks.
Prevent infection	Use aseptic technique when caring for catheter.
	Do *not* routinely change dressing over site.
	Change tubing every 24 hours or per agency policy.
Monitor for respiratory depression	Monitor vital signs, especially respirations, per policy.
	Use pulse oximetry and apnea monitoring when necessary.
	Maintain head of bed at 30 to 45 degrees.
Prevent undesirable complications	Assess for pruritus (itching) and nausea and vomiting.
	Administer antihistamines and antiemetics as ordered.
	Verify that tubing is connected to epidural catheter; label appropriately.
Maintain urinary and bowel function	Monitor intake and output.
	Assess bladder and bowel for distention.
	Assess for discomfort, frequency, and urgency.

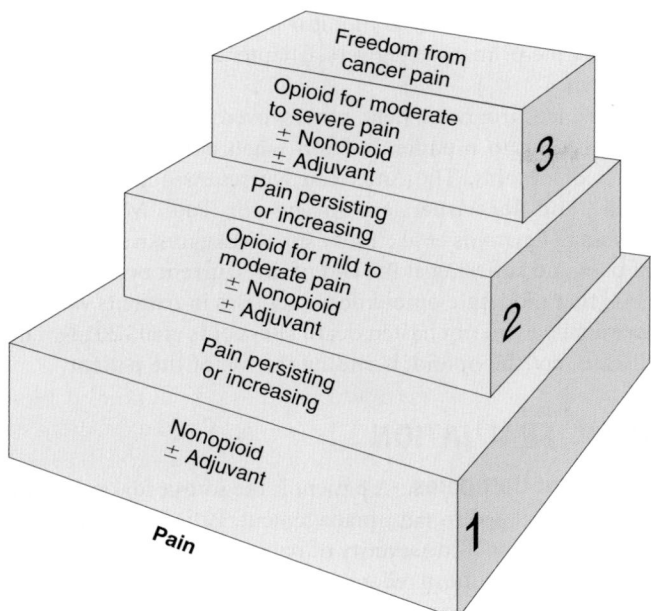

FIG 34.9 World Health Organization analgesic ladder is a three-step approach to treating cancer pain. (From http://www.who.int/cancer/palliative/painladder/en/.)

When a patient with cancer first has pain, it is best to begin with a higher dosage than what will be routinely needed. This provides a patient with immediate pain relief. The health care provider then slowly decreases the dosage to the amount that successfully controls pain. Patients receiving long-term opioids often develop a drug tolerance. Therefore they require higher dosages to attain pain relief. Higher dosages are not dangerous because most patients also develop tolerance to life-threatening side effects (Burchum and Rosenthal, 2016).

For patients with cancer, the aim of drug therapy is to anticipate and prevent or minimize pain. Therefore you give required analgesic dosages regularly, even when pain subsides. Regular administration maintains blood levels for ongoing pain control. However, patients still have flares of pain or "breakthrough pain" that require additional bolus doses of medication (rescue doses). Breakthrough pain is a transient flare of moderate-to-severe pain superimposed on continuous or persistent pain. A decrease in the duration of pain relief or an increase in the intensity of pain relief provided by the regular analgesia therapy and the need for an increased number of rescue doses are indications that a patient needs a higher opioid dose (Burchum and Rosenthal, 2016). A transmucosal fentanyl "unit" given buccally is available to treat breakthrough pain in opioid-tolerant patients.

Transdermal drug systems administer drugs via a patch placed on the skin. Patches are useful when patients are unable to take drugs orally. Self-adhesive patches deposit the opioid into the subcutaneous tissue. The subcutaneous tissue releases the drug slowly at predetermined rates for 72 hours.

This results in effective analgesia throughout the day and night. Inform patients that it sometimes takes 12 to 24 hours for analgesia to take effect when they first begin to use an analgesic patch (Burchum and Rosenthal, 2016). Therefore it is important for you to obtain an order for an immediate-release opioid for any breakthrough pain. Because heat causes more rapid drug absorption, warn patients to avoid external heat sources such as heating pads, hot showers, and prolonged exposure to the sun while using patches. Patients who have chronic stable pain are candidates for the fentanyl patch.

Another measure for treating severe persistent cancer pain is morphine given by continuous IV drip or intermittently by a PCA pump. Continuous infusions provide uniform pain control at lower dosages. Thus there are fewer side effects. Continuous-drip morphine is given in acute care settings and the home. An infusion control pump delivers morphine intravenously to ensure safe and accurate administration. Each agency has guidelines for morphine dose and infusion rates.

When a patient receives continuous-drip morphine, assess the IV site to ensure that it is patent and without complications (e.g., no redness, swelling, or drainage). A central line catheter such as a Groshong or Hickman catheter, an implanted venous access port, or a peripherally inserted central catheter (PICC) is usually best for long-term IV infusion. When a patient starts on continuous IV morphine, you need to monitor for and prevent overdose and central nervous system depression. Record baseline blood pressure and respiratory rates before the infusion begins. Monitor the patient frequently and closely per agency policy. If the patient's blood pressure or respirations decrease, reduce the infusion rate per the health care provider's order or agency policy. Small IV doses of naloxone can be ordered for severe respiratory depression and to increase respiratory rate and depth but not to reverse the pain relief. Patients who are placed on continuous analgesic infusions become opioid tolerant; thus respiratory depression is rare.

Restorative and Continuing Care. Patients in need of restorative care for pain usually have chronic persistent pain that is unrelenting. You continue to use nonpharmacological measures; however, additional pharmacological measures designed to give patients better long-term pain control are required. The goal is to use a comprehensive approach in supporting the patient and family.

Opioid Infusions. In the home or extended care settings, patients use ambulatory infusion pumps for opioid infusions. The pumps are lightweight and compact and allow free movement. A pump is battery powered and worn in a pouch attached to a belt or harness. The bag of parenteral fluid with medication fits inside the pump. A dose of opioid, delivered continuously over 24 hours, is slowly infused intravenously through a PICC or a central line catheter (see Chapter 18). Both catheters can be left in place for an extended period of time. Sometimes pain medication is infused subcutaneously with a small catheter that the patient inserts into subcutaneous tissue and replaces every 72 hours. The ambulatory pumps differ from PCA devices, which deliver only small, preset doses of medication. The patient and family caregiver learn to manage the pump, observe for drug side effects, and maintain function of the catheter that delivers the medication. Because the patient is managed initially on the opioid in the hospital before going home, the risk for side effects is not as great. A home care nurse routinely visits to be sure that patients and family caregivers manage the pump correctly.

Palliative Care. Palliative care offers treatments to help patients live perhaps years with a variety of incurable conditions including persistent pain. The goals of palliative care are to relieve suffering and support the best possible quality of life for patients with chronic and life-threatening conditions and their family members (ONS, 2016). Palliative care is not the same as end-of-life or hospice pain management.

Patients with chronic pain require a different approach to pain management than patients with acute pain. Health care providers cannot eliminate all pain, and learning to live with daily pain is difficult. It is important for patients with chronic pain to gain control of their pain versus allowing the pain to control them. Consider making a referral to the palliative care team when you care for patients diagnosed with incurable conditions that have persistent pain. These teams are composed of a variety of health care professionals who help patients achieve the level of pain control that allows them to function and enjoy life (ONS, 2016). The patient is an active participant in pain management. Without patient involvement, adequate pain control is not possible.

Hospice. Hospice programs care for patients who are terminally ill by helping them continue to live at home in comfort and privacy with the help of a health care team. The emphasis is on quality of life over quantity, and pain control is a priority. Under the guidance of hospice nurses,

family caregivers learn to monitor a patient's symptoms and become the primary caregivers. Chapter 27 discusses hospice in detail.

Hospice programs help nurses overcome their fears of contributing to a patient's death when administering large doses of opioids. The American Nurses Association (ANA, 2015) and the American Society for Pain Management Nursing (Reynolds et al., 2013) support aggressive treatment of pain and suffering at the end of life. Current evidence suggests that moderate opioid dose increases in patients who are terminally ill do not hasten death (Reynolds et al., 2013). The disease, not the opioid, is ending the life of the patient.

■■■ EVALUATION

Patient Outcomes. A patient is the source for evaluating outcomes related to pain management. Patients are the only ones who know if the severity of pain has lessened and which therapies bring most relief. To evaluate the effectiveness of nursing interventions, compare baseline pain assessments before treatments with ongoing evaluation findings during and after treatment. Similarly evaluate whether a patient's response to pain (e.g., positioning and body movements or ability to socialize or perform self-care) has changed (Box 34.12). Compare actual outcomes with expected outcomes to determine if your patient met his or her goal. Is the patient now able to perform the activities that pain had prevented? Continuous evaluation allows you to determine whether a patient needs new or revised therapies and interventions and if new nursing problems have developed. For example, if pain is not relieved to the patient's stated goal, does the medication, dose, or route need to be changed? If constipation results from use of opioids, you need to ensure that a bowel regimen is added to the plan of care. It is important to discuss a patient's ongoing pain management needs

---

BOX 34.12 EVALUATION

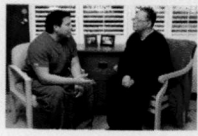

Two weeks after his last visit, Jim returns to evaluate Mrs. Ellis' progress. Her niece is visiting. Mrs. Ellis reports that she saw her health care provider, who prescribed an NSAID for her arthritis pain. She has not filled the prescription yet and is still taking her aspirin. She continues to have some gastrointestinal irritation after taking the aspirin. Jim has the chance to observe Mrs. Ellis use a warm compress on her hands and wrists. She applies the heat correctly, and the niece helps correctly. After 15 minutes Mrs. Ellis rates her pain on the FACES pain scale as 3. She states that the heat is soothing. During the visit Mrs. Ellis gets up to go to the kitchen using her walker, which she obtained from the physical therapist. Jim notes that although it takes her time to stand, her gait is steadier. He confirms that the niece can be called when Mrs. Ellis needs help at home. Mrs. Ellis shows

Jim that she has her niece's phone number posted in the kitchen next to the phone. She also states that her neighbor has offered to help with shopping.

DOCUMENTATION NOTE

"Reports receiving some pain relief from using moist heat on hands. Rates pain at level 3 on FACES pain scale after applying warm compresses. Niece is able to help correctly with procedure. Appears less fatigued and is ambulating with steadier gait using walker. Continues to have gastric irritation following use of aspirin. Identified her niece as one whom she can call when she needs assistance, and her neighbor will help with shopping. Recommended that she have her niece pick up NSAID prescription at pharmacy as soon as possible. Explained why she needs to replace aspirin with NSAID. Will evaluate effectiveness of NSAID at next visit in 2 weeks."

NSAID, nonsteroidal antiinflammatory drug.

with family caregivers and health care providers who will be involved in the patient's care after discharge or transfer.

Patient Expectations. Subtle behaviors such as a gentle smile or a sigh of relief indicate the level of a patient's satisfaction with pain relief. However, it is important for you to *ask* patients if you have met their expectations. Do not ask them if they are satisfied with their pain management because patients often answer "yes" even when their pain is severe. Instead say to a patient, "Tell me how well you think your pain medicine is helping you," or "You agreed to try relaxation to lessen your abdominal pain. Tell me, how has this worked for you?" If a patient's expectations have not been met, you need to spend more time understanding his or her desires. Working closely with a patient enables you to help the patient set realistic expectations that will be met within the limits of his or her condition and treatment plan. It is also important to review the current pain management plan and suggest changes as appropriate.

The Hospital Consumer Assessment of Healthcare Providers and Services (HCAHPS) survey is a national, standardized, publicly reported survey of patients' perspectives of hospital care. Data from the HCAHPS survey provide a standard for comparing hospitals. HCAHPS survey scores influence how hospitals are reimbursed by the Centers for Medicare and Medicaid Services (CMS). Two questions on the HCAHPS survey focus on patients' perceptions of how well hospital staff managed their pain (CMS, 2015). Hospitals, health care providers, and nurses use the results of HCAHPS surveys to evaluate their pain management practices. Poor or declining scores are analyzed for opportunities to improve current pain interventions.

SAFETY GUIDELINES FOR NURSING SKILLS

To ensure patient safety, communicate clearly with members of the health care team, assess and incorporate a patient's priorities of care and preferences, and use the best evidence when making decisions about your patient's care. When performing the skill in this chapter, remember the following points to ensure safe, individualized patient care:

- Be vigilant during the entire process of medication administration. Ensure that your patients receive the appropriate medications by following the six rights (see Chapter 17). Know why each medication is ordered for your patient, and explain the actions and side effects of the medication to your patient. Understand what you need to do before, during, and after medication administration. Evaluate the effectiveness and assess for adverse effects after your patients take their medications.
- Take care of yourself. You think as clearly and critically as possible if you are healthy. Healthy behaviors such as getting adequate sleep, making healthy food choices, and coping with stress in positive ways help you better process information and make safe decisions during medication administration.
- Set up and prepare medications in distraction-free areas.

SKILL 34.1 PATIENT-CONTROLLED ANALGESIA

View Video!

DELEGATION CONSIDERATIONS

The skill of administration of patient-controlled analgesia (PCA) cannot be delegated to nursing assistive personnel (NAP). The nurse directs the NAP to:

- Notify the nurse if the patient has a change in status including unrelieved pain or oversedation.
- Notify the nurse if the patient has questions about the PCA process or equipment.
- Never administer a PCA dose for the patient, and notify the nurse if anyone other than the patient is observed administering a dose for the patient.

EQUIPMENT

- PCA system and tubing
- Identification label and time tape (may come attached and completed by pharmacy)
- Needleless connector
- Alcohol swab
- Adhesive tape
- Clean gloves (when applicable)
- Equipment for vital signs and pulse oximeter, capnography (carbon dioxide) monitoring equipment

STEP	RATIONALE
ASSESSMENT	
1. Check accuracy and completeness of MAR or computer printout with health care provider's order for patient's name, name of medication, dose, frequency of medication (continuous or demand or both), and lockout period.	Health care provider order required for administration of opioid medication. Ensures patient receives right medications.
2. Check medical record for patient's history for drug allergies and typical reactions.	Avoids placing patient at risk for allergic reaction.

SKILL 34.1 PATIENT-CONTROLLED ANALGESIA—cont'd

View Video!

STEP	RATIONALE
3. Review medication information in drug reference manual or consult with pharmacist if uncertain about any medications to be administered.	Understanding medications before administering them prevents medication errors (Adhikari et al., 2014).
4. Perform hand hygiene. Assess severity and character of patient's pain. Use a standard pain scale. If patient is unable to provide a self-report, select an appropriate scale for assessing pain in patients who are nonverbal or not cognitively alert.	Reveals source and nature of pain and factors that may increase pain.
5. Assess environment for factors that could contribute to pain (e.g., noise, room temperature).	Elimination of irritating stimuli may help to reduce pain perception.
6. Assess for conditions that predispose patients to unwanted effects from opioids. Known, untreated, or unknown obstructive sleep apnea (OSA) poses a significant risk for respiratory depression Use the STOP-BANG questionnaire to assess for OSA (Lockhart et al., 2013) (see Chapter 33 and agency policy).	Assessment should be completed preoperatively by anesthesia. Identification allows treatment teams (surgeon, respiratory therapy, anesthesia) to take appropriate precautions such as making continuous positive airway pressure or bi-level positive airway pressure ventilation devices available.
7. Perform hand hygiene. Apply clean gloves. Assess patency of IV access and surrounding tissue for inflammation or swelling.	Reduces transmission of infection. IV line needs to be patent for safe administration of pain medication. Confirmation of placement of IV catheter and integrity of surrounding tissues ensures that medication is administered safely.
8. If patient had surgery, inspect incision while still wearing clean gloves. Gently palpate around area for tenderness. Use sterile gloves if necessary to place hand directly on incision. Remove gloves and perform hand hygiene.	Reveals evidence of tissue trauma or damage, which stimulates peripheral pain receptors to transmit impulses to cortex to create conscious awareness of pain.

Clinical Decision Point. Be aware that nausea is not an allergic reaction and it can be treated; pruritus alone is not an allergic reaction and is common to opioid use. Pruritus is treatable and does not rule out the use of PCA.

9. Assess patient's knowledge and perceived effectiveness of previous pain management strategies, especially previous PCA use.	Response to pain control strategies helps identify learning needs and affects patient's willingness to try therapy.

PLANNING

1. Collect appropriate equipment. Draw curtains around patient's bed or close door to room.	Aids in organization. Maintains patient privacy.
2. Prepare and organize equipment.	
3. Explain procedure to patient and family.	Reduces anxiety and fear.

IMPLEMENTATION

1. Perform hand hygiene.	Reduces transmission of infection.
2. Obtain PCA analgesic in cartridge prepared by pharmacy. Check label of medication against the MAR two times: when removing from storage and when preparing for assembly.	Follows the six rights of medication administration to be sure of correct medication. *This is the first and second check for accuracy.*
3. At the bedside, identify patient using at least two identifiers (e.g., name and birthday or name and medical record number) according to agency policy. Compare identifiers with information on patient's MAR or medical record.	Minimizes risk for medication error and harm to patient. Ensures correct patient. Complies with The Joint Commission standards and improves patient safety (TJC, 2018).
4. At the bedside, compare the MAR or computer printout with the name of medication on the drug cartridge. Have a second RN confirm health care provider's order and correct setup of the PCA. The second RN checks the order and the device independently and does not just look at existing setup.	Ensures the correct patient receives the right medication. *This is the third check for accuracy.*

STEP	RATIONALE
5. Before initiating analgesia, explain purpose and demonstrate function of PCA to patient and family as follows:	Allows patient participation in care and independence in pain control. Preoperative education about PCA therapy improves postoperative pain relief (Pasero and McCaffery, 2011).
a. Explain type of medication in device.	
b. Explain that device safely administers self-initiated small but frequent amounts of medication when needed to provide comfort and minimizes side effects from analgesia.	
c. Explain that self-dosing will aid in repositioning, walking, or coughing and deep breathing.	
d. Explain that device is programmed to deliver ordered type and dose of pain medication, lockout interval, and 1- to 4-hour dosage limits. Explain how lockout time prevents overdose.	
e. Demonstrate to patient how to push medication demand button (see illustration).	
f. Instruct patient to notify a nurse for possible side effects, problems in gaining pain relief, changes in severity or location of pain, alarm sounding, or questions.	
6. Apply clean gloves. Check infuser and patient-controlled module for accurate labeling or evidence of leaking.	Avoids medication error and injury to patient.
7. Position patient comfortably to be sure venipuncture or central line site is accessible.	Ensures unimpeded flow of infusion.
8. Insert drug cartridge into infusion device (see illustration) and prime tubing.	Locks system and prevents air from infusing into IV tubing.
9. Attach needleless adapter to tubing adapter of patient-controlled module.	Needed to connect with IV line.
10. Wipe injection port of maintenance IV line vigorously with alcohol or antiseptic for 15 seconds and allow to dry.	Minimizes entry of surface microorganisms during needle insertion, reducing risk of catheter-related bloodstream infection.
11. Insert needleless adapter into injection port nearest patient (at Y-site of peripheral IV or central line, or connect to its own IV site). There should not be a chance to use the PCA tubing for administering an IV push with another drug.	Establishes route for medication to enter main IV line. Needleless systems prevent needlestick injuries. Prevents medication interaction and incompatibility.

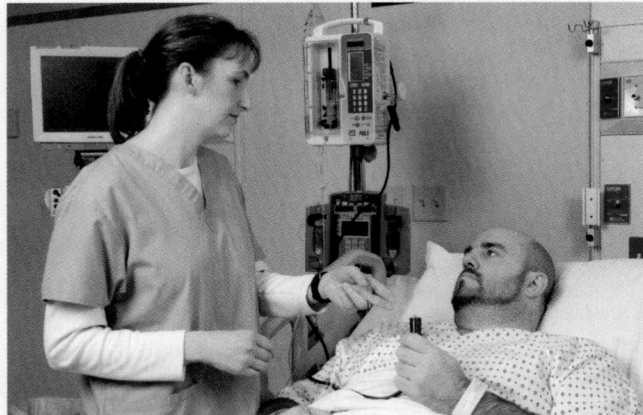

STEP 5e Patient learns how to press PCA device button.

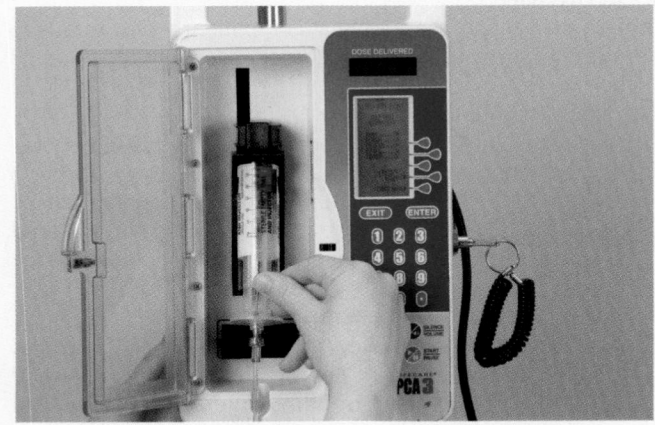

STEP 8 Nurse inserting drug cartridge into PCA device.

SKILL 34.1   PATIENT-CONTROLLED ANALGESIA—cont'd

View Video!

STEP	RATIONALE
12. Secure connection and anchor PCA tubing with tape. Label PCA tubing.	Prevents dislodging of needleless adapter from port. Facilitates patient's ability to ambulate. Label prevents error from connecting tubing from different device to PCA.
13. Program computerized PCA pump as ordered to deliver prescribed medication dose and lockout interval. Have second RN check setting. (**Note:** Recheck with oncoming RN during shift hand-off to ensure line reconciliation.)	Ensures safe, therapeutic drug administration. With appropriate dose intervals (e.g., 10 minutes), usually an appreciable analgesic effect and/or mild sedation is achieved before the patient can access the next dose, and thus there is a lower chance for oversedation and respiratory depression (Burchum and Rosenthal, 2016).
14. Administer loading dose of analgesia as prescribed. Manually give a one-time dose or turn on pump and program dose into pump.	Establishes initial level of analgesia.
15. Remove and discard gloves and supplies in appropriate containers. Dispose of empty cassette or syringe in compliance with institutional policy. Perform hand hygiene.	Reduces transmission of microorganisms. The Federal Controlled Substances Act regulates control and dispensation of opioids for all institutions.
16. If experiencing pain, have patient demonstrate use of PCA system; if not, have patient repeat instructions given earlier.	Repeating instructions reinforces learning. Checking patient's understanding through return demonstration helps you determine patient's level of understanding and ability to manipulate device.
17. Be sure venipuncture or central line site is protected, and recheck before leaving patient. Perform hand hygiene.	Ensures patency of IV line. Reduces transmission of infection.
18. **To discontinue PCA:**	
a. Check health care provider order for discontinuation. Obtain necessary PCA information from pump for documentation; note date, time, amount infused, and amount of drug wasted, and reason for wastage.	Ensures correct documentation of a schedule II drug. Two RNs must witness waste of opioids (narcotics) and document to meet requirements of the Controlled Substances Act for scheduled drugs. **Note:** Some agencies have a specific controlled substance disposal program (CSRx), which facilitates disposal of controlled substances in a safe, efficient manner and prevent diversion (check agency policy).
b. Perform hand hygiene and apply clean gloves. Turn pump off. Disconnect PCA tubing from primary IV line, but maintain IV access.	Reduces transmission of infection. Ensures continuation of IV.
c. Dispose of empty cartridge, tubing, and gloves according to agency policy. Perform hand hygiene.	

EVALUATION

1. Use pain rating scale to evaluate patient's pain intensity after treatments and procedures according to agency policy.	Determines response to PCA dosing. Documenting "PCA in use" or "PCA effective" is not an adequate record of patient's pain level.
2. Observe patient for nausea or pruritus.	Common side effects of opioid.
3. Monitor patient's level of sedation, vital signs, and pulse oximetry or capnography every 1 to 2 hours for the first 12 hours. Monitor more often at the start, during first 24 hours, and at night when hypoventilation and hypoxia tend to occur (Burchum and Rosenthal, 2016). Follow agency policy.	Patient is at highest risk the first 24 hours of use. Excess sedation (difficult to arouse) precedes respiratory depression.
4. Have patient demonstrate dose delivery.	Evaluates skill in use of PCA.
5. According to agency policy, evaluate number of attempts (number of times patient pushed the button), delivery of demand doses (number of times drug actually given and total amount of medication delivered in a particular time frame), and basal dose if ordered.	Assists in evaluating effectiveness of PCA dose and frequency in relieving pain. Maintains compliance with Controlled Substances Act.
6. Observe patient initiate self-care.	Demonstrates pain relief.

STEP	RATIONALE
7. **Use Teach-Back:** "I want to be sure I explained how PCA will help with your pain and how you should use the device. Explain to me how you should use the PCA device. What will you do if you find PCA is not relieving your pain?" Revise your instruction now or develop a plan for revised patient/family caregiver teaching if patient/family caregiver is not able to teach back correctly.	Determines patient's/family caregiver's level of understanding of instructional topic.

RECORDING AND REPORTING

- Record drug, concentration, dose (basal and/or demand), time started, lockout time, and amount of IV solution infused and remaining solution in nurses' notes in electronic health record (EHR) or chart. Many agencies have special PCA documentation forms.
- Document your evaluation of patient/family caregiver learning.

- Record regular assessment of patient response to analgesia on PCA medication form, in nurses' notes in EHR, on pain assessment flow sheet, or on other documentation according to agency policy. Assessment includes vital signs, oximetry or capnography, sedation status, pain rating, and status of vascular access site.

UNEXPECTED OUTCOMES AND RELATED INTERVENTIONS

- Patient verbalizes continued or worsening discomfort or displays nonverbal behaviors indicative of pain.
  - Perform complete pain reassessment.
  - Assess for possible complications other than pain.
  - Inspect IV site for possible catheter occlusion or infiltration.
  - Evaluate number of attempts and deliveries initiated by patient.
  - Check that maintenance IV fluid is running continuously.
  - Evaluate pump for operational problems.
  - Consult with health care provider.
- Patient is sedated and not easily aroused.
  - Stop PCA and notify health care provider.
  - Elevate head of bed 30 degrees unless contraindicated.
  - Instruct patient to take deep breaths.
  - Apply oxygen at 2 L/minute per nasal cannula (if ordered).

  - Assess vital signs.
  - Evaluate amount of opioid delivered within past 4 to 8 hours.
  - Ask family members if they pressed the button without patient's knowledge.
  - Review MAR for other possible sedating drugs.
  - Prepare to administer opioid-reversing agent.
  - Observe patient frequently (Burchum and Rosenthal, 2016).
- Patient is unable to manipulate PCA device to maintain pain control.
  - Consult with health care provider regarding alternative medication route or possibly a basal (continuous) dose.
  - If agency allows, determine if reliable family caregiver can responsibly manipulate PCA device (Pasero and McCaffery, 2011).

▌ KEY POINTS

- Acute pain, a protective mechanism that warns a person of tissue injury, is completely subjective.
- Misconceptions about pain lead to undertreatment.
- A patient's age, gender, anxiety, culture, previous experience, and meaning of pain influence the pain experience.
- The difference between acute and chronic pain involves the duration of discomfort, physical signs and symptoms, and the patient's perceptions regarding relief.
- A comprehensive assessment of a patient's pain must be performed to understand the extent to which pain affects the patient's ability to function.
- The patient's family and friends are a key resource in pain assessment.

- Eliminating sources of painful stimuli is a basic nursing measure for promoting comfort.
- Nonpharmacological therapies are effective in altering a patient's perception of pain, promoting muscle relaxation, and giving the patient control over pain.
- When administering opioids, know that respiratory depression is clinically significant only if there is a decrease in the rate and depth of respirations from a patient's baseline assessment. Give IV naloxone (Narcan) to reverse respiratory depression.
- For patients unable to self-report pain, be alert for subtle behaviors that indicate pain.
- Using a regular around-the-clock (ATC) schedule for analgesic administration is more effective than an as-needed schedule.

- A patient-controlled analgesia (PCA) device gives patients pain control with a low risk for overdose.
- Your primary role in caring for a patient who receives local anesthesia is to protect the patient from injury.
- The goal of therapy for patients with chronic pain is to anticipate and prevent pain.
- When a patient is receiving epidural analgesia, do not administer supplemental doses of opioids or sedatives because of possible additive central nervous system effects.

REFLECTIVE LEARNING

- Think about a patient you cared for who experienced pain. Was your assessment comprehensive?
- What pain medications were ordered for your patient, and how did you ensure the six rights of medication administration before administering them?
- Describe the monitoring you did and the side effects you observed for with the ordered medications. How did you determine if the patient's pain management plan was effective?

REVIEW QUESTIONS

1. A 79-year-old patient with a history of stroke 8 years ago resulting in aphasia (inability to verbally express thoughts) returns to the surgical unit after removal of a mass from his neck. The surgeon ordered pain medication every 4 hours as needed (prn) for postoperative pain. What should the nurse do next to help manage the patient's pain?
   1. Administer the pain medication every 4 hours around the clock
   2. Administer the pain medication when the patient becomes restless
   3. Wait until the patient verbalizes that he is experiencing pain to administer the pain medication
   4. Assess the patient's level of pain with the FACES pain scale

2. A nurse administered the first dose of an IV opioid to a patient who had surgery an hour ago. Which assessment finding requires immediate action by the nurse?
   1. Oxygen saturation of 95%
   2. Respiratory rate of 6 breaths/minute
   3. Heart rate 70 beats/minute
   4. Blood pressure 128/72 mm Hg

3. A patient is being discharged home on an around-the-clock opioid for chronic back pain. What additional medication would the nurse anticipate for this patient?
   1. Antihypertensive
   2. Antibiotic
   3. Laxative
   4. Stool softener

4. A patient was just admitted to your care after surgery. She states that her pain level is 6 on a 0-to-10 pain scale. She received a dose of IV pain medication 15 minutes ago. Which interventions may be beneficial for this patient at this time? (Select all that apply.)
   1. Reposition her for comfort.
   2. Massage her back.
   3. Tell her that she cannot have any more pain medication at this time because it is too soon.
   4. Take a few minutes to speak calmly with her to reduce her anxiety.
   5. Return to her room to reassess her pain when it is time for her next dose.

5. You receive a new order to administer morphine to your patient by patient-controlled analgesia (PCA). Arrange the steps for this procedure in the correct order.
   1. Explain to the patient how the PCA will help to control pain.
   2. Program the PCA pump to deliver medication dose and lockout time.
   3. Identify patient using at least two identifiers.
   4. Insert and secure needleless adapter into injection port nearest patient.
   5. Administer loading dose of morphine as ordered.
   6. Insert drug reservoir into pump and prime tubing.

evolve

Additional Review Questions, as well as rationales for all Review Questions, can be found on the Evolve website.

1. 4; 2. 2; 3. 3; 4. 1, 2, 4, 5; 5. 3, 1, 6, 4, 2, 5.

REFERENCES

Adhikari RJ, et al: A multi-disciplinary approach to medication safety and the implication for nursing education and practice, *Nurse Educ Today* 34(2):185, 2014.

Ali S, et al: An evidence-based approach to minimizing acute procedural pain in the emergency department and beyond, *Pediatr Emerg Care* 32(1):36, 2016.

American Nurses Association (ANA): *Code of ethics for nurses with interpretive statements*, 2015, http://www.nursingworld.org/MainMenuCategories/EthicsStandards/CodeofEthicsforNurses/Code-of-Ethics-For-Nurses.html.

Arthritis Foundation: *Arthritis medication*, n.d., http://www.arthritis.org/living-with-arthritis/treatments/medication/.

Beyer J, et al: The creation, validation, and continuing development of the Oucher: a measure of pain intensity in children, *J Pediatr Nurs* 7(5):335, 1992.

Burchum JR, Rosenthal LD: *Lehne's pharmacology for nursing care*, St Louis, 2016, Elsevier.

Centers for Medicare and Medicaid Services (CMS): *HCAHPS fact sheet*, 2015, http://

hcahpsonline.org/Files/HCAHPS_Fact_Sheet_June_2015.pdf.

Cheatle MD: Assessing suicide risk in patients with chronic pain and depression, *Current Pain Perspectives* 63(6):S6, 2014.

Chou R, et al: Guidelines on the management of postoperative pain, *J Pain* 17(2):131, 2016.

Cole LC, LoBiondo-Wood G: Music as an adjuvant therapy in control of pain and symptoms in hospitalized adults: a systematic review, *Pain Manag Nurs* 15(1):406, 2014.

Cooney MF, et al: American Society for Pain Management Nursing Position Statement with Clinical Practice Guidelines: authorized agent controlled analgesia, *Pain Manag Nurs* 14(3):176, 2013.

Dowell D, et al: CDC Guideline for prescribing opioids for chronic pain—United States, 2016, *MMWR Recomm Rep* 65(RR-1):1, 2016.

Herdman TH, Kamitsuru S: *NANDA International nursing diagnoses: definitions and classification, 2015-2017*, Oxford, 2014, Wiley Blackwell.

Huether SE, McCance KL: *Understanding pathophysiology*, St Louis, 2017, Elsevier.

Institute of Medicine (IOM): *Relieving pain in America: a blueprint for transforming prevention, care, education, and research*, Washington, DC, 2011, National Academies Press.

Krauss BS, et al: Current concepts in management of pain in children in the emergency department, *Lancet* 387:83, 2016.

Lewis SL, et al: *Medical-surgical nursing: assessment and management of clinical problems*, ed 9, St Louis, 2014, Elsevier.

Lockhart E, et al: Obstructive sleep apnea screening and postoperative mortality in a large surgical cohort, *Sleep Med* 14(5):407, 2013.

Mendell LM: Constructing and deconstructing the gate theory of pain, *Pain* 155(2):210, 2014.

National Cancer Institute (NCI): *Cancer pain (PDQ)–health profession version*, 2017, https://www.cancer.gov/about-cancer/treatment/side-effects/pain/pain-hp-pdq.

National Comprehensive Cancer Network (NCCN): *Adult cancer pain*, 2017, https://www.nccn.org/professionals/physician_gls/pdf/pain.pdf.

Oliver J, et al: American Society for Pain Management Nursing Position Statement: pain management in patients with substance use disorders, *Pain Manage Nurs* 13(3):169, 2012. Available at http://www.aspmn.org/documents/PainManagementinthePatientwithSubstanceUseDisorders_JPN.pdf.

Oncology Nursing Society (ONS): *Palliative care for people with cancer*, 2016, https://www.ons.org/advocacy-policy/positions/practice/palliative-care.

Oncology Nursing Society (ONS): *Cancer pain management*, 2017, https://www.ons.org/advocacy-policy/positions/practice/pain-management.

Pasero C, McCaffery M: *Pain assessment and pharmacologic management*, St Louis, 2011, Mosby.

Reynolds J, et al: American Society for Pain Management Nursing Position Statement: pain management at the end of life, *Pain Manag Nurs* 14(3):172, 2013.

Ruest S, Anderson A: Management of acute pediatric pain in the emergency department, *Curr Opin Pediatr* 28(3):298, 2016.

The Joint Commission (TJC): *Pain management*, 2017, https://www.jointcommission.org/topics/pain_management.aspx.

The Joint Commission (TJC): *2018 National Patient Safety Goals*, Oakbrook Terrace, IL, 2018, https://www.jointcommission.org/standards_information/npsgs.aspx.

Wong-Baker FACES Foundation: *Wong-Baker FACES Pain Rating Scale*, 2016, http://www.WongBakerFACES.org.

35

Nutrition

evolve MEDIA RESOURCES

http://evolve.elsevier.com/Potter/essentials
- Audio Glossary
- QSEN Activity and Review Questions Answers and Rationales
- Video Clip

OBJECTIVES

- Recognize the significance of essential nutrients in human nutrition.
- List the end products of digestion for carbohydrate, protein, and lipids.
- Describe the basic food groups and their use in planning meals for balanced nutrition.
- Explain the importance of a balance between energy intake and energy output.
- Summarize the dietary guidelines used in the United States.

- Discuss the major areas of nutrition assessment.
- Identify patients at risk for nutritional problems.
- Recognize a plan of care that meets the nutritional needs of a patient.
- Identify methods for feeding patients who require oral intake assistance.
- Describe the procedure for initiating and maintaining enteral tube feedings.
- Describe the procedure for initiating and maintaining parenteral nutrition.

KEY TERMS

amino acids, p. 973
anabolism, p. 975
anthropometry, p. 982
basal metabolic rate (BMR), p. 975
body mass index (BMI), p. 979
carbohydrates, p. 973
catabolism, p. 975
dietary reference intakes (DRIs), p. 975
dysphagia, p. 983
enteral nutrition (EN), p. 984

gluconeogenesis, p. 975
glycogenesis, p. 975
ideal body weight (IBW), p. 982
jejunostomy tube, p. 995
lipids, p. 974
medical nutrition therapy (MNT), p. 999
metabolism, p. 975
minerals, p. 974
monounsaturated fatty acids, p. 974
nitrogen balance, p. 974

nutrient, p. 973
omega-3 fatty acid, p. 974
omega-6 fatty acid, p. 974
parenteral nutrition (PN), p. 984
polyunsaturated fatty acids, p. 974
saturated fatty acids, p. 974
unsaturated fatty acids, p. 974
vitamins, p. 974
xerostomia, p. 982

Nutrition is a key component of health and is essential for normal growth and development, tissue maintenance and repair, cellular metabolism, and organ function. The human body needs an adequate supply of all nutrients for essential functions of cells.

Scientific principles regarding nutrition and the role of various nutrients in metabolism and health form a basis for the nutrition plan of care that you and the dietitian develop with your patients. Age, gender, activity level, medications, and disease processes all affect the use of nutrients and nutritional requirements.

CASE STUDY *Mrs. Gonzalez*

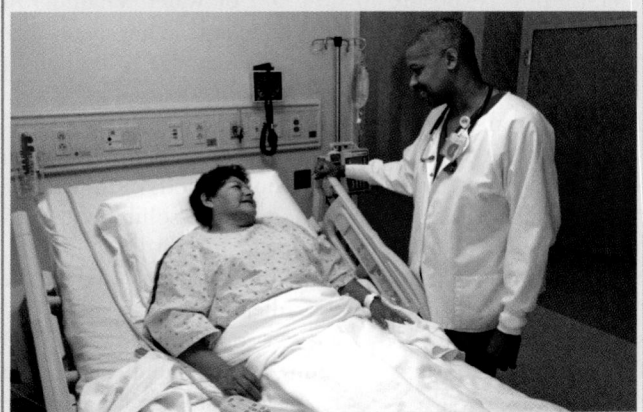

Mrs. Gonzalez is 65 years of age and came to the emergency department with slurred speech, right facial droop, and weakness in her upper and lower right-side extremities. She is admitted to the hospital with a diagnosis of acute stroke. Mrs. Gonzalez lives alone in a senior apartment complex. She has a daughter and two teenage grandchildren who live in another town nearby.

Mrs. Gonzalez is awake and alert and has drooping of the right side of her mouth. When she speaks, her voice sounds wet, and she has difficulty clearing her airway when she coughs. The physician ordered nothing by mouth (NPO) because Mrs. Gonzalez has trouble swallowing with oropharyngeal dysphagia. The evaluation by the speech-language pathologist (SLP) indicates inadequate clearance of food and liquid from the vocal folds and aspiration of thickened liquids. The SLP recommends enteral nutrition (EN) feedings and speech and swallowing therapy.

Matt is a nursing student assigned to Mrs. Gonzalez. As he prepares to assess her, he recalls information about the effect of dysphagia on nutrition and rehabilitation. He will begin by assessing Mrs. Gonzalez's current weight, weight history, diet history, and cultural customs. Matt knows to consult with a registered dietitian nutritionist (RDN) (also known as a registered dietitian [RD]) to assess Mrs. Gonzalez's nutrition status and help with nutrition interventions. Matt and the RDN will work as team members along with the SLP and physician to help Mrs. Gonzalez with her speech and swallowing rehabilitation.

Matt will begin the tube feedings for Mrs. Gonzalez after inserting a small-bore nasogastric (NG) feeding tube. The RDN outlines a feeding plan that will meet Mrs. Gonzalez's nutritional needs. Matt will continue to work with the RDN to prevent problems and monitor for safe and effective delivery of her EN feeding.

SCIENTIFIC KNOWLEDGE BASE

Principles of Nutrition

The body requires food to provide nutrients for growth and development, cellular metabolism, synthesis and repair of tissues, organ function, movement, and maintenance of body temperature. The gastrointestinal (GI) system allows for the nourishment of the body following food ingestion. Each organ or structure in the GI tract has a specific function aimed toward preparing food for the digestion and absorption of its nutrients.

Nutrients. A nutrient is a chemical substance that provides nourishment and affects metabolic and nutritive processes. The essential nutrients include carbohydrates, proteins, lipids, vitamins, minerals, and water. Only carbohydrates, proteins, and lipids provide energy and are thus known as the energy-yielding nutrients. Although not a *nutrient*, alcohol also provides energy. Vitamins and minerals serve as catalysts or coenzymes necessary for the use of nutrients for energy. Minerals and water regulate many body processes.

Carbohydrates. Carbohydrates are composed of carbon, hydrogen, and oxygen. They are starches and sugars obtained mainly from plant foods, with the exception of lactose, which is found only in milk of animal origin (e.g., cow's milk, goat milk). Carbohydrates provide 4 kilocalories per gram (kcal/g).

Fiber, a type of carbohydrate, is the structural part of plants and is sometimes called *nonstarch polysaccharides.* It also includes some nonpolysaccharides such as lignins and tannins. Human digestive enzymes cannot break down fiber. Therefore it does not contribute calorically to the diet. However, it does provide several benefits. Fiber is categorized as either soluble or insoluble. Soluble fiber becomes a gel in water and delays GI transit time; because of this, soluble fiber helps prevent diarrhea in patients receiving tube feedings. Insoluble fiber does not change in water and accelerates intestinal transit; this helps to prevent or relieve constipation.

Proteins. Amino acids are the building blocks of proteins and are made of hydrogen, oxygen, carbon, and nitrogen. They are vital for the synthesis of body tissue in growth, maintenance, and repair. The body synthesizes some amino acids. These are known as dispensable amino acids, meaning that they are *dispensable in the diet.* Amino acids that the body cannot synthesize are referred to as indispensable amino acids (formerly referred to as essential amino acids). Indispensable amino acids must be obtained from food sources. Protein can be used as a source of energy when carbohydrates and fatty acids are not available. Protein provides 4 kcal/g.

The required daily intake of protein (per kg of body weight) varies according to age and growth rates. For example, rapidly growing infants younger than 6 months of age require 2.2 g/kg daily. Adolescents require 1 g/kg daily. Most healthy adults require only about 0.8 g/kg of ideal body weight per day. Women who are pregnant or lactating need 25 g more than the usual daily need (Food and Nutrition Board [FNB], Institute of Medicine [IOM], 2002). Other factors that influence the body's need for protein include tissue repair, dietary quality of the protein consumed, and illness or disease state. For example, in patients with major burns, protein requirements often double or triple.

Protein is composed of 16% nitrogen. The body uses nitrogen for building, repairing, and replacement of body tissues. Nitrogen balance is achieved when nitrogen intake equals that of nitrogen output. When nitrogen intake is greater than output, the patient is in positive nitrogen balance. The body needs a positive nitrogen balance for growth (including pregnancy and muscle building) and wound healing. Negative nitrogen balance occurs when the output of nitrogen is greater than the intake. Negative nitrogen balance occurs in states of infection, sepsis, fever, burns, starvation, and trauma. Protein provides energy; however, because of the essential roles of protein, a balanced diet provides adequate kilocalories from nonprotein sources thus sparing protein from being used for energy. When there are insufficient carbohydrates in the diet to meet the energy needs of the body, protein stores are broken down and used for energy.

Fats. Fats (lipids) are insoluble in water but soluble in organic solvents such as ethanol and acetone. Fatty acids are the building blocks of fat. Lipids are a source of energy, providing 9 kcal/g.

Triglycerides are made up of three fatty acids attached to glycerol. Most lipids in foods and the human body are triglycerides. High blood levels of triglycerides in the blood are a risk factor for cardiovascular diseases.

Saturated fatty acids are saturated with as much hydrogen as they can hold. Monounsaturated fatty acids have a single double bond, and polyunsaturated fatty acids have two or more double bonds. Most animal fats have a high proportion of saturated fatty acids, whereas most vegetable fats have higher amounts of unsaturated fatty acids. For example, olive oil contains 14% saturated fatty acids, 77% monounsaturated fatty acids, and 9% polyunsaturated fatty acids. Trans fatty acids are created when vegetable oils are hydrogenated during food processing. The *2015–2020 Dietary Guidelines for Americans* recommends a diet low in both *trans* fats and saturated fats for optimal health (U.S. Department of Health and Human Services [USDHHS] and U.S. Department of Agriculture [USDA], 2015). Diets high in *trans* fats are associated with cardiovascular disease and mortality (de Souza et al., 2015).

The two essential fatty acids (EFAs) in human nutrition are linoleic acid (an omega-6 fatty acid) and linolenic acid (an omega-3 fatty acid). EFAs have many roles in the body, including producing cell membranes and hormones and regulating blood pressure, blood clot formation, and immune response. Studies indicate there is a reduction in cardiovascular disease risk when people replace dietary sources of saturated fats with polyunsaturated fats (Sanders, 2014).

Vitamins. Vitamins are organic substances present in small amounts in food and are essential for life. They generally serve as coenzymes or catalysts in cellular enzyme reactions. The body is unable to synthesize vitamins in adequate amounts and depends on regular dietary intake. The exception to this is vitamin K. A significant portion of the body's vitamin K needs is supplied by the bacteria found in the intestines; the rest is supplied by consuming dark, leafy green vegetables. Food processing, storage, and preparation all affect the bioavailability of vitamins. The bioavailability is usually highest in foods that are fresh and used quickly after minimal exposure to heat, air, or water. Vitamins A, C, and E are also important antioxidants. They neutralize *free radicals,* which produce oxidative damage to body cells and tissues.

Vitamins are categorized as either water-soluble or fat-soluble. Water-soluble vitamins (C and B complex vitamins) are stored in limited amounts for short periods of time in the body, requiring daily consumption. Water-soluble vitamins are absorbed easily from the GI tract.

Fat-soluble vitamins (A, D, E, and K) are stored in the body for longer periods; however, dietary intake is still necessary. In addition, the body produces some needed vitamin D through a series of steps beginning with sunlight exposure to the skin. Because the body has a high storage capacity for fat-soluble vitamins, toxicity is possible, particularly from excess supplementation. For this reason, always ask patients if they are taking supplements and in what quantities.

Minerals. Minerals are inorganic elements that catalyze biochemical reactions. They are classified as macrominerals when the daily requirement is 100 mg or more and microminerals or trace elements when the body needs less than 100 mg daily. Minerals have many functions and are required for most of the body's metabolic processes. Interactions occur among some minerals. For example, zinc absorption is inhibited with large doses of iron supplements.

Vitamins and minerals are best obtained from a healthy diet of varied food choices. When deficiencies exist, these nutrients can also be provided through supplementation. However, dietary supplements should not contain more than 100% of the recommended dietary allowance (RDA) for any nutrient unless specifically prescribed by a health care provider. Excessively high doses may be toxic.

Water. Normal cell function depends on an aqueous environment. Water is an essential nutrient with many functions in the body including transporting nutrients and waste products; providing a structure to large molecules (protein, glycogen); promoting metabolic reactions; serving as solvent, lubricant, and cushion; regulating body temperature; and maintaining blood volume.

Water makes up 60% to 70% of the total body weight. Infants have the greatest percentage of total body weight as water, and older adults have the least percentage of total body weight as water. Subsequently, infants and older adults are the most vulnerable to water deprivation and water loss. Muscle tissue is about 75% water, whereas fat tissue is only about 10% water. Thus a lean person contains a higher percentage of water in the body than an obese person does.

The human body requires approximately 1 to 1.5 mL of water for every kilocalorie of energy used (FNB, IOM, 2004). Ingesting liquids and solid foods such as fresh fruits and vegetables helps meet fluid needs. The body also produces water when food is oxidized during digestion.

Thirst is a protective mechanism that alerts an oriented person to the need for fluids. It is less reliable in infants and patients who are confused because they are unable to communicate that they are thirsty.

Digestion. The process of digestion begins in the mouth, where mastication, or chewing, breaks down food into smaller particles, and salivary amylase begins to digest starch. Mucus lubricates food particles for their passage through the esophagus into the stomach. Churning movements of the stomach mix food particles with hydrochloric acid. The acidic environment of the stomach deactivates salivary amylase. Gastric cells also release small amounts of gastric lipase (*tributyrinase*) to begin chemical digestion of fat. Most chemical digestion takes place in the small intestines, where a series of nutrient-specific enzymes break food particles into a simpler form.

Absorption. The small intestine is the primary site of nutrient absorption. It is lined with villi, which project into the lumen and greatly increase the surface area. The large intestine absorbs electrolytes and water. During bouts of increased intestinal motility (i.e., diarrhea), the nutrients move through the intestine too quickly for complete digestion or absorption of nutrients to take place.

Elimination. Intestinal contents move by peristaltic action into the large intestine. The body excretes unabsorbed nutrients as waste products. The end products of digestion include cellulose and similar fibrous substances that the body is unable to digest. The body also eliminates sloughed cells from the intestinal walls, mucus, digestive secretions, water, and microorganisms.

Metabolism. Metabolism refers to all bodily biochemical and physiological processes. Through metabolism, nutrients are converted into necessary substances required for cell function. The two types of metabolism are anabolism and catabolism. Anabolism is the building of more complex substances from smaller particles (e.g., synthesis of proteins from amino acids). Catabolism is the breakdown of large substances into simpler units (e.g., breaking down stored glycogen to yield individual units of glucose). Although catabolism produces some energy, both processes ultimately require energy, which must come from food or stored sources.

All macronutrients (carbohydrate, protein, and fat) produce chemical energy and maintain a dynamic balance of tissue buildup and breakdown. The chemical energy produced by metabolism is converted to other types of energy for use throughout the body. Muscle contraction uses mechanical energy, the nervous system uses electrical energy, and the mechanisms of heat production use thermal energy.

The major metabolic processes occur in the liver. The liver also regulates energy through its control of glucose metabolism. Glucose is the primary, and preferred, fuel for the body. Liver and muscle tissues store glucose in the form of glycogen via an anabolic process called glycogenesis. Lipogenesis is the anabolic process of converting excess energy from any macronutrient to fat for storage. Insulin and glucagon act as regulatory hormones to maintain blood glucose levels. Insulin promotes glucose use, and glucagon promotes glucose storage. During states in which glucose needs exceed glycogen

availability, the body breaks down fat and amino acids for conversion to glucose via a process called gluconeogenesis.

The basal metabolic rate (BMR) represents the energy needs of a person at complete physiological, mental, thermal, and emotional rest after awakening. Total energy needs are based on BMR plus energy needs for activity, energy required to break down food, and energy required for healing during illness. Energy balance occurs when energy intake equals energy output (or requirements). When energy intake is consistently less than energy needs (negative energy balance), a person loses weight. If energy intake consistently exceeds energy needs (positive energy balance), a person gains weight.

Storage. The body has a limited capacity to store carbohydrates as glycogen in the liver and muscle tissue for short-term energy needs. Remaining excess energy intake is stored as fat in adipose tissue. Protein is not stored; it is either used or converted to fat. When total energy demands exceed dietary sources, the body relies on stored energy (fat and glycogen). Fat-soluble vitamins are also stored in limited reserves (a few months), and the body releases them to meet the needs when dietary intake is insufficient. Most water-soluble vitamins are stored for only a few days.

Dietary Guidelines

Several agencies and organizations in the United States regularly publish and update dietary guidelines based on current scientific evidence. The guidelines change as nutrition researchers discover new knowledge.

Dietary Reference Intakes. In 1997 the Food and Nutrition Board of the National Institute of Medicine/National Academy of Sciences, in partnership with Health Canada, initiated the dietary reference intakes (DRIs) project. The DRIs are nutrient reference values that serve as a guide for good nutrition and provide the scientific basis for the development of food guidelines, such as the MyPlate Guidelines. There are four components to the DRIs: estimated average requirement (EAR), RDAs, adequate intakes (AIs), and tolerable upper intake levels (ULs). The EAR is the recommended amount of a nutrient that appears sufficient to maintain a specific body function for 50% of the population based on age and gender. The RDA is the average needs of 97.5% of the population, not the exact needs of an individual. The AI is the suggested intake for individuals based on observed or experimentally determined estimates of nutrient intakes by groups and is provided when there is insufficient evidence to set RDAs. The tolerable UL is the highest level that likely poses no risk for adverse health events. It is not a recommended level of intake (Institute of Medicine [IOM], n.d.).

MyPlate Guidelines and *2015–2020 Dietary Guidelines for Americans*. The U.S. Department of Agriculture (USDA) developed the ChooseMyPlate program (Fig. 35.1) to replace the food pyramid (USDA, n.d.). The MyPlate Guidelines help Americans choose healthier foods by providing a basic, visual guide for making food choices. The USDA also

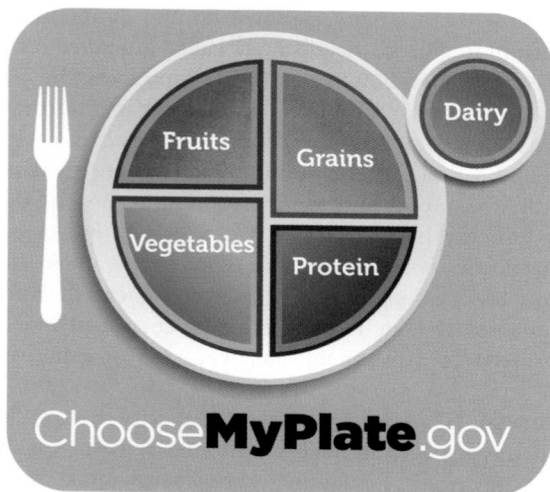

FIG 35.1 ChooseMyPlate. (From U.S. Department of Agriculture: ChooseMyPlate, 2011.)

developed educational tools that are freely accessible through their website (www.choosemyplate.gov). ChooseMyPlate and the *2015–2020 Dietary Guidelines for Americans* (USDHHS and USDA, 2015) place a strong emphasis on reducing calorie consumption and increasing physical activity to promote and maintain a healthy weight (Box 35.1). The *2015–2020 Dietary Guidelines* are intended for Americans older than 2 years of age. The Dietary Guidelines offer an excellent set of principles in the selection of food. To plan healthy diets, however, it is important to match the Dietary Guidelines with the food preferences of a specific individual and his or her cultural, socioeconomic, and personal inclinations.

Healthy People 2020. In 1997 the U.S. Department of Health and Human Services (USDHHS) and the Public Health Service (PHS) began a consensus process that establishes goals and objectives to promote health and reduce chronic disease related to diet and other lifestyle choices. The goals are updated every 10 years, and they are all available on the website at www.healthypeople.gov. The current initiative is titled *Healthy People 2020* with the aim of supporting "a society in which all people live long, healthy lives" (USDHHS, 2010). Box 35.2 provides some examples of the goals and objectives specific to nutrition. All health care professionals play a key role in promoting healthy dietary and lifestyle practices.

NURSING KNOWLEDGE BASE

There are sociological, cultural, psychological, and emotional aspects to eating and drinking in all societies. Holidays and events are celebrated with food, food is brought to individuals who are grieving, and food is used for medicinal purposes. There are cultural and religious food differences (Box 35.3). Food is incorporated into family traditions and rituals, and appearance is often associated with eating behaviors. An understanding of your patient's preferences, values, beliefs,

---

BOX 35.1   2015–2020 DIETARY GUIDELINES FOR AMERICANS

Summary Recommendations

FOLLOW A HEALTHY EATING PATTERN ACROSS THE LIFE SPAN
- All food and beverage choices matter.
- Choose a healthy eating pattern at an appropriate calorie level to help achieve and maintain a healthy body weight, support nutrient adequacy, and reduce the risk of chronic disease.
- A healthy eating pattern includes fruits, vegetables, protein, dairy, grains, and oils.
- A healthy eating pattern limits saturated fats and *trans* fats, added sugars, and sodium.

FOCUS ON VARIETY, NUTRIENT DENSITY, AND AMOUNT
- To meet nutrient needs within calorie limits, choose a variety of nutrient-dense foods across and within all food groups in recommended amounts.

LIMIT CALORIES FROM ADDED SUGARS AND SATURATED FATS AND REDUCE SODIUM INTAKE
- Consume an eating pattern low in added sugars, saturated fats, and sodium.
- Cut back on foods and beverages higher in these components to amounts that fit within healthy eating patterns.

SHIFT TO HEALTHIER FOOD AND BEVERAGE CHOICES
- Choose nutrient-dense foods and beverages across and within all food groups in place of less healthy choices.
- Consider cultural and personal preferences to make these shifts easier to accomplish and maintain.

SUPPORT HEALTHY EATING PATTERNS FOR ALL
- Everyone has a role in helping to create and support healthy eating patterns in multiple settings nationwide, from home to school to work to communities.

Data from U.S. Department of Health and Human Services (USDHHS) and U.S. Department of Agriculture (USDA): *2015-2020 dietary guidelines for Americans,* ed 8, 2015, https://health.gov/dietaryguidelines/2015/.

---

and attitudes about food and how those values affect food purchase, preparation, and intake will allow you to better support your patients in making healthy food choices.

Nutritional requirements depend on many factors. Individual caloric and nutrient requirements vary by stage of development, body composition, activity levels, conditions such as pregnancy and lactation, and the presence of disease. RDNs may use predictive equations that consider each of these factors as a starting point for estimating a patient's nutritional requirements.

Alternative Food Patterns

Individuals' patterns of food intake are based on religion, cultural background, ethics, health beliefs, concern about the environment, or any number of other reasons. A patient's

BOX 35.2 EXAMPLES OF FOOD AND NUTRITION OBJECTIVES FOR HEALTHY PEOPLE 2020

WEIGHT STATUS

- Increase proportion of adults who are at a healthy weight (BMI 18.5 to 24.9 kg/m²)
- Reduce proportion of adults who are obese
- Reduce proportion of children and adolescents 2 to 19 years of age who are obese
- Prevent inappropriate weight gain in youth and adults

FOOD AND NUTRIENT CONSUMPTION

- Increase contribution of fruits to diets of population 2 years of age and older
- Increase variety and contribution of vegetables to diets of population 2 years of age and older
- Increase contribution of whole grains to diets of population 2 years of age and older
- Reduce consumption of calories from solid fats and added sugars in population 2 years of age and older
- Reduce consumption of saturated fat in population 2 years of age and older
- Reduce consumption of sodium in population 2 years of age and older
- Increase consumption of calcium in population 2 years of age and older

IRON DEFICIENCY AND ANEMIA

- Reduce iron deficiency among young children and women of childbearing age
- Reduce iron deficiency among pregnant women

HEALTHIER FOOD ACCESS

- Increase number of states with nutrition standards for foods and beverages provided to preschool-age children in child care
- Increase proportion of schools that offer nutritious foods and beverages outside of school meals
- Increase number of states that have state-level policies that incentivize food retail outlets to provide foods that are encouraged by the *Dietary Guidelines for Americans*

FOOD INSECURITY

- Eliminate very low food security among children
- Reduce household food insecurity and in doing so reduce hunger

FOOD SAFETY

- Reduce infections caused by key pathogens transmitted commonly through food
- Reduce number of outbreak-associated infections caused by Shiga toxin–producing *Escherichia coli* O157 or *Campylobacter, Listeria,* or *Salmonella* species associated with food commodity groups
- Reduce severe allergic reactions to food among adults with food allergy diagnosis
- Increase proportion of consumers who follow key food safety practices

Data from U.S. Department of Health and Human Services (USDHHS): *Healthy people 2020,* Washington, DC, 2010, U.S. Government Printing Office, www.healthypeople.gov/2020/topics-objectives.

⊕ BOX 35.3 PATIENT-CENTERED CARE

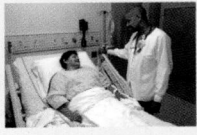

Matt reads about the influence of culture on an individual's nutrition status and choices. This includes ethnic food preferences; personal meaning of certain foods; availability of food by geographical area; economic resources for food preferences; and social norms that influence when, what, and how much a person eats. Foods often have symbolic meanings and are associated with births, deaths, religion, and social occasions. Special ethnic dishes or foods are served at ceremonies, holidays, and family celebrations. Recipes for these special dishes or foods are passed from generation to generation. Regular use of traditional foods is seen more frequently in older members of a family than in younger members. Younger family members use these foods more on holidays or for special events.

Matt wants to know more about Mrs. Gonzalez's food preferences and eating patterns. Eventually she will return to oral feeding as her swallowing becomes safer. He learns from her family that they typically get their protein from dry beans, cheeses, meats, fish, and eggs. Their grain intake is generally

corn made into tamales and tortillas. Rice and wheat products supply additional carbohydrates and fiber. They frequently eat chili peppers and deep-green and yellow vegetables along with a variety of fruits such as guava, papaya, mango, and other citrus fruits. Matt and the dietitian identify foods that Mrs. Gonzalez enjoys that will help provide a balanced diet as her ability to swallow improves.

IMPLICATIONS FOR PRACTICE

- Matt asks Mrs. Gonzalez about food she likes to prepare and serve at home and gathers input from her daughter as well.
- Matt identifies fluids that Mrs. Gonzalez enjoys despite the current need to thicken them.
- Matt works with the dietitian to incorporate some of Mrs. Gonzalez's favorite foods into her diet within the guidelines of her restrictions.
- Matt helps Mrs. Gonzalez identify ways to decrease fat intake and increase vegetables and fruit in her daily meals to ensure that she receives a well-balanced diet.

food preferences and choices may not meet nutrition recommendations based on ChooseMyPlate or the Dietary Guidelines for Americans. Optimal nutrition intake depends on balanced consumption of all required nutrients. The vegetarian diet is an example of a dietary pattern that is commonly consumed because of religious beliefs or personal preferences. There are several types of vegetarian diets, which are primarily plant based and eliminate many animal-based foods. Ovolactovegetarians avoid meat, fish, and poultry but eat eggs and milk products. Lactovegetarians consume milk and milk products but avoid eggs and other animal-based foods. Ovovegetarians consume egg products but avoid all other animal-based foods. Vegans eat only foods of plant origin. Individuals consuming a vegan diet are more susceptible to vitamin B_{12} deficiency, as this vitamin is found only in animal products. However, with the abundance of fortified and enriched plant-based foods (e.g., B_{12} and calcium fortified plant-based milk), it is not a limitation to this diet. Vegans consuming a comprehensive vegan diet score higher on the Healthy Eating Index compared with those who eat vegetarian diets (Clarys et al., 2014).

Developmental Needs

Infants Through School Age. Infancy is marked by rapid growth requiring high protein, vitamin, mineral, and energy availability. Infants need an energy intake of approximately 108 kcal/kg of body weight in the first half of infancy and 98 kcal/kg in the second half (FNB, IOM, 2002). Infants from birth to 12 months of age need approximately 700 to 800 mL/day of fluid because a large portion of total body weight is water (FNB, IOM, 2004).

Breastfeeding. The American Academy of Pediatrics (AAP), World Health Organization (WHO), and Institute of Medicine (IOM) recommend exclusive breastfeeding for approximately 6 months, with the continuation of breastfeeding for at least 1 year or as long as mutually desired by mother and infant (AAP, 2012). The benefits include an enhanced immune system, reduced food allergies and intolerances, reduced infant morbidity and mortality, and easier digestion. In addition, breast milk is convenient, fresh, always the correct temperature, and economical. Breastfeeding provides increased time for mother and infant bonding.

Breast Milk Substitutes. Commercially available infant formulas contain the approximate nutrient composition of human milk and are an acceptable alternative. Infants should not have regular cow's milk during the first year of life. Cow's milk does not meet infants' nutrient needs and has excessive sodium, potassium, and protein. Such high solute loads are dangerous to an infant's GI tract and renal system.

Introduction to Solid Food. Breast milk, or breast milk substitute, remains the major source of nutrition throughout the entire first year of life. However, the nutrient needs and physiological development of the infant warrants the introduction of solid foods to the basic diet of breast milk beginning around 6 months of age. Iron-fortified cereals are usually the first semisolid food introduced and are an important nonmilk source of protein and iron. Ideally, new foods are introduced one at a time, approximately 4 to 7 days apart, to identify and remove any allergens from the diet. Teach your patients to introduce new foods immediately before giving milk to increase acceptance and avoid satiety. Honey and corn syrup are potential sources of botulism toxin and should not be used in an infant's diet before the age of 1 year.

The growth rate slows during toddler years, requiring fewer kilocalories per kg of body weight. Toddlers are naturally intuitive eaters, and their appetite reflects these changing energy needs. Toddlers often exhibit strong food preferences and may become picky eaters. They are not able to consume enough volume of food to meet their nutrient needs in only three meals per day. Snacks are an important part of the overall diet for toddlers and should consist of high–nutrient density foods to help improve the quality of the diet. Data from *What We Eat in America* indicates that snacks provide 30% of total energy, 22% of protein intake, and about 25% of all vitamins and minerals in the diets of children 2 to 5 years of age (USDA Agricultural Research Service [ARS], 2014).

Toddlers (over 1 year of age) should drink full-fat milk or a milk substitute until the age of 2 years to ensure adequate intake of fatty acids necessary for brain and neurological development. Certain foods such as hot dogs, hard candy, nuts, grapes, chopped raw vegetables, and popcorn increase the risk for choking and should be avoided or consumed only with supervision. Preschoolers' (3 to 5 years of age) dietary requirements are similar to those of toddlers. They consume slightly more volume than toddlers, and nutrient density continues to be a very important aspect of their diet.

School-age children (6 to 12 years of age) grow at a slower and steadier rate, with a gradual decline in energy requirements per unit of body weight. Despite the better appetites and more diverse food intake of school-age children, you still need to assess their diets carefully for balance and variety. There is no room for excess intake of empty calories at this age. The intake of sugar-sweetened beverages prevents the intake of nutrient-dense foods and beverages. Although there are many contributing factors to obesity, diet and lifestyle are two readily modifiable factors. Researchers continue to find that the key to childhood obesity prevention is to increase current levels of physical activity and ensure a well-balanced diet for children (Wang et al., 2015; Kumar and Kelly, 2017).

Adolescents. Throughout the adolescent years, energy and protein requirements increase to meet greater metabolic demands of growth. Calcium is essential for rapid bone growth, and girls need a continuous source of iron to replace menstrual losses. Boys also need adequate iron for muscle development. B-complex vitamins are necessary to support heightened metabolic activity. Figure-conscious adolescents are susceptible to dieting, meal skipping, and subsequent nutrient deficiencies during the period of puberty and body changes. In extreme circumstances, eating disorders can develop. Snacks continue to be an important source of nutrient intake for teenagers, providing approximately 25% of their total dietary intake (USDA ARS, 2014). Fast food is commonly eaten during this stage of life and adds excess salt, fat, and often "empty" kilocalories.

Young and Middle-Age Adults. Adults need nutrients for energy, maintenance, and tissue repair. Energy needs usually decline over the years along with the metabolic rate. Adults who do not adjust their energy intake in response to a slowing metabolism will likely gain weight. Obesity is one of the most significant health care problems in the United States with 69.5% of adults (older than 20 years of age) currently overweight or obese (as defined by a body mass index [BMI] 25 kg/m² or higher) (National Center for Health Statistics [NCHS], 2016).

Pregnancy. Poor nutrition and inadequate maternal weight gain during pregnancy contribute to low birth weight in infants, preterm birth, and poor pregnancy outcomes (Han et al., 2011). The nutrition status of a mother at the time of conception is critically important to the developing embryo. Energy requirements during pregnancy are related to the mother's body weight, activity level, and stage of pregnancy. On average, a pregnant woman needs 15% to 20% more kilocalories than she needs when not pregnant. This is equal to approximately 340 kcal/day extra beginning in the second trimester and 450 kcal/day extra during the third trimester (FNB, IOM, 2002). Protein requirements throughout pregnancy increase by 25 g over nonpregnancy needs (FNB, IOM, 2002). Iron needs increase dramatically during pregnancy to provide for increased maternal blood volume, fetal blood storage, and blood loss during delivery. Most women benefit from taking supplemental iron.

The active form of folate, tetrahydrofolic acid, is particularly important for DNA synthesis and cell division. Inadequate intake is associated with increased risk of neural tube defects such as spina bifida and anencephaly (Copp and Greene, 2013). It is recommended that all women of childbearing age consume 400 mcg of folic acid daily, increasing to 600 mcg daily during pregnancy (FNB, IOM 1998).

Lactation. A woman needs an additional 330 to 400 kcal/day and 25 g of protein above her usual requirements to meet the nutrient demands of milk production (FNB, IOM, 2002). The increase in food consumption usually meets the increased needs for most vitamins and minerals. Women who are breastfeeding should drink about 3 L of fluid daily while limiting caffeine and avoiding alcohol and drugs because they are excreted in the breast milk. Remind women to talk with their health care provider about prescription drugs that may be excreted in breast milk.

Older Adults. Adults 65 years of age and older have similar needs for vitamins and minerals as younger adults but a decreased need for calories because of a slowing metabolic rate. This makes it even more important that older adults have well-balanced diets and ingest foods with high nutritional value. Numerous physiological and socioeconomic factors influence the nutrition status of older adults. For example, living on a fixed income may limit funds available to purchase food. Older adults are more likely to have a chronic disease that requires a therapeutic diet and medications and increases the risk for drug-nutrient interactions. They may have difficulty eating because of physical symptoms, lack of teeth, or dentures. Changes in cognition may limit an older adult's ability to select nutritious foods and to prepare meals. Some older adults need a vitamin and mineral supplement (Box 35.4).

The Administration on Aging, part of the Administration for Community Living (ACL) in the USDHHS (ACL, 2017) requires states to provide nutrition screening services for

---

BOX 35.4 CARE OF THE OLDER ADULT

Dietary Teaching

- Eat a balanced diet that contains a variety of foods. Avoid too much fat, cholesterol, sugar, and sodium.
- Eat foods that have adequate amounts of starch and fiber such as fruits and vegetables and whole-grain cereals and breads.
- Consult with a pharmacist about the potential for medication and food-nutrient interactions.
- Drink adequate fluids because the thirst sensation diminishes with age. Water requirements do not decrease with age.
- If unable to eat meat because of cost or difficulty chewing, find alternative sources of protein.
  - Cream soups and meat-based vegetable soups are nutrient-dense sources of protein.
  - Cheese, eggs, and peanut butter are also useful high-protein alternatives.
- Drink milk or fortified milk-substitute products for calcium and vitamin D to protect against osteoporosis. Provide calcium supplements if lactose intolerance is present or the patient declines to consume fortified milk-substitute products (e.g., soy milk, rice milk, almond milk).
- Take vitamin and nutrient supplements as recommended.

---

older adults who use home-delivered meal services. Adults with chronic illnesses have additional nutritional risks, especially if they live alone with few or no social or financial resources to help them obtain or prepare nutritionally sound meals. Vigilant nutrition screening by a home-health nurse provides early recognition of potential nutrient deficiencies and necessary interventions.

Overweight and Obesity

The problems associated with obesity are at epidemic levels in the United States. From 1998 to 2014, the number of adults who are obese increased from 22.9% to 36.4% of the population (NCHS, 2016). A combination of factors contributes to obesity including energy imbalance, lifestyle choices, genetics, socioeconomic disparities, and inadequate health care. **Body mass index (BMI)** is a reliable indicator of health based on weight status. BMI is calculated by dividing weight in kilograms (kg) by height in meters squared (m²). A BMI range of 18.5 to 24.9 kg/m² is associated with optimal health. A BMI greater than 24.9 is classified as overweight, and a BMI greater than 29.9 is classified as obese. On average, individuals who are obese die about 10 years earlier than individuals with a BMI in the optimal range because of various weight-related chronic diseases (Greenberg, 2013).

As with adults, the prevalence of overweight and obesity in children has drastically increased over the past several decades. In the United States, 17.5% of children 6 to 11 years of age are classified as obese, and 20.5% of adolescents 12 to 19 years of age are obese (NCHS, 2016). Childhood obesity contributes to costly medical problems related to the early development of chronic diseases such as type 2 diabetes mellitus, hypertension, dyslipidemia, obstructive sleep apnea, and nonalcoholic fatty liver disease (Kumar and Kelly, 2017). Prevention of childhood obesity is considered the best approach to reverse this trend. Childhood obesity is a strong predictor of adult obesity, and family education is an important component of decreasing the prevalence of this chronic disease. As a health care provider, teach about and encourage healthy food choices and eating in moderation along with increased physical activity in your patients.

CRITICAL THINKING

Synthesis

Patient care requires you to apply what you know about a patient, your knowledge base, experience, and critical thinking attitudes and standards. Your synthesis of this information allows you to make sound decisions as you apply the nursing process. Critical thinking synthesis involves combining all available information to obtain a clear picture needed to provide patient-centered care (Box 35.5).

Knowledge. Application of knowledge from nutrition principles and the basic and social sciences form your knowledge base related to nutrition care. Information that comes from interviewing and observing a patient and the responses you obtain during nursing interventions guide you toward application of knowledge. For example, your patient avoids cabbage. Possible reasons may include physiological discomfort (gas-forming food), psychological issues (forced to eat cabbage as a child), sociological reasons (associated with lower socioeconomic class), ethnicity (not readily available in the country of origin), teaching-related or learning-related reasons (never taught how to prepare cabbage), or mythology (a food that contains harmful chemicals). Consider these factors when helping your patient to plan a nutritious diet.

Experience. Multiple factors influence dietary patterns. In helping a patient change dietary patterns, draw on examples from your own experience (either personal experience or from past patients). Perhaps you attempted to change a dietary practice or have a family member who requires a special diet. Previous experiences with therapeutic diets or behavioral changes help you identify nursing interventions that may be successful for the patient.

Attitudes. Use the critical thinking skills of integrity and discipline during nutrition assessment and counseling. Although you will likely encounter patients whose dietary practices are different from yours, your role is to help patients attain a nutritionally balanced diet. You will also care for patients whose dietary patterns are not ideal. Changes in dietary practices occur over time. Perseverance is necessary in educating patients to understand the impact of unhealthy food choices.

Standards. The use of standards such as DRIs, the USDA MyPlate Guidelines, *2015–2020 Dietary Guidelines for*

BOX 35.5 SYNTHESIS IN PRACTICE

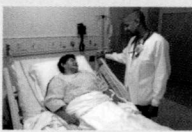

As Matt prepares to assess Mrs. Gonzalez, he recalls information about nutrition and its effect on rehabilitation, especially the importance of adequate calorie, protein, and fluid intake in patients who have had a stroke. He focuses on Mrs. Gonzalez's need for adequate nutrition, which for now is safely delivered via an enteral feeding tube, and he monitors her tolerance of the therapy. He wants to ensure that enteral nutrition is providing the energy she needs to heal and adequately rehabilitate to come as close to her norm as possible. He collaborates with a registered dietitian nutritionist to make sure that the regimen is meeting Mrs. Gonzalez's needs for essential nutrients.

Matt visits with the speech-language pathologist to assess the progress Mrs. Gonzalez is making in terms of swallowing safely. He explores whether it is expected that she will be able to resume oral intake soon or whether longer-term enteral feeding through a gastrostomy tube will be needed. A video swallow study demonstrates safe swallowing of a dysphagia diet with nectar-thick liquids. Matt acknowledges that Mrs. Gonzalez has little interest in oral intake; therefore he explores with her foods that she finds appealing and is interested in trying. Experience has taught Matt that economic and cultural preferences influence food choices. He is aware that Mrs. Gonzalez may not receive the fluid she needs as her fluids must be thickened for her safety in swallowing. Matt also knows that as the tube feeding is decreased and oral intake improves, Mrs. Gonzalez may still need to have fluid delivered via her feeding tube to make sure that she receives adequate fluid.

Americans, and the *Healthy People 2020* objectives provide general guidelines for assessing a patient's nutrition status. Other nutrition standards are also available from professional organizations such as the Academy of Nutrition and Dietetics, American Heart Association, American Diabetes Association, American Cancer Society, and American Society for Parenteral and Enteral Nutrition. These standards are evidence-based and are updated from new research findings.

NURSING PROCESS

■■■ ASSESSMENT

Screening. Nutrition screening is part of your initial assessment of a patient. Standardized nutrition screening tools are a quick method of identifying malnutrition. Nutrition screening tools commonly include objective measures such as age, BMI, weight change, and the presence of acute disease. A single objective measure alone does not predict a person's nutritional risk. Combine multiple objective and subjective measures related to nutrition to screen for nutritional risk. Health care institutions commonly use the initial nursing assessment as a nutrition screening. Certain nutritional risk factors such as unintentional weight loss, a modified diet, or the presence of GI symptoms (i.e., nausea, vomiting, diarrhea, constipation) are triggers for a nutrition consultation.

Several standardized nutrition screening tools are available to use in the inpatient and outpatient setting. One example is the Malnutrition Universal Screening Tool (MUST), a validated clinical method that uses current BMI, unintentional weight loss, and the presence of compromised nutrient intake for more than 5 days because of acute disease. The MUST is a simple, inexpensive tool that highly correlates to the medical diagnostic criteria for malnutrition (Poulia et al., 2017).

Nutrition Assessment. Refer patients at risk for nutritional problems to an RDN for a more in-depth nutrition assessment. Nutrition assessment is different from nutrition screening. The RDN completes a nutrition assessment, which includes an in-depth exploration of medical history, dietary history, physical examination, anthropometric measurements, and laboratory data (Table 35.1). Nutrition assessment determines nutrient and energy needs. In an acute care setting the RDN is available to make these calculations. In an outpatient setting, make a referral if an RDN is not available on-site.

Diet History. A diet history focuses on usual intake of food and liquids along with information about preferences, allergies, and digestive problems (Box 35.6). Open-ended questions encourage a patient to provide more information on food intake during the interview. For example, ask a patient who reports avoiding dairy products, "Tell me what led you to avoid dairy products?" The patient's answer to this question leads to physiological, psychological, sociological, religious, cultural, or food preference factors that you can further explore.

When indicated, the RDN will ask the patient to keep a detailed record of food intake over 3 days, including one weekend day, to determine a typical eating pattern and whether routine intake meets nutrient DRIs. The 3-day food record requires the use of measuring cups and scales. Instruct your patients to record the specific type of foods and the exact amounts ingested. Information on a patient's activity level and the presence of disease is necessary to estimate energy needs. For example, a patient who has a fever or has experienced severe trauma has high caloric demands, even though the activity level is limited. Estimated energy need, as calculated through prediction equations, is compared with actual caloric intake, obtained through calorie counts. A calorie count uses records of observed amounts of food consumed from a patient's meal trays as documented by the nursing or nutrition staff to estimate total calories and protein consumed daily. Consult with an RDN to determine a calorie count or energy requirements.

Medication History. Prescribed and over-the-counter medications have the potential for drug-nutrient interactions. Consultation with a pharmacist determines the specific risks for nutrient-drug interactions for your patients.

TABLE 35.1 FOCUSED PATIENT ASSESSMENT

FACTORS TO ASSESS	QUESTIONS	PHYSICAL ASSESSMENT
Food and nutrient intake	How many meals and snacks a day do you eat? What times do you normally eat meals and snacks? What portion sizes do you eat at each meal? Are you on a special diet because of a health problem? Who purchases and prepares the food?	Observe percentage of food consumed from meal tray. Inspect condition of skin, hair, and nails. Inspect oral cavity for signs of malnutrition such as cheilosis, stomatitis, and dry lesions at corners of mouth.
Patterns and dietary history	Which types of food do you like? Are you allergic to any foods? What type of problems do you have with these foods? Have you noticed any changes in taste? Do you have any problems with chewing or swallowing?	Observe patient swallowing. Inspect oral cavity for physical barriers to eating (e.g., tooth decay, poor-fitting dentures).
Changes in weight	Has your appetite changed? What is your normal weight? Have you noticed a change in your weight? Was this change anticipated (e.g., were you on a weight-reduction diet)? Over what period of time did your weight change?	Weigh patient and analyze for changes. Observe patient's muscle tone.
Skin	Have you noticed any changes in your skin such as scaliness, dryness, rashes, or bruising? Do you use skin moisturizers regularly?	Observe skin for color, moisture, changes in pigment, or bruising. Assess skin turgor.

BOX 35.6   DIET HISTORY

A trained nutrition professional interviews the patient about the number and timing of meals and snacks eaten per day, the patient's appetite and food dislikes, the presence or absence of gastrointestinal distress, the use of dietary supplements (vitamins, minerals, and herbal products), and other lifestyle choices. A trained interviewer can assess usual nutrient intake, seasonal changes in food choices, and data about all nutrients consumed.

Other information contained in a diet history includes the following:

- Specific foods consumed for breakfast, lunch, dinner, and snacks
- Food preferences, allergies, and aversions
- Use of enteral or parenteral nutrition
- Dietary restrictions or medically prescribed and/or modified-consistency diets
- Use of weight-reduction, vegetarian, macrobiotic, vegan, fad, or other diets
- Foods that cause indigestion, diarrhea, or gas
- Impact of any functional disabilities or limitations (e.g., food shopping, preparation, self-feeding, socioeconomic limitations)
- Potential drug-nutrient interactions including drug dose and treatment duration
- Chewing or swallowing difficulties (e.g., use of dentures, dysphagia, xerostomia, mucositis, mouth sores, tooth decay)
- Usual bowel movements; presence and duration of constipation or diarrhea
- Symptoms of malabsorption such as clay-colored or frequent fatty stools
- Weight history including percentage of weight lost over period of time lost

Older Adult Considerations. Multiple age-related factors may affect nutrition status in older adults. The presence of chronic illness, anorexia, slowed digestion and peristalsis, decreased physical and cognitive function, ability to feed self, medication side effects, loss of dentition, and xerostomia all may contribute to development of malnutrition.

The Mini Nutritional Assessment (MNA) is a nutrition screening tool developed specifically for adults older than 65 years of age. It is a more sensitive tool than other universal tools such as the MUST in the geriatric population for early identification of malnutrition or risk for malnutrition (Donini et al., 2016). The MNA contains six questions related to patient mobility; neuropsychological problems; current BMI; and the presence of a decline in food intake, weight loss, psychological stress, or acute disease over the past 3 months. The MNA is also a useful tool to predict pressure injury development in older adult patients (Yatabe et al., 2013). Early identification of pressure injury risk allows you to plan interventions to improve nutrition status and overall outcome. Go to the MNA interactive website for a tutorial at www.mna-elderly.com.

Patients at Risk for Nutritional Problems. Assess patients for conditions that may interfere with the ability to ingest, digest, or absorb adequate nutrients. Use a standardized tool to assess nutritional risks when possible. Congenital anomalies and surgical revisions of the GI tract interfere with normal function. Patients receiving only IV infusions of 5% to 10% dextrose are at risk for nutrient deficiencies. Older adults, infants, and patients who are malnourished are at greatest risk.

Physical Examination. Examine a patient for signs of actual or potential nutrition complications (Table 35.2). You can conduct a portion of the examination while performing or assisting the patient with hygiene. The skin and hair are primary areas that reflect nutrient and hydration deficiencies. Be alert for rashes; dry, scaly skin; poor skin turgor; skin lesions; hair loss; easily pluckable hair; hair without luster; and excessively dry or scaly scalp.

Anthropometry. Anthropometry is a systematic measurement of the size and makeup of the body using height and weight as the principal measures. Height and weight measurements typically are obtained during a patient's admission to any health care setting. If a patient is unable to stand, estimate height by measuring the patient's length with a tape measure while the patient lies supine. Assess weight with bed scales, and then compare height and weight with usual measurements, called *usual body weight (UBW)*, and standard norms for normal height-weight relationships, called ideal body weight (IBW). Serial measures of weight over time provide more useful information than one measurement. When collecting serial measurements of weight, weigh a patient at about the same time each day, on the same scale, and with the same amount of clothing. Unintentional changes in body weight indicate a risk factor for malnutrition. Refer patients who have lost 5% or more of their body weight in 1 month or 10% or more of their body weight over any amount of time for unknown reasons to an RDN for a nutrition evaluation.

Laboratory Values. No single laboratory or biochemical test is diagnostic for malnutrition. Factors that frequently alter test results include fluid balance, liver function, kidney function, and the presence of disease. Laboratory values useful in nutrition assessment include complete blood count, albumin, prealbumin, electrolytes, blood urea nitrogen (BUN), 24-hour urine urea nitrogen (UUN), creatinine, glucose, cholesterol, and triglycerides. Individual laboratory measures alone are not specific enough to indicate nutritional risk; therefore, they are combined with multiple objective measures to determine malnutrition risk. A low red blood cell count and low hemoglobin value indicate anemia. Hemoglobin, hematocrit, electrolyte, and BUN values also help to reflect the state of hydration. Serum proteins such as prealbumin and albumin levels are affected by acute inflammation, injury, and illness and are not sensitive to protein or energy deprivation until the point of overt starvation (e.g., BMI less than 12 kg/m^2) in an otherwise healthy individual (Lee et al., 2015). Thus, albumin and prealbumin levels should not be used alone as indicators of nutrition status. Nitrogen balance, which is

TABLE 35.2 PHYSICAL SIGNS OF NUTRITION STATUS

BODY AREA	INDICATORS OF MALNUTRITION
General appearance	Easily fatigued, no energy, falls asleep easily, looks tired, apathetic, cachectic
Weight	Overweight, obese, or underweight (special concern for underweight); unplanned weight loss over period of time
Posture	Poor posture, sagging shoulders, sunken chest, humped back
Muscles	Flaccid, weak, poor tone, tender; "wasted" appearance; impaired mobility
Mental status	Inattentive, irritable, confused
Neurological function	Burning and tingling of hands and feet (paresthesia), loss of position and vibratory sense, decrease or loss of ankle and knee reflexes
Gastrointestinal function	Anorexia, indigestion, constipation or diarrhea, symptoms of malabsorption, liver or spleen enlargement, abdominal distention
Cardiovascular function	Tachycardia, abnormal rhythm, elevated blood pressure
Hair	Stringy, dull, brittle, dry, thin and sparse, depigmented
Skin (general)	Rough, dry, scaly, pale, pigmented, irritated; bruises; petechiae
Face and neck	Swollen; skin dark over cheeks and under eyes
Lips	Dry, scaly, swollen; redness and swelling at corners of mouth (cheilosis); angular lesions at corners of mouth; fissures or scars (stomatitis)
Mouth, oral mucous membranes	Swollen, deep red oral mucous membranes; oral lesions
Gums	Spongy, bleed easily, inflamed, receding
Tongue	Swollen, scarlet and raw, magenta color, beefy (glossitis)
Teeth	Missing teeth, broken teeth
Eyes	Eye membranes pale (pale conjunctivae), redness of membrane (conjunctival injection), dryness or infection
Nails	Spoon-shaped (koilonychia), brittle, ridged
Legs and feet	Edema, tender calf, tingling, weakness, lesions
Skeleton	Bowlegs, knock-knees, chest deformity at diaphragm, beaded ribs, prominent scapulae

Data from Jelliffe DB: The assessment of the nutritional status of the community, *WHO Monograph No. 53*, Geneva, 1966; Clinical Assessment of Nutritional Status, *Am J Public Health* 63(11 Suppl):18, 1973, http://ajph.aphapublications.org/doi/pdf/10.2105/AJPH.63.11_Suppl.18; and Williams SR: Nutritional assessment and guidance in prenatal care. In Worthington-Roberts BS, Williams SR: *Nutrition in pregnancy and lactation,* ed 5, New York, 1993, McGraw-Hill.

measured through laboratory analysis of 24-hour UUN, is important to establish adequacy of protein and calorie intake.

Dysphagia. Dysphagia refers to difficulty with swallowing. It occurs because of damage to muscles and nerves or physical obstruction (Box 35.7). Physiological consequences of dysphagia include dehydration, malnutrition, and pneumonia; other consequences include increased length of hospital stay, health care cost, morbidity, and mortality (Sura et al., 2012).

Signs of dysphagia include coughing during or after a swallow, difficulty or painful chewing or swallowing, change in voice, unintentional weight loss, frequent clearing of throat, and recurrent chest infections (i.e., pneumonia) (Malhi, 2016). Other signs are abnormal gag, delayed swallowing, incomplete oral clearance or pocketing, regurgitation, pharyngeal pooling, drooling, delayed or absent trigger of swallow, and inability to speak consistently. Patients with dysphagia do not always exhibit overt signs such as coughing when food enters the airway. *Silent aspiration,* or aspiration that occurs without a cough, is a common cause of complications.

BOX 35.7 CAUSES OF DYSPHAGIA[a]

MYOGENIC (MUSCLE)
- Aging-related changes
- Muscular dystrophy
- Myasthenia gravis
- Myopathy
- Polymyositis

NEUROGENIC (NERVE)
- Amyotrophic lateral sclerosis (Lou Gehrig disease)
- Cerebral palsy
- Diabetic neuropathy
- Guillain-Barré syndrome
- Huntington disease
- Multiple sclerosis
- Parkinson disease
- Stroke
- Traumatic brain injury

OBSTRUCTIVE
- Anterior mediastinal masses
- Benign peptic stricture
- Candidiasis
- Cervical spondylosis
- Head and neck cancer
- Inflammatory masses
- Lower esophageal ring
- Trauma/surgical resection

OTHER
- Connective tissue disorders
- Gastrointestinal or esophageal resection
- Rheumatological disorders
- Vagotomy

[a]This is not an exhaustive list. Other disorders may lead to dysphagia.

Dysphagia often results in decreased food intake, which may then lead to malnutrition caused by inability to consume an adequate volume of food. Malnutrition resulting from inadequate protein, calorie, and micronutrient intake significantly slows down recovery. Early nurse-initiated screening with a dysphagia screening protocol improves patient outcome by reducing the risk for inpatient deaths and respiratory infections (Hines et al., 2016).

Dysphagia Screening. Dysphagia screening quickly identifies problems with swallowing so that you can refer at-risk patients for a more in-depth assessment (see Skill 35.1). Dysphagia screening includes medical record review and observation of a patient at a meal for change in voice quality, posture, and head control; percentage of meal consumed; eating time; drooling of liquids and solids; cough during and/or after a swallow; facial or tongue weakness; difficulty with secretions; pocketing; and presence of voluntary and dry cough. Bedside screening tools are designed for multidisciplinary use by RNs, RDNs, physicians, or SLPs. However, the gold standard for diagnosis is videofluoroscopy, as current bedside assessment protocols are not sufficiently sensitive (O'Horo et al., 2015). Refer at-risk patients to the SLP. The SLP administers trials of several consistencies of foods and fluids to obtain a comprehensive assessment of a patient's phases of swallowing to determine the degree of dysfunction and aspiration risk.

Patient Expectations. Patients who need help with nutritional problems have many expectations. It is important for you to learn what a patient expects in terms of resuming a normal diet or learning to adjust to a therapeutic diet. Patients with upper-arm immobility often require assistance with activities such as preparing meals, setting up the meal tray or plate, or feeding. Other patients expect information on the availability and use of assistive devices to increase independence with meals. A consultation with occupational therapy helps patients obtain assistive devices and provides education on their proper use. You may need to teach patients who have impaired vision how to feed themselves. A commonly used technique is to identify food locations by their placement according to a clock face (e.g., bread is at 12 o'clock, potatoes are at 3 o'clock, chicken is at 6 o'clock, vegetables are at 9 o'clock).

■ ■ ■ NURSING DIAGNOSIS

Following nursing assessment, cluster relevant defining characteristics to determine whether actual or potential nutritional problems exist. A decline in nutrition status will occur when the body does not ingest a nutrient in sufficient quantity, when it poorly digests or does not completely absorb nutrients, or when total daily caloric needs are deficient or excessive. The following are examples of nursing diagnoses appropriate for patients with compromised nutrition:

- *Deficient Knowledge (Nutrition)*
- *Diarrhea*
- *Feeding Self-Care Deficit*

- *Imbalanced Nutrition: Less Than Body Requirements*
- *Impaired Swallowing*
- *Obesity*
- *Overweight*
- *Risk for Aspiration*

During your assessment, identify the probable cause or related factor for the nutritional problem. Make sure that the nursing diagnosis is as precise as possible. Related factors need to be accurate so that you will select the appropriate interventions. For example, you suspect a patient who is overweight has nutrient deficiencies. The nursing assessment identifies dietary patterns that contributed to obesity. A more focused assessment examines the adequacy of all food groups and finds that the patient consumes excess high-fat foods but inadequate amounts of fruits and vegetables. You identify the nursing diagnosis *Imbalanced Nutrition: Less Than Body Requirements related to intake of nutrient-deficient foods.* Interventions include providing appropriate balanced diets and supplements or specialized nutrition support during episodes of acute illness. In contrast, if the assessment revealed the related factor to be associated with inadequate physical activity, the diagnosis is *Imbalanced Nutrition: Less Than Body Requirements related to lack of physical activity in proportion to caloric intake.* Your interventions then focus on proper diet as well as an exercise program.

■ ■ ■ PLANNING

During planning you select nursing interventions intended to improve a patient's nutrition status and the monitoring and evaluation to determine the effectiveness of your interventions. The input of all involved health care disciplines is necessary for planning successful patient-centered nutrition interventions. Reflect on the causes of a patient's malnutrition or risk for malnutrition. Individualize all interventions to the patient's needs and take into consideration the patient's comfort and preferences. Although variables exist between and among patients, common nutrition goals include symptom management, establishing and maintaining goal weight, and preservation of functional status. Modified diets, oral nutritional supplements, or more complex and costly enteral nutrition (EN) or parenteral nutrition (PN) is sometimes required to improve nutrition status. Consider the cost of these modifications and patient and family caregiver abilities before beginning an intervention. Social workers are very helpful in situations in which patients are unable to afford an intervention or need help planning how interventions will be carried out if the patient or family member is unable to do so.

Goals and Outcomes. The goal in caring for patients with compromised nutrition is to first prevent any further decline in status (i.e., maintain current status) and, if possible, to improve their nutrition status. Consider the association between the various nursing diagnoses of your patient when determining appropriate goals and outcomes (Fig. 35.2). If the nutrition diagnosis is *Imbalanced Nutrition: Less*

CONCEPT MAP

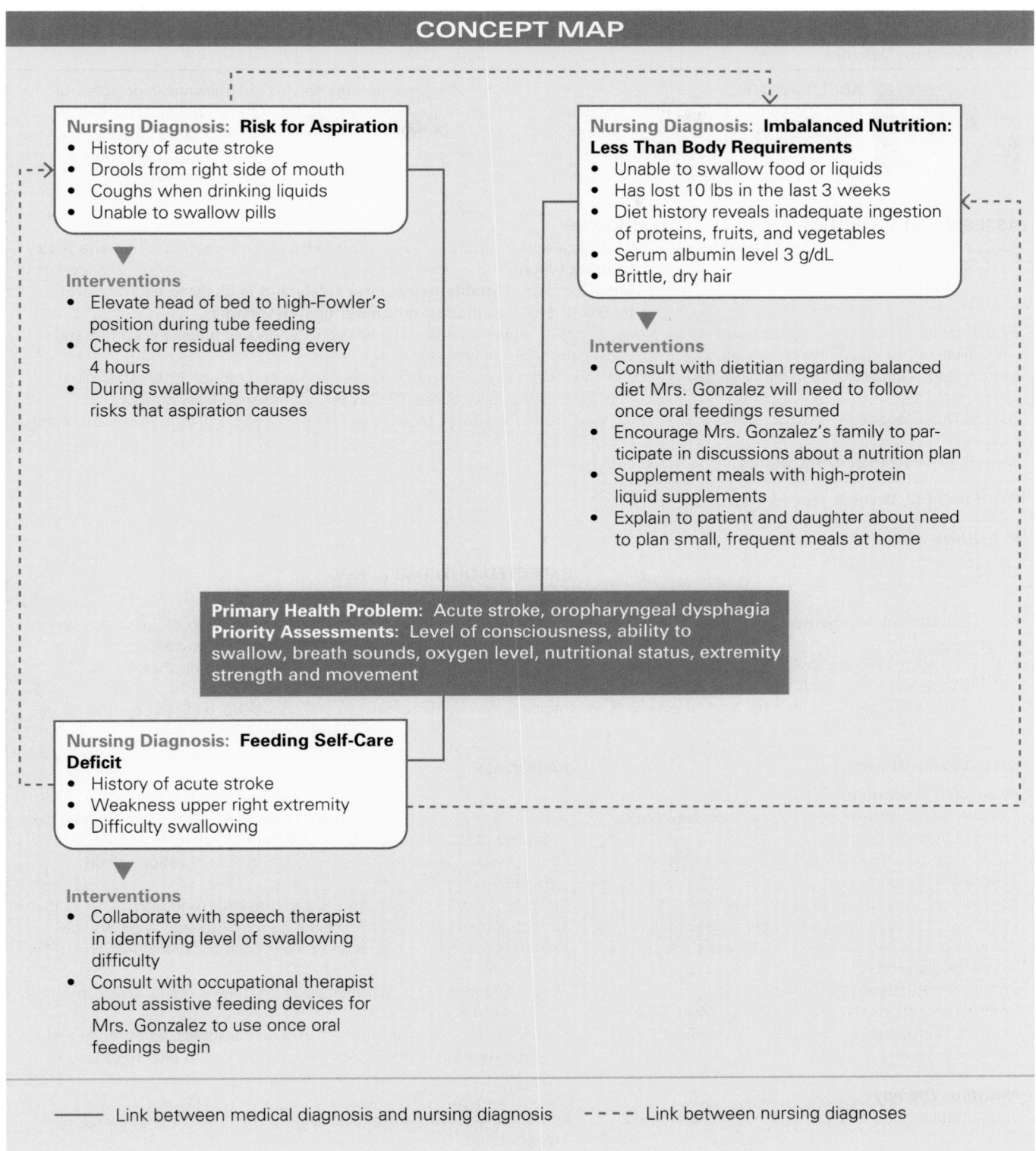

Nursing Diagnosis: Risk for Aspiration
- History of acute stroke
- Drools from right side of mouth
- Coughs when drinking liquids
- Unable to swallow pills

Interventions
- Elevate head of bed to high-Fowler's position during tube feeding
- Check for residual feeding every 4 hours
- During swallowing therapy discuss risks that aspiration causes

Nursing Diagnosis: Imbalanced Nutrition: Less Than Body Requirements
- Unable to swallow food or liquids
- Has lost 10 lbs in the last 3 weeks
- Diet history reveals inadequate ingestion of proteins, fruits, and vegetables
- Serum albumin level 3 g/dL
- Brittle, dry hair

Interventions
- Consult with dietitian regarding balanced diet Mrs. Gonzalez will need to follow once oral feedings resumed
- Encourage Mrs. Gonzalez's family to participate in discussions about a nutrition plan
- Supplement meals with high-protein liquid supplements
- Explain to patient and daughter about need to plan small, frequent meals at home

Primary Health Problem: Acute stroke, oropharyngeal dysphagia
Priority Assessments: Level of consciousness, ability to swallow, breath sounds, oxygen level, nutritional status, extremity strength and movement

Nursing Diagnosis: Feeding Self-Care Deficit
- History of acute stroke
- Weakness upper right extremity
- Difficulty swallowing

Interventions
- Collaborate with speech therapist in identifying level of swallowing difficulty
- Consult with occupational therapist about assistive feeding devices for Mrs. Gonzalez to use once oral feedings begin

——— Link between medical diagnosis and nursing diagnosis   - - - - Link between nursing diagnoses

FIG 35.2 Concept map.

Than Body Requirements, a goal will be for the patient to gain weight or to ingest adequate nutrients. If a patient is obese, a goal of care is to safely achieve weight reduction. Determine specific, individualized goals by identifying patient behaviors that have led to the compromised nutrition state (see Care Plan). Correction of poor dietary patterns is a long-term, rather than a short-term, goal. Short-term goals usually involve achieving calorie or nutrient targets on a daily or weekly basis. Explore patients' feelings about their weight and food and help them set realistic and achievable goals. Goals

⊚ CARE PLAN

Risk for Aspiration

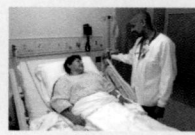

ASSESSMENT

Matt knows that strokes often cause dysphagia, increasing the risk for aspiration. Mrs. Gonzalez's diet history reveals that she ate balanced meals three times daily, including at least three servings of fruits and vegetables, before her stroke. Her diet maintained her weight. Her health care provider orders tube feedings through a nasally inserted feeding tube. Mrs. Gonzalez states, "I just don't know about a tube. I wish my doctor would just let me eat."

ASSESSMENT ACTIVITIES

Assess Mrs. Gonzalez's ability to swallow safely and the risk for aspiration.

Evaluate Mrs. Gonzalez's physical status, emphasizing her gastrointestinal status.

Monitor Mrs. Gonzalez's respiratory status.

Assess Mrs. Gonzalez's nutrition status and needs.

FINDINGS[a]

Mrs. Gonzalez was diagnosed with **acute stroke.** She **coughs when she tries to drink water.** The speech-language pathologist's (SLP) evaluation shows that Mrs. Gonzalez is **unable to swallow safely and is likely to aspirate oral intake.** The SLP diagnosed **oropharyngeal dysphagia.**

Mrs. Gonzalez's abdomen is soft and nondistended. She denies diarrhea and constipation. Her bowel sounds are active.

Lung sounds are clear. Respirations are regular at a rate of 12 breaths/minute. She has no shortness of breath. Oxygen saturation is 96% on room air.

Baseline albumin, blood glucose, renal function, and electrolyte levels are within normal limits.

[a]**Defining characteristics/risk factors** are shown in **bold** type.

NURSING DIAGNOSIS: Risk for Aspiration

PLANNING

GOAL

Mrs. Gonzalez will receive adequate nutrition by discharge.

Mrs. Gonzalez will regain swallowing ability assisted by speech therapy training by discharge.

EXPECTED OUTCOMES (NOC)[b]

Nutrition Status: Nutrient Intake

Mrs. Gonzalez's weight at discharge is within 2 lb of admission weight.

Mrs. Gonzalez does not exhibit signs of aspiration before discharge.

Mrs. Gonzalez progresses to an oral diet before discharge to the restorative care agency.

[b]Nursing outcomes classification label from Moorhead S, et al, editors: *Nursing outcomes classification (NOC),* ed 5, St Louis, 2013, Mosby.

INTERVENTIONS (NIC)[c]

Aspiration Precautions

Position Mrs. Gonzalez with head of bed elevated to minimum of 30 degrees.

Check tube placement before each use and at least every 4 to 6 hours.

Monitor tolerance of EN feedings (e.g., physical examination, abdominal radiographs, evaluation of risk factors for aspiration) every 4 to 6 hours and prn for signs of discomfort.

Continue with speech therapy and follow recommendations per provider order. Make sure that patient is properly positioned and supervised during oral intake trials.

Nutrition Therapy

Insert feeding tube and initiate feedings as ordered.

Advance tube feeding to goal rate, monitoring for tolerance.

RATIONALE

Head of bed elevated to minimum of 30 to 45 degrees decreases risk for aspiration (AACN, 2016a; McClave et al., 2016).

Feeding tube misplacement increases risk for aspiration (AACN, 2016b).

Critically ill patients receiving EN are at risk for regurgitation, aspiration, and pneumonia. Regularly monitoring for GI tolerance allows the nurse to identify problems and prevent complications (AACN, 2016b).

Regularly provided speech therapy helps patient regain ability to swallow foods and liquids.

Speech therapy includes trials of various consistencies of foods and liquids. Aspiration of food and liquids can lead to pneumonia.

Enteral tube feeding provides nutrients safely while swallowing is rehabilitated.

In the absence of critical illness (including metabolic or systemic complications), enteral feedings can advance to goal rate within 24 to 48 hours. Signs of GI intolerance include symptoms such as abdominal distention, vomiting, large gastric residual volume, and diarrhea (McClave et al., 2016).

[c]Nursing intervention classifications labels from Bulechek GM, et al, editors: *Nursing interventions classification (NIC),* ed 6, St Louis, 2013, Mosby.

CARE PLAN—cont'd

Risk for Aspiration

EVALUATION

NURSING ACTIONS	PATIENT RESPONSE/FINDING	ACHIEVEMENT OF OUTCOME
Monitor Mrs. Gonzalez's respiratory status.	Mrs. Gonzalez's lung sounds are clear, and she has no symptoms of aspiration.	Mrs. Gonzalez's lungs remain free of signs of aspiration.
Weigh Mrs. Gonzalez weekly.	Mrs. Gonzalez's weight is ½ lb less than her admission weight.	Mrs. Gonzalez's weight is maintained.
Monitor laboratory values.	Prealbumin remains 20 mg/dL, and albumin is 4 g/dL.	Prealbumin and albumin values are maintained within normal limits.

are achieved through diet planning, patient education, and helping a patient develop new behaviors that will enable him or her to achieve an optimal state of nutrition health.

Individualized planning for nutrition is critical. Mutually planned goals among the patient, RDN, and nurse ensure success. Patients often have unrealistic expectations about nutritional needs or dieting in reference to weight gain or loss. Help them understand this concept by asking them to reflect on their rate of weight gain or loss. Changes in weight usually occur over months or years unless an acute illness has occurred. People often become discouraged when they do not see rapid achievement of weight goals. Help your patients set realistic outcomes. For example, the following outcomes focus on reasonably achieving a weight-loss goal:

- Patient loses ½ to 1 lb per week.
- Patient consumes 64 oz of water instead of sugared beverages.
- Patient increases fruit and vegetable servings in diet to five servings per day.
- Patient achieves a negative energy balance of 500 kcal per day through reduced kilocalorie intake and increased energy expenditure.

Setting Priorities. Patients at risk for compromised nutrition have a plan of care aimed at improving nutrition status. However, many factors can influence the priorities of a patient's overall care. For example, if a patient is on oral intake, symptom control may be a priority (e.g., nausea or pain) before the patient feels comfortable to eat. Psychological factors such as fear or depression often influence a person's willingness or desire to eat. In this situation, discussing a patient's concerns takes precedence over starting mealtime. Food is important for all people, but when illness or circumstances disrupt appetite or the ability to eat, anticipate what is most important to achieve good nutrition.

Collaborative Care. Patients' nutritional needs extend beyond the acute hospital setting and into the home or rehabilitation care setting, requiring collaboration of the health care team, the patient, and the family and caregivers. Family and caregivers are often involved in food purchase and preparation. The nutrition plan of care will not succeed without their commitment to, involvement in, and understanding of nutrition goals.

Professionals who help provide nutrition support include the RDN, nutrition support clinical nurse specialist, pharmacists, and medical health care providers. Consult with an SLP, RDN, pharmacist, social worker, or occupational therapist when discharge planning includes ongoing nutrition assessment and interventions to meet nutritional needs. Some patients with severe cases of malnutrition require EN or PN to meet fluid, electrolyte, and nutrient needs.

Patients and family members need to learn the skills to administer nutrition therapies safely and effectively. Home care nurses play an important role in helping patients and families with the need for dietary changes and administration concerns, monitoring and problem prevention related to EN and PN feeding, and related lifestyle changes. Long-term nutrition management is a challenge, and effective collaborative relationships are essential to success.

■ ■ ■ ■ IMPLEMENTATION

Health Promotion. All health care providers play important roles in promoting healthy dietary practices. Although the RDN is the nutrition expert on the team responsible for nutrition plans, it is actually your frequent contact with the patient that will make the most lasting impression. Using free tools such as ChooseMyPlate (www.choosemyplate.gov) helps patients with their food choices, menu planning, and dietary patterns. Educate patients about food labels and their meanings, as well as product claims that are misleading; for example, some "reduced-fat" foods still have significant amounts of fat, some "lite" foods still contain considerable calories, and "low cholesterol" does not always mean low fat.

A high percentage of patients who attempt to lose weight are unsuccessful, regaining lost weight over time. However, research has shown that when a physician officially diagnoses a patient as overweight, weight loss efforts are more successful (Singh et al., 2010). Diet and exercise compliance affects success with weight loss. Many individuals are willing to pay for weight-loss programs if the program meets individual needs. Information on weight-loss diets is available everywhere, from the bookstore to the Internet. However, there is a lack of reliable evidence evaluating the effectiveness of commercial weight-loss programs. A successful weight-loss plan involves sustainable lifestyle modifications that include physical activity, self-monitoring, portion control, and knowledge of energy content of food.

One diet that is effective in maintaining weight loss, reducing blood pressure, and promoting health is the Dietary Approaches to Stop Hypertension (DASH) eating plan, which is based on research by the National Heart, Lung and Blood Institute (NHLBI) (Garvey et al., 2016). This diet effectively reduces blood pressure and is based on fruits, vegetables, fat-free or low-fat dairy products, whole grain products, fish, poultry, and nuts. It is also rich in protein and fiber. The DASH diet offers menus and recipes for two levels of daily sodium intake (2300 mg/day and 1500 mg/day) and several levels of total kilocalorie intake (1200 to 3100 kcal/day). The lower 1500-mg sodium DASH diet lowers blood pressure more quickly than the diet with higher levels of sodium (Bray et al., 2004). The DASH diet helps to reduce a person's risk for cardiovascular disease by helping to reduce blood pressure, total cholesterol, low-density lipoprotein cholesterol, and body weight (Siervo et al., 2015).

Food safety is a commonly overlooked aspect of health promotion. Contaminated and undercooked food products, especially eggs and meats, may result in severe debilitating and even fatal illnesses (Table 35.3). Patient education is one method of improving safe food practices for patients and their families (Box 35.8). Food safety is also an important nursing consideration if EN tube feeding is used to provide nutrition for the patient in the home setting.

Acute Care. It is common for oral intake to decrease during periods of stress and acute illness. This occurs because of the anorexic effects of stress-induced hormones. It is important to monitor a patient's nutrient intake, identify influences that reduce appetite, and plan interventions to manage stress and support nutrient needs.

Some patients have decreased intake in acute care settings due to diagnostic testing. Some blood and radiographic studies require a patient to receive nothing by mouth (NPO) until testing is completed. This disrupts mealtimes, and sometimes patients must wait for extended periods of time to eat or experience discomfort related to the test. Continue to assess a patient's nutrition status. Nutritional support is recommended when patients are NPO and receive only standard IV fluids for more than 5 to 7 days (Academy of Nutrition and Dietetics [AND], 2016).

Emotional stress also influences food intake. Patients who are worried about their families, finances, employment, or illness are not always able to eat or eat well enough to compensate for the effect of stress on metabolism.

Medications may also affect dietary intake and in some cases the body's use of nutrients. Some medications cause reduced appetite, slowed motility and constipation, anorexia, or malabsorption. For example, opioids (e.g., morphine sulfate, codeine) used for pain relief usually cause constipation. Medication-induced and condition-related nausea, vomiting, and diarrhea have a significant impact on nutrient intake. This is common with chemotherapy for cancer treatment. Taste changes often occur with chemotherapy, diuretics, and mineral preparations such as zinc. Work with an RDN to help a patient select foods that are tolerated and do not worsen the nausea or other symptoms. Sometimes

---

BOX 35.8 PATIENT TEACHING

Food Safety

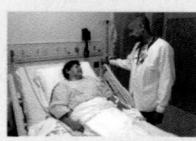 As Matt discusses measures he is taking to maintain safety during Mrs. Gonzalez's feeding, her daughter Maria asks Matt questions about food safety in general. Matt recognizes that very young patients, older-adult patients, patients with chronic illness, and patients who are immunosuppressed are at increased risk for foodborne illnesses (see Table 35.3). As Mrs. Gonzalez improves and begins to tolerate oral feedings, Matt consults with the registered dietitian nutritionist, and together they develop a teaching plan regarding food safety for the foods that Mrs. Gonzalez's family will be preparing at home.

OUTCOME
At the end of the teaching session Mrs. Gonzalez's family will state measures to reduce foodborne illnesses.

TEACHING STRATEGIES
Instruct Mrs. Gonzalez's family on ways to avoid foodborne illnesses, such as the following:
- Wash hands, food-preparation surfaces, and utensils with hot, soapy water.

- Cook meat, poultry, fish, and eggs until well done (180° F).
- Wash fresh fruits and vegetables thoroughly.
- Do not consume raw meat or unpasteurized milk or juices.
- Do not use food past expiration date.
- Refrigerate foods at 40° F within 2 hours of cooking.
- Keep foods properly refrigerated.
- Thaw frozen foods in the refrigerator.
- Discard food that you suspect is spoiled.
- Do not use wooden cutting boards. Instead use plastic laminate or solid surface cutting boards that can be disinfected.
- Wash dishcloths, dishtowels, and sponges regularly with bleach or use paper towels.
- Clean inside of refrigerator and microwave regularly with bleach or disinfectant soap.

EVALUATION
- Use the principles of teach-back to evaluate patient/family caregiver learning:
  - "State six measures to prevent foodborne illnesses."
  - "Describe one change you will make to reduce the chance of obtaining a foodborne illness."

TABLE 35.3 FOOD SAFETY

FOODBORNE DISEASE	ORGANISM	FOOD SOURCE	SYMPTOMS[a]
Botulism	*Clostridium botulinum*	Improperly canned foods, especially home-canned vegetables; fermented fish, baked potatoes in aluminum foil	Vomiting, diarrhea, blurred vision, double vision, difficulty swallowing, muscle weakness; can result in respiratory failure and death Onset: 12–72 hours Duration: variable
Escherichia coli infection	*E. coli*–producing toxin	Water or food contaminated with human feces	Watery diarrhea, abdominal cramps, some vomiting Onset: 1–3 days Duration: 3–7 days or longer
Hemorrhagic colitis or *E. coli* O157:H7 infection	*E. coli* O157:H7	Undercooked beef (especially hamburger), unpasteurized milk and juice, raw fruits and vegetables (e.g., sprouts), contaminated water	Severe (often bloody) diarrhea, abdominal pain and vomiting; usually little or no fever is present; more common among children 4 years of age or younger; can lead to kidney failure Onset: 1–8 days Duration: 5–10 days
Hepatitis	Hepatitis A	Raw produce, contaminated drinking water, uncooked foods and cooked foods that are not reheated after contact with infected food handler, shellfish from contaminated waters	Diarrhea, dark urine, jaundice, flulike symptoms (i.e., fever, headache, nausea, abdominal pain) Onset: 15–50 days Duration: variable, 2 weeks to 3 months
Listeriosis	*Listeria, Listeria monocytogenes*	Unpasteurized milk, soft cheeses made with unpasteurized milk, ready-to-eat deli meats	Fever, muscle aches, and nausea or diarrhea; women who are pregnant may have mild flulike illness, and infection can lead to premature delivery or stillbirth; patients who are elderly or immunocompromised may develop bacteremia or meningitis Onset: 9–48 hours Duration: variable
Clostridium perfringens food poisoning	*C. perfringens*	Meats, poultry, gravy, dried or precooked foods that are not promptly served or refrigerated	Intense abdominal cramps, watery diarrhea Onset: 8–16 hours Duration: usually 24 hours
Salmonellosis	*Salmonella*	Eggs, poultry, meat, unpasteurized milk or juice, cheese, contaminated raw fruits and vegetables, shellfish	Diarrhea, fever, abdominal cramps, vomiting Onset: 6–48 hours Duration: 4–7 days
Shigellosis or bacillary dysentery	*Shigella*	Raw produce, contaminated drinking water, uncooked foods and cooked foods that are not reheated after contact with an infected food handler	Abdominal cramps, fever, diarrhea; stools may contain blood and mucus Onset: 4–7 days Duration: 24–48 hours
Staphylococcal food poisoning	*Staphylococcus, Staphylococcus aureus*	Unrefrigerated or improperly refrigerated meats, potato and egg salads; cream pastries	Sudden onset of severe nausea and vomiting, abdominal cramps; diarrhea and fever may be present Onset: 1–6 hours Duration: 24–48 hours
Vibrio parahaemolyticus infection	*V. parahaemolyticus*	Undercooked or raw seafood such as shellfish	Watery (occasionally bloody) diarrhea, abdominal cramps, nausea, vomiting, fever Onset: 4–96 hours Duration: 2–5 days
Vibrio vulnificus infection	*V. vulnificus*	Undercooked or raw seafood such as shellfish (especially oysters)	Vomiting, diarrhea, abdominal pain, bloodborne infection, fever, bleeding within the skin, ulcers that require surgical removal; can be fatal to patients with liver disease or weakened immune systems Onset: 1–7 days Duration: 2–8 days

[a]Symptoms are generally most severe for the youngest and oldest age-groups.
Data from U.S. Department of Health and Human Services and U.S. Food and Drug Administration: *Foodborne illnesses: what you need to know,* www.fda.gov/Food/ResourcesForYou/Consumers/ucm103263.htm.

medications need to be provided to decrease nausea or pain, and other medications can be changed or their administration dose or timing altered.

Symptoms associated with illness often have a major effect on appetite. Pain, nausea, and shortness of breath make it difficult for patients to chew, swallow, and tolerate stomach filling. Patients may refuse to eat to avoid discomfort. Patients who are ill, have had surgery, or have been NPO for a long period of time often have specialized dietary needs. The lack of taste in low-sodium or low-fat diets may lead to reduced dietary intake or reduced compliance. In this situation you need to consider the benefits associated with the therapeutic diet against the detrimental effects of weight loss and malnutrition. Table 35.4 describes commonly prescribed diets for patients in health care settings.

Food presentation also affects appetite. Hot foods that are cold or cold foods that are warm are not appetizing. Overcooked or undercooked foods are generally unappealing. A meal tray balanced on a crowded, soiled over-bed table does not support an appetite. Removing the tray lid outside of a patient's room helps to decrease distress in patients who are sensitive to odors (e.g., patients with nausea). Support your patient's appetite through environmental adaptations, meal scheduling, attention to food preferences and patient symptoms, consultation with an RDN, and patient and family counseling.

Providing a Comfortable Environment. Provide an environment conducive to eating. Offer hand hygiene and make sure that a patient's room is free of reminders of treatments and odors. Provide mouth care when necessary to remove unpleasant tastes. Plan to administer analgesics or antiemetics early enough so that patients are more comfortable to eat at mealtime. Position a patient comfortably so that the meal is more enjoyable. If a patient refuses part of the meal, replace it with a suitable alternative.

Assisting Patients With Feeding. Some patients are unable to feed themselves adequately because of the severity of their illness, fatigue, or debilitation of their condition. Improve patient feeding by carefully protecting their dignity and actively involving them in the eating process. Encourage the patient to eat a small amount of food at a comfortable pace when helping with feeding. Provide independence using adaptive devices (Fig. 35.3) or finger foods. Position the patient in a chair or high-Fowler's position to improve swallowing and digestion. Allow the patient time to empty the mouth after every spoonful, attempting to match the speed of feeding to the patient's readiness. Encourage patients to direct the order in which they wish to eat food items. Mealtime is a good time to instruct patients and their families about a balanced diet and the selection of appropriate foods.

Patients with visual deficits also need special assistance. Patients with decreased vision are often able to feed themselves independently when they are given adequate information. Identify the food location on the plate as if it were a clock (e.g., meat at 9 o'clock and vegetable at 3 o'clock). Tell the patient where the beverages are located in relation to

the plate. Be sure that other care providers set the meal tray and plate in the same manner. Patients with impaired vision may be more independent during mealtimes with the use of large-handled adaptive utensils, which are easier to grip and manipulate.

TABLE 35.4	THERAPEUTIC DIETS
DIET	**DESCRIPTION**
Clear liquid	Broth, bouillon, coffee, tea, carbonated beverages, clear fruit juices, gelatin, popsicles
Full liquid	As for clear liquid with addition of smooth-textured dairy products (e.g., ice cream, yogurt drinks, milk), custards, very thin refined cooked cereals, vegetable juice, pureed vegetables, all fruit juices
Mechanical soft	As for full liquid with addition of ground or finely diced meats, flaked fish, cottage cheese, cheese, rice, potatoes, pancakes, light breads, cooked vegetables, cooked or canned fruits, bananas, soups, peanut butter
Fiber-restricted	Addition of easily digested foods such as pastas, casseroles, tender well-cooked meats (without added fat), and canned or cooked fruits and vegetables (without skin); desserts, cakes, cookies without nuts or coconut
High fiber	Addition of fresh uncooked fruits, steamed vegetables, bran, oatmeal, dried fruits
Low sodium	4-g, 2-g, 1-g, or 500-mg sodium diets; vary from no added salt (4-g sodium diet) to severe sodium restriction (500-mg sodium diet) that requires selective food purchases
Low cholesterol	300 mg/day or less cholesterol, in keeping with American Heart Association guidelines for serum lipid reduction
Diabetic	Nutrition recommendations by American Diabetes Association: focus on total energy and balanced intake of carbohydrates from fruits, vegetables, whole grains, legumes, and low-fat milk; fats; and proteins; caloric recommendations vary to accommodate patients' metabolic demands
Gluten free	Eliminates wheat, barley, rye, and their derivatives
Dysphagia diet	National Dysphagia Diet has three stages depending on patient's swallowing capacity; foods included vary according to stage
Regular	No restrictions unless specified

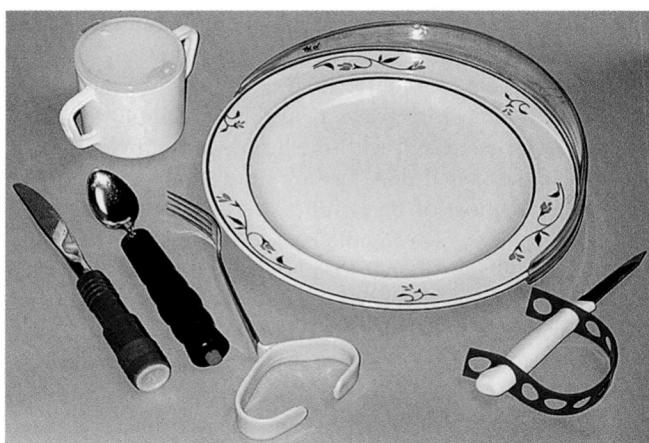

FIG 35.3 Assist devices for self-feeding.

Dysphagia. Effective dysphagia management, usually led by the SLP and RDN, requires an interprofessional approach. The SLP makes treatment recommendations that may include *any* or *all* of the following: strengthening exercises, oral and thermal stimulation techniques, various swallowing maneuvers, postural adjustments, and dietary modification by altering the consistency of foods and liquids (Wirth et al., 2016). The RDN ensures that appropriate food choices and recommendations are individualized and balanced with the nutrient and caloric needs of their patients.

Dysphagia Diet Management. In October 2002 the American Dietetic Association (now known as the Academy of Nutrition and Dietetics) published the National Dysphagia Diet Task Force (NDDTF) National Dysphagia Diet (NDDTF, 2002). The National Dysphagia Diet provides guidelines and standard terminology for food and texture modifications. There are three levels of solid foods: dysphagia pureed, dysphagia mechanically altered, and dysphagia advanced. The four levels of liquid are thin liquids (low viscosity), nectarlike liquids (medium viscosity), honeylike liquids (viscosity of honey), and spoon-thick liquids (viscosity of pudding) (NDDTF, 2002; AND, 2016).

Thickened liquids are commonly prescribed to prevent aspiration pneumonia. However, thickening agents alter the flavor and texture qualities of food. The period of adjustment to new dietary restrictions and the rehabilitation period may reduce intake for long periods of time, subsequently reducing quality of life and further increasing the risk for malnutrition and dehydration, particularly in the elderly (Cichero, 2013; Takeuchi et al., 2014; Swan et al., 2015).

The specified thickness of a liquid depends on a patient's swallowing deficit. Always use foods and fluids with the appropriate viscosity as determined by the SLP. Thin fluids (e.g., water) are generally the most difficult to swallow properly. Read the label directions carefully when modifying liquids to prepare the desired thickness correctly. Instructions are not universal for all thickening agents. Excessive thickness also has consequences. The risk of postswallow residue in the pharynx will increase with high-viscosity liquids (Steele et al., 2015).

Before each meal, position the patient in a chair or raise the head of the bed to an upright, seated position (Malhi, 2016). Have the patient slightly flex the head to a chin-down position to help prevent aspiration. If a patient has unilateral weakness, teach the patient and caregiver to place food in the stronger side of the mouth. Feed a patient with dysphagia slowly, provide small bites, and allow the patient to chew thoroughly and swallow the bite before taking another. Frequently assess the patient's chewing and swallowing throughout the meal. Allow the patient time to empty the mouth after each spoonful, matching the speed of feeding to the patient's readiness. If the patient begins to cough or choke, remove the food immediately.

Patients With Disabilities. Allow patients with disabilities to do as much as possible for themselves. When necessary, prepare the meal tray by cutting food into bite-size pieces, buttering bread, and pouring liquids. Use special eating utensils if necessary or as recommended by the occupational therapist. Patients with decreased motor skills may be more independent during mealtimes with the use of large-handled adaptive utensils. Some patients become fatigued during a meal, leading to poor intake. Provide help at the end of meals as needed. Evaluate the results of self-feeding. Recognize and commend patient success.

Interventions for Patients Unable to Meet Nutritional Needs Orally. Evidence-based guidelines help the RDN set goals and plan care for the patient who is unable to maintain adequate nutrition by the oral route (AND, 2016). These guidelines focus on enhancing oral nutrition as a priority. To improve intake, modify food choices to increase the nutrient value of food ingested, manage symptoms, administer medication to relieve nausea or pain if it interferes with oral intake, adjust mealtimes, or help with the process of eating. When these interventions fail to improve voluntary oral intake or when oral intake is not deemed safe, EN is considered to maintain adequate nutrition. PN is considered only when nutrition support via the GI tract is not physiologically possible, when the bowel must be rested, or when nutrient needs cannot otherwise be met. EN is preferred over PN because it maintains the structure and function of the gut and the gut-associated lymphoid tissue, prevents bacteria translocation, decreases the risk for infection, and is less expensive (AND, 2016; McClave et al., 2016). Work with the patient, family caregiver, and other health care team members to maintain adequate nutrition in the safest, most physiological, and most cost-effective manner possible.

Enteral Tube Feedings. EN refers to the use of the GI tract for the intake of nutrition. According to this definition, oral intake is also a form of EN. However, in a clinical setting EN refers only to when nutrients and fluids are administered into the stomach or GI tract via a feeding tube. NG feedings are delivered through a feeding tube introduced through the nose and into the stomach. Nasointestinal feedings are delivered through a feeding tube inserted through the nose and passed through the stomach to the small intestine (duodenum or jejunum). When patients have nasopharyngeal obstructions or are not candidates for nasally placed tubes or when the need for EN is anticipated to be longer than 4 to 6 weeks, feeding tubes may be inserted directly into the stomach (gastrostomy) or jejunum (jejunostomy) (Table 35.5). A variety of enteral feeding formulas are available including products either with or without fiber. Special enteral formulas are designed to meet the nutrient needs of certain diseases (e.g., diabetes, kidney disease, hepatic failure). However, there is little evidence that supports the use of such formulas. The American Society for Parenteral and Enteral Nutrition (ASPEN) guidelines are to use standard polymetric formulas when initiating EN (McClave et al., 2016). When provided in amounts to meet a patient's protein and calorie needs, products will usually also meet the patient's DRIs for micronutrients. As a rule, enteral formulas do not meet most patients' needs for fluid. After accounting for water provided through tube flushes, additional water must be provided to meet hydration needs. Consult with an RDN to ensure a patient's nutrient and fluid needs are met. The skills presented in this chapter focus on the administration of nutrition feedings directly into the GI tract with the goal of restoring and maintaining the patient's nutrition status.

Skill 35.2 describes insertion of a small-bore feeding tube. Feeding tubes are usually referred to as being nasally placed because that is the route most frequently used. The nose provides natural stability for tubes and it is the least invasive route. However, feeding tubes are sometimes placed orally if there has been trauma to the nose or if a patient already has an endotracheal tube placed in the mouth. Use the smallest gauge tube that is appropriate for a patient for comfort and to avoid irritation to the nasopharyngeal and esophageal mucosa. Occasionally the large-bore tube, initially inserted for gastric decompression, is used to initiate enteral feeding because it is already in place. If feeding continues for more than a few days, consult with the health care provider about placing a softer small-bore feeding tube (Miller et al., 2014). For an adult, most of these tubes are 8 to 12 Fr and 43 to 55 inches long. A stylet is often used during insertion of a small-bore tube to stiffen it for placement purposes and then removed when the correct position of the tube is confirmed.

Initiating Tube Feedings. When making the decision regarding enteral access, the health care provider considers the patient's rate of gastric emptying, GI anatomy and functionality, risk for gastric reflux and aspiration, anticipated duration of requirement for enteral access, and disease state. The prolonged use of NG tubes is associated with inconvenience, discomfort, psychological stress, and displacement requiring reinsertion (Gomes et al., 2015). It is not recommended to use them for long-term enteral access (AND, 2016). Feeding tubes that end in the stomach are used for gravity bolus or continuous infusion feedings. The small intestine does not have the storage capability of the stomach, and therefore a tube feeding administered into the small intestine is delivered more slowly and continuously with an infusion pump.

Aspiration into the lung can occur from secretions or other material in the oral pharyngeal area, or it may occur as a result of reflux of gastric contents including tube feeding formula. Aspiration irritates the bronchial mucosa and provides growth material for pneumonia or other infections.

TABLE 35.5	COMPARISON OF ENTERAL FEEDING TUBES	
TUBE	**FEATURES**	**NURSING CONSIDERATIONS**
Gastrostomy	Placed surgically (laparoscopic or open) with endoscope or fluoroscopy Held in place internally with balloon or semisolid "bolster"- or "bumper"-type end Uses external disc to prevent tube from migrating internally Uses low-profile tubes for patients who are conscientious of their body image or may be prone to pull at tube	Monitor external tube length as guide for placement. Internal migration can block pylorus, leading to gastric retention, patient discomfort, and emesis or large residual volumes. Check for tube tightness if person gains weight or is bloated or distended. If external disc is too tight, circulation is restricted, and skin breakdown often occurs. Use small gauze dressing under external disc. It may be used for stomach decompression. Usual gastric returns are expected. If tube is placed high in stomach, repositioning patient may help obtain returns. Use adapter for administration through low-profile tubes.
Jejunostomy	Placed surgically with endoscope or fluoroscopy Held in place by sutures, Dacron cuff, or small-volume balloon	Ability to use for gravity bolus feeding (meal-like feedings) is limited because jejunum lacks storage capacity of stomach. Monitor external tube length to watch for internal or external migration. High gastric-like residual volumes are not expected.
Gastrojejunostomy	Has gastric and small-bowel ports Low-profile gastrojejunostomy tubes that have small-bowel access may be used	Label port to be used for feeding and medications. Gastric port typically is used for decompression. Jejunal port is used for feeding. Monitor gastric returns. Gastric returns may indicate that jejunal port has flipped into stomach and is no longer appropriate for jejunal feeding.

Specific factors that increase a patient's risk for aspiration include neuromuscular or structural interference with swallowing (e.g., dysphagia, intubation), nasoenteric tubes (especially large-bore tubes), incorrectly placed feeding tube, inadequate nursing staff, delayed gastric emptying, vomiting, prolonged supine position, sedation, and advanced age (Elke et al., 2015). To reduce the risk of aspiration, keep the head of the bed elevated to a minimum of 30 degrees and monitor tolerance to EN daily by physical examination, radiological evaluation, presence of abdominal distention, and patient-reported pain or discomfort (McClave et al., 2016). Most health care providers order measurement of gastric residual volume (GRV) every 4 to 6 hours in patients receiving continuous feedings and immediately before a feeding in patients receiving intermittent feedings. However, the amount of GRV in a patient's stomach is not a sensitive indicator of aspiration risk (McClave et al., 2016).

The Society for Critical Care Medicine and ASPEN made the following recommendations regarding GRV: (1) do not use GRV as part of routine care to monitor patients in the intensive care unit (ICU) receiving EN; (2) in cases where GRV is still used, evaluate the patient for aspiration, and use nursing measures to reduce the risk for aspiration if GRV is between 200 mL and 500 mL; and (3) do not withhold feedings when GRV is less than 500 mL and there are no other signs of EN intolerance (McClave et al., 2016). Inadequate nutrient delivery through EN is a significant problem, particularly in patients in the ICU, when feedings are stopped without proper evidence of intolerance.

Ensure that enteral feedings are correctly connected to an enteral feeding tube (Box 35.9). The bedside method of testing feeding tube placement by injecting air into the tube while listening over the stomach with a stethoscope is ineffective and no longer used. The gold standard for determining tube location is x-ray confirmation. Monitor the tube location every 4 hours by assessing the color and pH of the gastric aspirate (Box 35.10), observe changes in the length of the tube that is external from the nose or abdomen, and review any available chest or abdominal x-ray reports for information about tube placement (American Association of Critical Care Nurses [AACN], 2016b).

Gastrostomy/Jejunostomy Tube Placement. When patients cannot tolerate nasally or orally placed tubes or when EN will be needed for more than several weeks, tubes may be placed into the GI tract through the abdomen. A surgeon inserts a gastrostomy tube through a small incision in the left upper quadrant of the stomach either laparoscopically or with an open surgical technique. The tube is held in place internally by a balloon, pigtail design, or other design. A *percutaneous endoscopic gastrostomy (PEG) tube* is placed with an endoscope. The design of the PEG tube holds it in place (Fig. 35.4). You administer feedings into the stomach via a gastrostomy tube using gravity bolus in small volumes or continuously by a slow infusion. Because gastrostomy tubes provide more options for feeding delivery and thus more freedom and flexibility for patients, they are used for longer-term feeding instead of jejunal tubes when possible (AND, 2016; Boullata et al., 2017).

BOX 35.9 EVIDENCE-BASED PRACTICE

PICO Question: In patients receiving enteral tube feeding, does the use of evidence-based strategies prevent inadvertent tubing misconnections?

SUMMARY OF EVIDENCE

Enteral feeding tube misconnections can result in solutions being delivered by the wrong route, causing serious consequences for patients. For example, the enteral feeding line can inadvertently be connected to central and peripheral intravascular catheters, peritoneal dialysis catheters, and tracheostomy tubes (The Joint Commission [TJC], 2014). The improper delivery of enteral tube feeding formula into any of these catheters can result in severe injury or fatal consequences. The Joint Commission issued a sentinel event alert to address this serious issue due to the number and potential consequences of reported misconnection errors (TJC, 2014). Following this alert, the International Organization of Standardization (IOS) released design standards for connectors that are exclusive to enteral feeding lines to prevent misconnections (IOS, 2016). The U.S. Food and Drug Administration supports and recommends using the IOS connectors to mitigate misconnections and increase patient safety (U.S. Department of Health and Human Services [USDHHS], 2015). Nurses must be vigilant to ensure that solutions are connected to the appropriate delivery devices and follow agency guidelines and procedures to prevent any adverse events that could lead to patient harm.

APPLICATION TO NURSING PRACTICE

- Ensure that all connections are appropriate; never force connections. The IOS-designed connectors will not fit any other connectors (TJC, 2014; IOS, 2016).
- Ensure that each device is clearly labeled (TJC, 2014; USDHHS, 2015).
- Trace tubing or catheter from the patient to the point of origin (TJC, 2014).
- Route tubes and catheters having different purposes in different, standardized directions (TJC, 2014).
- Do not rely on color coding to identify connections because color coding is not universal (USDHHS, 2015).
- Do not modify or adapt intravenous or feeding devices. Use equipment only as it is intended to be used (TJC, 2014).
- Ensure accurate communication during patient handoffs and trace all connections (Durfee et al., 2014; TJC, 2014).
- Make sure that staff (and patients as indicated) are properly educated about new devices (Durfee et al., 2014; Guenter, 2014; TJC, 2014).
- Educate patients, visitors, and nonclinical staff to seek clinical assistance to reconnect lines (TJC, 2014).
- Follow agency policy and procedure for reporting any near misses or adverse events (TJC, 2014).

BOX 35.10   PROCEDURAL GUIDELINES

Verifying Enteral Tube Placement by Obtaining Gastrointestinal Aspirate for pH Measurement via Large-Bore and Small-Bore Feeding Tubes: Intermittent and Continuous Feeding

DELEGATION CONSIDERATIONS

The verification of tube placement is the responsibility of the nurse and cannot be delegated to nursing assistive personnel (NAP). The nurse directs the NAP to immediately inform the nurse if:

- The patient's respirations change or patient complains of shortness of breath, coughing, or choking.
- The patient vomits or the NAP notices vomitus in patient's mouth during oral hygiene.
- Nasal skin irritation or excoriation is present.
- A change in the external length of the tube occurs, which could indicate displacement of the tube.

EQUIPMENT

60-mL ENfit syringe, stethoscope, clean gloves, pH indicator strip (scale of 1.0 to 11.0), small medication cup, water (tap water or sterile [see agency policy]) in a dated and initialed container at patient's bedside

STEPS

1. Identify patient using at least two identifiers (e.g., name and birthday or name and medical record number) according to agency policy.
2. Review agency policy and procedures for frequency and method of checking tube placement. *Do not insufflate air into tube to check placement.*
3. Observe for signs and symptoms of respiratory distress such as coughing, choking, or reduced oxygen saturation during feeding.
4. Identify conditions that increase risk for spontaneous tube migration or dislocation (e.g., altered level of consciousness or agitation, retching or vomiting, nasotracheal suction).
5. Observe external portion of tube for movement of ink or tape mark away from mouth or naris.
6. Review patient's medication record for orders for continuous feeding or a gastric acid inhibitor (e.g., cimetidine [Tagamet], ranitidine [Zantac], famotidine [Pepcid AC], nizatidine [Axid]) or a proton pump inhibitor (e.g., omeprazole [Prilosec]).
7. Review patient's medical record for history of prior tube displacement.
8. Explain procedure to patient and/or family caregivers.
9. Prepare equipment at patient's bedside, perform hand hygiene, and apply clean gloves.
10. Verify tube placement at the following times:
    a. For intermittently tube-fed patients, test placement immediately before each feeding (usually a period of at least 4 hours will have elapsed since previous feeding) and before medications (AACN, 2016b).
    b. Follow agency policy regarding when to test pH for patients receiving continuous tube feeding. Tube feed-

ings should never be stopped exclusively for the purpose of pH testing (AACN, 2016b). If feedings have been interrupted for more than a few hours, testing of the pH at this time may be useful in distinguishing placement (Bourgault et al., 2015).
    c. Wait to verify placement at least 1 hour after medication administration by tube or mouth.
11. *Continuous feeding:* Turn off or place feeding on hold. Clamp or kink feeding tube and disconnect from nasogastric (NG) or nasointestinal (NI) tube.
    Intermittent feedings: Remove plug at end of tube.
    Draw up 30 mL of air into a 60-mL ENfit syringe. Place tip of syringe into end of NG or NI tube. Flush NG or NI tube with 30 mL of air before attempting to aspirate fluid. Repositioning patient from side to side is helpful. In some cases, more than one bolus of air is necessary.
12. Draw back on syringe slowly and obtain 5 to 10 mL of gastric aspirate. Observe appearance of aspirate (see illustration). Aspirates from nasogastric tubes of continuously tube-fed patients often look like curdled enteral formula. During fasting, gastric aspirates from tube-fed patients are typically grassy green or clear. Small-bowel fluid is often bile stained. If gastric aspirates are bile stained, it may indicate that intestinal fluid has refluxed into the stomach (AACN, 2016b).
13. Gently mix aspirate in syringe. Expel a few drops into clean medicine cup. Measure pH of aspirated gastrointestinal contents by dipping pH strip into fluid or by applying a few drops of fluid to strip. Compare color of strip with color on chart (see illustration) provided by manufacturer.
    a. Gastric fluid from patient who has fasted for at least 4 hours usually has pH range of 5.0 or less.
    b. Fluid from tube in small intestine of fasting patient usually has pH greater than 6.0.

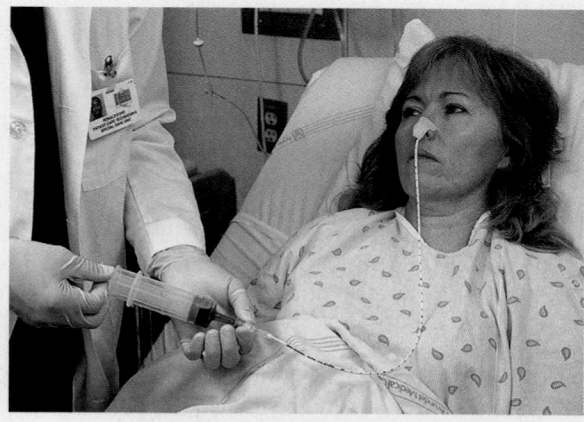

STEP 12 Obtain gastric aspirate.

BOX 35.10   PROCEDURAL GUIDELINES—cont'd

Verifying Enteral Tube Placement by Obtaining Gastrointestinal Aspirate for pH Measurement via Large-Bore and Small-Bore Feeding Tubes: Intermittent and Continuous Feeding

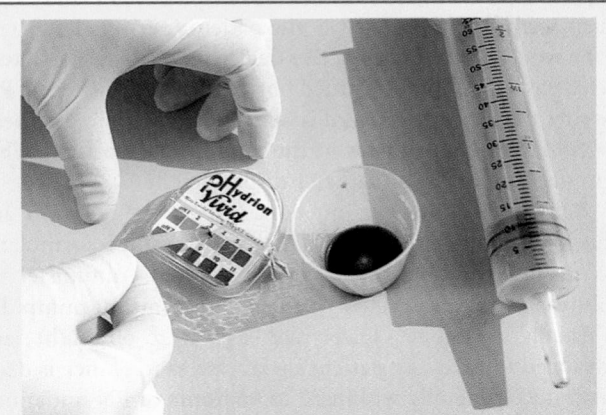

STEP 13 Compare color on test strip with color on pH chart.

14. Consider the use of radiographic confirmation of tube if the bedside techniques used raise doubt about the location of the tube (AACN, 2016b).
15. Irrigate tube.
16. Remove and dispose of gloves and supplies in appropriate receptacle. Perform hand hygiene.
17. Observe patient for signs of respiratory distress including persistent gagging, paroxysms of coughing, drop in oxygen saturation, and respiratory patterns (e.g., rate and depth) that are inconsistent with baseline measures.
18. Verify that external length of tube, pH, and appearance of aspirate are consistent with initial tube placement.
19. Use the principles of teach-back to evaluate patient/family caregiver learning. To determine that the patient and family understand about tube placement confirmation, state, "I want to make sure you understand what I explained earlier. Tell me why it is important for me to test gastric pH and the color of the gastric secretions before feedings."

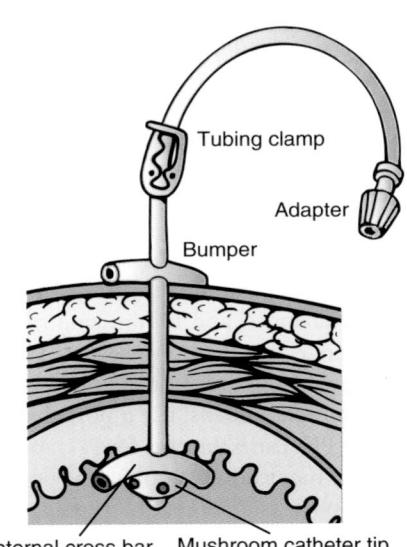

FIG 35.4 Percutaneous endoscopic gastrostomy tube.

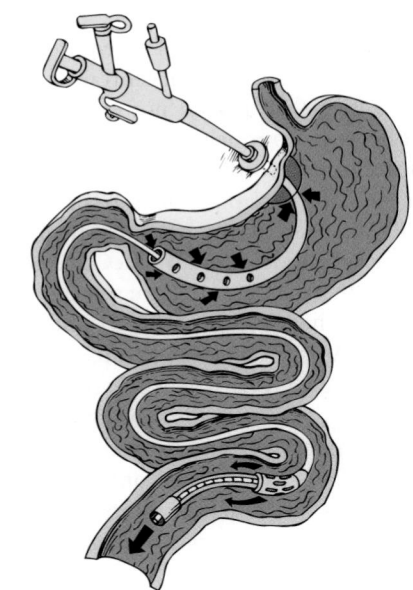

FIG 35.5 Endoscopic insertion of jejunostomy tube.

When patients have delayed gastric emptying or gastric resection or other surgery in the upper GI tract such as a pancreatectomy, a **jejunostomy tube** may be inserted to deliver nutrition (see Skill 35.3). Feedings delivered via a jejunostomy tube are usually delivered even more slowly (e.g., over a period of hours overnight) because the jejunum lacks the storage and regulated emptying capacity of the stomach. Jejunostomy tubes are inserted either directly into the small intestine through a percutaneous incision or through a gastrostomy opening into the small intestine. Gastrojejunostomy tubes provide access to both the stomach and the small intestine. The gastric port may be used for decompression of accumulated stomach content while feeding is delivered into

the jejunal port (Fig. 35.5). You need to know which port is gastric and which port is jejunal.

It is important to prevent and monitor for feeding tube displacement. Gastrostomy tubes that migrate internally sometimes block the pylorus or exit from the stomach to the small intestine. This results in increased GRV, discomfort, emesis, or leaking around the tube. An external disk helps prevent migration of a gastrostomy tube. Tubes that are too tight impair circulation between the external disc and the insertion site and quickly lead to breakdown of the site. Perform site care and assess the insertion site daily. Daily cleaning and evaluation of the site detects problems. Prevent displacement of a feeding tube by taping it to the abdomen

QSEN   QSEN ACTIVITY *Safety*

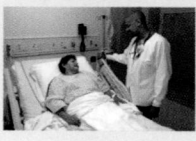

Matt is currently doing his clinical rotation on a medical nursing unit that cares for many patients with feeding tubes. He observes a nurse on the unit who is not following the agency protocol for checking feeding tube placement.

• What should Matt do in this situation?

evolve   Answers to QSEN Activities can be found on the Evolve website.

or tucking it into clothing for security as indicated or applying an abdominal binder if necessary. Displaced tubes can lead to infusion of fluid into the peritoneal space, which leads to serious complications (check agency policy).

Parenteral Nutrition. PN administers a solution of glucose, amino acids, minerals, electrolytes, and vitamins through a peripherally inserted venous catheter or central venous catheter (CVC). PN is used when the GI tract cannot be used or cannot digest and absorb nutrients in sufficient amounts to provide adequate nutrition. Patients are at an increased risk for infection because PN requires intravascular access and because of the high concentration of glucose in PN solutions. Patients on PN do not experience the many physiological benefits from being fed from the GI tract. PN is also significantly more costly than EN. The health care team evaluates the need for PN on a daily basis. The goal is to discontinue PN as soon as the patient can tolerate greater than 60% of energy needs enterally (McClave et al., 2016).

PN solutions that contain 10% or greater dextrose are hyperosmolar (i.e., highly concentrated) and irritate small peripheral veins. As a result, PN at this concentration is administered through CVCs where the blood flow is very rapid. This is called *central PN.* PN solutions with osmolality less than 900 mOsm may be administered through peripheral veins. Peripheral PN is usually used only for a short period (10 to 14 days or less) because it is still irritating to the blood vessels. In addition, it is challenging to meet a patient's nutritional needs with less concentrated solutions. A PN solution meets a patient's specific nutritional needs and is adjusted based on a patient's laboratory values and metabolic and nutrition status. Some PN solutions contain fat emulsions (lipids) with concentrations ranging from 10% to 30%. They are mostly composed of omega-6 fatty acids.

Fat emulsions can be combined with the other nutrients in a PN prescription to make a total nutrient admixture (TNA), or they can be provided in a separate bag via IV piggyback. Do not administer TNA if you observe oil droplets or an oily or creamy layer on the surface of the solution. Administer lipid emulsions peripherally or via a larger blood vessel (centrally).

Initiating Parenteral Nutrition. PN therapy requires a CVC inserted into the superior vena cava via the subclavian vein or, less ideally, the jugular vein. PN can also be administered via a peripherally inserted central catheter (PICC).

Nurses assist physicians during CVC insertion. Specially trained nurses insert PICCs (see agency policy and Chapter 18) (DiMaria-Ghalili et al., 2016). A chest x-ray confirms the location of the CVC after initial placement and when misplacement is suspected. Some patients needing long-term PN have a central venous access device (CVAD) such as a tunneled catheter or an implanted port. When administering PN, be sure the formula ordered is being delivered into a catheter or CVAD that terminates in the appropriate position. Thus you need to assess for catheter displacement.

Before beginning an infusion, inspect the solution and check the contents carefully to make sure that it is formulated according to the health care provider order. Administer the solution at the prescribed rate using an infusion pump. PN is usually started at a lower rate (e.g., 40 to 60 mL/hr) and advanced to meet the patient's goal rate as tolerance is demonstrated (generally within 72 to 96 hours of PN initiation). Reactions to lipid infusion include dyspnea, cyanosis, vomiting, headache, and chest pain. If a reaction occurs, stop the infusion and notify the health care provider immediately.

Caring for the Patient Receiving Parenteral Nutrition. Nursing care for the patient receiving PN focuses on seven major nursing goals: (1) preventing infection; (2) maintaining the PN system; (3) preventing metabolic, electrolyte, or fluid balance complications; (4) ensuring that the patient's nutrient and fluid needs are being met; (5) evaluating the continued need for PN or if oral intake or EN may be initiated; (6) planning for home PN if this is indicated; and (7) supporting the patient and family during major lifestyle changes.

Infection prevention includes strict aseptic management of the catheter hub, proper care of the CVC and dressing, maintaining policy recommendations for frequency of tubing and filter changes, and minimizing manipulation of the catheter (Ayers et al., 2014). Make sure PN solutions do not exceed their 24-hour infusion limit. If you are using a CVC that has multiple lumens, use a port that is exclusively dedicated for the PN. Label the port for PN, and do not infuse other solutions or medications through the port, unless clinical evidence supports the compatibility and stability of the combination (Boullata et al., 2014). During CVC dressing changes, always wear a mask to reduce the risk of introducing airborne contaminants. Assess the insertion site for signs of infection. Wear sterile gloves if you need to touch the site. Change the CVC dressing per institution policy and anytime it becomes wet, loose, or contaminated. Chlorhexidine gluconate (CHG)–impregnated dressings and cleaning solutions are preferred for skin antisepsis because they reduce the risk for CVAD-related bloodstream infections (Ullman et al., 2016). Scrub the catheter hub or port with 70% alcohol solution, tincture of iodine, or CHG using friction every time the system is entered. An in-line 0.22-mcg filter is typically used to remove air and particulate matter such as bacteria. Because fat molecules are large, you need to bypass the filter or use a larger filter (0.5 mcg) if a patient is receiving a fat emulsion.

Closely assess patients receiving PN for tolerance, the need for adjustments to the solution, and efficacy of the nutrition provided. Analyze laboratory findings for metabolic or electrolyte abnormalities and assess fluid balance, weight trends, and the ability to heal during administration. Laboratory monitoring includes frequent blood glucose testing because the high dextrose (glucose) content of the solution easily leads to hyperglycemia. Some patients need supplemental insulin (Box 35.11) (Ayers et al., 2014). Stopping the high-dextrose solution suddenly often leads to hypoglycemia. To reduce the risk of hypoglycemia, taper the solution before it is discontinued, especially if the patient is not currently receiving another source of carbohydrate. Be alert for changes in vital signs, changes in fluid balance, and laboratory results that indicate osmotic diuresis and dehydration, infection (e.g., an increased temperature or white blood cell count), electrolyte

---

BOX 35.11 PROCEDURAL GUIDELINES

Blood Glucose Monitoring

DELEGATION CONSIDERATIONS

When a patient's condition is stable, the skill of obtaining and testing a sample of blood for blood glucose level can be delegated to NAP. The nurse informs the NAP by:

- Explaining appropriate sites to use for puncture and when to obtain glucose levels.
- Reviewing expected blood glucose levels and when to report unexpected glucose levels to the nurse.

EQUIPMENT

Antiseptic swab; cotton ball; lancet device, either self-activating or button activated; blood glucose meter (e.g., Accucheck III, OneTouch); blood glucose test strips appropriate for meter brand used; clean gloves; paper towel

STEPS

1. Identify patient using at least two identifiers (e.g., name and birthday or name and medical record number) according to agency policy.
2. Assess patient's understanding of procedure and purpose of blood glucose monitoring. Determine if patient understands how to perform test and its importance in glucose control.
3. Determine if specific conditions need to be met before or after sample collection (e.g., fasting, postprandial, after certain medications, before insulin doses). In addition, determine if risks exist for performing skin puncture (e.g., low platelet count, anticoagulant therapy, bleeding disorders).
4. Assess area of skin to be used as puncture site. Inspect fingers or forearms for edema, inflammation, cuts, or sores. Avoid areas of bruising and open lesions. Do not use the hand on the side of a mastectomy or dialysis graft.
5. Review health care provider's order for time or frequency of measurement.
6. For patient with diabetes who performs test at home, assess ability to handle skin-puncturing device.
7. Explain procedure and purpose to patient and/or family. Offer patient and family opportunity to practice testing procedures, and provide resources/teaching aids.
8. Perform hand hygiene. Instruct patient to perform hand hygiene including forearm (if applicable) with soap and water. Rinse and dry.
9. Position patient comfortably in chair or in semi-Fowler's position in bed.
10. Remove reagent strip from vial and tightly seal cap. Check code on test strip vial. Use only test strips recommended for glucose meter. Some newer meters do not require code and/or have disk or drum with 10 or more test strips.

11. Insert strip into meter (refer to manufacturer directions [see illustration]). Do not bend strip. Meter turns on automatically.
12. Remove unused reagent strip from meter and place on paper towel or clean, dry surface with test pad facing up (refer to manufacturer directions).
13. Meter displays code on screen that must match code from test strip vial. Press proper button on meter to confirm matching codes. Meter is ready for use.
14. Perform hand hygiene and apply clean gloves. Prepare single-use lancet or multiple-use lancet device. **Note:** Some meters recommend that this step be completed before preparing test strip. Remove cap from lancet device; insert new lancet. Some lancet devices have disk or cylinder that rotates to new lancet.
    a. Twist off protective cover on tip of lancet. Replace cap of lancet device.
    b. Cock lancet device, adjusting for proper puncture depth.
15. Obtain blood sample.
    a. Wipe patient's finger or forearm lightly with antiseptic swab and allow to dry. Choose vascular area for puncture site. Select lateral side of finger. Avoid central tip of finger, which has a denser nerve supply (Pagana and Pagana, 2017).
    b. Hold area to be punctured in dependent position. Do not milk or massage finger site.
    c. Hold tip of lancet device against area of skin chosen for test site (see illustration). Press release button on device. Some devices allow you to see blood sample forming. Remove device.

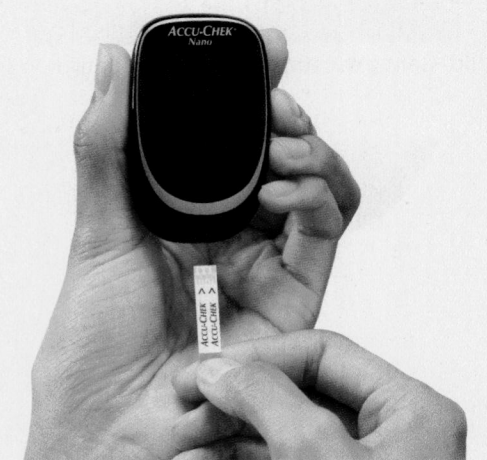

STEP 11 Load test strip into meter. (Courtesy Accucheck Glucometer.)

Continued

BOX 35.11   PROCEDURAL GUIDELINES—cont'd

Blood Glucose Monitoring

d. With some devices a blood sample begins to appear. Otherwise gently squeeze or massage fingertip until drop of blood forms (see illustration).
16. Obtain test results.
   a. Be sure that meter is still on. Bring test strip in meter to drop of blood. Blood will be wicked onto test strip (see illustration). Follow specific meter instructions to be sure that you obtain adequate sample.

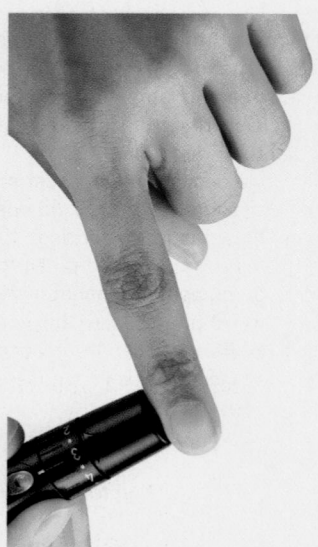

STEP 15c Prick side of finger with lancet. (Courtesy Accu-check Glucometer.)

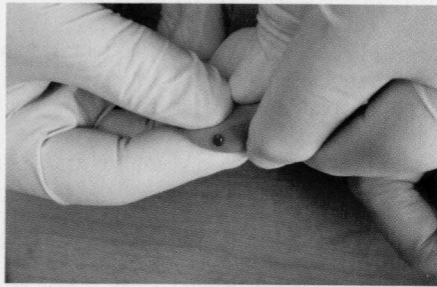

STEP 15d Gently squeeze puncture site until drop of blood forms.

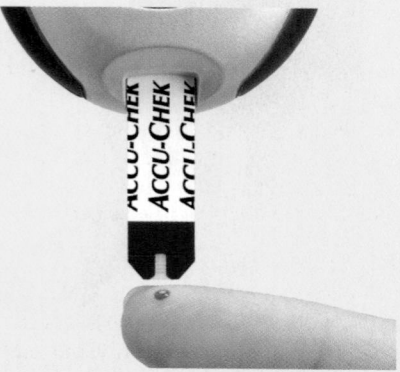

STEP 16a Touch test strip to blood drop. Blood wicks onto test strip. (Courtesy Accucheck Glucometer.)

Clinical Decision Point. Do not scrape blood onto the test strips or apply it to the wrong side of the test strip. This prevents accurate glucose measurement.

---

   b. Blood glucose test result will appear on screen (see illustration). Some devices "beep" when completed.
17. Turn meter off. Some meters turn off automatically. Dispose of test strip, lancet, and gloves in proper receptacles.
18. Perform hand hygiene.
19. Inspect puncture site for bleeding or tissue injury.
20. Compare glucose meter reading with normal blood glucose levels and previous test results.
21. Document glucose results and describe response including presence or absence of pain or excessive oozing of blood at puncture site.
22. Discuss test results with patient and encourage questions and participation in care.
23. Report blood glucose levels out of target range and take appropriate action for hypoglycemia or hyperglycemia.
24. Use the principles of teach-back to evaluate patient/family caregiver learning. State, "I want to be sure I explained how to obtain a blood glucose reading. Can you repeat the steps back to me?" Revise your instruction now or develop plan for revised patient teaching if patient is unable to teach back correctly.

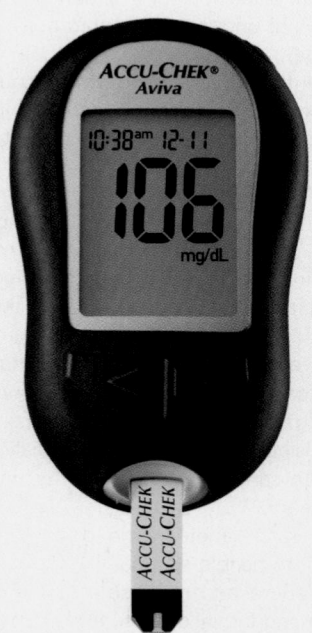

STEP 16b Results appear on meter screen. (Courtesy Accucheck Glucometer.)

imbalance or hyperglycemia, and clinical symptoms of high or low blood glucose. Report any unusual symptoms to the health care provider.

Restorative and Continuing Care

Diet Therapy in Disease Management. Patients discharged from a hospital with diet prescriptions often need dietary education to plan meals that meet specific therapeutic requirements. Restorative care includes immediate postsurgical, posthospitalization, and routine medical care.

Medical Nutrition Therapy. Optimal nutrition is important. Optimal nutrition is patient-centered and individualized. Medical nutrition therapy (MNT) is the diagnosis, therapy, and counseling services provided by an RDN for disease management. Patients with specific diseases often need to modify their diet to achieve balanced nutrition. These include GI diseases such as irritable bowel syndrome and malabsorption syndromes, metabolic disorders such as diabetes mellitus and hypoglycemia, cardiovascular disease, renal disease, liver disease, and cancer. Diet modifications need to correspond with the body's ability to metabolize certain nutrients, correct nutritional deficiencies, and eliminate harmful foods from the diet. Always work with the health care provider and RDN when planning and implementing modified diets. MNT includes the four steps of the Nutrition Care Process: nutrition assessment, nutrition diagnosis, nutrition intervention, and nutrition monitoring and evaluation (AND, 2016).

Home Care. When patients use EN or PN at home, the health care provider needs to verify that the home environment supports the use of nutritional support. A patient's medical suitability, rehabilitation potential, learning ability, and reimbursement sources are also determined (Durfee et al., 2014). The feeding regimen must meet the patient's nutrient and fluid needs and be compatible with the type of feeding tube and the patient's lifestyle. For example, administer bolus feedings over the length of time of a comfortable meal (e.g., 20 to 30 minutes if the tube terminates in the stomach) or deliver the feeding over 10 to 12 hours at night for jejunal feedings to free the patient of a pump during the day. Patients receiving PN at home often administer the entire daily solution over 10 or 12 hours at night. This allows the patient to disconnect from the infusion each morning, flush the central line, and have independent mobility during the day.

Home care nurses often see the patient on a regular basis. You teach patients or family caregivers how to administer PN or EN; assess the catheter or feeding tube; assess tolerance and adequacy of the nutrition and fluid regimen by monitoring weight, hydration status, or glucose level; watch for signs of infection; and help with troubleshooting and problem prevention. GRVs are typically not measured in adult patients receiving EN at home. You can withdraw gastric contents if the patient is very uncomfortable to avoid emesis and if indicated by the health care provider. If you do this, assess the patient's bowel status.

You help a patient transition to oral intake according to the health care provider's order. Help the patient be as independent and in control of his or her own life as much as possible, while maintaining safety and a therapeutic regimen. The need for nutrition support at home often results in significant lifestyle changes for both the patient and the family. For example, if a patient needs assistance with the feeding equipment, someone will need to be available at those specified times. The social aspect of sharing meals together may be disrupted. Be a patient advocate by investigating the options that best fit your patient's lifestyle.

■■■■ EVALUATION

Patient Outcomes. Ongoing evaluation measures the effectiveness of a patient's plan of care in meeting nutritional needs. Allow adequate intervals to evaluate your patient's progress; nutritional improvements take time.

Evaluation of clinical progress includes objective data such as weight status or improved laboratory parameters and subjective data such as a patient reporting improvement in food choices or self-reporting improved intake (Box 35.12). When clinical progress does not occur as expected, determine whether the interventions were not effective, not done or accepted by the patient, not realistic or appropriate, or affected by unanticipated or unidentified factors (see Care Plan).

If outcomes are not met, reassess the patient to determine if you missed important data. Some patients need reeducation if they have forgotten or misunderstood essential skills or knowledge. Validate that the patient and family caregiver are in agreement with the goals and are able to follow the nutrition plan of care.

Patient Expectations. Successful nutrition interventions often depend on a patient's willingness and ability to change

---

BOX 35.12 EVALUATION

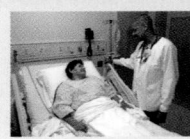

As Mrs. Gonzalez begins to eat again, Matt encourages her to eat first and then infuses her feeding right after meals. Her feeding volumes decrease as her oral intake increases. Matt also encourages her to ingest adequate volumes of fluid so that her feeding tube is no longer needed. Over time, Mrs. Gonzalez is able to consume all her required fluid and nutrients with a ground diet and nectar-thickened liquids. Matt removes the feeding tube in preparation for her transport to a restorative care facility.

Matt advises Mrs. Gonzalez to continue the current plan of care and emphasizes that it is important to continue speech therapy. He discusses the importance of compliance with diet modifications until swallowing function returns completely.

DOCUMENTATION NOTE
"Swallows without signs of aspirating. Oral intake of mechanically altered diet and fluid meets 100% of estimated needs according to dietitian. To be followed by restorative care facility."

existing behavior patterns and adapt to new patterns. If a patient is not committed to the expected changes, the interventions will not be successful. Some patients find it difficult to change their behavior and lose motivation over time. It is important to remember to individualize the nutrition care plan, focus on the patient, and refer back to the RDN when indicated.

Most patients respond to the opportunity to make informed choices. Explaining the reasons for behavioral changes and providing a patient with options for how to achieve the change help a patient make changes. If necessary, provide education over several brief sessions to maximize retention of information.

SAFETY GUIDELINES FOR NURSING SKILLS

Ensuring patient safety is an essential role of the nurse. To ensure patient safety, communicate clearly with members of the health care team, assess and incorporate the patient's priorities of care and preferences, and use the best evidence when making decisions about your patient's care. When performing the skills in this chapter, remember the following points to ensure safe, individualized care:

- Verify tube position and connector type (current or ENFit) at the beginning of each initial nursing assessment and before administration of feedings or medications and as needed (prn) (Boullata et al., 2017). The ENFit device will not be compatible with a Luer-Lok connection or any other type of small-bore medical connector, thus preventing misadministration of an enteral feeding (Institute for Safe Medication Practices [ISMP], 2015).
- Label enteral equipment with patient information, formula type, enteral access delivery site/access, administration method, individuals responsible for preparing and hanging the formula, and time and date formula is prepared and hung (Boullata et al., 2017).
- Ensure "right patient, right formula, right tube" by matching formula and rate to feeding order and verifying that enteral tubing set connects formula to feeding tube (see the ASPEN *Be ALERT* safety campaign for enteral feeding at www.nutritioncare.org).
- Elevate the head of the bed a minimum of 30 to 45 degrees for patients receiving enteral feedings unless medically contraindicated (AACN, 2016a; McClave et al., 2016).
- Trace all lines and tubing back to the patient to ensure that you have only enteral-to-enteral connections and that they are secure (Boullata et al., 2017).

- Monitoring tube placement is essential in early detection of tube misplacement. Auscultation is not a reliable method for verification of NG or nasointestinal tube placement because a tube inadvertently placed in the lungs, pharynx, or esophagus transmits a sound similar to that of air entering the stomach (AACN, 2016b).
- Food safety is especially important in providing EN. Feeding products and equipment used to deliver them are good growth media for bacteria. Clean, dry, and store syringes as two pieces to prevent moisture accumulation. Keep other equipment clean and dry, and change according to agency protocol.
- Refer to manufacturer guidelines to determine hang time for enteral feedings. Maximum hang time for formula is 8 hours in an open system and 24 hours in a closed, ready-to-hang system (if it remains closed) (Boullata et al., 2017). There is increased risk for bacterial growth in feedings that exceed the recommended hang time.
- To prevent tube clogging, flush tube with at least 30 mL of water (for adults without volume restriction) following enteral feedings. Use freshly obtained tap water as the flush and fluid administration solution unless normal saline is ordered or agency protocol is to use sterile water for patients who are immunocompromised (Boullata et al., 2017).
- Use liquid medications whenever possible or crush and adequately dilute medications administered via the feeding tube. Do not mix medications. Flush tube with at least 15 mL of water before, between, and after each medication administration in adult patients without volume restriction (Boullata et al., 2017).
- Administer continuous EN and PN with an infusion pump.

SKILL 35.1   ASPIRATION PRECAUTIONS

DELEGATION CONSIDERATIONS
The skill of following aspiration precautions while feeding a patient can be delegated to nursing assistive personnel (NAP). However, the nurse is responsible for the ongoing assessment of a patient's risk for aspiration and determination of positioning and any special feeding techniques. The nurse directs the NAP to:

- Position patient upright (preferably 45 to 90 degrees) or according to medical restrictions during and after feeding.
- Use aspiration precautions while feeding patients who need assistance.
- Immediately report any onset of coughing, gagging, a change in voice, or pocketing of food to the nurse.

EQUIPMENT
- Chair or bed that allows patient to sit upright
- Thickening agents as designated by speech-language pathologist (SLP)—rice, cereal, yogurt, gelatin, commercial thickener
- Tongue blade
- Penlight
- Oral hygiene supplies
- Suction equipment
- Clean gloves

STEP	RATIONALE

ASSESSMENT

1. Identify patient using at least two identifiers (e.g., name and birthday or name and medical record number) according to agency policy.

Ensures correct patient. Complies with The Joint Commission standards and improves patient safety (TJC, 2018).

2. Review results of nutrition screening in medical record.

Reveals risk patterns (e.g., patients with dysphagia may alter their eating patterns or choose foods that are easy to swallow but do not provide adequate nutrition).

3. Ask patient or family caregiver if patient has difficulties with chewing or swallowing various food textures.

Patients are likely to aspirate certain foods more than others.

4. Assess for conditions that cause dysphagia and thus present risk for aspiration (see Box 35.7). Also assess signs and symptoms of dysphagia (e.g., coughing, voice change, food pocketing). Use dysphagia screening tool if available.

Patients with neurological or neuromuscular disease and patients with trauma to or surgery of the oral cavity or throat are at increased risk.

5. Assess mental status including alertness, orientation, and ability to follow simple commands (e.g., open your mouth; stick out your tongue).

Dementia and cognitive impairment increase risk for dysphagia and aspiration (Rösler et al., 2015).

6. Assess patient's oral cavity, level of dental hygiene, missing teeth, or poorly fitting dentures (apply clean gloves if needed).

Poor oral hygiene can result in decayed teeth, plaque, and periodontal disease; these increase the risk for aspiration and pneumonia in patients with dysphagia (Sørensen et al., 2013).

7. Observe patient during mealtime for signs of dysphagia such as coughing, voice change, or fatigue. Observe patient attempt to feed self; note type of food consistencies and liquids patient is able to swallow.

Detects a change in eating habits or abnormal eating patterns that indicate a risk for dysphagia (AND, 2016; Hines et al., 2016; Malhi, 2016).

8. Indicate on patient's electronic medical record (EMR), chart, or Kardex that dysphagia/aspiration risk is present. *Option:* Some agencies use different-colored meal trays to signify patients at risk for aspiration.

Identifying a patient as having dysphagia reduces the risk that patient will receive improperly prepared oral nutrition without supervision.

9. Assess patient and family caregiver knowledge of aspiration precautions.

Encourages cooperation, minimizes risks and anxiety, and identifies teaching needs.

PLANNING

1. Provide patient rest time before meals.

Some practitioners recommend rest time before meals (Metheny, 2012). Muscle weakness and fatigue may increase risk of aspiration.

2. Explain to patient why you are observing him or her while eating.

Signs or symptoms associated with aspiration indicate need for further swallowing evaluation such as fluoroscopic examination.

3. Explain to patient and family caregiver about the aspiration precautions you are implementing.

Increases patient cooperation and prepares family caregiver for being able to assist.

IMPLEMENTATION

1. Perform hand hygiene and have patient or family caregiver (if going to assist with feeding) perform hand hygiene.

Prevents transmission of microorganisms. Educates patient and family caregiver about need to maintain infection control practices.

2. Apply clean gloves. Provide thorough oral hygiene including brushing of tongue before meal.

Intensified oral hygiene reduces risk for aspiration pneumonia (Sørensen et al., 2013).

3. Position patient in chair or raise head of the bed to upright, seated position (45- to 90-degree angle or highest position allowed by medical condition during meal).

Upright position aids safe swallowing and helps prevent aspiration (AACN, 2016a; Malhi, 2016).

4. Using penlight and tongue blade, gently inspect mouth for pockets of food.

Pockets of food found inside the cheeks may indicate that a patient has difficulty moving food from mouth into the pharynx to swallow. Food pocketing because of impaired swallowing increases risk for aspiration (Jeng et al., 2001).

5. Add thickener to thin liquids to create desired consistency per SLP assessment.

For patients unable to safely control swallowing of thin liquids, thickening agents slow the process of swallowing and increase safety by helping to prevent aspiration (Newman et al., 2016).

SKILL 35.1 ASPIRATION PRECAUTIONS—cont'd

View Video!

STEP	RATIONALE
6. Objectively measure viscosity of liquids to ensure consistency with recommendation by SLP.	Different thickening agents yield variable consistencies. Subjective measurements of viscosity are unreliable. Only thickening agents with reliable viscosity data should be used (Nita et al., 2013).
7. Have patient assume chin-tuck position. Remind patient to not tilt head backward when eating or while drinking.	Hyperextension of neck makes it easier for food to enter airway. Chin-tuck or chin-down position reduces aspiration in some patients. Patients need a minimum of 17.5 degrees of neck flexion to achieve a beneficial effect (Ra et al., 2014).
8. Provide tactile and temperature stimulation techniques if recommended by the SLP. Examples include increasing pressure on the tongue by a spoon during feeding and using cold utensils to stimulate oral cavity.	Provides tactile cue to food being eaten and may promote effective swallowing (Wirth et al., 2016).
9. Provide verbal coaching. Remind patient to chew and think about swallowing: • "Open your mouth" • "Feel the food in your mouth" • "Chew and taste the food" • "Raise your tongue to the roof of your mouth" • "Think about swallowing" • "Close your mouth and swallow" • "Swallow again" • "Cough to clear your airway"	Verbal cueing and positive reinforcement help patients focus on steps of normal swallowing. Instructing patients to repeat-swallow or practice effortful swallowing may help clear remaining food from the airway (Park et al., 2016).
10. Monitor swallowing and observe for throat clearing, coughing, choking, change in voice, and drooling of food; suction airway as needed.	Detects abnormal eating patterns that indicate a risk for aspiration from dysphagia (Hines et al., 2016; Malhi, 2016).
11. Minimize distractions and do not rush the patient through a meal. Allow time for adequate chewing and swallowing. Provide rest period as needed during meal.	Environmental distractions and conversations during mealtime may increase the risk for aspiration.
12. Ask patient to remain sitting upright for at least 30 to 60 minutes after meal.	Allows additional time for food particles in pharynx to clear.
13. Provide thorough oral hygiene after meal.	Oral hygiene reduces plaque and secretions containing bacteria that can cause pneumonia (Sørensen et al., 2013).
14. Remove gloves if worn. Return patient's tray to appropriate place and perform hand hygiene.	Reduces spread of microorganisms.

EVALUATION

1. Throughout meal observe patient's ability to swallow food and fluids of various textures and thickness without choking.

   Indicates if there is ease with swallowing and absence of signs related to aspiration. The ability to swallow safely may improve or deteriorate over time and within a single meal.

2. Monitor patient's intake and output (I&O), calorie count, and food intake.

   Aids in detection of malnutrition and dehydration resulting from dysphagia.

3. Weigh patient daily or weekly.

   Determines if weight is stable and reflects nutrition status.

4. Observe patient's oral cavity after meal.

   Determines presence of food pockets after meal.

5. **Use Teach-Back:** "We talked about why your loved one is at risk to aspirate food. Tell me the things to watch for that indicate trouble swallowing. What should you do if these things happen?" Revise your instruction now or develop a plan for revised patient/family caregiver teaching if patient/family caregiver is not able to teach back correctly.

   Determines patient's/family caregiver's level of understanding of instructional topic.

RECORDING AND REPORTING

- Document in patient's electronic health record (EHR) or chart assessment findings, patient's tolerance of liquids and food textures, amount of assistance required, position during meal, absence or presence of any symptoms of dysphagia during feeding or fluid intake, and total amount eaten.

- Document your evaluation of patient/family caregiver learning.
- Report any coughing, choking, voice changes, or other swallowing difficulties to health care provider.
- Communicate with other health care staff that patient has dysphagia during hand-off communication.

UNEXPECTED OUTCOMES AND RELATED INTERVENTIONS

- Patient coughs, gags, complains of food "stuck in throat," and has wet quality to voice when eating.
  - Stop feeding immediately and place patient on NPO. Notify health care provider, and suction as needed.
  - Schedule consultation with SLP for swallowing exercises and techniques to improve swallowing.

- Patient experiences weight loss over next several days/weeks.
  - Discuss findings with health care provider and registered dietitian nutritionist (RDN). Determine if increasing frequency or quality of foods is needed.
  - Nutritional supplements may be needed.

SKILL 35.2 INSERTING A NASOGASTRIC OR NASOINTESTINAL FEEDING TUBE

DELEGATION CONSIDERATIONS
The skill of feeding tube insertion cannot be delegated to nursing assistive personnel (NAP). However, NAP may help with patient positioning and comfort measures during tube insertion.

EQUIPMENT
Insertion
- Small-bore nasogastric (NG) or nasoenteric tube with or without stylet (select the smallest diameter possible to enhance patient comfort)
- 60-mL ENFit syringe
- Stethoscope, pulse oximeter, capnography *(optional)*
- Hypoallergenic tape, semipermeable (transparent) dressing, or tube fixation device
- Tincture of benzoin or other skin barrier protectant
- pH indicator strip (scale 1.0 to 11.0)

- Cup of water and straw or ice chips (for patients able to swallow)
- Water-soluble lubricant
- Emesis basin
- Towel or disposable pad
- Facial tissues
- Clean gloves
- Suction equipment in case of aspiration
- Penlight to check placement in nasopharynx
- Tongue blade

Removal
- Disposable pad
- Tissues
- Clean gloves
- Disposable plastic bag
- Towel

STEP	RATIONALE
ASSESSMENT	
1. Identify patient using at least two identifiers (e.g., name and birthday or name and medical record number) according to agency policy.	Ensures correct patient. Complies with The Joint Commission standards and improves patient safety (TJC, 2018).
2. Verify health care provider's order for type of tube and enteric feeding schedule. Also check order to determine if health care provider wants a prokinetic agent (e.g., metoclopramide) given before tube placement.	Health care provider's order is needed to insert a feeding tube. Prokinetic agent given before tube placement may help advance the tube into intestine.
3. Assess patient's knowledge of procedure.	Encourages cooperation, reduces anxiety, and minimizes risks. Identifies teaching needs.
4. Perform hand hygiene.	Reduces transmission of microorganisms.
5. Have patient close each nostril alternately and breathe. Examine each naris for patency and skin breakdown (apply clean gloves if drainage present).	Sometimes nares are obstructed or irritated, or a septal defect or facial fractures are present. Place tube in most patent nostril.
6. Review patient's medical history (e.g., for basilar skull fracture, nasal problems, nosebleeds, facial trauma, nasal-facial surgery, head or neck cancer, deviated septum, anticoagulant therapy, coagulopathy).	History of these problems may require you to consult with the health care provider to change route of nutrition support. Passage of tube intracranially can cause morbid complications (Miller et al., 2014).

SKILL 35.2 INSERTING A NASOGASTRIC OR NASOINTESTINAL FEEDING TUBE—cont'd

STEP	RATIONALE

Clinical Decision Point. If a patient is at risk of intracranial passage of the tube, avoid the nasal route. Oral placement or placement under medical supervision using fluoroscopic direct visualization is preferable. Insertion of a gastrostomy or jejunostomy tube is another alternative.

STEP	RATIONALE
7. Assess patient's height, weight, hydration status, electrolyte balance, caloric needs, and I&O.	Provides baseline information to measure nutrition improvement and metabolic parameters after enteral feedings are instituted (Boullata et al., 2017).
8. Assess patient's level of consciousness, presence of cough and gag reflex, ability to sit upright, obstructive or restrictive lung disease, and presence of mechanical ventilation.	These are risk factors for inadvertent tube placement into tracheobronchial tree (Sparks et al., 2011).

Clinical Decision Point. Recognize situations in which blind placement of a feeding tube poses an unacceptable risk for placement. Devices designed to detect pulmonary intubation such as carbon dioxide (CO_2) sensors or obtaining a radiograph enhances patient safety. To avoid insertion complications from blind placement in high-risk situations, clinicians trained in the use of radiographic confirmation should place tubes (AACN, 2016b).

STEP	RATIONALE
9. Perform physical assessment of abdomen. Perform hand hygiene, and remove and dispose of gloves (if worn).	Abdominal pain, tenderness, or distention may indicate medical problem that contraindicates feedings.
10. Assess patient and family caregiver knowledge of procedure for NG feeding tube insertion.	Encourages cooperation, minimizes risks and anxiety, and identifies teaching needs.

PLANNING

1. Provide privacy and prepare bedside environment for patient safety.	Preparing the environment helps the nurse think about the steps in the procedure; removing clutter from over-bed or bedside table removes barriers to insertion.
2. Prepare and organize equipment needed for insertion of NG feeding tube.	Ensures an organized approach for insertion of NG feeding tube.
3. Explain procedure to patient including sensations (e.g., discomfort or burning sensation in nasal passages) that will be felt during insertion.	Increases patient's cooperation with tube insertion procedure and helps lessen anxiety.
4. Explain to patient how to communicate during intubation by raising index finger to indicate gagging or discomfort.	Patient must have a way of communicating to alleviate stress and enhance cooperation.

IMPLEMENTATION

1. Perform hand hygiene. Prepare supplies at bedside.	Reduces transmission of microorganisms. Ensures organized procedure.
2. Stand on same side of bed as naris chosen for insertion and position patient upright in high Fowler's position (unless contraindicated). If patient is unresponsive, raise head of bed as tolerated in semi-Fowler's position with head tipped forward, using a pillow chin to chest. If necessary, have an NAP help with positioning of confused or unresponsive patients. If patient is forced to lie supine, place in reverse Trendelenburg's position.	Allows for easier manipulation of tube. An upright position aids safe swallowing and helps prevent aspiration (AACN, 2016a; Malhi, 2016). Forward head position assists with closure of airway and passage of tube into esophagus.
3. Apply pulse oximeter/capnograph and measure vital signs.	Provides baseline for objective assessment of respiratory status during tube insertion.
a. If patient has an increase in end-tidal CO_2 or decrease in oxygen saturation, do not insert tube until you determine patient's stability.	CO_2 detectors are helpful in detecting when the tube is placed in the tracheobronchial tree. However, x-ray confirmation of placement is necessary (AACN, 2016b).
4. Place bath towel over patient's chest. Keep facial tissues within reach.	Prevents soiling of gown. Insertion of tube frequently produces tearing.
5. Determine length of tube to be inserted and mark location with tape or indelible ink.	
a. Measure distance from tip of nose to earlobe to xyphoid process of sternum (see illustration). Mark this distance on tube with tape.	Length approximates distance from nose to stomach. Tip of NG tube must reach stomach to avoid risk for pulmonary aspiration, which increases when tubes terminate in the esophagus (AACN, 2016a).

STEP	RATIONALE
b. Measure distance from tip of nose to earlobe to midumbilicus for pediatric patient.	
c. Add additional 20 to 30 cm (8 to 12 inches) for nasojejunal tubes.	Length approximates distance from nose to jejunum.
6. Prepare NG or nasojejunal tube for intubation. **Note:** Do not ice tubes.	Iced tube becomes stiff and inflexible, causing trauma to nasal mucosa.
a. Obtain order for stylet tube and check agency policy for trained clinician to insert tube.	
b. If tube has a guidewire or stylet, inject 10 mL of water from ENFit syringe into tube.	Activates lubrication of tube for easier passage and ensures that tube is patent. Aids in guidewire or stylet removal. ENFit devices are not compatible with any other type of small-bore medical connector, thus preventing inappropriate connections and misadministration of an enteral feeding (ISMP, 2015).
c. If using stylet, make certain that it is positioned securely within tube.	Promotes smooth passage of tube into gastrointestinal (GI) tract. Improperly positioned stylet can cause tube to kink or injure patient. Once tube insertion is confirmed, have trained clinician remove stylet.
7. Prepare tube fixation materials. Cut hypoallergenic tape 10 cm (4 inches) long or prepare membrane dressing or other tube fixation device.	Used to secure tubing after insertion. Fixation devices allow tube to float free of the nares, thus reducing pressure on the nares and preventing medical device–related pressure injury.
8. Apply clean gloves.	Reduces transmission of microorganisms.
9. *Option:* Dip tube with surface lubricant into glass of room-temperature water or apply water-soluble lubricant (see manufacturer directions).	Activates lubricant to facilitate passage of tube into naris and GI tract.
10. Hand an alert patient a cup of water with straw (if able to swallow).	Patient is asked to swallow water to facilitate tube passage.
11. Explain the next steps and gently insert tube through nostril to back of throat (posterior nasopharynx). This may cause patient to gag. Aim back and down toward ear (see illustration).	Natural contours facilitate passage of tube into GI tract.
12. Have patient take deep breath and relax and flex head toward chest after tube has passed through nasopharynx.	Closes off glottis and reduces risk for tube entering trachea.
13. Encourage patient to swallow small sips of water. Advance tube as patient swallows. Rotate tube gently 180 degrees while inserting.	Swallowing facilitates passage of tube past oropharynx. Distinct tug may be felt as patient swallows, indicating that tube is following expected path.
14. Emphasize need to breathe through mouth and swallow during insertion.	Helps facilitate passage of tube and decreases patient's anxiety reaction during procedure.
15. Do not advance tube during inspiration or coughing because it is more likely to enter the respiratory tract. Monitor oximetry and capnography.	Can cause tube to inadvertently enter patient's airway, which will be reflected in changes in oxygen saturation and/or capnography.

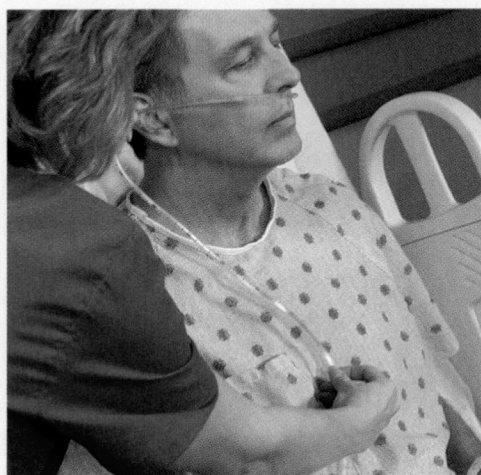

STEP 5a Measure to determine length of tube to insert.

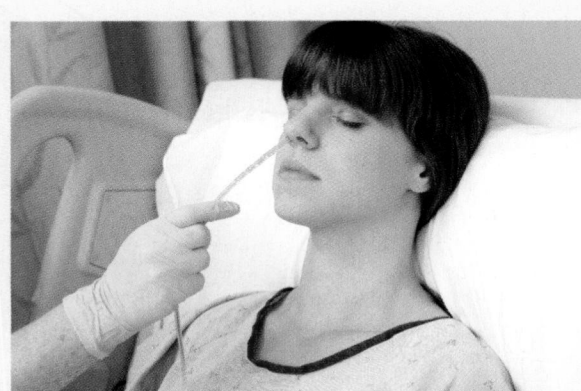

STEP 11 Insert tube through nostril to back of throat.

SKILL 35.2 INSERTING A NASOGASTRIC OR NASOINTESTINAL FEEDING TUBE—cont'd

STEP	RATIONALE
16. Advance tube each time patient swallows until desired length has been reached (see illustration).	Reduces discomfort and trauma to patient. Helps facilitate tube passage.

Clinical Decision Point. Do not force the tube or push against resistance. If patient starts to cough, experiences a drop in oxygen saturation, or shows other signs of respiratory distress, withdraw the tube into posterior nasopharynx until normal breathing resumes.

STEP	RATIONALE
17. Check for position of tube in back of throat using penlight and tongue blade.	Tube may be coiled, kinked, or entering trachea.
18. Temporarily anchor tube to nose with small piece of tape.	Movement of tube stimulates gagging. Allows assessment of general position before anchoring tube more securely.
19. Keep tube secure and check placement of tube by aspirating stomach contents to measure gastric pH. Also, assess amount, color and quality of return.	Proper tube position is essential before initiating feeding. (Confirm by radiograph before feeding is initiated.)

Clinical Decision Point. Insufflation of air into tube while auscultating abdomen is not a reliable means to determine position of feeding tube tip (AACN, 2016b).

STEP	RATIONALE
20. Anchor tube to patient's nose, avoiding pressure on nares. Mark exit site on tube with indelible ink. Select one of the following options for anchoring:	Marking tube can alert nurses to possible displacement of tube (AACN, 2016b; Boullata et al., 2017). Properly secured tube allows patient more mobility and prevents trauma to nasal mucosa.
a. Apply membrane dressing or tube fixation device.	Permits longer securement without need to change dressing.
(1) Membrane dressing:	
(a) Apply tincture of benzoin or other skin protectant to patient's cheek and area of tube to be secured.	Allows membrane to adhere to skin and protects skin.
(b) Place tube against patient's cheek and secure tube with membrane dressing, out of patient's line of vision.	Eliminates application of tape around naris. Decreases risk for inadvertent extubation.

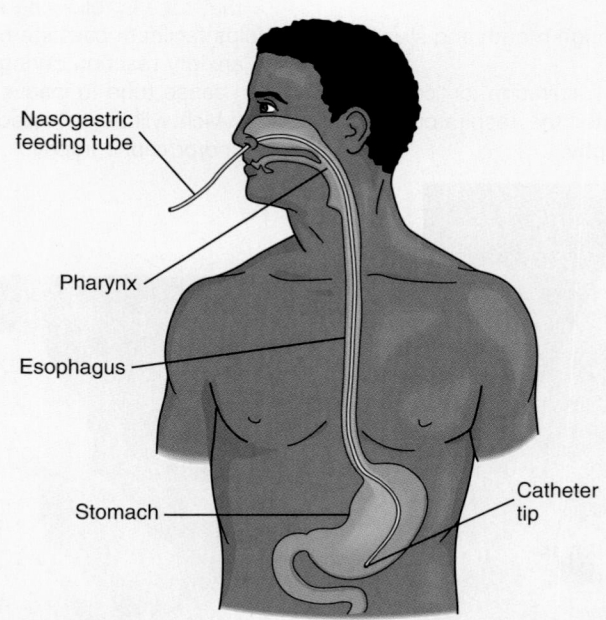

STEP 16 Nasogastric tube inserted through nasopharynx and esophagus into stomach.

STEP	RATIONALE

(2) Tube fixation device:

    (a) Apply wide end of patch to bridge of nose (see illustration).

Secures tube and reduces friction on naris.

    (b) Slip connector around feeding tube as it exits nose (see illustration).

b. Apply tape:

Prevents pulling of tube. May require frequent change if tape becomes soiled.

(1) Apply tincture of benzoin or other skin adhesive on tip of patient's nose and allow it to become "tacky."

Helps tape adhere better. Protects skin.

(2) Remove gloves and tear two horizontal slits on each side of tape at ⅓ and ⅔ length. Do not split tape. Fold middle sections forward.

Creates gap in tape that will allow tube to float and exert less pressure on naris.

(3) Tear vertical strip at bottom of tape. Print date and time on nasal portion of the tape.

Secures tube firmly. Documents when tube and tape were applied.

(4) Place intact end of tape over bridge of patient's nose. Wrap each strip around tube as it exits (see illustration).

Tube is free floating in the naris with this taping method, resulting in movement of tube in the pharynx. Securing tape to naris in this way reduces pressure on naris and reduces risk for medical device–related pressure injury (Markowitz et al., 2013).

21. Fasten end of tube to patient's gown using clip (see illustration) or piece of tape. Do not use safety pins to secure tube to gown.

Reduces traction on naris if tube moves, which can cause medical device–related pressure injury. Safety pins become unfastened and cause injury to patients.

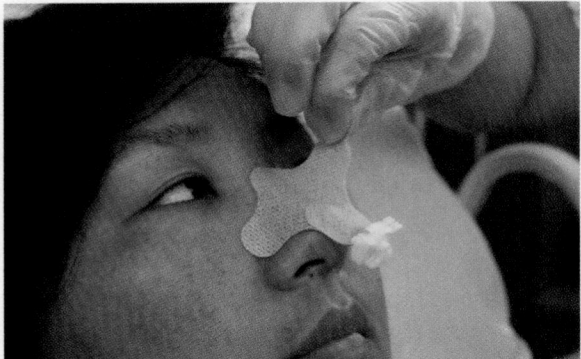

STEP 20a(2)(a) Applying tube fixation device to bridge of nose.

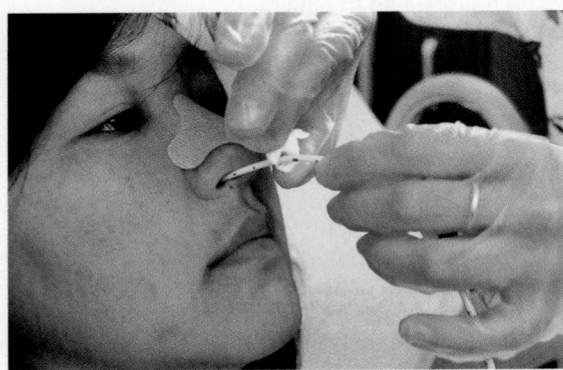

STEP 20a(2)(b) Slip connector around feeding tube.

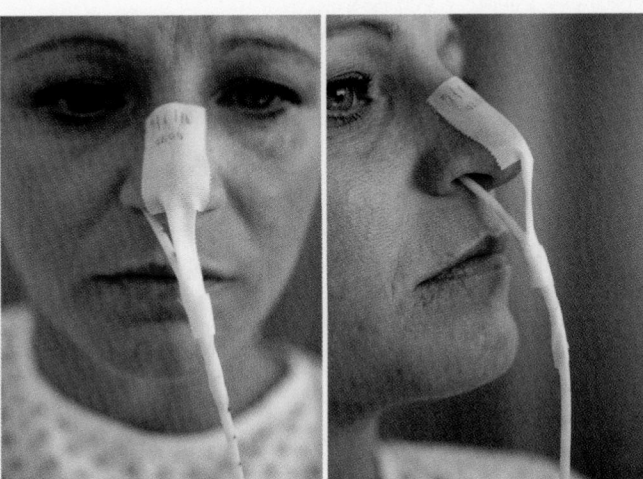

STEP 20b(4) Securing tape to nose.

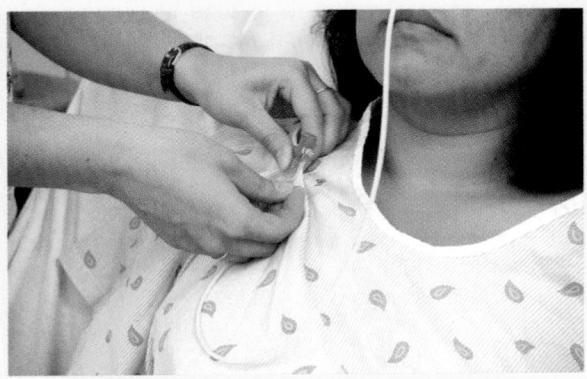

STEP 21 Fastening feeding tube to patient's gown.

SKILL 35.2 INSERTING A NASOGASTRIC OR NASOINTESTINAL FEEDING TUBE—cont'd

STEP	RATIONALE
22. Assist patient to comfortable position, but keep head of bed elevated at least 30 degrees (preferably 45 degrees) unless contraindicated. For intestinal tube placement, place patient on right side when possible until correct placement is confirmed by radiograph.	Promotes patient comfort and lowers risk of aspiration should patient receive tube feeding (Metheny and Frantz, 2013; AACN, 2016a). Placing patient on right side promotes passage of tube into small intestine.
23. Remove gloves and perform hand hygiene.	Reduces transmission of microorganisms.

Clinical Decision Point. Leave stylet in place until correct position is verified by x-ray film. Never try to reinsert a partially or fully removed stylet while feeding tube is in place. This can cause perforation of tube and injure patient.

STEP	RATIONALE
24. Contact radiology to obtain x-ray film of chest/abdomen.	Radiographic examination is the most accurate method to determine feeding tube placement (AACN, 2016b; Boullata et al., 2017).
25. Perform hand hygiene. Apply clean gloves and administer oral hygiene. Clean tubing at nostril with washcloth dampened in mild soap and water.	Reduces transmission of microorganisms. Promotes patient comfort and integrity of oral mucous membranes.
26. Remove gloves, dispose of equipment, and perform hand hygiene.	Reduces transmission of microorganisms.

TUBE REMOVAL

1. Verify health care provider's order for tube removal.	Health care provider's order is needed to remove feeding tube.
2. Gather equipment.	Ensures organized procedure.
3. Explain procedure to patient.	Encourages cooperation, reduces anxiety, and minimizes risks. Identifies teaching needs.
4. Perform hand hygiene. Apply clean gloves.	Reduces transmission of microorganisms.
5. Position patient in high Fowler's position unless contraindicated.	Reduces risk for pulmonary aspiration in the event patient vomits.
6. Place disposable pad or towel over patient's chest.	Prevents mucous and gastric secretions from soiling patient's clothing.
7. Disconnect tube from feeding administration set (if present) and clamp or cap end.	Prevents formula from spilling from tube as it is removed.
8. Remove tape or tube fixation device from patient's nose. Unclip tube from patient's gown.	Allows tube to be removed easily.
9. Instruct patient to take deep breath and hold it. Then as you kink end of tube securely (folding it over on itself), completely withdraw tube by pulling it out steadily and smoothly onto towel or disposable bag. Dispose of it into appropriate receptacle.	Prevents inadvertent aspiration of gastric contents while tube is removed. Kinking prevents leakage of fluid from tube. Promotes patient comfort. Reduces transmission of microorganisms.
10. Offer tissues to patient to blow nose.	Clears nasal passages of remaining secretions.
11. Offer mouth care.	Promotes patient's comfort.
12. Remove gloves; perform hand hygiene.	Reduces transmission of microorganisms.

EVALUATION

1. Observe patient's response to tube placement. Assess lung sounds; have patient speak; check vital signs; note any coughing, dyspnea, cyanosis, or decrease in oxygen saturation or capnography.	Symptoms may indicate placement in respiratory tract. Auscultation of crackles or wheezes, dyspnea, or fever may be delayed response to aspiration. Capnography indicates change in CO_2 concentration.
2. Confirm x-ray results with health care provider.	Verifies position of tube before initiating enteral feeding.
3. Remove stylet after radiographic verification of correct placement.	If placement needs adjustment, stylet is still in place.
4. Routinely check condition of nares, location of external exit site marking on tube, and color and pH of fluid aspirated from tube.	Routine evaluation ensures no formation of medical device–related pressure injury and correct placement of tube.
5. After removal, assess patient's level of comfort.	Provides for continued comfort of patient.

STEP	RATIONALE
6. **Use Teach-Back:** "I want to be sure that I explained to you what you can do during insertion of the nasogastric tube so that you can communicate with me. Tell me what you are going to do to communicate with me during tube insertion." Revise your instruction now or develop a plan for revised patient/family caregiver teaching if patient/family caregiver is not able to teach back correctly.	Determines patient's/family caregiver's level of understanding of instructional topic.

RECORDING AND REPORTING

- Record type and size of tube placed, location of distal tip of tube, patient's tolerance of procedure, condition of naris, and confirmation of tube position by x-ray.
- Document your evaluation of patient/family caregiver learning.

- Record removal of tube, condition of naris, and patient's tolerance.
- Report any type of unexpected outcome and the interventions performed.

UNEXPECTED OUTCOMES AND RELATED INTERVENTIONS

- Aspiration of stomach contents into respiratory tract (delayed response or small-volume aspiration), evidenced by auscultation of crackles or wheezes, dyspnea, or fever.
  - Report change in patient's condition to health care provider; if a chest x-ray film has not been recently obtained, suggest ordering one.
  - Position patient on side to protect airway.
  - Suction nasotracheally and orotracheally.
  - Prepare for possible initiation of antibiotics.

- Displacement of feeding tube to another site (e.g., from duodenum to stomach) possibly occurs when patient coughs or vomits.
  - Aspirate GI contents and measure pH.
  - Remove displaced tube, and insert and verify placement of new tube.
  - If there is a question of aspiration, obtain chest x-ray film.

SKILL 35.3 ADMINISTERING ENTERAL NUTRITION VIA NASOENTERIC, GASTROSTOMY, OR JEJUNOSTOMY TUBES

DELEGATION CONSIDERATIONS

The skill of administration of nasoenteric tube feeding can be delegated to nursing assistive personnel (NAP) (refer to agency policy). An RN or licensed practical nurse (LPN) must first verify tube placement and patency. The nurse directs the NAP to:

- Elevate head of bed to a minimum of 30 degrees (preferably 45 degrees) or sit patient up in bed or in a chair.
- Infuse the feeding as ordered; do not adjust the feeding rate.
- Report any difficulty infusing the feeding or any discomfort voiced by patient.

- Report any gagging, paroxysms of coughing, or choking.
- Provide frequent oral hygiene.

EQUIPMENT

- Disposable feeding bag, tubing, or ready-to-hang system
- ENFit syringe 60 mL or larger
- Stethoscope, pulse oximeter, capnography *(optional)*
- Enteral infusion pump for continuous feedings
- pH indicator strip (scale 1.0 to 11.0)
- Prescribed enteral formula
- Clean gloves
- ENFit connector

STEP	RATIONALE
ASSESSMENT	
1. Identify patient using at least two identifiers (e.g., name and birthday or name and medical record number) according to agency policy.	Ensures correct patient. Complies with The Joint Commission standards and improves patient safety (TJC, 2018).
2. Assess patient's clinical status to determine potential need for tube feedings: decreased level of consciousness, nutrition deficits, head or neck surgery, facial trauma, or impaired swallowing. Consult with nutrition support team and health care provider.	Identify candidates for enteral nutrition (EN) before they become nutritionally depleted. Health care provider order is necessary for feedings.
3. Assess patient for food allergies.	Prevents patient from developing localized or systemic allergic responses to feeding.

SKILL 35.3 ADMINISTERING ENTERAL NUTRITION VIA NASOENTERIC, GASTROSTOMY, OR JEJUNOSTOMY TUBES—cont'd

STEP	RATIONALE
4. Perform physical assessment of abdomen. Objective measures for assessing tolerance include changes in bowel sounds, expanding girth, tenderness and firmness on palpation, increasing nasogastric tube output, and vomiting.	These symptoms may indicate intolerance for feeding (McCarthy and Martindale, 2015). Report findings to health care provider to determine if tube feeding can proceed safely (Boullata et al., 2017).
5. Obtain baseline weight. Assess patient for fluid volume excess or deficit, electrolyte abnormalities, and metabolic abnormalities (e.g., hyperglycemia).	Enteral feedings should restore or maintain patient's nutrition status. Measures provide objective data and baseline to determine selection of formula and measure effectiveness of feedings.
6. Verify health care provider's order for type of formula, rate, route, and frequency.	Ensures that correct formula will be administered in appropriate volume. Enteral formulas are not interchangeable.
7. Assess patient's and family caregiver's knowledge of the rationale for and the administration of enteral feedings.	Encourages cooperation, minimizes risks and anxiety, and identifies teaching needs.

PLANNING

1. Provide privacy and prepare bedside environment for patient safety.	Preparing the environment helps the nurse think about the steps needed; removing clutter from over-bed or bedside table removes barriers to administration of feeding.
2. Prepare and organize equipment for enteral feeding administration.	Ensures organized approach for administration of feedings.
3. Explain enteral feeding administration procedure to patient and/or caregiver.	Decreases patient anxiety. Promotes patient cooperation and increases compliance.

IMPLEMENTATION

1. Perform hand hygiene. Apply clean gloves.	Reduces transmission of microorganisms and potential contamination of enteral formula.
2. Obtain formula to administer.	
a. Verify correct formula and check expiration date; note condition of container.	Ensures that correct therapy is to be administered and checks integrity of formula.
b. Provide formula at room temperature.	Cold formula may cause gastric cramping and discomfort because liquid is not warmed by mouth and esophagus.
3. Prepare formula for administration, following manufacturer's guidelines.	
a. Use aseptic technique when manipulating components of feeding system (e.g., formula, administration set, connections).	Bag, connections, and tubing must be free of contamination to prevent bacterial growth (Boullata et al., 2017).
b. Shake formula container well. Clean top of canned formula with alcohol swab before opening it.	Ensures integrity of formula; prevents transmission of microorganisms (Boullata et al., 2017).
c. For closed systems, connect administration tubing to container. If using open system, pour formula from brick pack or can into administration bag (see illustration).	Formulas are available in closed-system containers that hold a 24- to 48-hour supply of formula or in an open system, in which formula must be transferred from brick packs or cans to a bag before administration.
4. Open roller clamp and allow administration tubing to fill. Clamp off tubing with roller clamp. Hang container on IV pole.	Prevents introduction of air into stomach once feeding begins.
5. Place patient in high-Fowler's position or elevate head of bed at least 30 degrees (preferably 45 degrees). For patient forced to remain supine, place in reverse Trendelenburg's position, which raises head.	Elevated head helps prevent pulmonary aspiration (AACN, 2016a).
6. Verify tube has remained in correct place. Observe appearance of aspirate and measure pH.	Verifies if tip of tube is in stomach or intestine based on pH value (AACN, 2016b). pH testing is not always a reliable indicator (e.g., continuous feedings or medications can alter pH) (Simons and Abdallah, 2012). See agency procedure guidelines regarding other verification methods.

STEP	RATIONALE
a. *Nasoenteric tube:* Attach ENFit syringe and aspirate gastric contents. Observe appearance of aspirate, and note pH.	Gastric fluid for a patient who has fasted for at least 4 hours usually has a pH of 1.0 to 4.0 (especially when patient is not receiving gastric acid inhibitor).
b. *Gastrostomy tube:* Attach ENFit syringe and aspirate gastric contents. Observe appearance of aspirate, and note pH.	Continuous administration of tube feeding elevates pH (Metheny and Stewart, 2002; Simons and Abdallah, 2012).
c. *Jejunostomy tube:* Attach ENFit syringe and aspirate intestinal secretions. Observe appearance and if significant amounts are returned or resemble gastric secretions, and note pH.	Presence of intestinal fluid indicates that end of tube is in small intestine. If fluid tests acidic on pH test or looks like gastric fluid, tube may be displaced into stomach (AACN, 2016b).
7. Check gastric residual volume (GRV) before each feeding for bolus and intermittent feedings and every 4 to 6 hours for continuous feedings per agency policy. Do not use GRV as part of routine assessment for EN tolerance in patients in the intensive care unit (ICU).	GRV may indicate if gastric emptying is compromised in patients who are not critically ill. Intestinal residual is usually very small. If there is a substantial increase in GRV, displacement of tube into stomach may have occurred (AACN, 2016b). Measuring GRV in critically ill patients is not validated as a means of measuring tolerance. Instead, use physical examinations, review of abdominal x-ray films, and evaluation of clinical risk factors for aspiration to monitor EN feedings in patients in the ICU (McClave et al., 2016).
a. Draw 10 to 30 mL of air into ENFit syringe and connect to end of feeding tube. Inject air slowly into tube. Pull back slowly and aspirate total amount of gastric contents you can aspirate.	GRV may not be easy to obtain from a small-bore feeding tube. A large-volume syringe (e.g., 60 mL) may prevent gastric tube collapse.
b. Return aspirated contents to stomach unless volume exceeds maximum GRV (see agency policy for maximum GRV).	Prevents loss of nutrients and electrolytes in discarded fluid. There is insufficient evidence to define an exact amount or the safety of returning aspirated contents to the patient. More research is needed.
c. GRV of 200 to 500 mL should raise concern and lead to implementation of measures reducing the risk of aspiration. Automatic cessation of feeding should not occur for GRV less than 500 mL in absence of other signs of intolerance.	Raising the cutoff value for GRV from a lower number to a higher number does not increase risk for regurgitation, aspiration, or pneumonia. However, you should take measures to reduce the risk for aspiration when GRV is high (McClave et al., 2016).
d. Flush feeding tube with 30 mL of water.	Prevents clogging of tubing.

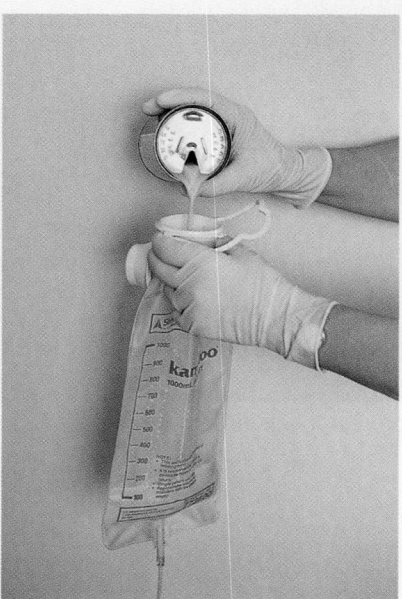

STEP 3c Pour formula into open feeding container.

SKILL 35.3   ADMINISTERING ENTERAL NUTRITION VIA NASOENTERIC, GASTROSTOMY, OR JEJUNOSTOMY TUBES—cont'd

STEP	RATIONALE
8. Use ENFit devices when administering enteral feedings.	These devices are not compatible with a Luer-Lok connection. Use of ENFit prevents misadministration of an enteral feeding or medication by the wrong route such as IV tubing (ISMP, 2015).
9. Intermittent feeding (administered at certain times during the day):	
a. Pinch proximal end of feeding tube and remove cap. Connect distal end of administration set tubing to ENFit device on feeding tube and release tubing.	Prevents excessive air from entering patient's stomach and leakage of gastric contents. Ensures feeding will be administered into correct tubing (ISMP, 2015).
b. Set rate by adjusting roller clamp on tubing or attach tubing to feeding pump. Allow bag to empty gradually over 30 to 45 minutes (the length of time of a comfortable meal). Label bag with tube-feeding type, strength, and amount. Include date, time, and initials.	Gradual emptying of tube feeding reduces risk for abdominal discomfort, vomiting, or diarrhea induced by bolus or too-rapid infusion of tube feedings. Labeling provides means to determine when to change administration set and confirms right patient is receiving feeding.

Clinical Decision Point. Use pumps designated for tube feeding, not IV fluids.

STEP	RATIONALE
c. Immediately follow feeding with water (per health care provider's orders or agency policy). Cover end of feeding tube with cap when not in use. Keep bag as clean as possible. Change administration set every 24 hours.	Prevents tube from clogging. Prevents air from entering stomach between feedings, and limits microbial contamination of system.
10. Continuous infusion method:	Method delivers prescribed hourly rate of feeding and reduces risk for abdominal discomfort.
a. Remove cap on tubing and connect distal end of administration set tubing to feeding tube using ENFit connector as in Step 9a.	Prevents excess air from entering patient's stomach and leakage of gastric contents. Ensures feeding will be administered into correct tubing (ISMP, 2015).
b. Thread tubing through feeding pump; set rate on pump and turn on (see illustration).	Delivers continuous feeding at steady rate and pressure. Feeding pump sounds alarm for increased resistance.

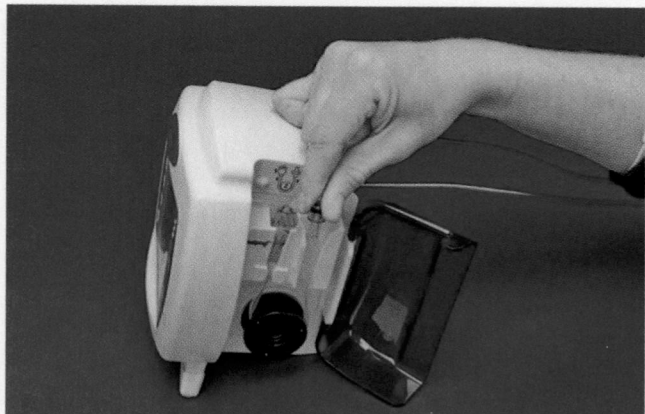

STEP 10b Connect tubing through infusion pump. (Image used with permission of Covidien. All rights reserved.)

STEP	RATIONALE
c. Advance rate of tube feeding (and concentration of feeding) gradually, as ordered.	Tube feeding can usually begin with full-strength formula. In the absence of critical illness (including metabolic or systemic complications), enteral feedings can advance to goal rate within 24 to 48 hours (McClave et al., 2016). Conservative initiation and advancement of EN depend on patient's age, medical condition, nutrition status, and expected patient tolerance (Kozeniecki and Fritzshall, 2015).

Clinical Decision Point. Maximum hang time for formula is 8 hours in an open system and 24 to 48 hours in a closed, ready-to-hang system (if it remains closed). The risk for contamination increases in formulas hanging more than 24 hours (Boullata et al., 2017). Refer to manufacturer guidelines.

STEP	RATIONALE
11. Flush tubing with 30 mL of water every 4 hours during continuous feeding (see agency policy) and before and after an intermittent feeding. Have registered dietitian recommend total free water requirement per day and obtain health care provider's order.	Provides patient with source of water to help maintain fluid and electrolyte balance. Clears tubing of formula.
12. Rinse bag and tubing with warm water whenever feedings are interrupted. Use new administration set every 24 hours.	Rinsing bag and tubing with warm water clears old tube feedings and reduces bacterial growth.
13. Dispose of supplies and perform hand hygiene.	Reduces transmission of microorganisms.

EVALUATION

1. Measure GRV per agency policy, usually every 4 to 6 hours, and ask if nausea or abdominal cramping is present.	Gastrointestinal tolerance of tube feedings must be closely monitored to avoid complications.
2. Monitor intake and output at least every 8 hours (or as ordered), and calculate daily totals every 24 hours.	Intake and output are indications of fluid balance—fluid volume excess or deficit.
3. Weigh patient daily until maximum administration rate is reached and maintained for 24 hours; then weigh patient 3 times per week.	Slow weight gain is indicator of improved nutrition status; however, sudden gain of more than 2 lb (0.9 kg) in 24 hours usually indicates fluid retention.
4. Monitor laboratory values as ordered by health care provider.	Determines correct administration of formula rate and strength.
5. Observe patient's respiratory status.	Change in respiratory status may indicate aspiration of tube feeding into respiratory tract. Symptoms may include coughing, dyspnea, tachypnea, change in oxygen saturation, crackles, and hoarseness.
6. Examine abdomen and auscultate bowel sounds.	Estimates status of gastric emptying and peristalsis.
7. For gastrostomy tubes, inspect site for signs of impaired skin integrity, symptoms of infection, injury, or tightness of tube.	Enteral tubes often cause pressure and excoriation at insertion site.
8. Observe nasoenteral tube insertion site at least daily (see agency policy). Note skin integrity and look for edema under device, excoriation, or presence of pressure injury.	Allows for early detection of excoriation that can progress to medical device–related pressure injury.
9. **Use Teach-Back:** "I want to be sure that I explained to you what you need to look out for that may tell us you are not tolerating your tube feeding. Tell me two things that may tell us that you are not tolerating your tube feedings." Revise your instruction now or develop a plan for revised patient/family caregiver teaching if patient/family caregiver is not able to teach back correctly.	Determines patient's/family caregiver's level of understanding of instructional topic.

RECORDING AND REPORTING

- Record amount and type of feeding, infusion rate, method of infusion, patient's response to tube feeding (e.g., GRV, cramping, bowel sounds, patency of tube, condition of skin at tube site).
- Document your evaluation of patient/family caregiver learning.

- Record volume of formula and any additional water on intake and output form.
- Report type of feeding, status of feeding tube, patient's tolerance, and adverse outcomes.

SKILL 35.3 ADMINISTERING ENTERAL NUTRITION VIA NASOENTERIC, GASTROSTOMY, OR JEJUNOSTOMY TUBES—cont'd

UNEXPECTED OUTCOMES AND RELATED INTERVENTIONS

- Feeding tube becomes clogged.
  - Attempt to flush tube with water.
  - Special products are available for unclogging feeding tubes; do not use carbonated beverages or juice.
  - Hold feeding and notify health care provider.
  - Maintain patient in semi-Fowler's position.
  - Contact pharmacist to change medications to liquid form and flush before and after intermittent feedings and medications (Kozeniecki and Fritzshall, 2015).
- Patient develops large amount of diarrhea (more than three loose stools in 24 hours).
  - Notify health care provider.
  - Consult dietitian about need to change formula to prevent malabsorption.
  - Identify and treat underlying medical/surgical issues and infections (Kozeniecki and Fritzshall, 2015).

- Provide perianal skin care after each stool.
- Determine other causes of diarrhea such as *Clostridium difficile* infection, contaminated tube feeding, or medication containing sorbitol.
- Patient develops nausea and vomiting.
  - Administer antiemetic as ordered.
  - Administer medications (ordered by health care provider) to increase gastric motility (e.g., prokinetic agents) and evaluate need for medications that slow gastric emptying (Kozeniecki and Fritzshall, 2015).
  - Ensure formula and water flushes are administered at room temperature (Kozeniecki and Fritzshall, 2015).
  - Temporarily reduce infusion rate or withhold tube feeding and notify health care provider.
  - Be sure that tube is patent; aspirate for residual.

KEY POINTS

- Digestion is the mechanical and chemical process by which food is broken down into its simplest form for absorption. Digestion and absorption occur mainly in the small intestine.
- Eating a balanced diet including carbohydrates, protein, lipids, vitamins, minerals, and water provides the essential nutrients to carry out the normal physiological functioning of the body.
- Ideal body weight (IBW) is maintained when energy intake in food or fluids equals energy output.
- Dietary reference intakes (DRIs) for macronutrients and micronutrients were formulated for population groups, not individuals.
- Guidelines for dietary change advocate (1) for a limitation of added sugars, saturated fats, and sodium intake; (2) for people to focus on variety, nutrient density, and amount; and (3) for a shift to healthier food and beverage choices.
- Age, developmental stages, and clinical conditions affect the requirements for essential nutrients. Periods of rapid growth increase the need for protein, vitamins, and minerals.
- Because improper nutrition affects all body systems, nutrition assessment includes a review of total physical assessment findings.
- Special hospital diets alter the composition, texture, digestibility, and residue of foods to meet a patient's needs.

- Enteral nutrition (EN) is for patients who are unable to ingest food safely or adequately but are able to digest and absorb nutrition via the gastrointestinal (GI) tract.
- EN preserves intestinal structure and function and maintains immunity.
- Parenteral nutrition (PN) supplies essential nutrients through a concentrated nutrient solution administered into the superior vena cava and is used when nutrition via the GI tract is not possible or cannot effectively meet patient needs.
- Medical nutrition therapy is a recognized treatment modality for both acute and chronic disease states.

REFLECTIVE LEARNING

- Consider a recent patient experience and describe any aspects of the patient's condition that may have nutritional implications.
- Consider a recent patient experience and describe cultural implications regarding nutrition recommendations that you applied or could have applied but may not have thought of during your encounter with the patient.
- Reflect on a patient you saw recently and list the questions that you asked the patient to assess the patient's nutrition health. Identify additional questions that you will ask next time in a similar situation to get an even more thorough perspective of a patient's nutrition status to help you implement a comprehensive patient-centered approach.

REVIEW QUESTIONS

1. Which food preparation information will the nurse provide to a patient with compromised immunity? (Select all that apply.)
   1. Cook meat, poultry, fish, and eggs until well done (180° F).
   2. Do not use food past expiration date.
   3. Refrigerate foods at 40° F within 2 hours of cooking.
   4. Thaw frozen foods on the kitchen counter overnight.
   5. Use wood cutting boards for chopping meat.
   6. Wash hands, food-preparation surfaces, and utensils with cold, clear water.

2. Which assessment finding in a 77-year-old patient alerts the nurse to a risk for impaired nutrition?
   1. Shellfish allergy
   2. History of lactose intolerance
   3. Unintentional weight loss of 18 lb in 6 months
   4. Wears dentures

3. Which nursing intervention is appropriate for a patient suspected to have dysphagia?
   1. Collaborate with speech-language therapist to identify level of swallowing difficulty.
   2. Offer antinausea medication after meals.
   3. Prepare patient for parenteral feedings.
   4. Have patient lie flat in the bed when eating.

4. Which nursing intervention ensures safety while a patient is receiving feeding via a nasally placed gastric feeding tube?
   1. Administer medications together to reduce the amount of fluid you need to flush the tube.
   2. Provide feeding and fluids that are congruent with what other patients of this age receive.
   3. Ensure that the tube is well secured, continually monitor the external length, and assess position at least every 4 hours.
   4. Listen while a bolus of air is injected to determine placement before administering medication into the tube.

5. The nurse is preparing to administer enteral nutrition (EN) via a jejunostomy tube. Place the steps below in the correct order to properly perform this skill.
   1. Obtain formula to administer.
   2. Perform hand hygiene and apply clean gloves.
   3. Place patient in high-Fowler's position.
   4. Prepare formula for administration.
   5. Verify tube placement.

evolve

Additional Review Questions, as well as rationales for all Review Questions, can be found on the Evolve website.

1. 1, 2, 3; 2. 3; 3. 1; 4. 3; 5. 2, 1, 4, 3, 5.

REFERENCES

Academy of Nutrition and Dietetics (AND): *Nutrition care manual*, 2016, www.nutritioncaremanual.org.

Administration for Community Living (ACL): *Administration on Aging*, 2017, https://www.acl.gov/about-acl/administration-aging.

American Academy of Pediatrics (AAP): Policy statement: breastfeeding and the use of human milk, *Pediatrics* 129(3): 496, 2012.

American Association of Critical Care Nurses (AACN): AACN Practice Alerts: prevention of aspiration in adults, *Crit Care Nurse* 36(1):e20, 2016a.

American Association of Critical Care Nurses (AACN): AACN Practice Alerts: initial and ongoing verification of feeding tube placement in adults, *Crit Care Nurse* 36(2):e8, 2016b.

Ayers P, et al: A.S.P.E.N. parenteral nutrition safety consensus recommendations, *JPEN J Parenter Enteral Nutr* 38(3):296, 2014.

Boullata JI, et al: A.S.P.E.N. clinical guidelines: parenteral nutrition ordering, order review, compounding, labeling, and dispensing, *JPEN J Parenter Enteral Nutr* 38(3):334, 2014.

Boullata JI, et al: ASPEN safe practices for enteral nutrition therapy, *JPEN J Parenter Enteral Nutr* 41(1):15, 2017.

Bourgault AM, et al: Methods used by critical care nurses to verify feeding tube placement in clinical practice, *Crit Care Nurse* 35:1, 2015.

Bray GA, et al: A further subgroup analysis of the effects of the DASH diet and three dietary sodium levels on blood pressure: results of the DASH-Sodium Trial, *Am J Cardiol* 94(2):222, 2004.

Cichero JA: Thickening agents used for dysphagia management: effect on bioavailability of water, medication and feelings of satiety, *Nutr J* 12:54, 2013.

Clarys P, et al: Comparison of nutritional quality of the vegan, vegetarian, semi-vegetarian, pesco-vegetarian and omnivorous diet, *Nutrients* 6:1318, 2014.

Copp AJ, Greene ND: Neural tube defects—disorders of neurulation and related embryonic processes, *Wiley Interdiscip Rev Dev Biol* 2(2):213, 2013.

de Souza RJ, et al: Intake of saturated and trans unsaturated fatty acids and risk of all cause mortality, cardiovascular disease, and type 2 diabetes: systematic review and meta-analysis of observational studies, *BMJ* 351:h3978, 2015.

DiMaria-Ghalili RA, et al: Standards of nutrition care practice and professional performance for nutrition support and generalist nurses, *Nutr Clin Pract* 31(4): 527, 2016.

Donini LM, et al: Mini-Nutritional Assessment, Malnutrition Universal Screening Tool, and Nutrition Risk Screening Tool for the Nutritional Evaluation of Older Nursing Home Residents, *J Am Med Dir Assoc* 17(10): 959.e11, 2016.

Durfee SM, et al: A.S.P.E.N. standards for nutrition support: home and alternate site care, *Nutr Clin Pract* 29(4):542, 2014.

Elke G, et al: Gastric residual volume in critically ill patients: a dead marker or still alive?, *Nutr Clin Pract* 30(1):59, 2015.

Food and Nutrition Board (FNB), Institute of Medicine (IOM): *Dietary reference intakes for thiamin, riboflavin, niacin, vitamin B6, folate, vitamin B12, pantothenic acid, biotin, and choline*, Washington, DC, 1998, National Academies Press.

Food and Nutrition Board (FNB), Institute of Medicine (IOM): *Dietary reference intakes for energy, carbohydrate, fiber, fat, fatty acids, cholesterol, protein, and amino acids*, Washington, DC, 2002, National Academies Press.

Food and Nutrition Board (FNB), Institute of Medicine (IOM): *Dietary reference intakes for water, potassium, sodium, chloride, and sulfate*, Washington, DC, 2004, National Academies Press.

Garvey WT, et al: American Association of Clinical Endocrinologists and American College of Endocrinology comprehensive clinical practice guidelines for medical care of patients with obesity, *Endocr Pract* 22(Suppl 3):1, 2016.

Gomes CA, et al: Percutaneous endoscopic gastrostomy versus nasogastric tube feeding for adults with swallowing disturbances, *Cochrane Database Syst Rev* (5):CD008096, 2015.

Greenberg JA: Obesity and early mortality in the United States, *Obesity (Silver Spring)* 21(2):405, 2013.

Guenter P: New enteral connectors raising awareness, *Nutr Clin Pract* 29(5):612, 2014.

Han Z, et al: Low gestational weight gain and the risk of preterm birth and low birthweight: a systematic review and meta-analyses, *Acta Obstet Gynecol Scand* 90(9):935, 2011.

Hines S, et al: Nursing interventions for identifying and managing acute dysphagia are effective for improving patient outcomes: a systematic review update, *J Neurosci Nurs* 48(4):215, 2016.

Institute for Safe Medication Practices (ISMP): *Safety Alert: ENFit enteral devices are on their way … Important safety considerations for hospitals*, 2015, www.ismp.org/newsletters/acutecare/showarticle.aspx?id=105.

Institute of Medicine (IOM): *DRI tables and application reports*, n.d., http://fnic.nal.usda.gov/dietary-guidance/dietary-reference-intakes/dri-tables-and-application-reports.

International Organization for Standardization (IOS): *ISO 80369-3:2016(en): Small-bore connectors for liquids and gases in healthcare applications—part 3: connectors for enteral applications*, Arlington, VA, 2016, Association for the Advancement of Medical Instrumentation.

Jeng C, et al: Clinical validation of the related factors and defining characteristics of impaired swallowing for patients with stroke, *J Nurs Res* 9(4):105, 2001.

Kozeniecki M, Fritzshall R: Enteral nutrition for adults in the hospital setting, *Nutr Clin Pract* 30(5):634, 2015.

Kumar S, Kelly AS: Review of childhood obesity: from epidemiology, etiology, and comorbidities to clinical assessment and treatment, *Mayo Clin Proc* 92(2):251, 2017.

Lee J, et al: Serum albumin and prealbumin in calorically restricted, nondiseased individuals: a systematic review, *Am J Med* 128(9):1023.e1, 2015.

Malhi H: Dysphagia: warning signs and management, *Br J Nurs* 25(10):546, 2016.

Markowitz J, et al: *Device-related pressure ulcers*, American Association of Critical Care Nurses (AACN) Clinical Scene Investigator Academy, 2013, www.aacn.org/wd/csi/docs/FinalProjects/IU%20Methodist%20ACC%20-%20Power%20Point%20Presentation.pdf.

McCarthy MS, Martindale RG: What's on the menu? Delivering evidence-based nutritional therapy, *Nursing* 45(8):36, 2015.

McClave SA, et al: Guidelines for the provision and assessment of nutrition support therapy in the adult critically ill patient: Society of Critical Care Medicine (SCCM) and American Society for Parenteral and Enteral Nutrition (A.S.P.E.N.), *JPEN J Parenter Enteral Nutr* 40(2):159, 2016.

Metheny NA: Preventing aspiration in older adults with dysphagia, *Best Practices in Nursing Care to Older Adults*, Issue No. 20, revised 2012.

Metheny NA, Frantz RA: Head-of-bed elevation in critically ill patients: a review, *Crit Care Nurse* 33(3):53, 2013.

Metheny NA, Stewart BJ: Testing feeding tube placement during continuous tube feedings, *Appl Nurs Res* 15(4):254, 2002.

Miller KR, et al: A tutorial on enteral access in adult patients in the hospitalized setting, *JPEN J Parenter Enteral Nutr* 38(3):282, 2014.

National Center for Health Statistics (NCHS): *Health, United States, 2015: with special feature on racial and ethnic health disparities*, Hyattsville, MD, 2016.

National Dysphagia Diet Task Force (NDDTF): *National Dysphagia Diet: standardization for optimal care*, Chicago, 2002, American Dietetic Association.

Newman R, et al: Effect of bolus viscosity on the safety and efficacy of swallowing and the kinematics of the swallow response in patients with oropharyngeal dysphagia: White Paper by the European Society for Swallowing Disorders (ESSD), *Dysphagia* 31(2):232, 2016.

Nita SP, et al: Matching the rheological properties of videofluoroscopic contrast agents and thickened liquid prescriptions, *Dysphagia* 28(2):245, 2013.

O'Horo JC, et al: Bedside diagnosis of dysphagia: a systematic review, *J Hosp Med* 10(4):256, 2015.

Pagana K, Pagana T: *Mosby's diagnostic and laboratory test reference*, ed 13, St Louis, 2017, Mosby.

Park JS, et al: Effects of neuromuscular electrical stimulation combined with effortful swallowing on post-stroke oropharyngeal dysphagia: a randomised controlled trial, *J Oral Rehabil* 43(6):426, 2016.

Poulia KA, et al: The two most popular malnutrition screening tools in the light of the new ESPEN consensus definition of the diagnostic criteria for malnutrition, *Clin Nutr* 36(4):1130, 2017.

Ra JY, et al: Chin tuck for prevention of aspiration: effectiveness and appropriate posture, *Dysphagia* 29(5):603, 2014.

Rösler A, et al: Dysphagia in dementia: influence of dementia severity and food texture on the prevalence of aspiration and latency to swallow in hospitalized geriatric patients, *J Am Med Dir Assoc* 16(8):697, 2015.

Sanders TA: Protective effects of dietary PUFA against chronic disease: evidence from epidemiological studies and intervention trials, *Proc Nutr Soc* 73(1):73–79, 2014.

Siervo M, et al: Effects of the Dietary Approach to Stop Hypertension (DASH) diet on cardiovascular risk factors: a systematic review and meta-analysis, *Br J Nutr* 113(1):1, 2015.

Simons SR, Abdallah LM: Bedside assessment of enteral tube placement: aligning practice with evidence, *Am J Nurs* 112(2):40, 2012.

Singh S, et al: Physician diagnosis of overweight status predicts attempted and successful weight loss in patients with cardiovascular disease and central obesity, *Am Heart J* 160(5):934, 2010.

Sørensen RT, et al: Dysphagia screening and intensified oral hygiene reduce pneumonia after stroke, *J Neurosci Nurs* 45(3):139, 2013.

Sparks DA, et al: Pulmonary complications of 9931 narrow-bore nasoenteric tubes during blind placement: a critical review, *JPEN J Parenter Enteral Nutr* 35(5):625, 2011.

Steele CM, et al: The influence of food texture and liquid consistency modification on swallowing physiology and function: a systematic review, *Dysphagia* 30(1):2, 2015.

Sura L, et al: Dysphagia in the elderly: management and nutritional considerations, *Clin Interv Aging* 7:287, 2012.

Swan K, et al: Living with oropharyngeal dysphagia: effects of bolus modification on health-related quality of life—a systematic review, *Qual Life Res* 24:2447, 2015.

Takeuchi K, et al: Nutritional status and dysphagia risk among community-dwelling frail older adults, *J Nutr Health Aging* 18(4):352, 2014.

The Joint Commission (TJC): Managing risk during transition to new ISO tubing connector standards, *Sentinel Event Alert* (53):2014.

The Joint Commission (TJC): *2018 National Patient Safety Goals*, Oakbrook Terrace, IL, 2018, The Commission. https://www.jointcommission.org/standards_information/npsgs.aspx.

Ullman AJ, et al: Dressing and securement for central venous access devices (CVADs): a Cochrane systematic review, *Int J Nurs Stud* 59:177, 2016.

U.S. Department of Agriculture (USDA): *ChooseMyPlate.gov*, n.d., www.choosemyplate.gov.

U.S. Department of Agriculture Agricultural Research Service (USDA ARS). *Snacks: percentages of selected nutrients contributed by food and beverages consumed at snack occasions, by gender and age, what we eat in America, NHANES 2011-2012*, 2014, https://www.ars.usda.gov/northeast-area/beltsville-md/beltsville-human-nutrition-research-center/food-surveys-research-group/docs/wweia-data-tables/.

U.S. Department of Health and Human Services (USDHHS): *Healthy people 2020*, Washington, DC, 2010, U.S. Government Printing Office.

U.S. Department of Health and Human Services (USDHHS), et al: *Safety considerations to mitigate the risks of misconnections with small-bore connectors intended for enteral applications: guidance for industry and Food and Drug Administration Staff*, 2015, www.fda.gov/downloads/MedicalDevices/DeviceRegulationandGuidance/GuidanceDocuments/UCM313385.pdf.

U.S. Department of Health and Human Services (USDHHS) and U.S. Department of Agriculture (USDA): *2015-2020 dietary guidelines for Americans*, ed 8, 2015, https://health.gov/dietaryguidelines/2015/.

Wang Y, et al: What childhood obesity prevention programmes work? A systematic review and meta-analysis, *Obes Rev* 16(7):547, 2015.

Wirth R, et al: Oropharyngeal dysphagia in older persons—from pathophysiology to adequate intervention: a review and summary of an international expert meeting, *Clin Interv Aging* 11:189, 2016.

Yatabe MS, et al: Mini nutritional assessment as a useful method of predicting the development of pressure ulcers in elderly inpatients, *J Am Geriatr Soc* 61:1698, 2013.

36

Urinary Elimination

evolve MEDIA RESOURCES

http://evolve.elsevier.com/Potter/essentials

- Audio Glossary
- Case Study Continuation

- QSEN Activity and Review Questions Answers and Rationales
- Video Clips

OBJECTIVES

- Explain the function and role of the urinary system in urine formation and elimination.
- Identify factors that influence urinary elimination.
- Discuss common urinary elimination alterations.
- Identify essential components to include in a nursing history from a patient with a urinary alteration.
- Describe how to perform a physical assessment that focuses on urinary elimination.
- Describe characteristics of normal and abnormal urine.
- Describe nursing responsibilities associated with common diagnostic tests of the urinary system.

- Prioritize nursing diagnoses associated with alterations in urinary elimination.
- Teach patients how to promote normal urination and control incontinence.
- Implement nursing measures to reduce urinary tract infections.
- Describe how to apply a condom catheter, insert an indwelling urinary catheter, and measure postvoid residual using a bladder scan.
- Measure intake and output to monitor bladder emptying, renal function, and fluid and electrolyte balance.

KEY TERMS

bacteremia, p. 1020
bacteriuria, p. 1020
catheter-associated urinary tract infection (CAUTI), p. 1025
catheterization, p. 1038
condom catheter, p. 1042
cystitis, p. 1020
dysuria, p. 1020
graduated measuring container, p. 1029

hematuria, p. 1019
micturition, p. 1020
postvoid residual, p. 1038
proteinuria, p. 1019
pyelonephritis, p. 1020
residual urine, p. 1037
stoma, p. 1023
suprapubic catheter, p. 1042
ureterostomy, p. 1023
urinal, p. 1037

urinalysis, p. 1031
urinary diversion, p. 1023
urinary incontinence (UI), p. 1021
urinary reflux, p. 1020
urinary retention, p. 1020
urinary tract infections (UTIs), p. 1020
urine hat, p. 1030
urometer, p. 1030
urosepsis, p. 1020
voiding, p. 1020

Providing effective nursing care requires you to support patients as they respond to alterations in their physical, psychological, spiritual, and emotional health. A basic human function is urinary elimination, which can be affected by a wide variety of illnesses and conditions. Many factors influ-

ence urine production, such as fluid intake, physical activity, and body temperature. Nurses support patients' urinary elimination needs by supporting normal micturition. Sometimes you will insert and maintain urinary catheters for close monitoring of urine output or to facilitate bladder emptying

CASE STUDY *Mrs. Vallero*

Mrs. Vallero is a 75-year-old woman who has been hospitalized for 4 days because of heart failure, fluid retention, and poorly controlled diabetes. She has a history of urinary incontinence and repeated episodes of urinary retention related to diabetic neuropathy. At the 3 p.m. shift report, Carly, a nursing student, learns that Mrs. Vallero's indwelling urinary catheter was removed 2 days ago and replaced within 12 hours because of frequent small-volume voiding of less than 100 mL, frequent episodes of small-volume incontinence, lower abdominal pain, and a postvoid residual of 600 mL. A second voiding trial was started this morning, with no recorded urine output since 7 a.m. when the catheter was removed. While making rounds, Carly talks with Mrs. Vallero, who states that she has only "dribbled" urine and is worried because "I thought this was all under control." Mrs. Vallero's nurse notified the health care provider of current assessment findings. A bladder scan revealed 400 mL of retained urine, and an order was obtained for intermittent catheterization. Mrs. Vallero was catheterized for 400 mL of pale, clear yellow urine.

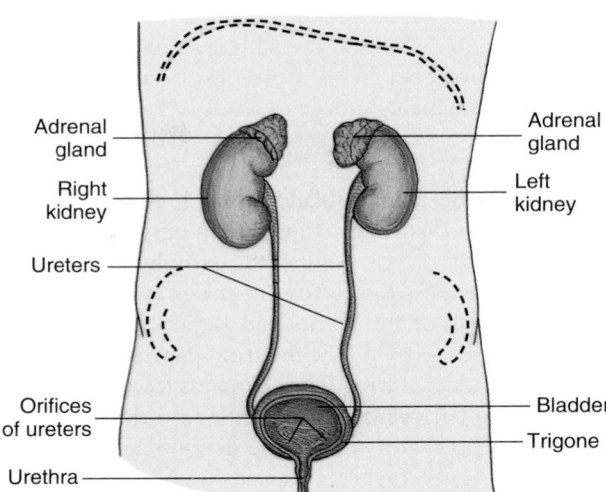

FIG 36.1 Organs of the urinary system.

brain allows the bladder to empty, the bladder contracts, the urinary sphincter relaxes, and urine leaves the body through the urethra (Huether and McCance, 2016).

Anatomy and Physiology of the Urinary Tract

Kidneys. The kidneys lie on either side of the vertebral column behind the abdominal peritoneum and against the deep muscles of the back level with the twelfth thoracic and third lumbar vertebrae. Normally the left kidney is higher than the right because of the anatomical position of the liver. Nephrons, the functional unit of the kidneys, remove waste products from the blood and play a major role in the regulation of fluid and electrolyte balance. Each nephron contains a cluster of capillaries called the *glomerulus*. The glomerulus filters water, glucose, amino acids, urea, uric acid, creatinine, and major electrolytes. Large proteins and blood cells do not normally filter through the glomerulus. Suspect glomerular injury when protein (**proteinuria**) or blood (**hematuria**) is found in the urine.

Not all glomerular filtrate is excreted as urine. Approximately 99% is resorbed into the plasma by the proximal convoluted tubule of the nephron, the loop of Henle, and the distal tubule. The remaining 1% is excreted as urine. The delicate balance of fluid and electrolytes is maintained during the resorption process (Huether and McCance, 2016). The kidneys normally produce 1 to 2 L of urine daily (Huether and McCance, 2016).

Ureters. A ureter is attached to each kidney pelvis and carries urinary wastes to the bladder. Urine draining from the ureters to the bladder is sterile. Peristaltic waves cause the urine to enter the bladder in spurts rather than steadily. Contractions of the bladder during micturition compress the lower portion of the ureters to prevent urine from back flowing into them (Huether and McCance, 2016). Obstruction of urine flow through the ureters such as by a kidney

when bladder function is impaired. Some patients require long-term urethral or suprapubic indwelling catheters when the bladder fails to empty effectively. You will consistently implement measures to minimize the risk for urinary tract infection (UTI) during the administration of nursing care. Nurses in all health care settings play a key role in teaching patients about bladder health.

SCIENTIFIC KNOWLEDGE BASE

Urinary elimination is the last step in the removal and elimination of excess water and the by-products of body metabolism. Adequate elimination depends on the coordinated function of the ureters, bladder, and urethra (Fig. 36.1). The kidneys filter waste products of metabolism from the blood. The ureters transport urine from the kidneys to the bladder. The bladder holds urine until the volume in the bladder triggers a sensation of urge, sending impulses to the sacral level of the spinal cord indicating the need to pass urine. When the stone can cause a back flow of urine (urinary reflux) into the ureters and pelvis of the kidney, causing distention (hydroureter/hydronephrosis), infection from stasis, and in some cases permanent damage to sensitive kidney structures and function.

Bladder. The urinary bladder is a hollow, distensible, muscular organ that holds urine. When empty, the bladder lies in the pelvic cavity behind the symphysis pubis. The bladder rests against the rectum in males and rests against the anterior wall of the uterus and vagina in females. The bladder expands as it fills with urine. Normally the pressure in the bladder during filling remains low; this prevents the dangerous backward flow of urine into the ureters and kidneys. In a pregnant woman, the developing fetus pushes against the bladder, reducing capacity and causing a feeling of fullness.

Urethra. Urine travels from the bladder through the urethra and passes to the outside of the body through the urethral meatus. The urethra passes through a thick layer of skeletal muscles called the *pelvic floor muscles.* These muscles stabilize the urethra and contribute to urinary continence. The external urethral sphincter, composed of striated muscles, contributes to voluntary control over the flow of urine (Huether and McCance, 2016). The female urethra is approximately 3 to 4 cm (1.18 to 1.5 inches) long, and the male urethra is approximately 18 to 20 cm (7 to 7.8 inches) long (Huether and McCance, 2016). The shorter length of the female urethra increases the risk for UTI because of close access to the bacteria-contaminated perineal area.

Act of Urination

Urination, micturition, and voiding all are terms that describe the process of bladder emptying. Micturition is a complex interaction between the bladder, urinary sphincter, and central nervous system. Several areas in the brain are involved in bladder control including the cerebral cortex, thalamus, hypothalamus, and brainstem. There are two micturition centers in the spinal cord; one coordinates inhibition of bladder contraction, and the other coordinates bladder contractility. As the bladder fills and stretches, bladder contractions are inhibited by sympathetic stimulation from the thoracic micturition center. Normal bladder capacity in adults is approximately 300 to 600 mL. With a strong sensation of urge and when in the appropriate place to void, the central nervous system sends a message to the micturition centers stopping sympathetic stimulation and starting parasympathetic stimulation from the sacral micturition center. The urinary sphincter relaxes, and the bladder contracts. When the time and place are inappropriate, the brain sends messages to the micturition centers to contract the urinary sphincter and relax the bladder muscle.

Factors Influencing Urination

Physiological factors, psychosocial conditions, and diagnostic or treatment-induced factors sometimes affect normal urinary elimination (Box 36.1). Understanding these factors helps you anticipate possible elimination problems and intervene when or before they develop.

Common Urinary Elimination Problems

The most common urinary elimination problems involve the inability to store urine or to fully empty urine from the bladder. Problems can result from infection; irritable or overactive bladder; obstruction of urine flow; impaired bladder contractility; or issues that impair innervation to the bladder, resulting in sensory or motor dysfunction.

Urinary Retention. Urinary retention is the inability to partially or completely empty the bladder. Acute or rapid-onset urinary retention stretches the bladder, causing feelings of pressure, discomfort and/or pain, and tenderness over the symphysis pubis; restlessness; and sometimes diaphoresis. Patients often have no urine output over several hours and in some cases experience frequency, urgency, small-volume voiding, or incontinence of small volumes of urine. Chronic urinary retention has a slow, gradual onset during which patients may report decreased voiding volumes, straining to void, frequency, urgency, incontinence, and sensations of incomplete emptying. Complete urinary retention occurs when there is no voiding; during partial retention, the bladder never empties completely. Incontinence caused by urinary retention is called *overflow incontinence.* The pressure in the bladder exceeds the ability of the sphincter to prevent the passage of urine, and the patient dribbles urine (Table 36.1). *In the case study, Mrs. Vallero has signs of urinary retention. She has had diabetes mellitus for more than 35 years, and it is likely that neuropathy is contributing to the inability of her bladder to empty completely.*

Urinary Tract Infections. Urinary tract infections (UTIs) are the most common health care–associated infections (HAI) (Galiczewski, 2016). The Centers for Disease Control and Prevention (CDC, 2017) reports that 75% of these infections result from the use of an indwelling urinary catheter. *Escherichia coli,* a bacterium commonly found in the colon, is the most common causative pathogen (Nicolle, 2014). Risk for a UTI increases when a patient has an indwelling catheter, urinary retention, urinary and fecal incontinence, or poor perineal hygiene practices.

Bacteriuria (bacteria in the urine) can lead to serious upper UTI (pyelonephritis) and life-threatening bloodstream infection (bacteremia or urosepsis). Symptoms of a lower UTI (bladder) include burning or pain with urination (dysuria) or irritation of the bladder (cystitis) characterized by urgency, frequency, incontinence, suprapubic tenderness, and foul-smelling, cloudy urine. In some cases, there is obvious blood in the urine (hematuria). If infection spreads to the upper urinary tract (pyelonephritis), patients frequently experience fever (39° C [102.2° F]), chills, diaphoresis, flank pain, and lower back pain (Casey, 2014). Older adults with a UTI often experience *delirium* (a change in mental status), new or increased

BOX 36.1 FACTORS INFLUENCING URINARY ELIMINATION

GROWTH AND DEVELOPMENT

- Children cannot voluntarily control voiding until 18 to 24 months of age when myelination is complete.
- Readiness for toilet training includes the ability to recognize the feeling of bladder fullness, hold urine for 1 to 2 hours, and communicate the sense of urgency.
- Some older adults experience a decrease in bladder capacity, increased bladder irritability, and increased frequency of bladder contractions during bladder filling.
- In older adults, the ability to hold urine between the initial desire to void and an urgent need to void decreases.
- Older adults are at increased risk for urinary incontinence as a result of chronic illnesses and factors that interfere with mobility, cognition, and manual dexterity.

SOCIOCULTURAL FACTORS

- Cultural and gender norms vary. North Americans expect toilet facilities to be private, whereas some cultures accept communal toilet facilities; gender-neutral bathrooms are becoming more common in the United States.
- Religious or cultural norms may dictate who is acceptable to assist in elimination practices.
- Social expectations (e.g., school recesses, work breaks) can interfere with timely voiding.

PSYCHOLOGICAL FACTORS

- Anxiety and stress sometimes affect a sense of urgency and increase frequency of voiding.
- Anxiety can impact bladder emptying because of inadequate relaxation of the pelvic floor muscles and urinary sphincter.
- Depression can decrease the desire for urinary continence.

PERSONAL HABITS

- The need for privacy and adequate time to void often influences the ability to adequately empty the bladder.

FLUID INTAKE

- If fluids, electrolytes, and solutes are balanced, increased fluid intake increases urine production.
- Alcohol decreases the release of antidiuretic hormones, thus increasing urine production.
- Fluids containing caffeine and other bladder irritants can prompt unsolicited bladder contractions, resulting in frequency, urgency, and incontinence.

PATHOLOGICAL CONDITIONS

- Diabetes mellitus, multiple sclerosis, and stroke can alter bladder contractility and the ability to sense bladder filling. Patients experience either bladder overactivity or deficient bladder emptying.
- Arthritis, Parkinson disease, dementia, and chronic pain can interfere with timely access to a toilet.
- Spinal cord injury or intervertebral disk disease (above S1) can cause the loss of urine control because of bladder overactivity and impaired coordination between the contracting bladder and the urinary sphincter.
- Prostatic enlargement (e.g., benign prostatic hyperplasia) can cause obstruction of the bladder outlet, which results in urinary retention.

SURGICAL PROCEDURES

- Local trauma during lower abdominal and pelvic surgery sometimes obstructs urine flow, requiring temporary use of an indwelling urinary catheter.
- Anesthetic agents and other agents given during surgery decrease bladder contractility and/or sensation of bladder fullness, often causing urinary retention (Woodward, 2015a).

MEDICATIONS

- Diuretics increase urinary output by preventing resorption of water and certain electrolytes.
- Some drugs change the color of urine (e.g., phenazopyridine—orange; riboflavin—intense yellow).
- Anticholinergics (e.g., atropine, overactive bladder agents) increase the risk for urinary retention by inhibiting bladder contractility (Rantell, 2014).
- Hypnotics and sedatives (e.g., analgesics, antianxiety agents) may reduce the ability to recognize and act on the urge to void.

DIAGNOSTIC EXAMINATIONS

- Cystoscopy may cause localized trauma of the urethra, resulting in transient (1 to 2 days) dysuria and hematuria.
- Whenever the sterile urinary tract is catheterized, there is a risk for infection.

---

incontinence, agitation or absence of normal behavior, decreased appetite, and deteriorating mobility resulting in increased falls.

Urinary Incontinence. Urinary incontinence (UI) is defined by the International Continence Society as the "any involuntary loss of urine" (Wilson, 2016). The highest incidence of UI occurs in older adults—17% of men older than 60 years of age and 30% to 50% of women older than 60 years of age (Testa, 2015). The most common forms of UI are urge or urgency UI and stress UI. Mixed UI occurs when both stress and urgency symptoms are present. Stress UI results from weakness or injury to the urinary sphincter or pelvic floor muscles. Urgency UI is caused by involuntary contractions of the bladder that cause leakage of urine. Overflow UI is associated with acute or chronic urinary retention. Involuntary loss of urine at night, or nocturnal enuresis, can be associated with overactive bladder, medication, or sleep apnea and is often referred to as bed-wetting. Functional UI is caused by factors that limit a patient's access to the toilet or other acceptable receptacle for urine (Bardsley, 2016). Functional UI may also be caused by poor motivation for continence, as seen when a patient has severe depression or has experienced cognitive decline that impairs the ability to sense

TABLE 36.1   TYPES OF URINARY INCONTINENCE

DEFINITION	CHARACTERISTICS	SELECTED NURSING INTERVENTIONS
Transient Incontinence Incontinence caused by medical conditions that in many cases are treatable and reversible	Common reversible causes include: • Delirium and/or acute confusion • Inflammation (e.g., UTI, urethritis) • Medications (diuretics) (Kehinde, 2016) • Excessive urine output (e.g., hyperglycemia, heart failure) • Mobility impairment • Fecal impaction • Depression • Acute urinary retention • Conditions that increase blood pressure or blood osmolality (e.g., dehydration) (Testa, 2015)	Look for reversible causes with new-onset or increased incontinence. Notify health care provider of any suspected reversible causes.
Functional Incontinence Loss of continence from causes outside the urinary tract; usually related to functional deficits such as altered mobility and manual dexterity, cognitive impairment, or environmental barriers impairing ability to reach or use toilet (Bardsley, 2016)	Toilet access restricted by: • Sensory impairments (e.g., vision) • Cognitive impairments cause poor motivation for or inability to attend to continence (e.g., delirium, dementia, severe retardation) • Altered mobility (e.g., hip fracture, arthritis, chronic pain, spastic paralysis associated with multiple sclerosis; slow movements associated with Parkinson disease, hemiparesis) • Altered manual dexterity (e.g., arthritis, upper-extremity fracture) • Environmental barriers (e.g., caregiver unavailable to help with transfers, pathway to bathroom not maneuverable with walker, tight clothing that is difficult to remove, incontinence briefs)	Ensure adequate lighting in bathroom. Provide individualized toileting program designed for degree of cognitive impairment: habit training program, scheduled toileting program, prompted voiding program. Provide mobility aids (e.g., raised toilet seats, toilet grab bars). Clear toilet area to allow access for walker or wheelchair. Suggest use of elastic waist pants without buttons or zippers. Stress that call bell always be within reach. Use incontinence containment product that patient can easily remove such as pull-up type pant or pad that can be moved aside easily for voiding.
Overflow Urinary Incontinence Involuntary loss of urine caused by overdistended bladder; often related to bladder outlet obstruction or poor bladder emptying caused by weak or absent bladder contractions	Distended bladder on palpation High postvoid residual Frequency Involuntary leakage of small volumes of urine Nocturia Common causes include neurological impairment, pelvic surgery, constipation, fecal impaction, pregnancy, prolapse, medication, and benign prostatic hyperplasia (Bardsley, 2016)	Interventions are individualized related to severity of urinary retention, ability of bladder to contract, and kidney damage. **Mild retention with some bladder function** • Timed voiding • Double voiding • Monitor postvoid residual per health care provider's direction • Intermittent catheterization **Severe retention, no bladder function** • Intermittent catheterization • Indwelling catheterization
Stress Urinary Incontinence Involuntary leakage of small volumes of urine associated with increased intraabdominal pressure and urethral hypermobility or weakness of or injury to urinary sphincter (e.g., weak pelvic floor muscles, trauma after childbirth, radical prostatectomy)	Small volume loss of urine with coughing, sneezing, laughing, exercise, walking, bending, lifting, or getting up from a chair Usually does not leak urine at night when sleeping	As directed by health care provider, instruct patient in pelvic muscle (Kegel) exercises: eight contractions performed 3 times a day (Bardsley, 2016).

TABLE 36.1 TYPES OF URINARY INCONTINENCE—cont'd

DEFINITION	CHARACTERISTICS	SELECTED NURSING INTERVENTIONS
Urge Urinary Incontinence Involuntary passage of urine often associated with strong sense of urgency related to overactive bladder (involuntary bladder contractions) caused by neurological problems, bladder inflammation, or bladder outlet obstruction	May experience one or all of the following symptoms: • Urgency • Frequency • Nocturia • Difficulty or unable to hold urine once urge to void occurs • Leaks on way to bathroom • Leaks larger volumes of urine, sometimes enough to wet outer clothing • Dribbling small amounts on way to bathroom • Strong urge/leaks when hears water running, washes hands, drinks fluids	Ask patient about symptoms of UTI. Avoid bladder irritants (e.g., caffeine, smoking tobacco, alcohol). Instruct patient in pelvic muscle (Kegel) exercises, urge inhibition exercises, or bladder training. If ordered by health care provider, monitor patient's symptoms and for presence of side effects of antimuscarinic medications.
Reflex Urinary Incontinence Involuntary loss of urine occurring at predictable intervals when patient reaches specific bladder volume related to spinal cord damage from C1 to S2.	Diminished or absent awareness of bladder filling and urge to void Leakage of urine without awareness May not completely empty bladder because of dyssynergia of urinary sphincter (i.e., inappropriate contraction of sphincter when bladder contracts, causing obstruction to urine flow) **Caution:** Patients with reflex incontinence are at risk for developing autonomic dysreflexia, a life-threatening condition that causes severe elevation of blood pressure and pulse rate and diaphoresis	Follow prescribed schedule for emptying bladder either through voiding or by intermittent catheterization. Use urine containment products: condom catheter, undergarments, pads, briefs. Monitor for signs and symptoms of urinary retention and UTI. Monitor for autonomic dysreflexia; this is a medical emergency requiring immediate intervention. Notify health care provider immediately.

UTI, Urinary tract infection.

and act on the urge to void in an appropriate manner. Functional incontinence sometimes develops when caregivers do not respond in a timely manner to requests for help with toileting. Table 36.1 summarizes the most common types, characteristics, and selected nursing interventions for UI.

Urinary Diversions. Patients who have their bladder removed (cystectomy) because of cancer or significant bladder dysfunction (e.g., related to radiation injury or neurogenic dysfunction with frequent UTI) require surgical procedures that divert urine to the outside of the body through an opening in the abdominal wall called a stoma. A urinary diversion is constructed from a section of intestine to create a storage reservoir or conduit for urine.

There are two types of continent urinary diversions. The continent urinary reservoir (Fig. 36.2A) is created from a distal portion of the ileum and proximal portion of the colon. The ureters are embedded in the reservoir, which is placed under the abdominal wall. A narrow segment of the ileum is brought out through the abdominal wall to form a small stoma. The ileocecal valve creates a one-way valve in the pouch. A catheter is inserted through the stoma to empty urine from the pouch. Patients catheterize the pouch 4 to 6 times a day for the rest of their lives.

The other type of continent urinary diversion, an orthotopic neobladder, uses an ileal pouch to replace the bladder. Anatomically the pouch is in the same position as the bladder was before removal, allowing a patient to void through the urethra using the Valsalva technique.

An ileal conduit or ureterostomy is a permanent incontinent urinary diversion created by transplanting the ureters into a closed-off portion of the intestinal ileum. The other end of the ureters come out onto the abdominal wall, forming a stoma (Fig. 36.2B). Patients have no sensation or control over the continuous flow of urine through the ileal conduit, requiring the effluent (drainage) to be collected in a pouch.

Nephrostomy tubes are small tubes tunneled through the skin into the renal pelvis to drain the renal pelvis when the

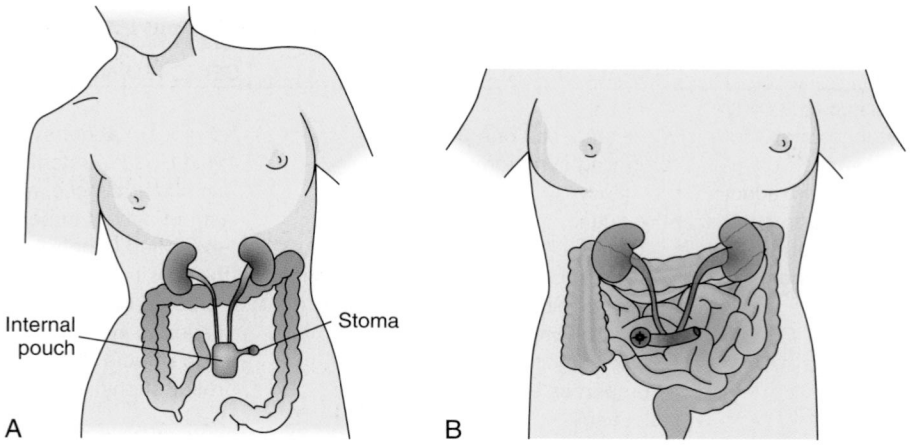

FIG 36.2 Types of incontinent and continent urinary diversions. **A,** Continent urinary reservoir. **B,** Urostomy (ileal conduit).

ureter is obstructed. Patients go home with these tubes and need careful teaching about site care and signs of infection.

NURSING KNOWLEDGE BASE

Urinary elimination is a basic body function that includes a variety of psychological and physiological needs. Physiological and psychosocial nursing care is essential when illness or disability interferes with meeting these needs. Patient-centered care requires an understanding beyond anatomy and physiology of the urinary system.

Infection Control and Hygiene

The urinary tract is sterile. Use infection control principles to help prevent the development and spread of UTIs. You need to follow the principles of asepsis when carrying out procedures involving the urinary tract or external genitalia. Perineal hygiene is always an essential component of care (see Chapter 31) and even more so when a patient has a urinary catheter or other alteration in the usual pattern of urinary elimination.

Developmental Considerations

A patient's ability to control micturition changes during the life span. The neurological system is not well developed until 2 or 3 years of age. Until this time a small child is not able to associate sensation of filling and urge with urination. When a child recognizes feelings of urge, can hold urine for 1 or 2 hours, and is able to communicate a need to eliminate, toilet training is much more likely to be successful. Continence training starts during daytime hours. Children who wet the bed at night without awakening from sleep have *nocturnal enuresis*. Some children experience this nighttime incontinence until late in childhood.

Pregnancy causes many changes in the body including the urinary tract. In early and late pregnancy, urinary frequency is common. Hormonal changes and the pressure of the growing fetus on the bladder cause increased urine production and shrinking bladder capacity.

Psychosocial Implications

Self-concept, culture, and sexuality all are closely related concepts that are affected when a patient has elimination problems. Self-concept changes over one's life span and includes body image, self-esteem, roles, and identity (see Chapter 24). Sometimes children resist urinating in the toilet and associate their urine and feces as extensions of self, thus not wanting to flush them away. The process of micturition is often a private event and requires you to be sensitive to a need for privacy. Incontinence is frequently devastating to self-image and self-esteem. When patients ask for help for this private and personal activity, they may feel embarrassed. Culture often dictates gender-specific roles when it comes to care of elimination issues. For example, in some cultures, it is not appropriate for a man to touch or talk about elimination matters with a woman (Box 36.2).

CRITICAL THINKING

Synthesis

Patient care requires you to apply what you know about a patient, your knowledge base, experience, and critical thinking attitudes and standards. Your synthesis of this information allows you to make sound decisions as you apply the nursing process. Critical thinking synthesis involves combining all available information to obtain a clear picture of the approach needed to provide patient-centered care. To make an appropriate nursing diagnosis and develop an individualized plan of care, all elements need to be integrated (Box 36.3).

Knowledge. During your patient's assessment, take into consideration your knowledge about the urinary system. Integrate knowledge from nursing and other disciplines. Many factors affect the urinary tract. For example, older adults often experience a change in mental status in response to UTIs; men experience stress UI caused by damage to the urinary sphincter after surgery for prostate cancer; and

BOX 36.2 PATIENT-CENTERED CARE

Urinary elimination is a private human activity. Incorporate sensitivity when caring for patients who have urinary elimination problems. Variations within a cultural group are common; thus assess and care for each patient individually. Many cultures have specific beliefs and practices related to elimination, privacy, and gender-specific care.

IMPLICATIONS FOR NURSING PRACTICE

- Ask patients to describe their beliefs and expectations about how to care for their elimination needs. Build mutual trust by adopting the patient's cultural beliefs and values (Collins, 2015).
- Privacy is important in many cultures; thus pay careful attention to closing doors, bedside curtains, and draping.
- Be certain that patients understand instructions and patient education when English is not their primary language (see Chapter 12). Provide a professional interpreter as needed.
- Certain cultures observe meticulous hygiene practices that designate the left hand to perform unclean procedures such as genitourinary hygiene. Perform hand hygiene before touching the patient and use your right hand when possible. Use the left hand to handle the urinal and/or secretions.
- Some cultures continue to practice female genital mutilation, which often includes removal of all or part of the clitoris, partial or complete removal of the labia minora, or total removal of the clitoris and labia minora and sewing together the labia majora for nonmedical reasons, leaving only a small opening for urine and menses (Clarke, 2016).

BOX 36.3 SYNTHESIS IN PRACTICE

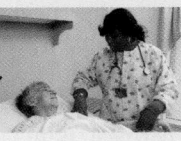 As Carly prepares to assess Mrs. Vallero, she remembers that urinary problems are common in older adults who have diabetes. Advanced age does not cause incontinence. She recalls that patients with urinary retention sometimes leak or "dribble" urine and are inaccurately diagnosed as incontinent. She knows that patients generally void at least every 6 hours and that Mrs. Vallero's recent catheterization, her decreased mobility, and history of diabetes increase her risk for urinary retention, incontinence of small amounts of urine, and urinary tract infection. In addition, she knows that she needs to assess if Mrs. Vallero feels the urge to urinate. She determines that no one has taken Mrs. Vallero to the bathroom recently. Carly also needs to find out more about her patient's urination patterns at home because Mrs. Vallero verbalized anxiety about her present voiding patterns.

Through previous clinical experiences, Carly learned that palpation of the abdomen over a distended bladder causes some discomfort, often creating an urge to urinate. Mrs. Vallero says she has a little *dolor* (pain) and grimaces slightly when Carly palpates her abdomen.

caffeine intake and the use of a diuretic frequently increase urinary urgency and frequency. Patients who are normally continent sometimes become incontinent after developing impaired mobility.

Experience. Urinary elimination problems are common in all health care settings. Reflect on previous and personal experiences to help you determine a patient's elimination needs. Perhaps you cared for an incontinent patient who developed a skin rash secondary to incontinence. Reflection on past experiences prompts you to start using a moisture barrier ointment as a preventive and protective skin care measure. Your experience with a UTI helps you understand a patient's frustration and embarrassment caused by frequency, urgency, and dysuria. Caring for other older adults with a functional disability helps you anticipate patient needs related to toileting.

Attitudes. Application of critical thinking attitudes is an important component of caring for a patient with urinary elimination problems. Approach patients with a confident attitude, but at the same time remain open to the opinions of other health care providers. An evidence-based approach to infection control principles when performing urinary catheterization decreases a patient's risk for **catheter-associated urinary tract infection (CAUTI)**. A CAUTI is defined as the development of a UTI in a patient in whom an indwelling urinary catheter was in place for greater than 2 days or within 2 days of urinary catheter removal (CDC, 2017). When assessing the needs of older adults with incontinence, persevere in getting the whole story, especially their continence status before acute care admission. This information makes a significant difference when designing an appropriate plan of care.

Standards. Apply standards of critical thinking when caring for patients with alterations in urinary elimination. When assessing and planning care for a patient with incontinence, it is important to identify patient needs accurately, determine relevant interventions, and ensure that the plan of care is broad enough to address the whole problem. Knowing that the UTI has aggravated the patient's incontinence, it is appropriate to administer an antibiotic for a UTI; however, the plan would not be complete without addressing problems with toilet access and patient teaching about UTI prevention. Use standards of care such as the *Guideline for Prevention of Catheter-Associated Urinary Tract Infections* (CDC, 2009) and the *ANA CAUTI Prevention Tool* (American Nurses Association [ANA], 2014).

NURSING PROCESS

■■■ ASSESSMENT

To identify urinary elimination problems and ensure patient-centered diagnosis and care, use your scientific and nursing knowledge, conduct a thorough nursing history of a patient's problem, perform a physical examination, assess a patient's urine, and review information from diagnostic tests and examinations.

Nursing History. The nursing history includes a review of a patient's elimination patterns, symptoms of urinary alterations, and assessment of factors affecting normal urination. Because urination is often considered a private matter, some patients find it difficult to talk about their voiding habits. Approach patients in a professional manner, and assure them that you will maintain their confidentiality.

Pattern of Urination. Information about a patient's normal pattern of urination establishes a baseline for comparison. Ask a patient about daily voiding patterns including frequency and times of day, normal volume at each voiding, and history of recent changes. Frequency of voiding varies among individuals depending on fluid intake, medications such as diuretics, and the intake of alcohol and caffeine. Be sure to ask if a patient is awakened from sleep with an urge to void and how many times this occurs. It is normal for hospitalized patients to experience an urge to void when they awaken at night because of noise, pain, or required treatments (e.g., nebulizer treatment).

Symptoms of Urinary Alterations. During assessment ask about the presence of symptoms listed in Table 36.2. Also determine whether a patient is aware of conditions or factors that precipitate or aggravate the symptoms.

Factors Affecting Voiding. Focused assessment enables you to gather data relevant to your patient's elimination pattern and identify factors that impact the ability to void normally (Table 36.3). Assess your patient's understanding of urinary problems, expectations of the care you will provide, and what the patient can do independently. Do not assume that patients with a diagnosis of cognitive impairment cannot understand or participate in care. Be aware of cultural differences related to the very private act of urination and how it affects nursing assessment and care.

Some patients (e.g., following surgery or receiving medications that affect bladder function) become concerned that something is wrong when you assess voiding amount and frequency every 2 hours. Patients receiving IV fluids do not always realize that they have an increased need for urination. Provide appropriate teaching so that patients understand that alterations in urination under these circumstances are to be expected.

Older Adult Considerations. Normal aging causes changes in the urinary system and the rest of the body that increase the risk for bladder dysfunction (see Box 36.1; Box 36.4). An enlarged prostate in older men obstructs urine flow from the bladder, resulting in incomplete bladder emptying, urgency, frequency, UTIs, and damage to the upper urinary tract from urinary retention. In older women, a decrease in estrogen results in urethral changes and decreased closing pressure. Aging and long-term neurological conditions such as multiple sclerosis, stroke, and dementia can also affect the urinary system and create elimination changes (Jones, 2015).

BOX 36.4   CARE OF THE OLDER ADULT

Bladder Dysfunction

- The prevalence of overactive bladder (OAB) (urgency, urge incontinence, frequency, and nocturia in the absence of UTI) increases with age (Rantell, 2014).
- The risk for urinary incontinence increases in patients as a result of aging, cognitive impairment, and chronic disease (Jones, 2015; Nazarko, 2015).
- Assess all possible causes of new-onset incontinence, which includes taking a comprehensive history for urinary incontinence (onset, duration, aggravating factors, characteristics, medical history, associated symptoms, attempted treatments, and severity) and performing a focused physical assessment of physical indicators within each body system (coughing, sensory impairment, skin breakdown) (Testa, 2015).
- Carefully assess older adults taking an antimuscarinic medication to treat urgency, urge incontinence, and OAB for mental status changes. Side effects of these medications include cognitive impairment, sedation, and inability to concentrate (Bardsley, 2016).
- Implement plans to maximize self-care and continence (e.g., toileting program, mobility aides, assistance with hygiene) when caring for older adults with impaired mobility and incontinence.
- Teach older women with stress incontinence about pelvic muscle (Kegel) exercises. There is no age limit on their effectiveness.
- The sensation of thirst decreases with aging. Remind older adults to drink adequate amounts of water.

These changes usually include decreased bladder capacity, decreased ability to delay voiding, loss of bladder contractility, and increased incidence of overactive bladder.

Physical Assessment. Assessment of the urinary system helps you identify signs and severity of urinary problems and monitor responses to medical and nursing interventions. The primary areas to assess include the kidneys, bladder, external genitalia, urethral meatus, and perineal skin (see Chapter 16).

Kidneys. When the kidneys are infected or inflamed, they become tender, and flank pain usually develops. You assess for tenderness by gently percussing the costovertebral angle (the angle formed by the spine and twelfth rib).

Bladder. In adults, the bladder rests below the symphysis pubis. When distended with urine, it rises above the symphysis pubis along the midline of the abdomen. A very full bladder extends to the umbilicus. On inspection you may observe a swelling or convex curvature of the lower abdomen. On gentle palpation of the lower abdomen, a full bladder will feel smooth and rounded, and a patient may report a sensation of urinary urge tenderness or pain. If you suspect an overfull bladder or incomplete emptying of the bladder, further assess the patient with a bladder scanner, a portable ultrasound machine that measures the volume of urine in the

TABLE 36.2 COMMON SYMPTOMS OF URINARY ALTERATIONS

DESCRIPTION	COMMON CAUSES
Urgency Immediate and strong desire to void that is not easily deferred	Full bladder UTI Inflammation or irritation of bladder Overactive bladder
Dysuria Pain or discomfort associated with voiding	UTI Inflammation of prostate Urethritis Trauma to lower urinary tract Urinary tract tumors
Frequency Voiding more than 8 times during waking hours and/or at decreased intervals such as less than every 2 hours	High volumes of fluid intake Alcohol intake Bladder irritants (e.g., caffeine) UTI Increased pressure on bladder (e.g., pregnancy) Bladder outlet obstruction (e.g., prostate enlargement, pelvic organ prolapse) Overactive bladder Uncontrolled diabetes mellitus or diabetes insipidus
Hesitancy Delay in start of urinary stream when voiding	Anxiety (e.g., voiding in public restroom or in front of others) Bladder outlet obstruction (e.g., prostate enlargement, urethral stricture)
Polyuria Voiding excessive amounts of urine	High volumes of fluid intake Uncontrolled diabetes mellitus Diabetes insipidus Diuretic therapy
Oliguria Diminished urinary output in relation to fluid intake	Fluid and electrolyte imbalance (e.g., dehydration) Kidney dysfunction or failure Increased secretion of ADH Urinary tract obstruction
Nocturia Awakened from sleep by urge to void	Excessive intake of fluids (especially coffee or alcohol before bedtime) Bladder outlet obstruction (e.g., prostate enlargement) Overactive bladder Medications (e.g., diuretic taken in the evening) Cardiovascular disease (e.g., hypertension) UTI
Dribbling Leakage of small amounts of urine despite voluntary control of micturition	Bladder outlet obstruction (e.g., prostatic enlargement) Incomplete bladder emptying Stress incontinence
Hematuria Presence of blood in urine Gross hematuria—blood easily seen in urine Microscopic hematuria—blood not visualized but detected on urinalysis	Tumors (e.g., kidney, bladder) Infection (e.g., glomerular nephritis, cystitis) Urinary tract calculi Trauma to urinary tract
Retention Acute retention: Suddenly unable to void when bladder is adequately full or overfull Chronic retention: Bladder does not empty completely during voiding, and urine retained in bladder	Bladder outlet obstruction (e.g., prostatic enlargement, urethral obstruction) Absent or weak bladder contractility (e.g., neurological dysfunction such as caused by diabetes, multiple sclerosis, lower spinal cord injury) Side effects of certain medications (e.g., anesthesia, anticholinergics, antispasmodics, antidepressants)

ADH, Antidiuretic hormone; *UTI,* urinary tract infection.

TABLE 36.3 FOCUSED PATIENT ASSESSMENT

FACTORS TO ASSESS	QUESTIONS	PHYSICAL ASSESSMENT
Fluid intake	Do you have any fluid restrictions? How much do you normally drink in 24 hours? Describe the types of fluids you drink. Are you decreasing your fluid intake because you need to use the toilet too often? How often do you drink beverages that contain caffeine or alcohol (e.g., coffee, tea, soft drinks, beer)?	Observe skin and mucous membranes for adequate hydration. Obtain intake and output over 24 hours.
Urinary symptoms (see Table 36.2)	Are you experiencing a sudden urge to urinate, burning or painful urination, frequent urination, difficulty urinating, excessive urination, the need to urinate at night, dribbling or blood in the urine, straining when you urinate, leaking urine on the way to the bathroom, or leaking urine when you cough or sneeze? Do you feel like you have completely emptied your bladder after you have urinated? When did you last urinate? How many times did you urinate in the last 24 hours?	Observe urine for: • Red color • Cloudiness • Foul odor • Amount with each voiding Assess vital signs for fever and tachycardia. Assess 24-hour intake and output. Start a bladder diary to record frequency and episodes of incontinence. Inspect the abdomen for distention. Inspect the perineal skin for evidence of incontinence-associated dermatitis. Palpate bladder for tenderness or distention. Determine postvoid residual by bladder scan if available.
Medication usage	Which medications including prescription, over-the-counter, and herbal supplements do you take, and how often do you take them? Do you take blood pressure medicine or a diuretic? Are you taking pain medicine?	Assess for signs of fluid and electrolyte disturbances (see Chapter 18). Inspect urine for pale color and dilute concentration. Start a bladder diary to record frequency and episodes of incontinence. Assess output for decreased frequency and amount. Palpate bladder for distention. Assess bowel pattern for constipation.
Functional ability	Do you have trouble getting to the bathroom or toilet on time? What type of help do you need when using the bathroom? Do you have trouble removing your clothing to use the toilet? Do you have difficulty cleaning yourself after urinating? Do you use a product to contain urine leakage (e.g., brief or incontinence pad)?	Observe patient's ability to get up or out of bed and walk safely to bathroom. Observe patient's ability to safely get on and off toilet. Observe patient's ability to remove clothing for toileting and perform hygiene. Assess patient's ability to understand instructions related to toileting (cognition, language, culture).
Environment	Does anything prevent you from getting to the bathroom on time? Do you use assistive devices in the bathroom (e.g., elevated toilet seat, handrails)?	Assess for adequate lighting in bathroom and need for assistive devices to facilitate safe toileting; easy access to nurse call system; clear path to bathroom, especially if a walker is used; and prompt response of nursing assistive personnel to patient requests for toileting.

TABLE 36.3 FOCUSED PATIENT ASSESSMENT—cont'd

FACTORS TO ASSESS	QUESTIONS	PHYSICAL ASSESSMENT
Medical history that possibly affects urinary system	Do you have a history of a UTI, urinary incontinence, urinary retention, kidney stones, prostate disease, pregnancy, neurological disease, pelvic organ prolapse, or diabetes mellitus? Do you have any difficulty feeling the need to urinate?	Start a bladder diary to record frequency, amount, and episodes of incontinence.
Recent surgery and critical illness (some anesthesia affects sensory and motor function of the bladder)	Do you feel the urge to urinate? Have you urinated since your surgery? Did you have a catheter before or after surgery?	Assess intake and output record for adequate frequency and amounts of voiding. Using a bladder scan, assess for urinary retention (see Box 36.5).

bladder. Using a bladder scanner minimizes unnecessary catheterization and associated risk for UTI (Box 36.5).

External Genitalia and Urethral Meatus. Careful and sensitive inspection of the external genitalia and urethral meatus yields important data. Normally there is no drainage or inflammation. To best examine a female patient, position her in the dorsal recumbent position to provide full exposure of the genitalia. Observe the labia majora for swelling, redness, tenderness, rashes, lesions, or evidence of scratching. Using a gloved hand retract the labial folds. The labia minora is normally pink and moist. The urethral meatus appears as an irregular opening or slit close to the vaginal opening. Look for drainage and lesions, and ask the patient if there is discomfort. If there is drainage, note the color and consistency. The vaginal tissue in postmenopausal women may be dryer and less pink than in younger women.

For men, examine the penis and look for any redness or irritation. If the patient is uncircumcised, retract the foreskin or ask him to do so. The foreskin normally moves easily back to expose the glans penis. In some cases, the foreskin becomes tight and cannot be retracted (a condition called phimosis), increasing risk for inflammation and infection. The urethral meatus is a slitlike opening just below the tip of the penis. Inspect the glans penis and meatus for discharge, lesions, and inflammation. Following inspection, return the foreskin to the unretracted position. Retracted foreskins cause dangerous swelling (called paraphimosis) of the penis (Steadman and Ellsworth, 2016).

Assess the urinary meatus of all patients with an indwelling catheter for infection such as catheter-related damage and presence of inflammation and discharge. Pulling and traction on catheters damages the urinary meatus by creating pressure on the urethra and meatus. In some severe cases the catheter erodes through the meatus to the vagina or through the glans and shaft of the penis. Early detection of trauma results in prompt intervention and prevention of further injury.

Perineal Skin. Regularly assess skin exposed to moisture, especially urine, for signs of incontinence-associated skin damage (IAD). Observe for erythema in areas exposed to moisture, which is most commonly noted in the labia in women, in the scrotum in men, and in the inner thigh and buttock region in both women and men (Voegeli, 2016). Be sure to thoroughly assess patients when they tell you they are experiencing burning, itching pain in these areas.

Assessment of Urine. To assess a patient's urine, measure a patient's fluid intake and urinary output (I&O), and observe the characteristics of the urine.

Intake and Output. You assess I&O to evaluate bladder emptying, renal function, and fluid and electrolyte balance. Although often written as part of a health care provider's order, placing a patient on I&O is also nursing judgment. Obtaining accurate I&O measurement often requires cooperation and assistance from a patient and family. Include all oral liquids and semiliquids, enteral feedings, and any parenteral fluids as intake (see Chapter 18). Include urine and any other fluid that leaves the body that can be measured, such as vomitus, gastric drainage in tubes, and wound drainage that is collected as output.

Urinary output is more than a key indicator of kidney and bladder function. A change in urine volume is significant, often indicating fluid imbalance, kidney dysfunction, or decreased blood volume. If a patient has an indwelling catheter after surgery, assess urinary output hourly to indirectly measure circulating blood volume. Continually assess your patient for signs of blood loss, and notify the health care provider if the urinary output falls below 30 mL/hour for more than 2 consecutive hours or if the patient has excessive urine output (called polyuria). Evaluate patients who have not voided for longer than 3 to 6 hours and have had fluid intake recorded for urinary retention. Assess for extreme increases or decreases in urine volume. Sometimes, just helping a patient to a normal position to void prompts urinary elimination.

Measure urine volume with containers that have volume measurement markings. Use a graduated measuring container after a patient voids in a bedside commode, bedpan, or urinal or after emptying urine from a catheter drainage

BOX 36.5   PROCEDURAL GUIDELINES

Using a Bladder Scanner to Measure Postvoid Residual

DELEGATION CONSIDERATIONS

The skill of measuring bladder volume by bladder scan can be delegated to nursing assistive personnel (NAP). The nurse determines the timing and frequency of the bladder scan measurement and interprets the measurements obtained. The nurse also assesses a patient's ability to toilet before measuring postvoid residual and the abdomen for distention if urinary retention is suspected. The nurse directs the NAP to:

- Follow manufacturer recommendations for use of the device.
- Measure postvoid residual volumes within 5 to 15 minutes after helping the patient void.
- Report and record bladder scan volumes.

EQUIPMENT

Bladder scanner (follow manufacturer instructions for use), ultrasound gel, cleaning agent such as an alcohol pad for scanner head, urethral catheterization tray with single-use catheter for straight/intermittent catheterization (see Skill 36.1)

STEPS

1. Identify patient using at least two identifiers (e.g., name and birthday or name and medical record number) according to agency policy (TJC, 2018).
2. Assess intake and output (I&O) record to determine urine output trends, and check the plan of care to verify correct timing of bladder scan measurement.
3. Perform hand hygiene and apply clean gloves.
4. Provide privacy by closing room door and bedside curtain.
5. Discuss procedure with patient. If the measurement is for postvoid residual, ask patient to void and measure voided urine volume. Measurement should be within 5 to 15 minutes of voiding.
6. Measurement of postvoid residual with bladder scan
   a. Help patient to supine position with head slightly elevated. Raise bed to appropriate working height. If side rails are raised, lower side rail on working side.
   b. Expose patient's lower abdomen.
   c. Turn on scanner per manufacturer guidelines.
   d. Set gender designation per manufacturer guidelines. Designate women who have had a hysterectomy as male.
   e. Wipe scanner head with alcohol pad or other cleaner and allow to air dry.
   f. Palpate patient's symphysis pubis (pubic bone). Apply generous amount of ultrasound gel (or a bladder scan gel pad if available) to midline abdomen 2.5 to 4 cm (1 to 1.5 inches) above symphysis pubis.
   g. Place scanner head on gel, ensuring that scanner head is oriented per manufacturer guidelines.
   h. Apply light pressure, keep scanner head steady, and point it slightly downward toward bladder. Press and release scan button (see illustration).

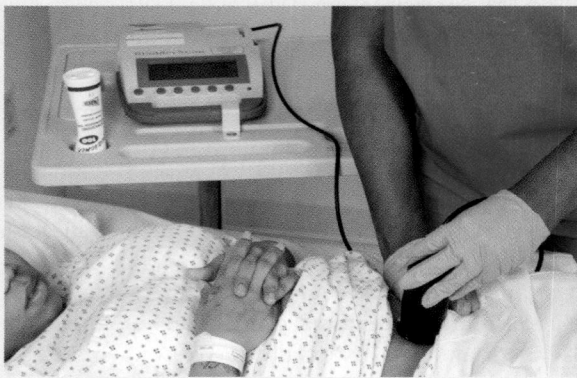

STEP 6h Placement of bladder scan head.

   i. Verify accurate aim (refer to manufacturer guidelines). Complete scan and print image (if needed).
   j. Remove ultrasound gel from patient's abdomen with paper towel.
   k. Remove ultrasound gel from scanner head and wipe with alcohol pad or other cleaner; allow to air-dry.
   l. Help patient to comfortable position. Lower bed and replace side rails accordingly.
   m. Remove gloves and perform hand hygiene.
7. Measurement of postvoid residual using straight/intermittent catheterization (see Skill 36.1).
8. Review health care provider's order to determine how often to assess residual urine.
9. Review I&O record to determine urine output trends.
10. **Use Teach-Back:** "We talked about the importance of using a bladder scan in your care. Tell me the purpose of using a bladder scan and how often a scan might be done." Revise your instruction now or develop a plan for revised patient/family caregiver teaching if patient/family caregiver is not able to teach back correctly.

---

bag. Each patient needs to have a graduated container for individual use to prevent potential cross-contamination. Label each container with the patient's name. Rinse the container after each use to minimize odor and bacterial growth. A **urine hat** (Fig. 36.3) collects urine in a toilet, allowing for patient privacy in the bathroom. Some catheters have a specialized drainage bag with a **urometer** attached between the drainage tubing and drainage bag that allows for accurate hourly urine measurement (Fig. 36.4). Empty drainage bags every 8 hours or as needed and record the output. When emptying catheter drainage bags, make sure that the drainage tube is reclamped and secured.

Characteristics of Urine. Inspect urine for color, clarity, and odor. Monitor and document any changes.

Color. Normal urine ranges in color from pale yellow (like straw) to amber depending on its concentration. Urine is usually more concentrated in the morning or in the presence of fluid volume deficits. As a patient drinks more fluids,

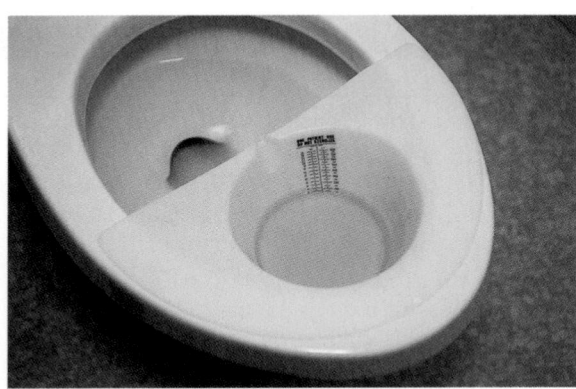

FIG 36.3 Urine hat.

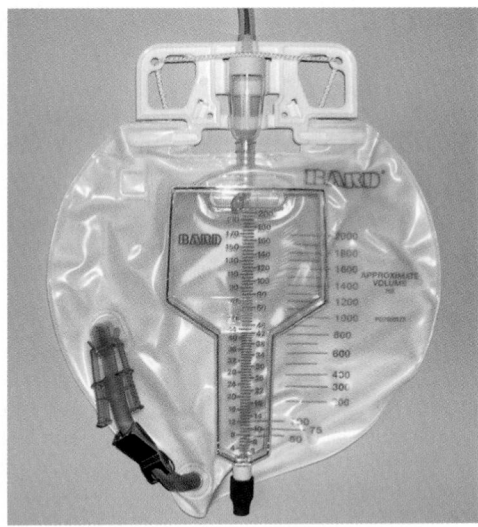

FIG 36.4 Urometer. (Courtesy Michael Gallager, RN, BSN, MSN, OSF, Saint Francis Medical Center, Peoria, IL.)

urine becomes less concentrated, and the color lightens. Patients taking diuretics commonly void dilute urine while the medication is active.

Hematuria, or blood in the urine, is never a normal finding. Bleeding from the kidneys or ureters usually causes urine to become dark red; bleeding from the bladder or urethra usually causes bright red urine. Hematuria and blood clots commonly cause urinary catheter blockage. Report these findings immediately to the patient's health care provider.

Various medications and foods can change the color of urine. Patients taking phenazopyridine, a urinary analgesic, void urine that is bright orange. Eating beets, rhubarb, and blackberries sometimes causes red urine. The kidneys excrete special dyes used in IV diagnostic studies, which discolor the urine. Patients with liver disease who have high concentrations of bilirubin (urobilinogen) often have dark amber urine. Report unexpected color changes to the health care provider.

Clarity. Normal urine appears transparent at the time of voiding. Urine that stands several minutes in a container becomes cloudy. Sometimes a patient's first voided urine of the day is cloudy because the urine is stored in the bladder overnight; urine normally clears on the next voiding. Patients with bacteria and white blood cells in their urine usually have thick and cloudy urine. In patients with renal disease, freshly voided urine often appears cloudy because of protein concentration.

Odor. Urine has a characteristic ammonia odor. The more concentrated the urine, the stronger the odor. As urine remains standing (e.g., in a collection device), more ammonia breakdown occurs, and the odor becomes stronger. A foul odor often indicates a UTI. Some foods such as asparagus and garlic can change the odor of urine.

Laboratory and Diagnostic Testing. You are responsible for collecting urine specimens for laboratory testing. The type of test determines the method of collection. Label all specimens at the bedside with the patient's name, date, time, and type of collection. Complete laboratory requisition forms with specific information required by the testing laboratory. Most urine specimens need to reach the laboratory within 2 hours of collection or be preserved according to the laboratory protocol (Pagana et al., 2017). Urine that stands in a container at room temperature without the required preservative grows bacteria and experiences changes that affect the accuracy of the test. Follow agency infection control policies and standard precautions when handling urine specimens (see Chapter 14). Urine specimens commonly collected include first morning specimen, random urine specimen, timed urine specimen, double voided specimen, and urine for culture and sensitivity. To obtain urine that is freshly voided, ask the patient to double void. Ask a patient to empty the bladder, then send the second voided specimen to the laboratory. To obtain urine as free of bacterial contamination as possible, a midstream, clean-catch urine specimen is sometimes required.

Urinalysis. When a routine urinalysis is ordered, collect a random or first morning specimen. A routine urinalysis requires no special preparation and is collected either by the patient voiding into an appropriate clean container or by urethral catheterization. You can obtain specimens from an indwelling catheter as long as you use the specimen port and not the drainage bag. Urinalysis includes a number of tests that are used for diagnostic screening for fluid and electrolyte disturbances, UTI, presence of blood, and other metabolic problems (Table 36.4). In some health care settings, you test urine using reagent strips. Follow manufacturer instructions when performing the test and reading the strips. Dip the reagent strip into fresh urine, and observe for color changes on the strip. Compare the colors on the strip with a color chart on the reagent strip container. Be sure to examine each color at the exact time indicated on the container.

Timed Urine Tests. Timed testing requires urine collection and testing either at a specific time of day or urine collected over a specific time period. These tests measure substances that may be excreted at higher levels at specific times of the day such as glucose 2 hours after a meal or

TABLE 36.4 ROUTINE URINALYSIS VALUES

MEASUREMENT (NORMAL VALUE)	INTERPRETATION
pH (4.6–8.0)	Indicates acid-base balance (average 6.0). Acid pH helps protect against bacterial growth. Urine that stands for several hours becomes alkaline from bacterial growth.
Protein (up to 8 mg/100 mL)	Protein is normally not present in urine. Presence of protein is a very sensitive indicator of kidney disease. Damage to glomerular membrane (such as in glomerulonephritis) allows for filtration of larger molecules such as protein to seep through.
Glucose (not normally present)	Patients with poorly controlled diabetes have glucose in the urine because of inability of tubules to resorb high serum glucose concentrations (greater than 180 mg/100 mL). Ingestion of high concentrations of glucose causes some glucose to appear in urine of healthy individuals.
Ketones (not normally present)	With poor control of type 1 diabetes, patients experience breakdown of fatty acids. End products of fatty acid metabolism are ketones. Patients with dehydration, starvation, high-protein diets, alcoholism, or excessive aspirin ingestion also have ketonuria.
Blood	A positive test for occult blood occurs when intact erythrocytes, hemoglobin, or myoglobin is present. Damage to glomerulus or tubules causes blood cells to enter urine. Trauma or disease of lower urinary tract also causes hematuria.
Specific gravity (1.005–1.030)	Measures concentration of particles in urine. High specific gravity reflects concentrated urine, and low specific gravity reflects diluted urine. Dehydration, reduced renal blood flow, and increase in ADH secretion elevate specific gravity. Overhydration, early renal disease, and inadequate ADH secretion reduce specific gravity.
Microscopic examination	
RBCs (up to 2)	Damage to glomeruli or tubules allows RBCs to enter the urine. Trauma, disease, presence of urethral catheters, or surgery of the lower urinary tract also causes RBCs to be present.
WBCs (0–4 per low-power field)	Elevated numbers indicate inflammation or infection.
Bacteria (not normally present)	Usually indicates infection or colonization (presence of bacteria and patient shows no symptoms of infection).
Casts (not normally present)	Casts are microscopic cylindrical bodies that look like objects within the renal tubule. There are two main categories of casts: acellular and cellular. Acellular casts include hyaline, granular, waxy, and fatty; cellular casts include WBC, RBC, bacterial, and epithelial cell casts. Their presence often indicates renal disease.
Crystals (not normally present)	Crystals indicate increased risk for development of renal calculi (stone). Some patients with high uric acid levels (gout) develop uric acid crystals. Patients with parathyroid abnormalities or malabsorption often develop phosphate and calcium oxalate crystals.

ADH, Antidiuretic hormone; *RBC,* red blood cell; *WBC,* white blood cell.
Data from Pagana TJ, et al: *Mosby's diagnostic and laboratory test reference,* ed 13, St Louis, 2017, Mosby.

substances that are to be measured over a specific time period such as sodium, potassium, and chloride as indicators of fluid and electrolyte disturbance (Pagana et al., 2017). For most 24-hour specimen collections, discard the first voided specimen and start collecting all urine with the next void for a 24-hour period in a special container that has a preservative added. Depending on the test, you need to keep the urine container cool by placing it in a container of ice. Provide patient education including an explanation of the test, an emphasis on the need to collect all urine voided during the prescribed time period, and how to avoid contaminating the specimen with stool or toilet paper. Carefully document the start and stop time of the test, as requested by the laboratory, to improve testing accuracy.

Clean-Catch Midstream Specimen. Collect a clean-catch midstream specimen when you want to obtain a specimen relatively free of contaminating microorganisms. A clean-catch urine specimen kit includes a sterile cup and disinfectant wipes. Illustrated instructions are often included. Teach the patient how to cleanse the urinary meatus effectively 2 to 3 times with a separate clean wipe each time, and remind female patients to clean the meatus by wiping front to back. Instruct male patients to retract their foreskin if not circumcised and to cleanse the meatus in a circular motion, moving from the center of the meatus to the outside. After cleansing, the patient opens the sterile urine cup. Caution your patient not to touch the inside of the cup. To collect the specimen, instruct the patient to start voiding in the toilet or other receptacle, stop the stream, position the sterile cup to collect urine, and then continue voiding into the cup. When finished, you or your patient puts the lid on the cup, and you send the specimen to the laboratory for testing.

Urine for Culture and Sensitivity. Urine specimens collected for culture and sensitivity determine the presence of bacteria and identify the appropriate antibiotic needed. Collect the specimen using clean-catheter midstream urine or by sterile catheterization (see Skill 36.1). Catheterize the stoma of a patient with a urinary diversion to obtain an accurate specimen. Sometimes a preliminary report is available in 24 hours, but usually 48 to 72 hours are needed for bacterial growth and sensitivity testing (Pagana et al., 2017).

Diagnostic Examinations. The urinary system is one of the few organ systems accessible to accurate diagnostic study by radiographic techniques. Studies are either simple and noninvasive or complex and invasive (Table 36.5). Before testing, nursing responsibilities include ensuring that a signed consent is completed (check agency policy). Assess whether the patient has allergies or has experienced a previous reaction to a contrast agent (Pagana et al., 2017). Administer bowel-cleansing agents as ordered; check agency policy. Ensure that the patient adheres to the appropriate pretest diet, which may be clear liquids or nothing by mouth (NPO). Nursing responsibilities after testing include assessing I&O and voiding and urine (color, clarity, presence of blood, dysuria, problems emptying). Also encourage fluid intake, especially if using radiopaque dye.

■ ■ ■ **NURSING DIAGNOSIS**

A thorough assessment of a patient's urinary elimination function reveals patterns of data that allow you to make relevant and accurate nursing diagnoses. Use critical thinking to reflect on knowledge of previous patients and the application of knowledge of urinary function. Identifying defining characteristics or risk factors leads you to select appropriate nursing diagnoses (see Chapter 9). You identify the relevant related factor for each problem-focused or health promotion diagnosis so as to select individualized nursing interventions (Ackley and Ladwig, 2017). For example, *Toileting Self-Care Deficit related to impaired transfer ability or impaired mobility* guides the selection of nursing interventions that remove barriers to toilet access. *Toileting Self-Care Deficit related to cognitive impairment* guides the selection of nursing interventions such as a prompted-voiding program or habit-training program. Following are some nursing diagnoses common in patients with urinary elimination problems:

- *Functional Urinary Incontinence*
- *Stress Urinary Incontinence*
- *Urge Urinary Incontinence*
- *Risk for Impaired Skin Integrity*
- *Risk for Infection*
- *Toileting Self-Care Deficit*
- *Impaired Urinary Elimination*
- *Urinary Retention*

■ ■ ■ **PLANNING**

Plan nursing care using a process that integrates your assessment of the patient's problem, your nursing knowledge related to the problem, and evidenced-based standards of nursing care (see Care Plan).

TABLE 36.5 COMMON DIAGNOSTIC TESTING

PROCEDURE	DESCRIPTION	SPECIAL NURSING CONSIDERATIONS
Noninvasive Procedures		
Abdominal radiograph (plain film; KUB or flat plate)	X-ray film of abdomen to determine size, shape, symmetry, and location of structures of lower urinary tract Common uses: Detect and measure size of urinary calculi	**Preparation:** • No special preparation. • Previous GI barium contrast study could alter results. • Contraindicated in pregnant patients.
CT scan	Noninvasive detailed three-dimensional real-time display imaging of abdominal structures provided by computerized reconstruction of cross-sectional images Common uses: Identify anatomical abnormalities, renal tumors, cysts, calculi, and obstruction of ureters	**Preparation:** • Follow bowel-cleansing protocol. • Assess for allergy to shellfish (iodine) or previous reaction to contrast media (if contrast agent is ordered). • Restrict food and fluid up to 4 hours before test (see agency protocol). **After procedure:** • Encourage fluids to promote excretion of dye. • Assess for delayed hypersensitivity reaction to contrast media. **Patient teaching:** • Explain that patient will be placed on a special bed that will move through a tunnel-like imaging chamber. Patient needs to lie still when instructed by the technician. Some patients feel claustrophobic and may need an order for a mild sedative.

Continued

TABLE 36.5   COMMON DIAGNOSTIC TESTING—cont'd

PROCEDURE	DESCRIPTION	SPECIAL NURSING CONSIDERATIONS
IVP	Imaging of urinary tract that views collecting ducts and renal pelvis and outlines ureters, bladder, and urethra; after IV injection of contrast media (iodine-based that converts to a dye), a series of x-ray films are taken to observe passage of urine from renal pelvis to bladder. Common uses: Detect and measure urinary calculi, tumors, hematuria, obstruction of urinary tract	**Preparation:** • Assess for allergies and dehydration. • Follow bowel-cleansing protocol. • Restrict food and fluid up to 4 hours before test (see agency protocol). **After procedure:** • Assess for delayed hypersensitivity to contrast media. • Encourage fluids after test to dilute and flush dye from patient. • Assess urine output; less than 30 mL/hr increases risk for contrast-induced nephropathy. **Patient teaching:** • Facial flushing and salty taste in the mouth is a normal response during dye injection. Patients also often feel dizzy, warm, or nauseated.
Ultrasound renal bladder	Imaging of kidneys, ureters, and bladder using sound waves. Identifies gross structural abnormalities and estimates volume of urine in bladder Common uses: Detect masses, cysts, obstruction, presence of hydronephrosis or hydroureter, abnormalities of bladder wall, and renal and pelvic calculi; measuring postvoid residual	**Preparation:** • Patients need to come to study with full bladder. • Fasting is not required. **Patient teaching:** • Test is completed in about 1 hour. • Patient will experience little or no discomfort during procedure.
Invasive Procedures Endoscopy-cystoscopy	Introduction of cystoscope through urethra into bladder to provide direct visualization, specimen collection, or treatment of bladder and urethra. Procedure is performed using local anesthesia in most cases, but under certain circumstances general anesthesia or conscious sedation may be used. Common uses: Microscopic hematuria; detect bladder tumors and obstruction of bladder outlet and urethra	**Preparation:** • Encourage patient to drink fluids several hours before procedure to ensure steady flow of urine and prevent infection. • When applicable, follow agency protocol for preoperative preparation (see Chapter 40). **During procedure:** • Instruct patient to lie still. • Patient may feel need to void as cystoscope passes bladder neck. **Patient teaching:** • Urine is sometimes tinged pink after test. Assess for signs and symptoms of UTI. Antibiotics are often ordered before and after procedure to reduce risk of UTI.

CT, Computed tomography; *GI,* gastrointestinal; *IVP,* intravenous pyelogram; *KUB,* kidney, ureter, bladder; *UTI,* urinary tract infection.
Data from Pagana TJ, et al: *Mosby's diagnostic and laboratory test reference,* ed 13, St Louis, 2017, Mosby.

Goals and Outcomes. Ensure goals and outcomes for urinary elimination problems are realistic and individualized. Patients often have more than one nursing diagnosis, and the diagnoses affect one another (Fig. 36.5). Assess the relationships among these diagnoses and establish patient-centered goals and outcomes in collaboration with the patient and family. For example, a realistic patient goal for a patient with *Toileting Self-Care Deficit related to impaired mobility* is: Patient will be able to independently use the toilet every 2 to 4 hours. An appropriate outcome is: Patient safely transfers to the toilet. To achieve this outcome, you identify a number of interventions such as ensuring that the nurse call system is within reach and providing assistive devices such as a raised toilet seat, support rails next to the toilet, and easy access to the urinal when in bed.

Setting Priorities. Establish priorities of care based on a patient's immediate physical and safety needs, patient expectations, and patient readiness to perform some self-care activities. For example, a patient with a long-term indwelling

◎ CARE PLAN

Urinary Retention

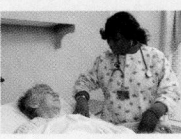

ASSESSMENT

Mrs. Vallero was unable to void 8 hours after catheter removal. A bladder scan showed retained urine. She underwent intermittent catheterization, and 500 mL of urine was obtained. It is now 4 hours since the catheterization. She has been drinking fluids including hot tea and water to increase her chances of urinating on her own.

ASSESSMENT ACTIVITIES	**FINDINGS**[a]
Verify the time patient's catheter was removed and post catheter urine obtained. Inspect the abdomen for distention and gently palpate for bladder distention every 2 hours on the even hours.	Palpation of bladder indicates **bladder distention.** During palpation patient states she has **sensation of bladder fullness.**
Assess patient's voiding pattern including volume at each voiding every 2 hours after straight catheterization completed.	Patient reports feeling pressure over her lower abdomen, has been **dribbling small amounts of urine,** and **is unable to urinate** following straight catheterization.

[a]**Defining characteristics/risk factors** are shown in **bold** type.

NURSING DIAGNOSIS: Urinary Retention related to recent removal of indwelling urinary catheter

---

PLANNING

GOAL	**EXPECTED OUTCOMES (NOC)**[b]
Mrs. Vallero will be able to void every 2 to 3 hours within 1 week.	**Urinary Elimination**
	Mrs. Vallero will void greater than 150 mL every 2 to 3 hours while awake.
	Urinary Continence
	Mrs. Vallero will verbalize no episodes of dribbling or incontinence within a week.
	Symptom Severity
	Mrs. Vallero will verbalize relief of lower abdominal discomfort within 2 to 3 hours.

[b]Outcome classification labels from Moorhead S, et al, editors: *Nursing outcomes classification (NOC)*, ed 5, St Louis, 2013, Mosby.

INTERVENTIONS (NIC)[c]	**RATIONALE**
Urinary Retention Care	
Remind Mrs. Vallero to use the toilet every 2 to 3 hours while awake (timed voiding), provide privacy for elimination, and allow 10 minutes for bladder emptying.	Timed or scheduled bladder training and providing time and privacy for voiding are effective interventions for all types of urinary incontinence (Roe et al., 2015; Testa, 2015)
Instruct Mrs. Vallero to keep a diary of her voiding time and amount including when she experiences urine leakage.	Keeping a record of voiding and times of urine leakage provides a way to monitor progress and individualize a voiding schedule (Testa, 2015).
Encourage Mrs. Vallero to use strategies that stimulate voiding such as drinking a warm beverage before voiding, taking a warm shower or bath, listening to running water when attempting to void, applying cold to the abdomen, stroking the inner thigh, or pouring warm water over the perineal area when on the toilet.	These strategies help relax the pelvic floor muscles and stimulate bladder contractions (Ackley and Ladwig, 2017).
Instruct Mrs. Vallero to double void.	Instructing patients to void and then change position or briefly stand before attempting to void for a second time allows for additional emptying of the bladder (Testa, 2015).
Measure postvoid residual by bladder scan at ordered intervals.	Monitoring postvoid residual after catheter removal can prevent dangerous and painful urinary retention (Bardsley, 2016).

[c]Intervention classification labels from Bulechek GM, et al, editors: *Nursing interventions classification (NIC)*, ed 6, St Louis, 2013, Mosby.

Continued

CARE PLAN—cont'd

Urinary Retention

EVALUATION

NURSING ACTIONS	PATIENT RESPONSE/FINDING	ACHIEVEMENT OF OUTCOME
Ask Mrs. Vallero about her urge to void, sensation of bladder fullness, and dribbling episodes.	Mrs. Vallero denies dribbling episodes, and she has a decreased urgency to urinate.	Dribbling episodes and sense of urgency relieved.
Evaluate Mrs. Vallero's urinary elimination log.	Mrs. Vallero's log shows most output is greater than 150 mL and she is able to void every 2 to 3 hours.	Urinary output is greater than 150 mL with each void.
Ask Mrs. Vallero if she continues to have lower abdominal pain.	Mrs. Vallero denies lower abdominal pain at this time. States that since she has urinated more at a time, she no longer has discomfort.	Lower abdominal discomfort is absent.

CONCEPT MAP

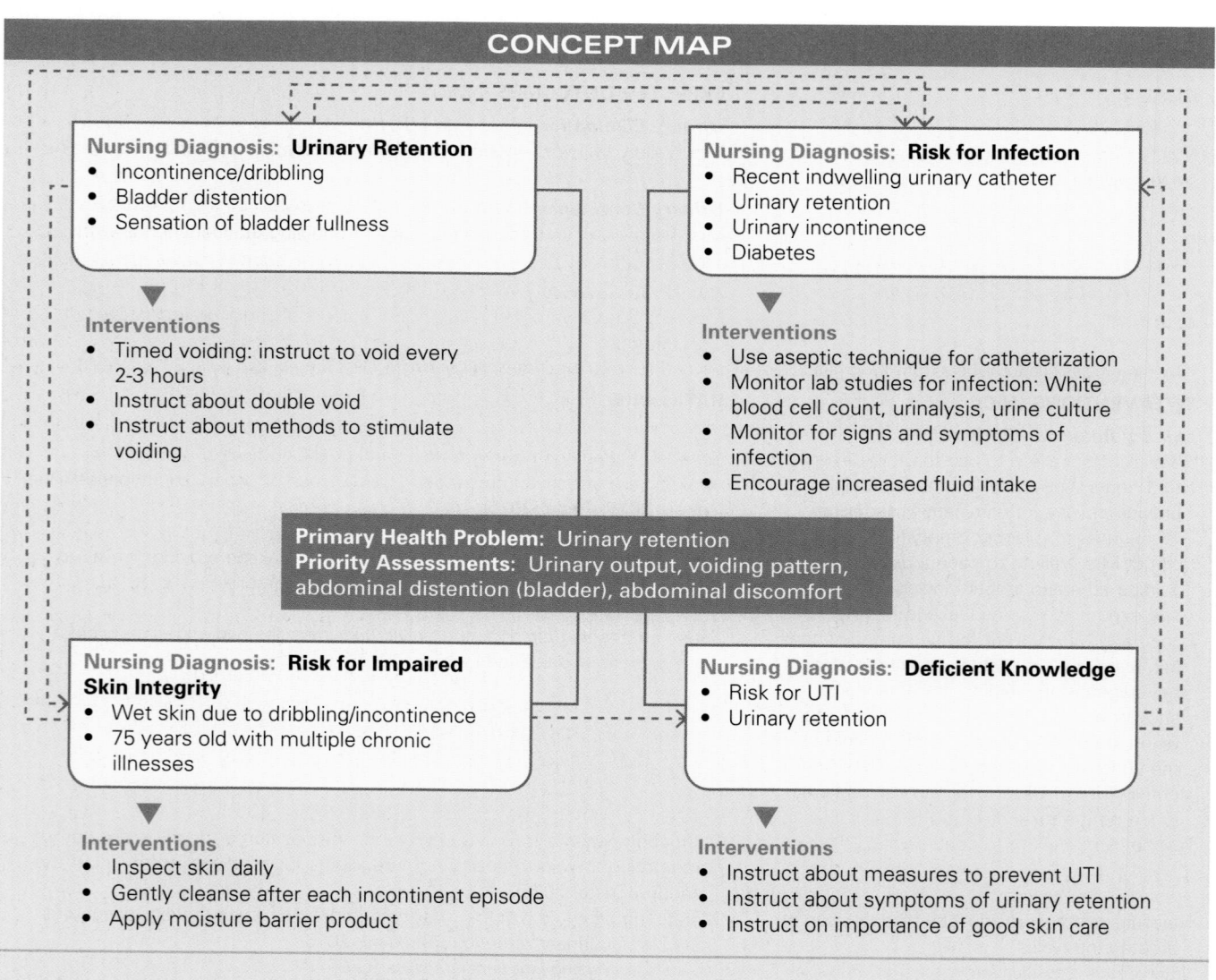

Nursing Diagnosis: Urinary Retention
- Incontinence/dribbling
- Bladder distention
- Sensation of bladder fullness

Interventions
- Timed voiding: instruct to void every 2-3 hours
- Instruct about double void
- Instruct about methods to stimulate voiding

Nursing Diagnosis: Risk for Infection
- Recent indwelling urinary catheter
- Urinary retention
- Urinary incontinence
- Diabetes

Interventions
- Use aseptic technique for catheterization
- Monitor lab studies for infection: White blood cell count, urinalysis, urine culture
- Monitor for signs and symptoms of infection
- Encourage increased fluid intake

Primary Health Problem: Urinary retention
Priority Assessments: Urinary output, voiding pattern, abdominal distention (bladder), abdominal discomfort

Nursing Diagnosis: Risk for Impaired Skin Integrity
- Wet skin due to dribbling/incontinence
- 75 years old with multiple chronic illnesses

Nursing Diagnosis: Deficient Knowledge
- Risk for UTI
- Urinary retention

Interventions
- Inspect skin daily
- Gently cleanse after each incontinent episode
- Apply moisture barrier product

Interventions
- Instruct about measures to prevent UTI
- Instruct about symptoms of urinary retention
- Instruct on importance of good skin care

——— Link between medical diagnosis and nursing diagnosis   - - - - Link between nursing diagnoses

FIG 36.5 Concept map.

catheter is admitted to the hospital with a severe UTI. The patient expects to resume self-care of the catheter. However, because of the severity of the infection and the patient's condition, remind the patient that you will perform all catheter care at this time. The priorities are to treat the infection, prevent reinfection, and teach the patient how to resume care of the catheter to prevent future infections.

Collaborative Care. Include all appropriate health care team members when planning individualized care for your patients. For example, when planning care for a patient with urge UI, you collaborate with a continence nurse specialist to help the patient learn techniques to inhibit urinary urge and strengthen pelvic floor muscles, an occupational therapist to help the patient learn efficient and safe toilet transfers, a physical therapist to help with strengthening exercises of the lower extremities, and a social worker to obtain assistive devices in the home. Include the family caregiver in planning when appropriate.

■ ■ ■ IMPLEMENTATION

Nursing care of patients with elimination alterations focuses on specific interventions that include patient education, promotion of normal voiding and complete bladder emptying, prevention of infection, and promotion of skin integrity and comfort.

Health Promotion. Health promotion helps a patient understand and participate in self-care activities to preserve and protect healthy urinary system function.

Patient Education. Success of therapies aimed at optimizing normal urinary elimination depends in part on thorough patient education. Although patients need to learn about all aspects of healthy urinary elimination, it is best to focus on a patient's specific elimination problem first. For example, a patient who has a UTI and poor hygiene practices benefits most from teaching focused on handwashing and proper perineal hygiene. Teach this patient about symptoms that indicate a UTI and the need to seek early treatment to prevent serious illness. Incorporate teaching about perineal hygiene when assisting a patient with bathing or performing catheter care.

Promoting Normal Micturition. Maintaining normal urinary elimination prevents many problems. Instruct patient to void at regular intervals, usually every 3 to 4 hours, depending on fluid intake. Teach patients to report to their health care provider any changes in bladder habits, frequency, urgency, pain when voiding, or blood in the urine. Many measures that promote normal voiding are independent nursing interventions.

Maintaining Elimination Habits. When in a hospital or long-term care facility, institutional routines often conflict with a patient's normal voiding routine. Create as much privacy as possible such as closing the door and bedside curtains; asking visitors to leave a room when a bedside commode, bedpan, or urinal is used; and masking the sounds of voiding with running water. Respond to requests for assistance with toileting as quickly as possible. Embarrassing accidents are easily avoided when help comes in time. Avoid the use of incontinence containment products unless needed for uncontrolled urine leakage. Some containment products are difficult to remove, increase the incidence of skin breakdown when not removed quickly, and interfere with prompt toilet access. Patients should avoid straining when voiding or moving the bowels. Encourage them to take enough time to empty the bladder completely, up to 5 to 10 minutes for some patients. Instruct patients to keep the bowels regular. A rectum full of stool irritates the bladder, causing urgency and frequency.

Maintaining Adequate Fluid Intake. A simple method to promote normal micturition is maintaining optimal fluid intake. A patient with normal renal function and no health problems requiring fluid restriction (e.g., heart failure) needs up to 2300 mL of fluid in a 24-hour period. Adequate fluid intake helps flush out solutes or particles that collect in the urinary system and decreases bladder irritability. Help patients increase their fluid intake by teaching the importance of adequate hydration, setting a schedule for drinking extra fluids, identifying fluid preferences, increasing high-fluid foods such as fruits, and encouraging frequent fluid intake in small volumes. Avoid or limit drinking beverages that contain caffeine (coffee, tea, chocolate drinks, soft drinks). Instruct patients to not limit fluids if experiencing incontinence. Concentrated urine often irritates the bladder and increases bladder symptoms. To prevent nocturia suggest that a patient avoid drinking fluids 2 hours before bedtime.

Promoting Complete Bladder Emptying. It is normal for a small volume of urine to remain in the bladder after micturition. When the bladder does not empty completely, and residual urine volumes are high, there is risk for incontinence and dangerous urinary retention. Excessive accumulation of urine in the bladder is painful for the patient; increases the risk for UTI; and can cause backward flow of urine into the ureters to the kidneys, causing kidney damage. Adequate bladder emptying depends on feeling an urge to urinate, contracting the bladder, and relaxing the urethral sphincter. Help patients into the normal position for voiding to promote relaxation and stimulate bladder contractions. Squatting is the normal anatomical position for female voiding. Women empty the bladder better when sitting on the toilet or bedside commode with the feet on the floor. If a female patient cannot use a toilet, position her on a bedpan (see Chapter 37). After bedpan use, help the patient perform perineal hygiene (see Chapter 31). A man voids more easily while standing. If the patient is unable to reach a toilet, have him stand at the bedside and void into a urinal (a plastic or metal receptacle for urine) (Fig. 36.6A). Always assess mobility status to determine if a male patient can stand safely, and implement safety measures such as having someone assist him if needed. If a patient is unable to stand at the bedside, help him use the urinal in bed. Some patients need help positioning the penis completely within the urinal and holding the urinal in place. Once the patient finishes voiding, carefully remove the urinal

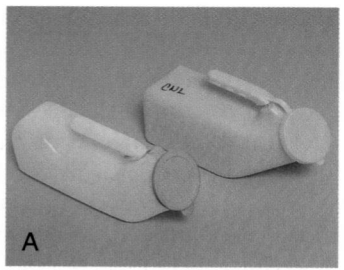

FIG 36.6 Types of male urinals **(A)** and female urinals **(B)**. (**B** courtesy Medegen Medical Products.)

and perform perineal hygiene (see Chapter 31). Most urinals are used by men, but some are specially designed for women (Fig. 36.6B). A female urinal has a larger opening at the top with a defined rim that helps position the urinal closely against the genitalia.

Educate your patients about ways to enhance their urinary health and improve bladder emptying (Box 36.6). To promote relaxation and stimulate bladder contractions, use sensory stimuli (e.g., turning on running water, putting a patient's hand in a pan of warm water, or stroking the female patient's inner thigh) and provide privacy. To improve bladder emptying, encourage patients to wait until the urine flow completely stops when voiding, and encourage them to attempt a second void (double voiding). Also encourage patients to attempt voiding according to the clock, not according to urge; this is called *timed voiding*. Do not implement the Credé method or manual compression of the bladder (i.e., placing the hands over the bladder and compressing it to assist in emptying) unless ordered by the health care provider. In the presence of a high postvoid residual or a complete inability of the bladder to empty, either intermittent or indwelling urinary catheterization is often required.

Preventing Infection. UTIs are one of the most common infections encountered in a primary care practice, accounting for 15% of antibiotic prescriptions that are ordered (Haddock, 2015). As a nurse, you play a key role in implementing evidenced-based practices to avoid this common and potentially dangerous infection. Some key interventions include promoting adequate fluid intake, perineal hygiene, and voiding at regular intervals. Encourage female patients to wipe from front to back after voiding and defecation; to avoid perfumed perineal washes and sprays, bubble baths, and tight clothing; to void before and after sexual intercourse; and to wear cotton underwear. If a patient has a problem with urine leakage, stress the importance of hygiene. Patients who use containment products need to use products that are designed for urine and wick wetness away from the body. Teach patients to avoid prolonged periods of urine wetness to prevent skin breakdown.

Acute Care. Patients with acute illness, surgery, or impaired urinary tract function usually require interventions that support urinary elimination.

BOX 36.6 PATIENT TEACHING

Urinary Retention Care

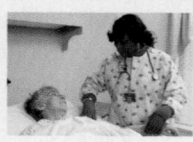

Mrs. Vallero is concerned about regaining her urinary function. Carly develops the following teaching plan.

OUTCOME
At the end of the teaching session, Mrs. Vallero will describe approaches to promote normal urinary elimination habits.

TEACHING STRATEGIES
- Establish rapport with Mrs. Vallero.
- Assess what Mrs. Vallero already knows about good practices for urinary health.
- Use the correct terms for parts of the anatomy while explaining their function.
- Provide appropriate visual diagrams and written materials.
- Instruct Mrs. Vallero how to monitor her own urinary output.
- Instruct about adequate fluid intake, incorporating fluid preferences.
- Describe the importance and technique of timed and double voiding.
- Reinforce correct perineal hygiene measures to reduce the risk for UTI.
- Provide Mrs. Vallero with pertinent signs and symptoms of UTI to report to her health care provider.

EVALUATION STRATEGIES
- Use the principles of teach-back to evaluate patient/family caregiver learning:
  - "I want to be sure you understand what we just discussed. Please describe strategies you can use at home to promote normal urination."
  - "Tell me how you will monitor your own urinary output."
  - "Describe the signs and symptoms of a UTI that you should report to your health care provider."

Catheterization. Urinary catheterization is the placement of a tube through the urethra into the bladder to drain urine. Because of the risk of CAUTIs the ANA developed an evidenced-based tool, the *ANA CAUTI Prevention Tool,* to guide the health care team with decision making regarding indwelling catheter insertion and care, maintenance of sterile technique, and best practices for timely catheter removal (Panchisin, 2016). Skill 36.1 lists steps for performing female and male urethral catheterization.

Patients can have urinary catheterization for short-term (up to 7 days), medium-term (up to 28 days) or long-term periods (up to a maximum of 12 weeks) (Yates, 2016). Conditions that require urinary catheter insertion include the need for accurate monitoring of urine output during some surgical procedures, critical illness, acute urinary retention, bladder outlet obstruction, and prolonged immobilization from spinal or multiple traumatic injuries. Catheterization should not be used routinely in surgical patients or in patients in nursing homes with incontinence (Gould et al., 2017). Indwelling catheters are also used for promotion of wound healing in sacral or perineal wounds and as a comfort measure in end-of-life care (Panchisin, 2016). Intermittent catheterization is used to measure postvoid residual when a bladder scanner is not available or as a way to manage chronic urinary retention.

Types of Catheters. Urinary catheters differ based on the number of catheter lumens. Some have balloons to keep the indwelling catheter in place, and some have a closed drainage system. Urinary catheters are made with one to three lumens (Fig. 36.7). You use single-lumen catheters (see Fig. 36.7A) for intermittent/straight catheterization (i.e., insertion of a catheter for one-time bladder emptying). Double-lumen catheters, designed for indwelling catheters, provide one lumen for urinary drainage and a second lumen that is used to inflate a balloon that keeps the catheter in place (see Fig. 36.7B). Use triple-lumen catheters (see Fig. 36.7C) for continuous bladder irrigation or when it is necessary to instill medications into a patient's bladder. One lumen drains the bladder, a second lumen inflates the balloon, and a third lumen delivers irrigation fluid into the bladder.

A health care provider chooses a catheter on the basis of factors such as latex allergy, history of catheter encrustation, and susceptibility to infection. Indwelling catheters are made of latex or silicone. Latex catheters with a special coating such as polytetrafluoroethylene reduce urethral irritation (Yates, 2016). All silicone catheters have a larger internal diameter

and are often helpful for patients who require frequent catheter changes because of encrustation. Antimicrobial catheters are coated with silver or an antibiotic. Current evidence shows silver-coated catheters may reduce the incidence of CAUTI for short-term use (Yates, 2016). Intermittent/straight catheters are made of rubber (softer and more flexible) or polyvinyl chloride. Patients who self-catheterize have a large selection of catheters, some with special coatings that do not require lubrication and others that are self-contained systems consisting of a prelubricated catheter and packaged with a preconnected drainage bag.

Catheter Sizes. The size of a urinary catheter is based on the French (Fr) scale, which reflects the internal diameter of the catheter. Use the smallest indwelling catheter size possible, 10 to 12 Fr for women and 12 to 14 Fr for men, to minimize trauma and risk for infection (Bardsley, 2015). Use of larger catheter diameters increases the risk for urethral trauma and bypassing, when the urine leaks between the urethral mucosa and the shaft of the catheter (Yates, 2016). Larger sizes may be used under special circumstances such as following urological surgery or in the presence of gross hematuria. Use smaller sizes for children: 5 to 6 Fr for infants, 8 to 10 Fr for children, and 10 to 12 Fr for adolescent girls.

Indwelling catheters come in balloon sizes ranging from 3 mL (for a child) to 30 mL for continuous bladder irrigation. The size of the balloon is usually printed on the catheter port (Fig. 36.8). The recommended balloon size for an adult is a 10-mL balloon (the balloon is 5 mL and requires 10 mL to fill completely) (Yates, 2016). Long-term use of larger balloons

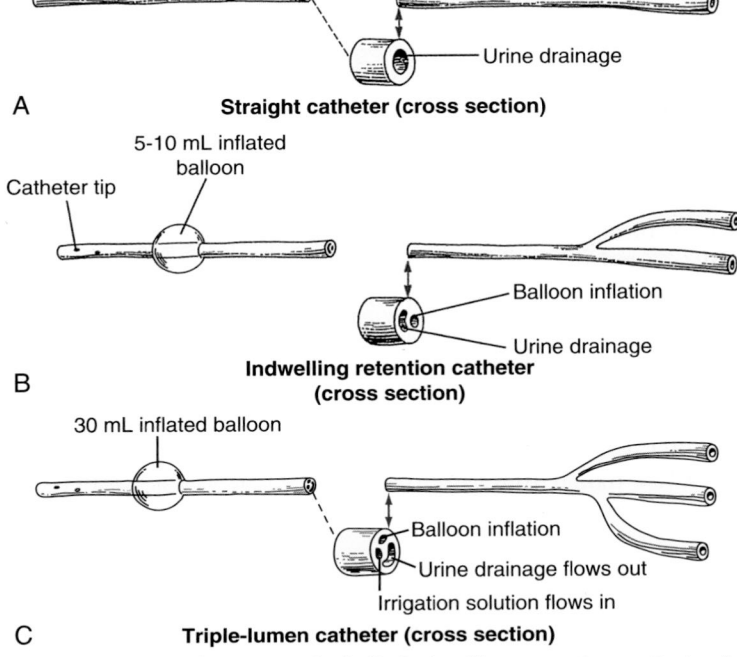

FIG 36.7 A, Straight catheter (cross section). **B,** Indwelling retention catheter (cross section). **C,** Triple-lumen catheter (cross section).

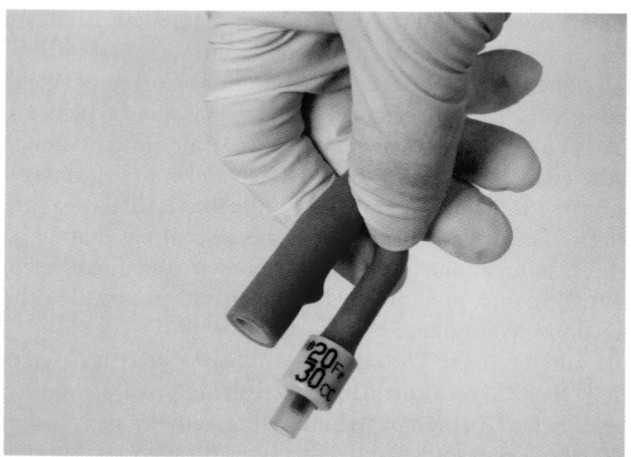

FIG 36.8 Size of catheter and balloon printed on catheter.

(30 mL) is associated with increased patient discomfort, irritation and trauma, increased risk of catheter expulsion, and incomplete emptying of the bladder because of urine that pools below the level of the catheter drainage eyes.

Catheter Changes. Use clinical indicators such as obstruction, prior treatment of a symptomatic infection, malfunction of the catheter, or compromise of the closed system to determine when to change long-term indwelling catheters and drainage bags (Gesmundo, 2016). In many cases you need to change catheters every 4 to 6 weeks. Change long-term catheters if they leak or become blocked and before obtaining a sterile specimen for urine culture. Avoid use of long-term catheterization because of the increased risk of CAUTI. Make every attempt to remove catheters as soon as a patient can void. See Boxes 36.7 and 36.8 for evidence-based nursing interventions to prevent CAUTI.

Closed Drainage Systems. An indwelling catheter is attached to a closed-system drainage bag to collect the continuous flow of urine. Do not separate the drainage system unless absolutely necessary to avoid introducing pathogens (Fig. 36.9). Always hang the bag below the level of the bladder on the bedframe or a chair so that urine drains down, out of the bladder. Do *not* let the bag touch the floor or secure it on a side rail. When a patient ambulates, carry the bag below the level of the patient's bladder. The only exception to this rule is when a patient has a catheter that is attached to a specially designed drainage bag (belly bag) worn across the abdomen. This system has a one-way valve to prevent the back flow of urine into the bladder. To keep the drainage system patent, check for kinks or bends in the tubing, avoid positioning the patient on the drainage tubing, prevent tubing from becoming dependent, and observe for clots or sediment that can cause blockage.

Routine Catheter Care. Patients with indwelling catheters require regular perineal hygiene (see Chapter 31), especially after bowel movements, to reduce the risk for CAUTI (Yates, 2016). In many institutions patients receive catheter care every 8 to 12 hours as the minimal standard of care.

BOX 36.7 PREVENTING CATHETER-ASSOCIATED URINARY TRACT INFECTIONS

- Use aseptic technique with sterile equipment when inserting urinary catheters into patients in an acute care setting.
- Secure indwelling catheters to prevent movement and pulling on the catheter.
- Maintain a closed urinary drainage system.
- Maintain an unobstructed flow of urine through the catheter, drainage tubing, and drainage bag.
- Keep the urinary drainage bag below the level of the bladder at all times.
- Avoid dependent loops in urinary drainage tubing.
- Prevent the urinary drainage bag from touching or dragging on the floor.
- When emptying the urinary drainage bag, use a separate measuring receptacle for each patient. Do not let the drainage spigot touch the receptacle.
- Before transfers or activity, drain all urine from tubing into bag and empty drainage bag.
- Empty the drainage bag when half full.
- Perform routine perineal hygiene daily and after soiling.
- Obtain urine samples using the sampling port. Cleanse the port with disinfectant. Use a sterile syringe/cannula.
- Ensure quality improvement programs alert providers when a patient has a catheter and include regular educational programming about catheter care.

Data from Centers for Disease Control and Prevention: *Guideline for prevention of catheter-associated urinary tract infections,* 2009, http://www.cdc.gov/hicpac/pdf/CAUTI/CAUTIguideline2009final.pdf.

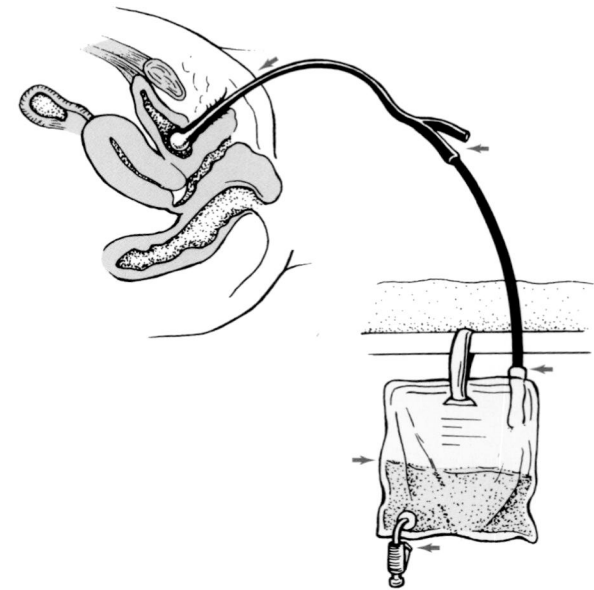

FIG 36.9 Potential sites *(arrows)* for introduction of infection.

Provide catheter care during perineal hygiene. You cleanse the catheter with the labia of a female patient separated or the foreskin of a male patient retracted so you can visualize the urethral meatus. Note any discharge, odor, or inflammation. Grasp the catheter with two fingers to prevent

BOX 36.8 EVIDENCE-BASED PRACTICE

PICOT Question: Does the implementation of evidence-based nursing protocols decrease the occurrence of catheter-associated urinary tract infections (CAUTIs) in hospitalized patients with indwelling urinary catheters?

SUMMARY OF EVIDENCE

CAUTIs account for nearly 40% or more of infections in acute care settings and increase length of hospital stay, morbidity, mortality, and costs (Quinn, 2015; Galiczewski, 2016). The *Guideline for Prevention of Catheter-Associated Urinary Tract Infections* from the Centers for Disease Control and Prevention (CDC, 2009) organizes evidence-based measures to reduce CAUTI into major areas that include appropriate use, proper insertion and maintenance techniques, quality improvement programs, and ongoing surveillance for CAUTIs and related causative factors (Andrade et al., 2016; Panchisin, 2016). A multiprotocol approach including detailed criteria for placement of a urinary catheter, daily assessment of catheter necessity, and a stop order to prevent use beyond medically necessary or early discontinuance within 7 days of insertion was successful in decreasing CAUTI rates (Galiczewski, 2016). Current evidence supports the effectiveness of nurse-driven protocols in reducing unnecessary catheter insertion, the duration of catheter use, and the incidence of CAUTI (Andrade et al., 2016; Quinn, 2015).

APPLICATION TO NURSING PRACTICE

- Become familiar with guidelines related to CAUTI prevention and care (Agency for Healthcare Research and Quality [AHRQ], 2015).
- Be aware of indications for catheter insertion, and advocate for a patient if the indications do not meet accepted guidelines (Bardsley, 2015).
- Collaborate with health care providers to remove catheters as early as possible when medical indications no longer exist (Dy et al., 2016).
- Develop nurse-driven protocols for CAUTI prevention (Andrade et al., 2016; Dy et al., 2016).

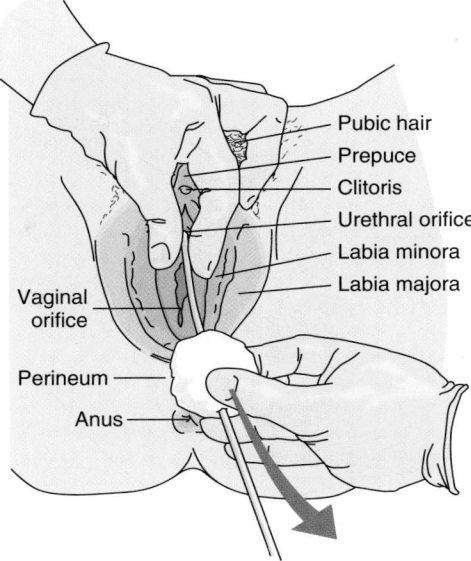

FIG 36.10 Cleansing the catheter during catheter care. (From Sorrentino SA, Remmert LA: *Mosby's textbook for nursing assistants,* ed 8, St Louis, 2012, Mosby.)

Labels: Pubic hair, Prepuce, Clitoris, Urethral orifice, Labia minora, Labia majora, Vaginal orifice, Perineum, Anus

steps to remove a catheter. Monitor a patient's voiding and urine output after catheter removal by using a voiding record, bladder diary, or I&O documentation. A bladder diary records the time and amount of each voiding including any incontinence. Use a bladder scan when needed to monitor bladder functioning and measure postvoid residual (see Box 36.5). Abdominal pain and distention, a sensation of incomplete emptying, incontinence, constant dribbling of urine, and voiding in very small amounts indicate possible inadequate bladder emptying, which requires intervention.

The risk of UTI increases with the use of an indwelling catheter (Carter et al., 2014). Symptoms of infection can develop 2 or 3 or more days after catheter removal. Patients need to be informed of the risk for infection, prevention measures, and signs and symptoms that need to be reported to a nurse and health care provider.

unnecessary traction. Using a clean washcloth, soap, and water, or a CHG bathing cloth, start cleansing the catheter close to the urinary meatus and move outward approximately 10 cm (4 inches) in a circular motion to remove any secretions that adhere to the catheter (Fig. 36.10). Remove all traces of soap and replace the foreskin if pulled back. Replace the catheter securement device as necessary (see Skill 36.1). Empty the drainage bag when it is three-quarters full, and record output. An overfull drainage bag creates tension and pulls on the catheter, resulting in trauma to the urethra and/or urinary meatus (Yates, 2016). See Boxes 36.7 and 36.8 for evidence-based nursing interventions to prevent CAUTI.

Catheter Removal. The Centers for Medicare and Medicaid Services (CMS) identified CAUTI as a never event (Galiczewski, 2016). Removing an indwelling catheter promptly after it is no longer needed is a key intervention that decreases the incidence and prevalence of CAUTI. See Skill 36.1 for the

QSEN QSEN ACTIVITY *Quality Improvement*

The patient care unit is evaluating a quality improvement (QI) project focused on reducing catheter-associated urinary tract infections (CAUTIs) (a never event). Urinary tract infections (UTIs) are common health care–associated infections (HAIs). A high percentage of HAI UTIs are caused by urinary catheterization, resulting in longer hospital stays, increased costs, and increased mortality.

- Which nursing care interventions would Carly, the nursing student, expect to find on the QI tool, and which data would indicate that the QI project was successful?

evolve Answers to QSEN Activities can be found on the Evolve website.

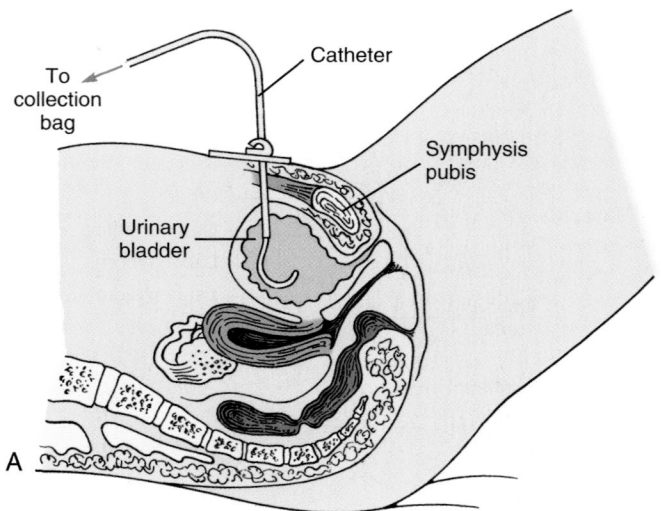

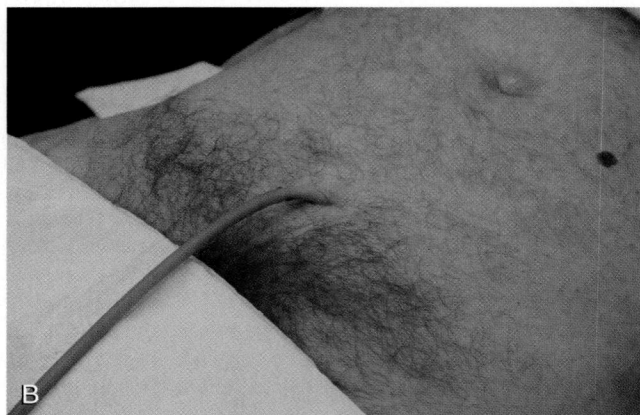

FIG 36.11 A, Placement of suprapubic catheter above the symphysis pubis. **B,** Suprapubic catheter without a dressing.

Suprapubic Catheters. A suprapubic catheter is a urinary drainage tube inserted surgically into the bladder through the abdominal wall above the symphysis pubis (Fig. 36.11). The catheter is sutured to the skin, secured with an adhesive material, or retained in the bladder with a fluid-filled balloon similar to an indwelling catheter.

Suprapubic catheters are placed when there is blockage of the urethra (e.g., enlarged prostate, urethral stricture, after urological surgery) and in situations when a long-term urethral catheter causes irritation or discomfort or interferes with sexual functioning. Because of the abdominal pressure on the catheter, the suprapubic catheter is usually size 16 Fr or larger (Yates, 2016).

Care of a suprapubic catheter involves daily cleansing of the insertion site and catheter. The same care for the tubing and drainage bag of a urethral catheter applies for a suprapubic catheter. Assess the insertion site for signs of inflammation and growth of overgranulation tissue. If insertion is new, expect slight inflammation as part of normal wound healing; however, monitor the site carefully because inflammation also indicates infection. Overgranulation tissue can develop at the insertion site as a reaction to the catheter. In some instances, intervention is needed. Site care follows principles of applying a dry dressing (see Chapter 38), and institutional policy indicates if aseptic or sterile technique is required.

Condom Catheters. An external catheter, also called a condom catheter, *penile sheath,* or *Texas catheter,* is a soft, pliable condomlike sheath that fits over the penis, providing a safe and noninvasive way to contain urine. Most external catheters are made of soft silicone that aids in reducing friction. They are clear to allow for easy visualization of skin under the catheter. Latex catheters are used by some patients. Verify that a patient does not have a latex allergy before applying this

type of catheter. Condom-type external catheters are held in place by either an adhesive coating of the internal lining of the sheath, a double-sided self-adhesive strip, brush-on adhesive applied to the penile shaft, or (in rare cases) an external strap. They may be attached to a small-volume (leg) drainage bag or a large-volume (bedside) urinary drainage bag, both of which need to be kept lower than the level of the bladder. A condom-type external catheter is suitable for patients who are incontinent and have complete and spontaneous bladder emptying. Condom catheters come in a variety of styles and sizes. Refer to manufacturer guidelines to ensure the best fit and correct application. See Box 36.9 for the steps in applying a condom catheter. Condom catheters are associated with less risk for UTI than indwelling catheters; thus they are an excellent option for a male patient with UI (Smart, 2014). Other externally applied catheters are available for men who cannot be fitted for a condom catheter. One type attaches to the glans penis using hydrocolloid strips that stay in place for multiple days and allows intermittent/straight catheterization (Woodward, 2015b). Another option available is a reusable condomlike device that is held in place by specially designed underwear.

Urinary Diversions. Immediately after surgery a patient with an incontinent urinary diversion wears a pouch to collect the urine (drainage). The pouch keeps the patient clean and dry, protects the skin from damage, and provides a barrier against odor. Urinary pouches with an antireflux flap are opaque or clear, drainable one-piece or two-piece pouches with cut-to-fit or precut wafers. Change the pouch every 5 to 7 days (National Institute of Diabetes and Digestive and Kidney Diseases [NIDDK], 2013). You can connect pouches to a bedside drainage bag for use at night.

When changing a pouch, gently cleanse the skin surrounding the stoma with warm tap water using a clean washcloth

BOX 36.9 PROCEDURAL GUIDELINES

Applying a Condom Catheter

DELEGATION CONSIDERATIONS

Assessment of the skin of a patient's penile shaft and determination of a latex allergy are done by a nurse before catheter application. The skill of applying a condom catheter can be delegated to nursing assistive personnel (NAP). The nurse directs the NAP to:

- Follow manufacturer directions for applying the condom catheter and securing device.
- Monitor intake and output (I&O) and record if applicable.
- Immediately report any redness, swelling, or skin irritation or breakdown of glans penis or penile shaft.

EQUIPMENT

Condom catheter kit (condom sheath of appropriate size, securement device [internal adhesive or strap], skin preparation solution [per manufacturer directions]); urinary collection bag with drainage tubing or leg bag and straps; basin with warm water and soap; towels and washcloths; bath blanket; clean gloves; scissors, hair guard, or paper towel

STEPS

1. Identify patient using at least two identifiers (e.g., name and birthday or name and medical record number) according to agency policy.
2. Review medical record and assess urinary pattern, ability to empty bladder effectively, and presence of urinary continence.
3. Assess patient's mental status, knowledge of purpose of using condom-type catheter, and ability to apply device. Include family caregivers as appropriate.
4. Review medical record for history of allergy to rubber or latex. Check patient's allergy wristband.
5. Perform hand hygiene. Provide privacy by closing room door and bedside curtain.
6. Raise bed to appropriate working height. Lower side rail on working side.
7. Apply gloves. Verify patient's size and type of condom catheter, or use manufacturer measuring guide. Prepare condom catheter, urinary drainage collection bag, and tubing (large-volume drainage bag or leg bag). Clamp off drainage bag port. Place nearby ready to attach to condom after applied.
8. Help patient into supine position or sitting position. Place bath blanket over upper torso. Fold sheets so that only penis is exposed.

9. Provide perineal care. Dry thoroughly before applying device. In uncircumcised patient ensure that foreskin has been replaced to normal position before applying condom catheter. Do not apply barrier cream.
10. Assess skin of penis for rashes, erythema, or open areas. (This may be deferred until just before catheter application.)
11. Clip hair at base of penis if necessary before application of condom sheath. If hair guard is available, place over penis before applying device. Remove hair guard after applying catheter. An alternative to a hair guard is to tear a hole in a paper towel, place it over penis, and remove after application of device (Woodward, 2015b).
12. Apply condom catheter. With nondominant hand grasp penis along shaft. With dominant hand, hold rolled condom sheath at tip of penis with head of penis in the cone. Smoothly roll sheath onto penis. Allow 2.5 to 5 cm (1 to 2 inches) of space between tip of glans penis and end of condom catheter (see illustration).
13. Apply appropriate securement device as indicated in manufacturer guidelines.
    a. Self-adhesive condom catheters: After application apply gentle pressure on penile shaft for 10 to 15 seconds to secure catheter.
    b. Outer securing strip–type condom catheters: Spiral wrap penile shaft with strip of supplied elastic adhesive. Strip should not overlap itself. Elastic strip should be snug, not tight (see illustration). **Caution:** Never use tape.
14. Remove hair guard if used. Connect drainage tubing to end of condom catheter. Be sure that condom is not twisted. If using large drainage bag, place excess tubing on bed and secure to bottom sheet.
15. Help patient to safe, comfortable position. Lower bed and place side rails accordingly.
16. Dispose of contaminated supplies, and remove and dispose of gloves. Perform hand hygiene.
17. Remove and reapply daily unless an extended-wear device is used. To remove condom, wash penis with warm, soapy water and gently roll sheath and adhesive off penile shaft.
18. **Use Teach-Back:** "We talked about what you need to do to prevent the drainage tube from blocking urine flow. Please tell me what you need to do."

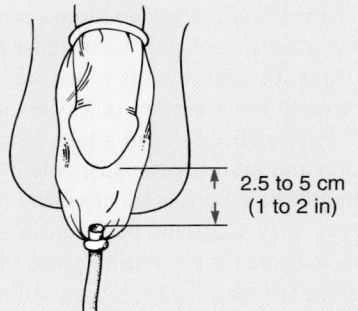

2.5 to 5 cm
(1 to 2 in)

STEP 12 Condom catheter.

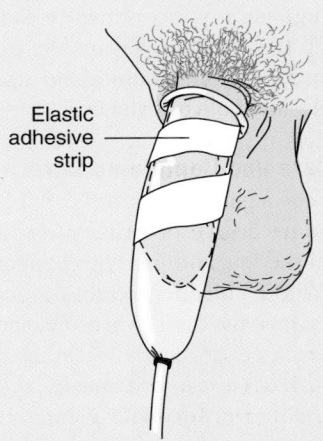

Elastic adhesive strip

STEP 13b Spiral application of adhesive strip.

and pat dry (Schreiber, 2016). Observe the appearance of the stoma and surrounding skin. The stoma is normally red and moist and is located in the right lower quadrant of the abdomen. Measure the stoma and cut the opening in the pouch. Remove the protective backing from the adhesive surface, and apply the pouch. Press firmly into place over the stoma. It is important for the patient to have the correct type and fit of an ostomy pouch. A specialty ostomy nurse is an essential resource when selecting the right appliance so that the pouch fits snugly against the surface of the skin around the stoma, preventing damaging leakage of urine (see Chapter 38).

Patients with continent urinary diversions do not wear external pouches. You or a nurse specialist will teach a patient how to intermittently catheterize the stoma. Patients need to catheterize 4 to 6 times a day for the rest of their lives. After creation of an orthotopic neobladder, patients have frequent episodes of incontinence until the neobladder slowly stretches and the urinary sphincter is strong enough to contain the urine (Leaver, 2016). The postoperative care of patients with continent urinary diversions varies widely with the surgical techniques used. Learn the surgeon's preferred routine and health care agency procedures before caring for these patients.

Medications. Some medications effectively treat urgency UI. The most commonly used are called *antimuscarinics* or *anticholinergics*. Oxybutynin (immediate release [IR]), tolterodine (IR), and darifenacin (modified release) are recommended as the first choice for treatment (Bardsley, 2016). The most common adverse effects of the antimuscarinics are dry mouth, constipation, and blurred vision. Current research finds use of 4 mg or 8 mg of fesoterodine improves urgency incontinence with very few cognitive changes (Wagg et al., 2015). Mirabegron, a beta-3-adrenoceptor agonist, is a newer agent that does not have the same adverse effects as the antimuscarinics but causes a small increase in blood pressure and heart rate in some patients (Rigby, 2015). Familiarize yourself with all the medications your patients take so that you can quickly identify potential side effects.

When caring for a patient starting an antimuscarinic, monitor the patient for a decrease in UI symptoms such as urgency, frequency, and urgency. A bladder diary that records the time of voiding and any incontinent episodes is one of the best ways to do this. Regularly assess the patient for side effects including constipation, straining during bowel movements, and changes in stool consistency.

Restorative Care and Continuing Care. Certain interventions can improve a patient's control over bladder emptying and restore some degree of urinary continence. These include behavioral therapy and lifestyle changes, pelvic floor muscle training (PFMT), bladder retraining, and a variety of toileting schedules. In some cases, when the bladder does not empty, patients or caregivers learn to catheterize intermittently. Whenever there is a risk for urine leakage, skin care is essential in the plan of care. Adequate urine containment and skin protection promote patient comfort and dignity.

Lifestyle Changes. Teach patients a number of lifestyle modifications to improve bladder function and decrease incontinence. In addition to health promotion interventions discussed earlier in this chapter, teach patients about foods and fluids that cause bladder irritation and increase symptoms of frequency, urgency, and incontinence. Teach patients to balance fluid intake throughout the day and to avoid caffeine, alcohol, and smoking tobacco to reduce symptoms of urinary leakage and bladder irritation (Testa, 2015). Constipation also frequently affects bladder symptoms; implement measures to promote bowel regularity (see Chapter 37). Encourage patients with obesity to lose weight and patients with edema to elevate their feet for a few hours in the afternoon to help reduce nighttime voiding frequency.

Pelvic Floor Muscle Training. Evidence supports that patients with urgency, stress, and mixed UI experience improvement and can eventually achieve continence when treated with PFMT. Teach patients who use PFMT how to identify and contract the pelvic floor muscles in a structured exercise program using Kegel exercises (Testa, 2015). The exercises work by increasing the pressure in the urethra, strengthening the pelvic floor muscles, and inhibiting unwanted bladder contractions. Many patients benefit from verbal instructions on how to do the exercises (Box 36.10).

Bladder Retraining. Bladder retraining is a behavioral therapy designed to help patients control bothersome urinary urgency and frequency. Patients learn about their bladder and techniques to suppress urgency. They collaborate with their health care providers to develop a toileting schedule based on their bladder diary. The toileting schedule slowly increases the interval between voiding. Patients need regular support and positive reinforcement during the retraining period. One technique called bladder inhibition helps patients inhibit the urge to void by taking slow, deep breaths to relax and then performing five or six quick strong pelvic muscle exercises (flicks) in quick succession to inhibit detrusor contraction (Testa, 2015). Only highly motivated and cognitively intact patients are candidates for this therapy. Support patients by reinforcing their schedule and providing emotional encouragement.

Toileting Schedules. A key component of any treatment plan for UI is regular toilet access. Individualize toileting schedules based on a patient's type of incontinence and functional disability (e.g., cognitive impairment). You can implement toileting schedules in any care setting. They are your first plan of action when you determine a patient is incontinent. Timed voiding or scheduled toileting is toileting based on a fixed schedule; it is not based on a patient's urge to void. You set the schedule based on a time interval (i.e., every 2 to 3 hours) or times of day such as before and after meals. It is very successful in adults with moderate-to-severe cognition and mobility impairments. Habit training is a toileting schedule based on a patient's usual voiding pattern. The usual times that a patient voids are identified from a bladder diary. The patient is toileted at these times. Prompted voiding is a program of toileting designed for patients with mild or moderate cognitive impairment. Caregivers ask the

BOX 36.10 PATIENT TEACHING

Pelvic Muscle (Kegel) Exercises

OUTCOME

At the end of the teaching session the patient will describe and demonstrate how to perform pelvic muscle (Kegel) exercises.

TEACHING STRATEGIES

- Use pictures to teach patient pelvic anatomy and the location of the pelvic muscles.
- Teach patient to identify and contract the correct muscle.
  - Women: Instruct the patient to squeeze the anus as if to hold in gas or to insert a finger into the vagina and feel the muscle squeeze around her finger.
  - Men: Instruct the patient to stand in front of a mirror, squeeze the anus as if to hold in gas, and watch to see if the penis moves up and down as he contracts the pelvic floor muscles.
  - Tell the patient to avoid contracting the abdomen, buttocks, or thighs when contracting the pelvic muscles.
- Teach pelvic muscle contraction exercises.
  - Quick flicks: Squeeze the muscle for 2 to 3 seconds and relax.
  - Sustained contractions: Squeeze the muscle for 5 to 10 seconds and relax after each contraction for 10 seconds.
- Teach patient to maintain a daily exercise schedule.
  - Perform 3 to 5 quick flicks followed by 5 to 10 sustained contractions.
  - Repeat these exercises 3 to 4 times a day.

EVALUATION STRATEGIES

- Use the principles of teach-back to evaluate patient/family caregiver learning:
  - "Tell me how you will perform pelvic muscle exercises."
  - "Describe your plan for exercise for the next week."

BOX 36.11 EVALUATION

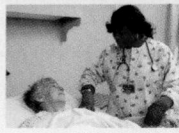 Carly talks with Mrs. Vallero the next evening. The patient's care plan incorporates timed voiding, oral fluids, and use of double voiding. She palpates Mrs. Vallero's bladder and then assists her to the toilet. After being sure that Mrs. Vallero is comfortable and leaving the nurse call system in place, Carly instructs her to double void. She returns to measure Mrs. Vallero's urinary output and evaluates for bladder residual using ultrasound bladder scan.

DOCUMENTATION NOTE

"Reports sensation of bladder fullness. Abdomen soft, sensation of bladder fullness over suprapubic area on light palpation. Assisted to bathroom. Gait slightly unsteady and slow. Breathing easy and regular. Double voiding technique reinforced. Voided 400 mL of clear, pale yellow urine. Stated, 'I don't feel so full now.' Returned to bed with nurse call system in reach. Postvoid residual volume 10 mL using portable ultrasound."

---

patient if he or she is wet or dry, give positive feedback for dryness, prompt the patient to toilet, and reward the patient for desired behavior. Although very successful, this toileting program often requires prompting by a consistent and motivated caregiver (Testa, 2015).

Intermittent Catheterization. Some patients experience chronic inability to completely empty the bladder because of neuromuscular damage related to multiple sclerosis, diabetes, spinal cord injury, and urinary retention. To minimize the risk of UTI, teach patients or family caregivers to catheterize the bladder using clean technique. In institutions where there is increased risk for exposure to multiple pathogens, intermittent catheterization follows the principles of sterile asepsis as discussed earlier in the chapter. Teach patients and family caregivers the importance of adequate fluid intake, signs of infection, and about their individualized catheterization schedule. The goal for intermittent catheterization is drainage of 400 mL of urine every 2 to 3 hours while awake. Individualize the schedule to meet this goal.

Skin Care. Incontinence-associated dermatitis (IAD) occurs in patients with urinary or fecal incontinence and manifests as reddened skin inflammation. Patients with extreme IAD often experience swelling and blisters (Voegeli, 2016). IAD is caused when urine irritates the skin as a result of skin overhydration and increased skin pH as a result of the higher alkaline in urine (Voegeli, 2016). Exposure to stool and urine increases the risk for skin injury. Key components for IAD prevention and treatment include gentle skin cleansing with a no-rinse pH balanced cleanser, skin moisturization, and application of a moisture barrier protectant (Beeckman et al., 2015). In some cases, patients develop a topical fungal infection that requires treatment with a steroid/antifungal cream or ointment. Patients often state they have intense itchiness in the perineal area. The problem is intensified in infants or adults who wear absorbent products to absorb urine.

■■■ EVALUATION

Patient Outcomes. To evaluate your patient's care plan, use the expected outcomes developed during planning to determine whether interventions were effective (Box 36.11). This evaluation process is dynamic. Use information gathered to modify the plan of care to meet expected outcomes. Evaluate for changes in a patient's voiding pattern and/or presence of symptoms such as dysuria, urinary retention, and UI. If a behavioral plan is in effect, evaluate patient/family caregiver compliance with the plan such as toileting according to the schedule or the number of incontinent episodes. Reinforce patient education, and explore potential barriers when your patient has difficulty following a behavioral plan.

Patient Expectations. Because patients are the best source for evaluation of outcomes and responses to nursing care, be sure to include your patients during evaluation. Encourage patients to express in their own words if their preferences and needs were met. Make revisions based on their feedback. Remember that urinary problems affect a patient physically, emotionally, psychologically, spiritually, and socially. You need to continually evaluate a patient's self-image, social interactions, sexuality, and emotional status throughout the duration of care.

SAFETY GUIDELINES FOR NURSING SKILLS

Ensuring patient safety is an essential role of the professional nurse. To ensure patient safety, communicate clearly with members of the health care team, assess and incorporate the patient's priorities of care and preferences, and use the best evidence when making decisions about your patient's care. When performing the skills in this chapter, remember the following points to ensure safe, individualized care:

- Follow principles of medical and surgical asepsis when performing catheterizations, helping patient with toileting needs, and handling urine specimens.
- Identify patients at risk for latex allergies.
- Identify patients with allergies to povidone-iodine (Betadine). Provide alternatives such as chlorhexidine.

SKILL 36.1   INSERTING AND REMOVING STRAIGHT/INTERMITTENT OR INDWELLING CATHETERS

DELEGATION CONSIDERATIONS
The skill of inserting a straight or indwelling urinary catheter cannot be delegated to nursing assistive personnel (NAP). The nurse directs the NAP to:
- Assist the nurse with patient positioning, focus lighting for the procedure, maintain privacy, empty urine from collection bag, and provide perineal care.
- Report postprocedure patient discomfort or fever to the nurse.
- Report abnormal color, odor, amount of urine in drainage bag, and if the catheter is leaking or causes pain.

EQUIPMENT
- Catheter kit containing sterile items (**Note:** Catheter kits vary)
  - Straight catheterization kit: single-lumen catheter, drapes (one fenestrated—has an opening in the center), sterile gloves, lubricant, cleansing solution incorporated in an applicator or to be added to cotton balls, and specimen container
  - Indwelling catheterization kit: drapes (one fenestrated—has an opening in the center), sterile gloves, lubricant, antiseptic cleansing solution incorporated in an applicator or to be added to cotton balls, specimen container, and prefilled syringe with sterile water (to inflate balloon); some kits contain a catheter with attached drainage bag; others contain only a catheter; others have no catheter
- Sterile drainage tubing and bag (if not included in indwelling catheter insertion kit)
- Device to secure catheter (catheter strap or other device)
- Extra sterile and clean gloves and catheter (optional)
- Basin with warm water, washcloth, towel, and soap for perineal care
- Flashlight or other additional light source
- Bath blanket, waterproof absorbent pad
- Measuring container for urine

STEP	RATIONALE
ASSESSMENT	
1. Identify patient using at least two identifiers (e.g., name and birthday or name and medical record number) according to agency policy.	Ensures correct patient. Complies with The Joint Commission standards and improves patient safety (TJC, 2018).
2. Review patient's medical record including health care provider's order and nurses' notes. Note previous catheterization including catheter size, response of patient, and time of catheterization.	Identifies purpose of inserting catheter (e.g., for measurement of postvoid residual, preparation for surgery, or specimen collection) and potential difficulty with catheter insertion.
3. Review medical record for any pathological condition that may impair passage of catheter (e.g., enlarged prostate gland in men, urethral strictures).	Obstruction of urethra may prevent passage of catheter into bladder.
4. Ask patient and check health record for allergies.	Identifies allergy to antiseptic, tape, latex, and lubricant.

STEP	RATIONALE
5. Assess patient's weight, level of consciousness, developmental level, ability to cooperate, and mobility.	Determines positioning for catheterization; indicates how much assistance is needed to properly position patient, ability of patient to cooperate during procedure, and level of explanation needed.
6. Assess patient's gender and age.	Determines catheter size.
7. Perform hand hygiene and apply clean gloves. Assess for pain and bladder fullness. Palpate bladder over symphysis pubis or use bladder scanner (if available).	Palpation of full bladder causes pain and/or urge to void, indicating full or overfull bladder.
8. Inspect perineal region, observing for perineal anatomical landmarks, erythema, drainage or discharge, and odor. Remove gloves and perform hand hygiene.	Assessment of female perineal landmarks improves accuracy and speed of catheter insertion.
9. Assess patient's knowledge, health literacy, prior experience with catheterization, and feelings about procedure.	Reveals need for patient instruction and/or support.

PLANNING

1. Provide privacy by closing room door and bedside curtain.	Promotes comfort and protects patient confidentiality.
2. Check patient's plan of care for size and type of catheter (if this is a reinsertion). Use smallest-size catheter possible. Collect all required equipment.	Ensures that patient receives correct size and type of catheter. Larger catheter diameters increase risk for urethral trauma (Yates, 2016). Small catheter allows for adequate drainage of periurethral glands.
3. Explain procedure to patient or family caregiver and arrange for extra personnel to help as necessary.	Promotes cooperation and informs patient about what to expect. Some patients are unable to assume positioning independently for procedure.

IMPLEMENTATION

1. Perform hand hygiene.	Reduces transmission of microorganisms.
2. Raise bed to appropriate working height. If side rails in use, raise side rail on opposite side of bed and lower side rail on working side.	Promotes good body mechanics. Use of side rails in this manner promotes patient safety.
3. Place waterproof pad under patient.	Prevents soiling of bed linen.

Clinical Decision Point. Obtain assistance to position and support patients who are weak, frail, obese, or confused.

---

4. Position patient:	
a. Female patient:	
(1) Help to dorsal recumbent position (on back with knees flexed). Ask patient to relax thighs so you can rotate hips.	Exposes perineum and allows hip joints to be externally rotated.
(2) Alternative female position: Position side-lying (Sims') position with upper leg flexed at knee and hip. Support patient with pillows if necessary to maintain position.	Alternative position is more comfortable if patient cannot abduct leg at hip joint (e.g., patient has arthritic joints or contractures).
b. Male patient:	
(1) Position supine with legs extended and thighs slightly abducted.	Comfortable position for patient aids in visualization of penis.
5. Drape patient:	Protects patient dignity by avoiding unnecessary exposure of body parts.
a. Female patient:	
(1) Drape with bath blanket. Place blanket diamond fashion over patient, with one corner at patient's midsection, side corners over each thigh and abdomen, and last corner over perineum (see illustration).	Protects patient dignity by avoiding unnecessary exposure of body parts.

SKILL 36.1   INSERTING AND REMOVING STRAIGHT/INTERMITTENT OR INDWELLING CATHETERS—cont'd

STEP	RATIONALE
b. Male patient:	
(1) Drape patient by covering upper part of body with small sheet or towel; drape with separate sheet or bath blanket so that only perineum is exposed (see illustration).	Protects patient dignity by avoiding unnecessary exposure of body parts.
6. Apply clean gloves. Cleanse perineal area with soap and water, rinse, and dry. Use gloves to re-examine patient and identify urinary meatus. Remove and discard gloves. Perform hand hygiene.	Perineal hygiene removes secretions, urine, and feces that could contaminate sterile field and increase risk for catheter-associated urinary tract infection (CAUTI) (Yates, 2016).
7. Position light to illuminate genitals or have assistant available to hold light source to visualize urinary meatus.	Adequate visualization of urinary meatus helps with speed and accuracy of catheter insertion.
8. Open outer wrapping of catheterization kit. Place inner wrapped catheter kit tray on clean, accessible surface such as bedside table or, if possible, between patient's open legs. Patient size and positioning dictate exact placement.	Provides easy access to supplies during catheter insertion.
9. Open inner sterile wrap covering tray containing catheterization supplies using sterile technique. Fold back each flap of sterile covering one at a time, with last flap opened toward patient.	Sterile wrap serves as sterile field.
a. Indwelling catheterization open system: Open separate package containing drainage bag, check to make sure that clamp on drainage port is closed, and place drainage bag and tubing in easily accessible location. Open outer package of sterile catheter, maintaining sterility of inner wrapper.	Open drainage bag systems have separate sterile packaging for sterile catheter, drainage bag and tubing, and insertion kit.
b. Indwelling catheterization closed system: All supplies are in sterile tray and are arranged in sequence of use.	Closed drainage bag systems have catheter preattached to drainage tubing and bag.
c. Straight catheterization: All needed supplies are in sterile tray that contains supplies and can be used for urine collection.	
10. Put on sterile gloves. (*Option:* Apply sterile drape with ungloved hands when drape is packed as first item. Touch only edges of drape. Then apply sterile gloves.)	Maintains surgical asepsis.

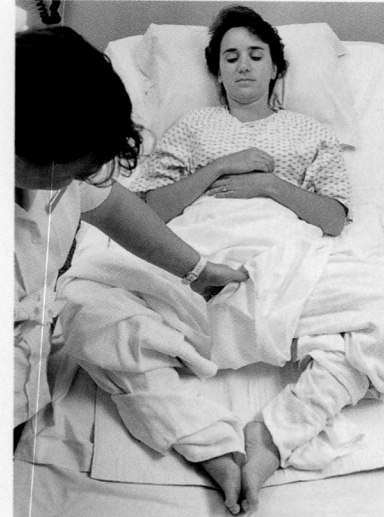

STEP 5a(1) Female patient draped and in dorsal recumbent position.

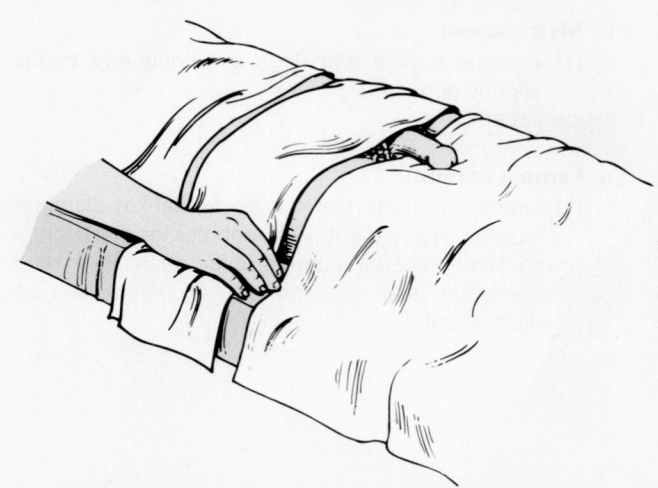

STEP 5b(1) Draping male patient with blankets.

STEP	RATIONALE
11. Drape perineum, keeping gloves and working surface of field sterile.	Sterile drapes provide sterile field over which you will work during catheterization.
a. Drape female patient:	
(1) Pick up square sterile drape touching only edges (2.5 cm [1 inch]).	When creating the cuff over sterile gloved hands, sterility of gloves and workspace is maintained.
(2) Allow drape to unfold without touching unsterile surfaces. Allow top edge of drape (2.5 to 5 cm [1 to 2 inches]) to form cuff over both hands.	
(3) Place drape with shiny side down on bed between patient's thighs. Slip cuffed edge just under buttocks as you ask patient to lift hips. Take care not to touch contaminated surfaces with sterile gloves.	
(4) Pick up fenestrated sterile drape out of tray. Allow drape to unfold without touching unsterile surfaces. Allow top edge of drape to form cuff over both hands. Apply drape over perineum, exposing labia (see illustration).	Opening in drape creates sterile field around labia.
b. Drape male patient:	
(1) Use of square drape is optional; you may apply fenestrated drape instead.	
(2) Pick up edges of square drape and allow to unfold without touching unsterile surfaces. Place over thighs, with shiny side down, just below penis.	
(3) Place fenestrated drape with opening centered over penis (see illustration).	
12. Move tray closer to patient. Arrange remaining supplies on sterile field, maintaining sterility of gloves. Place sterile tray with cleaning medium (premoistened swab sticks or cotton balls, forceps, and solution), lubricant, catheter, and prefilled syringe for inflating balloon (indwelling catheterization only) on sterile drape.	Provides easy access to supplies during catheter insertion and helps to maintain aseptic technique. Appropriate placement is determined by size of patient and position during catheterization.
a. If kit contains sterile cotton balls, open package of sterile antiseptic solution and pour over cotton balls. Some kits contain a package of premoistened swab sticks. Open end of package for easy access (see illustration).	Use of sterile supplies and antiseptic solution reduces risk of CAUTI (Galiczewski, 2016).

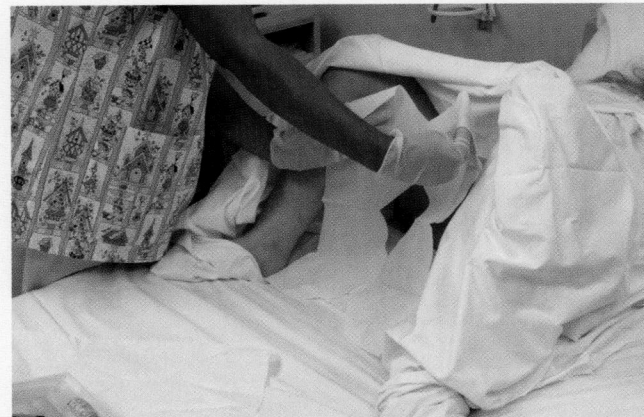

STEP 11a(4) Place sterile fenestrated drape (with opening in center) over perineum of female patient.

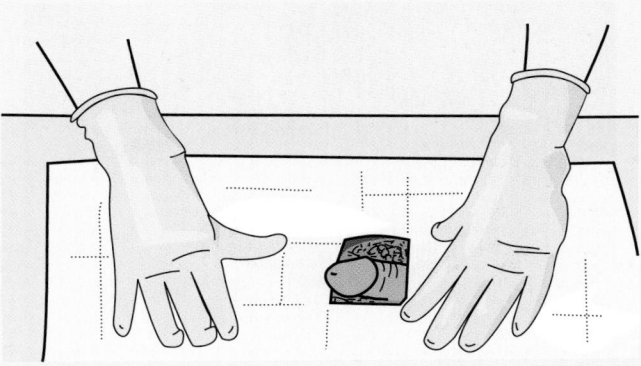

STEP 11b(3) Draping male patient with fenestrated drape.

SKILL 36.1 INSERTING AND REMOVING STRAIGHT/INTERMITTENT OR INDWELLING CATHETERS—cont'd

STEP	RATIONALE
b. Open sterile specimen container if specimen is to be obtained.	Makes container accessible to receive urine from catheter if specimen is needed.
c. For indwelling catheterization, open sterile wrapper of catheter and leave catheter on sterile field. If part of a closed system kit, remove tray with catheter and preattached drainage bag and place on sterile drape. Make sure that clamp on drainage port of bag is closed. If needed and if part of sterile tray, attach catheter to drainage tubing.	Indwelling catheterization trays vary. Some have preattached catheters; others need to be attached but are part of the sterile tray; others do not have catheter or drainage system as part of tray.
d. Open packet of lubricant and squeeze out on sterile field. Lubricate catheter tip by dipping it into water-soluble gel 2.5 to 5 cm (1 to 2 inches) for women and 12.5 to 17.5 cm (5 to 7 inches) for men (see illustration).	Lubrication minimizes trauma to urethra and discomfort during catheter insertion. Male catheter needs enough lubricant to cover length of catheter inserted.

Clinical Decision Point. Pretesting a balloon on an indwelling catheter by injecting fluid from the prefilled sterile water syringe into the balloon port is no longer recommended. Testing the balloon may distort and stretch it and lead to damage, causing increased trauma on insertion.

13. Clean urethral meatus:

a. Female patient:

(1) Separate labia with fingers of nondominant hand (now contaminated) to fully expose urethral meatus.	Optimal visualization of urethral meatus is possible.
(2) Maintain position of nondominant hand throughout procedure.	Closure of labia during cleaning means that area is contaminated and requires cleaning procedure to be repeated.
(3) Holding forceps in dominant hand, pick up one moistened cotton ball or pick up one swab stick at a time. Clean labia and urinary meatus from clitoris toward anus. Use new cotton ball or swab for each area that you clean. Clean by wiping far from labial fold, near labial fold, and directly over center of urethral meatus (see illustration).	Front-to-back cleaning moves from area of least contamination toward highly contaminated area. Follows principles of medical asepsis. Dominant gloved hand remains sterile.

b. Male patient:

(1) With nondominant hand (now contaminated) retract foreskin (if uncircumcised) and gently grasp penis at shaft just below glans. Hold shaft of penis at right angle to body. Nondominant hand remains in this position for remainder of procedure.	When grasping shaft of penis, avoid pressure on dorsal surface to prevent compression of urethra. Losing grasp during cleaning means that area is contaminated and requires cleaning procedure to be repeated.

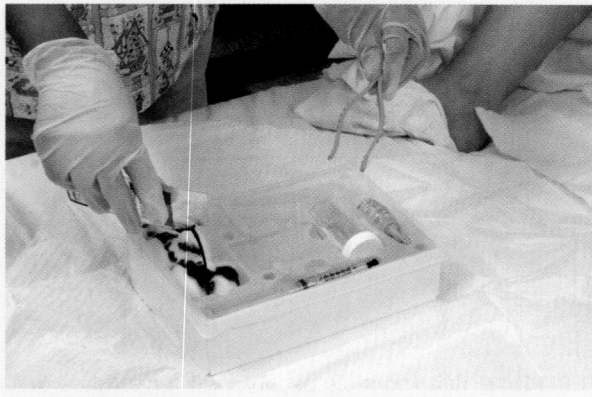

STEP 12a Sterile kit includes antiseptic swabs.

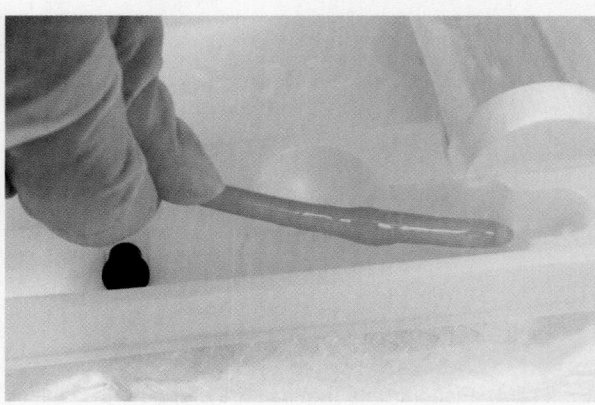

STEP 12d Lubricating catheter.

STEP	RATIONALE

(2) Using uncontaminated dominant hand, clean meatus with cotton balls or swab sticks, using circular strokes, beginning at the meatus and working outward in a spiral motion.

Circular cleaning pattern follows principles of medical asepsis.

(3) Repeat cleansing 3 times using clean cotton ball or swab stick each time (see illustration).

14. Pick up and hold catheter 7.5 to 10 cm (3 to 4 inches) from catheter tip with catheter loosely coiled in palm of hand. If catheter is not attached to drainage bag, make sure to position urine tray so that end of catheter can be placed there once insertion begins.

Holding catheter near tip allows for its easier manipulation during insertion. Coiling catheter in palm prevents distal end from striking nonsterile surface.

15. Insert catheter. Explain to patient that a feeling of burning, pinching, or pressure may be experienced as the catheter is inserted into the urethra. This sensation is normal and will go away quickly.

Information on what to expect during procedure helps reduce patient anxiety.

a. Female patient:

(1) Ask patient to bear down gently, and slowly insert catheter through urethral meatus (see illustration).

Bearing down may help visualize urinary meatus and promotes relaxation of external urinary sphincter, aiding in catheter insertion.

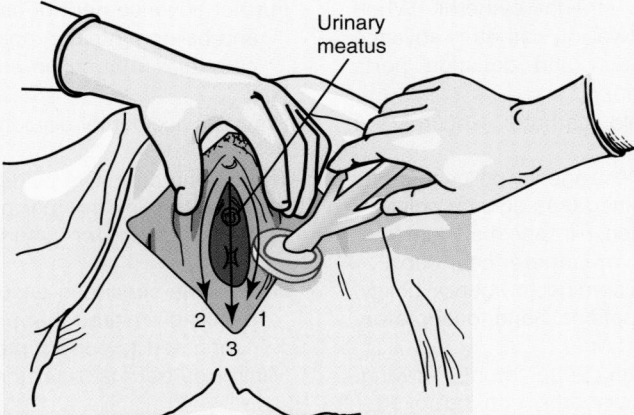

STEP 13a(3) Cleaning perineum of female patient.

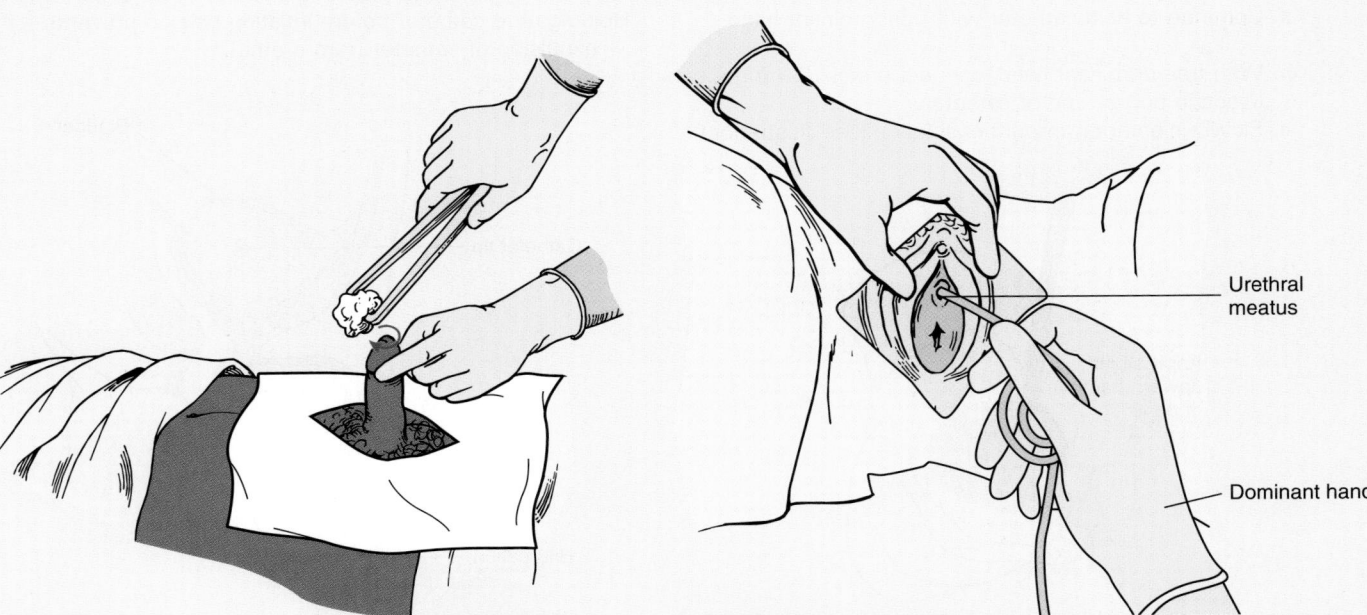

STEP 13b(3) Cleaning urinary meatus of male patient.

STEP 15a(1) Inserting catheter into urinary meatus of female patient.

SKILL 36.1   INSERTING AND REMOVING STRAIGHT/INTERMITTENT OR INDWELLING CATHETERS—cont'd

STEP	RATIONALE
(2) Advance catheter 5 to 7.5 cm (2 to 3 inches) or until urine flows out of catheter. When urine appears, advance catheter another 2.5 to 5 cm (1 to 2 inches). Do not use force to insert catheter.	Urine flow indicates that catheter tip is in bladder or lower urethra.
(3) Release labia and hold catheter securely with nondominant hand.	Prevents accidental dislodgment of catheter.
b. Male patient:	
(1) Lift penis to a position perpendicular (90 degrees) to patient's body and apply gentle upward traction (see illustration).	Straightens urethra to ease catheter insertion.
(2) Ask patient to bear down as if to void and slowly insert catheter through urethral meatus.	Relaxation of external sphincter aids in insertion of catheter.
(3) Advance catheter 17 to 22.5 cm (7 to 9 inches) or until urine flows out end of catheter.	There are variations in length of male urethra. Flow of urine indicates that tip of catheter is in bladder or urethra but not necessarily that the balloon portion of an indwelling catheter is in bladder.
(4) Stop advancing with a straight catheter. When urine appears in an indwelling catheter, advance it to bifurcation (inflation and deflation ports exposed) (see illustration).	Further advancement of catheter to bifurcation of drainage and balloon inflation port ensures that balloon portion of catheter is not still in prostatic urethra.
(5) Lower penis and hold catheter securely in nondominant hand.	Prevents accidental dislodgment of catheter.
16. Allow bladder to empty fully unless agency policy restricts maximum volume of urine drained (see agency policy).	There is no definitive evidence regarding whether there is benefit in limiting maximal volume drained.
17. Collect urine specimen as needed. Fill specimen container to 20 to 30 mL by holding end of catheter over cup.	Sterile specimen for culture analysis can be obtained.
a. Label and bag specimen according to agency policy. Label specimen in front of patient. Send to laboratory as soon as possible.	Fresh urine specimen ensures more accurate findings. Labeling ensures that diagnostic results will be connected to correct patient.
18. Straight catheterization: When urine stops flowing, withdraw catheter slowly and smoothly until removed.	Minimizes trauma to urethra.
19. **Indwelling catheter:** Inflate catheter balloon with amount of fluid designated by manufacturer.	Avoid using a balloon larger than 10 mL (Yates, 2016). Indwelling catheter balloons should not be underinflated.
a. Continue to hold catheter with nondominant hand.	Holding onto catheter before inflating balloon prevents expulsion of catheter from urethra.
b. With free dominant hand, connect prefilled syringe to injection port at end of catheter.	
c. Slowly inject total amount of solution (see illustration).	

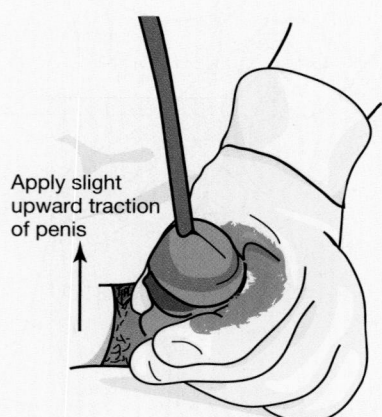

STEP 15b(1) Inserting catheter into urinary meatus of male patient.

Apply slight upward traction of penis

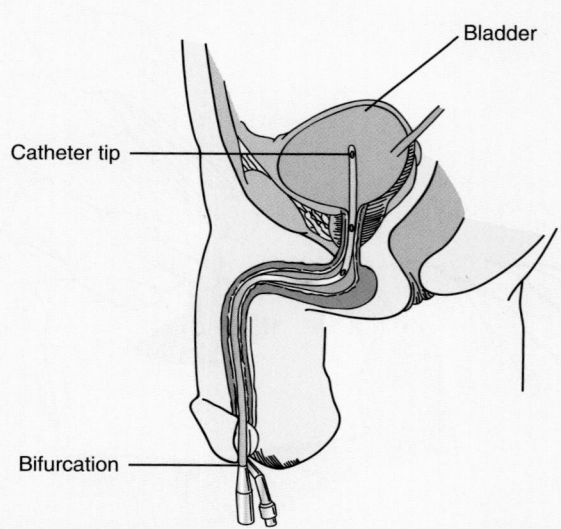

Bladder

Catheter tip

Bifurcation

STEP 15b(4) Male anatomy with correct catheter insertion to bifurcation.

STEP	RATIONALE

Clinical Decision Point. If patient reports sudden pain during inflation of a catheter balloon or resistance is felt when inflating the balloon, stop inflation, allow the fluid from the balloon to flow back into the syringe, advance catheter further, and reinflate balloon. The balloon may have been inflating in the urethra. If pain continues, remove catheter and notify the health care provider.

d. After inflating catheter balloon, release catheter from nondominant hand. *Gently* pull catheter until resistance is felt. Then advance catheter slightly.	By moving catheter slightly back into bladder, pressure on bladder neck is avoided.
e. Connect drainage tubing to catheter if it is not already preconnected.	
20. Secure indwelling catheter with catheter strap or other securement device. Leave enough slack to allow leg movement. Attach securement device at tubing just above catheter bifurcation.	Securing the catheter prevents traction on the catheter and ensures the balloon is not pulled into the neck of the bladder (Yates, 2016). Attachment of securement device at catheter bifurcation prevents occlusion of catheter.
a. Female patient:	
(1) Secure catheter tubing to inner thigh, allowing enough slack to prevent tension (see illustration).	
b. Male patient:	
(1) Secure catheter tubing to upper thigh (see illustration) or lower abdomen (with penis directed toward chest). Allow slack in catheter so that movement does not create tension on catheter.	Anchoring catheter reduces pulling and unnecessary pressure on the bladder neck, urethral-penile-scrotal junction, and urinary meatus (Ansell, 2016).
(2) If retracted, replace foreskin over glans penis.	Leaving foreskin retracted can cause discomfort and dangerous edema.

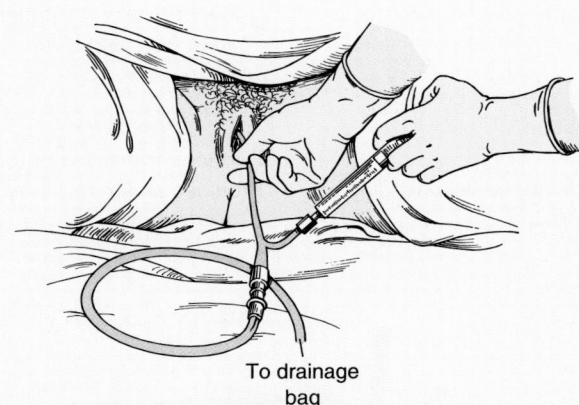

To drainage bag

STEP 19c Inflating balloon (indwelling catheter).

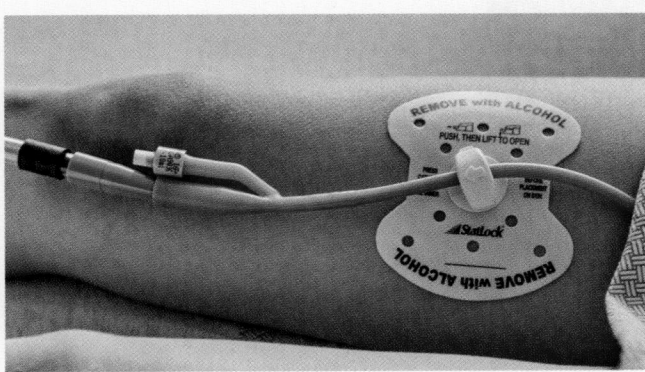

STEP 20a(1) Securing indwelling catheter on female patient with adhesive securement device.

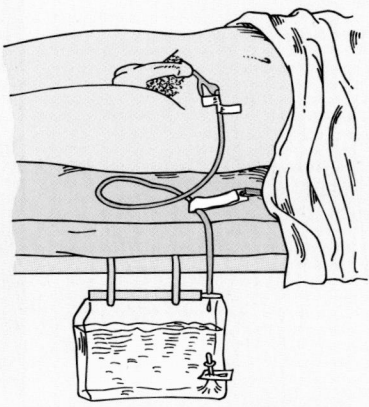

STEP 20b(1) Securing indwelling catheter on male patient with tape.

SKILL 36.1   INSERTING AND REMOVING STRAIGHT/INTERMITTENT OR INDWELLING CATHETERS—cont'd

STEP	RATIONALE
21. Clip drainage tubing to edge of mattress. Position drainage bag lower than bladder by attaching to bedframe. Do not attach to side rails of bed (see illustration) or place on the floor.	Drainage bags that are below level of bladder ensure free flow of urine to prevent reflux and contamination decreasing risk for CAUTI (Yates, 2016; Gould, 2017). Bags attached to movable objects such as a side rail increase risk for urethral trauma because of pulling or accidental dislodgment.
22. Check to ensure that there is no obstruction to urine flow. Coil excess tubing on bed and fasten to bottom sheet with clip or other securement device.	Obstruction to flow of urine increases risk for CAUTI (Nicolle, 2014; Gould et al., 2017).
23. Provide hygiene as needed. Help patient to comfortable position.	
24. Dispose of supplies in appropriate receptacles.	Reduces transmission of microorganisms.
25. Measure urine and record. If specimen collected, label container for culture, place in biohazard container, and send to laboratory.	Provides baseline for urine output and ensures prompt diagnostic analysis of urine.
26. Remove and dispose of gloves. Perform hand hygiene.	Reduces transmission of microorganisms.
27. **Removal of indwelling Foley catheter:**	
a. Close room door and bedside curtain.	Provides patient privacy.
b. Perform hand hygiene.	Reduces transmission of microorganisms.
c. Raise bed to appropriate working height. If side rails are raised, lower side rail on working side.	Promotes use of proper body mechanics.
d. Organize equipment for perineal care and/or removal of catheter.	Increases efficiency of procedure.
e. Position patient with waterproof pad under buttocks and cover with bath blanket, exposing only genital area and catheter. (1) Female patient in dorsal recumbent position. (2) Male patient in supine position.	Shows respect for patient dignity by exposing only genital area and catheter.
f. Apply clean gloves.	Reduces transmission of microorganisms.
g. Remove catheter securement device while maintaining connection with drainage tubing.	Provides ability to easily clean around catheter or to remove it.

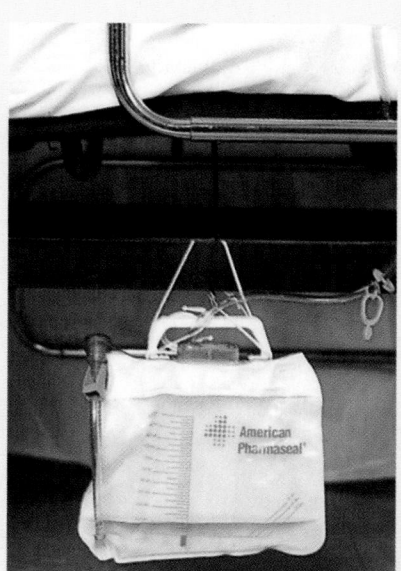

STEP 21 Drainage bag below level of bladder.

STEP	RATIONALE
h. Move syringe plunger up and down to loosen and then pull back plunger to 0.5 mL. Insert hub of syringe into inflation valve (balloon port). Allow balloon fluid to drain into syringe by gravity. Syringe should fill. Make sure that entire amount of fluid is removed by comparing removed amount with volume needed for inflation.	Partially inflated balloon can traumatize urethral wall during removal. Passive drainage of catheter balloon prevents formation of ridges in balloon. These ridges can cause discomfort or trauma during removal.
i. Pull catheter out smoothly and slowly. Examine it to ensure that it is whole. Catheter should slide out easily. Do not use force. If you note any resistance, repeat Step 27h to remove remaining water.	Nonwhole catheter means that pieces of catheter may still be in bladder. Notify health care provider immediately.
j. Wrap contaminated catheter in waterproof pad. Unhook collection bag and drainage tubing from bed.	Prevents transmission of microorganisms.
k. Reposition patient and provide hygiene as needed. Lower level of bed and position side rails accordingly.	Promotes patient comfort and safety.
l. Empty, measure, and record urine present in drainage bag.	Documents urinary output.
m. Encourage patient to maintain or increase fluid intake (unless contraindicated).	Maintains normal urine output.
28. Initiate voiding record or bladder diary. Instruct patient to tell you when need to empty bladder occurs and that all urine needs to be measured. Make sure that patient understands how to use collection container.	Evaluates bladder function.
29. Explain that many patients experience mild burning, discomfort, or small-volume voiding with first voiding, which soon subsides.	Burning results from urethral irritation.
30. Inform patient to report any signs of UTI.	
31. Ensure easy access to toilet, commode, bedpan, or urinal. Place urine hat on toilet seat if patient is using toilet. Place call bell within easy reach.	Reduces incidence of falls during toileting. Urine hat collects first voided urine.
32. Dispose of all contaminated supplies in appropriate receptacle, remove gloves, and perform hand hygiene.	Reduces transmission of microorganisms.

EVALUATION

1. Palpate bladder for distention or use bladder scan.	Determines if distention is relieved.
2. Ask patient to describe level of comfort.	Determines if patient's sensation of discomfort or fullness has been relieved.
3. Indwelling catheter: Observe character and amount of urine in drainage system.	Determines if urine is flowing adequately.
4. Indwelling catheter: Ensure that there is no urine leaking from catheter or tubing connections.	Prevents injury to patient's skin and ensures closed sterile system.
5. Observe time and measure amount of first voiding after catheter removal.	Indicates return of bladder function after catheter removal.
6. Evaluate patient for signs and symptoms of UTI.	Any patient who has recently had catheter removed is at risk for UTI.
7. Use principles of teach-back to evaluate patient/family caregiver learning. State, "I want to be sure I explained information about your urinary catheter. What can you do to ensure the urine flows out of the catheter?" Revise your instruction or develop plan for revised patient teaching if patient is unable to teach back correctly.	Determines patient and family caregiver level of understanding of instructional topic.

RECORDING AND REPORTING

- Record and report the reason for catheterization, type and size of catheter inserted, amount of fluid used to inflate balloon, specimen collection (if applicable), characteristics and amount of urine, patient's response to procedure, and education provided in nurses' notes in the electronic health record (EHR) or chart.
- Record amount of urine on intake and output (I&O) flow sheet record in EHR or chart.
- Report persistent catheter-related pain, inadequate urine output, and discomfort to health care provider.

- Record time for catheter care and appearance of urine; describe condition of meatus and catheter in EHR or chart.
- Record and report time of catheter removal, amount of water removed from balloon, and condition of urethral meatus and catheter as well as time, amount, and characteristics of first voided urine in EHR or chart.
- Record teaching and patient response related to catheter care, catheter removal, and fluid intake in EHR or chart.
- Report hematuria, dysuria, inability or difficulty voiding, and any new incontinence after catheter is removed.

UNEXPECTED OUTCOMES AND RELATED INTERVENTIONS

- Catheter goes into vagina.
  - Leave catheter in vagina.
  - Clean urinary meatus again. Using another catheter kit, reinsert sterile catheter into meatus (check agency policy). **Note:** If gloves become contaminated, start procedure over.
  - Remove catheter in vagina after successful insertion of second catheter.
- Patient has fever, chills, burning, flank pain, back pain, hematuria, painful urination, urgency, frequency, lower abdominal pain, change in mental status, and lethargy (Haddock, 2015).
  - Assess for bladder distention and tenderness.

- Monitor vital signs and urine output.
- Report findings to health care provider; signs and symptoms may indicate UTI.
- Patient is unable to void after catheter removal, has sensation of not emptying, strains to void, or experiences small voiding amounts with increasing frequency.
  - Assess for bladder distention.
  - Help to normal position for voiding and provide privacy.
  - Perform bladder ultrasound to assess for excessive urine volume in bladder.
  - If patient is unable to void within 6 to 8 hours of catheter removal and/or experiences abdominal pain, notify health care provider.

▊ KEY POINTS

- Voiding is a complex interaction that takes place among the bladder, urinary sphincter, and central nervous system.
- Many factors affect voiding such as growth and development, sociocultural implications, personal habits, fluid intake, pathological conditions, surgical procedures, medications, and diagnostic examinations.
- When completing a nursing history, collect data from a patient about patterns of urination, symptoms of urinary alterations, and factors affecting voiding.
- Normal urine is pale yellow to amber, is free of hematuria, appears transparent at time of voiding, and is free from odor. Medications and certain foods can alter normal urine characteristics.
- Nursing interventions to promote normal urination and control incontinence include educating patients to have adequate hydration, develop good voiding habits, maintain regular bowel movements, reduce or eliminate smoking, and report changes in bladder function to health care providers.
- Use the smallest catheter size with a 10-mL balloon to minimize trauma and risk for infection when inserting an

indwelling Foley catheter. Any patient with an indwelling catheter or who has recently had a catheter is at risk for a catheter-associated urinary tract infection (CAUTI).
- Use of a bladder scanner to measure postvoid residual avoids unnecessary catheterization and decreases the risk for developing a urinary tract infection (UTI).
- Monitoring a patient's intake and output is a common health care provider order or can be initiated per nursing judgment to evaluate bladder emptying, renal function, and fluid balance.

▊ REFLECTIVE LEARNING

- Reflect on a time when you cared for a patient with a Foley catheter. What approaches did you use to prevent infection? What challenges did you face with catheter care?
- Discuss cultural factors that you needed to consider before inserting a Foley catheter in one of your patients.
- Reflect on a patient you have cared for who had dementia. Describe how you completed your focused patient assessment of the urinary system.

REVIEW QUESTIONS

1. Place the following steps for application of a condom catheter to a male patient in appropriate order.
   1. Apply clean gloves, provide perineal care, and dry thoroughly.
   2. Identify patient using at least two identifiers.
   3. Assess penis for erythema, rashes, or open areas.
   4. Secure condom catheter according to manufacturer directions.
   5. Apply condom catheter.
   6. Clip hair at base of penile shaft as necessary.
   7. Connect drainage tubing to end of condom catheter.
   8. Perform hand hygiene, prepare condom catheter, and help patient to a supine or sitting position.

2. The nurse instructs a female patient how to perform Kegel exercises. Which patient statement indicates she can perform the exercises correctly?
   1. "I squeeze the anus as if I am holding in gas for 2 or 3 seconds"
   2. "I push like I need to have a bowel movement"
   3. "I squat down and squeeze my thighs together for 5 to 10 seconds"
   4. "I contract my abdomen and buttocks for 2 or 3 seconds"

3. Which of these is a nursing safety consideration before insertion of a Foley catheter? (Select all that apply.)
   1. Identify if patient is at risk for a latex allergy.
   2. Identify if patient has an allergy to povidone-iodine (Betadine).
   3. Follow asepsis principles when performing catheter insertion.
   4. Teach the patient Kegel exercises.
   5. Discard the first voided specimen.

4. The nurse is assessing intake and output for an alert patient at the end of shift and notes red-colored urine. Which nursing action is appropriate?
   1. Immediately call the health care provider
   2. Collect a clean-catch urine specimen
   3. Review the patient's dietary history for the past 24 hours
   4. Review the patient's most recent urinalysis laboratory report

5. A nurse is caring for a patient with a history of urinary retention. Which findings indicate the need to use a bladder scanner to measure postvoid residual? (Select all that apply.)
   1. Dribbling urine while experiencing urgency
   2. Absence of voiding in more than 6 hours
   3. Reports of pain with palpation of the bladder
   4. Swelling over the lower abdomen extending to the umbilicus
   5. Visible hematuria noted with the patient's last void

evolve

Additional Review Questions, as well as rationales for all Review Questions, can be found on the Evolve website.

1, 2, 8, 1, 3, 6, 5, 4, 7; 2, 1; 3, 1, 2, 3; 4, 3; 5, 1, 2, 3, 4.

REFERENCES

Ackley BJ, Ladwig GB: *Nursing diagnosis handbook: a guide for planning care,* ed 11, St Louis, 2017, Mosby.

Agency for Healthcare Research and Quality (AHRQ): *Toolkit for reducing CAUTI in hospitals,* 2015. https://www.ahrq.gov/sites/default/files/wysiwyg/professionals/quality-patient-safety/hais/cauti-tools/impl-guide/implementation-guide.pdf.

American Nurses Association (ANA): *ANA CAUTI prevention tool,* 2014. http://www.nursingworld.org/MainMenuCategories/ThePracticeofProfessionalNursing/Improving-Your-Practice/ANA-CAUTI-Prevention-Tool.

Andrade VLF, et al: Prevention of catheter-associated urinary tract infection, *Rev Lat Am Enfermagem,* 2016. https://www.ncbi.nlm.nih.gov/pmc/articles/PMC4809180/.

Ansell T: Indwelling urinary catheters: should we secure them? *Br J Nurs* 25(18):S22, 2016.

Bardsley A: Safe and effective catheterization for patients in the community, *Br J Community Nurs* 20(4):166, 2015.

Bardsley A: An overview of urinary incontinence, *Br J Nurs* 25(18):S14, 2016.

Beeckman D, et al: Incontinence-associated dermatitis (IAD): an update, *Dermatological Nursing* 14(4):32, 2015.

Carter N, et al: An evidenced-based approach to the prevention of catheter-associated urinary tract infections, *Urol Nurs* 34(5):238, 2014.

Casey G: Understanding urinary tract infections, *Nurs N Z* 20(5):20, 2014.

Centers for Disease Control and Prevention (CDC): *Guideline for prevention of catheter-associated urinary tract infections,* 2009. http://www.cdc.gov/hicpac/pdf/CAUTI/CAUTIguideline2009final.pdf.

Centers for Disease Control and Prevention (CDC): *Urinary tract infection (catheter-associated urinary tract infection [CAUTI] and non-catheter-associated urinary tract infection [UTI]) and other urinary system infection [USI]) events,* 2017. https://www.cdc.gov/nhsn/PDFs/pscManual/7pscCAUTIcurrent.pdf.

Clarke E: Female genital mutilation: a urology focus, *Br J Nurs* 25(18):1022, 2016.

Collins J: Nursing cultural competencies: improving patient care quality and satisfaction, *Ohio Nurses Rev* 90(1):10, 2015.

Dy S, et al: A nurse-driven protocol for removal of indwelling urinary catheters across a multi-hospital academic healthcare system, *Urol Nurs* 36(5):243, 2016.

Galiczewski J: Interventions for the prevention of catheter associated urinary tract infections in intensive care units: an integrative review, *Intensive Crit Care Nurs* 32:1, 2016.

Gesmundo M: Managing indwelling urinary catheters, *Nurs N Z* 22(6):14, 2016.

Gould CV, et al: *Guideline for prevention of catheter-associated urinary tract infection 2009*, update February 15, 2017. https://www.cdc.gov/infectioncontrol/pdf/guidelines/cauti-guidelines.pdf.

Haddock G: Improving the management of urinary tract infection, *Nursing and Residential Care* 17(1):22, 2015.

Huether SE, McCance KL: *Understanding pathophysiology*, ed 6, St Louis, 2016, Mosby.

Jones ML: Elimination of urine and incontinence of urine, *British Journal of Healthcare Assistants* 9(8):375, 2015.

Kehinde O: Common incontinence problems seen by community nurses, *Journal of Community Nursing* 30(4):46, 2016.

Leaver R: Managing the aftercare of patients with a Mitrofanoff pouch, *Journal of Community Nursing* 30(1):40, 2016.

National Institute of Diabetes and Digestive and Kidney Diseases (NIDDK): *Urinary diversion*, 2013. https://www.niddk.nih.gov/health-information/urologic-diseases/urinary-diversion.

Nazarko L: Person-centered care of women with urinary incontinence, *Nurse Prescribing* 36(6):288, 2015.

Nicolle L: Catheter-related urinary tract infection: practical management in the elderly, *Drugs Aging* 31:1, 2014.

Pagana TJ, et al: *Mosby's diagnostic and laboratory test reference*, ed 13, St Louis, 2017, Mosby.

Panchisin T: Improving outcomes with the ANA CAUTI Prevention Tool, *Nursing* 46(3):55, 2016.

Quinn P: Chasing zero: a nurse-driven process for catheter-associated urinary tract infection reduction in a community hospital, *Nurs Econ* 33(6):L6, 2015.

Rantell A: Pharmacological management of overactive bladder in women, *Nurse Prescribing* 12(5):232, 2014.

Rigby D: Mirabegron—promising new drug for overactive bladder syndrome, *Aust N Z Continence J* 21(2):40, 2015.

Roe B, et al: Systematic review of systematic reviews for the management of urinary incontinence and promotion of continence using conservative behavioural approaches in older people in care homes, *J Adv Nurs* 71(7):1464, 2015.

Schreiber M: Ostomies: nursing care and management, *Medsurg Nurs* 25(2):127, 2016.

Smart C: Male incontinence: using the urinary sheath, *Nursing and Residential Care* 16(10):568, 2014.

Steadman B, Ellsworth P: To circ or not to circ: indications, risks, and alternatives to circumcision in the pediatric population with phimosis, *Urol Nurs* 26(3):181, 2016.

Testa A: Understanding urinary incontinence in adults, *Urol Nurs* 35(2):82, 2015.

The Joint Commission (TJC): *2018 National Patient Safety Goals*, Oakbrook Terrace, IL, 2018, The Commission, http://www.jointcommission.org/standards_information/npsgs.aspx.

Voegeli D: Incontinence-associated dermatitis: new insights into an old problem, *Br J Nurs* 25(5):256, 2016.

Wagg A, et al: Review of the efficacy and safety of fesoterodine for treating overactive bladder and urgency urinary incontinence in elderly patients, *Drugs Aging* 32:103, 2015.

Wilson M: Urinary incontinence: considering the physical and psychological implications, *Br J Community Nurs* 21(5):222, 2016.

Woodward S: Intermittent catheterization for postoperative urinary retention, *Br J Nurs* 24(14):732, 2015a.

Woodward S: Selecting and fitting a penile sheath, *Br J Nurs* 24(5):290, 2015b.

Yates A: Indwelling urinary catheterization: what is best practice?, *Br J Nurs* 25(9):84, 2016.

Bowel Elimination

evolve MEDIA RESOURCES

http://evolve.elsevier.com/Potter/essentials
- Audio Glossary
- QSEN Activity and Review Questions Answers and Rationales
- Video Clips

OBJECTIVES

- Explain the physiology of digestion, absorption, and bowel elimination.
- Discuss physiological and psychological factors that influence bowel elimination.
- Describe common physiological alterations in bowel elimination.
- Assess a patient's bowel elimination pattern.

- Perform a fecal occult blood test.
- List nursing diagnoses related to alterations in bowel elimination.
- Describe the steps used in the nursing interventions that promote normal elimination and defecation.
- Evaluate outcomes of bowel elimination interventions.

KEY TERMS

cathartics, p. 1076
colon, p. 1061
colonoscopy, p. 1070
constipation, p. 1062
defecation, p. 1061
diarrhea, p. 1063
enema, p. 1079

fecal impaction, p. 1063
fecal incontinence, p. 1064
fecal occult blood test (FOBT), p. 1070
feces, p. 1061
flatus, p. 1061
hemorrhoids, p. 1064

ileus, p. 1079
laxatives, p. 1076
melena, p. 1068
ostomy, p. 1065
peristalsis, p. 1060
stoma, p. 1064

Regular bowel elimination is essential to maintain a healthy body. Alterations in bowel elimination are often early signs or symptoms of problems within either the gastrointestinal (GI) or other body systems. Bowel function depends on the balance of several factors such as age, diet, fluid intake, activity level, and medications. Elimination patterns and habits vary among individuals.

Individuals of any age are at risk for changes in intestinal activity. These changes are the result of illness, medications, diagnostic testing, or surgical intervention. Aging when accompanied by chronic illness, cognitive decline, decreased mobility, and a decrease in food and fluid intake changes digestive system function; however, aging alone does not necessarily alter the digestive process. Alterations in intestinal elimination respond to both preventive and supportive nursing care.

SCIENTIFIC KNOWLEDGE BASE

Anatomy and Physiology of the Gastrointestinal Tract

The GI tract is a series of hollow mucous membrane–lined muscular organs that begin at the mouth and end at the anal

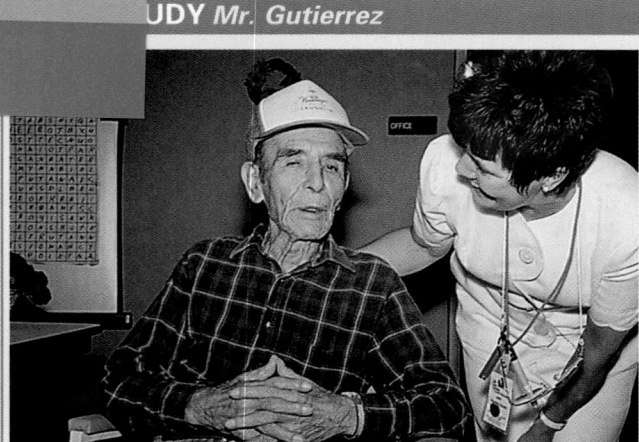

Mr. Gutierrez resides in an assisted-living apartment of a long-term care center. He keeps busy in his small garden plot and enjoys other activities of the center such as nightly card or bingo games and outings to major league baseball games and local museums. He is 82 years old and widowed and has lived in this area of the care center for more than 3 years. His family, with whom he is quite close, is scattered across the country. He has one niece who lives in the same town. Mr. Gutierrez believes that he is in good health. As long as he eats green chili peppers every day, he believes that he will remain healthy. Because he has a small kitchen in his apartment, he is able to make some of his favorite foods. His diet consists of flour and corn tortillas, beans, and rice. He likes most meats, but he prefers chicken and *asado* (made with pork). For breakfast he usually has huevos rancheros (corn tortillas with eggs and chili sauce). He has been hospitalized only twice, once for the flu and once for placement of a pacemaker. He presently takes three medications: digoxin, lisinopril, and Metamucil.

This afternoon Mr. Gutierrez has telephoned his niece for the fourth time. He reports, "My bowels are locked up and haven't moved in the last 2 days." He ate a big meal the previous evening and now reports feeling "all gassed up." His niece tried to explain about eating foods containing fiber and more vegetables. She reminded Mr. Gutierrez that the nursing student was coming later this afternoon and he could talk to the student about his problem.

Vickie is the nursing student assigned to Mr. Gutierrez. She has been seeing him once a week for 5 weeks as a part of a home health care clinical experience. They have developed a good rapport. Mr. Gutierrez's self-identified problems with his bowels are a frequent topic of conversation.

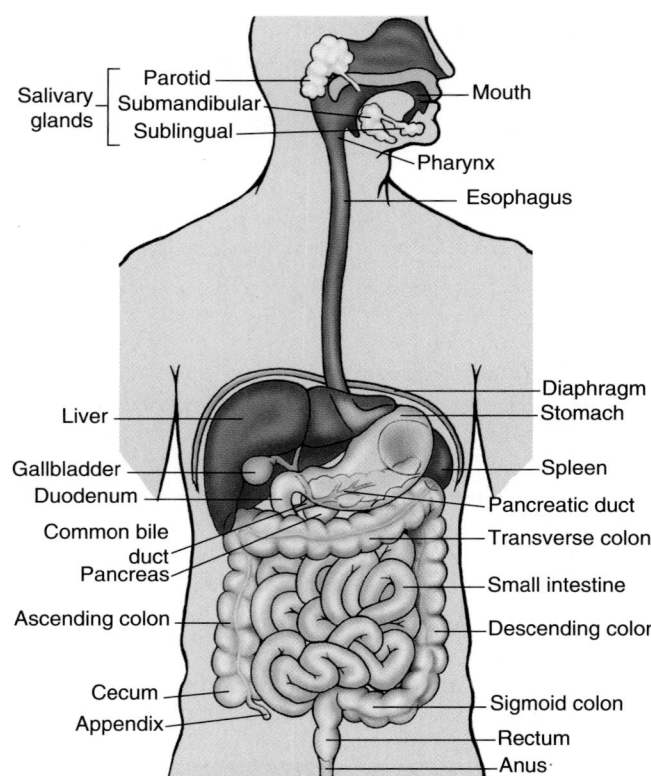

FIG 37.1 Gastrointestinal system. (From Monahan FD, Neighbors M: *Medical-surgical nursing,* ed 2, Philadelphia, 1998, Saunders.)

and softens the food in the mouth for easier swallowing. Enzymes in saliva begin the breakdown of food.

Esophagus. As food enters the upper esophagus, it passes through the upper esophageal sphincter, a circular muscle that prevents air from entering the esophagus and food from refluxing into the throat. The bolus of food travels down the esophagus with the aid of **peristalsis,** which is a contraction that propels food through the length of the GI tract. The food moves down the esophagus and reaches the cardiac sphincter, which lies between the esophagus and the upper end of the stomach. The sphincter prevents reflux of stomach contents back into the esophagus.

Stomach. The stomach performs three tasks: storing swallowed food and liquid, mixing food with digestive juices, and regulating emptying of its contents into the small intestine. The stomach produces and secretes hydrochloric acid (HCl), mucus, the enzyme pepsin, and intrinsic factor. Pepsin and HCl facilitate the digestion of protein. Mucus protects the stomach mucosa from acidity and enzyme activity. Intrinsic factor is essential in preparing vitamin B_{12} for absorption in the ileum.

Small Intestine. Movement within the small intestine, occurring by peristalsis, facilitates both digestion and absorption. Food comes into the small intestine as a semifluid

orifice. The functions of the GI tract are to break down ingested food for use as energy by body cells and promote the absorption of fluid and nutrients. It is a complex system, and changes in any one part can alter the function of other parts (Fig. 37.1).

Mouth. The mouth mechanically and chemically breaks down nutrients into usable size and form. The teeth chew food, breaking it down into a size suitable for swallowing. Saliva, produced by the salivary glands in the mouth, dilutes material and mixes with digestive juices. Resorption in the small intestine is so efficient that by the time the fluid reaches the end of the small intestine, it is semisolid in consistency. The small intestine is divided into three sections: the duodenum, the jejunum, and the ileum.

The duodenum is approximately 8 to 11 inches long and continues to process the fluid from the stomach. The second section, the jejunum, is approximately 8 feet long and absorbs carbohydrates and proteins. The ileum is approximately 12 feet long and absorbs water, fats, and bile salts. The duodenum and jejunum absorb most nutrients and electrolytes in the small intestine. The ileum absorbs certain vitamins, iron, and bile salts. Digestive enzymes and bile enter the small intestine from the pancreas and liver to further break down nutrients into a form usable by the body.

When small intestine function is impaired, it greatly alters the digestive process. Conditions such as inflammation, infection, surgical resection, or obstruction disrupt peristalsis, reduce absorption, or block the passage of the fluid. Electrolyte and nutrient deficiencies then develop.

Large Intestine. The lower GI tract is called the *large intestine* because it is larger in diameter than the small intestine. However, its length (1.5 to 1.8 m [5 to 6 feet]) is much shorter. The large intestine is divided into the cecum, ascending colon, transverse colon, descending colon, sigmoid colon, and rectum (see Fig. 37.1). It is the primary organ of bowel elimination.

The digestive fluid enters the large intestine by waves of peristalsis through the ileocecal valve, a circular muscle layer that prevents regurgitation back into the small intestine. The muscular tissue of the colon allows it to accommodate and eliminate large quantities of waste and gas (flatus). The colon has three functions: absorption, secretion, and elimination. It resorbs a large volume of water (up to 1.5 L) and significant amounts of sodium and chloride daily. The amount of water absorbed depends on the speed at which colonic contents move. Normally the fecal matter becomes a soft, formed solid or semisolid mass. If peristalsis is abnormally fast, there is less time for water to be absorbed, and the stool is watery. If peristaltic contractions slow, water continues to be absorbed, and a hard mass of stool forms, resulting in constipation.

Peristaltic contractions move contents through the colon. Intestinal content is the main stimulus for contraction. Mass peristalsis pushes undigested food toward the rectum. These mass movements occur only 3 or 4 times daily, with the strongest during the hour after mealtime.

The rectum, located at the end of the large intestine, is normally empty of waste products (feces) until just before defecation. It contains vertical and transverse folds of tissue that help to control expulsion of fecal contents during defecation. Each fold contains veins that can become distended from pressure during straining. This distention results in hemorrhoid formation.

Anus. The body expels feces and flatus from the rectum through the anus. Contraction and relaxation of the internal and external sphincters, which are innervated by sympathetic and parasympathetic nerves, aid in the control of defecation. The anal canal contains a rich supply of sensory nerves that allow people to sense when there is solid, liquid, or gas that needs to be expelled and aids in maintaining continence.

Defecation. The physiological factors essential to bowel function and defecation include normal GI tract function, sensory awareness of rectal distention and rectal contents, voluntary sphincter control, and adequate rectal capacity and compliance (Steele et al., 2016). Normal defecation begins with movement in the left colon, moving stool toward the anus. When stool reaches the rectum, the distention causes relaxation of the internal sphincter and an awareness of the need to defecate. At the time of defecation, the external sphincter relaxes, and abdominal muscles contract, increasing intrarectal pressure and forcing the stool out. Normally defecation is painless, resulting in passage of soft, formed stool. Straining while having a bowel movement indicates that the patient may need changes in diet or fluid intake or that there is an underlying disorder in GI function.

NURSING KNOWLEDGE BASE

To manage your patient's elimination problems, you need to understand normal elimination and factors that promote, impede, or cause alterations in elimination such as constipation, diarrhea, and fecal incontinence (Box 37.1). Supportive nursing care respects each patient's privacy and emotional needs and includes interventions designed to promote normal bowel elimination while minimizing discomfort.

Alterations in bowel elimination are embarrassing for patients. Because of the sensitivity that many patients experience with bowel elimination and its associated sounds and odors, be very sensitive about how you communicate, especially nonverbally. A patient may perceive changes in facial expression as disgust. Be aware of a patient's need for privacy during elimination.

Patients with chronic diseases of the GI system often have numerous hospitalizations, perhaps multiple surgeries, and significant changes in eating habits and lifestyles. They are often on complicated medication schedules that are taxing both physically and financially. Their desire for wellness sometimes leads them to consider alternative forms of medical treatment such as vitamin or herbal supplements. Remain nonjudgmental regarding a patient's health care choices.

Some patients with chronic GI diseases require an ostomy, which involves the surgical creation of a stoma on the abdomen for the passage of stool. An ostomy results in body image changes and loss of control over a very basic body function. It takes time to adjust to an ostomy. Learning how to care for an ostomy and having a reliable pouching system that prevents leakage of the fecal output and odor can help a patient to make this adjustment. An ostomy nurse with specialized training should be asked to see the patient with a new ostomy if one is available.

BOX 37.1   FACTORS INFLUENCING BOWEL ELIMINATION

AGE

- Infants have a smaller stomach capacity, less secretion of digestive enzymes, and more rapid intestinal peristalsis. The ability to control defecation does not occur until 2 to 3 years of age.
- Adolescents experience rapid growth of the large intestine and increased secretion of gastric acids to dissolve food fibers and act as a bactericide against swallowed organisms.
- Older adults may have decreased chewing ability. Partially chewed food is not digested as easily. Peristalsis declines, and esophageal emptying slows. This impairs absorption by the intestinal mucosa. Muscle tone in the perineal floor and anal sphincter weakens, causing difficulty in controlling defecation (National Institute of Diabetes, Digestive and Kidney Diseases [NIDDK], 2016).

DIET

- Regular daily food intake promotes peristalsis.
- High-fiber foods (e.g., fruits, greens, and other vegetables) and whole grains (cereals and breads) promote peristalsis and defecation by creating bulk.
- Low-fiber foods (e.g., pasta, white rice, white bread, cheese) slow peristalsis.
- Gas-producing foods (e.g., broccoli, cauliflower, onions, dried beans) stimulate peristalsis.
- People with lactose intolerance lack the enzyme lactase, which is needed to digest the simple sugars in milk. Lactose intolerance leads to diarrhea and cramping.
- People with gluten intolerance experience pain, bloating, diarrhea, or constipation.

POSITION DURING DEFECATION

- A sitting position allows a person to lean forward, exert intraabdominal pressure, and contract thigh muscles for normal defecation.
- Older adults and patients with chronic pain or immobility may have difficulty sitting down on or rising from a toilet seat. An elevated toilet seat and chairs with arms on the sides of the toilet help to promote defecation.
- Patients required to use a bedpan while lying down cannot contract muscles to defecate.

PREGNANCY

- As pregnancy advances and a fetus enlarges, this exerts pressure on the rectum. Constipation commonly occurs.

DIAGNOSTIC TESTS

- Examinations involving visualization of GI structures require the emptying of bowel contents. Patients receive nothing by mouth (NPO) or only clear liquids, bowel evacuants, and enema administration to cleanse the bowel before the test. This is called *bowel prep* and temporarily interferes with normal elimination.
- Barium examinations require ingestion of barium, a mixture that can cause constipation unless the barium is eliminated soon after a test.

FLUID INTAKE

- When there is adequate fluid intake (1.5 to 2 L/day), the body absorbs fluid into the fecal mass and increases bulk for easier passage.
- Warm beverages and fruit juices soften stool and increase peristalsis.
- Caffeinated drinks in moderation may stimulate peristalsis.

ACTIVITY

- Immobilization depresses colon motility, whereas regular physical exercise promotes peristalsis.

PSYCHOLOGICAL FACTORS

- Stress, anxiety, or fear initiates parasympathetic impulses, causing the acceleration of digestion and peristalsis. Diarrhea and gaseous distention result.
- Emotional depression decreases peristalsis and leads to constipation.

PERSONAL HABITS

- Failing to respond to the need to defecate and lack of privacy interfere with normal elimination patterns and lead to constipation.
- Hospitalized patients often share toilet facilities or use bedpans or bedside commodes. The resulting embarrassment causes them to ignore the urge to defecate.

PAIN

- Hemorrhoids, rectal surgery, and abdominal surgery cause a patient to suppress defecation because of pain; constipation develops.

MEDICATIONS

- Laxatives and cathartics soften stool and promote peristalsis.
- Antidiarrheal agents inhibit peristalsis.
- Opiates and anticholinergic drugs depress peristalsis and cause constipation.
- Antibiotics alter normal bowel flora and often produce diarrhea.
- Drugs that contain iron sometimes turn the stool black. Antacids cause a white discoloration. Anticoagulants can cause frank or occult blood in the stool.

SURGERY AND ANESTHESIA

- General anesthetics slow or halt peristalsis.
- Surgery involving bowel manipulation may temporarily stop peristalsis, creating a condition called *paralytic ileus*, which lasts for hours or days and resolves spontaneously.

Bowel Elimination Problems

Alterations in bowel elimination are caused by a variety of factors.

Constipation. Constipation is defined as having fewer than three bowel movements per week, but based on the American Society of Gastroenterologists recommendations, health care providers now also define constipation as one or more of the following: (1) hard or dry stools, (2) decreased frequency of stooling, (3) sensation of incomplete evacuation following a bowel movement, and (4) pain or straining associated with stool elimination (Steele et al., 2016).

Constipation is commonly caused by changes in diet, medications, mobility, inflammation, environmental factors (e.g., unavailability of toilet facilities or lack of privacy), and lack of knowledge about regular bowel habits. It is not a physiological response to aging, but changes in mobility and comorbidities that occur with aging make this condition more prevalent in older adults (Steele et al., 2016). Regardless of cause, intestinal motility slows, causing prolonged exposure of the feces to the intestinal wall. Liquid from the feces continues to be absorbed, leaving the stool hard and dry (Box 37.2).

BOX 37.2 COMMON CAUSES OF CONSTIPATION

- Irregular bowel habits and ignoring the urge to defecate
- Chronic illnesses (e.g., Parkinson disease, multiple sclerosis, rheumatoid arthritis, chronic bowel diseases, depression, eating disorders)
- Low-fiber diet high in animal fats (e.g., meats and carbohydrates); low fluid intake
- Stress (e.g., illness of a family member, death of a loved one, divorce)
- Physical inactivity
- Medications, overuse of laxatives
- Changes in life or routine such as pregnancy, aging, and travel
- Neurological conditions that block nerve impulses to the colon (e.g., stroke, spinal cord injury, tumor)
- Chronic bowel dysfunction (e.g., colonic inertia, irritable bowel)

Data from National Institute of Diabetes, Digestive and Kidney Diseases (NIDDK): *Health information,* 2016, https://www.niddk.nih.gov/health-information.

Constipation has significant health implications. Straining during defecation causes problems for patients with recent abdominal, gynecological, or rectal surgery. An effort to pass a stool can cause stress and pain in the surgical site. Patients with cardiovascular disease, diseases causing elevated intraocular pressure (glaucoma), and increased intracranial pressure need to prevent constipation and avoid straining to have a bowel movement.

Impaction. Fecal impaction results from unrelieved constipation. A patient is unable to expel the hardened feces retained in the rectum. In severe impaction the hardened fecal mass extends up into the sigmoid colon. Patients at greatest risk for impaction include those who are confused, weak, unconscious, or unaware of the need to defecate and patients who have an interruption in nerve supply to the bowel. An obvious sign of impaction is the inability to pass a stool for several days, despite a repeated urge to defecate. Continuous oozing of liquid stool after several days with no fecal output may indicate an impaction. Loss of appetite, abdominal distention and cramping, nausea and/or vomiting, and rectal pain can also occur.

Diarrhea. Diarrhea is an increase in the number of stools and the passage of liquid, unformed stools (Table 37.1). It is associated with disorders affecting digestion, absorption, and secretion in the GI tract. Intestinal contents pass too quickly through the small intestine and colon to allow for the usual absorption of fluid and nutrients. Dehydration leading to fluid and electrolyte and acid-base imbalances can result. Older adults and very young children are at the greatest risk for dehydration (Box 37.3). Persistent diarrhea may cause skin breakdown in the perianal region.

TABLE 37.1 CONDITIONS THAT CAUSE DIARRHEA

CONDITION	PHYSIOLOGICAL EFFECTS
Intestinal infection (streptococcal or staphylococcal enteritis)	Inflammation of intestinal mucosa, increased mucus secretion
Food allergies	Abnormal digestion of food elements, increased mucus secretion
Food intolerance (lactose, gluten, high fat, coffee, alcohol, spicy foods)	Abnormal digestion of food elements, increased mucus secretion
Tube feedings	Hyperosmolarity of some enteral solutions results in diarrhea because hyperosmolar fluids draw fluids into the GI tract
Medications	
Iron supplements	Irritation of intestinal mucosa
Antibiotics	Loss of normal flora, susceptibility to opportunistic infection
Laxatives (short term)	Increased intestinal motility and irritability
Inflammatory bowel disease (colitis, Crohn disease)	Inflammation and ulceration of intestinal walls, reduced absorption of fluids, increased intestinal motility
Surgical alterations	
Gastrectomy	Loss of reservoir function of stomach, improper absorption because food moves into duodenum too quickly
Intestinal resection	Reduced length of intestine, reduced amount of absorptive surface
Emotional stress (anxiety)	Increased intestinal motility

GI, Gastrointestinal.

BOX 37.3 SIGNS OF DEHYDRATION

Signs of dehydration in adults include the following:	Signs of dehydration in infants and young children include the following:
• Thirst • Less frequent urination than usual • Dark-colored urine • Dry skin • Fatigue • Dizziness • Light-headedness	• Dry mouth and tongue • No tears when crying • No wet diapers for 3 hours or more • Sunken eyes, cheeks, or soft spot in the skull • High fever • Listlessness or irritability

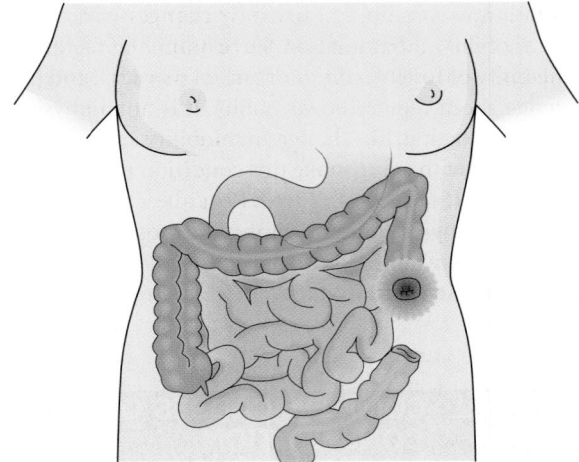

FIG 37.2 Sigmoid colostomy.

A common cause of diarrhea in health care facilities is *Clostridium difficile*; symptoms of *C. difficile* infection range from mild to severe diarrhea. This infection is acquired by use of antibiotics that depress natural intestinal flora, allowing an overgrowth of *C. difficile,* and by contact with the *C. difficile* organism. The best ways to prevent the occurrence and spread of *C. difficile* is cautious use of antibiotics and rigorous hand hygiene with soap and water (Mayo Clinic, 2016). Communicable foodborne pathogens also cause diarrhea. Thorough handwashing after using the bathroom and before and after meal preparation and careful cleansing and storing of fresh produce and meats help to reduce foodborne illnesses.

Fecal Incontinence. Fecal incontinence is the temporary or permanent inability to control the passage of feces and gas from the anus. Fecal incontinence is underreported because of shame or a sense that nothing can be done about it, yet it affects up to 20% of community-living adults and nearly 50% of nursing home residents (Callan and Wilson, 2016). It is embarrassing and may cause social isolation and loss of intimacy. It is often assumed that a loss of cognitive function is the primary reason that an older person is unable to remain continent; however, a person may be mentally alert but physically unable to avoid uncontrolled defecation. Impairment of anal sphincter function or control may cause incontinence. Conditions that create frequent, large-volume, watery stools predispose to fecal urgency and incontinence. Similar to diarrhea, incontinence predisposes a patient to skin breakdown. Management of fecal incontinence requires a complete understanding of the causes.

Flatulence. Flatulence (accumulated gas) is one of the most common GI disorders. It is a sensation of bloating and abdominal distention accompanied by excess gas. As gas accumulates in the lumen of the intestines, the bowel wall stretches and distends. Normally intestinal gas escapes through the mouth (belching) or the anus. However, when intestinal motility is reduced as a result of medications, general anesthetics, abdominal surgery, or immobilization, flatulence may become severe, causing abdominal distention and sharp pain.

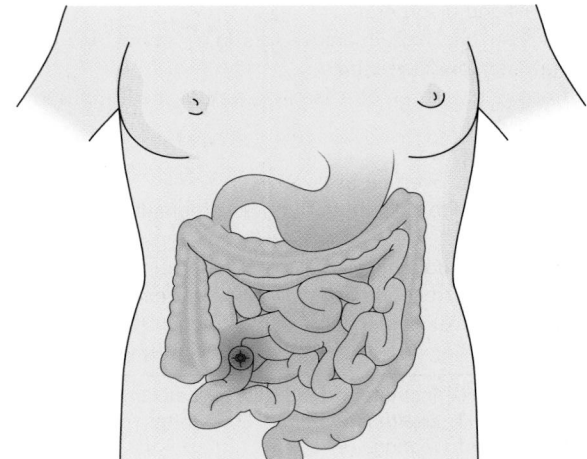

FIG 37.3 Ileostomy.

Hemorrhoids. Hemorrhoids are dilated, engorged veins in the lining of the rectum. Increased venous pressure resulting from straining at defecation, pregnancy, and chronic illnesses such as congestive heart failure and chronic liver disease are causative factors. A hemorrhoid forms either within the anal canal (internal) or through the opening of the anus (external). Passage of hard stool causes hemorrhoid tissue to stretch and bleed. Hemorrhoid tissue becomes inflamed and tender, and patients may report itching and burning. Because pain worsens during defecation, the patient sometimes ignores the urge to defecate, resulting in constipation.

Intestinal Diversions/Ostomies. Certain diseases or surgical alterations make the normal passage of intestinal contents throughout the small and large intestine difficult or inadvisable. When these conditions are present, a temporary or permanent opening (stoma) is surgically created by bringing a portion of the intestine out through the abdominal wall. These surgical openings are called an *ileostomy* or *colostomy,* depending on which part of the intestinal tract is used to create the stoma (Figs. 37.2 and 37.3). Newer surgical techniques allow more patients to have portions of their small and large intestine removed and the remaining portions to be reconnected so that they can continue to defecate through the anal canal.

The location of an ostomy determines stool consistency. The more intestine remaining, the more formed and normal the stool. For example, an ileostomy bypasses the entire large intestine, creating frequent, liquid stools. A person with a sigmoid colostomy has a more formed stool.

Loop ostomies are performed on an emergency basis and are reversible stomas that may be constructed in the ileum or the colon. The surgeon pulls a loop of intestine onto the abdomen and places a plastic rod, bridge, or rubber catheter temporarily under the bowel loop to keep it from slipping back. The surgeon then opens the bowel and sutures it to the skin of the abdomen. The loop ostomy has two openings through the stoma. The proximal end drains fecal effluent, and the distal portion drains mucus.

An end colostomy consists of a stoma formed by bringing a piece of intestine out through a surgically created opening in the abdominal wall, turning it down like a turtleneck and suturing it to the abdominal wall (see Fig. 37.2). The intestine distal to the stoma is either removed or sewn closed (called *Hartmann pouch*) and left in the abdominal cavity. End ostomies may be permanent or reversible. The rectum may be left intact or removed.

Managing a stoma that produces frequent passage of liquid stool (e.g., an ileostomy) can be challenging. Skin protection is important because of the liquid and caustic nature of the output, which may cause irritant dermatitis. The more common peristomal skin problems are contact dermatitis, fungal infections, or folliculitis (Salvadalena, 2016). An ostomy is managed with an odor-proof pouch with a skin barrier surrounding the stoma. Empty the pouch when it is $\frac{1}{3}$ to $\frac{1}{2}$ full. If the pouch becomes full of gas, open the pouch and expel the air. Change the pouching system approximately every 3 to 7 days, depending on the patient's individual needs.

Other Diversion Procedures. The ileoanal pouch anastomosis is a surgical procedure that is an option for some patients who need to undergo a colectomy (removal of the colon) for treatment of ulcerative colitis or familial polyposis. In this procedure the colon is removed, a pouch is created from the end of the small intestine, and the pouch is attached to the anus (Fig. 37.4). The ileoanal pouch provides for collection of waste material in a fashion similar to that of the rectum. The patient is continent of stool because stool evacuates via the anus. When surgeons create the ileal pouch, they also make a temporary ileostomy to allow the pouch anastomosis to heal.

A continent ileostomy involves creating a pouch from the small intestine. This procedure is rarely done now; however, some patients may have had this procedure in the past. The pouch has a continent stoma on the abdomen created with a valve that can be drained only when the patient places a large catheter into the stoma. The patient empties the pouch several times a day.

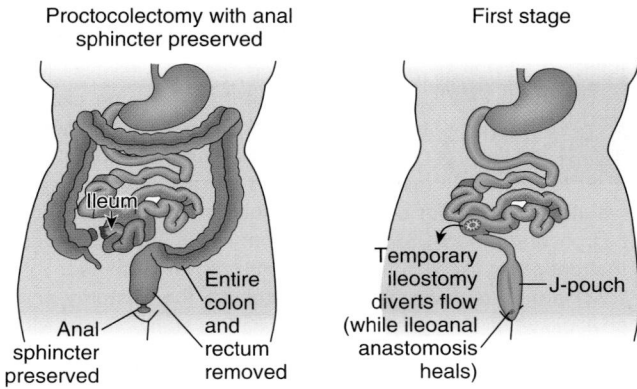

FIG 37.4 Ileal pouch anal anastomosis.

CRITICAL THINKING

Synthesis

Patient care requires you to apply what you know about a patient, your knowledge base, experience, and critical thinking attitudes and standards. Your synthesis of this information allows you to make sound decisions as you apply the nursing process. Critical thinking synthesis involves combining all available information to obtain a clear picture of the approach needed to provide patient-centered care (Box 37.4).

Knowledge. Reflect on knowledge regarding normal anatomy and physiology of the GI tract and specific GI alterations. This information helps you more accurately focus your nursing assessment and identify alterations when they exist. Even insignificant alterations in bowel elimination produce significant health problems for patients. For example, diarrhea often leads to electrolyte imbalances, dehydration, and rectal soreness.

Abdominal pain is one of the most common reports of patients who seek health care. Apply knowledge of the nature of pain (see Chapter 34) and pain assessment to analyze elimination problems. This helps to determine if the pain causes the symptoms associated with altered bowel elimination or if the bowel elimination problem results in pain or discomfort.

Bowel disorders affect a patient's body image and can cause embarrassment, a change in social habits, and general discomfort. It is important that you apply the knowledge from the psychosocial sciences and communication to understand and consider the psychological aspects associated with these diseases to provide patient-centered care.

The intake of certain foods reflects a patient's culture or beliefs. Foods in various cultures have different status relating to religion, availability, cost, and tradition. Understand the patient's cultural heritage and the role diet plays in health promotion and maintenance (see Chapters 21 and 35). When caring for patients from other cultures and ethnic groups, modifications of care are frequent, particularly when you care for patients' elimination needs (Box 37.5).

BOX 37.4 **SYNTHESIS IN PRACTICE**

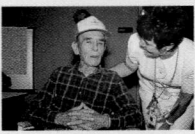

As Vickie prepares to assess Mr. Gutierrez, she reflects back on experiences with other patients in the home setting. She recalled one patient in particular who had elimination problems resulting from a diet consisting mainly of high-fat and high-carbohydrate foods. She believes that her involvement with that patient is likely to help in the care of Mr. Gutierrez.

Vickie also reviews her class notes on the anatomy and physiology of the gastrointestinal (GI) system. Given Mr. Gutierrez's age, Vickie reviews the physiological changes that aging produces within the digestive system. These changes include loss of teeth, taste bud atrophy, decreased secretion of gastric acid, and a slight decrease in small intestine motility.

Vickie thoroughly assesses Mr. Gutierrez's dietary intake by using a 24-hour diet recall. Being familiar with Mr. Gutierrez's Hispanic heritage, Vickie anticipates certain food preferences and needs to assess these. She knows that Mr. Gutierrez does not like the food served at the long-term care center and frequently requests "home-cooked" tortillas and green chili peppers from his niece.

The symptoms that Mr. Gutierrez exhibits (i.e., no bowel movement in 2 days and a feeling of bloating) are associated with several different problems. Vickie plans a thorough and precise assessment, being sure to rule out any abdominal discomfort or other symptoms expected from elimination problems. Because problems with bowel elimination have been an ongoing concern for Mr. Gutierrez, Vickie uses her assessment to identify nursing diagnoses and outline goals of care. She needs to avoid preconceived ideas regarding constipation in older adults. She must remain open to all the possibilities concerning changes in GI functioning.

BOX 37.5 **PATIENT-CENTERED CARE**

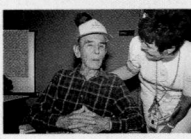

As Vickie prepares to care for Mr. Gutierrez, she learns that people from different cultures have different beliefs and practices. She knows that Mr. Gutierrez observes many of his cultural practices, and it is important that she understand early in his care how his culture and customs may impact the care plan. Elimination needs are very personal, and Vickie knows that she needs to respect and be sensitive to her patient's elimination practices.

IMPLICATIONS FOR PRACTICE

- When assisting a patient with bowel elimination needs or if the patient has an ostomy, accommodate the need for gender-congruent care if a patient expresses modesty and a need for privacy. Learn each patient's expectations.
- For all patients the presence and care of an ostomy presents unique challenges. New ostomies require monitoring and observation. A patient's cultural orientation may make the procedure more invasive and embarrassing.
- Most patients consider bowel and urinary secretions as not fit for public display. However, for some patients exposure of the lower torso is considered very private as well. Exposing the lower torso is necessary for ostomy care and may make the care and patient education more embarrassing. Covering as much of this area as possible and providing privacy by closing curtains and doors is important in decreasing this discomfort.
- Provide for distinct hygienic practices observed by certain cultures that designate the left hand to perform unclean procedures such as bowel elimination. Wash your hands thoroughly before touching the patient.
- Promote patients' understanding of the procedure to be done. Apply health literacy principles.
- Use an interpreter if needed.
- Repeat explanations because patients' anxiety about the loss of privacy can pose a distraction.

Experience. Elimination alterations are common for many patients who seek health care. In the acute care environment numerous variables including diet changes, medications, fluid restrictions, decreased activity, and diagnostic tests and surgery cause major alterations to bowel function. You provide better care to patients by reflecting on your previous experiences involving patients with similar alterations and lifestyle habits affecting elimination.

Attitudes. Apply all the attitudes of critical thinking when caring for patients with elimination problems (see Chapter 8). Creativity and perseverance come into play when patients need adjustments in their diet and exercise planning or when caring for patients with an intestinal diversion. Perseverance is also important in selecting effective diet therapies or finding the right medication regimen for patients with constipation or diarrhea. Confidence is an important factor in providing care to patients with bowel diversions or resections. Often these patients are very ill and in significant pain. Your confidence with moving and positioning a patient, managing ostomy care, and managing pain places the patient at ease and promotes their recovery.

Standards. To establish regular bowel habits, patients require consistency in bowel care and training for self-management. It is possible to establish regular bowel habits by setting standards for appropriate nutritional and elimination support. For example, the Association for Parenteral and Enteral Nutrition (ASPEN) has specific guidelines for nutritional support (see Chapter 35). The Wound, Ostomy and Continence Nurses Society (Goldberg et al., 2016) has specific standards for ostomy care. Regardless of age or disease state, maintenance of bowel function and integrity is essential to well-being.

When assessing a patient's abdominal pain, make sure that your findings are reported and documented clearly, accurately, and in a timely manner. Although the intellectual standards for critical thinking apply to all symptoms, thorough pain assessment is difficult because it is subjective in nature but essential. Numerous problems are detectable based on the nature of abdominal pain. Collaborate with health care providers as you assess your patients and identify appropriate plans of care.

Patients with alterations in bowel elimination, especially incontinence, are frequently embarrassed and need to be treated with respect by all health care providers. It is your responsibility to ensure that each patient's privacy is carefully protected and their physical care is provided in a respectful, competent, and timely manner.

NURSING PROCESS

The needs and problems of patients experiencing alterations in bowel elimination are distinct and numerous. Incorporate a caring approach and use appropriate communication techniques throughout the nursing process.

■■■ ASSESSMENT

Assessment of bowel elimination requires you to focus on any problems a patient has affecting the GI system. A patient's ability to chew food, recent intake of both solids and liquids, personal eating habits, and level of stress all influence bowel function. Include this information in your assessment.

Health History. Remember that each individual defines "normal (usual) bowel habits" uniquely and differently. Apply this knowledge in preparing questions for the patient interview to determine the presence and extent of GI alterations. Family members are usually helpful if the patient is unable to provide necessary information. Organize the nursing history around factors that affect bowel elimination including the following (Ball et al., 2015):

1. Determine your patient's usual pattern of bowel elimination. Usual frequency and time of day are important, but also determine if any changes in elimination patterns have occurred. Ask the patient why he or she thinks the bowel elimination change occurred. Get the patient's description of usual stool characteristics. Determine if the stool is normally watery or formed and soft or hard and the typical color. Ask the patient to describe the shape of a normal stool and the number of stools per day. Use a scale such as the Bristol Stool Form Scale to obtain an objective measure of stool characteristics (Blake et al., 2016) (Fig. 37.5).

2. Identify specific routines followed to promote normal elimination and manage constipation (e.g., drinking warm liquids, taking laxatives or enemas, eating specific foods, or trying to defecate at the same time each day). Ask how often the patient uses these strategies. If your patient uses an appropriate routine, consider incorporating the routine in your plan of care.

3. Determine if patient has an ostomy. Assess the frequency of fecal drainage, character of feces, type of pouching system used, and which routine of care works well for the patient.

4. Identify changes in appetite. Include changes in your patient's eating patterns and a change in weight, either

The Bristol Stool Form Scale

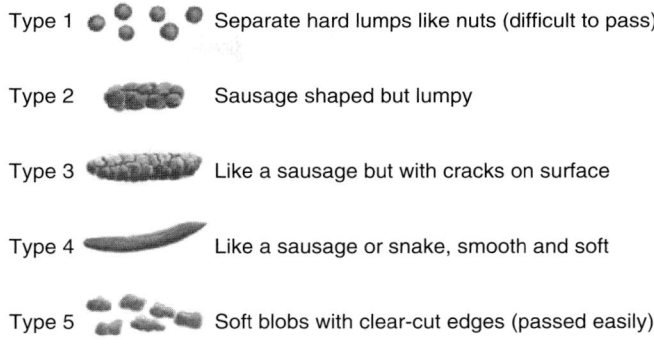

Type 1   Separate hard lumps like nuts (difficult to pass)

Type 2   Sausage shaped but lumpy

Type 3   Like a sausage but with cracks on surface

Type 4   Like a sausage or snake, smooth and soft

Type 5   Soft blobs with clear-cut edges (passed easily)

Type 6   Fluffy pieces with ragged edges, a mushy stool

Type 7   Watery, no solid pieces (entirely liquid)

FIG 37.5 Bristol Stool Form Scale. (Used with permission. *Bristol Stool Form Scale guideline,* 2013, http://aboutconstipation. org/site/about-constipation/treatment/stool-form-guide.)

loss or gain. If a change in weight is reported, inquire if the patient planned the weight change such as weight loss with a diet.

5. Gather a diet history including the patient's dietary preferences. Is mealtime regular or irregular? Does the patient eat certain foods infrequently? This enables you to determine the intake of grains, fruits, meats, and vegetables.

6. Obtain a daily fluid intake including the type and amount of fluid. Have the patient estimate the amount using common household measurements. Ask the patient to give you a 24-hour diet recall during your assessment. You may also want to ask the patient to complete a 72-hour food intake diary for the next visit.

7. Obtain a history of surgery or illnesses affecting the GI tract. This information often helps to explain if a patient has the ability to maintain or restore normal elimination patterns and if there is a family history of cancer involving the GI tract (Box 37.6).

8. Review patient's medications, including over-the-counter and herbal medications or preparations. Does the patient take anything that could alter defecation or fecal characteristics?

9. Assess a patient's emotional state including tone of voice and mannerisms, which reveal significant behaviors indicating stress.

10. Assess a patient's exercise history, including a description of the type, frequency, and amount of daily exercise.

11. Gather a history of pain or discomfort. Ask the patient whether there is a history of abdominal or anal pain. The location and nature of pain help to locate the source of a problem (see Chapter 34).

12. If a patient reports diarrhea, determine the number of stools per day, the consistency, and how long the problem

BOX 37.6 SCREENING FOR COLORECTAL CANCER

RISK FACTORS (ACS, 2017)

- Age: Older than 50
- Family history: Colorectal cancer, familial adenomatous polyposis, hereditary nonpolyposis colon cancer (Lynch syndrome)
- Personal history: Colorectal cancer or colorectal polyps, inflammatory bowel disease
- Race: African Americans have highest colon cancer rates
- Diet: High intake of animal fats or red meat and low intake of fruits and vegetables
- Obesity and physical inactivity
- Smoking and heavy alcohol consumption
- Type 2 diabetes

WARNING SIGNS

- Change in bowel habits (e.g., diarrhea, constipation, narrowing of stool lasting more than a few days)
- Rectal bleeding or blood in stool
- Sensation of incomplete evacuation
- Unexplained abdominal or back pain

AMERICAN CANCER SOCIETY SCREENING GUIDELINES FOR EARLY DETECTION OF COLORECTAL CANCER IN AVERAGE-RISK ASYMPTOMATIC PEOPLE[a]

Men and women 50 years of age and older[b]	Fecal occult blood test done on multiple samples at home	Annually starting at age 50[c]
	Fecal immunochemical test done on multiple samples at home	Annually starting at age 50[c]
	Flexible sigmoidoscopy	Every 5 years starting at age 50[c]
	Double-contrast barium enema	Every 5 years starting at age 50[c]
	Computed tomography, colonography	Every 5 years starting at age 50[c]
	Colonoscopy	Every 10 years starting at age 50

[a]These procedures are ordered by a health care provider depending on availability of resources and patient needs.
[b]Screening for high-risk individuals should begin earlier than 50 years of age. The American Cancer Society has specific recommendations at their website.
[c]Colonoscopy should be done if test results are positive.
Data from American Cancer Society (ACS): *American Cancer Society recommendations for colorectal cancer early detection,* 2017, http://www.cancer.org/cancer/colonandrectumcancer/moreinformation/colonandrectumcancerearlydetection/colorectal-cancer-early-detection-acs-recommendations.

has been present. Ask about causative factors such as recent illness, new medications, and dietary changes or travel outside the country in the past month. Assess for signs and symptoms of dehydration.

13. Assess the patient's mobility and dexterity. Determine your patient's ability to toilet independently or whether the patient needs assistive devices. Does the patient rely on a family caregiver in the home?

Older Adult Considerations. When assessing older adults, know and understand the changes that occur because of the aging process. Nurses often do not acknowledge an older adult's problems with intestinal elimination as an important consideration in their care. Remember that what appears at the outset to be a trivial complaint may be a significant problem physically and/or psychologically.

Physical Assessment. Assess the status of GI function to detect factors that affect elimination. Focus your patient assessment to identify problems associated with bowel elimination (Table 37.2). Conduct an examination of the oral cavity, abdomen, and external anal opening. If fecal impaction is suspected, a rectal examination may be done (see Chapter 16). When a digital examination is necessary, inspect the fecal material on the glove for several characteristics (Table 37.3). If there are no feces on the glove, ask the patient to describe a typical stool, noting recent changes. The patient or family caregiver is the most knowledgeable about changes. Also determine if the patient passes a large amount of gas or little gas.

Laboratory and Diagnostic Examinations

Laboratory Tests. There are no blood tests to specifically diagnose most GI disorders, but hemoglobin and hematocrit may be done to determine if anemia from GI bleeding is present. Liver function tests and serum amylase to assess for hepatobiliary diseases and pancreatitis may be ordered.

Fecal Specimens. Analysis of fecal contents detects alterations in GI functioning. Careful handling of a specimen is important to prevent exposure to infectious microorganisms. Follow standard precautions (see Chapter 14) when collecting and sending specimens to the laboratory. A patient is often capable of obtaining the specimen without assistance if properly instructed. Make sure that the patient understands not to mix feces with urine or water. The patient defecates into a clean, dry bedpan or special container placed under the toilet seat.

Laboratory tests for blood in the stool, ova and parasites, and stool cultures require only a small sample. Blood in the stool or melena causes stool to turn black and sticky like tar—hence the term *tarry stools*. Collect approximately 1 inch of formed stool or 15 to 30 mL of liquid diarrhea stool. Tests for measuring the output of fecal fat require a patient to collect stools for 3 to 5 days. You need to save all fecal material throughout the test period. Stool specimen tests for ova and parasites may require a chemical fixative. Fresh specimens are best for revealing parasites or larvae; therefore collected specimens should be taken directly to the laboratory for immediate examination. A stool culture to test for bacteria in the feces should also go to the laboratory quickly for the most accurate result.

After obtaining a specimen, tightly seal the container, place in the proper biohazard bag, complete laboratory requisition forms at the patient's bedside, and record all specimen collections in the patient's medical record. Avoid delays in sending specimens to the laboratory. Some tests require

TABLE 37.2 FOCUSED PATIENT ASSESSMENT

FACTORS TO ASSESS	QUESTIONS	PHYSICAL ASSESSMENT
Chewing	Do you have difficulty chewing? Do you have any mouth pain? Do you wear any dental devices such as dentures or partial replacement of teeth?	Inspect condition of teeth, tongue, gums, and mouth. Observe for fit of dentures or other dental devices, observing for sores or pressure areas from these devices. Observe patient eating meal; determine patient's ability to eat all types of foods.

Mobility	In Ambulatory Patients
	   Do you exercise regularly?
	   How often do you exercise?
	   What type of exercise do you do?
	   How active are you?
	 For Patients With Restricted Mobility
	   Are you able to use the toilet independently?
	   How much help do you need for toileting?
		Observe patient's gait.
		 Observe patient's ability to help with transfer, sit down on and get up from toilet, and activity.

Abdomen	Do you have gas, feel bloated, or have any pain or discomfort? Can you point to the area of pain or discomfort on your abdomen? Is the pain or discomfort always in the same place?	Observe all four abdominal quadrants, noting the presence of scars, masses, venous patterns, stomas, lesions, and peristaltic waves. Auscultate all four quadrants for the presence of bowel sounds; note if sounds are normal (gurgling), absent, or abnormal (high-pitched, or tinkling). Gently palpate all four quadrants, noting areas of distention, masses, or pain. When pain is present, note location.
Anal sphincter function	Can you feel if you are distended?	Inspect anal sphincter at rest and perform digital examination while asking patient to contract and relax sphincter. **Note:** A small amount of stool is normal; large amount of stool or hard stool indicates impaired emptying of bowel.

TABLE 37.3 FECAL CHARACTERISTICS

CHARACTERISTIC	NORMAL	ABNORMAL	ABNORMAL CAUSE
Color	Infant: Yellow Adult: Brown	White or clay Black or tarry (melena) Red Pale and oily	Absence of bile Iron ingestion or GI bleeding GI bleeding, hemorrhoids, ingestion of beets Malabsorption of fat
Odor	Malodorous; may be affected by certain foods	Noxious change	Blood in feces or infection
Consistency	Soft, formed	Liquid Hard	Diarrhea, reduced absorption Constipation
Frequency	Varies: Infant 4–6 times daily (breastfed) or 1–3 times daily (bottle-fed) Adult twice daily to 3 times a week	Infant more than 6 times daily or less than once every 1 to 2 days Adult more than 3 times a day or less than once a week	Hypermotility or hypomotility
Shape	Resembles diameter of rectum	Narrow, pencil shaped	Obstruction, increased peristalsis
Constituents	Undigested food, dead bacteria, fat, bile pigment, cells lining intestinal mucosa, water	Blood, pus, foreign bodies, mucus, worms Oily stool Mucus	Internal bleeding, infection, swallowed objects, irritation, inflammation, infestation of parasites Malabsorption syndrome, enteritis, pancreatic disease, surgical resection of intestine Intestinal irritation, inflammation, infection, or injury

GI, Gastrointestinal.

the stool to be warm. When stool specimens stand at room temperature, bacteria can grow in the specimen and alter test results.

A **fecal occult blood test (FOBT)**, or guaiac test, measures microscopic amounts of blood in the feces (Box 37.7). It is a useful screening test for colon cancer as recommended by the American Cancer Society (ACS) but is not conclusive, as other GI disorders can also cause bleeding (see Box 37.6). Two types of FOBT are approved by the U.S. Food and Drug Administration (FDA) to screen for colorectal cancer (NCI, 2016). With both types of FOBT, stool samples are typically collected by a patient using a kit, and the samples are returned to the doctor:

- The guaiac FOBT uses a chemical to detect heme, a component of the blood protein hemoglobin. Because the guaiac FOBT can also detect heme in some foods (e.g., red meat), certain foods need to be avoided before having this test.
- The fecal immunochemical test (FIT) uses antibodies to detect human hemoglobin protein specifically. Dietary restrictions are typically not required for FIT.

You or the patient need to repeat an FOBT test at least 3 times on three separate bowel movements while the patient refrains from ingesting foods and medications that cause a false-positive or false-negative result. The FOBT is done in the patient's home or health care provider's office. All positive tests should be followed up with flexible sigmoidoscopy or colonoscopy (ACS, 2017).

Instruct patients who are going to have an FBOT to avoid eating red meat for 3 days before testing. Although the health care provider should be consulted before asking a patient to stop any medication, if there are no contraindications the patient should be instructed to stop taking aspirin, ibuprofen, naproxen, or other nonsteroidal antiinflammatory drugs for 7 days because these could cause a false-positive test result. Vitamin C supplements and citrus fruits and juices should be stopped 3 days before the test because they can cause a false-negative result (ACS, 2017).

Diagnostic Examinations. Various radiological and diagnostic tests are used in patients experiencing alterations in the GI system (Box 37.8). Some of these examinations such as a **colonoscopy** require bowel preparation (bowel prep) for the test to be completed successfully. A bowel cleansing program usually includes a clear liquid diet and several types of laxatives taken for 12 to 24 hours before the test. It may be difficult or unpleasant for a patient, and the nurse needs to explain the importance of having the intestine free of fecal contents so that the provider doing the test can see any abnormalities or indications of disease. The nurse may want to remind the patient that completing the bowel cleansing program as directed will ensure optimal test results and avoid the possibility that the bowel cleansing program and test may have to be repeated at a later date.

Patient Expectations. When you assess a patient's expectations of care, always anticipate the patient's need for privacy and respect it. Bowel elimination problems are embarrassing for some patients. Ask the patient what is important to ensure that you give care in a personal and professional way.

When determining a patient's expectations, consider his or her normal bowel pattern. Some patients wish to have activities planned to maintain their normal routines. If what is "normal" to a patient is unhealthy or promotes negative health practices, educate the patient and work with him or her to adopt healthier routines. Because there is a direct link between nutrition and bowel elimination, consider the patient's cultural choices of foods and fluids. Sometimes the patient has to determine whether or not to consume favorite or special foods that cause symptoms. Methods of preparation are also a concern, especially if tradition, access, and cost are deciding factors.

■ ■ ■ ■ NURSING DIAGNOSIS

Gather data from the nursing assessment, validate the data, and analyze clusters of defining characteristics and risk factors to identify relevant nursing diagnoses. Reflecting on each of your data sources is necessary to determine the correct diagnosis. Defining characteristics and risk factors identified during your assessment often apply to more than

---

BOX 37.7 PROCEDURAL GUIDELINES

Measuring Fecal Occult Blood

DELEGATION CONSIDERATIONS

The skill of testing stool for occult blood can be delegated to nursing assistive personnel (NAP). The nurse is responsible for assessing the significance of the findings. The nurse informs the NAP to:

- Report immediately if blood is detected and not to discard stool from a positive test so the nurse may repeat the testing.

EQUIPMENT

Soap, water, washcloth, and towel; paper towel; clean gloves; wooden applicators; guaiac fecal occult blood test (gFOBT) kit or immunochemical fecal occult blood test (iFOBT, or FIT) kit

STEPS

1. If nurse is performing test: Identify patient using at least two identifiers (e.g., name and birthday or name and medical record number) according to agency policy.
2. Assess patient's or family member's understanding of need for stool test.
3. Explain procedure to patient and/or family member. Discuss reason for specimen collection and how patient can help or perform. Explain that feces must be free of urine and toilet tissue.
4. Perform hand hygiene and apply clean gloves.

BOX 37.7 PROCEDURAL GUIDELINES—cont'd

View Video!

Measuring Fecal Occult Blood

5. Use tip of wooden applicator to obtain small portion of feces. Obtain uncontaminated stool specimen and place in clean, dry container not contaminated with urine, water, or toilet tissue.

6. Measure for occult blood.
   a. **To perform gFOBT test:**
      (1) Open flap of test slide. Apply thin smear of stool on paper in first box.
      (2) Obtain second fecal specimen from different portion of stool and apply thinly to second box of slide (see illustration).
      (3) Close slide cover and turn slide over to reverse side. Open cardboard flap and apply 2 drops of developing solution on each box of guaiac paper (see illustration).
      (4) Read results of test after 30 to 60 seconds. Note color changes.
      (5) Dispose of test slide in proper receptacle.
   b. **To perform immunochemical fecal occult blood test (iFOBT or FIT):**
      (1) Read manufacturer's directions.
      (2) Use special spoon or other device provided in kit to collect a sample of stool.
      (3) Place in collection container that comes with the test kit.

7. If patient performs gFOBT or FIT test at home:
   a. Have patient flush the toilet before having a bowel movement.
   b. After passing stool, have patient put the used toilet paper in the waste bag provided. DO NOT put it into the toilet bowl.
      (1) gFOBT test: Have patient collect a stool sample from each of two or three bowel movements in a clean container, usually on consecutive days. Use the applicator stick to apply a smear of stool to a specific area of the test card. After the samples are dry, have patient return them to their doctor (directly or by mail).
      (2) FIT test: Have patient use the brush from the kit to brush the surface of the stool, and then dip the brush into the toilet water. Touch the brush on the space indicated on the test card. Add the brush to the waste bag and throw it away. Have patient return test card to doctor (directly or by mail).

Clinical Decision Point. Instruct patient to not perform test if patient has bleeding hemorrhoids; there is blood in the urine; it is during or within 3 days of menstrual period; there is any bleeding cuts or wounds on patient's hands; the test card has passed its expiration date; the test kit is damaged, dirty, or appears to have been tampered with in any way; or toilet water is saltwater or rusty.

---

8. Wrap wooden applicator or collection device in paper towel, grasp in nondominant hand, remove gloves over wrapped applicator. Discard in proper receptacle. Perform hand hygiene.
9. Record the results of the test; note color changes in guaiac paper. Note character of stool specimen.
10. **Use Teach-Back:** "You will need to check your stool two more times for blood when you go home. I want to be sure I explained the procedure correctly. Please repeat the steps back to me." Revise your instruction now or develop a plan for revised patient/family caregiver teaching if patient/family caregiver is not able to teach back correctly.

Clinical Decision Point. A single positive test result does not confirm bleeding or indicate colorectal cancer. To confirm positive results, test must be repeated while patient is on meat-free, high-residue diet with more in-depth diagnosis (Van Leeuwen et al., 2015).

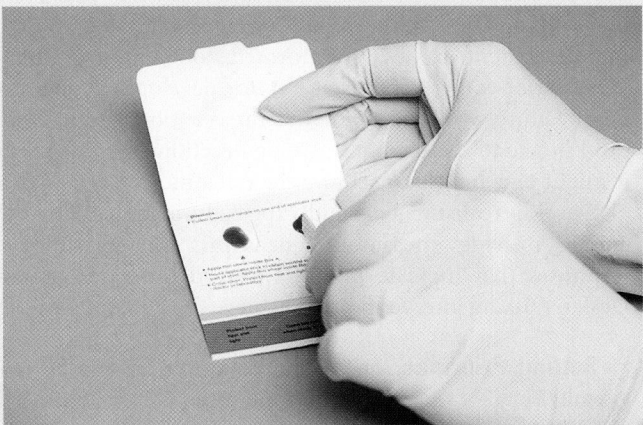

STEP 6a(2) Application of stool specimen to both spots on Hemoccult slide.

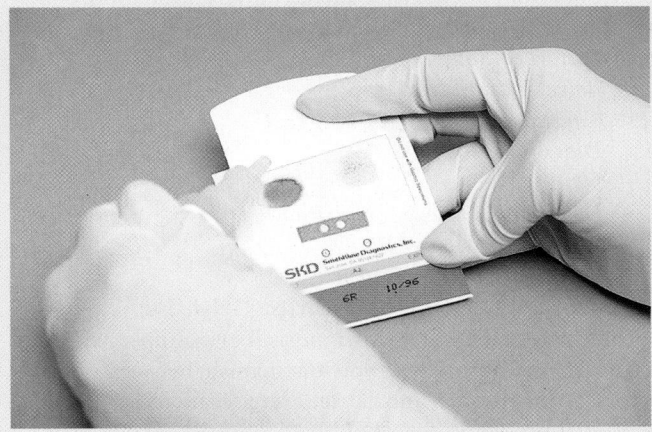

STEP 6a(3) Application of developing solution.

BOX 37.8 RADIOLOGICAL AND DIAGNOSTIC TESTS

DIRECT VISUALIZATION
Endoscopy
Examinations such as gastroscopy or colonoscopy use a lighted fiber optic tube to directly visualize the upper gastrointestinal (GI) tract (upper endoscopy) or large intestine (colonoscopy). The fiber optic tube contains a lens, forceps, and brushes for biopsy. If an endoscopy identifies a lesion such as a polyp, the polyp can be removed, and a biopsy will be done. These tests are done under sedation, usually in outpatient centers. Patients receive instructions about the preparation needed for the tests at the time they are scheduled for the procedure. Bowel preparation is necessary before a colonoscopy.

INDIRECT VISUALIZATION
Anorectal Manometry
Measures the pressure activity of internal and external anal sphincters and reflexes during rectal distention, relaxation during straining, and rectal sensation.

Plain Film of Abdomen/Kidneys, Ureter, Bladder (KUB)
Simple x-ray film of the abdomen requiring no preparation.

Barium Swallow/Enema
X-ray film examination using an opaque contrast medium (barium, which is swallowed) to examine the structure and motility of the upper GI tract including pharynx, esophagus, and stomach.

Barium instilled through the anal opening via an enema provides visualization of the structures of the lower GI tract. Usually a bowel preparation with laxatives is ordered before the procedure.

Ultrasound Imaging
Technique that uses high-frequency sound waves to echo off body organs, creating a picture of GI tract.

Computed Tomography (CT) Scan (Virtual Colonoscopy)
X-ray film examination of the body from many angles using a scanner analyzed by a computer. An oral contrast solution for the patient to drink may be ordered before the test. IV contrast solution may be injected during the test to improve visualization. This does not replace a colonoscopy because it does not allow for removal of polyps and biopsies.

Colonic Transit Study
A patient swallows a capsule containing radiopaque markers. The patient maintains a high-fiber diet for 5 days and refrains from medications that affect bowel function. On the fifth day x-ray film examination is performed.

Magnetic Resonance Imaging
Noninvasive examination that uses magnet and radio waves to produce a picture of the inside of the body.

---

one diagnosis; therefore be clinically skillful in determining patterns that reveal the diagnosis that best fits the patient's situation.

For example, a patient reports not having a bowel movement for several days. This defining characteristic applies to the problem-focused diagnoses of *Constipation* and *Perceived Constipation*. The difference is that on examination the patient with *Constipation* has a dry, hard stool with abdominal or rectal fullness. In contrast, the patient with *Perceived Constipation* has an expectation of having a stool daily when in fact the stools are normal. A variety of nursing diagnoses are relevant for patients with altered bowel elimination. Some examples are as follows (NANDA International, 2014):

- *Disturbed Body Image*
- *Bowel Incontinence*
- *Constipation*
- *Diarrhea*
- *Nausea*
- *Deficient Knowledge (Nutrition)*
- *Acute Pain*
- *Toileting Self-Care Deficit*

It is important to establish the correct "related to" factor for a problem-focused nursing diagnosis. For example, with the diagnosis of *Constipation* you distinguish between related factors of nutritional imbalance, exercise, medications, and emotional problems. Selection of the correct related factors for each diagnosis ensures that you implement the appropriate nursing interventions.

■■■ PLANNING

Goals and Outcomes. After you identify nursing diagnoses, determine how they are related to one another and to the patient's current status (Fig. 37.6). You and the patient set goals and expected outcomes to direct interventions. When possible these goals and outcomes incorporate the patient's elimination routines or habits as much as possible and reinforce routines that promote health. In addition, consider the patient's preexisting health concerns. For example, one method of reducing the risk for constipation is to achieve the goal of "establishing a normal defecation pattern" by increasing fluids and bulk in the patient's diet. An outcome would be that the patient "passes a soft, formed stool within 48 hours." However, if your patient is at risk for developing congestive heart failure, you will tailor the intervention of increasing fluid intake to the patient's cardiac function. For this reason it might take longer to achieve the outcome.

Develop realistic goals and expected outcomes. The outcomes provide measurable behaviors or physiological responses that indicate progress toward the goals of care. Design nursing interventions to achieve the outcomes of care.

Setting Priorities. Defecation patterns vary among individuals. For this reason, you and the patient work together to plan effective interventions to meet elimination needs and priorities (see Care Plan). A realistic time frame to establish a normal defecation pattern for one patient is sometimes very different for

CONCEPT MAP

Nursing Diagnosis: Constipation
- States "my bowels are locked up"
- Reports has not had a bowel movement in 2 days
- Stove is broken, and he has not been able to prepare rice or beans for 2 days

Interventions
- Consult with niece about getting Mr. Gutierrez's stove fixed
- Add bran flakes, bran, or fiber supplement to Mr. Gutierrez's diet
- Encourage Mr. Gutierrez to try to establish a routine time for defecation, preferably after breakfast or other meal

Nursing Diagnosis: Deficient Knowledge regarding diet
- Believes that eating green chili peppers every day will keep him healthy
- Diet consists of flour and corn tortillas with high intake of cheese and low intake of fruit
- Reports frequently taking laxatives
- Normally drinks about 800 mL of fluid a day

Interventions
- Educate Mr. Gutierrez about increasing fluids in his diet
- Instruct Mr. Gutierrez to drink eight 8-oz glasses of fluids per day
- Help Mr. Gutierrez develop a weekly meal plan that includes well-balanced meals with increased fiber
- Instruct Mr. Gutierrez on proper use of laxatives

Primary Health Problem: Constipation
Priority Assessments: Bowel elimination pattern, abdomen, comfort, dietary history

Nursing Diagnosis: Impaired Comfort
- Reports feeling "all gassed up"
- Reports not having "passed wind" for 2 days
- States has not felt like eating today
- Abdomen slightly distended

Interventions
- Teach Mr. Gutierrez to lie on his left side with knees flexed
- Encourage Mr. Gutierrez to increase his daily walking
- Have patient avoid foods that produce gas

Nursing Diagnosis: Dysfunctional Gastrointestinal Motility
- Hard, brown stool 2 days ago
- Abdomen slightly distended

Interventions
- Teach Mr. Gutierrez about time frame for resolution of constipation
- Encourage Mr. Gutierrez to increase his daily walking
- Instruct Mr. Gutierrez to discuss laxative use with health care provider

——— Link between medical diagnosis and nursing diagnosis   - - - - Link between nursing diagnoses

FIG 37.6 Concept map.

◎ CARE PLAN

Constipation

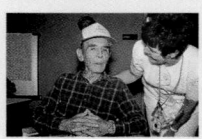

ASSESSMENT

Vickie and Mr. Gutierrez have been able to communicate without difficulty. Mr. Gutierrez complains of feeling "full of gas" but has not "passed any wind" in the last 2 days. His stove has not been working well, and he has been unable to prepare rice and beans.

ASSESSMENT ACTIVITIES

Determine when Mr. Gutierrez had his last bowel movement.
Determine Mr. Gutierrez's medication history.
Establish Mr. Gutierrez's dietary habits.

FINDINGS[a]

Mr. Gutierrez had his **last bowel movement 2 days ago. The stool was brown in color and hard.** "I took a laxative last night, and I think I need an enema."
A medication history shows that Mr. Gutierrez **frequently resorts to taking laxatives.**
Mr. Gutierrez eats a high intake of corn tortillas and cheese and a low intake of fruits. He drinks about 800 mL of fluid daily. Mr. Gutierrez also states, "I really haven't felt like eating today and have not eaten much for the last 4 days, and I need to move my bowels."

[a]**Defining characteristics/risk factors** are shown in **bold** type.

NURSING DIAGNOSIS: Constipation related to less than adequate fluid and dietary intake and chronic laxative use

---

PLANNING

GOAL

Mr. Gutierrez will establish and maintain a normal defecation pattern within 1 month.

Mr. Gutierrez will identify practices that reduce risk for or prevent constipation within 2 weeks.

EXPECTED OUTCOMES (NOC)[b]

Bowel Elimination
Mr. Gutierrez has a bowel movement within 48 hours.
Mr. Gutierrez's abdomen is soft, nondistended, and nontender within 24 hours.
Mr. Gutierrez passes soft, formed stools at least every 2 days.

Nutritional Status: Food and Fluid Intake
Mr. Gutierrez identifies need to increase the fiber content of his diet within 1 week.
Mr. Gutierrez discontinues laxative use and uses fiber supplements when needed.
Mr. Gutierrez identifies need to drink eight 8-ounce glasses of fluids a day within 3 days.

[b]Outcomes classification labels from Moorhead S, et al, editors: *Nursing outcomes classification (NOC)*, ed 5, St Louis, 2013, Mosby.

INTERVENTIONS (NIC)[c]

Constipation/Impaction Management

Instruct Mr. Gutierrez in a weekly menu plan including foods high in fiber: brown rice, beans and rice, tomatoes, and wheat tortillas.

Add wheat bran quinoa, vegetables high in insoluble fiber, or fiber supplement such as psyllium to Mr. Gutierrez's diet.

Consult with Mr. Gutierrez's niece and long-term care center to have his stove repaired.

Educate Mr. Gutierrez about use of liquids to promote softening of stool and defecation.

Encourage Mr. Gutierrez to establish a routine time for defecation (e.g., after breakfast or other meal).

RATIONALE

High-fiber foods increase the bulk of the fecal contents and add water to the stool.

Insoluble fiber foods increase peristalsis and improve the movement of intestinal contents through the gastrointestinal tract (Steele et al., 2016).

Cooking facilities are necessary for preparation of selected food preferences.

Fluids help to keep fecal mass soft and increase stool bulk, creating a laxative effect (Steele et al., 2016).

With aging there may be some normal changes in rectal sensation, and the body needs larger volumes to elicit the sensation to defecate. The normal mass-movement response to eating, which results in movement of colon contents approximately 1 hour after a meal, helps to establish routine bowel habits (Steele et al., 2016).

[c]Intervention classification labels from Bulechek GM, et al, editors: *Nursing interventions classification (NIC)*, ed 6, St Louis, 2013, Mosby.

CARE PLAN—cont'd

Constipation

EVALUATION

NURSING ACTIONS	PATIENT RESPONSE/FINDING	ACHIEVEMENT OF OUTCOME
Review Mr. Gutierrez's diary of foods and ask him about his intake.	Mr. Gutierrez describes likes and dislikes but admits to eating high-fat foods and few fruits and vegetables. Fluid intake averages 1400 mL daily for a week.	Mr. Gutierrez's intake of high-fiber foods is still limited. Fluid intake is improving.
Ask Mr. Gutierrez about his pattern of elimination over the last 2 weeks and laxative use.	Mr. Gutierrez says, "I'm not having so much trouble going." He states that he thinks he now goes about every 2 days.	He has bowel movements approximately every 2 days. He is successfully avoiding use of laxatives.
During follow-up visit examine Mr. Gutierrez's abdomen and observe stool (if possible).	Mr. Gutierrez has not used any laxatives for a week. Patient reports that stool is formed but is "not hard like before." Abdomen is soft and nontender with no distention.	Stool is softer. His abdomen is less distended.

another. In addition, if the patient has a new ostomy resulting from cancer, the priority of coping with cancer and its treatment precedes the patient's need to become independent in managing the care of the bowel diversion. In addition, when a bowel diversion is necessary, coping with changes in body image is a high priority for both the patient and the family.

Collaborative Care. Other health care team members are important resources for the patient and family. You sometimes refer a patient with chronic constipation to a dietitian to plan a nutritionally balanced diet that incorporates the patient's food preferences and lifestyle. Involving the family in the plan of care is important. When patients are disabled or debilitated, family members often become the primary caregivers. Patient and family education is important to promote understanding of ways to establish normal bowel function. If access to proper nutrition is a concern, referrals to community organizations that deliver meals to the home (e.g., Meals on Wheels and church groups) or provide transportation for patients are beneficial.

A clinical nurse specialist or wound, ostomy, and continence nurse specialist provides guidance in the care and management of ostomies and problems involving incontinence or skin breakdown. Use professionals from a variety of health care disciplines to provide safe, effective care.

■■■ IMPLEMENTATION

Health Promotion. Factors that normally promote bowel elimination are appropriate interventions for helping patients develop normal bowel habits. It is important to teach your patient about the benefits and effects of a balanced diet, regular exercise, and stress management and how to integrate each into a bowel routine. Teach your patients to develop a routine time for bowel evacuation. A good time is after a morning or evening meal when your patient does not feel rushed. Establishing a consistent time for bowel hygiene is just one practice to avoid constipation (Box 37.9).

Diet. A well-balanced diet that includes several servings of fruits and vegetables and whole grain foods daily and an

BOX 37.9 HEALTH PROMOTION

Bowel Hygiene

Helping patients and their families in healthy food selection and preparation practices reduces the risks of gastrointestinal (GI) disorders. There is increasing evidence that weight control with a body mass index of 25 or below; a diet rich in fruits, vegetables, and whole grains and low in fat and red meat; and daily exercise reduce risk for colorectal cancers, digestive diseases, and other cancers (ACS, 2017). Consider whether a patient is able to afford the foods recommended. In addition to solid foods, a patient with elimination problems needs to drink 1.5 to 2 L of fluids daily if not contraindicated by other medical conditions.

APPLICATION TO NURSING PRACTICE

- Recommend fluid intake of at least 1.5 L per day.
- Teach patients to limit alcohol because of its diuretic properties and not to count any alcoholic beverage as part of their daily intake of fluids.
- Suggest a high-fiber diet (25 to 30 g per day) to reduce constipation; as fiber passes through the colon, it retains fluid. As a result, bulkier and softer stools develop. In addition, the waste moves through the colon more easily and results in more regular bowel movements.
- Teach patients to use a combination of insoluble and soluble fiber (e.g., bran, fruits, and vegetables) to prevent constipation.
- Assess patient's ability to afford foods.
- Encourage physical activity in combination with adequate fluid intake and high-fiber diet to manage constipation. Walking once or twice a day for 30 minutes is sufficient.
- Explain need to use laxatives with caution. A stepwise progression of laxatives is recommended: first bulk-forming laxatives, followed by stool softeners and osmotic stimulants. Use suppositories and/or enemas if diet, fluid, and laxative regimen is not successful.

adequate fluid intake (1.5 to 2 L/day) promotes normal bowel function. Patients with colostomies have no diet restrictions based on their food tolerance. A patient with an ileostomy may need a low-residue diet (see Chapter 35) if he or she has a high output of fecal effluent. A good reminder for ostomy patients is to encourage drinking an 8-ounce glass of fluid when they empty their pouches. Patients with GI disorders or food intolerances need the help of a dietitian to devise a diet that meets their specific needs and promotes normal bowel function.

Exercise. An age-specific exercise program also helps patients maintain a healthy bowel pattern. Regular exercise such as walking, biking, or swimming daily promotes normal GI motility (Steele et al., 2016). Have patients who experience any level of immobilization from illness ambulate as soon as possible within the activity restrictions set by the health care provider (see Chapter 28).

Timing and Privacy. An important habit you teach your patients regarding bowel habits is to take time for defecation. Ignoring the urge and not taking time to defecate completely are common causes of constipation. To establish regular bowel habits, a patient needs to respond to the urge to defecate. Prompt response helps the patient reduce episodes of constipation.

Defecation is most likely to occur after meals. If a patient attempts to defecate during the time when mass colonic peristalsis occurs, the chances of successfully evacuating the rectum are greater. If a patient is restricted to bed or requires assistance in ambulating, recommend use of a bedside commode or a bedpan or have a caregiver help the patient reach the bathroom. Patients need prompt assistance before the urge disappears.

Some patients have previously established routines to promote defecation. When patients are hospitalized, health promotion habits become disrupted. Encourage patients to maintain as many of their regular practices as possible. Privacy is often a concern for patients. Health care providers should knock before entering a patient's room. Privacy curtains should be used, especially for patients who reside in semiprivate rooms or shared living areas. Remain acutely aware of the patient's need for modesty and privacy.

Promotion of Normal Defecation. To help patients evacuate contents normally and without discomfort, recommend interventions that stimulate the defecation reflex or increase peristalsis. Helping a patient into an upright sitting position increases pressure on the rectum and facilitates use of intraabdominal muscles. Patients who have had surgery or have muscular weakness or mobility limitations benefit from the use of elevated toilet seats. Regular toilets may be too low for patients to lower themselves to a sitting position because of pain or altered mobility. With an elevated seat the patient exerts less effort to sit and stand.

Acute Care. When patients become acutely ill the GI system is often affected. Simple changes in activity levels, sleeping patterns, diet, and medications directly affect regular bowel habits. Surgical intervention creates additional elimination problems for the patient in acute care (e.g., discomfort from an abdominal incision, absent or decreased GI peristalsis, or increased accumulation of intestinal gas following surgery). Whenever possible help the patient to the toilet or bedside commode and allow for privacy for a bowel movement. This facilitates the return of normal bowel habits.

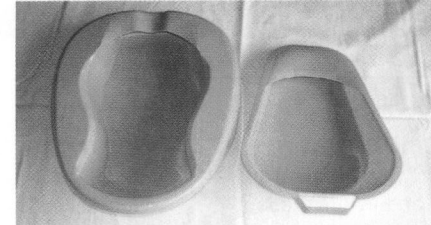

FIG 37.7 Types of bedpans. *From left:* Regular bedpan and fracture pan.

Positioning on Bedpan. A patient restricted to use of a bedpan for defecation usually needs help. Sitting on a bedpan is uncomfortable and awkward. Help position a patient comfortably. Two types of bedpans are available (Fig. 37.7). The regular bedpan, made of hard plastic, has a curved smooth upper end and a sharper-edged lower end and is about 5 cm (2 inches) deep. A fracture pan is used for patients with low-extremity fractures or any patient for whom raising the hips to get on a bedpan is too painful. It has a shallow upper end about 2.5 cm (1 inch) deep. The shallow end of the pan fits under the buttocks toward the sacrum, and the deeper end goes just under the upper thighs. The pan needs to be high enough so that the stool can enter the pan.

When positioning or assisting patients on bedpans, focus on preventing muscle strain and discomfort (Box 37.10). Never place a patient on a bedpan and then leave the bed flat unless activity restrictions demand it. This forces the patient to hyperextend the back to lift the hips onto the pan (Fig. 37.8A). It is often necessary to have the bed flat when placing a patient on a bedpan. Rolling the patient onto the bedpan is the most comfortable way to position a patient with impaired mobility. After it is positioned under the patient, raise the head of the bed 30 to 45 degrees (Fig. 37.8B). Patients who have overhead trapeze frames are able to lift themselves by grasping the trapeze bar. Always be sure to come back to the patient frequently to see if he or she is ready to get off. The patient who is sedated or cognitively impaired could fall asleep on the bedpan and develop serious pressure injury to the buttocks if left on it for a prolonged period of time.

For the more mobile patient a bedside commode is a safe, effective alternative to a bedpan. Its use is less exhausting and allows the patient to assume a more normal or familiar position for defecation.

Medications. Medications that initiate and facilitate stool passage include laxatives and cathartics, which have the short-term action of emptying the bowel. These agents are also used to cleanse the bowel for patients undergoing GI tests and abdominal surgery. Although the terms *laxative* and *cathartic* are often used interchangeably, cathartics generally have a stronger and more rapid effect on the intestines.

Although patients usually take medications orally, laxatives prepared as suppositories may act more quickly because of their stimulant effect on the rectal mucosa. Suppositories such as bisacodyl act within 30 minutes. Give the suppository shortly before a patient's usual time to defecate or

BOX 37.10   PROCEDURAL GUIDELINES

Assisting Patient On and Off a Bedpan

DELEGATION CONSIDERATIONS

The skill of providing a bedpan can be delegated to nursing assistive personnel (NAP). The nurse instructs the NAP how to:

- Correctly position patients with mobility restrictions or patients who have therapeutic equipment such as wound drains, IV catheters, or traction.
- Provide perineal and hand hygiene for patient as necessary after using a bedpan.

EQUIPMENT

Clean gloves; bedpan (regular or fracture) (see Fig. 37.7); bedpan cover; toilet tissue; specimen container (if necessary); plastic bag clearly labeled with date, patient's name, and identification number; basin, washcloths, towels, and soap; waterproof, absorbent pads (if necessary); clean drawsheet (if necessary)

STEPS

1. Perform hand hygiene. Assess patient's level of mobility, strength, ability to help, and presence of any condition (e.g., orthopedic) that interferes with use of bedpan.
2. Review medical record to determine need for stool specimen.
3. Explain procedure that you will use in turning and positioning, and include patient self-help tips (e.g., how to use a trapeze, how to move hips).
4. Obtain assistance from additional nursing personnel as warranted.
5. Apply clean gloves.

> **Clinical Decision Point. Use a fracture pan if patient has had a total hip replacement. An abduction pillow must be placed between the legs when turning to prevent dislocation of new joint.**

6. Provide privacy by closing door of room or curtains around bed.
7. Lower side rail on side of bed where you are standing. Raise bed horizontally according to your height. Position patient high in bed with head of patient's bed raised 30 to 45 degrees (as tolerated) (see Chapter 29).

> **Clinical Decision Point. Observe for the presence of drains, dressings, IV fluids, and traction. These devices make it difficult for a patient to assist with positioning, and you will likely need more personnel to help place patient on a bedpan.**

8. Fold back top linen to patient's knees, but do not expose patient. Place bedpan on bed.
9. **Positioning a patient who can help on a bedpan:**
   a. Raise side rail and instruct patient to grasp both side rails
   b. Have patient flex knees and lift hips upward.
   c. Place your hand closest to patient's head palm up under patient's sacrum to help lift. Ask patient to bend knees and raise hips. As patient raises hips, use other hand to slip bedpan under him or her (see illustration and Fig. 37.8). Be sure that open rim of bedpan is facing toward foot of bed. Do not force pan under patient's hips. (*Optional:* Have patient use overhead trapeze frame to raise hips.)
   d. *Optional:* If using fracture pan, slip it under patient as hips are raised (see illustration). Be sure that deep, open, lower end of bedpan is facing toward foot of bed.
10. **Positioning patient who is immobile or has mobility restrictions on a bedpan.**
    a. Lower head of bed flat or raise head slightly (if tolerated by medical condition).
    b. Help patient roll onto side with back toward you. Place bedpan firmly against patient's buttocks and down into mattress. Be sure that open rim of bedpan is facing toward foot of bed (see illustrations).

> **Clinical Decision Point. If patient has had a total hip replacement, use a fracture pan. Make sure that abduction pillow remains between the patient's legs while patient is transferring to and from and using the fracture pan.**

    c. Keep one hand against bedpan; place other around far hip of patient. Ask patient to roll back onto bedpan, flat in bed. Do not force pan under patient.
    d. Raise patient's head 30 degrees or to a comfortable level (unless contraindicated).
    e. Have patient bend knees (unless contraindicated).
11. Maintain patient's comfort, privacy, and safety. Cover patient for warmth. Place small pillow or rolled towel under lumbar curve of back.

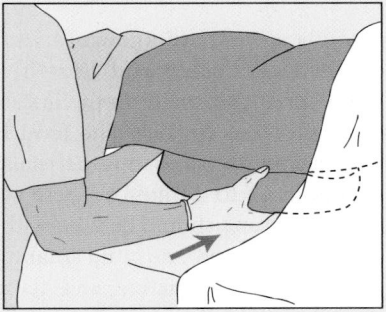

STEP 9c Placing bedpan under patient's hips.

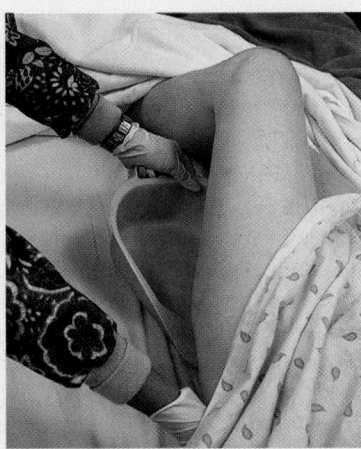

STEP 9d Patient lifts hips as fracture pan is positioned.

Continued

BOX 37.10 **PROCEDURAL GUIDELINES—cont'd**

Assisting Patient On and Off a Bedpan

12. Have call bell and toilet tissue within reach for patient. Give patient time to defecate.
13. Ensure that bed is in lowest position and raise side rails. Give patient time to defecate.
14. Remove and discard gloves and perform hand hygiene.
15. Remove bedpan.
    a. Perform hand hygiene and apply clean gloves
    b. Place patient's bedside chair close to working side of bed. Place towel on chair seat.
    c. Maintain privacy; determine if patient is able to wipe own perineal area. If you clean perineal area, use several layers of toilet tissue or disposable washcloths. For female patients clean from mons pubis toward rectal area. Deposit contaminated tissue in bedpan if no specimen or intake and output (I&O) is needed.
    d. Remove gloves and perform hand hygiene. Reapply gloves.
    e. **For mobile patient:** Ask patient to flex knees, placing body weight on lower legs, feet, and upper torso; lift buttocks up from bedpan. At same time place hand farther from patient on side of bedpan to support it (prevent spillage) and place other hand (closer to patient) under sacrum to help lift. Have patient lift and remove bedpan. Place bedpan on draped bedside chair and cover.
    f. **For immobile patient:** Lower head of bed. Help patient roll onto side away from you and off bedpan. Hold

bedpan flat and steady while patient is rolling off; otherwise spillage will occur. Place bedpan on draped bedside chair and cover.
16. Assist patient to comfortable position. Allow patient to perform hand hygiene. Change soiled linens, remove and dispose of gloves.
17. Place bed in its lowest position. Ensure that call bell, phone, drinking water, and desired personal items (e.g., books) are within easy access.
18. *Optional:* Obtain stool specimen as ordered (see Box 37.7). Wear gloves when emptying contents of bedpan into toilet or in special receptacle in utility room. Use spray faucet attached to most institution toilets to rinse bedpan thoroughly. Use disinfectant if required by agency, then store pan. Remove gloves.
19. Perform hand hygiene.
20. Assess characteristics of stool. Note color, odor, consistency, frequency, amount, shape (see Fig. 37.5), and constituents. Assess characteristics of urine if patient voided in bedpan. Document findings.
21. **Use Teach-Back:** "Since your leg is immobilized, I want to make sure you are comfortable getting off and on the bedpan by using the trapeze to pull your torso off the bed. Show me how you will position your arms on the trapeze." Revise your instruction now or develop a plan for revised patient/family caregiver teaching if patient/family caregiver is not able to teach back correctly.

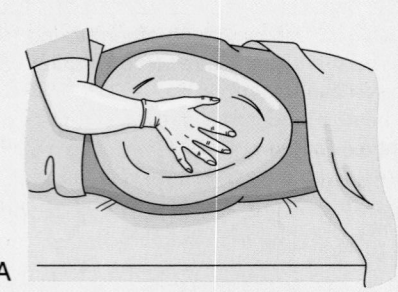 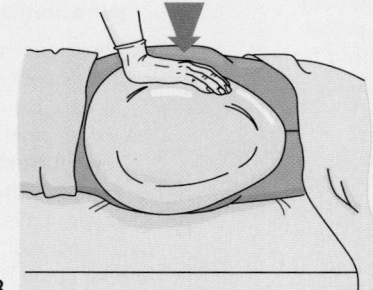 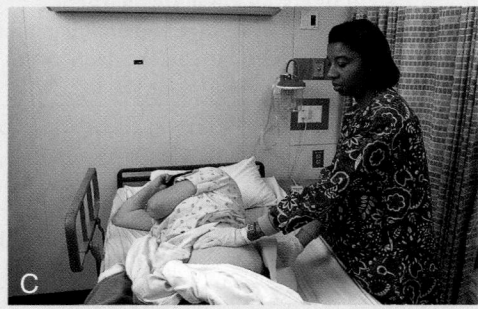

STEP 10b A, Position patient on one side and place bedpan firmly against buttocks. **B,** Push down on bedpan and toward patient. **C,** Nurse places bedpan in position. (**A** and **B** from Sorrentino SA, Remmert LN: *Mosby's textbook for nursing assistants,* ed 9, St Louis, 2017, Elsevier.)

---

immediately after a meal. Teach patients about the potential harmful effects of overuse of laxatives such as impaired bowel motility and decreased response to sensory stimulus. Make sure that a patient understands that laxatives are not to be used long term for maintenance of bowel function.

Before administering a laxative, assess for signs of a fecal impaction. The impaction must be removed before laxative therapy is initiated.

Laxatives and cathartics are classified by the method by which the agent promotes defecation. They are listed here in the order in which they should be used with patients.

- Bulk-forming agents, also known as *fiber supplements,* are considered the safest and least irritating to the intestine. They absorb water in the intestine and make the stool softer and bulkier. The fecal bulk stretches the intestinal walls, stimulating peristalsis. Passage of stool occurs in 12 to 24 hours. These agents must be taken with water and should be used with patients who have an adequate food and fluid intake. Patients may note increased gas formation and flatus when they first start taking these laxatives, but this will abate after 4 to 5 days.

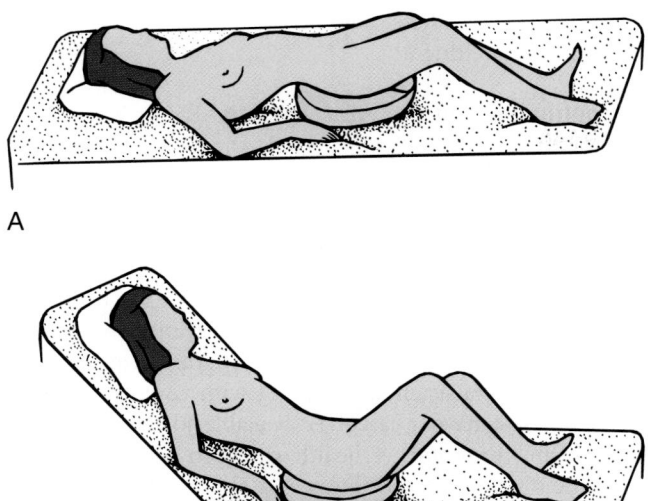

FIG 37.8 Positions on bedpan. **A,** Improper positioning of patient. **B,** Proper position reduces patient's back strain.

- Emollient laxatives soften the fecal mass and make it easier to evacuate. These agents are also called *stool softeners.*
- Osmotic laxatives pull fluid into the bowel to soften the stool and distend the bowel to stimulate peristalsis. Some are saline based; others contain lactulose, sorbitol, and polyethylene glycol.
- Stimulant laxatives cause local irritation to the intestinal mucosa, increase intestinal motility, and inhibit resorption of water in the large intestine. The rapid movement of feces causes retention of water in the stool. The drugs usually contain bisacodyl or senna and cause formation of a soft to fluid stool in 6 to 8 hours.

There are newer drugs for chronic constipation or motility disorders. It is too soon to tell if these medications will be effective and safe for long-term treatment, but they are not used for the relief of occasional constipation.

The most commonly used antidiarrheal agents are loperamide or diphenoxylate with atropine. Antidiarrheal agents decrease intestinal muscle tone to slow the passage of feces. As a result the body absorbs more water through the intestinal walls. However, the cause of diarrhea must be determined before effective treatment can be ordered by the health care provider. For example, if an infection is the causative factor, an antibiotic may be used for treatment; if inflammation is the cause, steroids may be given.

Nasogastric Tube for Gastric Decompression. At times following abdominal or pelvic surgery an **ileus** or temporary cessation of peristalsis occurs. A patient cannot eat or drink fluids without causing abdominal distention, nausea, and vomiting. The insertion of a nasogastric (NG) tube into the stomach serves to decompress the stomach, keeping it empty until normal peristalsis returns (see Skill 37.1). An NG tube is a pliable tube that is inserted through the patient's nose,

through the nasopharynx, and into the stomach. The tube has a hollow lumen that allows the removal of gastric secretions and the introduction of solutions into the stomach. The Levin and Salem sump tubes are most commonly used for stomach decompression. The Levin tube is a single-lumen tube with holes near the tip. You connect the tube to a drainage bag or an intermittent suction device to drain stomach secretions. The Salem sump tube is preferable for stomach decompression. The tube has two lumens: one for removal of gastric contents and one to provide an air vent. A blue "pigtail" is the air vent that connects with the second lumen. When you connect the main lumen of the sump tube to suction, the air vent permits free, continuous drainage of secretions. *Never clamp the air vent if the tube is connected to suction, and never use for irrigation.*

NG tube insertion is done using clean technique. The procedure is uncomfortable; patients experience a burning sensation as the tube passes through the sensitive nasal mucosa. One of the greatest nursing care challenges is keeping the patient comfortable because the tube is a constant irritation to mucosa and can cause a pressure injury. Routinely assess the condition of the nares and mucosa for inflammation and excoriation. Supportive care includes changing soiled tape or fixation devices daily when they become soiled, keeping the nares lubricated and clean, and providing frequent mouth care to minimize dehydration from mouth breathing.

Enemas. An **enema** is an instillation of a solution into the rectum and sigmoid colon to primarily promote defecation by stimulating peristalsis. The volume of fluid instilled breaks up the fecal mass, stretches the rectal wall, and begins the defecation reflex. Enemas are also used to administer drugs that exert a local effect on rectal mucosa. For example, sodium polystyrene sulfonate (Kayexalate) is used to treat patients with dangerously high serum potassium levels.

The most common use for an enema is temporary relief of constipation. Other indications include removing impacted feces, emptying the bowel before diagnostic tests and some surgical procedures, and beginning a program of bowel training. Discourage patients from relying on enemas at home to maintain bowel regularity. Enemas do not treat the cause of constipation. As with overuse of laxatives, frequent use may affect normal defecation reflexes.

Cleansing enemas promote complete evacuation of feces from the colon. They act by stimulating peristalsis through the infusion of a large volume of solution or through local irritation of the mucosa of the colon. Cleansing enemas include tap water, normal saline, low-volume hypertonic saline, and soapsuds solution. Each solution exerts a different osmotic effect, causing the movement of fluids between the colon and interstitial spaces beyond the intestinal wall. Infants and children should be given only normal saline enemas because they are at greater risk for fluid imbalance (Hockenberry and Wilson, 2014).

Tap water is hypotonic and exerts a lower osmotic pressure than fluid in interstitial spaces. After infusion into the colon, tap water escapes from the bowel lumen into interstitial spaces. The net movement of water is low; the infused volume stimulates defecation before large amounts of water leave the bowel. Do not repeat tap-water enemas because water toxicity or circulatory overload develops if the body absorbs large amounts of water.

Physiologically normal saline is the safest solution to use because it exerts the same osmotic pressure as fluids in interstitial spaces around the bowel. The volume of infused saline stimulates peristalsis. Giving normal saline enemas does not create the danger of excess fluid absorption. At times a soap solution is ordered to be added to tap water or saline to create the additional effect of intestinal irritation. Only pure castile soap is safe because harsh soaps or detergents cause bowel inflammation.

Hypertonic solutions infused into the bowel exert osmotic pressure that pulls fluids into the colon. The colon fills with fluid, and the resultant distention promotes defecation. Patients unable to tolerate large volumes of fluid benefit most from this type of enema. A hypertonic solution of 120 to 180 mL (4 to 6 oz) is usually effective.

A health care provider sometimes orders a high or low cleansing enema. The terms *high* and *low* refer to the height and pressure with which you deliver the fluid. You give high enemas to clean the entire colon. A low enema cleans only the rectum and sigmoid colon. After you infuse the enema, ask the patient to turn from the left lateral to the dorsal recumbent and over to the right lateral position. The position changes help fluid reach the large intestine.

Oil-retention enemas lubricate the rectum and colon. The feces absorb the oil and become softer and easier to pass. To enhance action of the oil, the patient retains the enema for several hours if possible. Skill 37.2 outlines the steps for enema administration.

Digital Removal of Stool. For patients with an impaction, the fecal mass is sometimes too large to pass voluntarily. If enemas fail, the mass needs to be broken up digitally. Patients with an impaction frequently have a continuous oozing of liquid stool because liquid passes around the impacted feces. Disimpaction is done only when all other measures have failed (Box 37.11).

The procedure is uncomfortable for the patient. Excess rectal manipulation irritates the mucosa and can cause bleeding. There is also risk of stimulation of the vagus nerve, which can result in a reflex slowing of the heart rate. Disimpaction in patients with spinal cord injury can cause autonomic dysreflexia (University of Michigan, 2013). Because of the potential complications of the procedure, some institutions restrict nurses from removing impactions digitally. Before you perform the procedure, check your agency policy regarding a health care provider's order.

Management of Patients With Fecal Incontinence or Diarrhea. You may apply a fecal collector around a patient's anal opening if the skin is intact. The devices are difficult to apply when there is a deep fold between the buttocks and there is hair in the area. There are fecal management systems available for short-term use with high-volume diarrhea. The devices have an intra-anal soft silicone catheter with a retention balloon, much like a Foley catheter for insertion into the rectal vault. The catheter connects to a drainage bag for collection of fecal effluent.

Continuing and Restorative Care. Before a patient is able to return home or is transferred to an extended care facility, you need to help establish regular elimination patterns.

Bowel Training. A bowel training program helps patients who still have some neuromuscular control to achieve normal defecation. The training program involves setting up a daily routine. By attempting to defecate at the same time each day and using measures that promote defecation, the patient gains control of bowel reflexes. The program requires time, patience, and consistency. A patient with cognitive impairment needs to have a caregiver available to devote time to the training program. A health care provider determines the patient's physical readiness and ability to benefit from bowel training.

Ostomy Care. Immediately after a surgical diversion it is necessary to place a pouch over the newly created stoma because in some ostomies output of effluent begins soon after surgery. The pouch collects all effluent and protects the skin from irritating dermatitis. A proper pouch fits comfortably, with its skin barrier covering the skin surface around the stoma and creating a good seal. The postoperative pouch is transparent to allow visibility of the stoma.

For up to 6 weeks the new stoma may be edematous. The stoma itself often has a series of small stitches around its perimeter. Apply a pouch and skin barrier that fits right around the stoma and protects the surrounding skin. Take care to avoid disrupting the suture line. It may be several days after surgery before bowel function returns. In the case of an ileostomy, the patient has frequent liquid stools when peristalsis returns. With a colostomy the fecal output may be loose in the first few days after surgery, but a more formed stool would be expected after the patient is eating again.

Many types of pouches and skin barriers are available (Colwell, 2016). Some pouches have skin barriers attached and are one-piece pouching systems (Fig. 37.9). Some of these one-piece pouches already are precut to size by the manufacturer, whereas others you custom cut to size for the patient's stoma measurement. Other systems have two separate pieces (Fig. 37.10). Attach the pouch to the skin barrier by attaching it to the flange (a plastic ring) on the barrier. Often you have to custom cut the skin barrier to the patient's specific stoma size. For two-piece systems use the skin barrier with flange corresponding to the size of the ring on the pouch, making sure that both pieces are from the same manufacturer. Understand how to use each of these different pouching systems before attempting to teach ostomy care to the patient. If possible, change the pouch when the stoma is less active, usually before meals.

Have patients participate in pouching because they need to learn to recognize the normal appearance of a stoma. It should be red and moist. By 6 weeks after surgery, the size should not change. If there are noticeable changes in the size of the stoma, either smaller or larger than normal, it should

BOX 37.11   PROCEDURAL GUIDELINES

Digital Removal of Stool/Fecal Impaction

DELEGATION CONSIDERATIONS

The skill of digitally removing a fecal impaction cannot be delegated to nursing assistive personnel (NAP). The nurse directs the NAP to:

- Help the nurse position a patient for the procedure.
- Observe the stool for color, consistency, rectal bleeding, or bloody mucus after the procedure and report immediately to the nurse.
- Provide perineal care following each bowel movement.

EQUIPMENT

Clean gloves; water-soluble local anesthetic lubricant (**Note:** Some agencies require use of water-soluble lubricant without anesthetic when nurse performs procedure); waterproof, absorbent pads; bedpan; bedpan cover (optional); bath blanket; basin, washcloths, towels, and soap; sphygmomanometer (optional)

STEPS

1. Identify patient using at least two identifiers (e.g., name and birthday or name and medical record number) according to agency policy.

   > **Clinical Decision Point. Because of the potential to stimulate the sacral branch of the vagus nerve, patients with a history of dysrhythmias or heart disease have a greater risk for changes in heart rhythm. Monitor patient's pulse before and during procedure. This procedure is often contraindicated in cardiac patients; if in doubt, verify with the health care provider.**

2. Perform hand hygiene. Pull curtains around bed, obtain patient's baseline vital signs, assess level of comfort, and palpate for abdominal distention before procedure.
3. Explain procedure to patient, including positioning and expected discomfort. Have patient demonstrate ability to take slow, deep breaths to relax.
4. Obtain assistance to help change patient's position if necessary. Raise bed horizontally to comfortable working height.
5. Lower side rail on patient's right side. Keeping far side rail raised, help patient to left side-lying position with knees flexed and back.
6. Drape patient's trunk and lower extremities with bath blanket and place waterproof pad under patient's buttocks.
7. Perform hand hygiene and apply clean gloves and place bedpan next to patient.

8. Lubricate gloved index finger and middle finger of dominant hand with anesthetic lubricant.
9. Instruct patient to take slow deep breaths during procedure. Gradually and gently insert gloved index finger and feel anus relax around finger. Insert middle finger. Gradually advance fingers slowly along rectal wall toward umbilicus.
10. Gently loosen fecal mass by moving fingers in scissors motion to fragment the fecal mass. Work fingers into hardened mass. Work stool downward toward end of rectum. Remove small sections of feces and discard into bedpan.
11. Observe patient's response and periodically assess heart rate and look for signs of fatigue.

   > **Clinical Decision Point. Stop procedure if heart rate drops or rhythm changes from patient's baseline or if patient has dyspnea or reports palpitations.**

   > **Clinical Decision Point. Patients who have a spinal cord injury and are unable to sense the need to defecate are at risk for autonomic dysreflexia from a full bowel. Rectal stimulation may aggravate this risk. Stop procedure if patient develops pounding headache, flushing of face, increased muscle spasms, blurred vision, and a blood pressure increase of 20 to 40 mm Hg. This is a medical emergency.**

12. Continue to clear rectum of feces allowing patient to rest at intervals.
13. After removal of impaction perform perineal hygiene.
14. Remove bedpan and inspect feces for color and consistency. Dispose of feces in toilet.
15. If needed, help patient to toilet or clean and store the bedpan. (Procedure may be followed by enema or cathartic.)
16. Remove gloves by turning them inside out and discarding in proper receptacle. Perform hand hygiene.
17. Record results of procedure by describing fecal characteristics and amount.
18. Reassess vital signs and compare with baseline values. Continue to monitor patient for 1 hour for bradycardia. Monitor blood pressure in patients with spinal cord injury.
19. **Use Teach-Back:** "I want to make sure you include high-fiber foods and fluids in your diet to help increase the passage of stool. Tell me what foods you will add to your diet." Revise your instruction now or develop a plan for revised patient/family caregiver teaching if patient/family caregiver is not able to teach back correctly.

be reported to the health care provider. Skill 37.3 describes the steps for pouching an ostomy.

A patient with an ostomy experiences a change in body image. The appearance of the stoma and accompanying effluent and odor can cause psychological stress. For the patient with a new ostomy, it is important for you to encourage self-care and acceptance of the ostomy (Box 37.12). Early involvement in self-care promotes confidence. Even simple tasks such as holding pieces of equipment during stoma pouching and learning to open and close the pouch help the patient

begin to adjust to bodily changes. Whenever possible, have an ostomy nurse provide care and teaching for the patient with a new stoma (Box 37.13). In addition, patients may benefit from information and encouragement from an ostomy support group.

Maintenance of Skin Integrity. The patient with diarrhea or fecal incontinence is at risk for skin breakdown when fecal contents remain on the skin (see Chapter 38). The same problem exists for the patient with an ostomy that drains liquid stool. Liquid stool is usually acidic and contains

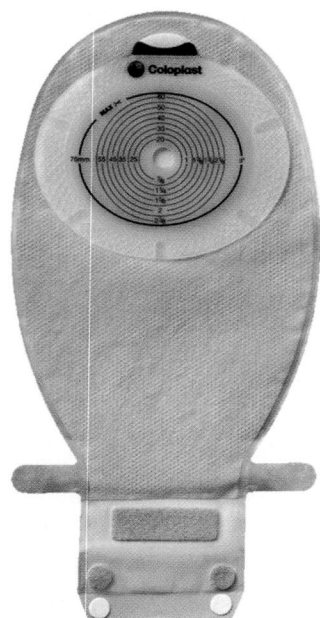

FIG 37.9 One-piece pouch with Velcro closure. (Courtesy Coloplast, Minneapolis, MN.)

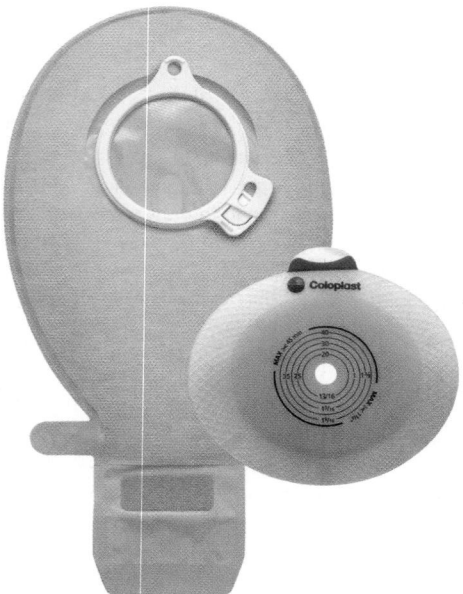

FIG 37.10 Two-piece pouch system with separate skin barrier and attachable pouch. (Courtesy Coloplast, Minneapolis, MN.)

digestive enzymes. Irritation from repeated wiping with toilet tissue causes skin breakdown. To prevent skin irritation, cleanse and dry the skin immediately after soiling occurs.

Instruct a patient or family caregiver about cleansing the perineal area with a no-rinse perineal cleanser and warm water or a prepackaged perineal wipe after each passage of stool. When caring for a patient who is debilitated, incontinent, and unable to ask for assistance, check frequently for

BOX 37.12 EVIDENCE-BASED PRACTICE

PICO Question: In adult patients with ostomies, what is the effect of patient education about ostomy care on the patient's quality of life?

SUMMARY OF EVIDENCE
Placement of an ostomy following colorectal cancer causes individuals to experience a change in body image. Individuals must adjust both physically and psychologically following the ostomy. Research found that quality of life was lowest 2 months after surgery but improved to almost preoperative levels at 12 months (Nichols, 2015). Nichols (2015) also found that physical, mental, emotional, and social adjustment was lower in individuals as they tried to incorporate ostomy care tasks into their daily life for the first 12 months after surgery. Some individuals continue to have concerns 5 or more years after an ostomy that impacts their adjustment and quality of life (Sun et al., 2013). These concerns include clothing adaptations, dietary concerns, activity limitations and adaptations, leakage, seal and adhesive issues, and skin and odor issues. Individuals with ostomies who receive ostomy care education look for ways to adjust their lives. Family caregivers also benefit from ostomy care education because they provide assistance to their loved ones (Goldberg, 2016).

APPLICATION TO NURSING PRACTICE
- Nurses with specialized knowledge and training can educate individuals before surgery to help with postoperative adjustment (Goldberg et al., 2016).
- Home health services during the first few months following ostomy placement improve individuals' adjustment.
- Help patients develop long-term support systems to cope with their ostomies (Sun et al., 2013).
- Provide long-term education and support for patients and family caregivers of individuals with ostomies (Goldberg et al., 2016).

(QSEN) QSEN ACTIVITY *Teamwork and Collaboration*

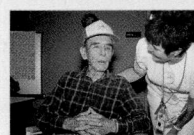

Vickie continued to keep in touch with Mr. Gutierrez's niece while he was in the hospital and visited him several times. He reluctantly agreed to go to a skilled nursing facility for a couple of weeks for continued ostomy care, teaching, and physical therapy. She learns that he is able to open and close his ostomy pouch and can empty the pouch with minimal assistance. Mr. Gutierrez and his niece have had several visits from the ostomy nurse at the hospital, and she gave them written instructions for his care and a follow-up appointment at the ostomy clinic in 1 week. The family requests that Vickie continue with her visits, as she has a good relationship with Mr. Gutierrez and he responds well to her.

- How can Vickie best prepare to continue caring for Mr. Gutierrez although she has little experience in ostomy care other than what she has received in her classroom learning?

evolve Answers to QSEN Activities can be found on the Evolve website.

BOX 37.13 PATIENT TEACHING

The Patient With an Ostomy

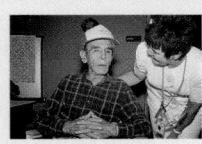

OUTCOME

Patient/caregiver can demonstrate changing an ostomy pouch.

TEACHING STRATEGIES

- Provide a comprehensive list of products needed to care for the ostomy.
- Provide patient/family caregiver with supplies to last 1 to 2 weeks and the contact number of the closest medical supply store.
- Demonstrate how to empty pouch and have patient/family caregiver begin emptying it while still in the hospital.
- Show patient/family caregiver the step-by-step approach for changing an ostomy pouch; provide at least one opportunity to change the ostomy pouch while patient is in hospital.
- Set up visits with an ostomy nurse or home care nurse and provide contact numbers.
- Provide detailed discharge instructions for skin care, driving, lifting, resuming exercise, and when to contact the health care provider.

EVALUATION

- Use the principles of teach-back to evaluate patient/family caregiver learning:
  - "Show me how you empty and change your ostomy pouch."
  - "Tell me the signs of peristomal skin irritation and how you would relieve it."
  - "Tell me about the type and amount of output that you should get from the stoma and when you need to call the health care provider."

BOX 37.14 EVALUATION

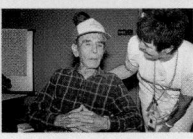

Vickie returns to see Mr. Gutierrez at home 2 weeks later. She is eager to determine if Mr. Gutierrez has made changes in his diet and if his problems with bowel elimination have been progressing. She is also eager to learn if the niece has helped to have Mr. Gutierrez's stove repaired.

Mr. Gutierrez tells Vickie that he has been eating bran cereal in the morning, has been eating rice and/or beans for dinner, and has added one fruit each day to his diet. He has been walking twice a day through the long-term care center. Although he does not have a bowel movement each day, his stools are much softer and easier to pass, and he says that he is less concerned. He has not taken a laxative since last talking with Vickie.

DOCUMENTATION NOTE

"Bowel elimination is improving. Abdomen is soft and non-distended. After discussing the teaching plan, has agreed to alter his eating habits to include more fiber, fruit, and fluids. Although concern over bowel habits has not ceased, does state he feels 'in better control' and has decreased laxative use. Niece assisted in having stove repaired."

defecation and cleanse the skin. Protect the skin around the anal area with barrier ointments. Baby powder or cornstarch is contraindicated because it does not provide a barrier to protect the skin. Check the skin for rashes that could indicate a yeast infection. Patients with incontinence who are taking antibiotics are particularly susceptible to yeast infections. This type of rash is raised and deep red with satellite lesions, and usually the patient will report itching. This rash should be reported promptly so that topical treatment can be started.

■ ■ ■ EVALUATION

Patient Outcomes. Evaluate the effectiveness of nursing interventions for the patient with alterations in bowel elimination by determining success in meeting the patient's expected outcomes and goals of care. Optimally the patient is to eliminate soft, formed stools regularly. In addition, the patient gains the information necessary to establish a normal elimination pattern (Box 37.14).

Evaluate success of the plan by having the patient describe his or her elimination pattern following therapy. Also make it a point to evaluate the character of the patient's stool. A return to a more normal, regular elimination pattern can take time. Periodically reevaluate the patient. The goals for patients should include defecation every 1 to 2 days; a soft, nondistended abdomen; and soft, formed stool.

Evaluate the adjustment of a patient to an ostomy during self-care. Inspect the patient's peristomal skin, looking for impairment in skin integrity. Your evaluation also includes observing the patient change and empty an ostomy pouch. Evaluate the stool formation in a patient with a colostomy because he or she may become constipated and should not have hard stools. A liquid to semiformed stool with an ileostomy is considered normal. Assess the patient's emotional state with regard to the ostomy and provide support as needed.

Patient Expectations. Using patient expectations identified during assessment, determine the patient's level of satisfaction with nursing care. Does the patient believe that you provided care respectfully, offering privacy and support when necessary? Is the patient satisfied with the elimination pattern established? Are stools easier to manage?

Your goal for the patient with an ostomy is to achieve a realistic level of self-care and maintain or reinforce a healthy body image. When discussing these issues with the patient, determine if the patient's participation in care helped him or her accept the ostomy. Were expectations of the patient unrealistic? Did the patient feel like a partner in care? Learning about the patient's level of satisfaction with care goes a long way toward helping future patients.

SAFETY GUIDELINES FOR NURSING SKILLS

Ensuring patient safety is an essential role of the professional nurse. To ensure patient safety, communicate clearly with the members of the health care team, assess and incorporate the patient's priorities of care and preferences, and use the best evidence when making decisions about your patient's care. When performing the skills in this chapter, remember the following points to ensure safe, individualized patient care:

- If a patient has cardiac disease or is taking cardiac or hypertensive medication, obtain a pulse rate before an enema because manipulation of rectal tissue stimulates

the vagus nerve and can cause a sudden decline in pulse rate, which can increase the patient's risk for fainting while on the bedpan, commode, or toilet.
- Instruct patients who self-administer enemas to use the side-lying position. Administering an enema with the patient sitting on the toilet is unsafe because it is impossible to safely guide the tubing into the rectum.
- Keep patient in sitting high-Fowler's position during nasogastric intubation to prevent aspiration (Shlamovitz and Shah, 2016).

SKILL 37.1   INSERTING AND MAINTAINING A NASOGASTRIC TUBE FOR GASTRIC DECOMPRESSION

DELEGATION CONSIDERATIONS

The skill of inserting and maintaining a nasogastric (NG) tube cannot be delegated to nursing assistive personnel (NAP). The nurse directs the NAP to:

- Measure and record the drainage from an NG tube.
- Provide oral and nasal hygiene measures.
- Perform selected comfort measures such as positioning or offering ice chips if allowed.
- Anchor the tube to patient's gown during routine care to prevent accidental displacement.
- Immediately report to the nurse any signs of redness or irritation to nares, abdominal pain, or blood in gastric drainage.

EQUIPMENT

- 14- or 16-Fr NG tube (smaller-lumen catheters are not used for decompression in adults because they must be able to remove thick secretions). **Option:** A dual purpose tube, one that is used for both gastric decompression and enteral feedings, may be ordered for selected patients.

- Water-soluble lubricant
- pH test strips (measure gastric aspirate acidity); use paper with a range of at least 1.0 to 11.0 or higher
- Tongue blade
- Flashlight
- Emesis basin
- Asepto bulb or catheter-tipped syringe
- 2.5-cm (1-inch)–wide hypoallergenic tape or commercial fixation device
- Safety pin and rubber band
- Clamp, drainage bag, or suction machine with pressure gauge if wall suction is to be used
- Towel
- Glass of water with straw
- Facial tissues
- Normal saline
- Tincture of benzoin *(optional)*
- Suction equipment
- Stethoscope, pulse oximeter/capnography device *(optional)*
- Clean gloves

STEP	RATIONALE
ASSESSMENT	
1. Identify patient using at least two identifiers (e.g., name and birthday or name and medical record number) according to agency policy.	Ensures correct patient. Complies with The Joint Commission Standards and improves patient safety (TJC, 2018).
2. Perform hand hygiene. (Apply gloves if risk of body fluid exposure). Inspect condition of patient's nares and nasal and oral cavity.	Documents if skin on nares is intact or irritated before NG tube insertion. Determines need for special nursing hygiene measures after tube placement.
3. Ask if patient has history of nasal surgery or congestion and allergies and note if deviated nasal septum is present.	Alerts nurse to potential obstruction. Insert tube into *uninvolved* nasal passage. Procedure may be contraindicated if surgery is recent.
4. Auscultate for bowel sounds. Palpate patient's abdomen for distention, pain, and rigidity. In presence of diminished or absent bowel sounds, auscultate abdomen at least 1 minute in each quadrant (Ball et al., 2015).	Documents baseline for any abdominal distention, gastrointestinal (GI) ileus, and general GI function, which later serves as comparison once tube is inserted.
5. Assess patient's level of consciousness and ability to follow instructions.	Determines patient's ability to assist in procedure.

Clinical Decision Point. If patient is confused, disoriented, or unable to follow commands, obtain assistance from another staff member to insert NG tube.

STEP	RATIONALE
6. Determine if patient had previous NG tube and, if so, which naris was used. Remove and dispose of gloves if worn. Perform hand hygiene.	Patient's previous experience complements any explanations and prepares patient for NG tube placement. Reduces transmission of microorganisms.
7. Verify health care provider order for type of NG tube to be placed and whether tube is to be attached to suction or drainage bag.	Requires order from health care provider. Adequate decompression depends on NG suction.
8. Assess patient's or family caregiver's knowledge of the procedure.	Encourages cooperation; minimizes risks and anxiety. Identifies teaching needs.

PLANNING

1. Provide privacy by closing curtains around bed or closing door and prepare bedside environment for patient safety.	Preparing the environment helps the nurse think about the steps needed; removing clutter from over-bed table removes barriers to completing procedure.
2. Prepare and organize NG tube insertion equipment at bedside.	Ensures organized approach for insertion of NG tube.
3. Inform patient that procedure may cause gagging and that there will be a burning sensation in nasopharynx as tube is passed. Develop hand signal with patient.	Increases patient's cooperation and ability to anticipate nurse's action. If patient is unable to tolerate procedure, use of hand signal will alert nurse.
4. Explain steps of insertion procedure to patient and family.	Promotes patient cooperation and increases compliance.

IMPLEMENTATION

1. Perform hand hygiene.	Reduces transmission of microorganisms.
2. Position patient upright in high-Fowler's position unless contraindicated. If patient is comatose, raise head of bed as tolerated in semi-Fowler's position with head tipped forward, chin to chest.	Promotes patient's ability to swallow during procedure. Good body mechanics prevent injury to nurse or patient.
3. Place bath towel over patient's chest; give facial tissues to patient. Allow patient to blow nose if necessary. Place emesis basin within reach.	Prevents soiling of patient's gown. Tube insertion through nasal passages may cause tearing and coughing with increased salivation.
4. Pull curtain around bed or close room door.	Provides privacy.
5. Wash bridge of nose with soap and water or alcohol swab.	Removes oils from nose to allow fixation devices to completely adhere.
6. Stand on patient's right side if right-handed or left side if left-handed. Lower side rail.	Allows easiest manipulation of tubing.
7. Instruct patient to relax and breathe normally while occluding one naris. Then repeat this action for other naris. Select nostril with greater airflow.	Tube passes more easily through naris that is more patent.
8. Measure distance from tip of patient's nose to earlobe to xiphoid process of the sternum (see illustration).	Length approximates distance from nose to stomach. The NEX (nose-earlobe-xiphoid) method is commonly used in clinical settings.

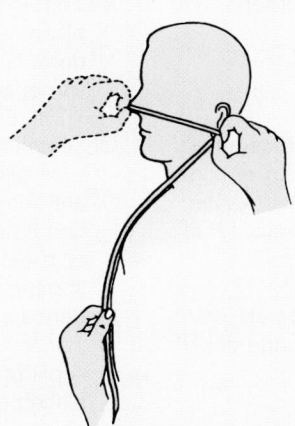

STEP 8 Determine length of tube to be inserted.

SKILL 37.1   INSERTING AND MAINTAINING A NASOGASTRIC TUBE FOR GASTRIC DECOMPRESSION—cont'd

STEP	RATIONALE
9. With small piece of tape placed around tube, mark length that will be inserted.	Indicates length of tube you will insert.
10. Prepare materials for tube fixation. Tear off a 3- to 4-inch length of hypoallergenic tape or open membrane dressing or other fixation device; see Step 24a(2).	Fixation devices allow tube to float free of nares, reducing pressure on nares and preventing device-related pressure injuries (Pittman et al., 2015).
11. Perform hand hygiene and apply clean gloves.	Reduces transmission of microorganisms.
12. Apply pulse oximetry/capnography device and measure vital signs.	Provides objective assessment of respiratory status during tube insertion.
13. *Option:* Dip tube with surface lubricant into a glass of room temperature water or lubricate 7.5 to 10 cm (3 to 4 inches) of end of tube with water-soluble lubricant (see manufacturer's directions).	Water activates lubricant and minimizes friction against nasal mucosa and aids in insertion of tube. Water-soluble lubricant is less toxic than oil-based lubricant if aspirated.
14. Hand an alert patient a cup of water if able to hold cup and swallow. Explain that you are about to insert the tube.	Swallowing water facilitates tube passage. Explanation decreases patient anxiety and increases patient cooperation.
15. Explain next steps. Insert tube gently and slowly through naris to back of throat (posterior nasopharynx). Aim back and down toward patient's ear (see illustration).	Natural contour facilitates passage of tube into GI tract and reduces gagging.
16. Have patient relax and flex head toward chest after tube as passed through nasopharynx.	Closes off glottis and reduces risk of tube entering trachea.
17. Encourage patient to swallow by taking small sips of water when possible. Advance tube as patient swallows, Rotate tube gently 180 degrees while inserting.	Swallowing facilitates passage of tube past oropharynx. A tug may be felt as patient swallows, indicating tube is following desired path.
18. Emphasize need to mouth breathe during procedure.	Helps facilitate passage of tube and alleviates patient's anxiety and fear during procedure.
19. Do not advance tube during inspiration of coughing because tube will likely enter the respiratory tract. Monitor oximetry/capnography.	When tube inadvertently enters airway, changes in oxygen saturation or end-tidal carbon dioxide (capnography) occur.
20. Advance tube each time patient swallows until you reach desired length.	Reduces discomfort and trauma to patient.

Clinical Decision Point. Do not force NG tube. If patient starts to cough or has a drop in oxygen saturation or increased carbon dioxide, withdraw tube into posterior nasopharynx until normal breathing resumes.

STEP	RATIONALE
21. Using penlight and tongue blade, check to be sure tube is not positioned in back of throat.	Tube could become coiled or kinked or enter trachea.
22. Temporarily anchor NG tube to nose with small piece of tape.	Securing tube prevents movement of tube and subsequent gagging. Allows for verification of tube placement.
23. Verify tube placement. Check agency policy for recommended methods of checking tube placement. a. Order bedside x-ray film of chest and abdomen.	Radiography is standard of care for verification of initial placement of NG tube (Tho et al., 2011). This must be done before any medication or liquid is administered (American Association of Critical Care Nurses [AACN], 2009; Emergency Nurses Association [ENA], 2015).
b. While waiting for x-ray, perform these procedures: Attach Asepto or catheter-tipped syringe to end of tube. Aspirate gently back on syringe to obtain gastric contents, observing amount, color, and quality of return (see illustration).	Observation of gastric contents is useful to determine initial tube placement. Gastric contents are usually green but are sometimes off-white, tan, bloody, or brown in color. Other common appearances of aspirate include yellow or bile-stained (duodenal placement) or possibly saliva-appearing (esophagus) (Walthen and Peyton, 2014).
c. Use pH test paper to measure aspirate for pH with color-coded pH paper. Be sure that paper range of pH is at least from 1 to 11 (see illustration).	Evidence supports pH test to be used as indicator for placement (Tho et al., 2011; Walthen and Peyton, 2014). A pH of 1.0 to 4.0 is a good indicator of gastric placement (Walthen and Peyton, 2014).

STEP	RATIONALE
24. Anchor NG tube with fixation device avoiding pressure on the nares. Select one of the following fixation methods.	Proper anchoring and marking of tube helps prevent migration of tube and pressure injury formation and identify change in placement of tube.
a. Apply tape:	
(1) Apply tincture of benzoin or other skin adhesive on bridge of patient's nose and allow it to become "tacky."	Helps tape adhere better. Protects underlying skin.
(2) Remove gloves. Tear small horizontal slits at ⅓ and ⅔ length of tape without splitting tape (see illustration). Fold middle sections toward one another to form a closed strip.	Positions tubing to lessen rubbing against soft palate and naris.
(3) Print date and time on tape and place top end of tape over bridge of patient's nose.	
(4) Wrap bottom end of tape around tube as it exits nose (see illustrations).	

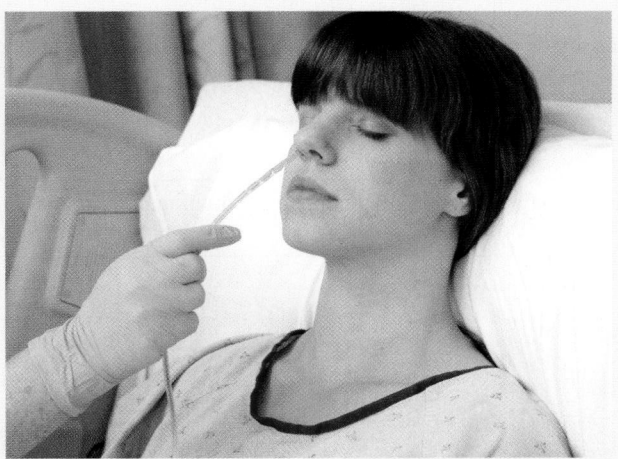

STEP 15 Insert nasogastric tube into patient's nares.

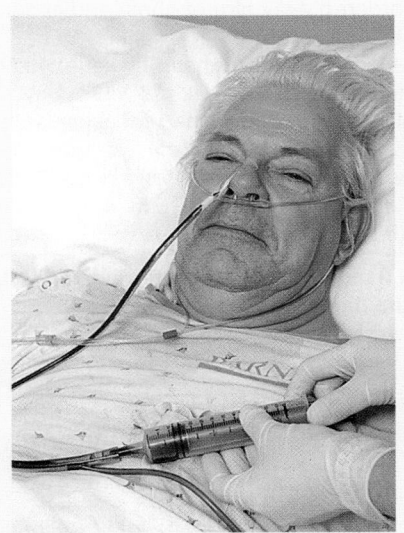

STEP 23b Aspiration of gastric contents.

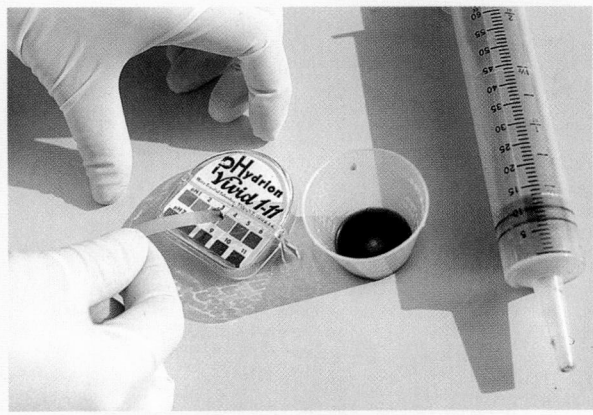

STEP 23c Checking pH of gastric aspirate.

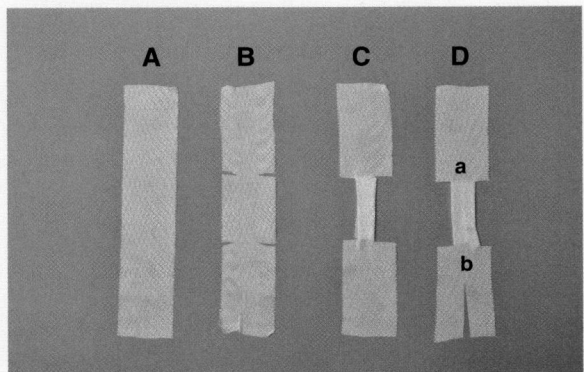

STEP 24a(2) Taping method. **A,** Start with a piece of tape. **B,** Make two slits on both sides of tape. **C,** Fold middle section inward. **D,** Tear a new slit in bottom of tape. The top part *(a)* should attach to the patient's nose, and the bottom part *(b)* should be wrapped around the tube.

SKILL 37.1   INSERTING AND MAINTAINING A NASOGASTRIC TUBE FOR GASTRIC DECOMPRESSION—cont'd

STEP	RATIONALE
b. Apply tube fixation device using shaped adhesive patch (see manufacturer's directions).	Secures tube and reduces friction on nares.
(1) Apply wide end of patch to bridge of nose (see illustration).	
(2) Slip connector around tube as it exits nose (see illustration).	
25. Fasten end of NG tube to patient's gown with a piece of tape. Do not use safety pins to fasten tube to gown.	
26. Keep head of bed elevated at least 30 degrees (preferably 45 degrees) unless contraindicated (Metheny and Franz, 2013).	Reduces risk for aspiration of stomach contents.

Clinical Decision Point. If inserting a Salem sump tube, keep the pigtail of the tube above level of the stomach. This prevents siphoning action that clogs tube.

27. Obtain ordered x-ray film of chest and abdomen.	Radiography is the standard of care for NG tube verification (Tho et al., 2011; Stewart et al., 2014).
28. Remove gloves, perform hand hygiene, and help patient to comfortable position.	Reduces transmission of microorganisms.
29. Once placement is confirmed measure amount of tube that is external and mark exit of tube at nares with indelible marker as a guide for any tube displacement. Record this information in patient's electronic health record (EHR) or chart.	The mark alerts nurses and other health care providers to possible tube displacement, which will require confirmation of tube placement.

Clinical Decision Point. Never reposition NG tube of a patient who has had gastric surgery because positioning can rupture the suture line.

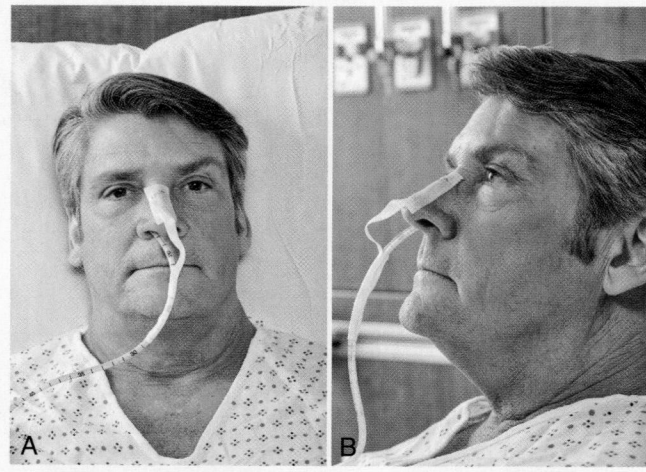

STEP 24a(4) **A,** Applying tape to anchor nasogastric tube. **B,** Nares are free of pressure from tape and tube.

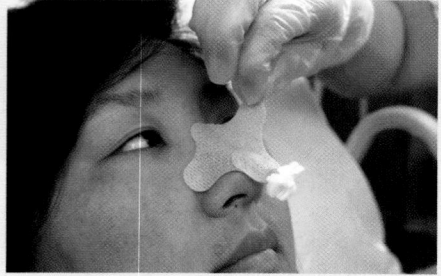

STEP 24b(1) Apply patch to bridge of nose.

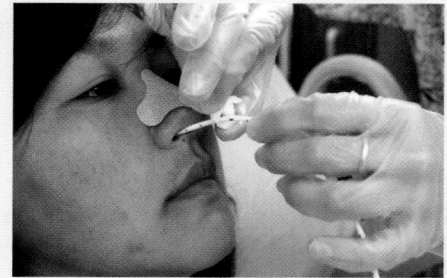

STEP 24b(2) Slip connector around nasogastric tube.

STEP	RATIONALE
30. Attach NG tube to suction as ordered.	Suction setting is usually ordered low intermittent, which decreases gastric irritation from NG tube.

Clinical Decision Point. If lumen of tube is narrow and secretions are thick, NG tube will not drain as desired. Irrigate tube (see Step 31). Consult with health care provider for higher suction setting if unable to irrigate tube because of thick secretions.

31. NG tube irrigation:	
a. Perform hand hygiene and apply clean gloves.	Reduces transmission of microorganisms.
b. Check for tube placement in stomach by disconnecting NG tube, connecting irrigating syringe, and aspirating contents (see Step 23b). Temporarily clamp tube or reconnect to connecting tube and remove syringe.	Prevents accidental entrance of irrigating solution into lungs.
c. Empty syringe of aspirate and use it to draw up 30 mL of normal saline.	Use of saline minimizes loss of electrolytes from stomach fluids.
d. Disconnect NG tube from connecting tubing and lay end of connection tubing on towel.	Reduces soiling of patient's gown and bed linen.
e. Insert tip of irrigating syringe into end of NG tube. Remove clamp (if present). Hold syringe with tip pointed at floor and inject saline slowly and evenly. Do not force solution.	Position of syringe prevents introduction of air into vent tubing, which causes gastric distention. Solution introduced under pressure causes gastric trauma.

Clinical Decision Point. Do not introduce saline through blue "pigtail" air vent of Salem sump tube.

f. If resistance occurs, check for kinks in tubing. Turn patient onto left side. Repeated resistance should be reported to health care provider.	Tip of tube may lie against stomach lining. Repositioning on left side may dislodge tube away from stomach lining. Buildup of secretions causes distention.
g. After instilling saline, immediately aspirate or pull back slowly on syringe to withdraw fluid. If amount aspirated is greater than amount instilled, record difference as output. If amount aspirated is less than amount instilled, record difference as intake.	Irrigation clears tubing so stomach should remain empty. Measure and document irrigation inserted in tube as intake.
h. Use irrigating syringe to place 10 mL of **air** into blue pigtail (not fluid).	Ensures patency of air vent.
i. Reconnect NG tube to drainage or suction. (Repeat irrigation if solution does not return.) Remove and dispose of gloves and perform hand hygiene.	Reestablishes drainage collection; may repeat irrigation or repositioning of tube until NG tube drains properly.
32. Removal of NG tube:	
a. Verify order to remove NG tube.	An order is required for procedure.
b. Perform hand hygiene. Auscultate abdomen for presence of bowel sounds.	Verifies return of peristalsis.
c. Explain procedure to patient and reassure that removal is less distressing than insertion.	Minimizes anxiety and increases cooperation during tube removal.
d. Apply clean gloves. Have towel accessible. Hand patient facial tissue.	Reduces transmission of microorganisms. Some patients wish to blow nose after tube is removed. Towel keeps gown from soiling. Temporary airway obstruction occurs during tube removal.
e. Turn off suction and disconnect NG tube from drainage bag or suction. With irrigating syringe, insert 20 mL of air into lumen of NG tube. Remove tape or fixation device from bridge of nose and from patient's gown.	Have tube free of connections before removal. Clears gastric fluids from tube to prevent aspiration of contents or soiling of clothing and bedding.
f. Instruct patient to take and hold breath.	Temporary airway obstruction occurs during tube removal.
g. Kink tubing securely and pull tube out steadily and smoothly into towel held in other hand while patient holds breath.	Kinking prevents tube contents from draining into oropharynx. Reduces trauma to mucosa and minimizes patient's discomfort. Towel covers tube, which is an unpleasant sight. Holding breath helps to prevent aspiration.
h. Inspect intactness of tube.	
i. Measure amount of drainage and note character of content. Dispose of tube and drainage equipment into proper container.	Provides accurate measure of fluid output. Reduces transfer of microorganisms.

SKILL 37.1 INSERTING AND MAINTAINING A NASOGASTRIC TUBE FOR GASTRIC DECOMPRESSION—cont'd

STEP	RATIONALE
j. Clean nares and provide mouth care.	Promotes comfort.
k. Position patient comfortably and explain procedure for drinking fluids if not contraindicated. Instruct patient to notify you if nausea occurs.	Sometimes patients are not allowed anything by mouth (NPO) for up to 24 hours. When fluids are allowed, orders usually begin with small amount of ice chips each hour and increase as patient is able to tolerate more.
l. Remove and discard gloves and perform hand hygiene.	Reduces transmission of microorganisms.
33. For all procedures, clean equipment and return to proper place. Place soiled linen in utility room or proper receptacle. Perform hand hygiene.	Proper disposal of equipment prevents spread of microorganisms and ensures proper exchange procedures.

EVALUATION

1. Observe amount and character of contents draining from NG tube. Ask if patient feels nauseated.	Determines if tube is decompressing stomach of contents.
2. Auscultate for presence of bowel sounds. Turn off suction while auscultating.	Determines return of peristalsis. Sound of suction apparatus is sometimes misinterpreted as bowel sounds.
3. Palpate patient's abdomen periodically. Note any distention, pain, and rigidity.	Determines success of abdominal decompression and return of peristalsis.
4. Inspect condition of nares and nose.	Evaluates onset of skin and tissue irritation.
5. Observe position of tubing.	Prevents tension applied to nasal structures.
6. Ask if patient feels sore throat or irritation in pharynx.	Evaluates level of patient's understanding.
7. **Use Teach-Back:** "I need to be sure I explained why you need the NG tube and the importance of letting me know if you are nauseated. Tell me why it is important for me to know if you feel nauseated." Revise your instruction now or develop a plan for revised patient/family caregiver teaching if patient/family caregiver is not able to teach back correctly.	Determines patient's/family caregiver's level of understanding of instructional topic.

RECORDING AND REPORTING

- Record length, size, and type of gastric tube inserted and in which naris it was inserted. In addition, record patient's tolerance of procedure, confirmation of tube placement, location of distal tip of tube, character of gastric contents, pH value, results of radiography, whether the tube is clamped or connected to drainage bag or to suction, and amount of suction supplied on flow sheet in nurses' notes in electronic health record (EHR) or chart.
- Document your evaluation of patient/family caregiver education and learning.
- Record difference between amount of normal saline instilled and amount of gastric aspirate removed on intake and output (I&O) sheet. Record amount and character of contents draining from NG tube every shift change.
- Record removal of tube "intact," patient's tolerance of procedure, and final amount and character of drainage.
- Report to health care provider any development of unexpected outcomes or presence of blood in gastric drainage.

UNEXPECTED OUTCOMES AND RELATED INTERVENTIONS

- Patient reports nausea or patient's abdomen is distended and painful.
  - Assess patency of tube. NG tube may not be in stomach.
  - Irrigate tube.
  - Verify that suction is on as ordered.
  - Notify health care provider if distention is unrelieved.
- Patient develops irritation or erosion of skin around naris.
  - Provide frequent skin care to area.
  - Use a taping method designed to reduce device-related pressure injury (see Steps 24a and 24b).
  - Consider switching tube to other naris.
- Patient develops signs and symptoms of pulmonary aspiration such as fever, shortness of breath, or pulmonary congestion.
  - Perform complete respiratory assessment.
  - Notify health care provider.
  - Obtain chest x-ray film as ordered.

SKILL 37.2 ADMINISTERING A CLEANSING ENEMA

DELEGATION CONSIDERATIONS

The skill of administering an enema can be delegated to nursing assistive personnel (NAP). **Note:** If a medicated enema is ordered, it must be administered by a nurse. The nurse directs the NAP about:

- How to properly position patients who have mobility restrictions or therapeutic equipment such as drains, IV catheters, or traction.
- Informing the nurse immediately about patient's new abdominal pain (*exception*: a patient reports cramping) or rectal bleeding.
- Informing the nurse immediately about the presence of blood in the stool or around the rectal area or any change in vital signs.

EQUIPMENT

- Clean gloves
- Water-soluble lubricant
- Waterproof, absorbent pads
- Toilet tissue
- Bedpan, bedside commode, or access to toilet
- Bath blanket
- Basin, washcloths, towel, and soap
- Stethoscope

Enema Bag Administration

- Enema container with tubing and clamp
- IV pole

- Appropriate-size rectal tube (adult: 22 to 30 Fr; child: 12 to 18 Fr)
- Correct volume of warmed (tepid) solution (adult: 750 to 1000 mL; adolescent: 500 to 700 mL). For pediatric patients the child's weight usually determines the volume for the enema, usually 5 to 10 mL/kg (Nurko and Zimmerman, 2014).

Prepackaged Enema

- Prepackaged enema container with lubricated rectal tip (Fig. 37.11)

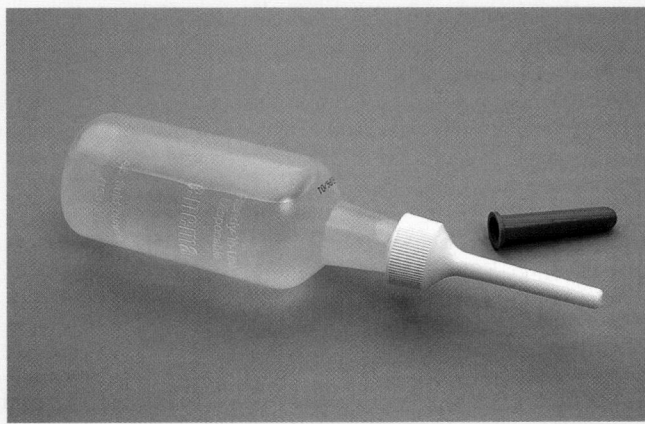

FIG 37.11 Prepackaged enema container with rectal tip.

STEP	RATIONALE

ASSESSMENT

1. Identify patient using at least two identifiers (e.g., name and birthday or name and medical record number) according to agency policy.

   Ensures correct patient. Complies with The Joint Commission Standards and improves patient safety (TJC, 2018).

2. Review health care provider's order for enema and clarify reason for administration.

   Health care provider order is usually required for hospitalized patient. The order states which type of enema the patient will receive.

3. Perform hand hygiene. Assess last bowel movement, normal versus most recent bowel pattern, presence of hemorrhoids, mobility, and presence of abdominal pain or cramping.

   Determines need for enema and type of enema used. Also establishes baseline for bowel function. Hemorrhoids may obscure rectal opening and cause discomfort or bleeding during evacuation.

4. Inspect abdomen for presence of distention and auscultate for bowel sounds.

   Establishes baseline for determining effectiveness of enema.

5. Assess patient's mobility and ability to turn and position on side. Perform hand hygiene.

   Determines if assistance is needed for positioning patient.

6. Assess patient for allergy to any active ingredients of Fleet enema.

   Reduces risk for allergic reaction.

7. Assess patient's level of understanding of purpose of enema.

   Allows for planning appropriate teaching measures.

Clinical Decision Point. "Enemas until clear" order means that you repeat enemas until patient passes fluid that is clear of fecal matter. The fluid the patient passes may be tinted and have small flecks of fecal matter. Check agency policy, but usually patient should receive only three consecutive enemas to avoid disruption of fluid and electrolyte balance. It is essential to observe contents of solution passed.

PLANNING

1. Provide privacy by closing curtains around bed or closing door and prepare bedside environment for patient safety.

   Preparing the environment early helps the nurse think about the steps needed; removing clutter from over-bed table removes barriers to completing procedure. Reduces embarrassment for patient.

SKILL 37.2 ADMINISTERING A CLEANSING ENEMA—cont'd

View Video!

STEP	RATIONALE
2. Prepare and organize equipment for enema at bedside.	Ensures organized approach for enema administration.
3. Explain to patient the steps of enema procedure.	Promotes patient cooperation and increases compliance.

IMPLEMENTATION

1. If enema is medicated, the skill may or may not be delegated to NAP (see agency policy). Check accuracy and completeness of each medication administration record (MAR) with health care provider's written order. Check patient's name, type of enema, and time for administration. Compare MAR with label of enema solution.	The order is most reliable source and only legal record of drugs or procedure that patient is to receive. Ensures that patient receives correct enema.
2. Place bedpan or bedside commode in easily accessible position. If patient will be expelling contents in toilet, ensure that toilet is available, and place patient's nonskid slippers and bathrobe in easily accessible position.	Bedpan is used if patient is unable to get out of bed. Nonskid slippers help prevent falling of patient who may be rushing to the bathroom. Extra gown provides modesty for patient.
3. Perform hand hygiene.	Reduces transmission of microorganisms.
4. With side rail raised on patient's right side and bed raised to appropriate working height, help patient turn onto left side-lying (Sims') position with right knee flexed. Encourage patient to remain in position until procedure is complete. Children are placed in dorsal recumbent position.	Allows enema solution to flow downward by gravity along natural curve of sigmoid colon and rectum, improving retention of solution.

Clinical Decision Point. Patients with poor sphincter control require placement of a bedpan under the buttocks. Administering enema with patient sitting on toilet is unsafe because curved rectal tubing can abrade rectal wall.

5. Apply clean gloves and place waterproof pad, absorbent side up, under hips and buttocks. Cover patient with bath blanket, exposing only rectal area, clearly visualizing anus.	Pad prevents soiling of linen. Blanket provides warmth, reduces exposure of body parts, and allows patient to feel more relaxed and comfortable.
6. Separate buttocks and examine perianal region for abnormalities including hemorrhoids, anal fissure, and rectal prolapse (protrusion of rectal tissue outside anus).	Findings influence approach for inserting enema tip. Prolapse contraindicates enema.
7. Administer enema.	
a. Administer prepackaged disposable enema:	
(1) Remove plastic cap from tip of container. Tip may already be lubricated. Apply more water-soluble lubricant as needed.	Lubrication provides for smooth insertion of rectal tube without causing rectal irritation or trauma. Extra lubricant provides added comfort in presence of hemorrhoids.
(2) Gently separate buttocks and locate anus. Instruct patient to relax by breathing out slowly through mouth.	Breathing out promotes relaxation of external rectal sphincter.
(3) Expel any air from enema container.	Introducing air into colon causes further distention and discomfort.
(4) Insert lubricated tip of container gently into anal canal toward umbilicus (see illustration).	Gentle insertion prevents trauma to rectal mucosa.

Adult: 7.5 to 10 cm (3 to 4 inches)
Adolescent: 7.5 to 10 cm (3 to 4 inches)
Child: 5 to 7.5 cm (2 to 3 inches)
Infant: 2.5 to 3.75 cm (1 to $1\frac{1}{2}$ inches)

Clinical Decision Point. If pain occurs or you feel resistance at any time during procedure, stop and discuss with health care provider. Do not force insertion.

(5) Roll plastic bottle from bottom to tip until all of solution has entered rectum and colon. Instruct patient to retain solution until urge to defecate occurs, usually 2 to 5 minutes.	Prevents instillation of air into colon and ensures that all solution enters rectum. Hypertonic solutions require only small volumes to stimulate defecation.

STEP	RATIONALE
b. Administer enema in standard enema bag:	
(1) Add warmed prescribed type of solution and amount to enema bag: Warm tap water as it flows from faucet, place saline container in basin of warm water before adding saline to enema bag, and check temperature of solution by pouring small amount of solution over inner wrist.	Hot water burns intestinal mucosa. Cold water causes abdominal cramping and is difficult to retain.
(2) If soapsuds enema (SSE) is ordered, add castile soap after water.	Reduces suds in enema bag.
(3) Raise container, release clamp, and allow solution to flow long enough to fill tubing.	Removes air from tubing.
(4) Reclamp tubing.	Prevents further loss of solution.
(5) Lubricate 6 to 8 cm (2½ to 3 inches) of tip of rectal tube with lubricant.	Allows smooth insertion of rectal tube without risk for irritation or trauma to mucosa.
(6) Gently separate buttocks and locate anus. Instruct patient to relax by breathing out slowly through mouth. Touch patient's skin next to anus with tip of rectal tube.	Breathing out and touching skin with tube promotes relaxation of external anal sphincter.
(7) Insert tip of rectal tube slowly by pointing it in direction of patient's umbilicus. Length of insertion varies.	Careful insertion prevents trauma to rectal mucosa from accidental lodging of tube against rectal wall. Insertion beyond proper limit can cause bowel perforation.

Clinical Decision Point. If tube does not pass easily, do not force. Consider allowing a small amount of fluid to infuse and then try to reinsert tube slowly. The instillation of fluid relaxes the sphincter and provides additional lubrication. If impaction is present, remove it before administering enema.

(8) Hold tubing in rectum constantly until end of fluid instillation.	Prevents expulsion of rectal tube during bowel contractions.
(9) Open regulating clamp and allow solution to enter slowly with container at patient's hip level.	Rapid infusion may stimulate evacuation of tubing and can cause cramping.
(10) Raise height of enema container slowly to appropriate level above anus: 30 to 45 cm (12 to 18 inches) for high enema; 30 cm (12 inches) for regular enema (see illustration); 7.5 cm (3 inches) for low enema. Instillation time varies with volume of solution administered (e.g., 1 L may take 10 minutes). You may use an IV pole to hold enema bag once you get a slow flow of fluid established.	Allows for continuous, slow instillation of solution. Raising container too high causes rapid instillation and possible painful distention of colon. High pressure causes rupture of bowel in infant.

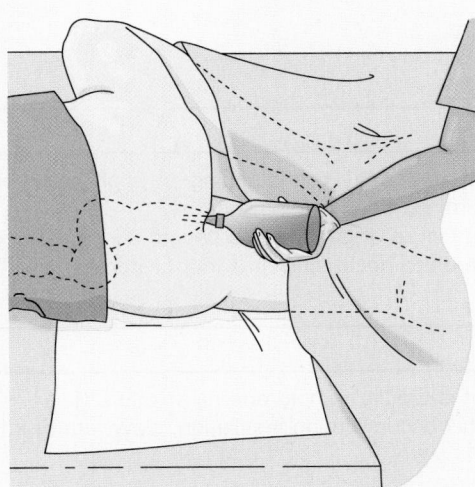

STEP 7a(4) With patient in left lateral Sims' position, insert tip of commercial enema into rectum. (From Sorrentino SA, Remmert LN: *Mosby's textbook for nursing assistants*, ed 9, St Louis, 2017, Elsevier.)

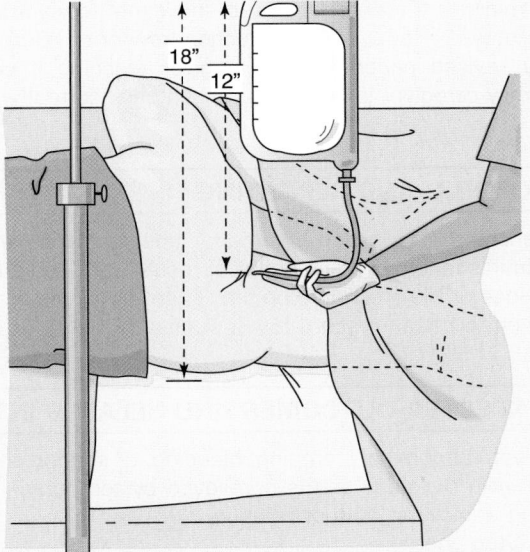

STEP 7b(10) IV pole is positioned so that the bottom of the enema bag is 18 inches above the anus.

SKILL 37.2 ADMINISTERING A CLEANSING ENEMA—cont'd

View Video!

STEP	RATIONALE

Clinical Decision Point. Temporary cessation of infusion minimizes cramping and promotes ability to retain solution. Lower container or clamp tubing if patient complains of cramping or if fluid escapes around rectal tube.

STEP	RATIONALE
(11) Instill all solution and clamp tubing. Tell patient that procedure is completed and that you will be removing tubing.	Prevents entrance of air into rectum. Patients may misinterpret sensation of removing tube as loss of control.
8. Place layers of toilet tissue around tube at anus and gently withdraw rectal tube and tip.	Provides for patient's comfort and cleanliness.
9. Explain to patient that some distention and abdominal cramping is normal. Ask patient to retain solution as long as possible until urge to defecate occurs. This usually takes a few minutes. Stay at bedside. Have patient lie quietly in bed if possible. (For infant or young child gently hold buttocks together for few minutes.)	Solution distends bowel. Length of retention varies with type of enema and patient's ability to contract rectal sphincter. Longer retention promotes stimulation of peristalsis and defecation.
10. Discard enema container or disposable bag and tubing in proper receptacle. Remove gloves and perform hand hygiene.	Reduces transmission and growth of microorganisms.
11. Help patient to bathroom or commode if possible. If using bedpan, help to as near normal position for evacuation as possible (wearing gloves).	Normal squatting position promotes defecation.
12. Observe character of stool and solution (caution patient against flushing toilet before inspection).	Determines if enema was effective.
13. Help patient as needed to wash anal area with warm soap and water (if nurse administers perineal care, use gloves).	Fecal contents irritate skin. Hygiene promotes patient comfort.
14. Remove and discard gloves and perform hand hygiene.	Reduces transmission of microorganisms.

EVALUATION

1. Inspect color, consistency, and amount of stool; odor; and fluid passed.	Determines if stool is evacuated or fluid is retained. Note abnormalities such as presence of blood or mucus.
2. Assess for abdominal distention.	Determines if distention is relieved.
3. **Use Teach-Back:** "I want to be sure I explained how to administer a Fleet enema to yourself. I want to be sure you understand the correct position for lying down to administer the enema. Please show me how you would lie down." Revise your instruction now or develop a plan for revised patient/family caregiver teaching if patient/family caregiver is not able to teach back correctly.	Determines patient's/family caregiver's level of understanding of instructional topic.

RECORDING AND REPORTING

- Record the type and volume of enema given, time of administration, characteristics of results, and patient's tolerance of the procedure on flow sheet or nurses' notes in electronic health record (EHR) or chart.
- Record patient's understanding through teach-back for self-administration of Fleet enema.
- Report failure of patient to defecate and any unexpected outcomes to health care provider or nurse.

UNEXPECTED OUTCOMES AND RELATED INTERVENTIONS

- Severe abdominal cramping, bleeding, or sudden abdominal pain develops and is unrelieved by temporarily stopping or slowing flow of solution.
  - Stop enema.
  - Notify health care provider.
  - Obtain vital signs.
- Patient is unable to hold enema solution.
  - If this occurs during instillation, slow rate of infusion.

View Video!

SKILL 37.3 POUCHING AN OSTOMY

DELEGATION CONSIDERATIONS

The skill of pouching a new ostomy should not be delegated to nursing assistive personnel (NAP). In some agencies care of an established ostomy (4 to 6 weeks or more after surgery) can be delegated to NAP. The nurse directs the NAP about:

- Expected amount, color, and consistency of drainage from an ostomy.
- Expected appearance of the stoma.
- Special equipment needed to complete a particular patient's pouching.
- Changes in a patient's stoma and surrounding skin integrity that should be reported.

EQUIPMENT

- Skin barrier/pouch—clear, drainable one-piece or two-piece, cut-to-fit or precut size
- Pouch closure device such as a clip if needed
- Ostomy measuring guide
- Adhesive remover *(optional)*
- Clean gloves
- Washcloth, towel or disposable waterproof barrier
- Basin with warm tap water
- Scissors
- Waterproof bag for disposal of pouch
- *Optional:* Gown or goggles if there is any risk of splashing when emptying pouch

STEP	RATIONALE

ASSESSMENT

1. Identify patient using at least two identifiers (e.g., name and birthday or name and medical record number) according to agency policy.

2. Perform hand hygiene and apply clean gloves.

3. Observe existing skin barrier and pouch for leakage and length of time in place. Pouch should be changed every 3 to 7 days, not daily (Colwell, 2016). If an opaque pouch is being used, remove it to fully observe stoma (dispose of pouch in proper receptacle).

Ensures patient safety. Complies with The Joint Commission Standards and improves patient safety (TJC, 2018).

Reduces transmission of microorganisms.

Assesses effectiveness of pouching system and detects potential for problems. To minimize skin irritation, avoid unnecessary changing of entire pouching system. When pouch leaks, skin damage from effluent causes more skin trauma than early removal of wafer.

> **Clinical Decision Point.** Repeated leaking may indicate need for different type of pouch or addition of products such as stoma putty. If pouch is leaking, change it. Taping or patching pouch to contain effluent leaves skin exposed to chemical or enzymatic irritation.

4. Observe amount of effluent in pouch and empty it if it is more than one-third to one-half full by opening pouch and draining it into a container for measurement of output. Note consistency of effluent and record intake and output.

5. Observe stoma for type, location, color, swelling, presence of sutures, trauma, and healing or irritation of peristomal skin. Determine if it is budded, flush with skin level, or retracted below skin level (see illustrations).

6. Observe placement of stoma in relation to abdominal contours or presence of scars or incisions. Remove and dispose of gloves, and perform hand hygiene.

Weight of pouch may disrupt seal of adhesive on skin. Monitors fluid balance and bowel function after surgery. Normal colostomy effluent is soft or formed stool, whereas normal ileostomy effluent is liquid.

Stoma characteristics influence selection of appropriate pouching system. Convexity in skin barrier is often necessary with flush or retracted stoma.

Determines if current pouching system is effective or if new selection is needed. Abdominal contours, scars, or incisions affect type of system and adhesion to skin surface. Reduces transmission of microorganisms.

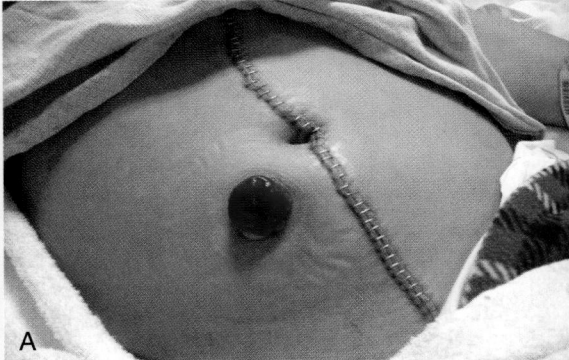 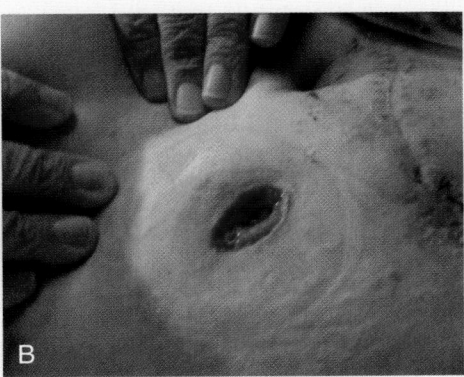

STEP 5 A, Budded stoma. **B,** Retracted stoma. (Courtesy Jane Fellows)

View Video!

SKILL 37.3 POUCHING AN OSTOMY—cont'd

STEP	RATIONALE
7. Explore patient's attitudes, perceptions, knowledge, and acceptance of stoma; discuss interest in learning self-care. Identify family caregiver who will be helping patient after leaving hospital.	Determines patient's willingness to learn. Facilitates teaching plan and timing of care to coincide with availability of family caregivers.

PLANNING

1. Provide privacy by closing curtains around bed or closing door and prepare bedside environment for patient safety.	Preparing the environment early helps the nurse think about the steps needed; removing clutter from over-bed table removes barriers completing procedure. Reduces embarrassment for patient.
2. Assemble equipment needed to change ostomy pouch.	Ensures organized approach for changing ostomy pouch.
3. Explain procedure to patient; encourage patient's interaction and questions.	Lessens patient's anxiety and promotes patient's participation.

IMPLEMENTATION

1. Have patient assume semi-reclining or supine position (same position assumed during assessment and pouching). (**Note:** Some patients with established ostomies prefer to stand.) If possible, provide patient with mirror for observation.	When patient is in semi-reclining position, there are fewer skin folds, which allows for ease of application of pouching system.
2. Perform hand hygiene and apply clean gloves.	Reduces transmission of microorganisms.
3. Place towel or disposable waterproof barrier under patient and across patient's lower abdomen.	Protects bed linen; maintains patient's dignity.
4. If not done during assessment, remove used pouch and skin barrier gently by pushing skin away from barrier. Use an adhesive remover to facilitate removal of skin barrier. Empty pouch and dispose of it in appropriate receptacle. Measure output if needed. **Note:** There may be no output at time of first pouch change.	Reduces skin trauma. Improper removal of pouch and barrier can cause peristomal skin irritation or breakdown.
5. Clean peristomal skin gently with warm tap water using washcloth; do not scrub skin. If you touch stoma, minor bleeding is normal. Pat skin dry. Have washcloth handy for additional cleansing if there is output from stoma while preparing pouch. Remove and dispose of gloves. Perform hand hygiene.	Soap leaves residue on skin, which may irritate skin. Pouch does not adhere to wet skin. Do not use products containing moisturizers, such as cleansers and baby wipes, because the pouch will not adhere well. Ileostomies have frequent output, especially after eating.
6. Measure stoma (see illustration). Expect size of stoma to change for first 4 to 6 weeks after surgery.	Allows for proper fit of pouch that will protect peristomal skin.
7. Trace pattern of stoma measurement on pouch backing or skin barrier (see illustration).	Prepares for cutting opening in pouch.

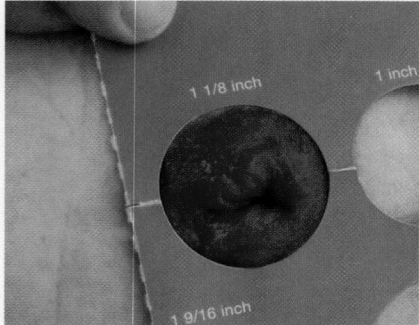

STEP 6 Measure stoma. (Courtesy Coloplast, Minneapolis, MN.)

STEP 7 Trace measurement on skin barrier. (Courtesy Coloplast, Minneapolis, MN.)

STEP	RATIONALE
8. Cut opening on backing or skin barrier wafer (see illustration). If using a moldable or shape to fit barrier, use fingers to mold the shape to fit the stoma.	Customizes pouch to provide appropriate fit over stoma.
9. Remove protective backing from adhesive backing or wafer (see illustration).	Prepares skin barrier for placement.
10. Apply gloves. Apply pouch over stoma (see illustration). Press firmly into place around stoma and outside edges. Have patient hold hand over pouch to apply heat to secure seal.	Pouch adhesives are heat and pressure sensitive and hold more securely at body temperature.
11. Close end of pouch with clip or integrated closure. Remove drape from patient. Assist patient to assume comfortable position.	Ensures pouch is secure. Contains effluent.
12. Remove and dispose of gloves and other disposables. Perform hand hygiene.	Reduces transmission of microorganisms.

EVALUATION

1. Observe condition of skin barrier and adherence of pouch to abdominal surface.	Determines presence of leaks.
2. Observe appearance of stoma, peristomal skin, abdominal contours, suture line, and presence of any flatus during pouch change.	Determines condition of stoma and peristomal skin and progress of wound healing.
3. Note if there is presence of any flatus during pouch change.	Determines if peristalsis is returning.
4. Observe patient's and family caregiver's willingness to view stoma and ask questions about procedure.	Determines level of adjustment and understanding of stoma care and pouch application. Allows planning for future education needs and progress toward acceptance of altered body image.
5. **Use Teach-Back:** "I want to be sure you understand what is involved in changing your ostomy pouch. Tell me what you should do to prevent your skin from becoming irritated and how often you should empty your pouch." Revise your instruction now or develop a plan for revised patient/family caregiver teaching if patient/family caregiver is not able to teach back correctly.	Determines patient's/family caregiver's level of understanding of instructional topic.

RECORDING AND REPORTING

- Record type of pouch and skin barrier applied; time of procedure; amount and appearance of effluent in pouch; location, size, and appearance of stoma; and condition of peristomal skin in nurses' notes in electronic health record (EHR) or chart.

- Document your evaluation of patient/family caregiver learning.
- Report to nurse and/or health care provider: abnormal appearance of stoma, suture line, peristomal skin, or character of output.

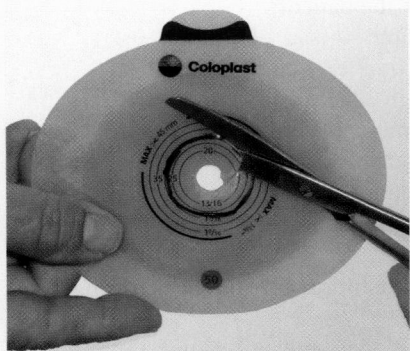
STEP 8 Cut opening in wafer. (Courtesy Coloplast, Minneapolis, MN.)

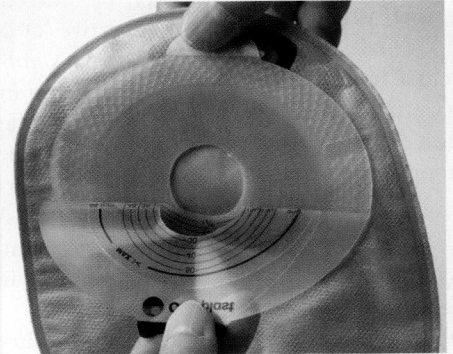
STEP 9 Remove protective backing. (Courtesy Coloplast, Minneapolis, MN.)

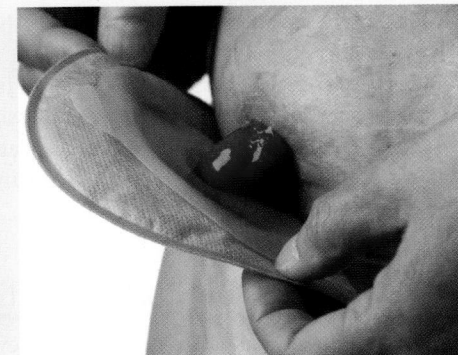
STEP 10 Apply pouch over stoma. (Courtesy Coloplast, Minneapolis, MN.)

SKILL 37.3   POUCHING AN OSTOMY—cont'd

UNEXPECTED OUTCOMES AND RELATED INTERVENTIONS

- Skin around stoma is irritated, blistered, or bleeding, or a rash is noted; may be caused by undermining of pouch seal by fecal contents causing irritant dermatitis, adhesive removal causing skin stripping, or fungal or other skin eruption.
  - Remove pouch more carefully.
  - Change pouch more frequently or use different type of pouching system.
  - Consult ostomy care nurse.
  - Avoid use of acetone-based products.

- Necrotic stoma may be bluish, purple, or black in color; dry instead of moist in texture; fail to bleed when washed gently; or show signs of tissue sloughing.
  - Report to nurse in charge or health care provider.
  - Document appearance.
- Patient refuses to view stoma or participate in care.
  - Obtain referral for ostomy care nurse.
  - Allow patient to express feelings.
  - Encourage family support.

KEY POINTS

- Mechanical breakdown of food elements, gastrointestinal (GI) motility, and selective absorption and secretion of substances by the large intestine influence the character of feces.
- Food high in fiber content and increased fluid intake keep feces soft.
- Daily exercise is important to maintenance of normal bowel function.
- The greatest dangers from diarrhea are dehydration and fluid and electrolyte imbalance.
- A patient with a fecal diversion (colostomy or ileostomy) requires teaching in the care of the stoma and support in adjusting to the change in body image and function.
- The location of an ostomy influences the consistency of stool.
- A fecal occult blood test (FOBT) or fecal immunochemical test (FIT) determines if blood is present in a stool sample. Both are screening tools for colon cancer for patients over 50 years of age.
- Consider frequency of defecation, fecal characteristics, effect of foods on GI function, and patient's food preferences when selecting a diet promoting normal elimination.
- Proper enema administration requires the slow instillation of the correct volume of a solution.
- Dangers during digital removal of stool include traumatizing the rectal mucosa and promoting vagal stimulation.
- Skin breakdown occurs after repeated exposure to liquid stool; prevention of this is an important nursing responsibility.

REFLECTIVE LEARNING

- You provided care for a patient with a new ileostomy today and he will be discharged from the hospital 2 days from now. He refused to look at his stoma or have teaching about ostomy care saying he was too tired because he did not sleep well last night. How will you prepare him for discharge when you see him tomorrow?
- Your postoperative patient will be going home on opioid pain medication. What patient education is necessary to prevent constipation, which is a common side effect of this medication?
- An elderly home care patient has diarrhea. You know that dehydration and perianal skin breakdown are risks with this condition. How will you teach caregivers to manage care to reduce these complications of diarrhea?

REVIEW QUESTIONS

1. When a patient has an ileostomy, the digestive process ends in the terminal ileum. Patient education by the nurse should include the need for the person to ingest more of which dietary component?
   1. More food
   2. Fluids and salt
   3. Less sugar and artificial sweetener
   4. Fiber to firm the stool
2. The nurse is providing care for a patient who reports no bowel movement for 5 days except for small amounts of liquid stool. Which immediate intervention will most likely be ordered for the patient?
   1. Laxatives at bedtime
   2. Manual removal of a fecal impaction
   3. Instruction in high-fiber diet
   4. Increase in her ambulation from 1 to 2 times a day
3. When caring for a patient with fecal incontinence, what is the best way for the nurse to protect the patient's skin?
   1. Cleanse the skin with a no-rinse cleanser and apply a barrier cream
   2. Scrub the skin with antimicrobial cleanser using a soft washcloth
   3. Cleanse skin with soap and water and apply talcum powder
   4. Wipe stool away with toilet paper and apply petrolatum ointment

4. A patient has a new ileostomy and needs to be taught how to care for the ileostomy. The nurse is seeing the patient on the first postoperative day. The patient has abdominal pain that is rated as 7 out of 10 and about 150 mL of dark green effluent in the ileostomy pouch. What skill would be best for the nurse to teach the patient at this time?
   1. Care of the peristomal skin
   2. Cutting and fitting the ostomy pouch
   3. Placing a new ostomy pouch
   4. Emptying the pouch

5. What lifestyle changes would the nurse include in a teaching plan for a patient who reports occasional constipation? (Select all that apply.)
   1. Daily laxative use
   2. Increased fluid intake
   3. Decreased fluid intake
   4. Regular exercise
   5. High-fiber diet
   6. More fruits and vegetables in the diet

evolve

Additional Review Questions, as well as rationales for all Review Questions, can be found on the Evolve website.

1, 2, 2; 3, 1; 4, 4; 5, 2, 4, 5, 6.

REFERENCES

American Association of Critical Care Nurses (AACN): *Practice alert. Initial and ongoing verification of feeding tube placement in adults,* 2009. The Association, http://www.aacn.org/wd/practice/docs/practicealerts/verification-feeding-tube-placement.pdf?menu=aboutus.

American Cancer Society (ACS): *American Cancer Society recommendations for colorectal cancer early detection,* 2017. http://www.cancer.org/cancer/colonandrectumcancer/moreinformation/colonandrectumcancerearlydetection/colorectal-cancer-early-detection-acs-recommendations.

Ball JW, et al: *Seidel's guide to physical examination,* ed 8, St Louis, 2015, Elsevier.

Blake MR, et al: Validity and reliability of the Bristol Stool Form Scale in healthy adults and patients with diarrhoea-predominant irritable bowel syndrome, *Aliment Pharmacol Ther* 44(7):693, 2016.

Callan L, Wilson M: Fecal incontinence: pathology, assessment and management. In Doughty D, Moore K, editors: *Wound Ostomy Continence Nursing Society core curriculum: continence management,* Philadelphia, 2016, Wolters Kluwer.

Colwell J: Selection of a pouching system. In Carmel J, et al, editors: *Wound Ostomy Continence Nursing Society core curriculum: ostomy management,* Philadelphia, 2016, Wolters Kluwer.

Emergency Nurses Association (ENA): *Clinical practice guideline, gastric tube placement verification,* 2015. https://www.ena.org/docs/default-source/resource-library/practice-resources/cpg/gastrictubecpg7b5530b71c1e49e8b155b6cca1870adc.pdf?sfvrsn=a8e9dd7a_8.

Goldberg M: Patient education following urinary/fecal diversion. In Carmel J, et al, editors: *Wound, Ostomy and Continence Nursing Society core curriculum: ostomy management,* Philadelphia, 2016, Wolters Kluwer.

Goldberg M, et al: *Best practice guideline: management of the patient with an ostomy,* Mt Laurel, NJ, 2016, Wound, Ostomy and Continence Nurses Society.

Hockenberry MJ, Wilson D: *Wong's nursing care of infants and children,* ed 10, St Louis, 2014, Mosby.

Mayo Clinic: C. difficile *infection,* 2016. http://www.mayoclinic.org/diseases-conditions/c-difficile/home/ovc-20202264.

Metheny NA, Franz RA: Head-of-bed elevation in critically ill patients: a review, *Crit Care Nurse* 33(3):53, 2013.

NANDA International: *NANDA International nursing diagnoses: definitions and classifications, 2015-2017,* Oxford, UK, 2014, Wiley-Blackwell.

National Cancer Institute: *Tests to detect colorectal cancer and polyps,* 2016. https://www.cancer.gov/types/colorectal/screening-fact-sheet.

National Institute of Diabetes, Digestive and Kidney Diseases (NIDDK): *Health information,* 2016. https://www.niddk.nih.gov/health-information.

Nichols T: Quality of life of US residents with ostomies as assessed using the SF36v2, *J Wound Ostomy Continence Nurs* 42(1):71, 2015.

Nurko S, Zimmerman LA: Evaluation and treatment of constipation in children and adolescents, *Am Fam Physician* 90(2):82, 2014.

Pittman J, et al: Medical device-related hospital-acquired pressure ulcers: development of an evidence-based position statement, *J Wound Ostomy Continence Nurs* 42(2):151, 2015.

Salvadalena G: Peristomal skin conditions. In Carmel J, et al, editors: *Wound Ostomy Continence Nursing Society core curriculum: ostomy management,* Philadelphia, 2016, Wolters Kluwer.

Shlamovitz G, Shah N: *Nasogastric intubation,* 2016. http://emedicine.medscape.com/article/80925-overview.

Steele S, et al: Motility disorders. In Carmel J, et al, editors: *Wound Ostomy Continence Nursing Society core curriculum continence management,* Philadelphia, 2016, Wolters Kluwer.

Stewart ML, et al: Interruptions in enteral nutrition delivery in the critically ill patients and recommendations for clinical practice, *Crit Care Nurse* 34: 14, 2014.

Sun V, et al: Surviving colorectal cancer: long-term, persistent ostomy-specific concerns and adaptations, *J Wound Ostomy Continence Nurs* 40(1):67, 2013.

The Joint Commission (TJC): *2018 National Patient Safety Goals,* Oakbrook Terrace, IL, 2018, The Commission, http://www.jointcommission.org/standards_information/npsgs.aspx.

Tho PC, et al: Implementation of the evidence-review on best practice for confirming the correct placement of nasogastric tube in patients in an acute care hospital, *Int J Evid Based Healthc* 9(1):51, 2011.

University of Michigan: *Troubleshooting autonomic dysreflexia,* 2013. http://www.med.umich.edu/1libr/SpinalCordInjuryProgram/AutomonicDysreflexia.pdf.

Van Leeuwen A, et al: *Davis's comprehensive handbook of laboratory and diagnostic tests with nursing implications,* ed 6, Philadelphia, 2015, Davis.

Walthen B, Peyton C: Pediatric nasogastric tube placement, *Nurs Crit Care* 9(3): 14, 2014.

CHAPTER

38

Skin Integrity and Wound Care

evolve MEDIA RESOURCES

http://evolve.elsevier.com/Potter/essentials

- Audio Glossary
- QSEN Activity and Review Questions Answers and Rationales
- Video Clips

OBJECTIVES

- Describe risk factors for pressure injury development.
- List the National Pressure Ulcer Advisory Panel (NPUAP) pressure injury stages.
- Describe guidelines for prevention of pressure injuries.
- Discuss the use of risk assessment tools in the assessment of pressure injuries.
- Discuss the response of the body during each phase of the wound-healing process.
- Describe wound assessment criteria: anatomical location, size, type and percentage of wound tissue, volume and color of wound drainage, and condition of surrounding skin.
- Differentiate healing by primary, secondary, and tertiary intention.
- Discuss common complications of wound healing.
- Explain factors that promote or impede wound healing.

- Describe the purposes of and precautions taken with applying dressings and binders.
- Describe the mechanism of action of wound care dressings.
- Describe the differences in therapeutic effects of heat and cold.
- Complete an assessment for a patient with risk for or actual impaired skin integrity.
- List nursing diagnoses associated with risk for or actual impaired skin integrity.
- Develop a nursing care plan for a patient with risk for or actual impaired skin integrity.
- Evaluate outcomes of nursing care using appropriate criteria for a patient with risk for or actual impaired skin integrity.

KEY TERMS

abrasion, p. 1114
binders, p. 1127
blanchable hyperemia, p. 1103
compress, p. 1135
debride, p. 1123
dehiscence, p. 1107
ecchymosis, p. 1114
eschar, p. 1101
evisceration, p. 1107

friction, p. 1105
granulation tissue, p. 1105
hematoma, p. 1107
hemostasis, p. 1107
induration, p. 1112
intertriginous dermatitis (ITD), p. 1101
laceration, p. 1105
maceration, p. 1120
nonblanchable hyperemia, p. 1103

pressure injury, p. 1101
primary intention, p. 1105
reactive hyperemia, p. 1103
secondary intention, p. 1105
shear, p. 1104
sitz bath, p. 1135
slough, p. 1101
tertiary intention, p. 1105
tissue ischemia, p. 1103

CASE STUDY *Mr. Martinez*

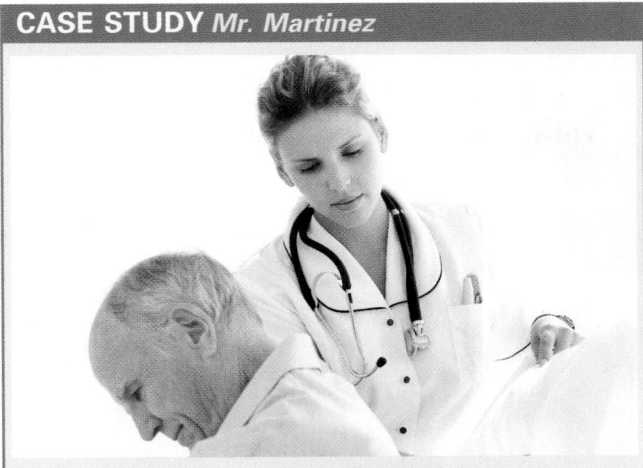

Copyright © Stockbyte/iStock/Thinkstock.

Mr. Louis Martinez, a 76-year-old retired accountant with a medical history of type 2 diabetes mellitus and hypertension, had coronary artery bypass surgery 6 months ago. While at home he became weak and rarely got out of his bed; he was unable to eat and has lost more than 20 lb over the last 2 months. He was diagnosed with pneumonia and is now hospitalized. Mr. Martinez is weak, having difficulty breathing, and experiencing limited mobility. Mr. Martinez lives in a one-family home with his wife. Their children and grandchildren live nearby and visit often. He states that his "bottom hurts" from lying in bed. Lynda is assigned to care for Mr. Martinez the week before his discharge.

SCIENTIFIC KNOWLEDGE BASE

Pressure Injuries

Pressure injury (formerly called pressure sore, *pressure ulcer, decubitus ulcer,* or *bedsore*) is localized damage to the skin and underlying soft tissue usually over a bony prominence or related to a medical or other device (Fig. 38.1). The injury can appear as intact skin or an open ulcer and may be painful. The injury occurs as a result of intense and/or prolonged pressure or pressure in combination with shear. The tolerance of soft tissue for pressure and shear may also be affected by microclimate, nutrition, perfusion, comorbid conditions, and condition of the soft tissue (Edsberg et al., 2016). The term *pressure injury* replaces *pressure ulcer* in the National Pressure Ulcer Advisory Injury Staging System (National Pressure Ulcer Advisory Panel [NPUAP], 2016). The updated staging definitions and change in terminology more accurately describe pressure injuries to both intact and ulcerated skin. In the previous staging system Stage 1 and deep tissue injury described injured intact skin, whereas the other stages described open ulcers. This led to confusion because the definitions for each of the stages referred to the injuries as "pressure ulcers." In addition to the change in terminology, Arabic numbers are now used in the names of the stages instead of Roman numerals. The term *suspected* has been removed from the deep tissue injury diagnostic label. The definitions from the 2016 NPUAP staging system follow (Edsberg et al., 2016).

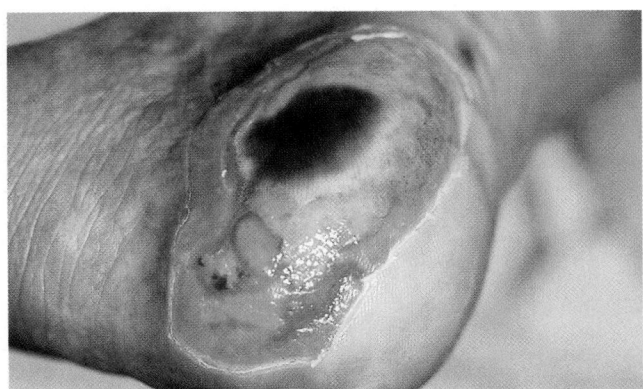

FIG 38.1 Pressure injury with tissue necrosis.

Pressure Injury Classification

- **Stage 1 Pressure Injury:** Intact skin with a localized area of nonblanchable erythema, which may appear differently in darkly pigmented skin. The presence of blanchable erythema or changes in sensation, temperature, or firmness may precede visual changes. Color changes do not include purple or maroon discoloration; these may indicate deep tissue pressure injury (Fig. 38.2A).

  Teaching points:
  - Stage 1 pressure injuries are often the first visible changes in the skin and have been historically referred to as the "heralding sign."
  - It is important that scar tissue and deep tissue pressure injury (DTPI) not be classified as a Stage 1 pressure injury.
  - The skin's blanching response can be assessed by pressing the skin with a finger to close the capillary bed. On release of pressure, the skin should immediately return to the native skin color. Diascopy, examination of the skin's blanch response through a color disc pressed on the skin, also may be used to assess the cutaneous blanche response.

- **Stage 2 Pressure Injury:** Partial-thickness skin loss with exposed dermis. The wound bed is viable, pink or red, and moist, or injury may manifest as an intact or ruptured serum-filled blister. Adipose (fat) is not visible, and deeper tissue is not visible. Granulation tissue, **slough** (soft, moist, devitalized tissue that may be yellow, tan, or green and either loose or firmly adherent), and **eschar** are not present. These injuries commonly result from adverse microclimate and shear in the skin over the pelvis and shear in the heel (Fig. 38.2B).

  Teaching points:
  - This stage should not be used to describe moisture-associated skin damage (MASD) including incontinence-associated dermatitis (IAD) and **intertriginous dermatitis (ITD)** (inflammation of skin where two surfaces rub such as groin, beneath breasts, and underarm area).
  - This stage should not be used to describe medical adhesive–related skin injury (MARSI) or traumatic wounds (skin tears, burns, abrasions).

Lightly Pigmented   Darkly Pigmented

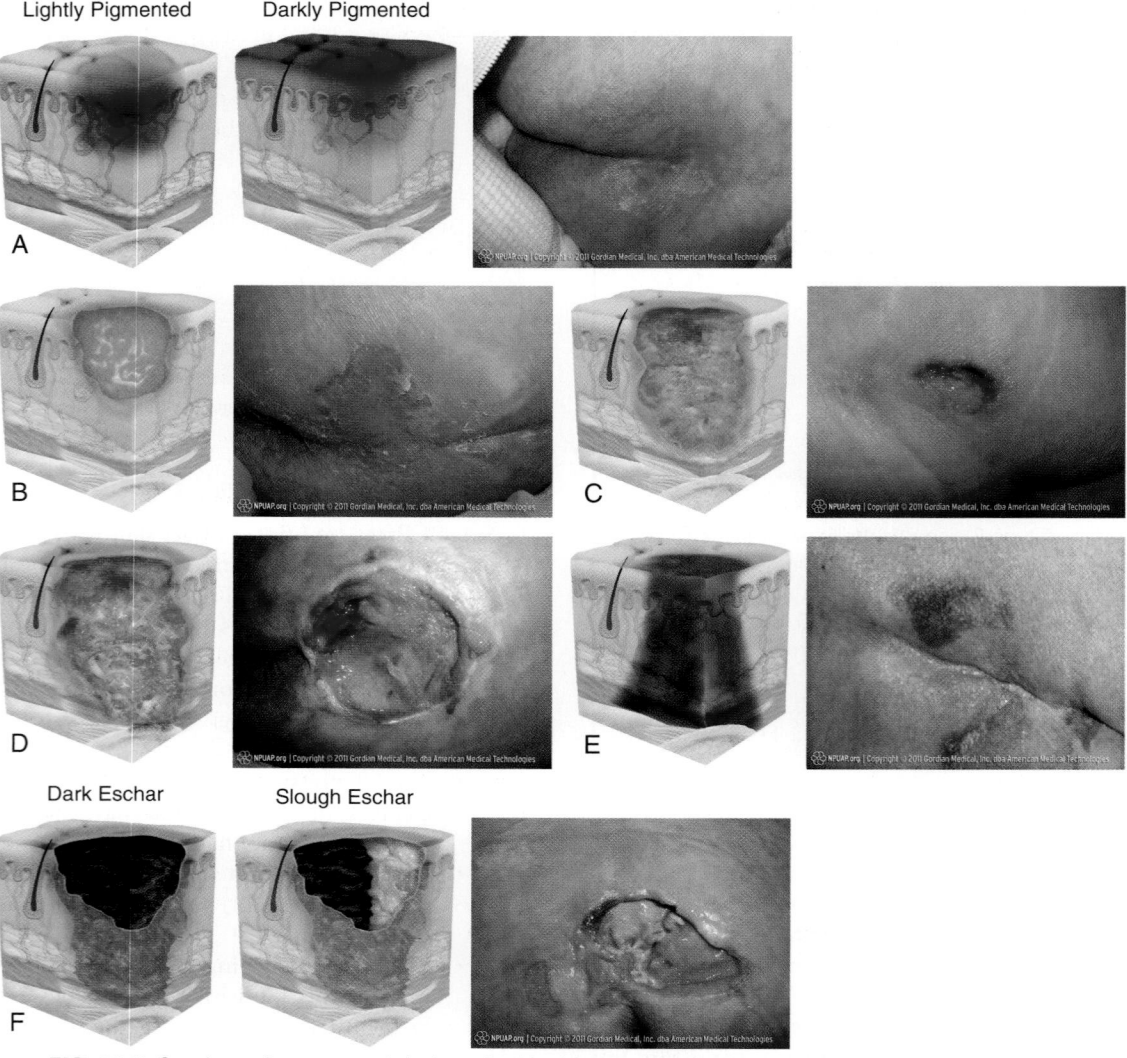

Dark Eschar   Slough Eschar

FIG 38.2 Staging of pressure injuries. **A,** Nonblanchable erythema of intact skin. **B,** Partial-thickness skin loss with exposed dermis. **C,** Full-thickness skin loss. **D,** Full-thickness skin and tissue loss. **E,** Persistent nonblanchable deep red, maroon, or purple discoloration. **F,** Obscured full-thickness skin and tissue loss. (Used with permission of the National Pressure Ulcer Advisory Panel. Copyright © NPUAP.)

- It is especially important if an injury is suspected of being a Stage 2 pressure injury that the presence or history of pressure and/or shear be confirmed.
- **Stage 3 Pressure Injury:** Full-thickness loss of skin, in which adipose (fat) is visible in the ulcer, and granulation tissue and epibole (rolled wound edges) are often present. Slough and/or eschar may be visible. The depth of tissue damage varies by anatomical location; areas of significant adiposity can develop deep wounds. Undermining (skin separates from the underlying tissue at the wound margins creating areas of tissue damage below the skin surface and less damage at the surface) and tunneling may occur. Fascia, muscle, tendon, ligament, cartilage, or bone is not exposed. If slough or eschar obscures the extent of tissue loss, this is an unstageable pressure injury (Fig. 38.2C).

Teaching points:
- Anatomical differences in body areas such as the buttocks versus the sacrum can result in very different depths of injury. Accurate staging is based on assessment of the extent of damage and visible tissue layer.
- For many years, slough was considered a nonviable tissue. However, research on biofilm has improved our understanding of the role of inflammation in chronic wounds. Slough is now recognized as an inflammatory exudate composed of proteinaceous tissue, fibrin, neutrophils, and bacteria, rather than nonviable tissues. The inflammatory exudate is often produced in response to biofilm. If the biofilm is not controlled, the slough will recur following debridement. Slough is usually light yellow/cream colored and moist and soft. Eschar is black/brown, dry, thick and leathery.

- With full-thickness skin loss, adipose (fat) is visible in the ulcer, and granulation tissue and epibole (rolled wound edges) are often present. Slough and/or eschar may be visible. The depth of tissue damage varies by anatomical location; areas of significant adiposity can develop deep wounds. Undermining and tunneling may occur.
- Fascia, muscle, tendon, ligament, cartilage, or bone is not exposed. If slough or eschar obscures the extend of tissue loss, that is an unstageable pressure injury.

- **Stage 4 Pressure Injury:** Full-thickness skin and tissue loss with exposed or directly palpable fascia, muscle, tendon, ligament, cartilage, or bone in the ulcer. Slough and/or eschar may be visible. Epibole (rolled edges), undermining, and tunneling often occur. Depth varies by anatomical location. If slough or eschar obscures the extent of tissue loss, this is an unstageable pressure injury (Fig. 38.2D).
  Teaching point:
  - Clinicians should assess for osteomyelitis, which may be present in Stage 4 pressure injuries.

- **Deep Tissue Pressure Injury:** Intact or nonintact skin with localized area of persistent nonblanchable deep red, maroon, or purple discoloration or epidermal separation revealing a dark wound bed or blood-filled blister. Pain and temperature change often precede skin color changes. Discoloration may appear differently in darkly pigmented skin. This injury results from intense and/or prolonged pressure and shear forces at the bone-muscle interface. The wound may evolve rapidly to reveal the actual extent of tissue injury or may resolve without tissue loss. If necrotic tissue, subcutaneous tissue, granulation tissue, fascia, muscle, or other underlying structures are visible, this indicates a full-thickness pressure injury (unstageable, Stage 3, or Stage 4). Do not use DTPI to describe vascular, traumatic, neuropathic, or dermatological conditions (Fig. 38.2E).
  Teaching points:
  - Confirm purple skin (appearing as ecchymosis or bruising) is due to pressure or shear and not a response to medication or trauma.
  - Attempt to identify the timing and setting of the pressure and shear that lead to DTPI for root cause analysis.
  - Document the evolution of DTPI following discovery (e.g., sloughing of epidermis to reveal deeper tissue damage and ultimately, if injury becomes full thickness, the stage of the resultant injury).

- **Unstageable Pressure Injury:** Full-thickness skin and tissue loss in which extent of tissue damage within the ulcer cannot be confirmed because it is obscured by slough or eschar. If slough or eschar is removed, a Stage 3 or Stage 4 pressure injury will be revealed. Stable eschar (i.e., dry, adherent, intact without erythema or fluctuance) on ischemic limb or heels should not be softened or removed (Fig. 38.2F).

Teaching points:
- When teaching others about unstageable pressure injury, clarify that this stage is unstageable because of the inability to visualize the wound base rather than the clinician's inability to determine the injury stage.
- Describe the role of eschar as the body's natural (biological) cover. Removing stable eschar in the poorly perfused area results in an open wound that may expose the limb to infection and tax the ability to heal.
- Treat stable eschar as dry gangrene, do not moisten or soften it. The most important intervention when managing an unstable pressure injury is pressure redistribution rather than eschar removal. As eschar loosens from the wound bed, trim the edges to avoid inadvertent removal.

Although a number of contributing or confounding factors are associated with pressure injuries, the significance of these factors is not fully understood. A patient with decreased mobility, inadequate nutrition, excessive skin moisture, decreased sensory perception, or decreased activity is at risk for development of pressure injury. Statistics vary, but in the United States pressure injury prevalence in acute care settings ranges from 0% to 15.8% (Pieper, 2016). Because pressure injuries often develop quickly when a patient becomes ill, it is important to identify patients who are at high risk to implement prevention interventions (Box 38.1).

Tissue ischemia (i.e., decreased blood flow to tissues) usually results in tissue death and occurs when capillary blood flow is obstructed, as in the case of pressure. When pressure is relieved in a relatively short time, reactive hyperemia occurs in an attempt to overcome the ischemic episode. **Reactive hyperemia** is a redness of the skin resulting from dilation of the superficial capillaries (Pieper, 2016). Reactive hyperemia blanches (turns light in color). Blanching erythema is an area of erythema that becomes white (blanches) when compressed by a finger (Fig. 38.3). This hyperemia usually resolves without tissue loss if pressure is reduced or eliminated. **Blanchable hyperemia** is more difficult to assess in patients with dark skin. The discoloration or redness is warm to touch and is often purple/blue or violet instead of red in darkly pigmented skin (Nix, 2016).

Nonblanchable hyperemia is redness that persists after palpation and indicates tissue damage (Fig. 38.4). When you press a finger against the red or purple area, it does not turn lighter in color. This indicates deep tissue damage and is commonly the first stage of pressure injury development. This stage of skin injury is sometimes reversible if the pressure is relieved and the tissue is protected.

Deeper tissue destruction occurs in some injuries. The skin separates from the underlying granulation tissue at the wound margins causing undermining. Undermining creates large areas of tissue damage below the surface of the skin and less damage at the surface. With continuous pressure over the area, deep tissue destruction continues, which often results in a larger pocket of necrotic tissue beneath the opening of the

BOX 38.1　EVIDENCE-BASED PRACTICE

PICO Question: Which interventions are most effective to reduce pressure injury development in patients who are hospitalized?

SUMMARY OF EVIDENCE

The development of pressure injuries is a serious quality-of-care issue in all health care settings. A patient with a pressure injury has an increased mortality risk compared with a patient with intact skin. The development of a pressure injury interferes with recovery, causes pain and infection, and often prolongs a patient's hospital stay. The Centers for Medicare and Medicaid Services (CMS) will no longer reimburse an acute care facility if a patient with intact skin develops a Stage 3 or Stage 4 pressure injury while hospitalized. Thus it is essential for hospitals to implement skin-care protocols from a quality and fiscal standpoint. Pressure injuries are preventable in many cases when hospitals develop and implement a comprehensive skin-care program (Padula et al., 2015). A comprehensive program includes skin and risk assessment on admission to the health care agency and on an ongoing basis. Skin assessment should be done daily in good lightening to determine changes in skin color, and areas of concern should be palpated using the back of your fingers (Nix, 2016). Validated risk screening scales such as the Braden Scale identify factors that place a patient at risk for developing a pressure injury (Bryant, 2016).

Quarterly analysis of the number of patients who have pressure injuries at a moment in time (prevalence) and the number of patients who acquire a pressure injury over a period of time (incident data) provide information used to develop evidence-based prevention and intervention education and care protocols that focus on reducing the incidence of pressure injuries (Maklebust and Magnan, 2016). Current evidence also supports the use of organized skin-care rounds, decision algorithms (e.g., skin-care protocols), product bundles, and ongoing education for the nursing staff (Kelleher et al., 2012; Barker et al., 2013; Padula et al., 2015).

APPLICATION TO NURSING PRACTICE

- Complete a thorough skin and risk assessment on all patients on admission to the health care setting, and continue assessments regularly throughout the hospital stay.
- Use the results of the skin and risk assessment to plan topical therapy based on evidence-based guidelines (Barker et al., 2013).
- Develop algorithms or protocols that help nurses use assessment information to develop the appropriate prevention care plan.
- Collect prevalence and incidence data about pressure injuries on nursing units to identify areas of practice that require attention.
- Consult with an interdisciplinary team to prevent pressure injuries and promote early treatment (Bryant and Nix, 2016a).

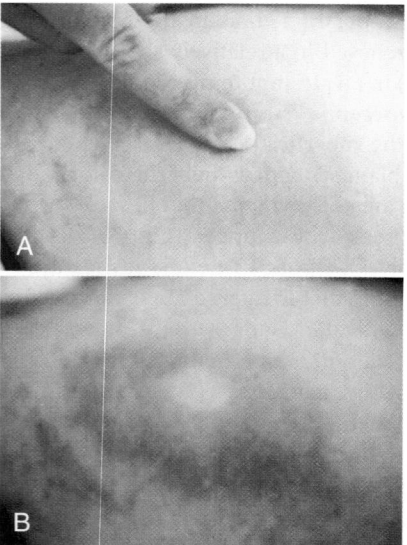

FIG 38.3 A, Check for blanching by applying fingertip pressure. **B,** Area of blanchable hyperemia.

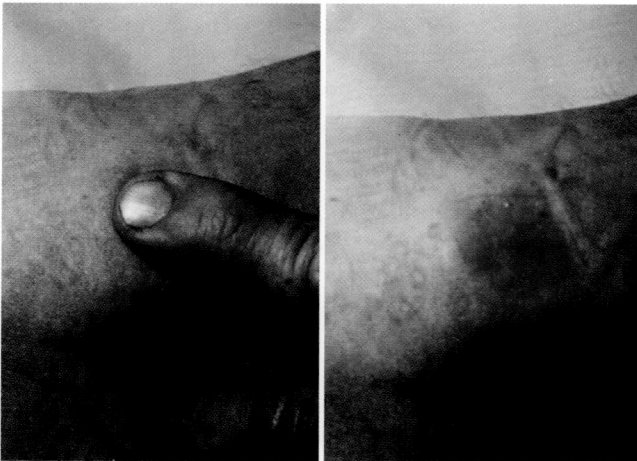

FIG 38.4 Nonblanchable hyperemia is darker than the surrounding skin and does not blanch with fingertip pressure.

main wound that resembles a tunnel; this is referred to as *tunneling.* Some wounds have more than one tunnel.

Factors Contributing to Pressure Injury Formation.
In addition to pressure, other factors increase a patient's risk for developing pressure injuries. External factors include shear, friction, and moisture; internal factors include nutrition and age.

Shear. The force exerted against the skin while the skin remains stationary and the bony structures move is called **shear.** For example, when the head of the bed is elevated, gravity causes the bony skeleton to pull toward the foot of

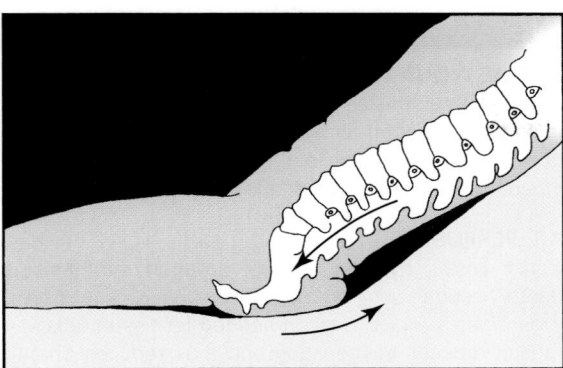

FIG 38.5 Shearing force.

the bed while the skin remains against the sheets (Fig. 38.5). The underlying tissue blood vessels become stretched and bent, impeding blood flow to the deep tissue. Injuries occur with large areas of undermining and less damage at the skin surface and may not be immediately visible at the skin surface because the injury occurs in deeper tissue (Maklebust and Magnan, 2016).

Friction. Friction is surface damage caused by the skin rubbing against another surface that often results in an abrasion. An abrasion is the loss of the epidermis, the top layer of the skin. The body surfaces most at risk for friction are the elbows and heels because abrasion of these surfaces occurs when they are rubbed against the sheets during repositioning. This type of damage alone should not be confused with or classified as a pressure injury, as friction alone is not an etiological factor for pressure injuries (Doughty and McNichol, 2016).

Moisture. Skin moisture increases the risk for injury formation. Moisture softens the skin and reduces its resistance to other physical factors such as pressure or shear. Moisture comes from many sources such as wound drainage, perspiration, and fecal and urinary incontinence. Skin moisture and wetness from incontinence frequently cause skin breakdown (Bryant, 2016).

Nutrition. Poor nutrition, specifically severe protein deficiency, increases the risk of the breakdown of soft tissue and alters fluid and electrolyte balance. Patients with protein loss have hypoalbuminemia. Low protein levels cause edema or swelling, which contributes to problems with the transportation of oxygen and nutrients (Pieper, 2016). When serum albumin levels fall drastically (e.g., to less than 3 g/100 mL), patients experience a shift of fluid from the extracellular fluid volume to the tissues, resulting in edema (Pieper, 2016).

Age. The dermis is thin in neonates and becomes thin in older adults. This makes the skin appear nearly transparent and increases the risk for skin tears. Thus neonates and young children (i.e., younger than 5 years of age) are at higher risk for pressure injury occurrence (Nix et al., 2016). An older patient's skin is more vulnerable to pressure, shear, and friction (Pieper, 2016).

Origins of Pressure Injuries. Sustained pressure exerted against the skin surface—for example, the compression of

skin between a bone and the bed surface—causes tissue and blood vessel compression that results in tissue ischemia and tissue death. However, pressure injuries also occur on any skin surface where pressure applied against the skin exceeds capillary closure pressure. Classic research identified that normal capillary pressure (i.e., the amount of pressure needed to keep the capillary open) ranges from 12 to 32 mm Hg, depending on the location in the capillary (Landis, 1930). When the intensity of the pressure exerted on the capillary exceeds 12 to 32 mm Hg, the vessel occludes, causing ischemic injury to the tissues. However, pressure to the tissue does not routinely result in pressure injury. Two other concepts, duration of the pressure and tissue tolerance, play a role.

High pressure over a short time and low pressure over a long time cause skin breakdown. Thus duration influences the effects of pressure; the longer pressure is applied, the more likely it is that tissue loss will occur. Tissue tolerance also plays an important role in pressure injury development. The integrity of the skin and the supporting structures influence the ability of the skin to redistribute the pressure. The factors mentioned previously (i.e., shear, friction, moisture, and internal factors such as nutrition and age) alter the ability of the skin and supporting tissue to respond to the pressure (Pieper, 2016).

Wound assessment (regardless of cause) includes the following parameters: anatomical location, extent of tissue involvement (full-thickness or partial-thickness loss), size (dimensions and depth of wound), tissue type (viable or nonviable) and percentage of wound tissue (e.g., viable versus nonviable), volume and color of wound exudate, and condition of surrounding skin (Nix, 2016). Staging a wound is done only if the etiology of the wound is pressure. These measures help evaluate the progress of the wound, drive decision making, and evaluate wound healing.

Wound-Healing Process

All wounds heal through an orderly series of integrated physiological responses. Multiple factors promote or impede wound healing (Box 38.2). A wound with little or no tissue loss such as a clean surgical incision heals by primary intention. The skin edges approximate, or close together, and the risk for infection is minimal.

In contrast, a wound involving loss of tissue such as a severe laceration or a chronic wound such as a pressure injury heals by secondary intention. The skin edges cannot come together because of the extensive tissue loss, and healing occurs gradually. A layer of granulation tissue, which is red, moist tissue consisting of blood vessels and connective tissue, covers the wound base; wound contraction brings the wound edges together; and the wound closes with scar formation.

There are also instances in which a surgical wound is initially closed in the deep tissue layers; however, the subcutaneous fat and skin layers are left open. This method of wound closure is called tertiary intention or delayed primary closure. The wound heals with a layer of granulation tissue at the edges and base, and several days after the initial wounding the health care provider brings the wound edges together

BOX 38.2 FACTORS INFLUENCING WOUND HEALING

AGE

- Blood circulation and oxygen delivery to the wound, clotting, and the inflammatory response are sometimes impaired in very young patients and older adult patients. Risk for infection is greater in these populations.
- Cell growth and differentiation in reconstruction are slower with advancing age.
- Scar tissue increases the risk for altered body part function in older adults.
- Age affects all phases of wound healing. A decline in the number of white blood cells places older adults at greater risk for a wound infection. A slowdown in the deposition of collagen in reepithelialization is common.

SCAR TISSUE

- Scar tissue never regains the tensile strength of noninjured skin, increasing the risk for further tissue injury and altered body part function.

NUTRITION STATUS

- Adequate nutrition status is critical for collagen synthesis, tensile strength, and immune function.
- Tissue repair and infection resistance depend on a balanced diet. Surgery, severe wounds, serious infections, and preoperative nutrition deficits increase nutritional requirements.

IMMUNOSUPPRESSION

- The repair process is more susceptible to infection.
- The body's ability to manifest signs of infection is compromised.

OBESITY

- Adipose tissue has a poor blood supply.
- Large volume of adipose tissue puts additional stress on incisional lines increasing the risk for dehiscence.
- Risk for infection is increased.

EXTENT OF WOUND

- Wounds with extensive tissue loss heal by secondary intention and remain open for a prolonged period of time.
- Sustained wound stress (e.g., vomiting, abdominal distention, coughing) disrupts wound layers and tissue repair.

TISSUE PERFUSION

- Chronic tissue hypoxia impairs collagen synthesis and reduces tissue resistance to infection.
- Oxygen fuels cellular function needed for tissue repair.
- Smoking reduces oxygenation and thus reduces fibroblast activity.

DIABETES MELLITUS AND PERIPHERAL VASCULAR DISEASES

- Patients with diabetes mellitus have small-vessel disease that impairs tissue perfusion; thus oxygen delivery is poor.
- An elevated blood glucose level (hyperglycemia) impairs macrophage function. Risk for infection is increased because of hyperglycemia and poor wound healing.
- Patients with diabetes demonstrate the following problems with wound healing: reduced collagen synthesis, decreased wound strength, and impaired white blood cell functioning. These adverse effects are at least in part caused by poor glycemic control.

RADIATION

- Radiation therapy, which eventually results in fibrosis and vascular scarring, interferes with postoperative wound healing when surgery is delayed more than 4 to 6 weeks and irradiated tissues become fragile and poorly perfused.

STRESS

- Stress increases production of corticosteroids, which impedes wound healing.
- The body's ability to show signs of infection is compromised.

Modified from Doughty DB, Sparks B: Wound healing physiology and factors that affect the repair process. In Bryant RA, Nix DP, editors: *Acute and chronic wounds: current management concepts,* ed 5, St Louis, 2016, Mosby.

with sutures or adhesive closures. An example of wound closure by delayed primary closure occurs when a patient has a ruptured appendix. In some cases the surgeon is unsure if the appendix had microperforations that caused subsequent spilling of the intestinal contents into the abdomen and wound. Thus the surgeon leaves the incision open for 4 to 5 days following surgery and then evaluates the wound. If after 4 to 5 days there are no clinical signs of infection, the surgeon closes the wound with either adhesive strips or sutures (Doughty and Sparks, 2016).

Wounds heal by one of two mechanisms: partial-thickness wound repair or full-thickness wound repair. Partial-thickness wound repair is necessary when there is loss of only the epidermis and/or part of the dermis such as wound healing by primary intention. Full-thickness wound repair is necessary when there is loss of the epidermis; loss of the dermis; and possible extension into subcutaneous layers, bone, and muscle.

Partial-Thickness Wound Repair. By resurfacing the wound with new epidermal cells, the body repairs wounds that heal by primary intention, shallow wounds that involve loss of only the epidermis and perhaps some of the dermis. The wounds go through several phases of wound healing, which are described next.

Inflammatory Response. Erythema and edema are the first response, bringing white blood cells (WBCs) to the site. The wounded area appears red and swollen. If the exudate, or discharge, that brings the WBCs to the area is allowed to dry, a scab forms. This response is brief and usually subsides in less than 24 hours (Doughty and Sparks, 2016).

Epidermal Repair. Epidermal cells begin migration across the wound, originating from the epidermal cells at the wound edges or the epidermal appendages. Peak epithelial proliferation occurs 24 to 72 hours after injury. Wounds kept in a moist environment heal in approximately 4 days, as opposed to 7 days when kept dry because new epithelial cells migrate across a moist surface. If a wound is dry, the cells need to find moisture below the skin surface (Doughty and Sparks, 2016).

Dermal Repair. The epidermis thickens, anchors to adjacent cells, and resumes normal function. The new epidermis is pink, dry, and fragile. If dermal repair is necessary, it occurs concurrently with epidermal repair.

Full-Thickness Wound Repair. Full-thickness wounds involve total loss of the skin layers (epidermis and dermis) and frequently involve the deeper tissue layers as well (subcutaneous tissue, muscle, and bone). A full-thickness wound is either acute (a surgical wound) or chronic (a pressure injury). Healing of a full-thickness acute wound such as a surgical incision proceeds by primary intention; healing of a full-thickness chronic wound such as a pressure injury proceeds by secondary intention. The key events differ between a chronic wound healing by secondary intention and an acute wound healing by primary intention.

Hemostasis Phase. A full-thickness wound healing by primary intention first goes through the hemostasis phase, which controls bleeding. Platelets cause coagulation and vasoconstriction. The platelets break down and release growth factors, which appear to initiate the entire wound-healing process (Beitz, 2016). Bleeding and hemostasis do not occur in wounds healing by secondary intention, thus compromising the repair process (Doughty and Sparks, 2016).

Inflammation Phase. The goal of this phase is to establish a clean wound bed and obtain bacterial balance. The inflammatory response brings WBCs to the area, cleaning up the site and releasing additional growth factors. This phase lasts approximately 3 days in an acute clean wound such as a surgical incision. However, in a chronic wound healing by secondary intention, this phase is prolonged and often lasts longer than 3 days.

Proliferative Phase. The key events in the proliferative phase are production of new tissue, epithelialization, and contraction. In wound healing by primary intention new capillary networks form to provide oxygen and nutrients for new tissue and contribute to the synthesis of collagen. As collagen fibers and capillary networks continue to synthesize and increase in size, the wound begins to contract. The last component of this phase is epithelialization, in which the epithelial cells migrate and cover the defect. Epithelialization occurs faster in a moist environment, supporting the role of moist wound dressings in wound care. In healing by secondary intention in a chronic wound such as a pressure injury, the proliferative phase is prolonged. As granulation tissue forms to fill in the wound bed, it is followed by contraction and epithelialization, the final phase. Contraction is much more important in secondary intention wounds because it reduces the amount of granulation tissue needed to fill the wound bed (Doughty and Sparks, 2016).

Remodeling Phase. The remodeling phase, which lasts up to 1 year, reorganizes the collagen to produce a more elastic, stronger collagen for the scar tissue. The tensile strength of the scar tissue is never more than 80% of the tensile strength

in nonwounded tissue (Doughty and Sparks, 2016). The remodeling process is the same for wounds healing by primary intention and secondary intention.

Complications of Wound Healing

Wound healing frequently has complications. When caring for patients with wounds, you need to assess a patient's wound-healing process while observing for complications.

Hemorrhage. Bleeding from an acute wound is normal during and immediately after initial trauma, but **hemostasis**, which is cessation of bleeding by vasoconstriction and coagulation, usually occurs within several minutes. Hemorrhage occurring later possibly indicates a slipped surgical suture, a dislodged clot, infection, or the erosion of a blood vessel by a foreign object (e.g., a drain). Hemorrhage is external or internal. Severe symptoms of internal hemorrhage are hypovolemic shock and swelling of the affected body part. Less severe internal hemorrhage symptoms include a **hematoma**, which is a localized collection of blood under the tissue, often appearing as a bluish swelling or mass. External hemorrhaging is obvious because dressings covering the wound quickly become saturated with blood.

Infection. Bacterial wound infection prevents healing by increasing tissue damage and altering the healing process. The chances of wound infection are greater when the wound contains dead or necrotic tissue, when foreign bodies are in or near the wound, and when the blood supply and local tissue defenses are lower than normal.

A contaminated or traumatic wound infection develops within 2 to 3 days; a surgical wound infection develops within 4 to 5 days. Locally drainage is often yellow, green, or brown and may be odorous, depending on the causative organism. The wound edges appear tense, swollen, and painful, with redness extending beyond the immediate wound edge. Systemic signs include fever, general malaise, and an elevated WBC count.

Dehiscence. When an acute wound fails to heal properly, the layers of skin and tissue separate. This most commonly occurs before collagen formation (3 to 11 days after injury). **Dehiscence** is the partial or total separation of layers of skin and tissue above the fascia in a wound that is not healing properly. Patients who are obese have a high risk for dehiscence because of constant strain on their wounds and the poor vascularity of fatty tissue. It occurs most often in abdominal surgical wounds after a sudden strain such as coughing, vomiting, or sitting up in bed. Patients often report feeling as though something has given way. When serosanguineous drainage increases from a wound, be alert for dehiscence.

Evisceration. **Evisceration** occurs when wound layers separate below the fascial layer and visceral organs protrude through the wound opening. It is a medical emergency requiring placement of sterile towels soaked in sterile saline over the extruding tissues to reduce chances of bacterial invasion and drying before surgical repair occurs.

NURSING KNOWLEDGE BASE

Maintenance of skin integrity and wound care is a nurse's major responsibility. Nursing research identifies risks for pressure injuries (e.g., pressure resulting from positioning, medical devices, and patients' individual risk factors). In addition, nursing research findings are important in developing guidelines for pressure injury prevention and care.

Prediction and Prevention

Guidelines for Prevention and Management of Pressure Ulcers from the Wound, Ostomy and Continence Nurses (WOCN) Society were recently reviewed and updated by nurse experts who performed extensive searches on the most up-to-date literature on pressure injuries (WOCN Society, 2016). The new guidelines provide the best available evidence in the prevention and management of pressure injuries. These

guidelines were accepted by the Agency for Healthcare Research and Quality (AHRQ). They include predictive tools that identify patients at highest risk for pressure injury development (WOCN Society, 2016). Patients identified to be at risk need a care plan to address and reduce identified risk factors.

The Braden Scale is one highly reliable tool that identifies patients at greatest risk for pressure injuries (Bergstrom et al., 1987a, 1987b, 1998). It is composed of six subscales: sensory perception, moisture, activity, mobility, nutrition, and friction and shear (Table 38.1). An adult in the hospital with a score of 16 or below or an older adult with a score of 18 or below is at risk for pressure injury development (Bergstrom et al., 1998; Ayello and Braden, 2002).

CRITICAL THINKING

Synthesis

Patient care requires you to apply what you know about a patient, your knowledge base, experience, and critical

TABLE 38.1	BRADEN SCALE FOR PREDICTING PRESSURE SORE RISK			
Sensory Perception Ability to respond appropriately to pressure-related discomfort	1. **Completely limited:** Unresponsive (does not moan, flinch, or grasp) to painful stimuli as a result of diminished level of consciousness or sedation *or* Limited ability to feel pain over most of body	2. **Very limited:** Responds only to painful stimuli Cannot communicate discomfort except by moaning or restlessness *or* Has sensory impairment that limits ability to feel pain or discomfort over half of body	3. **Slightly limited:** Responds to verbal commands but cannot always communicate discomfort or need to be turned *or* Has some sensory impairment, which limits ability to feel pain or discomfort in one or two extremities	4. **No impairment:** Responds to verbal commands Has no sensory deficit that limits ability to feel or voice pain or discomfort
Moisture Degree to which skin is exposed to moisture	1. **Constantly moist:** Skin kept moist almost constantly (e.g., by perspiration, urine) Dampness detected every time patient is moved or turned	2. **Very moist:** Skin often but not always moist Linen must be changed at least once a shift	3. **Occasionally moist:** Skin occasionally moist, requiring an extra linen change approximately once per day	4. **Rarely moist:** Skin usually dry; linen change only required at routine intervals
Activity Degree of physical activity	1. **Bedfast:** Confined to bed	2. **Chairfast:** Ability to walk severely limited or nonexistent Cannot bear own weight and/or must be assisted into chair or wheelchair	3. **Walks occasionally:** Walks occasionally during day, but for very short distances, with or without assistance Spends majority of each shift in bed or chair	4. **Walks frequently:** Walks outside room at least twice a day and inside room at least once every 2 hours during waking hours

TABLE 38.1   BRADEN SCALE FOR PREDICTING PRESSURE SORE RISK—cont'd

Mobility
Ability to change and control body position

1. **Completely immobile:**	2. **Very limited:**	3. **Slightly limited:**	4. **No limitations:**
Does not make even slight changes in body or extremity position without assistance	Makes occasional slight changes in body or extremity position but unable to make frequent or significant changes independently	Makes frequent though slight changes in body or extremity position independently	Makes major and frequent changes in position without assistance

Nutrition
Usual food intake pattern

1. **Very poor:**	2. **Probably inadequate:**	3. **Adequate:**	4. **Excellent:**
Never eats a complete meal Rarely eats more than one-third of any food offered Eats two servings or less of protein (meat or dairy products) per day Takes fluids poorly Does not take a liquid dietary supplement *or* Is NPO and/or maintained on clear liquids or IV feeding for more than 5 days	Rarely eats a complete meal and generally eats only about half of any food offered Protein intake includes only three servings of meat or dairy products per day Occasionally takes a dietary supplement *or* Receives less than optimal amount of liquid diet or tube feeding	Eats over half of most meals Eats a total of four servings of protein (meat, dairy products) each day Occasionally refuses a meal but usually takes a supplement if offered *or* Is on a tube-feeding or TPN regimen that probably meets most nutritional needs	Eats most of every meal Never refuses a meal Usually eats a total of four or more servings of meat and dairy products Occasionally eats between meals Does not require supplementation

Friction and Shear

1. **Problem:**	2. **Potential problem:**	3. **No apparent problem:**	
Requires moderate to maximal assistance in moving Complete lifting without sliding against sheets impossible Frequently slides down in bed or chair, requiring frequent repositioning with maximal assistance Spasticity, contractions, or agitation leads to almost constant friction	Moves feebly or requires minimal assistance During a move skin probably slides to some extent against sheets, chair, restraints, or other devices Maintains relatively good position in chair or bed most of the time but occasionally slides down	Moves in bed and chair independently and has sufficient muscle strength to sit up completely during move Maintains good position in bed or chair at all times	

IV, Intravenous; *NPO,* nothing by mouth; *TPN,* total parenteral nutrition.
Instructions: Score patient in each of the six subscales; add all subscales for overall score. Level of risk: not at risk, greater than 18; mild risk, 15–18; moderate risk, 13–14; high risk, 10–12; and very high risk, less than 9.
Copyright 1988. Used with permission of Barbara Braden, PhD, RN, Professor, Creighton University School of Nursing, Omaha, Nebraska, and Nancy Bergstrom, Professor, University of Texas–Houston, School of Nursing, Houston, Texas.

thinking attitudes and standards. Your synthesis of this information allows you to make sound decisions as you apply the nursing process. Critical thinking synthesis involves combining all available information to obtain a clear picture of the approach needed to provide patient-centered care. When you care for patients who are at risk for or who have pressure injuries, integrate information from all health-related sciences and knowledge from courses, experiences, and appropriate standards of practice into the management of your patient's wounds (Box 38.3).

Knowledge. Performing a pressure injury risk assessment requires you to use a validated risk assessment tool, such as the Braden Scale. Understanding the importance of risk factors that lead to pressure injury development allows you to plan appropriate interventions to reduce or eliminate risk factors to pressure injury development.

BOX 38.3 SYNTHESIS IN PRACTICE

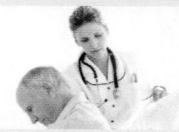

Copyright © Stockbyte/
iStock/Thinkstock.

Lynda reviews the nursing admission assessment and finds that Mr. Martinez was admitted with a pressure injury. The injury is classified as Stage 2 and is a partial-thickness wound over his sacral area that measures 1 × 2 inches (2.5 × 3.5 cm) × ⅛ inch deep. There is no necrotic tissue; the wound bed has red, moist tissue. Mr. Martinez has some dark pigmentation.

When Lynda prepares to conduct a skin assessment on Mr. Martinez, she recalls information about how pressure injuries develop and guidelines for skin assessment for patients with darkly pigmented skin. She focuses on assessing for changes in Mr. Martinez's skin integrity.

During a previous experience in an extended care facility, Lynda observed care of a patient with a Stage 4 pressure injury. From that experience, she gained knowledge about the debilitating effects of pressure injuries. In addition, she was able to practice various skin assessment techniques for Stage 4 pressure injuries and how to correctly assess adjoining skin and underlying tissues.

Knowing normal anatomy of the skin and underlying structures and the physiology of wound healing lets you implement appropriate nursing measures to facilitate healing. In addition, knowledge of the normal healing process helps you recognize complications requiring intervention. In choosing interventions consider the type of wound, the pain associated with it, conditions that promote or impede healing, and a patient's psychological well-being.

Experience. You are better able to assess a patient's wound when you are able to draw from your experiences and recognize normal and abnormal characteristics of wound healing. This is especially important when a patient has factors that impede wound healing such as peripheral vascular disease, poor nutrition, or reduced mobility. When caring for a patient who develops problems with wound healing, learn the clinical signs of complications. This is especially important when caring for a patient with darkly pigmented skin (Box 38.4).

Attitudes. Be vigilant in skin assessment when caring for all types of patients including patients who are acutely and chronically ill and patients in home care or extended care. Although respiratory and cardiac status are priorities, never overlook assessment of skin and wound integrity. Assume responsibility and ensure that you include meticulous skin assessment and pressure injury prevention measures in a patient's plan of care. Assess and routinely inspect skin and underlying tissue according to agency policy or nursing care

---

🌐 BOX 38.4 PATIENT-CENTERED CARE

Skin assessment is an important element in early detection of the development of pressure injuries. Changes in skin color that are easily identified in light-colored skin may not be easily observed in patients with darker pigmentation. Erythema also may be hard to detect in dark-skinned patients. In a light-skinned patient, irritation may cause redness. In a dark-skinned patient, skin irritation may cause an increase or decrease in pigmentation with no visible redness. Include a thorough assessment in all patients, but especially patients with darkly pigmented skin. Changes in sensation, temperature, or tissue consistency may precede visual skin changes (WOCN Society, 2016).

IMPLICATIONS FOR PRACTICE

- Use natural lighting, but note that visual inspection techniques to identify pressure injuries are ineffective. Thus you need to include assessment of temperature, edema, and changes in tissue consistency (WOCN Society, 2016). If possible, avoid fluorescent lighting.
- Assess localized skin color changes. Any of the following may appear:
  - Color remains unchanged when pressure is applied.
  - Color changes that differ from patient's usual skin color occur at site of pressure.

- If patient previously had a pressure injury, that area of skin may be lighter than the original skin color.
- A localized area of skin may be purple/blue or violet instead of red. Purple or maroon discoloration may indicate deep tissue injury (WOCN Society, 2016).
- Circumscribed area of intact skin may be warm to touch. As tissue changes color, intact skin will feel cool to touch. **Note:** Gloves may decrease nurses' sensitivity to changes in patient skin temperature.
- Localized heat (inflammation) is detected by making comparisons to surrounding skin. Localized area of warmth eventually will be replaced by area of coolness, which is a sign of tissue devitalization.
- Edema may occur with induration of more than 15 mm in diameter, and skin may appear taut and shiny.
- Palpate tissue consistency in surrounding tissues to identify any changes in tissue consistency between area of injury and normal tissue.
- Patients may have discomfort at a site that is predisposed to pressure injury development (e.g. bony prominence, under medical devices).

Adapted from Nix DP: Skin and wound inspection and assessment. In Bryant RA, Nix DP, editors: *Acute and chronic wounds: current management concepts*, ed 5, St Louis, 2016, Mosby; and Wound, Ostomy and Continence Nurses (WOCN) Society: *Guideline for prevention and management of pressure ulcers*, WOCN Clinical Practice Guidelines Series, Mount Laurel, NJ, 2016, The Society.

plan (WOCN Society, 2016). Be aware that skin breakdown is sometimes unavoidable. However, the sooner you assess for and identify the risk factors for skin breakdown and plan interventions, the less severe the impaired skin integrity should be.

In the immediate postoperative period some patients require well-thought-out modifications of wound care techniques. You usually do not change the initial dressing, but you are responsible for ensuring that the dressing remains dry and intact. With knowledge about pressure injuries, wounds, and normal wound healing, use creative measures to reduce the risks of impaired skin integrity and promote wound healing.

Standards. The WOCN Society publishes pressure injury guidelines to support clinical practice by providing consistent research-based clinical decisions (Box 38.5). In addition, wound care protocols such as surgical wound management vary by agency policy. Know your agency policy and practices regarding the use of skin-care products, dressing materials, and frequency of dressing change.

BOX 38.5 PRESSURE INJURY PREVENTION POINTS

ASSESSMENT

- Assess individual risk for developing pressure injuries.
- Perform pressure injury risk assessment using a validated tool such as the Braden Scale on all patients who have one or more risk factors when admitted to an acute care facility, home care, hospice, or extended care facility (NPUAP, EPUAP, and PPPIA, 2014; WOCN Society, 2016).
- Assess for intrinsic and extrinsic risk factors such as general medical conditions (e.g., diabetes, stroke, cardiopulmonary disease, other peripheral vascular diseases), significant weight loss, poor nutrition, increased length of stay in a health care agency, and stay in the intensive care unit because of critical illness.
- Inspect skin and bony prominences at least daily.
- Assess for history of prior pressure injury and/or presence of current injury because this places patient at increased risk for additional pressure injuries.

SKIN CARE AND EARLY TREATMENT

- Continue preventive measures even when a patient has a pressure injury to prevent pressure injury stage from advancing or additional pressure areas from developing.
- Clean and dry skin after each incontinent episode, using skin barriers such as cream, ointment, or paste to protect and maintain intact skin. Risk for skin injury is increased by prolonged skin moisture and wetness from urinary and fecal incontinence (Thayer et al., 2016).
- Minimize or eliminate pressure from medical devices such as oxygen tubing, catheters, cervical collars, casts, and restraints. Heat and humidity develop between the device and the skin, changing the microclimate of the skin. Prompt routine assessment of the skin under and surrounding the device reduces the risk for pressure injuries (Pittman et al., 2015).
- Turn and reposition a patient often to redistribute pressure from the superficial capillaries and allow tissues to compensate for temporary ischemia. Use safe patient-handling measures to turn and reposition patients every 1 to 2 hours as their condition allows. Proper positioning helps minimize formation of pressure injury.
- Use approaches to minimize friction and shear. Use lift sheets and devices when repositioning patients to reduce rubbing skin against the sheets. Raise head of bed no more than 30 degrees or at the lowest level of elevation consistent with patient's medical condition to prevent sliding and shear injury (WOCN Society, 2016).
- Avoid vigorous massage over bony prominences.

SUPPORT SURFACES AND PRESSURE REDISTRIBUTION

- Place patients at risk on a pressure-redistribution surface (McNichol et al., 2015; WOCN Society, 2016).
- Schedule regular and frequent turning and repositioning for patients who are bed-bound or chair-bound, taking into consideration the condition of the patient and the pressure redistribution support surface in determining repositioning strategy.
- Position sitting patients with special attention to the individual's anatomy, postural alignment, distribution of weight, and support of the feet.

NUTRITION

- Offer patients with nutritional and pressure injury risks a minimum of 30 to 35 kcal/kg body weight of protein per day with 1.25 to 1.5 g/kg/day protein and 1 mL of fluid intake per kcal per day (Stotts, 2016b).
- Provide prescribed doses of vitamin A (1000 to 2000 retinol equivalents), vitamin C (100 to 100 mcg), vitamin B (200% recommended dietary allowance), zinc (15 to 30 mg), iron (20 to 30 mg), and glutamine (0.3 to 0.4 g) and a daily multivitamin (Stotts, 2016b).
- Refer patients with nutritional and pressure injury risks to a registered dietitian.

PATIENT AND FAMILY CAREGIVER EDUCATION

- Educate patient and family caregiver about causes and risk factors for developing pressure injuries and ways to minimize risk.
- Include information on the following:
  - Etiology of and risk factors for pressure injuries
  - Importance of performing regular inspection of the skin, especially over bony prominences
  - Keeping the skin clean and dry
  - Selection and use of support surfaces
  - Measures to reduce friction from the sheet such as lifting rather than dragging across the bed
  - Demonstration of positioning to decrease risk for tissue breakdown
  - Promptly reporting health care changes and nutritional problems to health care providers

Data adapted from Wound, Ostomy and Continence Nurses (WOCN) Society: *Guideline for prevention and management of pressure ulcers,* WOCN Clinical Practice Guidelines Series, Mount Laurel, NJ, 2016, The Society.

NURSING PROCESS

■■■□ ASSESSMENT

Baseline and continual focused assessment data provide critical information about a patient's skin integrity and the increased risk for pressure injury development or impaired wound healing (Table 38.2). Although multiple factors affect skin integrity, it is important that you identify and assess the factors relevant for your patients.

Pressure Injuries. Use agency-approved skin assessment tools and perform assessment of a patient for risk of development of pressure injuries on admission to the agency, 24 to 48 hours after admission, at regular intervals, and when there is a significant change in a patient's condition. Follow agency guidelines for ongoing assessment, which is important because a patient's condition may change quickly. Subsequent assessments identify changes that increase a patient's risk for pressure injury development. In addition to assessing for potential risk factors, perform a thorough skin assessment on a daily basis to identify problems early and develop patient-centered interventions (see Skill 38.1). Prompt identification of patients at risk for or with skin integrity problems helps nurses use resources appropriately and reduce patients' risks. When patients are identified as being at risk for pressure

injuries, specific prevention and injury treatment strategies are included in the plan of care.

Skin. Assessment for tissue pressure damage includes visual and tactile inspection of the skin. Baseline assessment determines a patient's normal skin characteristics and any actual or potential areas of breakdown. This is especially important with high-risk patients such as patients with diabetes, stroke, or serious malnutrition. Note the presence of medical devices such as a nasogastric (NG) tube, oxygen equipment, and artificial airways and areas exposed to casts, traction, or splints (Pittman et al., 2015). In addition, the skin of an older adult patient is more fragile and has an increased risk for skin breakdown (Box 38.6).

Assess all areas of the skin from head to toe, paying attention to any reddened areas or breaks in skin integrity. Document the assessment. When you notice hyperemia, document location, size, and color, and reassess the area after 1 hour. If you suspect nonblanchable hyperemia, outline the affected area with a marker to make reassessment easier. Nonblanchable hyperemia is an early indicator of impaired skin integrity, but damage to the underlying tissue is sometimes more progressive. Palpate the tissues next to the observed area to gather further data about **induration** (hardening of tissue caused by edema or inflammation) and damage to the skin and underlying tissues.

TABLE 38.2   FOCUSED PATIENT ASSESSMENT

FACTORS TO ASSESS	QUESTIONS	PHYSICAL ASSESSMENT
Adequacy of patient's sensory perception	Do you feel me pinching the skin on your left hip? Can you feel me rubbing your left lower leg?	Apply painful stimuli to various body locations. If patient is unable to respond by affirming that he or she feels the stimuli, the patient has limited sensory perception.
Moisture	Does the bed sheet under your buttocks feel moist?	Routinely observe patient's bed linens for moisture. Observe patient's skin, noting if it is dry (rarely moist) or seldom damp (occasionally moist) or if skin is often but not always wet (moist). Observe for wound drainage.
Activity	Can you get out of bed by yourself to use the toilet? Are you able to get out of the bed or chair by yourself? Are you able to change your position in bed by yourself?	Check whether patient is incontinent of urine and stool. Assess patient's ability to walk at least once every 2 hours while awake (walks frequently) or whether patient is able to ambulate only short distances and if assistance is needed. Observe if patient is able to independently change positions in bed.
Nutrition	Were you able to eat the entire tray of food at mealtime? Assess last 2 meals. Are you hungry at mealtime?	Observe patient eating: Does patient need assistance? Assess amount of food the patient eats at meals for adequate nutrition, such as whether patient finishes over half of meals or is on tube feedings or TPN.
Friction and shear	When you are sitting up in the bed, do you find that you slide down toward the foot of the bed? Do you need assistance in moving up in bed or chair?	Assess if patient moves in bed and chair independently and maintains a good position at all times. Determine if the patient requires any assistance in moving up in bed and/or chair.

Copyright © Stockbyte/iStock/Thinkstock.

TPN, Total parenteral nutrition.

BOX 38.6 CARE OF THE OLDER ADULT

Issues Related to Skin Integrity

- There is decreased barrier function and less protection from excessive moisture, shear, friction, and pressure.
- Aging skin experiences decreased epidermal turnover; thus healing requires more time.
- The dermis is not as thick and the skin over the legs and arms is especially thin. This predisposes an older adult's skin to tearing.
- Decreased subcutaneous tissue reduces padding protection over bony prominences.
- There is decreased inflammatory reaction and more susceptibility to infection.
- Sensory perception is reduced; thus ability to detect pain on initial injury is lessened.

Data from Wysocki A: Anatomy and physiology of skin and soft tissue. In Bryant RA, Nix DP, editors: *Acute and chronic wounds: current management concepts,* ed 5, St Louis, 2016, Mosby.

Assess patients with lightly pigmented skin for blanching with return to normal skin tones. Also note changes in color, temperature, and hardness of the surrounding skin and tissues. Use visual and tactile inspection over the body areas most frequently at risk for pressure injury development. Pressure injuries occur most commonly over bony prominences such as the sacrum, ischial tuberosity, and trochanter. In addition the skin under medical devices, such as endotracheal tubes, oxygen tubing, casts, traction, and splints, is also at risk. When a patient lies in bed or sits in a chair, pressure occurs over bony prominences. Body surfaces subjected to the greatest weight or pressure such as the sacrum or ischium are at increased risk for pressure injury formation (Fig. 38.6).

Mobility. Assessment includes documenting level of mobility, the potential effects of impaired mobility on skin integrity, and data regarding the quality of muscle tone and strength. For example, determine if a patient is able to lift the weight off the ischial tuberosities and roll to a side-lying position. Some patients have adequate range of motion to independently move into a more protective position, but others do not. Finally assess the patient's activity tolerance (see Chapter 28).

Nutrition Status. Malnutrition is associated with overall morbidity and mortality. Perform a nutrition assessment when a patient enters a new health care setting and whenever there is a change in the patient's condition (Box 38.7) (see Chapter 35) (WOCN Society, 2016). Inadequate caloric intake causes weight loss and a decrease in subcutaneous tissue, allowing bony prominences to compress and restrict circulation. Assess nutrition status using a variety of approaches (e.g., monitoring intake and output, completing a 3-day calorie count, assessing serum albumin) to identify patients who need nutrition support.

Wounds. Assessment of a patient's wound varies from one health care setting to another. Consistent wound assessment over time reveals patterns and trends that indicate improvement or deterioration in a wound (Nix, 2016).

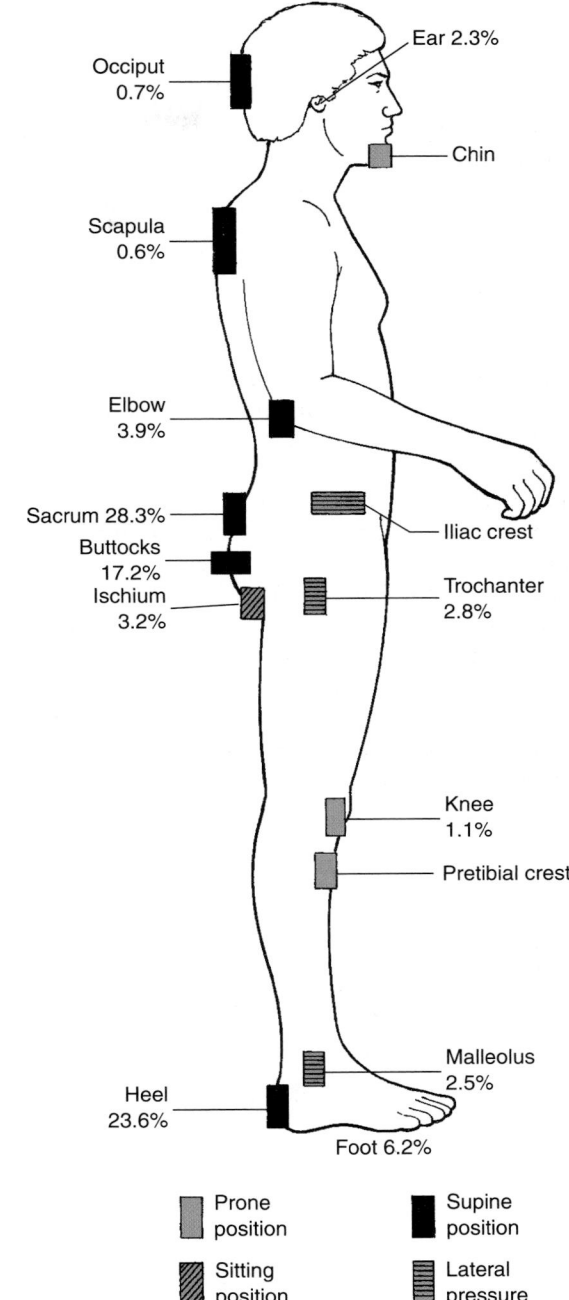

FIG 38.6 Sites for pressure injuries and frequency of ulceration per site. Note that sites for device-related pressure injuries, which may not involve bony prominences, are not included. (Data from VanGilder C, et al: Results of the 2008-2009 International Pressure Ulcer Prevalence Survey and a 3-year, acute care, unit specific analysis, *Ostomy Wound Manage* 55(11):39, 2009. In Bryant RA, Nix DP: *Acute and chronic wounds: current management concepts,* ed 5, St Louis, 2016, Elsevier.)

| BOX 38.7 | NUTRITION ASSESSMENT AND MANAGEMENT OF PRESSURE INJURIES: WOUND, OSTOMY AND CONTINENCE NURSES (WOCN) SOCIETY RECOMMENDATIONS |

Screen for nutritional deficiencies at admission to care setting and if patient's condition changes (see Chapter 35). Include the following parameters in assessment:

- Current and usual weight
- History of unintentional weight loss or gain: 5% or more in 30 days or 10% or more in 180 days
- Nutritional intake versus needs, incorporating protein, calorie, and fluid needs
- Adequacy of nutritional intake (i.e., calories, protein, and fluid)
- Signs of dehydration (i.e., skin turgor, urine output, elevated sodium)
- Medical/surgical history or interventions that influence nutritional intake or absorption of nutrients
- Psychosocial factors affecting food intake: ability to obtain and pay for food, facilities for cooking and environment for eating, and food preferences

Data from Wound, Ostomy and Continence Nurses (WOCN) Society: *Guideline for prevention and management of pressure ulcers,* WOCN Clinical Practice Guidelines Series, Mount Laurel, NJ, 2016, The Society.

Emergency Setting. In an emergency the type of wound determines the criteria for inspection. After you stabilize a patient's cardiopulmonary status (see Chapter 32), inspect the wound for bleeding. An abrasion, or loss of the dermis, is usually superficial with little bleeding but some weeping (plasma leakage from damaged capillaries). A laceration is damage to the dermis and epidermis and is a torn, jagged wound. The depth and location of the laceration affect the extent of bleeding, with serious bleeding possible in lacerations greater than 5 cm (2 inches) long or 2.5 cm (1 inch) deep.

Puncture wounds bleed in relation to the depth and size of the wound; internal bleeding and infection are the primary dangers. Inspect a wound for contaminant material such as soil, broken glass, shreds of cloth, and foreign substances clinging to penetrating objects. Next assess the size of the wound and the need for suturing or surface protection. When an injury results from trauma from a dirty penetrating object, determine if the patient has received a tetanus toxoid injection within the last 10 years.

Stable Setting. Once an acute wound is stable after surgery or treatment, assess progress toward healing. If a dressing covers the wound and there are orders not to change it, inspect the dressing and any external drains (see Chapter 40). If a dressing appears saturated with drainage, reinforce the secondary dressing and notify the health care provider immediately. Saturated dressings provide an excellent environment for bacterial growth; you need to inform the health care provider of the color, odor, and estimated amount of drainage.

When you plan a dressing change, consider giving the patient an analgesic at least 30 minutes before exposing a wound. Refer to notes documenting pain levels during previous dressing changes. Discuss pain levels at previous dressing changes with your patient to determine the appropriate pain-management interventions. Avoid accidentally removing or displacing underlying drains.

First inspect the appearance of the wound, noting the anatomical location; size; approximation of wound edges; presence and quality of exudate; type of tissue in an open wound; skin integrity around the wound; and signs of dehiscence, evisceration, or infection. Measure the length, diameter, and depth of every wound with a centimeter measuring guide. Note any ecchymosis, skin discoloration, or bruising caused by blood leakage into subcutaneous tissues after trauma to underlying vessels. The outer edges of a wound normally appear inflamed for the first 2 to 3 days, but this slowly disappears. When an infection develops, the wound edges are usually brightly inflamed, warm, tender, and swollen.

Next assess the character of wound drainage by noting the amount, color, odor, and consistency. The amount of drainage depends on the location and extent of the wound. A simple method for estimating the volume of wound drainage is to report the number and type of dressings used and saturated over an interval of time. The color and consistency of drainage vary, depending on its components. Types of drainage include the following:

1. *Serous:* Clear, watery plasma
2. *Sanguineous:* Fresh bleeding
3. *Serosanguineous:* Pale, more watery, a combination of plasma and red cells; may be blood streaked
4. *Purulent:* Thick, yellow, green, or brown, indicating the presence of dead or living organisms and WBCs

If drainage has a pungent or strong odor, an infection is likely. Document the integrity of the wound and the character of the drainage, describing the appearance by observable characteristics.

The presence of a drain is another important assessment. A drain is used in a surgical wound if a health care provider expects a large amount of drainage. Drains lie within tissue, extend from the skin, and are connected to a drainage bag or suction apparatus or allowed to drain into a dressing. Most drains attach to a collection device. First observe the security of the drain and its location with respect to the wound. Next note the character and amount of drainage if there is a collecting device. Pay particular attention to the flow of drainage through the tubing, and notify the health care provider of any sudden decrease that indicates a blocked drain or an increase indicating bleeding or infection (see Chapter 40).

In the case of a surgical wound, inspect the staples, sutures, or wound closures for irritation, and note whether the wound edges are intact. After the first few days when normal swelling around closures usually has subsided, continued swelling sometimes indicates closures that are too tight, which increases the risk for wound separation or dehiscence.

When a wound exhibits swelling, separation of its edges, or redness in the periwound area, it is important to evaluate for the presence of cellulitis. Use light palpation to detect localized areas of tenderness or collection of drainage. Wearing gloves, gently place your fingertips along the wound edges. If pressure causes fluid to be expressed from the wound, note the character of the drainage and collect a wound culture if needed. Sensitivity to such palpation is normal, but extreme tenderness indicates infection.

Pain assessment is an important component of wound assessment for detecting complications and planning for future wound care (see Chapter 34). Serious discomfort during inspection or palpation of the wound suggests underlying problems, whereas discomfort related to dressing removal or application calls for administration of analgesics before future dressing changes.

Wound Cultures. Collection of a wound culture is indicated if you detect clinical symptoms that suggest a wound infection such as increased erythema; increase in the amount and/or change in character of exudate; odor; increased local warmth; or systemic signs of infection such as fever, chills, or an increased WBC count. The swab technique is most commonly used. Cultures are obtained to direct antibiotic selection (Stotts, 2016a). Never collect a wound culture sample from old drainage because resident colonies of bacteria grow in the exudate. Aerobic organisms grow in superficial wounds exposed to the air, whereas anaerobic organisms tend to live in body cavities. Box 38.8 describes the procedure you use to collect an aerobic specimen. To collect an anaerobic specimen deep in a body cavity, use a sterile 10-mL syringe with a 22-gauge needle. Aspirate 5 mL of air into the syringe. After cleaning the skin with a disinfectant and allowing it to dry, insert a needle into the wound and aspirate wound drainage while moving the needle back and forth in two to four areas of the wound. Withdraw the needle from the wound and expel any air from the syringe. Inject contents from the syringe into a special vacuum container with culture medium. In some institutions you place a cork over the needle to prevent entrance of air and send the syringe to the laboratory.

BOX 38.8 RECOMMENDATED PROCEDURE FOR AEROBIC SWAB WOUND-CULTURE TECHNIQUE

1. Prepare to collect specimen using sterile technique (before administering antibiotics).
2. Clean wound surface 1 cm^2 with an antiseptic solution.
3. Moisten swab with normal saline.
4. While applying pressure, rotate applicator within 1 to 2 cm^2 of clean wound tissue (try to draw out tissue fluid).
5. When tip is saturated, insert into appropriate sterile container.
6. Complete laboratory slip providing clinical data, which includes wound site, time collected, and prior antibiotics.
7. Transport specimen within 1 hour to laboratory to keep the specimen stable.

From Stotts NS: Wound infection: diagnosis and management. In Bryant RA, Nix DP, editors: *Acute and chronic wounds: current management concepts*, ed 5, St Louis, 2016, Mosby.

Patient Expectations. Treatment for a pressure injury or a chronic wound is often costly and lengthy. Because patients and family caregivers need to be involved in their care, you need to know their expectations. A patient who actively participates in pressure injury prevention strategies may have an unrealistic expectation that a pressure injury will never occur. A patient with a wound may unrealistically expect rapid wound healing and become easily discouraged. Knowing these expectations helps you provide individualized care and helps a patient and family caregiver modify expectations as needed.

QSEN QSEN ACTIVITY *Evidence-Based Practice*

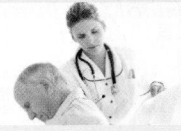

Copyright © Stockbyte/ iStock/Thinkstock.

Lynda finished her assessment and is working with Claudia, an experienced nurse. They are caring for Mr. Martinez, who has a Stage 2 pressure injury in his sacral region. Lynda and Claudia discuss different pressure injury prevention and treatment options, and Lynda plans to go to the library that evening to investigate which interventions would be most effective in preventing and treating Mr. Martinez's pressure injuries.

- Which possible key terms could Lynda use to search an online database to find research studies and professional guidelines to help her develop evidence-based nursing interventions?

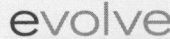 Answers to QSEN Activities can be found on the Evolve website.

■■■■ NURSING DIAGNOSIS

Use critical thinking to formulate nursing diagnoses for patients with actual problems or risks for impaired skin integrity. Assessment reveals clusters of data that indicate whether actual or a risk for *Impaired Skin Integrity* exists. After gathering appropriate assessment data, cluster defining characteristics to establish nursing diagnoses. For example, the destruction of the surface of the skin clearly allows you to make a problem-focused nursing diagnosis of *Impaired Skin Integrity*.

Some patients are at risk for impaired skin integrity; thus you need to assess for risk factors when a patient does not have an actual pressure injury. For example, a patient with intact skin who has decreased peripheral vascular circulation, is overweight, and is resistant to position change has a nursing diagnosis of *Risk for Impaired Skin Integrity* and needs specific nursing measures to reduce the risk for pressure injury. The identification of nursing diagnoses related to impaired skin integrity and wound healing helps you anticipate the need for supportive or preventive care. Nursing diagnoses are potentially relevant to a patient who requires wound care including the following:

- *Risk for Infection*
- *Impaired Bed Mobility*
- *Impaired Physical Mobility*
- *Imbalanced Nutrition: Less Than Body Requirements*
- *Acute Pain*
- *Impaired Skin Integrity*
- *Risk for Impaired Skin Integrity*
- *Ineffective Peripheral Tissue Perfusion*

Assess for related factors that contribute to each diagnostic statement. Risk diagnoses do not have related factors, so a patient with *Risk for Impaired Skin Integrity* would not have a "related to" statement.

When your patient has a problem-focused or health promotion diagnosis, related factors become the focus of your interventions. For example, the patient with *Impaired Skin Integrity related to a surgical incision* requires a different set of interventions than the patient with *Impaired Skin Integrity related to pressure and nutritional deficiency.*

■ ■ ■ PLANNING

Plan therapeutic interventions for your patients with actual problems or potential risks to skin integrity (Care Plan and Fig. 38.7). Design your therapies according to severity of problems or risks to the patient. Individualize the plan according to the patient's developmental stage and level of health.

Goals and Outcomes. Develop patient-centered goals aimed at preventing or reducing impaired skin integrity and/or promoting wound healing. Individualize care planning for the patient, taking into consideration his or her most immediate needs. Assess all patients for the risk for skin breakdown, and perform skin and wound assessments daily. Integrate information from the pressure injury risk and skin assessments into the plan of care and write attainable goals such as "Patient will not develop further skin breakdown" and "Patient's wounds will demonstrate healing." Include the patient and family caregiver in the assessment process so they see their contribution to reducing risk factors.

Setting Priorities. When planning care, establish priorities based on comprehensive assessment data, goals, and expected outcomes. In addition, consider a patient's everyday activities and family factors. Acute needs are immediate. Prioritize preventive interventions and implement them in a timely manner. Maintaining skin integrity and promoting wound healing prevent additional health care issues. Skin and wound priorities include performing ongoing assessment of pressure injury risk and wound status and providing interventions to control or eliminate contributing factors of pressure, shear, friction, moisture, and infection. Collaborate with other health care team members, such as registered dietitians and physical or occupational therapists, as needed.

Collaborative Care. With the trend toward earlier discharge from health care settings, it is important to consider a patient's plan for discharge. Discharge planning begins when a patient enters the health care system. Anticipating a patient's

---

◎ CARE PLAN

Impaired Skin Integrity

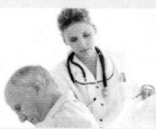

Copyright © Stockbyte/
iStock/Thinkstock.

ASSESSMENT

Mr. Martinez has limited activity tolerance. He does not tolerate position changes and wants to stay in a semi-Fowler's position at all times. He complains of a painful, burning sensation in his sacral region. A pressure injury is present that measures 1 × 2 inches with a depth of ⅛ inch.

ASSESSMENT ACTIVITIES	FINDINGS[a]
Determine if Mr. Martinez can tolerate small shifts of his body weight while in bed.	Mr. Martinez **thinks that he cannot tolerate positions that redistribute pressure.** Mr. Martinez says, "I'm uncomfortable in any position except when I'm sitting up in bed."
Inspect and palpate wound.	Wound assessment: 1 × 2–inch partial-thickness injury over sacral area with a red, moist base, Stage 2 pressure injury. Reddened skin around wound that is indurated.
Conduct a calorie count.	Mr. Martinez is eating less than 1600 calories daily.

[a]**Defining characteristics/risk factors** are shown in **bold** type.

NURSING DIAGNOSIS: Impaired Skin Integrity related to pressure over bony prominence in sacral region

PLANNING

GOAL	EXPECTED OUTCOMES (NOC)[b]
	Tissue Integrity: Skin and Mucous Membranes
Mr. Martinez's wound will show progress toward healing in 2 weeks.	Wound decreases in diameter in 7 days. There is no evidence of further wound progression or formation in 3 days.

[b]Outcomes classification label from Moorhead S, et al, editors: *Nursing outcomes classification (NOC),* ed 5, St Louis, 2013, Mosby.

◎ CARE PLAN—cont'd

Impaired Skin Integrity

INTERVENTIONS (NIC)[c]	RATIONALE
Pressure Management	
Post and implement a turning schedule. Inform Mr. and Mrs. Martinez about importance of maintaining the turning schedule.	Repositioning redistributes amount and duration of pressure (Bryant and Nix, 2016a; WOCN Society, 2016).
Obtain and place a low-air-loss overlay over patient's mattress.	Specialized beds and overlays redistribute pressure over entire body surface to prevent excess pressure on bony prominences (Nix and Mackey, 2016).
Wound Care	
Cleanse wound and skin around wound; dry skin.	Removes debris and exudate from wound bed without damaging healthy tissue (Bryant and Nix, 2016b).
Apply hydrocolloid dressing to wound per order; extend dressing 1½ inches beyond wound edges.	Hydrocolloid dressings support moist wound healing and protect the wound (Bryant, and Nix, 2016b).
Nutrition Management	
Collaborate with registered dietitian to determine appropriate number of calories and types of nutrients needed to promote wound healing.	Adequate nutrition such as increased calorie count, protein intake, and vitamins aids in wound healing (WOCN Society, 2016).

[c]Intervention classification labels from Bulechek GM, et al, editors: *Nursing interventions classification (NIC),* ed 6, St Louis, 2013, Mosby.

EVALUATION

NURSING ACTIONS	PATIENT RESPONSE/FINDING	ACHIEVEMENT OF OUTCOME
Observe wound to determine healing progress: measure wound diameter and depth; note condition of skin around wound; observe appearance of wound drainage and tissue at each dressing change.	Pressure injury is 1 × 1½ inch. Serous drainage is present. Wound tissue remains red and moist.	Reduction in wound size.
Palpate skin around wound.	Skin around wound remains intact with no palpable tissue change.	No evidence of advancing pressure injury or tissue damage.
Review calorie count over last week.	Calorie count denotes steady increase in daily calorie consumption.	Nutrition intake is improved.

discharge from an acute care institution and referral to a skilled nursing care facility or home care agency is necessary to help a patient remain mobile or regain mobility at home.

Patients and their families often need to continue wound management after discharge. Thus they need to discuss the likelihood that the patient will return home needing the assistance of skilled family members, home health nurses, or transfer to a skilled nursing facility for more care and observation.

Consult with a case manager to plan for the necessary resources for support once a patient is discharged. Include a physical therapist for evaluation of a patient's ability to transfer and walk upstairs (if there are stairs in the home). Consult with a registered dietitian to assess a patient's nutrition status and help with nutrition interventions.

■ ■ ■ IMPLEMENTATION

Health Promotion. Early identification of patients' risk factors helps prevent pressure injuries. Prevention minimizes the effect of risk factors and contributing factors on pressure injury development (see Box 38.5). Nursing interventions for prevention of pressure injuries include positioning, topical skin care, nutrition support, and the use of support surfaces.

Positioning. Repositioning is moving a patient to another position to relieve pressure off a particular part of the body or to redistribute the pressure on a body part (Maklebust and Magnan, 2016). Positioning interventions reduce pressure (Box 38.9). Repositioning frequency is determined by tissue tolerance, level of activity and mobility, general medical condition, overall treatment objectives, and support surface (European Pressure Ulcer Advisory Panel [EPUAP] and National Pressure Ulcer Advisory Panel [NPUAP], 2014). Therefore a standard turning interval of 1 to 2 hours does not prevent pressure injury development in some patients. The WOCN Society (2016) recommends reducing shear by maintaining the elevation of the head of the bed at 30 degrees or less for the supine position, using assistive devices when

CONCEPT MAP

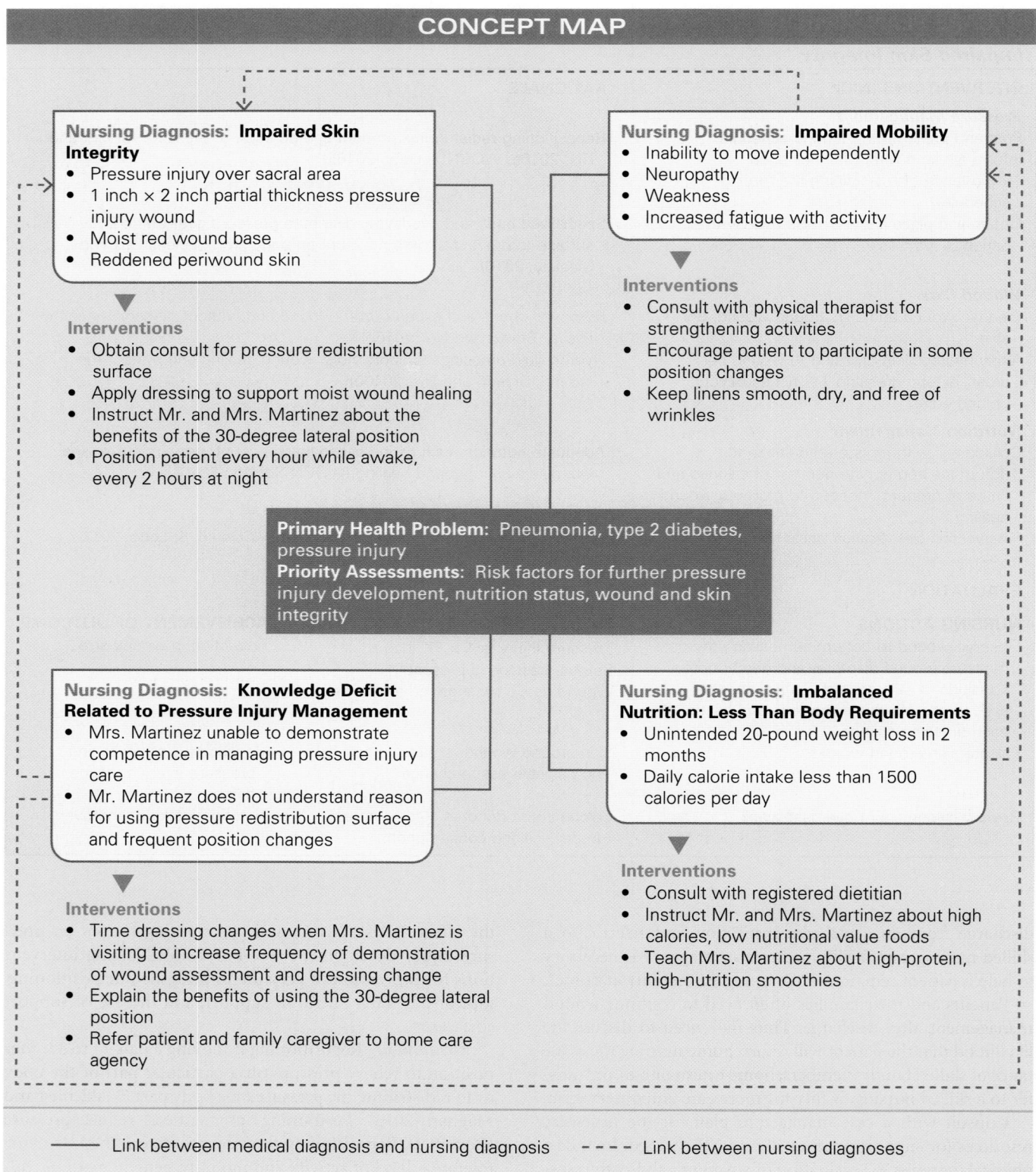

Nursing Diagnosis: Impaired Skin Integrity
- Pressure injury over sacral area
- 1 inch × 2 inch partial thickness pressure injury wound
- Moist red wound base
- Reddened periwound skin

Interventions
- Obtain consult for pressure redistribution surface
- Apply dressing to support moist wound healing
- Instruct Mr. and Mrs. Martinez about the benefits of the 30-degree lateral position
- Position patient every hour while awake, every 2 hours at night

Nursing Diagnosis: Impaired Mobility
- Inability to move independently
- Neuropathy
- Weakness
- Increased fatigue with activity

Interventions
- Consult with physical therapist for strengthening activities
- Encourage patient to participate in some position changes
- Keep linens smooth, dry, and free of wrinkles

Primary Health Problem: Pneumonia, type 2 diabetes, pressure injury
Priority Assessments: Risk factors for further pressure injury development, nutrition status, wound and skin integrity

Nursing Diagnosis: Knowledge Deficit Related to Pressure Injury Management
- Mrs. Martinez unable to demonstrate competence in managing pressure injury care
- Mr. Martinez does not understand reason for using pressure redistribution surface and frequent position changes

Interventions
- Time dressing changes when Mrs. Martinez is visiting to increase frequency of demonstration of wound assessment and dressing change
- Explain the benefits of using the 30-degree lateral position
- Refer patient and family caregiver to home care agency

Nursing Diagnosis: Imbalanced Nutrition: Less Than Body Requirements
- Unintended 20-pound weight loss in 2 months
- Daily calorie intake less than 1500 calories per day

Interventions
- Consult with registered dietitian
- Instruct Mr. and Mrs. Martinez about high calories, low nutritional value foods
- Teach Mrs. Martinez about high-protein, high-nutrition smoothies

———— Link between medical diagnosis and nursing diagnosis   - - - - Link between nursing diagnoses

FIG 38.7 Concept map.

turning or transferring patients, and using the 30-degree lateral position (Fig. 38.8).

When a patient can sit in a chair, reposition the patient every hour and limit sitting to 2 hours (EPUAP and NPUAP, 2014). In the sitting position the pressure on the ischial tuberosities is greater than when in the supine position. In addition, assist or teach patients with the ability to shift weight to reposition every 15 minutes. The patient should sit on gel or an air cushion to redistribute weight, decreasing the amount of weight on the ischial tuberosities.

BOX 38.9 WOUND, OSTOMY AND CONTINENCE NURSES (WOCN) SOCIETY RECOMMENDATIONS FOR PRESSURE REDUCTION AND RELIEF

- Use turn sheets, trapeze bars, and lift equipment to help with mobility.
- Maintain elevation of the head of the bed to 30 degrees or less for the supine position to prevent shear and subsequent tissue injury.
- Reposition and turn regularly and frequently.

- Use positioning devices to avoid placing the patient on the pressure injury or other areas at risk for pressure injury.
- When side lying, use a 30-degree laterally inclined position to relieve pressure over the trochanter.
- Continue to turn and reposition patient when support surfaces are in use.

Data adapted from Wound, Ostomy and Continence Nurses Society: *Guideline for prevention and management of pressure ulcers,* WOCN Clinical Practice Guidelines Series, Mount Laurel, NJ, 2016, The Society.

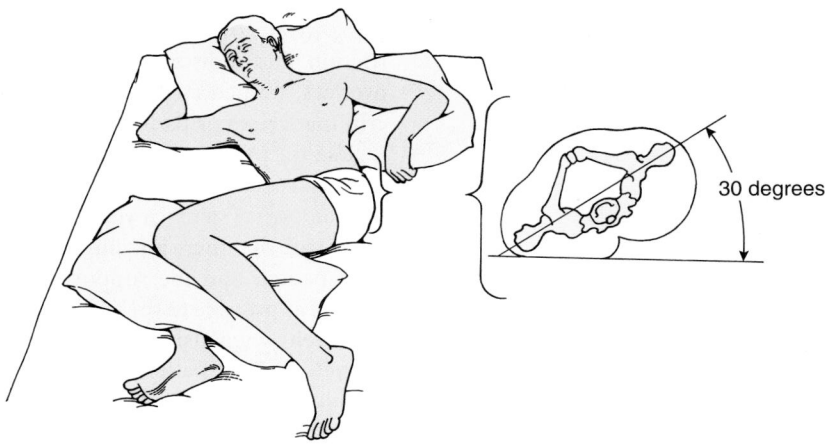

FIG 38.8 Thirty-degree lateral position. (Adapted from Bryant RA, Nix DP: *Acute and chronic wounds: current management concepts,* ed 5, St Louis, 2016, Elsevier.)

A patient's heels are an area of concern because of the small surface area (Fig. 38.9). Keep heels off the bed by using a pillow, support surfaces, and heel suspension devices to float the heels. When using pillows, position them under the calf muscle with slight knee flexion while preventing the heels from contacting the bed surface (Bryant and Nix, 2016a).

Topical Skin Care. Assess the skin daily, paying special attention to bony prominences. Do not massage reddened areas because reddened areas indicate tissue injury. Massage to these areas further injures the tissue by causing damage to the tissue capillaries. Examine your patient's skin for signs of dryness, cracking, edema, or excessive moisture.

Use a mild cleansing agent when cleansing intact skin. Soap causes dryness, which increases the risk for skin infection. Skin lubrication helps keep the skin intact; consider using a moisturizer on a routine basis (WOCN Society, 2016). Because intact skin is the initial defense for preventing skin breakdown, keep your patient's skin clean and dry. Many types of products are available for skin care; match their uses to the specific needs of your patient.

Use an incontinence cleanser for a patient who is incontinent of stool or urine. To protect the skin apply a moisture-barrier product (generally petrolatum or dimethicone based) liberally to the exposed area. The moisture barrier provides

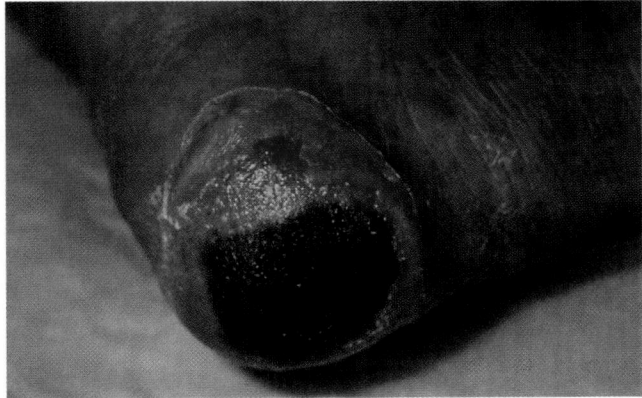

FIG 38.9 Formation of pressure injury on heel resulting from external pressure from mattress of bed. (Courtesy Janice Colwell, RN, MS, CWOCN, FAAN, Clinical Nurse Specialist, University of Chicago Medicine.)

skin protection from the irritating effects of stool or urine and allows you to clean the next incontinent episode easily. Apply the moisture-barrier ointment after each cleansing. For skin that has become exposed or stripped from incontinence, use a barrier paste that adheres to the irritated area and will not be removed with each cleansing. Offer a patient frequent access to the toilet to prevent fecal and urinary incontinence. You can contain fecal incontinence with a fecal incontinence collector when a patient is experiencing frequent liquid bowel movements and has intact perianal skin. (Fig. 38.10). An adhesive skin barrier is attached to a drainable pouch that is applied around the anus to collect liquid stool. Other external collection devices include male external catheters applied to the shaft of the penis to collect urine.

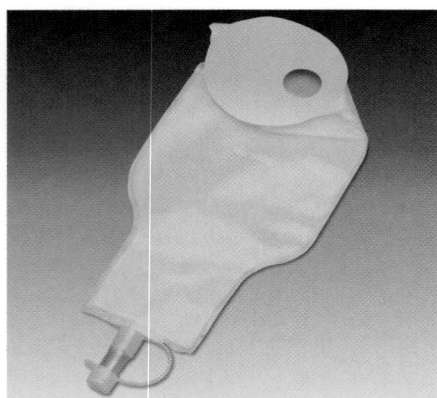

FIG 38.10 Hollister Fecal Incontinence Collector. (Permission to use this copyrighted material has been granted by the owner, Hollister Inc.)

When providing skin care to a patient who is incontinent, the health care team first assesses and treats the cause of the incontinence and then decides on protection and/or collection interventions. Underpads and diapers can protect skin in patients incontinent of stool and urine. Avoid using underpads and diapers with a plastic outer lining that holds moisture against the skin, which causes maceration (softening of the skin caused by moisture) (WOCN Society, 2016). Instead, select underpads or diapers that are absorbent and wick incontinence moisture away from the skin rather than trap it against the skin.

Support Surfaces. Support surfaces redistribute pressure exerted over bony prominences by maximizing contact (allowing the body to touch the entire surface) and redistributing weight over a large area. They also often reduce shear, friction, and moisture. Support surfaces include mattresses, overlays, framed specialty beds, chair pads, table pads, and crib mattresses or pads (Table 38.3).

Use the WOCN Society's evidence- and consensus-based support surface algorithm (Fig. 38.11) to help you select the best support system for your patients (McNichol et al., 2015). Make sure that there are minimal layers of bed linens between your patient and the support surface to keep your patient as close as possible to the surface for it to be effective. Remember, even when using a support surface, you still need to reposition your patient. Once a support surface is in use, reevaluate patients on a frequent basis to determine the

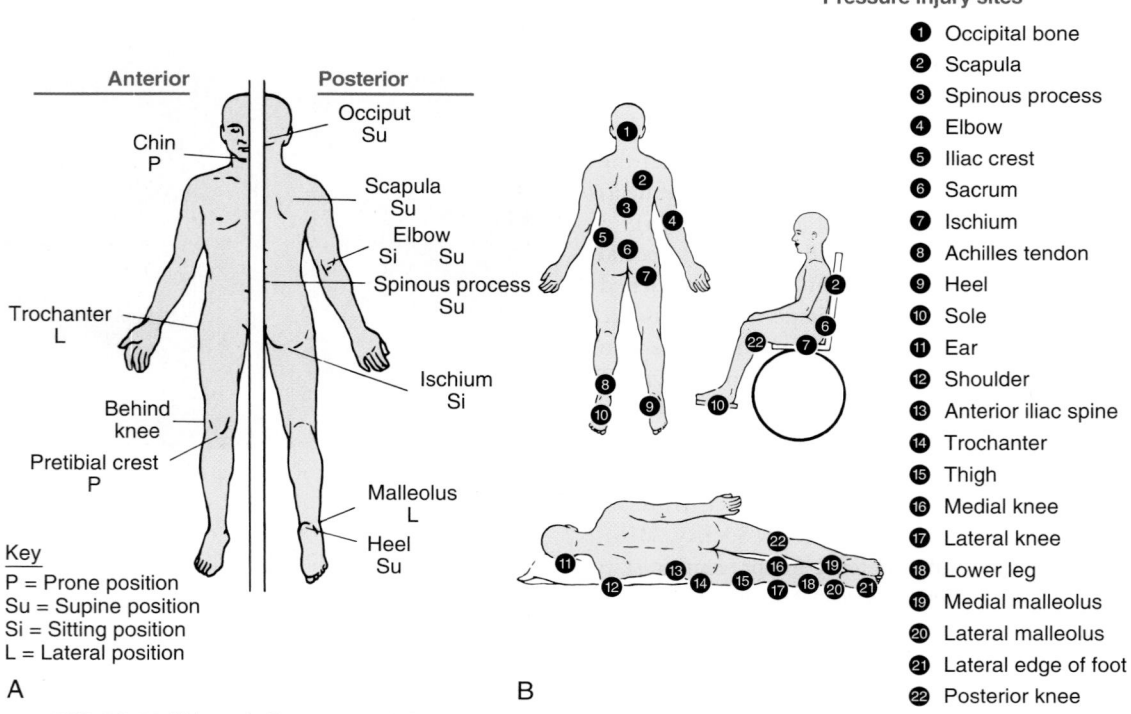

Pressure injury sites

1. Occipital bone
2. Scapula
3. Spinous process
4. Elbow
5. Iliac crest
6. Sacrum
7. Ischium
8. Achilles tendon
9. Heel
10. Sole
11. Ear
12. Shoulder
13. Anterior iliac spine
14. Trochanter
15. Thigh
16. Medial knee
17. Lateral knee
18. Lower leg
19. Medial malleolus
20. Lateral malleolus
21. Lateral edge of foot
22. Posterior knee

Key
P = Prone position
Su = Supine position
Si = Sitting position
L = Lateral position

A   B

FIG 38.11 Wound, Ostomy and Continence Nurses (WOCN) Society evidence- and consensus-based support surface algorithm. (From Trelease CC: Developing standards for wound care, *Ostomy Wound Manage* 20:46, 1988.)

TABLE 38.3 SUPPORT SURFACES

CATEGORY AND MECHANISM OF ACTION	INDICATIONS FOR USE	ADVANTAGES	DISADVANTAGES
Support Surfaces and Overlays			
Foam Overlay (Available as an Overlay or in a Full Mattress)			
Reduces pressure; the cover (top) can reduce friction and shear. Base height of 7.5–10 cm (3–4 inches); see manufacturer guidelines regarding amount of body weight supported.	Use for patients with moderate to high risk.	One-time charge No setup fee Cannot be punctured Available in various sizes (e.g., bed, chair, operating room table) Little maintenance Does not need electricity	Elevated body temperature Hot and may trap moisture Limited life span Plastic protective sheet needed for incontinent patients or patients with draining wounds Not indicated for patients with existing Stage 3 or Stage 4 pressure injuries
Water Overlay (Available as an Overlay or in a Full Mattress)			
Reduces pressure and pressure points because surface provides flotation with pressure reduction by redistributing patient's weight evenly over entire support surface.	Use for patients with high risk.	Readily available Some control over motion sensations Easy to clean	Easily punctured Heavy Fluid motion may make procedures (e.g., dressing changes, CPR) difficult Maintenance needed to prevent microorganism growth Patient transfers out of bed are difficult Difficult to raise and lower head of bed
Gel Overlay			
Reduces pressure and pressure points because surface provides flotation by redistributing patient's weight evenly over entire support surface.	Use for patients with moderate to high risk. Use for patients who are wheelchair dependent.	Low maintenance Easy to clean Multiple-patient use Impermeable to needle punctures	Heavy Expensive Lacks airflow for moisture control Variable friction control
Nonpowered Support Surface			
Reduces pressure by lowering mean interface pressure between patient's tissue and mattress.	Use for patients with moderate to high risk. Use for patients who can reposition themselves.	Easy to clean Multiple-patient use Low maintenance Potential repair of some air-filled products Durable	Damaged by punctures from needles and sharps Requires routine monitoring to determine adequate inflation pressure Patient transfers out of bed are difficult
Low-Air-Loss Overlay (Available as an Overlay or in a Full Mattress)			
Maintains constant and slight air movement against patient's skin, also assists in managing heat and humidity (microclimate) of the skin.	Use for patients with moderate to high risk.	Easy to clean Maintains constant inflation Deflates to facilitate transfer and CPR Moisture control Fabric covering overlay is air permeable, bacteria impermeable, and waterproof Reduces shear and friction Setup provided by manufacturer	Damaged by needles and sharps Noisy Requires electricity, but some are available with short backup battery In home may need to purchase backup generator in case of loss of electrical power

Continued

TABLE 38.3 SUPPORT SURFACES—cont'd

CATEGORY AND MECHANISM OF ACTION	INDICATIONS FOR USE	ADVANTAGES	DISADVANTAGES
Specialty Beds			
Air-Fluidized Bed			
Bed frame contains silicone-coated beads and provides pressure redistribution by the fluidlike medium that is created by forcing air through beads resulting in immersion and envelopment of patient.	Use for patients at high risk. Use for patients with Stage 3 or Stage 4 pressure injuries or burns.	Less frequent turning or repositioning Improved patient comfort Quickly becomes firm for CPR or other treatments when device is turned "off" Reduces shear, friction, and edema to site May facilitate management of copious wound drainage or incontinence Setup provided by manufacturer	Continuous circulation of warm, dry air may increase patient risk for dehydration Possible increase in room temperature Patient may experience disorientation Patient transfer difficult Heavy Expensive May not be wide enough for use with obese patients or patients with contractures Patient cannot lie prone because of risk of suffocation
Low-Air-Loss Bed			
Bed frame with series of connected air-filled pillows. Flow of air controls the amount of pressure in each pillow and assists in managing heat and humidity (microclimate) of the patient's skin.	Use for patients who need pressure relief, who cannot be repositioned frequently, or who have skin breakdown on more than one surface. Contraindicated in patients with unstable spinal column.	Can raise and lower head and foot of bed Easy transfer in and out of bed Less frequent turning schedule Pillows can be transferred to stretcher with patient Setup provided by manufacturer	Portable motor is noisy Bed surface material is slippery; patients can easily slide down mattress or out of bed when being transferred
Kinetic Therapy			
Provides continuous passive motion to promote mobilization of pulmonary secretions and low air loss, which provides pressure relief.	Use primarily for patients needing spinal stabilization. Should not be used when the patient is hemodynamically unstable.	Reduces pulmonary complications associated with restricted mobility Reduces risk for urinary stasis and urinary tract infections Reduces venous stasis	Does not reduce shear or moisture Cannot be used with cervical or skeletal traction Possible motion sickness initially Possible sensations of claustrophobia

CPR, Cardiopulmonary resuscitation.
Data from Doughty D, McNichol L: *Wound, Ostomy, and Continence Nurses Society core curriculum: wound management,* Philadelphia, PA 2016, Wolters Kluwer; and Wound Ostomy and Continence Nurses (WOCN) Society: *Guideline for prevention and management of pressure ulcers,* WOCN Clinical Practice Guidelines Series, Mount Laurel, NJ, 2016, The Society.

continued need and the effectiveness of the product. Patient and caregiver education on the importance and use of the support product is essential (Box 38.10).

Nutrition. Nutrition is fundamental to normal cell activity and tissue repair and regeneration. Although nutrition is important for all patients, it is of particular importance for a patient with a wound to prevent severe or prolonged depletion of nutrients that can impact healing (Stotts, 2016b). Complete a nutrition assessment on a patient who has a wound, collecting important data such as relevant patient history and

---

BOX 38.10 GUIDELINES FOR PATIENT EDUCATION REGARDING THERAPEUTIC SURFACES

- Explain the rationale for use of support surfaces. Be sure that patient and family caregiver know that this reduces pressure on the bony prominences by redistributing pressure between the surface and patient's skin.
- Teach patient and family caregiver the importance of using minimal layers of linen or absorbent pads between patient and surface.
- Explain the importance of frequent position changes even while on the support surfaces.
- Demonstrate to patient and family caregiver how to shift weight while on support surface.
- Demonstrate to patient and family caregiver how to use the 30-degree angle lateral position and pillows to support various positions.

BOX 38.11 WOUND-HEALING PRINCIPLES

- Control or eliminate causative factors.
  - Offload pressure.
  - Reduce friction and shear.
  - Protect from moisture.
- Provide systemic support to reduce existing and potential cofactors.
  - Optimize nutrition.
  - Provide adequate hydration.
  - Reduce edema.
  - Control blood glucose levels.
- Maintain physiological wound environment.
  - Prevent and manage infection.
  - Cleanse wound.
  - Remove nonviable tissue (debridement).
  - Maintain appropriate level of moisture.
  - Eliminate dead space.
  - Control odor.
  - Eliminate or minimize pain.
  - Protect periwound skin

From Bryant RA, Nix DP: Topical management. In Bryant RA, Nix, DP, editors: *Acute and chronic wounds: current management concepts*, ed 5, St Louis, 2016, Elsevier.

---

laboratory data. Normal wound healing requires adequate intake of protein, fat, and carbohydrates. Consider consulting with a registered dietitian to obtain a thorough evaluation of a patient's nutrition status and identify related interventions to improve nutritional intake.

Acute Care

Pressure Injuries. Address wound-management principles in an orderly fashion (Box 38.11). Provide appropriate wound management including managing pressure, shear, friction, and moisture (see Skill 38.2). Provide systemic support to enhance your patient's wound healing. Co-morbidities such as cardiovascular or pulmonary disease decrease the amount of oxygen-rich hemoglobin available for delivery to injured tissue. Oxygen is necessary for wound healing and resistance to infection. Interventions that maximize oxygen levels include pulmonary hygiene interventions and administering low-flow supplemental oxygen (see Chapter 32).

Wound healing also depends on adequate nutrition. Protein intake is necessary to support the development of new blood vessels and collagen synthesis. Carbohydrates, fats, and vitamins provide energy for cellular function. Interventions to support adequate nutrition intake include a nutrition referral and appropriate dietary supplements.

Certain medications (e.g., steroids) and medical conditions (e.g., diabetes) negatively influence wound healing. Because hyperglycemia impairs wound healing, blood glucose control is essential.

A stable wound environment and appropriate treatment are necessary to promote healing (Table 38.4). To maintain an environment to support healing it is important to control infection, **debride** (remove) necrotic tissue, provide exudate management, control dead space, and provide wound protection. Assess a patient with a pressure injury for signs and symptoms of a wound infection such as redness, warmth of surrounding tissue, odor, and the presence of exudate. If any of these signs is present, consult with the health care team to determine if you need to culture the wound and if systemic or topical antibiotics are indicated.

Cleanse pressure injuries at each dressing change to remove wound debris from the wound surface (WOCN Society, 2016). Cleanse dirty wounds by irrigation. Clean wounds require gentle flushing with normal saline solution.

Necrotic tissue slows wound healing because it is a source for infection and a barrier for epithelialization. After consulting with a health care provider or wound care specialist, plan a method of debridement. Types of debridement include mechanical, chemical, sharp, and autolytic (Ramundo, 2016).

A moist wound environment supports wound healing; however, excessive wound moisture macerates the wound edges, which puts the wound at risk for increasing in size and interferes with wound healing. Select a dressing that absorbs excessive moisture while providing the wound with necessary hydration. Eliminate dead space by loosely filling all cavities with dressings. Lightly fill wound cavities to support the growth of granulation tissue and discourage infection. Overfilling a wound with gauze places pressure within the wound bed and prevents development of granulation tissue.

Involve a patient's family or caregiver in management of pressure injuries and their treatment. Frequently patients require dressing changes after discharge. A patient's family or caregiver is an excellent source for dressing support and identification of possible wound-healing complications (Box 38.12).

Wounds

First Aid for Wounds. When a patient sustains a traumatic wound, first-aid interventions include promoting hemostasis, cleansing the wound, and protecting the wound from further injury.

TABLE 38.4   TREATMENT OPTIONS BY PRESSURE INJURY STAGE

INJURY STAGE	INJURY STATUS	DRESSING	COMMENTS[a]	EXPECTED CHANGE	TREATMENTS
1	Intact	None Transparent dressing Hydrocolloid	Allows visual assessment. Protects from shear. Do not use in the presence of excessive moisture. Does not allow visual assessment.	Resolves slowly without epidermal loss over 7–14 days.	Turning schedule. Support hydration. Nutrition support. Pressure redistribution mattress or chair cushion.
2	Clean, granular base	Composite film Hydrocolloid Hydrogel	Limits shear. Change when seal of dressing breaks, maximal wear time 7 days. Provides moist environment.	Heals through reepithelialization.	See previous stage. Manage incontinence.
3	Clean, granular base	Hydrocolloid Hydrogel covered with foam Calcium alginate Gauze Growth factors	Change when seal of dressing breaks, maximum wear time 7 days. Apply over wound to protect and absorb moisture. Apply over wound to protect and absorb moisture. Use when there is significant exudate. Cover with secondary dressing. Use with normal saline or other prescribed solution. Wring out excess solution; unfold to make contact with wound. Used with gauze per manufacturer instructions	Heals through granulation and reepithelialization.	See previous stages. Evaluate pressure redistribution needs.
4	Clean	Hydrogel covered with foam dressing Calcium alginate Gauze	See Stage 3, clean. Used with significant exudate; must cover with secondary dressing. See Stage 3 clean.	Heals through granulation and reepithelialization.	Surgical consultation often necessary for closure. See Stages 1, 2, and 3.
Unstageable	Wound covered with eschar	Adherent film Gauze plus ordered solution Enzymes None	Facilitates softening of eschar. Delivers solution and wicks wound drainage. Breaks down eschar, providing debridement. Rarely, if eschar is dry and intact, no dressing is used, allowing eschar to act as physiological cover.	Eschar lifts at edges as healing progresses. Eschar softens. Eschar loosens over time.	See previous stages. Surgical consultation may be considered for debridement.

[a]As with *all* occlusive dressings, wounds should *not* be clinically infected.

BOX 38.12 PATIENT TEACHING

Pressure Injury Dressing Change

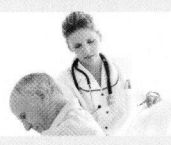

In preparation for Mr. Martinez's discharge, Lynda develops a teaching plan for Mrs. Martinez to teach her how to change Mr. Martinez's pressure injury dressing.

Copyright © Stockbyte/
iStock/Thinkstock.

OUTCOME

At the end of the teaching session Mrs. Martinez changes Mr. Martinez's dressing correctly.

TEACHING STRATEGIES

- Avoid using words and medical terminology that Mrs. Martinez will not understand.
- Provide a brief description of what you will teach. Include Mr. Martinez in all the teaching, even though he is unable to see the wound.
- Bring an extra dressing to the bedside to show Mr. and Mrs. Martinez what the dressing looks like; explain how it works and how to apply it.
- Use pictures of a pressure injury to help Mrs. Martinez understand what the wound looks like and how it will change in appearance as it heals or worsens.
- Allow Mrs. Martinez to watch at least one demonstration of you cleansing the wound and applying the dressing.
- Have Mrs. Martinez change the dressing with your supervision, allowing for return demonstrations.

EVALUATION

- Use the principles of teach-back to evaluate patient/family caregiver leaning:
  - While observing Mrs. Martinez changing the dressing, ask her, "Explain the steps you are taking to clean the wound and change the dressing."
  - "Tell me what information about the wound you need to report to the home health nurse."

Hemostasis. After assessing the type and extent of the wound, control bleeding from a laceration by applying direct pressure to the wound with a sterile or clean dressing. After bleeding subsides, an adhesive dressing strip or gauze dressing taped over the laceration allows skin edges to close and a blood clot to form. If a dressing becomes saturated with blood, add another layer of dressing, continue to apply pressure, and elevate the affected part. A health care provider sutures serious lacerations in an emergency clinic or hospital.

If a penetrating object such as a knife blade is in a patient's body, do not remove the object. Removal causes massive, uncontrolled bleeding. Apply pressure by rolling sterile gauze taped in place around the object but not on it or on surrounding tissues.

Cleansing. Gentle cleansing of a wound removes contaminants that serve as sources of infection. However, vigorous cleaning causes bleeding or further injury. For abrasions, minor lacerations, and small puncture wounds, rinse the wound in running water, gently cleanse with mild soap and water, rinse, and apply an over-the-counter antiseptic. When a laceration is bleeding profusely, only brush away surface contaminants and concentrate on hemostasis until the patient reaches a clinic or hospital.

Protection. Protect a wound by applying a sterile or clean dressing and immobilize the body part. A light dressing applied over minor wounds prevents entrance of microorganisms. In the case of small abrasions, it is acceptable to leave the wound open to air so that a scab forms.

The more extensive the wound, the larger the dressing required. In a home emergency a clean towel or diaper is often the best dressing. A bulky dressing applied with pressure minimizes movement of underlying tissues and helps to immobilize the entire body part. A dressing or cloth wrapped around a penetrating object immobilizes it adequately.

Dressings. The use of dressings requires an understanding of wound healing and factors influencing healing. A variety of dressing materials are available commercially. The choice of dressing and how it is applied influence wound healing. The proper dressing does not allow a full-thickness wound to become dry with scab formation. When this occurs, the dermis dehydrates and crusts. As a result a barrier forms against normal epidermal cell growth, slowing wound healing. Furthermore, dryness increases discomfort. Ideally a dressing provides a moist environment to promote normal epidermal cell migration. The proper dressing also absorbs drainage to prevent bacterial growth and wound drainage from coming in contact with intact skin.

For surgical wounds that heal by primary intention, dressings are commonly removed as soon as drainage stops. Frequently the health care provider removes the dressing 24 to 48 hours after surgery, which coincides with initial epithelialization.

Purpose. A dressing serves several purposes. It minimizes exposure to microorganisms. In wounds with minimal drainage, the natural formation of a fibrin seal eliminates the need for a dressing. A pressure dressing promotes hemostasis by exerting localized, downward pressure over an actual or potential bleeding site. A moist dressing lightly packed into the wound fosters normal healing by eliminating dead space in underlying tissues. Assess skin color, temperature, pulses in distal extremities, patient comfort, and any changes in sensation to ensure that dressings do not interfere with circulation.

A dry dressing promotes healing by allowing the wound to heal by primary intention and absorbing minimal oozing of wound drainage. When a wound is healing by secondary intention, use a dressing to provide a moist environment. Moisten the gauze with a solution, usually normal saline, wring it out, and unfold and lightly pack it into the wound. The purpose of a moist gauze dressing is to act as a sponge, absorbing excessive wound drainage while providing a moist environment. Change the dressing when it is saturated or if it begins to dry out. Always cover a moist dressing with a dry, secondary dressing.

A firmly taped or wrapped dressing supports or immobilizes a body part, minimizing movement of the underlying incision and traumatized tissues. Finally a dressing promotes thermal insulation to the wound surface and protects it from the dehydrating effects of air.

Type. Dressings vary by type of material and mode of application (dry or moist). Gauze is the most common dressing type. It does not interact with wound tissue and thus causes little wound irritation. It is available in different textures and shapes such as square, rectangle, and rolls of various lengths and widths. Moist or dry gauze dressings are best for wounds with moderate drainage, deep wounds, undermining, and tunnels. Saturate a moist gauze dressing with the prescribed solution, wring it out, then open and place it onto the wound tissue. The moistened gauze increases the ability of the dressing to absorb exudate. Cover the moist gauze with a secondary layer of dry gauze. Be sure that the moist gauze does not cover normal skin to prevent maceration. The moist dressing is changed on a scheduled basis to prevent drying of the gauze.

Transparent film dressings are clear sheets coated on one side with an adhesive. The adhesive side does not stick to the wound because of the moisture and traps moisture over the wound bed, providing a moist environment. The film is impermeable to fluid but semipermeable to oxygen. This type of dressing is used as a primary dressing in wounds with minimal tissue loss that have very little wound drainage. The dressing is applied to extend approximately $1\frac{1}{2}$ inches beyond the wound to allow for adherence. Change the dressing when the seal is broken.

Hydrocolloid dressings are made of gelling agents and have an adhesive wound surface. They come in a variety of sizes and shapes and are used to cover wounds, extending the hydrocolloid dressing at least $1\frac{1}{2}$ inches beyond the wound margin. Hydrocolloids form a gel as they interact with the wound surface. Because they are occlusive, they protect the wound from surface contaminants, and you can leave them over a wound for several days. When removed, you will note a gel over the wound base; the gel maintains a moist environment to support healing and washes away during wound cleansing.

Hydrogel dressings are available in sheets, spray bottles, or a gel in a tube (amorphous). They contain a high percentage of water and are used when wounds require moisture—either a wound with granulation (maintaining the moist wound environment needed for healing) or a wound that has a high percentage of necrotic tissue (the hydrogel facilitates debridement by softening the dead tissue). Hydrogels maintain moisture in some wounds for 1 to 3 days.

Alginate dressings are highly absorptive dressings made of spun fibers of seaweed. They absorb and hold exudate, maintain a moist environment, and are available in sheets or ropes. They are indicated for moderately to highly exudative wounds (Bryant and Nix, 2016b).

Negative-pressure wound therapy (NPWT) uses a combination dressing (foam and transparent film) with negative pressure via suction to help wound healing (Fig. 38.12). NPWT supports wound healing by evacuating wound fluids,

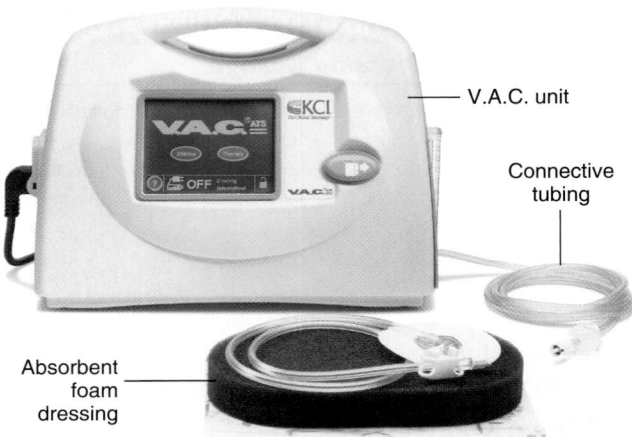

FIG 38.12 The vacuum-assisted closure (V.A.C.) ATS negative-pressure wound therapy system. *(Top to bottom)* V.A.C. system, connective tubing to go between V.A.C. system and dressing, absorbent foam dressing. (Courtesy KCI Licensing, San Antonio, TX.)

stimulating granulation tissue formation, reducing the bacterial burden of a wound, and maintaining a moist wound environment (Netsch et al., 2016). Before applying NPWT assess your patient's level of comfort. Some patients may require analgesia.

Apply NPWT by fitting the foam or dressing to the shape of the wound and placing a drainage/suction tube in the interior or on top of the dressing. Seal the dressing and the tube with a transparent dressing and connect the tube to a prescribed amount of negative pressure, which creates suction. The suction pulls all air out of the wound and creates an airtight seal. This therapy provides removal of excess wound fluid to stimulate granulation tissue and decrease wound bacteria (see Skill 38.3). Connect the suction tubing to a container that collects the wound fluid. NPWT is changed on a scheduled basis, usually every 48 hours. Current evidence shows that this therapy often reduces healing time in chronic wounds and results in early grafting of wounds (Netsch et al., 2016).

Changing Dressings. To prepare to change a dressing, you need to know the type of dressing, any underlying drains used, and the type of supplies needed for wound care. You adjust the type and amount of dressings if the amount of drainage changes or a wound becomes deeper. Notifying the health care provider of any change is essential.

The order for changing a dressing usually indicates the dressing type, frequency of changing, and solution or ointment you will apply. An order to "reinforce dressing prn" (add dressings without removing existing ones as needed) is common immediately after surgery when a health care provider does not want accidental disruption of the suture line or loss of hemostasis. A patient's medical or operating room record usually reveals whether drains are present. After the initial dressing change, communicate on the care plan the type of dressing materials and solutions to use and the type and location of drains. Skill 38.4 outlines the steps for applying moist saline dressings.

Use aseptic technique during dressing change procedures (see Chapter 14). It is also essential for a patient to understand the steps of the procedure beforehand to reduce anxiety. Describe normal signs of the healing process and answer questions about the procedure or wound.

If a patient needs to care for a wound at home, demonstrate dressing changes and provide an opportunity for the patient and family caregiver to practice. In the home, patients and family caregivers usually need to learn clean technique. Make sure that the patient is able to change a dressing independently or with assistance from a family caregiver before discharge unless home care will be provided.

Securing Dressings. Use tape, ties, or cloth binders to secure a dressing over a wound site. Binders are dressings made of large pieces of material to fit a specific body part. An arm sling is an example of a binder. A binder reduces stress on a wound.

The choice of anchoring depends on wound size, location, drainage, frequency of dressing changes, and patient's level of activity. You most often use tape to secure dressings if a patient does not react to tape. Hypoallergenic paper, plastic, and woven fabric tapes minimize skin reactions.

Tape comes in various widths. Choose a size that secures the dressing sufficiently. Make sure that the tape crosses the dressing and adheres to several inches of skin on each side. When securing the dressing, gently press the tape, exerting pressure away from the wound. Never apply tape over irritated skin. Apply a skin barrier to the skin around the wound to secure the tape to the skin barrier rather than to sensitive skin. To remove tape safely, loosen the end and gently release the tape from the patient's skin by pressing the skin away from the tape.

To avoid repeated removal of tape from sensitive skin, secure dressings with reusable Montgomery ties (see Skill 38.4, Step 13b). Each tie consists of a long strip; half contains an adhesive backing to apply to the skin, and the other half folds back and contains a cloth tie that you tie across a dressing and untie at dressing changes. A long dressing requires two or more sets of Montgomery ties. To provide even support to a wound and immobilize a body part, apply elastic gauze or cloth dressings and binders over a dressing.

Comfort Measures. Any wound can be painful, depending on the extent of tissue injury. Interventions for pain reduction during dressing changes include analgesia before the procedure, allowing "time-outs" during painful procedures, soaking dried dressings before removal, avoiding aggressive packing, positioning and supporting the wound area for comfort, and considering using low adhesive or nonadhesive dressings (Hopf et al., 2016).

Wound Cleansing. Wound cleansing removes surface bacteria, preventing the invasion of healthy tissue. Normal saline effectively cleans when delivered to the wound site with adequate force to agitate and wash away bacteria (Bryant and Nix, 2016b). Do not use povidone-iodine (Betadine),

hydrogen peroxide, and acetic acid to irrigate a clean, granular wound. These solutions are toxic to fibroblasts, a key cellular component in wound healing. Apply the following concepts when cleaning wounds:

1. Cleanse in a direction from the least contaminated area to the most contaminated such as from the wound or incision to the surrounding skin or from an isolated drain site to the surrounding skin (See Skill 38.4, Steps 9b and 9c).
2. Use light friction when applying antiseptics locally to the skin.
3. When irrigating, allow the solution to flow from the least contaminated to the most contaminated area.

Wound Irrigation. Irrigation is a way of cleansing wounds of exudate and debris. You use an irrigating syringe to flush the area with a constant flow of solution. Irrigations clean open, deep wounds and sensitive or inaccessible body parts. Administer the prescribed solution (usually normal saline) at body temperature to enhance comfort and provide local cleansing application.

When irrigating a clean wound, use sterile technique and an irrigation system with a safe level of pressure (4 to 15 psi) to prevent trauma to the newly formed granulation tissue (WOCN Society, 2016). This method provides an ideal solution pressure for cleansing wounds while minimizing tissue trauma (Fig. 38.13). Make sure that the syringe tip is over but not sticking into the wound. Skill 38.5 lists the steps for wound irrigation.

Suture Care. A health care provider closes a wound by bringing the edges as close together as possible to reduce the formation of scar tissue while minimizing trauma and tension and controlling bleeding. Sutures are threads or wires made of silk, steel, cotton, nylon, and polyester (Dacron) and are used to sew body tissues together. Dacron sutures minimize scar formation. Surgeons frequently use steel staples, a type of outer skin closure, because they result in less tissue trauma while providing extra strength (Fig. 38.14). Wounds can also be closed with Steri-Strips, a sterile tape applied along both sides of a wound to keep the edges closed (Fig. 38.15).

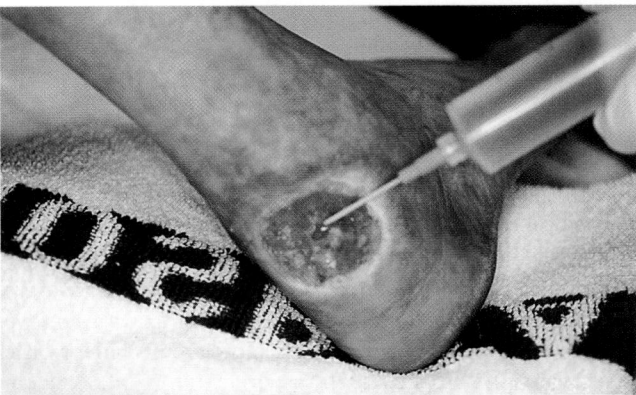

FIG 38.13 Wound irrigation using 35-mL syringe to facilitate removal of necrotic tissue.

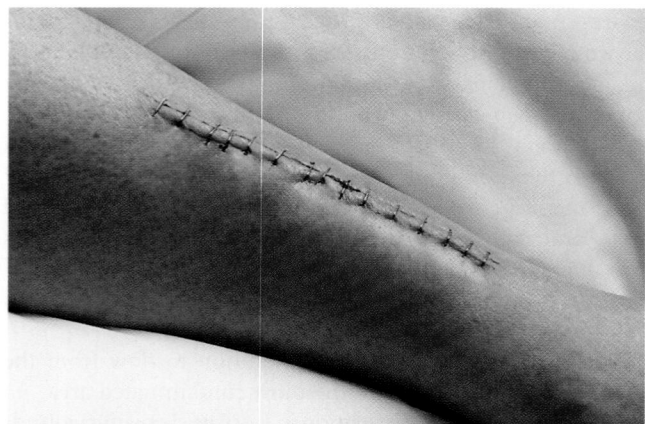

FIG 38.14 Wound closed with staples.

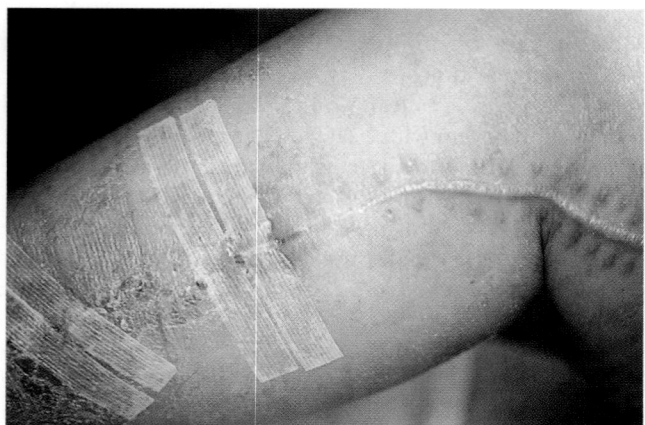

FIG 38.15 Steri-Strips placed over incision for closure.

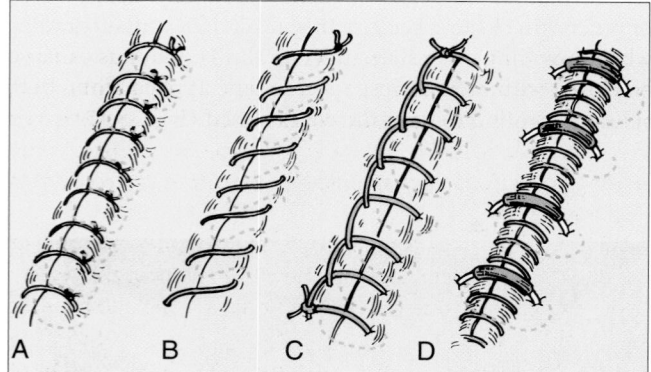

FIG 38.16 Examples of suturing methods. **A,** Intermittent. **B,** Continuous. **C,** Blanket continuous. **D,** Retention.

Be familiar with the types of suture methods (Fig. 38.16). Policies vary among institutions as to who removes sutures. If you remove sutures, a health care provider's order is necessary.

Drainage Evacuation. When drainage interferes with healing, drainage evacuation is achieved by using a drain or

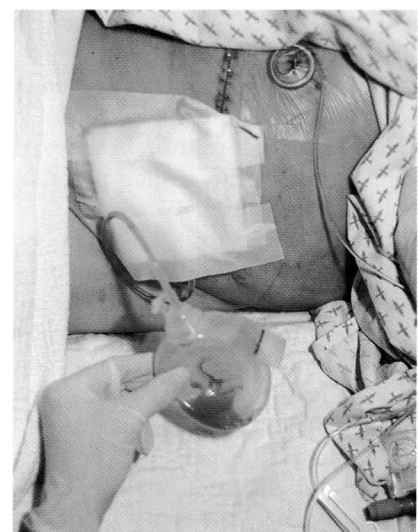

FIG 38.17 Jackson-Pratt drain and reservoir.

a drainage tube with continuous suction. Drainage evacuators are convenient, portable units that connect to tubular drains within a wound bed and exert a safe, constant, low-pressure vacuum to remove and collect drainage (Fig. 38.17). Ensure that suction is exerted and that all connection points between the evacuator and tubing are intact. The evacuator collects drainage that is assessed for volume and character. When the evacuator fills, measure output by emptying the contents into a graduated cylinder and immediately reset the evacuator to apply suction.

Bandages and Binders. A simple gauze dressing is often not enough to immobilize or provide support to a wound. Bandages and binders applied over or around dressings provide extra protection and therapeutic benefits by creating pressure over a body part, immobilizing a body part, supporting a wound, reducing or preventing edema, securing a splint, or securing dressings.

Dressings are available in rolls of various widths and materials including gauze, elasticized knit, and elastic webbing. Gauze dressings are lightweight, mold easily around contours of the body, and permit air circulation to underlying skin to prevent maceration. Elastic dressings conform well to body parts but are also used to exert pressure over a body part.

Principles for Application of Bandages and Binders. Correctly applied dressings and binders do not cause injury to underlying or nearby body parts or create discomfort for the patient. Before applying a dressing or binder, perform the following steps:

1. Inspect the surrounding skin for abrasions, edema, discoloration, or exposed wound edges.
2. Inspect the condition of underlying dressings and change if soiled.
3. Cover exposed wounds or open abrasions with a sterile dressing.
4. Assess the skin of underlying body parts that are distal to the dressing for signs of circulatory impairment

TABLE 38.5 PRINCIPLES FOR BANDAGE AND BINDER APPLICATION

PRINCIPLE	RATIONALE
Position body part you will be dressing in comfortable position of normal anatomical alignment.	Dressings cause restriction in movement. Immobilization in normal functioning position reduces risks of deformity or injury.
Prevent friction between and against skin surfaces by applying gauze or cotton padding.	Skin surfaces in contact with one another (e.g., between toes, under breasts) rub against one another to cause abrasion or chafing. Dressings over bony prominences rub against skin to cause breakdown.
Apply dressings securely to prevent slippage during movement.	Friction between dressing and skin causes skin breakdown.
When bandaging extremities, apply dressing first at distal end and progress toward trunk.	Gradual application of pressure from distal toward proximal portion of extremity promotes venous return and minimizes risk for edema or circulatory impairment.
Apply dressings firmly, with equal tension exerted over each turn or layer. Avoid excessive overlapping of dressing layers.	Equal tension prevents unequal pressure distribution over dressing body part. Localized pressure causes circulatory impairment.
Position pins, knots, or ties away from wound or sensitive skin areas.	Pins and ties used to secure dressings and binders exert localized pressure and irritation.

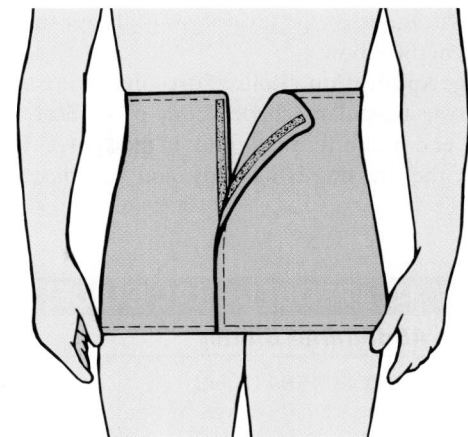

FIG 38.18 Abdominal binder secured with Velcro.

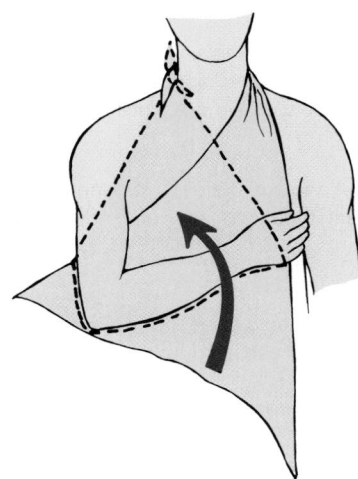

FIG 38.19 Application of a sling.

(coolness, pallor or cyanosis, diminished or absent pulses, swelling, numbness, and tingling) to provide a means for comparing changes in circulation after dressing application.

Table 38.5 outlines the principles of dressing and binder application. After you apply a dressing, assess, document, and immediately report any changes in circulation, comfort level, body function such as ventilation, and skin integrity. Explain to the patient that any dressing or binder will feel relatively firm or tight; assess the dressing carefully to be sure that it is applied properly and is providing therapeutic benefit, readjust it as necessary, and replace dressings when they become soiled. Seek an order before loosening or removing a dressing applied by a health care provider.

Binder Application. Binders are especially designed for the body part to be supported. The most common types of binders are an abdominal binder and sling (Box 38.13).

Abdominal Binder. An abdominal binder supports large incisions that are vulnerable to stress when the patient moves or coughs. It is a rectangular piece of cotton or elasticized material with many tails attached to the two longer sides or long extensions on each side to surround the abdomen (Fig. 38.18).

Slings. Slings support arms with muscular sprains or fractures. Commercially made slings have a long sleeve that extends to the elbow and a strap that fits around the neck. In the home patients can use a large triangular piece of cloth as a sling. The patient sits or lies supine for a sling application (Fig. 38.19). Instruct the patient to bend the affected arm, bringing the forearm straight across the chest. The open sling fits under the patient's arm and over the chest, with the base of the triangle under the wrist and the point of the triangle at the elbow. One end of the sling fits around the back of the neck. Bring the other end up over the affected arm while supporting the extremity. Tie the two ends at the side of the neck so that the knot does not press against the cervical spine. You can fold the loose fold at the elbow evenly around the elbow and pin it. To prevent the formation of dependent edema, make sure that the lower arm is always supported at a level above the elbow.

Bandage Application. Rolls of dressing secure or support dressings over irregularly shaped body parts. Each roll has a free outer end and a terminal end at the center. The rolled portion of the dressing is its body, and you place its outer surface against the patient's skin or dressing. Box 38.14 describes essential points when applying an elastic bandage.

Heat and Cold Therapy. Locally applying heat and cold to an injured body part provides therapeutic benefits. However, before using these therapies, understand normal body responses to local temperature variations, assess the integrity

---

BOX 38.13 PROCEDURAL GUIDELINES

Applying Abdominal Binder

DELEGATION CONSIDERATIONS

The skill of applying a binder can be delegated to nursing assistive personnel (NAP). A nurse assesses the condition of any incision, the skin, and the patient's ability to breathe before binder application. The nurse directs the NAP about:
- How to modify the skill such as special wrapping or manner of securing the binder.
- Reporting patient's complaint of pain, numbness, tingling, or difficulty breathing after applying abdominal binder or any changes in patient's skin color or temperature.

EQUIPMENT

Clean gloves if wound drainage present, gauze bandage as needed, correct type and size of binder, closures for cloth binder

STEPS

1. Identify patient using at least two identifiers (e.g., name and birthday or name and account number) according to agency policy.
2. Review medical record for order for binder (check agency policy).
3. Determine patient's level of comfort using a scale of 0 to 10. Administer prescribed analgesic 30 minutes before dressing change.
4. Gather necessary data regarding size of patient and appropriate binder to use (see manufacturer guidelines) to ensure proper fit.
5. Observe patient who needs support of thorax or abdomen; observe patient's ability to breathe deeply, cough effectively, and turn or move independently.
6. Perform hand hygiene and inspect skin for actual or potential alterations in integrity. Observe for irritation, abrasion, and skin surfaces that rub against one another.
7. Inspect any surgical dressing for intactness, presence of drainage, and coverage of incision. Change any soiled dressing before applying binder (using clean gloves). Remove gloves and perform hand hygiene.
8. Determine patient's knowledge of purpose of binder.
9. Close curtains or room door.
10. Perform hand hygiene and apply clean gloves (if likely to contact wound drainage).
11. Apply abdominal binder:
    a. Position patient in supine position with head slightly elevated and knees slightly flexed.
    b. Help patient roll on side away from you toward raised side rail while firmly supporting abdominal incision and dressing with hands. Fanfold far side of binder toward midline of binder.

c. Place binder flat on bed, right side up.
d. Place fan folded ends of binder under patient.
e. Instruct patient or help him or her roll over folded binder. For obese patients consider asking nurse colleague to assist.
f. Unfold and stretch ends out smoothly on far side of bed. Then stretch out ends on near side of bed.
g. Instruct patient to roll back into supine position.
h. Adjust binder so that supine patient is centered over binder, using symphysis pubis and costal margins as lower and upper landmarks.
i. If patient is very thin, pad iliac prominences with gauze bandage.
j. Close binder. Pull one end of binder over center of patient's abdomen. While maintaining tension on that end of binder, pull opposite end of binder over center and secure with Velcro closure tabs or metal fasteners. Provides continuous wound support and comfort.

Clinical Decision Point. After binder is in place, assess patient's ability to breathe deeply and cough effectively. When applied correctly, an abdominal binder over midline abdominal incisions has no effect on the patient's pulmonary function.

---

12. Assess patient's comfort level and adjust binder as necessary.
13. Remove gloves and perform hand hygiene.
14. Ask patient to rate pain on scale of 0 to 10.
15. Remove binder and surgical dressing to assess skin and wound characteristics at least every 8 hours.
    a. Evaluate patient's ability to ventilate properly including deep breathing and coughing every 4 hours to determine presence of impaired ventilation and potential pulmonary complications.
    b. Record baseline and post-binder condition of skin, circulation, integrity of underlying dressing, and patient's comfort level. Also record type of bandage applied.
    c. Report any complications (e.g., pain, skin irritation, impaired ventilation) to nurse in charge.
16. **Use Teach-Back:** "I want to be sure I explained your abdominal binder correctly. Describe how you will change your dressing using the binder at home." Revise your instruction now or develop a plan for revised patient/family caregiver teaching if patient/family caregiver is not able to teach back correctly.
17. Report reduced ventilation (e.g., pulse oximetry, pulmonary function tests) to health care provider immediately.

of the body part, determine the patient's ability to sense temperature variations, and ensure proper operation of equipment. You are legally responsible for the safe administration of all heat and cold applications.

Body Responses to Heat and Cold. Exposure to heat and cold causes systemic and local responses. Systemic responses occur through heat-loss mechanisms (sweating or vasodilation) or mechanisms promoting heat conservation (vasoconstriction or piloerection) and heat production (shivering) (see Chapter 15). Local responses to heat and cold occur through stimulation of temperature-sensitive nerve endings within the skin.

BOX 38.14   PROCEDURAL GUIDELINES

Applying Elastic Bandages

DELEGATION CONSIDERATIONS

The skill of applying an elastic bandage for compression cannot be delegated to nursing assistive personnel (NAP). A nurse assesses the condition of any wound or dressing before applying a bandage. The skill of applying bandages to secure non-sterile dressings can be delegated to NAP (refer to agency policy). The nurse instructs the NAP about:

- Modifying the bandage application such as with special taping.
- Reviewing what to observe and report back to the nurse (e.g., patient's complaint of pain, numbness, or tingling after application or changes in patient's skin color or temperature).

EQUIPMENT

Correct width and number of gauze or elastic bandages, clips or adhesive tape, clean gloves if wound drainage is present, pillow (optional)

STEPS

1. Identify patient using at least two identifiers (e.g., name and birthday or name and account number) according to agency policy.
2. Review patient's medical record for specific orders related to application of gauze or elastic bandage. Note area to be covered, type of bandage required, frequency of change, and previous response to treatment.
3. Assess patient's level of comfort (pain scale of 0 to 10). Administer prescribed analgesic as needed before dressing change.
4. Perform hand hygiene Apply clean gloves if drainage or break in skin is present. Observe adequacy of circulation by palpating temperature of skin and pulses, presence of edema, and sensation (distal to area to be bandaged). Observe skin color and movement of body part to be wrapped. **Note:** Impaired circulation may result in pain, coolness to touch compared with the opposite side of the body, cyanosis or pallor of skin, diminished or absent pulses, edema or localized pooling, and numbness and/or tingling of body part.
5. Inspect skin of area to be bandaged for alterations in integrity as indicated by presence of abrasion, discoloration, or chafing. Pay close attention to areas over bony prominences.
6. Inspect the condition of any wound for appearance, size, and presence and character of drainage and be sure that it is covered with a proper dressing. If not, reapply dressing (check agency policy for type of gloves to use). Remove clean gloves and perform hand hygiene.

7. Assess for size of bandage.
   a. *Gauze or basic elastic bandage to secure a dressing:* Assess size of area to be covered. Each successive roll of gauze or elastic should overlap previous layer. Use smaller widths for upper extremities and larger widths for lower extremities.
   b. *Elastic bandage to provide simple compression:* Assess circumference of lower extremity before or shortly after patient gets out of bed in the morning or after patient has been in bed for at least 15 minutes. Select width that will cover and overlap without bulkiness.
8. Identify patient's and family caregiver's knowledge level and ability to manipulate bandage if bandaging will be continued at home.
9. Close room door or curtains. Position patient comfortably in an anatomically correct supine position in bed.
10. Perform hand hygiene and apply clean gloves if drainage is present.
11. Apply gauze or elastic bandage to secure dressings.
    a. Elevate dependent extremity for 15 minutes before applying elastic bandage to promote venous return.
    b. Make sure that primary dressing over wound is securely in place.
    c. Begin elastic bandage application at the distal body part. Hold roll of bandage in your dominant hand and use other hand to lightly hold beginning layer.
    d. Apply even tension during application and begin with two circular turns to anchor bandage. Continue to maintain even tension and transfer roll to dominant hand as you wrap bandage (see illustration).

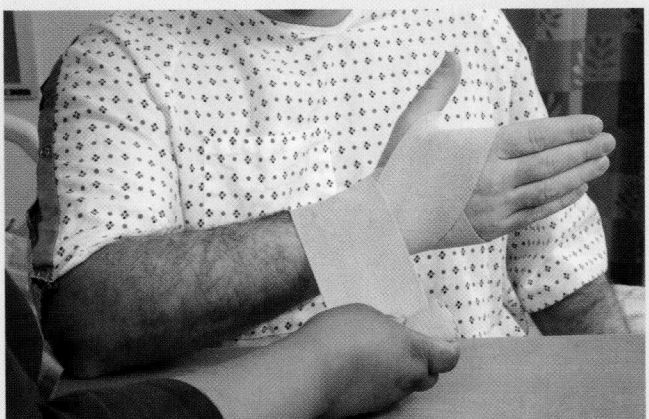

STEP 11d Hold elastic bandage in dominant hand and apply with circular turns.

Continued

BOX 38.14   PROCEDURAL GUIDELINES—cont'd

Applying Elastic Bandages

e. Apply bandage from distal point toward proximal boundary (see illustration), using appropriate turns to cover various shapes of body parts. Patients requiring elastic bandages for amputated limbs require specific bandage turns (see Step 12). Roll gauze, overlapping each layer by one-half to two-thirds the width of the bandage.

f. Double-check your tension and ensure that bandage is snug but not tight and that primary dressing or splint is positioned correctly. A tight bandage may cause numbness and tingling from impaired circulation and/or pressure on peripheral nerves.

g. While unrolling an elastic bandage, stretch bandage slightly. Explain to patient that smooth, even pressure will be applied to improve circulation, reduce swelling, immobilize body part, and provide pressure.

h. End bandage with two circular turns; secure end of gauze or elastic bandage to outside layer of bandage, not skin, with tape or clips (see illustration).

> **Clinical Decision Point. Keep toes or fingertips uncovered and visible for follow-up circulatory assessment except in cases in which toes or fingers are treated because of wounds.**

12. Apply elastic bandage over stump (see illustrations).
    a. Elevate stump with pillow or support it with the assistance of another person.
    b. Secure bandage by wrapping it twice around proximal end of stump or patient's waist (depending on size of stump). Make half turn with bandage perpendicular to its edge.

c. Bring body of bandage over distal end of stump.
d. Continue to fold bandage over stump, wrapping from distal to proximal points.
e. Secure with metal clips, Velcro if provided, or tape.

13. Remove gloves if worn and perform hand hygiene.
14. Assess degree of tightness of bandage, wrinkles, looseness, and presence of drainage.
15. Evaluate distal circulation when bandage application is complete, at least twice during next 8 hours, and then at least every shift.
    a. Observe skin color for pallor or cyanosis.
    b. Palpate skin for warmth.
    c. Palpate distal pulses and compare bilaterally.
    d. Ask patient to rate any pain on scale of 0 to 10 and to describe numbness, tingling, or other discomfort to evaluate for neurological and vascular changes.
16. Observe mobility of extremity.
17. **Use Teach-Back:** "I want to be sure I explained how to apply the elastic roll to your sprained ankle. Show me how you would apply this elastic roll to your ankle." Revise your instruction now or develop a plan for revised patient/family caregiver teaching if patient/family caregiver is not able to teach back correctly.
18. Record in electronic health record (EHR), chart, or flow sheets patient's level of comfort, circulation status, type of bandage applied, presence of swelling, and range of motion at baseline and after bandage application.
19. Report any changes in neurological or circulatory status to health care provider.

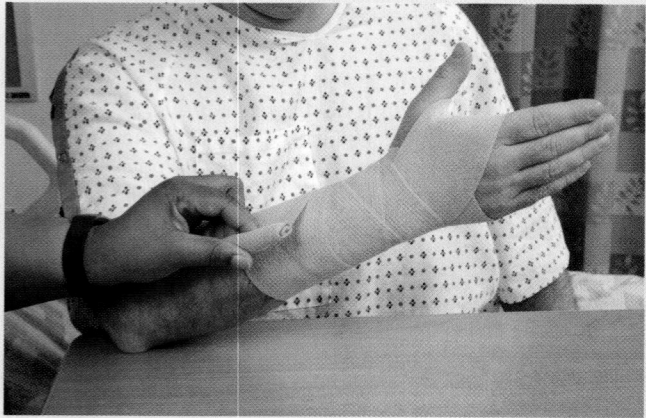

STEP 11e Apply bandage from distal to proximal.

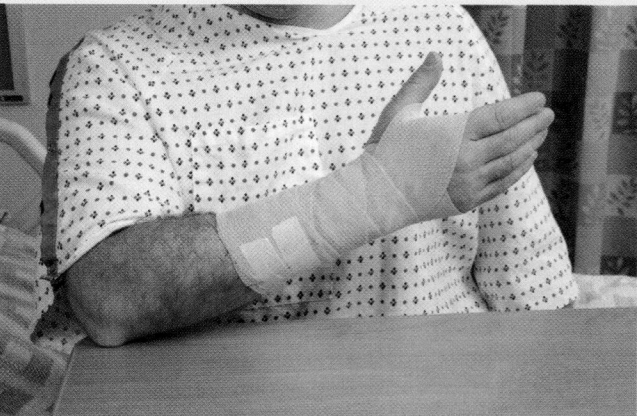

STEP 11h Secure with tape or closure device.

The adaptive ability of the body creates the major problem in protecting patients from injury resulting from temperature extremes. A person initially feels an extreme change in temperature but within a short time hardly notices the temperature variation. This phenomenon is dangerous because a person insensitive to heat and cold extremes is at risk for serious tissue injury. Recognize patients most at risk for injuries from heat and cold applications (Table 38.6).

Local Effects of Heat and Cold. Heat and cold stimuli create different physiological responses. The choice of heat or cold therapy depends on the local responses desired for wound healing (Table 38.7).

BOX 38.14 PROCEDURAL GUIDELINES—cont'd

Applying Elastic Bandages

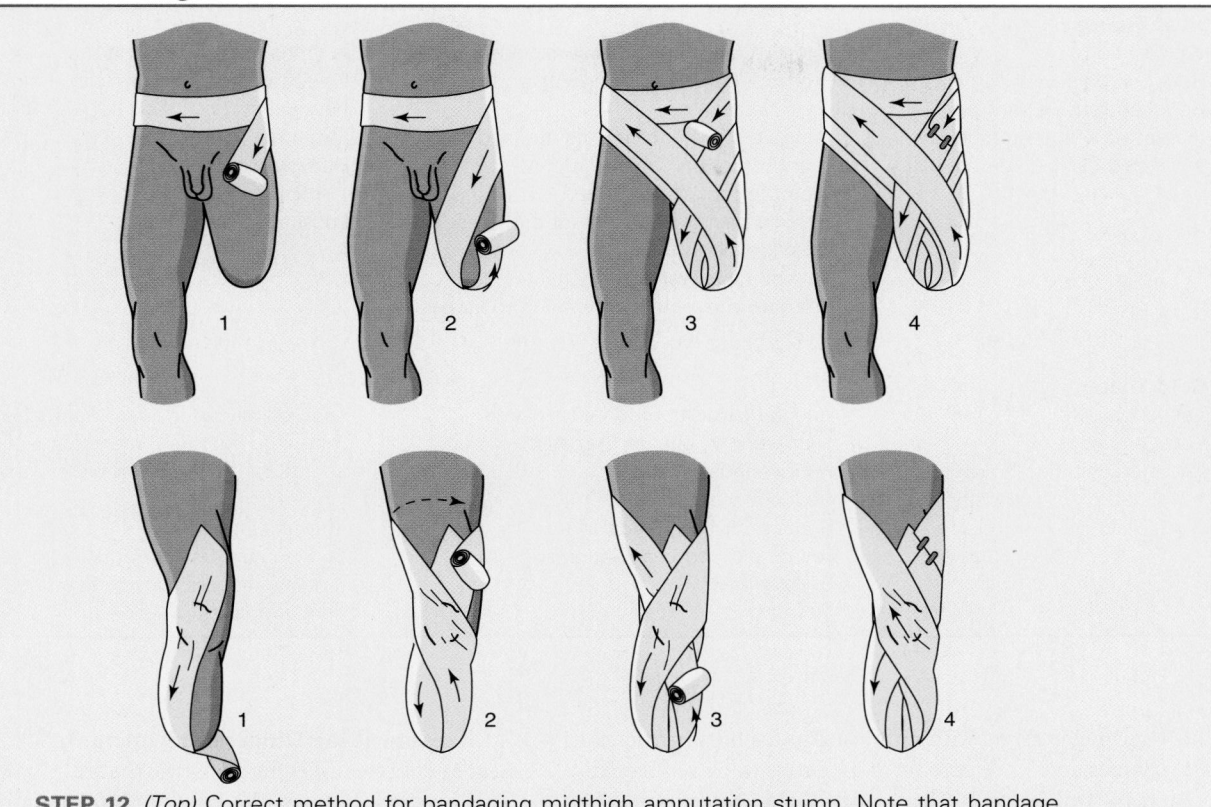

STEP 12 *(Top)* Correct method for bandaging midthigh amputation stump. Note that bandage must be anchored around patient's waist. *(Bottom)* Correct method for bandaging midcalf amputation stump. Note that bandage need not be anchored around waist. (From Monahan F, et al: *Phipps' medical-surgical nursing: health and illness perspectives,* ed 8, St Louis, 2006, Mosby.)

TABLE 38.6 CONDITIONS THAT INCREASE RISK FOR INJURY FROM HEAT AND COLD APPLICATION

CONDITION	RISK FACTORS
Very young; older adults	Thinner skin layers in children and older adults increase risk for burns; damage from cold; older adults have reduced sensitivity to pain.
Open wounds, broken skin	Subcutaneous tissue is more sensitive to temperature variations.
Areas of edema or scar formation	Scar tissue and edema have reduced sensation to temperature.
Peripheral vascular disease (e.g., diabetes, arteriosclerosis)	Body extremities are less sensitive to temperature and pain stimuli because of decreased peripheral circulation and/or local tissue injury. Cold applications further compromise blood flow.
Confusion or unconsciousness	There is reduced perception of sensory or painful stimuli. Patient may be unable to move away from or indicate discomfort from the heat or cold application.
Spinal cord injury	Alterations in nerve pathways prevent reception of sensory or painful stimuli.

Heat, especially moist heat, is generally therapeutic. However, prolonged heat application (e.g., for 1 hour or more) causes reflex vasoconstriction and reduces blood flow as the body attempts to control heat loss from the area. The periodic removal and reapplication of local heat restores vasodilation. Continuous exposure to heat damages epithelial cells, causing redness, localized tenderness, and even blistering of the skin.

Prolonged exposure of the skin to cold results in a reflex vasodilation. The inability of the cell to receive adequate blood flow and nutrients results in tissue ischemia. The skin initially takes on a reddened appearance, followed by a

TABLE 38.7   THERAPEUTIC EFFECTS OF HEAT AND COLD APPLICATIONS

PHYSIOLOGICAL RESPONSE	THERAPEUTIC BENEFIT	EXAMPLES OF CONDITIONS TREATED
Heat Therapy		
Vasodilation	Improve blood flow to injured body part	Arthritis or degenerative joint disease
Reduced blood viscosity	Promote delivery of nutrients and removal	Localized joint pain or muscle strains
Reduced muscle tension	of wastes	Low back pain
Increased tissue metabolism	Improve delivery of leukocytes and	Menstrual cramping
Increased capillary permeability	antibiotics to wound site	Hemorrhoid, perianal, and vaginal
	Promote muscle relaxation	inflammation
	Reduce pain from spasm or stiffness	Local abscesses
	Increase blood flow	
	Provide local warmth	
	Promote movement of waste products	
	and nutrients	
Cold Therapy		
Vasoconstriction	Reduce blood flow to injured site,	Immediately after direct trauma (e.g., sprains,
Local anesthesia	preventing edema formation	strains, fractures, muscle spasms)
Reduced cell metabolism	Reduce inflammation	Superficial laceration or puncture wound
Increased blood viscosity	Reduce localized pain	Minor burn
Decreased muscle tension	Reduce oxygen needs of tissues	After injections
	Promote blood coagulation at injury site	Chronic pain from arthritis, joint trauma, or
	Relieve pain	delayed-onset muscle soreness;
		inflammation

bluish-purple mottling with numbness and a burning type of pain. Tissues actually freeze from exposure to extreme cold.

Factors Influencing Heat and Cold Tolerance. The response of the body to heat and cold therapies depends on the following factors:

1. *Duration of application:* A person is better able to tolerate short exposures to heat or cold treatments.
2. *Body part:* The neck, inner aspect of the wrist and forearm, and perineal regions are more sensitive to temperature variations. The foot and the palm of the hand are less sensitive.
3. *Damage to body surface:* Exposed skin layers are more sensitive to temperature variations. Protect the skin when applying heat or cold therapies. Burns and skin injuries sustained from hot or cold therapies are serious reportable events and are preventable (National Quality Forum [NQF], 2016). Injuries from these therapies have functional applications; because they are viewed as preventable events, there is a potential that the related treatment health care costs are not reimbursable.
4. *Prior skin temperature:* The body responds best to minor temperature adjustments.
5. *Body surface area:* A person is less tolerant of temperature changes over a large area of the body.
6. *Age and physical condition:* Very young children and older adults are most sensitive to heat and cold. If a patient's physical condition reduces the reception or perception of sensory stimuli, the tolerance to temperature extremes is high, but the risk for injury is also high.

Assessment for Temperature Tolerance. Before applying heat or cold therapies, first observe the area that you will treat. This observation provides baseline information so that you can evaluate therapy-related skin changes. Alterations in skin integrity such as abrasions, open wounds, edema, bruising, bleeding, or localized areas of inflammation increase the risk for thermal injury. Identify conditions that contraindicate heat or cold therapy. *Do not* apply heat over an active area of bleeding (risk for continued bleeding) or an acute localized inflammation such as appendicitis (risk for rupture). Cold is contraindicated if the site of injury is edematous or the patient has impaired circulation or is shivering (may intensify shivering and reduce blood flow).

Assess the patient's sensory function and ability to recognize when heat or cold becomes excessive. If a patient has paralysis or peripheral vascular disease, observe circulation to the extremities. If a patient is confused or unresponsive, observe skin temperature, circulation, and integrity frequently after therapy begins. Finally assess the condition of all equipment used, checking for cracked cords, frayed wires, damaged insulation, exposed heating components, leaks, and evenness of temperature distribution.

Patient Education and Safety. Before applying heat or cold therapy, make sure that the patient and family caregiver understands its purpose, the symptoms of temperature exposure, and the precautions taken to prevent injury. Box 38.15 provides safety guidelines for applying heat and cold therapy.

Applying Heat and Cold. A prerequisite to using heat or cold application is a health care provider's order, which includes the body site to be treated and the type, frequency,

BOX 38.15 SAFETY GUIDELINES FOR APPLYING HEAT OR COLD THERAPY

- Explain the sensations that patient will feel during the procedure.
- Instruct patient and/or family caregiver to report changes in sensation or discomfort immediately.
- Provide a timer, clock, or watch so that patient can help you time the application.
- Be sure nurse call system is in an accessible location within patient's reach.
- Refer to institution policy and procedure manual for safe temperatures and duration of therapy.
- Do not allow patient to adjust temperature settings.
- Do not allow patient to move an application or place his or her hands on the wound site.
- Do not place patient in a position that prevents movement away from the temperature source.
- Do not leave patient who is unable to sense temperature changes or move from the temperature source unattended.

and duration of application. The correct temperature to use for heat and cold applications varies according to agency policy.

Choice of Moist or Dry. You administer heat and cold applications in dry or moist forms. Consider the type of wound or injury, location of the body part, and presence of drainage or inflammation when selecting dry or moist applications.

Warm Moist Compresses. A warm, moist compress improves circulation, relieves edema, and promotes concentration of pus and drainage. Moist heat is also beneficial in increasing muscle and ligament flexibility, relaxation, and healing and relieving muscle spasm and joint stiffness following the acute phase of a musculoskeletal injury (Petrofsky et al., 2013). A compress is a piece of gauze dressing moistened in a prescribed warmed solution. A pack is a larger cloth or dressing applied to a larger body area.

Heat from warm compresses evaporates quickly. To maintain a constant temperature, change the compress frequently or apply a waterproof heating pad over the compress. Because moisture conducts heat, make sure that the temperature setting of the device is lower for a moist compress than for a dry application. A layer of plastic wrap or a dry towel insulates the compress and retains heat. Moist heat promotes vasodilation and evaporation of heat from the surface of the skin. For this reason a patient feels chilly. Control drafts and keep the patient covered with a blanket or robe.

Warm Soaks. Immersion of a body part in a warmed solution promotes circulation, lessens edema, increases muscle relaxation, and allows application of medicated solution. You also administer a soak by wrapping the body part in dressings and saturating them with the warmed solution.

Position the patient comfortably, place waterproof pads under the area you plan to treat, and heat the solution to the patient's tolerance. Check the temperature by placing a small amount of solution on the inside of your forearm. Adjust the temperature if the solution is too warm or not warm enough before applying it to a patient. After immersing the body part, cover the container and extremity with a towel to reduce heat loss. It is usually necessary to remove the cooled solution and the body part and add heated solution after about 10 minutes. The challenge is to keep the solution at a constant temperature. Never add a hotter solution while the body part remains immersed. After any soak, dry the body part thoroughly to prevent maceration.

Sitz Bath. The patient who has had rectal surgery or an episiotomy during childbirth or who has painful hemorrhoids or vaginal inflammation benefits from a sitz bath, a bath in which only the pelvic area is immersed in warm fluid. The patient sits in a special tub or chair or in a basin that fits on the toilet so the legs and feet remain out of the water. Immersing the entire body causes widespread vasodilation and negates the effect of local heat to the pelvic area.

The desired temperature for a sitz bath depends on whether the purpose is to promote relaxation or clean a wound. It is often necessary to carefully add warm water during the procedure, which usually lasts 20 minutes. A disposable basin contains an attachment that resembles an enema bag and allows the gradual introduction of warmer water.

Prevent overexposure by draping bath blankets around the patient's shoulders and thighs and controlling drafts. Make sure that the patient is able to sit in the basin or tub with feet flat on the floor and without pressure on the sacrum or thighs. Because exposure of a large portion of the body to heat causes extensive vasodilation, assess the patient's pulse and facial color and ask whether he or she feels light-headed or nauseated.

Commercial Hot Packs. Commercially prepared, disposable hot packs apply warm, dry heat to an injured area. Striking, kneading, or squeezing the pack mixes chemicals that release heat. Package directions recommend the time for heat application.

Aquathermia and Dry Heat. A water-flow pad such as an aquathermia pad, electric heating pads, and commercial heat packs are common forms of dry heat therapy. A new product, an air-activated wearable heat wrap, maintains a temperature of 40° C (104° F) and can be worn 8 to 10 hours (Fig. 38.20). The aquathermia pad (water-flow pad) used in health care settings consists of a waterproof rubber or plastic pad connected by two hoses to an electrical control unit that has a heating element and motor. Distilled water circulates through hollowed channels in the pad to the control unit where water is heated (or cooled).

Hot-Water Bottles. The hot-water bottle is an economical means of applying heat to an injured body part. Many patients still use them in the home. Provide the following instructions about the safe use of water bottles:

1. Ensure that there are no leaks. Fill the bottle with warm tap water, secure the cap, and turn the bottle upside down.

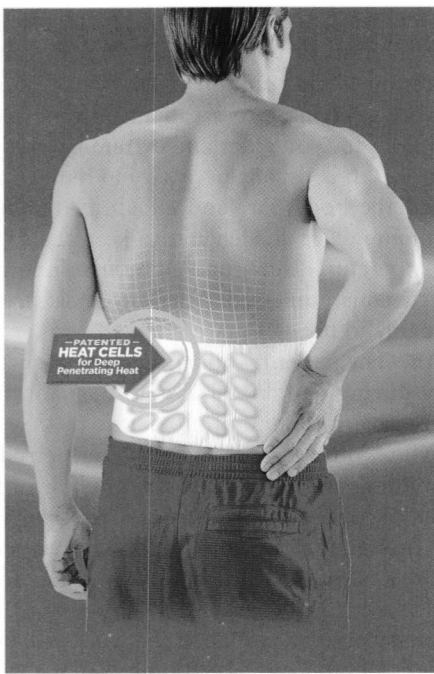

FIG 38.20 Dry heat wrap. (Image used with permission, Therma Wrap, Pfizer Consumer Healthcare. All rights reserved.)

2. Fill the bag only two-thirds full, expel air at the top, and secure the cap. The bag is then easier to mold over a body part.
3. Wipe off moisture on the outside of the bag.
4. Never apply a water bottle directly to the skin surface. Cover it with a towel or pillowcase.
5. Keep the bottle in place for 20 to 30 minutes.

Electric Heating Pads. Another conventional form of heat therapy is the heating pad, an electric coil enclosed within a waterproof pad covered with cotton or flannel cloth. The pad is connected to an electric cord that has a temperature-regulating unit for a high, medium, or low setting. Instruct patients to cover the pad with a flannel cover, towel, or pillowcase and to never apply pad directly to the skin. Remind patients to never use the high setting and to never lie on the pad. Last, advise the patient not to insert a safety pin through a heating pad to avoid electrical shock.

Cold Moist Compresses. The procedure for applying cold moist compresses is the same as that for warm compresses. Apply cold compresses for 20 minutes at a temperature of 15° C (59° F) to relieve inflammation and swelling. Compresses are clean or sterile. Observe for adverse reactions such as burning or numbness, mottling of the skin, redness, extreme paleness, or a bluish skin discoloration.

Cold Soaks. The procedure for preparing cold soaks and immersing a body part is the same as for warm soaks. The desired temperature for a 20-minute soak is 15° C (59° F). Take precautions to protect the patient from chilling.

Ice Bag or Collar. For a patient who has a muscle sprain, localized hemorrhage, or hematoma or has undergone dental surgery, an ice bag is ideal to prevent edema formation,

control bleeding, and anesthetize the body part. Use the bag correctly as follows:

1. Fill the bag with water, secure the cap, invert to check for leaks, and pour out the water.
2. Fill the bag two-thirds full with crushed ice so that it molds easily over a body part.
3. Release air from the bag by squeezing its sides before securing the cap (because excess air interferes with conduction of cold).
4. Wipe off excess moisture.
5. Cover the bag with a flannel cover, towel, or pillowcase.
6. Apply the bag to the injury site for 20 to 30 minutes; you may reapply it in an hour.

Commercial Cold Packs. Commercially prepared, single-use ice packs come in various sizes and shapes. When you squeeze or knead the pack, an alcohol-based solution is released inside to create the cold temperature. The soft outer coverings are usually safe to apply directly to the skin surface.

Restorative and Continuing Care. Some chronic wounds are the result of underlying pathological conditions that continue long after wound healing occurs. Healing for a pressure injury or a chronic wound is lengthy and requires continuity of care from the acute care setting to the restorative care setting. In this setting you use many of the principles and interventions detailed in the acute care section. Continue diligent assessment to identify patients at risk for impaired skin integrity and institute preventive measures as needed.

Despite efforts with wound care, wound healing will not occur if the patient is malnourished (see Chapter 35). Tissue repair requires more protein, carbohydrates, fats, vitamins, minerals, water, and oxygen than normal tissue metabolism (Stotts, 2016b). In addition, the delivery of nutritional substances to tissues depends on a healthy circulatory system. Malnutrition causes an insufficient supply of the necessary nutritional elements and alterations in blood vessel integrity. Work closely with registered dietitians to provide a well-balanced diet and educate patients about the importance of good dietary habits. A patient having surgery who is well nourished and has no complications requires at least 0.8 g/kg body weight of protein daily for nutritional maintenance; with injury protein needs may increase to 1.25 to 1.5 g/kg daily (National Pressure Ulcer Advisory Panel [NPUAP], European Pressure Ulcer Advisory Panel [EPUAP], and Pan Pacific Pressure Ulcer Injury Alliance [PPPIA], 2014; Stotts, 2016b). Patients weakened or debilitated by illness need supportive nutritional therapies. Supplemental tube feedings (enteral feedings) introduce nutrients directly into the gastrointestinal tract. If a patient is unable to tolerate enteral feedings, a health care provider often orders parenteral (intravenously administered) nutrition.

A patient with a wound that restricts mobility or has the potential to compromise the function of a joint sometimes requires additional physical and/or occupational therapy.

BOX 38.16 EVALUATION

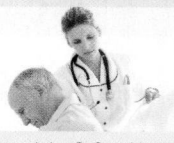

Copyright © Stockbyte/
iStock/Thinkstock.

Mr. Martinez's pressure injury is still present, but it is reduced in size and demonstrates progress toward healing. No other sites of nonblanchable erythema are noted, and the rest of his skin remains intact. He is scheduled for discharge to his home in 2 days. Lynda taught and observed Mrs. Martinez how to do the dressing changes and how to assess her husband's skin for signs of increased risk for or actual further skin breakdown. Lynda's clinical instructor also observed Mrs. Martinez perform the dressing change and agreed that the family caregiver teaching was complete and Mrs. Martinez was performing the skill correctly.

On her last day of this clinical experience, Lynda referred Mr. Martinez to a home care agency. With the help of her instructor, Lynda devised a plan of care for the home; Lynda and her instructor are meeting with the home care nurse today when she visits Mr. and Mrs. Martinez in the hospital.

DOCUMENTATION NOTE

"Small amount of serous drainage from Stage 2 pressure injury on sacrum. Wound is 1 × 1 inch × ½ inch deep, with red tissue. Mrs. Martinez cleansed wound with normal saline and applied hydrocolloid dressing. Maintained aseptic technique and correctly assessed skin. Mrs. Martinez reminds her husband to change his position every 1½ to 2 hours. Awaiting visit from home care nurse."

Work closely with a physical therapist to monitor a patient's activity and tolerance for exercise. It is important to optimize activity within a patient's physical limitations and return function as rapidly as possible.

■■■ EVALUATION

Patient Outcomes. Evaluate nursing interventions for reducing and treating pressure injuries and wound healing by determining a patient's response to nursing therapies and determining whether your patient achieved the desired goals and outcomes (Box 38.16). The primary goals are to prevent injury to the skin and tissues, reduce further injury to the skin and underlying tissues, and restore skin integrity. Evaluate specific interventions designed to promote skin integrity. Evaluate the patient and family caregiver's learning regarding prevention of pressure injuries and specific wound-healing interventions. In addition, identify and evaluate the need for additional support services for a patient and family and initiate the referral process.

Patient Expectations. Collect evaluation data about a patient's perception of wound care management. Patients with chronic wounds often receive care in their home and have certain expectations about their level of comfort, lifestyle, independence, and privacy. Determine if you respected and met your patient's expectations.

SAFETY GUIDELINES FOR NURSING SKILLS

Ensuring patient safety is an essential role of the professional nurse. To ensure patient safety, communicate clearly with members of the health care team, assess and incorporate the patient's priorities of care and preferences, and use the best evidence when making decisions about your patient's care. When performing the skills in this chapter, remember the following points to ensure safe, individualized patient care:

- When changing wound dressings, follow proper aseptic technique. Keep a plastic bag within reach to discard dressings and prevent cross-contamination. Keep extra gloves within reach in case of contamination or additional wound assessment.
- Routinely assess patients for individual risks for development of pressure injuries. Select and use a risk assessment tool; the Braden Scale is one of the most widely used and researched scales (Bryant and Nix, 2016a).
- Inspect skin at least daily or according to agency policy, and note and document all pressure points. Modify frequency of skin and wound assessment and frequency of skin care practices based on patient's risk factors and/or wound condition.
- Perform pressure injury risk assessment on all patients who have one or more risk factors when admitted to an acute care facility, home care, hospice, or extended care facility (NPUAP, EPUAP, and PPPIA, 2014; WOCN Society, 2016).
- Use approaches to minimize friction and shear. Use lift sheets when repositioning patients to reduce rubbing skin against sheets. Raise the head of the bed no more than 30 degrees (unless medically contraindicated) to prevent sliding and shear injury (WOCN Society, 2016).
- When a patient has a previous history of pressure injury or skin damage, the healed area presents a greater risk for skin breakdown than healthy, unwounded skin.
- Modify the frequency of wound assessment based on wound condition.
- Chronic diseases, especially vascular disease and diabetes, increase a patient's risk for pressure injury development and impede healing of wounds.

SKILL 38.1 ASSESSMENT OF PATIENT FOR PRESSURE INJURY: RISK AND SKIN ASSESSMENT

DELEGATION CONSIDERATIONS

The skill of pressure injury risk assessment cannot be delegated to nursing assistive personnel (NAP). The nurse instructs the NAP to:

- Report any changes to patient's skin such as redness, blistering, abrasion, or cuts to the nurse for further assessment.
- Keep patient's skin dry and provide hygiene after fecal or urinary incontinence.
- Frequently change patient's position according to patient's nursing care plan.
- Avoid trauma to patient's skin from tape, medical devices, pressure, friction, or shear. Report to the nurse any blistering, redness, or break in patient's skin.
- Report any abrasion from medical devices.

EQUIPMENT

- Risk assessment tool (use agency approved tool; see agency policy)
- Documentation record
- Pressure-redistribution mattress, bed, or chair cushion as needed
- Positioning aids
- Clean gloves

STEP	RATIONALE
ASSESSMENT	
1. Identify patient using at least two identifiers (e.g., name and birthday or name and medical record number) according to agency policy.	Ensures correct patient. Complies with The Joint Commission standards and improves patient safety (TJC, 2018).
2. Review medical record to assess patient's risk for pressure injury formation:	Determines need to administer preventive care and identifies specific factors that place patient at risk (NPUAP, EPUAP, and PPPIA, 2014).
a. Paralysis or immobilization	Patient is unable to turn or reposition independently to relieve pressure.
b. Presence of medical device such as nasogastric (NG) tube, oxygen equipment, artificial airway, drainage tubing, or mechanical devices (Doughty and McNichol, 2016)	Medical devices have the potential to exert pressure on the patient's nares or ears or on tissue adjacent to artificial airways or drainage tubes (Pittman et al., 2015).
c. Sensory loss (e.g., hemiplegia, spinal cord injury)	Patient is unable to feel discomfort from pressure and does not independently change position.
d. Circulatory disorders (e.g., peripheral vascular diseases, vascular changes from diabetes mellitus, neuropathy)	Reduce perfusion of tissue layers of skin.
e. Fever	Increases metabolic demands of tissues. Accompanying diaphoresis leaves skin moist.
f. Anemia	Decreased hemoglobin level reduces oxygen-carrying capacity of blood and amount of oxygen available to tissues.
g. Malnutrition	Inadequate nutrition leads to weight loss, muscle atrophy, and reduced tissue mass. Nutrient deficiencies result in impaired or delayed healing (Stotts, 2016b).
h. Fecal or urinary incontinence	Skin becomes exposed to moist environment that contains bacteria. Excessive moisture macerates skin (Bryant, 2016).
i. Heavy sedation and anesthesia	Patient is not mentally alert and does not turn or change position independently. Sedation alters sensory perception.
j. Age	Neonates and very young children are at high risk with the head being most common site of pressure injury occurrence (WOCN Society, 2016). There is a loss of dermal thickness in older adults, impairing ability to distribute pressure (Pieper, 2016).
k. Dehydration	Results in decreased skin elasticity and turgor.
l. Edema	Edematous tissues are less tolerant of pressure, friction, and shear.

STEP	RATIONALE
m. Existing pressure injuries	Limit surfaces available for position changes, placing available tissues at increased risk.
n. History of pressure injury	Tensile strength of skin from previously healed pressure injury is 80% or less; therefore this area cannot tolerate pressure as much as undamaged skin (Doughty and Sparks, 2016).
3. Select agency-approved risk assessment tool such as the Braden Scale or Norton Scale. Perform risk assessment when patient enters health care agency and repeat on regularly scheduled basis or when there is a significant change in patient's condition (WOCN Society, 2016).	Valid and reliable risk assessment tools evaluate patient's risk for developing a pressure injury (WOCN Society, 2016). Identifying risk factors that contribute to potential for skin breakdown allows you to target specific interventions for decreasing risk for skin breakdown.
4. Review assessment tool and levels of risk scores.	Risk cutoff score depends on instrument used. The score involves identifying risk factors that contributed to it and minimizing those specific deficits (Ayello and Braden, 2002; Ayello, 2012).
5. Perform hand hygiene. Assess condition of patient's skin over regions of pressure (see Fig. 38.11). Apply gloves as needed with open and/or draining wounds. Also assess tissue adjacent to medical devices, drainage tubes, and artificial airways.	Body weight against bony prominences places underlying skin at risk for breakdown. Medical devices exert pressure directly on the skin or underlying tissue (Black et al., 2010, 2015).
a. Inspect for skin discoloration (redness in light-toned skin; purplish or bluish in darkly pigmented skin) and tissue consistency (firm or boggy feel) and/or palpate for abnormal sensations (Nix, 2016).	Indicates that tissue is under pressure; hyperemia is a normal physiological response to hypoxemia in tissues.
b. Palpate discolored area on skin and under and around medical devices, release your fingertip, and look for blanching.	If on palpation an area of redness blanches (lightens in color), this indicates normal reactive hyperemia; the tissue is not at risk for skin breakdown. Tissue that does not blanch when palpated indicates abnormal reactive hyperemia, an indication of possible ischemic injury.
c. Inspect for pallor and mottling.	Persistent hypoxia in tissues that were under pressure; an abnormal physiological response.
d. Inspect for absence of superficial skin layers.	Represents early pressure injury formation, usually a partial-thickness wound that may have resulted from friction and/or shear.
e. Inspect for localized heat, edema, or induration, especially in individuals with darkly pigmented skin.	Localized heat, edema, and induration have been identified as warning signs for pressure injury development. As it is not always possible to see signs of redness on darkly pigmented skin, these additional signs should be considered in assessment (NPUAP, EPUAP, and PPPIA, 2014).
6. Assess skin around and beneath medical devices every nursing shift for additional areas of potential pressure injury caused by medical devices (Table 38.8) (Black et al., 2015).	Patients at high risk have multiple sites for pressure necrosis from medical devices in areas other than bony prominences (Coyer et al., 2014; Makic, 2015). Pressure points around medical devices (e.g., nares, oxygen cannula and masks, drainage tubing) can cause pressure injury to underlying tissue, which can become full-thickness pressure injuries (Black et al., 2015; Pittman et al., 2015; Stechmiller et al., 2016).
a. Nares: NG tube, oxygen cannula	Pressure to nares occurs from tape and other materials used to secure NG tube. Patients' ears and tips of nares are at risk for pressure from nasal cannula (Black et al., 2015; Schallom et al., 2015).
b. Tongue and lips: oral airway, endotracheal (ET) tube	Pressure results from artificial airway and materials used to secure airway (Black et al., 2015).
c. Ears: oxygen cannula, pillow	
d. Drainage or other tubing	Stress and pressure against tissue at exit site or from tubing lying under any part of patient's body (Black et al., 2015).

SKILL 38.1 ASSESSMENT OF PATIENT FOR PRESSURE INJURY: RISK AND SKIN ASSESSMENT—cont'd

View Video!

TABLE 38.8 STRATEGIES TO PREVENT MEDICAL AND IMMOBILIZATION DEVICE–RELATED PRESSURE INJURY

DEVICE	PRESSURE AREAS	PREVENTION STRATEGIES[a]
Nasogastric tubes	Nares Skin on nasal bridge	Secure tube using pressure-relieving techniques, which direct pressure from tube away from nares (see Chapters 35 and 37). Reposition tube.
Endotracheal tubes	Lips Tongue	Remove securing device daily and inspect for pressure injury (Branson et al., 2014). Rotate tube every shift or more often.
Nasotracheal tube	Nose/nasal bridge Nares	Remove securing device daily and inspect for pressure injury (Branson et al., 2014). Reposition.
Tracheostomy tubes	Front of neck and stoma site Back of neck	Remove securing device daily. Increase stoma care. Apply dressing to back of neck.
Oxygen cannula and tubing	Ears Nose	Apply dressing to external ear. Periodically remove cannula to relieve pressure and inspect for pressure injury (Schallom et al., 2015).
NIPPV/BiPAP	Forehead Nose/nasal bridge	Pretreat bridge of nose with dressing before application of mask. If possible remove mask for a few minutes.
Drainage tubing	Area immediately next to drainage tube Adjacent area during patient position changes	Apply appropriate dressing around drainage tube. Check tubing placement with each position change. Instruct patient not to lie on tubing (Pittman et al., 2015).
Indwelling catheter	Thighs Female: urethra, labia Male: tip of penis	Provide meticulous perineal care. Anchor and secure catheter to reduce pressure.
Orthopedic devices	All areas where device comes in contact with patient's skin and tissues	When possible and not contraindicated inspect under device.
Neck collar	Neck and occipital region Scalp	Remove hard collar as soon as possible and replace with softer collar (Black et al., 2015). Inspect scalp daily.
Compression stockings	Calf Behind knee Heel Toes	Verify proper fit. To reduce pressure and risk of injury to skin and underlying tissues remove stockings twice daily for at least 1 hour (Black et al., 2015).
Immobilization devices	Wrists Ankles	Apply dressing between patient's skin and immobilizer (Black et al., 2015). Verify space between immobilizer and patient's skin. With assistive personnel present remove restraint one at a time to inspect skin.

BiPAP, Bi-level positive airway pressure; *NIPPV*, noninvasive positive pressure ventilation.
[a]In addition to routine inspection and cleansing of skin under and around medical device.

STEP	RATIONALE
e. Wound drainage	Wound drainage increases risk for skin breakdown because it is caustic to skin and underlying tissues. Tubing from drainage devices (e.g., Jackson-Pratt, Hemovac) causes pressure under device and on adjacent skin (Black et al., 2015).

STEP	RATIONALE
f. Indwelling urethral (Foley) catheter	For female patients the catheter can put pressure on the labia, especially when edematous. For male patients pressure from a catheter not properly anchored can put pressure on the tip of the penis and urethra (Black et al., 2015).
g. Orthopedic and positioning devices such as casts, neck collars, or splints	Applied devices have the potential to cause pressure to underlying and adjacent skin and tissue (Black et al., 2015).
h. Compression stockings.	Compression stockings have the potential to cause pressure, especially if they are poorly fitting or rolled down (Black et al., 2015).
i. Immobilization device and restraints	If device is too tight or poorly placed or patient strains, pressure points occur under device.
7. Remove and dispose of gloves and perform hand hygiene.	Reduces transmission of organisms.
8. Observe patient for preferred positions when in bed or chair.	Preferred positions result in weight of body being placed on certain bony prominences. Presence of contractures may result in pressure exerted in unexpected places.
9. Observe ability of patient to initiate and help with position changes.	Potential for friction and shear increases when patient is completely dependent on others for position changes.
10. Assess patient and family caregiver understanding of risks for development of pressure injuries.	Determines baseline knowledge for pressure injury risk and identifies areas for patient teaching.

PLANNING

1. Provide privacy and prepare bedside environment for patient safety.	Providing privacy and preparing environment before the procedure helps to ensure a clean and distraction-free area for organizing procedure-related equipment.
2. Prepare and organize equipment. Be sure you have correct risk assessment tool at patient's bedside.	Facilitates smooth completion of assessment.
3. Explain procedure and purpose to patient and family caregiver.	Relieves anxiety and provides opportunity for education.

IMPLEMENTATION

1. Implement prevention guidelines adapted from *Guideline for Prevention and Management of Pressure Ulcers* (WOCN Society, 2016).	Reduces patient's risk for developing a pressure injury.
2. Perform hand hygiene and apply clean gloves if patient has open, draining wounds.	Use of standard precautions prevents accidental exposure to body fluids.
3. Inspect skin at least once a day.	
a. Observe patient's skin; pay particular attention to bony prominences and areas around and under medical devices and tubes. If you find a reddened area, gently press the area with a gloved finger to check for blanching. If the area does not blanch, suspect tissue injury and recheck in 1 hour. Discoloration may vary from pink to a deep red.	Monitoring the skin on a routine basis provides a "watch" for changes that deviate from baseline data (Nix, 2016). Persistent redness when lightly pigmented skin is pressed can indicate tissue injury. If an area of redness blanches (lightens in color), this indicates that skin is not at risk for breakdown.

Clinical Decision Point. Do not massage reddened areas because doing so may cause additional tissue trauma. Reddened areas indicate blood vessel damage, and massaging can further damage the vessel (Bryant and Nix, 2016a).

b. If patient has darkly pigmented skin, look for color changes that differ from patient's normal skin color such as red, blue, or purple tones.	Darkly pigmented skin may not blanch. Although the skin may not show direct changes in color, the color may differ from the surrounding area (see Box 38.4) (NPUAP, EPUAP, and PPPIA, 2014).
4. Each shift, check all treatment and assistive devices (e.g., catheters, feeding tubes, casts, braces) for potential pressure points (see Table 38.8). Remove gloves and perform hand hygiene.	Pressure from these devices increases the risk on bony prominences and other areas.
a. Verify that device is correctly sized, positioned, and secured.	Incorrect size, placement, and securing of a medical device can cause excessive pressure and rubbing by the device on the underlying skin (Makic, 2015).

SKILL 38.1   ASSESSMENT OF PATIENT FOR PRESSURE INJURY: RISK AND SKIN ASSESSMENT—cont'd

STEP	RATIONALE
b. Consider shielding the underlying at-risk skin with protective dressing (silicone, hydrocolloid).	These dressings absorb moisture from the body and reduce pressure to the underlying skin (Black et al., 2015; Makic, 2015).

Clinical Decision Point. Inspect skin around and beneath orthopedic devices (e.g., cervical collar, braces, cast). Note any abrasions or warmth in areas where devices can rub against the skin (Pittman et al., 2015; Schallom et al., 2015).

STEP	RATIONALE
5. Review patient's pressure injury risk assessment score.	Risk scores aid in identifying interventions to lessen or eliminate present risk factors.
6. If immobility, inactivity, or poor sensory perception is a risk factor for patient, consider one of the following interventions:	Immobility and inactivity reduce patient's ability or desire to independently change position. Poor sensory perception decreases patient's ability to feel the sensation of pressure or discomfort.
a. Reposition patient on a scheduled basis, and frequently assess the skin condition to help to identify early signs of pressure damage. If skin changes occur, reevaluate plan.	Reduces duration and intensity of pressure. Some patients may require more frequent repositioning (NPUAP, EPUAP, and PPPIA, 2014).
b. When patient is in side-lying position in bed, use 30-degree lateral position (see illustration). Avoid a 90-degree lateral position.	Reduces direct contact of trochanter with support surface.
c. When needed use pillow bridging (see illustration).	Use of pillows prevents direct contact between bony prominences.

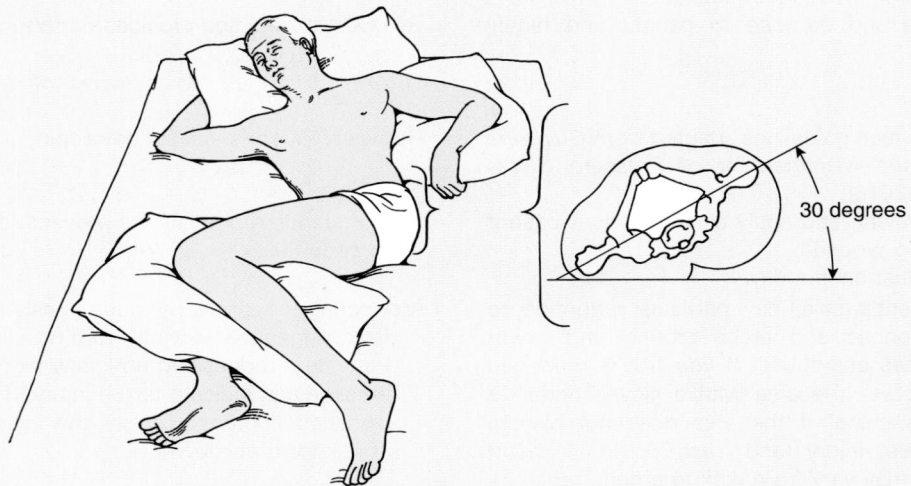

STEP 6b Thirty-degree lateral position with pillow placement.

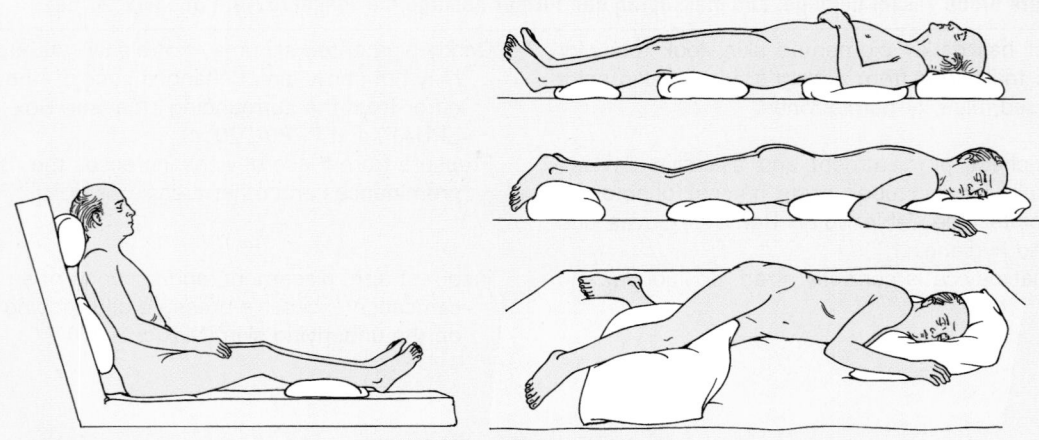

STEP 6c Pillow bridging.

STEP	RATIONALE
d. Place patient (when lying in bed) on a pressure redistribution surface.	Reduces amount of pressure exerted on tissues.
e. Place patient (when in a chair) on a pressure redistribution device and shift the points under pressure at least every hour (WOCN Society, 2016).	Reduces amount of pressure on sacral and ischial areas.
7. If friction and shear are identified as risk factors, consider the following interventions:	Friction and shear damage underlying skin.
a. Use two nurses and a pull sheet to reposition patient. Use a slide board to transfer patient from bed to stretcher.	Proper repositioning of patient prevents dragging along the sheets. Slide board provides slippery surface to reduce friction.
b. Ensure that heels are free from the surface of the bed by using a pillow under the calves to elevate the heels or use a heel suspension device; knees should be in 5- to 10-degree flexion (Baath et al., 2016; WOCN Society, 2016).	"Floating" the heels from the bed surface offload the heel completely and redistribute the weight of the leg along the calf without applying pressure on the Achilles tendon (Baath et al., 2016).
c. Maintain head of bed at 30 degrees or lower or at lowest elevation consistent with patient's condition (do not lower head of bed if patient is at risk for aspiration) (WOCN Society, 2016).	Decreases potential for patient to slide toward foot of bed and incur shear injury.
8. If patient receives a low score on a moisture subscale, consider one of the following interventions:	Continual exposure of body fluids on patient's skin increases risk for skin breakdown and pressure injury development.
a. Apply clean gloves. Clean and dry the skin after each incontinent episode. Apply moisture-barrier ointment to perineum and surrounding skin after each incontinent episode (WOCN Society, 2016).	Protects the skin from fecal or urinary incontinence.
b. If skin is denuded, use a protective barrier paste after each incontinent episode.	Provides a barrier between the skin and stool and/or urine, allowing for healing.
c. If moisture source is from wound drainage, consider frequent dressing changes, protective barriers for skin, or collection devices.	Frequent exposure of skin to wound drainage is avoided.
9. If friction and shear are risk factors and patient is chair bound:	Relief of pressure by changing from lying to sitting position is insufficient if sitting is prolonged. The maximum amount of time a patient can sit before there is a need to reposition is unknown (WOCN Society, 2016).
a. Perform hand hygiene and apply clean gloves as needed. Tilt patient's chair seat to prevent sliding forward, and support arms, legs, and feet to maintain proper posture (NPUAP, EPUAP, & PPPIA, 2014).	
b. Limit amount of time patient spends in a chair without pressure relief (NPUAP, EPUAP, & PPPIA, 2014).	
c. For patients who can reposition themselves while sitting, encourage pressure relief every 15 minutes using chair push-ups, forward lean, or side to side (WOCN Society, 2016).	
10. Remove gloves and discard in appropriate receptacle. Perform hand hygiene.	Reduces transmission of microorganisms.
11. Educate patient and family caregiver regarding pressure injury risk and prevention (WOCN Society, 2016).	Assists in adhering to interventions to reduce pressure injury risk.

EVALUATION

1. Observe patient's skin for areas at risk for tissue damage, noting change in color, appearance, or texture.	Enables you to evaluate success of prevention techniques.
2. Observe tolerance of patient for position change by measuring level of comfort on a pain scale.	Position changes sometimes interfere with patient's sleep and rest pattern.
3. Compare subsequent risk assessment scores and skin assessments.	Provides ongoing comparison of patient's risk level to facilitate appropriateness of plan of care.

View Video!

SKILL 38.1 ASSESSMENT OF PATIENT FOR PRESSURE INJURY: RISK AND SKIN ASSESSMENT—cont'd

STEP	RATIONALE
4. **Use Teach-Back:** "I want you to understand why we need to assess your skin on an ongoing basis. Tell me why we will be checking your skin on a regular basis." Revise your instruction now or develop a plan for revised patient/family caregiver teaching if patient/family caregiver is not able to teach back correctly.	Determines patient's/family caregiver's level of understanding of instructional topic.

RECORDING AND REPORTING

- Record in nurses' notes in electronic health record (EHR), chart, or flow sheets any skin changes, patient's risk score, and skin assessment. Describe positions, turning intervals, pressure-redistribution devices, and other prevention measures. Note patient's response to interventions.

- Document your evaluation of patient/family caregiver understanding of need for frequent skin and pressure injury assessment.
- Report need for additional consultations for high-risk patient to health care provider.

UNEXPECTED OUTCOMES AND RELATED INTERVENTIONS

- Skin becomes mottled, reddened, purplish, or bluish.
  - Refer patient to wound, ostomy, and continence nurse (WOCN); registered dietitian; clinical nurse specialist (CNS); nurse practitioner (NP), or physical therapist as necessary. Reevaluate position changes and bed surface.

- Areas under pressure develop persistent discoloration, induration, or temperature changes.
  - Refer patient to WOCN; registered dietitian; CNS; NP; or physical therapist as necessary.
  - Modify patient's positioning and turning schedule.

SKILL 38.2 TREATING PRESSURE INJURIES

DELEGATION CONSIDERATIONS

The skill of treatment of pressure injuries and dressing changes cannot be delegated to nursing assistive personnel (NAP). The nurse instructs the NAP to:
- Report immediately to the nurse pain, fever, or any wound drainage.
- Report immediately to the nurse any change in skin integrity.
- Report any potential contamination to existing dressing (e.g., patient incontinence, dislodgment of dressing).

EQUIPMENT
- Protective equipment: clean gloves, goggles, cover gown (if splash is a risk)
- Clean gloves

- Sterile gloves *(optional)*
- Plastic bag for dressing disposal
- Measuring device
- Sterile cotton-tipped applicators (check agency policy for use of sterile applicators)
- Topical agent (as ordered)
- Cleansing agent (as ordered)
- Sterile solution container
- Dressing of choice based on patient wound characteristics
- Hypoallergenic tape (if needed)
- Documentation records
- Scale for assessing wound healing
- Washbasin

STEP	RATIONALE
ASSESSMENT	
1. Identify patient using at least two identifiers (e.g., name and birthday or name and medical record number) according to agency policy.	Ensures correct patient. Complies with The Joint Commission standards and improves patient safety (TJC, 2018).
2. Review accuracy of health provider's order for topical agent and/or dressing.	Ensures administration of proper medication and treatment.

Clinical Decision Point. Determine if order is consistent with established wound care guidelines and outcomes for a patient. If order is not consistent with guidelines or varies from the identified outcome for a patient, review with health care team.

3. Determine if patient has allergies to topical agents.	Topical agents could contain ingredients that cause localized skin reactions.

STEP	RATIONALE
4. Assess for factors affecting wound healing: poor perfusion, immunosuppression, or preexisting infection.	Factors will affect treatment and wound healing.
5. Assess patient's nutrition status. Clinically significant malnutrition is present if (1) serum albumin level is less than 3.5 g/dL, (2) lymphocyte count is less than 1800/mm^3, or (3) body weight decreases more than 15% (see illustration) (WOCN Society, 2016).	Delayed wound healing occurs in patients with poor nutrition status.

Clinical Decision Point. When you suspect malnutrition, consider a nutrition consultation to modify patient's diet to promote wound healing.

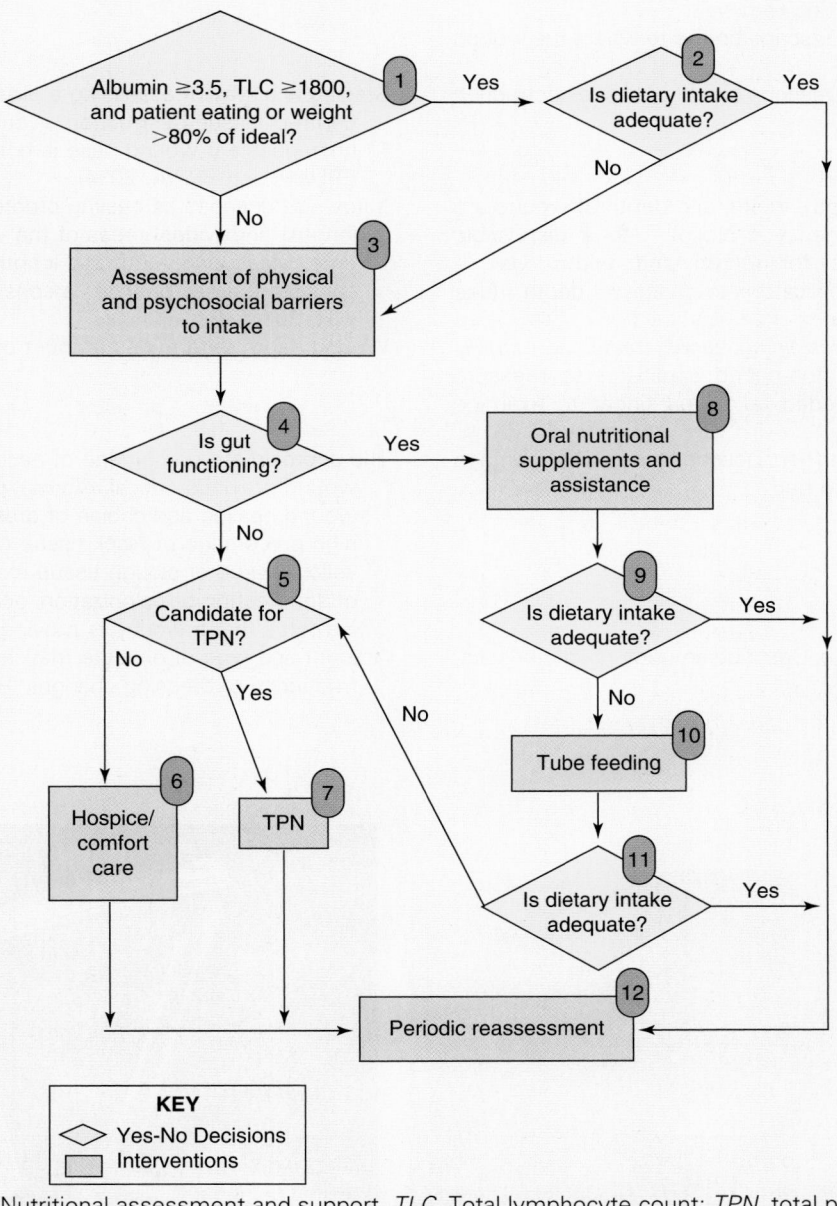

STEP 5 Nutritional assessment and support. *TLC*, Total lymphocyte count; *TPN*, total parenteral nutrition. (From Bergstrom N, et al: *Treatment of pressure ulcers*, AHCPR Pub. No. 95-0652, Rockville, MD, 1994, Agency for Health Care Policy and Research, Public Health Service, U.S. Department of Health and Human Services.)

SKILL 38.2   TREATING PRESSURE INJURIES—cont'd

STEP	RATIONALE
6. Assess patient's level of comfort on a pain scale of 0 to 10. If patient is in pain, determine if a prn pain medication has been ordered and administer.	Dressing change should not be a traumatic event for patient; evaluate wound pain before, during, and after wound care management (Hopf et al., 2016).
7. Close room door or bedside curtains.	Provides privacy.
8. Position patient to allow dressing removal and position plastic bag for dressing disposal.	Provides accessible area for dressing change. Proper disposal of old dressing promotes proper handling of contaminated waste.
9. Perform hand hygiene and apply clean gloves. Remove and discard old dressing.	Reduces transmission of microorganisms and prevents accidental exposure to body fluids.
10. Assess patient's wounds using wound parameters, and continue ongoing wound assessment per agency policy. **Note:** This wound assessment may be done during procedure after dressing removal.	Determines effectiveness of wound care and guides treatment plan of care (WOCN Society, 2016).
a. *Wound location:* Describe body site where the wound is located.	
b. *Stage of wound:* Describe extent of tissue destruction (see Fig. 38.2).	Staging is a way of assessing a pressure injury based on depth of tissue destruction. Wounds are documented as unstageable if wound base is not visible (NPUAP, EPUAP, and PPPIA, 2014).
c. *Wound size:* Length, width, and depth of wound are measured per agency protocol. Use a disposable measuring guide for length and width. Use a cotton-tipped applicator to assess depth (see illustrations).	Injury size changes as healing progresses; therefore the longest and widest areas of the wound change over time. Measuring width and length by measuring consistent areas provides a consistent measurement (Nix, 2016).
d. *Presence of undermining, sinus tracts, or tunnels:* Use a sterile cotton-tipped applicator to measure depth and, if needed, a gloved finger to examine wound edges.	Wound depth determines amount of tissue loss.
e. *Condition of wound bed:* Describe type and percentage of tissue in wound bed.	The approximate percentage of each type of tissue in the wound provides critical information on the progress of wound healing and choice of dressing. A wound with a high percentage of black tissue requires debridement, yellow tissue or slough tissue may indicate the presence of an infection or colonization, and granulation tissue indicates that a wound is moving toward healing.
f. *Volume of exudate:* Describe amount, characteristics, odor, and color.	Amount and type of exudate may indicate type and frequency of dressing changes (Bryant and Nix, 2016b).

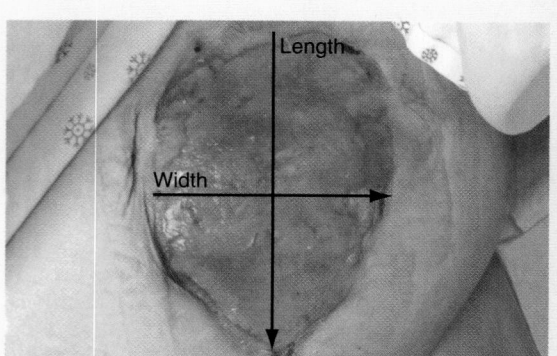
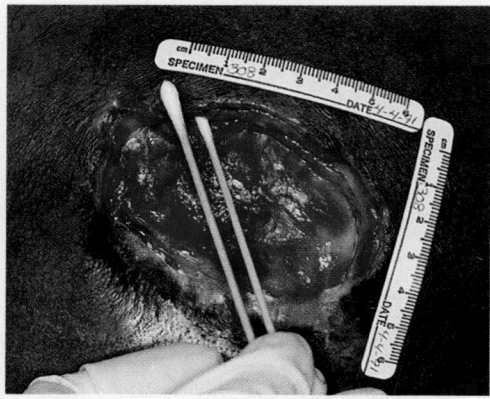

STEP 10c Measuring wound width, length, and undermining of skin. (Left image from Bryant RA, Nix DP, editors: *Acute and chronic wounds: current management concepts,* ed 5, St Louis, 2016, Elsevier.)

STEP	RATIONALE
g. *Condition of periwound skin:* Examine the skin for breaks; dryness; and the presence of a rash, swelling, redness, or warmth. Modify assessment based on patient's skin color (see Box 38.4).	Impaired skin condition at the edge of an injury indicates progressive tissue damage. Maceration on periwound skin shows a need to alter the choice of wound dressing.
h. *Wound edges:* Examine edges for rolled edges, signs of moisture-associated skin damage, redness.	Provides information regarding epithelialization, chronicity, and etiology.
11. Assess periwound skin; check for maceration, redness, denuded tissue.	Determines if skin barrier is needed to protect periwound area.
12. Remove gloves, discard appropriately, and perform hand hygiene.	Reduces transmission of microorganisms. Repeated hand hygiene is needed as you assess other pressure areas. Different organisms contaminate different wounds.
13. Assess patient's and family caregiver's understanding of prevention, treatment, and factors contributing to recurrence of pressure injuries (WOCN Society, 2016).	Patient and caregiver need to partner with health care providers to prevent further skin breakdown.

PLANNING

STEP	RATIONALE
1. Provide privacy and prepare bedside environment for patient safety.	Providing privacy and preparing the environment before the procedure helps to ensure a clean and distraction-free area for organizing procedure-related equipment.
2. Prepare and organize the following necessary equipment and supplies:	
a. Wash basin, warm water, equipment, and supplies	
b. Normal saline or other wound-cleansing agent in sterile solution container	Clean wound surface before applying topical agents and new dressing.

Clinical Decision Point. Use only noncytotoxic agents to clean wounds.

STEP	RATIONALE
c. Prescribed topical agent:	
(1) Enzyme debriding agents (follow specific manufacturer directions for frequency of application) *Or*	Enzymes debride dead tissue to clean wound surface. Enzymes are not applied to healthy tissue.
(2) Topical antibiotics	Topical antibiotics decrease bioburden of wound and should be considered for a 2-week course of treatment for nonhealing wounds (WOCN Society, 2016).
d. Prepare appropriate dressing based on stage of pressure injury, wound characteristics, principles of wound management, health care provider orders, and patient care setting (see Table 38.4). Dressing options include:	Dressing should maintain moist environment for wound while keeping surrounding skin dry (Bryant and Nix, 2016b).
(1) Gauze. Apply as a moist dressing, a dry cover dressing when using enzymes or topical antibiotics, or as a means to deliver solution to a wound.	Gauze delivers moisture to a wound and is absorptive.
(2) Transparent film dressing. Apply over superficial wounds with minimal or no exudate and skin subjected to friction.	Maintains a moist environment and offers intact skin protection.
(3) Hydrocolloid dressing	Maintains moist environment to facilitate wound healing while protecting wound base.
(4) Hydrogel—available in a sheet or in tube	Maintains moist environment to facilitate wound healing.
(5) Calcium alginate	Highly absorbent of wound exudate in heavily draining wounds.
(6) Foam dressings	Protective and prevents wound dehydration; also absorbs moderate-to-large amounts of drainage.
(7) Silver-impregnated dressings/gels	Controls bacterial burden in wound.
(8) Wound fillers	Fills shallow wounds, hydrates, and absorbs.
e. Obtain hypoallergenic tape or adhesive dressing sheet.	Used to secure nonadherent dressing. Prevents skin irritation and tearing.
3. Explain procedure to patient and family caregiver. Individualize teaching plan for older adults, considering normal aging changes that affect learning.	Preparatory explanations relieve anxiety, correct any misconceptions about the wound and treatment, and offer an opportunity for patient and family education.

SKILL 38.2 TREATING PRESSURE INJURIES—cont'd

STEP	RATIONALE
IMPLEMENTATION	
1. Perform hand hygiene and apply clean gloves. Open sterile packages and topical solution containers. Keep dressings sterile. Wear goggles, mask, and moisture-proof cover gown if potential for contamination from spray exists when cleaning wound.	Reduces transmission of microorganisms.
2. Lower side rails and position patient.	
3. Remove bed linen and arrange patient's gown to expose wound and surrounding skin. Keep remaining body parts draped.	Prevents unnecessary exposure of body parts.
4. Clean wound thoroughly with normal saline or prescribed wound-cleansing agent from least contaminated to most contaminated area. For deep wounds clean with an irrigating syringe, as ordered. Remove gloves and discard.	Cleansing wound removes wound exudate and/or dressing residue and reduces surface bacteria.
5. Perform hand hygiene and apply clean or sterile gloves.	Maintains aseptic technique during cleaning, measuring, and applying dressings. With some chronic wounds clean versus sterile gloves are appropriate (WOCN Society, 2011). Refer to agency policy regarding use of clean or sterile gloves.
6. Apply topical agents to wound using cotton-tipped applicators or gauze as ordered:	
a. Enzymes	Follow manufacturer directions for method and frequency of application. Be aware of which solutions inactivate enzymes and avoid their use in wound cleaning.
(1) Apply small amount of enzyme debridement ointment directly to necrotic areas in pressure wound. *Do not apply enzyme to surrounding skin.*	Thin layer absorbs and acts more effectively than a thick layer. Excess medication irritates surrounding skin (Bryant and Nix, 2016b). Proper distribution of ointment ensures effective action.

Clinical Decision Point. If using an enzymatic debriding agent, do not use wound-cleansing agents with metals.

STEP	RATIONALE
(2) Place moist gauze dressing directly over wound and tape in place. Follow specific manufacturer recommendation for type of dressing material to use to cover a pressure injury when using enzymes. Tape dressing in place.	Protects wound and prevents removal of ointment during turning or repositioning.
b. Antibacterials (examples include bacitracin, metronidazole, and silver sulfadiazine)	Reduces bacterial growth.
7. Apply prescribed wound dressing:	
a. Hydrogel	Hydrogel dressings are designed to hydrate and donate moisture to the wound (Bryant and Nix, 2016b).
(1) Cover surface of wound with thick layer of the amorphous hydrogel, or cut a sheet to fit wound base.	Provides moist environment to facilitate wound healing.
(2) Apply secondary dressing such as dry gauze; tape in place.	Holds hydrogel against wound surface because amorphous hydrogel (in tube) or sheet form does not adhere to wound and requires a secondary dressing to hold it in place.
(3) If using impregnated gauze, pack loosely into wound; cover with secondary gauze dressing and tape.	A loosely packed dressing delivers the gel to the wound base and allows any wound debris to be trapped in the gauze.
b. Calcium alginate	Alginate dressings absorb serous fluid or exudate forming a nonadhesive hydrophilic gel that conforms to the shape of the wound (Bryant and Nix, 2016b). Use in heavily draining wounds.
(1) Lightly pack wound with alginate using sterile cotton-tipped applicator or gloved finger.	The dressing swells and increases in size; tight packing can compromise blood flow to the tissues.
(2) Apply a secondary dressing and tape in place.	

STEP	RATIONALE
c. Transparent film dressing, hydrocolloid, and foam dressings	

Clinical Decision Point. Use transparent dressings for autolytic debridement of noninfected superficial pressure injuries. Use a hydrocolloid to protect skin from friction. Some brands have custom shapes available for specific anatomical parts such as heels, elbows, and sacrum.

STEP	RATIONALE
8. Reposition patient comfortably off pressure injury.	Prevents pressure to injury.
9. Remove gloves and dispose of soiled supplies. Perform hand hygiene.	Reduces transmission of microorganisms.

EVALUATION

STEP	RATIONALE
1. Observe skin surrounding injury for inflammation, edema, and tenderness.	Determines progress of wound healing.
2. Inspect dressings and exposed wounds observing for drainage, foul odor, and tissue necrosis. Monitor patient for signs and symptoms of infection: fever and elevated white blood cell (WBC) count.	Wounds can become infected.
3. Compare subsequent wound measurements using one of the scales designed to measure wound healing such as Pressure Ulcer Scale for Healing (PUSH) Tool or Bates-Jensen Wound Assessment Tool (BWAT).	Use one scale consistently, as this allows for comparison of serial measurements to evaluate wound healing. Use of a standard scale provides a method for consistent data collection to document wound progress or lack thereof.
4. **Use Teach-Back:** "I want to be sure that you understand why we will examine your pressure injury on an ongoing basis. Tell me why we measure your wound and examine the tissue surrounding the wound at each dressing change." Revise your instruction now or develop a plan for revised patient/family caregiver teaching if patient/family caregiver is not able to teach back correctly	Determines patient's/family caregiver's level of understanding of instructional topic.

RECORDING AND REPORTING

- Record in nurses' notes in electronic health record (EHR) or chart type of wound tissue present, wound measurements, periwound skin condition, character of drainage or exudate, type of topical agent used, and dressing applied. Note patient's response to dressing change.
- Document your evaluation of patient and family caregiver understanding for frequent observation and measuring of wound.
- Report any deterioration in wound appearance to nurse in charge or health care provider.

UNEXPECTED OUTCOMES

- Skin surrounding wound becomes macerated.
  - Reduce exposure of surrounding skin to topical agents and moisture.
  - Select a dressing that has increased moisture-absorbing capacity.
- Wound becomes deeper with increased drainage and/or development of necrotic tissue.
  - Review current wound care management.
  - Consult with multidisciplinary team regarding changes in wound care regimen.
  - Obtain wound cultures.
- Pressure injury extends beyond original margins.
  - Monitor for systemic signs and symptoms of poor wound healing such as abnormal laboratory results (WBC count, levels of hemoglobin/hematocrit, serum albumin, serum prealbumin, total proteins), weight loss, and fluid imbalances.
  - Assess and revise current turning schedule.
  - Consider further pressure-redistribution devices.

SKILL 38.3 NEGATIVE-PRESSURE WOUND THERAPY

DELEGATION CONSIDERATIONS

The skill of negative-pressure wound therapy (NPWT) cannot be delegated to nursing assistive personnel (NAP). The nurse directs the NAP to:

- Use caution in positioning or turning patient to avoid tubing displacement.
- Report any change in dressing shape or integrity to the nurse.
- Report any change in patient's temperature or comfort level to the nurse.
- Report any wound fluid leakage around the edges of the adhesive drape.

EQUIPMENT

- NPWT unit (requires health care provider's order). For this skill the vacuum-assisted closure (V.A.C.) unit is used for illustration; several other systems are available, and their applications may differ (see manufacturer instructions).
- NPWT dressing (gauze or foam [see manufacturer recommendations], transparent dressing, adhesive drape)
- NPWT suction device
- Tubing for connection between NPWT unit and NPWT dressing
- Three pairs of gloves, clean and sterile
- Scissors, sterile
- Waterproof biohazard bag for disposal
- Skin preparation, skin barrier protectant, hydrocolloid dressing, skin barrier
- Moist washcloths
- Linen bag
- Protective equipment: gown, mask, goggles (used when splashing from wound is a risk)

STEP	RATIONALE
ASSESSMENT	
1. Identify patient using at least two identifiers (e.g., name and birthday or name and medical record number) according to agency policy.	Ensures correct patient. Complies with The Joint Commission standards and improves patient safety (TJC, 2018).
2. Review health care provider's orders for frequency of dressing change, amount of negative pressure, type of foam or gauze to use, and pressure cycle (intermittent or continuous).	Determines frequency of dressing change, negative pressure setting, and special instructions. Health care provider's order is also necessary for reimbursement.
3. Review electronic health record (EHR) for signs and symptoms related to condition of patient's wound.	Provides baseline to compare your findings with previous dressing change assessments and reflects wound-healing progress.
a. Assess patient's level of comfort on a pain scale of 0 to 10.	Serves as baseline to measure response to dressing therapy.
b. Administer prescribed analgesic as needed 30 minutes before dressing change.	A comfortable patient will be less likely to move suddenly, causing wound or supply contamination.
4. Perform hand hygiene and apply clean gloves. Assess location, appearance, and size of wound. Remove and dispose of gloves. Perform hand hygiene.	Provides information regarding status of wound healing, presence of complications, and proper type of supplies and assistance needed.
5. Assess patient's and family caregiver's knowledge of purpose of dressing and whether they will participate in dressing wound.	Identifies patient's learning needs. Prepares patient and family if dressing will need to be changed at home.
PLANNING	
1. Provide privacy and prepare bedside environment for patient safety.	Providing privacy and preparing the environment before the procedure helps to ensure a clean and distraction-free area for organizing procedure-related equipment.
2. Prepare and organize equipment.	Organizes procedure.
a. Verify that suction tubing is intact and suction device is working properly.	Ensures that when the nurse has prepared the wound for negative pressure, the equipment is in working order. This further increases wound care efficiency.
3. Explain procedure to patient and family caregiver.	Relieves anxiety and promotes understanding of healing process.
IMPLEMENTATION	
1. Perform hand hygiene and put on clean gloves. If risk for spray exists, don protective gown, goggles, and mask.	Reduces transmission of infectious organisms from soiled dressings to nurse's hands.
2. Position patient comfortably and drape to expose only wound site. Instruct patient not to touch wound or sterile supplies.	Promotes patient's cooperation and smooth completion of procedure. Prevents contamination of sterile supplies.

STEP	RATIONALE
3. Cuff top of disposable waterproof biohazard bag and place within reach of work area.	Cuff prevents accidental contamination of top of outer bag.
4. Follow manufacturer directions for removal and replacement of wound filler and dressing.	Each NPWT unit varies slightly with wound fillers, dressing, and reattachment of suction. Knowing your agency's specific NPWT directions facilitates a smooth dressing change.
a. Turn off NPWT unit by pushing therapy on/off button.	Deactivates therapy and allows for proper drainage of fluid in drainage tubing.
b. Keeping tube connectors attached to NPWT unit, raise tubing connectors; disconnect tubes from one another, and drain fluids into drainage collector.	Prevents backflow of any drainage in tubing back into wound.
c. Before lowering, tighten clamp on canister tube, and disconnect canister and dressing tubing at connection points.	Prevents drainage from exiting tubing when removed.
5. Remove transparent film by gently stretching transparent film and slowly pull away from skin.	Prevents injury to wound tissue. Protects periwound skin breakdown from transparent adhesive.
6. Remove old dressing one layer at a time and discard in bag. Observe drainage on dressing. Use caution to avoid tension on any drains that are present.	Determines type and amount of dressings needed for replacement. Prevents accidental removal of drains.
7. Perform wound assessment. Observe surface area and tissue type, color, odor, and drainage within wound. Measure length, width, and depth of wound as ordered.	Determines condition of wound and need for replacement of dressing. Measurement of wound is necessary to assess wound healing progression and justify continuation of NPWT for third-party payers (Netsch et al., 2016).

Clinical Decision Point. This is a time when a wound care nurse or physician might debride the wound. Debridement of eschar or slough, if present, should be performed for removal of devitalized tissue to prepare wound bed (Netsch et al., 2016).

STEP	RATIONALE
8. Remove and discard gloves in waterproof bag. Avoid having patient see old dressing because sight of wound drainage may be upsetting. Perform hand hygiene.	Reduces transmission of microorganisms. Lessens patient anxiety during procedure.
9. Clean wound.	Irrigation removes wound debris and cleans wound bed.
a. Apply sterile or clean gloves depending on agency policy and wound status.	Cleaning periwound is essential for an airtight seal. With some chronic wounds clean versus sterile gloves are appropriate (WOCN Society, 2011).
b. If ordered, irrigate wound with normal saline or other solution ordered by health care provider (see Skill 38.5). Gently blot periwound with gauze to dry thoroughly.	

Clinical Decision Point. Health care providers may order wound cultures routinely. However, when drainage looks purulent or has a foul odor or if there is a change in amount or color, obtain wound culture. This may be an indication that the wound may need to be treated for an infection and the NPWT may need to be discontinued (Netsch et al., 2016).

STEP	RATIONALE
10. Apply skin protectant, barrier film, solid skin barrier sheet, or hydrocolloid dressing to periwound skin.	Maintains airtight seal needed for NPWT. Protects periwound skin from moisture-associated skin damage.
11. Fill any uneven skin surfaces (e.g., creases, scars, skin folds) with skin barrier product (e.g., paste, strip).	Further helps to maintain airtight seal (Netsch et al., 2016).
12. Remove and discard gloves. Perform hand hygiene.	Prevents transmission of microorganisms.
13. Depending on type of wound, apply sterile or new clean gloves (see agency policy).	Fresh sterile wounds require sterile gloves. Chronic wounds require clean technique (WOCN Society, 2011).

SKILL 38.3   NEGATIVE-PRESSURE WOUND THERAPY—cont'd

STEP	RATIONALE
14. Apply NPWT.	
a. Prepare NPWT filler dressing. Consult with wound care expert for appropriate type.	Filler dressing depends on NPWT used and can include foam or gauze dressings with or without antimicrobials such as silver. The type of dressing may be adjusted based on undermining, tunneling, or sinus tracts present (Netsch et al., 2016).
(1) Measure wound and select appropriate size dressing.	Establishes baseline for wound size. Black polyurethane foam has larger pores and is most effective in stimulating granulation tissue and wound contraction. White soft foam is denser with smaller pores and is used when the growth of granulation tissue needs to be restricted (Netsch et al., 2016).
(2) Using sterile scissors, cut filler dressing foam to wound size, making sure to fit exact size and shape of wound including tunnels and undermined areas.	Proper size of foam dressing maintains negative pressure to entire wound (Netsch et al., 2016).

Clinical Decision Point. In some instances an antimicrobial product such as silver-impregnated gauze or topical antibiotic is order. These products help reduce the bioburden of the wound.

STEP	RATIONALE
b. Place filler dressing in wound following manufacturer instructions. Be sure filler dressing is in contact with entire wound base, margins, and tunneled and undermined areas. Count number of filler dressings, and document in patient's chart.	Maintains negative pressure to entire wound. Edges of foam dressing must be in direct contact with patient's skin. Dressing count provides nurse who removes dressing with number of filler dressings that should be removed.
c. Place suction device per manufacturer instructions.	
d. Apply NPWT transparent dressing over foam wound dressing.	
(1) Trim dressing so that it will cover wound and extend onto periwound skin approximately 2.5 to 5 cm (1 to 2 inches).	Prepares dressing of appropriate size for wound.
(2) Apply transparent dressing, keeping it wrinkle-free (see illustration).	Ensures that wound is properly covered and negative-pressure seal can be achieved. Dressing should be airtight with no tunnels or gaps to ensure a good seal when suction is activated.
(3) Secure tubing to transparent film, aligning drainage holes to ensure occlusive seal. Do not apply tension.	Excessive tension may compress foam dressing and impede wound healing. It also produces pressure and/or shear force on periwound area (Netsch et al., 2016).
(4) Secure tubing several centimeters away from dressing, avoiding pressure points.	Drainage tubes over bony pressure prominences can cause medical device–related pressure injuries (Pittman et al., 2015; Netsch et al., 2016).

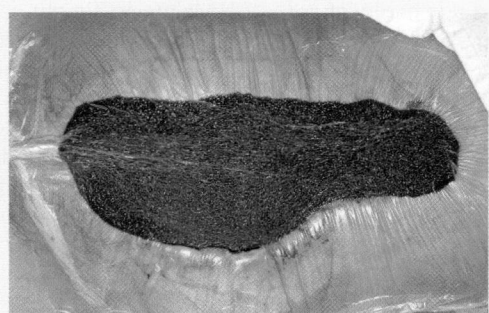

STEP 14d(2) Foam wound filler, transparent dressing over existing wound. (Courtesy KCI Licensing, San Antonio, TX.)

STEP	RATIONALE
15. After wound is completely covered, connect tubing from dressing to tubing from canister and NPWT unit and set at ordered suction level.	Continuous therapy delivered at 125 mm Hg is most routinely used; lower levels of pressure (75 to 80 mm Hg) can be used to reduce pain without compromising effectiveness (Netsch et al., 2016).
a. Remove canister from sterile packing and push unit until you hear a click. **Note:** An alarm sounds if canister is not properly engaged.	
b. Connect dressing tubing to canister tubing. Make sure that both clamps are open.	Facilitates suctioning needed for NPWT.
c. Place on level surface or hang from foot of bed. **Note:** Will deactivate therapy.	Unit alarms and deactivates therapy if it is tilted beyond 45 degrees.
d. Press power button (commonly this is a green-lit button) and set pressure as ordered.	Activates system.
16. Inspect NPWT system.	
a. Verify that system is on. This is different for each type of NPWT unit. For example, on some units the display screen shows "Therapy On." Check agency policy and procedure for specific information.	
b. Verify that all clamps are open and all tubing is patent.	
c. Examine the system to be sure that seal is intact and therapy is working.	Negative pressure is achieved when a tight seal is present (Netsch et al., 2016).
d. If a leak is present, use strips of transparent film to patch areas around edges of wound.	
17. Record initials and date and time on new dressing.	Provides reference for next dressing change.
18. Help patient to comfortable position.	Enhances patient comfort and relaxation.

Clinical Decision Point. Unless patient's diagnosis contraindicates activity, patients may ambulate with NPWT. Ambulation will improve patient's exercise tolerance and muscle strength.

STEP	RATIONALE
19. Discard gloves, dispose of any dressing material, and perform hand hygiene.	Prevents transmission of microorganisms.

EVALUATION

1. Inspect condition of wound on ongoing basis. Use agency wound-healing scale noting wound size, drainage, and odor.	Documents progression of wound healing.
2. Ask patient to rate pain using scale of 0 to 10.	Determines patient's level of comfort after procedure.
3. Verify airtight dressing seal and correct negative-pressure setting.	Determines effective negative pressure being applied.
4. Measure wound drainage output in canister on regular basis.	Monitors fluid balance and wound drainage.
5. **Use Teach-Back:** "I want to be sure I explained clearly how to place the filler dressing into the wound before you are discharged. Show me how to place the filler dressings into your wound." Revise your instruction now or develop a plan for revised patient/family caregiver teaching if patient/family caregiver is not able to teach back correctly.	Determines patient's/family caregiver's level of understanding of instructional topic.

SKILL 38.3 NEGATIVE-PRESSURE WOUND THERAPY—cont'd

UNEXPECTED OUTCOMES AND RELATED INTERVENTIONS

- Wound appears inflamed and tender, drainage has increased, and odor is present.
  - Notify health care provider.
  - Obtain wound culture.
  - Increase frequency of dressing changes.
- Patient reports increase in pain.
  - Patient may need more analgesia.
  - Instill normal saline to moisten foam and other filler dressings to allow them to loosen from granulation tissue.

- If using black foam, switch to polyvinyl alcohol white soft foam.
  - Decrease pressure setting.
  - Change from intermittent to continuous cycling.
  - Change type of NPWT system.
- Patient or family caregiver is unable to perform dressing change.
  - Provide additional teaching and support.
  - Obtain services of home care agency.

RECORDING AND REPORTING

- Record in nurses' notes in electronic health record (EHR), chart, or flow sheets appearance of wound, characteristics of drainage, placement of NPWT (type of dressing, pressure mode and setting), and patient response to dressing change.

- Document your evaluation of patient/family caregiver learning.
- Report brisk bright red bleeding, evidence of poor wound healing, evisceration or dehiscence, and possible wound infection to health care provider immediately.

SKILL 38.4 APPLYING DRESSINGS: DRY, DAMP-TO-DRY, AND TRANSPARENT

DELEGATION CONSIDERATIONS

The skill of applying dry, damp to-dry, and transparent dressings may sometimes be delegated to nursing assistive personnel (NAP) if the wound is chronic (see agency policy and Nurse Practice Act). The nurse is responsible for wound assessments, care of acute new wounds, wound care requiring sterile technique, and evaluation of wound healing. The nurse directs the NAP about:

- Any unique modifications of the dressing change such as the need for use of special tape or taping techniques to secure the dressing.
- Reporting pain, fever, bleeding, change in wound color, or wound drainage to the nurse immediately.

EQUIPMENT

- Clean gloves
- Sterile gloves *(optional)*
- Sterile dressing set (scissors, forceps) *(optional*; check agency policy)

- Sterile drape *(optional)*
- Sterile dressings: 4 × 4–inch gauze, abdominal pads
- Sterile basin *(optional)*
- Antiseptic ointment (as prescribed)
- Wound cleanser (as prescribed)
- Sterile normal saline or prescribed solution
- Debriding gel as ordered
- Tape, Montgomery ties, or hydrocolloid dressing as needed (include nonallergenic tape if necessary)
- Skin barrier *(optional* if using Montgomery ties)
- Protective waterproof underpad
- Biohazard bag
- Adhesive remover *(optional)*
- Measurement devices *(optional)*: cotton-tipped applicator, measuring guide, camera
- Personal protective equipment (PPE): gown, goggles, mask as needed
- Additional lighting if needed (e.g., flashlight, treatment light)

STEP	RATIONALE
ASSESSMENT	
1. Identify patient using at least two identifiers (e.g., name and birthday or name and account number) according to agency policy.	Ensures correct patient. Complies with The Joint Commission standards and improves patient safety (TJC, 2018).
2. Review accuracy of health care providers' orders for type of dressing.	Indicates dressing supplies needed.
3. Review previous nurses' notes and electronic health record (EHR).	Helps to plan for proper dressing type, securement, and supplies needed and if assistance is needed during dressing procedure.
4. Assess patient for allergies, especially antiseptics, tape, or latex, and acquire specific orders for dressing change.	Reduces risk for localized or systemic allergic reactions to these supplies.

STEP	RATIONALE
5. Ask patient to rate his or her level of pain using a pain scale of 0 to 10 and assess character of pain. Administer prescribed analgesic as needed 30 minutes before dressing change.	Superficial wounds with multiple exposed nerves may be intensely painful, whereas deeper wounds with destruction of dermis should be less painful (Krasner, 2016). A comfortable patient is less likely to move suddenly, causing wound or supply contamination. Serves as baseline to measure response to dressing therapy.
6. Identify patients with risks for wound-healing problems including aging, premature infant, obesity, diabetes mellitus, circulation disorders, nutrition deficit, immunosuppression, radiation therapy, high levels of stress, and use of steroids.	Physiological changes resulting from aging, chronic illness, poor nutrition, medications that affect wound healing, and cancer treatments have potential to affect wound healing (Doughty and Sparks, 2016).
7. Assess patient's and family caregiver's knowledge of purpose of dressing change and readiness and willingness of patient or family caregiver to participate in dressing wound.	Determines level of support and explanation required. Identifies teaching needs to prepare patient or family caregiver to provide dressing changes at home.
PLANNING	
1. Provide privacy and prepare bedside environment for patient safety.	Providing privacy and preparing the environment before the procedure helps to ensure a clean and distraction-free area for organizing procedure-related equipment.
2. Prepare and organize equipment.	
a. Place disposable biohazard bag within reach of work area (see illustration).	Ensures easy disposal of soiled dressings.
b. Prepare dressing materials.	Provides for smooth organized dressing change.
3. Explain procedure to patient and family caregiver including type of dressing and frequency of dressing change.	Decreases patient's and family caregiver's anxiety.

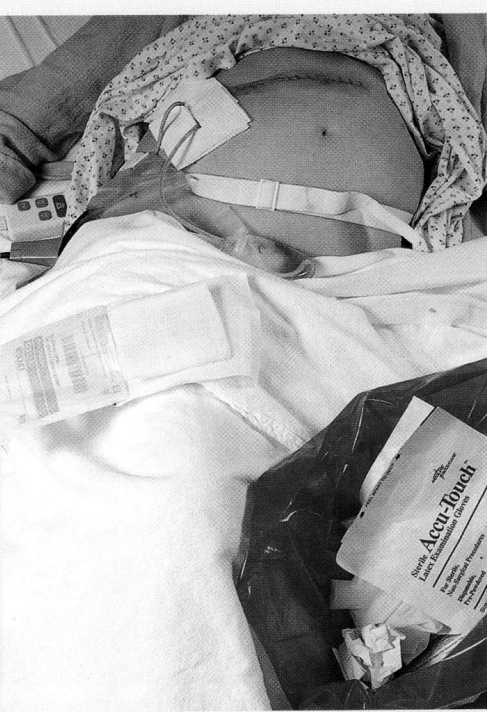

STEP 2a Disposable waterproof bag placed near dressing site.

SKILL 38.4 APPLYING DRESSINGS: DRY, DAMP-TO-DRY, AND TRANSPARENT—cont'd

STEP	RATIONALE

IMPLEMENTATION

1. Perform hand hygiene and apply clean gloves. Apply gown, goggles, and mask if risk for splashing exists.

   Reduces transmission of microorganisms.

2. Lower side rail and position patient comfortably and drape to expose only wound site. Instruct patient not to touch wound or sterile supplies.

   Draping provides access to wound while minimizing exposure. Dressing supplies become contaminated when touched by patient's hand.

3. Gently remove tape, bandages, or ties: use nondominant hand to support dressing and with dominant hand pull tape parallel to skin and toward dressing. If dressing is over hairy area, remove in direction of hair growth. Get patient permission to clip area (check agency policy). Remove any adhesive from skin.

   Pulling tape toward dressing reduces stress on suture line or wound edges and reduces irritation and discomfort.

4. With gloved hand or forceps remove dressing one layer at a time, observing appearance of drainage on dressing. Carefully remove outer secondary dressing first; then remove inner primary dressing that is in contact with wound bed. If drains are present, slowly and carefully remove dressings, avoiding tension on any drainage devices. Keep soiled undersurface from patient's sight.

   Purpose of primary dressing is to remove necrotic tissue and exudate. Appearance of drainage may be upsetting to patient. Avoids accidental removal of drain.

   a. If dressing adheres to wound, moisten with normal saline and remove.

   Prevents injury to wound surface and periwound during dressing removal.

5. Inspect wound and periwound for appearance, color, size (length, width, and depth), drainage, edema, presence and condition of drains, approximation (wound edges are together), granulation tissue, and odor. Use measuring guide or ruler to measure size of wound; see Skill 38.2, Step 10c. Gently palpate wound edges for bogginess or patient report of increased pain.

   Assesses condition of wound and periwound condition. Indicates status of healing.

6. Fold dressings with drainage contained inside and remove gloves inside out. With small dressings remove gloves inside out over dressing (see illustrations). Dispose of gloves and soiled dressing according to agency policy. Cover wound lightly with sterile gauze pad and perform hand hygiene.

   Contains soiled dressings, prevents contact of nurse's hands with drainage, and reduces cross-contamination.

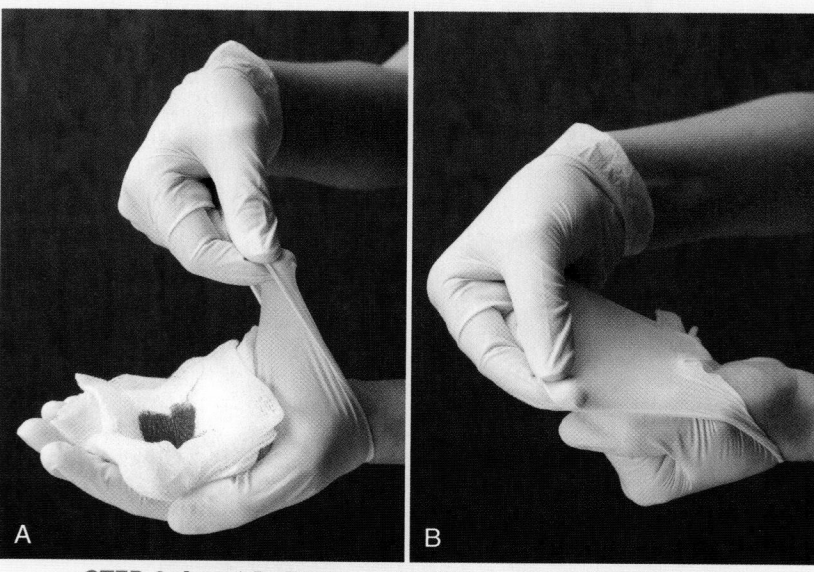

STEP 6 A and **B,** Dispose of soiled dressings by placing in gloved hand and pulling glove off over dressing and then off hand.

STEP	RATIONALE
7. Describe appearance of wound and any indicators of wound healing to patient.	Wounds may be unsettling and frightening to patients. It helps patient to know that wound appearance is as expected and whether healing is taking place.
8. Create sterile field with sterile dressing tray or individually wrapped sterile supplies on over-bed table (see Chapter 14). Pour any prescribed solution into sterile basin.	Sterile dressings remain sterile while on or within sterile surface. Preparation of all supplies before dressing change prevents break in technique during dressing change.
9. Cleanse wound.	
a. Perform hand hygiene and apply clean gloves. Use gauze moistened in saline or antiseptic swab (per health care provider order) for each cleansing stroke or spray wound surface with wound cleanser.	Prevents transfer of organisms from previously cleaned area.
b. Clean from least to most contaminated area (see illustration).	Cleaning in this direction prevents introduction of organisms into wound.
c. If a drain is present, remove split gauze (see illustration A). Clean around any drain (if present) using circular strokes starting near drain and moving outward and away from insertion site (see illustration B).	Correct aseptic technique in cleaning prevents contamination.

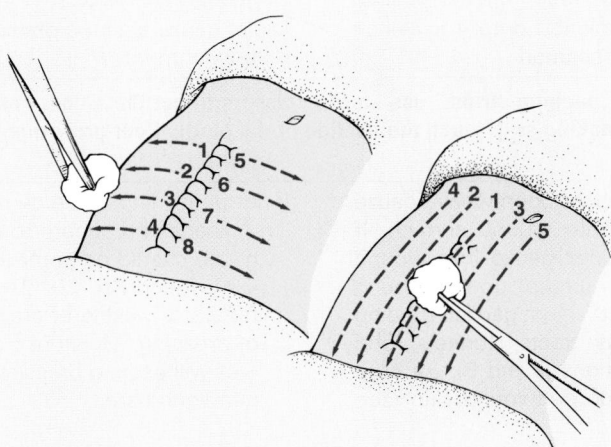

STEP 9b Methods for cleansing a wound, cleansing from least to most contaminated.

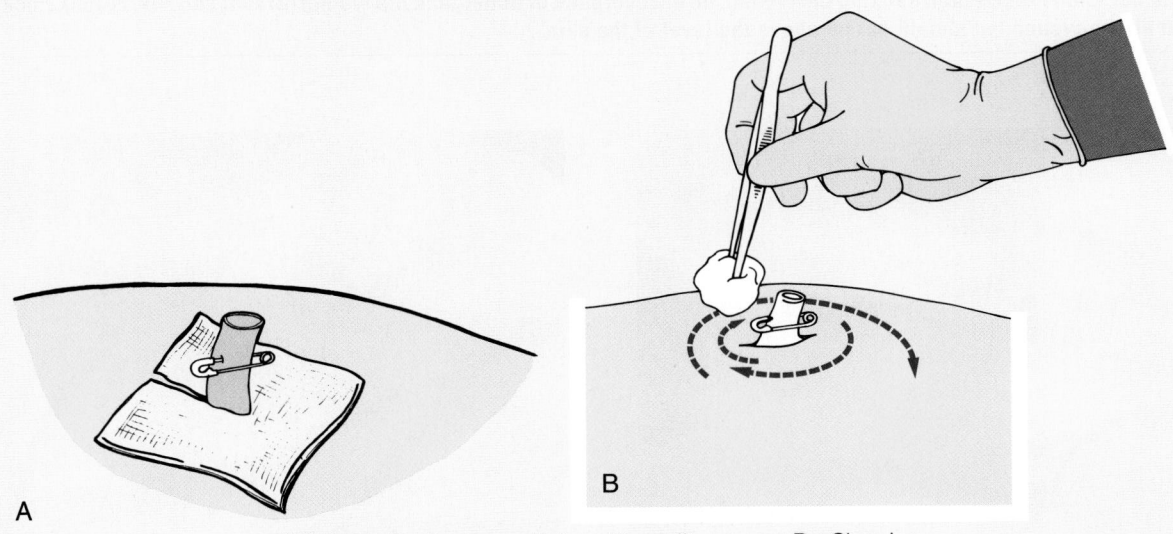

STEP 9c A, Penrose drain with split gauze. **B,** Cleaning around a drain site.

SKILL 38.4 APPLYING DRESSINGS: DRY, DAMP-TO-DRY, AND TRANSPARENT—cont'd

STEP	RATIONALE
10. Use sterile dry gauze to blot wound bed.	Drying reduces excess moisture, which could eventually harbor microorganisms.
11. Apply antiseptic (if ordered) with sterile cotton-tipped applicator or gauze along wound edges. Dispose of gloves. Perform hand hygiene.	Helps reduce growth of microorganisms.
12. Apply dressing (see agency policy).	
a. Dry sterile dressing:	
(1) Apply clean gloves (see agency policy).	Some agencies or condition of wounds may require sterile gloves.
(2) Apply loose woven gauze as contact layer (see illustration).	Promotes proper absorption of drainage.
(3) If drain is present, apply precut, split 4 × 4–inch gauze around drain (see Step 9c).	Secures drain and promotes drainage absorption at site.
(4) Apply additional layers of gauze as needed.	Ensures proper coverage and optimal absorption.
(5) Apply thicker woven pad (e.g., Surgipad, abdominal [ABD] pad) (see illustration).	This dressing is used on postoperative wounds when there is excessive drainage.
b. Damp to dry dressing:	
(1) Apply sterile or clean gloves (see agency policy).	Reduces transmission of infection.
(2) Pour prescribed sterile solution onto 4 × 4–inch gauze. Wring out excess solution.	Moist gauze absorbs drainage and maintains a moist environment.

Clinical Decision Point. If using "packing strips," use sterile scissors to cut the amount of dressing that you will use to pack the wound. Do not let the packing strip touch the outside of the bottle. Pour prescribed sterile solution over packing strip. Wring out excess solution.

(3) Unfold gauze and apply moist open-weave gauze as single layer directly onto wound surface. If wound is deep, gently pack gauze into wound with sterile gloved hand or forceps until all wound surfaces are in contact with moist gauze including dead spaces from sinus tracts, tunnels, and undermining (see illustrations A and B). Be sure that gauze does not touch periwound skin (see illustration C).	Inner gauze should be damp, not dripping wet, to absorb drainage and adhere to debris. When packing a wound, gauze should conform to base and side of wound (Bryant and Nix, 2016b). Wound is loosely packed to facilitate wicking of drainage into absorbent outer layer of dressing. Moisture from a dressing that is excessively wet will escape dressing and often macerates periwound area.

Clinical Decision Point. Be sure to count how many pieces of gauze are packed in the wound, especially deep wounds. This ensures that all gauze from previous dressing change are removed from wound.

Clinical Decision Point. When packing the wound, do not overpack or underpack the wound (Bryant and Nix, 2016b). Packing should fill the wound but should not be above the level of the skin.

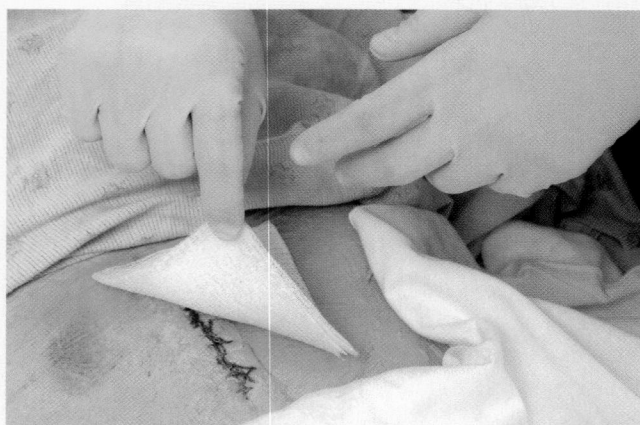

STEP 12a(2) Placing dry gauze dressing over simple wound.

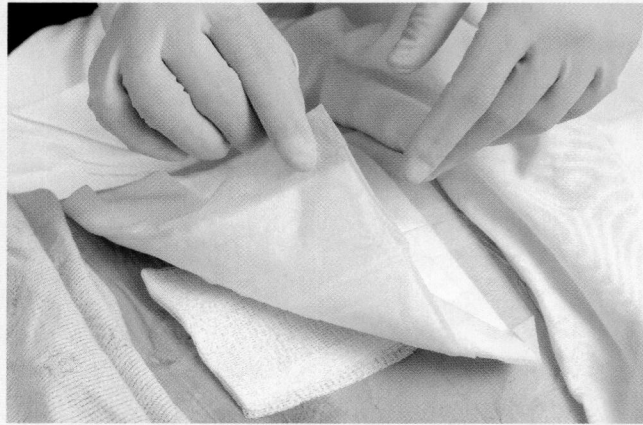

STEP 12a(5) Placing abdominal pad over gauze dressing.

STEP	RATIONALE
(4) Apply dry sterile 4 × 4–inch gauze over moist gauze.	Dry layer absorbs excessive moisture from wound.
(5) Cover with ABD pad, Surgipad, or gauze.	Protects wound from entrance of microorganisms.
13. Secure dressing.	
a. Tape: Apply tape over gauze and 1 to 2 inches (2.5 to 5 cm) beyond dressing. Use nonallergenic tape when necessary.	Supports and helps dressing remain in place.
b. Montgomery ties (see illustrations):	Prevents skin irritation. Ties allow for repeated dressing changes without removal of tape.
(1) Be sure that skin is clean and dry. Application of skin barrier under adhesive tape is recommended.	A solid skin barrier protects intact skin from stretch and tension of adhesive tape.
(2) Remove paper backing from adhesive surface and apply to skin 1 to 2 inches from the wound.	
(3) Place ties on opposite sides of dressing over skin or skin barrier.	
(4) Secure dressing by lacing ties across dressing snugly enough to hold it secure but without placing pressure on skin.	

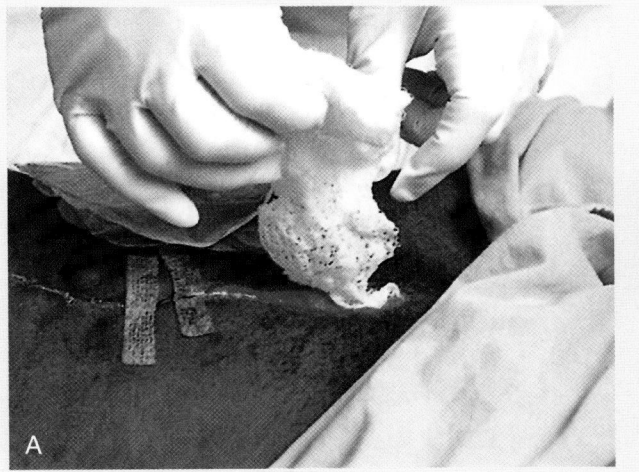
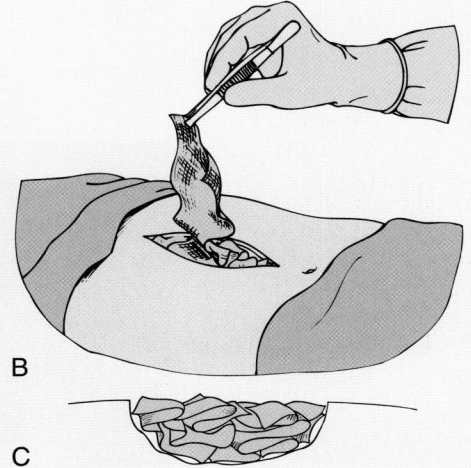

STEP 12b(3) **A** and **B,** Packing wound with fine-mesh gauze. **C,** Cross section of deep wound packed loosely with gauze roll.

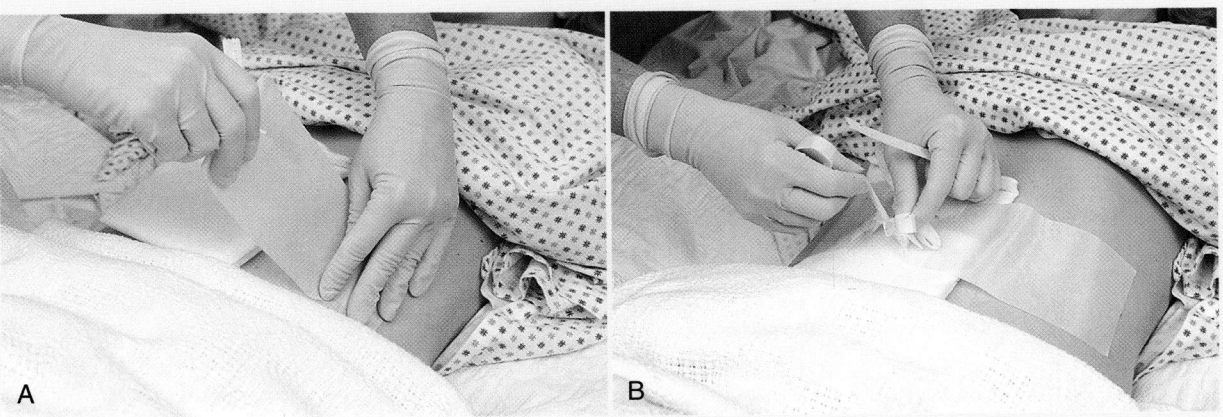

STEP 13b Montgomery ties. **A,** Each tie is placed at side of gauze dressing. **B,** Securing ties encloses dressing.

SKILL 38.4 APPLYING DRESSINGS: DRY, DAMP-TO-DRY, AND TRANSPARENT—cont'd

STEP	RATIONALE
c. For protective window:	A protective window is an alternative to Montgomery ties for smaller wounds. There is less skin irritation by placing tape on window strips.
(1) Cut strip of hydrocolloid pad into four strips used to form a "window" around the wound.	
(2) Use skin barrier to wipe areas of skin where strips will be applied.	
(3) Apply adhesive strips to frame a "window" around the wound (see illustration).	
(4) Apply dressing and then secure tape ends to adhesive strips.	
d. For dressing an extremity, secure with roller gauze (see illustration) or elastic net.	Roller gauze conforms to contour of foot or hand.
14. Dispose of all dressing supplies. Remove cover gown and goggles, and remove gloves inside out; dispose of all items according to agency policy.	Reduces transmission of microorganisms. Clean environment enhances patient comfort.
15. Label tape over dressing with your initials and date dressing is changed.	Provides timeline for when next dressing change is to be scheduled.
16. Help patient to comfortable position.	Promotes patient's sense of well-being.
17. Perform hand hygiene.	Reduces transmission of microorganisms.

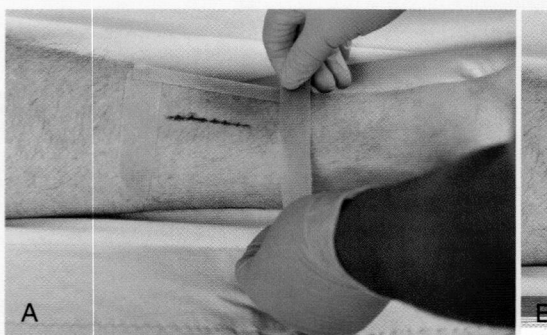
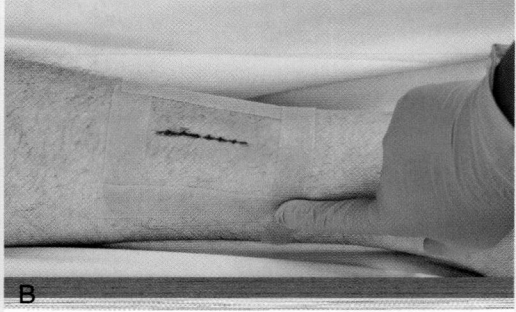

STEP 13c(3) **A** and **B,** Apply adhesive strips to frame a "window" around the wound.

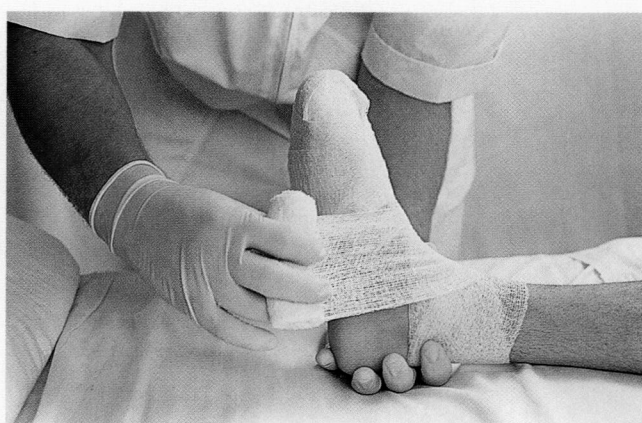

STEP 13d Wrap roller gauze around extremity to secure dressing.

STEP	RATIONALE

EVALUATION

1. Observe appearance of wound for healing: measure size of wound; observe amount, color, and type of drainage and periwound erythema or swelling.

Determines rate of healing.

2. Ask patient to rate pain using a scale of 0 to 10.

Increased pain is often indication of wound complications such as infection or result of dressing pulling tissue.

3. Inspect condition of dressing at least every shift.

Determines status of wound drainage.

4. **Use Teach-Back:** "I want to be sure I explained why and how often you need to continue these dressing changes in the hospital and at home. Tell me why it is important to change your dressing and how often to do so." Revise your instruction now or develop a plan for revised patient/family caregiver teaching if patient/family caregiver is not able to teach back correctly.

Determines patient's/family caregiver's level of understanding of instructional topic.

RECORDING AND REPORTING

- Record in nurses' notes in electronic health record (EHR), chart, or flow sheets relevant observations such as appearance and size of wound, characteristics of drainage, presence of necrotic tissue, type of dressing applied, patient's response to dressing change, and level of comfort.

- Document your evaluation of patient and family caregiver learning.
- Report any unexpected appearance of wound drainage, accidental removal of drain, bright red bleeding, or evidence of wound dehiscence or evisceration.

UNEXPECTED OUTCOMES AND RELATED INTERVENTIONS

- Wound appears inflamed and tender, drainage is evident, or odor is present.
  - Monitor patient for signs of infection (e.g., fever, increased white blood cell count).
  - Notify health care provider.
  - Obtain wound cultures as ordered.
  - If there is yellow, tan, or brown necrotic tissue, notify health care provider to determine need for debridement.
- Wound bleeds during dressing change.
  - Observe color and amount of bloody drainage. If excessive, may need to apply direct dressing.
  - Inspect area along dressing and directly underneath patient to determine amount of bleeding.

- Obtain vital signs as needed.
- Notify health care provider.
- Patient reports sensation that "something has given way under the dressing."
  - Observe wound for increased drainage or dehiscence (partial or total separation of wound layers) or evisceration (total separation of wound layers and protrusion of viscera through wound opening).
  - If dehiscence or evisceration occurs, protect wound. Cover with sterile moist dressing.
  - Instruct patient to lie still.
  - Stay with patient to monitor vital signs.
  - Notify health care provider.

SKILL 38.5 PERFORMING WOUND IRRIGATION

View Video!

DELEGATION CONSIDERATIONS

The skill of sterile wound irrigation cannot be delegated to nursing assistive personnel (NAP). However, in some settings you can delegate the cleansing of chronic wounds using clean technique. It is the nurse's responsibility to assess and document wound characteristics and evaluate wound care interventions before any delegation. The nurse directs the NAP to:

- Report any changes in patient's comfort level, wound drainage, increased temperature, or any bright red drainage.
- Report to the nurse wound color, presence of bleeding, or change in drainage when wound is cleansed.

SKILL 38.5 PERFORMING WOUND IRRIGATION—cont'd

View Video!

EQUIPMENT

- Irrigant/cleansing solution (volume 1.5 to 2 times the estimated wound volume)
- Irrigation delivery system (per order), depending on amount of pressure desired
- Sterile irrigation: It is often helpful to use a 35-mL syringe with a 19-gauge angiocatheter to facilitate optimal pressure for cleansing with minimal risk for tissue injury (Bryant and Nix, 2016b) or handheld shower.

- Protective equipment: sterile gloves, gown, and goggles if splash/spray risk exists
- Waterproof underpad if needed
- Dressing supplies
- Disposable waterproof biohazard bag
- Extra towels and padding (to use to protect bed)
- Wound assessment supplies

STEP	RATIONALE
ASSESSMENT	
1. Identify patient using at least two identifiers (e.g., name and birthday or name and medical record number) according to agency policy.	Ensures correct patient. Complies with The Joint Commission standards and improves patient safety (TJC, 2018).
2. Review health care provider's order for irrigation of open wound and type of solution to be used.	Open-wound irrigation requires medical order including type of solution to use.
3. Assess patient's level of comfort using a pain scale of 0 to 10. If patient is uncomfortable, offer an analgesic at least 30 to 45 minutes before procedure.	Provides baseline to determine tolerance to procedure.
4. Review medical record for signs and symptoms related to patient's open wound:	Provides ongoing data to indicate change in wound status (Nix, 2016).
a. Extent of impairment of skin integrity including size of wound	
b. Number of drains present	Awareness of drain position facilitates safe dressing removal and determines need for special dressings.
c. Drainage including previous amount, color, consistency, and odor	Drainage should decrease in healing wound. When drainage increases, it is often related to infection. The presence of an odor also indicates a wound infection (Doughty and Sparks, 2016).
d. Wound color	Color represents balance between necrotic tissue and new scar tissue. Proper selection of wound care products on the basis of wound color facilitates removal of necrotic tissue and promotes new tissue growth (Nix, 2016).
e. Culture reports	An infected wound is colonized with bacteria. Culture reports identify type of bacteria and proper treatment. Ongoing wound cultures document resolution of infectious process (Stotts, 2016b).
f. Assessment of old dressing (e.g., dry and clean; drainage color, amount, and odor; bleeding).	Provides data of wound drainage on existing dressing.
5. Assess patient for history of allergies to antiseptics, solutions, medications, tapes, or dressing material.	If known allergies, apply a sample of prescribed wound treatment as skin test before flushing wound with large volume of solution or select different tape or dressing material.
PLANNING	
1. Administer analgesic 30 to 45 minutes before starting wound irrigation procedure.	Promotes pain control and permits patient to move more easily and be positioned to facilitate wound irrigation (Krasner, 2016).
2. Provide privacy and prepare bedside environment for patient safety.	Maintains privacy.
3. Prepare and organize appropriate supplies for wound irrigation and dressing.	
a. Cuff waterproof bag.	Cuffing helps to maintain large opening, permitting placement of contaminated dressing without touching waste bag itself.
4. Explain procedure to patient and family members.	Promotes cooperation and reduces anxiety.
5. Perform hand hygiene, and position patient.	Frequent hand hygiene reduces microorganisms.

STEP	RATIONALE
6. Position patient comfortably to permit gravitational flow of irrigating solution over wound and into collection receptacle (see illustration).	Directing solution from top to bottom of wound and from clean to contaminated area prevents further infection. Position patient during planning stage, keeping in mind bed surfaces needed for later preparation of equipment.
a. Position patient so that wound is vertical to collection basin. Irrigant should be room temperature.	Room temperature solution increases comfort and reduces vascular constriction response in tissues.
b. Place padding or extra towel on bed under area where irrigation will take place.	Protects bedding from becoming wet.
c. Place padding or extra towel in the bed.	Protects bedding.
d. Expose only the wound.	Prevents patient from becoming chilled.

IMPLEMENTATION

STEP	RATIONALE
1. Perform hand hygiene.	While cleansing a wound, use meticulous hand hygiene and proper infection control procedures before and after removing soiled dressings to limit the risk for health care–acquired infection (Jaszarowski and Murphree, 2016).
2. Apply gown, mask, and goggles as indicated. Apply clean gloves and remove old dressing. Discard old dressing and gloves in biohazard bag. Perform hand hygiene.	Reduces transmission of microorganisms. Protects nurse from splashes or sprays of blood and body fluids.
3. Apply clean or sterile gloves (check agency policy). Use sterile precautions when sterile gloves are needed. Perform wound assessment and examine recent charted assessment of patient's open wound (see Skill 38.1).	Provides ongoing wound-healing data.
4. Expose area near wound only.	Provides privacy and prevents chilling of patient.
5. To irrigate wound with wide opening:	
a. Fill 35-mL syringe with irrigation solution.	Irrigating wound uses a mechanical force, which helps with separation and removal of necrotic debris and surface bacteria (Jaszarowski and Murphree, 2016). Flushing wound helps remove debris and facilitates healing by secondary intention.
b. Attach 19-gauge angiocatheter.	Catheter lumen delivers ideal pressure for cleansing and removing debris (Ramundo, 2016). Mechanical debridement may include irrigation, which can be done through the use of a 35-mL syringe with a 19-gauge angiocatheter with irrigation pressures delivered between 4 and 15 psi (WOCN Society, 2016).
c. Hold syringe tip 2.5 cm (1 inch) above upper end of wound and over area being cleansed.	Prevents syringe contamination. Careful placement of syringe prevents unsafe pressure of flowing solution.
d. Using continuous pressure, flush wound; repeat Steps 5a to 5c until solution draining into basin is clear.	Flushing wound helps to remove debris; clear solution indicates removal of all debris.
6. Irrigate deep wound with very small opening:	
a. Attach soft catheter to filled irrigation syringe.	Catheter permits direct flow of irrigant into wound. Expect wound to take longer to empty when opening is small.
b. Gently insert tip of catheter into opening about 1.3 cm (0.5 inch).	Prevents tip from touching fragile inner wall of wound.

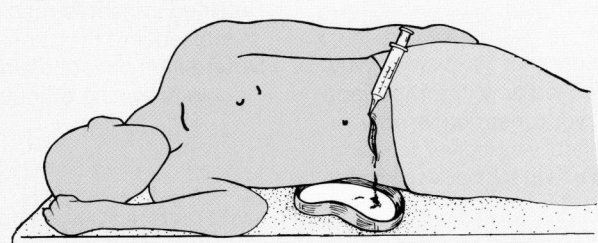

STEP 6 Patient position for wound irrigation.

SKILL 38.5 PERFORMING WOUND IRRIGATION—cont'd

View Video!

STEP	RATIONALE
Clinical Decision Point. Do not force catheter into wound because this will cause tissue damage.	
c. Using slow, continuous pressure, flush wound.	Use of slow mechanical force of stream of solution loosens particulate matter on wound surface and promotes healing (Ramundo, 2016).
Clinical Decision Point. Pulsatile high-pressure lavage is often the irrigation of choice for necrotic wounds. Pressure settings should be set per provider order, usually between 4 and 15 psi, and should not be used on skin grafts, exposed blood vessels, muscle, tendon, or bone. Use with caution if patient has coagulation disorder or is taking anticoagulants (Ramundo, 2016).	
d. While keeping catheter in place, pinch it off just below syringe.	Avoids contamination of sterile solution.
e. Remove and refill syringe. Reconnect to catheter and repeat until solution draining into basin is clear. Remove gloves and discard.	
7. Perform hand hygiene and apply clean gloves. Cleanse wound with handheld shower.	
a. With patient seated comfortably in shower chair or standing if condition allows, adjust spray to gentle flow; make sure that water is warm.	Useful for patients able to shower with assistance or independently. May be done at home.
b. Shower for 5 to 10 minutes with shower head 30 cm (12 inches) from wound.	Ensures that wound is thoroughly cleansed.
8. When indicated, obtain cultures after cleansing with nonbacteriostatic saline.	WOCN Society (2016) recommends using quantitative bacterial cultures (tissue biopsy or swab cultures). The most common types of wound cultures are swab technique, aspirated wound fluid, or tissue biopsy (Stotts, 2016a).
Clinical Decision Point. Obtain wound culture if indicated by the presence of inflammation around the wound, purulent odor or drainage, new drainage, or fever in patient.	
9. Dry wound edges with gauze; dry patient after shower.	Prevents maceration of surrounding tissue from excess moisture.
10. Apply appropriate dressing and label with time, date, and nurse's initials.	Maintains protective barrier and healing environment for wound.
11. Remove mask, goggles, and gown.	Prevents transfer of microorganisms.
12. Dispose of equipment and soiled supplies, remove gloves, and perform hand hygiene.	Reduces transmission of microorganisms.
13. Help patient to comfortable position.	

EVALUATION

1. Have patient rate level of comfort on scale of 0 to 10.	Patient's pain should not increase as a result of wound irrigation.
2. Observe type of tissue in wound bed.	Identifies wound-healing progress and determines type of wound cleansing and dressing needed.
3. Inspect dressing periodically (see agency policy).	Determines patient's response to wound irrigation and need to modify plan of care.
4. Evaluate periwound skin integrity.	Determines if extension of wound has occurred or signs of infection are present (warm red periwound skin).
5. Observe for presence of retained irrigant.	Retained irrigant is medium for bacterial growth and subsequent infection.
6. **Use Teach-Back:** "I want to be sure that I explained why the wound was irrigated today. Tell me why it is important to irrigate your wound." Revise your instruction now or develop a plan for revised patient/family caregiver teaching if patient/family caregiver is not able to teach back correctly.	Determines patient's/family caregiver's level of understanding of instructional topic.

RECORDING AND REPORTING

- Record in nurses' notes in electronic health record (EHR), chart, or flow sheets wound assessment before and after irrigation; amount, color, and odor of drainage on dressing removed; amount and type of solution used; irrigation device used; patient's tolerance of procedure; and type of dressing applied after irrigation.

- Document your evaluation of patient and family caregiver learning.
- Immediately report to health care provider any evidence of fresh bleeding, sharp increase in pain, retention of irrigant, or signs of shock.

UNEXPECTED OUTCOMES AND RELATED INTERVENTIONS

- Bleeding or serosanguineous drainage appears.
  - Flush wound during next irrigation using less pressure.
  - Notify health care provider of bleeding.
- Retained fluid and debris appear.
  - Increase amount of fluid during irrigation.
  - Increase amount of pressure when flushing wounds.
  - Make sure that wound is clear of retained fluid and debris before applying new dressing.

- Suture line opening extends.
  - Notify health care provider.
  - Reevaluate amount of pressure to use for next wound irrigation.

KEY POINTS

- Wounds with partial-thickness tissue loss heal by epidermal repair, and full-thickness wounds heal by forming scar tissue.
- A clean surgical incision with little tissue loss heals by primary intention.
- When there is extensive tissue loss, a wound heals by secondary intention.
- Healing of full-thickness wounds proceeds through four overlapping phases: hemostasis, inflammation, proliferation, and remodeling.
- The chances of wound infection are greater when the wound contains dead or necrotic tissue, when foreign bodies lie on or near the wound, and when blood supply and tissue defenses are reduced.
- Physical stress from vomiting, coughing, or sudden muscular contraction can cause separation of wound edges (dehiscence).
- Wound assessment includes anatomical location, size (dimensions and depth of wound), type and percentage of wound tissue, volume and color of wound drainage, and condition of surrounding skin.
- Wound drains remove secretions within tissue layers to promote wound closure.
- Never collect a wound culture from old drainage.
- Principles of wound management include controlling or eliminating the cause, providing systemic support to reduce existing and potential cofactors, and maintaining a physiological wound environment.

- A moist environment supports wound healing.
- When cleaning wounds or drain sites, clean from the least to the most contaminated area.
- Apply a dressing or binder in a manner that does not impair circulation or irritate the skin.
- The safe use of heat or cold therapy requires an assessment of the patient's sensory function, identification of risk factors, and understanding of the physiological effects of heat and cold.
- An acute sprain, fracture, or bruise responds best to cold applications.
- Warm applications are effective for improving circulation to wound sites and promoting muscle relaxation.

REFLECTIVE LEARNING

- Reflect on a patient you have cared for who experienced a pressure injury. Discuss your findings when you assessed your patient's pressure injury. How confident did you feel in staging the injury and describing the type and quality of the wound tissue?
- What response did you receive when you asked the patient and family about how the pressure injury developed and what they can do to prevent this from occurring in the future?
- How confident were you in planning your patient's care to prevent further skin breakdown and support healing of the wound?

REVIEW QUESTIONS

1. A nurse is planning care for a patient who has a red area over a bony prominence that blanches when assessed. Which of the following interventions are appropriate? (Select all that apply.)
   1. Massage the area to improve the local circulation.
   2. Reposition the patient off the area.
   3. Reassess the area after the patient is off the area for 1 hour.
   4. Request nonbleached sheets for this patient's bed.
   5. Place a cold pack under the area and reassess in 1 hour.

2. When obtaining a wound culture specimen to determine the presence of a wound infection, the nurse correctly collects the specimen from the:
   1. Necrotic tissue.
   2. Wound drainage.
   3. Wound circumference.
   4. Cleansed wound.

3. Two days after undergoing abdominal surgery, a patient with a closed abdominal wound reports a sudden "pop" after coughing. When the nurse examines the surgical wound site, the sutures are no longer holding the incisional edges together, there is a gap in the incision, and pieces of small bowel are noted at the bottom of the now opened wound. What is the correct intervention?
   1. Allowing the area to be exposed to air until all drainage has stopped
   2. Placing several cold packs over the area, protecting the skin around the wound
   3. Covering the area with sterile saline-soaked towels and immediately notifying the surgical team
   4. Covering the area with sterile gauze, placing a tight binder over the area, and asking the patient to remain in bed for 30 minutes

4. Nursing interventions to manage a patient who is experiencing frequent fecal and urinary incontinence include which of the following? (Select all that apply.)
   1. Frequent perineal and sacral skin assessments
   2. Using a large absorbent diaper, changing when saturated
   3. Keeping the buttocks exposed to air at all times
   4. Using an incontinence cleanser, followed by application of a moisture-barrier ointment
   5. Offering frequent ambulation and help to the toilet

5. Place the following steps in correct order for performing a wound irrigation.
   1. Use slow continuous pressure to irrigate wound.
   2. Attach 19-gauge angiocatheter to syringe.
   3. Fill syringe with irrigation fluid.
   4. Assess wound.
   5. Position angiocatheter over wound.

evolve

Additional Review Questions, as well as rationales for all Review Questions, can be found on the Evolve website.

1. 2, 3; 2. 4; 3. 3, 4. 1, 4, 5; 5. 4, 3, 2, 5, 1.

REFERENCES

Ayello EA: Predicting pressure ulcer risk, *Best Pract Nurs Care Older Adult* 5:1, 2012. https://www.nhqualitycampaign.org/files/Try_This_Issue_5_-_Predicting_Pressure_Ulcer_Risk.pdf.

Ayello EA, Braden B: How and why do pressure risk assessment, *Adv Skin Wound Care* 15(3):125, 2002.

Baath C, et al: Prevention of heel pressure ulcers among older patients from ambulatory care to hospital discharge. A multicenter randomized controlled trial, *Appl Nurs Res* 30:170, 2016.

Barker AL, et al: Implementation of pressure prevention best practice recommendations in acute care: an observational study, *Int Wound J* 10(3):313, 2013.

Beitz JM: Wound healing. In Doughty D, McNichol L, editors: *Wound Ostomy and Continence Nurses Society core curriculum: wound management*, Philadelphia, 2016, Wolters Kluwer.

Bergstrom N, et al: A clinical trial of the Braden Scale for predicting pressure sore risk, *Nurs Clin North Am* 22(2):417, 1987a.

Bergstrom N, et al: The Braden Scale for predicting pressure sore risk, *Nurs Res* 36:205, 1987b.

Bergstrom NL, et al: Predicting pressure risk: a multisite study of the predictive validity of the Braden Scale, *Nurs Res* 47(5):261, 1998.

Black J, et al: Medical device-related pressure ulcers in hospitalized patients, *Int Wound J* 7(5):358, 2010.

Black J, et al: Use of wound dressings to enhance prevention of pressure ulcers caused by medical devices, *Int Wound J* 12(3):322, 2015.

Branson RD, et al: Management of the artificial airway, *Respir Care* 59(6):974, 2014.

Bryant RA: Types of skin damage and differential diagnosis. In Bryant RA, Nix DP, editors: *Acute and chronic wounds: current management concepts*, ed 5, St Louis, 2016, Mosby.

Bryant RA, Nix DP: Developing and maintaining a pressure ulcer prevention program. In Bryant RA, Nix DP, editors: *Acute and chronic wounds: current management concepts*, ed 5, St Louis, 2016a, Mosby.

Bryant RA, Nix DP: Principles of topical management. In Bryant RA, Nix DP, editors: *Acute and chronic wounds:*

current management concepts, ed 5, St Louis, 2016b, Mosby.

Coyer FM, et al: A prospective window into medical device-related pressure ulcers in intensive care, *Int Wound J* 11(6):656, 2014.

Doughty DB, McNichol LL: General concepts related to skin and soft tissue injury caused by mechanical factors. In Doughty D, McNichol L, editors: *Wound Ostomy and Continence Nurses Society core curriculum: wound management*, Philadelphia, 2016, Wolters Kluwer.

Doughty DB, Sparks B: Wound healing physiology and factors that affect the repair process. In Bryant RA, Nix DP, editors: *Acute and chronic wounds: current management concepts*, ed 5, St Louis, 2016, Mosby.

Edsberg LE, et al: Revised National Pressure Ulcer Advisory Panel Pressure injury staging system revised pressure injury staging system, *J Wound Ostomy Continence Nurs* 43(6):585, 2016.

European Pressure Ulcer Advisory Panel (EPUAP) and National Pressure Ulcer Advisory Panel (NPUAP): *Prevention of pressure ulcers: quick reference guide*, Washington, DC, 2014, National Ulcer Advisory Panel, http://www.epuap.org/guidelines-/.

Hopf HW, et al: Managing wound pain. In Bryant RA, Nix DP, editors: *Acute and chronic wounds: current management concepts*, ed 5, St Louis, 2016, Mosby.

Jaszarowski KA, Murphree RW: Wound cleansing and dressing selection. In Doughty D, McNichol L, editors: *Wound Ostomy and Continence Nurses Society core curriculum: wound management*, Philadelphia, 2016, Wolters Kluwer.

Kelleher AD, et al: Peer-to-peer nursing rounds and hospital-acquired pressure ulcer prevalence in a surgical intensive care unit: a quality improvement project, *J Wound Ostomy Continence Nurs* 39(2):152, 2012.

Krasner DL: Wound pain impact and assessment. In Bryant RA, Nix DP, editors: *Acute and chronic wounds: current management concepts*, ed 5, St Louis, 2016, Mosby.

Landis EM: Micro-injection studies of capillary blood pressure in human skin, *Heart* 15:209, 1930.

Makic MBF: Medical device-related pressure ulcers and intensive care patients, *J Perianesth Nurs* 30(4):336, 2015.

Maklebust J, Magnan MA: Pressure ulcer prevention. In Doughty D, McNichol LL,

editors: *Wound Ostomy and Continence Nurses Society core curriculum: wound management*, Philadelphia, 2016, Wolters Kluwer.

McNichol L, et al: Identifying the right surface for the right patient at the right time: generation and content validation of an algorithm for support surface selection, *J Wound Ostomy Continence Nurs* 42(1):19, 2015.

National Pressure Ulcer Advisory Panel (NPUAP): *National Pressure Ulcer Advisory Panel (NPUAP) announces a change in terminology from pressure ulcer to pressure injury and updates the stages of pressure injury*, 2016, http://www.npuap.org/national-pressure-ulcer-advisory-panel-npuap-announces-a-change-interminology-from-pressure-ulcer-to-pressure-injury-and-updates-the-stages-of-pressure-injury.

National Pressure Ulcer Advisory Panel (NPUAP), European Pressure Ulcer Advisory Panel (EPUAP), and Pan Pacific Pressure Ulcer Injury Alliance (PPPIA): Haseler E, editor: *Prevention and treatment of pressure ulcers: clinical practice guideline*, Osborne Park, Western Australia, 2014, Cambridge Media.

National Quality Forum (NQF): *Patient Safety 2015 final report*, 2016, http://www.qualityforum.org/Publications/2016/02/Patient_Safety_2015_Final_Report.aspx.

Netsch DS, et al: Negative pressure wound therapy. In Bryant RA, Nix DP, editors: *Acute and chronic wounds: current management concepts*, ed 5, St Louis, 2016, Mosby.

Nix DP: Skin and wound inspection and assessment. In Bryant RA, Nix DP, editors: *Acute and chronic wounds: current management concepts*, ed 5, St Louis, 2016, Mosby.

Nix DP, Mackey DM: Support surfaces. In Bryant RA, Nix DP, editors: *Acute and chronic wounds: current management concepts*, ed 5, St Louis, 2016, Mosby.

Nix DP, et al: Skin care needs of the neonatal and pediatric patient. In Bryant RA, Nix DP, editors: *Acute and chronic wounds: current management concepts*, ed 5, St Louis, 2016, Mosby.

Padula WV, et al: Factors influencing adoption of hospital-acquired pressure ulcer prevention programs in US academic medical centers, *J Wound Ostomy Continence Nurs* 42(4):327, 2015.

Petrofsky JS, et al: Effect of heat and cold on tendon flexibility and force to flex the

human knee, *Med Sci Monit* 19:661, 2013.

Pieper B: Pressure ulcers: impact, etiology, and classification. In Bryant RA, Nix DP, editors: *Acute and chronic wounds: current management concepts*, ed 5, St Louis, 2016, Mosby.

Pittman J, et al: A. Medical device–related hospital-acquired pressure ulcers: development of an evidence-based position statement, *J Wound Ostomy Continence Nurs* 42(2):151, 2015.

Ramundo JM: Wound debridement. In Bryant RA, Nix DP, editors: *Acute and chronic wounds: current management concepts*, ed 5, St Louis, 2016, Mosby.

Schallom M, et al: Pressure ulcer incidence in patients wearing nasal-oral versus full-face noninvasive ventilation masks, *Am J Crit Care* 24(4):349, 2015.

Stechmiller JK, et al: Bottom up (pressure shear) injuries. In Doughty D, McNichol L, editors: *Wound Ostomy and Continence Nurses Society core curriculum: wound management*, Philadelphia, 2016, Wolters Kluwer.

Stotts NA: Wound infection: diagnosis and management. In Bryant RA, Nix DP, editors: *Acute and chronic wounds: current management concepts*, ed 5, St Louis, 2016a, Mosby.

Stotts NA: Nutritional assessment and support. In Bryant RA, Nix DP, editors: *Acute and chronic wounds: current management concepts*, ed 5, St Louis, 2016b, Mosby.

Thayer DM, et al: Top down injuries prevention and management of moisture associated skin damage, medical adhesive-related skin injury and skin tears. In Doughty D, McNichol L, editors: *Wound Ostomy and Continence Nurses Society core curriculum: wound management*, Philadelphia, PA, 2016, Wolters Kluwer.

The Joint Commission (TJC): *2018 National Patient Safety Goals*, Oakbrook Terrace, IL, 2018, The Commission. https://www.jointcommission.org/standards_information/npsgs.aspx.

Wound, Ostomy and Continence Nurses (WOCN) Society: *Clean vs. sterile dressing techniques for management of chronic wounds: a fact sheet*, Mount Laurel, NJ, 2011, WOCN.

Wound, Ostomy and Continence Nurses (WOCN) Society: *Guideline for prevention and management of pressure ulcers*, WOCN Clinical Practice Guidelines Series, Mount Laurel, NJ, 2016, The Society.

39

Sensory Alterations

evolve MEDIA RESOURCES

http://evolve.elsevier.com/Potter/essentials
- Audio Glossary

- QSEN Activity and Review Questions Answers and Rationales

OBJECTIVES

- Differentiate the processes of reception, perception, and reaction to sensory stimuli.
- Compare the relationship of sensory function with an individual's level of wellness.
- Discuss common causes and effects of sensory alterations.
- Discuss common sensory changes that occur with aging.
- Identify factors to assess in determining a patient's sensory status.
- Describe behaviors indicating sensory alterations.

- Develop a plan of care for patients with sensory deficits.
- Describe nursing interventions with rationales that promote effective communication with patients who have sensory alterations.
- Describe conditions in the health care agency or patient's home that you adjust to promote meaningful sensory stimulation.
- Discuss ways to maintain a safe environment for patients with sensory alterations.

KEY TERMS

accommodation, p. 1170
age-related macular degeneration, p. 1169
auditory, p. 1168
cataracts, p. 1169
diabetic retinopathy, p. 1169
glaucoma, p. 1169

gustatory, p. 1168
Meniere's disease, p. 1171
olfactory, p. 1168
ototoxic, p. 1170
presbycusis, p. 1170
presbyopia, p. 1170
proprioception, p. 1168

refractive errors, p. 1179
sensory deficits, p. 1169
sensory deprivation, p. 1169
sensory overload, p. 1169
tactile, p. 1168
tinnitus, p. 1170

People are unique because they are able to sense a variety of stimuli in their environment. Stimulation comes from many sources inside and outside of the body, particularly through the senses of sight (visual), hearing (auditory), touch (tactile), smell (olfactory), and taste (gustatory). Additional senses include pressure, pain, temperature, vibration, and position (proprioception) (Meiner, 2015). People learn about the environment from healthy sensory organs. Patients need to adapt to their environment when their sensory function is altered. As a nurse, you will learn to recognize when

patients are at risk for developing sensory problems and help meet their needs when they have sensory alterations. Your nursing care helps patients learn to alter their environment for improved safety.

SCIENTIFIC KNOWLEDGE BASE

Normal Sensation

People feel and react to sensations when their nervous systems are intact. Perception or awareness depends on a

CASE STUDY *Mrs. Alicea*

Mrs. Alicea is a 73-year-old woman who is at the senior health center for her routine 6-month checkup. She has been visiting the senior center on a regular basis for the past 8 years. She has lived alone since her husband died 1 year ago. She lives in a single-story, four-room home a few miles away from the health center. Her son, Rico, lives 5 minutes away. Rico drives Mrs. Alicea to her health care visits. Six months ago Mrs. Alicea reported progressive hearing loss. Today when she enters the clinic she reports "having trouble seeing."

Peter Morris, a nursing student assigned to the senior health center, is learning to conduct assessments and develop health promotion plans for patients at the senior center. For the past month Peter has been attending his clinical rotation at the center and participating in teaching health promotion activities. He enjoys this rotation because he is learning more about geriatric nursing and finding that older adults are very independent and have productive lives.

region of the cerebral cortex where specialized brain cells interpret the quality and nature of each sensory stimulus. Sensory experiences include reception, perception, and reaction. People react to stimuli that are most meaningful to them. Sensory alterations occur when people attempt to react to every stimulus within their environment, when stimuli are lacking, and when stimuli cannot be received.

Types of Sensory Alterations

Many factors influence the capacity to receive or perceive sensations (Box 39.1). In your nursing experience you care for patients with a variety of sensory problems such as sensory deficits, sensory deprivation, and sensory overload. When patients have more than one sensory alteration, their ability to function and relate within the environment becomes impaired.

Sensory Deficits. A sensory deficit occurs when problems with sensory reception or perception exist (Box 39.2). Patients are not able to receive certain stimuli (e.g., light

and sound), or stimuli are distorted (e.g., blurred vision from cataracts and abnormal taste sensation from xerostomia). A sudden sensory loss can be caused by injury or as a side effect to medications (Box 39.3). When a deficit is chronic or develops gradually, a patient learns to rely on unaffected senses. Some senses become more acute to compensate for an alteration. For example, a patient who is blind develops an acute sense of hearing and learns to use a cane to adapt to visual challenges, whereas a patient who cannot hear "bluffs" his way through a conversation instead of admitting that he did not hear what was said.

Sensory deficits such as low vision and blindness are very common forms of disability. Four major diseases that frequently cause impaired vision in Americans 40 years of age and older are age-related macular degeneration, glaucoma, cataracts, and diabetic retinopathy (Touhy and Jett, 2016). Sensory deficits frequently cause patients to change their behaviors in adaptive or maladaptive ways. For example, some patients withdraw socially to cope with the loss (Touhy and Jett, 2014).

Sensory Deprivation. Sensory deprivation occurs when inadequate quality or quantity of stimuli impairs perception. It has different causes such as reduced sensory input (hearing loss), confusion, and a restricted environment (bed rest). Sensory deprivation sometimes produces cognitive changes such as the inability to solve problems, poor task performance, and disorientation. It also can cause affective changes (e.g., boredom, restlessness, increased anxiety, emotional lability) and/or perceptual changes (e.g., reduced attention span, disorganized visual and motor coordination, confusion of sleeping and waking states).

Children often become more anxious, displaying restlessness, difficulty with problem solving, and depression when they experience sensory deprivation (Hockenberry and Wilson, 2015). In adults the symptoms of sensory deprivation are similar to those of psychological illness, confusion, severe electrolyte imbalance, or the influence of psychotropic drugs. Thus accurate diagnosis of sensory deprivation is crucial.

Sensory Overload. When a person receives multiple sensory stimuli, the brain has difficulty distinguishing the stimuli, leading to sensory overload. A person with sensory overload no longer perceives the environment in a way that makes sense. Overload prevents a meaningful response to stimuli. As a result, thoughts race, attention moves in many directions, and restlessness occurs. The patient demonstrates panic, confusion, and aggressiveness. The patient may have loss of sleep or altered sleeping patterns (daytime drowsiness). Sensory overload causes a state similar to that of sensory deprivation.

Patients of all ages who are acutely ill easily develop sensory overload in the health care environment. Constant pain; noise from equipment; and nursing activities of turning, repositioning, and administering treatments

BOX 39.1   FACTORS THAT INFLUENCE SENSORY FUNCTION

AGE
Infants
- Binocular vision begins at 6 weeks and is well established by 4 months. During the second year of life infants discriminate shapes, objects, and colors.
- Neonates respond to loud noises. Within a year infants visually locate the source of noises.
- Newborns react to strong odors such as alcohol and vinegar by turning their heads. They can identify their own mother's milk.

Children
- Refractive errors are the most common types of visual disorders in children and are treated with corrective lenses.
- Serious visual impairment affects a child's ability to play and socialize.
- Children are usually frightened and confused by a sudden or progressive loss of sight. Parents and children need support to help them adjust to a disability (Hockenberry and Wilson, 2015).

Adults
- Visual changes include **presbyopia** and the need for glasses for reading (ages 40 to 50). In addition, the cornea, which helps with light refraction to the retina, becomes flatter and thicker. These aging changes lead to astigmatism.
- Pigment is lost from the iris; collagen fibers build up in the anterior chamber, which increases the risk for glaucoma by decreasing the resorption of intraocular fluid.

Older Adults
- Atrophy of the cerumen glands causes thicker and dryer cerumen, which is more difficult to remove and may completely obstruct the auditory canal (Touhy and Jett, 2014).
- Obstructive hearing loss is reversible, but changes in the structure and function of the inner ear that occur as older adults grow older are not.
- Age-related hearing changes include **presbycusis,** characterized by decreased hearing acuity, speech intelligibility, and pitch discrimination. Low-pitched sounds are easiest to hear, but it is difficult to hear conversation over background noise. It is also difficult to discriminate consonants (*f, s, th, ch, sh, b, p, k,* and *t*). Speech sounds are distorted, and there is a delayed reception and reaction to speech.
- Visual changes include reduced visual fields, increased glare sensitivity, impaired night vision, reduced **accommodation,** reduced depth perception, and reduced color discrimination. Symptoms occur because the pupils in the older adult take longer to dilate and constrict secondary to weaker iris muscles. Color vision decreases because the retina is duller and the lens yellows. Older adults may require 3 times as much light to see things as they did when they were in young adulthood (Touhy and Jett, 2014).
- Olfactory changes begin around age 50 and include a loss of cells in the olfactory bulb of the brain and a decrease in the number of sensory cells in the nasal lining. Reduced sensitivity to odors is common.
- A small decrease in the number of taste cells occurs with aging, beginning around age 60. Reduced sour, salty, and bitter taste discrimination is common. The ability to detect sweet tastes seems to remain intact (Touhy and Jett, 2014).
- Proprioceptive changes include increased difficulty with balance, spatial orientation, and coordination. These changes make it difficult to avoid obstacles and prevent an accident from happening when fast action is necessary. The automatic response to protect and brace oneself when falling is slower.
- Tactile changes are common including declining sensitivity to pain, pressure, and temperature secondary to peripheral vascular disease and neuropathies.

MEDICATIONS
- **Ototoxic** medications (see Box 39.3) such as analgesics, antibiotics, or diuretics affect hearing acuity, balance, or both, with the most common symptom being **tinnitus** (ringing in the ears). Ototoxicity causes a progressive or continuing hearing loss that in many patients goes unnoticed until the ability to understand speech is affected (Cone et al., 2016). Hearing loss is not always permanent, depending on the extent of damage and the length of time that the drug is given. Patients with renal failure have an increased sensitivity to ototoxic drugs.

ENVIRONMENT
- Excessive environmental stimuli result in sensory overload marked by confusion, disorientation, and inability to make decisions. Restricted environmental stimulation leads to sensory deprivation. Poor quality of environment worsens sensory impairment.

PREEXISTING ILLNESSES
- Disorders such as peripheral vascular disease and stroke alter peripheral tissue perfusion and affect tactile information. Diabetic neuropathy is a common complication of diabetes and can result in retinal edema, detachment, and blindness (Meiner, 2015).

SMOKING
- Chronic tobacco use atrophies the taste buds and affects olfactory function.

NOISE LEVELS
- Constant exposure to high noise levels causes hearing loss.

---

overwhelm patients with stimuli. Some patients such as patients in critical care settings are at a greater risk for sensory overload than others. Behavioral changes are easily confused with mood swings or disorientation. Constant reorientation and control of excessive stimuli become an important part of a patient's care.

NURSING KNOWLEDGE BASE

In the United States nearly half of adults older than 75 years of age have a hearing impairment; the incidence increases with age (National Institute of Deafness and Other Communication Disorders [NIDCD], 2016). Approximately 80% of

BOX 39.2   COMMON SENSORY DEFICITS

VISUAL

- Presbyopia: Gradual decline in ability of the lens to accommodate or to focus on close objects. Reduces ability to see near objects clearly.
- Cataract: Clouding of the lens in the eye that interferes with passage of light through the lens and reduces the light that reaches the retina. Cataracts usually develop gradually and often result in cloudy or blurry vision, glare, double vision, and poor night vision (National Eye Institute [NEI], 2015).
- Dry eyes: Result when tear glands produce too few tears, resulting in itching, burning, or reduced vision.
- Glaucoma: A slowly progressive increase in intraocular pressure that causes progressive pressure against the optic nerve. At first vision stays normal, and there is no pain. If left untreated, there may be a loss of peripheral (side) vision (Touhy and Jett, 2014).
- Diabetic retinopathy: Pathological changes of the blood vessels of the retina secondary to increased pressure, resulting in hemorrhage, macular edema, and reduced vision or vision loss.
- Age-related macular degeneration: Occurs when the macula (specialized portion of the retina responsible for central vision) degenerates as a result of aging and loses its ability to function efficiently. An early sign includes distortion that causes edges or lines to appear wavy. The disease causes the progressive loss of central vision. Peripheral vision remains intact (Touhy and Jett, 2014).

HEARING

- Presbycusis: A common progressive hearing disorder in older adults (see Box 39.1).
- Cerumen accumulation: Buildup and hardening of earwax in the external auditory canal causes conduction deafness.

BALANCE

- Dizziness and disequilibrium: Common condition in older adults, usually resulting from vestibular dysfunction and precipitated by change in position of the head to the rest of the body.
- Meniere's disease: Caused by pressure in the inner ear as a result of excessive fluid. Cause of the excessive fluid is unknown. Diagnosis is based on medical history interview, physical examination, and clinical symptoms of vertigo, tinnitus, and a full feeling or pressure in the affected ear (Meiner, 2015).

TASTE

- Xerostomia: Decrease in salivary production that leads to thicker mucus and a dry mouth. Interferes with the ability to eat and leads to appetite and nutritional problems.

NEUROLOGICAL

- Peripheral neuropathy: Most commonly associated with diabetes. Other causes include alcoholism, peripheral vascular disease, traumatic injury, medication effects, infections, and immune system diseases. Characterized by symptoms that include numbness and tingling of the affected area and stumbling gait.
- Hemiplegia: Caused by a thrombus, hemorrhage, or embolus affecting a blood vessel leading to or within the brain. Creates altered proprioception with marked incoordination and imbalance. Loss of sensation and motor function in extremities controlled by the affected area of the brain also occurs.

BOX 39.3   EXAMPLES OF MEDICATIONS REPORTED TO CAUSE OTOTOXICITY

ANTIBIOTICS
- Aminoglycosides
- Macrolides
- Vancomycin

SALICYLATES
- Aspirin

NONSTEROIDAL ANTIINFLAMMATORY DRUGS
- Ibuprofen

DIURETICS
- Ethacrynic acid
- Furosemide
- Bumetanide

ANTINEOPLASTIC AGENTS
- Cisplatin
- Carboplatin

From Mudd PA, Meyers AD: *Ototoxicity,* 2016, http://emedicine.medscape.com/article/857679-overview#a1.

adults older than 85 years of age have hearing loss (Touhy and Jett, 2016). In addition, 285 million people are visually impaired, and 39 million are blind worldwide (World Health Organization [WHO], 2014). Older people are at increased risk of several eye diseases including age-related macular degeneration, cataracts, and glaucoma. It is estimated that the number of people older than 60 years of age will increase from 10% to 22% by 2050 (Touhy and Jett, 2016). Therefore it is important as a nurse to understand the impact of sensory alterations, as age-related sensory decline will continue to increase among patients. The loss of major sensory input usually has profound consequences on patients' independence. As a nurse, stay informed of new health care and nursing knowledge as it pertains to the older adult population and the effects of diverse sensory changes.

Vision and hearing alterations affect the function and quality of life of older adults. A loss of sensory input often creates feelings of grief, anger, depression, and loss of self-esteem (Touhy and Jett, 2014). Self-esteem disturbances frequently lead to social isolation and withdrawal from social activities (Meiner, 2015). Patients with dual sensory losses experience less social contact compared with patients with unisensory loss or intact sensory acuity. Interventions to improve social contact in older adults with sensory impairment may lead to improvements in their mental health (Heine and Browning, 2015). Your knowledge about the effects of sensory loss on your patients allows you to promote their healthy aging.

BOX 39.4   EVIDENCE-BASED PRACTICE

PICO Question: Do patients who are critically ill sleep better when a "quiet-time" protocol versus standard care is implemented in an intensive care unit (ICU)?

SUMMARY OF EVIDENCE

Sound levels in the ICU have been found to be consistently above levels recommended by the World Health Organization (Tainter et al., 2016). Excessive noise levels have negative physical and psychological effects on hospitalized patients (Fillary et al., 2015). The number of patients, patient acuity, design of the unit, building ventilation system, and staff and visitor conversations influence noise levels in health care facilities (Konkani et al., 2014). Frequent nursing activities and medical equipment alarms are other noise sources in the ICU. Current evidence supports that implementing protocols that require periods of time during which nurses reduce light and other environmental stimuli is important to critical care patients and nurses (Maidl et al., 2014; Riemer et al., 2015). Quiet-time protocols have been found to promote patient rest, improve the quality of sleep, reduce patient anxiety levels, and reduce stress levels among nurses (Maidl et al., 2014; Riemer et al., 2015; McAndrews et al., 2016). Although it is challenging to create times without distractions in a busy ICU, implementation of a quiet-time protocol can benefit patients.

APPLICATION TO NURSING PRACTICE

- Assess all patients for signs of sensory overload such as anxiety and restlessness.
- Identify sources of noise on the unit such as equipment and machines.
- Develop strategies to reduce noise to an acceptable level.
- Modify your work flow to establish a restful environment for patients to sleep.
- Establish a routine for patient care.
- Collaborate with hospital staff to provide patients with quiet time.
- Educate patients and families about the goal of quiet time to create a peaceful and healing environment.

BOX 39.5   SYNTHESIS IN PRACTICE

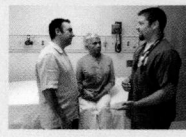

While Peter prepares to assess Mrs. Alicea, he recalls what he has learned about the pathophysiology of eye disorders. He focuses on the "warning signs" of eye problems, determining which, if any, of the signs Mrs. Alicea has experienced. Because Mrs. Alicea reports hearing and visual losses, Peter considers the communication approaches best suited for conducting a successful assessment. He plans to position himself so that Mrs. Alicea is able to see his face clearly. Peter also will speak slowly and enunciate words clearly, giving time for Mrs. Alicea to respond to questions. Avoiding questions answered by "yes" or "no" will require Mrs. Alicea to provide more detailed answers, ensuring that she heard Peter's questions correctly.

Peter respects Mrs. Alicea's cultural background and explores implications for the delivery of culturally sensitive care. Some Mexican-Americans engage in "small talk" when beginning the interview before discussing the serious aspects of the interview because being direct is considered rude and self-disclosure is for people whom the individual knows well (McMurry et al., 2017). It will thus be important for Peter to express caring and respect for Mrs. Alicea and be prepared to provide time for small talk to be successful in gathering a complete assessment. Family is often highly valued and is the main focus of social identification within the Mexican culture (McMurry et al., 2017). Thus Peter plans to determine if Rico is the primary individual who helps Mrs. Alicea complete instrumental activities of daily living (IADLs) and other activities.

Peter's own grandmother has bilateral cataracts. He reflects on how she adjusted to her visual loss to continue activities she enjoys. He learned in class that you can make a variety of adaptations to maximize the sensory functions that a patient still has. Peter plans to discover if Mrs. Alicea has made any adaptations in her home environment. Creativity is an important attitude to exercise.

Managing patients with sensory alterations challenges you to apply nursing research and information from your practice to help patients participate in their environment, remain socially interactive, and continue to be productive. In addition, your application of critical thinking principles helps you promote patients' sensory function and protect them from possible injury (Box 39.4).

CRITICAL THINKING

Synthesis

Patient care requires you to apply what you know about a patient, your knowledge base, experience, and critical thinking attitudes and standards (Box 39.5). Your synthesis of this information allows you to make sound decisions as you apply the nursing process. Critical thinking synthesis involves combining all available information to obtain a clear picture of the approach needed to provide patient-centered care.

Knowledge. A number of factors cause sensory alterations. Knowledge of these factors and of the anatomy and physiology and the normal components of a sensory experience helps you understand how a particular alteration affects a patient's function. Knowing the pathophysiological changes of specific sensory organ disorders also helps you anticipate how sensory changes affect a patient. When you identify characteristics of sensory alterations and the interventions to minimize them, you are able to implement a comprehensive and individualized plan of care.

Depending on a patient's problem, use your knowledge of communication principles (see Chapter 11) to select the best communication method. Patients with hearing impairments require different communication approaches to obtain a complete and accurate nursing assessment and deliver interventions effectively. You also need to have a working knowledge of pharmacology because a variety of medications affect sensory function. Being able to anticipate the side effects of medications allows you to prepare patients for possible sensory changes.

Experience. Many of us have experienced altered sensory function personally or while interacting with family, friends, or patients. Previous personal or clinical experiences with sensory changes help you anticipate a patient's care needs. How do individuals adapt to hearing aids and glasses? What adjustments do they make to function safely in their homes? Which communication techniques are necessary when speaking to individuals with hearing impairment? Such experiences help you choose successful nursing interventions when caring for patients in a variety of health care settings.

Attitudes. Critical thinking attitudes lead you to become a more disciplined thinker. Creativity is often necessary to find the right solutions for your patient's problems. For example, living in a nonstimulating home environment can cause sensory deprivation. Work with your patient to develop changes in the home to improve the quality of stimulation and reduce the patient's risk for injury. Curiosity applies when a patient shows unexplained behavioral changes. Asking why and being curious help you assess a less obvious sensory problem.

Standards. An important ethical standard to follow when assisting patients with sensory alterations is preservation of autonomy (see Chapter 6). For a patient to regain independence, do not override autonomy with the principle of beneficence. Although professionals believe they know what is best, remember patients have to live with the sensory alteration and adapt to the consequences of their own choices. The Joint Commission (TJC), along with the Americans with Disabilities Act (ADA), requires health care institutions to address the needs of patients with sensory alterations and provide interpretation services as necessary to establish understanding and maintain confidentiality (TJC, 2017). Evidence-based standards of care and practice such as standards from the American Academy of Ophthalmology (AAO, 2015) and the American Speech-Language-Hearing Association (ASHA, 2016) provide criteria for screening sensory problems and establishing standards for competent, safe, effective care and practice.

NURSING PROCESS

■ ■ ■ ASSESSMENT

When assessing your patients, consider all factors that influence sensory function. Collect a complete nursing history by examining how a sensory deficit affects your patient's self-concept, lifestyle, self-care ability, psychosocial adjustment, health promotion habits, safety, and ability to communicate

and function in the everyday world. Your assessment also needs to focus on the quality and quantity of stimuli within a patient's environment.

Sensory Status. Include an assessment of the nature and characteristics of sensory alterations in the nursing history (Table 39.1). Assessment categories include the type and extent of sensory impairment, the onset and duration of symptoms, and whether there are factors that aggravate or relieve symptoms. Often you observe such characteristics by watching a patient perform routine activities of daily living (ADLs) in the home or health care setting.

Physical Examination. Patients with known or suspected sensory deficits resulting from visual and hearing losses, spinal cord injury, or peripheral neuropathies require complete and detailed sensory examinations (see Chapter 16). Assessing the extent of sensory loss allows you to focus your review on behaviors of sensory deficits (Table 39.2). If your examination suggests a sensory alteration, observation during history taking, physical examination, or care provides additional information about a person's condition. Observe a patient's physical appearance, measure cognitive ability, and assess emotional stability. At this time also remember that factors other than sensory alterations cause impaired perception (e.g., medications, pain, or electrolyte imbalances).

Patients at Risk. A sensory assessment is a priority for any patient at risk for sensory alterations. Patients at high risk for hearing loss include patients who work in areas with high noise levels such as airports, construction, and farm workers. For patients found to be at risk for noise exposure, encourage them to participate in annual screening and to attend hearing conservation classes. Occupational health nurses perform regular audiometric testing to promote hearing conservation.

A sensory assessment is particularly important for older adults and adults living in a confined environment such as a nursing home or patients who are hospitalized and on protective isolation. Older adults are a high-risk group because of normal physiological changes associated with aging. However, be careful not to automatically assume that a patient's sensory problem is related to advancing age. For example, adult sensorineural hearing loss is often caused by exposure to excess and prolonged noise or metabolic, vascular, and other systemic alterations. Some older patients are unaware of sensory changes or are reluctant to share information for fear of the consequences (Touhy and Jett, 2016). In this case, you may need to gather information from a family caregiver.

Although most nursing homes or centers offer meaningful stimulation through group activities, environmental design, and mealtime gatherings, there are exceptions. Patients isolated in a health care setting or at home because of conditions such as active tuberculosis or severe immune system depression are often isolated in a private room and frequently

TABLE 39.1 FOCUSED PATIENT ASSESSMENT

FACTORS TO ASSESS	QUESTIONS	PHYSICAL ASSESSMENT
Sensory status	Tell me about any problems you have with your ears, hearing, balance, vision, or sensing touch. When did the difficulty begin? Did it begin gradually or suddenly? Is it constant, or does it come and go? How would you describe it? What are your preferences for treatment? If appropriate, would you wear glasses to improve your vision or hearing aids to improve communication?	Assess patient's hearing, balance, vision, and sense of touch (see Chapter 16). Observe patient behaviors during conversation and while watching patient perform IADLs and ADLs.
Self-care management in home and community care settings	For patients with visual alterations: Tell me how you prepare a meal or write a check? For patients with hearing impairments: Is there a certain pitch that you have trouble hearing such as conversation on the telephone or the telephone ringing? For patients with decreased tactile sensation: Tell me how you dress or bathe safely using warm water.	Observe patient in the home, in the kitchen while preparing a meal. Observe patient's ability to communicate effectively. Observe patient during dressing and bathing.
Health promotion practices	Describe for me how you clean your ears. Do you have difficulty caring for your glasses, hearing aids, or contact lenses? Do you wear safety glasses, eye shields, or ear noise protective gear when appropriate?	Observe ear/eye routine care. Find out when patient last had an eye or ear screening. Check for appropriate eye protection with eye shields and safety glasses or face shields.

ADLs, Activities of daily living; *IADLs,* instrumental activities of daily living.

TABLE 39.2 BEHAVIORS INDICATING SENSORY DEFICITS

BEHAVIOR INDICATING DEFICIT (CHILDREN)	BEHAVIOR INDICATING DEFICIT (ADULTS)
Vision Self-stimulation including eye rubbing, body rocking, sniffing, arm twirling; hitching (using legs to propel while in sitting position) instead of crawling	Poor coordination, squinting, underreaching or overreaching for objects, persistent repositioning of objects, impaired night vision, accidental falls
Hearing Frightened when unfamiliar people approach, no reflex or purposeful response to sounds, failure to be awakened by loud noise, slow or absent development of speech, greater response to movement than to sound, avoidance of social interaction with others	Blank looks, decreased attention span, lack of reaction to loud noises, increased volume of speech, positioning head toward sound, smiling and nodding head in approval when someone speaks, using other means of communication such as lip reading or writing, complaints of ringing in ears
Touch Inability to perform developmental tasks related to grasping objects or drawing, repeated injury from handling harmful objects (e.g., hot stove, sharp knife)	Clumsiness, overreaction or underreaction to painful stimulus, failure to respond when touched, avoidance of touch, sensation of pins and needles, numbness
Smell Difficult to assess until child is 6 or 7 years old; difficulty discriminating unpleasant odors	Failure to react to noxious or strong odors, increased body odor, decreased sensitivity to odors
Taste Inability to tell whether food is salty or sweet, possible ingestion of strange-tasting things	Change in appetite, excessive use of seasoning and sugar, complaints about taste of food, weight change
Position Sense Clumsiness, extraneous movement, excessive arm swinging in children with hyperactivity or learning difficulty	Poor balance and spatial orientation, shuffling gait, reduced response to bracing self when falling, more precise and deliberate movements

experience sensory deprivation. Other patients who are immobilized by bed rest, physical impediments (e.g., casts or traction), or chronic disability are unable to experience all the normal sensations of free movement and are at risk for sensory deprivation. Be alert for any behavioral changes common to sensory deprivation.

Hospital environments are full of sensory stimuli. This does not mean that all patients in the hospital experience sensory overload. Carefully assess patients subjected to high stress levels (e.g., intensive care unit [ICU] environment, long-term hospitalization, and multiple therapies). Be aware that patients can have a combination of a sensory deficit and overload simultaneously. For example, a patient in the ICU experiences sensory deficit because the room has no windows but also experiences sensory overload from noise that occurs around the clock at the nurse's station.

Patient's Lifestyle. Learn about a patient's perception of a sensory loss to find out how his or her quality of life has been influenced. Ask patients to describe problems that a sensory alteration creates for their normal daily routines and lifestyle. Does a sensory alteration change your patient's ability to retain social relationships, continue performing at work or school, or function within the home?

Socialization. The amount and quality of contact with family members or friends determines whether a patient with sensory alterations becomes isolated. Assess if a patient lives alone and whether family, friends, or neighbors frequently visit. The absence of visitors to the home or a health care setting creates a sense of monotony that contributes to social isolation. Also assess a patient's involvement in social groups, social skills, and level of satisfaction in the support given by family and friends.

Self-Care Management. A patient's functional ability incorporates ADLs (e.g., grooming, bathing, dressing, toileting) and instrumental activities of daily living (IADLs) (e.g., grocery shopping, yard maintenance, money management, using a phone). If a sensory alteration impairs your patient's functional ability, planning for discharge from a health care setting and providing resources within the home become necessary. Include in your assessment the activities that patients normally do for themselves, how the sensory alteration impairs their functioning, and whether a family caregiver is available for support.

If a patient uses an assistive aid such as glasses or a hearing aid, assess how the patient routinely cleans and stores the device. Does the patient use the proper solutions and store cleaned devices correctly? Have the patient demonstrate cleaning of a device when you are in the home or clinic setting. Some patients are reluctant to wear hearing aids. When patients report that they have hearing aids but do not wear them, investigate potential reasons such as the appearance of the hearing aid, poor fit, difficulty in seeing or working with a small object, and lack of patient knowledge about care and use of the hearing aid. If a patient requires assistance in caring for an aid, assess how well a family caregiver is able to perform this function.

Psychosocial Adjustment. Because some patients are unaware of or unwilling to discuss behavioral changes, family caregivers and friends are often the best resources when determining if sensory changes have altered a patient's behavior. Assess if the patient has shown any recent mood swings such as outbursts of anger, depression, or fear. Does the patient avoid interactions with others? Sensory alterations also often cause changes in orientation and ability to concentrate.

Health Promotion Practices. Assess the daily routines that patients follow in maintaining sensory function including hygiene measures. The information determines a patient's need for education or referral to appropriate resources. Also assess if a patient has routine eye and hearing examinations and when the last examination was completed.

Hazards. Make sure that the home environment is healthy, comfortable, and safe. Information from a home safety assessment, which screens for the presence of risks in rooms and spaces within a home, helps you identify hazards in the patient's living environment. A home safety checklist is usually available in most home care agencies, and the findings will give you options to make the home safe. Assess the home setting including the outdoors and all rooms in the home for hazards that increase the risk for injury (e.g., poorly lit stairs, obstacles in walking paths, uneven sidewalks). The type of sensory alteration makes some home features more hazardous than others. Patients with impaired vision require more light. Patients who are blind often need information written in braille. Patients with hearing deficits sometimes require safety alarms with visual signals. Patients with severe hearing impairments need to have a telecommunication device for the deaf (TDD). The TDD has a keyboard and displays numbers and letters that provide messages from another TDD to the person who has a hearing impairment. The ADA requires any health care agency that receives Medicare funding to have TDDs (Touhy and Jett, 2014).

Assess for any factors in a health care setting that will be dangerous to the patient. Assess a patient's hospital room for clutter, unnecessary equipment, and obstacles in the path leading to the bathroom. Also ask the patient about barriers or obstacles that the patient perceives as potentially dangerous such as wet floors or equipment lines.

Meaningful Stimuli. Meaningful stimuli reduce the incidence of sensory deprivation. In the home check for the use of bright colors, comfortable furnishings, adequate lighting, good ventilation, and clean surroundings. Also observe for the presence of pets, family pictures, television, a clock, or a calendar. Note if patients have roommates, visitors, or any personal items such as pictures. A patient becomes disoriented in a barren environment that gives few signals for normal sensory perception. Meaningful stimuli influence the patient's alertness and the ability to participate in self-care.

Environmental Stimuli. Excessive environmental stimuli cause sensory overload. In an acute care setting the frequency of observations, tests, and procedures is often stressful to a patient. Assess the location of a patient's room. If it is near repetitive or loud noises (e.g., nurses' station or supply room), the patient is at risk for sensory overload. In addition, explore for the presence of a loud television, a talkative roommate or one with multiple visitors, or a bright room light as possible contributing factors. Patients who are in pain, traction, or restricted by a cast are at risk for excessive stimulation. Your responsibility as a nurse is to identify, reduce, or eliminate excessive stimuli.

Communication Methods. Assess if patients have trouble speaking, understanding, reading, or writing to understand the quality of their communication. Next, ask patients which communication method they prefer. Patients with existing sensory deficits often develop alternative ways of communicating. Some patients with hearing impairments read lips, use sign language, wear a hearing aid, or read and write notes. Patients with visual impairments learn to detect voice tones and inflections to identify the emotional tone of a conversation. To assess communication methods, sit facing the patient, speaking in a normal tone. Disorganized speech, a long period of silence, or a patient who continually asks you to repeat your sentences indicates a sensory deficit. Some patients also show signs and symptoms of confusion or respond in an inappropriate manner because of their hearing impairment.

Patient Expectations. When conducting an assessment, review a patient's expressed needs and expectations. Many patients have a definite plan as to how they want their care delivered. Some expect you to provide equipment for them so that they can properly care for their eyeglasses or hearing aids. Asking patients what they expect helps you to initiate effective strategies and provide access to resources. Eliciting patient values and preferences is also an essential skill of patient-centered care (Box 39.6). Some patients request that family members or friends help with their care. Begin by asking, "What do you expect from the nursing staff to feel that you are receiving good care?" and "Now that I better understand what affects your ability to see/hear, what do you expect in the care that we will be providing for you?"

■ ■ ■ NURSING DIAGNOSIS

After assessment, review all available data and look critically for patterns of risk factors and defining characteristics that suggest a health problem relating to sensory alterations. For example, defining characteristics of the problem-focused diagnosis *Social Isolation* include seeking to be alone; being uncommunicative; verbalization or observation of discomfort in social situations; and a sad, dull affect. Validate your findings to ensure accuracy of the diagnosis. Examples of nursing diagnoses that apply to patients with sensory alterations include the following:

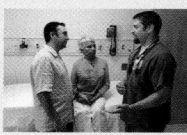

⊕ BOX 39.6 PATIENT-CENTERED CARE

Peter is aware that people who are from a Hispanic/Latino culture are the largest minority group in the United States. However, he is uncertain if disparities in sensory alteration exist across ethnicities. Therefore before he meets with Mrs. Alicea on his next clinical day, he takes some time to read about the incidence of sensory alterations in different ethnic groups in the United States.

Peter learns that although visual disabilities occur in people of all ethnic groups, by 2050 the highest prevalence of visual impairment will be in the Hispanic/Latino population (Varma et al., 2016). Visual field loss has a negative impact on health-related quality of life (Crews et al., 2014). Peter uses this information to develop a patient-centered plan of care that focuses on Mrs. Alicea's visual impairment.

IMPLICATIONS FOR PRACTICE
- Assess what Mrs. Alicea already knows about her condition.
- Ask Mrs. Alicea, "What questions do you have about your condition?"
- Encourage Mrs. Alicea to discuss the effect of her visual impairment on her health-related quality of life.
- Ask Mrs. Alicea how she is coping with visual alterations.
- Ask Mrs. Alicea about her social networks and supportive relationships.
- Elicit and respect Mrs. Alicea's preferences in her plan of care.
- Ask Mrs. Alicea to teach back or demonstrate what was taught.

- *Anxiety*
- *Fear*
- *Impaired Physical Mobility*
- *Risk for Injury*
- *Deficient Knowledge*
- *Impaired Social Interaction*
- *Bathing Self-Care Deficit*
- *Risk for Falls*

When a problem-focused diagnosis has been identified, determine the related factor that likely is associated with the patient's health problem. The etiology or "related to" factor of a problem-focused nursing diagnosis needs to be accurate to ensure that you select appropriate interventions. For example, if impacted cerumen is the cause of a patient's hearing alteration, following a protocol for cerumen removal improves auditory perception (Touhy and Jett, 2014). If a patient's auditory alteration is related to altered sensory reception from nerve deafness, nursing interventions of alternative communication methods are more successful in minimizing the patient's hearing impairment. When a risk diagnosis has been identified, be sure you have identified the risk factors for which you can intervene.

■ ■ ■ PLANNING

Patients with sensory alterations have many needs (Fig. 39.1). The plan of care you develop depends on your assessment of a patient's sensory status, perception and acceptance of the sensory alteration, and how well the patient has adjusted to the loss (see Care Plan).

Goals and Outcomes. During planning develop an individualized plan of care incorporating each nursing diagnosis. Partner with your patient to develop a realistic plan that incorporates what you know about the patient's sensory problems and the extent to which the patient can maintain or improve sensory function. Make sure that goals not only meet a patient's immediate needs but also strive toward

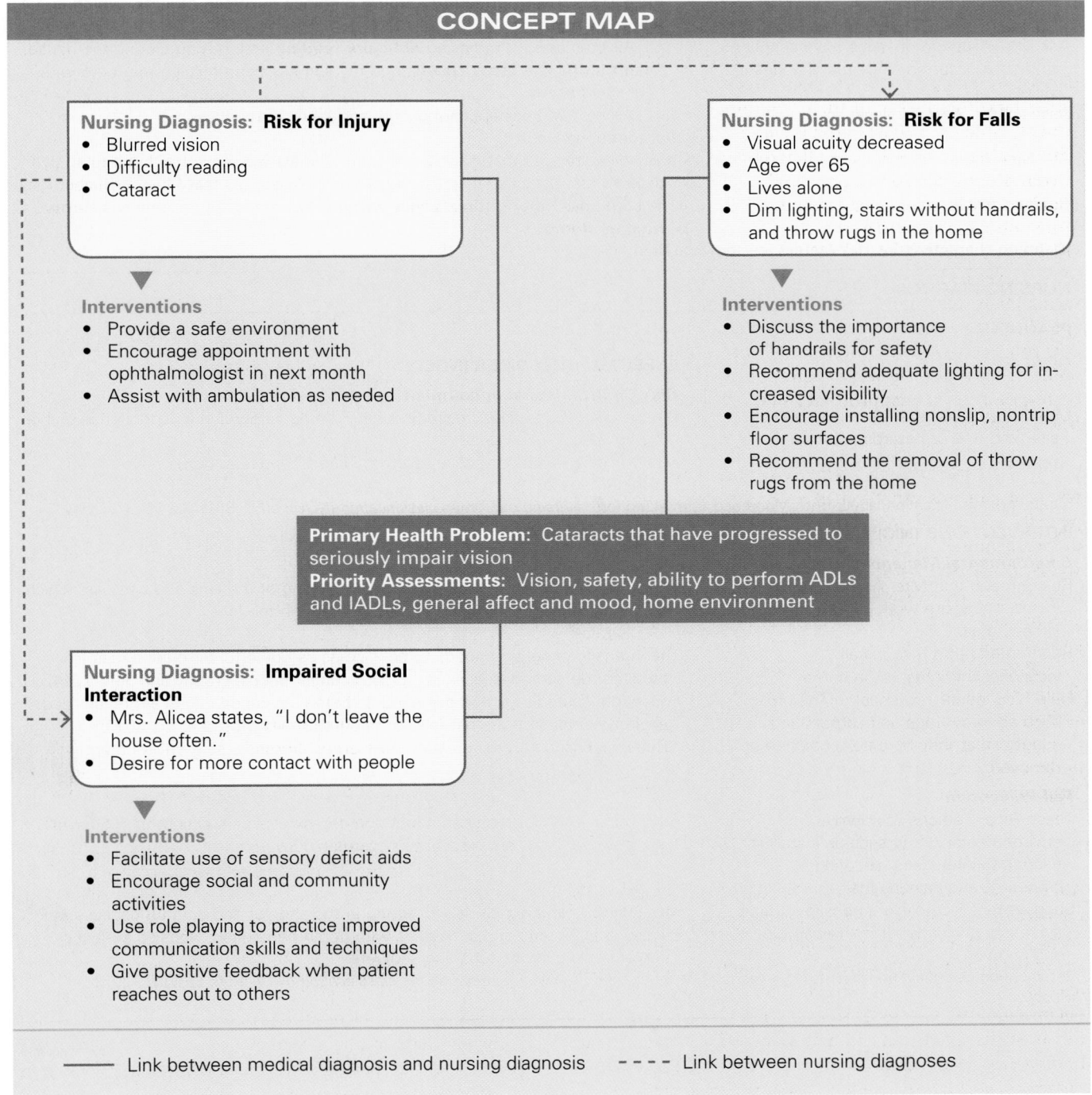

CONCEPT MAP

Nursing Diagnosis: Risk for Injury
- Blurred vision
- Difficulty reading
- Cataract

Interventions
- Provide a safe environment
- Encourage appointment with ophthalmologist in next month
- Assist with ambulation as needed

Nursing Diagnosis: Risk for Falls
- Visual acuity decreased
- Age over 65
- Lives alone
- Dim lighting, stairs without handrails, and throw rugs in the home

Interventions
- Discuss the importance of handrails for safety
- Recommend adequate lighting for increased visibility
- Encourage installing nonslip, nontrip floor surfaces
- Recommend the removal of throw rugs from the home

Primary Health Problem: Cataracts that have progressed to seriously impair vision
Priority Assessments: Vision, safety, ability to perform ADLs and IADLs, general affect and mood, home environment

Nursing Diagnosis: Impaired Social Interaction
- Mrs. Alicea states, "I don't leave the house often."
- Desire for more contact with people

Interventions
- Facilitate use of sensory deficit aids
- Encourage social and community activities
- Use role playing to practice improved communication skills and techniques
- Give positive feedback when patient reaches out to others

——— Link between medical diagnosis and nursing diagnosis   - - - - Link between nursing diagnoses

FIG 39.1 Concept map. *ADLs,* Activities of daily living; *IADLs,* instrumental activities of daily living.

◎ CARE PLAN

Risk for Injury

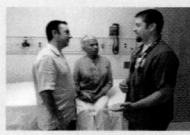

ASSESSMENT

Mrs. Alicea comes to the clinic reporting "having trouble seeing." Peter notes that Mrs. Alicea appears unsteady when standing. He knows that people with vision impairments are at risk for impaired balance and slow reaction time, contributing to a greater fall risk. Peter plans to assess Mrs. Alicea's changes in vision more closely to identify interventions to decrease her risk for injury.

ASSESSMENT ACTIVITIES	FINDINGS[a]
Ask Mrs. Alicea to describe her vision changes.	Mrs. Alicea states, "When I try to read or sew, my **vision is blurred,** even with my glasses. I have **difficulty judging distance between objects, which is worse at night.**"
Ask Mrs. Alicea to describe any changes that have occurred since the changes in vision.	Mrs. Alicea states, "I'm having **difficulty reading** and moving around the house. **I can't judge the steps clearly,** and my son has been helping me more with household chores."
Assess Mrs. Alicea's visual acuity.	Mrs. Alicea's corneas appear opaque, and there is a reduction in accommodation.
Ask Mrs. Alicea the results of her last visit with the ophthalmologist.	Mrs. Alicea reports that it has been about 2 years since she has been to an eye doctor. Mrs. Alicea states, "At my last visit, I was told that I had a cataract."
Conduct a home hazard assessment.	The home has **dim lighting, stairs without handrails,** and **numerous throw rugs on floors.**

[a]**Defining characteristics/risk factors** are shown in **bold** type.

NURSING DIAGNOSIS: Risk for injury

PLANNING

GOAL	EXPECTED OUTCOMES (NOC)[b]
	Risk Control: Visual Impairment
Mrs. Alicea's home environment will be safe and free of hazards within 4 weeks.	Mrs. Alicea reports an increased sense of home safety and independence within 2 weeks.
	Mrs. Alicea and her son make recommended changes to home environment within 4 weeks.

[b]Outcomes classification labels from Moorhead S, et al, editors: *Nursing outcomes classification (NOC),* ed 5, St Louis, 2013, Mosby.

INTERVENTIONS (NIC)[c]	RATIONALE
Environmental Management: Safety	
Recommend that Mrs. Alicea's son Rico install a nonglare work surface in the kitchen area.	Sensitivity to glare increases because of clouding of the lens and vitreous, which results in scattering of light that passes through the lens.
Recommend that Rico install incandescent lights in the home.	The intensity of lighting needs to be 3 times as powerful for older adults to produce the same visual acuity as for younger people (Touhy and Jett, 2014).
Help Rico identify potential trip hazards such as throw rugs and carpets and suggest that they be either modified or removed.	Loose, unsecured rugs and damaged carpets with curled edges are recognized environmental hazards that may contribute to falls (Rosen et al., 2013). Removal of trip hazards prevents falls and promotes a safe environment.
Fall Prevention	
Teach Rico methods to improve environmental safety such as installing handrails along stairs, securing carpeting, and painting stairs.	A decrease in visual acuity and depth perception places a patient at risk for falls in the presence of environmental hazards (Touhy and Jett, 2016).
Suggest that Rico place a nonslip surface such as a nonskid mat in the bathtub and shower.	Mrs. Alicea is at a higher risk for falling in the shower and bathtub because of visual impairments and difficulties with depth perception. Nonskid surfaces prevent falling in bathtubs and showers.

[c]Intervention classification labels from Bulechek GM, et al, editors: *Nursing interventions classification (NIC),* ed 6, St Louis, 2013, Mosby.

◎ **CARE PLAN—cont'd**

Risk for Injury

EVALUATION

NURSING ACTIONS	PATIENT RESPONSE/FINDING	ACHIEVEMENT OF OUTCOME
During her next visit to the health center, ask Mrs. Alicea if she has experienced any trips or falls since modifications to her home were made. Ask Rico if his mother is having any difficulties moving through her home.	Mrs. Alicea states that she has not fallen or tripped since Rico made the suggested modifications to her home. Rico states his mother is able to walk through her home with a steady, purposeful gait.	Outcome met.
Conduct a home visit and reassess the home environment.	Rico has changed all light bulbs in the halls and stairways. He removed all throw rugs and painted edges of stairs bright white. Kitchen work surface has not changed yet.	Home environment has improved. Rico needs help identifying contractors to help him change the work surface in the kitchen to decrease glare.

---

rehabilitation. Goals and outcomes need to be realistic and measurable. Some sensory alterations are short term, requiring only temporary interventions. Permanent sensory alterations require long-term goals, with a series of outcomes that the patient reaches over time. For example, if a patient sustains an injury causing blindness, the long-term goal of "managing self-care within the home" requires numerous short-term outcomes and outcomes that show progressive advancement. Examples of such outcomes include "Patient ambulates safely within the home in 2 weeks" and "Patient performs ADLs with minimal assistance within 4 weeks."

Setting Priorities. You determine the type and extent of sensory alteration affecting a patient when determining priorities of care. The patient also helps prioritize aspects of care. Generally you rank diagnoses and the nursing interventions you select in order of importance based on a patient's safety, personal desires, and needs. For example, making plans for a patient's *Risk for Injury* may be an initial priority over the diagnosis of *Social Isolation*. When setting priorities, safety is always a top priority. Sometimes it becomes necessary for a patient to make major changes in self-care activities, communication, and socialization. Helping patients learn about ways to communicate more effectively or use adaptive equipment promotes safety and allows patients to participate in favorite activities.

Collaborative Care. Review all resources available to patients when you develop a plan of care and make appropriate referrals to other health care professionals. Referrals to occupational therapist, speech-language pathologist, and social services ensure a multidisciplinary approach. Referral to home care is another option. The family plays a key role in providing meaningful stimulation and learning ways to help a patient adjust to limitations when the patient returns home. Teach hospitalized patients and their families how to adapt interventions to their lifestyles. Community resources such as the American Foundation for the Blind, the American Red Cross, and the Lions Club provide information to help patients and families with discharge planning and home needs.

■■■ **IMPLEMENTATION**

Collaborate with your patients and their family members to develop interventions that allow a patient to maintain a safe, pleasant, and stimulating sensory environment. Effective interventions help a patient with sensory alterations function safely with existing deficits and continue a normal lifestyle.

Health Promotion. Good sensory function begins with promoting the health of sensory organs and maximizing existing sensory function. When a patient seeks health care, provide interventions that reduce risk for sensory losses. Also recommend relevant visual and hearing guidelines.

Screening and Prevention. Preventable blindness is a worldwide health issue that begins with children and requires appropriate screening. Four recommended interventions are (1) screening for rubella, syphilis, chlamydia, and gonorrhea in women who are considering pregnancy; (2) advocating adequate prenatal care to prevent premature birth (with the danger of exposure of the infant to excessive oxygen); (3) administering eye prophylaxis in the form of erythromycin ointment approximately 1 hour after an infant's birth; and (4) periodic screening of all children, especially newborns through preschoolers, for congenital blindness and visual impairment caused by refractive errors and strabismus (Hockenberry and Wilson, 2015).

The most common visual problem during childhood is a refractive error such as nearsightedness. A school nurse is usually responsible for vision testing of school-age and adolescent children and has the role of detection, education, and referral. Parents need to know the signs of visual impairment in the infant such as failure to react to light and reduced eye contact. Instruct parents to report signs of visual impairment to their health care provider. Trauma from flying or penetrating objects is a common cause of blindness in children. Parents and children need education about ways to avoid eye trauma such as avoiding use of toys with long, pointed projections and instructing children not to run while carrying pointed objects. Instruct patients that they can find safety equipment in sports and department stores.

Adults also need routine visual screenings. If left undetected and untreated, glaucoma leads to permanent visual loss. The AAO (2015) recommends that individuals at any age with symptoms of eye disease or individuals at risk for eye disease (such as individuals with a family history of eye disease, diabetes, or high blood pressure) see an ophthalmologist to determine how frequently their eyes should be examined. In the absence of symptoms or risk factors for disease, the AAO recommends a baseline eye examination at 40 years of age. Follow-up examinations are based on risk factors for disease and the results of the initial screening. Adults 65 years of age and older need examinations every 1 to 2 years (AAO, 2015). Individuals of African American and Hispanic descent need close follow-up because they are at risk for an earlier onset, higher incidence, and more rapid progression of glaucoma.

Hearing impairment is one of the most common disabilities in the United States. At-risk children include children with a family history of childhood hearing impairment, perinatal infection (rubella, herpes, or cytomegalovirus), low birth weight, chronic ear infections, and Down syndrome. Advise pregnant women of the importance of early prenatal care, avoidance of ototoxic drugs, and testing for syphilis and rubella.

Chronic middle ear infections are also a common cause of hearing impairment in children. Children who have frequent ear infections need periodic auditory testing. Warn parents of the risk and encourage them to seek medical care when their child has symptoms of an earache or respiratory infection. Exposure to loud noise is common for children and young adults who use cellular phones and music players routinely. Advise both children and parents to use earplugs or earphones to block high-decibel sounds.

The ASHA (2016) recommends that adults have hearing screenings at least every decade through 50 years of age and every 3 years thereafter. Once a patient reports a hearing loss, regular testing also becomes necessary.

Managing Environmental Hazards. Occupational hearing loss is one of the most common work-related illnesses in the United States and results in about 22 million U.S. workers being exposed to hazardous noise levels at work (Centers for Disease Control and Prevention [CDC], 2016). Occupational safety and health professionals use the Hierarchy of Control to determine how to implement feasible and effective controls in a work environment. For example, eliminating noise is the most effective step, but if this is not possible, buying quiet equipment and tools and isolating workers from noise hazards are environmental control measures (CDC, 2016). Advise adults who work in high-risk occupational areas to follow work site safety guidelines and wear hearing protectors.

The CDC (2013) reported that each day about 2000 U.S. workers sustain a job-related eye injury that requires medical treatment. About one-third of the injuries are treated in hospital emergency departments, and more than 100 of these injuries result in 1 or more days away from work (CDC, 2013). Adults are also at risk for eye injury while playing sports. Eye injuries occur from striking or scraping the eye, injury from penetrating objects, and chemical or thermal burns. As a nurse, encourage patients at risk for injury to wear eye protection such as goggles, face shields, safety glasses, or full face respirators. The Occupational Safety and Health Administration (OSHA, n.d.) has guidelines for workplace safety.

Use of Assistive Aids. Patients with sensory deficits often wear corrective lenses, eyeglasses, or hearing aids and need to keep them accessible, functional, and clean (see Box 31.15 in Chapter 31). Sometimes a family caregiver or friend also needs to know how to clean and care for the assistive aids. Reinforce proper lens and hearing aid care in any health maintenance discussions. Patients who wear contact lenses who do not clean their lenses appropriately, use contaminated lens storage cases or contact lens solutions, or use homemade saline are at risk for serious eye infections. Reinforce proper lens care and how this prevents infection. Patient education about prevention and treatment of diseases affecting vision and hearing, available social services, assistive devices, and the need for annual physical examinations helps provide a patient with better coping abilities and health maintenance.

A wide variety of cosmetically acceptable hearing aids is currently available. Patients often need encouragement and support to explore the assistive device best suited to their unique needs. Because hearing aids are expensive, explore potential financial resources with your patients. Offer patients printed information on hearing loss, the benefits of hearing aid use, and how to use the hearing aid (Meiner, 2015). Family members or friends who support the use of the aid often positively influence the patient to use the aid as instructed. When a patient has a new hearing aid, provide adequate education. Patients usually begin wearing the hearing aid for 15 to 20 minutes and gradually increase the time until they can wear it for 10 to 12 hours. If your patient is having problems tolerating a hearing aid, refer the patient to an audiologist and suggest that he or she explore other types of hearing aids.

Promoting Meaningful Stimulation. You help patients make their environments more stimulating by making adaptations that incorporate the normal physiological changes that accompany sensory deficits (Box 39.7). For example, as patients age, their pupils lose the ability to adjust, creating a sensitivity to glare. You reduce this sensitivity by recommending that family members install nonglare surfaces in the home.

Some patients experience reduced tactile sensations in a limited portion of their body. Touch therapy helps to stimulate existing function. If the patient is willing to be touched, hair brushing and combing, a backrub, passive range of motion, and touching the arms or shoulders increase tactile contact. Turning and positioning also improve the quality of tactile sensation.

BOX 39.7 PROMOTING SENSORY STIMULATION

- Reduce glare by eliminating waxed floors and shiny surfaces exposed to bright sunlight, installing tinted glass or sheer curtains over large windows, and using soft and diffused lighting.
- Teach use of assistive devices to improve visual acuity (e.g., pocket magnifiers, telescopic-lens eyeglasses, large-print books, clocks and watches with large numbers).
- Recommend introducing brighter colors (e.g., red, orange, yellow) into the home environment so patients are able to differentiate between surfaces and room objects.
- Explain how to maximize hearing reception or minimize effects of hearing loss by increasing amplification on televisions or radios and playing recorded music in low-frequency sound.
- Promote sense of taste through good oral hygiene, serving well-seasoned and differently textured foods, chewing food thoroughly, and avoiding blending or mixing foods.
- Enhance the sense of smell by removing unpleasant odors from the environment and introducing pleasant smells such as mild room deodorizers or fragrant flowers.

QSEN QSEN ACTIVITY *Safety*

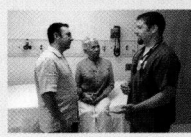

At the end of his clinical day Peter is leaving the senior health center when he observes a loose throw rug at the top of the stairway at the entrance. Peter discussed home safety interventions with Mrs. Alicea; however, he is concerned about environmental modifications needed to make the senior health center safer for patients with sensory deficits. Peter considers who he should talk to and whether his actions will make a difference. He decides to communicate his observations and concerns to his nursing instructor. Together they complete an environmental risk assessment, outline a plan to create a safer senior health center, and communicate their observations and strategies to the health care team.

- Did Peter display the knowledge, skills, and attitudes of what it means to be a competent nurse? Explain your answer. How did Peter's critical thinking attitude affect patient safety?

evolve Answers to QSEN Activities can be found on the Evolve website.

Establishing Safe Environments. Patients become less secure within their home and workplace when they have a sensory alteration. Make recommendations for improving safety within a patient's living environment without restricting independence. The nature of an actual or potential sensory loss determines the necessary safety precautions. Security is necessary for a person to feel independent. Inform patients that organizing informal network agreements with neighbors often have a positive effect on home safety and security concerns (Touhy and Jett, 2016).

Visual Adaptations. Safety is a concern when patients experience decreases in visual acuity, peripheral vision, adaptation to the dark, or depth perception. With reduced peripheral vision a patient cannot see panoramically because the outer visual field is less discrete. With reduced depth perception, a person is unable to judge how far away objects are located. This is a special danger when the patient walks down stairs or over uneven surfaces. Have patients or family caregivers remove clutter such as footstools or electrical cords. Encourage the installation of thresholds over uneven floor surfaces between rooms. Rearrange furniture to allow a patient to move about more easily without fear of tripping or running into objects. Make sure that all flooring in a patient's home is in good repair, and be sure to remove all throw rugs. Stairwells need to be well lighted, and securely fastened handrails extending the full length of both sides of the stairs are preferred.

Front and back entrances to the home and work areas need good lighting. Light fixtures need high-wattage bulbs with wider illumination. A light switch located at the top and bottom of stairwells is an additional safety element. Have the patient replace fluorescent lighting with incandescent lights.

Driving is a particular safety hazard for patients with visual alterations. A sensitivity to glare creates a problem for driving at night with headlights. Reduced peripheral vision prevents a driver from seeing cars in the next lane. Reduced vision, a decrease in reaction time, reduced hearing, and decreased strength in the legs and arms frequently limit older adults' driving skills. To minimize risk, encourage older patients to drive only in familiar areas and not during rush hour. Urge older adults to drive defensively and avoid driving at night or at dusk. Older adults need to drive slowly but not so slowly that they create a safety hazard for other drivers.

Some patients have problems seeing dials or controls on electrical appliances and equipment. Use color contrasts such as tape, paint, or fingernail enamel to highlight dials. Have patients describe their usual daily activities to find opportunities for color coding to prevent accidents related to visual impairments.

Hearing Adaptations. Individuals need to hear environmental sounds such as fire alarms, alarm clocks, phones, or doorbells. Change or amplify the sound of these devices to a more low-pitched, buzzerlike quality. Signaling devices such as a flashing light on a phone allow patients with hearing impairments greater independence. Lamps designed to turn on in response to sounds such as doorbells, burglar alarms, smoke detectors, and babies crying are also available. Advise family and friends who call the patient regularly to let the phone ring for a longer period.

Smell and Tactile Adaptations. The patient with a reduced sensitivity to odors is often unable to smell leaking gas, a smoldering cigarette, fire, or tainted food. Encourage the patient to use smoke detectors and take precautions such as checking ashtrays or placing cigarette butts in water. Also advise the patient to check food package dates and inspect the appearance of food. Patients with reduced tactile sensation need to use hot and cold applications (see Chapter 38) cautiously and *never* use a high setting. Make sure that the temperature on the home water heater is no higher than 120° F. With reduced tactile sensation to the feet, inform patients to wear shoes at all times to protect the feet from injury.

Communication. It is important for individuals to be able to interact with people around them. The type of sensory loss influences the methods and styles of communication you use during interactions with patients. Some patients with hearing impairments are able to speak normally. To communicate clearly with patients who have hearing impairments, family and friends need to learn to move away from background noise, rephrase rather than repeat sentences, be positive, and have patience. Some patients who are deaf have serious speech alterations. Patients who are deaf use sign language, read lips, write with pad and pencil, or use a computer for communication (Box 39.8).

Acute Care. Some patients are hospitalized to treat sensory deficits (e.g., acute eye infection), and some have preexisting sensory problems. You need to know a patient's health history to appropriately support self-care activities while promoting a safe environment.

Orientation to the Environment. Completely orient patients with sensory impairments to the immediate health care environment. Always keep your name tag visible, address the patient by name, explain the patient's location, and frequently include the time and date in conversations. Reduce the tendency for patients to become confused by offering short and simple, repeated explanations and reassurance. Encourage family and friends not to argue with or contradict a confused patient but to explain calmly their location, identity, and time of day.

Patients with serious visual impairments need to feel comfortable knowing the boundaries of their environment. Have a patient walk through a room and feel the walls to establish a sense of direction. Remember to approach a patient who is blind from the front. Explain the location of objects within the room such as chairs or equipment. It is important to keep all objects in the same place and position. Moving an object even a short distance creates a safety hazard. Reorient the patient frequently by describing the location of key items. Place necessary objects such as the nurse call system, patient-controlled analgesia (PCA) button, glasses, water, or facial tissue in front of patients to prevent falls caused by reaching. Ask a patient how he or she prefers to arrange objects so that ambulation is easier. Remove clutter and unnecessary equipment. Always keep the path to the bathroom clear.

Safety Measures. Help patients with acute visual impairments walk (Fig. 39.2). Stand on the patient's dominant, stronger, or uninjured side. The patient grasps your elbow or upper arm. You then walk one-half step ahead and slightly to the patient's side. The patient's shoulder is directly behind your shoulder. Relax and walk at a comfortable pace. Warn the patient when approaching doorways and tell him or her

whether the door opens in or out. Do not leave a patient with visual impairment alone in an unfamiliar area. If the patient has unstable mobility, use a gait belt during walking (see Chapter 28).

Communication. Strategies to enhance communication include providing adequate lighting and rearranging furniture or a mobile computer so that you can face a patient while talking. When communicating with patients, actively listen and provide adequate time for patients with sensory

---

BOX 39.8 PATIENT TEACHING

Communication Strategies for Interacting With Patients Who Have Hearing Impairments

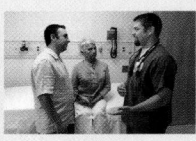 Rico tells Peter that he is concerned about communicating with his mother now that she has both hearing and vision deficits. Peter understands that hearing impairment is a debilitating problem for many older adults; however, interventions by health care providers, family, and friends help patients maintain communication. Peter investigates strategies for interacting with patients who have dual impairments. Using this information, he develops the following teaching plan for Rico.

OUTCOME

At the end of the teaching session, Rico verbalizes four strategies that he can use to improve communication with his mother.

TEACHING STRATEGIES

- Explain to Rico that he needs to speak clearly and use face-to-face communication throughout the interaction (Contrera et al., 2016).
- Inform Rico to speak at a reasonable speed and not to shout (NIDCD, 2016).
- Inform Rico to watch his mother's facial expressions or gestures to help him understand her better (NIDCD, 2016).
- Explain to Rico that he should rephrase a misheard statement rather than repeat it (Contrera et al., 2016).
- Teach Rico to make sure that his mother's hearing aids are in place and she is wearing her glasses when needed (Touhy and Jett, 2014).
- Tell Rico to pause between sentences or phrases to confirm understanding (Touhy and Jett, 2014).
- Tell Rico that he should be patient and stay positive and relaxed (National Institute on Deafness and Other Communication Disorders, 2016).
- Explain to Rico that his mother will hear more clearly when background noise is minimized or eliminated (Contrera et al., 2016).

EVALUATION

- Use the principles of teach-back to evaluate patient/family caregiver learning:
  - "I want to be sure you understand the ways to talk with your mother so that she can understand you. Tell me three ways to talk with your mother so that she hears you clearly."

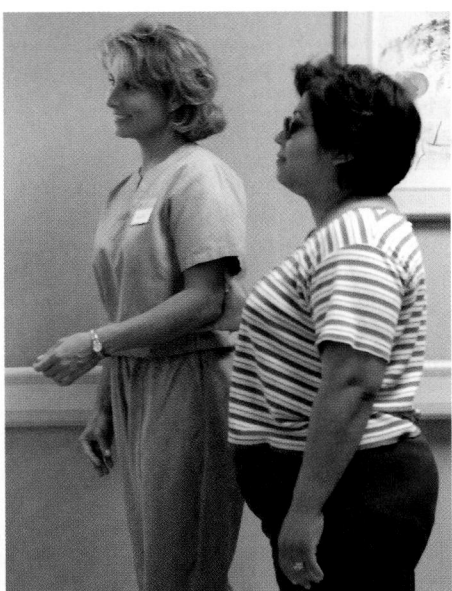

FIG 39.2 A nurse assists a patient with a visual impairment ambulate. (From Sorrentino SA, Remmert LN: *Mosby's textbook for nursing assistants,* ed 8, St Louis, 2012, Mosby.)

BOX 39.9 INTRODUCING STIMULI INTO THE CARE SETTING

VISUAL
- Open the drapes to the patient's room.
- Raise the head of the bed and draw back dividing curtains or partitions.
- Provide attractive decorations on tables or cabinets such as fresh flowers, plants, a picture, or greeting cards.
- Provide audiobooks and large-print reading material.

AUDITORY
- Sit down and speak with the patient. Make the conversation meaningful.
- Turn on a radio with the type of music the patient enjoys. A favorite radio or television program is stimulating.

TASTE AND SMELL
- Provide attractive, taste-appealing meals. Be sure that tableware and glasses are clean. Make sure that warm foods are served warm and cold foods are served cold.
- Provide a variety of textures, aromas, and flavors to enhance the patient's appetite.

---

deficits to respond (Touhy and Jett, 2014). Alert the entire multidisciplinary team when a patient has a sensory alteration. Report the most effective way to communicate with the patient in the patient's medical record.

Controlling Sensory Stimuli. Patients need time for rest and freedom from stress caused by frequent monitoring and repeated tests. Reduce sensory overload by organizing the plan of care to control for excessive stimuli. Combining activities such as dressing changes, bathing, and vital sign assessment in one visit prevents a patient from becoming overly fatigued. Coordination with other departments reduces the time needed for tests and examinations. A patient needs time for rest and quiet. Perform routine nursing procedures as quietly as possible. Encourage a family member to sit quietly with a patient or involve the family member in an undemanding repetitive activity such as combing hair.

Try to control extraneous noise in and around a patient's room such as television volume and visitors. Turn off bedside equipment not in use. Close a patient's room door if necessary. Hospital staff need to control loud laughter or conversation at the nurses' station. In addition to controlling excess stimuli, try to introduce meaningful stimulation that makes the environment pleasing and comfortable (Box 39.9).

Restorative and Continuing Care. After patients have experienced a sensory loss, they need to adjust to continue a normal lifestyle. Many of the interventions previously discussed under health promotion are adaptable for the home setting. Similar to the health care environment, the home environment needs to be healthy, comfortable, and safe. Use data from your assessment of home setting hazards to suggest changes in a person's home environment.

Promoting Self-Care. Patients who have had surgery related to a sensory deficit need a plan of care that allows them to return safely to their home environment. Most patients have same-day surgical procedures (see Chapter 40). Family members or friends need to understand how the patient's sensory impairment affects the ability to perform ADLs and IADLs and the factors that lessen or worsen sensory problems. IADLs require a higher level of cognitive and physical functioning than ADLs (Touhy and Jett, 2016). Community resources discussed in the planning section are useful.

Patients with sensory impairments are often able to continue independent self-care activities. For meals you arrange food on the plate and condiments, salad, or drinks around the plate according to numbers on the face of a clock (Fig. 39.3). The patient becomes oriented to the items after the family member explains the location of each. Patients need help to arrange self-care items such as clothing, hygiene, food supplies, and utensils in a consistent location to continue managing daily care activities.

A patient with visual impairments also needs help to reach the bathroom safely. Safety bars need to be installed near the toilet. A bar that is a different color from the wall is easier to see. Never allow patients to place towels on safety bars because this interferes with a person's grasp.

If tactile sense is decreased, zippers or Velcro strips, pullover sweaters or blouses, and elasticized waists are easier for a patient to use. If a patient has a partial paralysis, you dress the affected side first. Some patients also need assistance with basic grooming such as brushing, combing, shaving, and shampooing hair. Make referrals to and collaborate with physical and/or occupational therapy to ensure that patients are able to function at an optimal level.

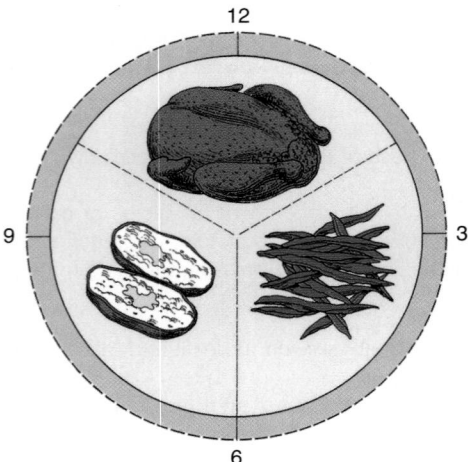

FIG 39.3 Arrange food on a plate and orient patient to placement based on numbers on a clock face.

BOX 39.10 CARE OF THE OLDER ADULT

Therapies to Reduce Loneliness

- Spend time with a person in silence or conversation.
- When it is acceptable to a patient, use physical contact such as holding a hand or embracing a shoulder to convey caring.
- Help older adults maintain contact with people important to them.
- Recommend alterations in living arrangements if physical isolation is a factor.
- Provide information about support groups or groups that provide assistive services.
- Link a person with organizations attuned to the social needs of older adults.
- Introduce the idea of bringing a companion such as a pet into the home when appropriate.

Socialization. Interacting with others becomes a burden for many patients with vision and hearing impairments. A patient with a hearing loss sometimes becomes embarrassed and exhausted after asking people to continuously repeat what they say. Patients often lose the motivation to engage in social activities, resulting in a deep sense of loneliness. Introduce therapies to reduce loneliness, particularly in older adults (Box 39.10). Family members need to learn to focus on a person's ability rather than his or her disability. Never assume that a person with a hearing or visual impairment does not wish to speak.

◼◼◼◼ EVALUATION

Patient Outcomes. It is important to evaluate whether care measures maintain or improve a patient's ability to interact and function within the environment (Box 39.11 and see Care Plan). The patient is the source for evaluating outcomes. The nature of a patient's sensory alterations influences how you evaluate the outcome of care. When caring for a patient with a hearing deficit, use proper communication techniques

---

BOX 39.11 EVALUATION

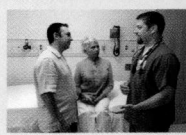 One month has passed since Mrs. Alicea's last visit to the senior health care center. Today Peter sits down and talks with both Mrs. Alicea and Rico. He learns that Mrs. Alicea is no longer having problems with glare because Rico changed the lights in the house to incandescent bulbs. Rico also reports that he plans to install sheer curtains that Mrs. Alicea chose last week in the living room. Mrs. Alicea also tells Peter that Rico has made a "few changes around the house" including rearranging furniture, securing some throw rugs while removing others, and removing the extension cords. After purchasing a magnifier at a local drug store, Mrs. Alicea is able to read the newspaper and medication labels more easily.

On examination Mrs. Alicea's visual acuity continues to reveal blurring when she tries to read an informational pamphlet. Her pupils continue to respond slowly to accommodation. Peter asks if she has made an appointment with her ophthalmologist. She confirms that the appointment is within the next 2 weeks.

Mrs. Alicea confides, "Overall I think the ideas we talked about last time helped me. I feel a little better about getting around the house and doing the things I like to do." When asked if he has noticed any changes in his mother's actions, Rico states, "She seems less fearful of falling."

DOCUMENTATION NOTE

"Visited clinic this morning as scheduled. Implemented measures at home to improve visual acuity and sensitivity to glare. Son supportive in making necessary home environment changes. Plans to make additional changes. Appointment with ophthalmologist in 2 weeks."

---

and then evaluate whether he or she has gained the ability to hear or interact more effectively. When a patient does not achieve expected outcomes, you need to change interventions or alter the patient's environment.

For all patients it is important to evaluate the integrity of the sensory organs and the ability to perceive stimuli. This often involves a simple vision or hearing evaluation by asking a patient to perform a self-care skill. Be sure to determine if patients understand and are following recommended therapies and meeting mutually set goals. Using teach-back is a good approach. If nursing care has been directed at improving or maintaining sensory acuity, asking a patient to explain or demonstrate a newly learned self-care skill is an effective evaluative measure.

Patient Expectations. It is important to learn if patients think they are receiving appropriate care. A sensory deficit is potentially embarrassing and threatens a person's self-image. Does the patient feel comfortable relating to you? Was the patient able to maintain the plan of care for assistive devices? Did the patient think you were exhibiting a caring, professional approach? Asking patients if nursing care successfully met their expectations provides valuable knowledge when you care for other patients with similar sensory problems.

KEY POINTS

- Sensory perception depends on a region in the cerebral cortex where specialized brain cells interpret the quality and nature of sensory stimuli.
- Because a patient learns to rely on unaffected senses after a sensory loss, you design interventions to preserve function of these senses.
- Aging results in a gradual decline of acuity in all senses.
- Environmental stimuli in a hospital such as in an intensive care unit place a patient at risk for sensory overload.
- The extent of support from family members and significant others influences the quality of sensory experiences.
- Assessment of sensory function includes a physical examination and measurement of functional abilities.
- The presence of cerumen in the external auditory canal is a common cause of hearing loss in older adults.
- Sensory losses create loneliness and impair the ability to socialize.
- An assessment of the environment includes identifying hazards, sources of meaningful stimulation, and the amount of stimuli.
- Prenatal screening and childhood immunizations prevent sensory alterations in the newborn and child.
- The care plan for patients with sensory alterations includes participation by family members.
- Patients with visual impairments need to learn boundaries within the environment to ambulate safely.
- Patients with existing hearing deficits are able to learn alternative ways to communicate.
- Nursing care for patients with sensory alterations includes using stronger sensory stimuli, compensating with other senses, and modifying the environment to maximize remaining sensory function.
- To prevent sensory overload, control stimuli, orient the patient to the environment, and promote rest by minimizing interruptions.
- Safety is a top concern when setting priorities for patients who experience sensory deprivation.

REFLECTIVE LEARNING

- Consider a patient experience you had today and describe how the patient's loss of sensory function affected his or her psychological and psychosocial health.
- Consider the multidisciplinary team involved in your patient's care today and discuss why a multidisciplinary approach produces the best results for patients with sensory impairments.
- Discuss the resources available in your community that you can share with patients with sensory impairments who can no longer drive or who need low-vision rehabilitation.

REVIEW QUESTIONS

1. Which of the following guidelines does the nurse follow when caring for patients with visual impairments? (Select all that apply.)
   1. Invite the patient's family to speak on their behalf.
   2. Introduce yourself and use face-to-face communication.
   3. Ask the patient about how he or she would like to be assisted.
   4. Speak louder to compensate for a dual sensory impairment.
   5. Orient the patient to the room and keep pathways clear of obstacles.

2. The nurse is performing an assessment on a young child recently diagnosed with a hearing impairment. What is the highest priority for the nurse at the onset of the interview?
   1. Perform a physical examination.
   2. Discuss risk and benefits of a cochlear implant.
   3. Ask the patient or family what helps the child hear best.
   4. Provide the patient's family with a list of community resources.

3. A patient in an intensive care unit is experiencing sleeplessness, irritability, and difficulty concentrating. Which interventions should the nurse implement to decrease stimulation? (Select all that apply.)
   1. Establish a routine of care.
   2. Move the patient to a semiprivate room.
   3. Teach self-stimulation methods such as singing.
   4. Provide a quiet environment to allow optimal sleep.
   5. Coordinate lighting with a normal day and night cycle.

4. The nurse is performing an assessment of a patient with a suspected diagnosis of cataracts. Which clinical sign would the patient most likely report?
   1. Cloudy or blurry vision
   2. Severe eye and head pain
   3. Reduced peripheral vision
   4. Progressive loss of central vision

5. The nurse recognizes that which patient is most likely at risk for experiencing sensory deprivation?
   1. A patient who is depressed and lives with her spouse in assisted living
   2. A patient with dual sensory impairments confined to bed in long-term care
   3. A patient who is acutely ill and has intrusive monitoring and treatment equipment
   4. A patient with a chronic illness who is having many diagnostic tests and treatments

evolve

Additional Review Questions, as well as rationales for all Review Questions, can be found on the Evolve website.

1, 2, 3, 5; 2, 3; 3, 1, 4, 5; 4, 1; 5, 2.

REFERENCES

American Academy of Ophthalmology (AAO): *Frequency of ocular examinations*, San Francisco, CA, 2015, American Academy of Ophthalmology.

American Speech-Language-Hearing Association (ASHA): *Who should be screened for hearing loss?* 2016. http://www.asha.org/public/hearing/Who-Should-be-Screened/.

Centers for Disease Control and Prevention (CDC): *Eye safety*, 2013. https://www.cdc.gov/niosh/topics/eye/.

Centers for Disease Control and Prevention (CDC): *Noise and hearing loss protection*, 2016. https://www.cdc.gov/niosh/topics/noise/reducenoiseexposure/noisecontrols.html.

Cone B, et al: *Ototoxic medications (medication effects)*, 2016. http://www.asha.org/public/hearing/Ototoxic-Medications/.

Contrera KJ, et al: Hearing loss health care for older adults, *J Am Board Fam Med* 29(3):394, 2016.

Crews DE, et al: Health-related quality of life among people aged ≥ 65 years with self-reported visual impairment: findings from the 2006-2010 behavioral risk factor surveillance system, *Ophthalmic Epidemiol* 21(5):287, 2014.

Fillary J, et al: Noise at night in hospital general wards: a mapping of the literature, *Br J Nurs* 24(10):536, 2015.

Heine C, Browning C: Dual sensory loss in older adults: a systematic review, *Gerontologist* 55(5):913, 2015.

Hockenberry MJ, Wilson D: *Wong's nursing care of infants and children*, ed 10, St Louis, 2015, Mosby.

Konkani A, et al: Reducing hospital ICU noise: a behavior-based approach, *J Healthc Eng* 5(2):229, 2014.

Maidl CA, et al: The influence of "quiet time" for patients in critical care, *Clin Nurs Res* 23(5):544, 2014.

McAndrews NS, et al: Quiet time for mechanically ventilated patients in the medical intensive care unit, *Intensive Crit Care Nurs* 35(22):22, 2016.

McMurry L, et al: Mexican Americans. In Giger JN, editor: *Transcultural nursing: assessment and intervention*, ed 7, St Louis, 2017, Mosby.

Meiner SE: *Gerontologic nursing*, ed 5, St Louis, 2015, Mosby.

National Eye Institute (NEI): *Facts about cataract*, 2015. https://nei.nih.gov/health/cataract/cataract_facts.

National Institute of Deafness and Other Communication Disorders (NIDCD): *Hearing loss and older adults*, 2016. https://www.nidcd.nih.gov/health/hearing-loss-older-adults.

Occupational Safety and Health Administration (OSHA): *Eye and face protection*, n.d. https://www.osha.gov/SLTC/eyefaceprotection/standards.html.

Riemer HC, et al: Decreased stress levels in nurses: a benefit of quiet time, *Am J Crit Care* 24(5):396, 2015.

Rosen T, et al: Slipping and tripping: fall injuries in adults associated with rugs and carpets, *J Inj Violence Res* 5(1):61, 2013.

Tainter CR, et al: Noise levels in surgical ICUs are consistently above recommended standards, *Crit Care Med* 44(1):147, 2016.

The Joint Commission (TJC): *2017 Hospital accreditation standards*, Oakbrook, IL, 2017, The Commission.

Touhy TA, Jett A: *Ebersole & Hess' Gerontological nursing and healthy aging*, ed 4, St Louis, 2014, Mosby.

Touhy TA, Jett A: *Ebersole & Hess' Toward health aging: human needs and nursing response*, ed 9, St Louis, 2016, Mosby.

Varma R, et al: Visual impairment and blindness in adults in the United States: demographic and geographic variations from 2015 to 2050, *JAMA Ophthalmol* 134(7):802, 2016.

World Health Organization (WHO): *Visual impairment and blindness*, 2014. http://www.who.int/mediacentre/factsheets/fs282/en/.

evolve MEDIA RESOURCES

http://evolve.elsevier.com/Potter/essentials
- Audio Glossary
- QSEN Activity and Review Questions Answers and Rationales
- Video Clip

OBJECTIVES

- Explain components of perioperative nursing care.
- Differentiate among classifications of surgery and types of anesthesia.
- List factors to include in preoperative, intraoperative, and postoperative assessment of a surgical patient.
- Design an evidence-based, patient-centered preoperative teaching plan.
- Discuss methods of preparing a patient for surgery.
- Compare and contrast providing care for a patient undergoing outpatient versus inpatient surgery.

- Outline the importance of safety initiatives applied throughout the perioperative patient experience.
- Describe intraoperative factors that affect a patient's postoperative care.
- Identify factors to assess in a patient in postoperative recovery.
- Construct an evidence-based plan of care designed to prevent postoperative complications.

KEY TERMS

Aldrete score, p. 1227
antiembolic stockings, p. 1208
atelectasis, p. 1188
bronchospasm, p. 1195
circulating nurse, p. 1209
conscious sedation, p. 1213
embolism, p. 1189
enhanced recovery after surgery (ERAS), p. 1219
general anesthesia, p. 1213

laryngospasm, p. 1195
malignant hyperthermia, p. 1193
moderate sedation/analgesia, p. 1213
multimodal analgesia, p. 1225
nasogastric (NG) tube, p. 1208
operating room (OR), p. 1209
outpatient, p. 1187
paralytic ileus, p. 1219
perioperative nursing, p. 1187

postanesthesia care unit (PACU), p. 1214
preanesthesia care unit, p. 1209
prehabilitation, p. 1190
preoperative teaching, p. 1192
presurgical care unit (PSCU), p. 1209
pulmonary hygiene, p. 1195
regional anesthesia, p. 1213
rhabdomyolysis, p. 1189
scrub nurse, p. 1209

Perioperative nursing includes care given before (preoperative), during (intraoperative), and after (postoperative) surgery. Surgery takes place in a variety of settings including hospitals, ambulatory surgery centers, clinics, health care providers' offices, and mobile units. Many surgeries are performed on an outpatient basis, with patients entering a health care setting, undergoing surgery, and being discharged the same day. Other surgical patients enter a health care setting as outpatients for preoperative screening and testing and are later admitted to a hospital after surgery.

CASE STUDY Mr. Korloff

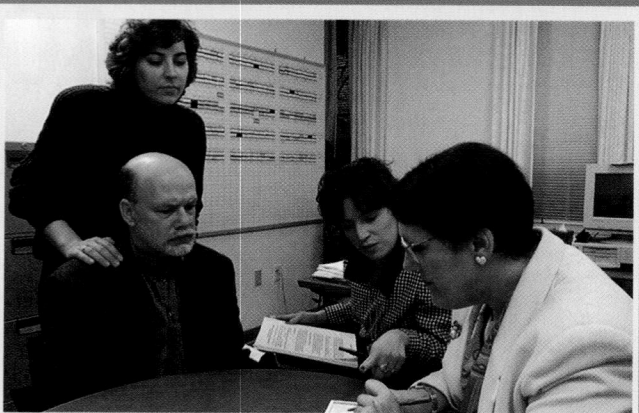

Mr. Korloff is a 53-year-old man who has had abdominal pain off and on for 2 months. Following a series of diagnostic tests, he is now scheduled for elective laparoscopic gallbladder surgery. Mr. Korloff is originally from Russia and has lived in the United States for 10 years. He speaks English relatively well but still speaks in Russian when family is present. He is a vice president for an international business firm. He is widowed and has two adult daughters; both were born in Russia. His daughters are married and live in the same neighborhood as Mr. Korloff. However, both have full-time jobs.

Sue is a nursing student assigned to the preadmission center at the local hospital where she has been working for 2 weeks. She is completing her last clinical rotation and will graduate in 1 month. She plans to seek employment in a hospital on a general surgery floor after graduation. Sue's father recently had surgery for prostate cancer.

Patients requiring extensive preoperative care may be admitted to a hospital before surgery. The principles of caring for perioperative patients are basically the same, regardless of the setting, except for the timing and extent of therapy.

SCIENTIFIC KNOWLEDGE BASE

Surgical procedures have evolved significantly over the last 20 years. Surgeries that once required hospitalization for 3 to 4 days are now performed on an outpatient basis. Hospitals across the United States are applying strategies to improve the preparation of patients before surgery and enhancing their recovery during the surgical stay. When scientific evidence is consistently applied, patients recover more quickly with better outcomes.

Classification of Surgery

Surgical procedures are classified according to the seriousness, urgency, and purpose of surgery (Table 40.1). For example, a breast biopsy, done for diagnostic purposes, is classified as urgent and done on an outpatient basis. Knowing the classification helps you to plan appropriate preoperative and postoperative care for each patient.

Surgical Risk Factors

Numerous factors create risks for a patient undergoing surgery. Knowledge regarding the physiology of the stress response (see Chapter 26) and factors that affect a patient's response to the stress of surgery is necessary to anticipate patient needs for preoperative preparation, teaching, counseling, and postoperative care.

Smoking. There is a significant association between smoking and postoperative pulmonary complications, specifically pneumonia and atelectasis. Chronic smoking increases the amount and thickness of mucus secretions in the lungs. After surgery a patient who smokes has greater difficulty clearing the airways of mucus and needs to practice deep breathing and coughing exercises even more vigorously than a nonsmoking patient (see Chapter 32). Smoking also increases the risk for circulatory and infectious complications (Claessen et al., 2016).

Age. Very young and older patients are at greater surgical risk because of immature or declining physiological states. Periods of extreme stress such as surgery and anesthesia can quickly physically decompensate older adults and make them susceptible to perioperative complications. Older adults have a greater incidence of complications than younger adults. The most common complications include heart failure, pneumonia, renal failure, infection, stroke, and delirium. Maintaining a patient's normal body temperature is a concern during surgery. Compared with adults, infants have a proportionately greater surface area and less subcutaneous fat, placing them at risk for wide temperature variations. Additionally, general anesthetics inhibit shivering, a protective reflex to maintain body temperature, and anesthetics cause vasodilation, which results in heat loss. During surgery an infant also has difficulty maintaining a normal circulatory blood volume. The total blood volume of infants is considerably less than that of older children and adults, creating a risk for dehydration and overhydration.

Nutrition. Normal tissue repair and resistance to infection depend on adequate nutrition. Surgery increases the need for nutrients. After surgery a patient requires at least 1500 kcal/day to maintain energy reserves. For proper wound healing, additional protein; carbohydrates; zinc; and vitamins A, B, C, and K are necessary (see Chapter 35). Of adults who are hospitalized, 20% to 70% are considered malnourished or at nutritional risk (Lewis et al., 2014). Patients who are malnourished are more likely to have poor tolerance of anesthesia, negative nitrogen balance, delayed postoperative recovery, infection, and delayed wound healing.

Obesity. Obesity is a complex medical disorder that often coexists with other medical problems (Rothrock, 2015). The patient with obesity may have reduced respiratory reserve because of the upward pressure against the diaphragm caused by an enlarged abdomen. Positioning is critical to maintain

TABLE 40.1 CLASSIFICATION FOR SURGICAL PROCEDURES

TYPE	DESCRIPTION	EXAMPLE
Seriousness		
Major	Involves extensive reconstruction or alteration in body parts; poses great risks to well-being	Coronary artery bypass, colon resection, removal of larynx, resection of lung lobe
Minor	Involves minimal alteration in body parts; often designed to correct deformities; minimal risks compared with major procedures	Cataract extraction, facial plastic surgery, tooth extraction
Urgency		
Elective	Performed on basis of patient's choice; not essential and is not always necessary for health	Bunionectomy, facial plastic surgery, breast reconstruction
Required	Necessary for patient's health; can prevent additional problems from developing (e.g., tissue destruction, impaired organ function); not necessarily an emergency	Excision of cancerous tumor, removal of gallbladder for stones, vascular repair for obstructed artery (e.g., coronary artery bypass)
Urgent	Requires prompt attention within 24–48 hours	Repair of fracture, incision and drainage of wound infection
Emergent	Surgery performed immediately to save life or preserve function of body part	Repair of perforated appendix, repair of traumatic amputation, control of internal hemorrhaging
Purpose		
Diagnostic	Surgical exploration used to confirm a diagnosis; sometimes involves removal of tissue for further diagnostic testing	Exploratory laparotomy (incision into peritoneal cavity to inspect abdominal organs), breast mass biopsy
Ablative	Amputation or removal of diseased body part	Amputation, removal of appendix, cholecystectomy
Palliative	Relieves or reduces intensity of disease symptoms; does not produce cure	Colostomy, removal of necrotic tissue, resection of nerve roots
Reconstructive/restorative	Restores function or appearance to traumatized or malfunctioning tissues	Internal fixation of fractures, scar revision
Procurement for transplant	Removal of organs and/or tissues from a person pronounced brain dead for transplantation into another person	Kidney, cornea, or liver transplant
Constructive	Restores function lost or reduced as result of congenital anomalies	Repair of cleft palate, closure of atrial septal defect in heart
Cosmetic	Improves personal appearance	Blepharoplasty to correct eyelid deformities; rhinoplasty to reshape nose

control of the patient's airway. The recumbent and supine positions required on the operating bed (table) for surgery limit a patient's ventilation. Trendelenburg's position is even more poorly tolerated. This position should be avoided until the patient is intubated and the airway is secure (Rothrock, 2015). There is also an increased risk for pressure injury, aspiration of pulmonary secretions, deep vein thrombosis (DVT), pulmonary embolism, and rhabdomyolysis (Rothrock, 2015) during the administration of anesthesia. The increased workload of the heart and atherosclerotic blood vessels often results in compromised cardiovascular function. Because of these physiological changes, patients who are obese often have difficulty resuming normal physical activity after surgery. Hypertension, coronary artery disease,

type 2 diabetes mellitus, hyperlipidemia, liver disease, and heart failure are common in this population. Patients who are obese are also more susceptible to developing embolism, atelectasis, and pneumonia after surgery than patients who are not obese.

In addition, excess weight placed on skin over bony prominences restricts blood flow and poses risk for impaired skin integrity. Obesity increases the risk of poor wound healing and wound infection because fatty tissue contains a poor blood supply, which slows the delivery of essential nutrients and antibodies needed for healing. It is more difficult to close a surgical wound because of the thick adipose layer. The risk for wound dehiscence and evisceration is increased because of these factors (see Chapter 38).

Obstructive Sleep Apnea. Obstructive sleep apnea (OSA) can have a profound effect on patient morbidity and mortality following surgery (Harrelson and Fencl, 2016). OSA is a syndrome of periodic complete or partial obstruction of the upper airway during sleep (see Chapter 33) (American Society of Anesthesiologists [ASA] Task Force on Perioperative Management of Patients With Obstructive Sleep Apnea, 2014). It increases the risk for perioperative respiratory complications such as oxygen desaturation and apnea. Many patients have undiagnosed OSA. Screen patients before surgery with simple questions regarding snoring, apnea during sleep, frequent arousals during sleep, morning headaches, daytime somnolence, and chronic fatigue (Helvig et al., 2014; Ganzberg, 2016). A risk assessment should be performed even in pediatric patients during the preoperative interview (Ogg, 2016). Always instruct patients diagnosed with OSA to bring their positive airway pressure machine for use after surgery.

Immunocompetence. Radiation and chemotherapeutic drugs used to treat cancer, immunosuppressive agents used to prevent rejection after organ transplantation, and steroids used to treat inflammatory conditions make the body vulnerable to infection. These therapies, in addition to disorders affecting the immune system such as acquired immunodeficiency syndrome (AIDS), suppress the immune system. Immunosuppression increases the risk for infection after surgery. For example, a patient with cancer has radiation therapy to reduce the size of a cancerous tumor before surgery to remove the tumor. Radiation causes fibrosis and vascular scarring in the radiated area. The tissues become fragile and poorly oxygenated, increasing the risk for wound infection. Irradiation treatments are required before surgery; ideally surgery takes place 4 to 6 weeks after treatment to avoid wound-healing problems.

Fluid and Electrolyte Balance. The body responds to surgery as a form of trauma. As a result of the adrenocortical stress response, hormonal reactions cause sodium and water retention and potassium loss within the first 2 to 5 days after surgery (see Chapter 18). Severe protein breakdown creates a negative nitrogen balance. The severity of the stress response influences the degree of fluid and electrolyte imbalance. More extensive surgery is associated with more severe physiological stress. Patients with preexisting renal, fluid and electrolyte, metabolic, gastrointestinal (GI), respiratory, or cardiovascular problems are at greater risk for operative complications. For example, a patient who is dehydrated from vomiting before surgery is at increased risk for hypovolemic shock.

Depression. Clinical depression is associated with suppression of the immune system, posing increased risk for patients to develop postoperative infections (Ghoneim and O'Hara, 2016). In addition, patients with preoperative depression experience poorer surgical recovery outcomes including higher incidence of medical complications during the 6 months following surgery (Poole et al., 2014). Depression is also commonly associated with cognitive impairment, which may worsen postoperatively and become a factor in reducing patient adherence to necessary medical therapies. There is evidence that acute postoperative pain causes depression, and depression lowers the threshold for pain, making pain management difficult in patients with depression (Ghoneim and O'Hara, 2016).

Pregnancy. When caring for a pregnant patient, consider the needs of both the pregnant woman and her unborn fetus. Surgery is reserved for urgent or emergent reasons such as appendicitis or trauma. The enlarged uterus displaces abdominal organs and distorts landmarks, making surgery more complex. Anesthetics and medications administered during the first trimester can cause fetal abnormalities. During pregnancy the following maternal physiological changes occur that increase the complexity of patient care (Rothrock, 2015):

1. Cardiac output and respiratory tidal volume increase to keep up with the increase in metabolism and blood pressure decreases, making interpretation of vital signs and recognition of hypovolemic shock more difficult.
2. The high level of progesterone relaxes the lower esophageal sphincter and decreases GI motility, which slows gastric emptying, resulting in an increased risk for aspiration of stomach contents.
3. There is an increase in white blood cells near term beyond the normal range for that of nonpregnant women who have no infection.
4. There is an increased risk for DVT as a result of increased fibrinogen levels and decreased clotting time.

In addition, a pregnant patient and her family experience increased psychological stress because of fear of fetal loss or complication. The perioperative team addresses these concerns.

Prehabilitation

Poor baseline physical performance capacity and poor nutritional status increase the risk of complications after major surgery and prolong recovery (McGill Perioperative Program, 2017). Poor physical health and fitness increases a patient's risk of complications and death after major elective surgery (Perry et al., 2016). Preadmission interventions to improve patients' health and fitness (referred to as prehabilitation) may reduce postoperative complications, decrease the length of hospital stays, and enhance a patient's recovery. A typical prehabilitation protocol usually has multiple components including exercise (endurance and strength training), diet, psychological, and evidence-based clinical (e.g., hydration and bowel management) components (Fournier et al., 2016; Perry et al., 2016). Appropriate and thorough preoperative education is also a component of prehabilitation to promotion desirable behavioral changes (e.g., adherence). Anxiety and worry also affect a patient's recovery, and many prehabilitation programs include psychological or counselor consultations to help patients learn relaxation and breathing exercises and anxiety reduction techniques (McGill Perioperative Program, 2017).

NURSING KNOWLEDGE BASE

Perioperative Communication

Perioperative nurses use the nursing process to provide continuity of care for surgical patients. In some settings perioperative nurses assess a patient's health status before surgery, identify specific patient needs, teach and counsel, attend to a patient's needs in the operating room (OR), and follow a patient's recovery. In other words, one nurse follows a patient throughout the operative experience. However, more commonly different nurses care for a patient during each phase of the surgical experience.

Communicating patient information between perioperative nurses during the transfer of care is essential to ensure continuity of care. Transitions from one care provider to another place patients at risk for injuries and errors. A standardized approach to hand-off communication in the highly complex, fast-paced perioperative environment involving the interdisciplinary team minimizes these risks (Garrett, 2016). A number of tools exist for perioperative team members including TeamSTEPPS, SBAR, briefing and debriefing, checklists, and clarifying questions (see Chapter 11). In addition to a standardized process, mistakes can be reduced through the use of effective communication skills such as using effective nonverbal behaviors, active listening, and understanding the effects and emotions of others in the OR setting (see Chapter 11).

Complication Prevention

Patients are at high risk for a variety of complications after surgery including surgical wound infection, hyperglycemia, respiratory and cardiac complications, and pressure injury. Nurses play a key role in prevention, and medical and nursing research has contributed to the knowledge of how to prevent many of these complications. Prevention of surgical complications requires critical thinking and knowledge of the anatomy and physiology of all major body systems. Assessment begins in the preoperative phase and continues through the postoperative period. You must conduct thorough assessments, anticipate and identify problems, consider a patient's risks, use appropriate resources, and make the decisions needed to take quick action to prevent complications.

Surgical Site Infection Prevention

Surgical site infection (SSI) prevention has been a major focus for health care providers since the Centers for Disease Control and Prevention published *Guideline for the Prevention of Surgical Site Infection* (Mangram et al., 1999). SSIs continue to be a leading component of nosocomial morbidity and mortality (Young et al., 2014), which make the reduction of SSIs a global priority for health care organizations (Love, 2016). Evidence-based strategies to prevent SSIs include antibiotic selection, dosing, and timing; appropriate preoperative hair removal; proper skin preparation; maintaining

normothermia; and glucose control (Anderson et al., 2014). Supplemental strategies include OR traffic control, preoperative bathing with chlorhexidine gluconate (CHG), and reducing unnecessary blood transfusions (Love, 2016).

Glycemic Control and Infection Prevention

There is a relationship between wound and tissue infection and blood glucose levels. There is a significant association between poorly controlled diabetes both preoperatively and postoperatively and SSI (Martin et al., 2016). Poor control of blood glucose levels (specifically hyperglycemia) during surgery and afterward increases the risk for wound infection and patient mortality in certain types of surgery (Tanner et al., 2015; Wukich, 2015). Perioperative nurses work with their medical colleagues to maintain normal glucose levels in the postoperative period to reduce the risk for wound and tissue infection. The American Diabetes Association (ADA, 2016) recommends a glycemic range of 80 to 180 mg/dL (4.4 to 10.0 mmol/L) for perioperative patients.

Respiratory and Cardiac Complications

General anesthesia and mechanical ventilation impair pulmonary function, even in healthy individuals, and result in decreased oxygenation following anesthesia (Karcz and Papadakos, 2013). Surgical patients will also experience a reduction in functional residual capacity of up to 50% of the preanesthesia value. Pulmonary atelectasis is a common finding in anesthetized patients, as it occurs in 85% to 90% of healthy adults (Karcz and Papadakos, 2013). These factors are further complicated by patients' preexisting comorbidities, the type and duration of surgery, and appropriate use of anesthetics and analgesics. Perioperative nursing care must focus on maximizing ventilation postoperatively, thinning and removing pulmonary secretions, and promoting activity as early as possible.

Each year more than 10 million adults (5% of surgeries) experience major cardiac complications in the first 30 days following noncardiac surgery (Devereaux and Sessler, 2015). These complications can lead to prolonged hospitalization, increased health care costs, and death.

Risk factors for cardiac complications include high-risk surgery, history of ischemic heart disease, history of congestive heart failure, history of cerebrovascular disease, preoperative treatment with insulin, and preoperative serum creatinine value greater than 2.0 mg/dL. As in the case of pulmonary complications, a thorough preoperative risk assessment is critical. Nurses conduct regular monitoring of vital signs, patient response to sedation and anesthesia, and oxygenation status to detect any cardiac problems that might develop postoperatively.

Pressure Injury Prevention

Surgical patients pose a unique challenge in preventing pressure injuries. Risk factors for pressure injuries intraoperatively include sustained pressure from positioning, the length and type of surgery, and lack of movement during the perioperative period. Pressure compresses skin and muscle between bones and the surface on which the patient is lying (stretcher, OR bed, hospital bed) resulting in tissue ischemia (see Chapter 38). Anesthetic agents lower blood pressure, altering tissue perfusion. Factors such as shear force from moving unconscious or debilitated patients, weight from multiple layers of drapes, and moisture on the OR bed (fluids used for skin cleansing and surgical site irrigation) further add to the risk for pressure injury formation (Engels et al., 2016). OR nurses prevent pressure injuries intraoperatively by conducting a careful preoperative assessment, using predictive tools such as the Munro scale and Scott triggers, using proper support surfaces and safe patient-handling equipment, and protecting bony prominences and areas of high pressure (Black et al., 2015; Spruce, 2017). Nurses perform a careful skin assessment before, during, and after surgery and intervene by using low-air-loss or pressure-reduction beds and mattresses and frequent repositioning for patients unable to move themselves.

CRITICAL THINKING

Synthesis

Patient care requires you to apply what you know about a patient, your knowledge base, experience, and critical thinking attitudes and standards. Your synthesis of this information allows you to make sound decisions as you apply the nursing process. Critical thinking synthesis involves combining all available information to obtain a clear picture of the approach needed to provide patient-centered care.

Knowledge. It is essential to have a strong knowledge base in anatomy and physiology, physical examination (see Chapter 16), principles of aseptic technique (see Chapter 14), pharmacology (see Chapter 17), and teaching-learning principles (see Chapter 12). In addition, understanding the effect that surgical procedures and medications have on different body systems is essential. It is also important to understand the normal stress response to anticipate potential complications during the perioperative experience (see Chapter 26). Effective preoperative teaching requires a knowledge base of teaching and communication principles (see Chapter 11) and the planned surgical procedure.

Experience. Any personal experience with surgery helps you understand the anxiety of patients and their families and explain some of the physical sensations that patients experience. Past experiences with surgical patients enable you to anticipate questions that a patient and family will ask and focus preoperative teaching. In addition, experience helps you recognize physiological changes in patients more quickly so you can initiate preventive and corrective measures early.

Attitudes. A key attitude for a perioperative nurse is responsibility. As a perioperative nurse, you are responsible for implementing perioperative care standards and advocating for each patient. When a patient consents to surgery and receives an anesthetic agent that alters the level of conscious-ness, health care providers have the responsibility to protect a patient. You are responsible for maintaining a patient's rights when the patient cannot speak on his or her own behalf.

Perioperative nurses think independently by considering a wide range of ideas and concepts in making decisions about patient care. One example is application of evidence in the plan of care to deal with individual patient differences. For example, to promote venous return, a nurse positions a pregnant patient on the operating table with a positioning wedge under the right hip to displace the uterus to the left. Assess each patient and use the most appropriate padding and positioning techniques possible to prevent injury.

Your attitude about using discipline when assessing patients and providing perioperative care is essential. Numerous routines are followed in preparation of a patient for surgery and for an efficient and optimal recovery. Systematically follow your organization policies and procedures and the current standards of practice to ensure high-quality care for each patient.

Standards. The application of critical thinking intellectual standards is important when caring for a patient having surgery, particularly if a patient has preexisting physical or psychological factors that may influence surgical outcomes. Be very precise, accurate, and complete in gathering assessment data, and use a logical, relevant, and well–thought out approach in making clinical decisions because a patient's condition can change quickly.

The Association of periOperative Registered Nurses (AORN) has established evidence-based guidelines for nurses in perioperative clinical practice. The guidelines, incorporated in the content of this chapter, cover practices to ensure patient safety, appropriate monitoring and evaluation, infection control practices, and timely and effective nursing interventions. As a perioperative nurse, you are responsible for following these guidelines (AORN, 2017a).

Recommendations for perioperative care are specifically addressed in The Joint Commission *2018 National Patient Safety Goals* (TJC, 2018). These recommendations include correct patient identification, relaying important test results, using medication safely, using alarms safely, preventing infection, and preventing mistakes in surgery (TJC, 2018). For example, perioperative nurses use evidence-based guidelines for performing a surgical time-out with the perioperative team, tracking and reporting critical results of tests and diagnostic procedures, labeling all medications both on and off a sterile field, administering antimicrobial agents for prophylaxis, preparing the operative site before an incision, and performing wound care after surgery.

PREOPERATIVE SURGICAL PHASE

The first phase of the perioperative experience is the preoperative surgical phase. Patients having surgery are at various stages of health. Some patients enter a health care agency feeling relatively healthy while awaiting elective surgery. Other patients enter in great distress when facing emergency surgery. Many tests and procedures often are necessary to ensure that surgery is indicated and that a patient is in an optimum condition, regardless of the setting where surgery is to take place. During these tests and procedures, a patient meets many health care personnel who play a role in his or her care and recovery. Family members or friends can play a role in providing support and education reinforcement, but they also face many of the same stressors as patients.

Some patients have preoperative diagnostic testing several days before surgery in a hospital, surgeon's office, or outpatient surgery center or laboratory. With this testing completed, patients usually enter a surgical facility (e.g., hospital, surgery center, clinic) the day that surgery is performed and return home on the same day. A patient sometimes enters the hospital the day before surgery. Be able to properly prepare a patient for surgery, regardless of where the patient enters the health care setting. Prehabilitation activities improve outcomes and reduce postoperative complications (Santa, 2015).

NURSING PROCESS

■■■ ASSESSMENT

Your preoperative assessment of a patient establishes a baseline before surgery and alerts you to special needs and potential intraoperative and postoperative complications the patient may encounter. The standards for the factors to include in an assessment are the same for inpatients as well as outpatients. Use effective communication skills to gather information and screen patients for potential risk factors for surgery.

Nursing History. The preoperative history includes key elements that are relevant to a patient's surgical risks and needs (Box 40.1). Interview family members or significant others if a patient is unable to relate all needed information. Use a professional interpreter if a patient is unable to speak or understand English (see Chapter 21). Also be sure to discuss advance directives. Ask if a patient has a durable power of attorney for health care and a living will (see Chapter 5) and include a copy in the chart. The law requires advance directive identification for patients of all ages and for all surgical procedures. Often directives are modified during the perioperative period but are reestablished after postoperative stabilization.

Medical History. A review of a patient's medical history includes the primary reason for seeking medical care and past illnesses and surgeries. The medical history screens surgical candidates for major medical conditions that increase the risk for complications (Table 40.2). If a patient is at increased risk, surgery as an outpatient may not be advisable. For example, ask women of childbearing age about the date of their last menstrual period (LMP), if their LMP was "typical" for them, and if they have had unprotected sex in the last month. Because many women do not know they are pregnant early in the first trimester, institutions require a pregnancy test when a patient of childbearing age is scheduled for surgery. Inquire about family history for anesthetic complications

BOX 40.1 SYNTHESIS IN PRACTICE

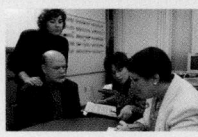

As Sue prepares to conduct Mr. Korloff's preadmission assessment, she recalls what she has learned regarding risk factors for patients undergoing surgery. Mr. Korloff has a history of heart disease. He was treated for a cardiac rhythm irregularity 5 years ago but has had no further problems. Sue applies the intellectual standards of being thorough and specific when questioning Mr. Korloff about any potential cardiac symptoms. She plans to have his daughters present during the discussion as well.

Sue's knowledge of laparoscopic surgery helps her anticipate the types of postoperative problems that Mr. Korloff is likely to develop such as food intolerance and abdominal or referred pain from the carbon dioxide gas used during laparoscopy. Sue's experience with prior patients helps her to explain some of the sensations that Mr. Korloff will experience such as a sore throat from the endotracheal (breathing) tube used for administering anesthesia. She informs Mr. Korloff and his daughters that he will have IV fluids infusing until he tolerates oral fluids and that he will likely experience mild discomfort from the surgical procedure. Mr. Korloff will be getting out of bed as soon as possible after surgery, following the nursing unit's early mobility evidence-based protocol. If all goes well, he will likely be discharged the next day.

because an adverse reaction called **malignant hyperthermia** is an inherited disorder. Malignant hyperthermia is a life-threatening complication resulting in high carbon dioxide levels, tachypnea, tachycardia, heart rhythm irregularities, and muscular rigidity with elevated temperature in the late stages (Denholm, 2015).

Previous Surgeries. Review of a patient's past experience with surgery will reveal if there are physical and psychological responses that may develop during the current planned procedure. Complications such as anaphylaxis or malignant hyperthermia during previous surgery alert you to the need for preventive measures. Be sure you know the location of emergency equipment in your work area. A history of postoperative complications such as persistent vomiting or uncontrolled pain alerts you to consult with the surgeon, as there may be a possible need for different medications. Reports of severe anxiety before a previous surgery identify the need for additional emotional support, preoperative teaching, and possibly antianxiety medications. Inform the surgeon and/or anesthesia care provider of your findings when you believe that intervention is indicated.

Knowledge. Assess what a patient knows about surgery in general and what specifically is known about the patient's planned surgery. Include an assessment of the patient's readiness and ability to learn (see Chapter 12). Patients who are uninformed or given incorrect information will require more extensive preoperative instruction. Include family members in this assessment when appropriate.

Medication History. Review if a patient is taking any medications that predispose the patient to surgical complications

TABLE 40.2   MEDICAL CONDITIONS THAT INCREASE THE RISKS OF SURGERY

TYPE OF CONDITION	REASON FOR RISK
Bleeding disorders (thrombocytopenia, hemophilia)	Increases risk for hemorrhaging during and after surgery.
Diabetes mellitus	Increases susceptibility to infection and impairs wound healing from altered glucose metabolism and associated circulatory impairment. Fluctuating blood glucose levels cause central nervous system alterations during anesthesia. Stress of surgery causes increases in blood glucose levels.
Heart disease (recent myocardial infarction, dysrhythmias, congestive heart failure) and peripheral vascular disease	Stress of surgery causes increased demands on myocardium to maintain cardiac output. General anesthetic agents depress cardiac function.
Hypertension	Increases risk for cardiovascular complications during anesthesia (e.g., stroke, reduced tissue oxygenation).
Upper respiratory infection	Increases risk for respiratory complications during anesthesia (e.g., pneumonia, spasm of laryngeal muscles).
Renal disease	Alters excretion of anesthetic drugs and their metabolites as well as acid-base balance, increasing risk for surgical complications.
Liver disease	Alters metabolism and elimination of drugs administered during surgery and impairs wound healing and clotting time because of alterations in protein metabolism.
Fever	Predisposes patient to fluid and electrolyte imbalances and often indicates underlying infection.
Chronic respiratory disease (emphysema, bronchitis, asthma)	Reduces patient's ability to compensate for acid-base alterations. Anesthetic agents reduce respiratory function, increasing risk for severe hypoventilation.
Immunological disorder (leukemia, acquired immunodeficiency syndrome [AIDS], bone marrow depression, organ transplantation, use of chemotherapeutic drugs)	Increases risk for infection and delays wound healing after surgery.
Abuse of alcohol and street drugs	Patients who abuse drugs sometimes have underlying disease (human immunodeficiency virus [HIV], hepatitis) and altered wellness, which affect healing. Alcohol addiction causes unpredictable reactions to anesthesia. Patients go into withdrawal during and after surgery.
Chronic pain	Regular use of pain medications often results in higher tolerance. Increased doses of opioids frequently are necessary to achieve postoperative pain control.

(Table 40.3). Many medications interact unpredictably with anesthetic agents during surgery (Burchum and Rosenthal, 2016). If a patient regularly uses prescription medications, over-the-counter (OTC) medications, or herbal supplements, the surgeon may temporarily discontinue them before surgery or adjust the dosages. Instruct patients to ask their surgeon whether they should take their usual medications the morning of surgery. If a patient is having inpatient surgery, all prescription drugs taken before surgery are automatically discontinued after surgery unless reordered. Be vigilant in reviewing a patient's preoperative orders so that you do not forget any medication that a patient needs to take before the operation. As a patient moves through different areas (e.g., holding area to OR), it is important that a complete list of the patient's medications is accurately communicated through medication reconciliation from nurse to nurse (see Chapter 17) (TJC, 2017).

Allergies. Allergies to medications, topical agents used to prepare the skin for surgery, and latex create significant risks for surgical patients. An allergic response to any agent is potentially fatal, depending on its severity. A latex allergy can manifest as redness, inflammation, pruritus, and blisters of the skin or as hay fever–like symptoms and anaphylaxis.

All health care workers need to know about their patient's allergies. In most agencies patients who have allergies receive an allergy identification band at the time of admission that remains on until discharge. Allergies may also be listed in patients' charts (either on a physical chart or on an electric health record [EHR]), on medical order sheets, and on patients' medication administration records (MARs). Verify allergies before, during, and after surgery.

Smoking Habits. A patient who smokes is at a greater risk for postoperative pulmonary complications than a patient who does not smoke. Smoking decreases ciliary movement of

TABLE 40.3	MEDICATIONS WITH SPECIAL IMPLICATIONS FOR SURGICAL PATIENTS
DRUG CLASS	**EFFECTS DURING SURGERY**
Antibiotics	Potentiate action of anesthetic agents. If taken within 2 weeks before surgery, aminoglycosides (gentamicin, tobramycin, neomycin) cause mild respiratory depression from depressed neuromuscular transmission.
Antidysrhythmics	Reduce cardiac contractility and heart rate and impair cardiac conduction during anesthesia.
Anticoagulants	Alter normal clotting factors, increasing risk for hemorrhage during and after surgery. Discontinue at least 48 hours before surgery. Aspirin is a common medication that alters clotting mechanisms.
Anticonvulsants	Long-term use of certain anticonvulsants (e.g., phenytoin, phenobarbital) alters metabolism of anesthetic agents.
Antihypertensives	Interact with anesthetic agents and cause bradycardia, hypotension, and impaired circulation. They inhibit synthesis and storage of norepinephrine in sympathetic nerve endings.
Corticosteroids	Prolonged use of corticosteroids causes adrenal atrophy, which reduces the ability of the body to withstand stress and results in hypotension during surgery. Dosages are sometimes temporarily increased before and during surgery.
Insulin	Patients with diabetes often need different insulin doses after surgery. Their nutritional intake is decreased immediately after surgery; however, stress response and IV administration of glucose solutions increase blood sugar. Regulating blood sugars with insulin after surgery is challenging.
Diuretics	Potentiate electrolyte imbalances (particularly potassium), increasing risk for dysrhythmias during and after surgery.
NSAIDs	Inhibit platelet aggregation and prolong bleeding time, increasing susceptibility to bleeding during and after surgery.

NSAIDs, Nonsteroidal antiinflammatory drugs.

mucus from the lower airways upward, increases mucus production, and causes bronchial constriction, thus increasing airway obstruction. After surgery, patients have greater difficulty clearing the airways of mucus secretions and are at increased risk for bronchospasm and laryngospasm. Use this information to plan aggressive postoperative pulmonary hygiene including more frequent turning, deep breathing, coughing, use of incentive spirometry, and chest physiotherapy if ordered. Smoking is associated with both coronary and peripheral artery disease (Lewis et al., 2014) and increased platelet aggregation, which also limits blood flow through the capillaries (Schroeder et al., 2016). Provide measures to decrease the risk for clot formation such as pneumatic compression stockings, deep breathing, leg exercises, anticoagulant therapy, and early ambulation.

Alcohol and Controlled Substance Use and Abuse. The surgical team needs to be aware of the use of alcohol and controlled substances by patients to prepare for adverse reactions such as withdrawal that may occur perioperatively. Increased tolerance to opioids occurs with chronic opioid use, resulting in an increased need for anesthesia and postoperative analgesics.

Family Support. Determine if and to what extent a patient will have support from family members or significant others. Surgery often results in temporary disability that requires direct care and assistance from family caregivers during recovery. Patients frequently underestimate the impact that surgery will have on them. They do not always immediately assume the same level of physical activity that they had before

surgery and often return home with dressings to change, pain to manage, or exercises to perform. Ask questions to determine the condition of a patient's home environment, the availability of family caregivers, and how a patient's expected limitations will affect his or her ability to perform activities of daily living. For example, a patient receives discharge instructions that state the need to use an incentive spirometer every 2 hours. When talking with the patient, you discover that he or she has difficulty using the device. In this case you educate the family caregiver to help the patient use the incentive spirometer until he or she demonstrates using the device without assistance.

Occupation. Surgery often results in physical alterations that prevent a patient from immediately returning to work. Assess a patient's occupational history to anticipate the effect that surgery will have on convalescence and eventual work performance. Explain any restrictions that a patient will have when returning to work. Early recognition of a problem may call for consultation with an occupational therapist.

Feelings. Surgery often causes anxiety and a feeling of loss of control for patients. Studies have shown that excessive preoperative anxiety increases intraoperative anesthetic requirement and can prolong recovery (Cao et al., 2017). Family members are often concerned about the ability of a patient to return to a productive life and the impact that recovery will have on the family unit. Assess a patient's feelings about having surgery from both verbal and nonverbal cues. Researchers are developing a user-friendly tool for the rapid assessment of state anxiety during the perioperative period that offers promise as a more objective measure of anxiety state (Cao et al., 2017). A patient who is fearful may ask many questions or be very quiet, may seem uneasy when strangers enter the room, or may actively seek the company of friends and relatives.

You have limited time to spend with a patient. As a nurse in an outpatient surgical program, telephone the patient at home before surgery or interview him or her during a preadmission testing visit. As a nurse in the hospital, choose a time for discussion with patients after preliminary admission procedures or diagnostic tests are complete. A patient's ability to share feelings depends in part on your willingness to ask questions, listen, be supportive, and clarify misconceptions.

Cultural Factors. Cultural beliefs, attitudes, and traditions affect how patients respond to any health care problem; surgery is no exception. Differences in the use of both verbal and nonverbal communication require you to assess and respond to cues with a patient and family (Box 40.2). This is especially important after you conduct the initial preoperative assessment and then look for changes in a patient's status after surgery. For example, patients from some cultures may remain silent out of respect, not fear. Learn how to form relationships that enable you to understand a person's culture and preferences. Use open-ended statements and questions such as, "Tell me about what this surgery means to you and your family." "Having surgery may make you feel afraid; tell me your concerns." In some cultures, women follow the directives of the significant male member of the family; therefore it is very important to explain everything to the husband, father, or brother of a female patient for her to participate in the plan of care (Giger, 2017). When doing this, make sure to have permission from the patient to share personal health information. Many cultural and religious taboos exist concerning the body, who cares for the physical needs of others, and treatments appropriate for healing; thus it is important to explore these issues with a patient and/or family member. Although it is important to recognize and plan for differences based on culture, remember that not all members of one family hold the same beliefs or practices (see Chapter 25). Asking relevant questions of each patient concerning his or her spiritual beliefs and expectations about surgery further individualizes your nursing care (see Chapter 22). Patients' spiritual beliefs help in coping with fears and anxieties related to the upcoming surgery. Assist a patient in obtaining the spiritual help requested before surgery. For example, contact the spiritual representative of the patient's choice before going to surgery.

Coping Resources. Assessment of patients' feelings and self-concept reveals whether they have the ability to cope with the stress of surgery. It is also valuable to ask patients about their stress management techniques (e.g., talking with others, listening to music, exercising). If a patient has had previous surgery, discuss the behaviors that helped to resolve past tension or nervousness. You will sometimes instruct a patient in relaxation exercises to help control anxiety (see Chapter 19).

Body Image. Surgical removal of a diseased tissue or organ may leave permanent disfigurement or alteration in body function. Concern over mutilation, change in sexuality, or loss of a body part adds to a patient's fears. Individuals react differently, depending on age, culture, occupation, self-image, and self-esteem. Encourage patients to express these concerns so that you can offer support (see Chapter 24).

Patient Expectations. It is important to identify the perceptions and expectations of a patient and family regarding surgery, recovery, and health care providers. This information allows you to plan interventions for teaching and emotional preparation and provides the basis for evaluation of care. For example, some patients have unrealistic expectations regarding pain control and the use of pain medications. Patients who are prepared to experience pain and know the proper use of pharmacological and nonpharmacological pain-relief measures tend to require less medication (Rothrock, 2015).

Patients and family members often have misconceptions about surgery. *For example, in the case study it is important for Sue to discuss with Mr. Korloff's daughters their understanding of his ability to perform activities at home that require lifting or moving heavy objects in the immediate postoperative period.*

⊕ BOX 40.2 PATIENT-CENTERED CARE

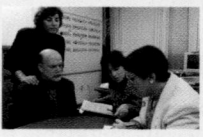

In preparing a preoperative plan of care, Sue explores Mr. Korloff's experiences, beliefs, and preferences about surgery. Studies have shown that some Russian Americans expect the nurse to be friendly, using open, inviting, nonverbal postures and a friendly smile. Sue learns that this is the case for Mr. Korloff by the way that he reacts to her communication. Sue must also learn if Mr. Korloff is willing to share his health problems with her. From his responses she determines he values receiving immediate information and answers from her and other health care workers. He follows health care instructions when he fully understands them. It is clear to Sue that Mr. Korloff has strong family ties and values. The Russian American father usually plays a primary role in the function of the family. Using this knowledge, Sue develops a patient-centered plan of care.

IMPLICATIONS FOR PRACTICE

- Assess Mr. Korloff's opinions about surgery first and then include his family.
- Assess Mr. Korloff's expectations of the level of involvement of the family in his surgical preparation and care.
- Provide preoperative teaching in a warm, caring, open manner using frequent smiles and hand gestures.
- Speak slowly and clearly in a low, calm voice using simple words.
- Provide an explanation of the importance of postoperative exercises so that Mr. Korloff understands why the exercises are important and will be more willing to do them after surgery.
- Determine if family members are close to Mr. Korloff and include them in the teaching session.

Sue learns that Mr. Korloff has a 40-lb older dog at home. He will not be able to lift the dog as he usually does when taking the dog in the car with him. When a patient is well prepared and knows what to expect in day-to-day activities, his or her knowledge is reinforced.

You have a professional obligation to provide clarification or more information when a patient is unaware of the actual reason for surgery. In such cases speak with the surgeon before revealing specific information related to the medical diagnosis to prevent confusion and identify the need for clarification.

Physical Examination. You conduct a physical examination (see Chapter 16) for all surgical patients preoperatively. The extent of any assessment depends on the patient's condition and the nature of the surgery. The assessment places emphasis on findings in a patient's medical history and on body systems that surgery or anesthesia will affect (Table 40.4).

General Survey. Gestures and body movements often reflect decreased energy or weakness caused by illness. Height and body weight are important indicators of nutritional status and are used to calculate medication dosages. Preoperative vital signs provide a baseline for intraoperative and postoperative comparison because anesthetic agents and medications can alter vital signs. Preoperative assessment of vital signs is also important to detect fluid and electrolyte abnormalities (see Chapter 18). An elevated temperature is cause for concern, as a fever can alter drug metabolism and increase the risk for fluid and electrolyte imbalances. If a patient has an underlying infection, elective surgery is often postponed until the infection is treated or resolved.

Head and Neck. Assessment of oral mucous membranes reveals the level of hydration. Dehydration increases the risk for the development of serious fluid and electrolyte imbalances during surgery. During the oral examination identify loose or capped teeth because there is a risk that they may become dislodged during endotracheal intubation. Note any dentures or partial plates that your patient uses; remove them when necessary and give to a family member to prevent loss or damage, and document this action in the patient record.

Inspection of the soft palate and nasal sinuses sometimes reveals sinus drainage indicative of respiratory or sinus infection. To rule out the possibility of local or systemic infection, palpate for cervical lymph node enlargement. Also inspect the jugular veins for distention. Excess fluid within the circulatory system or failure of the heart to contract efficiently frequently leads to jugular vein distention. A patient with heart disease or fluid overload is at risk for cardiovascular complications during surgery.

Skin. Thoroughly inspect a patient's skin, especially over bony prominences. Focus particularly on areas of the skin that will be under pressure during surgery, as a patient often lies in a fixed position for several hours. Nurses in the OR will position patients to avoid pressure over bony prominences and to protect vulnerable areas. A patient is susceptible to skin breakdown if the skin is thin, is dry, or has poor turgor (see Chapter 38).

Thorax and Lungs. A decline in ventilatory function, assessed through breathing pattern and chest excursion,

---

TABLE 40.4 FOCUSED PATIENT ASSESSMENT

Preoperative Assessment

FACTORS TO ASSESS	QUESTIONS	PHYSICAL ASSESSMENT
Significant medical history and previous surgeries	Do you have any bleeding disorders; diabetes; heart, lung, kidney, or liver disease; or any immune disorder?	Monitor vital signs and note any abnormalities.
		Inspect neck for jugular vein distention (cardiac disease, fluid overload).
	Have you had a recent fever or upper respiratory infection?	Inspect skin for turgor, dryness, rashes, skin breakdown.
		Auscultate heart and lungs for abnormal sounds (murmurs, congestion, bruits).
	Tell me if you have any pain.	Perform pain assessment with pain tool including severity, location, description, measures used to relieve.
		Assess extremities for decreased sensation, hair loss, clubbed fingers, deformed nails, sluggish capillary reflex, color.
Medication history and allergies	Which prescription, over-the-counter, and herbal medications are you currently taking?	Inspect any medication containers brought in by patient or family.
	What instructions were you given from your surgeon about taking or omitting medications before surgery?	
	Do you have any personal and/or family history of allergies to medications (including anesthetics), latex, foods, or anything you put on your skin?	Monitor laboratory values for any evidence of side effects of medications or drug levels, if ordered.

indicates a patient's risk for respiratory complications. Serious pulmonary congestion often causes postponement of surgery. For example, narrowing of the airways, as occurs with chronic lung disease, also called chronic obstructive pulmonary disease (COPD), increases the risk for airway obstruction because of bronchospasm related to endotracheal intubation and anesthesia.

Heart and Vascular System. If a patient has heart disease, assess the apical pulse rate and rhythm to establish a baseline with which to compare postoperatively. Assessment of peripheral pulses, color, and temperature of extremities is particularly important for a patient undergoing vascular or orthopedic surgery and when applying constricting bandages or casts to an extremity after surgery. Postoperative changes in skin color and sensation or development of a weak or absent pulse in a patient who had adequate circulation before surgery indicates impaired circulation.

Abdomen. Alterations in GI function after surgery often result in decreased or absent bowel sounds and abdominal distention. Assessment of a patient's usual abdominal anatomy is useful to assess for distention. Assessment of preoperative bowel sounds and normal elimination pattern is useful as a baseline. If surgery requires manipulation of portions of the GI tract or if a general anesthetic is used, normal peristalsis sometimes does not return immediately, and bowel sounds may be absent or diminished for hours to several days.

Neurological Status. A patient's level of consciousness, speech, and attention changes as a result of general anesthesia. After the effects of anesthesia disappear, expect a patient to normally return to his or her preoperative level of responsiveness. However, postoperative delirium is a common complication in older adults; risk factors include age older than 65 years, chronic cognitive decline or dementia, poor vision or hearing, severe illness, and the presence of infection (American Geriatrics Society [AGS], 2015). Thus a thorough assessment is required for patients at risk including patient's level of arousal, orientation, speech, emotions, and perceptual status (see Chapter 16).

Spinal or epidural anesthesia causes temporary paralysis of the lower extremities. Be aware of preexisting weakness or impaired mobility of the lower extremities to avoid becoming alarmed when full motor function does not return immediately after a procedure.

Risk Factors. Knowledge of preoperative risk factors discussed earlier enables you to take necessary precautions in planning care.

Diagnostic Screening. Patients undergo diagnostic test screening for preexisting abnormalities before surgery. Patients scheduled for elective surgery have testing as an outpatient either several days before or on the morning of surgery. If tests reveal abnormal values, the surgeon or anesthesia care provider may cancel surgery until the condition stabilizes. As the preoperative nurse, coordinate the completion of tests and verify that a patient is prepared properly. Review diagnostic results when available, alert the surgeon

and/or anesthesia care provider to findings, and intervene as appropriate.

Screening tests depend on a patient's condition and the nature of the surgery. Table 40.5 summarizes routine screening tests. In addition, a patient will require a blood type and screen in the event a transfusion becomes necessary during surgery. Additional preoperative tests include a urinalysis screen for urinary tract infections (UTIs), renal disease, or diabetes mellitus and a 12-lead electrocardiogram (ECG) to analyze heart rate and rhythm.

Older Adult Considerations. Older patients are at greater surgical risk as a result of physiological changes related to aging (see Chapter 23). A chest x-ray film to assess the size and shape of the heart, presence of lung lesions and chest wall abnormalities, and position of the diaphragm and aorta is a common preoperative test for older adult patients and patients with cardiovascular or pulmonary abnormalities. An older patient's physical capacity to adapt to the stress of surgery lessens because of deterioration of certain body functions (Table 40.6).

■ ■ ■ □ NURSING DIAGNOSIS

After you obtain assessment data, cluster defining characteristics and risk factors to identify appropriate nursing diagnoses. A nursing diagnosis establishes direction for care during one or all phases of surgery. The nature and type of surgery and a patient's age and health status suggest defining characteristics for problem-focused nursing diagnoses. For example, a patient's restlessness, poor eye contact, and expressed concern about the results of surgery point to the diagnosis of *Anxiety*. However, you need to validate the assessment to avoid misdiagnosis. In the foregoing assessment restlessness may also indicate *Acute Pain*.

Risk factors in a patient's history such as obesity, history of smoking, or preexisting conditions such as diabetes may result in a risk diagnosis such as *Risk for Infection*. Risk diagnoses allow you to plan preventive interventions. You need to ensure that you identify the nursing diagnosis that best fits your patient's problems. Possible nursing diagnoses for the preoperative patient include the following:

- *Anxiety*
- *Compromised Family Coping*
- *Ineffective Coping*
- *Fear*
- *Risk for Imbalanced Fluid Volume*
- *Risk for Infection*
- *Deficient Knowledge*
- *Risk for Imbalanced Nutrition: Less Than Body Requirements*

A problem-focused diagnosis and its related factors offer direction to the most effective nursing interventions for a patient. Ensure that related factors are accurate to avoid inappropriate interventions. For example, *Anxiety related to deficient knowledge of perioperative routines* requires you to offer thorough instruction before surgery and immediately after

TABLE 40.5 COMMON LABORATORY BLOOD TESTS (ADULT VALUES)

TEST	NORMAL VALUES[a]	SIGNIFICANCE	
		LOW	HIGH
Complete Blood Count (CBC)			
Hemoglobin (Hgb)	Female: 12–16 g/dL; male: 14–18 g/dL	Anemia	Polycythemia (elevated red blood cell count)
Hematocrit (Hct)	Female: 37%–47%; male: 42%–52%	Fluid overload	Dehydration
Platelet count	150,000–400,000/mm^3	Decreased clotting	Increased risk of blood clot
White blood cell count	5000–10,000/mm^3	Decreased ability to fight infection	Infection
Blood Chemistry			
Sodium (Na)	136–145 mEq/L	Fluid overload	Dehydration
Potassium (K)	3.5–5.0 mEq/L	Cardiac rhythm irregularities	Cardiac rhythm irregularities
Chloride (Cl)	98–106 mEq/L	Follows shifts in sodium blood levels	Follows shifts in sodium blood levels
Carbon dioxide (CO_2)	23–30 mEq/L	Affects acid-base balance in blood	Affects acid-base balance in blood
Blood urea nitrogen (BUN)	10–20 mg/dL	Liver disease/fluid overload	Renal disease/dehydration
Glucose	74–106 mg/dL fasting; 80–180 mg/dL recommended for surgical patient (ADA, 2016); older adult: 82–115 mg/dL	Insulin reaction, inadequate glucose intake	Diabetes mellitus and stress of surgery
Creatinine	Female: 0.5–1.1 mg/dL; male: 0.6–1.2 mg/dL	Malnutrition	Renal disease
Coagulation Studies			
International normalized ratio (INR)	0.76–1.27	Risk of clot	Risk of bleeding
Prothrombin time (PT)	11–12.5 sec; 85%–100%	Risk of clot	Risk of bleeding
Partial thromboplastin time (PTT)	60–70 sec	Risk of clot	Risk of bleeding
Activated PTT (APTT)	30–40 sec	Risk of clot	Excess heparin; risk of spontaneous bleeding

[a]Normal ranges vary slightly among laboratories.
From Pagana KD, et al: *Mosby's diagnostic and laboratory test reference,* ed 13, St Louis, 2017, Mosby.

surgery. However, *Anxiety related to threat of ineffective role performance* requires counseling and coaching during perioperative care.

■■■ PLANNING

Always include a patient and family in any discussions before surgery. Patient-centered care planning integrates patient and family preferences and values in how you teach and inform. For example, if a patient speaks a language different from yours, have a professional interpreter available to provide preoperative instruction (see Chapter 21). Involving the patient and family early can improve a patient's motivation to recover. This is especially important when patients are placed on prehabilitation programs. In a recent study involving patients scheduled for colorectal surgery, patients who received a home-based intervention of moderate aerobic and resistance exercises, nutritional counseling with protein supplementation, and relaxation exercises 4 weeks before surgery had better functional status postoperatively compared with patients who did not have prehabilitation (Santa, 2015; Gillis et al., 2014). Motivation to participate in prehabilitation is critical. Patients and family members must understand the plan and the outcomes that can be achieved when the plan is followed.

Informing patients and families during planning also minimizes surgical risks and postoperative complications because they can inform you of factors to monitor and

TABLE 40.6 PHYSIOLOGICAL FACTORS THAT PLACE OLDER ADULTS AT RISK DURING SURGERY

ALTERATIONS	RISKS	NURSING IMPLICATIONS
Cardiovascular System		
Degeneration of myocardium and valves Long-term use of medications (i.e., levodopa, bromocriptine, tricyclic antidepressants) Preexisting cardiac disease	Reduced cardiac reserve; hypotension; heart failure and dysrhythmias	Assess baseline vital signs, patient's fluid volume status, medication history. Use caution in administering IV fluids as first-line treatment.
Rigid arteries and reduction in sympathetic and parasympathetic innervation to heart	Predisposes patient to postoperative hemorrhage and hypertension	Instruct patient in techniques for performing leg exercises and proper turning.
Increase in calcium and cholesterol deposits within small arteries; thickened arterial walls	Increases risk for clot formation in lower extremities	Apply antiembolism stockings and mobile or sequential compression devices (see Chapter 29) postoperatively.
Integumentary System		
Decreased subcutaneous tissue and increased fragility of skin	Patient prone to pressure injury and skin tears	Assess skin every 2 hours or more often; pad all bony prominences during surgery. Turn or reposition every 2 hours if possible using safe patient-handling techniques.
Pulmonary System		
Decline in pulmonary reserve, increased ventilation/perfusion (V̇/Q̇) mismatch Diminished hypoxic and hypercapnic ventilatory drive Altered pharmacology of anesthetic drugs intraoperatively, causing residual/prolonged effects Decreased laryngeal reflexes makes patients more prone to aspiration (Iskandar et al., n.d.)	Reduced vital capacity; reduced coughing reflex	Instruct patient in proper technique for coughing, deep breathing, splinting incision, and use of incentive spirometer.
Reduced range of movement in diaphragm	Greater residual capacity or volume of air left in lung after normal breath, reducing amount of new air brought into lungs with each inspiration	When possible have patient participate in early mobility.
Stiffened lung tissue and enlarged air spaces	Reduces blood oxygenation levels	Provide supplemental oxygen when ordered postoperatively.
Decreased ability to cough and clear upper airway	Increases risk for postoperative pulmonary infection	Have patient cough, deep breathe, and use incentive spirometer every 2 hours postoperatively.
Renal System		
Reduced blood flow to kidneys	Increases risk for damage to renal tissues	For patients hospitalized before surgery, determine baseline urinary output for 24 hours.
Reduced glomerular filtration rate and excretory times	Limits ability to eliminate drugs or toxic substances	Maintain adequate hydration. Consider placing Foley catheter (per order) in at-risk patients to monitor urine output throughout perioperative period.
Reduced bladder capacity	Voiding frequency increases, and larger amount of urine stays in bladder after voiding Sensation of need to void sometimes does not occur until bladder is full	Instruct patient to notify nurse immediately when sensation of bladder fullness develops. Keep nurse call system and bedpan in an accessible location within patient's reach.

TABLE 40.6	PHYSIOLOGICAL FACTORS THAT PLACE OLDER ADULTS AT RISK DURING SURGERY—cont'd		
ALTERATIONS	**RISKS**	**NURSING IMPLICATIONS**	
Neurological System			
Deficit in cholinergic transmission; acetylcholine plays important roles in attention, consciousness, and memory (Iskandar et al., n.d.)	Delirium manifested by inattention, disorganized thinking, alteration in consciousness, cognitive deficit (memory, orientation, executive functions), hallucinations	Perform thorough assessment of baseline cognitive impairment; MMSE, DEAR score (age, cognition, ADLs, hearing/visual impairment, chemical use); consider geriatric consultation in at-risk patients (Iskandar et al., n.d.)	
Sensory losses including reduced tactile sense and increased pain tolerance	Patient less able to respond to early warning signs of surgical complications	Orient patient to surrounding environment. Observe for nonverbal signs of pain.	
Decreased reaction time	Patient becomes easily confused after anesthesia	Reorient frequently. Round on patient frequently. Keep side rails up and room free from clutter.	
Metabolic System			
Reduced number of red blood cells and hemoglobin levels	Reduces ability to carry adequate oxygen to tissues	Administer necessary blood products. Monitor blood test results.	
Change in total amounts of body potassium and water volume	Increases risk for fluid or electrolyte imbalance	Monitor fluid and electrolyte levels.	

ADLs, Activities of daily living; *MMSE,* Mini-Mental State Examination.

consider. Structured preoperative teaching reduces the amount of anesthesia and postoperative pain medication needed, decreases the occurrence of postoperative urinary retention, promotes an earlier return to normal oral intake, and decreases length of hospital stay (Rothrock, 2015). Patients who understand what to expect about their surgical experience are less likely to be fearful and are better prepared for expected outcomes.

Goals and Outcomes. The plan of care begins in the preoperative phase, and you modify it as needed during the intraoperative and postoperative phases (see the Care Plan). The goals of care for the surgical patient include the following:

- Understanding the physiological and psychological responses to surgery
- Understanding intraoperative and postoperative events
- Achieving early mobilization postoperatively
- Achieving emotional and physiological comfort and rest
- Achieving return of normal physiological function after surgery (e.g., return of normal vital signs, fluid and electrolyte balance, muscle function)
- Remaining free of surgical wound infection
- Remaining safe from harm during the perioperative period

Outcomes established for each goal of care provide measurable ways to determine a patient's progress toward meeting stated goals. For example, in the case of "understanding intraoperative and postoperative events," outcomes may include "patient describes postoperative exercises" and "patient explains positioning during surgery."

Setting Priorities. Establish individualized care by prioritizing nursing diagnoses and interventions based on the assessed needs of each patient. Setting priorities requires clinical judgment. For example, your patient has two nursing diagnoses, *Anxiety* and *Deficient Knowledge.* You determine the priority nursing diagnosis is *Deficient Knowledge* for this patient because, in this case, patient instruction will likely relieve the anxiety. Be thorough in your plan and be sure that it reflects your understanding of the implications of a patient's age, physical and psychological health, educational level, previous experience with surgery, cultural beliefs and practices, and stated and/or written wishes concerning advance directives.

Collaborative Care. Perioperative care requires collaboration with other health care disciplines. Consider which members of the health care team (e.g., dietitians, occupational therapists) you need to involve while planning patient care. For example, patients who require aggressive pulmonary rehabilitation such as patients having thoracic surgery may require a referral to a respiratory therapist. Many patients and their families benefit from referral to pastoral care, especially if the procedure is emergent or life threatening. You anticipate patient and family caregiver discharge needs based on information learned in the initial assessment.

The preoperative planning phase for ambulatory surgical patients usually occurs in an outpatient setting before or on the morning of surgery. Ideally it begins in the surgeon's office and continues in the home. This gives a patient and family time to reflect on the surgical experience, make necessary physical preparations (e.g., prehabilitation), and ask

◎ CARE PLAN

Deficient Knowledge

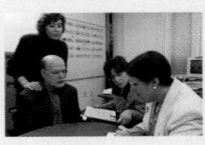

ASSESSMENT

As Mr. Korloff enters the preadmission center for testing, Sue greets him and his daughters. She explains the need to gather a history and asks Mr. Korloff if he wishes to have his daughters join him. He smiles and says, "Yes, my daughters will be my nurses for a few days." The nursing staff report that Mr. Korloff's daughters have been calling on the phone and asking many questions about intraoperative and postoperative events. Mr. Korloff is alert and attentive and answers appropriately. His vision and hearing are normal. This will be his first experience having surgery.

ASSESSMENT ACTIVITIES

Ask Mr. Korloff what he has been told regarding surgery by his surgeon.

Ask Mr. Korloff what he understands about preoperative preparation and what to expect after surgery.

Ask Mr. Korloff what concerns him about having surgery.

FINDINGS[a]

He states that **he knows very little about the surgery.**

He says **he knows few specifics and asks if he will have "a needle in my arm to give me fluids?"**

He repeatedly says, "Oh, I'm not worried," but then **asks many questions, often repeatedly.**

[a]**Defining characteristics/risk factors** are shown in **bold** type.

NURSING DIAGNOSIS: Deficient Knowledge regarding implications of surgery (cholecystectomy) related to first surgical experience and inadequate preparation

---

PLANNING

GOAL	EXPECTED OUTCOMES (NOC)[b]
	Knowledge: Treatment Procedure
Mr. Korloff will understand preoperative, intraoperative, and postoperative events before the day of surgery.	On the day before surgery, Mr. Korloff and his daughters describe events that commonly occur in the holding area and operating room.
	On the day of admission, Mr. Korloff and his daughters describe routine postoperative nursing procedures.
	On the day of admission, Mr. Korloff and his daughters describe ways to participate in postoperative care.

[b]Outcome classification labels from Moorhead S, et al, editors: *Nursing outcomes classification (NOC),* ed 5, St Louis, 2013, Mosby.

INTERVENTIONS (NIC)[c]	RATIONALE
Teaching: Procedure/Treatment	
Give Mr. Korloff a copy of the teaching booklet *Your Surgical Experience* or offer options such as video and web-based programs.	Preoperative teaching increases patient satisfaction regarding knowledge of the perioperative process (Ortiz et al., 2015). Teaching decreases stress, fear, and anxiety and reduces length of hospitalization, development of complications, and recovery time after discharge (Lewis et al., 2014). Web-based programs to deliver patient education in preoperative areas have increased patient satisfaction with instruction (Nahm et al., 2012).
Provide planned teaching session for Mr. Korloff and his daughters after preadmission testing. Explain events that will occur in holding area (e.g., insertion of IV catheter, vital sign check) and in operating room (e.g., positioning, anesthesia). Use visual aids to help Mr. Korloff understand the laparoscopic procedure.	Teaching focused on information that patient will need to know on morning of admission decreases anxiety and allows patient and family to better participate in care.
Allow Mr. Korloff to express his feelings and fears related to surgery.	Expressing feelings and fears decreases anxiety related to the surgical experience for patient teaching to be more effective.
Provide planned teaching session on day of admission to counsel Mr. Korloff and his daughters on common events that occur after surgery, importance of early ambulation, and participation in postoperative exercises. Use demonstration of exercises. Answer questions.	Preoperative counseling along with instruction and support about physiotherapy can foster early mobilization among patients (Samnani et al., 2014). Preoperative teaching improves patient's ability to participate in care activities and resume activities of daily living after surgery. Demonstration is an effective method in teaching psychomotor skills.
Have Mr. Korloff perform return demonstration of postoperative exercises.	Return demonstration verifies that learning has occurred and patient is able to correctly perform exercises to reduce postoperative complications.

[c]Intervention classification labels from Bulechek GM, et al, editors: *Nursing interventions classification (NIC),* ed 6, St Louis, 2013, Mosby.

CARE PLAN—cont'd

Deficient Knowledge

EVALUATION

NURSING ACTIONS	PATIENT RESPONSE/FINDING	ACHIEVEMENT OF OUTCOME
Ask Mr. Korloff and his daughters to identify the basic purpose of the surgery and changes to expect afterward.	Mr. Korloff describes the surgical procedure and explains why he needs the surgery.	Mr. Korloff demonstrates a good understanding of the surgery.
Ask Mr. Korloff and his daughters to identify routine types of postoperative monitoring and treatment. Observe Mr. Korloff perform postoperative exercises.	Mr. Korloff describes postoperative exercises to perform after surgery but is not able to discuss monitoring activities. Mr. Korloff demonstrates coughing, deep breathing, and use of leg exercises. Has difficulty using incentive spirometer. Mr. Korloff's daughters remind him to hold his breath for 2 to 3 seconds with use of incentive spirometer.	Mr. Korloff describes postoperative exercises. Requires further instruction on monitoring activities. Mr. Korloff demonstrates coughing, deep breathing, and leg exercises appropriately. Requires further demonstration and assistance from his daughters in use of incentive spirometer.

questions about postoperative procedures. Well-planned preoperative care ensures that a patient and family caregiver are well informed and actively participate during recovery.

■■■ IMPLEMENTATION

Preoperative nursing interventions focus on patient education and physical preparation of a patient for surgery.

Informed Consent. A surgeon cannot legally perform surgery and an anesthesia care provider cannot administer an anesthetic until a patient understands the need for the procedure and the steps, risks, expected results, and alternative treatments involved. Chapter 5 summarizes issues and guidelines for informed consent. Patients need to sign all consent forms before you administer any preoperative medications that alter their consciousness. The primary responsibility for informing a patient rests with the surgeon and anesthesia care provider. If a patient is confused or uncertain about a procedure, you are professionally and ethically obligated to contact the surgeon and/or anesthesia care provider so that further discussion and clarification are offered. A patient always has the right to refuse surgery or treatment even after giving written consent.

Health Promotion. Health promotion activities during the preoperative phase focus on prevention of complications, health maintenance, and support of possible rehabilitation needs after surgery.

Prehabilitation. Surgeons and clinicians are beginning to recognize that prehabilitation during the preoperative period may represent a more appropriate time than the postoperative period to implement preventive interventions. Components of a prehabilitation program will vary by the surgical procedure and the condition and age of a patient. Common components include the following (McGill Perioperative Program, 2017):

1. Medical optimization: Patients who have comorbidities such as high blood pressure, diabetes, or arthritis may require adjustments in medication doses and frequencies and monitoring of vital signs.
2. Physical activity: It is common for patients who are facing surgery to have a sedentary lifestyle. A physical activity program aims to increase aerobic capacity and muscle and core strength. Aerobic and resistive exercises are common program components.
3. Nutrition plan: A patient who is undernourished before surgery has greater risk of morbidity and mortality. The primary goal of nutrition therapy is to optimize nutrient stores preoperatively and provide adequate nutrition to compensate for the catabolic response of surgery postoperatively.
4. Strategies to reduce anxiety: Patients may meet with a counselor or psychologist to focus on learning relaxation and breathing exercises and anxiety reduction techniques.

Preoperative Teaching. Patient education relieves anxiety, increases patient satisfaction, speeds recovery, decreases the amount of perceived pain, and facilitates a more rapid return to work or normal functioning (Lewis et al., 2014). Systematic, structured, and interactive preoperative teaching positively influences patient recovery. Structured teaching, when successful, helps patients gain knowledge and skills needed to influence the following postoperative factors:

1. Ventilatory function: Exercises improve the ability and willingness to deep breathe and cough effectively.
2. Physical functional capacity: Knowledge of benefits of exercise increases understanding and willingness to ambulate and resume activities of daily living.
3. Sense of well-being: Patients who are prepared for surgery experience less anxiety and report a greater sense of psychological well-being.
4. Length of hospital stay: Participation in postoperative activities frequently reduces a patient's length of

hospital stay by preventing or minimizing postoperative complications.

5. Anxiety about pain and amount of pain medication needed for comfort: Patients who learn before surgery about pain and ways to relieve it are less anxious about the pain, ask for what they need, and actually require less pain medication after surgery (Pinar et al., 2011).

The most effective type of teaching program for surgical patients covers the entire surgical experience. Box 40.3 outlines the parameters for perioperative preparation. Preoperative teaching occurs in the home, surgeon's office, or preadmission unit. Offer printed literature (large print when appropriate), web-based programs, DVDs, or videotapes to patients. It is a common practice for the preoperative nurse to call patients before surgery to provide education and clarify questions.

Always include family caregivers in preoperative preparation if the patient has given permission to do so. They are frequently the coaches for postoperative exercises when a patient returns from surgery. If family caregivers do not understand routine postoperative events, their anxiety heightens a patient's fears or concerns. Reduce misunderstanding and anxiety with thoughtful preparation.

Timing. Preoperative teaching is most useful when started the week before admission (or earlier if a patient is in a prehabilitation program) and reinforced immediately before surgery. Teaching performed when a patient is less anxious results in more effective learning because anxiety and fear are barriers to learning. Always present information in a logical sequence beginning with preoperative events and advancing to intraoperative and postoperative routines. Preoperative teaching checklists offer helpful guidelines for presenting patients with a comprehensive set of instructions. Teaching includes information on what patients can expect and how to participate fully in their own plan of care such as preoperative fasting and proper use of medications and herbal supplements (Rothrock, 2015).

Surgical Procedure. After the surgeon explains the basic purpose of the surgical procedure and its steps, a patient may ask you additional questions. While answering questions, use familiar terminology and avoid using technical medical terms because this adds to a patient's confusion. Avoid saying anything that contradicts the surgeon's explanation. One way to avoid contradictions is to first ask what the surgeon told a patient. If a patient has little or no understanding about the surgery, refer the patient back to the surgeon for additional information.

Preoperative Routines. Explain the preoperative routines that a patient will undergo. For example, explain to a patient why an IV infusion is necessary. Knowing which tests and procedures are planned and why increases a patient's sense of control.

The anesthesia care provider visits with a patient to complete a preanesthesia assessment either during the preoperative admission process or in the presurgical care unit. A patient and family need to know about this visit in advance so that they can ask any questions and be prepared to provide

---

BOX 40.3 PATIENT TEACHING

Perioperative Patient Preparation

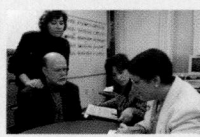 Sue plans time after completing Mr. Korloff's assessment to discuss the planned surgery with him and his daughters. She begins by asking Mr. Korloff to describe what he thinks the procedure will involve, share any concerns, and identify the type of information he wants to understand. This shows Sue's cultural sensitivity, which makes teaching more patient-centered.

OUTCOME
At the end of the teaching session Mr. Korloff will be able to:
- Describe preoperative, intraoperative, and postoperative procedures to anticipate for a laparoscopic procedure
- Demonstrate postoperative exercises

TEACHING STRATEGIES
Preoperative Procedures
- State time to arrive at agency and time of surgery (approximate time or if his case is "to follow" a previous surgery).
- Explain extent and purpose of food and fluid restrictions.
- Explain or review informed consent.
- Teach about physical preparation required (e.g., bowel or skin preparation).
- Explain about procedures performed in preanesthesia just before transport to operating room (IV line insertion, urinary catheterization or voiding, preoperative medications).

Intraoperative Procedures
- Describe preanesthesia care environment and activities.
- Describe operating room environment.
- Explain about the roles of circulating nurse, scrub nurse, and anesthesia care provider.

Postoperative Procedures
- Describe postanesthesia care environment and activities.
- Teach about pain control and other comfort measures.
- Explain purpose of any anticipated tubes, drains, or IV lines.
- Emphasize importance of postoperative exercises (see Skill 40.1).
- Demonstrate exercises and have patient perform return demonstration.
- Encourage Mr. Korloff and family to verbalize any concerns.
- Assess Mr. Korloff and his family's understanding of perioperative preparation and respond appropriately.

EVALUATION
- Use the principles of teach-back to evaluate patient/family caregiver learning:
  - "Describe your understanding of preoperative, intraoperative, and postoperative procedures."
  - "Demonstrate coughing, deep-breathing, and turning exercises."

necessary information such as history of allergies and previous experience with anesthesia.

Explain to a patient and family the importance of the patient following oral intake instructions for food and liquids as provided by the surgeon and anesthesia care provider. During the use of general anesthesia, the muscles relax, and gastric contents can reflux into the esophagus. The anesthetic eliminates a patient's ability to gag. Therefore a patient is at risk for aspiration of food or fluids from the stomach into the lungs.

The American Society of Anesthesiologists (ASA) provides recommendations on fluid and food intake before procedures requiring general anesthesia, regional anesthesia, or sedation/analgesia. These recommendations include fasting from intake of clear liquids for 2 or more hours, breast milk for 4 hours, formula and nonhuman milk for 6 hours, and a light meal of toast and clear liquids for 6 hours. A patient also cannot have any meat or fried foods 8 hours before surgery, unless explicitly specified by the anesthesia care provider or surgeon (ASA Committee on Standards and Practice Parameters, 2011). Despite these regulations, many agencies still have patients maintain nothing by mouth (NPO) after midnight. Ensure that you follow the health care provider's orders. The surgeon's orders also provide additional guidance for routines to explain to a patient (e.g., intravenous therapy, preoperative medications, or insertion of a urinary catheter or nasogastric [NG] tube).

Intraoperative Routines. The scheduled operative time is only an estimated time. Unanticipated delays occur for many reasons that have nothing to do with your patient. Emphasize that the scheduled time is a rough estimate and the actual time can be sooner or later. Most surgical waiting areas give family members pagers so that they can be contacted by the surgical staff for updates (e.g., when surgery begins and time patient arrives in recovery). Tell family members where to wait and inform them that the surgeon will speak to them when the surgery is completed. Communicate any excessive delays that occur to the family.

Postoperative Routines. A patient and family want to know about postoperative events. If they understand routine postoperative vital sign monitoring, they are less likely to worry when nurses perform these assessments. If a patient is to be placed on an early mobility protocol, patients and families need to understand that the patient is not being rushed unnecessarily but that early mobility prevents hospital deconditioning (see Chapter 28). Also explain if a patient is to have IV lines, dressings, or drainage tubes. Do not overprepare or underprepare a patient and family. You cannot predict all of a patient's requirements, and a patient may be misinformed about a therapy that may not be initiated. Contradictions between your explanations and reality cause anxiety.

Sensory Preparation. Provide a patient with information about sensations typically experienced before, during, and after surgery. Preparatory information helps patients anticipate the steps of a procedure and form a realistic image of the surgical experience. When sensations occur as predicted, a patient is better able to cope with the experiences. For example, warn that the OR room is very bright and cool. Explain that you will apply a cuff for a noninvasive blood pressure monitor to the patient's arm. This monitor makes a hum and a beep, and the cuff tightens around the arm. Informing a patient about these and other sensations in the OR reduces anxiety before the patient is anesthetized, which helps to decrease the amount of anesthetic needed for induction. Other postoperative sensations to describe include blurred vision from ophthalmic ointment, dryness of the mouth or the sensation of a sore throat resulting from an endotracheal tube, pain at the incision site, tightness of the dressings, and feeling cold.

Pain Relief. One of the surgical patient's greatest fears is pain. The family is also concerned about a patient's comfort. Preoperative preparation regarding pain and pain-control measures helps patients know what to expect and anticipate how to cope with pain. Patient-controlled analgesia (PCA) is common and provides patients with control over pain. Explain to a patient how to operate a PCA pump and the importance of administering medication as soon as pain becomes persistent postoperatively (see Chapter 34). This applies also to patients who have epidural analgesia postoperatively. Additionally, patients who receive epidural or regional analgesia need a thorough understanding of how the medication affects movement and sensation.

Oral and parenteral analgesics do not provide adequate pain relief if a patient waits until the pain becomes excruciating before using or requesting an analgesic. Even though around-the-clock (ATC) analgesia is more effective, most patients still have analgesics ordered prn (as needed). Pain control is essential for a surgical patient to recover quickly. Encourage a patient to use analgesics as needed and not be fearful of any dependence on them following surgery. Explain the schedule for administration of all analgesics. If analgesics are not ordered continuous or ATC, encourage a patient to inform nurses as soon as pain becomes a persistent discomfort. Offering pain medication when it is due can maintain low levels of discomfort for the patient. A patient needs to know that it takes time for a drug to act and that the drug may not entirely eliminate all the discomfort. Inform a patient and family of other therapies available for pain relief such as focused breathing and relaxation, distraction such as listening to music (Palmer et al., 2016), and the use of heat or cold compresses.

Postoperative Exercises. Preoperative teaching programs frequently include explanation and demonstration of postoperative exercises including diaphragmatic breathing, incentive spirometry, controlled coughing, turning, and leg exercises (see Skill 40.1). Diaphragmatic breathing improves lung expansion and oxygen delivery without using excess energy. A patient learns to use the diaphragm during deep breathing to take slow, deep, and relaxed breaths. Eventually a patient's lung volume improves. Deep breathing also helps to clear any anesthetic gases used during surgery from the airways. To facilitate deep breathing a health care provider often orders an incentive spirometer for a patient (see Chapter 32). Incentive spirometry encourages forced inspiration. The therapy is effective in preventing atelectasis after surgery.

Coughing helps to remove retained mucus in the airways. A deep, productive cough is more beneficial than merely clearing the throat. A patient needs to anticipate postoperative discomfort and understand the importance of coughing even when it is difficult. Teach a patient to splint an abdominal or thoracic incision to minimize pain during coughing. Pain control is essential for effective deep breathing and coughing; educate a patient to ask for pain medications as needed.

Leg exercises and turning improve blood flow to the extremities and reduce venous stasis, reducing the risk for clot formation and subsequent pulmonary emboli. Contractions of lower leg muscles promote venous return, making it difficult for clots to form. Turning helps to mobilize pulmonary secretions and increases ventilation and perfusion of the lungs. After explaining each exercise, demonstrate it. Then, while acting as a coach, ask a patient to demonstrate each exercise. Show family members how they can become coaches as well. Also explain that a patient is likely to have compression hose stockings after surgery to reduce risk of DVT.

Early Mobility and Activity Resumption. Many surgical protocols now include early mobility guidelines that are designed to minimize or prevent hospital-acquired deconditioning (see Chapter 28). Early mobility protocols are associated with improved outcomes such as reduced DVT, reduced length of stay in patients with community-acquired pneumonia, and maintained or improved functional status from admission to discharge in older adult patients and patients who undergo major surgery (Pashikanti and Von Ah, 2012). Explain to patients and family members how quickly patients will begin activities such as range of motion, sitting on the side of the bed, assisted ambulation, and distance to walk. Also assure patients that appropriate mobility aids will be used and assistance by nursing staff will ensure their safety.

Some patients will not be able to initiate early mobility until their conditions have stabilized. Explain that it is normal for a patient to progress gradually in activity. If a patient tolerates activity, activity levels progress more quickly.

Promotion of Nutrition. A surgical patient is vulnerable to fluid and electrolyte imbalances as a result of inadequate preoperative intake, excessive fluid loss during surgery, and the stress response. A patient is usually NPO for several hours before surgery to reduce risks for vomiting and aspirating emesis during surgery. Instruct a patient to eat and drink sufficient amounts before fasting to ensure adequate fluid and nutrient intake. Some patients will have followed prehabilitation nutritional diets. Make sure that the patient's diet includes foods high in protein with sufficient amounts of carbohydrates, fat, and vitamins. Instruct a patient and family members regarding preoperative fasting requirements and oral medication use. Notify the surgeon and anesthesia care provider as soon as possible if a patient eats or drinks during the fasting period.

For patients who are hospitalized, remove all fluids and solid foods from the bedside and post a sign in a highly visible location to alert hospital personnel and family members about fasting restrictions. Instruct patients to rinse their mouths with water or mouthwash and brush their teeth but not to swallow anything, even clear liquids. Patients may take oral medications with sips of water if ordered by the health care provider. Notify the dietary department to cancel meals. A patient who is at home the evening before surgery needs to understand the importance of not taking food or fluids, when to start fasting, and be willing to follow restrictions.

Promotion of Rest. Rest is essential for normal healing. Anxiety about surgery may interfere with the ability of a patient to relax or sleep. During preoperative instruction give the patient and family time to express feelings about surgery and ask questions either together or separately. A patient's level of anxiety influences the frequency of discussions, and you need to encourage expression of these concerns. If a patient is ordered to take a sedative hypnotic or antianxiety medication the night before surgery, explain the purpose and encourage its use. Also, if the patient is hospitalized the night before, use interventions that normally promote sleep in the home (see Chapter 33).

Acute Care. The degree of preoperative physical preparation depends on a patient's health status, the surgery, and the surgeon's preferences. You will tailor nursing interventions accordingly to the type of surgery, the setting in which the surgery is done, and the needs of each individual patient.

Minimize Risk for Surgical Wound Infection. The risk for developing a surgical wound infection depends on the amount and type of microorganisms contaminating a wound, the susceptibility of the host, and the condition of the wound at the end of the operation (Box 40.4). All three factors interact, determining the risk for infection (see Chapter 14). The skin is the most common site for microorganisms to grow and multiply. Without proper skin preparation, the risk for postoperative wound infection is high. Many surgeons have patients take a bath or shower with an antimicrobial soap such as CHG the evening before surgery. However, evidence is still not conclusive that preoperative bathing with agents such as CHG reduce bacterial colonization of the skin (Anderson et al., 2014). Adequate levels of CHG must be achieved and maintained on the skin by allowing CHG to dry completely. Often patients are instructed to bathe or shower more than once, whereas others are instructed to give special attention to cleansing the proposed operative site with special cleansing pads. If the surgical procedure involves the head, neck, or upper chest area, a patient also is required to shampoo the hair. Surgeons generally order hair removal only if the hair has the potential to interfere with exposure, closure, or dressing of the surgical site. Remove hair as close to the time of surgery as possible (AORN, 2017a). Instruct patients not to shave the surgical area because shaving leaves nicks that can harbor infectious microorganisms.

Prevention of Bowel Incontinence and Contamination. Historically, mechanical bowel preparation, or the

BOX 40.4 EVIDENCE-BASED PRACTICE

PICO Question: Does the implementation of bundled strategies compared with standard nursing care reduce surgical site infections?

SUMMARY OF EVIDENCE

Surgical site infections (SSIs) are associated with considerable morbidity costs as well as a number of negative experiences including pain, loss of earnings, frequent hospitalizations, and altered quality of life. Implementation of bundled strategies to control the environment during the perioperative experience decreases the risk for infection (Anderson et al., 2014). Handwashing is the most effective tool in preventing infection. Everyone is responsible for safe patient-centered care, regardless of his or her role (Kiernan, 2015). Specific interventions to prevent surgical wound infection include not removing hair at the surgical site unless hair will interfere with surgery (clipping is appropriate), disinfection of the skin with an alcohol-containing antiseptic immediately before the incision is made, administration of a prophylactic antibiotic preoperatively and discontinued within 24 hours postoperatively, glycemic control, maintenance of normothermia (35.5° C or more) perioperatively, and skin adhesive or antimicrobial dressings (Anderson et al., 2014; Spencer and Christie, 2014; Tanner et al., 2015). Evidence demonstrates a direct relationship between the use of these preventive measures and decreased postoperative wound infection (Anderson et al., 2014; Tanner et al., 2015). Nurses working in perioperative areas play a significant role in preventing and detecting postoperative wound infection, as they ensure that key interventions are implemented for all patients in all situations.

APPLICATION TO NURSING PRACTICE
- Conduct ongoing monitoring postoperatively for clinical signs of SSI (Kiernan, 2015).
- Administer antibiotics on time as ordered and inform health care provider if antibiotics are not discontinued within 24 hours postoperatively (Anderson et al., 2014).
- If hair is clipped, do so outside the operating room.
- Maintain normothermia (temperature of 35.5° C or more) during the perioperative period (Anderson et al., 2014).
- Attend education regarding the outcomes associated with SSI, risks for SSI, and methods to reduce risk to all patients, patients' families, surgeons, and perioperative personnel.

administration of osmotic agents, stimulant cathartics, and regimens that involve a combination of these agents, have been used to "cleanse" the bowel to clear the colon of stool, make it easier for surgeons to handle the colon, and reduce pressure at the site of a colon anastomosis (Kumar et al., 2013). Enemas were also given for the same purposes. However, evidence now suggests that mechanical bowel preparation is no longer needed for most patients and procedures (Kumar et al., 2013). Surgical patients have been shown to have good outcomes without such preparation. For example, there have been reports of earlier return of bowel function and shorter hospital stays among patients who did not have mechanical bowel preparation before surgery (Kumar et al.,

2013). However, surgeons are sometimes slow to adopt new evidence. The administration of cathartics, laxatives, and enemas is still common in many health care agencies.

Interventions on Day of Surgery. On the morning of surgery complete the routine procedures discussed in the following sections before releasing a patient for surgery.

Documentation. Before a patient goes to the OR, check the medical record to be sure that all relevant laboratory and test results are present. Check all consent forms for completeness and accuracy of information. Some agencies use a checklist based on the World Health Organization (WHO) checklist to ensure compliance with best practices to improve surgical patient safety (WHO, 2017). A preoperative checklist provides guidelines for ensuring completion of all nursing interventions. Check the nurses' notes to be sure that documentation is current, especially if a patient experienced unpredicted problems the night before surgery.

Assessment of Vital Signs. Make a final assessment of vital signs and document them on the preoperative flow sheet or checklist and in the nurses' notes. If any of the vital signs are abnormal, notify the surgeon.

Hygiene. Basic hygiene measures including bathing and hair care remove skin contamination and increase a patient's comfort. Some surgeons will order a bath using an antimicrobial agent. Because a patient cannot wear personal nightwear to the OR, provide a clean hospital gown and instruct the patient to remove all other articles of clothing including undergarments. After being NPO throughout the night, a patient may have a very dry mouth. Offer mouthwash and toothpaste and caution a patient not to swallow anything.

Preparation of Hair and Removal of Cosmetics. During major surgery the anesthesia care provider positions a patient's head to put an endotracheal tube into the airway (see Chapter 32). This involves manipulation of the hair and scalp. To avoid injury, ask a patient to remove hairpins, clips, wigs, or hairpieces. Patients can braid long hair and wear disposable hats to contain hair before entering the OR. Many hair products are flammable. When the surgical site is the head or neck, it is important to ensure that these are removed before using electrocautery to reduce the risk for fire.

During and after surgery the anesthesia care provider and nurses assess skin and mucous membranes to determine a patient's level of oxygenation, circulation, and fluid balance. A pulse oximeter is often applied to a finger to monitor oxygen saturation of the blood (see Chapter 15). Anesthesia care providers also use end-tidal carbon dioxide, by way of capnography, to assess patients' physiological stability. Have patients remove all makeup (lipstick, powder, blush, nail polish) and at least one artificial fingernail to expose normal skin and nail coloring. Anything in or around the eye irritates or injures the eye during surgery. Have patients remove contact lenses, false eyelashes, and eye makeup. Eyeglasses usually remain in the room or you can give them to a family member immediately before a patient enters the OR.

Removal of Prostheses. It is easy for any type of prosthetic device to become lost or damaged during surgery. Have patients remove all removable prosthetics for safekeeping. If a patient has a brace or splint, check with the surgeon to determine whether it should remain with a patient to be reapplied after surgery. Although patients need to remove hearing aids, eyeglasses, and contact lenses, do not have them do this until just before the surgery. Allowing patients to wear these aids facilitates communication and increases a patient's sense of control. Refer to agency policies for clarification.

Give a patient privacy when he or she has to remove dentures. Place dentures in special containers and label with the patient's name for safekeeping to prevent breakage or give the dentures to a family member. Assess a patient for loose teeth. A broken tooth can become dislodged during insertion of an endotracheal tube and obstruct the airway.

Inventory and secure all prosthetic devices. Give prosthetics to family members or keep the devices at a patient's bedside. Follow agency policy and document the location of devices.

Preparation of Bowel and Bladder. If a patient does have an enema or cathartic ordered for the morning of surgery (see Chapter 37), give it at least 1 hour before a patient leaves for surgery, allowing time for a patient to defecate without rushing.

Instruct a patient to void just before leaving for the OR. If a patient is unable to void, document this on the preoperative checklist. An empty bladder minimizes incontinence and injury to the bladder during surgery. An empty bladder also makes abdominal organs more accessible. The surgeon orders an indwelling catheter if the surgery is long or the incision is in the lower abdomen (see Chapter 36).

Application of Antiembolism Devices. Many surgeons order antiembolic stockings or compression devices for patients to wear during or after surgery. When correctly sized and properly applied, these devices reduce the risk for DVT (see Chapter 29). Antiembolic stockings maintain compression of small veins and capillaries of the lower extremities. The constant compression forces blood into larger vessels, promoting venous return and preventing venous stasis. Sequential compression and continuous compression devices are attached to an air pump that inflates and deflates compression sleeves. A sequential compression device applies intermittent pressure sequentially from the ankle to the knee and alternating calves, mimicking the venous return process of walking. A continuous compression device such as the ActiveCare+S.F.T. (MCS Inc., Concord, MA) identifies a patient's normal venous blood flow pulses and actively synchronizes compression to the natural pulse rhythm.

Promotion of Patient's Dignity. During preoperative preparations it is important to maintain a patient's privacy, to reduce sources of anxiety, and not to depersonalize your interactions with the patient. Patients admitted for ambulatory and same-day surgery often sit in a waiting room before surgery. Once inside the preoperative setting, protect patients' modesty, allow them to wear underclothes when possible, and provide cover robes. Ensure hospitalized patients their privacy by closing room curtains or doors during preoperative preparation. Allow the family to stay until a patient goes to the OR.

Performing Special Procedures. Sometimes a patient's condition requires special interventions before surgery. Anticipate that the surgeon may order IV infusions (see Chapter 18), insertion of a Foley catheter (see Chapter 36), insertion of a nasogastric (NG) tube for gastric decompression (see Chapter 37), or administration of medications such as antibiotics and sedatives (see Chapter 17).

Safeguarding Valuables. Give family members any patient valuables or secure items for safekeeping in a designated location. Many agencies require patients to sign a release to free the institution of responsibility for lost valuables. Document the description of items in the patient's chart, and give a copy of the listed valuables to a designated family member. Patients are often reluctant to remove wedding rings or religious medals. Tape a wedding band in place; however, do not create a tourniquet with the tape. If there is a risk that a patient will experience swelling of the hand or fingers, remove the band.

Administering Preoperative Medications. The surgeon or anesthesia care provider may order preoperative drugs for you to give before a patient leaves for the OR. Complete all nursing interventions before giving the preoperative medications. Preoperative drugs such as benzodiazepines, opioids, antiemetics, and anticholinergics can cause dry mouth, drowsiness, and dizziness. Keep the patient's bed side rails in the up position, the bed in the low position, and the nurse call system within easy reach of the patient. The Centers for Disease Control and Prevention (CDC) recommend administration of antibiotics for prevention of SSI postoperatively (CDC, n.d.). The recommendations follow evidence-based standards and guidelines for specific procedures. Guidelines recommend administering within 1 hour before incision (2 hours for vancomycin and fluoroquinolones). Note that antibiotics may thus be given in the holding area.

Instruct a patient to remain in bed until the surgical nursing assistant or transporter arrives to take the patient to the OR and to call for assistance if there is a need to get out of bed. A patient may not realize how significantly impairing preoperative medication can be, which can lead to falls if the patient tries to ambulate without assistance. Never allow a patient to sign an informed consent document while under the influence of an opioid or sedative.

■■■■ EVALUATION

Evaluation of the preoperative goals and outcomes of the plan of care begins before surgery and extends into the postoperative period, providing direction for future interventions. For some patients surgery is an emergency. Others require procedures up until surgery. Conduct an evaluation that corresponds with established goals and outcomes for any surgical patients.

Patient Outcomes. Determine if a patient and family have adequate preoperative preparation by asking the patient to describe the surgical procedure, its purpose, and the expected postoperative care (Box 40.5). This allows you to

BOX 40.5 EVALUATION

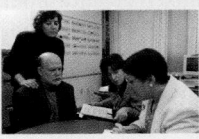

It is the morning of Mr. Korloff's surgery, and Sue and the primary nurse admit him to the hospital with the help of one of his daughters. She checks that the informed consent has been signed and witnessed. She completes his physical assessment, which focuses on assessing breath sounds, condition of his skin, and vital signs. Sue also completes the preoperative checklist. She asks Mr. Korloff if he has any questions about the nature or purpose of the surgery. At times he still seems a bit anxious about what to expect. Sue also reviews with Mr. Korloff and his daughter the events that will occur in the holding area and the postanesthesia care unit. She asks if they have any concerns about any aspect of the procedure or routine, and she addresses these concerns. Sue then reviews the exercises that were in the booklet he received in the preadmission testing center. She has Mr. Korloff demonstrate coughing and deep breathing while reinforcing its importance once surgery is over. She then gives Mr. Korloff a hospital gown and cover-up and shows him to the changing area. After he has removed his clothes and put on the hospital gown, Sue accompanies Mr. Korloff and his daughter to the holding area.

DOCUMENTATION NOTE

"Admitted for scheduled laparoscopic cholecystectomy. Blood pressure, 142/84 mm Hg; pulse, 88 beats/min; respirations, 18 breaths/min; temperature, 98.9° F. Lungs clear to auscultation bilaterally with normal excursion. Skin warm and dry; no evidence of lesions. Remained NPO during the night. Reviewed instructions on postoperative exercises and demonstrates coughing and deep breathing. Has some difficulty holding incentive spirometer in mouth. Daughter will be in waiting area during procedure."

evaluate the patient's understanding of the physiological and psychological responses expected from surgery. Evaluate adequacy of preoperative teaching by asking a patient to demonstrate exercises. Evaluate anxiety by monitoring pulse and blood pressure, facial expressions, and verbal interactions. In addition, ask a patient if he or she remains anxious or fearful of any aspect of the surgery.

Patient Expectations. Determine if expectations of the patient and family have been met up to this point. Spend time talking with them to assess if they are satisfied with their preparation. Knowing this information allows you to help a patient redefine realistic expectations. In emergency situations, it is important to evaluate this in a timely, condensed manner. The family often becomes the focus of the evaluation if a patient is unable to respond or is in a condition that prevents a meaningful discussion.

Transport to the Operating Room

Personnel in the **operating room (OR)** notify the nursing unit or preoperative surgery holding area when it is time to transport the patient to the OR. In many hospitals a nursing assistant or a transporter brings a wheelchair or stretcher for transporting patients. The transporter checks the patient's identification bracelet against the patient's medical record to be sure that the correct person is going to surgery. When using a stretcher to transport a patient, the nurses and transporter help the patient safely transfer from bed to stretcher.

Give the family the opportunity to visit before a patient goes to the OR. Then direct the family to the appropriate waiting area. If a patient has been hospitalized before surgery and will be returning to the same nursing unit, prepare the bed and room for his or her return to be better prepared for postoperative care. Include the following in a postoperative bedside unit:

1. Sphygmomanometer, stethoscope, and thermometer
2. Emesis basin
3. Clean gown
4. Washcloth, towel, and facial tissues
5. IV pole and pump
6. Suction equipment (if needed)
7. Oxygen equipment (if ordered)
8. Extra pillows for positioning patient comfortably
9. Bed pads to protect bed linen from drainage
10. PCA (see Chapter 34) pump and tubing (if ordered)
11. Bed raised to stretcher height, bed linen turned back, and furniture moved to accommodate the stretcher

Preanesthesia Care Unit. In most hospitals a patient enters a **preanesthesia care unit** or **presurgical care unit (PSCU)** (sometimes called a *holding area*) outside the OR, where preoperative preparations are completed. Nurses in the PSCU are part of the OR staff. If an IV catheter is not already present, a nurse or anesthesia care provider inserts a catheter to establish a route for fluid replacement, IV drugs, or blood or blood products. The nurse or anesthesia care provider also administers preoperative medications and/or conscious sedation at this time and provides a warming device such as a forced-air blanket to maintain normothermia during surgery.

If a patient needs to have hair removed around the surgical site, perform this procedure in a private area near the OR immediately before surgery. AORN recommended practices include the use of electric or battery-operated clippers for preoperative hair removal (AORN, 2017a). Clippers minimize the risk for irritation and small cuts, which predispose a patient to infection. Follow manufacturer guidelines if you use a depilatory to remove hair.

INTRAOPERATIVE SURGICAL PHASE

Care of a patient during surgery requires careful preparation and knowledge of the events that will occur during a surgical procedure.

NURSE'S ROLE DURING SURGERY

A nurse will assume one of two roles in the OR: **circulating nurse** or **scrub nurse** (Fig. 40.1). The circulating nurse, who is a licensed RN, is responsible for care of the patient in the OR by completing a preoperative assessment, establishing and implementing the intraoperative plan of care, evaluating the care, and providing for the continuity of care after surgery while serving as the patient advocate. The circulating nurse assists the anesthesia care provider with endotracheal intubation, calculating blood loss and urinary output, and administering blood. This nurse monitors sterile technique of surgical team members and contributes to maintenance of a

safe OR environment. The circulating nurse assists the surgeon and scrub nurse by operating nonsterile equipment, providing additional instruments and supplies; maintaining accurate and complete documentation; and tracking sponge, needle, and instrument counts.

The scrub nurse is an RN, a licensed practical nurse (LPN), or a surgical technologist. Similar to the surgeon, the scrub nurse performs surgical hand antisepsis and applies sterile gown and gloves for a procedure. The scrub nurse maintains the sterile field during a surgical procedure and adheres to strict surgical asepsis. This individual assists with applying surgical drapes over the surgical field and anticipates and hands the surgeon instruments, sponges, sutures, and other supplies.

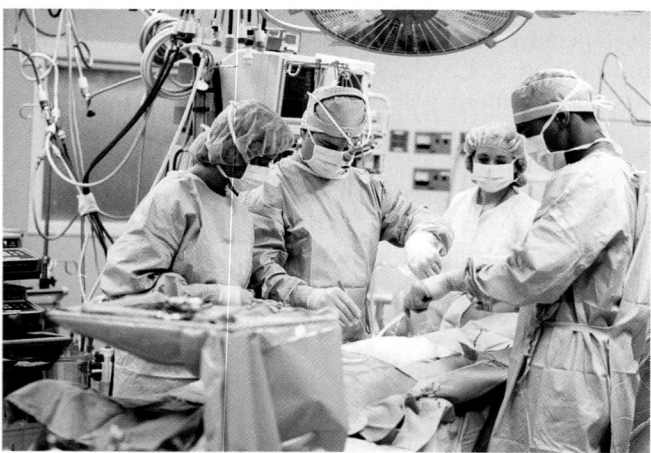

FIG 40.1 Nurses in operating room. (© 2011 Jupiterimages Corporation.)

NURSING PROCESS

■■■■ ASSESSMENT

As a circulating nurse, conduct a special preoperative assessment to verify that a patient is ready for surgery and to plan intraoperative care. Ask a patient his or her name and date of birth and compare the response with the identification band and medical record. Review consent forms, allergies, medical history, physical assessment findings, and test results. Verify with a patient the type of surgery and the surgical site (Table 40.7). Pay special attention to a patient's psychological comfort. Also perform an assessment of key body systems.

TABLE 40.7	FOCUSED PATIENT ASSESSMENT
Intraoperative Assessment		

FACTORS TO ASSESS	QUESTIONS	PHYSICAL ASSESSMENT
Right patient	What is your full name and birth date?	Ask patient to state name and birth date. Inspect patient identification band for patient name and date of birth and compare with medical record.
Right surgical procedure on right body part	What surgery are you going to have done today? Point to the location (site) of your surgery for me. Compare answer with operative permit.	Inspect and palpate body part to add any physical evidence of need for surgery (redness, edema, pain). Sometimes there is none depending on the nature of the surgery. Observe for surgical site marking if laterality of body part involved (i.e., right ankle marked with "yes"). Marking is performed by surgeon or surgical assistant usually in the PSCU (TJC, 2018).
Right set of data in chart	Verify and clarify with patient any medical, surgical, medication, and allergy history found in preoperative assessment. Review findings from laboratory reports, diagnostic tests, x-ray films, and ECG.	Inspect skin for stated surgical scars, signs of pressure injury, scrapes or other nonintact skin. Observe for presence and patency of ordered tubes and lines (NG, Foley, IV).
Right frame of mind of patient	What do you expect as an outcome of surgery? How do you feel about surgery? If patient changes mind about surgery, notify surgeon. Surgery will be canceled or postponed.	Observe for signs of fear and anxiety. Monitor vital signs for indications of excessive anxiety.

ECG, Electrocardiogram; *NG,* nasogastric; *PSCU,* presurgical care unit.

The AORN (2017b) recommends a comprehensive assessment to ensure proper positioning of patients on an OR bed. Assessment should include the type of procedure, estimated length of procedure, desired procedural position, and required positioning equipment and devices.

■■■ NURSING DIAGNOSIS

Review preoperative nursing diagnoses and modify them to individualize the care plan in the OR. Add diagnoses and related factors based on a patient's condition, specific surgical intervention, and method and type of anesthesia. Nursing diagnoses for the intraoperative patient often include the following:

- *Risk for Aspiration*
- *Decreased Cardiac Output*
- *Risk for Deficient Fluid Volume*
- *Impaired Gas Exchange*
- *Risk for Infection*
- *Risk for Perioperative-Positioning Injury*
- *Impaired Skin Integrity*
- *Risk for Latex Allergy Response*

Nursing care in the OR routinely includes monitoring for *Latex Allergy Response* and prevention of *Risk for Perioperative-Positioning Injury*. These diagnoses provide direction for the intraoperative and postoperative care of patients.

■■■ PLANNING

Goals and Outcomes. Some preoperative patient-centered outcomes extend into the intraoperative phase. These include remaining free of infection and intraoperative injury and achieving psychological and physical comfort. Additional goals include maintaining skin integrity, therapeutic body temperature, and fluid and electrolyte balance. You will measure goal achievement through outcome criteria such as the ongoing presence of intact skin, without redness or irritation; body temperature within a patient's normal range; stable vital signs; and adequate urinary output. The circulating nurse gathers outcome measures. Being able to monitor skin condition is difficult if the patient cannot be moved while on the surgical bed. Some patients are placed on gel mattresses. Do not slide patients across these surfaces.

Setting Priorities. Priority setting and continuity of care come from the plan of care, which should include any additional information from oral and written reports of the preadmission area and/or the PSCU. However, a patient's condition can change quickly during surgery.

Collaboration. Planning in the OR involves communication and cooperation among the team to anticipate specific patient challenges (e.g., patient has obesity, COPD, or rheumatoid arthritis). These factors influence the equipment to be used in the OR and having adequate staff members to transfer and position patients on the OR bed.

■■■ IMPLEMENTATION

A major focus of intraoperative care is to prevent injury and complications related to anesthesia, surgery, positioning, and use of equipment. As the perioperative nurse advocate for patients during surgery, protect patients' dignity and rights at all times.

Acute Care

Admission to the Operating Room. After assessing a patient in the PSCU, the circulating nurse transfers a patient into the OR. A patient is usually still awake and notices health care providers wearing surgical masks, protective eyewear, and gowns. Carefully assist with transfer of a patient to the operating bed, being sure that the stretcher and bed are locked in place and enough staff are available for a safe transfer. After a patient is transferred to the bed, the OR team secures the patient with a safety strap. Just before starting the surgical procedure, the surgical team takes a time-out for a final verification of the right patient, right procedure, and right site. When possible, involve the patient in the verification process. This final time-out is part of The Joint Commission *Universal Protocol for Eliminating Wrong Site, Wrong Procedure, and Wrong Person Surgery* (TJC, 2018).

Attaching Monitoring. After securing a patient safely, first apply small plastic electrodes on the chest and extremities for continuous ECG monitoring during surgery. A monitor displays the electrical activity of the heart. Next apply a blood pressure cuff around a patient's arm for the anesthesia care provider to measure the blood pressure. Attach a pulse oximeter sensor or probe to a patient's finger or forehead for measurement of oxygen saturation of the blood to forewarn clinicians about the development of hypoxemia (see Chapter 15) (Jubran, 2015).

Electrosurgical Precautions. Some procedures involve the use of high-frequency ultrasound or argon beam electrical currents to heat and cut tissue with great precision. Electrosurgical devices present risks for patient injury, the most common being burns at the dispersive electrode site (Spruce and Braswell, 2012). The AORN (Spruce and Braswell, 2012) outlines the standards for how to use the devices correctly and protect patients from injury. OR staff are at risk for injury, as electrosurgical devices can cause fires, electrical shock, or explosions. Know your agencies policies and procedures.

Intraoperative Warming. Intraoperative warming prevents hypothermia during surgery and thus prevents postoperative complications such as shivering, cardiac arrest, need for blood transfusion, and pressure injuries. The AORN (2017a) has evidence-based guidelines for prevention of unplanned patient hypothermia. The guidelines include performing a preoperative assessment, continuous monitoring of the patient's temperature intraoperatively, and implementing evidence-based interventions such as the use of active and passive warming methods based on the procedure, patient position, IV access sites, and warming-equipment constraints (AORN, 2017a). The use of warming devices (Fig. 40.2)

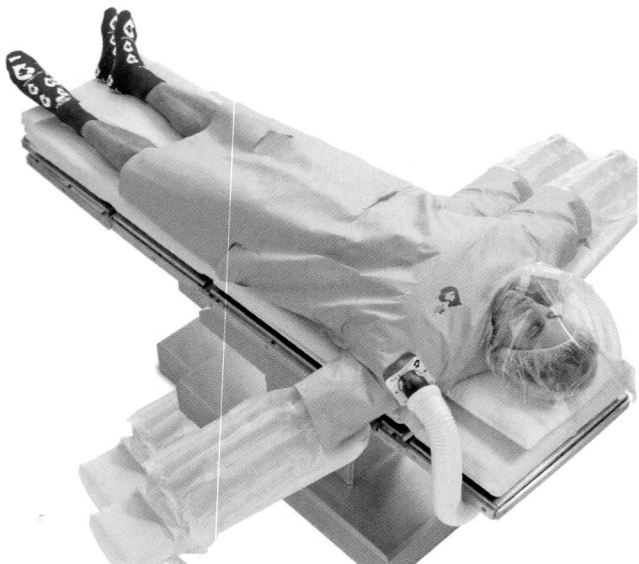

FIG 40.2 3M Bair Hugger perioperative warming device. (Reproduced with permission. Copyright © 2017 3M. All rights reserved.)

reduces postoperative pain levels and SSI, offers thermal comfort, and reduces treatment costs.

Psychological Support. Entering the OR is stressful for most patients. Reassure a patient and remain at the patient's side until after anesthesia is induced. Offering a hand to hold is often helpful. If a patient is awake during surgery, give support throughout the surgical procedure.

Positioning. Patient positioning typically occurs after full muscle relaxation from anesthesia has been achieved. When using general anesthesia, the nursing personnel and surgeon usually do not position a patient until the anesthesia care provider has successfully intubated the patient and achieved the stage of complete relaxation. The AORN (2017b) has issued new guidelines for positioning patients. An injury to the skin, soft tissues, joints, ligaments, bones, eyes, nerves, and blood and lymph vessels can occur from improper positioning. Proper positioning includes the following components: ensuring patient comfort and dignity, maintaining homeostasis, protecting anatomical structures and avoiding complications and injuries, promoting access to the surgery site, promoting access for the administration of IV fluids and anesthetic agents, and promoting access of OR surgical equipment. The aim is to achieve these components with the patient in good body alignment and with circulatory and respiratory function maintained.

The AORN recommends positioning patients on surfaces that redistribute pressure including foam, gel, air, fluid, or a combination. If a high-risk patient undergoes surgery, high-specification reactive foam surfaces are now recommended (AORN, 2017b).

Consider a patient's comfort and safety. It is sometimes difficult for a patient to understand why he or she feels a

TABLE 40.8	INTRAOPERATIVE NURSING CARE
OUTCOMES	**INTERVENTIONS**
Patient is free of infection.	Comply with current hand hygiene guidelines. Maintain standard precautions. Monitor surgical asepsis during surgical case (all members of OR team). Practice aseptic technique if circulating nurse. Perform surgical skin scrub if scrub nurse.
Patient is free of pressure injuries.	Use appropriate pressure-relieving strategies in OR, especially for high-risk patients (e.g., very obese, nutritionally depleted, long surgical procedure). Strategies include repositioning patients every 2 hours during lengthy procedures, repositioning devices such as face masks and nasal/oral tubes when possible, and using gel pads with a foam base custom fit for an OR table.
Patient is free of injury.	Apply sterile surgical drapes. Perform accurate sponge, needle, and instrument counts. Provide grounding for electrosurgical cautery. Provide eye protection when using a laser.
Patient maintains body temperature.	Monitor body temperature. Warm irrigating solutions. Apply warming blanket or garment intraoperatively.
Patient maintains fluid and electrolyte balance.	Monitor blood loss, NG tube drainage, and urinary output. Provide blood products as ordered. Monitor type and flow rate of IV fluids.

NG, Nasogastric; *OR*, operating room.

wide range of discomfort after surgery. If a joint is extended too far in an alert person, pain stimuli warn the individual that muscle and joint strain is too great and the person changes position. Normal defense mechanisms do not protect an anesthetized patient. A patient's muscles are so relaxed that it is relatively easy to place the patient in a position that he or she normally does not assume while awake. A patient often remains in the same position for several hours. Once the patient awakens, musculoskeletal pain can be significant. Intraoperative nursing care includes interventions to prevent infection and injury to a patient, maintain fluid and electrolyte balance, and control a patient's temperature (Table 40.8).

TABLE 40.9 EXAMPLES OF COMPLICATIONS OF ANESTHESIA

TYPE	COMPLICATIONS
General anesthesia	Aspiration of vomitus, cardiac irregularities, decreased cardiac output, hypotension, hypothermia, hypoxemia, laryngospasm, malignant hyperthermia, nephrotoxicity, respiratory depression
Regional anesthesia Epidural Spinal	Hypotension Hypothermia Injury to spinal cord, injury to numb legs, respiratory paralysis, spinal headache
Local anesthesia	Anaphylactic shock, hives, rash
Conscious sedation	Aspiration, decreased level of consciousness, hypoxemia, respiratory depression

Introduction of Anesthesia. The nature and extent of a patient's surgery and current physical status influence the type of anesthesia administered in surgery. It is important after surgery that you know the complications to anticipate after a patient receives anesthesia (Table 40.9).

General Anesthesia. Under general anesthesia a patient loses all sensations, consciousness, and reflexes including gag and blink reflexes. A patient's muscles relax, and the patient experiences amnesia. General anesthesia is administered during major procedures requiring extensive tissue manipulation or any time that analgesia, muscle relaxation, immobility, and control of the autonomic nervous system are required. This includes minor procedures, especially with children.

Regional Anesthesia. Regional anesthesia involves loss of sensory and/or motor function of a specific portion or dermatome of the body by temporarily interrupting normal nerve conduction (Nordquist and Halaszynski, 2014). This type of anesthesia is accomplished by injecting a local anesthetic along the pathway of a nerve exiting from the spinal cord (Rothrock, 2015). Administration techniques include peripheral nerve, spinal, epidural, and caudal (common in children) blocks.

Benefits of regional anesthesia include improved acute perioperative pain management, reduced use of opioids, achievement of skeletal muscle relaxation limiting need and risks of IV muscle relaxants, continued presence of protective upper airway reflexes, and ability of patients to remain conscious during a procedure. A patient requires careful monitoring during and immediately after regional anesthesia for return of sensation and movement distal to the regional anesthesia. Be sure that the patient is protected from harm until full sensation and motor function have returned.

Local Anesthesia. Local anesthesia is the administration of an anesthetic agent into the part of the body where the incision is to be made. It involves local infiltration by injection or topical application. There is a loss of sensation at the desired surgical site by inhibiting peripheral nerve conduction. Local anesthetics are used during minor procedures in ambulatory surgery. Local anesthetics are also used along with general or regional anesthesia. Long-acting local anesthetics are sometimes injected into the incision at the end of a patient's surgery for postoperative pain relief (see Chapter 34). The perioperative nurse caring for a patient with local anesthesia receives education and competency verification. The perioperative nurse assesses the patient, monitors vital signs, observes for symptoms of toxicity, and provides education and supportive care during the procedure (AORN, 2017a).

Moderate Sedation (Conscious Sedation). IV moderate sedation/analgesia or conscious sedation is routinely used for diagnostic or therapeutic procedures (e.g., colonoscopy or certain laparoscopies) that do not require complete anesthesia but simply a decreased level of consciousness. Explain to a patient that he or she will receive moderate sedation/analgesia to achieve mood alteration, continued consciousness, enhanced cooperation, elevated pain threshold, minimal variation of vital signs, some degree of amnesia, and rapid and safe return to activities of daily living. Perioperative nurses performing this function have additional training and have demonstrated competencies in administering medications to achieve moderate sedation/analgesia and in monitoring patients (Rothrock, 2015).

The ability to assess, diagnose, and intervene if a complication arises is essential for all nurses caring for sedated patients. This includes skills in airway management, oxygen delivery, and use of resuscitation equipment (AORN, 2017a). The RN should monitor and document vital signs, oxygen saturation, assessment of breath sounds and heart rhythm, and level of consciousness every 15 minutes or per protocol during the procedure and the immediate recovery period (see agency policy) (AORN, 2017a).

Support any patient who remains awake by explaining procedures, encouraging questions, and warning a patient when unpleasant sensations will be experienced. Alternative therapies may be used to support the patient during this time. For example, music therapy may serve as a cost-effective means of reducing anxiety for both adult and pediatric patients throughout the perioperative experience (Palmer et al., 2016).

Documentation of Intraoperative Care. During the intraoperative phase continue the established plan of care and modify it as needed. Document all patient care activities and procedures performed by OR personnel throughout the surgical procedure. This documentation provides useful data for the nurses who care for the patient after surgery.

■■■ EVALUATION

Evaluation of many interventions implemented during the intraoperative phase occurs in the postoperative phase

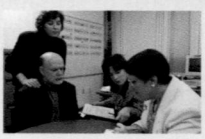

BOX 40.6   EVALUATION

Mr. Korloff's surgery is complete, and he is transferred to the postanesthesia care unit (PACU). Sue accompanies him into the PACU. She reviews the operative record. Mr. Korloff received general anesthesia, and the procedure was uneventful. Mr. Korloff did not receive any blood or blood products. He received Ringer's lactate solution intravenously via a catheter in the left lower forearm. Sue examines the IV site, and it is without signs of phlebitis or infiltration. Small gauze dressings were applied to the four small abdominal puncture wounds, with no drainage noted. Sue positions Mr. Korloff to maintain a patent airway and notes that his respirations are 12 breaths/min and unlabored. Airway is clear of secretions. There are no signs of pressure over bony prominences.

because complications (e.g., surgical wound infection, deep pressure injuries) can arise days after surgery.

Patient Outcomes. After surgery perform a postoperative evaluation of a patient before the patient leaves the OR (Box 40.6). Inspect the skin carefully for areas of the skin where equipment or positioning has exerted pressure. Examine the condition and intactness of the surgical dressing. Monitor body temperature immediately after surgery to assess thermoregulation. Obtain vital signs and auscultate lung sounds to assess pulmonary and fluid and electrolyte status. Check the status of all IV lines, catheters, or drainage tubes before transfer to the postanesthesia care unit (PACU).

Patient Expectations. During a procedure when a patient remains conscious, ask the patient about pain, numbness, and perceived room temperature. This determines if the analgesia is adequate and if a patient is comfortable in regard to position and temperature. When a patient is having major surgery, it is very important to keep the family informed. Typically, family members want to know if surgery is progressing without problems. Most hospitals either provide phones within waiting areas or use family members' cell phones to allow nursing staff to reach families and explain the progress of the surgery. If the patient has given permission for you to talk with family members, provide updates and support to the family in a private environment.

POSTOPERATIVE SURGICAL PHASE

Following surgery a patient's postoperative course involves two phases: the immediate recovery period and convalescence. The immediate recovery period following ambulatory surgery normally lasts 1 to 2 hours, and convalescence occurs at home. For a hospitalized patient the immediate postoperative period often lasts a few hours, with convalescence lasting 1 or more days, depending on the extent of surgery and a patient's response.

RECOVERY

During recovery it is important to be very conscientious in monitoring a patient and making the clinical judgments necessary to determine if the patient is progressing as expected. This is a time when a patient's condition can change very quickly. Immediately after surgery the patient goes to the postanesthesia care unit (PACU) for close monitoring. Before the patient arrives, the PACU nurse receives a hand-off report from the surgical team in the OR to relay the patient's most current status, nursing care priorities, and the need for special equipment. The report includes information about anesthetic agents given during surgery, IV fluids and blood products administered, status of the wound including the presence of drainage devices, and whether the patient had any surgical complications such as excessive blood loss. Many hospitals now use standardized handoff checklists to ensure clear communication and prevent adverse events. While a patient is in the PACU, conduct ongoing assessments every 15 minutes or per protocol.

POSTANESTHESIA CARE IN AMBULATORY SURGERY

The postanesthesia care of patients having ambulatory surgery occurs in two phases. Phase 1 is essentially the same as described for hospitalized patients in the PACU. Phase 2 prepares patients for discharge and self-care. A patient receiving only local anesthesia is usually admitted directly to the phase 2 area. In phase 2 encourage a patient to gradually sit up on the stretcher or recliner and begin to take ice chips, sips of water, or other clear liquids after regaining full alertness.

Phase 2 postanesthesia care occurs in a room equipped with medical recliner chairs, side tables, and footrests. Kitchen facilities for preparing light snacks and beverages may be in the area, along with restrooms. The phase 2 environment promotes comfort and well-being of a patient and family until discharge. Continue to monitor a patient during this phase and initiate postoperative teaching with patients and family members (Box 40.7). When a patient's condition remains stable in the sitting position and there is no nausea or dizziness, he or she is discharged.

RECOVERY PHASE

Once a patient is stable, usually within 2 to 3 hours, the anesthesia care provider or surgeon transfers the hospitalized patient to a postoperative nursing unit, whereas the ambulatory surgical patient returns home. Unstable patients remain in the PACU or go to an intensive care unit for more intense monitoring and care. During recovery or convalescence consider the goals of care established during the preoperative and intraoperative phases to help a patient return to baseline physiological function. In addition, direct your nursing care toward facilitating a patient's smooth transition home. Encourage family participation (when appropriate) in a patient's plan of care. The family can provide the patient

BOX 40.7 **INFORMATION GIVEN TO AMBULATORY SURGICAL PATIENTS**

- Health care provider's office telephone number (24-hour answer)
- Telephone number for surgery center
- Follow-up appointment date and time
- Review of prescribed medications, discussion of when to take and common side effects
- Guidelines related to specific surgery and surgeon's preference: dressing and wound care, bathing allowed, activity restrictions or exercises to perform
- Guidelines related to anesthesia: diet and fluid resumption, activity restrictions (e.g., driving)
- Warning signs of more common complications

coaching during postoperative exercises and important psychosocial support.

NURSING PROCESS

■■■ ASSESSMENT

The parameters you assess for a patient following surgery are essentially the same during recovery and convalescence. When patients enter the PACU, perform an assessment of the respiratory and circulatory status and attach electronic monitors. Conduct assessments while considering patients' surgical risks and the type of surgery performed. For example, if a patient has a history of smoking and had abdominal surgery involving a high abdominal incision, focus on his or her respiratory status. A patient's pain could potentially reduce ventilation, leading to the development of atelectasis.

Once a patient reaches a postoperative nursing unit, perform vital sign measurements and assessments less often, usually every 15 to 30 minutes initially, then hourly, and then less often per surgeon or health care provider orders. Follow institutional policy on vital signs after surgery. Table 40.10 summarizes a focused postoperative assessment. Table 40.11 alerts you to common postoperative complications that can occur in various body systems.

Respiration. Assess the quality of a patient's respirations and the patency of the airway. A patient receiving a general anesthetic often has an artificial airway still in place when arriving in the PACU. Certain anesthetic agents and opioids often continue to affect ventilation, so be especially alert for slow, shallow breathing. Assess respiratory rate, rhythm, depth, and quality of ventilatory movement. Auscultate the lungs for adventitious sounds such as crackles that do not clear with coughing and for wheezing, which results from air squeezed through passageways narrowed almost to closure from secretions (Jarvis, 2016). If breathing is unusually shallow, place your hand over a patient's face or mouth to feel exhaled air. Normally oxygen saturation is greater than 95%;

oxygen saturation less than 90% is a clinical emergency (WHO, 2011).

Once a patient is on a surgical nursing unit, respirations have usually stabilized. Frequent auscultation of lung sounds is important because a patient is at risk for developing pneumonia unless he or she follows postoperative exercises routinely. Remember that pain control is important during convalescence so that a patient is able to cough and deep breathe with relative ease.

Circulation. A patient is at risk for cardiovascular complications from actual or potential blood loss at the surgical site, side effects of anesthesia, electrolyte imbalances, and depression of normal circulatory regulating mechanisms. Continuous ECG monitoring is routine in the PACU to detect rhythm and rate disturbances. Assessment of heart rate and rhythm and blood pressure compared with preoperative values assesses a patient's cardiovascular status and thus determines the patient's status and progress.

Assess circulatory perfusion, especially for patients who have had procedures that impair circulation such as vascular surgery, use of a tourniquet, or application of casts or tight dressings. Always be alert to the amount of bleeding that occurs after surgery and the possibility of hemorrhage. The risk for hemorrhage continues for several days after surgery. Blood loss occurs externally through a drain or incision or internally within the surgical site. Either type of hemorrhage is indicated by a decrease in blood pressure; elevated heart and respiratory rates; a thready pulse; cool, clammy, pale skin; and restlessness.

Temperature Control. The more common use of intraoperative warming devices reduces the occurrence of hypothermia. However, the OR and PACU environments are cool, and a patient's depressed level of body function may lower metabolism with a drop in body temperature. When patients begin to awaken in the PACU, assess if they feel cold or uncomfortable. Shivering is not always a sign of hypothermia but rather a side effect of certain anesthetic agents. Assess body temperature to plan for interventions. Monitoring body temperature on a surgical unit is important for detecting early occurrence of infection (e.g., wound or lung). If a patient develops a fever, report it to the surgeon immediately.

Neurological Function. A patient is usually drowsy in the PACU but reacts to verbal commands. However, drugs, electrolyte and metabolic changes, pain, delirium, reduced oxygen saturation, and emotional factors influence level of consciousness. Normally as anesthetic agents are metabolized, a patient's reflexes return, the patient regains muscle strength, and a normal level of orientation returns. Assess level of consciousness and orientation, and check for pupillary and gag reflexes, hand grasp, and movements of the extremities (see Chapter 16). If a patient had surgery involving a portion of the neurological system, conduct a more thorough neurological assessment.

TABLE 40.10 FOCUSED PATIENT ASSESSMENT

Postoperative Assessment

FACTORS TO ASSESS	QUESTIONS/RECORD REVIEW	PHYSICAL ASSESSMENT
Respirations	Ask if patient feels short of breath or has discomfort during breathing. Review medical history for conditions involving respiratory system, medications taken, and any allergies. Review report of type of anesthesia and agents used during surgery. Review report of any medications given during surgery or in PACU that affect respiratory function (analgesics, antianxiety agents).	Monitor respiratory rate, rhythm, and depth every 15 min × 4 or until stable, then every 30 min × 2, and then every hour × 4. Compare with baseline findings. Observe for symmetry of chest wall movements, color of skin and mucous membranes. Auscultate breath sounds for rales, wheezing, decreased or absent sounds. Apply pulse oximeter to detect oxygen saturation.
Circulation	Review baseline heart rate for current comparison. Review report of amount of blood loss and any replacement blood products in OR and PACU. Review current IV orders as to type of fluid and infusion rate. Ask if patient is having any dizziness or visual disturbances when changing positions.	Monitor pulse rate and rhythm and blood pressure at same frequency as respiratory rate or more often as patient's condition warrants. Maintain continuous ECG monitoring if ordered. Assess level of consciousness and symptoms of restlessness or altered mental status. Observe skin, nail beds, and mucous membranes for color and hydration. Palpate peripheral pulses distal to surgical site, tight dressing, or cast if present. Inspect for amount of bleeding on dressing, in drainage systems (NG suction, Hemovac, Jackson-Pratt drain, Foley catheter), and underneath patient.
Infection control	Review patient's risk factors for infection and poor wound healing (contaminated surgical site, history of diabetes mellitus, smoking, HIV, or use of immunosuppressive drugs [e.g., prednisone]). Ask if patient is having any burning or pain with urination. Ask if patient is having extreme tenderness at wound site.	Monitor patient temperature and white blood cell count as indicated. Inspect urine output. Note color, consistency, and odor. Observe surgical wound for redness, edema, warmth, drainage, and dehiscence. Note character of drainage (e.g., color, odor, consistency).
Gastrointestinal function	Review report for history of problems with gastrointestinal function. Are you having any nausea or abdominal cramping? How's your appetite? Have you passed any gas or had a bowel movement today? How was the stool compared with your normal stool?	Inspect for abdominal distention. Auscultate for bowel sounds in all four quadrants at least every shift until discharge. Palpate abdomen for firmness. Monitor NG tube for patency and NG tube output for color and amount of drainage (if present). Observe patient's ability and willingness to tolerate fluids and food.
Comfort	Review symptoms of pain before surgery, type of anesthesia, location of surgery, and expected level of pain associated with this type of surgery. Review history of alcohol or illicit drug use. Ask patient to rate pain on a 0-to-10 scale. Inquire about pain level before and after each administration of pain medication.	Observe for signs and symptoms of discomfort (restlessness, elevated pulse, respirations, blood pressure, grimaces, guarding). Assess for any side effects of pain medication (altered mental status, depressed respirations, bradycardia, orthostatic hypotension, nausea or vomiting, urinary retention, constipation). Observe patient's expressions, body position, ability to rest or sleep.

ECG, Electrocardiogram; *HIV*, human immunodeficiency virus; *NG*, nasogastric; *OR*, operating room; *PACU*, postanesthesia care unit.

TABLE 40.11   COMMON POSTOPERATIVE COMPLICATIONS

COMPLICATION	CAUSE
Respiratory System	
Atelectasis: Collapse of alveoli with retained mucus secretions. Signs and symptoms: elevated respiratory rate, dyspnea, fever, crackles over involved lobes of lungs, productive cough.	Caused by inadequate lung expansion. Greater risk in patients with upper abdominal surgery who have pain during inspiration and repress deep breathing.
Pneumonia: Inflammation of alveoli caused by infectious process. Usually develops in lower dependent lobes of lung if patient is immobilized. Signs and symptoms: fever, chills, productive cough, chest pain, purulent mucus, dyspnea.	Caused by poor lung expansion with retained secretions. *Streptococcus pneumoniae,* a resident bacterium in respiratory tract, causes most cases of pneumonia.
Hypoxemia: Inadequate concentration of oxygen in arterial blood. Signs and symptoms: restlessness, dyspnea, hypertension, tachycardia, diaphoresis, cyanosis.	Respirations depressed by anesthetics or analgesics. Increased retention of mucus with impaired ventilation occurs from pain, poor positioning, or poor coughing and deep breathing.
Pulmonary embolism: Clot blocks pulmonary artery and disrupts blood flow to one or more lobes of lung. Signs and symptoms: dyspnea, sudden chest pain, cyanosis, tachycardia, hypotension.	Patients who are immobilized and have preexisting circulatory or coagulation disorders are at high risk. Patients with pelvic and abdominal cancer surgeries are at higher risk.
Circulatory System	
Hemorrhage: Loss of large amount of blood externally or internally in short period of time. Signs and symptoms: hypotension, weak and rapid pulse, cool and clammy skin, rapid breathing, restlessness, reduced urine output.	Slipping of suture or dislodged clot at incisional site. Patients with coagulation disorders are at higher risk.
Hypovolemic shock: Reduced perfusion of tissues and cells from loss of circulatory fluid volume. Signs and symptoms: same as for hypovolemic shock.	Hemorrhage usually causes hypovolemic shock after surgery.
Thrombophlebitis: Inflammation of vein (usually in leg), often accompanied by clot formation. Signs and symptoms: swelling and inflammation of involved site, aching or cramping pain. Vein feels hard, cordlike, and sensitive to touch.	Venous stasis is aggravated by prolonged sitting or immobilization, trauma to vessel wall, and hypercoagulability of blood.
Thrombus: Formation of clot attached to interior wall of vein or artery, which occludes vessel lumen. Symptoms include localized tenderness along vein, swollen calf or thigh in affected leg. Decreased pulse below thrombus (if arterial).	Venous stasis and vessel trauma. Venous injury is usually common after surgery of legs, abdomen, pelvis, and major vessels. Patients with major surgery or trauma to these areas are at risk for thrombus formation.
Embolus: Piece of thrombus that has dislodged and circulates in bloodstream until it lodges in another vessel, commonly lungs, heart, or brain.	Thrombi also form from increased coagulability of blood.
Gastrointestinal System	
Paralytic ileus: Nonmechanical obstruction of bowel caused by physiological, neurogenic, or chemical imbalance; it may be associated with decreased peristalsis. Common in initial hours after surgery.	Handling of intestines during surgery can lead to loss of peristalsis for a few hours to several days.
Abdominal distention: Retention of air within intestines. Signs and symptoms: increased abdominal girth, complaint of fullness and "gas pains."	Caused by slowed peristalsis from anesthesia, bowel manipulation, or immobilization.
Nausea and vomiting: Symptoms of improper gastric emptying or chemical stimulation of vomiting center. Patient complains of gagging or feeling full or sick to stomach.	Caused by severe pain, abdominal distention, fear, medications, eating or drinking before peristalsis returns, and initiation of gag reflex.

Continued

TABLE 40.11	COMMON POSTOPERATIVE COMPLICATIONS—cont'd
COMPLICATION	**CAUSE**
Genitourinary System	
Urinary retention: Involuntary accumulation of urine in bladder as result of loss of muscle tone. Signs and symptoms: inability to void, restlessness, and bladder distention occurring 6–8 hours after surgery.	Caused by effects of anesthesia, opioid analgesics; local manipulation of tissues surrounding bladder; and poor positioning of patient, which impairs voiding reflex.
Urinary tract infection caused by bacteria or yeast entering through urethra. Possible symptoms: pain, itching, burning, urgency, and frequency.	Health care–acquired urinary tract infection can occur after bladder catheterization, with poor adherence to catheter care, and if catheter remains in place too long.
Integumentary System	
Wound infection: An invasion of deep or superficial wound tissues by pathogenic microorganisms. Signs and symptoms: warm, red, and tender skin around incision; fever and chills; purulent drainage. It usually appears 3–6 days after surgery.	Caused by poor aseptic technique intraoperatively or during postoperative dressing changes, contaminated wound before surgical exploration. Patients who are chronically ill, obese, or immunosuppressed are at high risk.
Wound dehiscence: Separation of wound edges at suture line. Signs and symptoms: increased drainage and appearance of underlying tissues occurring 6–8 days after surgery.	Caused by malnutrition, obesity, preoperative radiation to surgical site, old age, poor circulation to tissues, and unusual strain on suture line from coughing, vomiting.
Wound evisceration: Protrusion of internal organs and tissues through incision. It usually occurs 6–8 days after surgery.	Develops following wound dehiscence (see above).
Nervous System	
Intractable pain: Pain that is not amenable to analgesia or pain-relief measures.	Related to wound healing, type of dressing, anxiety, or patient positioning.

Once a patient returns to a surgical nursing unit, a sudden change in consciousness is not normal. However, routine detailed neurological assessment is unnecessary unless a patient is slow to awaken fully or has had surgery involving the neurological system.

Fluid and Electrolyte Balance. Because of a risk for fluid and electrolyte abnormalities, assess the patient's hydration status and cardiac and neurological function for signs of electrolyte alterations (see Chapter 18). Routinely inspect the IV catheter and insertion site to verify patency; absence of signs of phlebitis, infection, and infiltration; and proper infusion of IV fluids. It is important that a good venous access is available in case a patient requires fluid and/or blood replacement. IV fluids are continued on the surgical nursing unit, sometimes for several days. Duration of IV catheter use depends on the type of surgery, the medications received, and how well a patient tolerates resumption of oral fluids and food.

Monitor and accurately record intake and output to assess fluid balance and renal and cardiac function. Measure all sources of input (e.g., IV fluids and oral intake) and output (e.g., NG tubes, drains, diarrhea, and urine), and consult with the surgeon if appropriate.

Skin Integrity and Condition of the Wound. Thoroughly assess the condition of a patient's skin. A rash may indicate a drug sensitivity or allergy. Abrasions or petechiae

can result from inadequate padding during positioning or securing on the operating bed. If a patient has new burns or serious injury to the skin, communicate this information by completing an incident or occurrence report (see Chapter 5).

The surgical wound sometimes has no dressing, or it is covered with gauze or transparent dressing that protects the wound site. For visible wounds, observe the appearance of the suture line and note the color, odor, and consistency of any drainage (see Chapter 38). Observe the incision for closure of wound edges; any evidence of pulling of sutures or separation of wound edges should be reported to the surgeon. Estimate the amount of drainage by noting the extent and area of the dressing covered (e.g., lower half of dressing saturated with sanguineous drainage). It is common to mark or draw around the drainage, writing the date and time on the dressing to track the amount of drainage over time. If a patient has a wound drainage system, monitor the output and character of drainage routinely. Keep the drainage tubes patent by removing any kinks. A sudden increase in drainage indicates possible hemorrhage.

If a wound becomes infected, it usually occurs 3 to 6 days after surgery. Ongoing observation of a wound includes inspection for redness, increased warmth, edema, and purulent drainage. A patient may have already been discharged from the hospital when infection develops. Instruct a patient or family caregiver on how to assess the wound at home and to immediately report any signs and symptoms of wound infection to the surgeon.

Genitourinary Function. Spinal anesthesia often prevents a patient from feeling bladder fullness or distention and may cause urinary retention for 6 to 8 hours. Palpate the lower abdomen just above the symphysis pubis for bladder distention. Use a bladder scanner or ultrasound to determine if urine has accumulated in the bladder (see Chapter 36). A full bladder is painful and often the cause of a patient's restlessness, agitation, or high blood pressure. If a patient has an indwelling urinary catheter, monitor urine output and expect at least 30 mL/hr in adults or 1 to 2 mL/kg/hr in infants and children. Observe the color and odor of urine. Surgery involving portions of the urinary tract normally causes bloody urine for at least 12 to 24 hours.

Gastrointestinal Function. Anesthetics slow GI motility and can cause nausea. Manipulation of the intestines during abdominal surgery further impairs peristalsis. Faint or absent bowel sounds are expected during the immediate recovery phase. Normal bowel sounds usually return in about 24 hours, unless major abdominal surgery was performed. Paralytic ileus (i.e., loss of function of the intestine), which causes abdominal distention, is always a possibility after abdominal surgery. Ask if the patient is passing flatus, an important sign indicating return of normal bowel function that may be more indicative of postoperative GI function return in patients undergoing abdominal surgery than presence of bowel sounds. Inspect the abdomen for distention caused by gas and development of internal bleeding in patients who have had abdominal surgery. If an NG tube is in place for decompression, assess the patency of the tube (see Chapter 37) and the color and amount of drainage.

Comfort. A fundamental tenet of good patient care is adequate pain management, one of the most important priorities in postoperative care (Simpson and Bruckenthal, 2016). As a patient awakens from general anesthesia, the sensation of discomfort often becomes prominent. Some patients perceive pain before regaining full consciousness. Acute incisional pain causes patients to become restless and frequently causes changes in heart rate and blood pressure. Appropriate pain management enables patients to deep breathe and cough more effectively and initiate early ambulation. If a patient has PCA or patient-controlled epidural analgesia (PCEA), have the patient begin using the device as soon as possible (see Chapter 34). The ASA (ASA Committee on Standards and Practice Parameters, 2012) recommends that a postoperative patient should receive systemic, as opposed to intramuscular, analgesics ATC and not prn.

A patient who has regional or local anesthesia usually does not experience pain initially because the incisional area is still anesthetized. You need to be skilled at assessing patients' extent and character of pain and the extent of reduced sensation to an anesthetized area. Pain scales are an effective method of initially assessing and then evaluating pain to determine the response to analgesics and objectively documenting the perceived severity of a patient's pain (see Chapter 34).

Patient education on what to expect regarding postoperative pain is important, and nurses play an integral role in providing this information. It has been demonstrated that patients receiving adequate instruction regarding management of their pain give higher satisfaction scores than patients who report they received inadequate counseling (Bruckenthal and Simpson, 2016).

■ ■ ■ NURSING DIAGNOSIS

Based on your assessment and information gathered from the reports of members of the surgical team, identify nursing diagnoses that apply to your patient. Nursing diagnoses that give direction to the continuing care of a patient in the PACU and on the surgical nursing unit after surgery include the following:

- *Ineffective Airway Clearance*
- *Anxiety*
- *Disturbed Body Image*
- *Ineffective Breathing Pattern*
- *Risk for Deficient Fluid Volume*
- *Risk for Infection*
- *Impaired Physical Mobility*
- *Nausea*
- *Acute Pain*
- *Delayed Surgical Recovery*

Analyze and validate assessment data. Cluster defining characteristics and risk factors to identify correct nursing diagnoses. For example, a finding of *Anxiety* manifested by restlessness, glancing about, or facial tension could be related to *Acute Pain, Urinary Retention,* or *Ineffective Peripheral Tissue Perfusion.* Further assessment (e.g., pain score, bladder fullness) and clustering of findings lead to the correct diagnosis and then the appropriate interventions. Remember any given symptom could be an indicator of a patient having multiple nursing diagnoses.

■ ■ ■ PLANNING

Because of the critical nature of the immediate postoperative period, the plan of care in the PACU involves close monitoring of a patient and frequent assessments to ensure stable physiological function. On the surgical nursing unit focus care on facilitating a patient's recovery (Box 40.8). More hospitals are adopting enhanced recovery after surgery (ERAS) protocols to better standardize care and apply best evidence to improve patient outcomes. The ERAS protocols include specific interventions that are to be completed at set time frames until a patient is discharged (e.g., early mobility to begin immediately, IV line discontinued in 12 hours, routine antinausea drugs). Base nursing care on your nursing assessment and the surgeon's postoperative orders or protocol. Typical postoperative orders include the following:

1. Frequency of vital signs monitoring and special assessments
2. Types of IV fluids and rate of infusion
3. Application of compression devices and stockings

BOX 40.8 SYNTHESIS IN PRACTICE
Postoperative Assessment and Planning

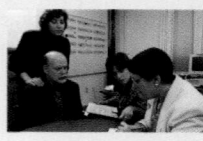

Mr. Korloff's stay in the postanesthesia care unit (PACU) is uneventful except for pain in the right shoulder. Sue explains to Mr. Korloff that air is injected into the abdominal cavity during a laparoscopy and can cause referred pain. In the PACU Mr. Korloff's pain was a 7 on a scale of 0 to 10.

It is the evening of the day of Mr. Korloff's surgery. Mr. Korloff is on the surgical nursing unit for an overnight stay because of his previous cardiac history. He performs deep-breathing and coughing exercises and, after a few demonstrations by Sue, uses the incentive spirometer as ordered. Because he is ambulating frequently in the hall with the assistance of his daughters, he is not performing postoperative leg exercises. The IV fluids were discontinued just before he left the PACU. Mr. Korloff tolerates a clear liquid diet and is passing flatus. He rates his pain as 5 on a scale of 0 to 10, continuing to note some discomfort in the shoulder area. His pain has been controlled with an oral pain medication, acetaminophen with codeine, which he receives every 3 to 4 hours around the clock. His vital signs are within normal limits compared with preoperative values, and his lungs are clear on auscultation. The four small abdominal puncture wounds are without drainage or redness.

4. Postoperative medications (including medications for pain, nausea, and DVT prophylaxis)
5. Oxygen therapy or incentive spirometry
6. Fluids and food allowed by mouth with progression of diet
7. Level of activity that a patient is allowed to resume
8. Position that patient is to maintain while in bed
9. Intake and output measures
10. Diagnostic tests and studies

Goals and Outcomes. Goals of care during recovery in the PACU include returning a patient to normal physiological functioning without complications and maintaining physical and psychological comfort. Examples of outcomes include stable vital signs within a patient's normal range, patent airway, palpable peripheral pulses, oxygen saturation greater than 95% (WHO, 2011), an intact closed incision with minimal wound drainage, and balanced intake and output. Another outcome is for a patient to be awake and oriented to the PACU environment with the ability to move all extremities and verbalize pain relief and decreased anxiety.

Once a patient is on the surgical nursing unit, more long-term goals are developed. Maintenance of pain control with improvement in physiological function is still a priority. Adequate wound healing without the presence of infection, restoration of nutrition, a patient's return to a functional state of health, and maintenance of self-concept and body image are additional goals. Examples of measurable outcomes include the following: patient states that level of pain relief is acceptable and appetite has improved; nutritional intake returns to previous or improved caloric intake; patient states willingness to participate in discharge instruction.

Setting Priorities. While in the PACU a patient's priorities usually center on physiological needs. As you review preoperative and intraoperative data and your ongoing assessments in the PACU, you determine how a patient is progressing and set priorities on developing needs. For example, if a patient begins to awaken without complications but urinary output is less than normal, consult with the surgeon or anesthesia care provider to determine if IV fluids need to be increased to prevent dehydration. Data indicating any immediate postoperative complications such as hemorrhage require alteration in the plan of care and implementation of necessary emergency measures.

A patient's physical status often changes on the surgical nursing unit; thus it remains important to be alert for developing complications. Focus priorities on returning a patient to preoperative functioning or better. Patients generally have many nursing diagnoses (Fig. 40.3). However, management of acute pain is often the priority of postoperative nursing care. If a surgical patient's pain is properly managed, ambulation begins earlier, deep breathing and coughing are less difficult, and the patient has a better sense of well-being. In addition, begin to prepare a patient for discharge by providing the patient and family caregiver necessary instruction and ensuring that adequate resources are available in the home. It is important to inform patients and families regarding what to do about pain and side effects after discharge. Patients place high importance on information about the pain experience, the pain-management plan after discharge, and management of side effects. Monitoring a patient for any psychosocial problems such as body image disturbance or altered coping is also important during convalescence.

Continuity of Care. Continuity of nursing care between the OR, the PACU, and the surgical nursing unit depends on good hand-off communication among all members of the nursing and surgical team. Nursing staff within each area must convey clear and accurate information about a patient's status, treatments, and medications to the next nurse who assumes care for a patient. For example, you need to thoroughly describe the condition of a wound so that each nurse knows what to anticipate during wound assessment and evaluation and care. In that way all staff are able to detect any signs of poor wound healing early.

An ambulatory surgical patient will likely be discharged home with family members or friends. It is essential that a patient and family understand the patient's continuing care needs. Usually the ambulatory surgery nursing staff has discharge instruction sheets available. When caring for patients on surgical nursing units, consider their continuing care needs in the home. For example, referral to home care services or a clinical nurse specialist in wound care or ostomy care provides valuable assistance.

CONCEPT MAP

Nursing Diagnosis: Deficient Knowledge
- First experience with surgery
- Primary language of Russian affects ability to understand medical terms
- Has questions about procedure

▼

Interventions
- Provide planned teaching sessions (including daughters) in preadmission
- Use visual teaching aids showing laparoscopy method and positioning in surgery
- Provide reinstruction morning of surgery, focusing on areas about which the patient and daughters remain uncertain

Nursing Diagnosis: Anxiety
- Expresses concerns about surgery
- States, "I am just worried about how this will affect me over the next few weeks."
- Requires repeat explanations on aspects of preoperative instruction

▼

Interventions
- After preadmission tests, sit down with the patient and daughters and discuss their specific concerns
- Teach relaxation exercise to the patient and have him return demonstrate
- Suggest to daughters the use of distraction by having conversations with the patient and bringing business magazines for the patient to read after surgery

Primary Health Problem: Elective laparoscopic surgery—cholecystectomy
Priority Assessments: Readiness to learn, level of knowledge, coping strategies, ability to understand questions

Nursing Diagnosis: Impaired Verbal Communication
- Sometimes looks away from nurse during discussion and turns to daughters instead
- Ability to speak in English reduced when discussing medical terms
- Hesitates to find words when asking questions

▼

Interventions
- Have a professional interpreter present when explaining medical procedures
- Ask the patient if there is anything about his culture that will influence his acceptance of postoperative care
- Incorporate the patient's values into how postoperative care is delivered: when to involve daughters, how to manage pain

——— Link between medical diagnosis and nursing diagnosis   - - - - Link between nursing diagnoses

FIG 40.3 Concept map.

■■■ IMPLEMENTATION

Critical thinking is important in the postoperative care of patients. Consider the interrelationship of all body systems and the effect of therapies. A patient remains at risk for a variety of postoperative complications (see Table 40.11) unless aggressive care is provided and a patient becomes actively involved in recovery and convalescence. Know the components of any ERAS protocol to ensure that your interventions are timely. Review a patient's perioperative teaching and reinforce as needed (Box 40.9). If a patient is an older adult, use gerontological nursing practice guidelines (Box 40.10).

Respiration. Following general anesthesia a patient in the PACU often has an oral or nasal airway present from the OR to maintain a patent airway until regular breathing at a normal rate resumes. This airway is not taped in place. As respiratory function returns, a patient pulls or spits out the airway. A patient's ability to do so signifies a return of a normal gag reflex.

One of the greatest concerns after surgery is airway obstruction resulting from weakness of pharyngeal or laryngeal muscle tone (from the effects of anesthetics); aspiration of emesis; accumulation of secretions in the pharynx, trachea, or bronchial tree; or laryngeal or subglottic edema. Often the tongue causes airway obstruction. The following measures maintain airway patency:

1. Position a patient on one side with the face downward and the neck slightly extended (Fig. 40.4). A small, folded towel supports the head. Neck extension prevents pharyngeal occlusion of the airway. When the face is angled downward, the tongue moves forward, and mucus secretions flow out of the mouth instead of accumulating in the pharynx. If the nature of the surgery prevents turning a patient on one side, elevate the head of the bed and slightly extend a patient's neck with the head turned to the side. Never position patients with arms over or across their chest because this reduces maximum chest expansion.
2. Suction the artificial airway and oral cavity for mucus secretions as necessary (see Chapter 32). Avoid continually eliciting the gag reflex, which causes vomiting. Before removing an airway, suction the back of the airway to remove any mucous plugs or mucus secretions.

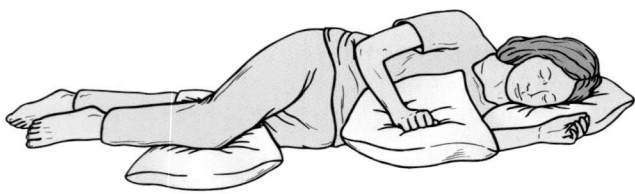

FIG 40.4 Position of patient during recovery from general anesthesia. (From Lewis SL, et al: *Medical-surgical nursing: assessment and management of clinical problems*, ed 8, St Louis, 2014, Mosby.)

3. Begin deep breathing and coughing exercises as soon as a patient responds to instructions.
4. Administer oxygen as ordered, and monitor oxygen saturation with a pulse oximeter.

Once a patient reaches a surgical nursing unit, begin aggressive pulmonary hygiene. A patient participates actively if preoperative instruction was effective. Remember to have the family help coach patients in completing their exercises.

BOX 40.9   PATIENT TEACHING

Postoperative Teaching

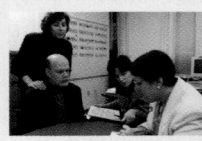

Mr. Korloff tells Sue that the plan is for discharge tomorrow and he hopes he will remember everything that she taught him before surgery. Sue develops the following teaching plan.

OUTCOME

At the end of the teaching session, Mr. Korloff will be able to:

- Verbalize understanding of pain-relief approaches
- Identify foods to include in a high-protein diet
- Describe wound care practices for home care and what problems to report

TEACHING STRATEGIES

- Reinforce the need to take pain medication before pain becomes severe.
- Encourage Mr. Korloff to avoid smoking because nicotine accelerates the metabolism of pain medication, resulting in shorter duration of effect.
- Teach nonpharmacological means of pain control such as slow deep breathing, progressive relaxation with music, and use of tactile stimulation such as back rubs (see Chapter 34).
- Teach the names, purpose, and timing of medications and possible side effects so that Mr. Korloff can continue medications safely at home.
- Teach signs and symptoms of hemorrhage and wound infection.
- Instruct in proper hand hygiene.
- Demonstrate wound care techniques that are necessary to keep laparoscopy wounds clean after discharge (see Chapter 38).
- Review high-protein foods within scope of Mr. Korloff's food preferences that are needed for wound healing.
- Have Mr. Korloff or a family member develop a 3-day meal plan.

EVALUATION

- Use the principles of teach-back to evaluate patient/family caregiver learning:
  - "Identify foods to include in your diet."
  - "Describe the pain medications you are to take each day and when."
  - "Describe the side effects of your prescribed medications."
  - "Describe wound care and what signs and symptoms of abnormal wound healing you should report to your health care provider."

Encourage diaphragmatic breathing exercises every hour while a patient is awake. Follow diaphragmatic breathing by having a patient use the incentive spirometer. Encourage a patient to reach the inspiratory volume achieved before surgery on the spirometer. Proper use of the spirometer ensures a maximum inspiration. Encourage regular turning and early ambulation (see Chapter 28). Walking stimulates an increased respiratory rate and improves circulation. Assist patients who are restricted to bed to turn from side to side every 1 to 2 hours while awake and to sit when possible. If a patient develops pulmonary secretions, encourage coughing exercises followed by deep breathing at least once an hour. Maintain pain control so that a patient achieves a full, productive cough. Provide frequent oral hygiene to help a patient

expectorate mucus easily. If a patient is NPO or on a limited fluid intake, the mouth easily becomes dry. Initiate postural drainage and suctioning if a patient is too weak or unable to cough secretions.

Circulation. In the PACU it is important to monitor for changes in blood pressure or heart rate. The surgeon usually writes an order indicating which changes to report. However, use critical thinking and notify the surgeon when there is a significant change or a continuous negative trend in vital signs. Hemorrhage is external if you observe increased bloody drainage on dressings or through drains. If a dressing becomes saturated, the blood oozes down a patient's sides and collects in a pool under bedclothes. Always check underneath a patient for drainage whether or not the dressing is saturated. When hemorrhage is internal, the operative site becomes swollen and tight, and a hematoma develops. Report the first signs of suspected hemorrhaging to the surgeon immediately. Maintain the IV infusion, monitor vital signs continuously, continue oxygen, and raise a patient's legs in a modified Trendelenburg's position (see Chapter 31) to promote venous return until a patient's condition stabilizes.

Early measures directed at preventing venous stasis are aimed at preventing DVT during convalescence. Begin the following interventions on the surgical nursing unit as soon as possible:

1. Encourage patients to perform leg exercises at least every hour while awake unless contraindicated by surgery.
2. Apply antiembolism stockings or a sequential compression device as ordered by the surgeon (see Chapter 29). Often you apply these devices on a patient in the OR. Remove the stockings or device every 8 hours and leave off for 1 hour. Thoroughly assess the skin of the legs at this time.
3. Encourage early ambulation. Hospitals have taken steps to increase activity and mobility levels of inpatients as soon as possible to prevent deconditioning and other complications of immobilization (see Chapter 29). The American Association of Critical Care Nurses (AHRQ, 2013) recommends an early progressive mobility protocol for critical care patients, and many hospitals are transitioning similar protocols to regular postoperative nursing units. The degree of activity allowed progresses as a patient's condition improves. Follow the protocol of your agency to ensure patient activity progresses. There are usually screening criteria (e.g., vital sign stability, neurological status) before a patient can be placed on an early mobility protocol. If vital signs are normal, first help a patient sit on the side of the bed to dangle. Dizziness is a sign of postural hypotension (see Chapter 15). Check a patient's blood pressure again and ensure that he or she is not dizzy to determine if ambulation is safe. Assist patient during ambulation by using a gait belt. During the first few times out of bed, a patient often walks only a few feet. Tolerance improves each time. Evaluate a patient's tolerance to activity by

---

BOX 40.10 CARE OF THE OLDER ADULT

Principles of Postoperative Care

- Design teaching strategies to incorporate any decline in cognitive and sensory functioning such as decision-making process, vision, and hearing. For example, use teaching materials with large print.
- Older adults are at greatest risk for complications related to transitions of care, especially in the ambulatory care setting. The likelihood of the older adult having multiple care providers and comorbidities can compromise safety.
- If a patient will be on bed rest for more than 24 hours, an order for subcutaneous heparin or enoxaparin is necessary to prevent deep vein thrombosis.
- Intake and output is maintained longer after surgery. Perfusion of kidneys is compromised, and older adults frequently decrease oral intake of fluids to minimize voiding frequency.
- Any fluid, electrolyte, or acid-base imbalance quickly alters mental status. Older adults often need to be closer to the nurses' station and monitored more frequently for possible delirium, confusion, disorientation, or decreased level of consciousness. Fall precautions are necessary.
- Patients with increased pain tolerance need to be medicated appropriately when they indicate that they have pain. Give them treatment options. Offer pain medications before painful procedures (e.g., dressing changes, walking in the hallway, getting up from a chair).
- Pain medication is more likely to cause altered mental status in older adults, increasing the need to monitor for confusion and disorientation.
- Metabolism of drugs is slowed in older patients; thus the effects of medication persist for a longer period of time.
- Nutritional deficits are common, and diets high in protein, calcium, and vitamins B and C are necessary for wound healing and positive nitrogen balance. Carbohydrate intake is essential for energy and to spare protein use for wound healing. Increase iron intake if a patient is anemic.
- Older adults have more difficulty with constipation because of decreased peristalsis, decreased activity, weakening of abdominal muscles, and risk for dehydration. Orders for a stool softener and/or extra fiber are accompanied by increased fluid intake despite the resulting increased need to void.

periodically assessing pulse rate and whether the patient has shortness of breath. Avoid positioning a patient in a manner that interrupts blood flow to the extremities. While a patient is in bed, do not place pillows or rolled blankets directly under the knees. Compression of the popliteal vessels causes a thrombus to form. When sitting in a chair, have a patient elevate the legs on a footstool, avoiding hyperextension of the knee. Never allow a patient to sit with one leg crossed over the other.

4. Administer anticoagulant drugs if ordered. Small doses of anticoagulants such as low-molecular-weight heparin given subcutaneously reduce risk for thrombus formation.

5. Promote adequate fluid intake orally or intravenously. Adequate hydration prevents the concentration of platelets and red blood cells and thus prevents formation of small clots within blood vessels. Adequate hydration also promotes tissue healing and liquefies respiratory secretions.

Temperature Control. A patient's temperature is usually maintained in the OR through use of perioperative warming devices. However, as a result of the cool temperature in the OR and evaporative heat loss, a patient may be cool when arriving in the PACU. If no device is in place, provide warmed blankets or other warming devices (e.g., heated air blankets). Patients often still feel cold when reaching a surgical nursing unit. Offer extra blankets or apply a loose-fitting pair of socks to the feet.

Neurological Function. Deep breathing and coughing help to expel retained anesthetic gases and increase a patient's return to a baseline level of consciousness. Try to arouse a patient by calling his or her name in a moderate tone of voice, noting whether the patient responds appropriately. If the patient remains asleep or is unresponsive, waken him or her through touch or by gently moving a body part. If you need a painful stimulus to wake a patient, notify the anesthesia care provider. Orientation to the environment is important in maintaining alertness. Explain that surgery is complete, and describe all procedures and nursing measures performed.

Be alert for patient behaviors or symptoms indicating postoperative delirium. Box 40.11 outlines common symptoms of delirium. A variety of measures can be used to manage or minimize the symptoms of delirium, including the following:

- Sensory enhancement (ensuring glasses, hearing aids, or listening amplifiers)
- Mobility enhancement (ambulating at least twice per day if possible)
- Cognitive orientation and therapeutic activities (tailored to the individual)

In addition, pain control, cognitive stimulation tailored to the individual's interests and mental status, simple communication approaches, nutritional and fluid enhancement, and sleep enhancement (daytime sleep hygiene, relaxation, nonpharmacological sleep protocol, and nighttime routine) can be effective (AGS, 2015).

BOX 40.11 SYMPTOMS ASSOCIATED WITH POSTOPERATIVE DELIRIUM

- Change in level of arousal: drowsiness or decreased arousal[a] or increased arousal with hypervigilance
- Delayed awakening from anesthesia[a]
- Abrupt change in cognitive function (worsening confusion over hours or days) including problems with attention, difficulty concentrating, new memory problems, new disorientation
- Difficulty tracking conversations and following instructions
- Thinking and speech that is more disorganized, difficult to follow, slow,[a] or rapid
- Quick-changing emotions, easy irritability, tearfulness, uncharacteristic refusals to engage with postoperative care
- New perceptual disturbances (e.g., illusions, hallucinations)
- Motor changes such as slowed or decreased movements,[a] purposeless fidgeting or restlessness, new difficulties in maintaining posture such as sitting or standing[a]
- Sleep/wake cycle changes such as sleeping during the day[a] and/or awake and active at night
- Decreased appetite[a]
- New incontinence of urine or stool[a]
- Fluctuating symptoms and/or level of arousal over the course of minutes to hours

[a]Hypoactive symptoms.
Adapted from American Geriatrics Society: Postoperative delirium in older adults: best practice statement from the American Geriatrics Society, *Journal of the American College of Surgeons* 220(2):136, 2015.

Fluid and Electrolyte Balance. A patient's only source of fluid intake immediately after surgery is IV; therefore it is important to maintain a patent IV catheter (see Chapter 18). You typically remove the IV catheter once a patient awakens after ambulatory surgery and can tolerate water without GI upset. A more seriously ill patient requires an IV catheter to receive fluids until hydration and electrolyte balance are achieved. Some patients require blood products depending on the amount of blood lost during surgery. A surgeon orders a prescribed solution and rate for each IV infusion. Infuse IV solutions through an infusion pump to ensure correct volume delivery.

Genitourinary Function. A full bladder is painful and causes a patient to become restless or agitated as the patient awakens from surgery. Some patients will have indwelling urinary catheters inserted until voluntary control of urination returns postoperatively. This includes patients undergoing urological surgery, undergoing anticipated lengthy surgeries, or requiring intraoperative monitoring of urine output (Meddings et al., 2014). If a catheter is in place and urinary output is less than 30 mL/hr in an adult patient or less than 1 to 2 mL/kg/hr in infants and children, check for catheter occlusion or kinking. Notify the surgeon if measured output does not improve.

In many hospital settings nurses now remove urinary catheters without a direct physician order. Nurse-led protocols for catheter removal have been effective in reducing catheter-associated infections (see Chapter 36) (Meddings et al., 2014). One protocol that has been effective is the *HOUDINI* protocol. The acronym outlines when *not* to remove an indwelling catheter: *h*ematuria, gross; *o*bstruction, urinary; *u*rological surgery; *d*ecubitus ulcer—open sacral or perineal wound in incontinent patient; *i*nput and output critical for patient management or hemodynamic instability; *n*o code, comfort care, hospice care; *i*mmobility because of physical constraints.

Nurses monitor urinary output and bladder distention regularly, and when patients do not meet the above-listed criteria the nurses remove the catheter and then assess for voiding every 6 hours. If a patient does not void in 6 hours, the nurse will perform bladder scanning and insert a straight catheter to drain the bladder. If the patient does not void after an additional 6 hours, the health care provider is notified (Adams et al., 2012). Always follow your agency protocol for prevention of catheter-associated urinary tract infections (CAUTIs).

Even if a patient has been NPO for hours, IV fluids give the renal system sufficient fluid to excrete urine. Continued difficulty in voiding may require reinsertion of an indwelling catheter, which increases the patient's risk for CAUTIs (see Chapter 36). Monitor intake and output, and if a patient's urine is dark and concentrated, notify the surgeon. The minimum urine output is 30 mL/hr in adults or 1 to 2 mL/kg/hr in infants and children. Notify the surgeon if output is less than these ranges.

Gastrointestinal Function. Minimize a patient's nausea during recovery in the PACU by avoiding sudden movement. If a patient has an NG tube, maintain tube patency per protocol or as ordered (see Chapter 37). Occlusion of an NG tube causes the accumulation of gastric contents in the stomach. Because stomach emptying slows under anesthesia, the accumulated contents cannot escape, and nausea and vomiting develop. Normally a patient does not receive fluids to drink in the PACU because of the risk for vomiting and altered mental status from general anesthesia. Use a moist swab to relieve dryness of a patient's lips and mouth. If a patient is nauseated, give prescribed medication to prevent vomiting and aspiration.

Interventions for preventing GI complications promote the return of normal elimination and faster resumption of normal nutritional intake. It may take several days for a patient who has GI surgery to resume a normal dietary intake. Normal peristalsis does not usually return for 24 to 48 hours. In contrast, a patient whose GI tract is unaffected directly by surgery simply recovers from the effects of anesthesia before resuming dietary intake. Follow these guidelines:

1. Maintain a gradual progression in dietary intake. Patients having ambulatory surgery can generally resume their diet immediately after surgery. Patients requiring an intraoperative IV line receive only IV fluids initially. Patients who have had abdominal surgery are usually NPO the first 24 hours or until the passage of flatus. Once a surgeon orders resumption of oral intake, first provide clear liquids such as water, apple juice, or decaffeinated tea or coffee after nausea subsides. Overloading with large amounts of fluids causes distention and vomiting. If a patient tolerates liquids without nausea, advance the diet to full liquids, followed by a light diet of solid foods and finally a regular diet, stressing the importance of foods that are high in protein and vitamin C. Poor pain control can reduce a patient's appetite. Good pain management is thus important. Patients who have had abdominal surgery are usually NPO the first 24 hours or until the passage of flatus.

2. Promote ambulation and exercise. Physical activity stimulates a return of peristalsis. A patient who experiences abdominal distention and "gas pain" often obtains relief while walking.

3. Maintain an adequate fluid intake. Fluids keep fecal material soft for easy passage and provide hydration.

4. Administer fiber supplements, stool softeners, and rectal suppositories as ordered. Constipation or distention often develops after surgery related to side effects of anesthetic agents, pain medication, and dehydration.

5. Stimulate a patient's appetite by removing sources of noxious odors, controlling pain, and providing small servings of nonspicy foods.

6. Help a patient sit (if possible) during mealtime to minimize pressure on the abdomen.

7. Provide frequent oral hygiene.

8. Provide meals when a patient is rested and free from pain. A patient often loses interest in eating if he or she is exhausted by activities such as ambulation before mealtime.

Comfort. The anesthesia care provider orders medications for pain management in the PACU. IV opioid analgesics such as morphine sulfate are often the drugs of choice for the immediate postoperative period. Titrate IV morphine as ordered until pain relief is achieved. Morphine can depress level of consciousness, respirations, and blood pressure, but at appropriate doses this is rare. Assess a patient for the proper dose of analgesic, and monitor for possible side effects. Once a patient is awake, a PCA or PCEA pump may be initiated. If a patient has had epidural or regional anesthesia, monitor carefully and follow safety guidelines in giving additional analgesics (see Chapter 34).

Too often opioids are the only analgesics used for perioperative pain. Opioids (a class of central-acting analgesics) provide powerful dose-dependent relief of pain delivering good analgesic effect (Nordquist and Halaszynski, 2014). However, opioids can alter central nervous system activity and lead to physical and psychological dependence with longer-term use, especially in elderly patients. Opioids can also cause adverse effects such as nausea, sedation, constipation, ileus, respiratory depression, and risk of abuse, so be observant for early development of these symptoms.

Nonopioid **multimodal analgesia** is a treatment option that can reduce reliance on unimodal therapy with opioids postoperatively (Nordquist and Halaszynski, 2014). More patients are receiving combinations of drugs with opioids including nonsteroidal antiinflammatory drugs (NSAIDs), which have been shown to reduce morphine requirements in PCA after major surgery (McDaid et al., 2010). Other adjuvants that are beneficial to use especially in elderly patients include acetaminophen (non-NSAID analgesic) and antidepressant medications, which improve a patient's sense of well-being, reduce fatigue, and do not disrupt the normal sleep cycle (Nordquist and Halaszynski, 2014).

A patient's pain increases as the effects of anesthesia wear off; this often occurs when a patient reaches the surgical nursing unit. A patient becomes more aware of surroundings and more perceptive of discomfort. The incisional area is only one source of pain. Irritation from drainage tubes, tight dressings, or casts and the muscular strains caused from positioning on the operating bed also cause discomfort. Air insufflation during laparoscopic surgery can cause significant discomfort, especially in the shoulder area.

Pain slows recovery. Assess a patient's pain thoroughly. When a patient requests pain medication, determine the location, nature, and character of the pain. Patients have the most surgical pain during the first 24 to 48 hours after surgery. Provide analgesics as often as allowed. IV or epidural PCA systems allow patients to administer analgesics from specially prepared pumps (see Chapter 34). A PCA device is attached to the IV line, or the analgesic is given via an epidural catheter, as with fentanyl or morphine. A patient controls the amount of analgesia received within set doses and times ordered by the surgeon or anesthesia care provider. Program the doses and frequencies of pain medication into the pump. PCA medication is delivered at a preprogrammed basal rate, a bolus dose at specified intervals as needed, or both. Continuous epidural analgesia is frequently used after surgery for thoracic and abdominal surgical procedures. Continuous epidural analgesia can provide superior pain relief in terms of less analgesic use, better postoperative pain relief, and faster return of GI function.

Notation of respirations and level of consciousness is important for a patient receiving pain medications through a PCA pump or an epidural catheter. The Joint Commission requires documentation of frequent objective pain assessments using a pain scale, appropriate nursing interventions, and evaluation of a patient's response (Baker, 2016).

Promoting Wound Healing. Surgical gauze dressings remain in place the first 24 hours after surgery to reduce the risk for infection. During this time add an extra layer of gauze on top of the original dressing if drainage develops. Mark or draw around the drainage on the dressing, and date and time the marking. This provides a means to monitor increasing amounts of drainage. Notify the surgeon if bleeding is excessive. In certain types of surgery the surgeon chooses to use no dressing at all (see Chapter 38) or a transparent dressing.

Closely observe the surgical wound to note any early signs and symptoms of infection. If a wound becomes infected, it usually occurs 3 to 6 days after surgery. Always use aseptic technique during dressing changes and wound care. Surgical drains need to remain patent so that accumulated secretions are removed from the incision site.

To ensure continuity of care be sure that all staff are aware of the proper materials to use in a dressing change. It is common for patients to feel discomfort during an extensive dressing change; therefore offer pain medication 5 to 30 minutes before a procedure. Time the procedure to begin when the pain medication begins to work. For example, oral pain medications take about 30 minutes to begin working; therefore give oral pain medication 30 minutes before a procedure. IV pain medications given IV push usually only take 5 to 10 minutes to work; therefore give IV pain medication 5 to 10 minutes before a dressing change.

A critical time for wound healing is 24 to 72 hours after surgery. A patient exerts physical stress on a wound from coughing, vomiting, or movement in bed. Inadequate nutrition, impaired circulation, and metabolic alterations further impair healing. Abdominal wound dehiscence can result in evisceration. Evisceration, which typically occurs several days after surgery, is a medical emergency. In the event of evisceration, cover any exposed abdominal contents with gauze soaked with sterile normal saline. Prepare an IV infusion set for rapid infusion of IV fluids.

If you anticipate that a patient will need to continue dressing changes after discharge, plan instruction when the patient is alert and comfortable and family caregivers are present. Before discharge, ensure that the patient knows how to obtain the needed supplies and that the patient or a family member can safely change the dressings.

QSEN QSEN ACTIVITY *Quality Improvement*

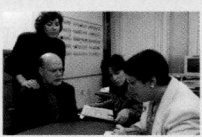

Sue is working on a surgical unit that is implementing a quality improvement (QI) project focused on prevention of postsurgical site infections. Sue's review of the literature reinforces the importance for all health care team members involved in a patient's postoperative care to implement multiple strategies to reduce the risk for surgical site infections (SSIs) (Burden, 2016; Leonard, 2016). She recognizes that she, along with other health care professionals of varying backgrounds and values, are part of system processes that affect the outcomes of care provided for patients and their families. Sue's additional review of the literature regarding QI projects reveals that consistent communication and implementation of the plan of care are imperative to obtain the expected outcome of prevention in the number of SSIs.

- How does Sue identify gaps between local and best practice? In what way might Sue apply communication principles to determine outcomes of the project?

evolve Answers to QSEN Activities can be found on the Evolve website.

Maintaining Self-Concept. During a patient's recovery, the appearance of wounds, bulky dressings, and extruding drains and tubes threaten the self-concept. The nature of the surgery often creates a permanent change in body image. If surgery leads to impairment in body function, the patient's role within the family and community often changes significantly. Observe the patient for alterations in self-concept (see Chapter 24). Some patients show revulsion toward their appearance by refusing to look at an incision or carefully covering dressings with bedclothes. The fear of not being able to return to a functional role in the family or to a previously held job may cause a patient to avoid participating in the care plan.

The family or significant other frequently plays an important role in efforts to improve a patient's self-concept. Help the family to accept the patient's feelings and still encourage independence. The following measures support a patient's self-concept:

1. Provide privacy during dressing changes or wound inspection by closing room curtains and draping a patient so that only the dressing and incisional area are exposed.
2. Maintain a patient's hygiene. A complete bath the first day after surgery usually makes a patient feel renewed. Offer a clean gown and washcloth if the gown becomes soiled. Keep a patient's hair neatly combed and offer frequent oral hygiene, every 2 hours while awake, especially for a patient who is NPO.
3. Prevent drains from overflowing. Measure drainage every 8 hours for output recording. Empty and measure them more often if drainage is excessive.
4. Maintain a pleasant environment. Store or remove all unused supplies, and keep the bedside orderly and clean.
5. Offer opportunities for a patient to discuss feelings about appearance. Patients worry about permanent scarring. When a patient chooses to look at an incision for the first time, make sure that the area is clean. Optimally the patient will care for the incision site by applying simple dressings or bathing.
6. Give the family opportunities to discuss ways to promote a patient's self-concept. Encouraging independence is difficult for a family member who has a strong desire to help a patient in any way. By knowing about the appearance of a wound or incision, family members can be supportive during dressing changes.

Restorative and Continuing Care. Promote a patient's independence and active participation in care to help the patient return to a functional state of health. When a patient continues to have pain or experiences postoperative complications, motivation for self-care is sometimes low. The goals set for the patient's involvement need to be realistic. It is unrealistic to involve the patient if movement or activity is restricted or if participation increases discomfort.

Keep the patient and family informed of progress made toward recovery. Many patients become depressed if they think recovery is slow. Explain the length of time expected to reach a level of maximal recovery. For some patients surgery also causes permanent physical limitations that require time to accept.

Plan care daily, keeping in mind the ultimate goals for recovery. From the moment a patient enters the hospital, anticipate and plan for the patient's return home. Involve family caregivers in the plan of care as long as permission is given by the patient to do so. Involvement of family members in the care plan facilitates early discharge and adequate care at home. Instruct family caregivers in care activities such as dressing changes, how to assist with ambulation, and medication management. If family members are unable to help a patient, work with the surgeon, social worker, or discharge planner for referrals to home care agencies to provide services at home.

■■■ EVALUATION

Patient Outcomes. In the PACU continuously evaluate the effectiveness of interventions and a patient's response. A patient's condition can change quickly. Evaluation of a patient's status involves ongoing measurement of vital signs, pulse oximetry, wound drainage, intake and output, and other physical assessments. Nurses use scales such as the Aldrete score and Richmond Agitation-Sedation Scale (RASS) to evaluate a patient's level of consciousness and return of motor function. Determine frequency of these assessments based on a patient's response to anesthesia. If evaluation reveals that a patient is recovering from anesthesia, the surgeon or anesthesia care provider discharges a patient from the PACU.

On the surgical nursing unit evaluate the effectiveness of care based on expected outcomes resulting from nursing interventions. Evaluation occurs over several days. It is important to evaluate a patient's clinical progress and readiness for discharge by observing participation in postoperative exercises, self-care activities, and ambulation (Box 40.12). Also evaluate if a patient feels prepared for discharge from the acute care facility. Is a patient able to explain the required care that is to be continued after discharge? Have a patient demonstrate procedures such as wound care or medication administration.

Evaluate outcomes of the ambulatory surgical patient by making a postoperative telephone call to the patient's home. The call, usually placed 24 hours after surgery, reassures a patient and allows for evaluation of recovery progress and the opportunity to answer any questions from a patient or family.

Patient Expectations. In the PACU some patients are not able to voice expectations. However, evaluation of pain is critical. Note a patient's movement and positioning because nonverbal behaviors indicate if a patient is comfortable. If the patient can verbalize, validate his or her perception of pain by frequently asking how the patient feels and using a

BOX 40.12 EVALUATION

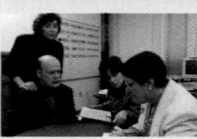

Mr. Korloff progressed well and is ready for discharge the day after surgery. He expresses relief that everything went well and that he will be able to return to work hopefully by next week. Sue continues to care for him on the surgical patient care unit. She explains how to remove the gauze on the puncture sites and tells him to bathe and shower tomorrow. Symptoms Mr. Korloff and his daughters need to watch for include redness, swelling, bile-colored drainage or pus from the abdominal wounds, severe abdominal pain, nausea, vomiting, and fever with a temperature greater than 37.7° C (100° F) or chills. Any symptoms need to be reported to Mr. Korloff's surgeon immediately. His daughters observed the puncture sites and can identify symptoms of complications. Mr. Korloff is ready for discharge and plans to stay with one of his daughters over the weekend. Sue makes a follow-up surgical appointment for Mr. Korloff and gives him the surgeon's phone number in case he has any questions or concerns once he returns home.

DOCUMENTATION NOTE

"Abdominal puncture sites dry and intact, without redness or tenderness. Discharge teaching provided to patient and daughters. Repeated signs and symptoms of complications; wound care instructions; activity restrictions; and follow-up appointment time, date, and place during teach-back. Patient and daughters verbalize understanding of all discharge instructions."

pain-assessment scale. If pain is not adequately relieved, change the dosage or type of medication. Evaluate a patient's level of anxiety by assessing the presence of any concerns or fears. Further explanation of postoperative progress and procedures reduces anxiety.

As a patient recovers, physical and psychological comfort continues to be a typical expectation of patients and families. Ask patients if they feel their expectations have been met, and if not, give a patient and family numerous opportunities to ask questions about what to anticipate when returning home.

SAFETY GUIDELINES FOR NURSING SKILLS

Ensuring patient safety is an essential role of the professional nurse. To ensure patient safety, communicate clearly with members of the health care team, assess and incorporate the patient's priorities of care and preferences, and use the best evidence when making decisions about your patient's care. When performing the skill in this chapter, follow these safety guidelines:

- Know if a patient will have any activity restrictions after surgery that prevent performance of postoperative exercises or require adaptation of skill.
- Be sure that patient uses proper body mechanics when performing exercises for turning.

SKILL 40.1 TEACHING POSTOPERATIVE EXERCISES

DELEGATION CONSIDERATIONS

The skills of preoperative teaching cannot be delegated to nursing assistive personnel (NAP). NAP can reinforce and assist patients in performing postoperative exercises. The nurse instructs the NAP about:

- Any precautions or safety issues unique to the patient (e.g., fall precautions, bleeding precautions, weight-bearing issues, dietary concerns).
- Informing the nurse of any identified concerns (e.g., patient is unable to perform exercises correctly).

EQUIPMENT

- Stretcher or bed
- Pillow
- Incentive spirometer
- Preoperative education flow sheet
- Positive expiratory pressure (PEP) device
- Stethoscope

STEP	RATIONALE
ASSESSMENT	
1. Identify patient using at least two identifiers (e.g., name and birthday or name and medical record number) according to agency policy.	Ensures correct patient. Complies with The Joint Commission standards and improves patient safety (TJC, 2018).

STEP	RATIONALE
2. Assess patient's risk for postoperative respiratory complications. Identify underlying lung conditions from medical record and review preoperative and postoperative orders.	General anesthesia predisposes patient to respiratory problems. The presence of underlying respiratory conditions increases patient's risk for pulmonary complications. Preoperative and postoperative orders often require adaptations in the way a patient performs exercises.
3. Perform hand hygiene. Ask about patient's previous experiences with surgery and anesthesia.	Allows for individualized teaching and addressing specific patient concerns.
4. Assess patient's cognitive level, primary language, and cultural factors that may influence approach to instruction: have patient read a phrase from an instructional leaflet; ask patient to describe meaning of surgery.	These factors may alter patient's ability to understand the meaning of surgery and the activities to participate in postoperatively. Also influences the approach needed to individualize instruction.
5. Determine patient's ability to perform deep breathing and coughing and inspiratory spirometer activity.	Patient's inability to perform postoperative respiratory exercises increases risk for pulmonary complications.
6. Assess patient's anxiety related to surgery.	Directs you to provide additional emotional support and indicates patient's readiness to learn.
7. Assess family caregiver's willingness to learn and support patient after surgery.	Family caregiver's presence after surgery can be a potential motivating factor for patient recovery. Caregiver can coach patient through postoperative exercise and observe for any postoperative problems.

PLANNING

STEP	RATIONALE
1. Prepare equipment as needed.	
2. Prepare health literacy–appropriate teaching materials.	Instructional materials written at appropriate reading level enhance patient's ability to learn.
3. Plan teaching sessions to occur when patient is not in pain.	Decreased levels of pain enhance patient learning.
4. Plan to explain postoperative exercises to patient and any family caregiver, including importance to recovery and physiological benefits.	Information allows patient to understand significance of exercises and motivates learning. Promotes patient cooperation and decreases anxiety.
5. Prepare room for teaching.	Environment needs to be conducive to learning (see Chapter 12).

IMPLEMENTATION

STEP	RATIONALE
1. Perform hand hygiene. Inform patient and family caregiver of date, time, and location of surgery; anticipated length of surgery; additional time in postanesthesia recovery area; and where to wait.	Reduces transmission of infection. Accurate information helps reduce stress associated with surgery.
2. Answer questions patient and family caregiver ask during instructional session.	Responding to patient and family caregiver questions helps to decrease anxiety and demonstrates your concern for them.
3. Instruct patient on preoperative bowel or skin preparations as needed. Check agency policy regarding use and number of preoperative showers and agent to be used for each shower (2% chlorhexidine gluconate is used most often) (Chlebicki et al., 2013). Following each preoperative shower, the skin should be rinsed thoroughly and dried with a fresh, clean, dry towel, and patient should don clean clothing.	Proper skin preparation is a critical element in preventing SSIs. Rinsing the skin removes residual antiseptic preparation that may cause skin irritation. After use, towels contain microorganisms that can grow in the presence of moisture. Using a fresh towel after each shower and donning clean clothing minimizes the risk of reintroducing microorganisms to clean skin (AORN, 2017a; Graling and Vasaly, 2013).
4. Instruct patient on extent and purpose of food and fluid restrictions for period specified before surgery (e.g., no oral intake for 2 hours before surgery; no meat or fried foods 8 hours before surgery, unless otherwise specified by surgeon or anesthesia care provider) (ASA Committee on Standards and Practice Parameters, 2011).	During general anesthesia, muscles relax, and gastric contents can reflux into esophagus, leading to aspiration. Anesthetic eliminates patient's ability to gag.

SKILL 40.1 TEACHING POSTOPERATIVE EXERCISES—cont'd

View Video!

STEP	RATIONALE
5. Describe perioperative routines (e.g., time-out, site marking, IV therapy, urinary catheterization, hair clipping or removal, laboratory tests, transport to operating room [OR]).	Allows patient to anticipate and recognize routine procedures, reducing anxiety.
6. Describe planned effect of preoperative medications.	Provides information about what to expect, decreasing anxiety.
7. Review which routine medications patients need to discontinue before surgery.	Some medications are discontinued before surgery to minimize effects that can cause surgical risks. Anticoagulants may increase bleeding and are usually discontinued several days before surgery. Insulin dosages are usually adjusted because of reduced intake of food before surgery.
8. Describe perioperative sensations to expect in holding area or OR (e.g., blood pressure cuff tightening, electrocardiogram leads, cool room, and beep of monitor).	Helps to relieve patient anxiety.
9. Describe pain-control methods to be used postoperatively. Discuss what pain is acceptable, explain that patient will not be pain-free, but the pain will be managed. Many patients have a patient-controlled analgesia (PCA) pump postoperatively.	Patients are fearful of postoperative pain. Explaining pain-management techniques reduces this fear.
10. Describe what patient will experience after surgery (e.g., where patient will be on awakening, frequent vital signs, turning, catheters, drains, tubes, alternating pressure from sequential compression device).	Provides a concrete description of what patient can expect after surgery so that patient is prepared.
11. **Teach turning:**	
a. Instruct patient on turning and sitting up (especially suited for abdominal and thoracic surgery).	Promotes circulation and ventilation.
(1) Turn onto right side: Have patient assume supine position and move to side of bed (in this case left side); instruct to flex knees, press heels against mattress, and lift buttocks to move up toward left side of bed (see illustration). Top side rails on both sides of bed should be in up position.	Positioning begins on side of bed so that turning to other side does not cause patient to roll toward edge of bed. Buttocks lift prevents skin shearing. If patient's bed has turn assist device, use it.
(2) Have patient splint incision with right hand or with right hand with pillow over incisional area; keep right leg straight and flex left knee up (see illustration); and grab right side rail with left hand, pull toward right, and roll onto right side. Reverse process to turn to left side.	Supports incision and decreases discomfort while turning.
(3) Instruct patient to turn every 2 hours from side to side while awake. Often patient will require assistance with turning postoperatively.	Reduces risk of vascular, pulmonary, and pressure injury complications.

Clinical Decision Point. Some patients such as patients with back surgery or vascular repair are restricted from flexing their legs after surgery. Some patients may be restricted from turning.

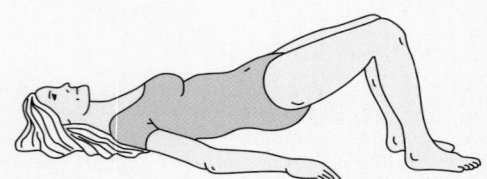

STEP 11a(1) Buttocks lift for moving to side of bed.

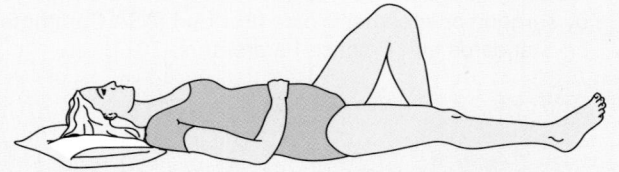

STEP 11a(2) Leg position when turning to right.

STEP	RATIONALE
(4) Sit up on right side of bed: Elevate head of bed and have patient turn onto right side. While lying on right side, patient pushes on mattress with left arm and swings feet over edge of bed with nurse's assistance. To sit up on left side of bed, reverse this process. Stay at patient's side.	Sitting position lowers diaphragm to permit fuller lung expansion. Staying with patient reduces fall risk.
12. Teach deep breathing and coughing:	Patient may be unable or reluctant to deep breathe because of weakness or pain, resulting in secretions remaining in the base of the lungs. Collection of secretions increases risk of pulmonary atelectasis and pneumonia.
a. Assist patient to high-Fowler's position in bed with knees flexed or have patient sit on side of bed or chair in upright position.	Sitting position facilitates diaphragmatic expansion.
b. Instruct patient to place palms of hands across from one another lightly along the lower border of the rib cage or upper abdomen (see illustration).	This allows patient to feel the rise and fall of abdomen during deep breathing (Lewis et al., 2014).
c. Have patient take slow, deep breaths, inhaling through nose. Explain that patient will feel normal downward movement of diaphragm during inspiration. Demonstrate as follows:	Helps to prevent hyperventilation or panting. Slow, deep breaths allow for more complete lung expansion.
(1) Have patient avoid using chest and shoulder muscles while inhaling.	Increases unnecessary energy expenditure and does not promote full lung expansion.
(2) Have patient take slow, deep breath; hold for count of 3 seconds; and slowly exhale through mouth as if blowing out a candle (pursed lips).	Resistance during exhalation helps to prevent alveolar collapse.
(3) Have patient repeat breathing exercise 3 to 5 times.	Repetition reinforces learning.
(4) Have patient take two slow, deep breaths, inhaling through nose and exhaling through pursed lips.	Deep breaths expand lungs fully so that air moves behind mucus to facilitate coughing.
(5) Have patient inhale deeply a third time and hold breath to count of 3. Cough fully for 2 to 3 consecutive coughs without inhaling between coughs.	Deep breathing moves up secretions in the respiratory tract to stimulate the cough reflex without voluntary effort on the part of patient (Lewis et al., 2014).
(6) Caution patient against just clearing throat.	Clearing throat does not remove mucus from deeper airways.
(7) Have patient practice several times. Instruct patient to perform turning, coughing, and deep breathing every 2 hours. Have family caregiver coach patient to exercise.	Ensures mastery of technique. Frequent pulmonary exercises and movement decrease risk of postoperative pneumonia (Lewis et al., 2014).

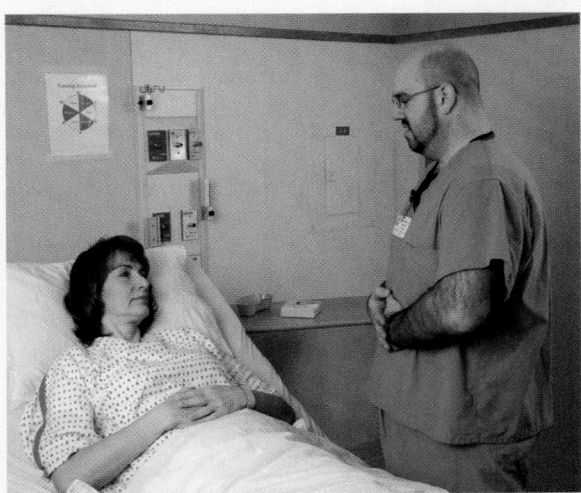

STEP 12b Deep-breathing exercise—placement of hands on upper abdomen during inhalation.

SKILL 40.1   TEACHING POSTOPERATIVE EXERCISES—cont'd

View Video!

STEP	RATIONALE
13. Instruct patient on use of incentive spirometer (see illustration):	Provides visual aid of respiratory effort. Encourages deep breathing to loosen secretions in lung bases.
a. Position patient in sitting position in chair or in reclining position with head of bed elevated at least 45 degrees.	Facilitates diaphragm lowering and lung expansion.
b. Instruct patient to exhale completely and place mouthpiece so that lips completely cover it and inhale slowly, maintaining constant flow through unit (see illustration).	Promotes complete inflation of lungs and minimizes atelectasis. Mouth position ensures proper seal and prevents loss of air.
c. After a maximum inspiration, patient should hold breath for 2 to 3 seconds and exhale slowly.	Promotes alveolar inflation.
d. Set marker on spirometer at maximum inspiration point achieved by patient to establish postoperative target.	Establishes measure of normal maximum breath for patient. Provides outcome measure to determine postoperative return to preoperative volumes.
e. Instruct patient to breathe normally for a short period and repeat process 10 times every hour while awake.	Prevents hyperventilation and fatigue.
14. Teach positive expiratory pressure therapy and "huff" coughing:	
a. Set PEP device for setting ordered.	Higher settings require more effort.
b. Instruct patient to assume semi-Fowler's or high-Fowler's position in bed or chair, and place nose clip on patient's nose (see illustration).	Promotes optimum lung expansion and expectoration of mucus.
c. Have patient place lips around mouthpiece. Instruct patient to take a full breath and then exhale 2 or 3 times longer than inhalation. Repeat pattern for 10 to 20 breaths.	Ensures that patient does all breathing through mouth. Ensures that patient uses device properly.
d. Remove device from mouth and have patient take a slow, deep breath and hold for 3 seconds.	Promotes lung expansion before coughing.
e. Instruct patient to exhale in quick, short, forced "huffs." Repeat exercise every 2 hours while awake.	"Huff" coughing, or forced expiratory technique, promotes bronchial hygiene by increasing expectoration of secretions.
15. Teach controlled coughing:	Position facilitates diaphragm excursion and enhances thorax and abdominal expansion.
a. Explain importance of maintaining an upright position.	Deep breaths expand lungs fully so air moves behind mucus and facilitates effective coughing.

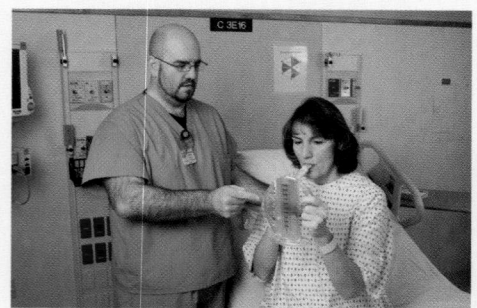

STEP 13 Patient demonstrates incentive spirometry.

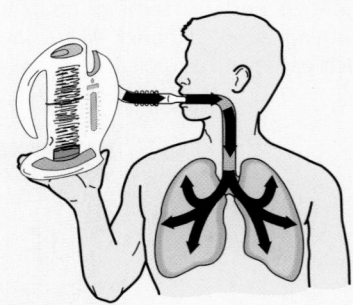

STEP 13b Diagram of use of incentive spirometer.

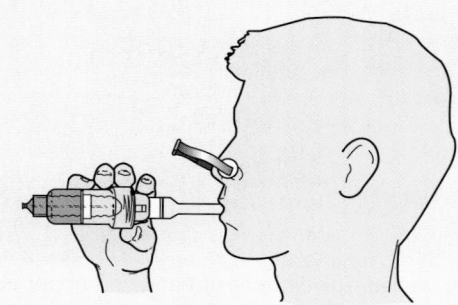

STEP 14b Diagram of use of positive expiratory pressure device.

STEP	RATIONALE
b. Demonstrate coughing. Take two slow, deep breaths, inhaling through nose and exhaling through (pursed lips) mouth.	Consecutive coughs help remove mucus more effectively and completely than one forceful cough.
c. Inhale deeply a third time and hold breath to count of three. Cough fully for 2 to 3 consecutive coughs without inhaling between coughs (see illustration). (Tell patient to push all air out of lungs.)	Clearing throat does not remove mucus from deeper airways.
d. Caution patient against just clearing throat instead of coughing deeply.	Clearing throat does not remove mucus from deeper airways.
e. If surgical incision is either thoracic or abdominal, teach patient to place either hands or pillow with hands over pillow over incisional area to splint incision (see illustration). During breathing and coughing exercises, press gently against incisional area for splinting and support.	Surgical incision cuts through muscles, tissues, and nerve endings. Deep-breathing and coughing exercises place additional stress on suture line and cause discomfort. Splinting incision with hands or pillow provides firm support and reduces incisional pulling and pain.
f. Patient continues to practice coughing exercises, splinting imaginary incision (see illustration). Instruct patient to cough 2 to 3 times every hour while awake.	Deep coughing with splinting effectively expectorates mucus with minimal discomfort.
g. Instruct patient to examine sputum for consistency, odor, amount, and color changes; notify nurse if any changes are noted.	Sputum consistency, odor, amount, and color changes indicate pulmonary complication such as pneumonia.
16. **Teach leg exercises:**	Promotes circulation, designed to reduce incidence of deep vein thrombosis (DVT).
a. Instruct and encourage patient to perform leg exercises every 1 to 2 hours while awake: ankle rotation, dorsiflexion and plantar flexion, leg extension and flexion, and straight leg exercises (unless activity restricted).	Facilitate venous return.
b. Position patient supine.	
c. Instruct patient to rotate each ankle in complete circle and draw imaginary circles with big toe 5 times (see illustration).	Promotes joint mobility.
d. Alternate dorsiflexion and plantar flexion while instructing patient to feel calf muscles tighten and relax. Repeat 5 times (see illustration).	Helps maintain joint mobility and promote venous return to prevent thrombus formation.

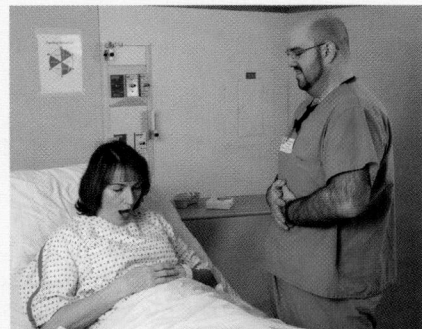

STEP 15c Controlled coughing with placement of hands on upper abdomen.

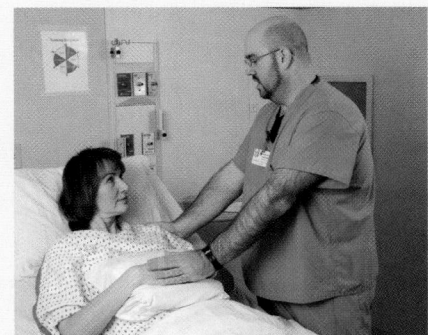

STEP 15e Patient splinting abdomen with pillow.

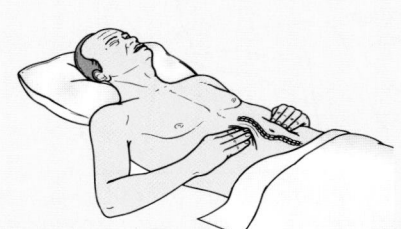
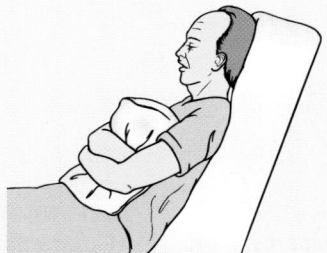
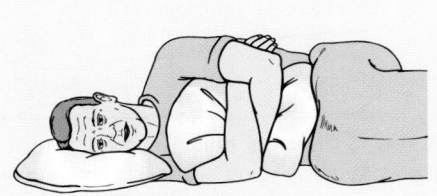

STEP 15f Techniques for splinting incisions. (From Lewis SL, et al: *Medical-surgical nursing: assessment and management of clinical problems*, ed 8, St Louis, 2011, Mosby.)

SKILL 40.1   TEACHING POSTOPERATIVE EXERCISES—cont'd

View Video!

STEP	RATIONALE

e. Perform quadriceps setting by tightening thigh and bringing knee down toward mattress and relaxing. Repeat 5 times (see illustration).

Quadriceps-setting exercises contract muscles of upper legs, maintain knee mobility, and improve venous return to heart.

f. Instruct patient to alternate raising legs straight up from bed surface. Leg should remain straight. Repeat 5 times (see illustration).

Causes quadriceps muscle contraction and relaxation that helps promote venous return (Lewis et al., 2014).

g. Instruct patient to perform these four leg exercises 10 to 12 times every 1 to 2 hours while awake.

Leg exercises stimulate circulation, which prevents venous stasis to help prevent formation of DVT (Lewis et al., 2014).

17. Have patient continue to practice exercises before surgery at least every 2 hours while awake. Teach patient to coordinate turning and leg exercises with diaphragmatic breathing and use of incentive spirometer or PEP.

18. Verify that patient's expectations of surgery are realistic and accurate.

Can prevent postoperative anxiety or anger.

19. Reinforce therapeutic coping strategies. If ineffective, encourage alternatives. Perform hand hygiene.

Therapeutic coping strategies promote postoperative compliance and recovery.

EVALUATION

1. Observe patient demonstrating splinting, turning and sitting, deep breathing, and leg exercises.

Validates patient's ability to perform postoperative exercises.

2. Ask family caregiver to identify location of waiting room and validate if correct.

Establishes family's knowledge of where they can wait for patient information.

3. Ask family caregiver to explain how to help prepare patient at home before surgery.

Establishes postoperative home care is in place for patient on discharge.

4. Observe level of emotional support family caregiver provides patient.

Identifies preoperative emotional support for patient.

5. **Use Teach-Back:** "I want to be sure I explained what you need to know about getting ready for surgery. Tell me the reason you will be doing turning and leg exercises after surgery. Show me how to turn." Revise your instruction now or develop a plan for revised patient/family caregiver teaching if patient/family caregiver is not able to teach back correctly.

Determines patient's/family caregiver's level of understanding of instructional topic.

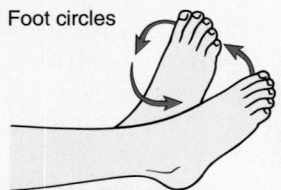

STEP 16c Foot circles. (From Lewis S, et al: *Medical-surgical nursing: assessment and management of clinical problems*, ed 9, St Louis, 2014, Mosby.)

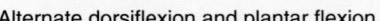
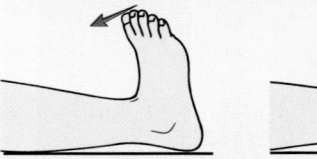
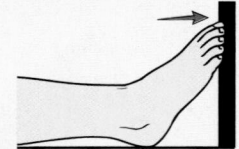

Alternate dorsiflexion and plantar flexion

STEP 16d Alternate dorsiflexion and plantar flexion (From Lewis S, et al: *Medical-surgical nursing: assessment and management of clinical problems*, ed 9, St Louis, 2014, Mosby.)

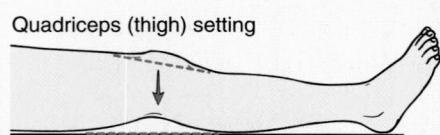

Quadriceps (thigh) setting

STEP 16e Quadriceps (thigh) setting. (From Lewis, S et al: *Medical-surgical nursing: assessment and management of clinical problems*, ed 9, St Louis, 2014, Mosby.)

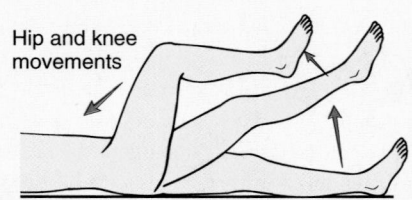

Hip and knee movements

STEP 16f Hip and knee movements. (From Lewis S, et al: *Medical-surgical nursing: assessment and management of clinical problems*, ed 9, St Louis, 2014, Mosby.)

RECORDING AND REPORTING

- Document all preoperative patient and family caregiver teaching and response to teaching in the nurses' notes in the electronic health record (EHR) or chart.

UNEXPECTED OUTCOMES AND RELATED INTERVENTIONS

- Patient identifies an incorrect procedure, site, date, or time of surgery.
  - Provide the correct information verbally and in writing for patient and family caregiver.
- Patient incorrectly performs postoperative exercises.
  - Explain and demonstrate correct exercise technique.
  - Explain the importance of each postoperative exercise.
  - Instruct patient to repeat demonstration.

KEY POINTS

- Previous illnesses and past surgeries affect a patient's ability to tolerate surgery.
- Older adult patients are at greater surgical risk because of the physiological changes associated with aging.
- All medications taken before surgery are automatically discontinued after surgery unless a health care provider reorders the drugs.
- Preadmission interventions to improve patients' health and fitness (referred to as prehabilitation) may reduce postoperative complications, decrease the length of hospital stays, and enhance a patient's recovery.
- Family members and significant others can assist patients with preoperative exercises and provide emotional support after surgery.
- Preoperative assessment of vital signs and physical findings provides a baseline with which to compare postoperative assessment data.
- Primary responsibility for informed consent rests with the surgeon.
- Structured preoperative teaching positively influences postoperative recovery.
- In ambulatory surgery, nurses use the limited time available to assess, prepare, and educate patients for surgery.
- Nurses within the operating room (OR) focus on protecting a patient from potential harm.
- Postoperative assessment centers on the body systems most likely affected by surgery.
- Because a surgical patient's condition may change rapidly during recovery, monitor a patient's status at least every 15 minutes until stable.
- Postoperative nursing interventions focus on prevention of complications.
- Use of enhanced recovery after surgery protocols apply evidence-based interventions to ensure better patient outcomes postoperatively.
- The risk for postoperative complications increases when a patient does not become actively involved in recovery.

REFLECTIVE LEARNING

- Reflect on either a patient you have cared for or one of your own family members who underwent surgery. How would you evaluate the patient's level of preparation for the surgical experience? In what way would you improve the patient's preparation?
- Think of three ways family members can support a patient who is scheduled for surgery. How can you as a nurse offer interventions to enable the family to be successful?
- Consider a patient you have recently cared for. What surgical risks would that patient have if he or she was scheduled for surgery involving general anesthesia?

REVIEW QUESTIONS

1. Communication between a nurse caring for a patient in the preoperative holding area and the circulating nurse in the operating room (OR) can best be enhanced by which of the following? (Select all that apply.)
   1. Documenting assessment findings in the medical record
   2. Using a standardized SBAR tool
   3. Being responsive in using nonverbal communication techniques
   4. Giving specific information to a transportation technician to convey to the OR nurse
   5. Listening to OR nurses' questions
2. Which of the following nursing interventions is a strategy for prevention of surgical site infections?
   1. Antibiotic selection
   2. Removal of hair by shaving over a surgical site
   3. Maintaining body temperature at 35.5° C or higher during surgery
   4. Cleansing the skin with chlorhexidine gluconate

3. A patient who returned from surgery 3 hours ago following a kidney transplant is reporting pain at a 7 on a scale of 0 to 10. The nurse has tried repositioning with no improvement in the patient's pain report. Unmanaged surgical pain can lead to which of the following problems? (Select all that apply.)
   1. Delayed ambulation
   2. Reduced ventilation
   3. Catheter-associated urinary tract infection
   4. Retained pulmonary secretions
   5. Reduced appetite
4. Which of the following factors place an older adult patient at risk during surgery? (Select all that apply.)
   1. Stiffened lung tissue
   2. Decline in pulmonary reserve
   3. Increased laryngeal reflexes
   4. Reduced blood flow to kidneys
   5. Increased cholinergic transmission

5. Match the nursing interventions on the left with the complication to be prevented on the right. An intervention may apply to more than one complication.

Nursing Intervention	Complication
___1. Offering glasses or hearing aid	a. Deep vein thrombosis
___2. Early ambulation	b. Wound infection
___3. Strict aseptic technique	c. Delirium
___4. Deep-breathing exercises	d. Pneumonia
___5. Hydration	

evolve

Additional Review Questions, as well as rationales for all Review Questions, can be found on the Evolve website.

1, 2, 3, 5; 2, 3; 3, 1, 2, 4, 5; 4, 1, 2, 4; 5, 1c, 2a,c, 3b, 4d, 5a,d.

REFERENCES

Adams D, et al: HOUDINI: Make that urinary catheter disappear—nurse-led protocol, *J Infect Prev* 13(2):446, 2012.

Agency for Healthcare Research and Quality (AHRQ): *Implementing the ABCDE bundle at the bedside*, 2013, https://innovations.ahrq.gov/qualitytools/implementing-abcde-bundle-bedside.

American Diabetes Association (ADA): Standards of medical care in diabetes—2016, *Diabetes Care* 39(Suppl 1):S1, 2016.

American Geriatrics Society (AGS): Postoperative delirium in older adults: Best Practice Statement from the American Geriatrics Society, *J Am Coll Surg* 220(2):136, 2015.

American Society of Anesthesiologists (ASA) Committee on Standards and Practice Parameters: Practice guidelines for preoperative fasting and the use of pharmacologic agents to reduce the risk of pulmonary aspiration: application to healthy patients undergoing elective procedures, *Anesthesiology* 114(3):495, 2011.

American Society of Anesthesiologists (ASA) Committee on Standards and Practice Parameters: Practice guidelines for acute pain management in the perioperative setting: an updated report by the American Society of Anesthesiologists Task Force on Acute Pain Management, *Anesthesiology* 116(2):248, 2012.

American Society of Anesthesiologists (ASA) Task Force on Perioperative Management of Patients With Obstructive Sleep Apnea: Practice guidelines for the perioperative management of patients with obstructive sleep apnea, *Anesthesiology* 120(2):268, 2014.

Anderson DJ, et al: Strategies to prevent surgical site infections in acute care hospitals: 2014 update, *Infect Control Hosp Epidemiol* 35(6):605, 2014.

Association of periOperative Registered Nurses (AORN): *Guidelines for perioperative practice*, Denver, 2017a, The Association.

Association of periOperative Registered Nurses (AORN): Guideline for positioning the patient, *AORN J* 105(4):8, 2017b.

Baker DW: *Joint Commission Statement on Pain Management*, 2016, https://www.jointcommission.org/joint_commission_statement_on_pain_management/.

Black J, et al: *Operating room ulcers: who is at risk? Can they be prevented?*, 2015, http://www.npuap.org/wp-content/uploads/2015/08/NPUAP-OR-Webinar-August-2015-Handouts.pdf.

Bruckenthal P, Simpson MH: The role of the perioperative nurse in improving surgical patients' clinical outcomes and satisfaction: beyond medication, *AORN J* 104(6):S17, 2016.

Burchum JR, Rosenthal LD: *Lehne's pharmacology for nursing care*, ed 9, St Louis, 2016, Elsevier.

Burden K: Using a change model to reduce the risk of surgical site infection, *Br J Nurs* 25(17):949, 2016.

Cao X, et al: A novel visual facial anxiety scale for assessing preoperative anxiety, *PLoS ONE* 12(2):e0171233, 2017.

Centers for Disease Control and Prevention (CDC): *Top CDC recommendations to prevent healthcare-associated infections*, n.d., https://www.cdc.gov/HAI/pdfs/hai/top-cdc-recs-factsheet.pdf.

Chlebicki MP, et al: Preoperative chlorhexidine shower or bath for prevention of surgical site infection: a meta-analysis, *Am J Infect Control* 41(2):167, 2013.

Claessen F, et al: What factors are associated with a surgical site infection after operative treatment of an elbow fracture?, *Clin Orthop Relat Res* 474(2):562, 2016.

Denholm B: Using a vulnerability theoretical model to assess the malignant hyperthermia susceptible population: implications for advanced practice emergency nurses, *Adv Emerg Nurs J* 37(3):209, 2015.

Devereaux PJ, Sessler DI: Cardiac complications in patients undergoing major noncardiac surgery, *N Engl J Med* 373:2258, 2015.

Engels D, et al: Pressure ulcers: factors contributing to their development in the OR, *AORN J* 103(3):271, 2016.

Fournier M, et al: Preoperative optimization of total joint arthroplasty surgical risk: obesity, *J Arthroplasty* 31(8):1620, 2016.

Ganzberg S: Obstructive sleep apnea and office-based surgery, *Anesth Prog* 63(2):53, 2016.

Garrett J: Effective perioperative communication to enhance patient care, *AORN J* 104(2):111, 2016.

Ghoneim MM, O'Hara MW: Depression and postoperative complications: an overview, *BMC Surg* 16:5, 2016.

Giger JN: *Transcultural nursing: assessment and intervention*, ed 7, St Louis, 2017, Mosby.

Gillis C, et al: Prehabilitation versus rehabilitation: a randomized control trial in patients undergoing colorectal resection for cancer, *Anesthesiology* 121(5):937, 2014.

Graling P, Vasaly FW: Effectiveness of 2% CHG cloth bathing for reducing surgical site infection, *AORN J* 97(5):547, 2013.

Harrelson DR, Fencl JL: Care of the patient with obstructive sleep apnea, *AORN J* 103(4):433, 2016.

Helvig A, et al: Postoperative management of patients with obstructive sleep apnea: implications for the medical-surgical nurse, *Medsurg Nurs* 23(3):171, 2014.

Iskandar M, et al: *Postoperative care of the geriatric patient*, n.d., http://studylib.net/doc/5591588/postoperative-care-in-the-geriatric-patient.

Jarvis C: *Physical examination and health assessment*, ed 7, St Louis, 2016, Saunders.

Jubran A: Pulse oximetry, *Crit Care* 19(1):272, 2015.

Karcz M, Papadakos PJ: Respiratory complications in the postanesthesia care unit: a review of pathophysiological mechanisms, *Can J Respir Ther* 49(4):21, 2013.

Kiernan M: Prevention of surgical site infection: compliance is key, *Br J Nurs* 24(17):856, 2015.

Kumar A, et al: Preoperative bowel preparation in children: polyethylene glycol versus normal saline, *Afr J Paediatr Surg* 10(3):235, 2013.

Leonard L: Continuing the fight in reducing the risk of surgical site infections in the perioperative environment, *J Perioper Pract* 26(5):6, 2016.

Lewis S, et al: *Medical-surgical nursing: assessment and management of clinical problems*, ed 9, St Louis, 2014, Mosby.

Love KL: Patient care interventions to reduce the risk of surgical site infections, *AORN J* 104(6):506, 2016.

Mangram AJ, et al: Guideline for prevention of surgical site infection, *Infect Control Hosp Epidemiol* 20(4):247, 1999.

Martin ET, et al: Diabetes and risk of surgical site infection: a systematic review and meta-analysis, *Infect Control Hosp Epidemiol* 37(1):88, 2016.

McDaid C, et al: Paracetamol and selective and non-selective non-steroidal anti-inflammatory drugs (NSAIDs) for the reduction of morphine-related side effects after major surgery: a systematic review, *Health Technol Assess* 14(17):1, 2010.

McGill Perioperative Program: *What is prehabilitation?*, 2017, https://www.mcgill.ca/peri-op-program/patient-information/what-prehabilitation.

Meddings J, et al: Reducing unnecessary urinary catheter use and other strategies to prevent catheter-associated urinary tract infection: an integrative review, *BMJ Qual Saf* 23(4):277, 2014.

Nahm E, et al: Effects of a web-based preoperative education program for patients undergoing ambulatory surgery: a preliminary study, *J Hosp Adm* 1(1):21, 2012.

Nordquist D, Halaszynski TM: Perioperative multimodal anesthesia using regional techniques in the aging surgical patient, *Pain Res Treat* 2014:902174, 2014.

Ogg M: Assessing a child for sleep apnea, *AORN J* 104(2):167, 2016.

Ortiz J, et al: Preoperative patient education: can we improve satisfaction and reduce anxiety?, *Braz J Anesthesiol* 65(1):7, 2015.

Palmer JB, et al: Collaborating with music therapists to improve patient care, *AORN J* 104(3):192, 2016.

Pashikanti L, Von Ah D: Impact of early mobilization protocol on the medical-surgical inpatient population: an integrated review of literature, *Clin Nurse Spec* 26(2):87, 2012.

Perry R, et al: Pre-admission interventions to improve outcome after elective surgery—protocol for a systematic review, *Syst Rev* 5:88, 2016.

Pinar G, et al: The efficacy of preoperative instruction in reducing anxiety following gyneoncological surgery: a case control study, *World J Surg Oncol* 9:38, 2011.

Poole L, et al: The combined association of depression and socioeconomic status with length of post-operative hospital stay following coronary artery bypass graft surgery: data from a prospective cohort study, *J Psychosom Res* 76(1):34, 2014.

Rothrock J: *Alexander's care of a patient in surgery*, ed 15, St Louis, 2015, Mosby.

Samnani SS, et al: Impact of preoperative counselling on early postoperative mobilization and its role in smooth recovery, *Int Sch Res Notices* 2014:250536, 2014.

Santa MD: Optimization of surgical outcomes with prehabilitation, *Appl Physiol Nutr Metab* 40(9):966, 2015.

Schroeder G, et al: The effect of smoking on patients having spinal surgery, *Curr Orthop Pract* 27(2):140, 2016.

Simpson MH, Bruckenthal P: The current state of perioperative pain management: challenges and potential opportunities for nurses, *AORN J* 104(6):S1, 2016.

Spencer MP, Christie J: A 7 S bundle approach to preventing surgical site infections, *Am J Infect Control* 42(6):S103, 2014.

Spruce L: Back to basics: preventing perioperative pressure injuries, *AORN J* 105(1):93, 2017.

Spruce L, Braswell ML: Implementing AORN recommended practices for electrosurgery, *AORN J* 95:373, 2012.

Tanner J, et al: Do surgical care bundles reduce the risk of surgical site infections in patients undergoing colorectal surgery? A systematic review and cohort meta-analysis of 8,515 patients, *Surgery* 158(1):66, 2015.

The Joint Commission (TJC): *2017 Hospital accreditation standards*, Oakbrook Terrace, IL, 2017, The Joint Commission.

The Joint Commission (TJC): *2018 National patient safety goals*, Oakbrook Terrace, IL, 2018, The Commission. https://www.jointcommission.org/standards_information/npsgs.aspx.

World Health Organization (WHO): *Surgical safety checklist*, 2017, http://www.who.int/patientsafety/safesurgery/checklist/en/.

World Health Organization (WHO): *Pulse oximetry training manual*, 2011, http://www.who.int/patientsafety/safesurgery/pulse_oximetry/who_ps_pulse_oximetry_training_manual_en.pdf.

Wukich DK: Diabetes and its negative impact on outcomes in orthopaedic surgery, *World J Orthop* 6(3):331, 2015.

Young H, et al: The effect of preoperative skin preparation products on surgical site infection, *Infect Control Hosp Epidemiol* 35(12):1535, 2014.

b indicates boxes, *f* indicates illustrations, and *t* indicates tables.

1239

PATIENT TEACHING

CARE OF THE OLDER ADULT

◎ CARE PLAN